Textbook of RADIOGRAPHIC POSITIONING and RELATED ANATOMY

4th Edition

Expanded Fourth Edition
With 2315 illustrations, 33 in full color

Kenneth L. Bontrager, MA, RT(R)

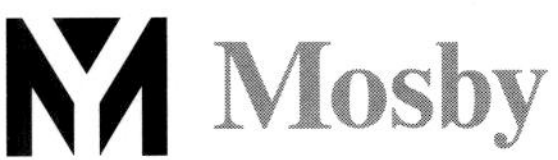

St. Louis Baltimore Boston Carlsbad Chicago Naples New York Philadelphia Portland
London Madrid Mexico City Singapore Sydney Tokyo Toronto Wiesbaden

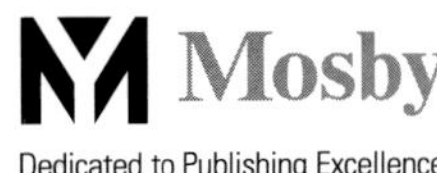

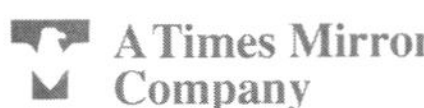

Editor: Jeanne Rowland

Developmental Editor: Lisa M. Potts

Project Manager: Mark Spann

Graphic Design and Typography: Neil A. Bontrager
Troy A. Bontrager
Komra Moriko

Illustrations: Debra Ravin
Joan Lapré
Sally Schmitt

Photography: Kenneth L. Bontrager

Facilities for Photography:
Energized Laboratory
Gateway Community College, Phoenix, Arizona

Phoenix Baptist Hospital and Medical Center
Phoenix, Arizona

St. Joseph's Hospital and Medical Center
Phoenix, Arizona

University of Iowa Hospitals and Medical Clinics
Iowa City, Iowa

Fourth Edition

Printed in the United States of America

Mosby-Year Book, Inc.
11830 Westline Industrial Drive, St. Louis, MO 63146

Library of Congress Cataloging in Publication Data

Bontrager, Kenneth L.
Textbook of radiographic positioning and related anatomy, fourth edition
Bibliography: p.
Includes index.
1. Radiography, Medical–Positioning.
2. Anatomy, Human
I. Title. (DNLM: 1. Technology, Radiologic.
WN 160 B722T)
RC 78.4.B66 1982 616.07'572 81-82006
ISBN 0-8151-0947-4

97 98 99 00 01 02 / 9 8 7 6 5 4 3 2 1

DEDICATION

I first dedicate this to my parents, to Andrew A. Bontrager for demonstrating to his children strong moral and Christian values, and a work ethic and drive to succeed; and in memory of Nora Yutzy Bontrager whose gentleness, love and unwavering faith and belief in me as a child and teenager provided the self-confidence I needed to pursue my education and reach for my dreams and goals. Her strong continuing influence and unspoken assurances have helped provide the will and perseverance I needed to complete a work of this type.

I also dedicate this to our sons, Neil and Troy, and our two new daughters-in-law, Kim and Robyn, all of whom I love very much. They, along with Mary Lou, my lifelong partner and helpmate, are the most important people in my life. In helping me reach my goals, I trust each of you has caught the vision and the inspiration to pursue your dreams, and I know you will make a difference and be a contributor in the careers you have chosen for your life work.

Last, I dedicate this to all those future students who will be learning from this text; to my former students; and to those many fellow technologists and educators who over the past years helped me, encouraged me, and even corrected me when needed. You have allowed me to experience a joy and satisfaction in life and the good feeling of fulfillment in knowing I had some small part in helping others pursue and reach their goals of entering a helping profession where they can achieve success and make their mark in life.

CONTRIBUTORS

Barry T. Anthony, RT(R) Swedish Medical Center, Englewood, CO.

Patrick Apfel, M.Ed, RT(R) University of Nevada, Las Vegas, NV.

Alex Backus, MS, RT(R) Gateway Community College, Phoenix, AZ.

Karen Brown, RT(R) St. Joseph's Hospital and Medical Center, Phoenix, AZ.

Claudia Calandrino, MPA, RT(R) Signa Health Plans of Calif., Los Angeles, CA.

Nancy Dickerson, RT(R)(M) Mayo Clinic, Rochester, MN.

Eugene D. Frank, MA, RT(R) FASRT Mayo Clinic, Rochester, MN.

Richard Geise, Ph.D. University of Minnesota Hospitals, Minneapolis, MN.

Cecilie Godderidge, BS, RT(R), Consultant and Lecturer in Pediatric Imaging, Boston, MA.

Jessie R. Harris, RT(R) Signa Health Plans of California, Los Angeles, CA.

John P. Lampignano, M.Ed, RT(R) Gateway Community College, Phoenix, AZ.

James D. Lipcamon, RT(R) Harbor-UCLA Diagnostic Imaging Center, Torrance, CA.

Kathy M. Martensen, BS, RT(R) University of Iowa Hospitals & Clinics, Iowa City, IA.

J. Fred Price, MS, RT(R) FASRT Garland County Community College, Hot Springs, AR.

Joan Radke, BS, RT(R) University of Iowa Hospitals and Clinics, Iowa City, IA.

E. Russel Ritenour, Ph.D. University of Minnesota Hospitals, Minneapolis, MN.

James A. Sanderson, BS, RT(R) St. Joseph's Hospital and Medical Center, Phoenix, AZ.

Mariane Tortorici, Ed.D, RT(R) University of Nevada, Las Vegas, NV.

PREFACE

Purpose and History

Early in my career as I was teaching, first at a hospital based program then at a city-wide college affiliated program in radiologic technology, I discovered that all the other allied health programs were far ahead of us in the type and quality of instructional media available in their fields of study. We had no audiovisuals or teaching ancillaries of any type, and many of our textbooks were outdated, incomplete and difficult to read and comprehend. Therefore, as I was completing my graduate degree in education and instructional media, I began developing audiovisuals and self-paced instructional programs for the classes I was teaching. Thus began my writing and publishing career. Beginning in the 1970s, we developed the first programmed audiovisual educational media in radiologic technology on **Radiographic Anatomy and Positioning**. I chose this subject for my initial writings because this was the one basic subject that **all** students needed to learn and master.

This comprehensive, 21 unit audiovisual series was soon being widely used throughout the United States and Canada. However, it became evident that students also needed a thorough, clearly written, easy to understand student textbook on this subject. Students were very frustrated trying to dig out and supplement relevant positioning information in the then existing references on the basic projections that were covered in our audiovisuals. Therefore, in the early 1980s the first edition of this textbook took form and soon was being widely used as a textbook to supplement our audiovisual self-paced instructional series, which then included over 1,500 slides, 48 audio cassettes, a three-volume student workbook and a five-volume set of instructor's manuals.

Distinctive of this Presentation

The strength and best feature of this textbook is its readability and ease of comprehension. This is largely due to the style and format used in presenting the information. We use extensive visuals throughout all portions of the book, always placing the visuals next to the printed text being discussed. This "show and tell" method of presenting information comes from experience in writing self-paced audiovisual media and adapting this style of writing to a textbook format. I have found that not only is comprehension increased with this style of writing, but retention is also increased because readers can readily visualize the information being presented. Most of us remember through mental images, and we know that we remember much more of what we see than what we hear (or read). When we see and hear at the same time, we maximize both our comprehension and retention.

Combining Anatomy and Positioning

When I first began teaching positioning courses, it was customary to teach positioning as a totally separate course from anatomy. I soon realized that a thorough understanding of pertinent anatomy was essential when learning positioning to prevent the tendency of rote memory of body positions, angles, and central ray locations. By thoroughly combining the anatomy and positioning in each chapter, as we have done in both the audiovisuals and this textbook, the reader is better able to conceptually visualize the shape and contours of each body part being radiographed and thus can change or adapt positioning routines as needed. The evaluation and critique of radiographs also require a good understanding of anatomy.

Expanded Fourth Edition

In planning for this new edition, much time and effort went into determining what should be added and what should be changed or deleted to provide both educators and students even better resources for teaching and learning the art and science of radiographic positioning. A comprehensive national survey was first completed, as described on the following pages, to determine what projections were considered essential by the clinical affiliates for all students to master. Additional surveys and conferences were carried out to help determine what new chapters or sections of chapters should be added and what should be deleted or changed.

New to this Edition

Educators universally agreed that more information on **mobile and trauma radiography** was needed to better prepare radiographers in these areas. As a result after many drafts and rewrites, a totally new comprehensive chapter on mobile and trauma radiography was completed. It includes basic trauma and mobile positioning principles, as well as trauma terminology and contemporary mobile and trauma equipment. Also included are trauma positioning demonstrations for **all** body parts, performed without moving the patient from a supine position.

The **mammography chapter** was revised and updated to include a new projection commonly performed today. Also added was information on the new Mammography Quality Standard Act and current terminology and abbreviations, all of which are vital information needed for ACR accreditation.

The **pediatric chapter** was updated to include a new section on the pediatric abdomen, including GI and urinary tract procedures.

The **skull and facial bones chapters** were revised to condense the anatomy into one chapter to reduce duplication and provide increased clarity. New illustrations were added, all of which are now in full color to better demonstrate all parts of the complex cranial anatomy.

The chapters on the **spine** were totally reorganized into a more logical order of information, beginning with the cervical spine and ending with the sacrum and coccyx.

Critique radiographs have been added at the end of the chapters to provide readers examples of radiographs to critique and determine what repeatable error is present on each radiograph. The student workbook and laboratory manual includes questions and answers on each of these critique radiographs. These exercises should be carried out by the students **prior to classroom time**. This will prepare them for classroom or lab discussions on each of these critique radiographs, as well as additional radiographs provided on slides for the instructors as part of the ancillary lecture slide set.

The **special procedures chapters** were updated to include new information on contemporary computed tomography and other special procedures equipment. Also added was a totally new section on those more common vascular and nonvascular interventional angiographic procedures being performed today.

Emphasis on Protection and Patient Dosages

As described in our code of ethics, radiologic technologists are responsible for controlling and "limiting the radiation exposure to the patient, self and others of the health care team".* This requires a good understanding and application of **radiation protection practices** and an **awareness of radiation dose ranges** received by the patient for each body part being radiographed. The relationship between patient doses and specific projections (AP or PA), and various combinations of exposure factors need to be understood. Also each radiographer should have an understanding of specific dose ranges to radiosensitive organs and the effect of area shielding to these doses. This awareness of specific dose ranges can also be an additional motivating factor for careful positioning and technique selection to prevent unnecessary repeats.

In the same way that positioning and related anatomy have been combined in this textbook, patient dosages and additional shielding emphasis is now also combined with positioning. This is achieved by more detailed shielding descriptions and by adding patient dose icon boxes on most positioning pages, indicating specific skin doses as well as midline and organ doses when such radiosensitive organs are in or near the primary x-ray beam.

KLB

*Code of Ethics, #7, page 46

ANCILLARIES

Student Workbook/Lab Manuals, Volumes I and II

Fourth edition student workbook/lab manuals, which are totally current with the fourth edition textbook, have also been completed. New emphasis has been placed on review exercises and self tests on each chapter with more critical thinking questions, as well as more questions based on specific clinical situations. I am also pleased that John Lampignano (one of the most able and effective educators I know) has joined me as coauthor of this two-volume set, bringing his extensive teaching experience and expertise to this project.

Lecture Slide Set and Instructors' Manuals, Volumes I and II

A new and updated lecture slide set is now available to provide a complete and up-to-date set of lecture slides to guide instructors through classroom presentations following each chapter of this textbook.

John Lampignano has also joined me as coauthor of the totally new two-volume instructor's manual, which provides a printout of each slide placed beside a lecture guide outline for that slide. Included in this lecture guide are some interactive student exercise suggestions as well as discussion questions to provide meaningful classroom learning experiences. Thus, more of the classroom presentations can be used for answering questions and to supplement what the students have already learned from the textbook and student workbook exercises, which should be completed prior to the classroom time.

We are pleased to once again offer a current total teaching package for learning radiographic positioning and related anatomy. New and updated multiple-choice unit evaluation exams are also provided with answers in the instructor's manual. The use of this total instructional package will ensure that all the necessary information has been presented and learning experiences provided so that students will be prepared to pass the registry examination and function as well-trained radiographers in today's demanding health care clinical setting.

KLB

ACKNOWLEDGMENTS

Determination of appropriate acknowledgments for this project is difficult because of the many persons who have contributed to this and earlier editions. I want to first acknowledge and thank **Barry Anthony,** RT, for his contributions in the areas of anatomy and special procedures for the first edition of both this text and the associated audiovisual series, which provided the foundation for this textbook. I also want to thank those contributors who made significant contributions in their areas of expertise as listed on a later page and to those reviewers who reviewed portions of initial drafts of this manuscript. I especially want to acknowledge and thank two persons who not only reviewed various drafts of new parts of this manuscript but who read every page of the final draft and who took the time to not only proof for accuracy but to also add positive and detailed suggestions of what should be added or deleted. These two persons are **David Hall,** MS, RT(R), Broward Community College, Davie, FL, and **John Lampignano,** MS, RT(R), Gateway Community College, Phoenix, AZ. I would also like to thank anatomists **David Lindsay,** PhD, and George Kendrick, PhD, for their thorough review and suggestions on the anatomy sections.

I am very grateful to **Jim Sanderson,** BS, RT and **Karen Brown,** RT, St. Joseph's Hospital and Medical Center and **Dell Hershberger**, RT, Phoenix Baptist Hospital and Medical Center, for those many evenings that they helped us with positioning photography and in locating and copying radiographs.

I thank **Jeanne Rowland**, **Mark Spann** and **Lisa Potts** from Mosby-Year Book, Inc. for their support and assistance with this total project.

I also thank **Debra Ravin** for her extra care in producing high quality drawings, and **Komra Moriko** and **Julie Salvante** of our production staff for their help and contributions with the art and graphics.

Last and most important to me I want to thank my wife, **Mary Lou** and our two sons, **Neil** and **Troy,** for their love and support during the past fifteen years since I began writing the first edition of this textbook. This has been a continuing family project, during which time both Neil and Troy have literally grown up with "the book" and for the last two editions they, along with Mary Lou, did most of the keying in of text and the graphic design and layout for their perfectionist dad and husband, who always found something that could be improved.

KLB

NATIONAL SURVEY INFORMATION

Initial Survey

In November 1989 a questionnaire was first sent to all accredited radiologic technology programs in the United States and to each of their clinical affiliates. The purpose of this survey was to determine a national standard or norm of procedures and/or specific projections or positions that are the minimum essentials that all students should master and demonstrate competency for prior to graduation. Based on the tabulated results of this survey, these basic procedures and minimum routines were then included in the third edition of this positioning textbook, with the recommendation that these be taught by all schools nationwide to prepare the students to function effectively in any region of the United States upon graduation.

Procedures and routines may differ in various provinces and regions of Canada, and no attempt was made to include all of these in this survey.

Updated Survey

In May 1995, as an initial step in planning and preparing for the fourth edition of this textbook, a second survey was conducted to provide updated information on the minimal standard of routine (basic) and special (optional) projections. In an effort to provide information as accurate as possible for minimum routines that should be included in this edition and be taught by all schools, this time only those responses completed by the **clinical facilities themselves** were included in the final survey tabulation. We wanted to determine what the clinical facilities wanted, which hopefully is the same as what the college educators think they should be teaching.

Description of Questionnaire

The survey questionnaires included a listing of possible projections for each body part. Respondents were asked to check those projections that were performed frequently enough in their department that, in their opinion, all students should master and demonstrate at least minimum proficiency levels before graduation. The first column was for **basic** or **routine** projections, which were defined as **"those projections which are routine or basic for your department, for all average helpful patients."** The second column was for checking those **special** (extra or optional) projections, which were defined as **"those additional projections which are not considered routine or basic in your department but which are sometimes taken as special or extra (optional) for demonstrating specific pathology, or for patients who cannot cooperate fully."** Projections that were not checked in either column indicated that these were done with such low frequency in their department that all students should not have to master them prior to graduation.

Survey Results

The results of the survey, as printed in each chapter of this text on the pages preceding the positioning section, indicate the percent of checks tabulated for each column for that projection. This allows you the reader to see what percentage of those completing the questionnaire indicated each projection to be either basic (routine) or special (extra) in their department. The 1989 results are included in parentheses to demonstrate changes in routines that have occurred during this 6-year time period.

All projections or positions checked by 18 to 20% or more of respondents were considered to be essential and are included in this text either as basic or as special projections. A few exceptions were made to include those newer special projections that, in the author's opinion, were significant enough to be included. Examples of this in the third edition were the **Merchant method** for the patellofemoral joint, and the **apical oblique** for the shoulder. Two such new projections for this fourth edition are the **mediolateral projection for the hip** (Sanderson method) and the **biplane angulation method for the trauma oblique cervical spine**, both of which are described in the new Chapter 19, Trauma and Mobile Radiography.

Survey Questionnaire Responses

A total of approximately 2,100 survey questionnaires were sent to all clinical affiliates of accredited radiologic technology programs in the United States. A total of 637 completed questionnaires were received and tabulated. These responses were divided into hospital based programs and college based programs. The response differences between college and hospital based programs were not significant. The difference in size of the hospitals was also not significant. However, the differences between regions of the United States were significant for certain projections as described in the Appendix A at the end of this text.

Summary of Survey Results

Total essential projections (as indicated by 18 to 20% or higher of responses).

Chart of Essential Projections	
Basic (routine) projections	145
Special (extra or optional) projections	76
Total	221

Note: These basic and special projections were only counted once if they are basically the same or very near the same projection even though used for different examinations with only slightly different centering. An example of this is the parietoacanthial (PA Waters) which was checked for facial bone routine as well as for nasal bones and optic foramina. The AP axial (Towne) and submentovertex (SMV) also were counted as only one projection even though used for different exams for the cranial and facial bones.

CONTENTS

Chapter 1 Principles, Terminology, and Radiation Protection **1**

Chapter 2 Chest **55**

Chapter 3 Abdomen **85**

Chapter 4 Upper Limb **101**

Chapter 5 Proximal Humerus and Shoulder Girdle **147**

Chapter 6 Lower Limb **171**

Chapter 7 Proximal Femur and Pelvis **221**

Chapter 8 Cervical and Thoracic Spine **247**

Chapter 9 Lumbar Spine, Sacrum and Coccyx **279**

Chapter 10 Bony Thorax–Sternum and Ribs **305**

Chapter 11 Skull and Cranium Bones **323**

Chapter 12 Facial Bones **359**

Chapter 13 Paranasal Sinuses, Mastoids and Temporal Bone **385**

Chapter 14 Upper Gastrointestinal System **411**

Chapter 15 Lower Gastrointestinal System **445**

Chapter 16 Gallbladder and Biliary Ducts **483**

Chapter 17 Urinary System **503**

Chapter 18 Mammography **529**

Chapter 19 Trauma and Mobile Radiography **545**

Chapter 20 Pediatric Radiography **581**

Chapter 21 Additional Imaging Procedures–Orthoroentgenography, Arthrography, Myelography and Conventional Tomography **611**

Chapter 22 Cranial Computed Tomography **633**

Chapter 23 Thoracic, Abdominal and Pelvic Computed Tomography **659**

Chapter 24 Angiography **679**

Chapter 25 Magnetic Resonance Imaging **723**

Bibliography **754**

Appendix A Survey Responses and Regional Differences **755**

Subject Index **757**

CHAPTER 1

Principles, Terminology and Radiation Protection

CONTRIBUTIONS BY:
Kathy Martensen, BS, RT (R)
E. Russel Ritenour, PhD
Richard Geise, PhD
Barry T. Anthony, RT (R)

CONTENTS

General, Systemic and Skeletal Anatomy and Arthrology

Structural organization **2**

Body systems **3**

Osteology **6**

Classification of bones **7**

Development of bones **9**

Classification of joints **10**

Radiographic Terminology

General terms **14**

Body planes, sections and lines **15**

Body surfaces and parts **16**

Positioning and body positions **17**

Specific body positions **18**

Radiographic projections **20**

Relationship terms **22**

Terms related to movement **24**

Summary of potentially misused terms **28**

Basic Imaging Principles

Evaluation criteria **29**

Positioning accuracy **29**

Film markers and patient ID **30**

Radiographic quality:
- Density **31**
- Contrast **32**
- Detail **33**
- Distortion **34**
- Anode heel effect **36**

Radiation Protection

Units of radiation **37**

Radiographer protection **37**

ALARA principles **38**

Patient doses:
- General diagnostic procedures **38**
- Sample patient dose chart **39**
- Fluoroscopic procedures **39**
- Worker protection during fluoroscopy **40**

Patient protection
(8 ways of reducing patient exposure) **41**

Positioning Principles

Professional ethics and patient care **46**

Protocol and order for
general radiographic procedures **47**

Positioning methods and steps **48**

Essential projections **50**

Principles for positioning routines **50**

Topographic positioning landmarks **52**

Body habitus **53**

Viewing radiographs, CT and MRI images **54**

General, Systemic and Skeletal Anatomy and Arthrology

General Anatomy

Anatomy is the science of the structure of the human body, while **physiology** deals with functions of the body, or how the body parts work. In the living subject, it is almost impossible to study anatomy without also studying some physiology. Radiographic study of the human body, however, is primarily a study of the anatomy of the various systems with lesser emphasis on the physiology. Consequently, anatomy of the human system will be emphasized in this radiographic anatomy and positioning textbook.

Note: Phonetic respelling of anatomical and positioning terms are included throughout this text to aid in correct pronunciation of those terms commonly used in medical radiography.*

STRUCTURAL ORGANIZATION

Several levels of structural organization compose the human body. The lowest level of organization is the **chemical level**. All of the chemicals necessary for maintaining life are composed of **atoms**, joined in various ways to form **molecules**. Various chemicals in the form of molecules are organized to form **cells**.

Cells

The cell is the basic structural and functional unit of the entire human being. Every single part of the body, whether muscle, bone, cartilage, fat, nerve, skin or blood, is composed of cells.

Tissues

Tissues are groups of similar cells which, together with their intercellular material, perform a specific function. The four basic types of tissues are:

*1. **Epithelial** (ep′ i-the′ le-al):* Tissue which covers internal and external surfaces of the body including lining of vessels and organs, such as the stomach and intestines.

*2. **Connective:*** Tissues which bind together and support the various structures.

*3. **Muscular:*** Tissues which make up the substances of a muscle.

*4. **Nervous:*** Tissues which make up the substance of nerves and nerve centers.

Organs

When various tissues are joined together to perform a specific function, the result is an organ. Organs usually have a specific shape. Some of the organs of the human body are the kidneys, heart, liver, lungs, stomach and brain.

System

A system consists of a group or association of organs that have a similar or a common function. The urinary system, consisting of kidneys, ureters, bladder and urethra, as described on page 4, is an example of a body system. There are **ten individual body systems** composing the total body.

Organism

All of the ten systems of the body functioning together constitute the total organism – one living being.

**Dorland's Illustrated Medical Dictionary*, 27th ed., Philadelphia: WB Saunders Co., 1988.

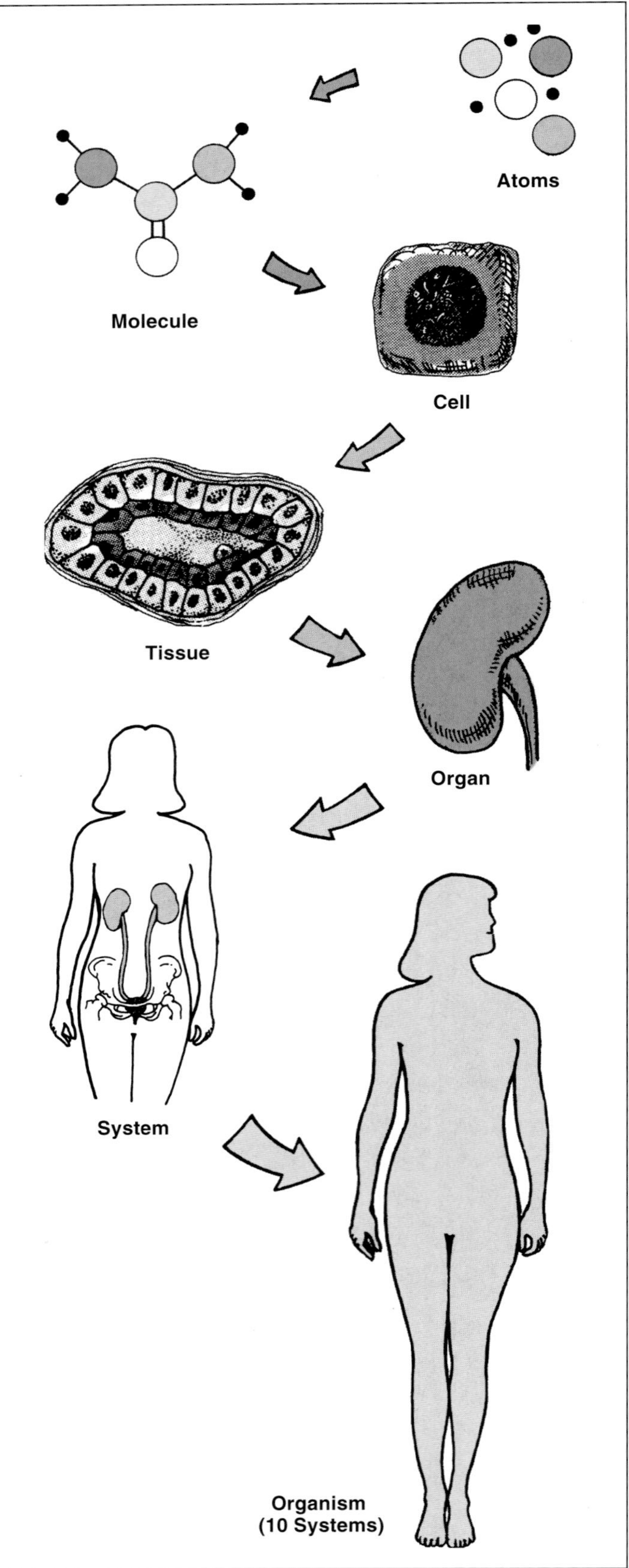

Fig. 1-1. Levels of human structural organization.

Systemic Anatomy

BODY SYSTEMS

The human body is a structural and functional unit made up of ten lesser units termed systems. These **ten systems** are: (1) skeletal, (2) circulatory, (3) digestive, (4) respiratory, (5) urinary, (6) reproductive, (7) nervous, (8) muscular, (9) endocrine, and (10) integumentary *(in-teg-u-men′ tar-e)*.

1. Skeletal System

The skeletal system is an important system to be studied by the radiographer. The skeletal system includes the **206 separate bones** of the body and their associated cartilages and joints. The study of bones is termed **osteology**, while the study of joints is termed **arthrology**.

Four functions of the skeletal system are to:

1. Support and protect the body.
2. Allow movement by interacting with the muscles to form levers.
3. Produce blood cells.
4. Store calcium.

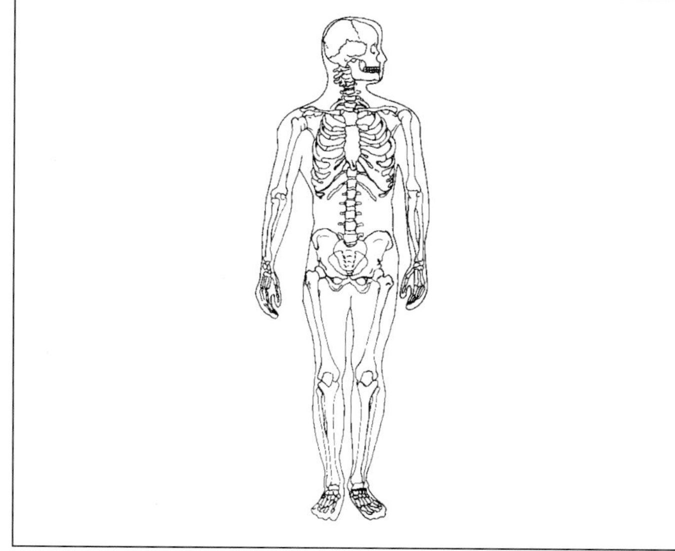

Fig. 1-2. Skeletal system.

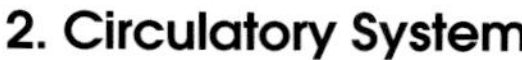

2. Circulatory System

The circulatory system is composed of the cardiovascular organs–heart, blood and blood vessels, and the lymphatic system–lymph nodes, lymph vessels and lymph glands.

Six functions of the circulatory system are to:

1. Distribute oxygen and nutrients to the cells of the body.
2. Carry cell waste and carbon dioxide from the cells.
3. Transport water, electrolytes, hormones and enzymes.
4. Protect against disease.
5. Prevent hemorrhage by forming blood clots.
6. Help regulate body temperature.

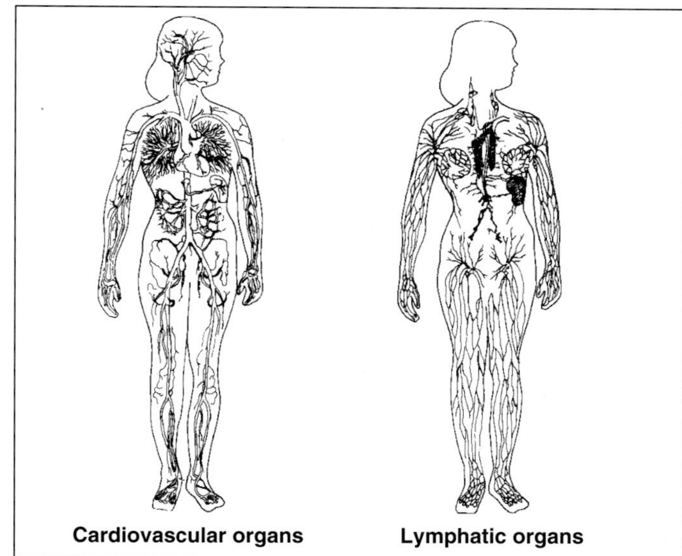

Fig. 1-3. Circulatory system.

3. Digestive System

The digestive system includes the alimentary canal and certain accessory organs. The alimentary canal is made up of the mouth, pharynx, esophagus, stomach, small intestine, large intestine and anus. Accessory organs of digestion include the salivary glands, liver, gallbladder and pancreas.

The twofold function of the digestive system is to:

1. Prepare food for absorption by the cells through numerous physical and chemical breakdown processes.
2. Eliminate solid wastes from the body.

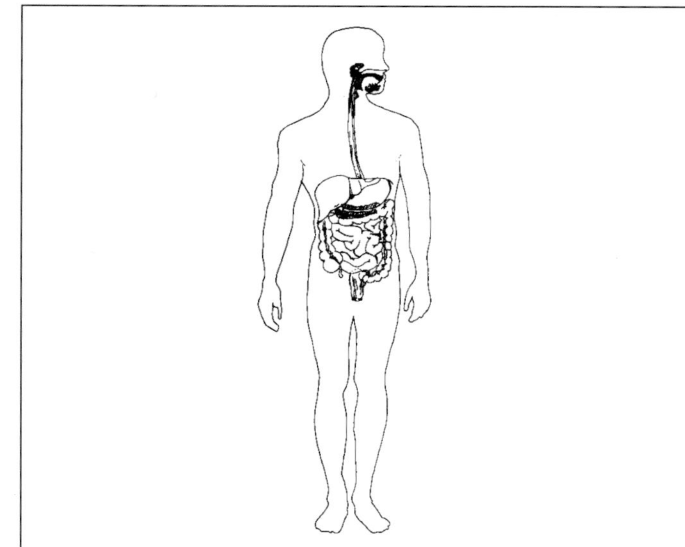

Fig. 1-4. Digestive system.

4. Respiratory System

The respiratory system is composed of two lungs and a series of passages connecting the lungs to the outside atmosphere. The structures making up the passageway from the exterior to the alveoli of the lung interior are the nose, mouth, pharynx, larynx, trachea and bronchial tree.

Three functions of the respiratory system are to:
1. Supply oxygen to the blood and eventually to the cells.
2. Eliminate carbon dioxide from the blood.
3. Assist in regulating the acid-base balance of the blood.

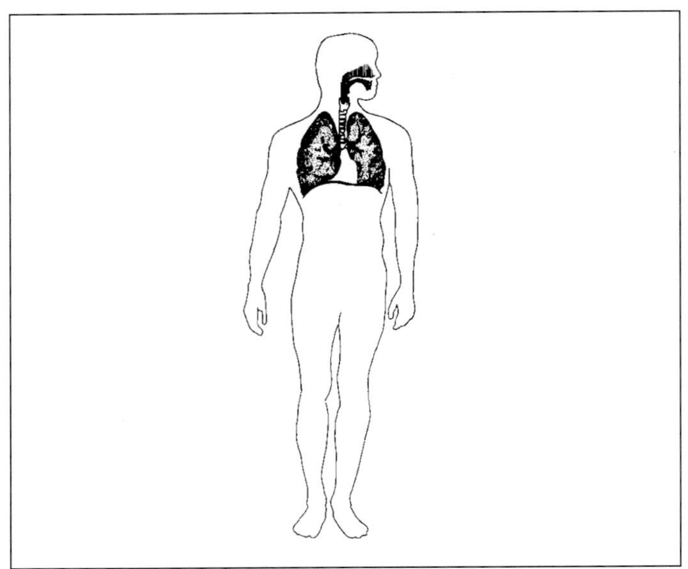

Fig. 1-5. Respiratory system.

5. Urinary System

The urinary system includes those organs that produce, collect and eliminate urine. The organs of the urinary system are the kidneys, ureters, bladder and urethra.

Four functions of the urinary system are to:
1. Regulate the chemical composition of the blood.
2. Eliminate many waste products.
3. Regulate fluid and electrolyte balance and volume.
4. Maintain the acid-base balance of the body.

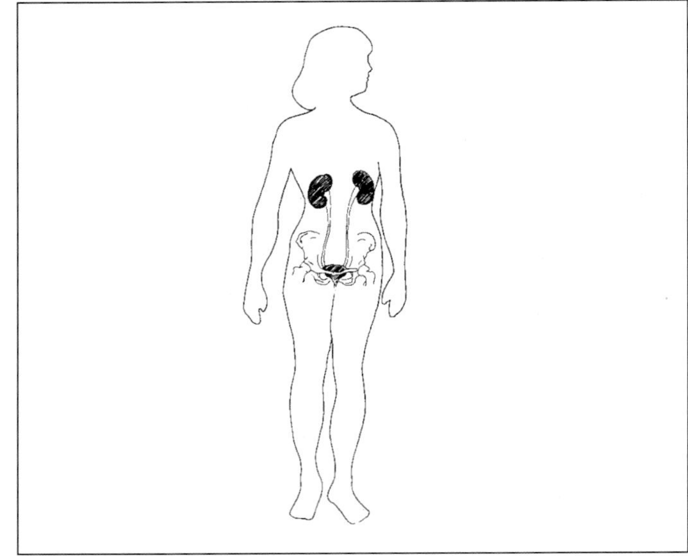

Fig. 1-6. Urinary system.

6. Reproductive System

The reproductive or genital system includes those organs that produce, transport and store the germ cells. The testes in the male and the ovaries in the female produce mature germ cells. Transport and storage organs of the male include the vas deferens, prostate gland and penis. Additional organs of reproduction in the female are the uterine tubes, uterus and vagina.

The function of the reproductive system is to reproduce the organism.

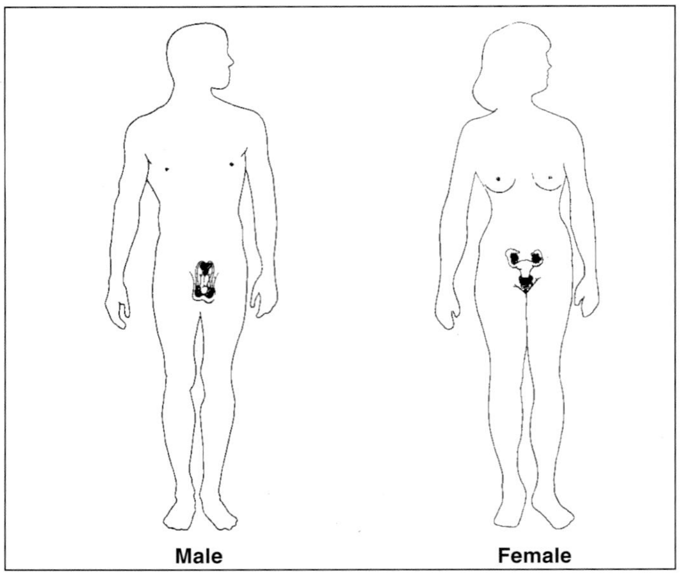

Male Female

Fig. 1-7. Reproductive system.

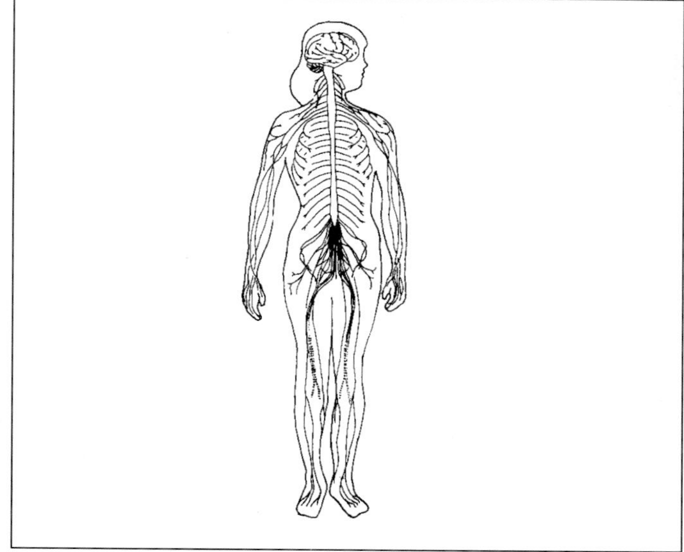
Fig. 1-8. Nervous system.

7. Nervous System

The nervous system is composed of the brain, spinal cord, nerves, ganglia and special sense organs such as the eyes and ears.

The function of the nervous system is to regulate body activities with electrical impulses traveling along various nerves.

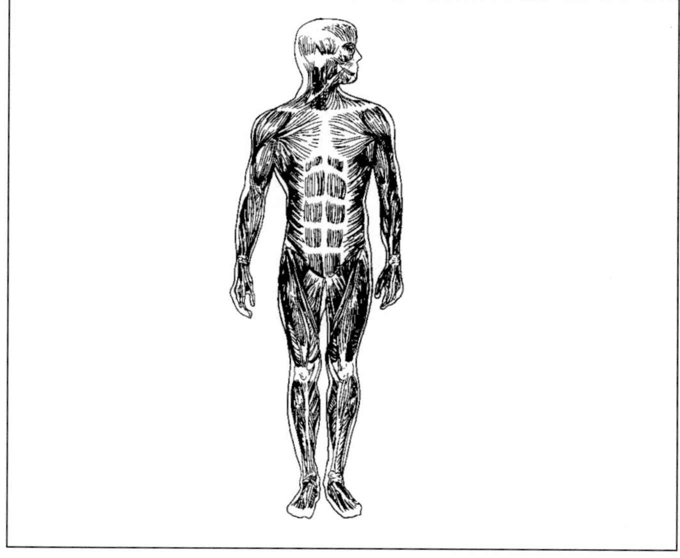
Fig. 1-9. Muscular system.

8. Muscular System

The muscular system includes all muscle tissues of the body and is subdivided into three types: (1) skeletal, (2) visceral, and (3) cardiac.

Most of the muscle mass of the body is skeletal muscle, which is striated and under voluntary control. The voluntary muscles act in conjunction with the skeleton to allow body movement. About 43% of the weight of the human body is composed of voluntary or striated skeletal muscle.

Visceral muscle, which is smooth and involuntary, is located in the walls of hollow internal organs such as blood vessels, stomach and intestines. These muscles are termed involuntary because their contraction is usually not under voluntary or conscious control.

Cardiac muscle is found only in the walls of the heart and is involuntary, but striated.

Three functions of muscle tissue are to:

1. Allow movement, such as locomotion of the body or movement of substances through the alimentary canal.
2. Maintain posture.
3. Produce heat.

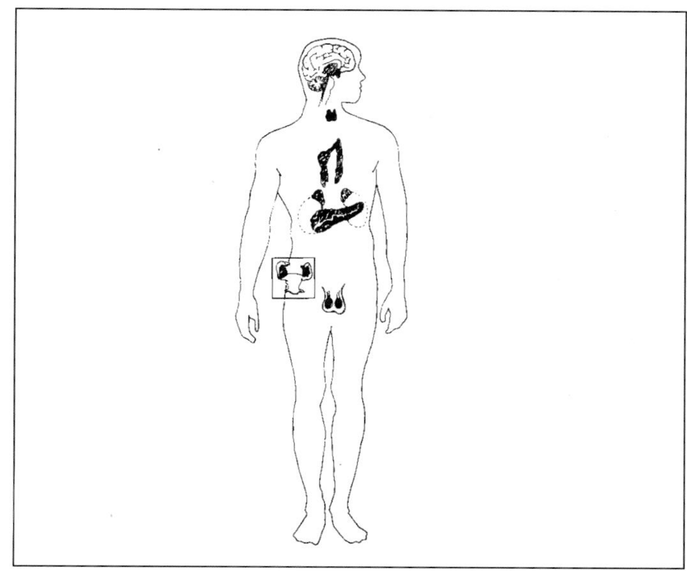
Fig. 1-10. Endocrine system.

9. Endocrine System

The endocrine system includes all of the ductless glands of the body. These glands include the testes, ovaries, pancreas, adrenals, thymus, thyroid, parathyroids, pineal and pituitary. The placenta acts as a temporary endocrine gland.

Hormones, which are the secretions of the endocrine glands, are released directly into the bloodstream.

The function of the endocrine system is to regulate bodily activities through the various hormones carried by the cardiovascular system.

10. Integumentary System

The tenth and final body system is the **integumentary** *(in-teg-u-men′tar-e)* system, which is composed of the skin and all structures derived from the skin. These derived structures include hair, nails, and sweat and oil glands.

The skin is an organ that is essential to life. In fact, the skin is the largest organ of the body, covering a surface area of approximately 7,620 square centimeters in the average adult.

Four functions of the integumentary system are to:
1. Regulate body temperature.
2. Protect the body.
3. Eliminate waste products through perspiration.
4. Receive certain stimuli such as temperature, pressure and pain.

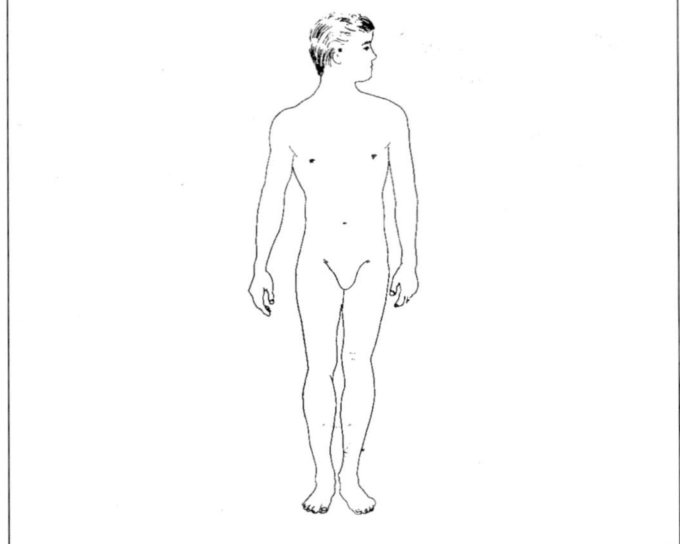

Fig. 1-11. Integumentary system.

Skeletal Anatomy

Since a large part of general diagnostic radiography involves examinations of the bones and joints, **osteology** *(os′te-ol′o-je)* (the study of bones) and **arthrology** *(ar-throl′o-je)* (the study of joints) are important subjects for the radiographer.

OSTEOLOGY

The adult skeletal system is composed of **206 separate bones**, forming the framework of the entire body. Certain cartilages, such as at the ends of long bones, are included in the skeletal system. These bones and cartilages are united by ligaments and provide surfaces to which the muscles attach. Since muscles and bones must combine to allow body movement, these two systems are sometimes collectively referred to as the locomotor system.

The adult human skeleton is divided into either the **axial skeleton** or the **appendicular skeleton**.

Axial Skeleton

The **axial** *(ak′se-al)* **skeleton** includes all bones that lie on or near the central axis of the body. The adult axial skeleton consists of **80 bones** and includes the skull, vertebral column, ribs and sternum (shaded regions of body skeleton in Fig. 1-12).

Adult Axial Skeleton		
Skull:	Cranium	8
	Facial bones	14
Hyoid		1
Auditory ossicles (small bones in each ear)		6
Vertebral column:	Cervical	7
	Thoracic	12
	Lumbar	5
	Sacrum	1
	Coccyx	1
Thorax:	Sternum	1
	Ribs	24
Total number of bones in adult axial skeleton		**80**

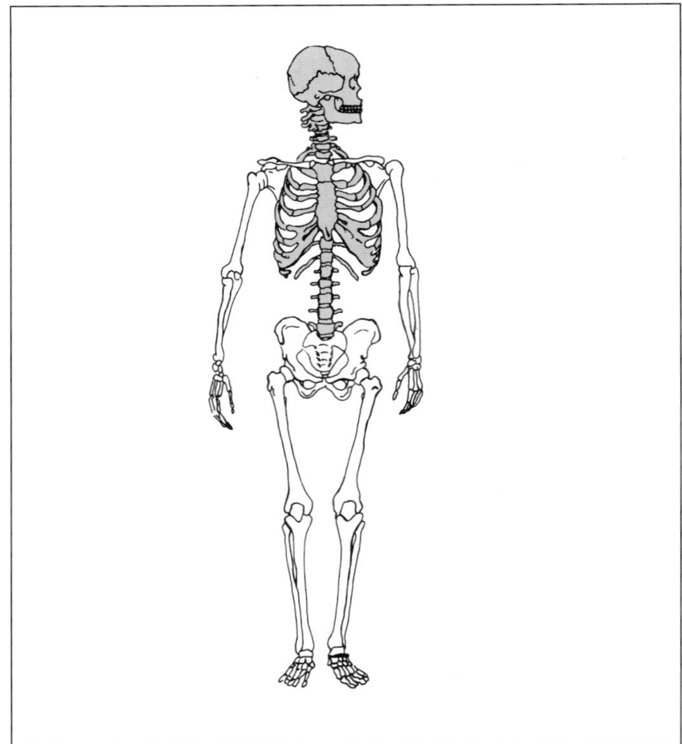

Fig. 1-12. Axial skeleton–80 bones.

Appendicular Skeleton

The second division of the skeleton is the **appendicular** *(ap′ en-dik′ u-lar)* portion. This division consists of all bones of the upper and lower limbs (extremities), as well as the shoulder and pelvic girdles (shaded regions in Fig. 1-13). There are **126 separate bones** in the adult appendicular skeleton.

Adult Appendicular Skeleton		
Shoulder girdles:	Clavicle	2
	Scapula	2
Upper limbs:	Humerus	2
	Ulna	2
	Radius	2
	Carpals	16
	Metacarpals	10
	Phalanges	28
Pelvic girdle:	Hip bone	2
Lower limbs:	Femur	2
	Tibia	2
	Fibula	2
	Patella	2
	Tarsals	14
	Metatarsals	10
	Phalanges	28
Total number of bones in appendicular skeleton		**126**

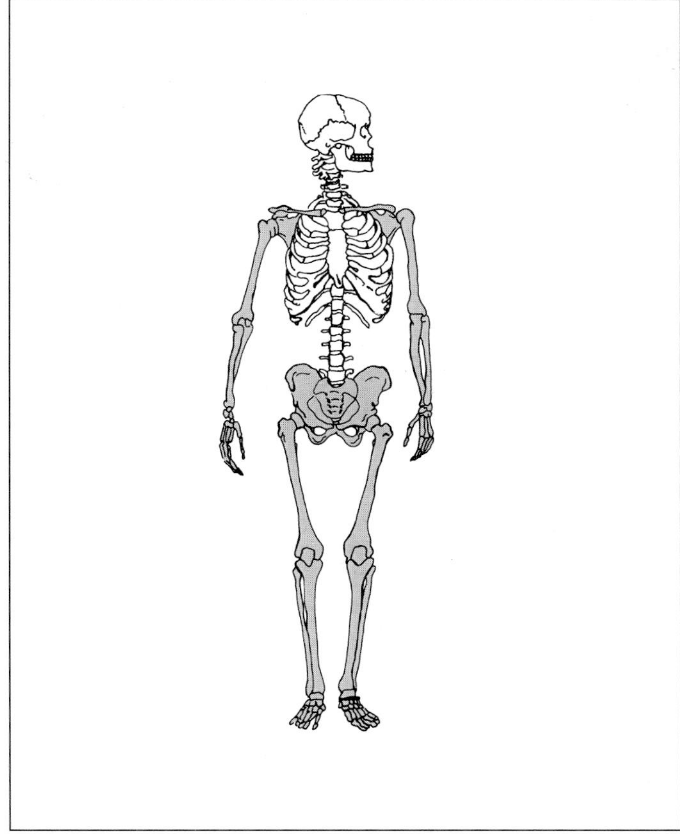

Fig. 1-13. Appendicular skeleton–126 bones.

CLASSIFICATION OF BONES

Each of the 206 bones of the body can be classified according to shape as a long bone, short bone, flat bone, or irregular bone.

Long Bones

Long bones consist of a **body** (shaft or diaphysis [*di-af′ i-sis*]), and two ends or extremities. The ends of long bones articulate with other bones; thus the ends are enlarged, smooth and covered with hyaline cartilage.

Hyaline *(hi′ ah-lin)*, meaning glassy or clear, is a common type of cartilage or connecting tissue, also known as gristle. Its name comes from the fact that it is not visible with ordinary staining techniques, thus appearing as "clear" or glassy in lab studies. It is present in many places, including the covering over ends of bones, where it is called **articular cartilage**.

Long bones are found only in the appendicular skeleton. Fig. 1-14 is a radiograph of a humerus, a typical long bone of the upper arm.

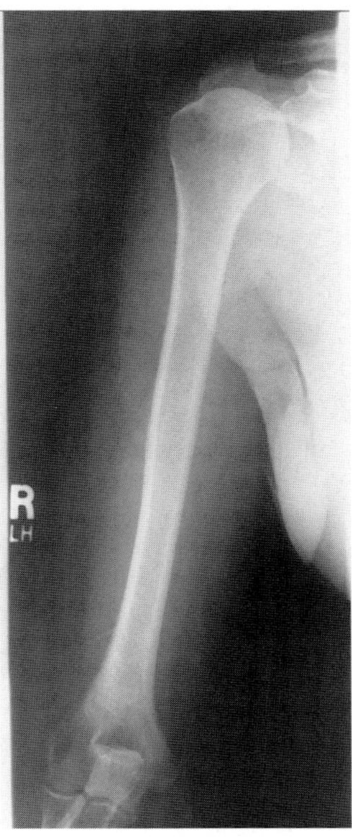

Fig. 1-14. Long bone (humerus).

Composition of Long Bones: The outer shell of most bones is composed of hard or dense bone tissue known as **compact bone** or **cortex**, meaning an external layer. Compact bone has few intercellular empty spaces and serves to protect and support the entire bone.

The **body** (shaft or diaphysis) contains a thicker layer of compact bone than the ends to help resist the stress of the weight placed on them.

Inside the shell of compact bone, and especially at both ends of each long bone, is found **spongy** or **cancellous bone**. Cancellous bone is highly porous and usually contains red bone marrow, which is responsible for production of red blood cells.

The body of a long bone is hollow. This hollow portion is known as the **medullary** *(med′ u-lar″ e)* **cavity**. In the adult the medullary cavity usually contains fatty yellow marrow. A dense fibrous membrane, the **periosteum** *(per″ e-os′ te-am)*, covers bone except at the articulating surfaces.

The articulating surfaces are covered with a layer of cartilage. The periosteum is essential for bone growth, repair and nutrition. Bones are richly supplied with blood vessels that pass into them from the periosteum. Near the center of the shaft of long bones, a **nutrient artery** passes obliquely through the compact bone via a **nutrient foramen** into the medullary cavity.

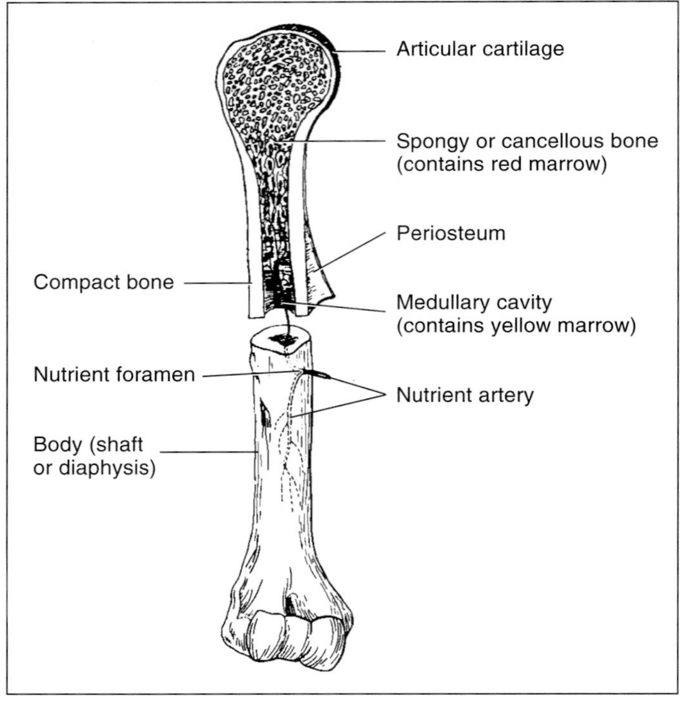

Fig. 1-15. Long bone.

Short Bones

Short bones are roughly cuboidal in shape and are only found in the wrists and ankles. Short bones consist mainly of cancellous tissue with a thin outer covering of compact bone. The eight **carpal bones** of each wrist and the seven **tarsal bones** of each foot are all short bones.

Flat Bones

Flat bones consist of two plates of compact bone with cancellous bone and marrow between them. Examples of flat bones are the bones making up the **calvarium** (skull cap), **sternum**, **ribs** and **scapulae**.

The narrow space between the inner and outer table of flat bones in the cranium is known as **diploe** *(dip′ lo-e)*. Flat bones provide either protection or broad surfaces for muscle attachment.

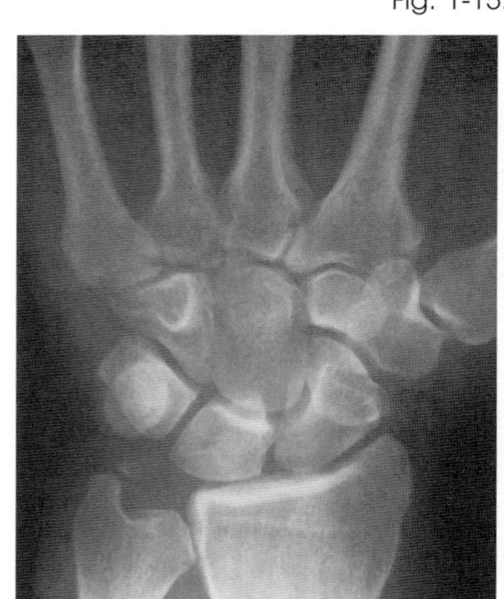
Fig. 1-16. Short bones (carpals).

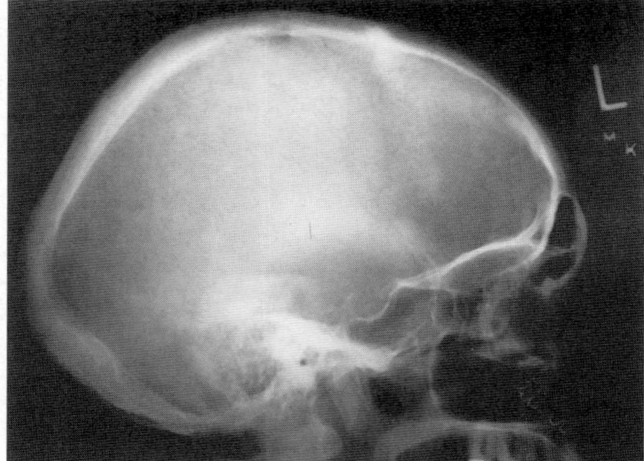

Fig. 1-17. Flat bones (calvarium).

Irregular Bones

Bones that have peculiar shapes are lumped into the final category of irregular bones. **Vertebrae**, **facial bones**, **bones of the base of the cranium** and **bones of the pelvis** are examples of irregular bones.

Blood Cell Production

It should be noted that in adults **red blood cells** (RBCs) are produced by the red bone marrow of certain flat and irregular bones such as the **sternum**, **ribs**, **vertebrae** and **pelvis**.

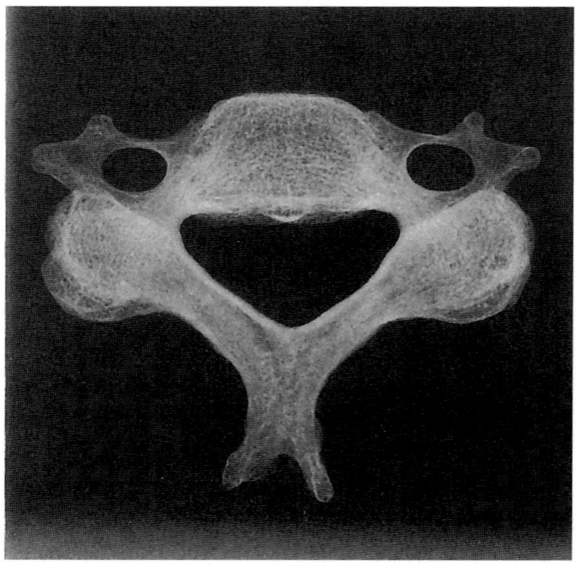
Fig. 1-18. Irregular bone (vertebra).

DEVELOPMENT OF BONES

The process by which bones form in the body is known as **ossification** *(os″ i-fi-ka′ shun)*. The embryonic skeleton is composed of fibrous membranes and hyaline cartilage. Ossification begins about the sixth embryonic week and continues until adulthood.

Two Kinds of Bone Formation

Two kinds of bone formation are known. When bone replaces membranes, the ossification is termed **intramembranous** *(in″ trah-mem′ brah-nus)*. When bone replaces cartilage, the result is **endochondral** *(en″ do-kon′ dral)* (intracartilaginous) ossification.

Intramembranous Ossification: Intramembranous ossification occurs rapidly and takes place in bones that are needed for protection, such as sutures of the flat bones of the skullcap, which are centers of growth in early bone development.

Endochondral Ossification: Endochondral ossification occurs much slower than intramembranous ossification and occurs in most parts of the skeleton, especially in the long bones.

Primary and Secondary Centers of Endochondral Ossification

The first center of ossification is termed the **primary center** and occurs in the mid body area. This primary center of ossification becomes the body (shaft or diaphysis).

Secondary centers of ossification appear near the ends of long bones. Most secondary centers appear after birth, while most primary centers appear before birth. Each secondary center of ossification is termed an **epiphysis** *(e-pif′ i-sis)*. Epiphyses of the distal femur and the proximal tibia are the first to appear and may be present at birth in the term newborn. Cartilaginous plates, termed **epiphyseal plates,** are found between the body and each epiphysis until skeletal growth is complete.

Growth in the length of bones is due to a longitudinal increase in these epiphyseal cartilaginous plates. This is followed by progressive ossification through endochondral bone development until all of the cartilage has been replaced by bone, at which time growth to the skeleton is complete. This process of epiphyseal fusion of the long bones occurs progressively from the age of puberty to **full maturity,** which is **about 25 years**. However, the time for each bone to complete growth varies for different regions of the body. In addition, the female skeleton usually matures more quickly than does the male skeleton. Extensive charts that list the normal growth patterns of the skeleton are available.

Radiograph Demonstrating Bone Growth

Fig. 1-20 shows a radiograph of the knee region of a six-year-old child. Primary and secondary centers of endochondral ossification or bone growth are well demonstrated and labeled.

Primary Centers: The primary centers of bone growth show well developed bone and include the **body** (A) (mid shaft or diaphysis) area.

Secondary Centers: The secondary centers of bone growth are the **epiphyses** (C), which are shown at the distal end of the femur and the proximal end of the tibia and fibula. These epiphyses are separated from the main bone by a space or joint called an **epiphyseal plate** (B). These are made up of cartilage that does not visualize on radiographs because there is no calcium in these areas at this stage of growth. Therefore, these epiphyseal plates disappear completely as cartilage and are replaced with calcium when growth is completed.

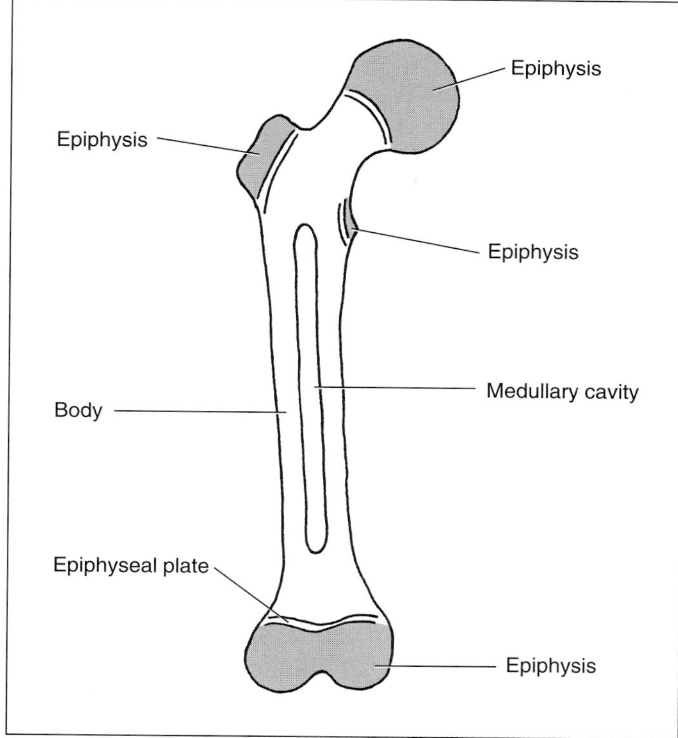

Fig. 1-19. Endochondral ossification.

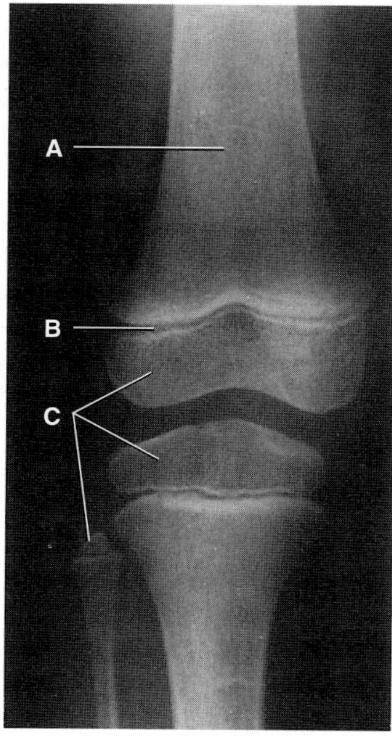

Fig. 1-20. Knee region (six-year-old-child).

Arthrology (Joints)

The study of joints or articulations is called **arthrology**. In studying joints of the skeletal system it is first important to understand that movement does not occur in all joints. Indeed the first types of joints to be described are primarily immovable joints held together by several fibrous layers. These are joints adapted for growth rather than for movement. The second grouping of joints includes most joints of the body, that is those adapted for movement.

CLASSIFICATION OF JOINTS

Functional

Joints are sometimes classified according to their function as to their mobility or lack of mobility. The three common functional classifications are as follows:

- **Synarthrosis** *(sin″ ar-thro′ sis)*–Immovable joint.
- **Amphiarthrosis** *(am″fe-ar-thro′ sis)*–Limited movement.
- **Diarthrosis** *(di″ ar-thro′ sis)*–Freely movable joint.

Structural

Sometimes all joints or articulations of the body are grouped or classified according to the above three functional classes. However, the primary classification system of joints, which is recognized by *NOMINA ANATOMICA* and which is used in this textbook, **is a structural classification** based on the **type of tissue that separates the ends of the bone**. Functional types (listed by description of movement type) are included under each of these structural classifications.

There are three structural classifications based on the **three types of tissues** that separate the ends of bones in the different joints. These three classifications by tissue types along with the subclasses are as follows:

- **Fibrous** *(fi′ brus)* **joints**:
  1. Syndesmosis *(sin″ des-mo′ sis)*
  2. Suture *(su′ tur)*
  3. Gomphosis *(gom-fo′ sis)*
- **Cartilaginous** *(kar″ ti-laj′ i-nus)* **joints**:
  1. Symphysis *(sim′fi-sis)*
  2. Synchondrosis *(sin″kon-dro′ sis)*
- **Synovial** *(si-no′ ve-al)* **joints**.

These three classes and their subclasses will be described and illustrated with examples beginning, with fibrous joints.

Fibrous Joints

Fibrous joints lack a joint cavity. The adjoining bones, which are nearly in direct contact with each other, are **held together by fibrous connective tissue**. Three types of fibrous joints are; **syndesmoses**, which are slightly movable; **sutures**, which are immovable; and **gomphoses**, a unique type of joint with only very limited movement (Fig. 1-21).

1. Syndesmoses

The only true syndesmosis joint in the body is the **distal tibiofibular joint**.* Fibrous ligaments hold the distal tibia and fibula together at this joint, which is only **slightly movable** or **amphiarthrodial.**

*Clemente, CD. *Gray's Anatomy*, 13th ed., Philadelphia: Lea and Febiger; 1985 (p. 322).

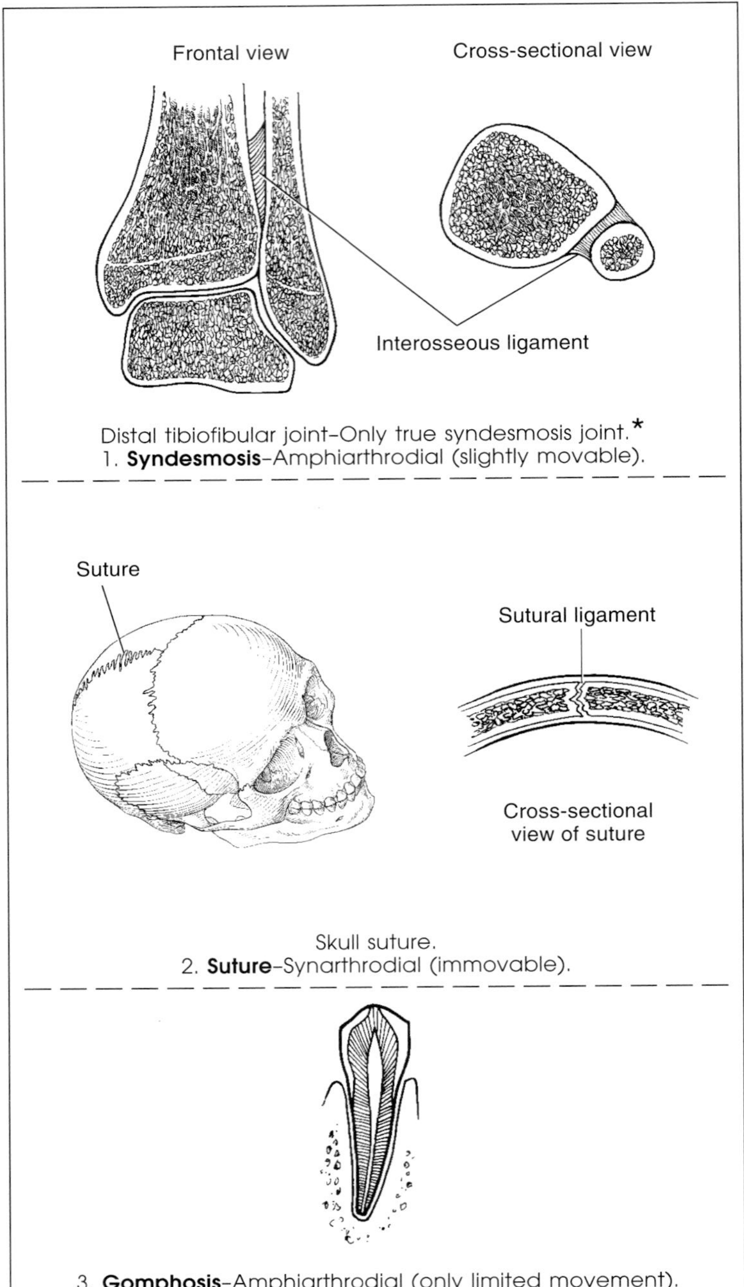

Fig. 1-21. Fibrous joints–Three types.

2. Sutures

Sutures are found between bones in the skull. These bones make contact with one another along interlocking or serrated edges and are held together by layers of fibrous tissue or ligaments. Therefore, there is very limited movement at these articulations, and on an adult they are considered **immovable** or **synarthrodial joints.**

Some limited expansion-compression type movement at these sutures can occur in the infant skull, such as during the birthing process, but upon reaching adulthood, active bone deposition partially or completely obliterates these suture lines.

3. Gomphoses

A **gomphosis** joint is a third unique type of fibrous joint in which a conical process is inserted into a socket-like portion of bone. This joint or fibrous union, which strictly speaking does not occur between bones but between the roots of the teeth and the alveoli of the mandible and maxillae, is a specialized type of articulation allowing only very limited movement.

Cartilaginous Joints

Cartilaginous joints also lack a joint cavity and the articulating bones are **held tightly together by cartilage**. Like fibrous joints they allow little or no movement. Therefore, these joints are either synarthrodial or amphiarthrodial and are held together by two types of cartilage. They are as follows:

1. Symphyses

The essential feature of a symphysis type joint is **the presence of a broad, flattened disc of fibrocartilage** between two contiguous bony surfaces. These fibrocartilage disks form relatively thick pads that are capable of being compressed or displaced, thereby allowing some movement of these bones, or **amphiarthrodial** (slightly movable).

Examples of such symphyses are the intervertebral disks (between bodies of the vertebrae), and the symphysis pubis (between the two pubic bones of the pelvis).

2. Synchondroses

A typical synchondrosis is a **temporary form of joint** wherein the connecting **hyaline cartilage** (which on long bones is called an epiphyseal plate) is converted into bone upon reaching adulthood. These temporary types of growth joints are considered **synarthrodial** or immovable.

Examples of such joints are the epiphyseal plates between the epiphyses and body (diaphyses) of long bones, and at the three-part union of the pelvis, which forms the "cup-shaped" acetabulum for the hip joint.

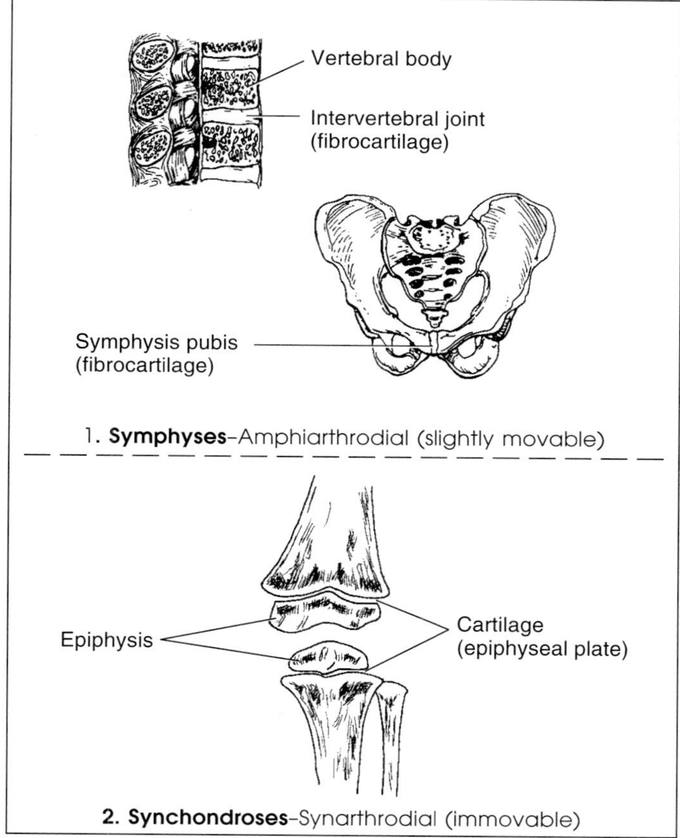

Fig. 1-22. Cartilaginous joints.

Synovial Joints

The third classification of joints are synovial joints, those freely movable joints, mostly of the upper and lower limbs, characterized by **a fibrous capsule containing synovial fluid.** The ends of the bones making up a synovial joint may make contact but are completely separate and contain a joint space or cavity, which allows for the wide range of movement at these joints. Synovial joints are generally diarthrodial or freely movable. (Exceptions to this are the sacroiliac joints of the pelvis, which are amphiarthrodial or slightly movable.)

The exposed ends of these bones contain thin protective type coverings of **hyaline articular cartilage**. The **joint cavity**, which contains a viscous lubricating **synovial fluid**, is enclosed and surrounded by a **fibrous capsule**, which is reinforced by strengthening **accessory ligaments**. These ligaments limit motion in undesirable directions. The inner surface of this fibrous capsule is thought to secrete the lubricating synovial fluid.

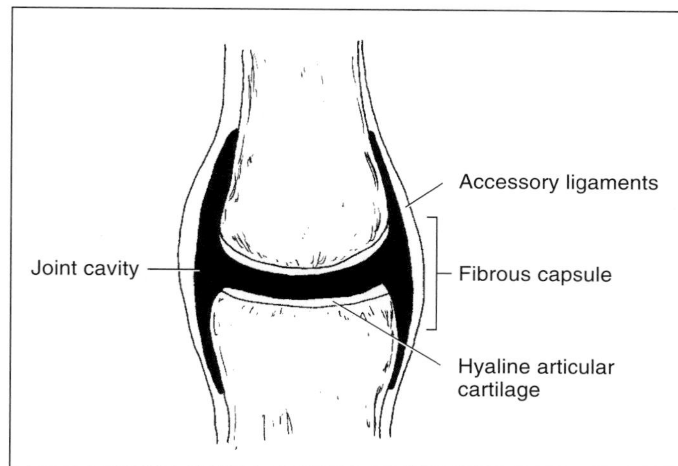

Fig. 1-23. Synovial joints–Diarthrodial (freely movable).

Movement Types of Synovial Joints

Synovial joints occur in considerable number and variety, and they are grouped according to the **six types of movements** they permit. These are listed in order from the least to the greatest permitted movement.

The preferred name is listed first followed by older terms or synonyms in parentheses. (This practice is followed throughout this textbook.)

1. Plane (Gliding) Joints

This type of synovial joint permits the least movement, which as the name implies, is **a sliding or gliding motion between the articulating surfaces**.

Examples of such joints are the **intermetacarpal**, **carpometacarpal** and **intercarpal** joints of the hand and wrist.

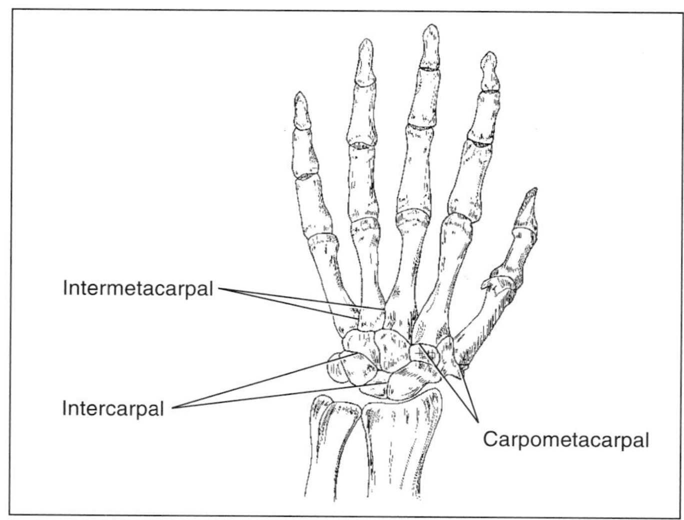

Fig. 1-24. Plane (gliding) joints.

2. Ginglymus (Hinge) Joints

The articular surfaces of a ginglymus *(jin′ glĭ-mus)* or hinge joint are molded to each other in such a way to permit **flexion and extension movements** only. The articular fibrous capsule on this type of joint is thin on those surfaces where bending takes place but strong collateral ligaments firmly secure the bones at the lateral margins of the fibrous capsule.

Examples of such joints are the **interphalangeal joints** of both fingers and toes, the **knee joint**, the **elbow joint** and the **ankle joint**.

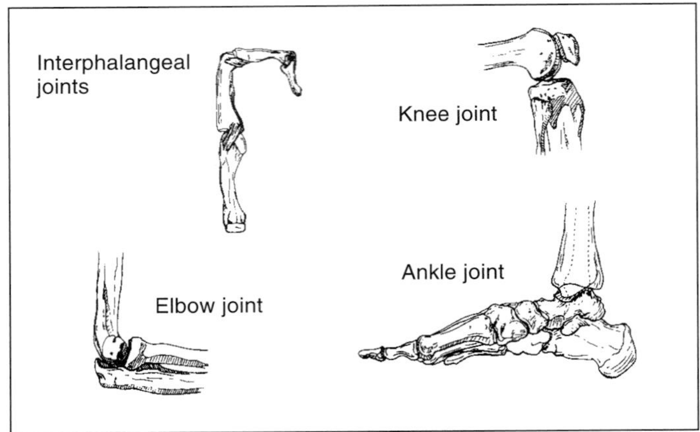

Fig. 1-25. Ginglymus (hinge) joints.

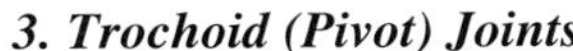

3. Trochoid (Pivot) Joints

The trochoid *(tro′ koid)*, or pivot, joint is formed by a bony pivot-like process that is surrounded by a ring of ligaments and/or bony structure. This allows **rotational movements** around a single axis.

Examples of such joints are the **proximal** and **distal radioulnar joints** of the forearm which demonstrate this pivot-like movement during rotation of the hand and wrist.

Another example is the joint **between first and second cervical vertebrae**. The dens of the axis (C2) forms the pivot, and the anterior arch of the atlas (C1), combined with posterior ligaments, forms the ring.

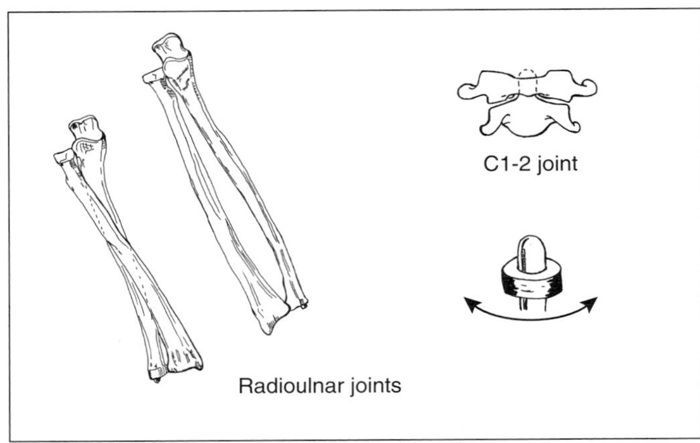

Fig. 1-26. Trochoid (pivot) joints.

4. Ellipsoid (Condyloid) Joints

In the ellipsoid *(e-lip′ soid)* or condyloid joint, movement occurs primarily in one plane combined with a slight degree of rotation at an axis which is at right angles to the primary plane of movement. The rotational movement is somewhat limited by associated ligaments and tendons.

This type of joint therefore allows primarily four directional movements of **flexion and extension,** along with **abduction and adduction**. **Circumduction** movement also occurs, which results from cone-like sequential movements of flexion, abduction, extension and adduction.

Examples of ellipsoid joints are the **2nd through 5th metacarpophalangeal joints of fingers**, the **wrist joint**, and the **metatarsophalangeal joints of the toes**.

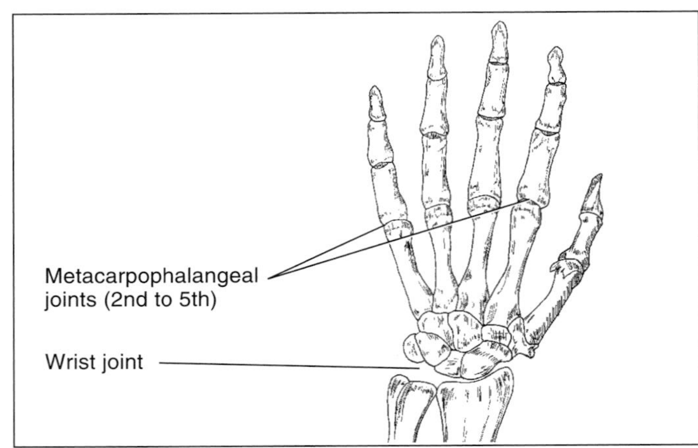

Fig. 1-27. Ellipsoid (condyloid) joints.

5. Sellar (Saddle) Joints

The term sellar *(sel′ ar)* or saddle describes this joint structure well in that the ends of the bones are shaped concavo-convex or opposite to one another as illustrated in Fig. 1-28 (two saddle-like structures fit into each other).

Movements of this biaxial type sellar joint are the same as for ellipsoidal joints, namely **flexion, extension, adduction, abduction** and **circumduction**.

The best example of a sellar joint is the first carpometacarpal joint of the thumb.

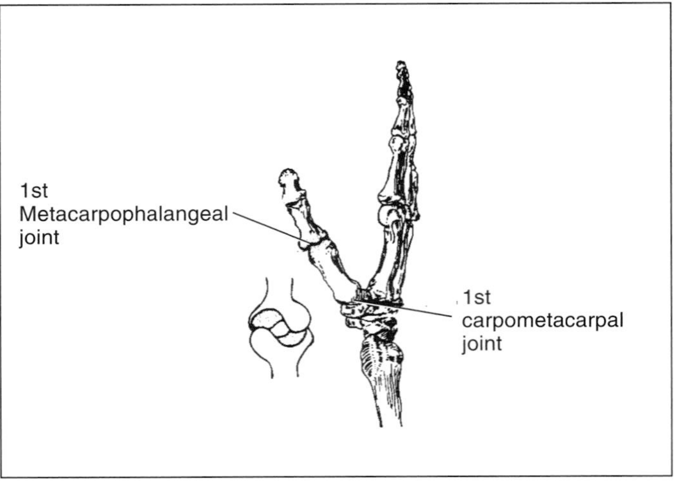

Fig. 1-28. Sellar (saddle) joints.

6. Spheroid (Ball and Socket) Joints

The spheroid *(sfe′ roid)* or ball and socket joint allows the greatest freedom of motion. The distal bone making up the joint is capable of motion around an almost indefinite number of axes, with one common center.

The greater the depth of the socket, the more limited the movement. The joint, however, is stronger and more stable. For example, the hip joint is a much stronger and more stable joint than the shoulder joint, but the range of movement is also more limited in the hip.

Movements of spheroid joints are **flexion, extension, abduction, adduction, circumduction, medial** and **lateral rotation.**

The two examples of ball and socket joints are the **hip joint** and the **shoulder joint**.

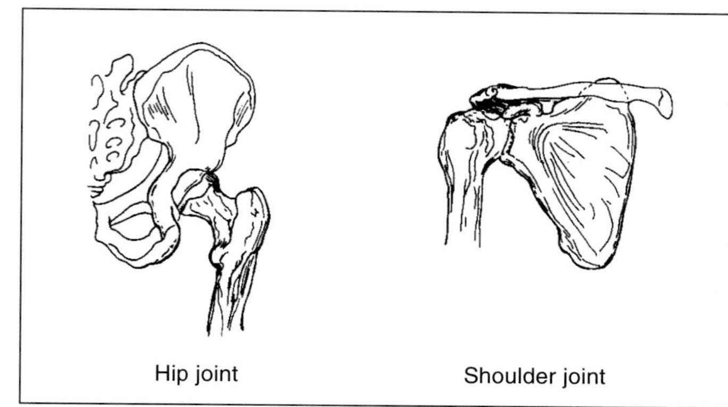

Fig. 1-29. Spheroid (ball and socket) joints.

Summary of Joint Classification

Joint classification	*Mobility classification*	*Movement types*	*Movement description*	*Examples*
A. Fibrous joints				
1. Syndesmoses	Amphiarthrodial (slightly movable)	—	—	–Distal tibiofibular joint
2. Sutures	Synarthrodial (immovable)	—	—	–Skull sutures
3. Gomphoses	Very limited movement	—	—	–Around roots of teeth
B. Cartilaginous joints				
1. Symphyses	Amphiarthrodial (slightly movable)	—	—	–Intervertebral disks –Symphysis pubis
2. Synchondroses	Synarthrodial (immovable)	—	—	–Epiphyseal plates of long bones, and between the three parts of the pelvis
C. Synovial joints	Diarthrodial (freely movable)	1. Plane (gliding)	–Sliding or gliding	–Intermetacarpal, intercarpal, and carpometacarpal joints
		2. Ginglymus (hinge)	–Flexion and extension	–Interphalangeal joints of fingers and toes, knee, ankle and elbow joints
		3. Trochoid (pivot)	–Rotational	–Proximal and distal radioulnar, and between C1 and C2 vertebrae
		4. Ellipsoid (condyloid)	–Flexion and extension –Abduction and adduction –Circumduction	–2nd to 5th metacarpophalangeal and wrist joints
		5. Sellar (saddle)	–Flexion and extension –Abduction and adduction –Circumduction	–First carpometacarpal of thumb
		6. Spheroid (ball and socket)	–Flexion and extension –Abduction and adduction –Circumduction –Medial and lateral rotation	–Hip and shoulder joints

Study of Arthrology Continues: Arthrology or the study of joints will continue throughout this text as specific anatomy, including all joints of the human body, is studied in more detail in following chapters.

Radiographic Terminology

It is essential that each person planning to work as a medical radiographer clearly understand the terminology commonly used in medical radiographic positioning. This part of Chapter 1 lists, describes and illustrates those commonly used terms consistent with the positioning and projection terminology as adopted and published by *The American Registry of Radiologic Technologists* in January 1990.* These terms are also generally consistent with those used in Canada, according to the *Canadian Association of Medical Radiation Technologists.*

Throughout this text the use of named positions (proper names of the person first describing a specific position or procedure) are referred to as a method, such as the Towne, Waters and Caldwell methods.

The anatomical terms used in this section and throughout this text are in agreement with the widely used standard as adopted in 1985 by the Twelfth International Congress of Anatomists in London, published in the sixth edition of *NOMINA ANATOMICA.*†

GENERAL TERMS

Terms commonly used in radiographic positioning are defined and illustrated (with examples) to clarify meanings and definitions.

1. Radiograph** (ra′de-o-graf)* ***vs. X-ray Film:

- A radiograph is an x-ray film containing a processed image of an anatomical part of a patient (produced by action of x-rays on x-ray film).

Radiography** (ra″de-og′rah-fe)* ***is the production of radiographs.

Note: In practice, the terms **radiograph** and **x-ray film** are often used interchangeably. The x-ray film specifically refers to the physical piece of material upon which the radiographic image is exposed. The term radiograph includes the x-ray film **and** the image that it contains.

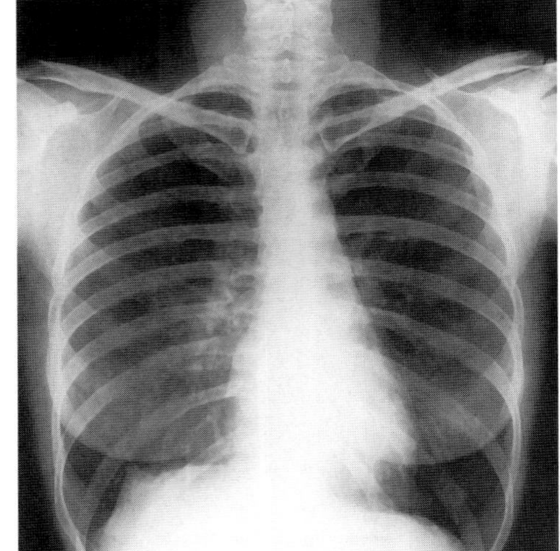

Fig. 1-30. Chest radiograph.

2. Radiographic Examination or Procedure:

- A radiographer is shown positioning the patient for a routine chest exam or procedure.

A radiographic examination of the chest includes five general functions as follows:
(a) Positioning of the body part; and CR (central ray) alignment.
(b) Selection of radiation protection measures.
(c) Selection of exposure factors (radiographic technique) on control panel of x-ray machine.
(d) Initiating or "making" the exposure.
(e) Processing (developing) of the film.

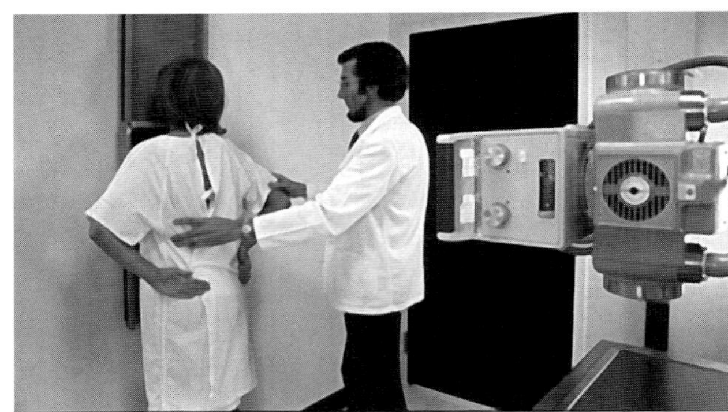

Fig. 1-31. Radiographic examination.

3. Anatomical** (an″ah-tom′e-kal)* ***Position:

- An **upright position, arms adducted** (down), **palms forward, head and feet directed straight ahead.**

This specific body position is used as a reference for other positioning terms.

Note: When referring to one part of the body in relationship to other parts, one must always think of the person as **standing erect in the anatomical position**, even when describing parts of a patient who is lying down, otherwise confusion as to the meaning of the description may result.

Viewing radiographs: A common general rule in viewing radiographs is to display them so that **the patient is facing the viewer**, with the patient in the **anatomical position**. This is described in more detail at the end of Chapter 1.

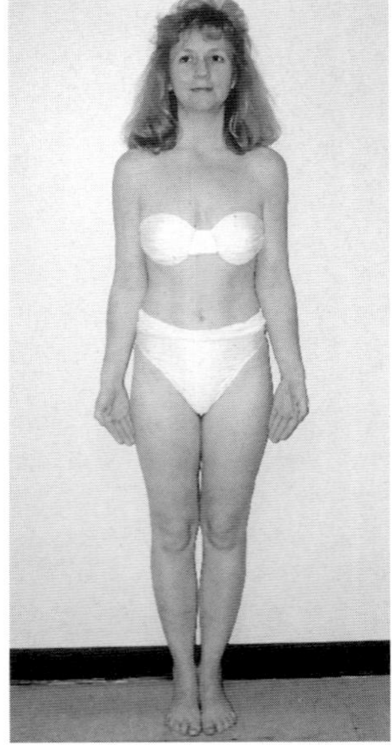

Fig. 1-32. Anatomical position.

**ARRT Educator's Handbook,* 3rd ed. The American Registry of Radiologic Technologists, St. Paul, 1990.
†*Nomina Anatomica,* 6th ed. Authorized by the Twelfth International Congress of Anatomists in London, 1985. Churchill Livingstone, Edinburgh London, 1989.

BODY PLANES, SECTIONS AND LINES

Positioning terms describing central ray angles or relationships between body parts are often related to **imaginary planes** passing through the body in the **anatomical position**. The study of CT (computed tomography) and MRI (magnetic resonance imaging) emphasizes sectional anatomy, which also involves the primary body planes and sections as follows:

Plane - A straight line surface connecting two points.

4. Sagittal (saj' i-tal) Plane:

- The vertical plane dividing the body into **right and left parts**.
- The **midsagittal plane**, also called the **median plane**, is a midline sagittal plane dividing the body into **equal right and left parts**. It passes approximately through the sagittal suture of the skull; therefore, any plane parallel to the median plane is called a sagittal plane.

  These can also be described as anteroposterior planes, which are parallel to the long axis of the body.

5. Coronal (ko-ro' nal) or Frontal Plane:

- The vertical plane dividing the body into **anterior and posterior parts.**
- The midcoronal plane divides the body into equal anterior and posterior parts. It is called a coronal plane because it passes approximately through the coronal suture of the skull. Therefore any plane parallel to the frontal or midcoronal plane is called a coronal plane.

  These planes can also be described as side-to-side or lateral planes that are parallel to the long axis of the body and perpendicular to the median or midsagittal plane.

6. Horizontal (Transverse or Axial) Plane:

- Any plane passing through the body at **right angles to the sagittal or coronal planes**, dividing the body into superior and inferior portions.

Section - A "cut" surface or "slice" of an organ.

7. Longitudinal Sections:

- Those sections running **lengthwise** in the direction of the long axis of the body or any of its parts, regardless of the position of the body (erect or recumbent).

  Longitudinal sections may be taken in the **sagittal** or **coronal** planes.

8. Transverse or Axial Sections (Cross-sections):

- Are taken **at right angles along any point of the longitudinal axis** of the body or its parts.

Note: **Oblique planes or sections** are those planes or sections that slant or deviate from any of the three body planes.

Sagittal, coronal and axial images: CT and MRI images are scanned (or taken) in these three orientations or views. The **sagittal image** is a sectional view through a sagittal plane (Fig. 1-35). A **coronal image** is seen through a coronal plane (Fig. 1-36). The **axial (cross-sectional) image** refers to a horizontal view at some point along the length of the body (Fig. 1-37).

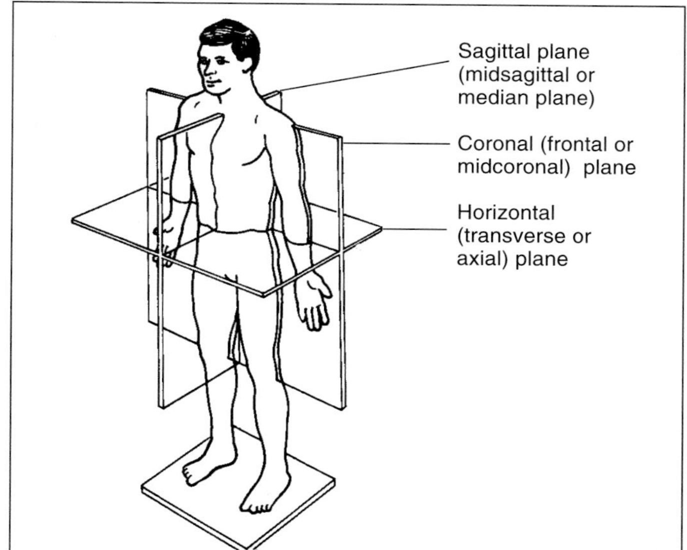

Fig. 1-33. Sagittal, coronal, and horizontal body planes.

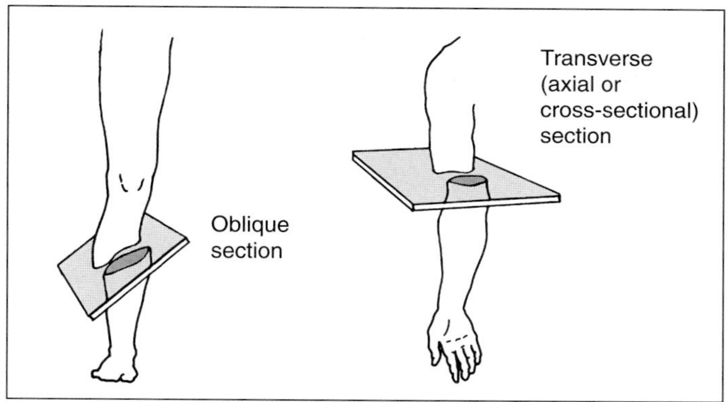

Fig. 1-34. Transverse (axial or cross-sectional) and oblique sections.

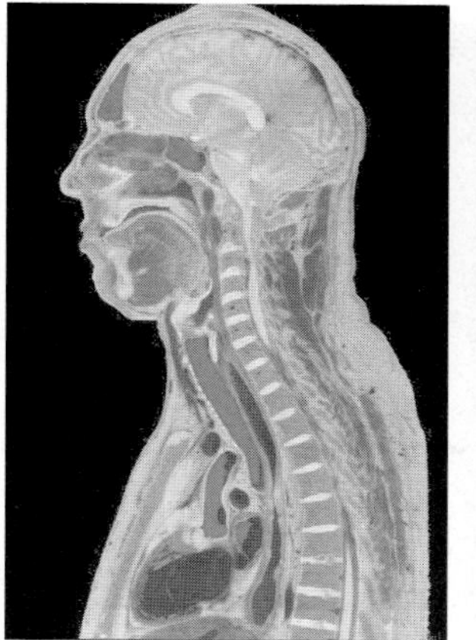

Fig. 1-35. Sagittal image.

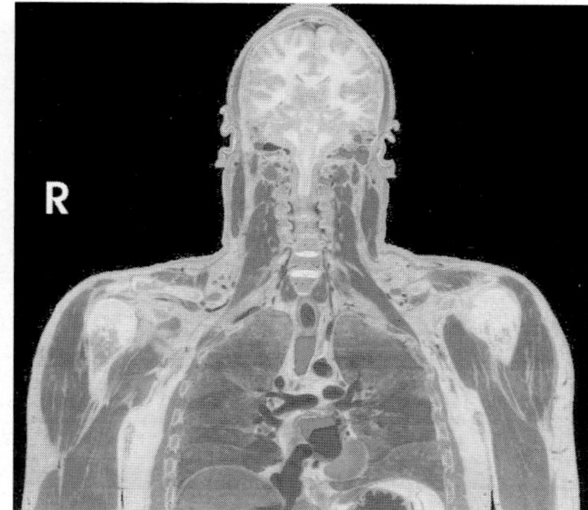

Fig. 1-36. Coronal image.

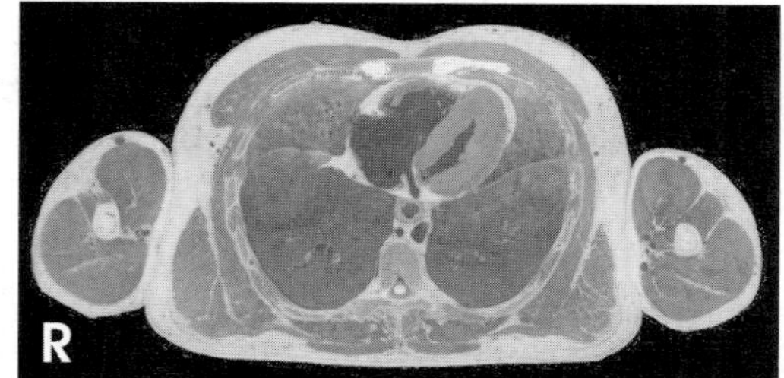

Fig. 1-37. Axial (cross-sectional) image–Mid-thorax.

Line–An imaginary straight line connecting two anatomical landmarks.*

9. ***Reid's** (rēdz)* ***Base Line**** ***(Infraorbitomeatal Line):***

- A **line** passing from the infraorbital margin (inferior edge of bony orbits) through the superior border of the external auditory meatus (EAM), to the mid occipital bone.
- In radiographic positioning this line is most commonly referred to as the **IOML** (infraorbitomeatal line).

Note: The EAM, also known as the auricular point, is the external opening of the ear.

Reid's base line is sometimes referred to as just the **"base line,"** sometimes also called the **anthropological base line** of the skull.

This line is used in cranial topography to measure and locate specific cranial points or structures. This is also commonly used as a reference line in skull positioning, as will be described in later chapters.

Base plane of skull: A transverse **plane** formed by connecting the base lines on each side of the skull. This is also sometimes called the **anthropological plane**, or the **Frankfort horizontal plane**.*

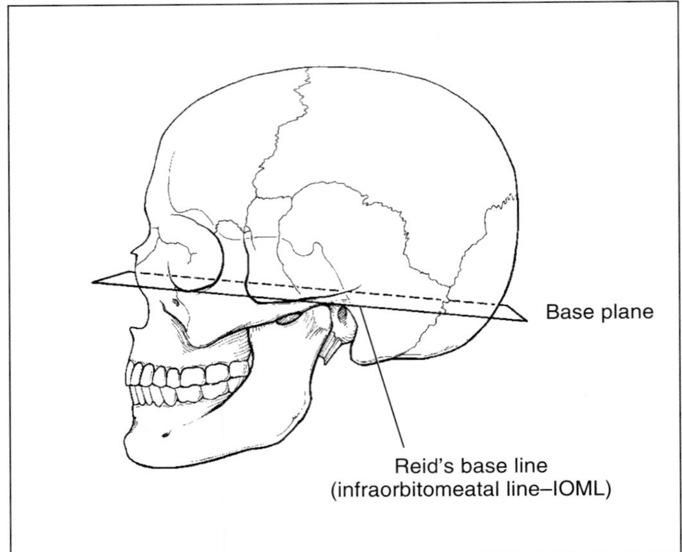

Fig. 1-38. Reid's base line. **-Infraorbitomeatal line-IOML.**

BODY SURFACES AND PARTS

Terms for the Back and Front Portions of the Body

10. ***Posterior** (pos-te' re-or)* ***or Dorsal** (dor' sal):*

- Refers to the **back half** of patient or that part of the body seen when viewing the person from the back. This includes the bottom of feet and the back of hands.

11. ***Anterior** (an-te' re-or)* ***or Ventral** (ven' tral):*

- Refers to **front half** of patient or that part seen when viewed from the front. This includes the tops of feet and the fronts or palms of hands.

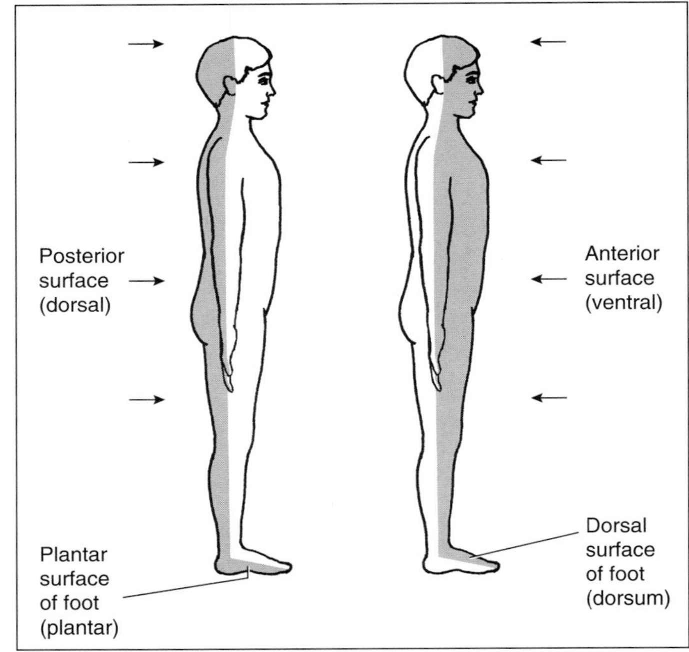

Fig. 1-39. Posterior vs. anterior.

Terms for Surfaces of the Hands and Feet

Three terms used in radiography to describe specific surfaces of the upper and lower limbs are:

12. ***Plantar** (plan' tar):*

- Refers to the **sole** or **posterior** surface of the foot.*†

13. ***Dorsum** (dor' sum):*

- Refers to the **top** or **anterior** surface of the foot.*

As described above, the term **dorsum or dorsal in general refers to the vertebral or posterior part** of the body. However, in human anatomy, when used in relationship with the foot, the term dorsum or dorsal specifically refers to the **anterior** or **top** of the foot.

14. ***Palmar** (pal' mar)* ***(Volar):***

- Refers to the **palm of the hand.*** In the anatomical position this would be the same as the **anterior or ventral** surface of the hand.

Note: The term **volar** is sometimes used to refer to the palm of the hand, the palmar surface. However, volar may also be used to refer to the sole of the foot. "Vola" literally means the hollow of the hand or foot.

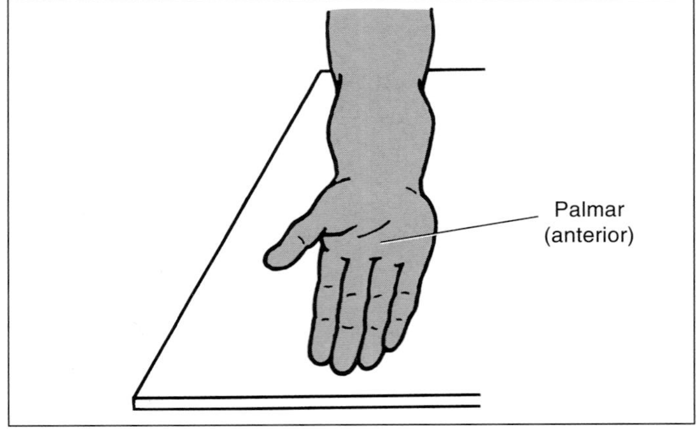

Fig. 1-40. Palmar (volar) surface.

**Dorland's Illustrated Medical Dictionary,* 27th ed., Philadelphia: WB Saunders Co.; 1988.
†Gray, H. *Gray's Anatomy,* 30th ed., Philadelphia: Lea and Febiger; 1984.

POSITIONING AND BODY POSITIONS

The term **positioning** or **radiographic positioning** as used in the title of this textbook in general refers to the science or study of positioning a patient in certain body positions to radiographically demonstrate or visualize specific body parts on film or other image receptors.

In radiography, the term **position** is used two ways, first as a **general body position** as described below (terms 15 through 21), and second as **specific body positions** (terms 22 through 31).

General Body Positions

15. Supine *(soo´pīn):*

- A general body position.
- **Lying on back** with face directed upward (anteriorly).

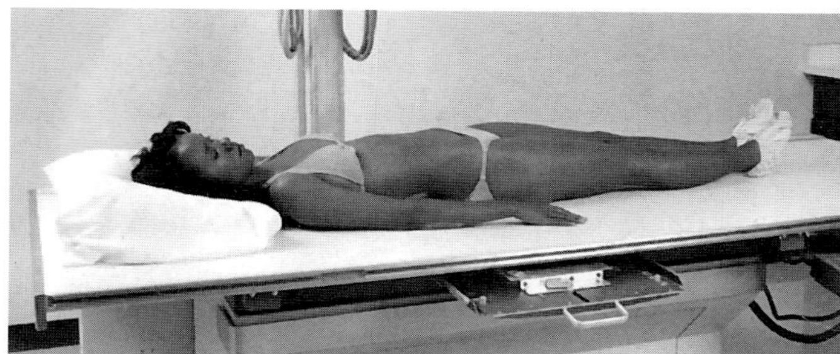

Fig. 1-41. Supine.

16. Prone *(prōn):*

- A general body position.
- **Lying on abdomen,** facing downward (head may be turned to one side).

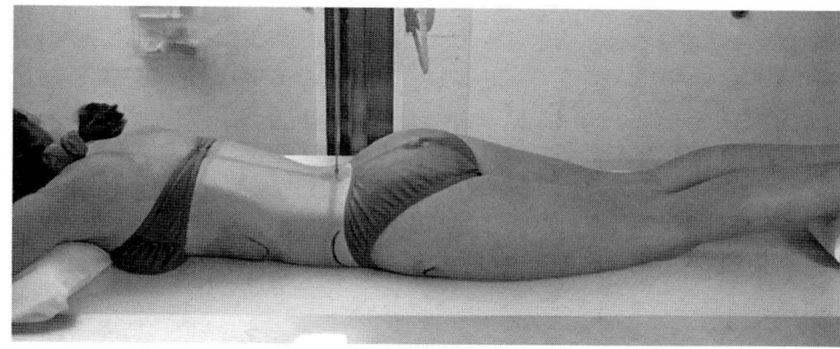

Fig. 1-42. Prone.

17. Erect *(i´reckt´):*

- A general body position.
- An **upright position,** to stand or sit erect.

18. Recumbent *(re-kum´bent)* ***(Reclining):***

- A general body position.
- **Lying down in any position** (prone, supine, on side etc.).

Dorsal Recumbent: Lying on back (supine).

Ventral Recumbent: Lying face down (prone).

Lateral Recumbent: Lying on side (right or left lateral).

19. Trendelenburg[*] *(tren-del´en-berg):*

- A general body position.
- A recumbent position with body plane tilted so **head is lower than feet.**

Note: In radiology, the term Trendelenburg is commonly used to refer to any supine position wherein the head is lower than the feet, even though certain references state a specific amount of tilt that varies from 30 to 40°.[†]

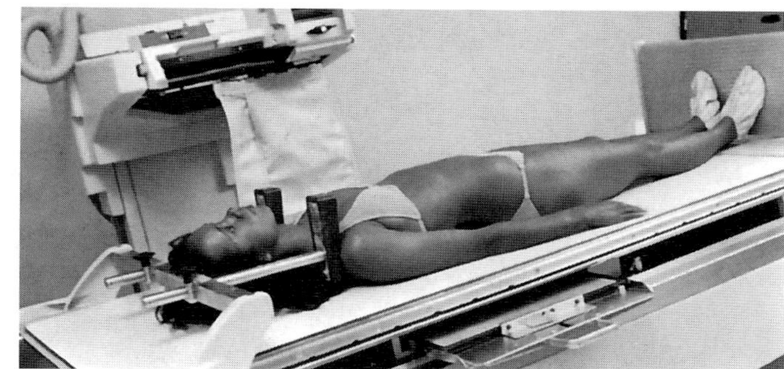

Fig. 1-43. Trendelenburg position–Head lower than feet.

20. Fowler's[††] *(fow´lerz)* ***Position:***

- A general body position
- A recumbent position with the body plane tilted so the **head is higher than the feet** (such as 18 to 20 inches or 45 to 50 cm higher, or ≈30° tilt).[†]

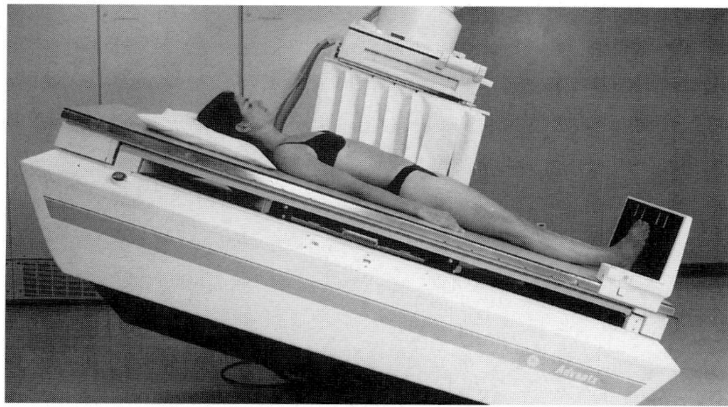

Fig. 1-44. Fowler's position–Feet lower than head.

21. Lithotomy *(lĭ-thot´o-me)* ***Position:***

- A general body position.
- A **recumbent** (supine) position with knees and hip flexed and thighs abducted and rotated externally, supported by leg and ankle supports.

Note: This term comes from litho (stone) and tome (cut), and is a position for surgical removal of a kidney stone. A slight modification of this position is illustrated on a special x-ray table as used in retrograde urography described in a later chapter on the urinary system.

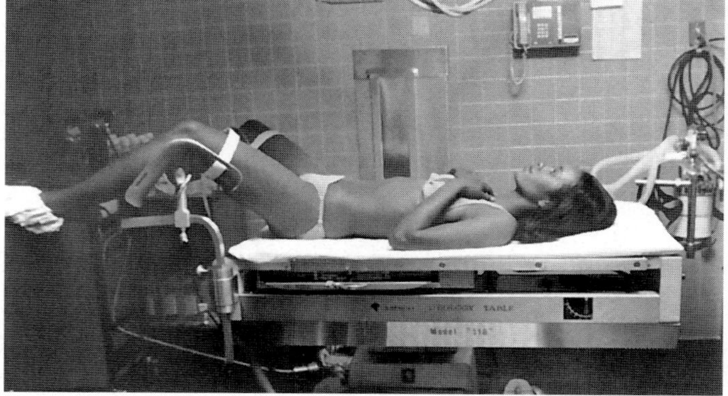

Fig. 1-45. Modified lithotomy position (for retrograde urography).

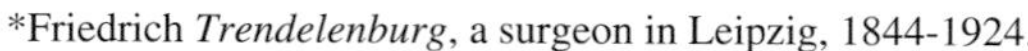

*Friedrich *Trendelenburg*, a surgeon in Leipzig, 1844-1924.

†*Dorland's Illustrated Medical Dictionary*, 27th ed.

††George Ryerson *Fowler*, an American surgeon, 1848-1906.

Specific Body Positions

The second way the term **position** is used in radiography is to refer to a specific body position described by **the body part closest to the film** (obliques and laterals) or by the **surface on which the patient is lying** (decubitus).

***22. Lateral** (lat′ er-al) **Position** (also see Lateral Projection, page 20):*

- A specific body position.
- Refers to the side of, a side view or "sideways."
- Specific lateral positions are described by **the part closest to the film or image receptor**, or **that body part from which the CR exits**, such as the specific lateral positions of Figs 1-46 and 1-47.

Note: A true lateral position will always be 90° or perpendicular or at a right angle to a true AP or PA projection. If it is not a true lateral it would be an oblique position.

23. Oblique** (ob-lēk′, or ob-līk′*) **Position:

- A specific body position.
- A slanting or angled position in which neither the median (sagittal) nor frontal (coronal) body plane is perpendicular or at a right angle to the film or image receptor.

Note: Oblique positions are described by **the part closest to the film or image receptor**, or that **body part from which the CR exits**, such as the oblique chest positions of Figs. 1-48 and 1-50.

24. Left Posterior Oblique (LPO) Position:

- Describes that specific oblique position in which the **left posterior** aspect of the body is closest to the film, or image receptor (Figs. 1-48 and 1-49).
- The x-ray beam exits from the left posterior aspect of the body.

Projections: These could also correctly be referred to as **AP oblique projections** since the CR enters an anterior surface and exits posteriorly. This, however, is not a complete description and, if used, also requires a specific position clarifier such as **LPO or RPO position**. Therefore throughout this text these body obliques will be referred to as **positions** and not projections **described by the part closest to the film.**

25. Right Posterior Oblique (RPO) Position:

- Describes that position in which the **right posterior** part of the body is closest to the film (not specifically illustrated).

26. Right and Left Anterior Oblique (RAO and LAO) Positions:

- Those oblique positions in which either the **right or left anterior** aspect of body is closest to the film or image receptor. These can be in erect or recumbent general body positions, as shown in Figs. 1-50 and 1-51.

Projections: These could also be described as **PA oblique projections** if a position clarifier is added such as an RAO or LAO **position**.

Note: It is **not** correct to use these oblique terms LPO, RPO, RAO or LAO as projections because they do not describe the path of the central ray (see page 20).

**(Ob-lēk′)* is the preferred pronunciation according to *Dorland's Illustrated Medical Dictionary* (27th Edition), *Webster's New World Dictionary* (3rd College Edition) and the *American College Dictionary*. *(Ob-līk′)* is the second pronunciation, as especially used in the military.

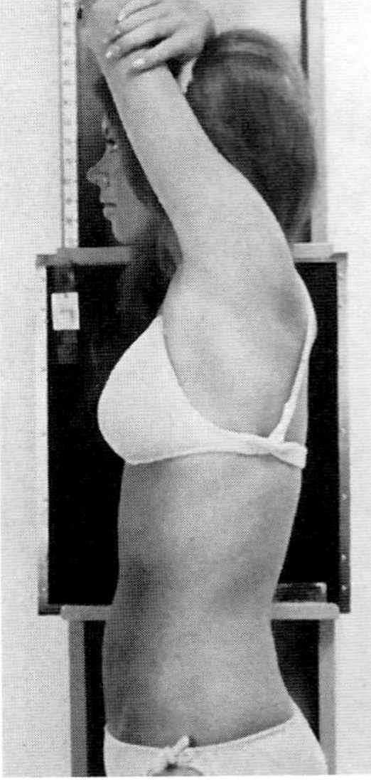

Fig. 1-46. Erect R lateral position.

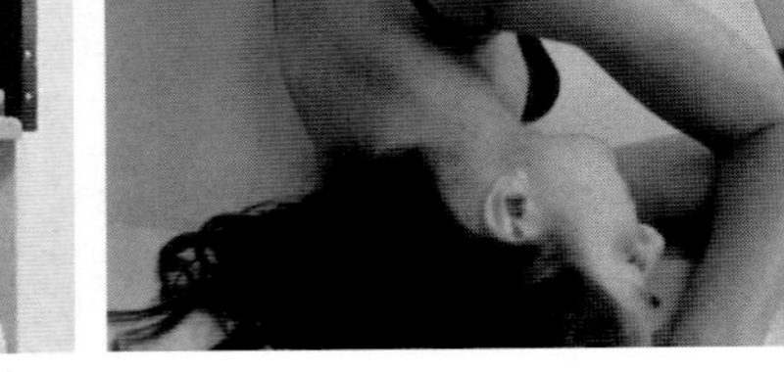

Fig. 1-47. Recumbent R lateral position.

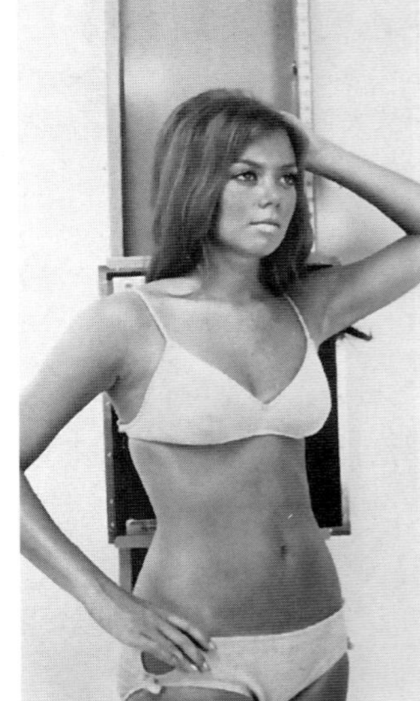

Fig. 1-48. Erect LPO position.

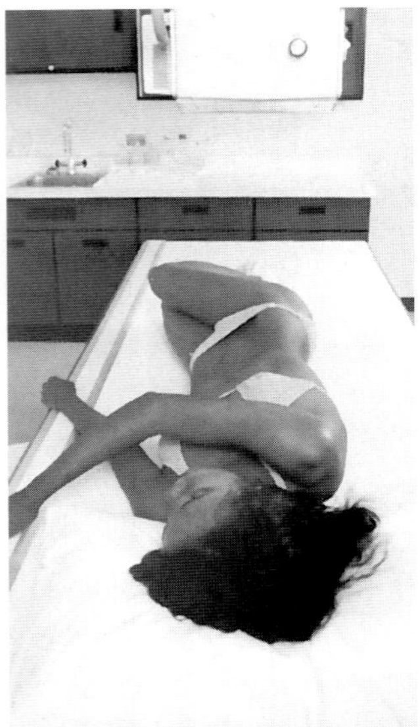

Fig. 1-49. Recumbent LPO position.

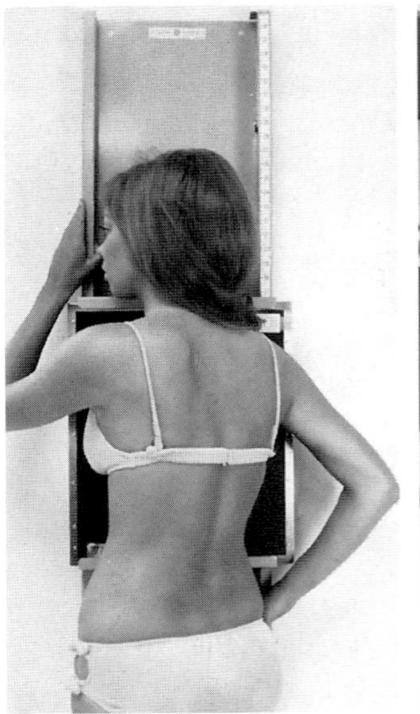

Fig. 1-50. Erect RAO position.

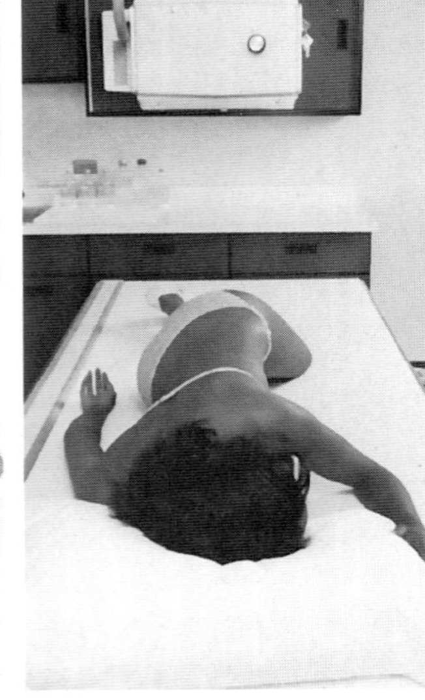

Fig. 1-51. Recumbent RAO position.

27. Decubitus (de-ku′ bi-tus) (Decub.) Position:

- Literally means to "lie down," or the position assumed in "lying down."*
- A body position meaning to **lie on a horizontal surface,** designated according to **that surface on which the body is resting**.

Therefore this refers to the patient **lying down** on one of the following body surfaces: back (dorsal), front (ventral), side (right or left lateral).

In radiographic positioning, decubitus is **always used with a horizontal x-ray beam**.

Note: In radiographic positioning, this term is used to denote **both** a specific recumbent body position and the use of a horizontal x-ray beam. Decubitus projections are essential to detect air-fluid levels or free air in a body cavity such as in the chest or abdomen.

28. Left Lateral Decubitus Position (AP Projection):

- That position wherein the patient **lies on her (his) left side** and the **x-ray beam is directed horizontally** from **anterior to posterior (AP)** (Fig. 1-52).

The AP in parenthesis is important as a qualifying term to denote the direction of the CR, which in Fig. 1-52 is anteroposterior (AP).

Note: This is similar to a recumbent left lateral body position except the x-ray beam is directed horizontally, making this a **left lateral decubitus position (AP projection)**.

29. Right Lateral Decubitus Position (PA Projection):

- That position wherein the patient lies on **her (his) right side** and the **x-ray beam is directed horizontally** from **posterior to anterior (PA)** (Fig. 1-53).

30. Dorsal Decubitus Position (Left Lateral):

- That position wherein the patient is **lying on her (his) dorsal** (posterior) surface with the **x-ray beam directed horizontally** and laterally, exiting from the left side, which is closest to the film or image receptor (Fig. 1-54).

Note: This is similar to a supine body position except the x-ray beam is directed horizontally with the x-ray beam exiting from the left side, indicating that this is a **dorsal decubitus left lateral position**.

31. Ventral Decubitus Position (Right Lateral):

- That position with the patient **lying on the ventral (anterior) surface** with the **x-ray beam directed horizontally** and laterally exiting from the right side, which is closest to the film or image receptor (Fig. 1-55).

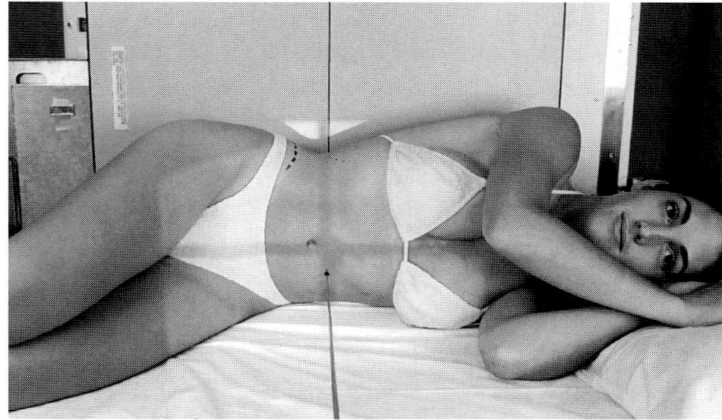

Fig. 1-52. Left lateral decubitus (AP).

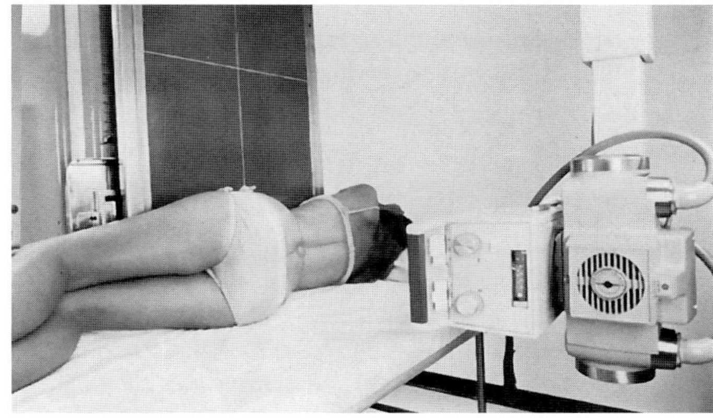

Fig. 1-53. Right lateral decubitus (PA).

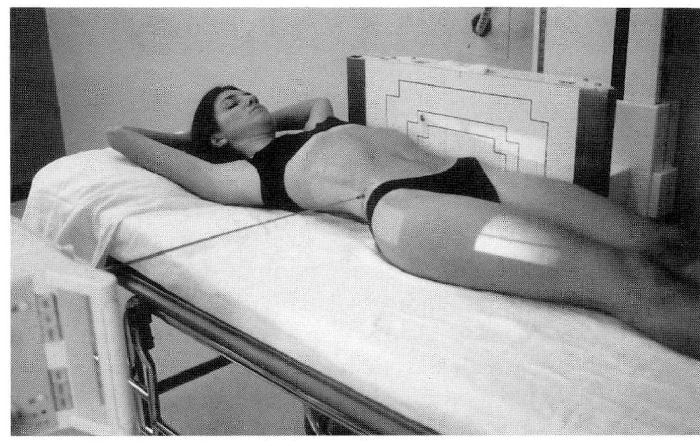

Fig. 1-54. Dorsal decubitus (L lat.).

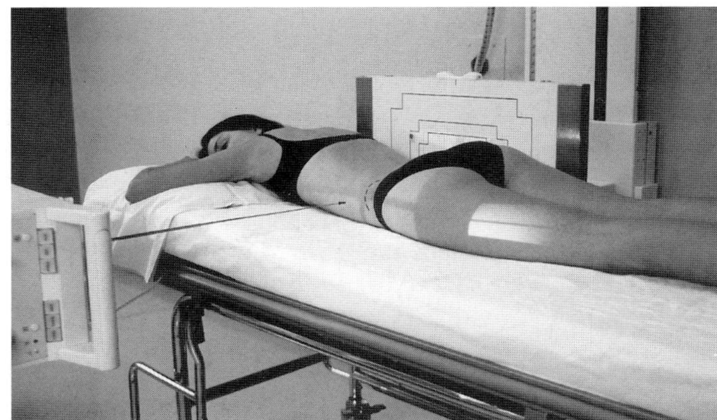

Fig. 1-55. Ventral decubitus (R lat.).

**Dorland's Illustrated Medical Dictionary*, 27th ed., Philadelphia: WB Saunders; 1988.

RADIOGRAPHIC PROJECTIONS

Projection is a positioning term that by definition describes the **direction or path of the x-ray beam** as it passes through the patient, projecting an image onto radiographic film or other image receptors. (The x-ray beam can also be described as the **central ray**, or **CR**).

According to the ARRT, the term **projection** should be "restricted to the discussion of the path of the central ray."*

32. Posteroanterior** (pos″ ter-o-an-te′ re-or) **(PA) Projection:

- A projection of the CR from **posterior to anterior.**
- Combines these two terms, posterior and anterior, into one word, abbreviated as PA. The CR enters at the posterior surface and exits at the anterior surface (PA projection).
- A PA projection is assumed to be a **true PA** without intentional rotation, which requires the CR to be perpendicular to the coronal body plane, and parallel to the sagittal plane, unless some qualifying oblique or rotational term is used to indicate otherwise.

Body position: The PA and AP projections as illustrated can be further described as an **erect anterior or posterior position** of the chest, describing the body part closest to the film or image receptor (that part of the body from which the x-ray beam exits). However, in practice it is more common to just call these PA and AP projections of the chest.

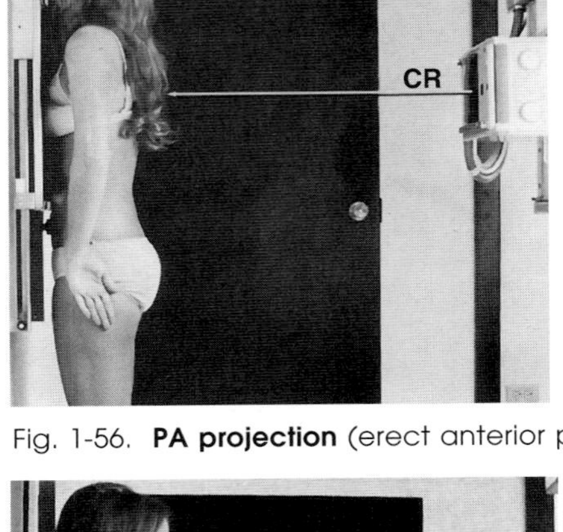

Fig. 1-56. **PA projection** (erect anterior position).

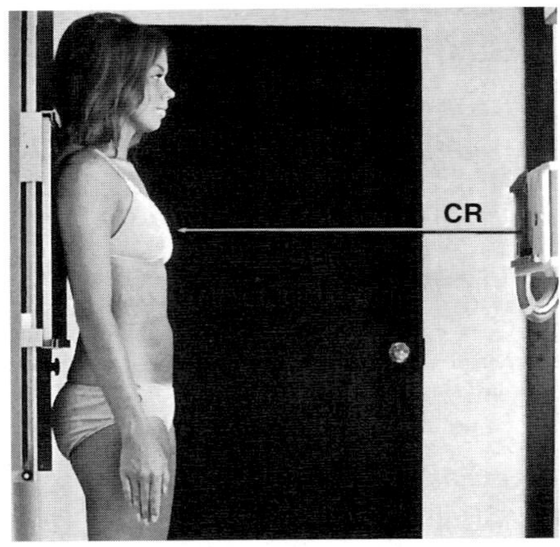

Fig. 1-57. **AP projection** (erect posterior position).

33. Anteroposterior** (an″ ter-o-pos-te′ re-or) **(AP) Projection:

- A projection of CR from **anterior to posterior**, the opposite of PA.
- Combines these two terms, anterior and posterior, into one word.
- Describes the direction of travel of the CR, which enters at an anterior surface and exits at a posterior surface (AP projection).
- Assumes a **true AP** without rotation unless a qualifier term is also used, indicating it to be an oblique projection.

AP or PA Oblique Projections:

- An AP or PA projection that is obliqued or rotated and not a true AP or PA.

  Must include a qualifying term describing the body position such as RAO, etc., or (for parts of upper and lower limbs) describes which way it is rotated, such as medial or lateral. (Fig. 1-58)

Summary: Oblique projections of the **thorax**, **abdomen** and **pelvis** can be most accurately and simply described as a **specific body position** without a qualifying positioning term and will be used as such throughout this text (terms 24 through 26). Oblique projections of **parts of the upper and lower limbs,** however, are most accurately described as **AP or PA oblique projections** with lateral or medial rotation.

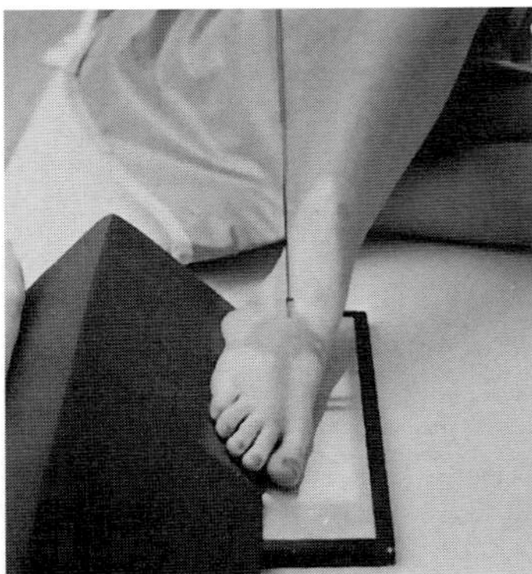
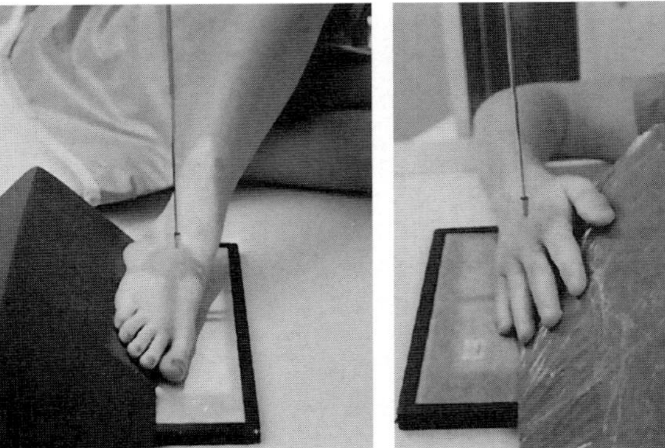

Fig. 1-58a. **AP oblique projection** -Medial rotation (foot).

Fig. 1-58b. **PA oblique projection** -Lateral rotation (hand).

34. Lateral Projection:

- A side-to-side projection of the CR described by the path of the CR, such as the **mediolateral ankle projection.** Determining medial and lateral sides is based on the patient in the **anatomical position**.

  If used as a general lateral side-to-side projection, it must include a qualifier position term such as **a right or left lateral position**.

Summary: Lateral can be used correctly as a **position**, such as an R or L lateral chest position, or it can be used correctly as a **projection** by describing the path of CR, such as a mediolateral or lateromedial projection of parts of an upper or lower limb.

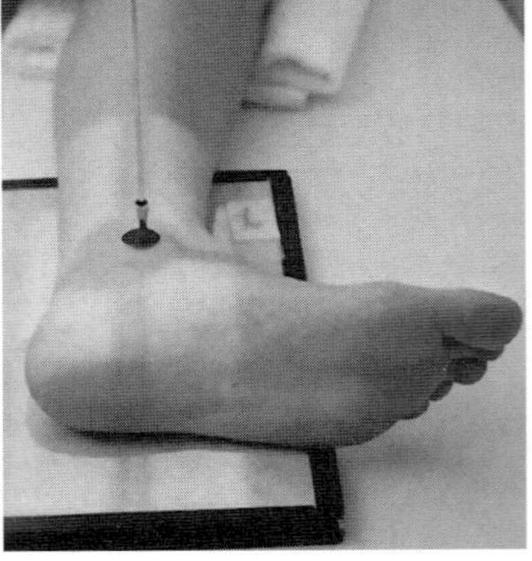

Fig. 1-59a. **Mediolateral projection** (ankle).

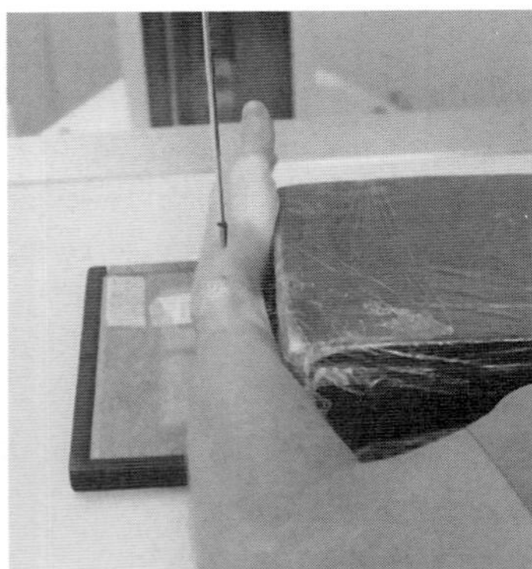

Fig. 1-59b. **Lateromedial projection** (hand).

**ARRT Educator's Handbook,* 3rd ed. ARRT, St. Paul, 1990.

ADDITIONAL SPECIAL USE PROJECTION TERMS

Following are some additional terms commonly used by practicing radiographers to describe projections. These terms, as shown by their definitions, also refer to the path or projection of the x-ray beam. A complete list of correct projection terms is included on the final terminology page 28.

35. Axial** (ak′ se-al) **Projection:

- Axial refers to the **long axis** of a structure or part (around which a rotating body turns or is arranged).

  The term **superoinferior** or **cephalocaudad** describes the x-ray beam directed along the long axis or center line of the human body from the head (cephalad) to the feet (caudad).

  Special application: In positioning, the term axial has traditionally been used to describe **any angle of the central ray more than a certain number of degrees along the long axis of the body**. It should be noted, however, in a true sense an axial projection would be directed along, or parallel to, the long axis of the body or part. The term "semi" axial, or "partly" axial more accurately describes any angle along the axis that is not truly along or parallel to the long axis. However, for the sake of consistency with other references, the term axial projection will be used throughout this text to describe both axial and semi-axial projections as defined above and as illustrated in Figs. 1-60 and 1-61.

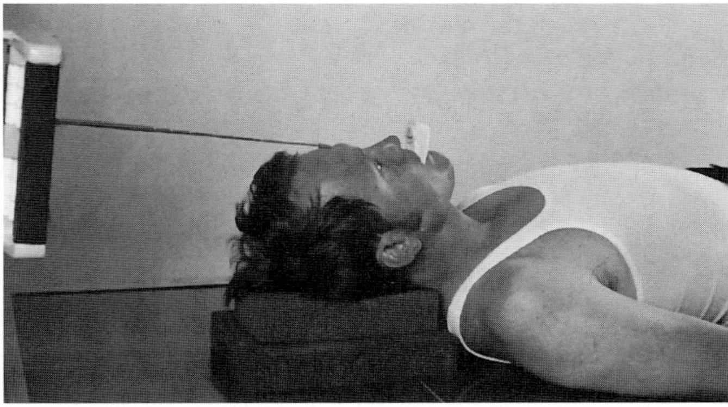

Fig. 1-60. Axial (superoinferior) projection.

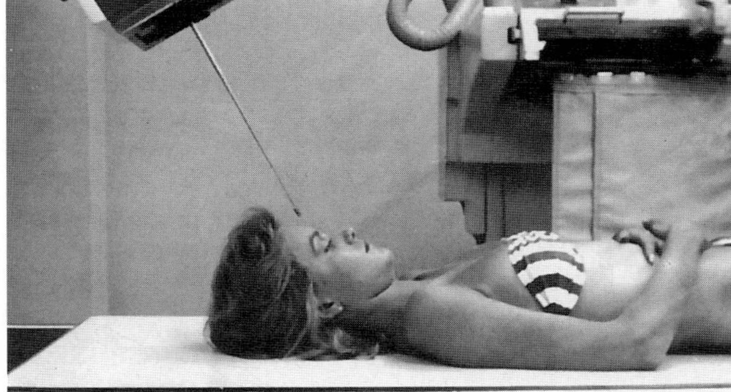

Fig. 1-61. AP axial (semi-axial) projection.

36. Tangential** (tan″ jen′ shal) **Projection:

- Means **touching a curve or surface at only one point.**
- A special use of the term projection to describe a projection that merely skims a body part to project that part into profile and away from other body structures.

  Examples: Following are three examples or applications of the term tangential as defined above:
  –Zygomatic arch projection (Fig. 1-62).
  –Trauma skull projection for demonstrating impacted skull fracture (Fig. 1-63).
  –Special projection of patella (Fig. 1-64).

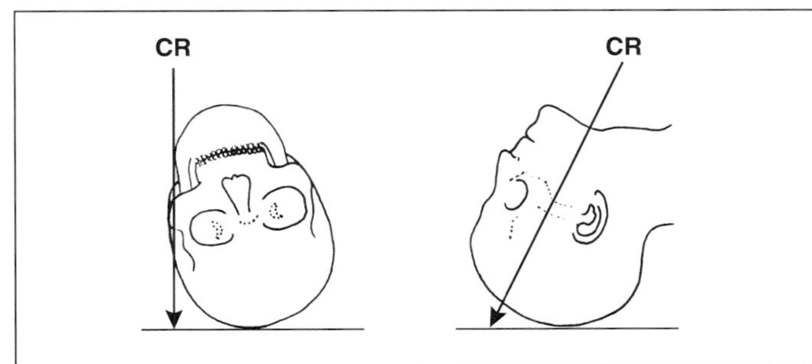

Fig. 1-62. Tangential projection.

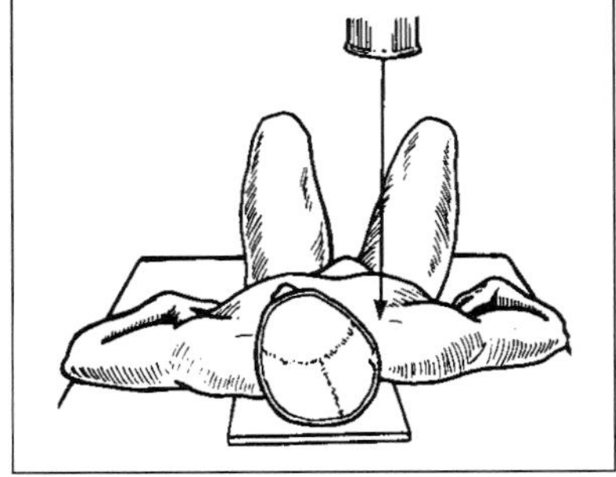

Fig. 1-63. Tangential projections. Fig. 1-64.

37. Apical AP Projection – Lordotic** (lor-dot′ ik) **Position:

- A **specific AP chest projection** for demonstrating the apices of the lungs without superimposition by the clavicles.
- The term **lordotic** comes from **lordosis**, a term denoting curvature of the cervical and lumbar spine. As the patient assumes this position (Fig. 1-65), the lumbar lordotic curvature is exaggerated making this a descriptive term for this special chest projection.

  Note: Lordosis, kyphosis and scoliosis are specific terms describing spinal curvatures (see Chapter 8).

38. Transthoracic Projection:

- A lateral or side-to-side projection through the thorax.
- Requires a qualifying positioning term to fully describe a specific position (Fig. 1-66).

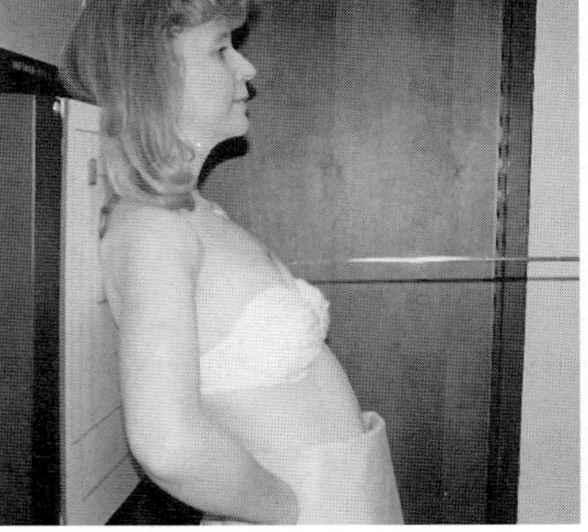

Fig. 1-65. AP chest lordotic projection.

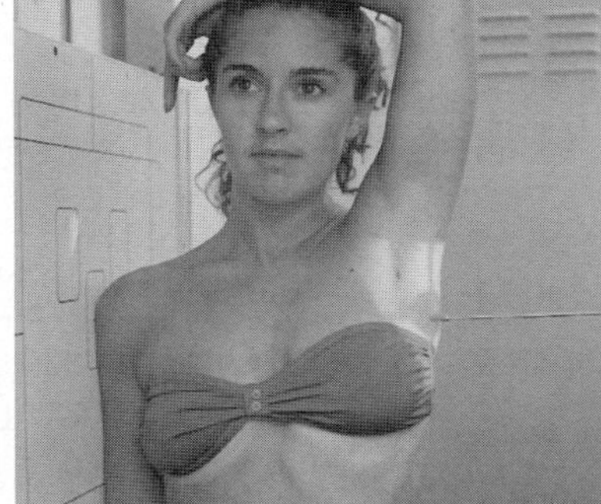

Fig. 1-66. Transthoracic lateral (R lateral shoulder position).

RELATIONSHIP TERMS

Following are paired positioning and/or anatomical terms describing relationships to parts of the body with opposite meanings:

***39. Medial** (me′ de-al) or **Mesial** (me′ ze-al):*

- **Toward the center,** or toward the median plane or midline.

Example: In the anatomical position, the medial aspect of the arm is the "inside" part closest to the median plane.

Lateral:

- This is another use of the term lateral meaning the opposite of medial, or **away from the center**, or **away from median plane or midline of body**.

Examples: In the anatomical position, the thumb is on the lateral aspect of the hand. The lateral part of the abdomen and thorax is that part away from the medial plane.

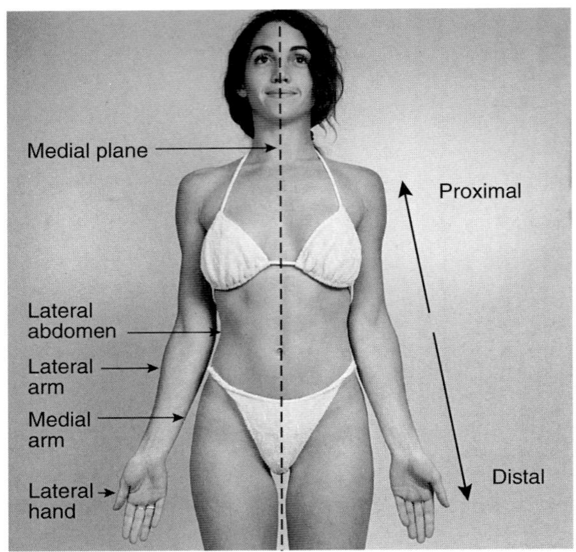

Fig. 1-67. Medial vs. lateral, proximal vs. distal.

***40. Proximal** (prok′ si-mal):*

- **Near the source** or beginning. In regard to the upper and lower limbs, it would be that part closest to the trunk, the source or beginning of that limb.

Example: The elbow is proximal to the wrist.

***41. Distal** (dis′ tal):*

- **Away from the source** or beginning or away from the trunk.

Example: The wrist is distal to the elbow.

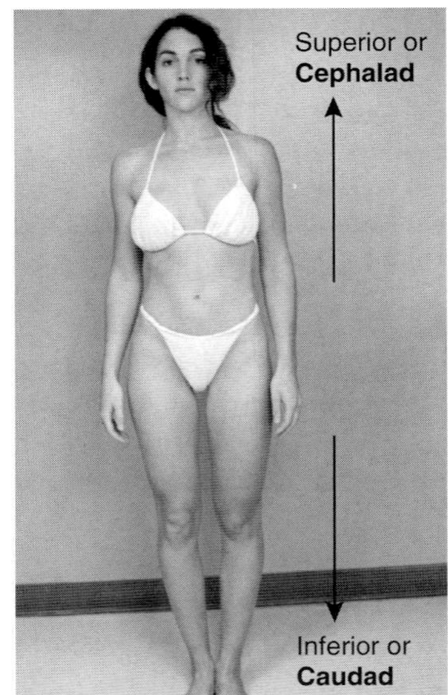

Fig. 1-68. Cephalad vs. caudad.

42. Cephalad** (sef′ ah-lad) or **Superior:

- **Toward head end** of body.
- A cephalad angle is an angle toward the head end of the body. Cephalad or cephalic is a word literally meaning head, or toward the head.*

  The term **superior** means higher or above, and is sometimes used rather than cephalad for an angle toward the head end of the body.

43. Caudad** (kaw′ dad) or **Inferior:

- **Away from head end** of body, toward the feet.
- Caudad or caudal comes from cauda, literally meaning "tail."* In human anatomy it is the same as inferior or away from the head, toward the feet.

  The term **inferior** literally means lower in place or position and can be used rather than caudad for an angle toward the feet.

Note: These two terms are correctly used to describe the direction of angle for axial projections along the entire body, not just related to the head. For example, a routine AP projection for the sacrum includes a CR angle of 15° cephalad or superior (toward the head). A routine AP projection of the coccyx includes a 10° caudad or inferior angle (toward the feet).

These terms can also be used to describe relationships of body parts to each other (Fig. 1-68).

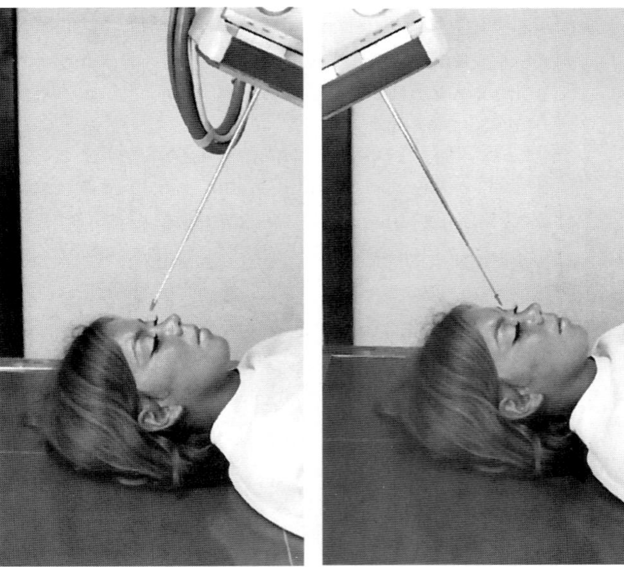

Fig. 1-69. Cephalad CR angle. Fig. 1-70. Caudad CR angle.

**Dorland's Illustrated Medical Dictionary*, 27th ed. Philadelphia: WB Saunders; 1988.

44. Ipsilateral (ip″ si-lat′ er-al):

- **On the same side** of the body or part.

45. Contralateral (kon″ trah-lat′ er-al):

- **On the opposite side** of the body or part.

Example: The right thumb and the right great toe are ipsilateral; the right knee and the left hand are contralateral.

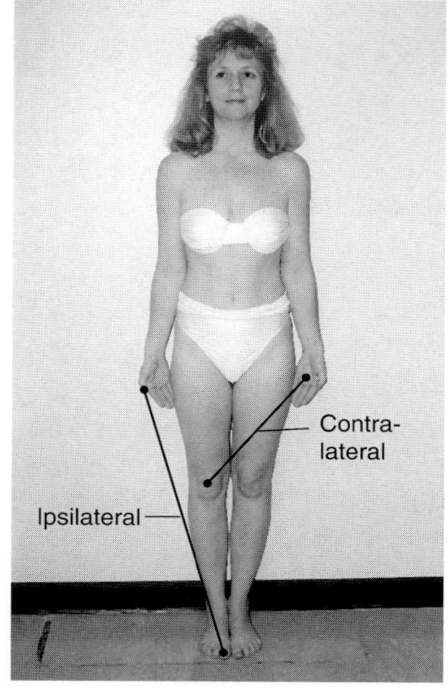

Fig. 1-71. Anatomical position.

46. Interior (Internal, Inside):

- **Inside** of something, **nearer to the center.**
- Prefix: **Intra**, meaning **within** or **inside.** (Intravenous–inside a vein.)
- Prefix: **Inter**, meaning situated **between something.** (Intercostal–located between the ribs.)

47. Exterior (External, Outer):

- Situated on or near the outside.
- Prefix: **Exo**, meaning **outside** or **outward**. (Exocardial–something developing or situated outside the heart.)

Note: Another example of the use of these two terms involves the circulatory system, wherein the internal carotid artery passes inside the cranium to the brain and the external carotid artery to the exterior parts of the head.

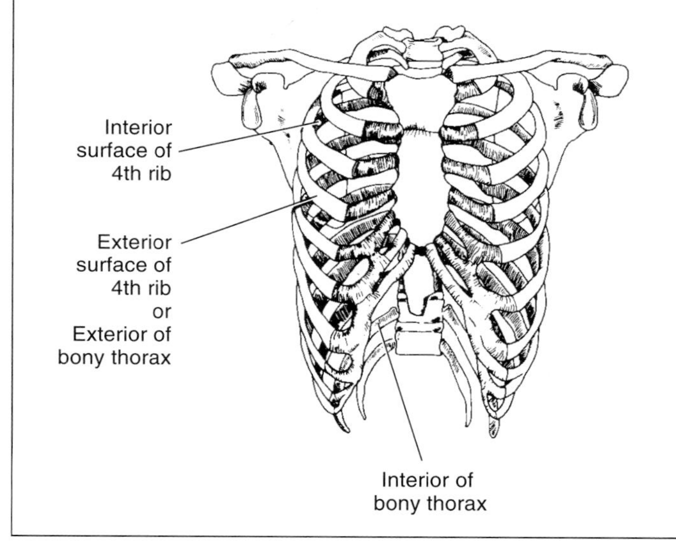

Fig. 1-72. Bony thorax.

48. Superficial:

- Nearer to the skin surface.

49. Deep:

- **Further from the skin surface** than other structures being compared.

Example: The cross-sectional drawing in Fig. 1-73 shows that the humerus is deep compared to the skin of the arm.

Another example would be a superficial tumor or lesion indicating that it is located near the surface, compared to a deep tumor or lesion located deeper within the body or part.

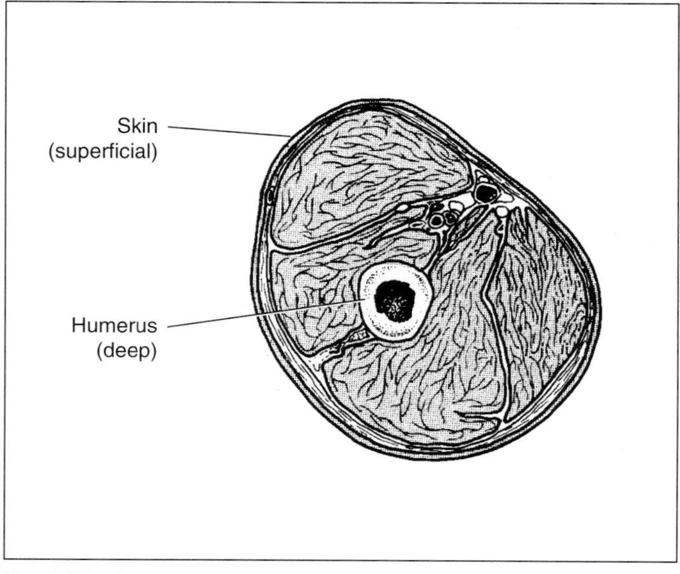

Fig. 1-73. Cross section of arm.

TERMS RELATED TO MOVEMENTS

The final group of positioning and related terms that every radiographer should know are those relating to various movements. Many of these are listed as paired terms describing movements in opposite directions.

50. Flexion:

- In flexing or bending a joint, **the angle** between parts **is decreased**.

51. Extension:

- In extending or straightening a joint, **the angle between parts is increased**.

  Extension is moving from a flexed to a straightened position.

52. Hyperextension:

- Extending a joint **beyond the straight or neutral position**.

  Example: A hyperextended elbow or knee results when the joint is extended beyond the straightened or neutral position. This is not a natural movement for these two joints and results in injury or trauma.

  Note: A special use of flexion and extension involves the spine. Flexion is bending forward and extension is returning to the neutral position. A backward bending beyond the neutral position is **hyperextension**. In practice, however, the terms flexion and extension are commonly used for these two extreme flexion and hyperextension projections.

  A second example of a special use of the term hyperextension is that of the wrist wherein the carpal canal or carpal tunnel view of the carpals is visualized by a special hyperextended wrist movement, also called dorsiflexion. (See Chapter 4 for the carpal canal projections.)

53. Ulnar Flexion of Wrist:

- To **decrease** the angle (flex) **between the hand and the ulnar side** of the forearm (this wrist position is used for a special projection for the scaphoid).

54. Radial Flexion of Wrist:

- To **decrease** the angle (flex) **between the hand and the radial side** of the distal forearm (flex toward thumb side).

  Note: The terms **ulnar deviation** and **radial deviation** are sometimes also used in medicine as being synonymous with flexion. Ulnar deviation therefore would be the same movement as ulnar flexion, and radial deviation would be the same as radial flexion. This is confusing, however, because the term deviation literally means to "turn aside" or "away from."* This would indicate that ulnar flexion would be a radial deviation, or a turning away from the radial side. By this definition, deviation is the opposite of flexion. Therefore to avoid confusion, the term deviation is not used in this text in reference to wrist movements even though these terms are sometimes used in practice as being synonymous with flexion.

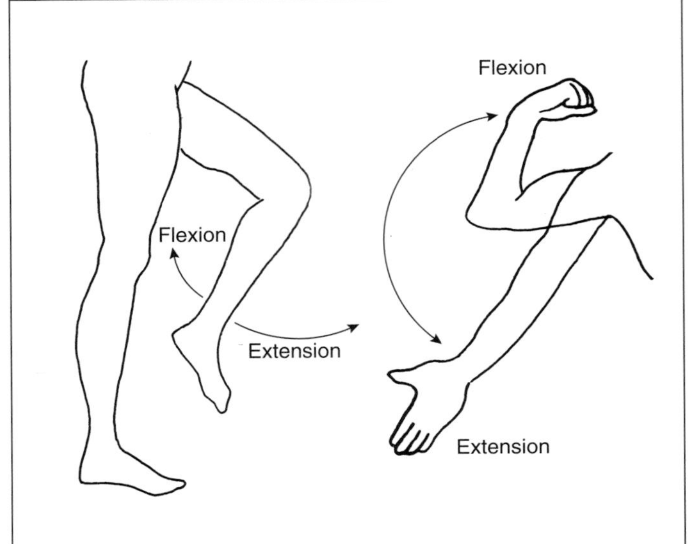

Fig. 1-74. Flexion vs. extension.

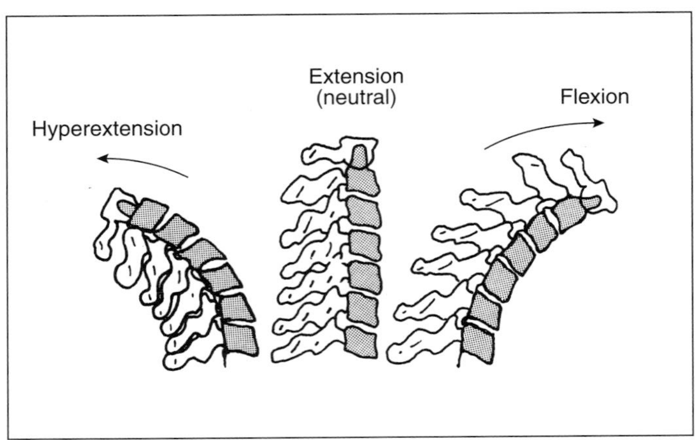

Fig. 1-75. Flexion, extension and hyperextension of spine.

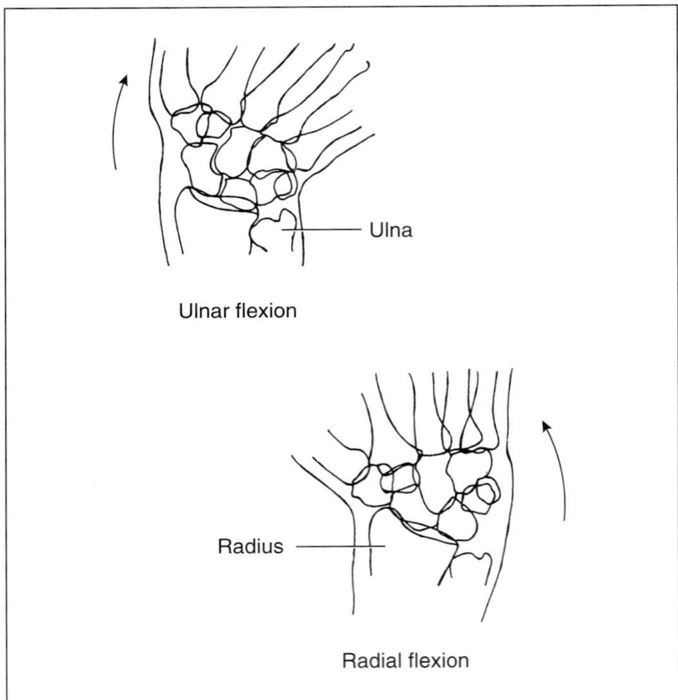

Fig. 1-76. Movements of wrist joint.

**Dorland's Illustrated Medical Dictionary*, 27th ed., Philadelphia: WB Saunders, 1988.

55. *Dorsiflexion* *(dor″ si-flek′ shun)* ***of Ankle:***

- To **decrease the angle** (flex) between the dorsum (top of foot) and the lower leg, moving foot and toes upward.

56. Plantar Flexion of Ankle:

- **Extending the ankle joint,** moving foot and toes downward from the normal position.

57. *Eversion* *(e-ver′ zhun):*

- An **outward stress movement** of the foot at the ankle joint applied to the calcaneus without rotation of the leg.

  The plantar surface (sole) of the foot is turned or rotated away from the median plane of the body (sole faces more laterally).

  The leg does **not** rotate, and stress is applied to the medial aspect of the ankle joint for evaluation of possible joint space (ankle mortise) widening.

Valgus *(val′ gus)* describes the bending of the part outward.* Valgus stress describes a deformity wherein the part is **angled away from the midline** of the body. Valgus is sometimes used to describe **eversion stress** of the ankle joint.

58. *Inversion* *(in-ver′ zhun):*

- An **inward stress movement** of the foot at the ankle joint without rotation of the leg.

  The plantar surface of foot (sole) is turned or rotated medially.

  The leg does **not** rotate, and stress is applied to the lateral aspect of the ankle joint.

  Note: Correctly used, these terms refer to stress movements as described, and **not** to the usual medial and lateral rotational movements used for oblique positioning of the ankle joint.

Varus *(va′ rus)* meaning "knock-kneed," describes the bending of a part inward or **toward the midline**.* The term **varus stress** is sometimes also used to describe **inversion stress** applied at the ankle joint.

Note: The terms valgus and varus are also used to describe the loss of alignment of bone fragments. Thus with valgus angulation, the bone fragment would be angled outward or away from the midline, and varus angulation inward or toward the midline. (See fracture term #6, Chapter 19.)

59. Medial Rotation (Internal Rotation):

- A rotation or turning of a body part, moving the **anterior** aspect of the part **toward the inside or median plane**.

60. Lateral Rotation (External Rotation):

- A rotation of an **anterior** body part **toward the outside or away from the median plane**.

  Note: Remember, in radiographic positioning these terms describe the movement of the **anterior** aspect of the part being rotated. Thus in the forearm movements (Fig. 1-80) the anterior aspect of the forearm moves medially or internally on medial rotation, and laterally or externally on lateral rotation.

  Another example is the medial and lateral obliques of the knee in which the **anterior** part of the knee is rotated medially and laterally respectively (Chapter 6).

Dorland's Illustrated Medical Dictionary, 27th ed., Philadelphia: WB Saunders, 1988.

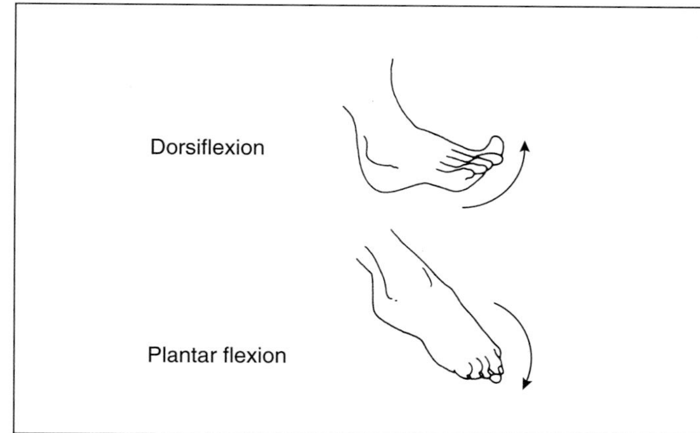

Fig. 1-77. Movements of ankle joint.

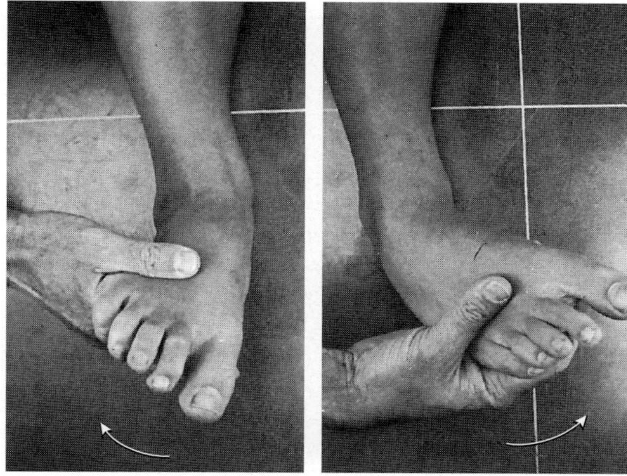

Fig. 1-78. Eversion. Fig. 1-79. Inversion.
Stress movements of ankle joint.

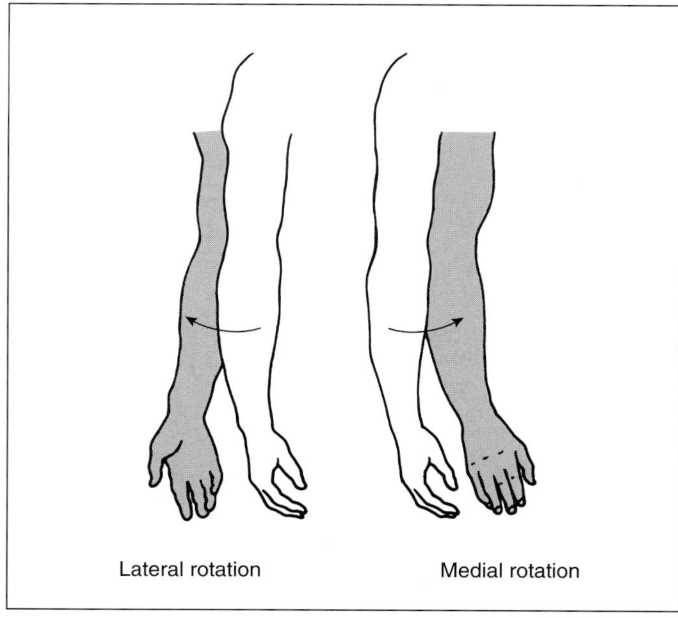

Fig. 1-80. Rotational movements.

61. Abduction *(ab-duk′ shun):*

- A movement of arm or leg **away** from body, a lateral movement (to draw away from).

  Another application of this term is the abduction of the fingers or toes, which means spreading them apart.

62. Adduction *(ah-duk′ shun):*

- A movement of arm or leg **toward** the body, to draw toward a center or medial line.

  Adduction of the fingers or toes means moving them together or toward each other.

Note: A memory aid is to associate the d in towar<u>d</u> with the d in a<u>d</u>duction.

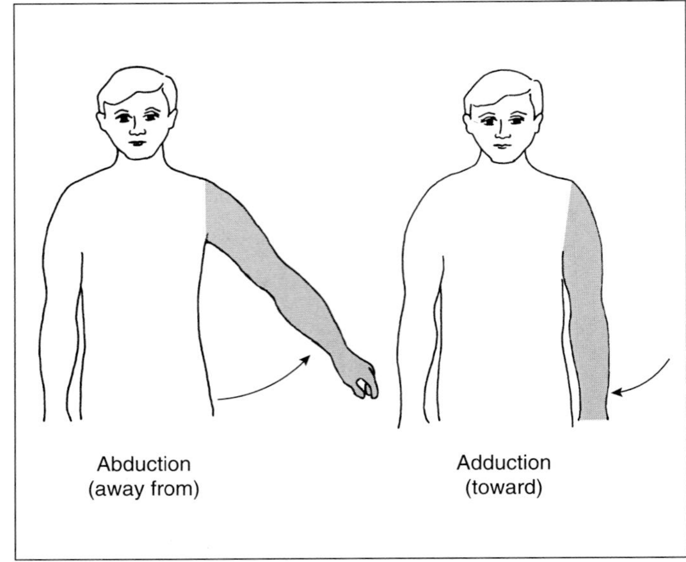

Fig. 1-81. Movements of limbs (extremities).

63. Supination *(su″ pi-na′ shun):*

- A rotational movement of the hand into the anatomical position (palm up in supine position or forward in erect position).

  This movement rotates the radius of the forearm laterally along its long axis.

64. Pronation *(pro-na′ shun):*

- A rotation of hand into the opposite of the anatomical position (palm down or back).

Note: To help remember these terms, relate them to the body positions of supine and prone. Supine or supination means face up or palm up, and prone or pronation means face down or palm down.

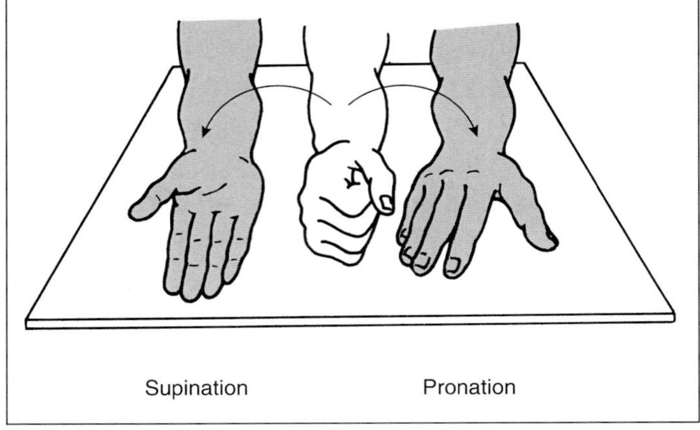

Fig. 1-82. Movements of hand.

65. Protraction *(pro-trak′ shun):*

- A **movement forward** from a normal position.

66. Retraction *(re-trak′ shun):*

- A **movement backward**, or the condition of being drawn back.

Example: Protraction is moving the jaw forward (sticking the chin out) or drawing the shoulders forward. Retraction is the opposite of this, moving the jaw backward or squaring the shoulders, as in a military stance.

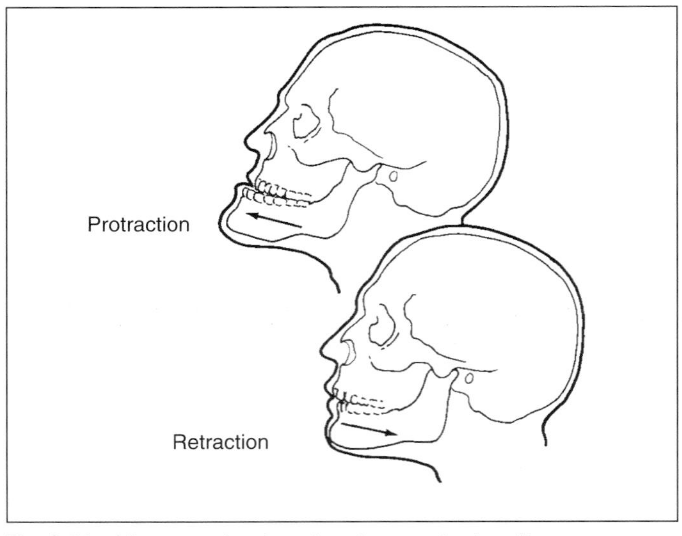

Fig. 1-83. Movements of protraction and retraction.

67. Elevation:

- **A lifting, raising** or **moving of a part superiorly**.

68. Depression:

- **A letting down, lowering** or **moving of a part inferiorly**.

Example: Shoulders are elevated when raising them, as occurs when shrugging the shoulders. Depressing the shoulders is lowering them, as in positioning them for a lateral cervical spine.

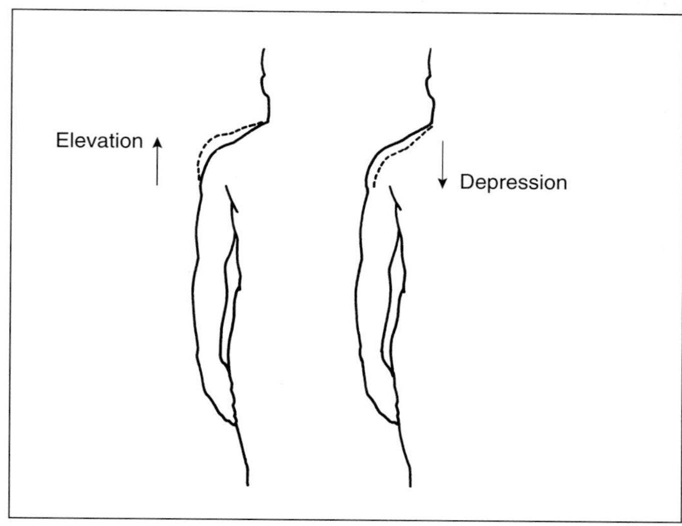

Fig. 1-84. Elevation and depression movements of shoulders.

69. Circumduction (ser″kum-duk′shun):

- To **move around in the form of a circle**.

These involve sequential movements of flexion, abduction, extension and adduction, resulting in a cone type movement at any joint with the four movements possible (e.g., fingers, wrist, arm or leg).

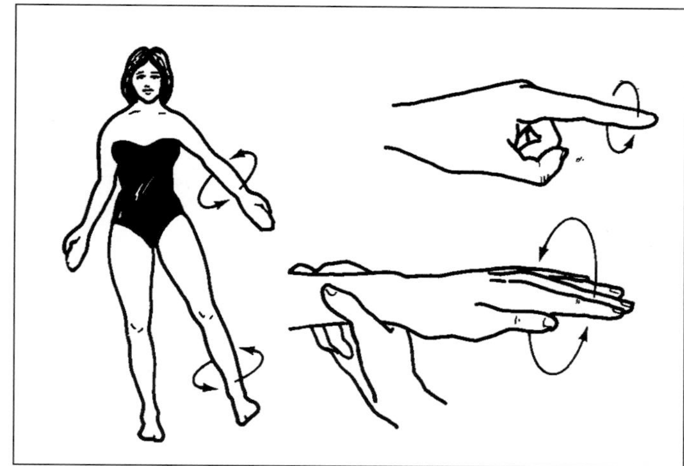

Fig. 1-85. Circumduction movements.

70. Tilt:

- A **slanting or tilting movement**.
- To move into a **slanting position with respect to the long axis**.

The body part is slanted or **tilted** 15° in the example in Fig. 1-86 such that the CR is **not** aligned with or parallel to the long axis, and the long axis of the head is **not** aligned with the long axis of the body.

Note: Observe that no rotation has occurred in relation to the long axis; however, the long axis of the head would **not** be parallel to the long axis of the body, even if the chin were pulled down as for an AP projection, thus the 15° tilt.

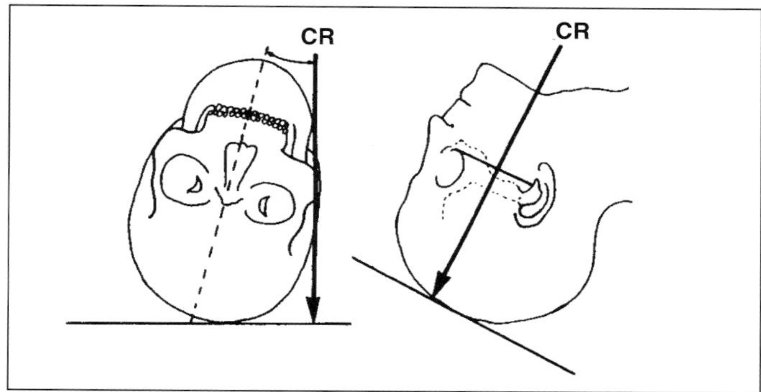

Fig. 1-86. 15° tilt (tangential projection for zygomatic arch).

71. Rotation:

- To **turn or rotate a body part on its axis**.
- A **rotational movement**.

The body part is **rotated** 37° from a PA projection in the example in Fig. 1-87.

Note: Observe that no tilting has occurred in that the long axis of the head is still aligned with or parallel to the long axis of the body.

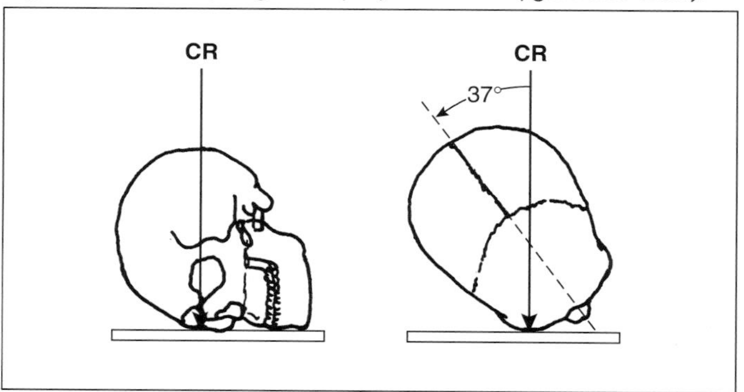

Fig. 1-87. 37° rotation from PA (parieto-orbital projection for optic foramen).

SUMMARY OF POTENTIALLY MISUSED TERMS

The three terms, **position**, **projection**, and **view**, are sometimes confusing and used incorrectly in practice. These terms should be understood and used correctly.

Position:

- Position is a term used to indicate the patient's **general physical position** such as **supine**, **prone**, **recumbent** or **erect**.
- Position is also used to describe **specific body positions** by that body part closest to the film or image receptor, such as **laterals** and **obliques** (Fig. 1-88 and 1-89).

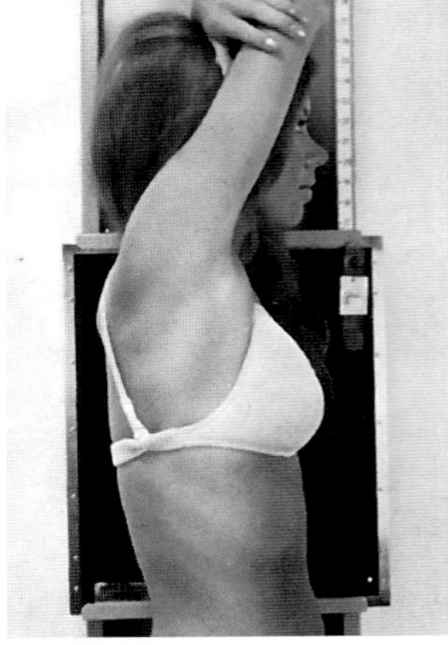

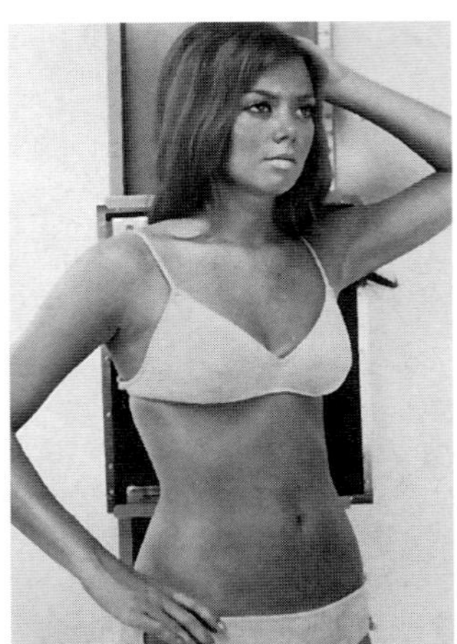

Fig. 1-88. L lat. position. Fig. 1-89. LPO position. -Specific body positions.

Projection:

- **A correct positioning term describing or referring to the path of the x-ray beam**, projecting an image onto radiographic film.

  Following is a list of terms with correct use of projection, which includes a specific description of the points of entrance and exit.

  –**AP or PA projection**: True AP or PA projections without intentional rotation of body part. If not a true AP or PA, the term oblique must be included and a qualifying position or rotational term must also be used.

  –**Dorsoplantar and plantodorsal projections**: AP and PA projections of foot (Fig. 1-90), see terms 12 and 13.

  –**Parietoacanthial projection** (special PA Waters skull projection): The CR enters at the parietal bone and exits at the acanthion (Fig. 1-91). The opposite of this is the **acanthioparietal** projection (reverse Waters).

  –**Mediolateral or lateromedial projections**: Specific lateral projections for parts of the upper and lower limbs, such as the foot or ankle (Fig. 1-92). (Also used for certain lateral mammography projections.)

  –**Submentovertex (SMV) projection**: CR enters below the chin or mentum and exits at the vertex or top of skull (Fig. 1-93). The opposite projection of this would be **verticosubmental** projection.

  –**Inferosuperior axial projection** (special shoulder and hip projections): CR enters below or inferiorly, and exits above or superiorly. The opposite of this is the **superoinferior** projection.

  –**Parieto-orbital or orbitoparietal projections**: Special facial bone projections. The CR passes through the skull entering at the parietal bone and exiting through the orbit on the parieto-orbital projection (also called the Rhese oblique or the Rhese method, Chapter 12, Facial Bones).

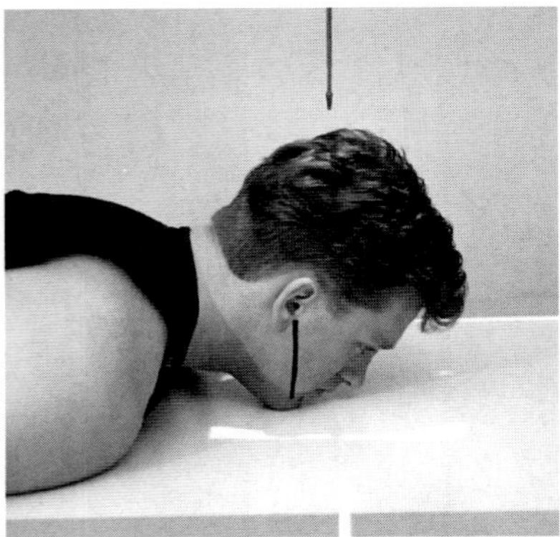

Fig. 1-90. AP (dorsoplantar) projection of foot.

Fig. 1-91. Parietoacanthial (PA Waters) projection.

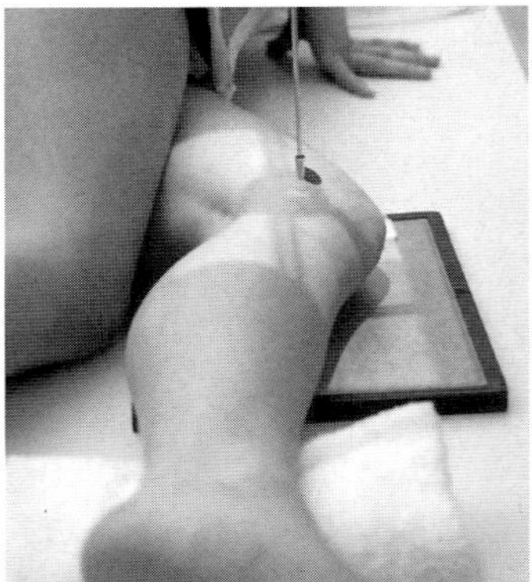

Fig. 1-92. Mediolateral projection–Knee.

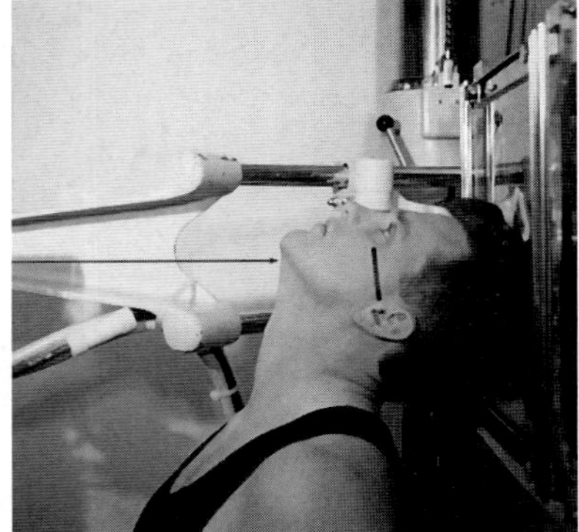

Fig. 1-93. Submentovertex (SMV) projection.

- Special positioning uses of the term projection:

  –**Axial** (or semi-axial): An "angled" projection along the long axis of the body.

  –**Tangential**: A projection wherein the CR merely touches a body part projecting that part away from other structures.

  –**Transthoracic**: A lateral side-to-side projection passing through the thorax.

View:

- Is **not** an accepted positioning term in the United States.
- Should **only** be used in discussing the radiograph or image.
- Represents the **radiographic image** as seen from the vantage of the film or other image receptor such as a fluoroscopic screen, or computer monitor.

Note: **View is the exact opposite of projection** and therefore becomes confusing when used as a positioning term.

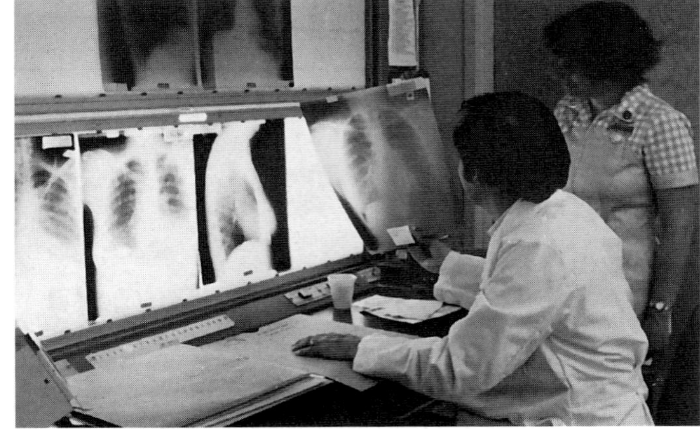

Fig. 1-94. Viewing radiographs.

Basic Imaging Principles

EVALUATION CRITERIA

The goal of every radiographer should not be just to take a "passable" or merely a "diagnostic" radiograph wherein only obvious pathological changes are evident, but the goal should be an optimum image which can be evaluated by a definable standard, as described under evaluation criteria.

The less than optimal radiograph may be considered passable if exposure factors are sufficient to result in a merely diagnostic image, but it may demonstrate sloppy and careless technique; the markers may not be placed correctly, or the centering or collimation may be off. Other carelessness may also be evident such as not being aligned to the long axis of the film, or unnecessary magnification or distortion evident by improper tube-part-film placement or alignment.

Therefore, it is imperative that the goal for every radiograph taken should be that optimal image as described under evaluation criteria. An example of evaluation criteria as used in this text for a lateral forearm is shown on the right.

Lateral Forearm Criteria

Evaluation Criteria

- The elbow should be flexed 90° and the forearm should be aligned to the long axis of the half of exposed film.
- The carpals should be visible distally, and the distal humerus proximally.
- **No rotation**: Ulnar head of distal ulna should be directly superimposed and centered over radius; humeral epicondyles should be directly superimposed.
- Radial head should superimpose coronoid process; radial tuberosity should not be seen in profile.
- Wrist and elbow joints will be only partially open due to beam divergence.
- Lateral collimation borders should be visible but borders at both ends should be minimal so as not to cut off essential anatomy of joints.
- Optimum exposure with no motion should visualize sharp bone margins and clear trabecular markings throughout. Densities should be similar at distal and proximal ends of forearm.

Fig. 1-95. Evaluation criteria (as listed in positioning pages).

POSITIONING ACCURACY

Part Placement on Film Holder

Positioning accuracy first includes correct placement of the part to be demonstrated on the cassette so that all of the anatomy to be visualized is within the collimated borders, but no unnecessary anatomy is irradiated. This means a large enough cassette must be selected and the collimation field must be opened large enough to include all of the body part being radiographed, but not so large as to expose body parts not required for diagnosis.

A general rule states that the long axis of the body part should be aligned with the long axis of the film as shown in Fig. 1-97. The exception to this general rule is in those cases where the body part needs to be angled on the cassette from corner to corner to ensure that both joints of the body part are included on the film. An example is the femur or leg on a large adult, which may need to be placed diagonally (corner to corner) on the 14 x 17 in. (35 x 43 cm) cassette to ensure that the joints at both ends are well visualized. When this is done, the collimation field must then also be rotated and aligned to the body part.

Also, when two or more projections are taken on the same film, such as an AP and lateral forearm taken on one 11 x 14 in. (28 x 35 cm) cassette, the long axis of the body part should always be aligned the same way with the parts running in the same direction.

Rotation

Positioning accuracy also requires that the part being radiographed be correctly positioned so that the specific projection or position being taken will visualize the body part precisely as planned. For example, the lateral forearm correctly positioned with no rotation will result in the ulnar head being directly superimposed and centered through the distal radius (see Evaluation Criteria, Fig. 1-95 and radiograph, Fig. 1-97).

Additional Factors Affecting Image Quality

Additional factors that affect image quality as indicated by the last evaluation criteria item are described later in this chapter under image quality.

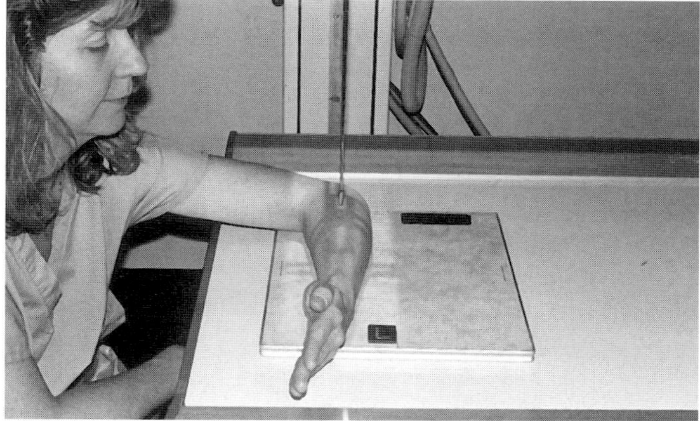

Fig. 1-96. Accurate positioning for lateral forearm.

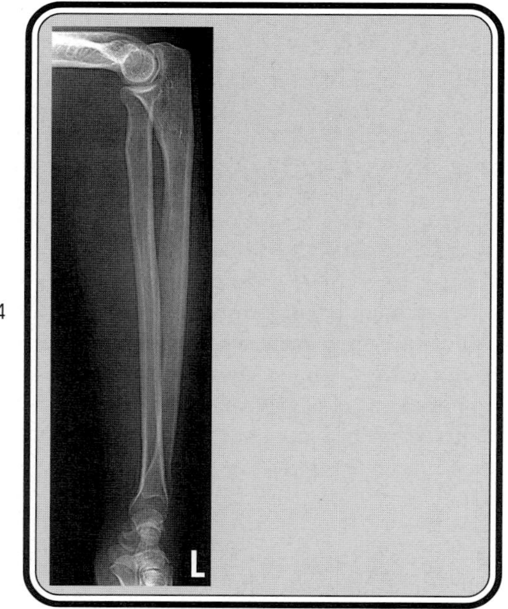

Fig. 1-97. Lateral forearm.

FILM MARKERS AND PATIENT IDENTIFICATION

A **minimum** of two types of markers should be imprinted in the emulsion of **every** radiograph. These are **patient identification and date,** and **anatomical side markers.**

Patient Identification and Date

Generally this patient information, which includes data such as name, date, case number, and institution, is provided on an index card, then photoflashed on the film in the space provided by a lead block in the film holder. Each cassette or film holder should have a marker on the exterior indicating this area where the patient ID, including the date, will be flashed (Fig. 1-98). Care must be taken so this area does not superimpose the essential anatomy being demonstrated.

Throughout this text the preferred location of this patient ID marker in relationship to the body part is shown, as well as the preferred place for the Right or Left marker. These are shown on each positioning page in the small box drawing indicating the correct film size and the film position orientation, lengthwise or crosswise.

A general rule is to place the patient ID information at the top margin of the film on chests, and on the lower margin on abdomens (see small arrows on Figs. 1-100 and 1-101). This marker should always be placed where it is the least likely to superimpose essential anatomy.

Anatomical Side Marker

In addition to the patient ID information, a right or left radiopaque marker must also appear on every radiograph correctly indicating the patient's right or left side, or to indicate which limb is being radiographed, the right or left. These may be either the word "Right" or "Left" or just the initials "R" or "L". This side marker should preferably be placed directly on the film holder alongside the collimated border of the side being identified with the placement such that the marker will not "cover up" or superimpose essential anatomy.

Remember, however, these are radiopaque markers and thus must be placed just within the collimation field so they will be exposed by the x-ray beam and imprinted in the film emulsion.

The two markers, the patient ID and anatomical side marker, must be correctly placed on **ALL** radiographs. Generally it is **not** an acceptable practice to write this information on the film after it is processed because of legal and liability problems from potential mismarkings. Generally unless contraindicated, **a radiograph taken without these two markers should be repeated,** which obviously results in unnecessary radiation to the patient, making this a serious error.

Additional Markers or Identification

Certain other markers or identifiers may also be used such as **radiographer initials**, which are generally placed on the R or L marker to identify the specific radiographer responsible for that exam. Sometimes the exam room number is also included. **Time indicators** are also commonly used noting the minutes of elapsed time in a series such as the 1 min., 5 min., 15 min. and 20 min. series of radiographs taken in an intravenous urogram (IVU) procedure.

Another important marker on all decubitus positions is a **decub** marker or some type of indicator such as an **arrow identifying which side is up.** A special type of R or L marker such as a mercury ball marker wherein the mercury ball drops to the down side of the marker may also be used to indicate erect or decub positions. If this type of R or L mercury ball marker is not used when the film is placed vertically, then an "**upright**" or "**erect**" marker and/or an arrow must be used to identify erect chest or abdomen positions compared to recumbent, and to indicate which side is up.

Inspiration (INSP) and **expiration** (EXP) markers are used for special comparison PA projections of the chest. **Internal** (INT) and **external** (EXT) markers may be used for rotation projections such as for the proximal humerus and shoulder. Sample markers are shown in Fig. 1-102.

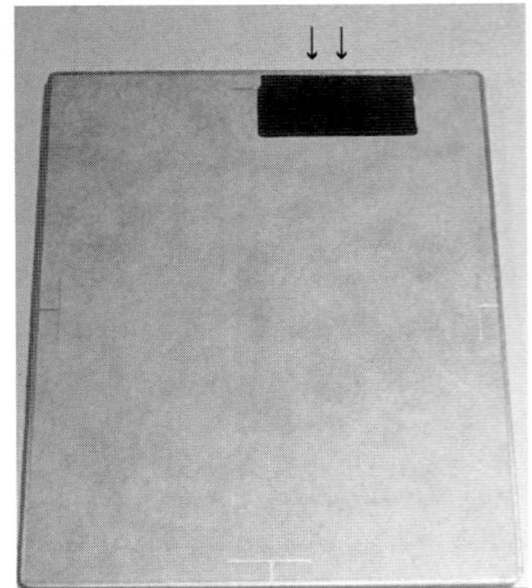

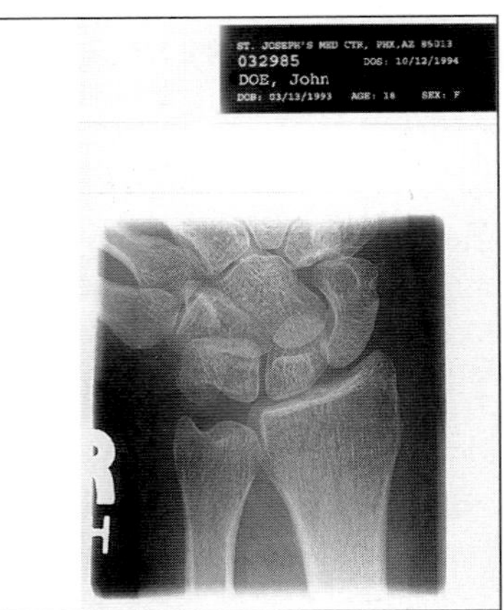

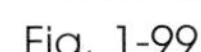

Fig. 1-98. Patient ID information. Fig. 1-99.

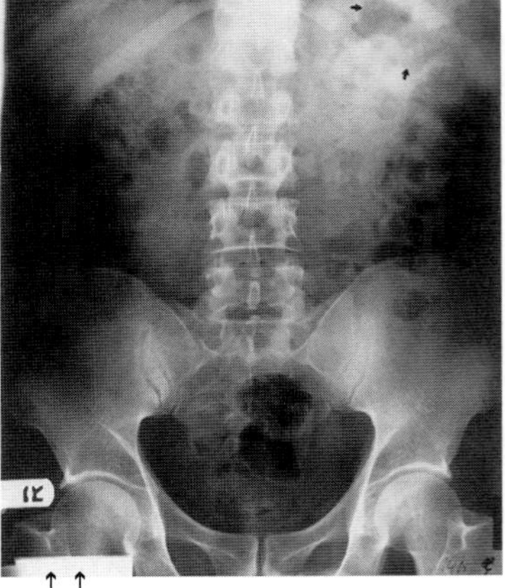

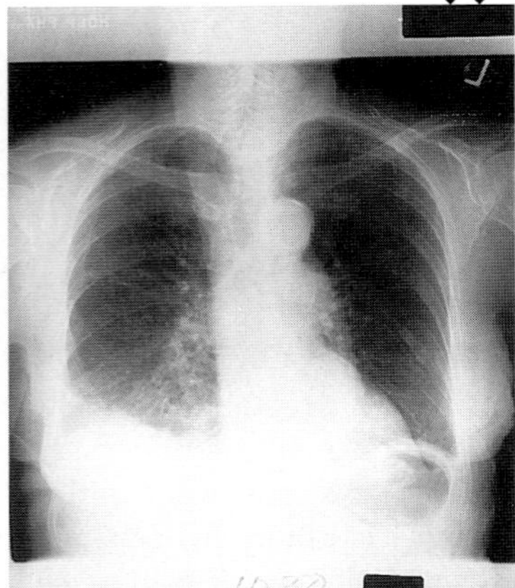

Fig. 1-100. Correctly placed side markers and patient ID info. Fig. 1-101. (Patient's right to viewer's left.)

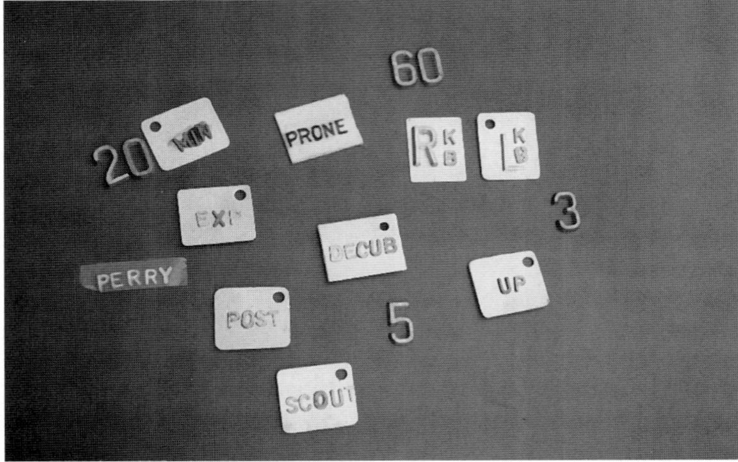

Fig. 1-102. Sample markers.

RADIOGRAPHIC TECHNIQUE AND IMAGE QUALITY

A study of radiographic technique and image quality includes all those factors or variables which relate to the precision or accuracy with which the structures and tissues being radiographed are reproduced on radiographic film or other image receptors. Certain of these factors or variables relate more directly to radiographic positioning and a discussion of the applied aspects of these factors follow.

Exposure Factors (Technique)

There are three exposure variables or factors that are set on the control panel of the x-ray machine by the radiographer each time a radiograph is produced (Fig. 1-103). These **three exposure variables** or factors, sometimes referred to as **technique factors**, are:

1. **Kilovoltage peak** (kVp)
2. **Milliamperage** (mA) } mAs
3. **Exposure time** (s)

Milliamperage (mA) and Time(s) (exposure time in seconds) are usually combined into milliampere seconds (mAs), which determine the quantity or amount of x-rays emitted from the x-ray tube each time an exposure is "made."

These exposure factors each have a controlling effect on the quality of the radiographic image. To produce that optimum quality image for each radiographic examination should be the goal of every radiographer. Therefore, in addition to being able to position the patient correctly, as will be described and illustrated throughout this positioning textbook, one must also understand certain image quality factors and their relationship to these exposure factors or variables.

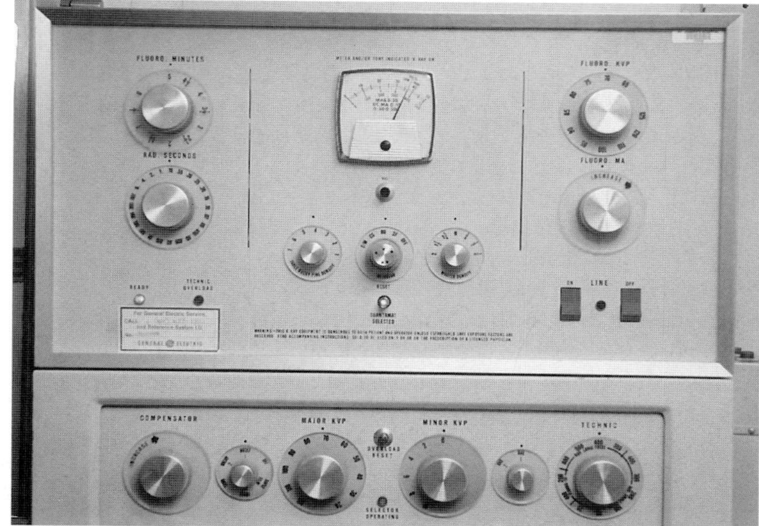

Fig. 1-103. KVp, mA and time(s) controls.

Image Quality Factors

Certain factors by which one evaluates the quality of a radiographic image are termed **image quality factors**. The four primary image quality factors are:

1. **Density**
2. **Contrast**
3. **Detail**
4. **Distortion**

Each of these four factors and how they can be controlled or affected will be described beginning with density.

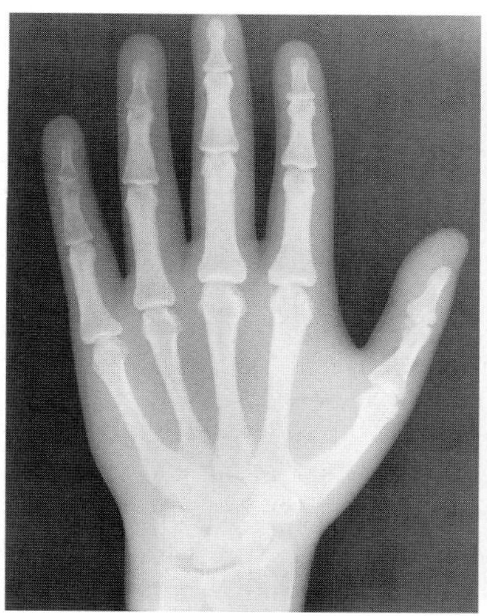
Fig. 1-104. 2.5 mAs (60 kVp) -Underexposed.

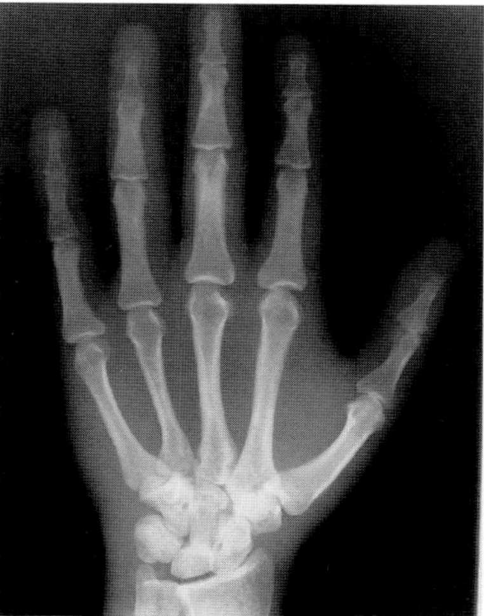
Fig. 1-105. 5 mAs (60 kVp) -Repeated, double mAs.

DENSITY

Definition

Radiographic density can be described as **the amount of blackening of the processed radiograph**. The higher the amount of blackening, the greater the density, and the less the amount of light which will pass through the radiograph when placed in front of an illuminator or light source.

Controlling Factors

The **primary controlling factor of density is mAs,** which controls density by directly controlling the quantity or amount of x-rays emitted from the x-ray tube during an exposure. Thus twice the mAs will double the quantity of x-rays emitted and double the density.

In addition to mAs as the controlling factor, the **distance** of the x-ray tube from the film, **source image receptor distance (SID),** also has an effect on radiographic density, according to the inverse square law. For example, twice the distance will reduce the intensity of the x-ray beam by one-fourth, which then reduces radiographic density by one-fourth. Distance, then, has a significant effect on density, but since a standard distance is generally used, **mAs becomes the variable used to either increase or decrease radiographic density.**

Density Change Rule

A general rule states that mAs must be changed at least **30 to 35%** to make a noticeable change in radiographic density. Therefore, if a radiograph is underexposed enough to be unacceptable, a 30 to 35% increase would make only a noticeable change, but generally would not be enough to correct the radiograph. A good general rule suggests that **doubling is generally the minimal change in mAs required to correct an underexposed radiograph** (one that is too light).

For example, if a hand taken with 2.5 mAs was too light or underexposed to a degree that warranted a repeat (Fig. 1-104), then the mAs should be increased to at least 5 mAs if kVp and other factors were not changed (Fig. 1-105). In the same way, an overexposed or too dark radiograph that warrants repeating generally requires cutting the mAs in half if other factors are not changed.

Summary: Adequate density must be present on the finished radiograph to accurately visualize those tissues or organs being radiographed. Too little density (underexposed) or too much density (overexposed) will not adequately visualize these tissues or structures.

CONTRAST

Definition

Radiographic contrast is defined as **the difference in density on adjacent areas of a radiograph or other image receptor**. This can also be defined as the **variation in density**. The greater this variation, the higher the contrast. The less this variation or the less difference between density on adjacent areas, the lower the contrast. This is demonstrated by the step wedge on the left in Fig. 1-106, which shows greater differences in densities between adjacent areas, thus **high** contrast.

Contrast can also be described as long scale or short scale contrast referring to the range of all optical densities from the lightest to the darkest parts of the radiograph. This is again demonstrated in Fig. 1-106 showing **high contrast** with greater differences in adjacent densities, and a **short scale contrast** because there are fewer different density steps.

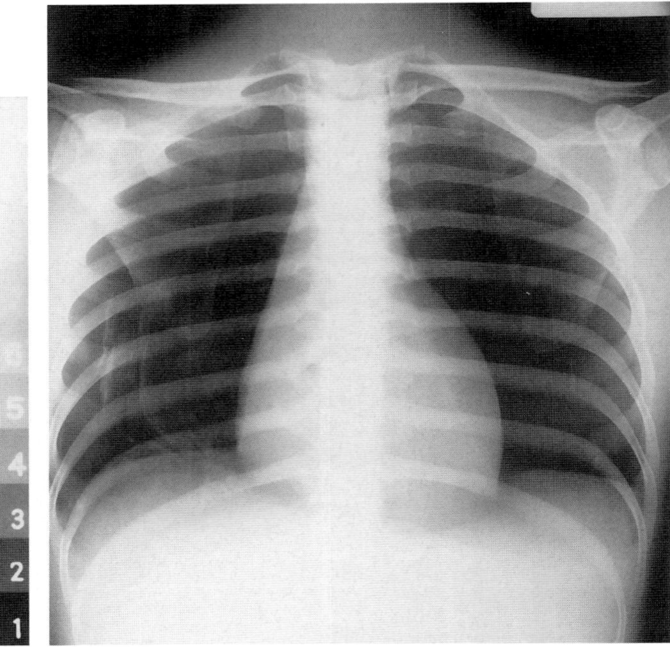

Fig. 1-106. **High** contrast, **short** scale 50 kVp, 800 mAs.

Purpose or Function

The purpose or function of contrast is to **make the anatomical detail of a radiograph more visible.** Therefore, optimum radiographic contrast is important, and an understanding of contrast is essential in evaluating radiographic quality.

Lower or higher contrast is not necessarily good or bad by itself. For example, lower contrast with less difference between adjacent densities (long scale contrast) is more desirable on certain exams, such as on chest radiographs where the many different shades of gray are needed to visualize the very fine lung markings. This is demonstrated by comparing the two chest radiographs in Figs. 1-106 and 1-107. The low contrast (long scale) chest in Fig. 1-107 demonstrates more shades of gray as evident by the faint outlines of the ribs and vertebrae visible through the heart and mediastinal structures. These shades of gray outlining the ribs and vertebrae are less visible through the mediastinum on the high-contrast chest radiograph in Fig. 1-106.

A higher contrast (short scale) may be more desirable for demonstrating certain skeletal structures where more difference in adjacent densities is needed to clearly visualize outlines or borders, such as for the upper or lower limbs. In general, however, radiographs with very high contrast (short scale) often lack information, and a lower or long-scale contrast radiograph demonstrating a greater number of different densities may result in more diagnostic information and thus, in general, may be more desirable. However, the preferred kVp range and the resultant contrast scale varies, based on radiologist preference. Suggested kVp ranges are included with each projection in the positioning pages of this textbook. Some departmental routines, however, will include lower kVp ranges than those suggested.

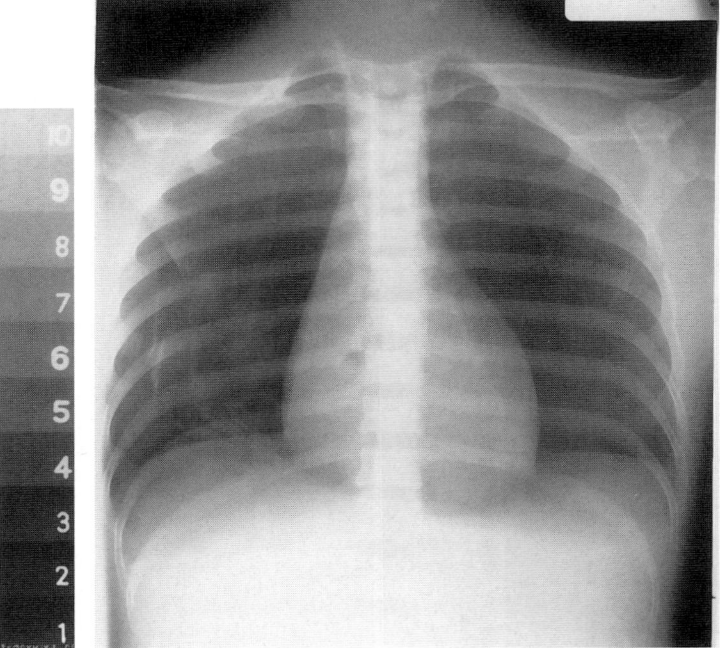

Fig. 1-107. **Low** contrast, **long** scale 110 kVp, 10 mAs.

Controlling Factors

The **primary controlling factor for contrast is kVp**. KVp controls the energy or penetrating power of the primary beam. The higher the kVp, the greater the energy and the more uniformly the x-ray beam penetrates the various mass densities of all tissues. Thus, higher kVp produces less variation in attenuation (differential absorption), resulting in lower contrast.

Kilovoltage (kVp) is also a **secondary controlling factor of density**. Higher kVp, resulting in both more x-rays and greater energy x-rays, will cause more x-ray energy to reach the film with a corresponding increase in overall density. A general rule of thumb states that a **15% increase in kVp will increase density the same as doubling the mAs**. Thus, in the lower kVp range such as at 50 to 70 kVp, an 8 to 10 kVp increase will double the density (equivalent to doubling the mAs). In the 80 to 100 kVp range, it requires a 12 to 15 kVp increase to double the density. The importance of this relates to radiation protection because as kVp is increased, mAs can be significantly reduced, resulting in less radiation to the patient.

Summary: A general rule states that the **highest kVp and lowest mAs which yield sufficient diagnostic information should be used on each radiographic examination.** This will both reduce patient exposure and in general result in radiographs with good diagnostic information.*

*Statkiewiez-Shere, M.A., Visconti, P.J., and Ritenour, E.R. *Radiation Protection in Medical Radiography,* 2nd ed., St. Louis; Mosby, 1993.

DETAIL

Definition

Detail, sometimes referred to as **recorded detail**, can be defined as **the visible sharpness of structures on the radiograph.** This sharpness of image detail is demonstrated by the clarity or sharpness of fine structural lines and borders of tissues or structures as visible on the radiographic image. Lack of detail is known as blur or unsharpness.

Controlling Factors

The optimum radiograph will display good image sharpness, as described for each exam in this text under Evaluation Criteria. The greatest deterrent to image sharpness as related to positioning is **motion**.

Additional factors that control or influence detail are **focal spot size**, **SID** (Source Image receptor Distance) and **OID** (Object Image receptor Distance). The use of the smaller focal spot results in less geometric unsharpness, thus a sharper image or better detail. (See page 35.) Therefore, the small focal spot, as selected on the control panel, should be used whenever possible.

Combined with a **small focal spot**, an **increase in SID** and a **decrease in OID** will result in less geometric unsharpness, which will **increase** detail, as described in the section which follows on distortion.

Two Types of Motion

There are two types of motion that influence radiographic detail. These are voluntary and involuntary motion.

Voluntary motion, from breathing or movement of body parts during exposure, can be avoided or at least minimized by certain factors during positioning. The use of support blocks, sandbags or other immobilization devices can be used effectively to reduce motion. These are most effective for exams of upper or lower limbs, as will be demonstrated throughout this text. Retention bands to support patients for exams of the chest or abdomen will also be demonstrated for weak or unsteady patients as a way to prevent patient movement during the exposure.

Involuntary motion, such as from peristaltic action of abdominal organs, is more difficult if not impossible to control completely. If image unsharpness is present due to motion, it is important to be able to determine from the radiograph if this blurring or unsharpness is due to voluntary or involuntary motion because there are different ways to control these two types of motion.

Difference Between Voluntary and Involuntary Motion

Voluntary motion, which is much easier to prevent, is characterized by **generalized blurring of linked structures,** such as the blurring of the diaphragm evident in Fig. 1-108.

Involuntary motion, such as from peristalsis, is more difficult to control and can be identified by **localized unsharpness** or blurring as demonstrated by the small arrows in the upper left abdomen (Fig. 1-109). Sometimes certain relaxing techniques, or in some cases careful breathing instructions, may help in reducing involuntary motion. **Short exposure time,** however, is the best and sometimes the only way to minimize image unsharpness due to involuntary motion.

A general rule to minimize image unsharpness due to voluntary motion is to **always use support devices when needed**, and **careful instructions on breathing control**.

For minimizing both kinds of motion, use **a faster film-screen combination** and as **short exposure time as possible**. In general, one should use as high mA and as short exposure time as possible within the limits of the specific equipment being used.

Summary: Loss of detail is most often caused by **motion**, either voluntary or involuntary, which is primarily **controlled by use of immobilization devices, breathing control** and use of **short exposure times**.

The use of the **small focal spot**, the **least possible OID,** and a **greater SID** also improve the recorded detail or definition on the radiograph as described and illustrated on the following pages.

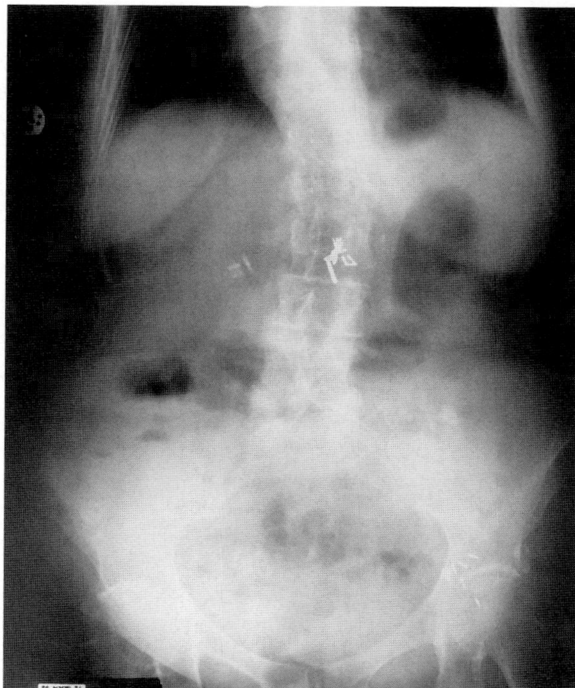

Fig. 1-108. Voluntary motion (breathing motion) –Blurring of diaphragm and overall unsharpness.

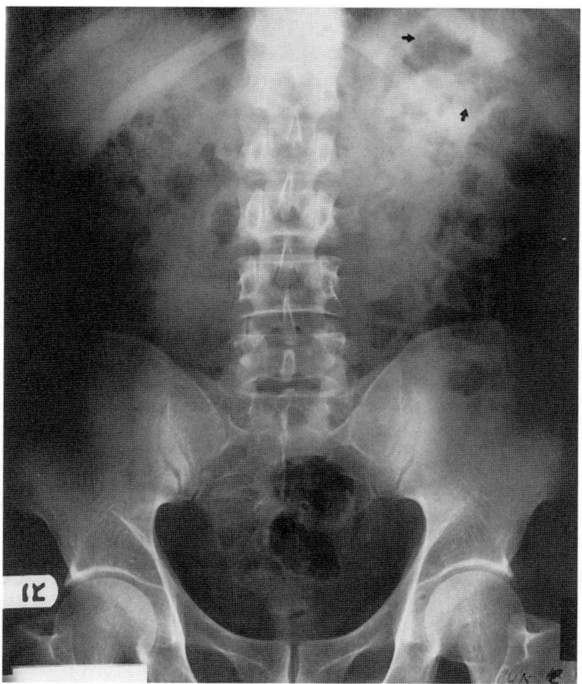

Fig. 1-109. Involuntary motion (from peristaltic action) –Localized blurring in upper left abdomen (see arrows).

Summary Chart for Controlling Detail	
1. Small focal spot	– Use small focal spot whenever possible to improve detail.
2. Shorter exposure time	– Use shortest exposure time possible to control voluntary and involuntary motion.
3. Film/screen speed	– Use faster film-screen speed to control voluntary and involuntary motion.
4. SID	– Use longer SID to improve detail.
5. OID	– Use shorter OID to improve detail.

DISTORTION

Definition:

The fourth and final image quality factor is **distortion,** which can be defined as **the misrepresentation of object size or shape as projected onto radiographic recording medium**. Magnification sometimes is listed as a separate factor but since it is a size distortion, it can be included along with shape distortion. Therefore, distortion, whether it is shape or size distortion, is a misrepresentation of the actual object and as such is undesirable.

However, no radiograph is an exact image of the body part being radiographed. This is impossible because there is always some magnification and/or distortion due to **OID** and **the divergence of the x-ray beam.** Therefore, distortion must be minimized and controlled.

X-ray Beam Divergence

This is a basic but important concept to understand in a study of radiographic positioning. X-ray beam divergence occurs because x-rays originate from a narrow source in the x-ray tube and diverge or spread out to cover the entire film or image receptor (Fig. 1-110).

The size of the x-ray beam is limited by adjustable collimators, which absorb periphery x-rays on four sides, thereby controlling the size of the collimation field. The larger the collimation field and the shorter the SID, the greater the angle of divergence at the outer margins. This increases the potential for distortion at these outer margins. In general, only the exact center point of the x-ray beam, the central ray (CR), has no divergence as it penetrates the body part and strikes the film at 90° or perpendicular to the plane of the x-ray film. This results in the least possible distortion at this point. All other aspects of the x-ray beam strike the film at some angle other than 90° with the angle of divergence increasing to the outermost portions of the x-ray beam.

The drawing in Fig. 1-110 demonstrates three points on the body part (marked A, B, and C) projected onto the film, demonstrating some magnification except at the point of the CR. Therefore, due to the effect of the divergent x-ray beam, combined with at least some OID, this type of size distortion is inevitable and its effect, as well as other types of shape distortion, must be controlled.

The x-ray beam divergence, combined with the size of the focal spot, also creates geometric unsharpness due to the penumbra effect as described on the following page.

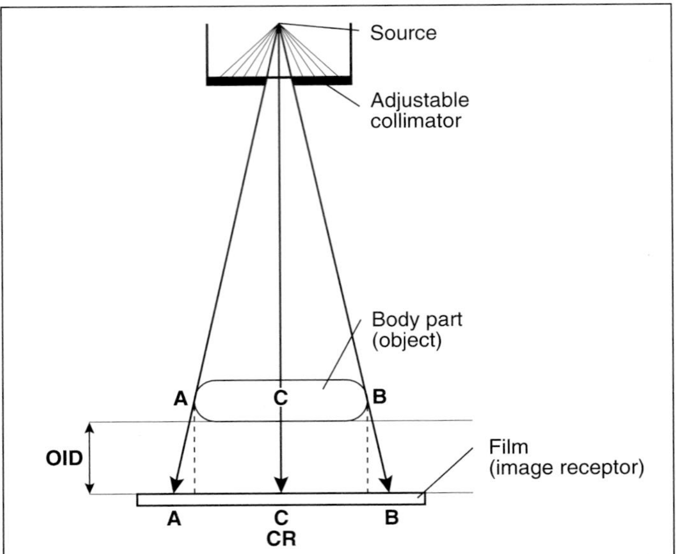

Fig. 1-110. X-Ray beam divergence.

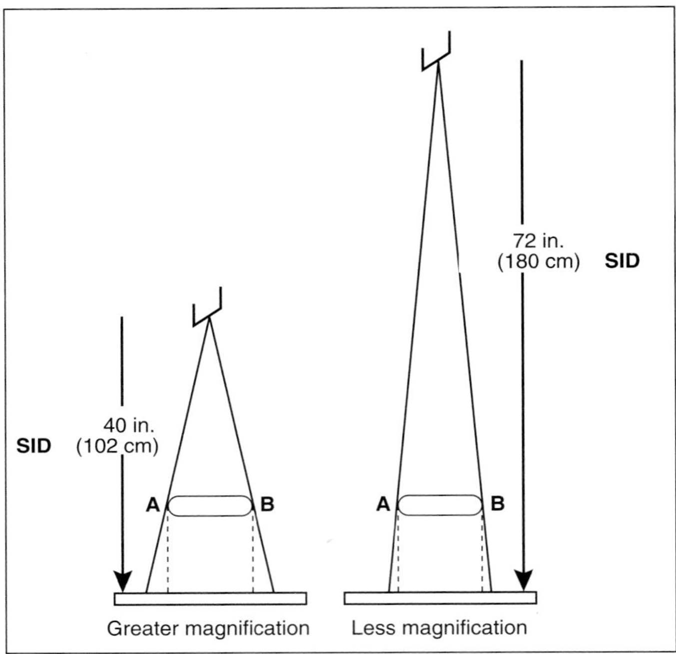

Fig. 1-111. Effect of SID.

Controlling Factors

Four primary controlling factors of distortion are (1) **SID**, (2) **OID**, **(3) object film alignment** and (4) **CR** (central ray) **alignment**.

1. SID: The effect of SID on size distortion is demonstrated in Fig. 1-111. Note that **at a greater SID there is less magnification than at a shorter SID**. This is a primary reason chest radiographs are taken at a minimum of 72 in. (183 cm) rather than at the more common minimum 40 in. (102 cm). A 72 in. (183 cm) SID results in less magnification of the heart and other structures within the thorax.

Minimum 40 in. (102 cm) SID: For many years it has been common practice to use 40 inches (102 cm) as the standard SID for most radiographic exams. However, in the interest of **decreasing patient exposure** and **improving recorded detail**, it is becoming more common to increase the standard SID to 42, 44 or even 48 inches (107, 112 or 122 cm). Studies have shown, for example, that increasing the SID from 40 to 48 inches will reduce the entrance dose to the patient by 12.5%.*

Also due to the x-ray beam divergence principle described above, this increase in SID has the added benefit of **decreasing** magnification and distortion, thus decreasing geometric unsharpness, which **increases** the recorded detail or definition.

Due to problems of shorter technologists not being able to reach the tube at the greater SID distances, and the increase in mAs required (50% increase in changing from 40 to 48 inches), many departments still use a standard 40 or 42 in. (102 cm) SID. Also, some departments use a 44 in. (112 cm) SID for Bucky tray procedures and 40 in. (102 cm) for table-top exams because the distance between the table-top and Bucky tray is 3 to 4 inches on most floating type tabletops. However, some of the newer x-ray tubes with steep anode angles require a greater than 40 in. (102 cm) SID for sufficient field coverage for the larger films.

Therefore, throughout this text, the suggested SID as listed on each positioning page is a **minimum** of 40 in. (102 cm). Departmental protocol concerning this will need to be determined by each radiographer.

Minimum 12 in. (30 cm) SOD: Radiation safety standards state the **absolute minimum SOD (Source Object Distance) shall be 12 in. (30 cm).** SOD refers to the distance from the source (focal spot of x-ray tube) to closest surface of the patient (object).

*Kebart, RC, Jame, CC. "Benefits of Increasing Focal Film Distance." *Radiologic Technology*: 1991; **62-6**:434-441.

2. OID: The effect of OID (Object Image receptor Distance) on magnification or size distortion is clearly illustrated in Fig. 1-112. **The closer the object being radiographed is to the image receptor, the less the magnification or distortion and the better the detail or definition.**

This is one advantage for taking radiographs of the upper and lower limbs table-top rather than Bucky. The cassette is placed under the patient on the table-top rather than in the Bucky tray. The Bucky tray in most floating type tabletops is from 3 to 4 in. (8-10 cm) below the table-top, which increases the OID. This not only increases magnification and distortion but also **decreases image sharpness**.

Focal spot size and image unsharpness: For purposes of describing the principle of x-ray beam divergence and the controlling factors of distortion, a point source has been used in the illustrations for the source of x-rays at the x-ray tube. In actuality the source of x-rays is from an **area** on the anode known as the **focal spot**. The size of the focal spot is determined by the **size of filament at the cathode,** and by the **angle of the target area** on the anode. The selection of the small focal spot on a dual-focus x-ray tube, or the use of a smaller angle anode x-ray tube, will result in **less blurring or unsharpness of the image** due to the penumbra effect of geometric unsharpness (Fig. 1-113).

The anode angle is determined by the equipment manufacturer and thus is not a variable controlled by the technologist. The selection of the smaller focal spot on a dual-focus x-ray tube is a variable controlled by the technologist. However, even with the smallest focal spot possible, some penumbra is present. The **effect of this geometric unsharpness is greatly increased or magnified when the OID is increased or the SID decreased**. Therefore, not only does an increase in OID and a decrease in SID result in an increase in size distortion or magnification of the image, but this also increases the overall blurring or unsharpness of the radiographic image.

3. Object Film Alignment: The third important controlling factor of distortion as related to positioning is object film alignment. This refers to the **alignment or plane of the object being radiographed in relationship to the plane of the x-ray film** or other image receptor. If the object plane is not parallel to the plane of the film, distortion occurs. The greater the angle of inclination of the object, the greater the amount of distortion.

The effect of improper object alignment is most obvious at the **joints or ends of bony structures.** This is best demonstrated on joints involving the upper and lower limbs. For example, if a finger being radiographed is not parallel to the film, the joint spaces between the phalanges will not be visualized as being open due to the overlapping of the ends of the bones as demonstrated (Fig. 1-114).

This is also demonstrated by the two oblique hand positions in Figs. 1-115 and 1-116. On the left the digits (fingers) are aligned and supported **parallel to the film**, resulting in open interphalangeal joints.

On the right wherein the digits are **not** parallel to the film, the interphalangeal joints of the digits would not be open, and possible fractures within these joint regions may not be visible on the resultant radiograph.

Summary: These examples demonstrate an important positioning principle. **Correct object alignment** (wherein the plane of the body part being x-rayed is as near parallel as possible to the plane of the film) **results in less distortion and more open joint spaces.**

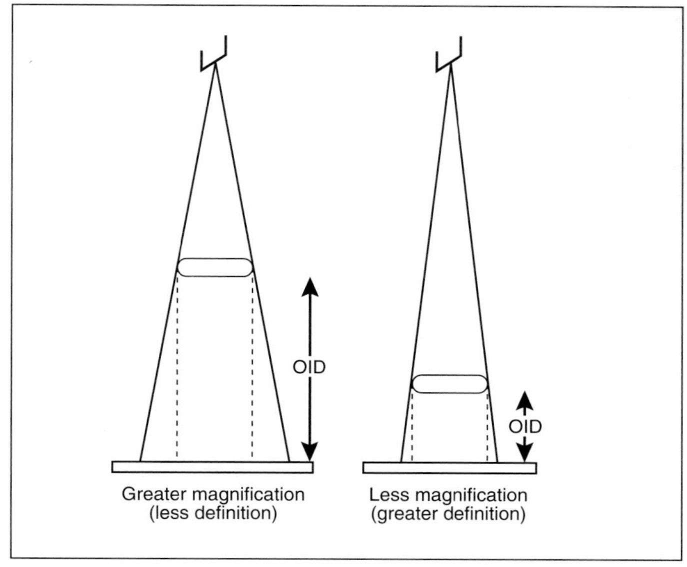

Fig. 1-112. Effect of OID.

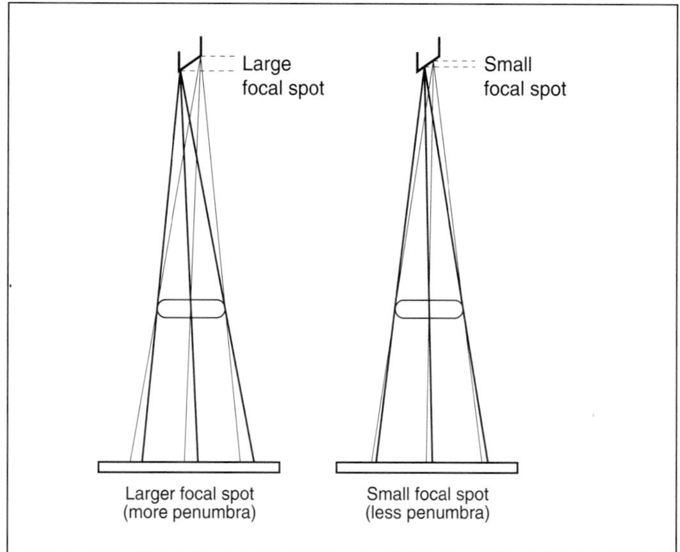

Fig. 1-113. Effect of focal spot size.

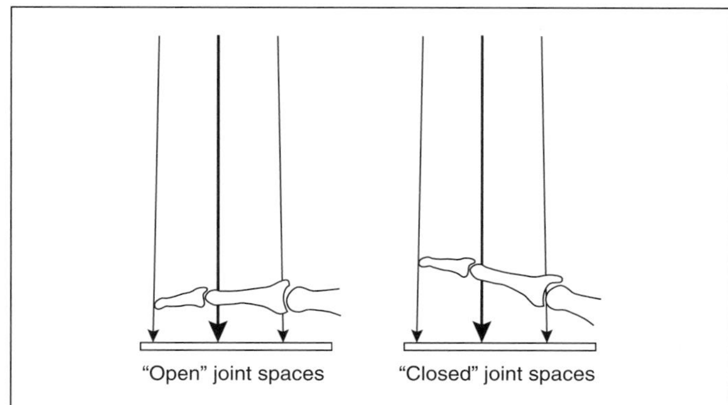

Fig. 1-114. Object alignment and distortion.

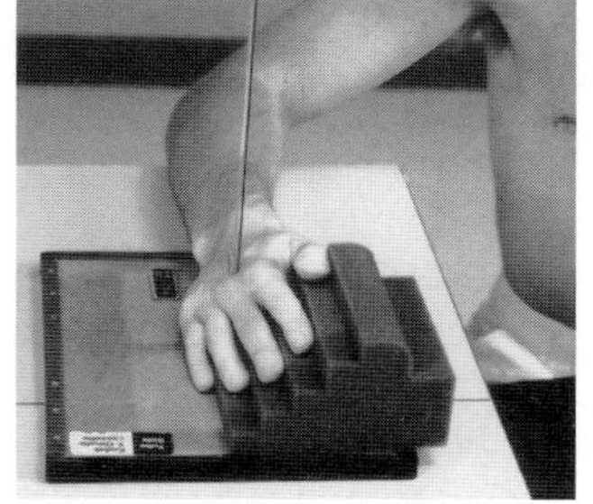

Fig. 1-115. Digits parallel –Joints open.

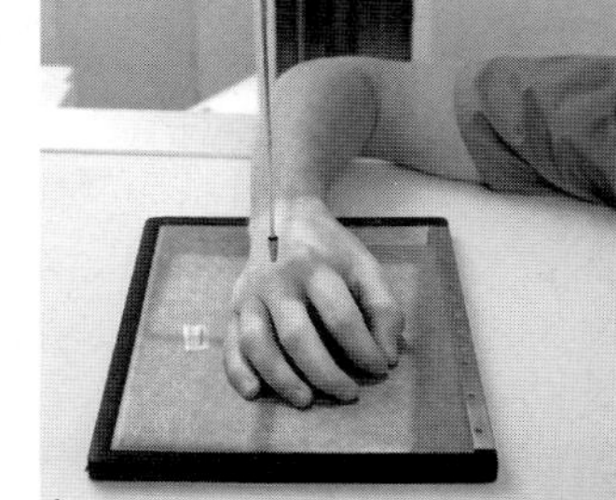

Fig. 1-116. Digits not parallel –Joints **not** open.

Controlling Factors continued

4. Central Ray (CR) Alignment: Another important principle in positioning, and the fourth controlling factor of distortion, is **correct use of the CR**. As already stated, in general only the exact center of the x-ray beam, the CR, has no divergence as it projects that part of the object at 90° or perpendicular to the plane of the film. Therefore, **there is the least possible distortion at the CR,** as x-rays can travel through a joint space at this point unimpeded. Distortion increases as the angle of divergence increases from the center of the x-ray beam to the outer edges. This is why correct centering or correct CR placement is important in minimizing image distortion.

An example of correct CR placement for an AP knee is shown in Fig. 1-117. The CR will pass through the knee joint space with minimal distortion and the joint space should appear open.

Fig. 1-118 demonstrates correct centering for an AP femur wherein the CR is directed to the area of the mid-femur. The knee joint, however, is now exposed by divergent rays (as shown by arrow), which will create distortion of knee joint structures. The knee joint space will therefore **not** appear open on this AP femur projection, and a second AP knee is required if knee joint detail is required.

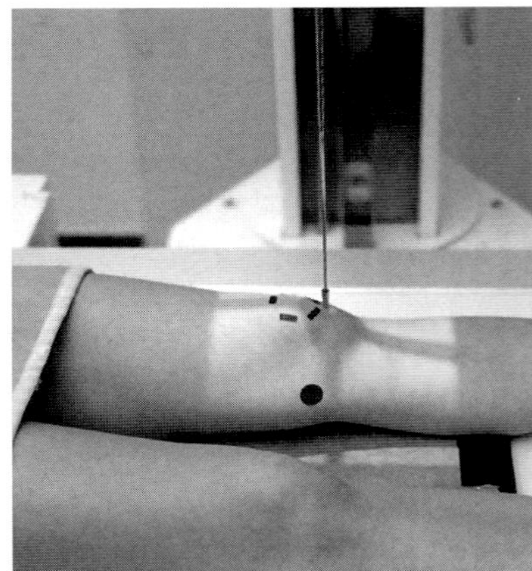

Fig. 1-117. Correct CR for AP knee.

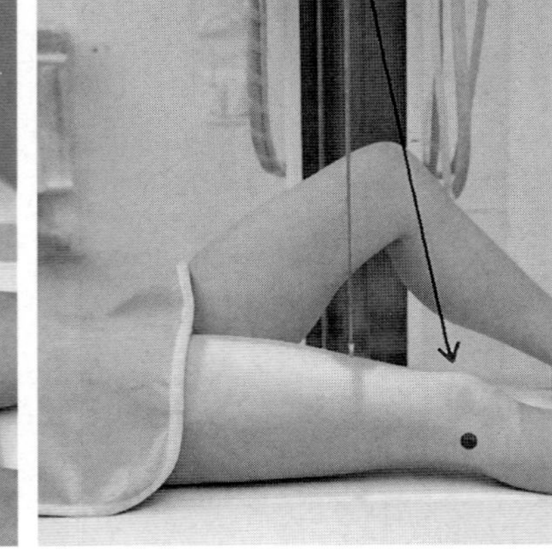

Fig. 1-118. Correct CR for femur (distortion occurs at knee).

Summary: Distortion, a misrepresentation of size and shape on the radiographic image, can be minimized by four controlling factors:

1. SID: Increase in SID decreases distortion (also increases detail).

2. OID: Decrease in OID decreases distortion (combined with small focal spot, decrease in OID also increases detail).

3. Object Alignment: Distortion is decreased with correct object film alignment (plane of object is parallel to plane of film).

4. CR: Correct CR placement decreases distortion in that the center-most portion of the x-ray beam with the least divergence is used to the best advantage.

ANODE HEEL EFFECT

The anode heel effect describes a phenomenon wherein **the intensity of the radiation emitted from the cathode end of the x-ray field is greater than that at the anode end.** This is due to the angle of the anode face in that there is greater attenuation or absorption of the x-rays at the anode end. The reason for this is those x-rays emitted from deeper within the anode must travel through more anode material before exiting at the anode end than those emitted in the direction of the cathode.

Studies show that the difference in intensity from the cathode to anode end of the x-ray beam can vary from 30 to 50%, depending on the target angle using a 17 in. (43 cm) film at 40 in. (102 cm) SID (Fig. 1-119).*

In general the smaller the focal spot, the greater the heel effect. This effect is also most pronounced at shorter SID, because as the SID is decreased, the angle or spread of beam that must be used to cover a given field size is increased as demonstrated in Fig. 1-119. Thus the **anode heel effect is most pronounced with a larger film using a smaller focal spot.**

Note: A sharper angle anode (less than 12°) will also increase the heel effect, but this is controlled by the manufacturer and not the radiographer.

*Gratale, P, Wright, DL, Daughtry, L. "Using the Anode Heel Effect for Extremity Radiography." *Radiologic Technology* 1990; 61-3:195-198.

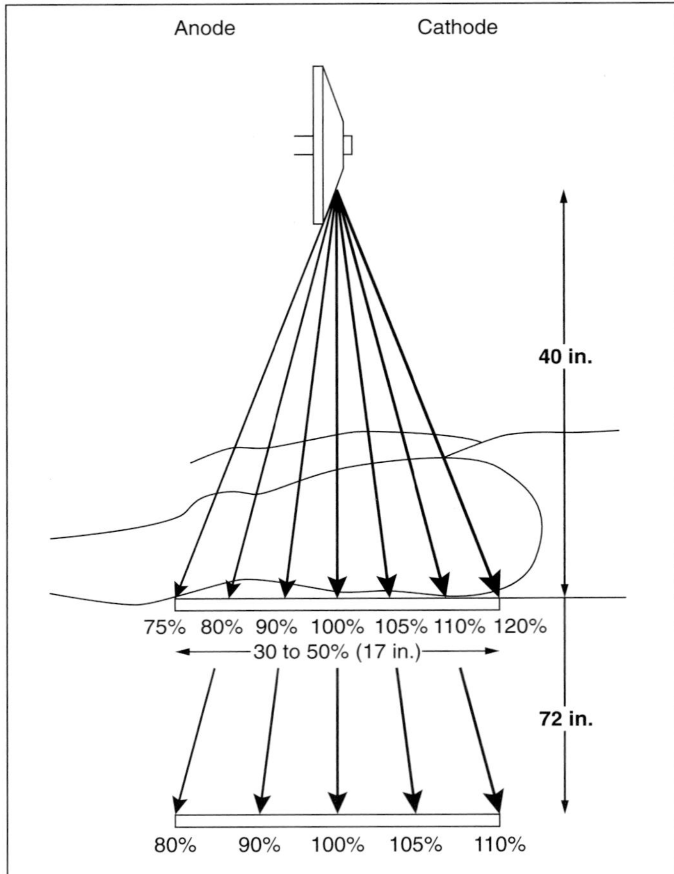

Fig. 1-119. Anode heel effect.

Positioning Considerations

Obtaining optimum exposures of certain body parts which have a significant variation in thickness along the axis of the x-ray beam should include correct use of this anode heel effect by **placing the thicker body part at the cathode end of the x-ray table** (the cathode and anode ends of the x-ray tube are usually marked on the protective housing).

The abdomen, spine and long bone limbs, such as the femur and tibia/fibula, are common examples of anatomic structures that vary enough in thickness or density that correct use of the anode heel effect is recommended for optimum radiographic images.

Exception: It should be noted that it is not always practical or even possible to take advantage of the anode heel effect (depending on the patient's condition or the arrangement of specific x-ray equipment in a room).

Radiation Protection

with Richard Geise, Ph.D.

INTRODUCTION

As a professional responsible for one's actions, the responsibility of radiation protection for the patient, one's self, and fellow workers is very important for radiologic technologists. A complete study and understanding of radiation protection is essential for every radiographer but is beyond the scope of this anatomy and positioning text. However, the application or applied principles of radiation protection is very much an essential part of a course in radiographic anatomy and positioning because it is the responsibility of every radiographer to **always ensure that the radiation dose to both the patient and the radiographer be kept as low as possible**.

UNITS OF RADIATION

Units of Radiation Exposure–Roentgen (R)

Roentgen is a measurement of **radiation exposure in air**, measured by the amount of ionization in a given unit of air.

Units of Radiation Dose–Rad and Rem

Rad and rem are units of **dose** (ionization within tissue, also described as energy absorbed by tissue). In diagnostic radiology using x-ray energy, the three units can be considered equivalent (1 R = 1 rad = 1 rem). **Rads** are used primarily for **patient doses,** and **rem** are used for **radiation protection** purposes, such as in reporting worker doses with film badges.

Traditional vs. SI Units

The SI (System Internationale) is the national standard for units of radiation measurement since 1958. However, just as the United States is slow in converting to the metric system for other measurements, conventional units of radiation measurements such as the **roentgen**, **rad** and **rem** are still in common use in the United States rather than SI units. Conversion and prefix tables are provided in Figs. 1-120 and 1-121 to facilitate conversions between traditional and SI systems, and to convert among units within the SI system.

RADIOGRAPHER PROTECTION

In January 1994, the Nuclear Regulatory Commission (NRC) changed some of the standards concerning maximum permissible doses. The correct term now for maximum permissible dose is **dose-limiting recommendations.** The dose-limiting recommendation for occupationally exposed workers is **5 rem (50 mSv) of whole body effective dose (ED) per year**. This 5 rem or 50 mSv is also sometimes referred to as the **annual effective dose limit** for whole body occupational exposure. The ED for occupationally exposed workers, such as radiographers, is much greater than the dose limit for the **general population,** which is **0.1 rem (1 mSv) per year** for continuous or frequent exposure, and **.5 rem (5 mSv) per year** for infrequent annual exposure.*

The maximum **quarterly** dose measurement is the same as the **annual** ED. For example, if the full 5 rem were received by a radiographer in one quarter, he (she) would have to be reassigned for the remainder of that year.

The cumulative lifetime ED limit for an occupationally exposed worker is **1 rem (10 mSv) times the years of age**. For example, a 50-year old radiographer has a maximum allowable accumulated dose of 50 rem (500 mSv). However, because of the small risk of long-term effects of low level radiation, it is important that radiographers limit their exposure to the **least amount possible**, or even less than the allowable 5 rem per year.

Exposure should be monitored for each occupationally exposed worker. If **0.1 rem (1 mSv)** or more of exposure could potentially be received per year, the area should be supervised by a qualified radiation protection officer.

To convert from (traditional units)	*to (SI units)*	*Multiply by*
Roentgen (R)	**C/kg** (Coulombs/kg of air)	2.58 x 10^{-4} (.000258)
Rad (radiation absorbed dose)	**Gray** (Gy)	10^{-2} (.01) (1 rad = .01 Gy)
Rem (radiation equivalent man)	**Seivert** (Sv)	10^{-2} (.01) (1 rem = .01 Sv)

Note: Patient doses throughout this textbook are given in mrads (1 mrad = 10^{-2} or .01 mGy, and 1 mGy = 100 mrad)

Dose limits are given in rem (Seivert, Sv) (1 rem = .01 Sv or 10 mSv, and 1 mSv = 0.1 rem)

Fig. 1-120. Conversion table–Traditional to SI units.

Summary and Conversion Examples:

1. Convert **rad** to **gray (Gy)**: Rad can easily be converted to grays by **dividing by 100.**

   Example: The dose to the male testes on an AP hip is: ≈**322 mrad** (.322 rad).

   Convert to SI units, milligray (mGy): 322 ÷ 100 = **3.22 mGy** (.00323 gray).

   To convert the other way from gray to rad (or mGy to mrad) **multiply by 100**.

2. Convert **rem** to **Sievert (Sv)**: Rem can easily be converted to Sievert by **dividing by 100**.

   Example: A 30-year-old radiographer has a cumulative lifetime ED of: **30 rem** (30,000 mrem).

   Convert to SI units, Sievert (Sv): 30 ÷ 100 = **.3 Sv** (300 mSv)

3. Convert **rem** to **mSv:** This is a common conversion for radiation protection purposes.

   Example: **Multiply by 10 (5 rem** x 10 = **50 mSv)**

Prefix	*Symbol*	*Exponential expression*	*Multiplication factor*
giga	G	10^9	1,000,000,000
mega	M	10^6	1,000,000
kilo	k	10^3	1,000
hecto	h	10^2	100
deca	da	10^1	10
BASE UNIT		10^0	1
deci	d	10^{-1}	0.1
centi	c	10^{-2}	0.01
milli	m	10^{-3}	0.001
micro	µ	10^{-6}	0.000,001
nano	n	10^{-9}	0.000,000,001

Fig. 1-121. SI prefixes and conversions.

*NCRP Reprint 116, *Limits of Exposure to Ionizing Radiation*, National Council of Radiologic Protection and Measurements; 1993

Minors

Minors under 18 years of age should not be employed in situations in which they are occupationally exposed. The ED limit for minors is that of the general public, which is 0.1 rem (1 mSv) per year.

Personnel Monitoring

Film badges or **TLD** (thermoluminescent dosimetry) **badges** must always be worn by all personnel who have the potential of receiving more than one fourth the maximum permissible dose. They must be worn **at the waist or chest level**, except in **fluoroscopy,** where they should be worn at the **collar area outside the lead apron**. Film badges, which are the most widely used, need to be changed and read every month, and TLD badges at least every 3 months.

Pregnant Radiographers

The pregnant radiographer and other occupationally exposed workers should take all precautions possible to keep exposure to the embryo/fetus as low as possible. The recommended maximum equivalent dose to the fetus is **.05 rem (0.5 mSv) during any 1 month**, and **0.5 rem (5 mSv)** for the **gestation period**.

Also, pregnant radiographers should wear a **second** film badge or other monitoring device at the abdomen area **under the lead apron**, in addition to the usual one worn outside the lead apron at the chest area. These monitoring devices must be clearly marked as to which is worn under the apron at the abdomen, and which is worn at the collar area.

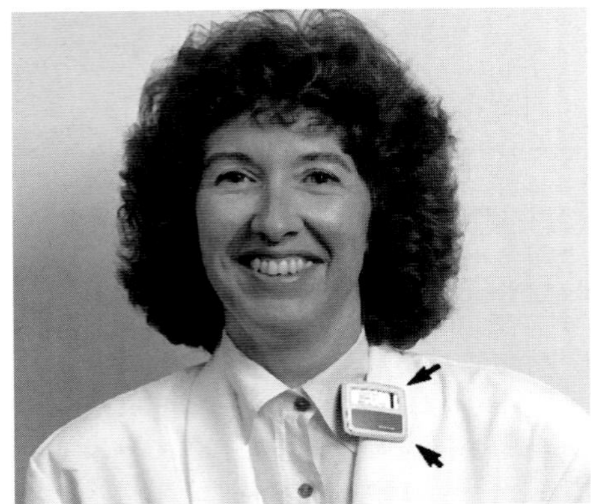

Fig. 1-122. Radiographer wearing a film badge.

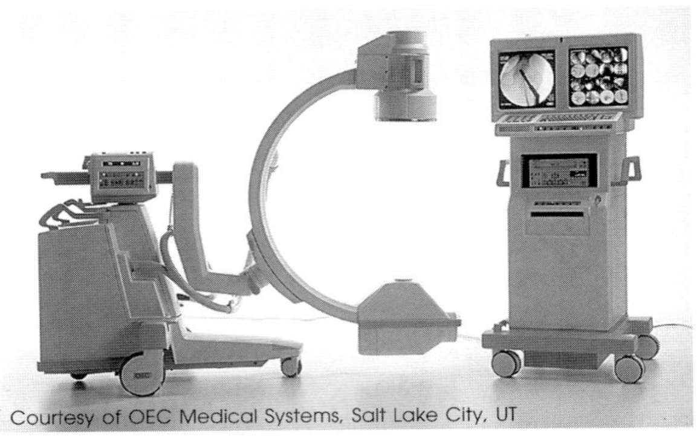

Courtesy of OEC Medical Systems, Salt Lake City, UT

Fig. 1-123. C-arm mobile digital fluoroscopy unit.

ALARA PRINCIPLES

There is a protection principle called **ALARA** that goes much further in protecting the worker than the ED level. This principle states that occupational exposure should be kept "**As Low As Reasonably Achievable**." This is an important principle that all radiographers should strive for, and following is a summary of four important ways this can be achieved:

1. **Always wear a film badge or other monitoring device**. Although the badge doesn't lower exposure of the wearer, long-term accurate records of badge readings are important for determining protection practices.
2. If restraining patients is necessary, it should be by **a person other than an occupationally exposed worker**. This person should never stand in the primary or useful beam and should always wear protective aprons and gloves. Restraint devices or retention bands should be used whenever possible, and only as a last resort should anyone stay in the room to restrain patients–this should **never** be radiology personnel.
3. Practice the use of **close collimation**, **filtration of primary beam**, **optimum kVp techniques**, **high-speed screens and film** and **minimum repeat exams**. Exposure of the radiographer is due primarily to scattered radiation from the patient and other sources. Therefore, reduction in patient exposure results in reduction in exposure of the radiographer as well.
4. Follow the **three-part cardinal rule** of radiation protection, the **time**, **distance** and **shielding** principle. The radiographer should minimize his/her **time** in an exposure field, stand **as far away** from the source as possible, and utilize **lead shielding** when in an exposure field.

   This is important in trauma and mobile radiography, especially with **mobile C-arm digital fluoroscopy units** (Fig. 1-123). These are used with orthopedic or biliary tract surgery, foreign body localization, pacemaker insertion and interventional vascular procedures. Protection from scatter is especially important for mobile fluoro units such as the C-arm due to the potential of increased patient and worker doses as described in detail in Chapter 19 on trauma and mobile radiography (page 557).

PATIENT DOSES

General Diagnostic Procedures

As already described, the amount of energy absorbed by a certain amount of tissue is the radiation absorbed dose (rad). For a particular x-ray examination, it is possible to talk about several different "doses" to the patient. The number most often quoted is the exposure to the skin in the region where the radiation first strikes the body, commonly called the skin entrance exposure, **SEE**. (This is sometimes referred to as entrance skin exposure, ESE.) This exposure is approximately the skin dose. The skin dose has the highest numerical value of all the doses but in radiography it has the least biological significance. As the radiation passes through the body on the way to the film, its intensity drops as much as several hundred times. The average doses to specific organs are useful for estimating the likelihood that those organs will develop cancer from radiation.

Effective Dose (ED or E): The effective dose (**ED**, sometimes referred to as just **E**) takes into account the dose to all organs and their relative risk or the weighting factors of becoming cancerous (or in the case of the gonads, the risk of genetic damage). The effective dose is the quantity that can be used to **compare average radiation to the whole body from a radiological procedure, with that received from natural background radiation**.

The patient dose chart on the next page, shows the **skin entrance exposure (SEE), specific organ doses**, and the **effective dose (ED)** for a standard size patient for a sampling of common radiographic projections.

The chart demonstrates the effects of using different kVp and compares doses of AP vs. PA projections. It also shows the effect of gonadal shielding and the total ED values for male and female.

This chart also reveals that for **males** the highest ED for these sample projections is #10, the **AP unshielded hip** (ED=84 mrem). This is primarily due to the high testes dose, which can be greatly reduced with gonadal shielding (ED is reduced to 14).

For the **female** the highest ED is #4, the **AP thoracic spine on a 14 x 17 in. film without breast shields** (ED=63). This is primarily due to the high breast dose, which can be reduced by breast shielding or collimation to a 7 x 17 in. size (ED reduced to 35).

Patient Dose Chart

Comparisons	Projection	kVp	mAs	SEE (mR)	Organ doses (mrad) rounded to the nearest mrad: testes	ovaries	thyroid	marrow	lung	breast	ED (mrem): male	female
1. AP *vs.*	AP chest (72" FFD)	120	2	12	0	0	4	1	7	10	2	5
PA	PA chest (72" FFD)	120	2	12	0	0	1	2	7	1	2	2
2. AP *vs.*	AP skull (10x12)	80	25	302	0	0	92	4	1	1	3	5
PA	PA skull (10x12)	80	25	302	0	0	8	10	0	0	3	3
3. AP *vs.*	AP esophagram	110	6	142	0	0	48	9	66	124	15	54
PA	PA esophagram	110	6	142	0	0	9	16	69	10	16	20
4. 14 x 17 *vs.*	AP thoracic spine	75	20	209	0	0	23	8	72	158	15	**63**
7 x 17	AP thoracic spine	80	20	241	0	0	26	5	34	94	6	35
5. 7 x 17 *vs.*	AP lumbar spine	80	40	483	2	74	0	10	16	4	10	29
14 x 17 *vs.*	AP lumbar spine	75	40	418	2	92	0	17	33	8	17	42
14 x 17 shielded	AP lumbar spine	75	40	418	1	92	0	17	33	8	17	42
6. AP *vs.*	AP upper GI	110	15	356	0	26	2	21	99	13	26	37
PA *vs.*	PA upper GI	110	15	356	0	14	2	43	90	9	28	34
Lateral	Lateral upper GI	110	30	1100	1	18	5	33	147	20	42	53
7. 80 kVp *vs.*	AP abdomen	80	22	266	6	68	0	13	4	1	10	26
70 kVp *vs.*	AP abdomen	70	41	365	6	80	0	13	4	1	13	31
70 kVp shielded	AP abdomen	70	41	365	2	80	0	13	4	1	11	31
8. AP *vs.*	AP barium enema	110	10	237	8	89	0	22	6	1	12	32
PA *vs.*	PA barium enema	110	10	237	5	78	0	51	5	1	15	34
PA shielded	PA barium enema	110	10	237	1	78	0	51	5	1	14	34
9. AP *vs.*	AP pelvis	80	40	483	45	100	0	23	1	0	26	39
AP shielded	AP pelvis	80	40	483	6	100	0	23	1	0	16	39
10. AP *vs.*	AP hip (one 10 x 12)	80	40	483	322	59	0	9	0	0	**84**	18
AP shielded	AP hip (one 10 x 12)	80	40	483	42	14	0	9	0	0	14	7

Notes: **SID** = 40 in. (102 cm) unless specified. **Film size** = 14 x 17 in. (35 x 43 cm) unless specified. **Film-screen speed = 400. "Shielded"** refers to male or female gonadal shield in place: –male gonadal shield, –female gonadal shield. **Patient thickness** = 20 cm AP or PA and 34 cm laterally. **The effective dose (ED)** can be compared with the U.S. average yearly background of 300 mrem. Organ dose estimates based on tables in *Handbook of Radiation Doses in Nuclear Medicine and Diagnostic X-ray,* J.G. Keriakes and M. Rosenstein, CRC Press, Boca Raton, 1980. Breast doses and ED estimates by authors.

Fig. 1-124. Patient dose chart.

Fluoroscopic Procedures

Typical patient exposures during several GI fluoroscopy procedures are shown in Fig. 1-125, which includes approximate skin entrance exposures (SEE) during fluoroscopy and spot filming. This does not include doses from overhead films for those exams that can be determined from the dose chart above. Fluoroscopic procedures generally involve **much higher patient doses** than conventional "overhead tube" diagnostic exams because of the need to penetrate the barium or iodine contrast media and the time required to manipulate the media in the patient. Fortunately, however, the volume of tissue exposed during fluoroscopy and spot filming is fairly small.

Using magnification mode in fluoroscopy generally increases the dose rate but decreases the volume of tissue exposed. Pulsed fluoroscopy may be used to reduce dose in proportion to the number of pulses used per second. Spot film doses also can be reduced by using photospot cameras or digital fluoroscopy (DF) as described in Chapter 14 on the upper GI system, page 426.

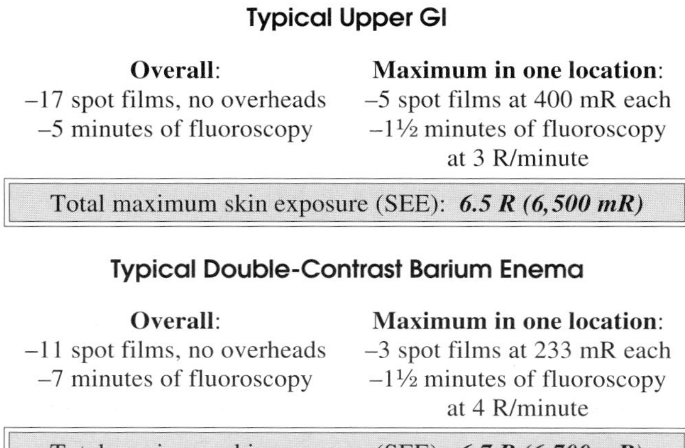

Typical Upper GI

Overall:	**Maximum in one location**:
–17 spot films, no overheads	–5 spot films at 400 mR each
–5 minutes of fluoroscopy	–1½ minutes of fluoroscopy at 3 R/minute

Total maximum skin exposure (SEE): ***6.5 R (6,500 mR)***

Typical Double-Contrast Barium Enema

Overall:	**Maximum in one location**:
–11 spot films, no overheads	–3 spot films at 233 mR each
–7 minutes of fluoroscopy	–1½ minutes of fluoroscopy at 4 R/minute

Total maximum skin exposure (SEE): ***6.7 R (6,700 mR)***

Fig. 1-125. Typical patient exposures during fluoroscopy and spot filming.

WORKER PROTECTION DURING FLUOROSCOPY

Exposure Patterns and Worker Protection

During routine fluoroscopy of the gastrointestinal tract, personnel are exposed to radiation scattered by the patient and other objects being irradiated. Exposure to this scatter radiation drops off with one over the square of the distance from the part of the patient being examined, so the dose drops dramatically as the workers move away from the patient and table. This is demonstrated in Fig. 1-126 showing estimated scatter radiation exposure fields directly beside the intensifier tower without tower drape shielding in place.

The intensifier tower, tower lead drapes, Bucky-slot shield, x-ray table, patient foot rest if present, and even the radiologist, all provide a source of shielding for the technologist (Fig. 1-127). The important **Bucky slot shield** closes the 2 or 3 inch space under the table-top when the Bucky is all the way to the end of the table-top (see Chapter 14, page 425). Note that the area "F" behind the radiologist and away from the patient and table has the lowest exposure rate of less than 25 mR per hour.

When the intensifier tower is lowered as close as possible to the patient, much of the scatter to the worker's eyes and neck region is eliminated. The vertical and lateral dimensions of the exposure field move in dramatically as the distance between the patient and the intensifier tower is reduced.

Older remote control systems, which are not shown here, with the x-ray tube over the table and the intensifier tower below are designed for remote use only due to greatly increased scatter radiation present with these systems. In these rooms, which are less commonly used today, technologists and fluoroscopists should operate behind a remote protective barrier.

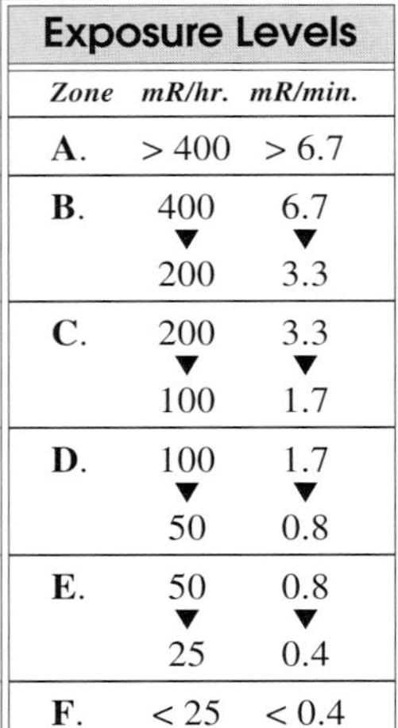

Exposure Levels

Zone	mR/hr.	mR/min.
A.	> 400	> 6.7
B.	400 ▼ 200	6.7 ▼ 3.3
C.	200 ▼ 100	3.3 ▼ 1.7
D.	100 ▼ 50	1.7 ▼ 0.8
E.	50 ▼ 25	0.8 ▼ 0.4
F.	< 25	< 0.4

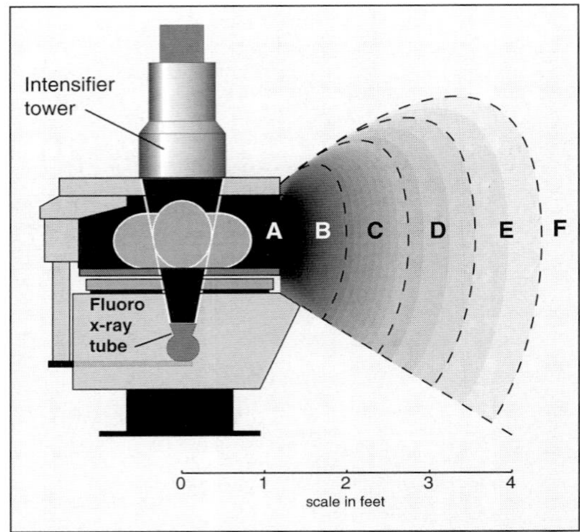

Fig. 1-126. Fluoroscopy exposure patterns **without tower drape shields in place.**

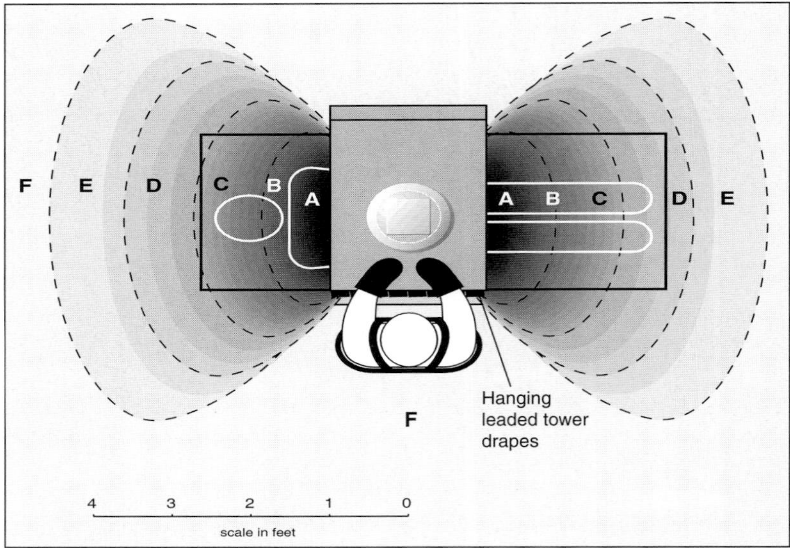

Fig. 1-127. Fluoroscopy exposure patterns during fluoroscopy **with tower drape shields in place** and with intensifier tower close to patient.

Worker Protection Practices

Even with correct shielding in place and the intensifier tower as close to the patient as possible, a certain amount of scatter radiation is present during routine fluoroscopy (Fig. 1-127).

Scatter is greatest in the immediate region of the patient close to the table on each side of the radiologist, who has the leaded tower drapes between himself and the patient. Therefore technologists and/or other workers in the room can reduce their exposure by **not standing close to the table** on either side of the radiologist, but staying back out of the higher scatter fields as much as possible.

Everyone involved in a fluoroscopic procedure **must wear lead aprons** as a protective measure. A 0.5 mm lead equivalent apron will reduce the scattered radiation to the majority of the body by typically ten or more times. This is usually enough to reduce risks to a reasonable level, well below maximum permitted levels. Typical doses behind aprons are less than 10 mrem per month (immeasurable by film badges) in low-use departments, and are almost never above 20 mrem per month for technologists involved in only GI fluoroscopy. At these levels it may not be necessary to reassign a pregnant technologist to keep fetal exposure from fluoroscopy below the maximum permitted levels. Reassignment, however, should be considered on an individual basis in the light of the ALARA principle.

One should be cautious if using "light weight" aprons or ones that have large cut-outs around the arms and low necklines. These allow more exposure to dose-sensitive organs such as the thyroid, lungs and even breasts at certain angles. It has been suggested that the protection of a 0.5 mm equivalent lead apron of this design is no better than a .25 mm lead equivalent apron that covers a larger area.

Many older aprons do not have specific thyroid shields. These can be either separate collar-type shields, which can be worn with the neck cutout type apron (Fig. 1-128), or they can be the newer type aprons, which include a raised collar-type extension for thyroid protection (Fig. 1-129).

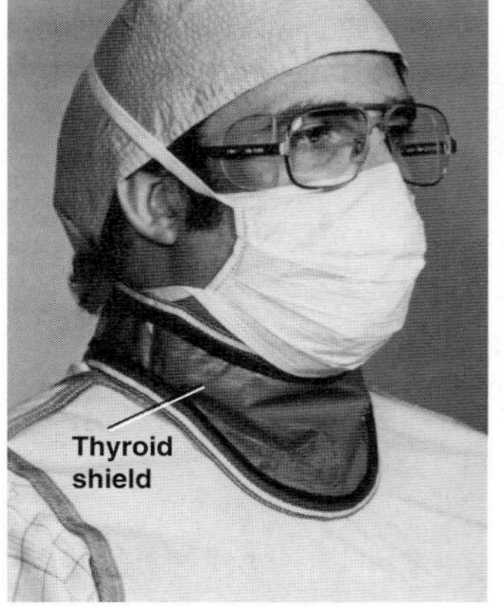

Fig. 1-128. Thyroid shields with regular neck cutout apron.

Courtesy of Nuclear Assoc., Carle, NY

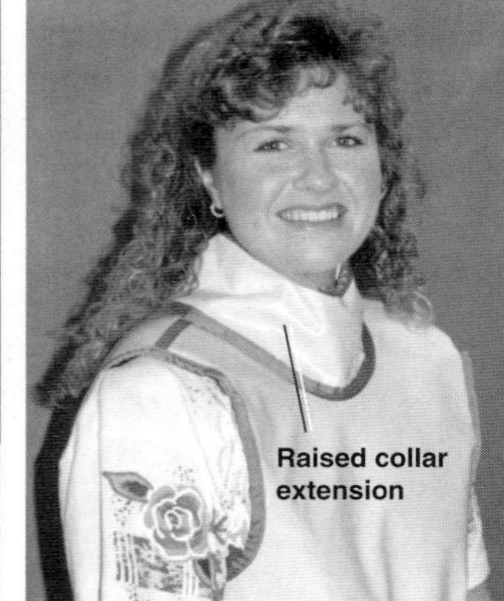

Fig. 1-129. Apron with raised collar extensions.

Courtesy of Shielding International, Inc., Madras, OR

Wearing thyroid shields when available is in keeping with the ALARA principle, but the overall reduction in effective dose and risk provided by thyroid shields is small. Also, additional lead protection provided by gloves and lead glasses is generally not needed by technologists during routine GI fluoroscopic duties if recommended practices are followed as described above.

Fluoroscopy Exposure Rates Limits: Due to the potential higher patient and worker doses during fluoroscopy, Federal standards set limits of exposure rates of intensified fluoroscopy units at **10 R/min**. With most modern equipment, however, the average fluoroscopy rate is between 3 or 4 R/min. as shown by the examples on page 39, Fig. 1-125.

PATIENT PROTECTION

Each professional radiographer subscribes to a code of ethics that includes responsibility for controlling and limiting the radiation exposure to patients under their care. This is a serious responsibility and each of the following eight specific ways of reducing patient exposure needs to be understood and consistently put into practice as described on the following pages. They are as follows:

1. Minimum repeat radiographs.
2. Correct filtration.
3. Accurate collimation.
4. Specific area shielding (gonadal and female breast shielding).
5. Protection for pregnancies.
6. Use of optimum exposure factors.
7. Use of high-speed screen-film combinations.
8. Minimize patient exposure by an awareness of patient (organ) dosage per exam and how these can be reduced. Examples are the correct use of gonadal and breast shields, the use of higher kVp, lower mAs techniques, and the use of PA rather than AP projections to reduce dose to thyroid, neck region and female breasts for upper thorax and head procedures.
   Note: Eye dose is not considered in effective dose determination as defined on page 38. Larger doses than those received in diagnostic radiology are required to cause cataract formation.

1. Minimum Repeat Radiographs

The first basic and most important way to prevent unnecessary radiation is to **avoid unnecessary repeat radiographs**. One of the primary causes for repeat radiographs is **poor communication** between the radiographer and the patient. Breathing instructions that are unclear and not understood are one of the common causes of motion and the need to repeat radiographs.

When procedures are not clearly explained, the patient can have added anxiety and nervousness because of the fear of the unknown. This stress from uncertainty and fear often increases the patient's state of mental confusion and ability to cooperate fully. To prevent this the radiographer must take the necessary time, even with heavy schedules and full work loads, to **carefully and fully explain the breathing instructions as well as the procedure in general in simple terms that the patient can understand.**

Patients need to be forewarned of any movements or strange noises by the equipment during the exposure. Also any burning sensation or other possible effects from injections during exposures should be explained to the patient.

Carelessness in positioning or **selection of incorrect exposure factors** are also common causes for repeats and should be avoided.

Correct and accurate positioning requires a good knowledge and understanding of anatomy because this allows the radiographer to visualize the size, shapes and locations of structures being radiographed. This is the reason for combining the anatomy with positioning in every chapter of this text.

2. Correct Filtration

Filtration of the primary x-ray beam reduces exposure to the patient by absorbing most of those lower energy "unusable" x-rays, which primarily expose the patient's skin and superficial tissue. The net effect of filtration is a "hardening" of the x-ray beam, resulting in an increase in the effective energy or penetrability of the x-ray beam.

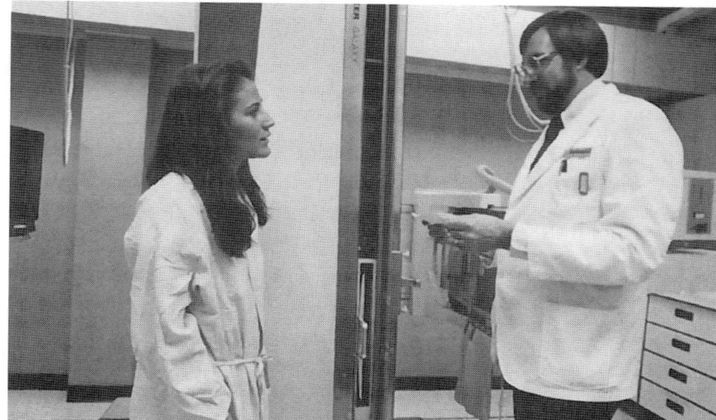

Fig. 1-130. Clear precise instructions help relieve patient anxieties to aid in avoiding unnecessary repeats.

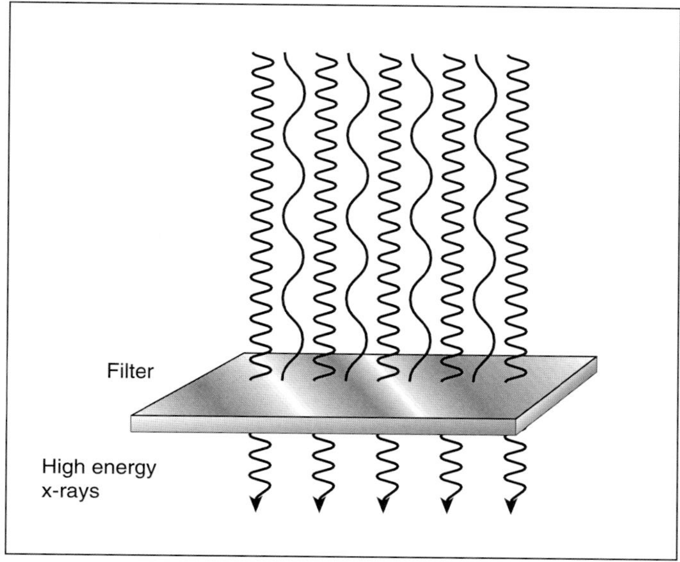

Fig. 1-131. Filtration removes low energy x-rays (which are not useful) from the beam by absorbing them while permitting higher energy x-rays to pass through.

Filtration is described in two ways. First is **inherent** or built-in filtration from the structures making up the x-ray tube itself. For most x-ray tubes this is approximately 0.5 mm aluminum (Al) equivalent.

Second and more important to radiographers is **added filtration**, which is the amount of filtration added between the x-ray tube and the collimator, and within the collimator itself.

Minimum total filtration (inherent plus added) is **2.5 mm Al equivalent** for equipment producing 70 kVp or greater.

Aluminum (Al) is the metal most commonly used for filters in diagnostic radiology, with molybdenum (Mo) often used in mammography. The amount of required added filtration as established by federal laws is dependent on the operating kVp range of the equipment. The manufacturers of x-ray equipment are required to meet these standards.

Periodic Checking of Filtration: The filtration of diagnostic imaging equipment should be checked yearly, and after a major equipment service such as replacement of the tube or collimator. This should be done by qualified personnel such as a medical physicist. The responsibility of the radiographer is to ensure that the proper filter material for each tube is checked when needed and that it remains in place.

3. Accurate Collimation

Accurate collimation is an essential way to reduce patient exposure by **limiting the size and shape of the x-ray beam to only the area of clinical interest**, or that area required to be visualized on the film or other image receptor. Careful and accurate collimation is emphasized and demonstrated throughout this textbook.

The adjustable collimator is commonly used for general diagnostic radiographic equipment. The illuminated light field defines the x-ray beam field on accurately calibrated equipment and can be used effectively to determine the tissue area being irradiated. Safety standards require that collimators be accurate to within **2% of the SID**.

The concept of divergence of the x-ray beam must be considered in accurate collimation. Therefore, the illuminated field size as it appears on the skin surface of the patient will appear smaller than the actual size of the anatomical area to which one is collimating. This is most evident on an exam such as a lateral thoracic or lumbar spine (Fig. 1-132) in which there is considerable distance from the skin surface to the film in the Bucky tray. In such cases the light field when collimated correctly to the area of interest will appear much too small unless one considers the divergence of the x-ray beam.

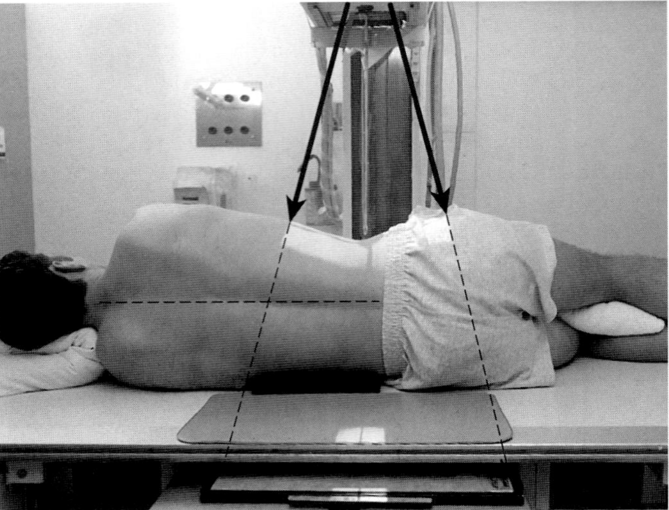

Fig. 1-132. Close four-sided collimation (collimation field may appear too small because of divergence of x-rays).

Collimation and Tissue Dose: Accurate and close collimation to the area of interest results in a dramatic drop-off in tissue dosage as one moves away from the border of the collimated x-ray field. For example, the dose at **3 cm** from the edge of the exposure field will be about **10%** of that received in the field. At a distance of **12 cm** the dose will be only about **1%** of that within the field.*

Note: These are average approximations of dose reductions. Specific percentages will be affected by body-part thicknesses, kVp range, equipment calibration and other factors.

Automatic Positive Beam Limitation (PBL): All general purpose x-ray equipment built between 1974 and 1993 in the United States and Canada require collimators with PBL features that automatically collimate the useful x-ray beam to the film size. (This requirement became optional after May 3, 1993, due to a change in FDA regulations.) The PBL feature consists of sensors in the film cassette holder which, when activated by placing a cassette in the cassette holder (Bucky tray), automatically signals the collimator to adjust the x-ray beam to that size film.

The PBL device can be deactivated or overridden with a key, but this should only be done under special conditions in which larger collimation by manual control is needed. A red warning light automatically comes on as a reminder that the PBL system has been deactivated, and regulations require that the key cannot be removed while the system is being overridden (Fig. 1-133).

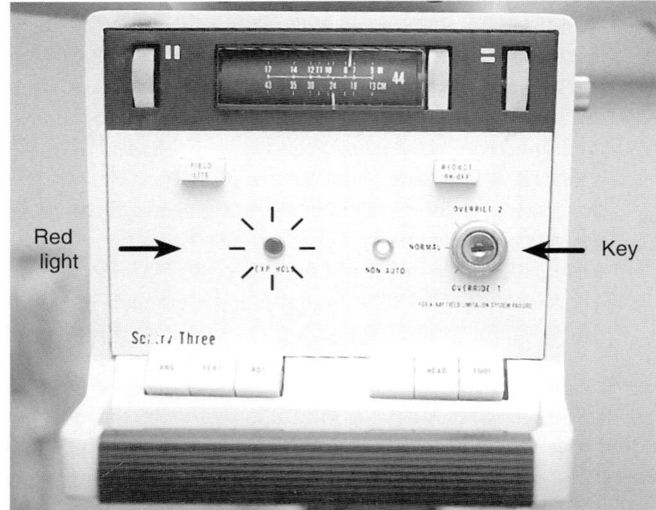

Fig. 1-133. Automatic collimation (PBL).

Manual Collimation: Even with automatic collimation, PBL, the operator can also manually reduce the collimation field size even further than that which is set automatically by the film size. This should be done for all exams in which the film size is larger than the critical area being radiographed. Accurate manual collimation also is required for exams of the upper and lower limbs taken table-top wherein the PBL device is not activated. Throughout the positioning pages of this textbook, collimation guidelines are provided to maximize patient protection by careful and accurate collimation.

This practice of close collimation to only the area of interest reduces patient exposure **two ways**. First, it **reduces the volume of tissue directly irradiated**, and second, it **reduces the accompanying scatter radiation**. This scatter radiation resulting from lack of accurate collimation or other shielding not only adds unnecessary increased patient exposure but also results in decreased image quality by the "fogging" effect of scatter radiation. (This is especially true in high-volume tissue areas such as the abdomen or chest.)

Three Reasons for Four-sided Collimation: In addition to (1) reducing patient exposure and (2) improving image quality, a third reason for this general rule of at least some visible collimation on all four sides is a **check system ensuring that maximum collimation did occur**. If there is no collimation border visible on the radiograph on any one or more sides on exams taken table-top where there is no automatic collimation, then there is no evidence that the primary beam was restricted at all.

An added benefit for at least some collimation on all four sides, if possible, is the ability to check the final radiograph for **correct central ray location**. This is done by placing a large imaginary X from the four corners of the collimation field as seen on the resultant radiograph. The exact center of this X indicates where the CR was located.

Collimation rule: A general rule followed throughout this text indicates that collimation should **limit the exposure field to only the area of interest,** and **collimation borders should be visible on the film on all four sides** if the film size is large enough to allow this without "cutting off" essential anatomy.

*Keriakes, JG, Rosenstein, M. *Handbook of Radiation Doses in Nuclear Medicine and Diagnostic X-ray*, Boca Raton, CRC Press; 1980.

4. Specific Area Shielding

Specific area shielding is required when radiosensitive tissue or organs such as the thyroid gland, breasts and gonads are in or near the useful beam. Examples of this type of area shielding are **breast** and **gonadal** shields, which can be used over female breasts and male or female gonads for certain examinations such as a scoliosis spine series (Figs. 1-135 and 1-136).

The most common and most important area shielding is **gonadal shielding**, used to protect the reproductive organs from irradiation when they are in or near the primary beam. The two general types of specific area shielding are **shadow shields** and **contact shields**.

Shadow Shields: As the name implies, shadow shields, which are attached to the tube head or collimator, are devices placed between the x-ray tube and the patient, thus casting a shadow of the shield over the specific areas being shielded. One such type of shield is shown in Fig. 1-134 wherein the shield is attached to a flexible arm which can be adjusted to cast a shadow from the collimator light over the gonads or other areas being shielded.

Another more common and newer type is shown in Fig. 1-135 wherein individual breast and gonad shields are attached with magnets directly to the bottom of the collimator. These may also be combined with clear lead compensating filters to provide a more uniform exposure for body parts that are not uniform in thickness or density, such as for a thoracic and lumbar spine scoliosis radiograph (Fig. 1-136).

Gonadal Contact Shields: Flat contact gonadal shields are most commonly used for patients in recumbent positions. Larger vinyl-covered lead shields of **.5 mm lead equivalent** placed over the gonadal area in general may be used **to absorb scatter and/or leakage radiation** (Fig. 1-137). These shields are usually made from the same lead-impregnated vinyl materials used for lead aprons.

Shields to absorb 95 to 99% of primary rays in the 50 to 100 kVp range require a minimum of 1 mm lead equivalent. Thus when used in the **primary x-ray field**, contact gonad shields should be **a minimum of 1 mm lead equivalent**. Examples of these may be smaller vinyl-covered lead material cut into various shapes to be placed directly over the reproductive organs as shown in Figs. 1-138 and 1-139).

Male: Gonadal shields for males should be placed distally to the symphysis pubis covering the area of the testes and scrotum (Fig. 1-138). The upper margin of the shield should be at the symphysis pubis. Suggested shapes of male shields are also shown. Smaller sizes should be used for smaller youth or children. These are slightly tapered at the top and wider at the bottom to better shield the testes and scrotum without obscuring pelvic and hip structures.

Female: Placement of gonadal shielding on females to cover the area of the ovaries, fallopian tubes and uterus is a little more difficult to determine. A general guideline for female adults is to shield an area 4½ to 5 in. (11 to 13 cm) proximal or superior to the symphysis pubis, and 3 to 3½ in. (8 to 9 cm) each way from the pelvic midline. The lower border of the shield should be at or slightly above the symphysis pubis, with the upper border extending just above the level of the ASIS (**A**nterior **S**uperior **I**liac **S**pines) (Fig. 1-139).

Various-shaped female ovarian shields may be used, but they should be wider in the upper region to cover the area of the ovaries, and narrower towards the bottom to offer less obstruction of pelvic or hip structures. The shielded area would be proportionally smaller on children. For example, a 1-year-old female would require a shield only about 2½ to 3 in. (6 to 7 cm) wide and 2 in. (5 cm) in height placed directly superior to the symphysis pubis.*

Gonadal shields, if placed correctly, will reduce the gonadal dose **50 to 90%,** if the gonads are in the primary x-ray field (see patient dose chart on page 39).

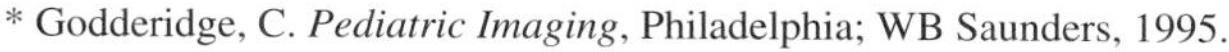

* Godderidge, C. *Pediatric Imaging*, Philadelphia; WB Saunders, 1995.

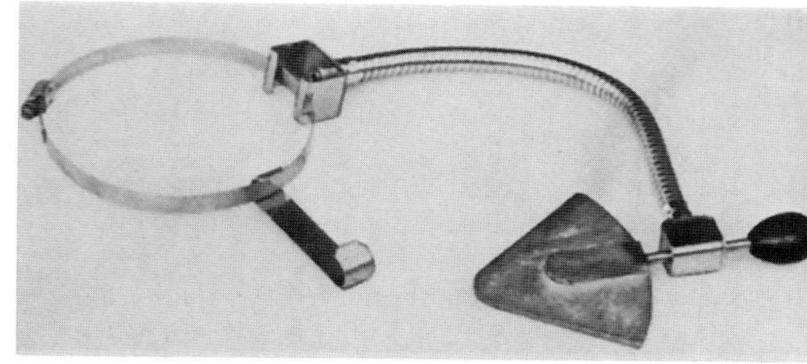

Fig. 1-134. Shadow shield on flexible arm.
(Courtesy of Nuclear Associates, Carle, NY)

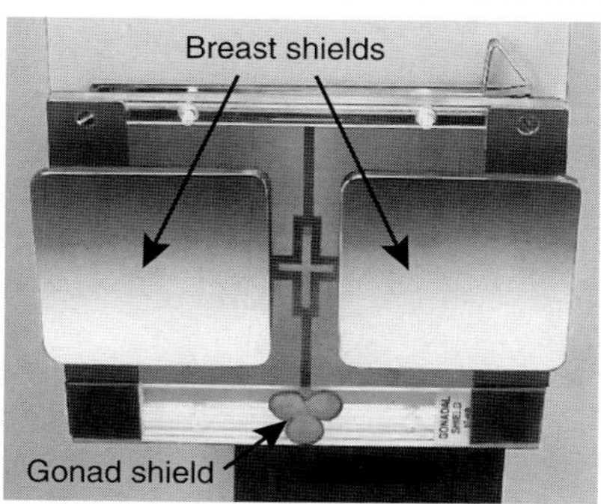

Fig. 1-135. Shadow shields in place under collimator (attached with magnets)
(Courtesy of Nuclear Associates)

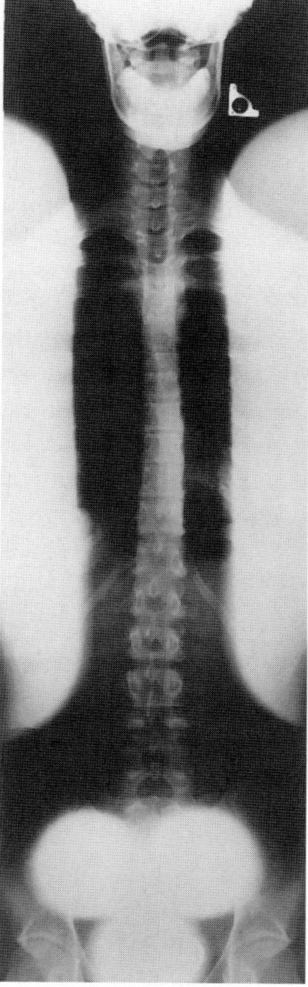

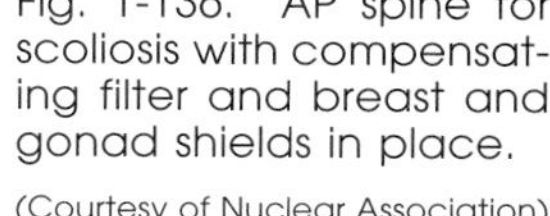

Fig. 1-136. AP spine for scoliosis with compensating filter and breast and gonad shields in place.
(Courtesy of Nuclear Association)

Fig. 1-137. Vinyl-covered lead shield in place over pelvis

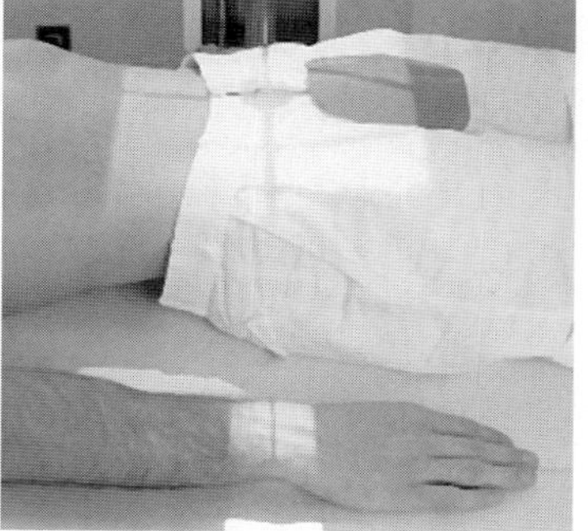

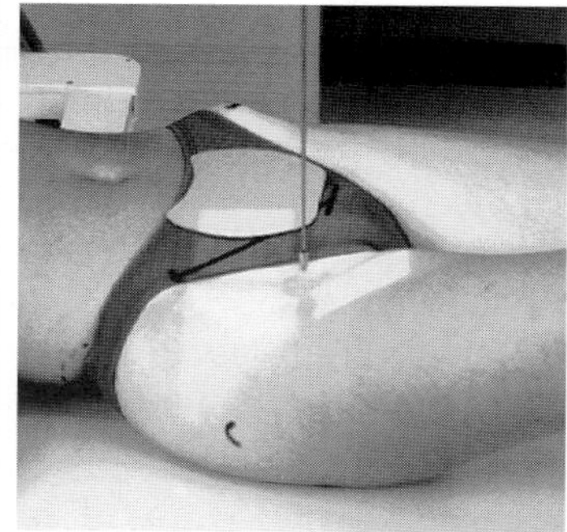

Fig. 1-138. AP pelvis -Flat contact shields- AP hip. Fig. 1-139.
(1 mm lead equivalent)

-Male gonadal shield

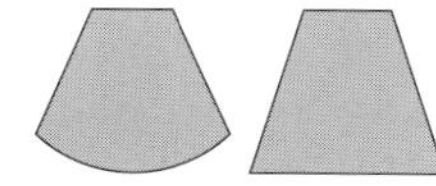

Possible shapes

-Female ovarian shield

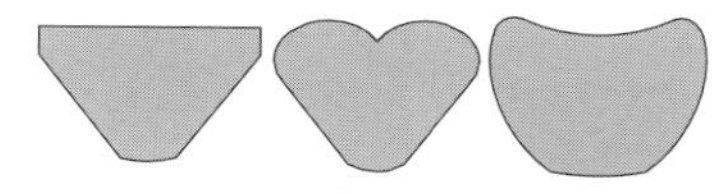

Possible shapes

Summary Rules for Specific Area Shielding: Consistent and correct use of specific area shielding is a challenge for each radiographer because of the added time and equipment required. The importance, however, of protecting radiation-sensitive organs and the gonads of children and adults of reproductive age from unnecessary radiation exposure should be sufficient motivation to consistently practice the following three rules for gonadal shielding:

1. **Should be used on all potentially reproductive age patients.** A common departmental policy is to include specific area shielding for all children and those adults of reproductive age. (A good policy followed in many departments is to shield gonads for all patients when possible).
2. **Should be used when the radiation sensitive areas lie within or near** (2 in. or 5 cm) **the primary beam unless such shielding obscures essential diagnostic information.**
3. **Accurate beam collimation** and careful positioning must accompany the use of such shielding. Specific area shielding is important, but this should always be a **secondary** protective measure and **not** a substitute for accurate collimation.

5. Protection for Pregnancies

Pregnancies and potential pregnancies require special consideration for all women of child-bearing age because of the evidence that the developing embryo is especially sensitive to radiation. This concern is particularly critical during the first two months of pregnancy when the fetus is most sensitive to radiation exposure and the mother is usually not yet aware of the pregnancy.

In the past, **the ten-day rule**, as stated by the ICRP (International Commission on Radiation Protection) was used as a safeguard for potential early pregnancies. This rule stated that all radiologic examinations involving the pelvis and lower abdomen be scheduled during the first 10 days following the onset of menstruation since no conception will have occurred during this time. More recently this rule is being abandoned as reported in various documents by both the ICRP and the American College of Radiology due to the potential harm of cancelling essential x-ray procedures during this 10-day period. Studies have shown that if x-ray exams are clinically indicated, they should be performed, even during this period. Exceptions to this are those higher dose exams of the pelvic area or fluoroscopy procedures that can be delayed a few weeks without compromising the health of the patient. However, posters or signs (Figs. 1-140 and 1-141) should be posted in examination rooms and waiting room areas reminding the patient to inform someone of their known pregnancy or potential pregnancy.

If x-ray procedures are performed during this period of potential pregnancy, it is important to use all those radiation protection practices already described, especially careful collimation.

For **known pregnancies**, the following exams result in higher doses to the fetus and embryo, and should require confirmation from the referring physician and the radiologist that the exam is indicated:

- Lumbar spine
- Sacrum and coccyx
- Intravenous urogram (IVU)
- Fluoroscopic procedures (abdomen)
- Pelvis
- Proximal femur and hip
- Gallbladder
- Computed tomography

6. Optimum Exposure Factors

A sixth important radiation protection practice involves the use of those optimum exposure factors that reduce patient exposure. The selection of optimum exposure factors should not only result in the highest quality radiograph possible yielding maximum diagnostic information, but should also result in the least possible patient dose. The use of high kVp techniques with lower mAs significantly reduces patient dose, as already described in this chapter.

IF YOU ARE PREGNANT
PLEASE TELL THE TECHNOLOGIST

SENORAS-SI ESTAN EMBARAZADAS FAVOR
DE NOTIFICAR A LOS TECHNOLOGISTAS

Fig. 1-140. Warning sign. (Courtesy of St. Joseph's Hospital, Phoenix, AZ)

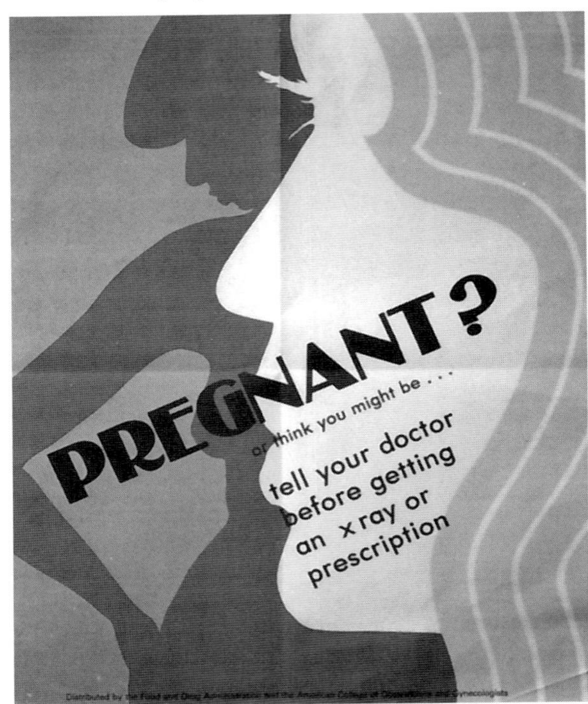
PREGNANT?
or think you might be . . .
tell your doctor before getting an x ray or prescription

Fig. 1-141. Warning poster.

7. Optimum Speed Screen-Film Combinations

The seventh protection practice involves the use of high-speed screen-film combinations, which reduces patient dose dramatically. For all screen-film combinations, over 99% of the radiographic image results from light emitted by the intensifying screens, and less than 1% from the primary rays themselves. Therefore, the speed of the intensifying screens has a great effect on the required x-ray exposure to the patient in producing radiographs.

Certain rare earth high-speed screens in common use today have speeds that are 4 times or more faster than that of the more commonly used 100-speed (par-speed) screens. Therefore, the patient exposure can be reduced by one quarter or more.

Some films with thicker emulsion or with different chemical dyes are also faster or more sensitive, thus reducing the amount of exposure required. The use of higher-speed screens and films, however, does result in some loss of image definition or sharpness of detail, and one must balance the reduction in patient exposure with the potential loss of detail in the resultant image. It is common practice to use slower 100 speed (detail) screens with table-top procedures, such as upper and lower limbs, when a grid is not used and optimum detail is important.

Faster-speed screens are commonly used for larger body parts when grids and higher exposure techniques are required.

Screen-Film Rule: Use the highest speed screen-film combination which results in diagnostically acceptable radiographs.

Note: Departmental protocol or routines generally indicate which speed film-screen combinations should be used for which types of procedures. This is not a decision generally made by individual radiographers.

8. Minimize Patient Exposure by an Awareness of Patient Doses Per Exam

The eighth and final way radiographers can reduce patient exposure as described in this text is to minimize patient exposure by an understanding and awareness of the amount of radiation radiographers are exposing the patient to each time they "make" an exposure. They should know the effect of various exposure combinations on patient dose, and the effect of accurate collimation and of correctly placed gonadal shields. They should know the effect of dose to the thyroid and female breasts on AP compared to PA projections for the head, neck and upper thorax region. In the same way that a good understanding of anatomy is important in learning positioning, some understanding of **patient dose ranges** is also important for each projection or radiographic procedure.

When a repeat is necessary due to a positioning or technique error, approximately how much additional dose is being given to the patient? What is the effect on dosage when the kVp is increased and mAs decreased? How much can the ovarian dose be reduced for certain projections such as a female hip if a correctly-placed ovarian shield is used? How much more dose to the testes does a male receive on an axiolateral or inferosuperior lateral hip, as compared to other lateral hip projections?

To answer these questions for radiographers, sample patient doses are listed in the patient dose chart on page 39, and are also included with each projection described in this textbook in a small icon box format as shown on the right and as described below:

Dose Calculations

Skin Dose (Sk): Skin entrance dose was determined by using certain adjustment factors with source-skin distance and backscatter considerations. Thus, the exposure in roentgens (R) as emitted from the x-ray tube is converted to absorbed dose units at the skin as measured in millirad (mrad).

Midline Dose (ML): Midline doses are similar to specific organ doses located in mid body regions. All doses as listed assume accurate collimation to the region of interest as shown in the shaded collimation field and cassette drawing on each positioning page of this text.

Gonadal Dose (Gon): Gonadal doses as listed for Male (M) and Female (F) assume no specific gonadal shields were used. These doses would be 50 to 90% less than those listed if correctly placed gonadal shields were used as described under gonadal contact shields on page 43.

These gonadal doses are given without shielding to remind the radiographer of the extreme importance of gonadal shielding whenever possible when the gonads are in or near the primary exposure field if such shielding does not cover essential anatomy.

Gonadal doses for certain upper and lower limb procedures and procedures of the head and neck region are indicated as NDC (No Detectable Contribution). This indicates that measurements were made, but the contribution to the gonadal dose was insignificant. Therefore, gonadal shielding for such exams is generally not essential for protection purposes. For these procedures involving the upper body, thyroid and/or breast doses will replace the gonadal dose when available.

Thyroid and/or Breast Doses: Certain projections of the head, neck and thorax include significant primary and/or scatter dose to the thyroid gland and/or female breasts, which are radiosensitive organs and should be shielded if possible. These doses will replace the gonadal doses where available to emphasize the need to shield these regions, or take PA rather than AP projections when possible.

Sample Exposure and Dose Icon Boxes
-AP Lumbar Spine, p 289

• Technique and dose–AP

	cm	kVp	mAs	Sk.	ML.	Gon.
@ 80 kVp:	17	80	15	242	62	M 1 F 27
@ 92 kVp:	17	92	8	176	51	M 1 F 21

mrad

Measurement and Techniques (Exposure Factors):

cm (17) –AP lumbar measurement for this model "patient" (see Note 1).
kVp (80 or 92) –Kilovoltage required for this "patient."
mAs (15 or 8) –mAs required at specified kVp.

Patient Doses in mrad @ 80 kVp, 15 mAs and @ 92 kVp and 8 mAs:

Sk. –Skin entrance dose
ML. –Midline dose
Gon. –Gonadal doses for the male (M) and female (F) with accurate collimation as indicated, assuming no specific gonadal shields were used.

(Thyroid and/or breast doses when available will be substituted for gonadal doses for projections involving the upper body where these doses become significant and gonadal doses are insignificant.)

Additional Factors:

- 40 in. (102 cm) SID
- Kodak 100-speed screens for table-top procedures
- Kodak 400-speed screens used with grids
- 12:1 Bucky grid and 6:1 portable grids.

Note 1: Some of the models as demonstrated in this textbook are smaller than the average adult patient, indicating that the kVp or mAs would be as much as two times higher on some patients, with corresponding **higher doses**.

Note 2: Exposure factors (kVp and mAs) are listed only to indicate the basis for the associated patient doses, and are not recommended technique factors that can be used in any department. Variables such as screen and film speed, grid ratio, film processing, SID, filters and equipment calibration will determine the technique factors required for specific equipment.

Note 3: All doses as calculated for this textbook are based on an output at one meter SID (100 cm or about 40 inches) of 6 mR/mAs at 80 kVp. This is for a three-phase generator with a half value layer of 3 mm aluminum at 80 kVp.

Note 4: Doses were calculated in part using tables in the CRC *Handbook of Radiation Doses in Nuclear Medicine and Diagnostic X-ray* by James Keriakes and Marvin Rosenstein, by CRC Press, Boca Raton, 1980.

Specific organ doses were calculated based on a "Computer Program for Tissue Doses in Diagnostic Radiology (CD13)" from the Center for Devices and Radiological Health, Rockville, Maryland.

Fig. 1-142. Explanations concerning exposure and patient dose icon boxes, as included on each positioning page of this text.

Positioning Principles

PROFESSIONAL ETHICS AND PATIENT CARE

The medical radiographer (radiologic technologist) is a medical professional and an important member of the health care team responsible in general for radiologic examination of patients. This requires not only a broad understanding of anatomy terminology used in this profession, an understanding of the basic imaging principles and radiation protection as covered in the first part of this chapter, but also an understanding of what it means to be a professional responsible for the patients under their care. This includes being responsible for one's actions under a specific code of ethics (shown on the right).

The term ethics in general refers to the moral principles of behavior of individuals. More specifically a **Code of Ethics** describes the **rules of acceptable conduct toward others,** as defined within certain professions.

As a medical professional responsible for the welfare of patients in their care, radiologic technologists must adhere to a strict code of conduct with absolute honesty in carrying out their tasks and responsibilities in a professional manner. They must also remember that they are a supporting member of the medical team, which includes radiologists and referring physicians.

The current code of ethics as printed on this page reflects the recognition of the radiologic technologist as a professional who "**practices ethical conduct appropriate to the profession, and protects the patient's right to quality radiologic technology care**" (principle 8). Principle 7 also emphasizes the added responsibilities as a professional who "**performs services in accordance with an accepted standard of practice, and demonstrates expertise in limiting the radiation exposure...**"

This code of ethics and the increased recognition of radiologic technology as a profession indicating responsibility for their actions and behavior, places additional responsibility on technologists in the areas of patient doses, radiation protection and optimum quality radiographs. Throughout this textbook, emphasis is given to knowing approximate patient doses for each projection and maximizing radiation protection for the patient. Thus patient doses, gonadal shielding and collimation notations are included on each positioning page for all projections.

Evaluation criteria sections are included with each projection or position that identifies a definable standard for each radiographic image described and illustrated.

Code of Ethics

1. *The Radiologic Technologist conducts himself/herself in a professional manner, responds to patient needs and supports colleagues and associates in providing quality patient care.*
2. *The Radiologic Technologist acts to advance the principle objective of the profession to provide services to humanity with full respect for the dignity of mankind.*
3. *The Radiologic Technologist delivers patient care and service unrestricted by concerns of personal attributes or the nature of the disease or illness, and without discrimination, regardless of sex, race, creed, religion, or socioeconomic status.*
4. *The Radiologic Technologist practices technology founded upon theoretical knowledge and concepts, utilizes equipment and accessories consistent with the purpose for which they have been designed, and employs procedures and techniques appropriately.*
5. *The Radiologic Technologist assesses situations, exercises care, discretion and judgment, assumes responsibility for professional decisions, and acts in the best interest of the patient.*
6. *The Radiologic Technologist acts as an agent through observation and communication to obtain pertinent information for the physician to aid in the diagnosis and treatment management of the patient, and recognizes that interpretation and diagnosis are outside the scope of practice for the profession.*
7. *The Radiologic Technologist utilizes equipment and accessories, employs techniques and procedures, performs services in accordance with an accepted standard of practice, and demonstrates expertise in limiting the radiation exposure to the patient, self and other members of the health care team.*
8. *The Radiologic Technologist practices ethical conduct appropriate to the profession, and protects the patient's right to quality radiologic technology care.*
9. *The Radiologic Technologist respects confidences entrusted in the course of professional practice, protects the patient's right to privacy, and reveals confidential information only as required by law or to protect the welfare of the individual or the community.*
10. *The Radiologic Technologist continually strives to improve knowledge and skills by participating in educational and professional activities, sharing knowledge with colleagues and investigating new and innovative aspects of professional practice. One means available to improve knowledge and skills is through professional continuing education*

Code of ethics as adopted by:
THE AMERICAN SOCIETY OF RADIOLOGIC TECHNOLOGISTS
THE AMERICAN REGISTRY OF RADIOLOGIC TECHNOLOGISTS
as revised in July 1994.

PROTOCOL AND ORDER FOR GENERAL DIAGNOSTIC RADIOGRAPHIC PROCEDURES

Each radiology department should establish an agreed-on protocol and order by which all general diagnostic radiographic procedures are performed. This is necessary for an orderly and effective working system whereby all radiographers (students or graduate technologists) follow the same order and procedure.

The specific items included, as well as the order of these various steps or procedures, will vary depending on the location, type and size of department. This may also vary depending on whether the radiographer is working solo or as a team with another technologist or student wherein certain duties are divided.

Following is a sample protocol for general diagnostic radiographic procedures as established and used by a midwestern U.S. university hospital.*

Protocol for General Diagnostic Radiographic Procedures
1. Read and assess requisition completely.
2. Determine which screen-film combination you will need.
3. Determine what size and number of cassettes you will need.
4. Stock passbox/cassette cabinet with proper amount and type of cassettes.
5. Prepare radiographic room.
6. Correctly identify the patient. (Check arm band or have patient repeat full name.)
7. Dress patient correctly. (Sometimes done by nurse or transaide.)
8. Explain to the patient what you will be doing and what is expected of them.
9. ASSIST the patient to position and place you want them for the first film.
10. Measure the part to be radiographed.
11. Determine the radiographic technique to be used and set on the machine.
12. Position the patient accurately.
13. Collimate the beam so that only the area of interest is included.
14. Identify right and left side of patient with the proper lead marker.
15. Restrain the patient if needed.
16. Use lead gonadal shielding on anyone under 50 years of age.
17. Provide lead aprons and lead gloves, if necessary, for EVERYONE assisting with restraint in the room.
18. Take exposure, while watching patient through window.
19. Repeat steps 8 through 18 for each radiographic view needed.
20. Patient is not to be left alone in the radiographic room unless restrained and holding a pull cord.
21. Explain that you are going to develop and view the films you have taken to determine if adequate radiographs have been taken.
22. Fog each exposed cassette with the patient's identification card.
23. Place exposed cassettes in a pass box to the darkroom.
24. Record the date, time, number of films, name, room number, technique used, and patient history on the requisition.
25. Properly critique radiographs. If no radiograph needs to be repeated, place in proper slot or send with patient if indicated.
26. Place a corrected patient exam card in the designated computer terminal completed box, including the time, room number, number of films and rejects.
27. Assist the patient from table to wheel chair, cart or walking position.
28. Open door for the patient.
29. Explain to outpatients where they are to go next. Take inpatients to the proper holding area and place a TO GO card in the transaide area.
30. Straighten up the radiographic room, change linens and clean off table with alcohol so room will be ready for the next patient.
31. Wash your hands.

Fig. 1-143. Sample protocol.

*Submitted by Kathy Martensen, BS, RT (R), University of Iowa Hospitals and Clinics, Iowa City, Iowa.

POSITIONING METHODS AND STEPS

Much of the work of a general diagnostic radiographer involves steps 9 to 13 of the sample protocol listed on the preceding page. This includes careful and accurate positioning of the patient in such a way as to demonstrate correctly on radiographic film or other image receptors, certain body parts as requested by a physician for diagnostic purposes. For the student radiographer, radiographic positioning skills become a central or core function or skill that every radiographer must learn and master.

Fixed vs. Floating Table-top

Factors influencing the positioning process or steps include the type of equipment being used. One example is the specific type of x-ray table, namely the economical **fixed table-top** type (more common in physicians' offices or clinics), versus the **floating table-top** type commonly used in radiology departments.

Most modern x-ray tables have a floating table-top, which allows the radiographer to easily move both the patient and table-top together in any direction without having to physically slide or move the patient with the sheet as is required on a fixed table-top. Some floating table-tops are moved manually by activating a release hand switch allowing the table-top to be manually moved either lengthwise or crosswise. Other table types, when used in combination with fluoroscopy, have motor-driven features that electrically move the table-top either crosswise or lengthwise when these switches are pressed. These switches or controls are on the front of the table and/or on the fluoro unit controls (Fig. 1-145).

Cassette Tray and Bucky Grid: Each of these table types has a pull-out cassette tray under the table, which includes a Bucky-type moving grid.

In general, the specific positioning method and steps as described in this text are the same with either the floating table-top and separate movable Bucky tray or the fixed table-top and movable Bucky tray combination.

Beam-Restricting Devices

Another significant improvement and change in x-ray equipment that has affected the specific steps or methods of positioning is the type of x-ray beam restricting devices used. Older equipment used primarily **metal cones** of various sizes and shapes. Modern equipment now includes an **illuminated adjustable collimator**, which allows careful and accurate restriction of the x-ray beam field-size in each of the four dimensions. Most adjustable collimators also include positive beam limitation (PBL) features that automatically collimate to the cassette size in the Bucky tray as described in a preceding section under radiation protection methods.

These adjustable collimators include a projected light field and central ray location as visible on the patient and on the partially pulled out Bucky tray and cassette as shown in Fig. 1-146. This allows for accurate visualization of the size and location of the actual projected x-ray beam in relationship to the specific part or area of the patient being radiographed. The lighted exposure field from the collimator also contains centering lines and a central circle or cross indicating the location of the central ray (CR) on the specific body part.

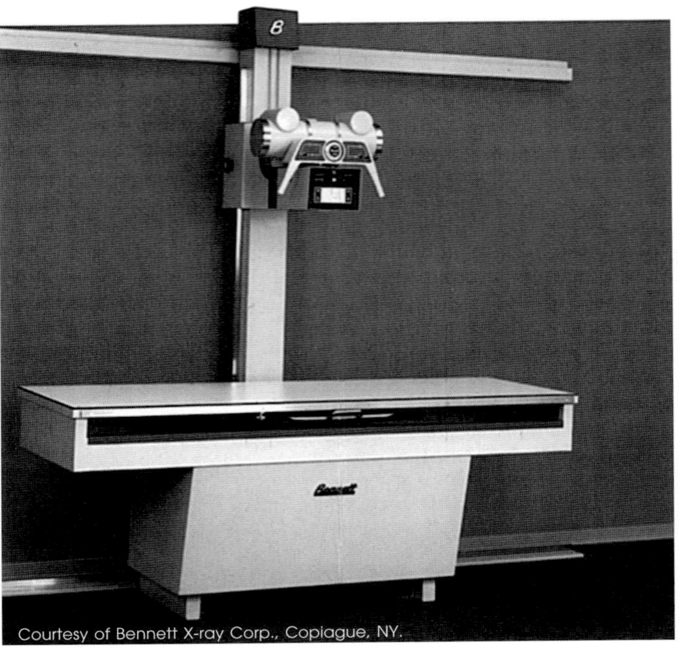

Courtesy of Bennett X-ray Corp., Copiague, NY.

Fig. 1-144. Fixed table-top with movable Bucky tray only (patient has to be physically moved on the table-top).

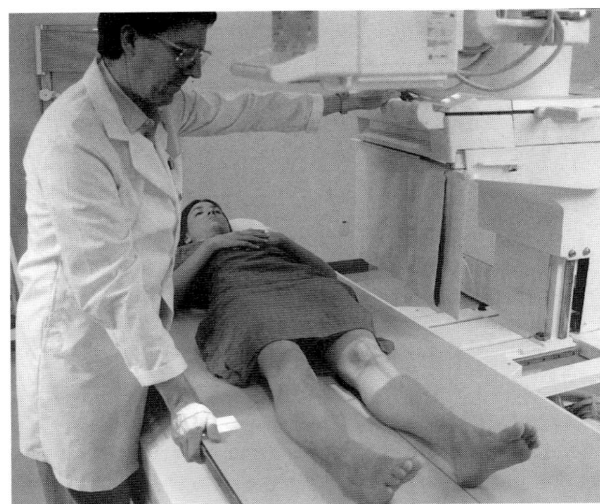

Fig. 1-145. Floating table-top and movable Bucky tray (patient and table-top move together).

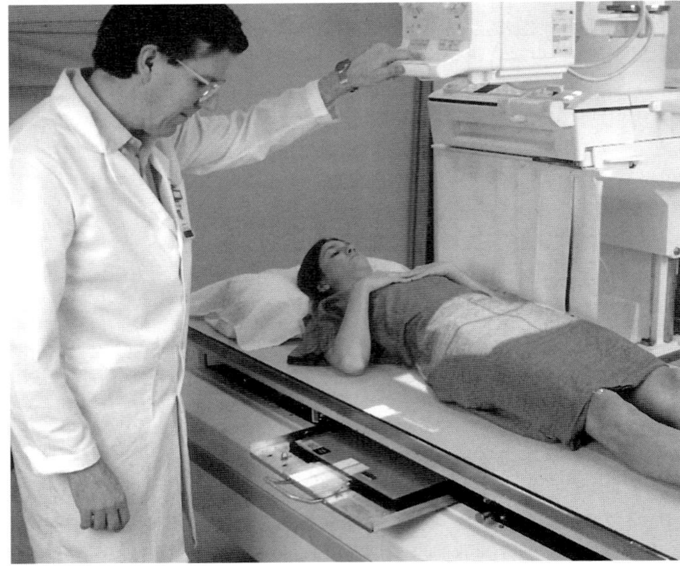

Fig. 1-146. Adjustable collimator (x-ray beam limitation device). Includes illuminated exposure field containing center-area CR lines and a CR indicator light projected onto the Bucky tray.

Positioning Sequence and Routine

With time and experience each radiographer will develop a sequence or positioning routine which works best for him or her with the specific equipment being used. However, for the student initially learning the steps and principles of radiographic positioning, an orderly and systemized step-by-step procedure for positioning is described below. This prevents the development of careless and inaccurate habits that may result in inconsistent and sloppy work as a radiographer.

After identifying and greeting the patient and carefully explaining the procedure (protocols #6 to 8, Fig. 1-143, page 47), the patient positioning process begins as follows:

Step 1. General Patient Positioning *(protocol #9):*
For an exam performed on the x-ray table, the positioning process begins by assisting the patient onto the x-ray table and into one of the following body positions: supine, prone, lateral, or oblique (Fig. 1-147).

The correct size cassette should be placed in the Bucky tray either lengthwise or crosswise; or under the part being radiographed for table-top exams.

Note: The x-ray tube should have been checked to ensure that the central ray (CR) of the collimator light is centered to the center line of the table when the table is in the center "notched" position. (This should be done before the patient is placed on the x-ray table.) This ensures that the CR and x-ray beam when used for part centering will be aligned correctly with the film when the cassette in the Bucky tray is pushed all the way in.

Step 2. Measuring Part Thickness *(protocol #10):*
The body part being radiographed is then measured, and the correct exposure factors (technique) are set on the control panel (protocol #11).

Note: Part measurement is not required if AEC (Automatic Exposure Control) is used.

Step 3. Part Positioning *(protocol #12):*
For most projections the specific body part being examined is first positioned in relationship to CR. This means for these projections, the **CR is first and/or primary in the positioning process**. The patient is turned and moved as needed to center the body part to the CR. In this example (Fig. 1-149) the patient and table-top (with floating-type table-top) is moved to align the correct body part (knee) to the CR as indicated by the "+" in the light field.

Step 4. Film Centering:
After the part has been centered to the CR, then the **film is also centered to the CR**. For table Bucky procedures, this is done by moving the cassette in the Bucky tray longitudinally to center the film (cassette) to the projected center light of the CR (Fig. 1-150).

CR Icon: This icon is included on each positioning page in this textbook for those projections wherein the **CR is of primary importance**, reminding the radiographer to pay special attention to the CR during the positioning process.

Accurate CR centering is especially important for upper and lower limbs wherein joints are the primary interest area, and the CR must be accurately directed to the mid-joint region.

Collimation: The collimator light borders are then adjusted or closed as needed to include only the essential anatomy (protocol #13).

Markers: The R or L marker is placed correctly to be in the exposure field without superimposing essential anatomy (protocol #14).

Final Positioning Step: As a final part positioning step, the overall body position and the centering is checked to ensure that the part is **accurately centered**, and that **all anatomical parts of interest are included** within both the light field borders and the film borders.

A final check for correct gonadal shield placement should also be done (protocol #16) before making the exposure with breathing instructions as needed (protocol #18).

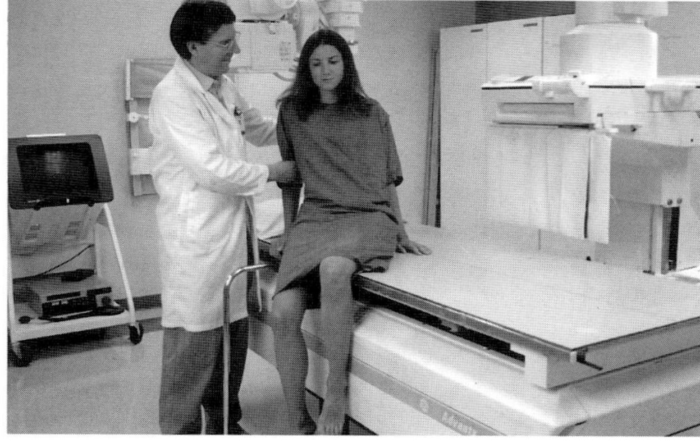

Fig. 1-147. **Step 1:** Patient positioning (onto x-ray table).

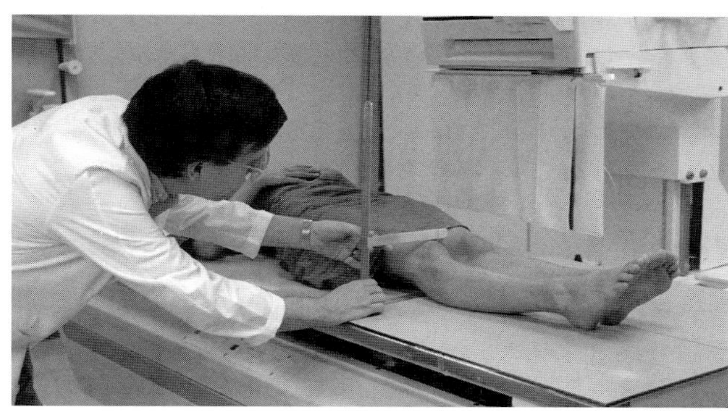

Fig. 1-148. **Step 2:** Part measured.

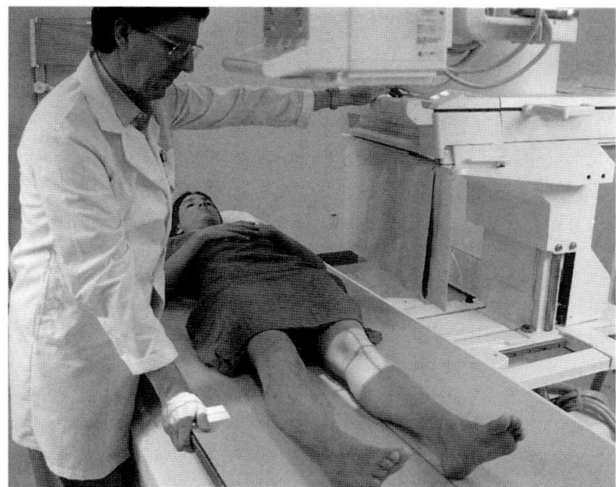

Fig. 1-149. **Step 3:** Part positioning –Part centered to CR (knee is being aligned to CR with floating table-top).

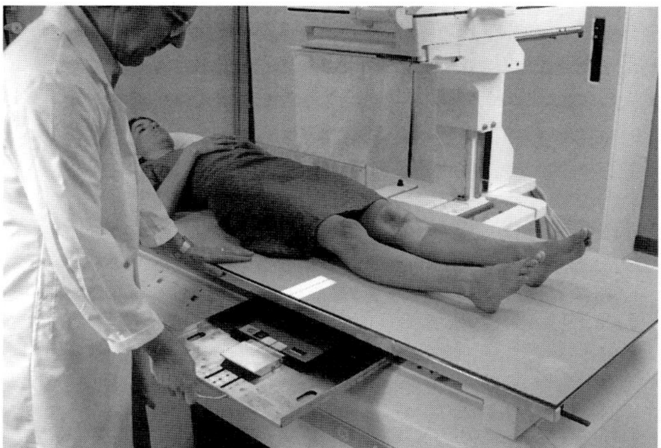

Fig. 1-150. **Step 4:** Film positioning –Film centered to CR (cassette in Bucky tray is aligned lengthwise to CR).

ESSENTIAL PROJECTIONS

Routine (Basic) Projections

Certain routine or basic projections are listed and described in this text for each radiographic examination or procedure commonly done throughout the United States and Canada. Routine or basic projections are defined as **those projections commonly taken on all average patients who are helpful and can cooperate fully**. This, of course, will vary depending on radiologist preference and between various parts of the country, as indicated by the national survey results included in each chapter and in the Appendix of this text.

Special (Alternate) Projections

In addition to the routine or basic projections, there are certain special or alternate projections also included for each examination or procedure described in this text. These are defined as **those projections most commonly taken to better demonstrate specific anatomical parts, or for certain pathological conditions, or those which may be necessary for patients who cannot cooperate fully**.

It is suggested by this author (based on the most recent survey results) that all students should learn and demonstrate proficiency for all essential projections as listed in this text. This includes all routine (basic) projections as well as all special (alternate) projections as listed and described in each chapter. An example of these basic and special projection boxes for Chapter 2 of the chest are shown in Fig. 1-151.

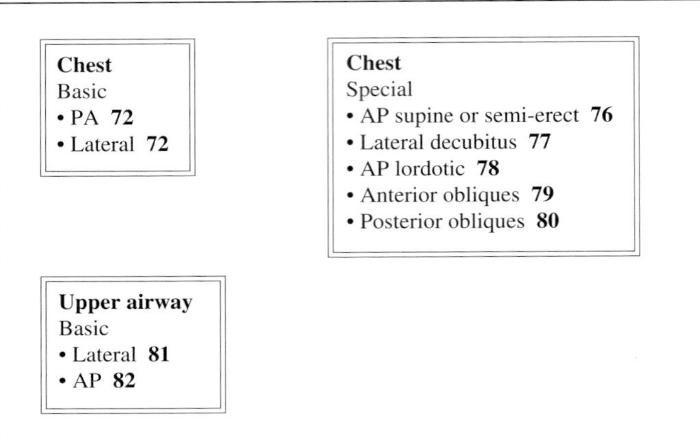

Chest
Basic
• PA **72**
• Lateral **72**

Chest
Special
• AP supine or semi-erect **76**
• Lateral decubitus **77**
• AP lordotic **78**
• Anterior obliques **79**
• Posterior obliques **80**

Upper airway
Basic
• Lateral **81**
• AP **82**

Fig. 1-151. Sample basic and special routines boxes for Chapter 2, Chest.

PRINCIPLES FOR DETERMINING POSITIONING ROUTINES

There are two general rules or principles which, if understood, will help one remember and understand why certain minimum projections are taken as routine or as basic for various radiographic examinations or procedures.

1. A Minimum of Two Projections (90° from each other)

A general rule in diagnostic radiology suggests that a minimum of two projections taken as near 90° from each other as possible are required for most radiographic procedures. Exceptions include mass chest screening which may include only a single PA projection, the KUB (kidneys, ureter, and bladder) of the abdomen, and an AP of the pelvis in which only one projection provides ample information.

The three reasons for this general rule of a minimum of two projections taken as near 90° from each other as possible are:

a. Problem of Anatomical Structures Being Superimposed: In general, a single projection should never be taken for any routine radiographic examination because of the superimposition of body parts. Certain pathological conditions such as some fractures, small tumors, etc., may not be visualized on one projection only.

b. Localization of Lesions or Foreign Bodies: A minimum of two projections, taken at 90° or as near right angles from each other as possible, are essential in determining the location of any lesion or foreign body (Fig. 1-152).

Example: Foreign bodies (the white densities are metallic fragments) embedded in tissues of the hand. Note that both the PA and lateral projections are necessary to determine the exact location of these metallic fragments in two dimensions.

c. Determination of Alignment of Fractures: Any fracture requires a minimum of two projections, taken at 90° or as near right angles as possible, both to visualize fully the fracture site and to determine alignment of the fractured parts (Figs. 1-153 and 1-154).

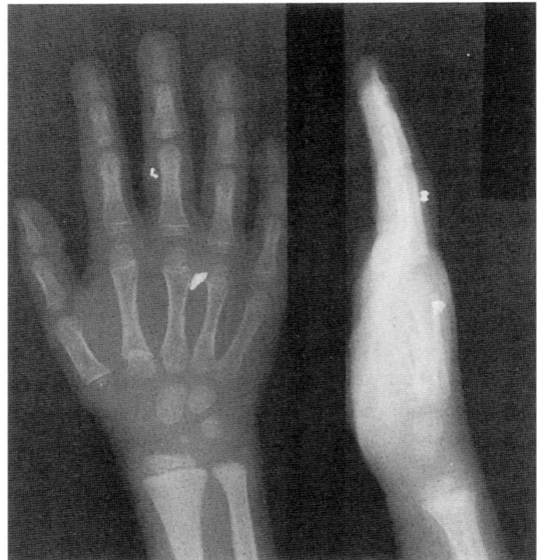

Fig. 1-152. Foreign bodies (metallic fragments in soft tissue posteriorly).

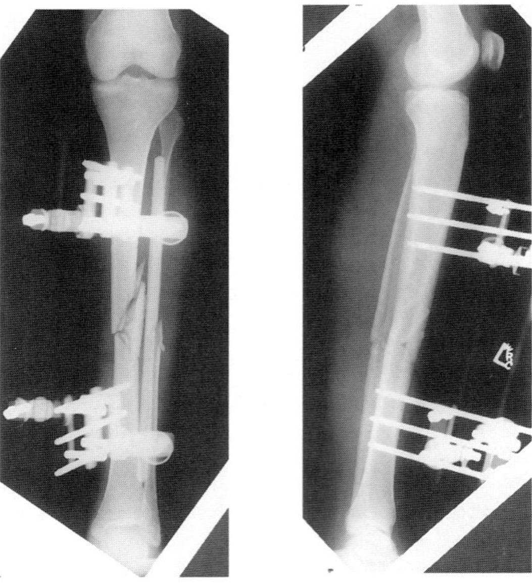

Fig. 1-153. For fracture alignment. Fig. 1-154.

2. A Minimum of Three Projections When Joints are in Prime Interest Area

This second general rule or principle suggests that all radiographic procedures of the skeletal system involving joints require a minimum of **three** projections rather than only two. These are **AP** or **PA, lateral** and **oblique**.

The reason for this is more information is needed than can be provided on only two projections. For example with the multiple surfaces and angles of the bones making up the joint, a small oblique chip fracture or other abnormality within the joint space may not be visualized on either the frontal or the lateral views but may be well demonstrated in the oblique position.

Examples of exams generally requiring **three** projections as routine or basic (joint is in prime interest area):

- Fingers
- Toes
- Hand
- Wrist
- Elbow
- Ankle
- Foot
- Knee

Examples of exams requiring **two** projections as routine or basic (long bones and chest):

- Forearm
- Humerus
- Femur
- Hips
- Tibia-fibula
- Chest
- Post-reduction upper and lower limbs (only two projections 90° from each other for alignment purposes, even if joint is in prime interest area).

Exception: Cranium (skull and/or facial bones). Routine or basic projections of the skull and/or various facial bones generally includes at least two projections, AP (PA) and lateral, but also may require additional projections with special CR angle projections or obliques to prevent superimposition of structures which need to be demonstrated.

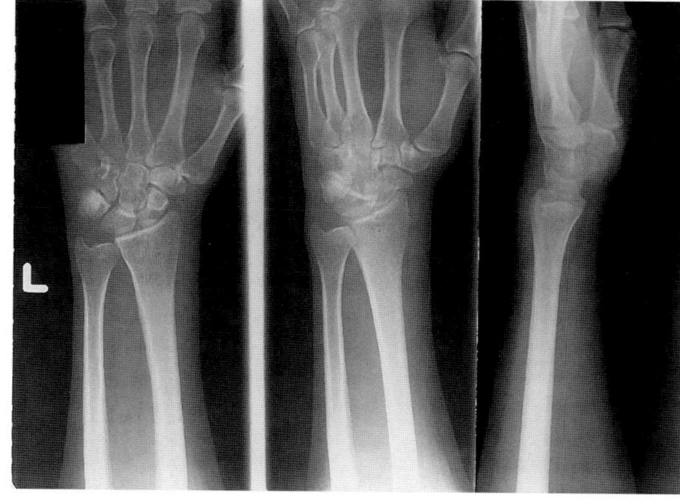

Fig. 1-155. Wrist–Requires three projections.

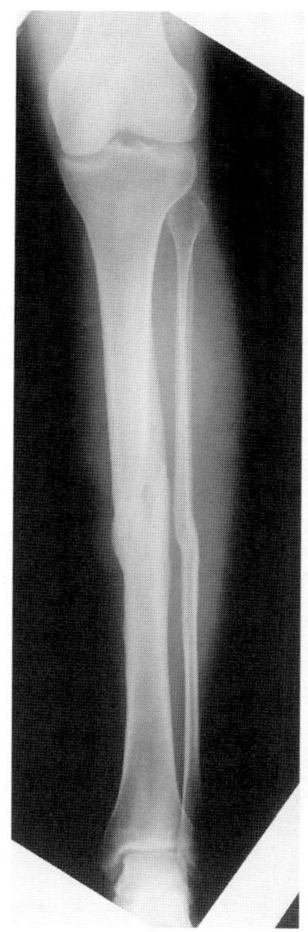

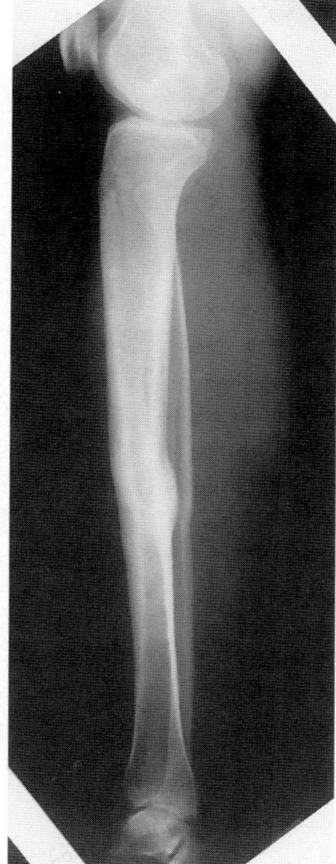

Fig. 1-156. Fig. 1-157.
Lower leg–Requires two projections/positions.

Note: This is the same patient as in Figs. 1-153 and 1-154 on preceding page, now demonstrating the healed fractures correctly aligned.

TOPOGRAPHIC POSITIONING LANDMARKS

Radiographic positioning requires the location of specific structures or organs within the body, many of which are not visible to the human eye from the exterior. Therefore certain landmarks which are parts of the bony skeleton as shown on these drawings can be located by gentle palpation and used to locate internal structures or organs.

Palpation: Palpation refers to the process of applying light pressure with the fingertips directly on the patient to locate these positioning landmarks. **This must be done gently** as the area being palpated may be painful or sensitive for the patient. Also, **the patient should always be informed of the purpose of this palpation prior to beginning this process**.

Positioning Bony Landmarks

Throughout this textbook, certain of these bony landmarks are described and demonstrated on models in those chapters wherein positioning is required of specific organs or structures.

This is the purpose of bikini-clad models in this text. On actual patients most of these landmarks are not visible under clothing or hospital gowns and palpation is required to locate these landmarks for accurate positioning.

Note: Palpation of certain of these landmarks such as the ischial tuberosity (10) and/or symphysis pubis (9) may be embarrassing for the patient, and radiographers with practice can use other related landmarks effectively as will be described in later chapters.

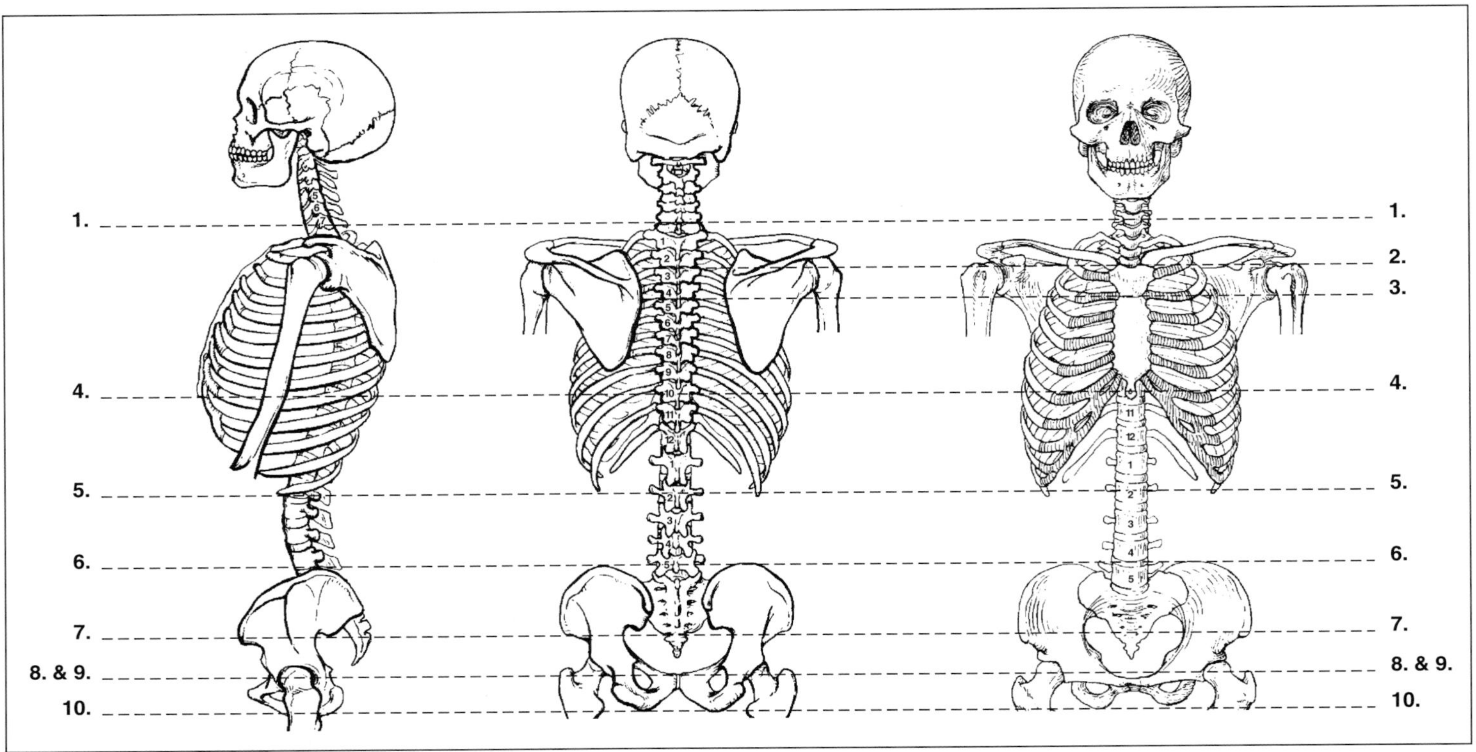

Fig. 1-158. Positioning landmarks.

Bony Landmarks

Landmark	*Used for positioning these body parts*	*Corresponding level of vertebral column*
1. Vertebra prominens (long spinous process of C7)	Upper margin of chest, C- or T-spine	C7-T1
2. Jugular notch (superior margin of sternum)	Chest, sternum, clavicle, T-spine	T2-3
3. Sternal angle (raised area of junction of manubrium and body of sternum)	Chest, sternum	T4-5
4. Xiphoid process (distal portion of sternum)	Sternum, stomach, gallbladder, T-spine, upper margin of abdomen	T9-10
5. Inferior costal (rib) margin (lateral inferior border of rib cage)	Stomach, gallbladder, ribs	L2-3
6. Iliac crest (uppermost margin of curved border of ilium portion of pelvis)	Mid abdomen, stomach, gallbladder, colon, L-spine, sacrum	L4-5 interspace
7. Anterior superior iliac spine (ASIS) (prominent anterior border of iliac crest)	Hips, pelvis, sacrum	S1-2
8. Greater trochanter (bony process of proximal femur, to locate requires firm palpation while rotating leg and femur)	Abdomen, pelvis, hip	Distal coccyx, or slightly inferior to
9. Symphysis pubis (anterior junction of pubic bones of pelvis)	Lower margin of abdomen, pelvis, hip, sacrum and coccyx	≈1 in. (2.5 cm) inferior to distal coccyx
10. Ischial tuberosity (lowermost, posteriorly located bony process of pelvis)	Prone abdomen, colon, coccyx	1 to 2 in. (2.5 to 5 cm) inferior to distal coccyx

BODY HABITUS

Radiographic positioning requires an understanding of the common variations in body form or shape (habitus). This variation in form or shape of the body has a significant effect on the shape and location of internal body organs. Therefore each radiographer must learn to recognize these body types and know the effect on internal organs as described in each chapter pertaining to the positioning of these organ systems.

The four common body types are illustrated by the drawings below, with appropriate percentages of the general population represented by each type.

Three photographs demonstrating the more common body types are also shown below.

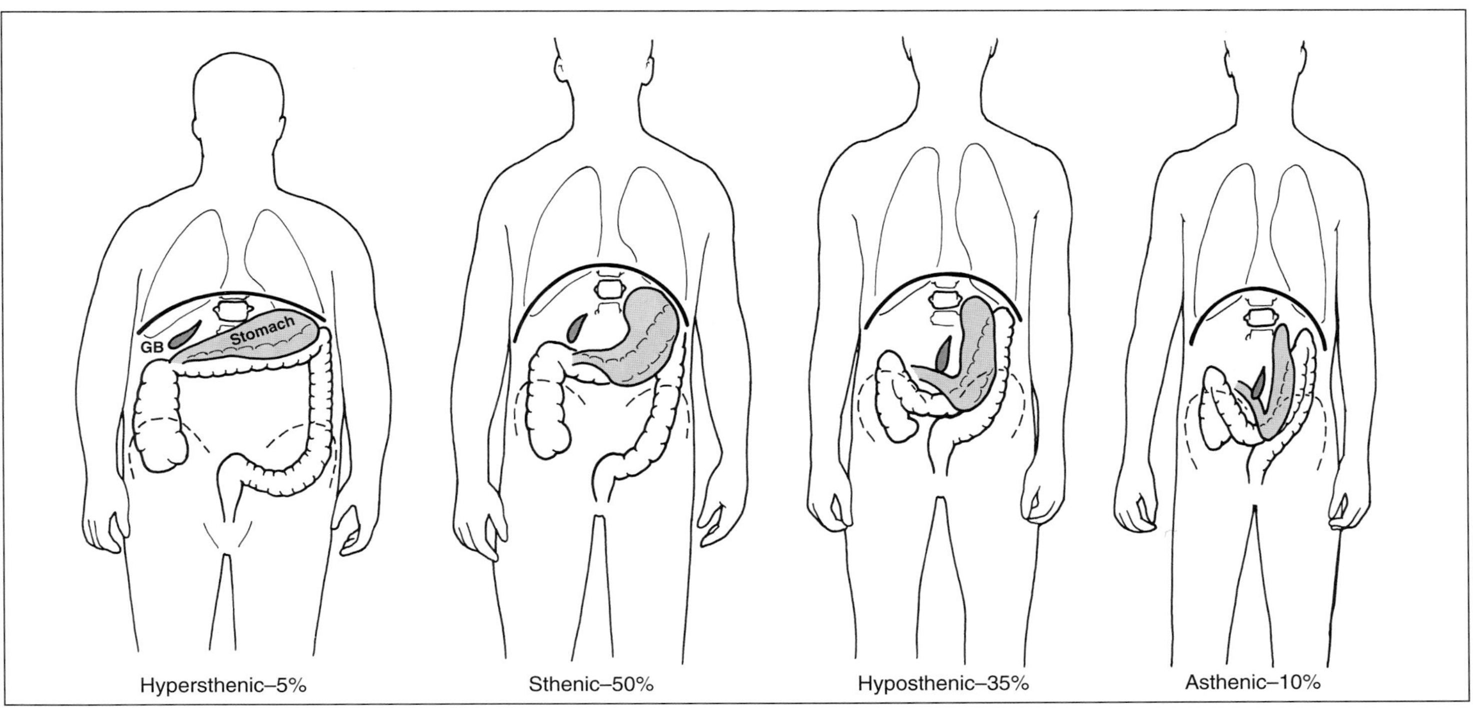

Fig. 1-159. Body habitus types.

Hypersthenic: This represents only 5% of the population of the most "stocky," massive built body-type. The thoracic cavity is wide and deep from front to back with a short vertical dimension, indicating a high diaphragm. This also makes the upper abdomen very wide, affecting the location of organs such as the gallbladder, stomach and colon as seen in this drawing and as described in later chapters.

Sthenic: This represents the nearer average, but slightly heavy-set and frequently more muscular type persons. The chest and abdominal organs are nearer average in shape and location but tend toward the hypersthenic, massive body type as seen on the above drawing.

Hyposthenic: This represents the nearer average but more slender and sometimes taller body type. The gall bladder and stomach are lower and nearer the centerline with the colon also located somewhat lower in the abdomen.

Asthenic: This is the more extreme slender body-type (10%) with a thoracic cavity that is narrow and shallow but with a long vertical dimension indicating a low diaphragm. The upper abdomen is also narrower on top and wider at its lower dimension, placing most of the abdominal organs low in the abdomen.

General Population and Body Types: The photographs on the left represent examples of different body types found among the general population.

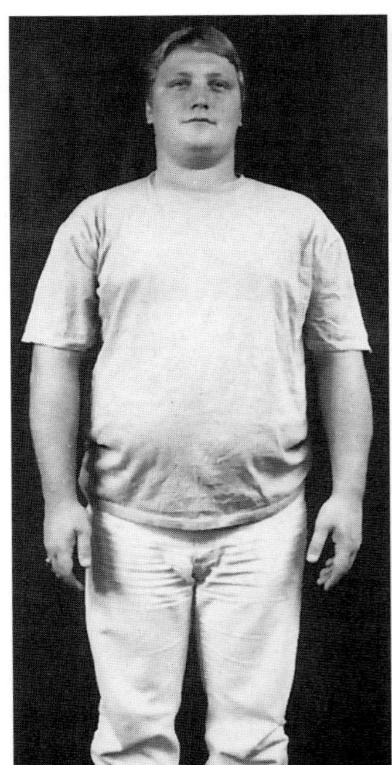

Fig. 1-160. Hypersthenic.

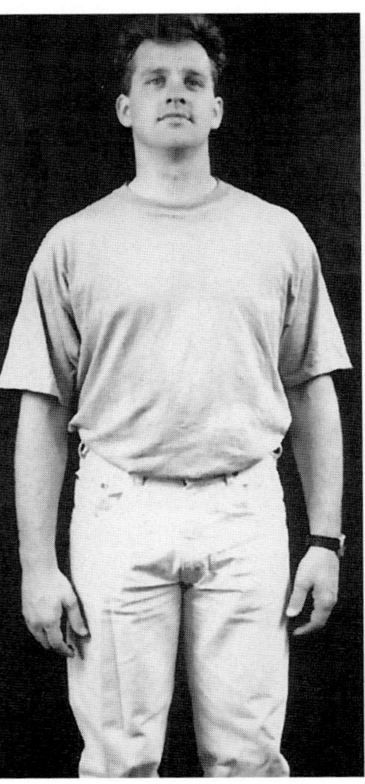

Fig. 1-161. Sthenic.

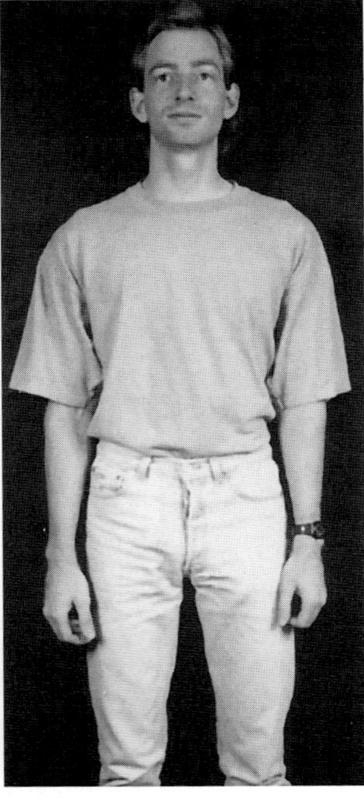

Fig. 1-162. Hyposthenic/asthenic.

VIEWING RADIOGRAPHS

The way radiographs are placed for viewing will depend on radiologist preference and what is most common in that part of the country. However, in the United States and Canada a common and accepted way to place radiographs on the view box or illuminator for viewing is to display them **so the patient is facing the viewer**, with the patient in the anatomical position (as if the viewer were ready to shake hands with the patient). **This always places the patient's left to the viewer's right**. This is true for **either AP or PA projections.** When displayed correctly, the R or L marker will appear to be right-side up on AP projections but will appear reversed on PA projections.

Lateral projections are marked by the side closest to the film (R or L). If the R or L is placed on the anterior aspect of the patient, they can be displayed the same as an AP or PA, with the left marker on the viewer's right and the right marker on the viewer's left. An exception is the chest for some radiologists who prefer them placed with the L marker to the viewer's left.

Decubitus chests and abdomens are generally viewed the way the x-ray tube "sees" them, placed crosswise with the upside of the patient also on the upper part of the view box.

Upper and lower limbs are viewed as projected by the x-ray beam onto the film, the R or L marker appears right-side-up, if it has been placed on the film correctly. Radiographs including the digits (hands and feet) are generally placed with the digits up. Other radiographs of the limbs, however, are viewed in the anatomical position with the limbs hanging down (Fig. 1-164).

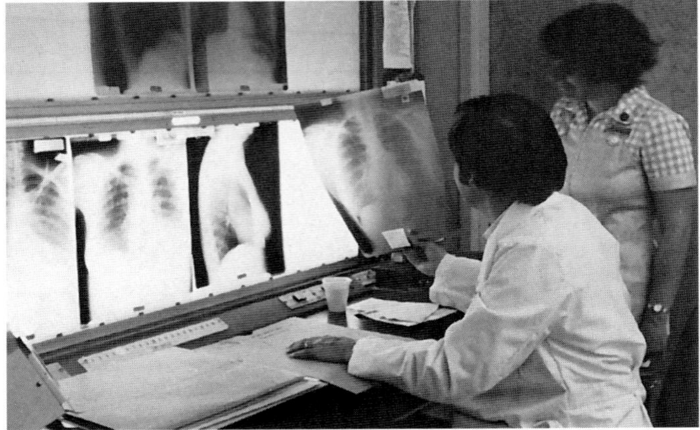

Fig. 1-163. Viewing chest radiographs (patient's right always to viewer's left, both PA and AP).

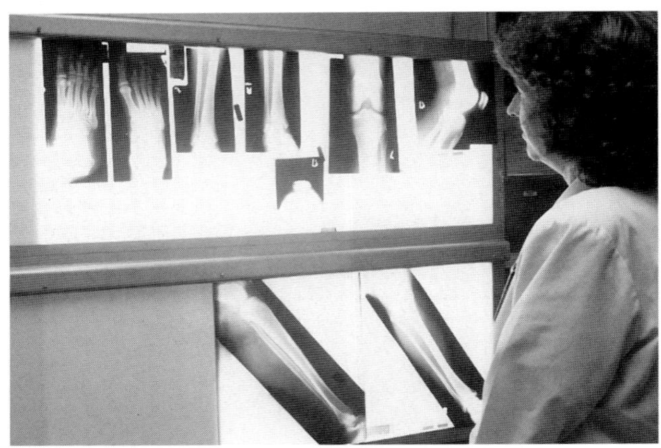

Fig. 1-164. Viewing upper or lower limb radiographs (hands and feet, digits up).

VIEWING CT OR MRI IMAGES

The generally accepted way of viewing all CT and MRI images is similar to conventional radiographs even though the image represents a thin "slice" or sectional view of anatomical structures. In general these images are again placed as if the patient were in the anatomical position and facing you, which **always places the patient's right to the viewer's left**.

Axial (Cross-sectional) Images (Fig. 1-165)

Axial or transverse (sometimes also called cross-sectional) images require a different orientation in thinking as to how these images are viewed. The most important thing to remember is that even with these cross-sectional "slice" type images, you again always place them as if you were facing the patient, with his or her right to your left.

Some also suggest that you view the image as if hypothetically you were "inside" the body looking upward. However in actuality it doesn't matter whether you were in a lower inside position looking up at the slice of anatomy, or if you were on top looking down because you only see a very thin slice of anatomy which looks the same on the "bottom" side as the "top" side. What does matter is how, hypothetically, you are turned with respect to the body when you are looking up or looking down inside the body. The same rule will apply–always stand as if you were facing the patient with the patient's right to your left.

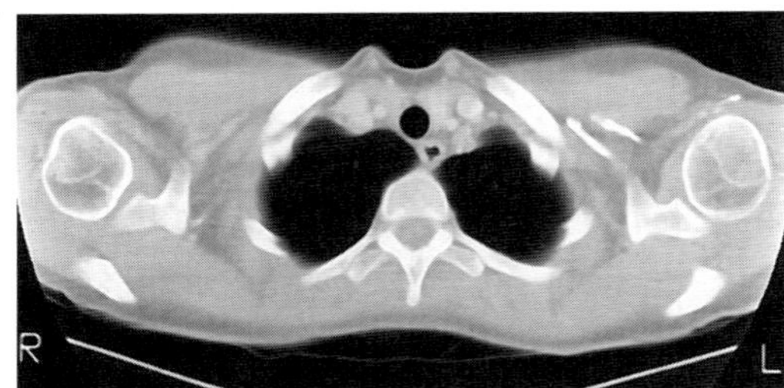

Fig. 1-165. Axial (cross-sectional) image (upper-thorax–Level of T3).

Coronal Images (Fig. 1-166)

Coronal images represent side-to-side sections or slices through the coronal (frontal) plane. Such images would be placed for viewing similarly to a conventional AP or PA radiograph, the patient's right to the viewer's left.

Sagittal Images (Fig. 1-167)

Sagittal images represent a front-to-back type section or slice through the sagittal plane. These can also be thought of as anteroposterior planes that are parallel to the midsagittal plane of the body. Therefore, a sagittal sectional image would be placed for viewing similarly to a conventional lateral projection radiograph.

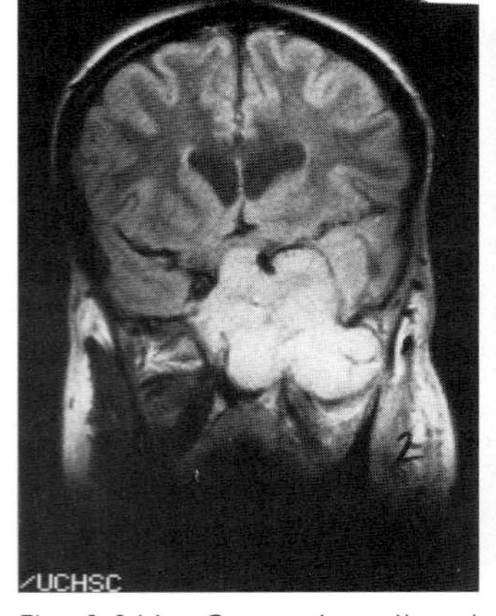

Fig. 1-166. Coronal sectional image (cranium).

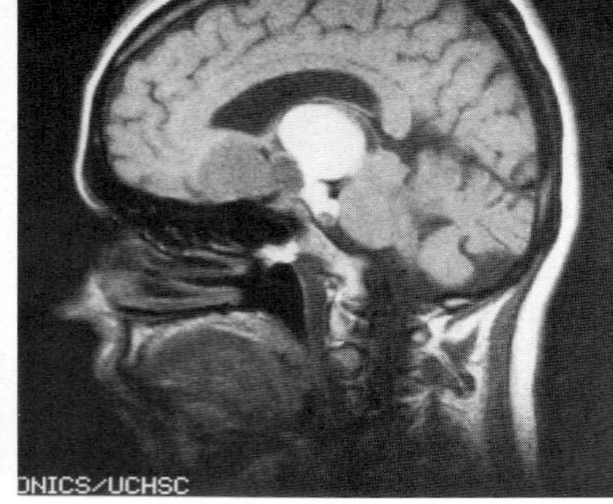

Fig. 1-167. Sagittal sectional image (cranium).

CHAPTER 2

Chest

CONTRIBUTIONS BY:
Karen Brown, RT (R)
Kathy Martensen, BS, RT (R)

CONTENTS

Radiographic Anatomy

Bony thorax **56**
Respiratory system **57**
Larynx **58**
Trachea **59**
Right and left bronchi **60**
Lungs **61**
Chest radiographs **62**
Mediastinum **63**

Radiographic Positioning

Body habitus and degrees of inspiration **64**
Positioning considerations **65**
Erect chest radiographs **66**
Evaluation criteria **67**
PA chest positioning **67**
Lateral chest positioning **68**
Central ray location and positioning method **69**
Lung dimensions and film holder placement **70**
Collimation guidelines **70**
Survey information **71**
Basic and special projections **71**
Chest (basic):
- PA **72**
- Lateral **74**

Chest (special):
- AP supine or semierect **76**
- Lateral decubitus **77**
- AP lordotic **78**
- Anterior oblique **79**
- Posterior oblique **80**

Upper airway (basic):
- Lateral **81**
- AP **82**

Appendix–CR location and printed ruler **83**
Radiographs for critique **84**

Radiographic Anatomy

Chest

Chest radiographic examinations are the most common of all radiographic procedures. It is common for student radiographers to begin their clinical experience taking chest radiographs. Before beginning such clinical experience, however, it is important to learn and understand chest anatomy well, including relative relationships of all anatomy within the chest cavity.

The **chest,** or **thorax,** is the upper part of the trunk between the neck and the abdomen. Radiographic anatomy of the chest is divided into three sections: the **bony thorax**, the **respiratory system proper**, and the **mediastinum**.

BONY THORAX

The **bony thorax** is that part of the skeletal system providing a protective framework for the parts of the chest involved with breathing and blood circulation. **Thoracic viscera** is the term used to describe these parts of the chest consisting of the lungs and the remaining thoracic organs contained in the mediastinum.

Anteriorly, the bony thorax consists of the **sternum** (breastbone), which is made up of three divisions. The superior portion is the **manubrium** *(mah-nu′ bre-um)*, the large center portion is the **body**, and the smaller inferior portion is the **xiphoid process**.

Superiorly, the bony thorax consists of the **two clavicles** (collarbones) connecting the sternum to the **two scapulae** (shoulder blades), the **twelve pairs of ribs** circling the bony thorax, and the **twelve thoracic vertebrae** posteriorly. A detailed description of all parts of the bony thorax is presented in Chapter 10.

Topographic Positioning Landmarks

Accurate and consistent radiographic positioning requires certain landmarks, or reference points, that one can use to center the film correctly to ensure that all essential anatomy is included on that specific projection. These topographic landmarks need to be parts of the body that are easily and consistently located on patients, such as parts of the bony thorax. For chest positioning two of these landmarks are the **vertebra prominens** and the **jugular notch**.

1. Vertebra Prominens (7th cervical vertebra)
This can be an important landmark for locating the central ray location on a PA chest projection. It can be readily palpated on most patients by applying light pressure with the finger tips at the base of the neck. The vertebra prominens is the first prominent process felt as you gently but firmly palpate down the back of the neck with the head dropped forward. With a little practice this landmark can be readily located on most patients, especially if the head and neck are flexed forward.

2. Jugular notch (manubrial or suprasternal notch)
The jugular notch is an important landmark for locating the central ray location on AP chest projections. This is easily palpated as a deep notch or depression on the superior portion of the sternum below the thyroid cartilage (commonly known as Adam's apple).

The mid thorax, at the level of T7 (7th thoracic vertebra), can easily be located from these two landmarks, as will be described later in this chapter.

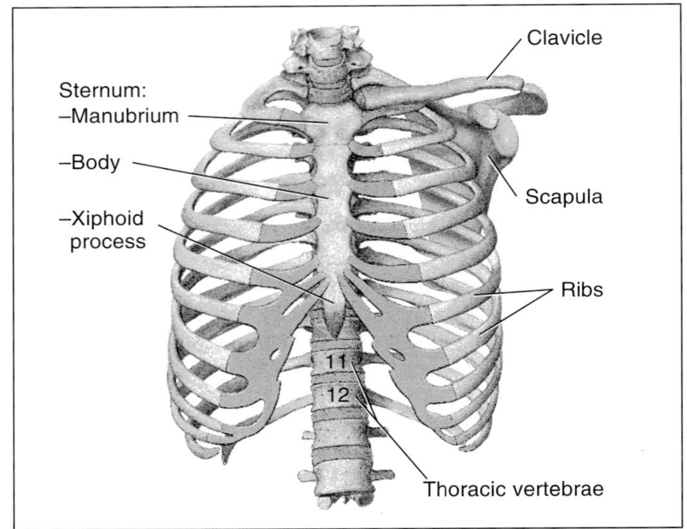

Fig. 2-1. Bony thorax.

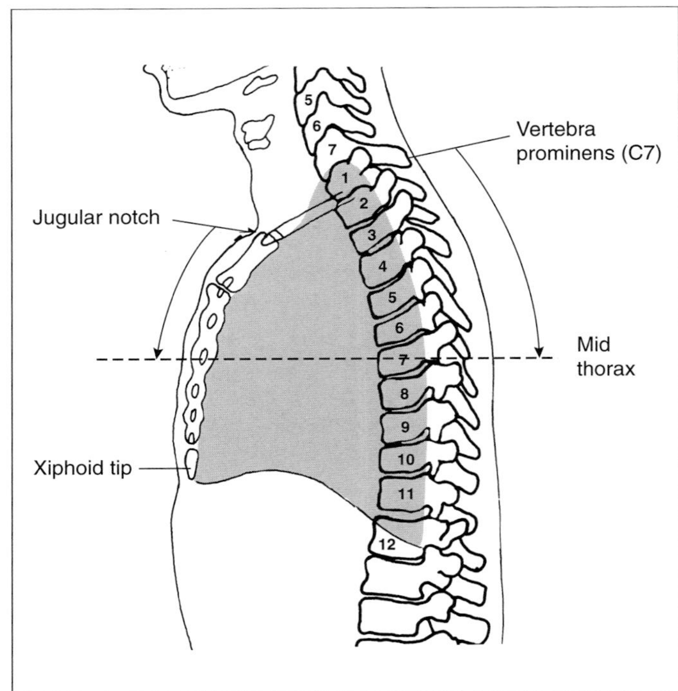

Fig. 2-2. Topographic landmarks.

Xiphoid tip: The inferior tip of the sternum, the **xiphoid tip**, which corresponds to the level of T9 or T10 (9th or 10th thoracic vertebra), can also be palpated. This corresponds to the approximate level of the anterior portion of the diaphragm, which separates the chest cavity from the abdominal cavity. However, this is not a reliable landmark for positioning the chest because of body habitus variations and the variable lower position of the posterior lungs, which may extend as far as T11 or T12 on inspiration, as shown in Fig. 2-2.

RESPIRATORY SYSTEM

Respiration is the exchange of gaseous substances between the air we breathe and the blood stream. This is brought about by the respiratory system, which consists of those parts of the body through which air passes as it travels from the nose and mouth into the lungs. Four general divisions of the respiratory system shown in Fig. 2-3 are the **pharynx**, **trachea**, **bronchi** and **lungs**.

An important structure of the respiratory system is the dome-shaped **diaphragm**, which is the chief muscle of inspiration. Each half of the diaphragm is termed a **hemidiaphragm** (hemi meaning half). As the dome of the diaphragm moves downward, it **increases** the volume of the thoracic cavity. This, along with certain other dimensional movements of the thorax described later in this chapter, **decreases** the intrathoracic pressure, creating a "sucking" action or negative pressure effect, resulting in air being drawn into the lungs through the nose and mouth, pharynx, larynx, trachea, and bronchi.

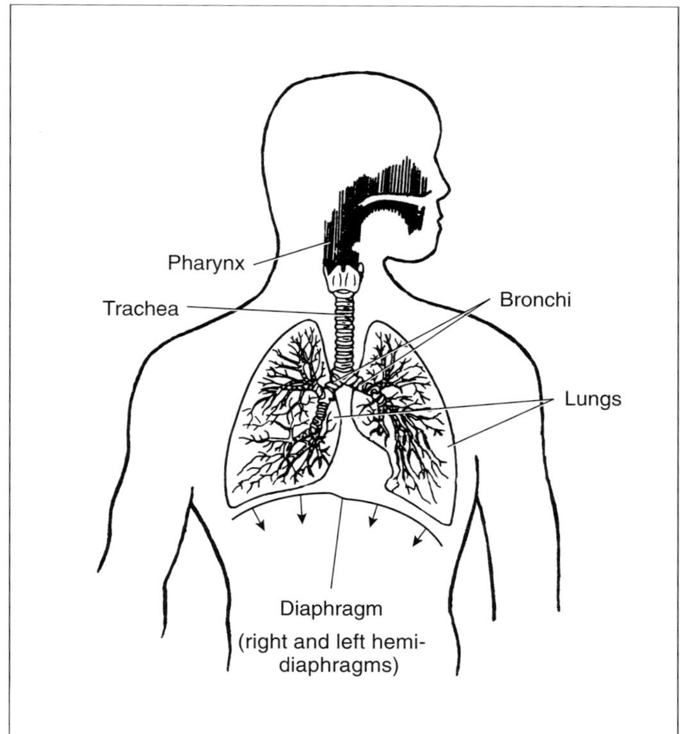

Fig. 2-3. Respiratory system.

Pharynx *(far′ inks)* (upper airway)

The **pharynx** is a structure or passageway important to the respiratory system because air must pass through it prior to entering the respiratory system proper, which begins with the larynx, or voice box. The pharynx, also referred to as the upper airway or the upper respiratory tract, is that posterior area between the nose and mouth above, and the larynx or voice box and the esophagus below. This is the area that serves as **a passageway for both food and fluids as well as air, thus making it common to both the digestive and respiratory systems**. For this reason it is **not** considered part of the respiratory system proper.

The pharynx has three divisions as shown in Fig. 2-4: the **nasopharynx** *(na″ zo-far′ inks)*, **oropharynx** *(o″ ro-far′ inks),* and **laryngopharynx** *(lah-ring″ go-far′ inks)*. The interior of the pharynx communicates posteriorly with certain cavities, the nose above (nasopharynx), the mouth (oropharynx), and the larynx below (laryngopharynx), as well as the esophagus. The **hard palate** and **soft palate** make up the roof of the oral cavity. The lower posterior aspect of the soft palate is called the **uvula** *(u′ vu-lah),* which marks the boundary between the nasopharynx and the oropharynx.

The laryngopharynx lies above and posterior to the larynx and extends from the upper border of the **epiglottis** *(ep″ i-glot′ is)* to where the laryngopharynx narrows to join the esophagus.

The freer upper portion of the epiglottis projects upward behind the tongue and acts as a lid for the slanted opening of the larynx. During the act of swallowing, the epiglottis flips down and covers the laryngeal opening, which prevents food and fluid from entering the larynx and bronchi.

Additional structures shown on this sectional lateral drawing are the **hyoid bone**, the **thyroid cartilage** of the larynx (Adam's Apple), the **thyroid gland**, and the **trachea**, which are described in more detail in the next section on the larynx or trachea.

Air Pathway: The dotted black lines indicate the pathway that air may take from the external environment to the trachea and eventually to the lungs. Note that air passing through either the nose or mouth must pass through at least some portion of the pharynx.

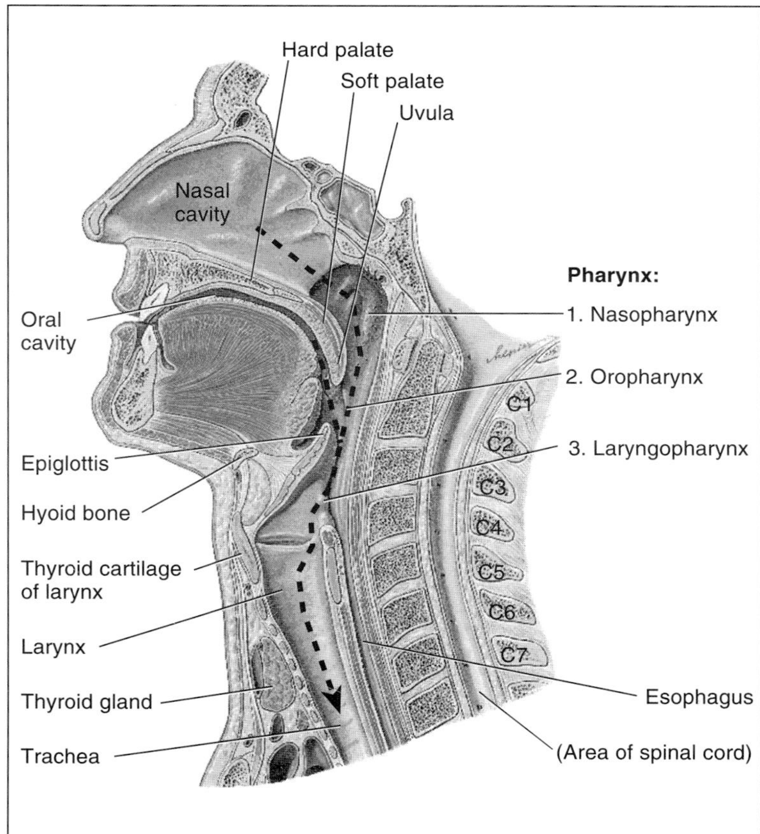

Fig. 2-4. Pharynx, upper airway (midsagittal section).

Esophagus

The **esophagus** is the part of the digestive system that connects the pharynx with the stomach. Note the relationship of the esophagus to both the pharynx and the larynx. It begins at the distal end of the laryngopharynx and continues downward to the stomach, **posterior to the larynx and trachea**. (Chapter 14 describes the esophagus in detail along with the upper digestive system.)

2

Four Parts of Respiratory System

The four parts of the respiratory system proper important in chest radiography are as follows:

1. **Larynx** *(lar′ inks)* (voice box)
2. **Trachea** *(tra′ ke-ah)*
3. **Right** and **left bronchi** *(bron′ chi)*
4. **Lungs**

The larynx, trachea and bronchi form a continuous, tubular structure through which air can pass from the nose and mouth into the lungs, as shown in Figs. 2-3 and 2-4 on the preceding page.

Note: Remember the pharynx serves as a passage for both air and food and thus is not considered part of the respiratory system proper.

1. Larynx (voice box)

The **larynx**, or voice box, is a cagelike, cartilaginous structure approximately 1½ to 2 inches (4 to 5 cm) in length in an adult. The larynx is in the anterior portion of the neck, suspended from a small bone called the **hyoid** (Fig. 2-5). The hyoid bone is found in the upper neck just below the tongue or floor of the mouth (Fig. 2-4). The hyoid bone is **not** part of the larynx.

The larynx serves as the organ of voice. Sounds are made as air passes between the **vocal cords** located within the larynx (Fig. 2-6). The upper margin of the larynx is at the approximate level of **C3**. Its lower margin, where the larynx junctions with the trachea, is at the level of **C6**.

The framework of the larynx consists of cartilages, connected by ligaments and moved by numerous muscles that assist in the complex sound-making or voice process. The largest and least mobile of these cartilages is the **thyroid cartilage**, which consists of two fused plate-like structures that form the anterior wall of the larynx. The prominent anterior projection of the thyroid cartilage is easily palpated and is known as the **laryngeal prominence**, or "Adam's apple." This prominent structure is an important positioning landmark because it is easy to locate. The laryngeal prominence of the thyroid cartilage located at approximately the level of **C5** is an excellent topographical reference for locating specific skeletal structures in this region.

The **cricoid** *(kri′ koid)* **cartilage** is a ring of cartilage forming the inferior and posterior wall of the larynx. It is attached to the first ring of cartilage of the trachea.

One of the cartilages making up the larynx is the uniquely-shaped **epiglottis**, which is shaped like a leaf with the narrow distal stem portion attached to a part of the thyroid cartilage. As described on the preceding page, the epiglottis flips down and covers the trachea during the act of swallowing (see arrows).

Axial (Cross-section) Image of Larynx: Due to the wide acceptance of CT (Computed Tomography) and MRI (Magnetic Resonance Imaging), it is important for the radiographer to recognize anatomical structures in cross section. Fig. 2-7 shows an axial (also called cross-sectional) view of the midportion of the larynx at the level of C5. Only major structures are labeled in this section. A more detailed study of the cross sectional anatomy of the chest is found in Chapter 23 on thoracic computed tomography.

Note: Conventional CT images such as seen here are commonly viewed as though one were facing the patient. Thus, the patient's right is to the viewer's left. This is the same way conventional radiographs are placed for viewing (see Chapter 1, page 54).

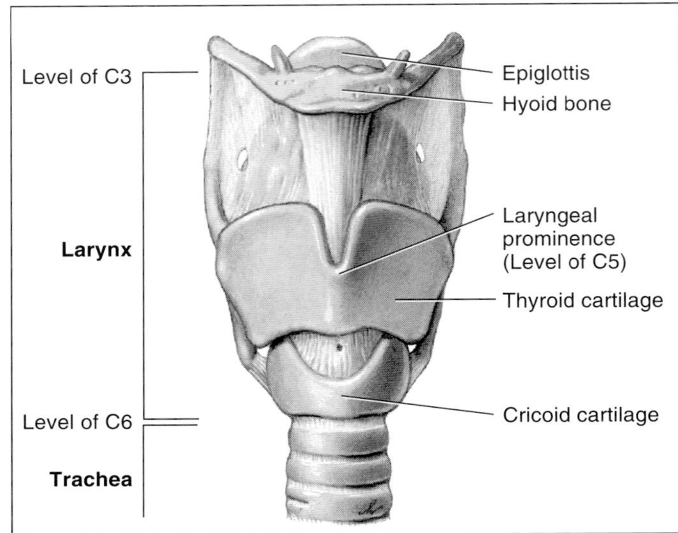

Fig. 2-5. Larynx (frontal view).

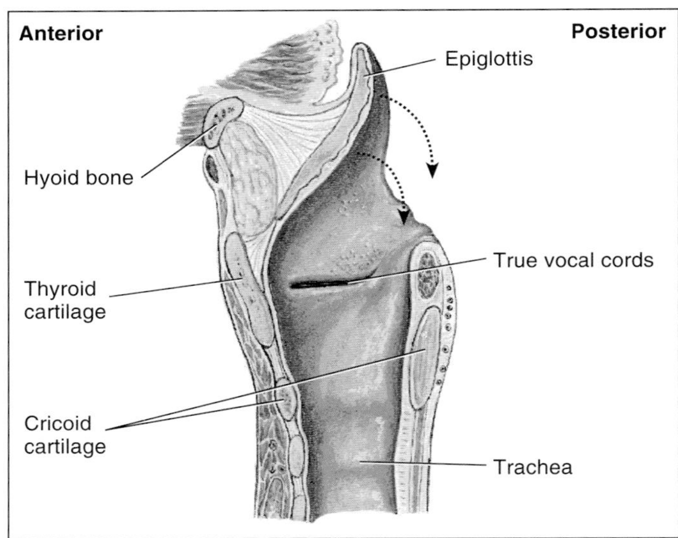

Fig. 2-6. Larynx (lateral view).

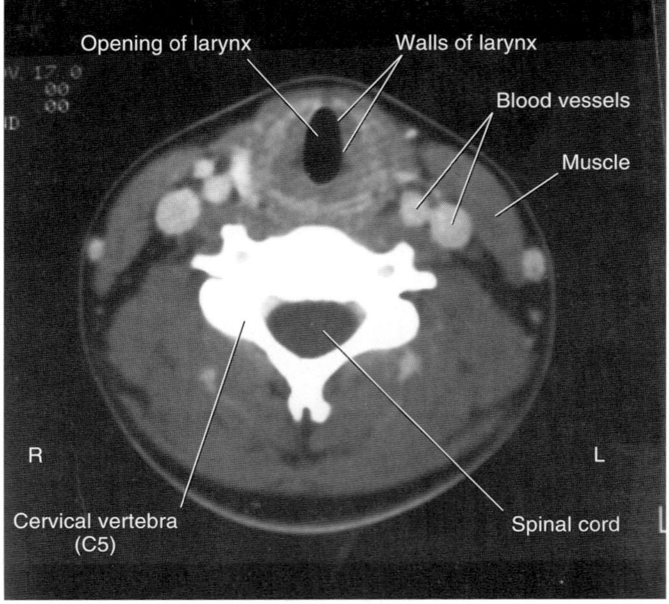

Fig. 2-7. CT image of neck through larynx–axial (cross) section at level of C5.

2. Trachea

Continuing from the larynx downward, the second division of the respiratory system proper is the **trachea**, or windpipe. It is a fibrous muscular tube about ¾ in. (2 cm) in diameter and 4½ in. (11 cm) long. Approximately 20 C-shaped rings of cartilage are embedded in its walls. These rigid rings keep the airway open by preventing the trachea from collapsing during inspiration.

The trachea, located just anterior to the esophagus, extends from its junction with the larynx at the level of **C6** (6th cervical vertebra) downward to the level of **T4** or **T5** (4th or 5th thoracic vertebra) where it divides into right and left primary bronchi.

Certain glands that need to be understood due to their location with respect to the respiratory system are the **thyroid**, **parathyroid**, and the **thymus glands**.

Thyroid Gland: The thyroid gland is a vascular organ located anteriorly in the neck region just below the larynx with its right and left lateral lobes lying on each side and distal to the proximal trachea (Fig. 2-8). In the adult it weighs 25 to 30 grams (almost one ounce) and has a very rich blood supply. As with other such glandular organs, the thyroid gland is more radiosensitive than many other body structures or organs. Therefore, knowing the relative size and location of this gland is important for radiographers to be able to reduce exposures to these regions as much as possible by shielding and by collimation of the x-ray beam.

One of the unique features of the thyroid gland is its ability to store certain hormones, then slowly release them to aid in the regulation of body metabolism. These hormones also help regulate body growth and development as well as activity of the nervous system, especially in children.

Parathyroid Glands: Parathyroid glands are small rounded glands embedded on the posterior surfaces of the lateral lobes of the thyroid gland. Usually there are two parathyroids attached to each lateral thyroid lobe as shown in Fig. 2-8. They store and secrete certain hormones that aid in specific blood functions, including blood calcium levels.

Thymus Gland: The thymus gland is located just distal to the thyroid gland and is demonstrated and described later in this chapter as part of mediastinal structures (Fig. 2-22).

Radiographs

The AP and lateral radiographs of the upper airway visualize the air-filled trachea and larynx. This AP radiograph (Fig. 2-9) demonstrates a column of air primarily in the upper trachea region as seen in the lower half of the radiograh (darkened area, see arrows). Certain enlargements or other abnormalities of the thymus or thyroid glands may be demonstrated on such radiographs, as well as pathology within the airway system itself.

The lateral radiograph (Fig. 2-10) demonstrates the air-filled trachea and larynx (A), the region of the esophagus (B), and shows the locations relative to each other. Note that the esophagus is located more posteriorly and the trachea anteriorly. The general locations of the thyroid gland (C) and the thymus gland (D) are also demonstrated.

Axial (Cross-section) Image of Trachea

Fig. 2-11 is a CT image through the upper chest at the approximate level of T3. Observe again that the trachea is located anteriorly to the esophagus, both of which are anterior to the thoracic vertebrae. The upper lungs are located to each side of the trachea and the thoracic vertebrae.

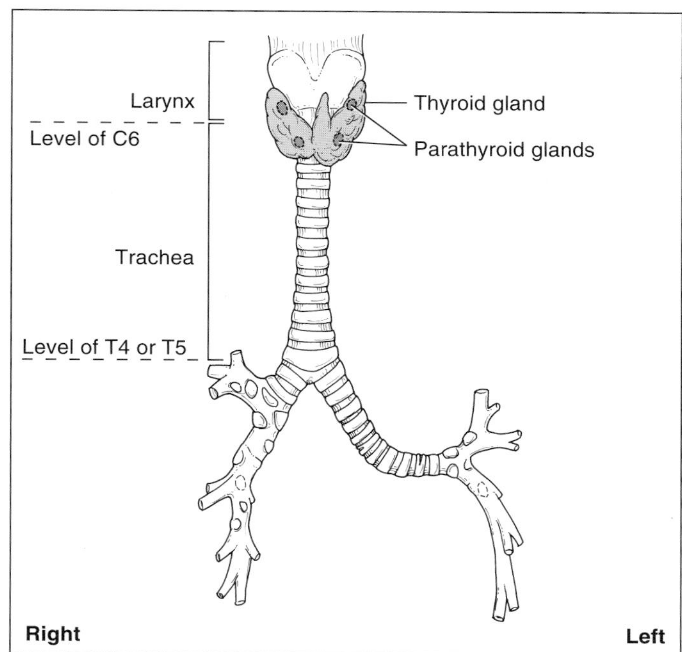

Fig. 2-8. Trachea.

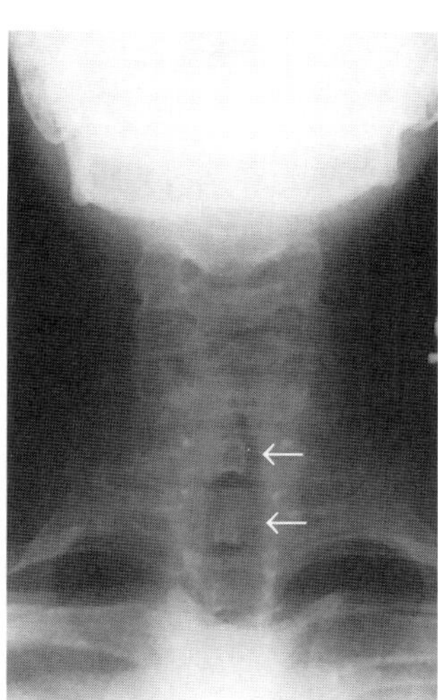

Fig. 2-9. AP upper airway.

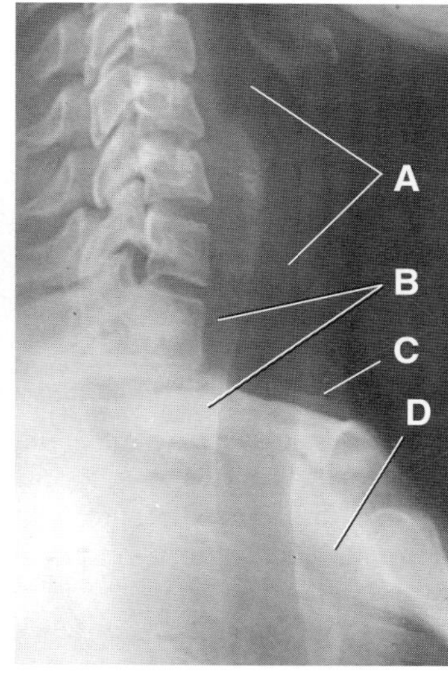

Fig. 2-10. Lateral upper airway.

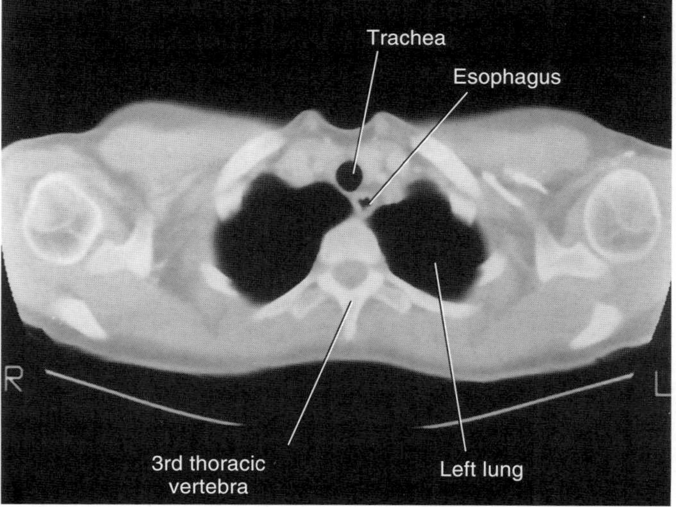

Fig. 2-11. Axial (cross) section at level of T3.

3. Right and Left Bronchi

The third part of the respiratory system consists of the **right** and **left primary bronchi,** also known as the right and left primary or main stem bronchi.

The **right primary bronchus** is **wider** and **shorter** than the left bronchus. The right primary bronchus is also more vertical; therefore the angle of divergence from the distal trachea is less abrupt for the right bronchus than for the left. This **difference in size and shape** between the two primary bronchi is important because food particles or other foreign objects that happen to enter the respiratory system are more likely to enter and lodge in the **right** bronchus.

The **right bronchus** is about 1 in. or 2.5 cm long and 1.3 cm in diameter. The angle of divergence of the right bronchus is only about 25°.

The **left bronchus** is smaller in diameter (1.1 cm) than the right, but about twice as long (2 in. or 5 cm). The divergent angle of the left bronchus is approximately 37°. This increased angle and the smaller diameter make food particles or other foreign matter **less** likely to enter the left bronchus compared with the right.

The **carina** *(kah-ri′nah)* is a specific prominence, or ridge, of the lowest tracheal cartilage as seen at the bottom and inside portion of the trachea, where it divides into right and left bronchi. As viewed from above through a bronchoscope, the carina is to the left of the midline, and the right bronchus appears more open than the left, which clearly demonstrates why particles coming down the trachea are more likely to enter the right bronchus.

The position of the carina, as shown in Fig. 2-12, is at the lower level of the division into the right and left primary bronchi. This is at the approximate level of T5 and is used as a specific reference point or level for computed tomography (CT) of the thorax, as described in Chapter 23.

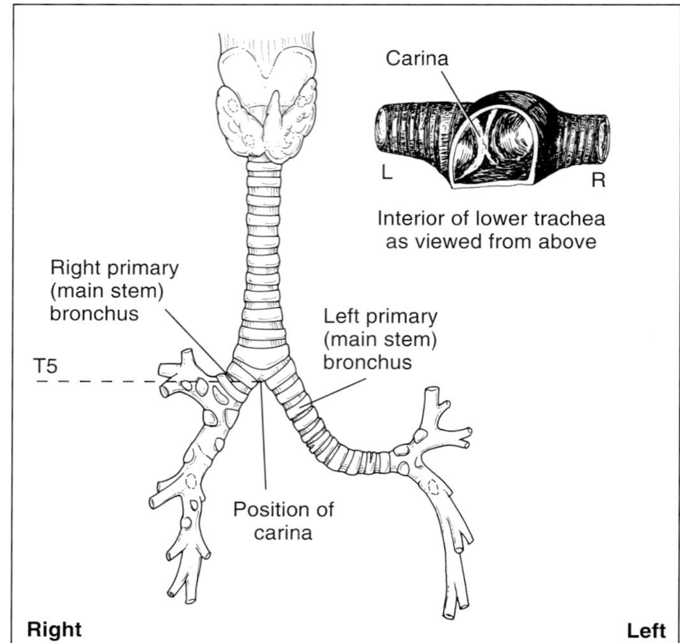

Fig. 2-12. Bronchi.

Secondary Bronchi, Lobes and Alveoli

In addition to the difference in size and shape between the right and left bronchi, another important difference is that the **right** bronchus divides into **three** secondary bronchi, but the **left** divides into only **two** with each entering individual lobes of the lungs. Thus the **right lung** contains **three lobes** and the **left** contains **two lobes**, as demonstrated in both Figs. 2-12 and 2-13. These secondary bronchi continue to subdivide into smaller branches, termed **bronchioles**, that spread to all parts of each lobe.

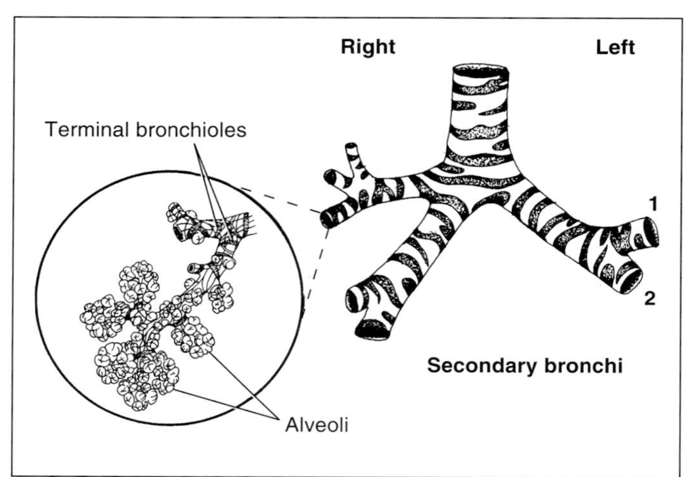

Fig. 2-13. Secondary bronchi and alveoli.

Each of these small **terminal bronchioles** terminates in very small air sacs or air spaces called **alveoli**. There are from 500 to 700 million alveoli within the two lungs. It is here that oxygen and carbon dioxide are exchanged in the blood through the thin walls of the alveoli.

Axial (Cross-section) Image of Bronchi and Lungs

Fig. 2-14 represents an axial (cross-sectional) image through the right and left primary or main stem bronchi at the approximate level of T7. This section is just below the termination of the trachea; thus the trachea is not shown, but the air-filled right and left bronchi are visualized.

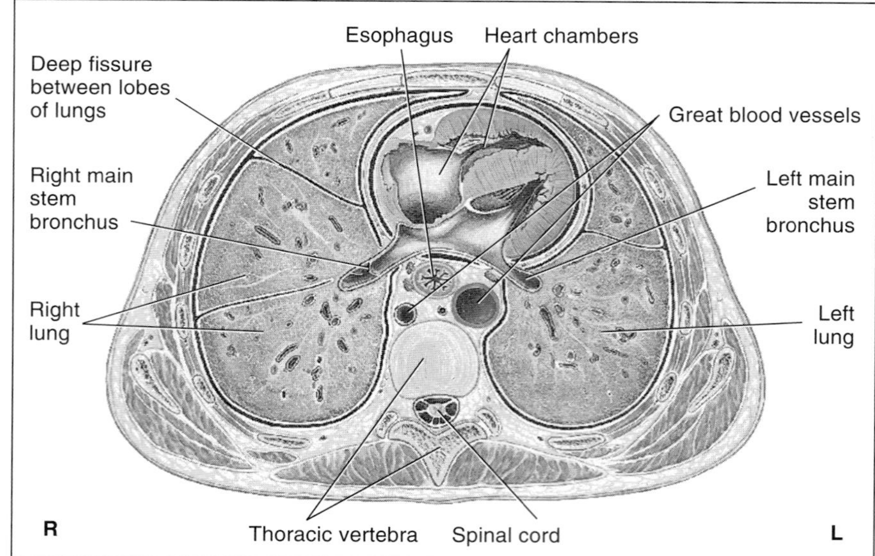

Fig. 2-14. Axial (cross-sectional) image of lungs and heart, level of T7.

4. Lungs

The fourth and last division of the respiratory system is made up of the two large, spongy **lungs**, located on each side of the thoracic cavity. The lungs fill all of the space not occupied by other structures. It is important to remember that the right lung is made up of **three** lobes, the **superior** (upper), **middle**, and **inferior** (lower) lobes, divided by **two deep fissures**. The left lung has only **two** lobes, the **superior** (upper) and **inferior** (lower) separated by a **single deep oblique fissure**.

The lungs are made up of a light spongy but highly elastic substance called **parenchyma** (*pah-reng′ ki-mah*). This allows for the breathing mechanism responsible for expansion and contraction of the lungs, which brings oxygen in and removes the carbon dioxide from the blood through the thin walls of the alveoli.

Each lung is contained in a delicate double-walled sac, or membrane, called the **pleura,** visualized in both the frontal view drawing (Fig. 2-15), and the cross-sectional drawing (Fig. 2-16). The outer layer of this pleural sac lines the inner surface of the chest wall and diaphragm and is called the **parietal pleura**. The inner layer covering the surface of the lungs, including dipping into the fissures between the lobes, is called the **pulmonary** or **visceral pleura** (Fig. 2-16).

The potential space between the double-walled pleura is called the **pleural cavity**, which contains a lubricating fluid allowing movement of one on the other during breathing. When a lung collapses or when air or fluid collects between these two layers, then this space may be visualized radiographically. Air or gas present in this pleural cavity results in a condition called a **pneumothorax,** wherein the air or gas pressure in the pleural cavity may cause the lung to collapse. Accumulation of fluid in the pleural cavity (pleural effusion) creates a condition called a **hemothorax**. Inflammation of the double-walled pleura membrane is called **pleurisy**, which causes friction and severe pain during breathing.

Pulmonary emphysema (which can be caused by smoking) is a pathological condition of the lungs characterized by **increased dimensions** of the lungs beyond normal. The terminal bronchioles become dilated and lose their effectiveness, and breathing becomes labored and difficult. Due to the increased air accumulation, **kVp and/or mAs must be decreased** to prevent overexposed or dark chest radiographs.

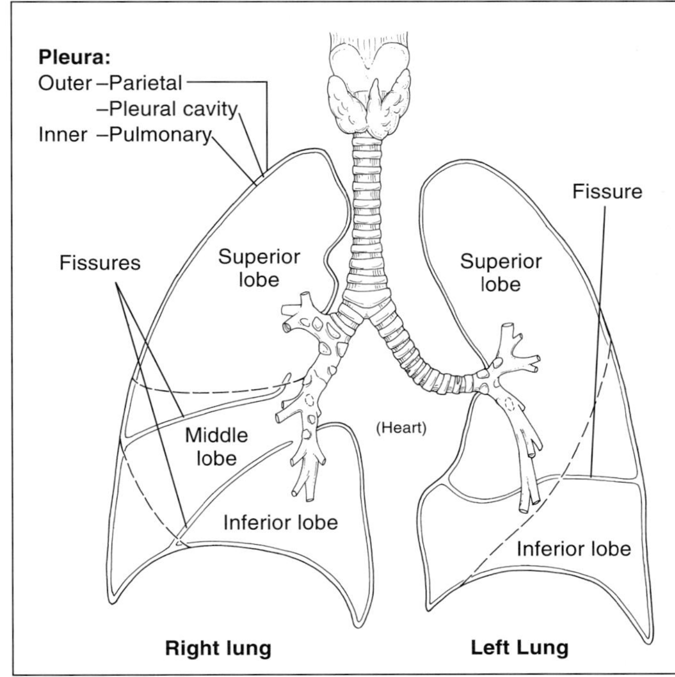

Fig. 2-15. Lungs.

Cross Section of Lungs and Heart

The drawing in Fig. 2-16 demonstrates a cross-sectional view through the lower third of the mediastinum and lungs. Clearly demonstrated is the double-walled membrane, the **pleura,** which completely encloses the lungs, including around the heart. The outer membrane, the **parietal pleura,** and the inner membrane, the **pulmonary** (or **visceral) pleura,** are clearly visible, as is the potential space between them, the **pleural cavity**.

The double-walled **pericardial sac**, which surrounds the heart, is also identified. This drawing demonstrates the relationship of the pericardial sac surrounding the heart with the pleural sac surrounding the lungs. The pleural and pericardial spaces or cavities are exaggerated on this drawing to better demonstrate these parts. Normally there is no space between the double walls of the pericardial sac or between the parietal and visceral pleura unless pathology is present.

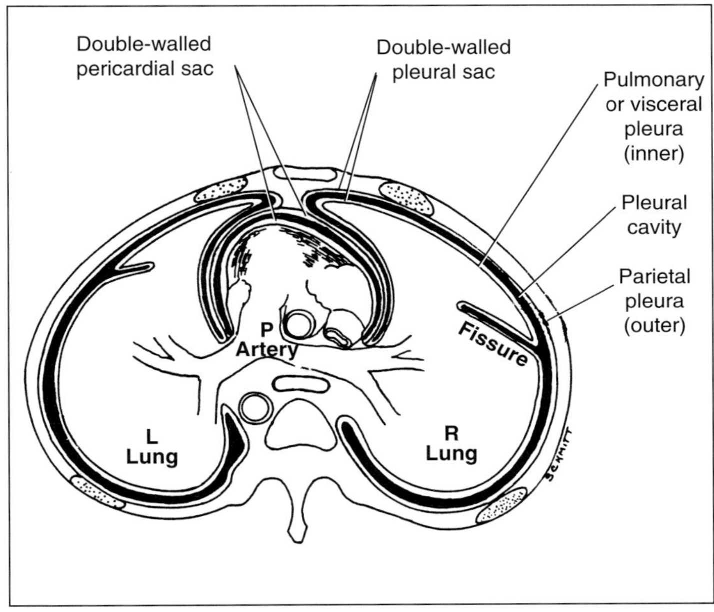

Fig. 2-16. Cross section of lower mediastinum and lungs.

CT Cross Sectional Image

The CT image in Fig. 2-17 at the level of T9 shows the relationship and relative size of the heart, descending aorta, and lungs. The heart is located slightly more to the **left** as can also be seen on a PA chest radiograph. The heart is shown to be located in the very **anterior** portion of the chest cavity directly behind the sternum. The esophagus is directly posterior to the heart, with the descending aorta between the esophagus and the thoracic vertebrae.

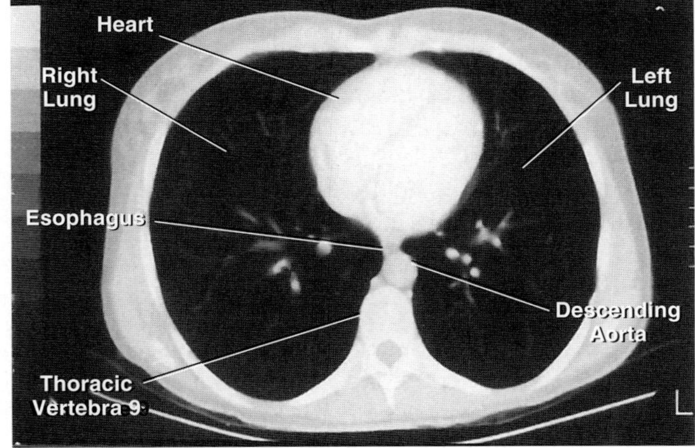

Fig. 2-17. CT image of lower thorax (level of T9).

PA Chest Radiograph

Enormous amounts of medical information can be obtained from a properly exposed and carefully positioned PA chest radiograph. Although the technical factors are designed to optimally visualize the lungs and other soft tissues, the bony thorax can also be seen. The clavicles, scapulae and ribs can be identified by carefully studying the chest radiograph in Fig. 2-18. The sternum and thoracic vertebrae are superimposed along with mediastinal structures, such as the heart and great vessels; therefore, the sternum and vertebrae are not well visualized on a PA chest radiograph.

The lungs and trachea (A, enhanced by a dotted outline) of the respiratory system are well shown, although usually the bronchi are not easily seen. The first portion of the respiratory system, the larynx, is usually above the top border of the radiograph and cannot be seen. The heart, the large blood vessels and the diaphragm are also well visualized.

The labeled parts on the radiograph are also demonstrated in Fig. 2-19, a frontal view of the thorax with the bony structures removed. The thyroid gland, large blood vessels and the thymus gland are also demonstrated in their relationship to the lungs and heart.

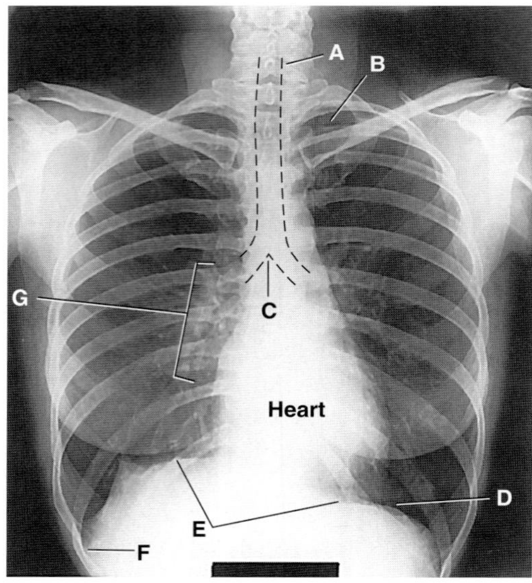

Fig. 2-18. PA chest radiograph.

Parts of Lungs

Parts of the lungs that are important radiographically are as follows:

The **apex** (B) of each lung is that **rounded upper area above the level of the clavicles**. As can be seen in Fig. 2-18, the apices of the lungs extend well up into the lower neck area to the level of T1 (first thoracic vertebra). This important part of the lungs must be included on chest radiographs.

The **carina** (C) is shown as the lowest margin of the separation of the trachea into the right and left bronchi.

The **base** (D) of each lung is the lower concave area of each lung that rests on the **diaphragm** (F). The diaphragm is a muscular partition separating the thoracic and abdominal cavities.

The **costophrenic angle** (E) refers to the extreme outermost lower corner of each lung where the diaphragm meets the ribs. In positioning for chest radiographs, it is important to know the relative locations of the uppermost and lowermost parts of the lungs, namely the apices and the costophrenic angles respectively, to ensure that these regions are included on every chest radiograph. Pathology, such as a small amount of fluid collection, would be evident at these costophrenic angles in the erect position.

The **hilum** (hilus) (G) , also known as the **root** region, is the central area of each lung where the bronchi, blood vessels, lymph vessels and nerves enter and leave the lungs.

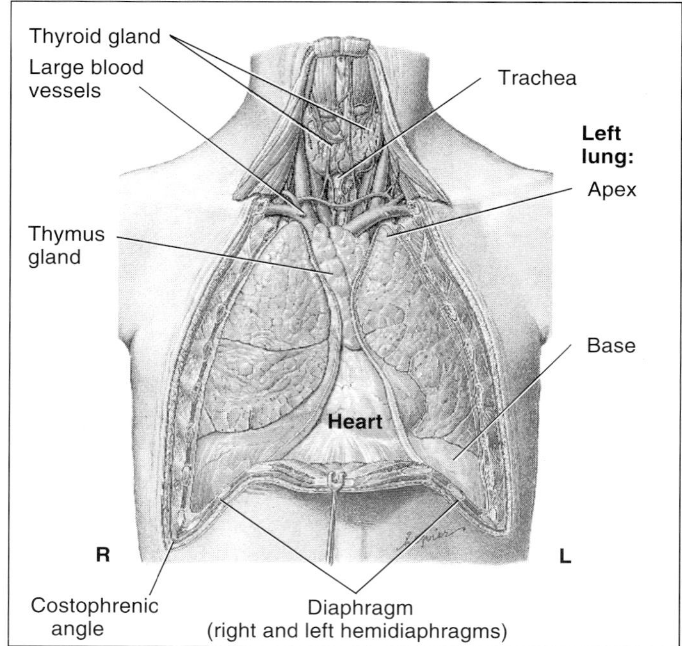

Fig. 2-19. Lungs.

Lateral Chest View

The lateral chest radiograph (Fig. 2-20) is marked to demonstrate the same parts as labeled in the adjoining drawing (Fig. 2-21). This drawing shows the left lung as seen from the medial aspect. Since this is the left lung, only two lobes are seen. Note that some of the **lower lobe** extends above the level of the **hilum** posteriorly, while some of the **upper lobe** extends below the hilum anteriorly. The posterior part of the **diaphragm** is the most inferior part of the diaphragm. The single deep **oblique fissure** dividing the two lobes of the left lung is again shown, as is the end-on view of a bronchus.

It is of significance, radiographically, to know that the right lung is usually about 1 inch shorter than the left lung. The reason for this difference is the large space-occupying liver located in the right upper abdomen, which pushes up on the **right hemidiaphragm**. The right and left hemidiaphragms (F) are seen on the lateral chest radiograph in Fig. 2-20. The more superior of the two is the right hemidiaphragm, as also seen on the PA chest radiograph (Fig. 2-18).

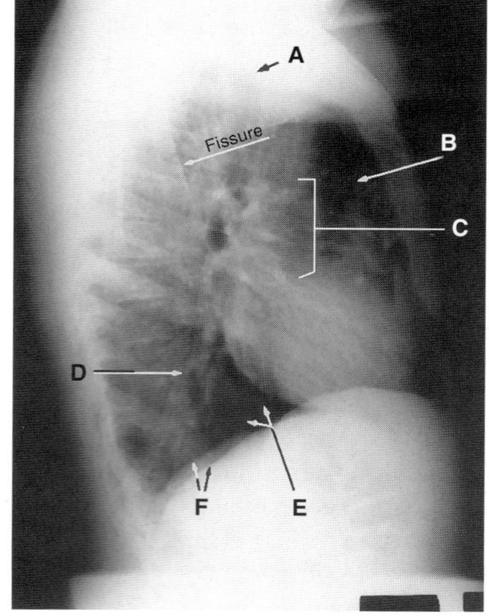

Fig. 2-20. Lateral chest radiograph.

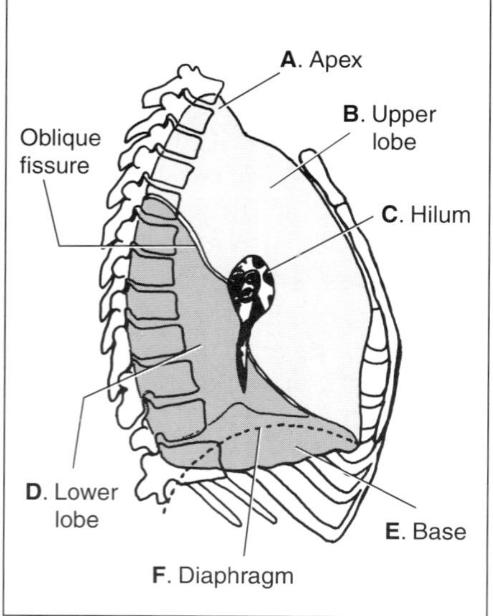

Fig. 2-21. Medial left lung.

MEDIASTINUM

The medial portion of the thoracic cavity between the lungs is called the **mediastinum**. The thyroid and parathyroid glands as described earlier in this chapter are **not** considered mediastinal structures because they are located more superiorly and are not within the mediastinum. The thymus gland, however, is located within the mediastinum, inferior to the thyroid gland and anterior to the trachea and esophagus (Fig. 2-22).

Four radiographically important structures located in the mediastinum are: the (1) **thymus gland,** the (2) **heart and great vessels**, the (3) **trachea**, and the (4) **esophagus**.

1. Thymus Gland

The thymus gland, located behind the upper sternum, is said to be a temporary organ because it is very prominent in an infant and reaches its maximum size of about 40 grams at puberty, then gradually decreases until it almost disappears in the adult. At its maximum size it would appear much larger than shown in Fig. 2-22. It may be visualized on chest radiographs of children but generally not for adults because the denser lymphatic tissue has been replaced by less dense fat. At its maximum development, the thymus gland lies above and anterior to the heart and pericardium.

The thymus gland functions primarily during childhood and puberty to aid with the functioning of certain body immune systems that help the body in its resistance to diseases. It is believed to contribute to the ability of the body to produce antibodies, which serve in rejecting foreign tissue and cells.

2. Heart and Great Vessels

The heart and the roots of the great vessels are enclosed in a double-walled sac called the pericardial sac, as demonstrated in an earlier drawing (Fig. 2-16). The heart is located posterior to the body of the sternum, and anterior to the 5th to 8th thoracic vertebrae. It lies obliquely in the mediastinal space, and approximately two thirds of the heart lies to the left of the median plane.

The **great vessels** in the mediastinum are the inferior and superior vena cava, aorta, and large pulmonary arteries and veins. The **superior vena cava** is a large vein that returns blood to the heart from the upper half of the body (Fig. 2-22). The **inferior vena cava** is a large vein returning blood from the lower half of the body.

The **aorta** is the largest artery in the body (≈1 in. or 2 to 5 cm in diameter in an average adult). It carries blood to all parts of the body through its various branches. The aorta is divided into three parts: the **ascending aorta**, coming up out of the heart, the **arch of the aorta**, and the **descending aorta**, which passes through the diaphragm into the abdomen where it becomes the abdominal aorta.

Various **pulmonary arteries and veins** that are present in the mediastinum are shown in Figs. 2-23 and 2-24. These supply blood and return blood to and from all segments of the lungs. The arterial network surrounds the small air sacs or alveoli, where oxygen and carbon dioxide are exchanged with the blood.

See Chapter 24 for more complete drawings of the heart and great vessels as part of the total body circulatory system including total body drawings of major arteries and veins.

3 & 4. Trachea and Esophagus

The trachea, within the mediastinum, separates into the right and left primary and secondary bronchi, as shown in Fig. 2-23.

The proximal esophagus is located posterior to the trachea and continues down through the mediastinum **anterior to the descending aorta** until it passes through the diaphragm into the stomach.

Note also in Fig. 2-24 that the heart is located in the very **anterior** aspect of the thoracic cavity, directly behind the sternum.

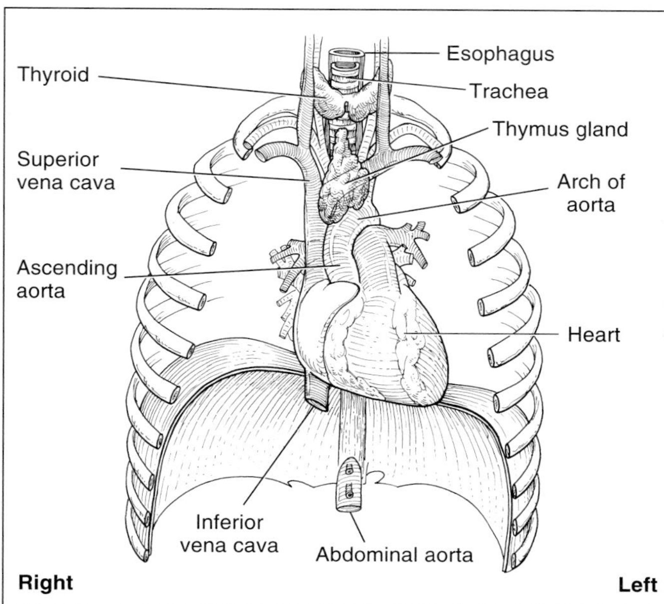

Fig. 2-22. Structures within mediastinum (anterior view).

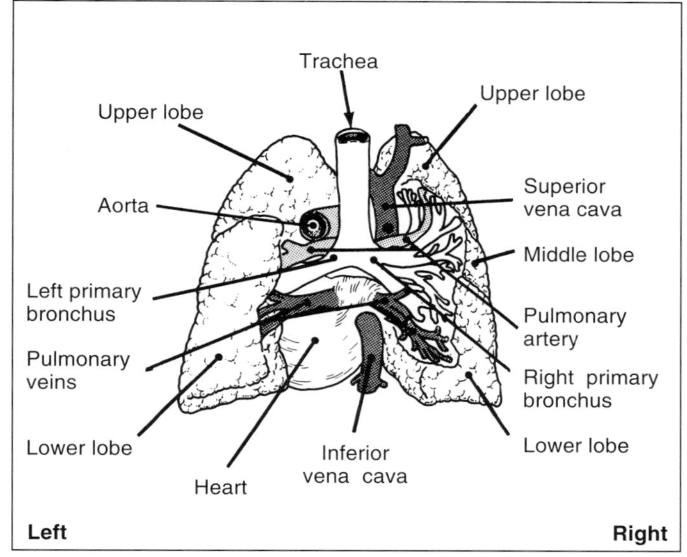

Fig. 2-23. Lungs and structure within mediastinum (posterior view).

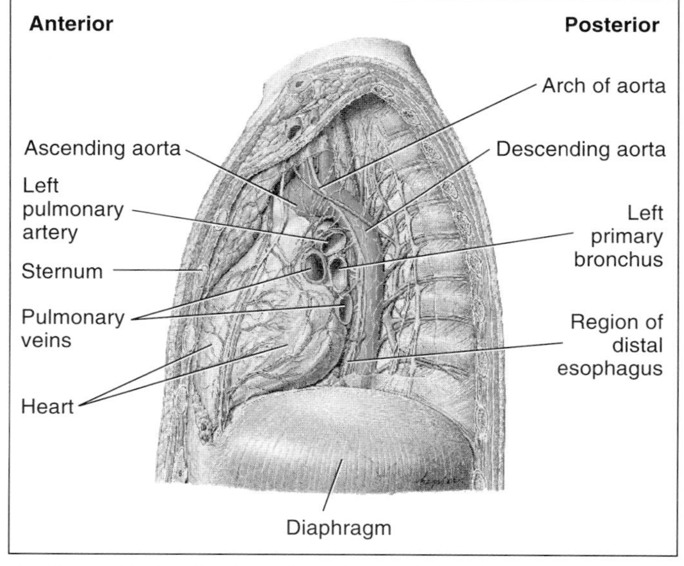

Fig. 2-24. Mediastinal relationships on left side with lung removed.

Radiographic Positioning

Body Habitus

Body habitus requires special consideration in chest radiography. For example, the massively built **hypersthenic** has a thorax that is very **broad** and very **deep** from front to back, but is **shallow** in vertical dimension as shown with the PA radiograph in Fig. 2-26. Therefore, care must be taken that the sides or the costophrenic angles are not cut off on a PA chest, which must be taken with the film placed crosswise. Careful centering is also required on the lateral projection to ensure that the anterior or posterior margins are included on the film.

The other extreme is the slender **asthenic**. This thorax is **narrow** in width and **shallow** from front to back, but is very **long** in its vertical dimension. Therefore, in positioning for such a chest, one must ensure that the film is long enough to include both the upper apex areas, which extend well above the clavicles, as well as the lower costophrenic angles. A nearer average **hyposthenic** type chest PA radiograph is shown in Fig. 2-27. Care in vertical collimation for such patients must also be exercised so that the costophrenic angles are not cut off on the lower margin.

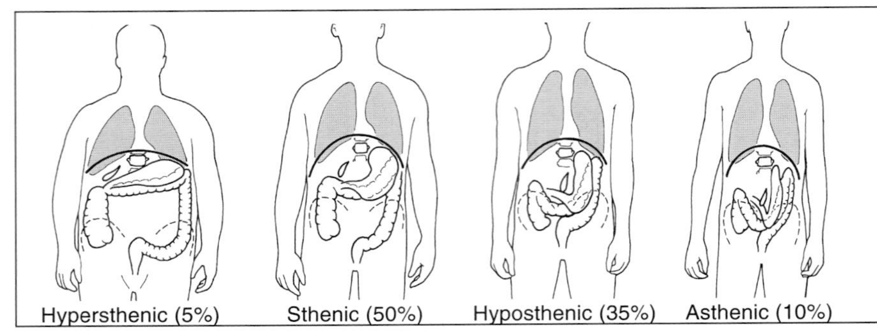

Fig. 2-25. Body habitus.

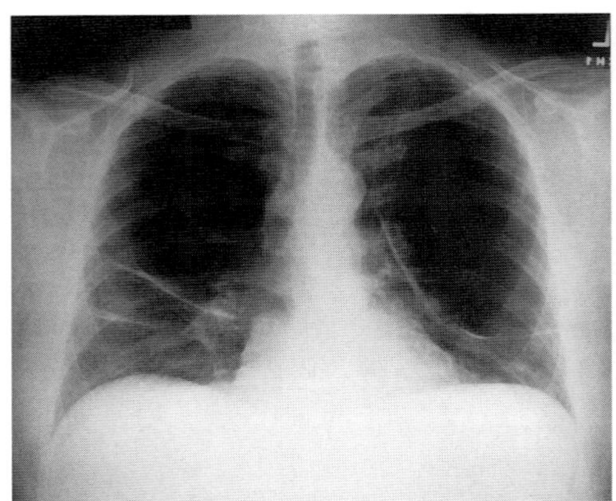

Fig. 2-26. PA (hypersthenic).

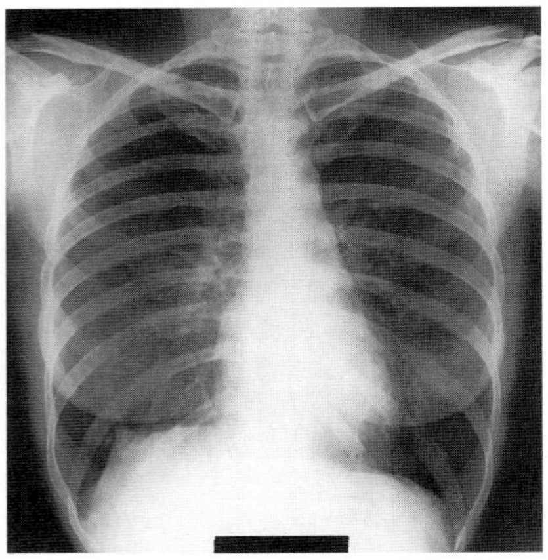

Fig. 2-27. PA (hyposthenic).

Breathing Movements

Movements of the bony thorax during inspiration (taking air in) and expiration (expelling air) greatly change the dimensions of the thorax, and thus the thoracic volume. To increase the volume of the chest during inspiration, the thoracic cavity increases in diameter in **three dimensions**.

The first of these is the **vertical diameter**, which is increased primarily by the diaphragm contracting and moving downward, thereby increasing the thoracic volume.

The **transverse diameter** is the second dimension increased during inspiration. The ribs swing outward and upward, which increases the transverse diameter of the thorax.

The third dimension to be increased is the **anteroposterior diameter**, also increased during inspiration by the raising of the ribs, especially the second through the sixth ribs. During expiration the elastic recoil of the lungs, along with the weight of the thoracic walls, causes the three diameters of the thorax to return to normal.

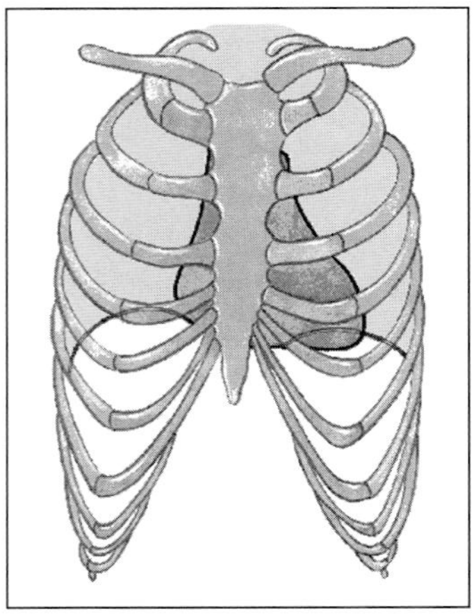

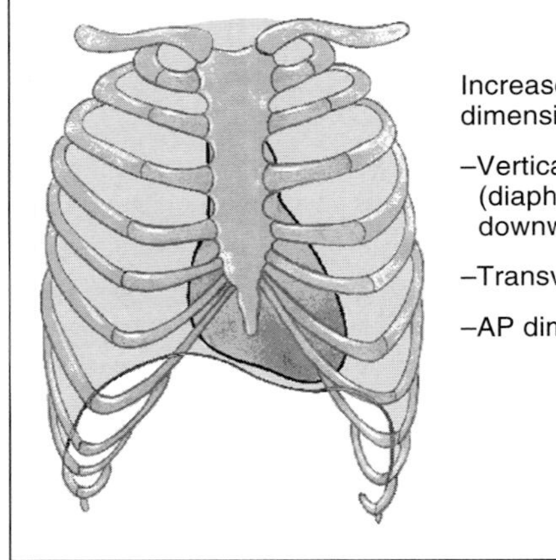

Fig. 2-28. Expiration.

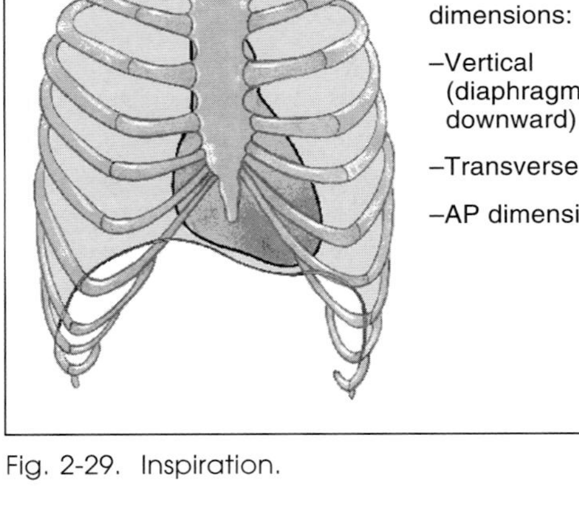

Fig. 2-29. Inspiration.

Degree of Inspiration

To determine the degree of inspiration in chest radiography, one should be able to identify and count the rib pairs on a chest radiograph. The first and second pairs are the most difficult to locate. When a chest radiograph is taken, it is important that the patient take as deep a breath as possible and then hold it to fully aerate the lungs.

The best way to determine the degree of inspiration is to observe how far down the diaphragm has moved by counting the pairs of ribs in the lung area above the diaphragm. A general rule for average adult patients is to "show" a **minimum of ten or eleven ribs** on a good PA chest radiograph. To determine this, start at the top with rib number one and count down to the tenth or eleventh rib posteriorly. The posterior part of each rib, where it joins a thoracic vertebra, is the most superior part of the rib. The diaphragm should always be checked to see that it is below the level of at least the tenth rib, as shown on the radiograph in Fig. 2-30. In this example, eleven posterior ribs are shown, which is expected on most healthy patients.

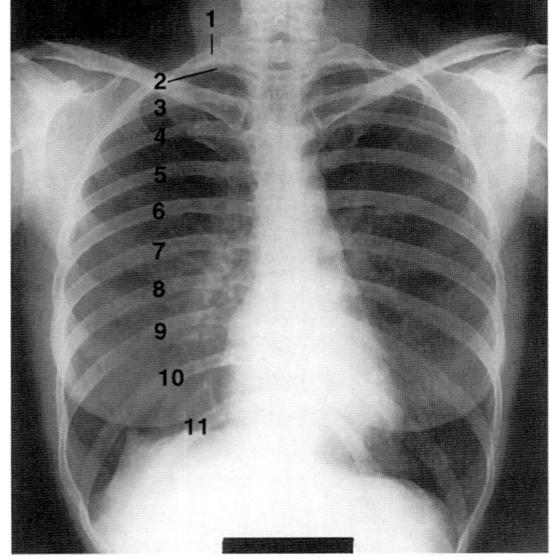

Fig. 2-30. Posterior ribs.

POSITIONING CONSIDERATIONS

Patient preparation for chest radiography includes the removal of all opaque objects from the chest and neck regions, including clothes with buttons, snaps, hooks or any objects that would be visualized on the radiograph as a shadow. To ensure that all such objects are removed from the chest region, the usual procedure is to ask the patient to remove all clothing, including bras, along with necklaces or other objects around the neck. The patient then puts on a hospital gown, which commonly has the opening in the back.

Long hair braided or tied together in bunches with rubber bands or other fasteners may cause suspicious shadows on the radiograph if it is left superimposing the chest area. Oxygen lines or pacemaker wires should be carefully moved to the side of the chest if possible.

Radiation Protection

Patients should be protected from unnecessary radiation for all diagnostic radiographic examinations. This is especially true for chest radiography because these are the most common of all radiographic examinations and are done repeatedly on persons throughout their lifetimes.

Repeat Exposures: Even though chest radiographic exams are often considered the simplest of all radiographic procedures, they also are the exam with the highest number of repeats in many radiology departments. Therefore, it is important to minimize unnecessary radiation exposure from repeat exposures by taking extra care in positioning and CR centering, and in the selection of correct exposure factors if AEC systems are not used. It is also important to reduce patient dose as much as possible through the use of correct radiation protection practices by way of close collimation and gonadal shielding.

Collimation: Careful collimation is important in chest radiography. Restricting the primary x-ray beam by collimation not only reduces patient dose by reducing the volume of tissue irradiated, but also reduces patient exposure by the accompanying reduction in scatter radiation.

Utilizing the collimation guidelines as described on the following positioning pages will allow for consistent optimum chest collimation.

Gonadal Shielding: In addition to careful collimation, a leaded gonadal shield should be used for the abdominal area below the lungs. This is especially important for children, pregnant women and for all those of childbearing age. A minimal rule is that **gonadal shielding should be used on all patients of reproductive age.** Many departments, however, have a general policy of gonadal shielding for all patients in chest radiography.

A common type of gonadal shield for chest radiography is some type of freestanding, adjustable mobile shield placed between the patient and the x-ray tube. A vinyl-covered lead shield that ties around the waist can also be used. Both of these types of shields should provide shielding from the level of the iliac crests or slightly higher, to the mid thigh area.

Back Scatter Protection: To protect the gonads from scatter and secondary radiation from the chest film holder device and the wall behind it, some references suggest a freestanding shield or a wraparound shield also be placed **between the patient and the chest board and wall.**

Technical Factors

Kilovoltage (kVp): Generally, kVp should be high enough to result in sufficient contrast to demonstrate the many shades of gray needed to visualize the finer lung markings. Thus, in general, chest radiography uses **low contrast**, described as a **long-scale contrast** with more shades of gray. This requires high kVp of 100 to 130.

Lower kVp, yielding high contrast, will not provide sufficient penetration to visualize well the fine lung markings in the areas behind the heart and at the lung bases. Too high contrast is evident when the heart and other mediastinal structures appear underexposed, even though the lung fields are sufficiently penetrated.

Patients with less dense, expanded lungs, such as with emphysema or hyperexpanded lungs, will require a decrease in kVp or other exposure factors.

As a general rule, in chest radiography, the use of high kVp (above 100) requires the use of grids. Either moving grids or fine-line focused fixed grids can be used.

Exceptions to this are some portable chests taken with equipment that is limited to 80-90 kVp, where screens may be used rather than grids.

Exposure Time and Milliamperage (mAs–milliampere seconds): Generally, chest radiography requires the use of high mA and short exposure times to minimize the chance of motion and resultant loss of sharpness.

Sufficient mAs should be used to provide for optimum density of lungs and mediastinal structures. A determining factor for this on PA chest radiographs is to be able to **see faint outlines of at least the mid and upper vertebrae and posterior ribs through the heart and other mediastinal structure shadows.**

Placement of Film Markers: Throughout the positioning sections of this text, the correct or best placement of patient ID information and film markers is indicated. The top portion of each positioning page includes a box drawing demonstrating the correct film holder size and placement (lengthwise or crosswise), and indicates the best location for patient ID blocker, as well as the location and type of film marker used for that specific projection or position. The use of a grid or screen film holder is indicated along with a suggested kVp range.

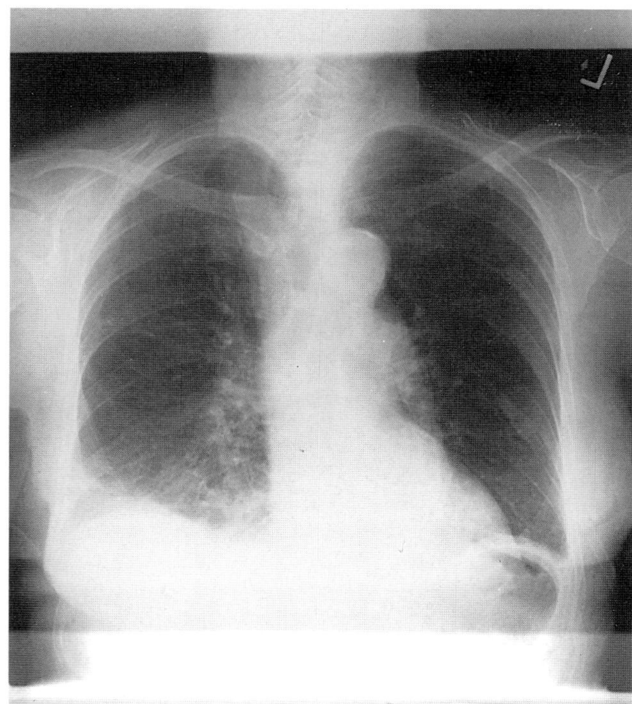

Fig. 2-31. PA chest (with correct collimation, exposure and film markers).

BREATHING INSTRUCTIONS

Breathing instructions are very important in chest radiography because any chest or lung movement occurring during the exposure will result in "blurring" of the radiographic image. It is also imperative that chest radiographs be taken on **full** inspiration to demonstrate the lungs as they appear fully expanded. However, the full inspiration should not be forced to the point of strain, causing unsteadiness. This needs to be explained to the patient prior to the exposure as the patient is being positioned.

Also, more air can be inhaled without too much strain on the **second** breath, compared to the first. Therefore, the patient should be asked to **hold the second full breath** rather than the first. It may be necessary to practice this breathing procedure with the patient before actually making the exposure.

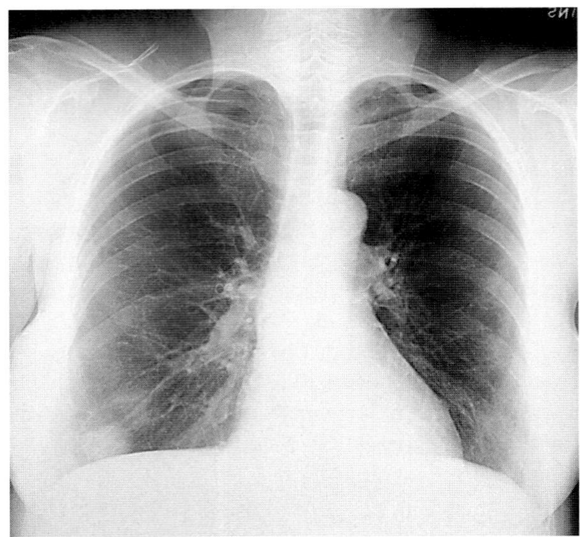

Fig. 2-32. Inspiration. (Courtesy of Llori Lundh)

Inspiration and Expiration

Occasionally there are exceptions to taking chest radiographs on full inspiration only. For certain conditions comparison radiographs are taken on both **full inspiration** and **full expiration**. One indicator for this is **atelectasis** *(at″e-lek′tah-sis)*, which is a condition of incomplete expansion of a lung or portion of a lung, or a collapse of a lung caused by various conditions.* Other indicators for comparison inspiration/expiration chest radiographs are a possible small pneumothorax (air or gas in the pleural cavity), fixation or lack of normal movement of the diaphragm, the presence of a foreign body, or to distinguish between an opacity in the rib or in the lung. When such comparison radiographs are taken, they should be labeled "inspiration" and "expiration." Note the pneumothorax of the upper right lung demonstrated in the chest radiograph in Fig. 2-33 (see arrows). This is not evident on the inspiration radiograph of the same patient taken at the same time in Fig. 2-32.

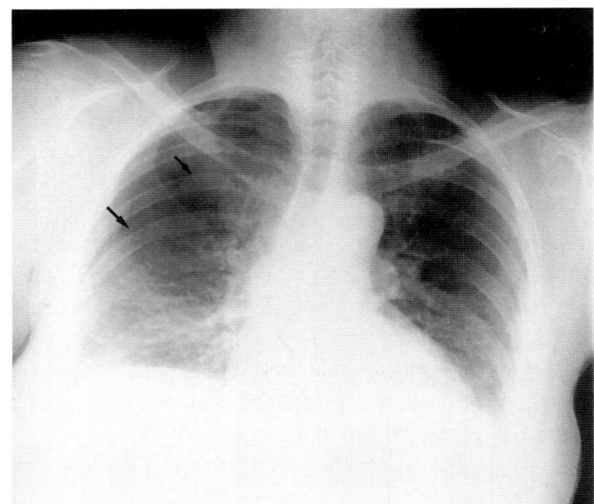

Fig. 2-33. Expiration. (Courtesy of Llori Lundh)

Erect Chest Radiographs

All chest radiographs should be taken in an erect position if the patient's condition allows. Three reasons for this are as follows:

1. To allow the diaphragm to move down farther.
An erect position causes the liver and other abdominal organs to drop, allowing the diaphragm to move farther down on full inspiration, thus allowing the lungs to fully aerate.

2. To show possible air and fluid levels in the chest.
If both air and fluid are present within a lung or within the pleural space, the heavier fluid, such as blood or serum, will gravitate to the lowest position while the air will rise. In the recumbent position, a pleural effusion will spread out over the posterior surface of the lung, resulting in a hazy appearance of the entire lung. In the upright position, fluid will locate near the base of the lung. The partially erect chest radiograph (Fig. 2-34) shows some fluid in the right lower thoracic cavity. The supine radiograph of the same patient (Fig. 2-35) shows a generalized hazy appearance of the entire right lung due to the presence of fluid now spread throughout the right thorax.

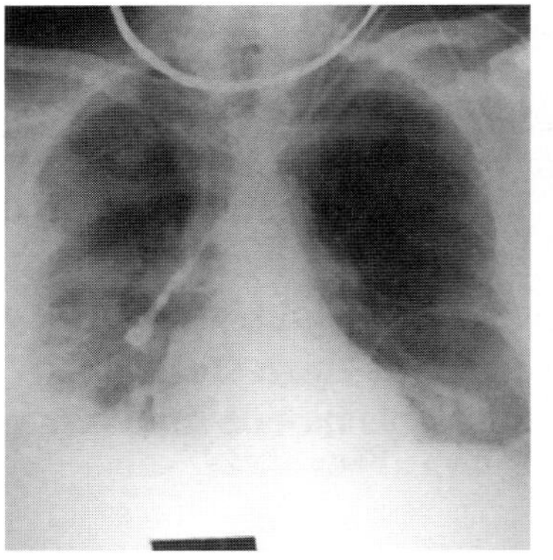

Fig. 2-34. Partially erect, some fluid evident in right lower lung.

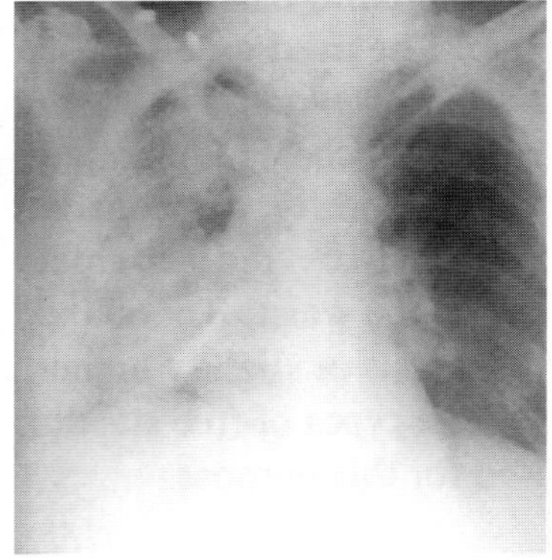

Fig. 2-35. Supine, 40" (same patient, shows fluid throughout right lung)

3. To prevent engorgement and hyperemia of pulmonary vessels.
The term **engorgement** literally means "distended or swollen with fluid."* **Hyperemia** *(hi″per-e′me-ah)* refers to an excess of blood, in part due to a relaxation of the distal small blood vessels or arterioles.*

An erect position in general tends to minimize engorgement and hyperemia of pulmonary vessels whereas a supine position will increase this, which can change the radiographic appearance of these vessels and the lungs in general.

PA Seventy-two inch (180 cm) SID: Chest radiographs taken AP at a minimum 40 in. (102 cm) rather than PA at 72 in. (180 cm) will cause **increased magnification of the heart shadow,** which complicates the diagnosis of possible cardiac enlargement. The **primary reason** for this is greater magnification due to **increased divergence** or angle of the x-ray beam at a shorter SID as described in Chapter 1. A longer SID, such as 72 in. or 180 cm, magnifies less because the x-ray beam diverges less.

A **second reason** for less magnification of the heart on a PA 72" chest is the **anterior location** of the heart within the mediastinum, placing it closer to the film on the PA, thus less magnification.

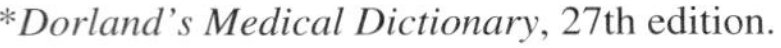

**Dorland's Medical Dictionary*, 27th edition.

EVALUATION CRITERIA

The description for each chest projection or position in this chapter includes an evaluation criteria section. In this section specific criteria are listed and described by which one can evaluate the resultant radiograph. The goal of every radiographer should be to take the "optimal" radiograph. These evaluation criteria provide **a definable standard** by which every chest radiograph can be evaluated to determine where improvements can be made.

Certain important evaluation criteria related to positioning, which are common to all routine PA and lateral chest radiographs, are as follows:

PA Chest Positioning

True PA, No Rotation: Even a slight amount of rotation on a PA chest projection will result in distortion of size and shape of the heart shadow since the heart is located anteriorly in the thorax. Therefore, it is important that there be **NO** rotation. To prevent rotation, ensure that the patient is standing evenly on both feet with both shoulders rolled forward and downward. Also, check the posterior aspect of the shoulders as well as the lower posterior rib cage and the pelvis to ensure no rotation. Scoliosis, or curvature of the thoracic spine, makes it more difficult to prevent rotation, and extra care is required to avoid rotation for such patients.

Rotation on PA chest radiographs can be determined by examining both sternal ends of the clavicles for a symmetrical appearance in relationship to the spine. On a true PA chest without any rotation, both the **right and left sternal ends of the clavicles will be the same distance from the spine.** Note the rotation evident in Fig. 2-37 by the difference in distance from the spinal column of the sternal end of the right clavicle as compared to the left.

The direction of rotation can be determined by which sternal end of the clavicle is closest to the spine. For example, in Fig. 2-37 the left side of the thorax is moved toward the film (right side moved away from film) which creates a slight LAO that will decrease the distance of the left clavicle from the spine.

Extending The Chin: Sufficient extension of the patient's chin will ensure that the chin and neck are not covering up or superimposing the uppermost lung regions, the apices of the lungs. This is demonstrated by the two radiographs in Figs. 2-38 and 2-39. Also, be sure the upper collimation border is high enough so that the apices are not cut off.

Minimizing Breast Shadows: The patient with large pendulous breasts should be asked to lift them up and outward, then remove her hands as she leans against the film holder to keep them in this position. This will lessen the effect of breast shadows over the lower lung fields. Remember, however, that depending on the size and density of the breasts, breast shadows over the lower lateral lung fields cannot be totally eliminated (Fig. 2-40).

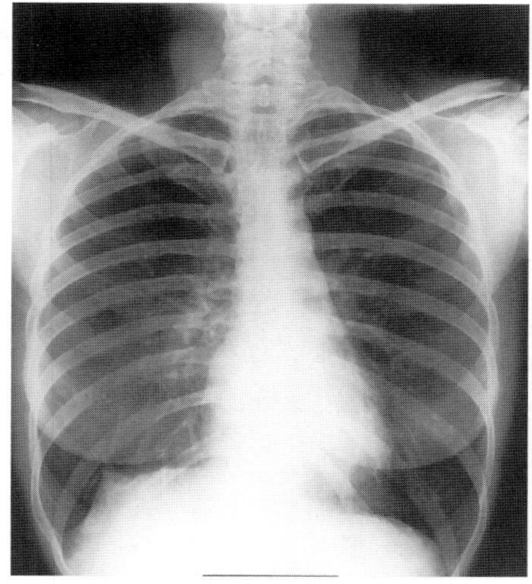
Fig. 2-36. Without rotation.

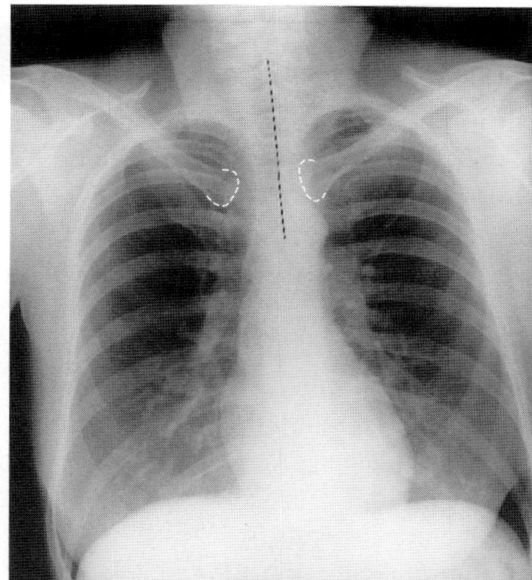
Fig. 2-37. With rotation (slight LAO).

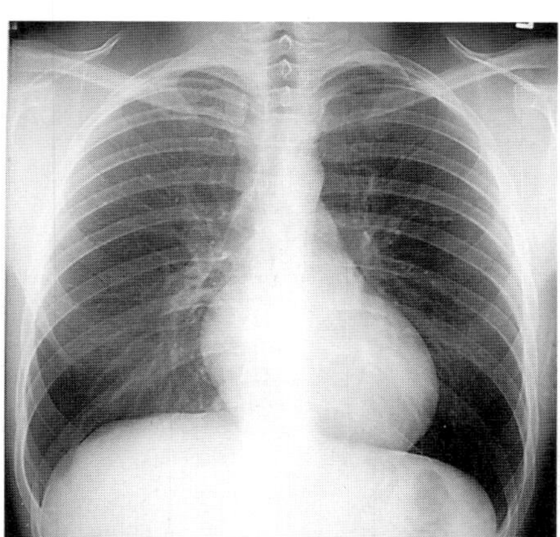
Fig. 2-38. Chin up.

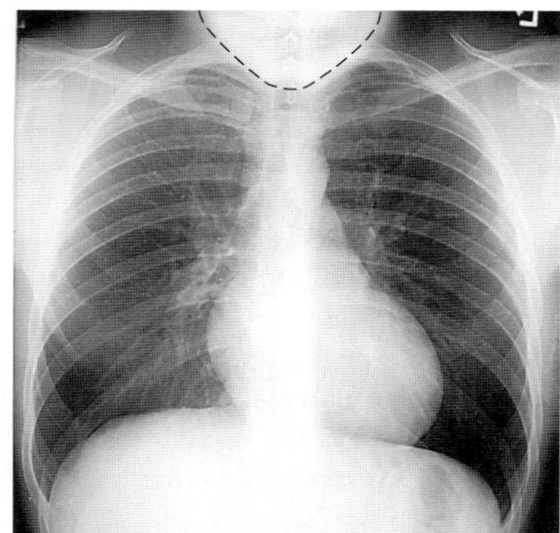
Fig. 2-39. Chin down.

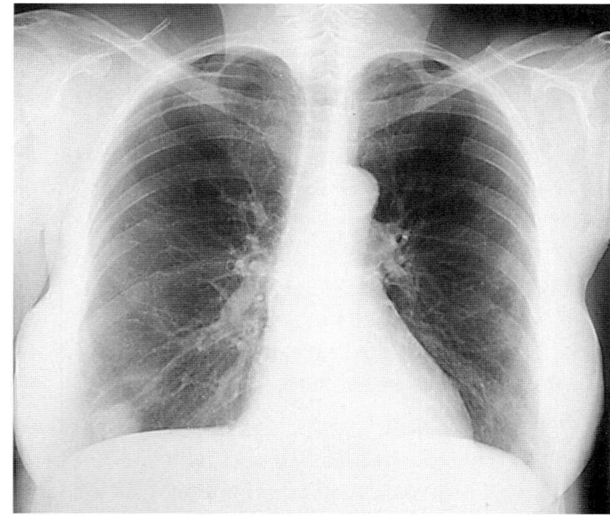
Fig. 2-40. Breast shadows evident.

Lateral Chest Positioning

Side Closest To Film: The patient's side closest to the film is best demonstrated on the finished radiograph. A **left lateral** should be done unless departmental protocol indicates otherwise, or unless certain pathology in the right lung indicates the need for a right lateral. A left lateral will better demonstrate the heart region because the heart is located primarily in the left thoracic cavity.

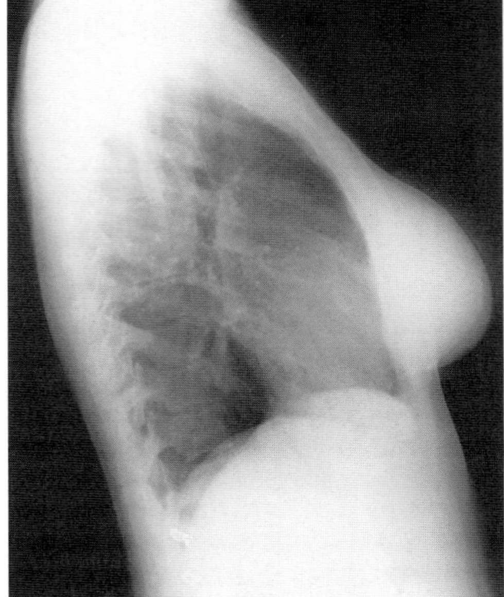

Fig. 2-41. Without excessive rotation.

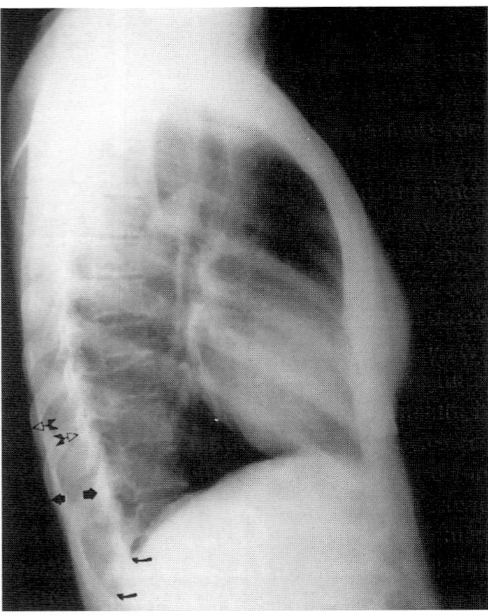

Fig. 2-42. With excessive rotation.

True Lateral, NO Rotation** or **Tilt: Ensure that the patient is standing straight with weight evenly distributed on both feet with arms raised. As a check against rotation, confirm that the posterior surfaces of the shoulder and the pelvis are directly superimposed and perpendicular to the film. Due to the divergent x-ray beam, the posterior ribs on the side farthest away from the film will be magnified slightly and also will be projected slightly posterior compared to the side closest to the film on a true lateral chest. This will be more noticeable on a broad-shouldered patient taken at 72" (183 cm.) SID. A longer SID of 120" (305 cm), as used in some departments, will result in less beam-divergence and therefore less separation of the posterior ribs. However, this separation of posterior ribs due to divergence of the x-ray beam at the commonly used 72 in. (183 cm) SID should only be ¼ to ½ inch or about 1 cm. Any more separation than this indicates rotation of the thorax from a true lateral position.*

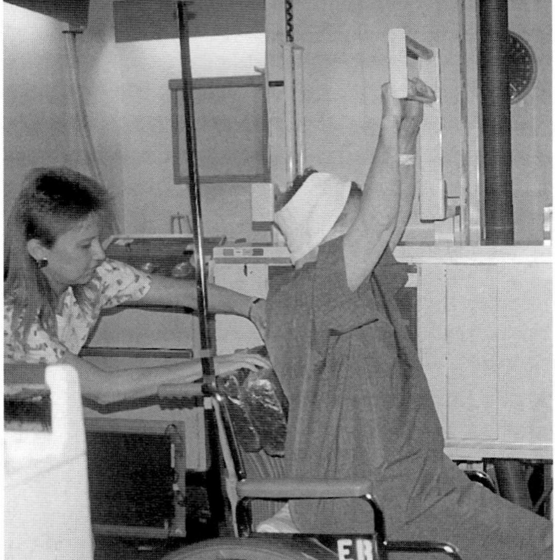

Fig. 2-43. Arms raised high.

Note: Some references, including previous editions of this textbook, suggest an intentional slight anterior rotation of the side away from the film so the posterior ribs would be directly superimposed. This may be preferred in some departments, but since the heart and most lung structures are nearer mid structures and thus not affected by the beam divergence, a preferred method may be a straight lateral with respect to the film, which will cause a slight separation of the posterior ribs and costophrenic angles.

Fig. 2-42 demonstrates a lateral chest with **excessive rotation**, as indicated by the **amount of separation of the right and left posterior ribs**, and **separation of the two costophrenic angles**. This represents a positioning error and would generally require a repeat.

Direction of Rotation: The direction of rotation on a lateral chest is sometimes difficult to determine on a radiograph. Frequently, however, this can be determined by identifying the left hemidiaphragm by the gastric air bubble in the stomach, or by the inferior border of the heart shadow, both of which are associated with the left hemidiaphragm.*

No tilt: There also should be **no tilt or "sideway leaning."** The **midsagittal plane must be parallel to the film.** This means that if the patient's shoulders are firmly against the film holder on a lateral chest, the lower lateral thorax and/or hips may be an inch or two away. This is especially true on broad-shouldered patients.

Arms Raised High: Ensure that the patient raises both arms sufficiently high to prevent superimposition on the upper chest field. Patients who are weak or unstable may need to grasp a support (Fig. 2-43).

When the patient's arms are not raised sufficiently, the soft tissues of the upper arm will superimpose portions of the lung field, as demonstrated in Fig. 2-44.

Note: Arrows demonstrate margins of soft tissues of the arms overlying upper lung fields. This would require a repeat and should be avoided.

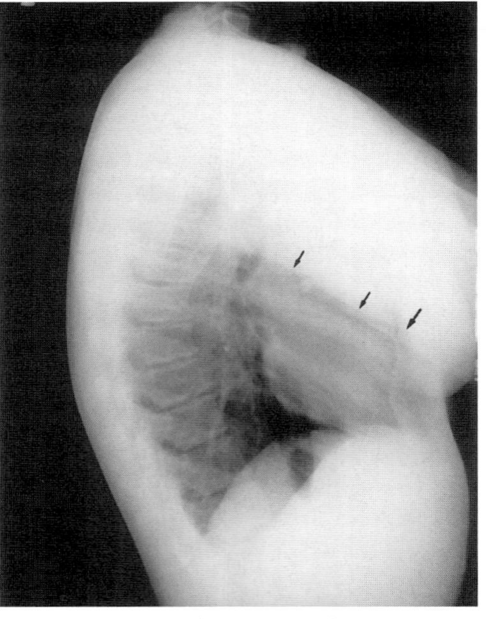

Fig. 2-44. Arms not raised–**Positioning error.**

*McQuillen-Martensen, K; *Radiographic Critique*; Philadelphia, WB Saunders; 1996.

CENTRAL RAY LOCATION

Traditionally, the top of the shoulder and the exterior borders of the thorax have been used as positioning landmarks for chest radiography. This method usually includes placing the top of the cassette about 2 inches above the shoulders and centering the CR to the center of the film. However, this positioning method is inconsistent, considering variations in lung field dimensions due to differences in body habitus, as demonstrated by comparing Figs. 2-45 and 2-46. The center of the lungs (indicated by "X") is shown to be near the center of the film for this male on the left, but is near the upper third of the film on this small and older female on the right. Therefore, the CR obviously was **not** centered to the lungs in Fig. 2-46, which also resulted in inaccurate collimation, exposing a large portion of the upper abdomen. This demonstrates the importance of a chest positioning method that **consistently centers the central ray to the center of the lung fields with accurate collimation on <u>both</u> top and bottom.**

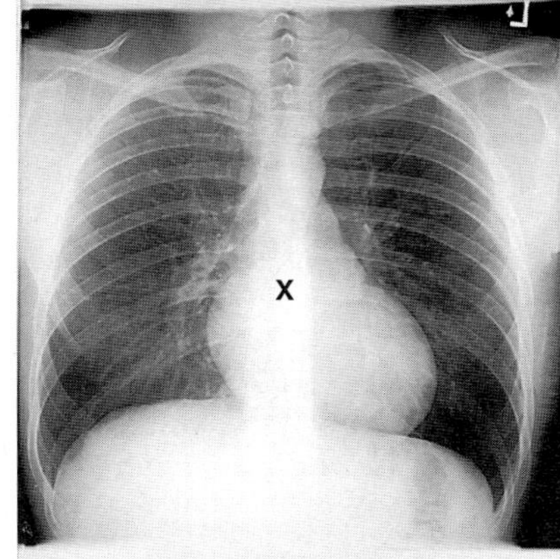

Fig. 2-45. Average sthenic/hyposthenic male (correct CR and collimation.)

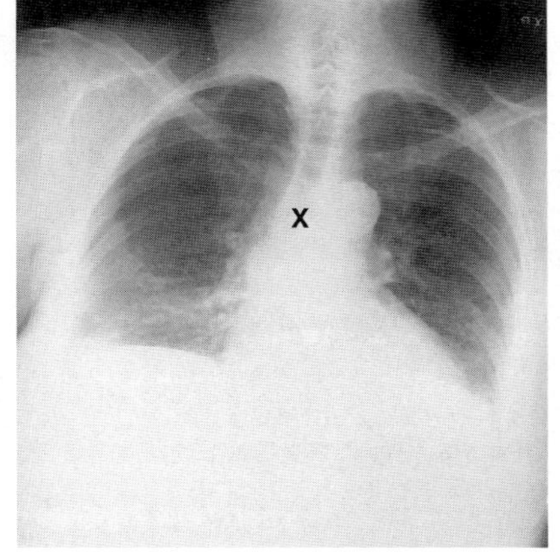

Fig. 2.46. Small and older female (**incorrect** CR and collimation).

Central Ray Chest-Positioning Method

As described in Chapter 1, accurate CR location to the center of the part being radiographed is important to prevent distortion of anatomical parts and for consistent exposures by AEC systems. This is especially true for chest radiographs.

Bony topographical landmarks are consistent and reliable as a means of determining CR locations. Two such specific landmarks for locating the center of the lung fields are as follows:

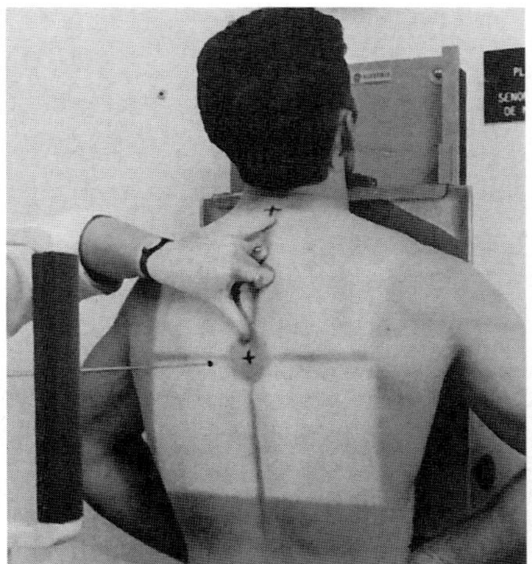
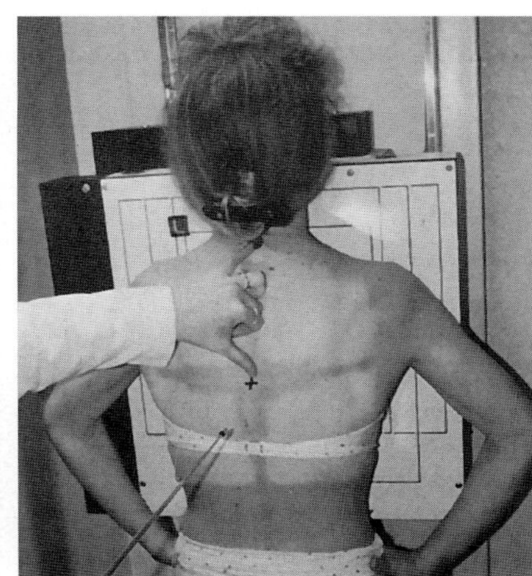
Fig. 2-47. Correct CR utilizing vertebra prominens. Fig. 2-48.

***Vertebra Prominens** (PA Chest):* The vertebra prominens corresponds to the level of the T1, and to the uppermost margin of the apex of the lungs. This topographical landmark, which can be palpated at the base of the neck, is the preferred landmark for locating the CR on a PA chest as shown in Figs. 2-47 and 2-48. For the average female, this is down about 7 in. (18 cm), and for the male about 8 in. (20 cm).

One way of determining this distance is by an average hand spread as shown. Most hands can reach 7 inches. The 8-inch distance can be determined by estimating an additional inch. If the hand spread method is used, one should practice with a ruler to consistently determine these distances (see ruler printed in Appendix A, page 84).

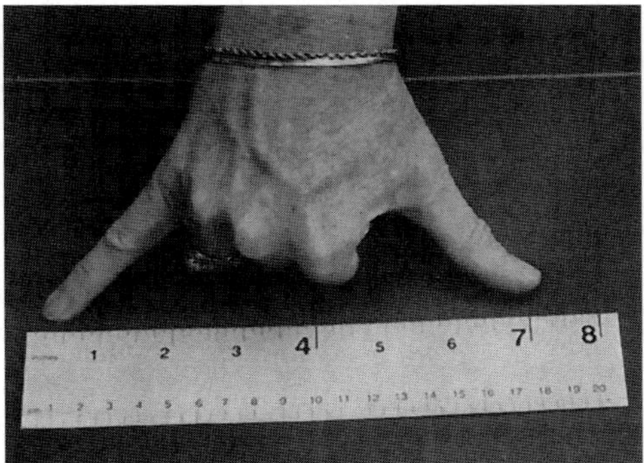

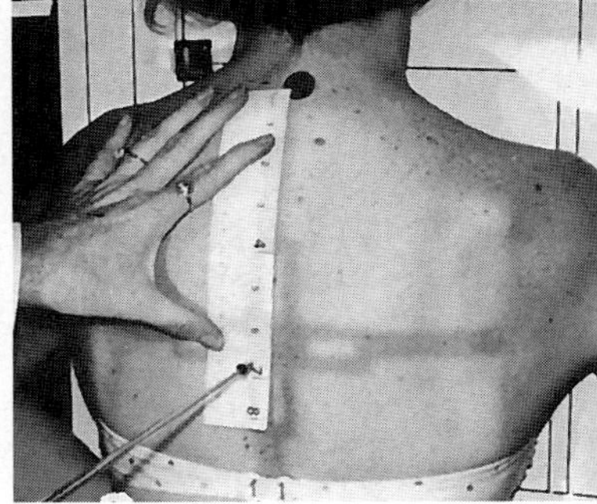
Fig. 2-49. Hand spread method–7 or 8 in. (18-20 cm). 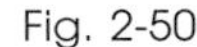 Fig. 2-50.

These differences between male and female are true for near-average body-types for the general population, with crossover exceptions in which certain larger athletic type females may also have longer lung fields, and some males shorter lungs. However, for purposes of chest positioning for the general population, these average measurements of **7 inches for a female** and **8 inches for a male** can be used as reliable guidelines.

Exceptions: Other exceptions in centering that each radiographer should learn to recognize are variations in body types. For example, the author found that 15 to 20% of the general male population were the well-developed athletic sthenic/hyposthenic type, which requires centering to nearer T8, or 9 in. (22 cm) down. Also, about 5 to 10% of the population are the hypersthenic type, which only requires from 6 to 7 in. (15 to 18 cm) down from the vertebra prominens.

Note: For most patients this CR level for PA chests is also near the level of the inferior angle of the scapula, but this varies some depending on the amount of downward slope of the shoulders and is not as reliable a landmark.

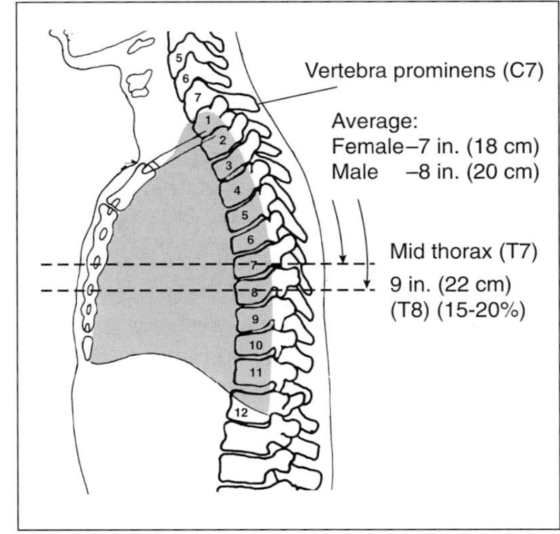

Fig. 2-51. Topographical landmarks for PA chest.

Central ray location continued

Jugular Notch *(AP Chest):* The easily palpated jugular notch is the recommended landmark for location of the CR for AP chest radiographs. The level of T7 on an average adult is 3 to 4 in. (8 to 10 cm) below the jugular notch. For most older or hypersthenic patients, this is approximately **3 in. (8 cm)**. For younger and/or sthenic/hyposthenic athletic types, this is nearer **4, or even 5 in. (10 to 12 cm).**

This distance can also be determined by the radiographer's hand width. The average-sized hand width with the fingers together is approximately 3 in. (8 cm). See Fig. 2-53.

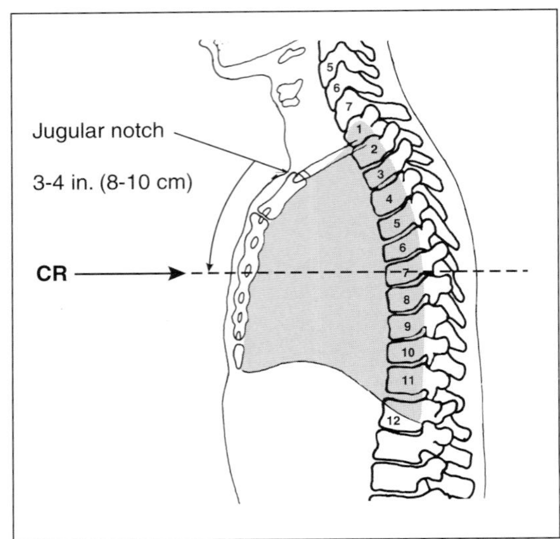

Fig. 2-52. Topographical landmark for AP chest.

Lung Dimensions and Film Holder Placement

PA or AP chest radiographs are most commonly taken with the cassette film holder placed lengthwise. However, contrary to common belief, **the width or horizontal dimension of the average PA or AP chest is greater than the vertical dimension** (see Appendix at the end of this chapter).

The study described in this appendix also shows that the width or horizontal dimension on a PA or AP chest exceeds 13 in. (33 cm) on 15 to 20% of patients. This requires that the 14 x 17 in. (35 x 43 cm) film holder be placed **crosswise** so as not to cut off lateral lung margins on these patients.

PA Chest: Most erect PA chests are done with dedicated chest units, which may not allow for this crosswise placement of the film. However, cassettes with portable stationary grids can be placed crosswise for this purpose.

As the patient is standing and facing the chest film holder, one can determine whether to place the film crosswise on larger patients by standing behind the patient and placing one's hands squarely on each side of the chest. **If there is any doubt that both sides of the chest can be included, the film holder should be placed crosswise, remembering that the height of the average lung field is less than the width.**

AP Chest: For AP chest radiographs (usually taken at less than 72 in. or 180 cm with an accompanying increase in divergence of the x-ray beam), the chance of the side borders of the lungs being cut off increases if the film is placed lengthwise. Therefore, it is recommended that for AP chest radiographs, the 14 x 17 in. (35 x 43 cm) film be placed **crosswise**, with the film and CR centered to a point 3 to 4 in. (8 to 10 cm) below the jugular notch (Fig. 2-53).

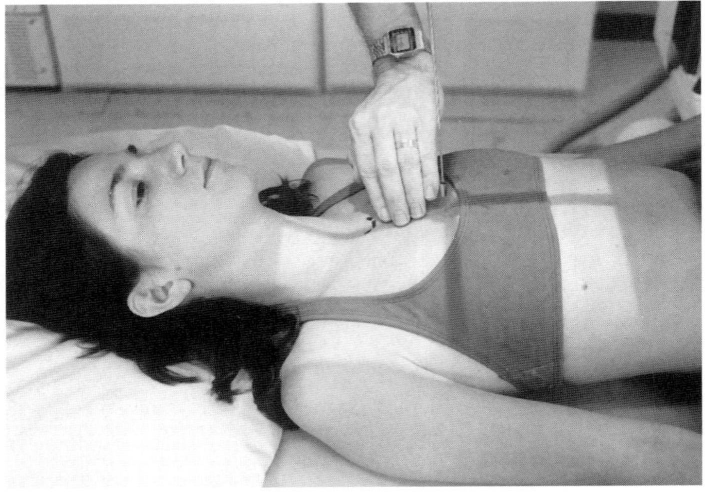

Fig. 2-53. Film crosswise, CR 3 to 4 in. (8 to 11 cm) below jugular.

Collimation Guidelines

Side collimation borders can easily be determined by adjusting the illuminated field margins to the **outer skin margins** on each side of the posterior chest surface (remembering that lungs expand during deep inspiration). The upper and lower collimation borders, however, are more difficult to determine because these lung margins are not visible externally.

A reliable method for upper and lower chest collimation is to adjust the upper border of the illuminated light field to the **vertebra prominens,** which with the divergent rays, will result in an upper collimation margin on the film of about 1½ in. or 4 cm above the vertebra prominens (Figs. 2-54 and 2-55). This will then also result in a lower collimation border of 1 to 2 in. (3 to 5 cm) below the costophrenic angles, if the CR was correctly centered. These distances above and below the lungs allow for some margin of error in CR placement without cutting off upper or lower lungs.

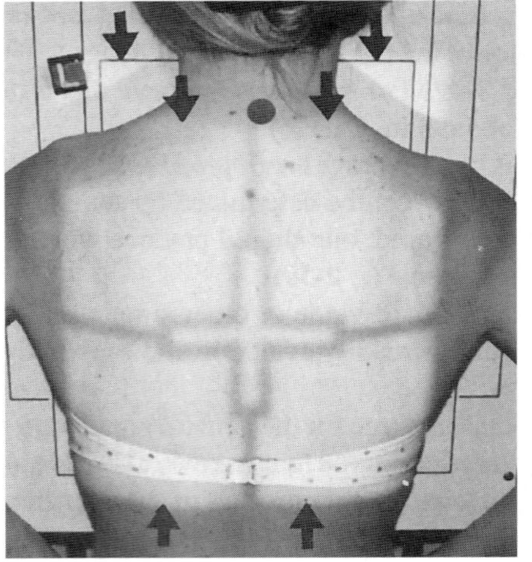

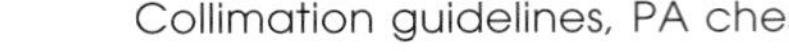

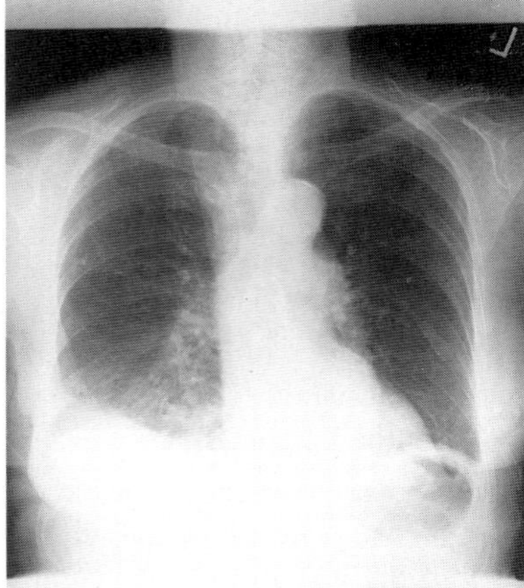

Fig. 2-54. Collimation guidelines, PA chest. Fig. 2-55.

CR -T7 or T8.
Sides -Outer skin margins.
Upper -Level of vertebra prominens.

NATIONAL SURVEY

Departmental standard and special operating procedures (departmental routines) for the chest are fairly consistent throughout the United States. This was determined by the results of a national survey completed in 1995 and 1989 to determine national norms for standard and special radiographic operating procedures for the chest and upper airway. The survey results for 1995 are compared with those of 1989, where comparison data are available. The numbers after the years along the top of the U.S. Average box indicate the number of responding institutions in 1995 and 1989.

Chest Routine

Chest	1995–637 (1989–529) U.S. Average	
	Basic 1995 (1989)	Special 1995 (1989)
• PA erect	99% (99%)	
• Lat. erect	98% (99%)	
• AP lordotic		72% (38%)
• Lat. decub.		68% (70%)
• Ant. obliques		46% (30%)
• Post. obliques		41% (30%)
• AP supine		45% (82%)

Upper Airway Routine

Upper Airway	1995–637 (1989–529) U.S. Average	
	Basic 1995 (1989)	Special 1995 (1989)
• Lateral	80% (99%)	
• AP	70% (75%)	
• Oblique		21% –

Summary

Chest: These results indicate that 99% of all departments throughout the United States responding to the survey for radiographic procedures of the chest include the PA and lateral projections as standard or routine.

The 1995 survey also indicates that the AP lordotic is performed as a special projection by an average of 72% of all responding institutions. This compares with only 38% in 1989, indicating a significant increase in the use of this projection. The Western states indicated less use of this projection (60%) as compared with the middle U.S. (75%) and Eastern states as shown in the appendix of this textbook.

The frequency of the AP supine chest as a special projection in 1995 (45%) was significantly less than in 1989 (82%). The reason for this is unknown but it may have been influenced by the way the question was stated in the survey of 1995 as compared with 1989.

Upper Airway: For the upper airway to demonstrate the air-filled larynx and trachea as well as the region of the thyroid and thymus glands, the survey results indicate that 80% in 1995 and 99% in 1989 of all departments include the lateral position as routine or standard, and 70% and 75%, respectively, include the AP projection.

The one special projection for this procedure was the oblique projection, but only an average of 21% of the respondents indicated this, and it is not described separately in this chapter.

STANDARD AND SPECIAL OPERATING PROCEDURES

Certain basic and special projections for the chest are demonstrated and described on the following pages as suggested standard or basic and as special departmental procedures which all student radiographers should master.

Basic Projections

Standard or basic projections, also sometimes referred to as routine projections or departmental routines, are those projections commonly taken on average patients who are helpful and can cooperate in performing the procedure.

Special Projections

Special projections are those more common projections taken as extra or additional projections to better demonstrate certain pathologic conditions or specific body parts, or when the patient is not able to cooperate fully.

Basic and Special Projections

Chest
Basic
• PA **72**
• Lateral **74**

Chest
Special
• AP supine or semierect **76**
• Lateral decubitus **77**
• AP lordotic **78**
• Anterior oblique **79**
• Posterior oblique **80**

Upper airway
Basic
• Lateral **81**
• AP **82**

PA Projection

Ambulatory patient

Chest
Basic
• PA
• Lateral

Structures Best Shown

Lungs, including both apices, air-filled trachea, bronchi, heart and great vessels, diaphragm to include costophrenic angles, and bony thorax.

Technical Factors

- Film size–14 x 17 in. (35 x 43 cm), lengthwise or crosswise (see Note).
- Moving or stationary grid.
- 110-125 kVp range.
- Technique and dose:

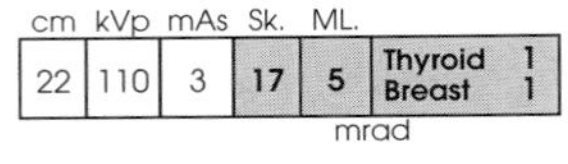

cm	kVp	mAs	Sk.	ML.	
22	110	3	17	5	Thyroid 1 Breast 1
				mrad	

or

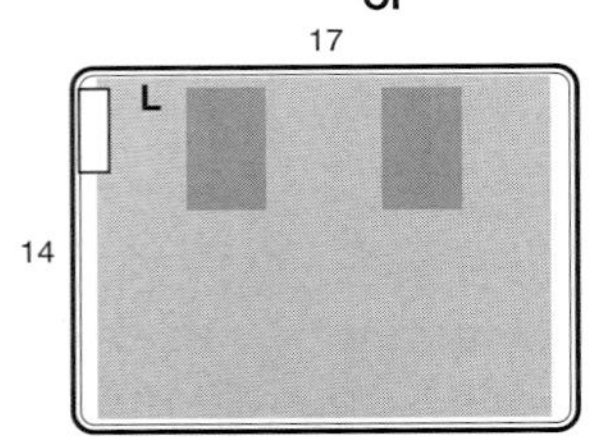

Dark boxes indicate AEC chamber selections

Shielding: Secure lead shield around waist or use an adjustable mobile shield on a stand behind patient.

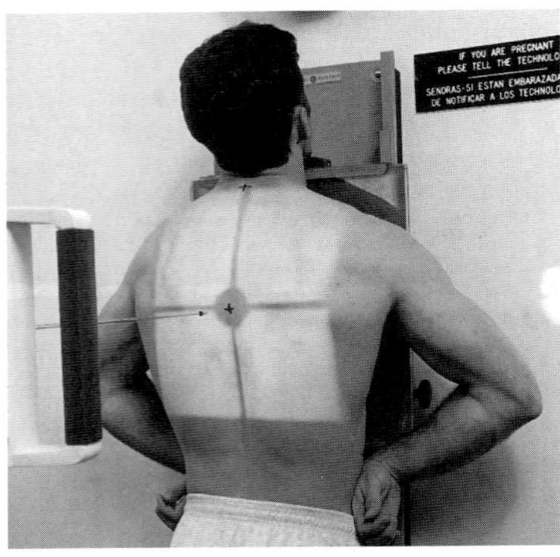

Fig. 2-56. PA chest.

Patient Position

- Patient erect, feet spread slightly, weight equally distributed on both feet.
- Chin raised, resting against film holder.
- Hands on lower hips, palms out, elbows partially flexed.
- Shoulders rotated forward against film holder to allow scapulae to move laterally clear of lung fields. Also depress shoulders downward to move clavicles below the apices.
- See page 67 for minimizing breast shadows.

Part Position

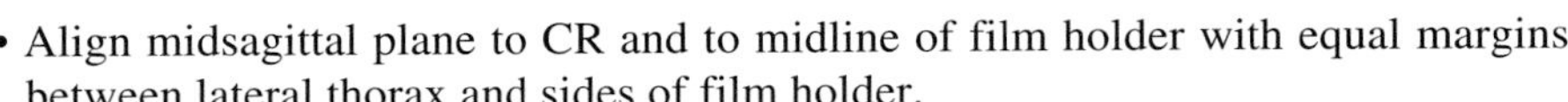

- Align midsagittal plane to CR and to midline of film holder with equal margins between lateral thorax and sides of film holder.
- Ensure **no rotation** of thorax.
- Raise or lower CR and film holder as needed to the level of T7 for average patient.

Central Ray

- CR perpendicular to the film and centered to the **midsagittal plane at the level of T7** (7 to 8 in. or 18 to 20 cm below vertebra prominens).
- Center cassette to CR.
- 72 in. (180 cm) SID.

Collimation: Collimate on four sides to area of lung fields. (Top border of illuminated field should be to level of vertebra prominens, and lateral borders to outer skin margins.)

Respiration: Exposure made at end of **2nd full inspiration**.

Note: Place cassette crosswise for larger or hypersthenic-type patients. See page 64 for further explanations.

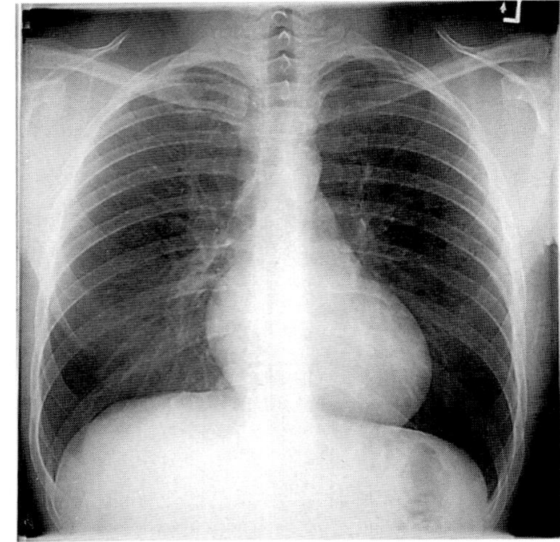

Fig. 2-57. PA chest.

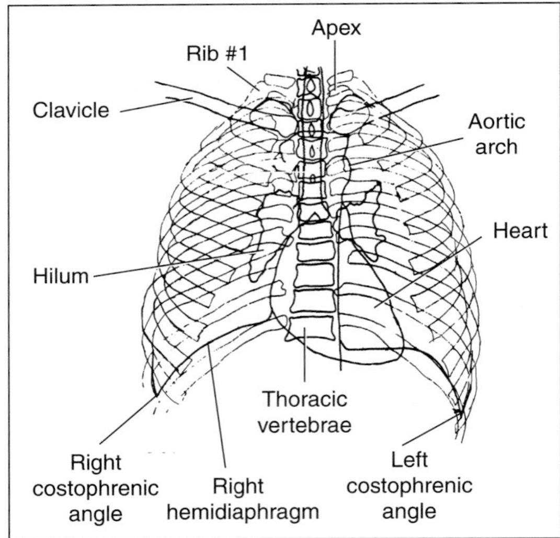

Fig. 2-58. PA chest.

Evaluation Criteria

- **No rotation**; both sternoclavicular joints should be the same distance from the vertebral column; the distance from the lateral borders of the ribs to the vertebral column should be the same on each side, from the upper to the lower rib cage.
- Scapulae should not superimpose the lungs if shoulders are rotated forward sufficiently.
- Collimation margins should appear on four sides on smaller patients. The center of the collimation field should be to area of T7 on average patients.
- Entire lungs should be included on film, superior apices to the lower costophrenic angles.
- Larger breast shadows should primarily be lateral to lung fields, with correct placement during positioning.
- **Full inspiration** should result in a minimum of 10 (11 on most patients) posterior ribs visualized above diaphragm.
- **No motion** should result in sharp outlines of diaphragm and heart borders.
- Optimum exposure and sufficient long contrast scale should visualize the fine vascular lung markings throughout lungs. **Faint outlines should be visible for at least the mid and upper thoracic vertebrae and posterior ribs through the heart and mediastinal structure shadows.**

PA Projection

On stretcher if patient cannot stand

Chest
Basic
• **PA**
• Lateral

Structures Best Shown

Lungs, including both apices, air-filled trachea, heart and great vessels, diaphragm to include costophrenic angles, and bony thorax.

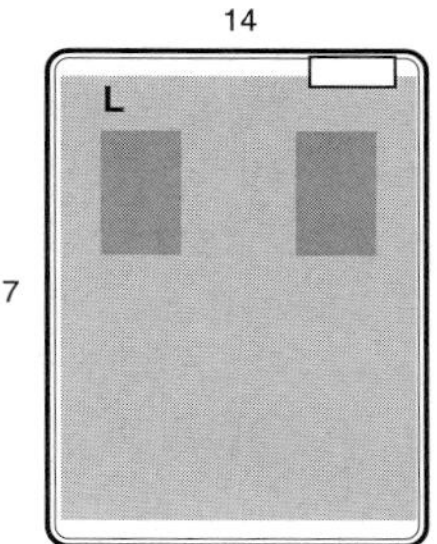

or

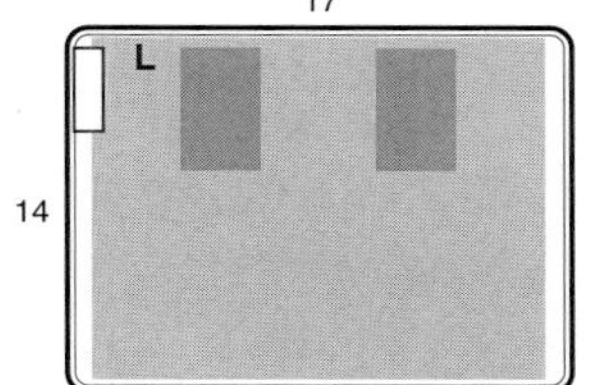

Technical Factors

- Film size–14 x 17 in. (35 x 43 cm) lengthwise or crosswise.
- Moving or stationary grid.
- 110–125 kVp range.
- Technique and dose:

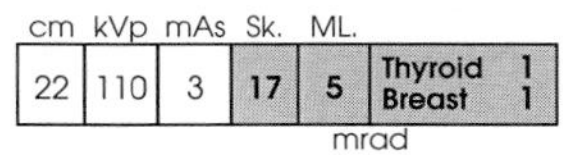

cm	kVp	mAs	Sk.	ML.	
22	110	3	17	5	Thyroid 1 Breast 1
			mrad		

Shielding: Secure lead shield around waist to shield gonads.

Patient Position

- Patient erect, seated on cart, legs over the edge.
- Arms around cassette unless a chest film holder is used, then position as for an ambulatory patient.
- Shoulders rotated forward and downward.
- **No rotation** of thorax.

Part Position 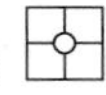

- Adjust the height of film holder so top of cassette is about 2 in. (5 cm) above top of shoulders and CR is at T7.
- If portable cassette is used because patient cannot be placed up against chest board, place pillow or padding on lap to raise and support cassette as shown, but keep cassette against chest for minimum OID (Fig. 2-60).

Central Ray

- CR perpendicular to the film and centered to the **midsagittal plane at the level of T7**, (7 to 8 in. or 18 to 20 cm below vertebra prominens).
- Center cassette to level of CR, if portable cassette is used.
- 72 in. (180 cm) SID.

Collimation: Collimate to area of lung fields. Upper border of illuminated field should be **to level of vertebra prominens**, which with divergent rays, will result in upper collimation border on film to about 1.5 in. or 4 cm above apex of lungs.

Respiration: Make exposure upon **2nd full inspiration**.

Note: Use compression band or other means to ensure that patient is stable and will not waver or move during exposure.

Evaluation Criteria

- Radiograph should appear similar to ambulatory PA chest as described on preceding page.

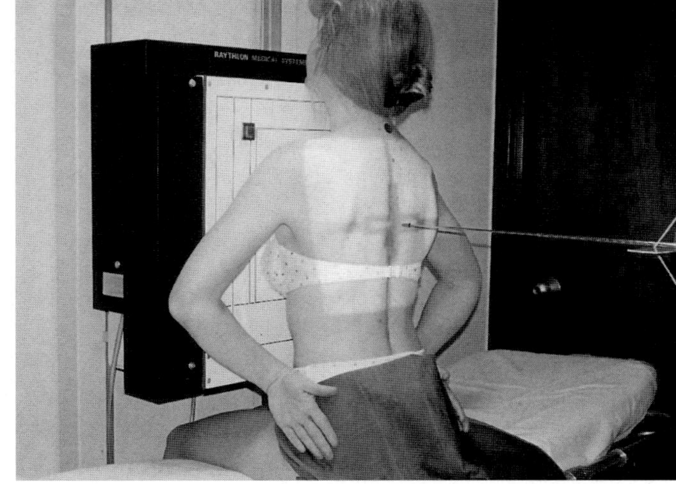

Fig. 2-59. PA chest (patient against chest board).

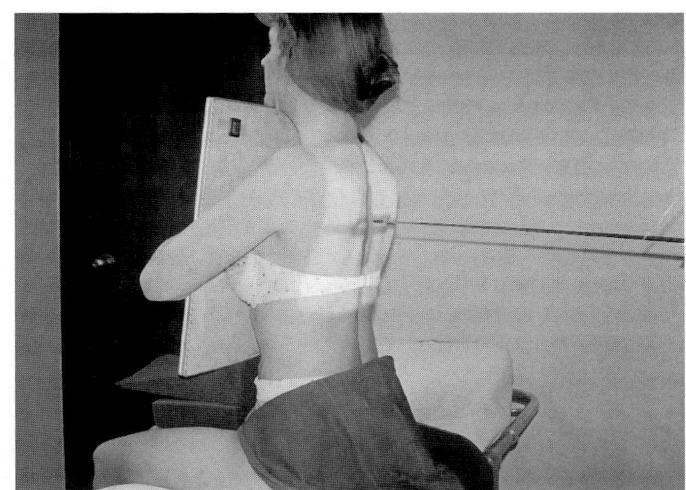

Fig. 2-60. PA chest (patient holding cassette).

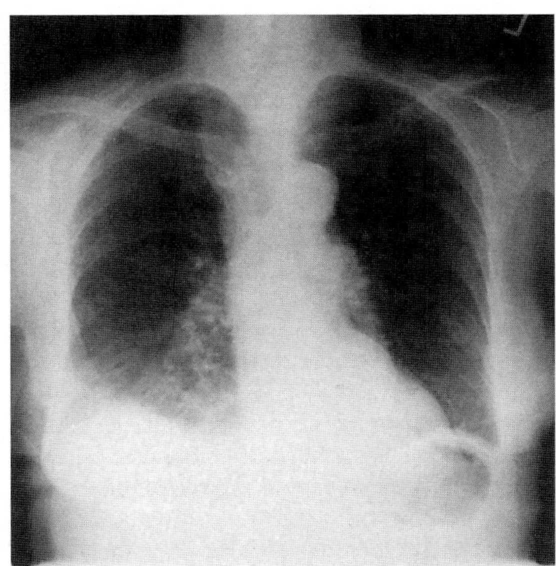

Fig. 2-61. PA chest.

Lateral Position
Ambulatory patient

Chest
Basic
• PA
• **Lateral**

Structures Best Shown

Lungs, trachea, heart and great vessels, diaphragm to include posterior costophrenic angles, and bony thorax.

Technical Factors

- Film size–14 x 17 in. (35 x 43 cm), lengthwise.
- Moving or stationary grid.
- 110-125 kVp.
- Technique and dose:

cm	kVp	mAs	Sk.	ML.	mrad
22	125	8	59	47	Thyroid 4, Breast 12

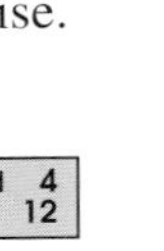

Shielding: Secure lead shield around waist or use mobile lead shield to protect gonads.

Patient Position

- Patient erect, **left side** against film unless patient's complaint is on right side; then do a right lateral if departmental protocol includes this option.
- Weight evenly distributed on both feet.
- Raise arms above head.
- Keep chin up.

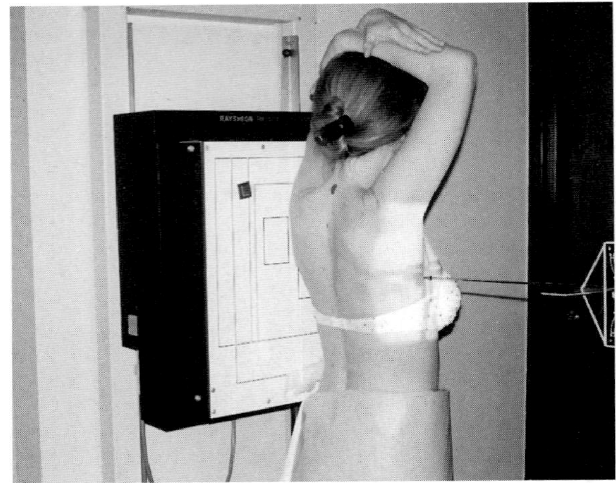

Fig. 2-62. Left lateral chest position.

Part Position

- Center patient to CR and to film anteriorly and posteriorly.
- Position in a **true lateral** position (Coronal plane is perpendicular, and sagittal plane is parallel to film holder).
- Lower CR and film holder slightly from PA if needed (see Note).

Central Ray

- CR perpendicular, directed to **mid thorax at level of T7** (3 to 4 in. or 8 to 10 cm below level of jugular notch).
- 72 in. (180 cm) SID.

Collimation: Collimate on four sides to area of lung fields (top border of light field to level of vertebra prominens).

Respiration: Exposure made at end of **2nd full inspiration**.

Note: Ensure that midsagittal plane is **parallel to film**, which for slender but broader shouldered patients will result in hips and lower thorax **not** being against film holder.

This increase in OID of the lower chest will also result in the costophrenic angles of the lungs being projected lower due to the divergence of the x-ray beam. Therefore, **the CR and film holder need to be lowered a minimum of 1 in. or 2 cm from the PA** on this type of patient to prevent cutoff of costophrenic angles.

If patient is weak and unsteady, take lateral on cart or in wheelchair as shown on following page.

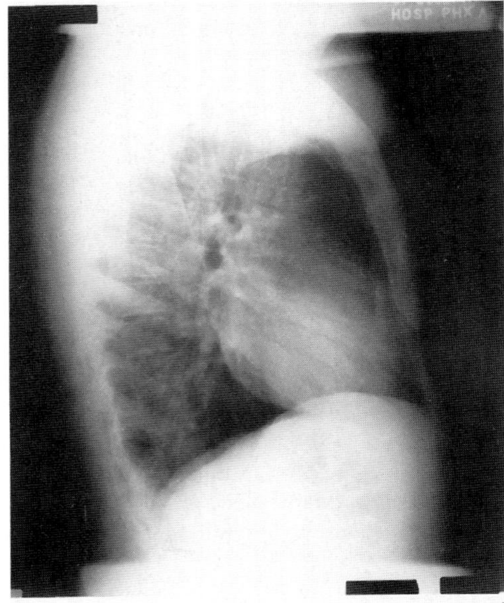

Fig. 2-63. Lateral chest.

Evaluation Criteria

- **No rotation**; posterior ribs and costophrenic angle on side away from film are projected slightly (¼-½ in. or 1-2 cm) posterior due to divergent rays. **Note**: For direction of rotation, see page 68 and critique radiographs on page 83.
- Chin and arms should be elevated sufficiently to prevent excessive soft tissues from superimposing apices.
- Image should include lung apices at the top and costophrenic angles on the lower margin of the film.
- Collimation margins should appear on all four sides on smaller patients. The center of the collimation field should be at the level of T7 on average patients.
- The hilum region should be in the approximate center of the film.
- **NO motion** should be evidenced by sharp outlines of the diaphragm and lung markings.
- Should have sufficient exposure and long scale contrast to **visualize rib outlines and lung markings through the heart shadow and upper lung areas** without overexposing other regions of the lungs.

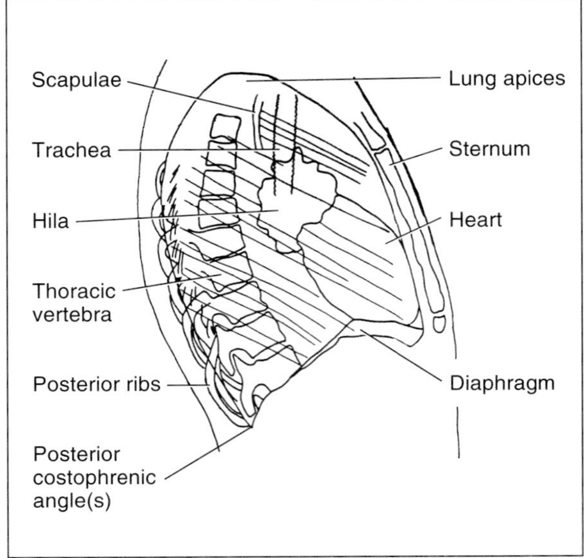

Fig. 2-64. Lateral chest.

Lateral Position

With a wheelchair or cart, if patient cannot stand

Chest
Basic
• PA
• Lateral

Structures Best Shown

Lungs, trachea, heart and great vessels, diaphragm including posterior costophrenic angles, and bony thorax.

Technical Factors

- Film size–14 x 17 in. (35 x 43 cm), lengthwise.
- Moving or stationary grid.
- 110-125 kVp.
- Technique and dose:

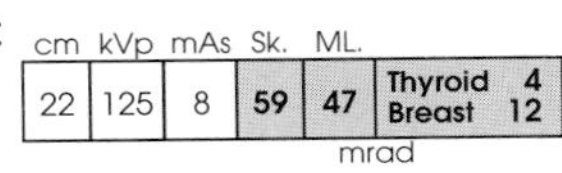

cm	kVp	mAs	Sk.	ML.	
22	125	8	59	47	Thyroid 4 Breast 12

mrad

Shielding: Secure lead shielding around waist to protect gonads.

Patient Position on Cart

- Patient seated on cart; legs over the edge if this is easier for patient (ensure that cart does not move).
- Arms crossed above head, or hold on to arm support.
- Keep chin up.

Patient Position in Wheelchair

- Place pillow or other support under smaller patients so arm rests of wheel chair do not superimpose lower lungs.
- Turn patient in wheel chair to lateral position as close to film holder as possible.
- Have patient lean forward and place support blocks behind back; raise arms above head and hold on to support bar–**keep arms high.**

Part Position

- Center patient to CR and to film by checking anterior and posterior aspects of thorax; adjust CR and film holder to level of T7.
- Ensure **NO** rotation by viewing patient from tube position.

Central Ray

- CR perpendicular, directed to **level of T7**. (3 to 4 in. or 8 to 10 cm below level of jugular notch.)
- 72 in. (180 cm) SID.

Collimation: Collimate on four sides to area of lung fields.

Respiration: Exposure made at end of **2nd full inspiration.**

Note: Always attempt to have patient sit completely erect in wheel chair or on cart if possible. However, if the patient's condition does not allow this, the head end of the cart can be raised as nearly erect as possible using a radiolucent support behind back (Fig. 2-67). All attempts should be made to get patient as nearly erect as possible.

Evaluation Criteria

Radiograph should appear similar to ambulatory lateral position as described under evaluation criteria on preceding page.

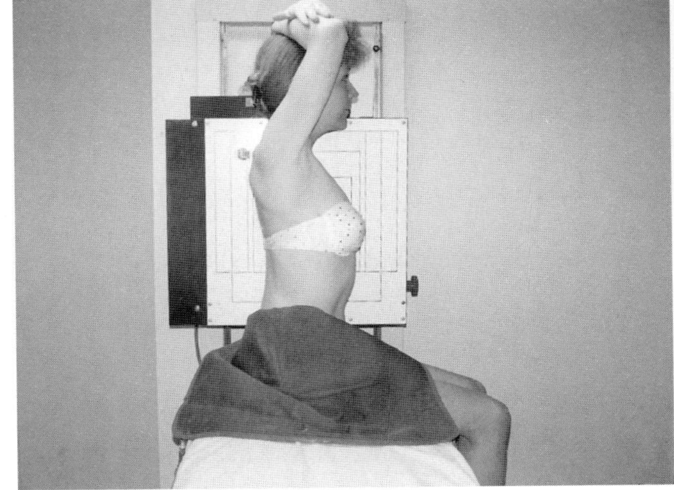

Fig. 2-65. Left lateral chest position on cart.

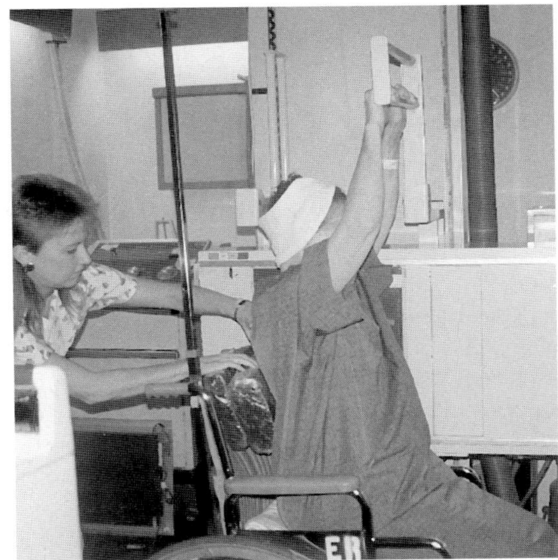

Fig. 2-66. Left lateral position in wheel chair. (arms up, support behind back)

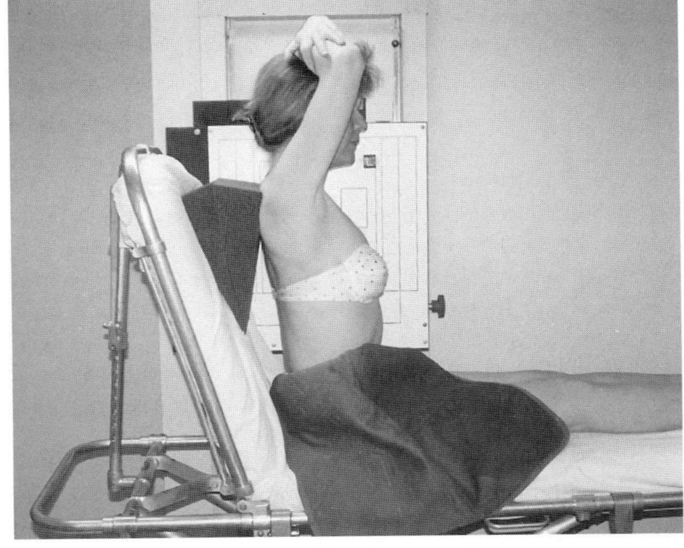

Fig. 2-67. Erect, supported left lateral position.

AP Projection

Supine or semierect (in department or as bedside portable)

Chest
Special
- **AP supine or semierect**
- Lateral decubitus (AP)
- AP lordotic
- Anterior oblique
- Posterior oblique

Structures Best Shown

Lungs, air-filled trachea, bony thorax, diaphragm including costophrenic angles, and heart and great vessels. Heart shadow will be magnified due to shorter SID and AP projection.

Fig. 2-68. AP supine.

Technical Factors

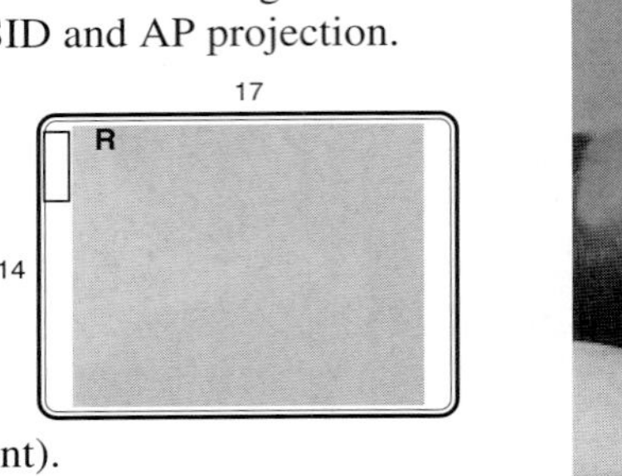

- Film size–14 x 17 in. (35 x 43 cm) crosswise (average to large).
- Screens or stationary grid. (Screens commonly used with portables at 70-80 kVp.)
- 80-100 kVp range with grid (large patient).
- Technique and dose: @ 40 in.

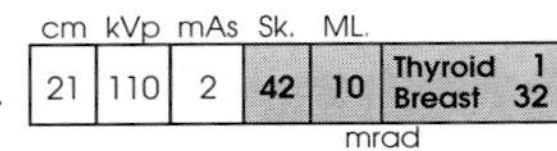

cm	kVp	mAs	Sk.	ML.	
21	110	2	42	10	Thyroid 1 Breast 32
			mrad		

Shielding: Place lead shield to shield gonads.

Patient Position

- Patient supine on cart; if possible, the head end of the cart or bed should be raised into a semierect position (see Notes below).
- Roll shoulders forward by rotating arms medially or internally.

Part Position

- Place film holder under or behind patient, align center of film to CR (top of film holder ≈2 in. or 5 cm above shoulders).
- Center patient to CR and to film holder; check by viewing patient from the top or near tube position.

Central Ray

- CR angled **caudad to be perpendicular to sternum** (requires ±5° caudad angle, prevents clavicles from obscuring the apices).
- CR to **level of T7**, 3 to 4 in. or 8 to 10 cm below jugular notch.
- For supine position, raise tube to at least a 40 in. (102 cm) SID, although more distance is preferred (prevents clavicles from obscuring the apices).

Collimation: Collimate to area of lung fields.

Respiration: Exposure made at end of **2nd full inspiration**.

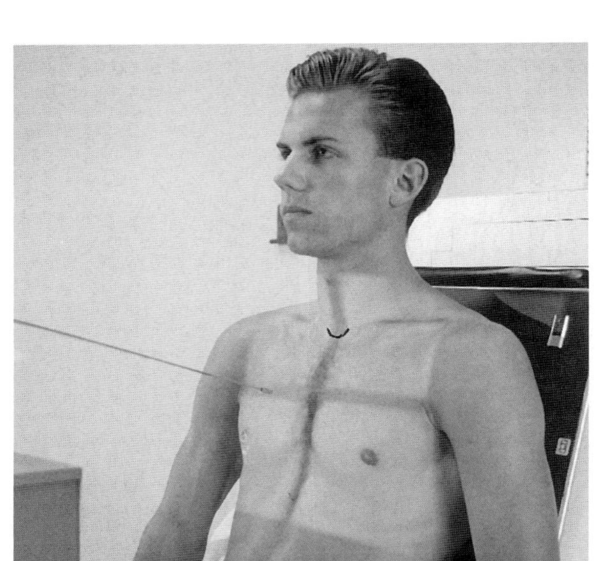

Fig. 2-69. AP semierect.

Notes: Crosswise film placement is recommended to minimize chance of lateral cutoff. This requires **accurate CR alignment to center of film** without caudal angle to prevent grid cutoff if grid is used.

For **semierect position**, use 60 in. (150 cm) or even 72 in. (180 cm) SID if this is possible to obtain. Always indicate the SID used; also indicate those projections obtained, such as AP supine or AP semierect.

Evaluation Criteria

- Evaluation criteria for those taken in supine or semierect positions should be similar to those for a PA projection described on a preceding page, with three exceptions.
  1. The heart will appear larger due to increased magnification from a shorter SID.
  2. Possible chest effusion and other potential pathologies for this type of patient will often obscure vascular lung markings when compared with a fully erect PA chest projection.
  3. Usually there will not be as full an inspiration, with only 8 or 9 posterior ribs visualized above diaphragm. Thus the lungs will appear more dense because the lungs are not fully aerated.

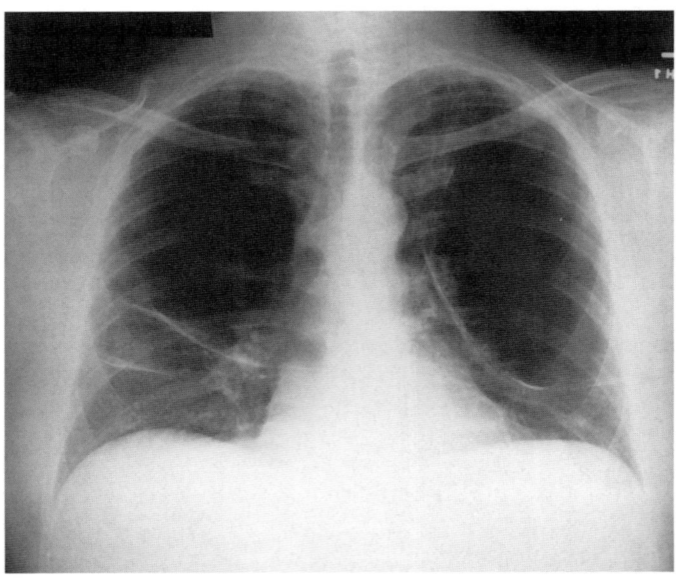

Fig. 2-70. AP.

Lateral Decubitus Position (AP Projection)

Chest
Special
- AP supine or semierect
- **Lateral decubitus** (AP)
- AP lordotic
- Anterior oblique
- Posterior oblique

Structures Best Shown

Small **pleural effusions** by demonstrating air-fluid levels in pleural space, or **small amounts of air** in pleural cavity for possible pneumothorax (see Notes.)

Technical Factors

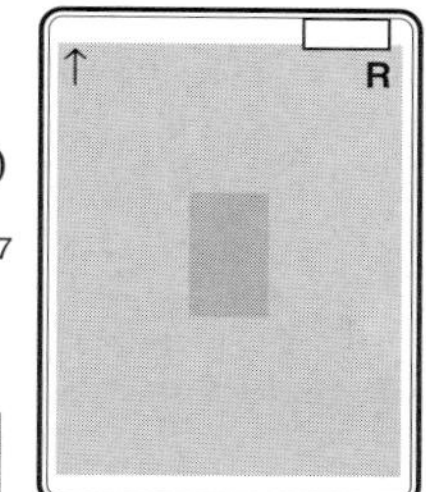

- Film size–14 x 17 in. (35 x 43 cm.), **crosswise**. (Crosswise with respect to patient.)
- Moving or stationary grid.
- 110-125 kVp range.
- Use decub marker (or arrow).
- Technique and dose:

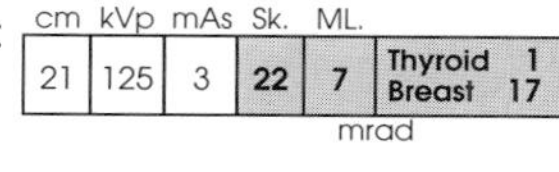

cm	kVp	mAs	Sk.	ML.	
21	125	3	22	7	Thyroid 1 Breast 17

mrad

Shielding: Place lead shield to shield gonads.

Patient Position

- Use a cardiac board on the cart or place a radiolucent pad under patient.
- Patient lying on right side for right lateral decubitus and on left side for left lateral decubitus (see Notes below).
- Raise both arms above head to clear lung field; place back of patient firmly against film holder. Secure stretcher to prevent patient from moving forward and possibly falling. Place pillow under head.
- Flex knees slightly and ensure that coronal plane is parallel to film with **no** body rotation.

Part Position

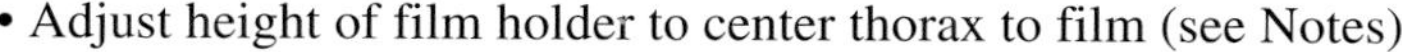

- Adjust height of film holder to center thorax to film (see Notes).
- Adjust patient and cart to center midsagittal plane and T7 to CR (top of film is about 2 in. or 5 cm above shoulders).

Central Ray

- CR horizontal, directed to center of film, to **level of T7,** 3 to 4 in. (8 to 10 cm) inferior to level of jugular notch**.** (A **horizontal** beam **must** be used to show air-fluid level or pneumothorax.)
- 72 in. (180 cm) SID.

Collimation: Collimate to area of lung fields (see Notes).

Respiration: Exposure made at end of **2nd full inspiration**.

Alternate Positioning: Some prefer that the head be 10° lower than the hips to reduce the apical lift caused by the shoulder, thereby allowing the entire chest to remain horizontal (requires support under hips).

Notes: Place appropriate marker to indicate which side of chest is up.

May be taken as a right or left lateral decubitus. For **possible fluid** in pleural cavity (pleural effusion), the suspected side should be **down**. Do **not** cut off that side of the chest.

For possible **small amounts of air** in pleural cavity (pneumothorax), the affected side should be **up** and care must be taken **not** to cut off this side of the chest.

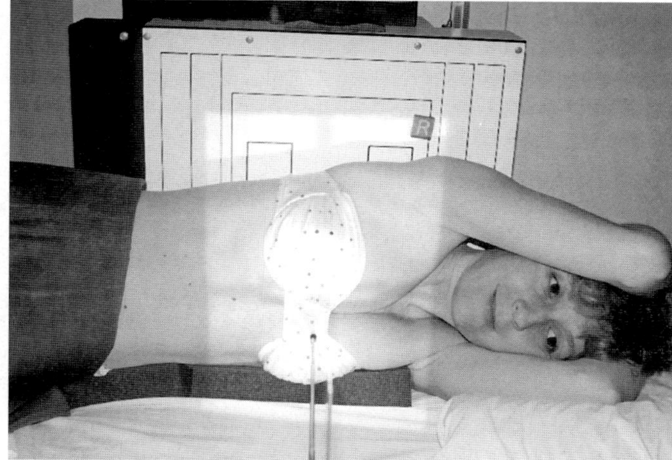

Fig. 2-71. Left lateral decubitus position (AP projection).

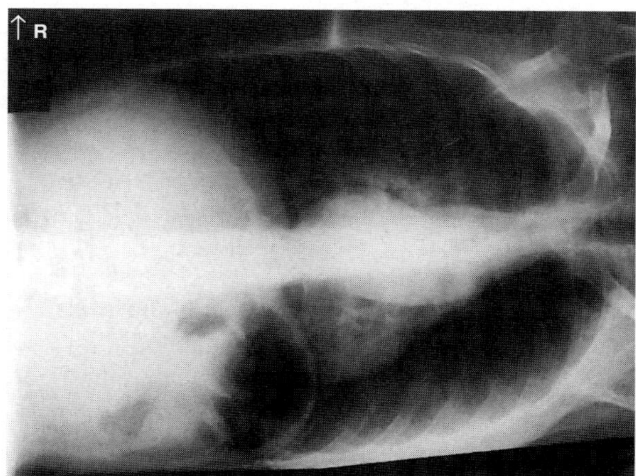

Fig. 2-72. Left lateral decubitus.

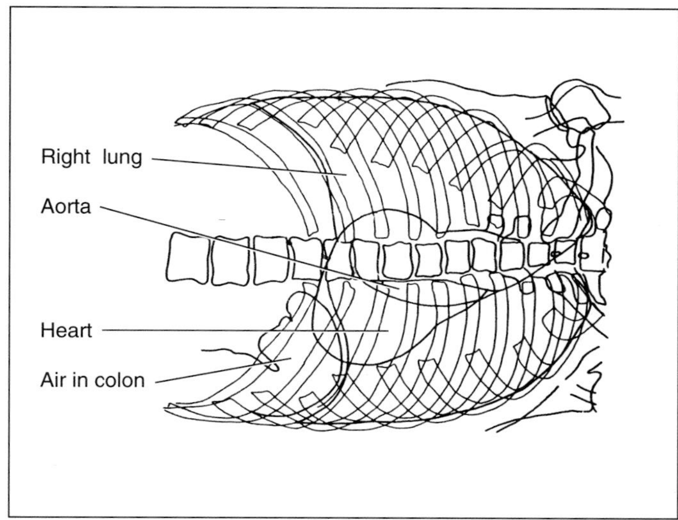

Fig. 2-73. Left lateral decubitus.

Evaluation Criteria

- **No rotation**, should have equal distance from vertebral column to the lateral borders of ribs on both sides; sternoclavicular joints should be same distance from the vertebral column.
- Entire lungs, including apices and both lateral borders, should be included.
- Center of collimation field should be to area of T7 on average-sized patients.
- Arms should not superimpose upper lungs.
- **No motion**; diaphragm and heart borders should appear sharp.
- Optimum contrast scale and exposure should result in **faint visualization of vertebrae and ribs through heart shadow.**

AP Lordotic Projection

Chest
Special
- AP supine or semierect
- Lateral decubitus (AP)
- **AP lordotic**
- Anterior oblique
- Posterior oblique

Structures Best Shown

Apices without clavicular superimposition and interlobar effusions. To rule out calcifications and masses beneath the clavicles.

Technical Factors

- Film size–14 x 17 in. (35 x 43 cm), lengthwise.
- Moving or stationary grid.
- 110-125 kVp range.
- Technique and dose:

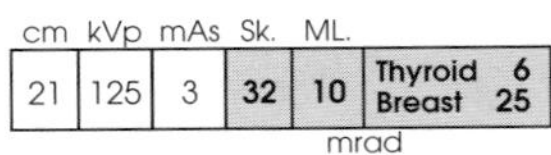

cm	kVp	mAs	Sk.	ML.	mrad
21	125	3	32	10	Thyroid 6 Breast 25

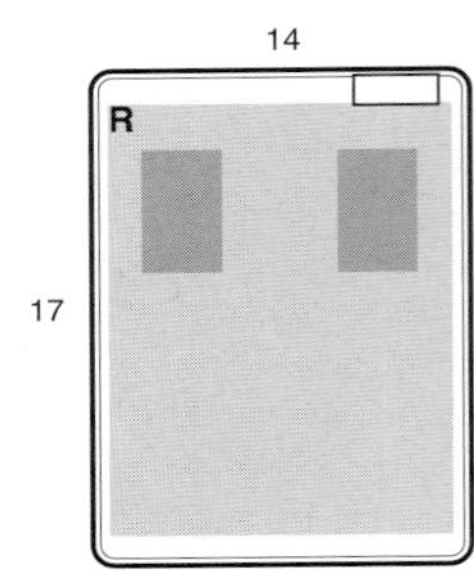

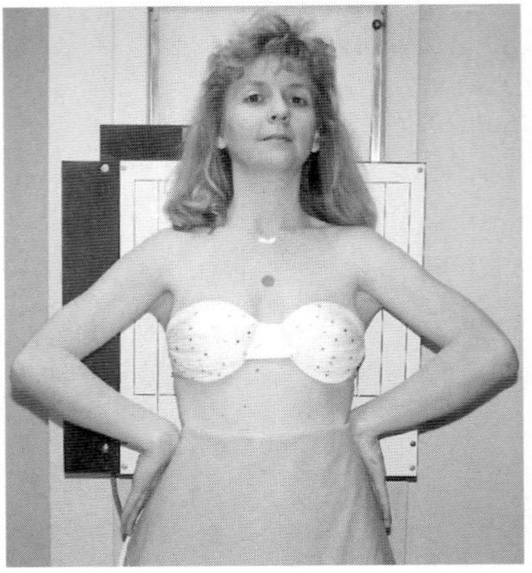

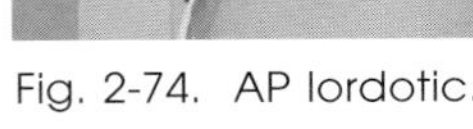
Fig. 2-74. AP lordotic.

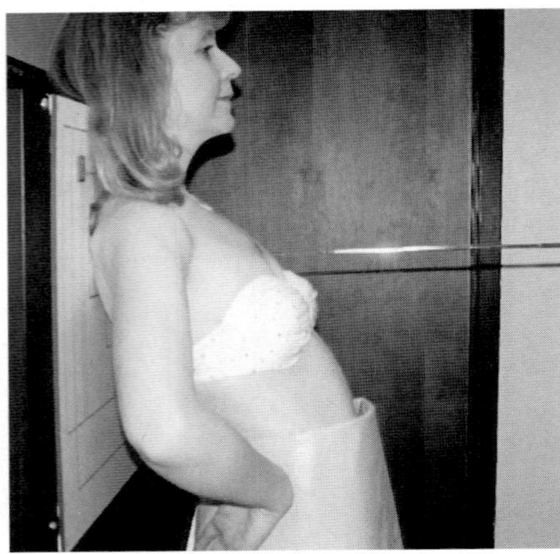
Fig. 2-75. AP lordotic.

Shielding: Secure lead shield around waist to shield gonads.

Patient Position

- Have patient stand about one foot away from film holder and lean back with shoulders, neck and back of head against film holder.
- Rest both hands on hips, palms out; roll shoulders forward.

Part Position

- Center midsagittal plane to CR and to centerline of film.
- Center cassette to CR. (Top of film should be about 3 or 4 in. [8 or 10 cm] above shoulders on average patient.)

Central Ray

- CR **perpendicular** to film, centered to **mid sternum** (3 to 4 in. or 9 cm below jugular notch).
- 72 in. (180 cm) SID.

Collimation: Collimate to area of lungs of interest.

Respiration: Exposure made at end of **2nd full inspiration.**

Exception (Fig. 2-76)

If patient is weak and unstable and/or is not able to assume the lordotic position, an **AP semi-axial projection** may be taken with the patient in an erect or supine position with back against table or film holder. Shoulders are rolled forward and arms positioned as for lordotic position.

The **CR** is directed **15 to 20° cephalad**, to the mid sternum.

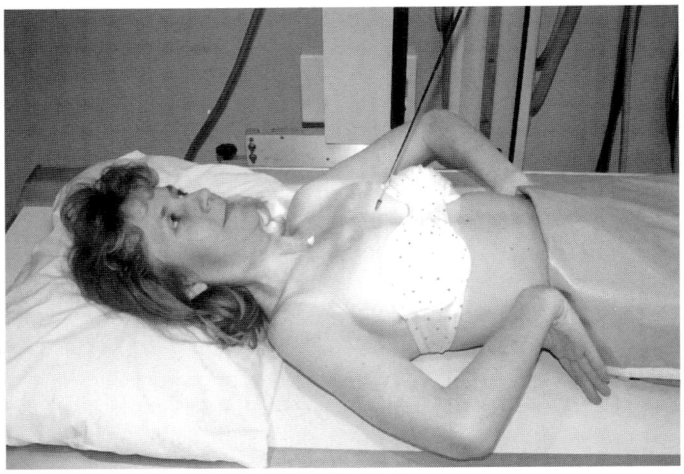

Fig. 2-76. Exception: Semi-axial AP.

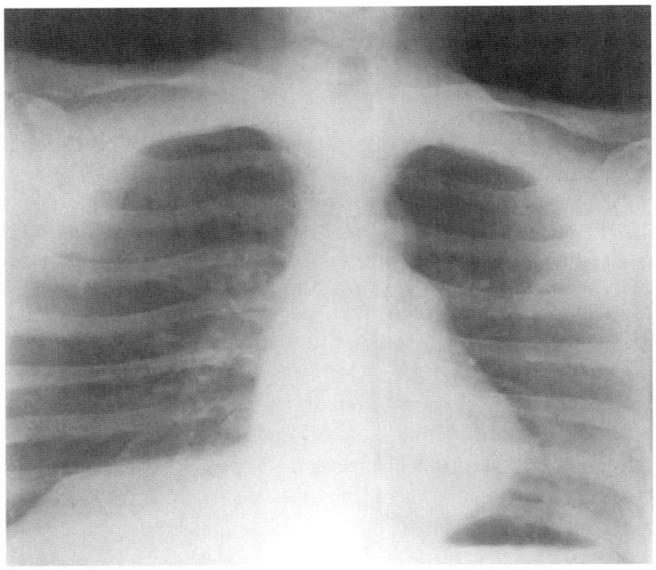

Fig. 2-77. AP lordotic.

Evaluation Criteria

- Clavicles should appear nearly horizontal and **above or superior to apices.**
- **No rotation**, sternal ends of the clavicles should be the same distance from vertebral column on each side. The lateral borders of the ribs on both sides should appear to be near equal distances from the vertebral column.
- Center of collimation field should be mid sternum with more collimation visible on the bottom.
- Ribs appear distorted with posterior ribs appearing nearly horizontal.
- **No motion**, diaphragm, heart and rib outlines should appear sharp.
- Optimum contrast scale and exposure should **visualize the faint vascular markings of lungs, especially in area of apices and upper lungs.**

Anterior Oblique Positions–RAO & LAO

Chest
Special
- AP supine or semierect
- Lateral decubitus (AP)
- AP lordotic
- **Anterior oblique**
- Posterior oblique

Technical Factors

- Film size–14 x 17 in. (35 x 43 cm), lengthwise.
- Moving or stationary grid.
- 110–125 kVp range
- Technique and dose:

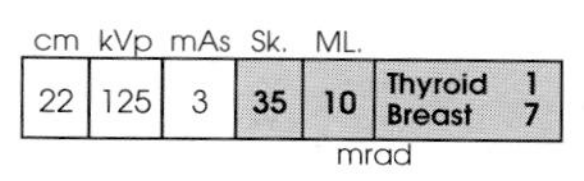

cm	kVp	mAs	Sk.	ML.		
22	125	3	35	10	Thyroid	1
					Breast	7
			mrad			

Structures Best Shown

LAO • Right lung, trachea, bony thorax with heart and aorta in front of vertebral column.

RAO • Left lung, trachea, bony thorax, with heart and aorta in front of vertebral column.

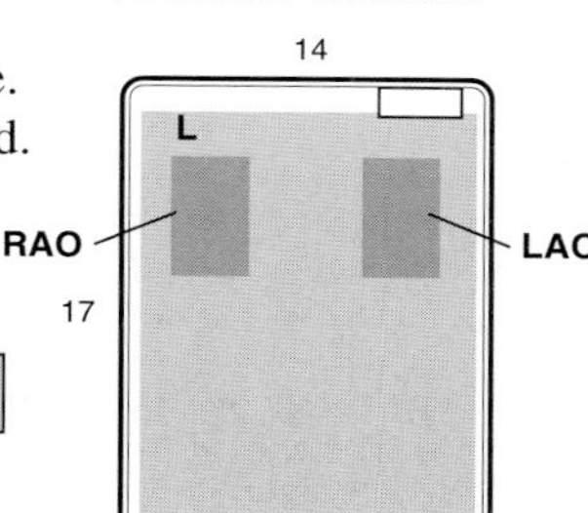

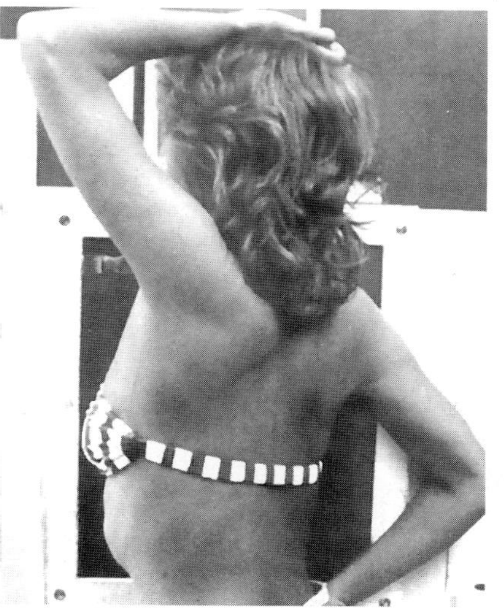
Fig. 2-78. 45° RAO position.

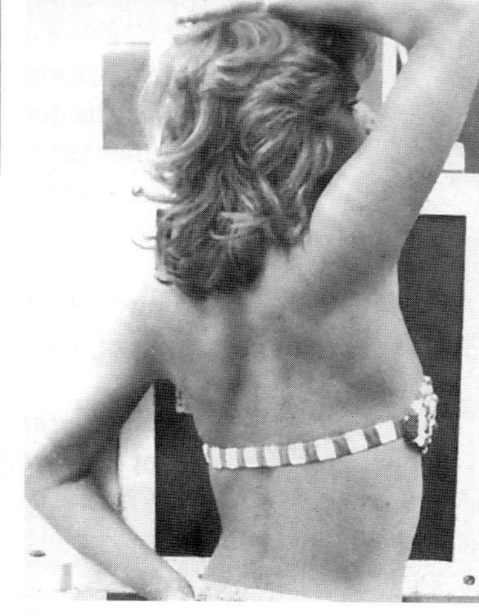
Fig. 2-79. 45° LAO position.

Shielding: Secure lead shield around waist to shield gonads.

Patient Position

- Patient erect, rotated 45° with left anterior shoulder against film holder for the LAO; and 45° with right anterior shoulder against film holder for the RAO. (See Notes for 60° LAO.)
- Flex the arm nearest film holder and place hand on hip, palm out.
- Raise opposite arm to clear lung field and rest hand on chest film holder for support, keeping arm raised as high as possible.
- Have patient look straight ahead; keep chin raised.

Part Position 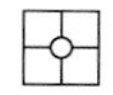

- As viewed from the x-ray tube, center the patient to CR and to film, with top of film about 1 inch (2.5 cm) above vertebra prominens.

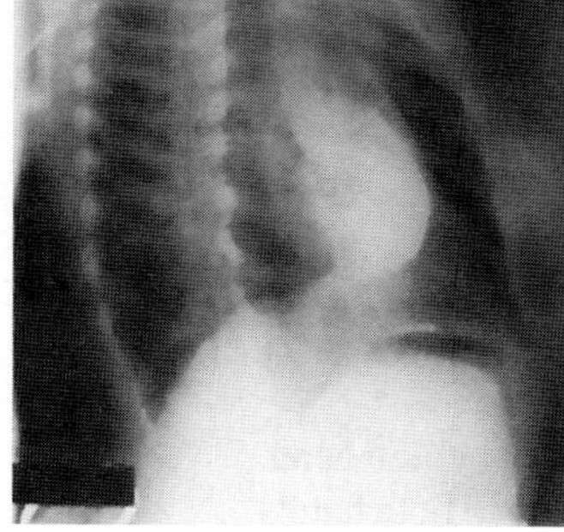
Fig. 2-80. 45° RAO position.

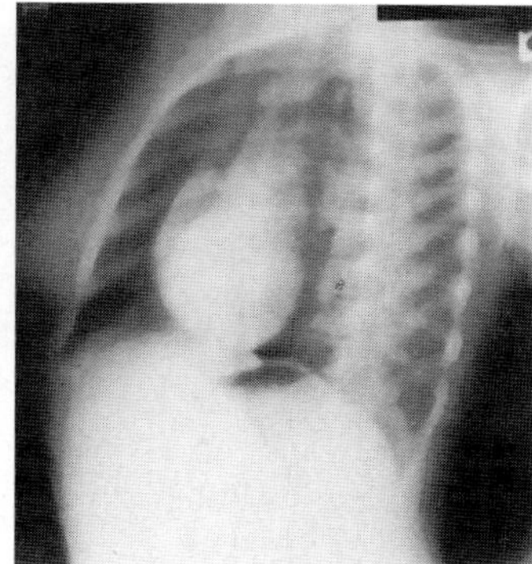
Fig. 2-81. 45° LAO position.

Central Ray

- CR perpendicular, directed **to level of T7**. (7 to 8 in. or 8 to 10 cm below level of vertebra prominens.)
- 72 in. (180 cm) SID.

Collimation: Collimate to area of lungs.

Respiration: Exposure made at end of **2nd full inspiration**.

Notes: For **anterior** obliques, the side of interest is generally the side **farthest** from the film. Thus the **RAO** will best visualize the **left** lung.

Certain positions for studies of the **heart** require an **LAO** with an increase in rotation to **60°**.

Less rotation (15 to 20°) may be of value for better visualization of the various areas of the lungs for possible pulmonary diseases.

Apex
Heart
Right costophrenic angle
Diaphragm

Fig. 2-82. 45° RAO position.

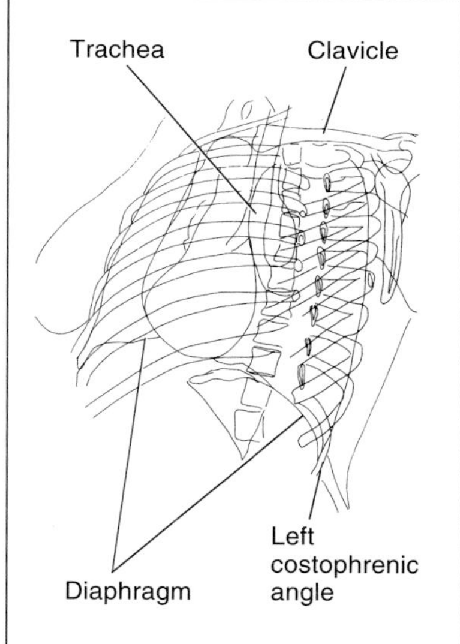

Fig. 2-83. 45° LAO position.

Evaluation Criteria

- To evaluate a 45° rotation, the distance from the outer margin of the ribs to the vertebral column on the side farthest from the film should be approximately twice the distance as the side closest to the film.
- Both lungs from the apices to the costophrenic angles should be included.
- Center of collimation field should be to the mid lung area at the level of T7.
- The air-filled trachea, great vessels and heart outlines are best visualized on a 60° LAO. (A 45° RAO will also visualize these structures.)
- **No motion**: The outline of the diaphragm and heart should appear sharp.
- Optimum exposure and sufficient, long contrast scale will result in **visualization of general vascular markings of the lungs and faint rib outlines throughout lungs, except through the most dense part of the heart shadow.**

Posterior Oblique Positions–RPO & LPO

Chest
Special
- AP supine or semierect
- Lateral decubitus (AP)
- AP lordotic
- Anterior oblique
- **Posterior oblique**

Exception: Posterior obliques can be taken if patient cannot assume an erect position for anterior obliques or if supplementary projections are required.

Structures Best Shown

LPO • Left lung, trachea, bony thorax, with heart and aorta in front of vertebral column.

RPO • Right lung, trachea, bony thorax, with heart and aorta in front of vertebral column.

Technical Factors

- Film size–14 x 17 in. (35 x 43 cm), lengthwise.
- Moving or stationary grid.
- 110-125 kVp range.
- Technique and dose:

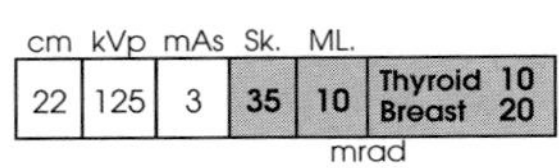

cm	kVp	mAs	Sk.	ML.	Thyroid / Breast (mrad)
22	125	3	35	10	Thyroid 10, Breast 20

14
R
LPO
RPO
17

Shielding: Secure lead shield around waist to shield gonads.

Patient Position (Erect)

- Patient erect, rotated 45° with right posterior shoulder against film holder for RPO, and 45° with left posterior shoulder against film holder for LPO.
- Raise the arm closest to the film and support behind head. Place other arm on hip with palm out, or place both hands on hips with palms out as shown.
- Have patient look straight ahead.

Recumbent Position

- If patient cannot stand or sit, posterior obliques on table can be taken.
- Place supports under head and under elevated hip and shoulder.

Part Position

- Top of film holder about 1 in. (2 cm) above vertebra prominens, or about 5 in. (12 cm) above level of jugular notch (2 in. or 5 cm above shoulders).
- Center thorax to CR and to film.

Central Ray

- CR perpendicular, to the **level of T7.**
- 72 in. (180 cm) SID.

Collimation: Collimate to area of lungs.

Respiration: Exposure made after **2nd full inspiration.**

Note: **Posterior** obliques best visualize the side **closest** to the film.

Posterior positions show the same anatomy as the opposite anterior oblique. Thus the LPO position corresponds to the RAO, and the RPO to the LAO.

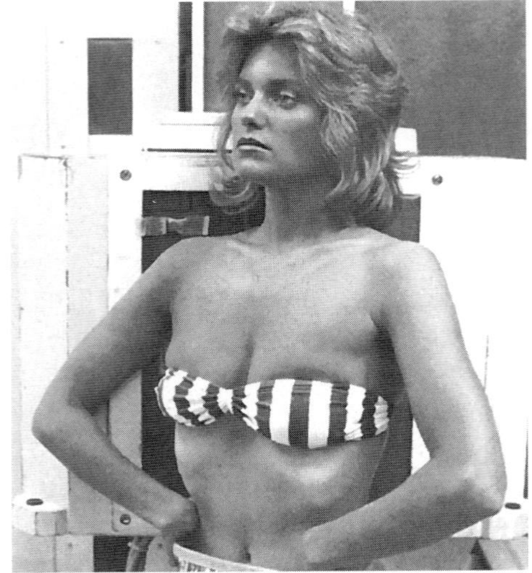

Fig. 2-84. RPO 45° position.

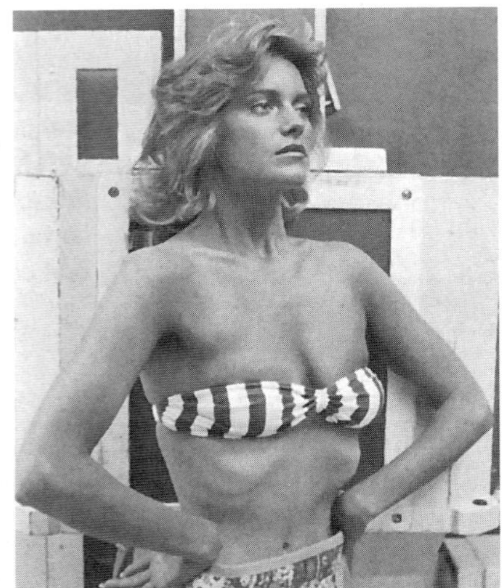

Fig. 2-85. LPO 45° position.

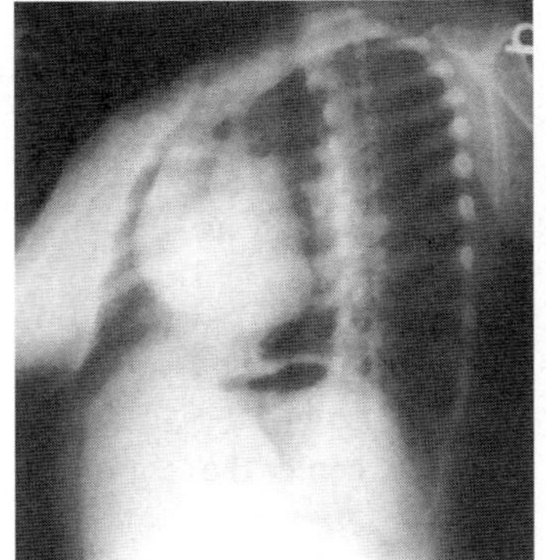

Fig. 2-86. 45° RPO position.

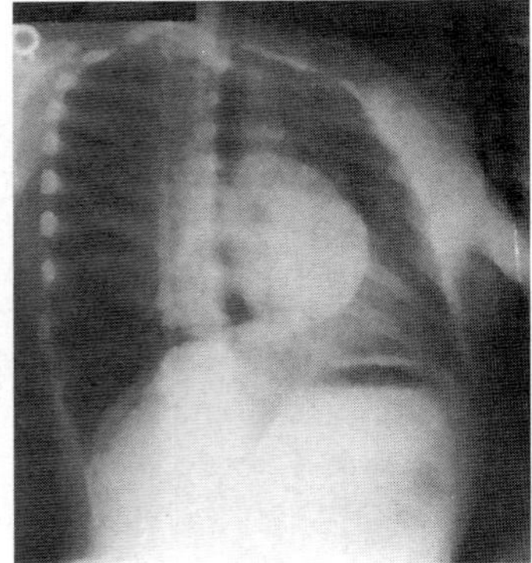

Fig. 2-87. 45° LPO position.

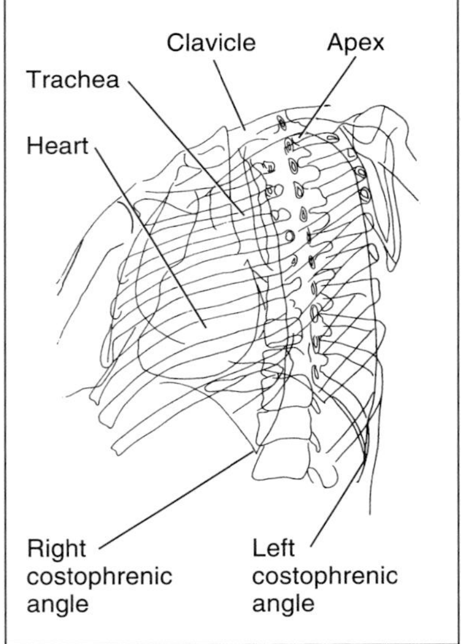

Fig. 2-88. 45° RPO position.

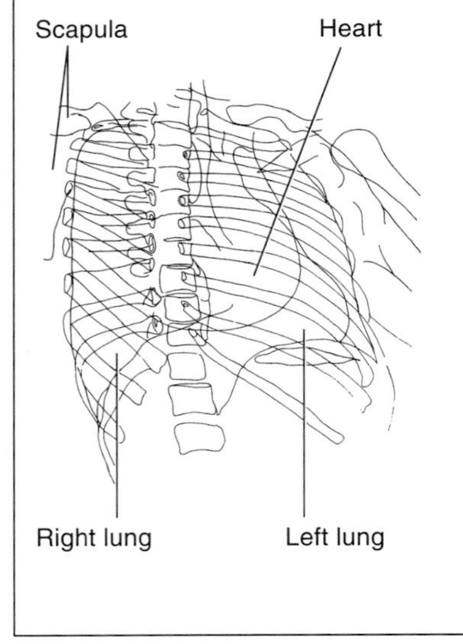

Fig. 2-89. 45° LPO position.

Evaluation Criteria

Positioning criteria are similar to those of anterior obliques described on previous page. However, due to increased magnification of anterior diaphragm, lung fields usually appear shorter on posterior obliques compared with anterior obliques. The heart and great vessels also appear larger on posterior obliques because they are farther from the film.

Lateral Position

Upper airway
Basic
• **Lateral**
• AP

Structures Best Shown

Air-filled larynx and trachea, the region of thyroid and thymus glands and upper esophagus if opaque.

Technical Factors

- Film size–10 x 12 in. (24 x 30 cm), lengthwise.
- Moving or stationary grid.
- 80±6 kVp range (see Note below).
- Technique and dose:

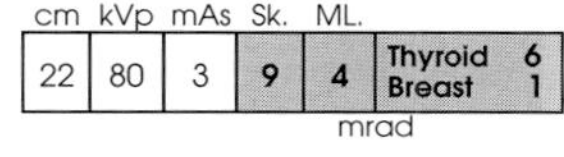

cm	kVp	mAs	Sk.	ML.	
22	80	3	9	4	Thyroid 6 Breast 1
			mrad		

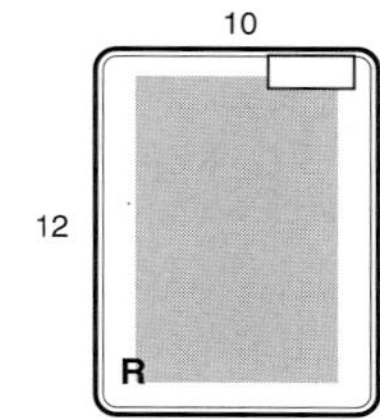

Shielding: Secure lead shield around waist to shield gonads.

Patient Position

- Upright if possible, seated or standing in a lateral position (may be taken in R or L lateral, and may be taken recumbent tabletop if necessary).

Part Position

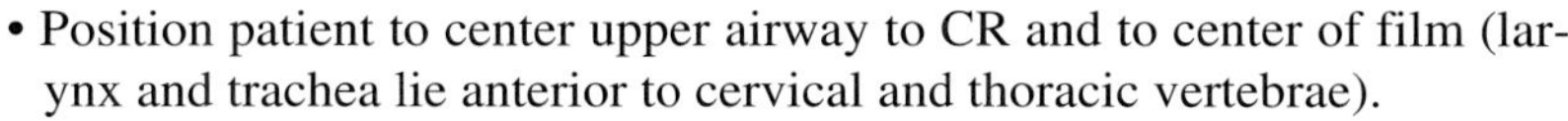

- Position patient to center upper airway to CR and to center of film (larynx and trachea lie anterior to cervical and thoracic vertebrae).
- Rotate shoulders posteriorly with arms hanging down clasping hands behind back.
- Raise chin slightly and have patient look directly ahead.
- Adjust film height to place top of film at level of EAM, (external auditory meatus), which is the opening of the external ear canal. (See Note if area of primary interest is the trachea rather than the larynx.)

Central Ray

- CR perpendicular to center of film **at level of C6 or C7**, midway between the laryngeal prominence of the thyroid cartilage and the jugular notch. (See Notes for lower centering if trachea is area of primary interest.)
- 72 in. (180 cm) SID if possible to minimize magnification.

Collimation: Collimate to area of interest.

Respiration: Exposure should be made **during a slow deep inspiration** to ensure filling trachea and upper airway with air.

Notes:

Exposure: Exposure for the lateral of the upper airway in the neck region should be that of a soft tissue lateral. If the trachea is the primary area of interest, the exposure should be approximately that of a lateral chest.

Centering for trachea area: If the primary interest area is the trachea, the film and CR should be lowered about 1.5 to 2 in. (4 to 5 cm) to center the entire trachea (C6 to T4 or T5) to the film, which places the CR at the jugular notch.

Evaluation Criteria

- The larynx and trachea should be filled with air and well visualized. Centering for the **upper airway** (larynx and proximal trachea) should include the EAM at the upper border of the film and T3 or T4 on the lower border. If the **trachea** is the primary area of interest, the centering should be lower to center the area of the trachea (C6 to T4 or T5) to the film.
- The shadows of the shoulders should primarily be posterior to and not superimpose the area of the trachea.
- Collimation borders should appear on both sides with ideally only minimal (⅛ in. or less) borders on top and bottom. The center of the collimation field should be to the CR location as described above.
- Optimum exposure includes a soft-tissue technique wherein the air-filled larynx and upper trachea are not overexposed. The cervical vertebrae will appear underexposed.

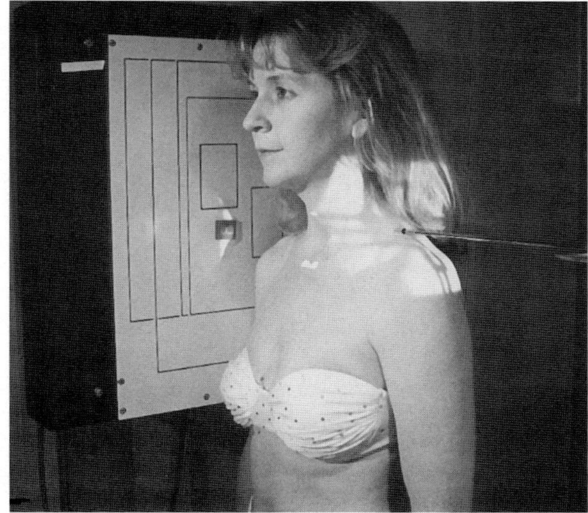

Fig. 2-90. Right lateral position–Upper airway.

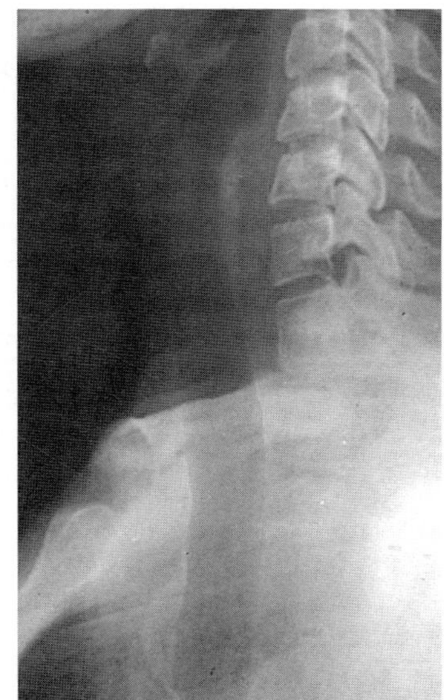

Fig. 2-91. Lateral –Upper airway.

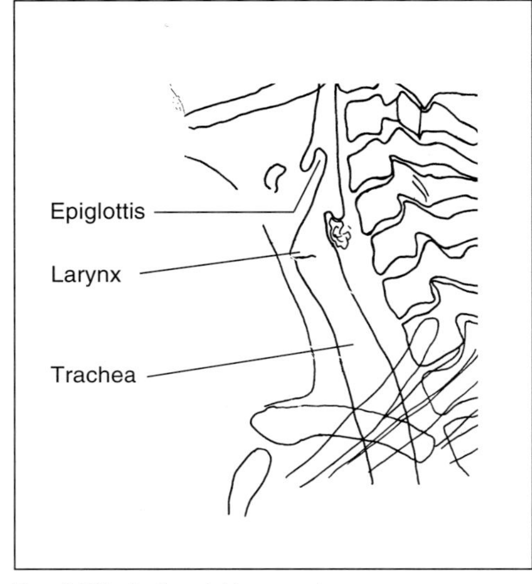

Fig. 2-92. Lateral–Upper airway.

AP Projection

Upper airway
Basic
• Lateral
• **AP**

Structures Best Shown

Air-filled larynx and trachea, the region of thyroid and thymus glands and upper esophagus if opacified.

Technical Factors

- Film size–10 x 12 in. (24 x 30 cm), lengthwise.
- Moving or stationary grid.
- 80±6 kVp range.
- Technique and dose:

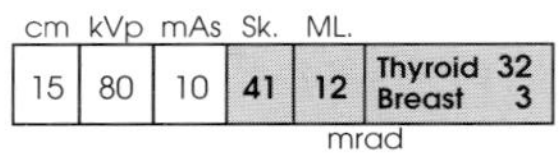

cm	kVp	mAs	Sk.	ML.	mrad
15	80	10	41	12	Thyroid 32 Breast 3

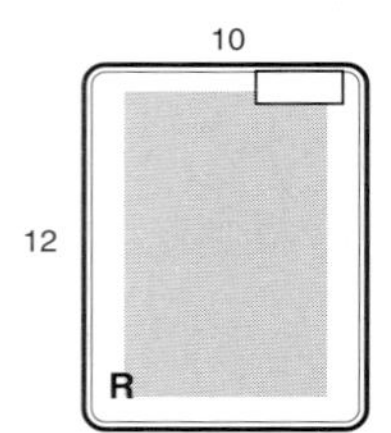

Shielding: Secure lead shield around waist to protect gonads.

Patient Position

- Upright if possible, seated or standing with back of head and shoulders against film holder. (May be taken recumbent tabletop if necessary.)

Part Position 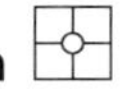

- Align midsagittal plane to CR and to midline of grid or table.
- Raise chin so that **acanthiomeatal line is perpendicular to the film** (line from the acanthion or area directly under the nose and the meatus or EAM); have patient look directly ahead.
- Adjust the film height to place top of film about 1 or 1½ in. (3 to 4 cm) below EAM. (See Note for explanation of centering.)

Central Ray

- CR perpendicular to center of film **at level of T1-2**, about 1 in. (2.5 cm) above the jugular notch.
- Minimum 40 in. (102 cm) SID.

Collimation: Collimate to area of interest.

Respiration: Exposure should be made **during a slow deep inspiration** to ensure filling trachea and upper airway with air.

Notes:

Exposure: Exposure for this AP projection should be approximately that of an AP of the cervical and/or thoracic spine.

Centering for upper airway and trachea: Centering for this AP projection is slightly lower than for the lateral position described on the previous page because the most proximal larynx area is not visualized on the AP due to the superimposed base of skull and mandible. Therefore, more of the trachea can be visualized.

Evaluation Criteria:

- The larynx and trachea should be filled with air and well visualized. (See Notes for centering explanation.) The area of the proximal cervical vertebrae (the lower margin of the shadow of the superimposed mandible and base of skull) to the mid thoracic region should be included.
- There should be no rotation as evidenced by the symmetrical appearance of the sternoclavicular joints.
- Collimation borders should appear on both sides with ideally only minimal (1/8 in. or less) borders on top and bottom. The center of the collimation field should be to area of T1-2.
- Optimum exposure should be dark enough to visualize the air-filled trachea through the cervical and thoracic vertebrae.

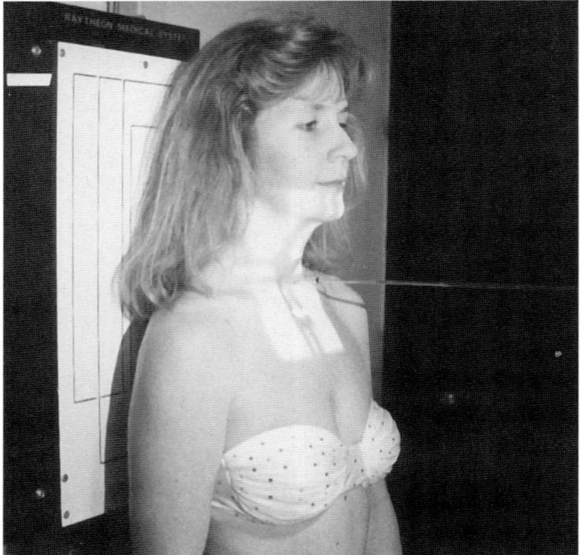

Fig. 2-93. AP–Upper airway.

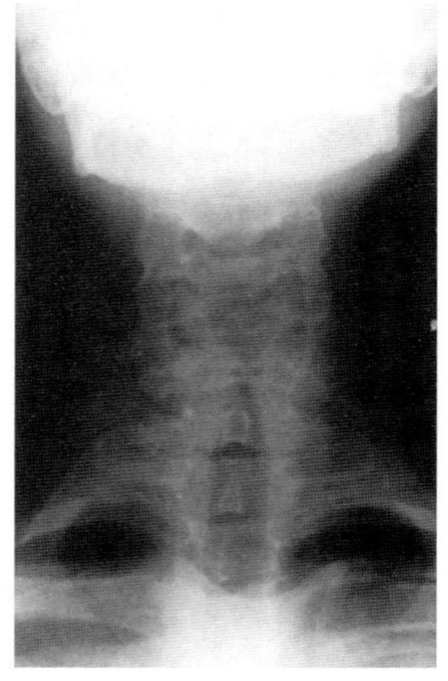

Fig. 2-94. AP–Upper airway.

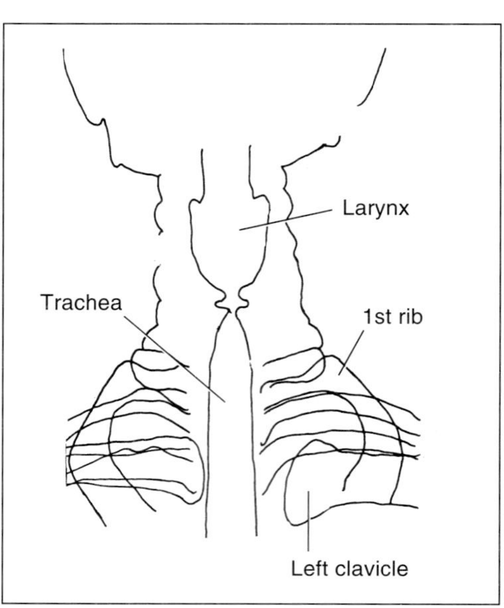

Fig. 2-95. AP–Upper airway.

Appendix–CR Location Chest Positioning Method*

A sample of a portion of the data sheet used to determine accurate CR locations for chest positioning with corresponding accurate collimation is shown below. Included are actual lung measurements from radiographs which are compared with the centering estimates used in positioning for the chest radiographs using the hand spread method. (The printed ruler on this page can be used to determine hand spread measurements.)

It should be noted that measurements "C" and "A" are greater than the corresponding measurements "D" or "B" on the radiograph because of the curvature of the thorax. This difference will be greater on older patients, with spinal curvature (kyphosis) and for those with more of a barrel shaped chest.

Note also in the total sample of 130 patients, the average height of the lungs was **10.4 in.** and the average width was **11.7 in.** (average width is 1.3 in. greater than height). It is also interesting to note that only 13 patients had lung height measurements greater than the width, and these were smaller patients weighing only an average of 131 lbs.

However, the 30 patients in this sample who weighed over 200 lbs. had an average lung width of **13 in.** Therefore, for most of these patients the film should be placed crosswise to prevent side cut-off. The average lung height on these larger patients was only **10.7 in.,** indicating that a 14 x 17 in. film can safely be placed crosswise without danger of lung cutoff on top or bottom.

It should be remembered, however, that these are averages and there are exceptions, such as larger, well-developed, athletic patients, for whom the height may be greater than the width.

Chest CR and Lung Measurement Study

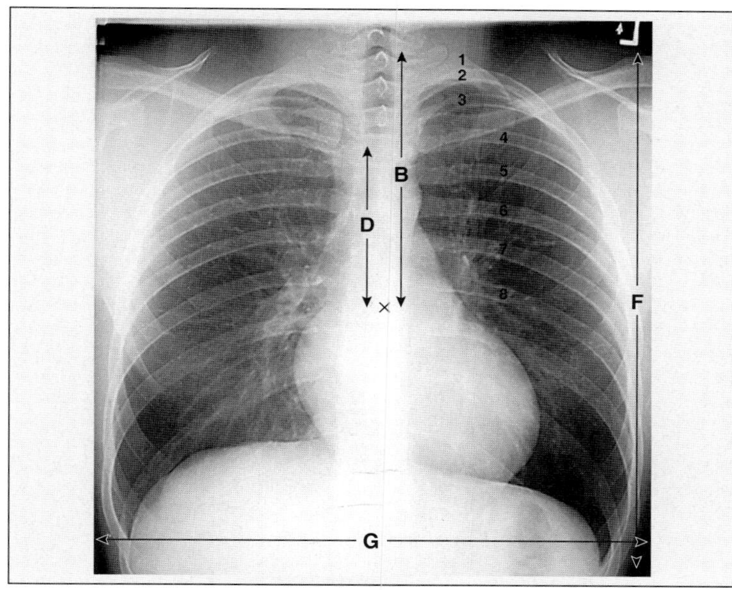

Fig. 2-96. Larger-than-average male, CR=T8.
Actual lung measurements: width (G) =13 in.
height (F)=12.5 in.

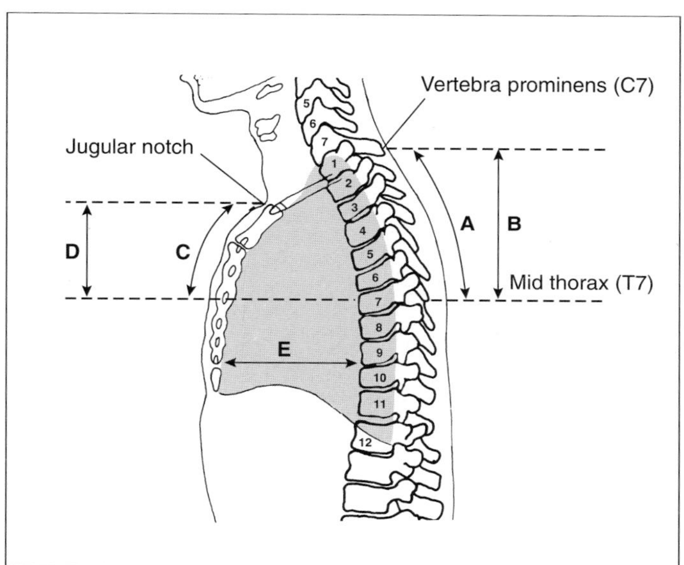

Fig. 2-97. CR and landmarks (average patient).

Patient Data					Centering Est. (Hand Spread Method)		Measurements of Lung Dimensions (from film)					Upper Collimation (from film)	Critique Remarks
					AP & Lat.	PA			Height	Depth	Width		
Case Number	Height	Weight	Age	M/F	C	A	D	B	F	E	G	H	
†Averages:	5'8"	162 lbs.	48	±50/50	3-4"	M=8" F=7"	2.7"	4.8"	10.4"	8.5"	11.7"	.98"	
(30 patients +200 lbs)		+200 lbs.							10.7"		13"		requires film crosswise
(13 patients F>G)		131 lbs.							11.4"		10.5"		height greater than width

†Total sample 130 adult patients

*Note: This CR location chest positioning method and the chest measurements quoted in this chapter were determined by the author in cooperation with Kathy Martensen, R.T., University of Iowa and Karen Brown, R.T., William Gize and Tonya Morisette, St. Joseph's Hospital, Phoenix, AZ.

Radiographs for Critique

Each of these chest radiographs demonstrates some errors which required a repeat. These as well as additional critique chest radiographs are also available as part of the accompanying lecture slide set and instructor's manual.

Questions and answers concerning each of these chest radiographs as to specific positioning errors and how they can be corrected and prevented are included in the student workbook/lab manuals which accompany this textbook.

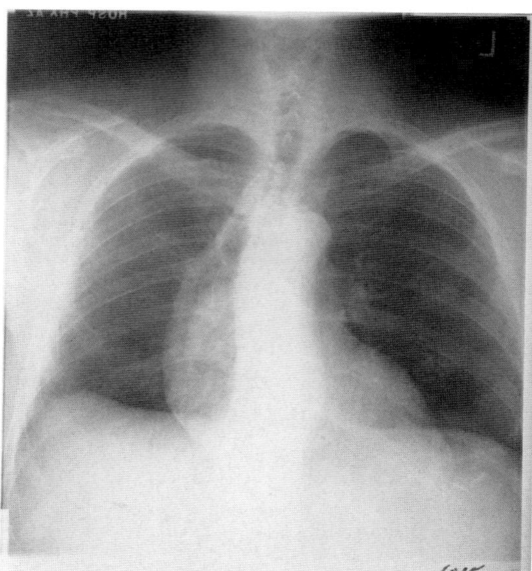

Fig. C2-98. PA chest, 43-year-old male.

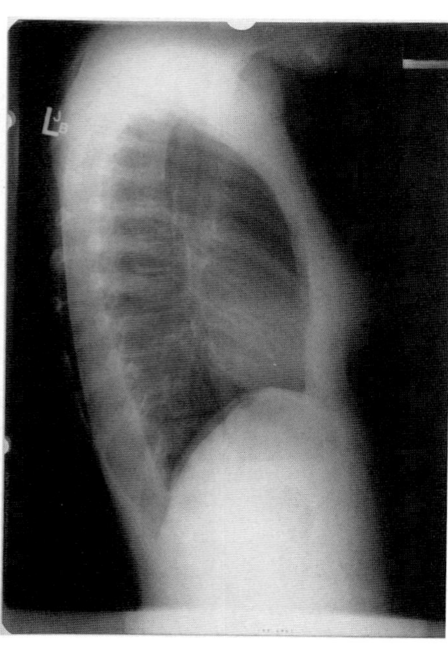

Fig. C2-99. Lateral chest, young female.

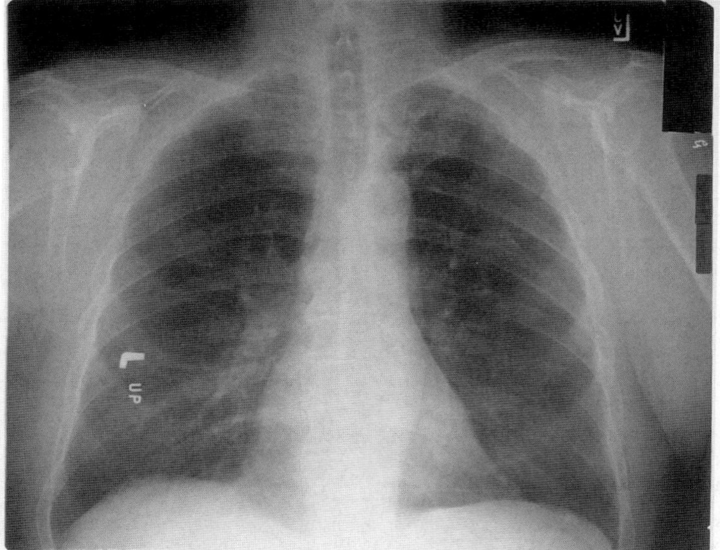

Fig. C2-100. PA chest, 74-year-old male

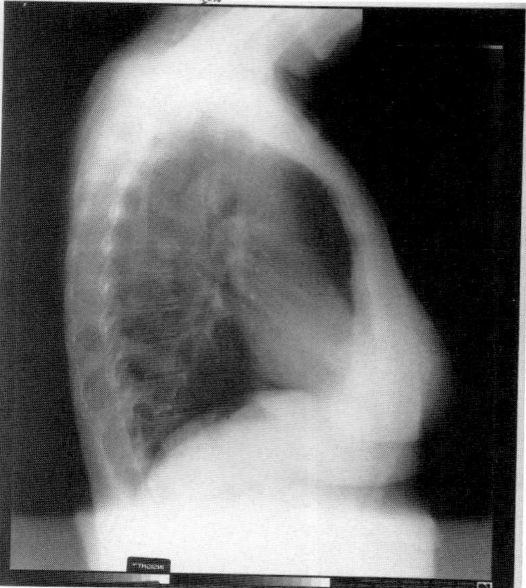

Fig. C2-101. Lateral chest, female.

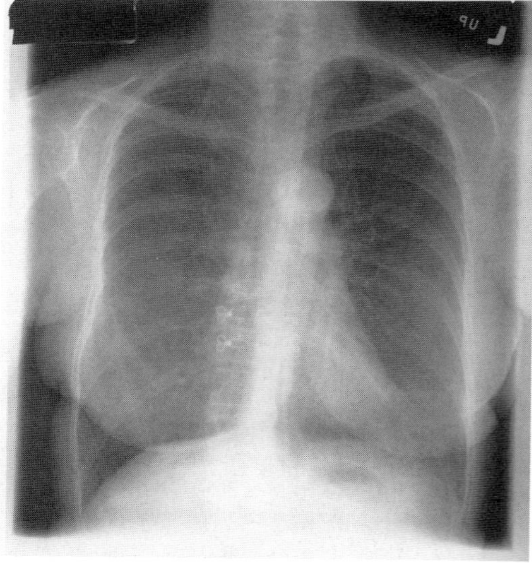

Fig. C2-102. PA chest, 73-year-old female.

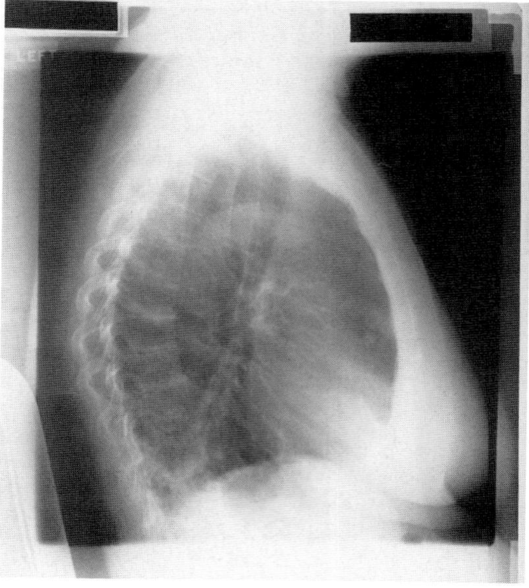

Fig. C2-103. Lateral chest, taken in wheelchair.

CHAPTER 3

Abdomen

CONTRIBUTIONS BY:
John P. Lampignano, M Ed, RT (R)
Kathy Martensen, BS, RT (R)
Barry T. Anthony, RT (R)

CONTENTS

Radiographic Anatomy

Abdominal radiography **86**

Acute abdominal series **86**

Abdominal muscles **86**

Abdominal organ systems **86**

Digestive system
(stomach, small intestine, large intestine) **86**

Accessory digestive organs
(pancreas, liver, gallbladder, spleen) **88**

Urinary system **88**

Abdominal cavity
(peritoneum, mesentery, omentum) **89**

Anatomical relationships
(retroperitoneal and infraperitoneal organs) **89**

Quadrants and regions **90**

Topographic landmarks **91**

Radiographic Positioning

Positioning considerations **92**

Survey information **93**

Basic and special projections **93**

Abdomen (basic):
- AP supine (KUB) **94**

Abdomen (special):
- PA prone **95**
- Lateral decubitus AP **96**
- Erect AP **97**
- Dorsal decubitus (lateral) **98**

Acute abdomen:
- Three-way series **99**
  or two-way series **99**

Radiographs for critique **100**

Radiographic Anatomy

ABDOMINAL RADIOGRAPHY

This chapter covers the anatomy and positioning for what are sometimes called "plain" films of the abdomen. The most common is an AP supine abdomen, also sometimes called a KUB (Kidneys, Ureters and Bladder). These are taken without injection of contrast media.

Plain radiographs of the abdomen (KUB) are commonly taken prior to performing abdominal examinations utilizing contrast media to rule out certain pathologies.

Acute Abdominal Series: Certain acute or emergency conditions of the abdomen may develop from conditions such as bowel obstruction, perforations involving free air (air outside the digestive tract) or fluid in the abdomen, or a possible intra-abdominal mass. These acute or emergency conditions require what is commonly called an "acute abdominal series," or a "two-way" or "three-way abdomen" series, wherein several abdominal radiographs are taken in different positions to demonstrate air fluid levels and/or free air within the abdominal cavity.

Abdominal radiography requires an understanding of anatomy and relationships of the organs and structures within the abdominopelvic cavity.

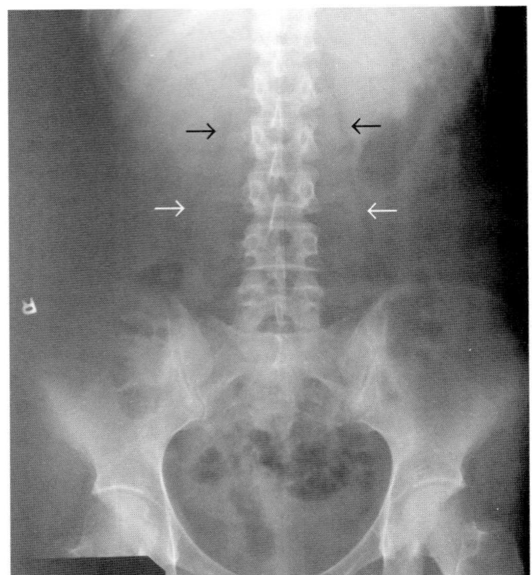
Fig. 3-1. AP abdomen (KUB).

Abdominal Muscles

There are many muscles associated with the abdominopelvic cavity. The three that are the most important in abdominal radiography are the diaphragm and the right and left psoas *(so´es)* major.

The **diaphragm** is an umbrella-shaped muscle separating the abdominal cavity from the thoracic cavity. The diaphragm must be perfectly motionless during radiography of either the abdomen or the chest. Motion of the patient's diaphragm can be stopped by providing appropriate breathing instructions.

The two **psoas major** muscles are located on either side of the lumbar vertebral column. The lateral borders of these two muscles should be visible on a diagnostic abdominal radiograph when correct exposure factors are utilized (see arrows, Fig. 3-1).

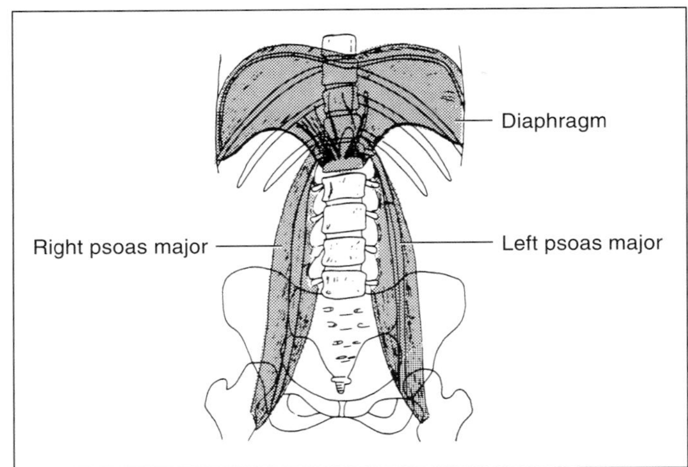

Fig. 3-2. Abdominal muscles.

ABDOMINAL ORGAN SYSTEMS

The various organ systems found within the abdominopelvic cavity are presented only briefly in this chapter. Each of these systems is described in greater detail in later chapters devoted to those specific systems.

Digestive System

The digestive system along with its accessory organs (the liver, gallbladder and pancreas) fill much of the abdominal cavity. The pancreas is located posterior to the stomach and not well visualized on this drawing.

The organs of the digestive system are listed as follows:

- Oral cavity
- Pharynx
- Esophagus
- Stomach
- Small intestine
- Large intestine

Mouth, Pharynx and Esophagus: The digestive system begins at the **mouth** and continues as the **pharynx** and **esophagus.** The esophagus is located in the mediastinum of the thoracic cavity.

Digestive Organs within Abdominal Cavity: The digestive organs within the abdominal cavity are the **stomach, small intestine** and **large intestine**. Each of these organs is described briefly in this chapter, with detailed specific anatomy covered in later chapters along with positioning for each of these gastrointestinal tract systems.

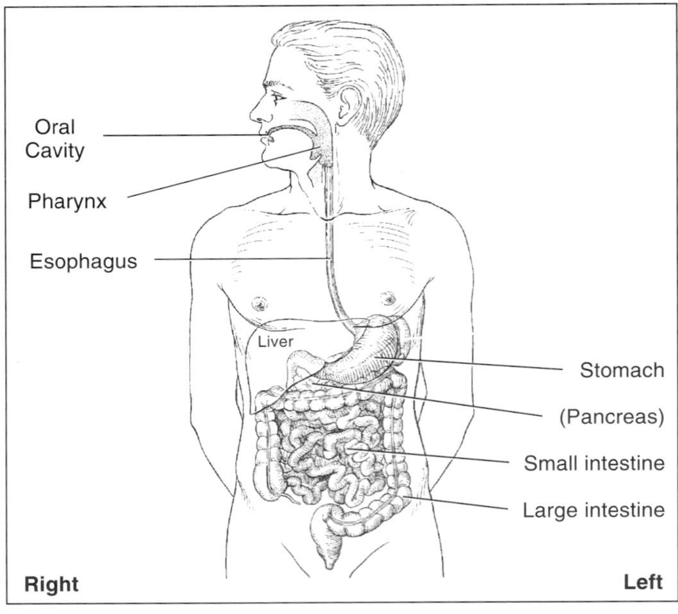

Fig. 3-3. Digestive tract.

Stomach

The stomach is the first organ of the digestive system located within the abdominal cavity. The stomach is an expandable reservoir for swallowed food and fluids. The size and shape of the stomach is highly variable depending on the volume of its contents and on the body habitus.

"Gastro" is a common term for stomach (Greek word "gaster" means stomach). Thus the term GastroIntestinal (GI) tract or system describes the entire digestive system starting with the stomach and continuing through the small and large intestines.

Small Intestine

The small intestine continues from the stomach as a long, tubelike convoluted structure about 15 to 18 feet (4.5 to 5.5 meters) in length. The three parts of the small intestine as labeled in Figs. 3-4 and 3-5 are:

A. Duodenum *(doo″ o-de′ num)*
B. Jejunum *(je-joo′ num)*
C. Ileum *(il′ eum)*

Duodenum (A): The first portion of the small intestine, the duodenum, is the shortest, but the widest in diameter of the three segments. It is about 10 inches or 25 cm in length. When filled with contrast medium, the duodenum looks like the letter C. The proximal portion of the duodenum is called the **duodenal bulb** or cap. It has a certain characteristic shape, usually well seen on barium studies of the upper GI tract. Ducts from the liver, gallbladder and pancreas drain into the duodenum.

Jejunum and Ileum (B and C): The remainder of the small bowel lies in the central and lower abdomen. The first two-fifths following the duodenum is termed the **jejunum**, while the distal three-fifths is called the **ileum**. (Note the spelling of the ileum as compared to the superior portion of the hip bone, which is spelled ilium.)

The orifice (valve) between the distal ileum and the cecum portion of the large intestine is called the **ileocecal valve**.

Radiograph of Stomach and Small Intestine (Fig. 3-5)

Air is seldom seen filling the entire stomach or small intestine on a plain abdominal radiograph of a healthy, ambulatory adult. The radiograph in Fig. 3-5 visualizes the stomach, small intestine and proximal large intestine because they are filled with radiopaque barium sulfate. Note the long convoluted loops of the three labeled parts of the small intestine located in the mid and lower abdomen.

Large Intestine

The large intestine begins in the right lower quadrant at the junction with the small intestine at the **ileocecal valve**. That portion of the large intestine below the ileocecal valve is a saclike area termed the **cecum**. The **appendix** is attached to the posteromedial aspect of the cecum. The vertical portion of the large bowel above the cecum is the **ascending colon**, which joins the **transverse colon** at the **right colic** (*kol′ ik*, referring to colon) **flexure**. The transverse colon joins the **descending colon** at the **left colic flexure**. Alternate names for the two colic flexures are **hepatic** and **splenic** flexures based on their proximity to the liver and spleen respectively.

The descending colon continues as the S-shaped **sigmoid colon** in the lower left abdomen. The **rectum** is the final 6 in. (15 cm) of the large intestine. The rectum ends at the **anus**, the sphincter muscle at the terminal opening of the large intestine.

As will be seen in body habitus drawings, the shape and location of the large intestine varies greatly with the transverse colon located high on wide hypersthenic types, and low in the abdomen on slender hyposthenic and asthenic types. This will be demonstrated in Chapters 14 and 15 of the upper and lower GI systems.

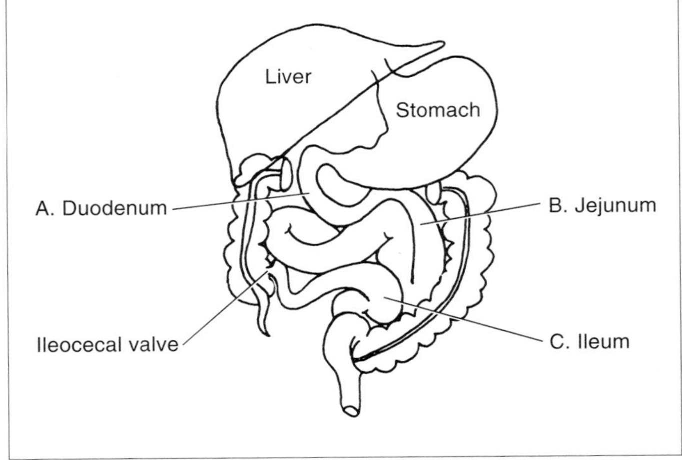

Fig. 3-4. Stomach and small intestine.

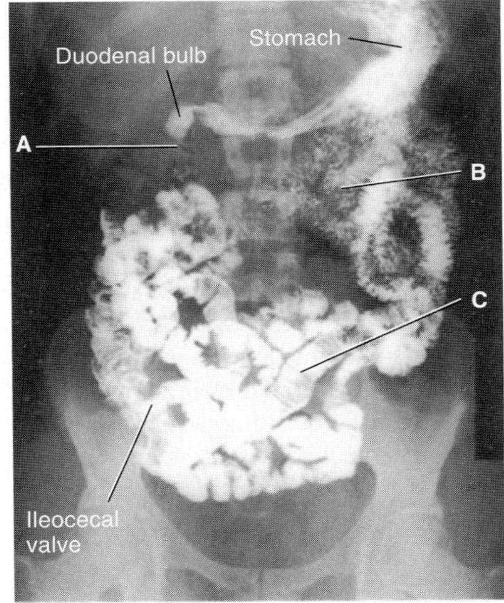

Fig. 3-5. Stomach and small intestine radiograph.

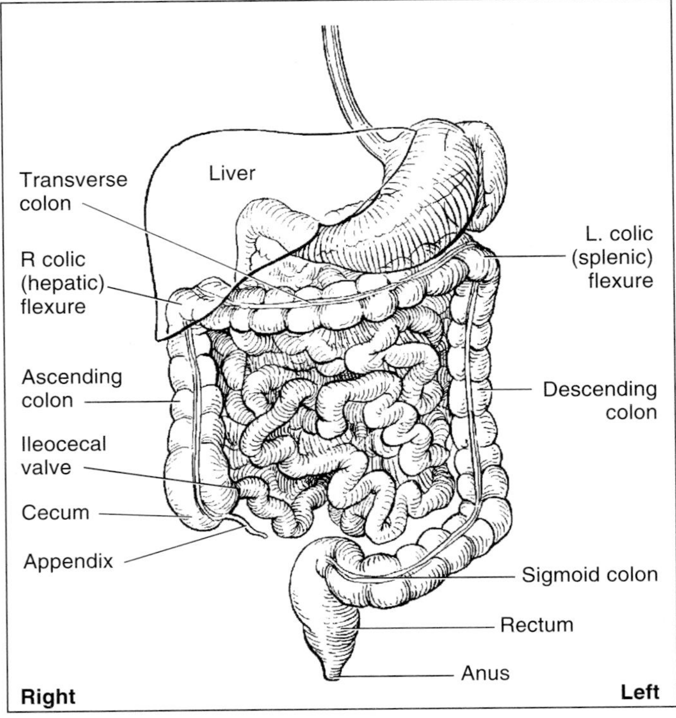

Fig. 3-6. Large intestine.

Accessory Digestive Organs

Three accessory organs of digestion, also located in the abdominal cavity, are: (1) Pancreas, (2) Liver, (3) Gallbladder.

(1) Pancreas: The pancreas, which is not seen on a plain abdominal radiograph, is an elongated gland located **posterior to the stomach** and near the posterior abdominal wall, between the duodenum and the spleen. The average length is about 6 inches (12.5 cm). Its head is nestled in the C-loop of the duodenum, and the body and tail of the pancreas extend toward the upper left abdomen.

The pancreas is part of the **endocrine** (internal) **secretion system**, and also part of the **exocrine** (external) **system**. The endocrine portion of the pancreas produces certain essential hormones such as insulin, which aids in controlling the blood-sugar level of the body. As part of its exocrine functions, it produces large amounts (up to 1½ qt. or 1500 ml daily) of digestive juices that move to the duodenum through a main pancreatic duct as needed for digestion.

(2) Liver: The liver is the largest solid organ in the body, occupying most of the **right upper quadrant**. One of its numerous functions is the production of bile, which assists in the digestion of fats. If bile is not needed for digestion, it is stored and concentrated for future use in the gallbladder.

(3) Gallbladder: The gallbladder is a pear-shaped sac located **below the liver**. The primary functions of the gallbladder are to store and concentrate bile, and to contract and release bile when stimulated by an appropriate hormone. The gallbladder in most cases cannot be visualized without contrast media as described in Chapter 16.

A CT cross-sectional image (Fig. 3-8) through the level of L1-2 (1st or 2nd lumbar vertebra) demonstrates anatomical relationships of abdominal structures, including the accessory digestive organs, in relationship to the stomach and duodenum.

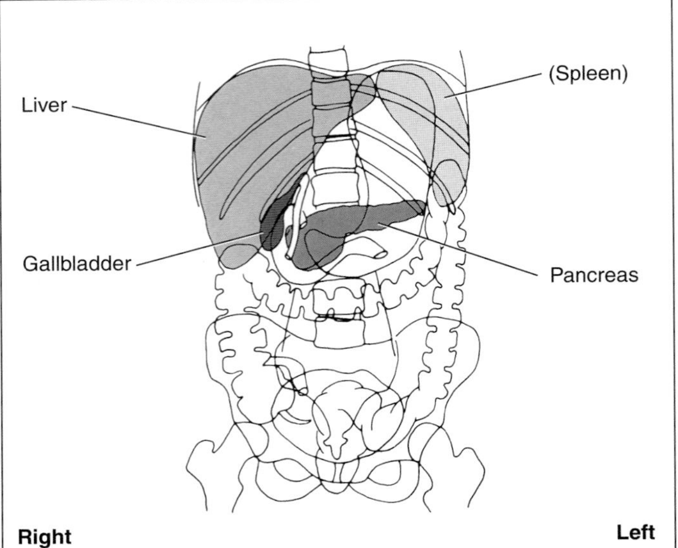

Fig. 3-7. Accessory organs of digestion and spleen.

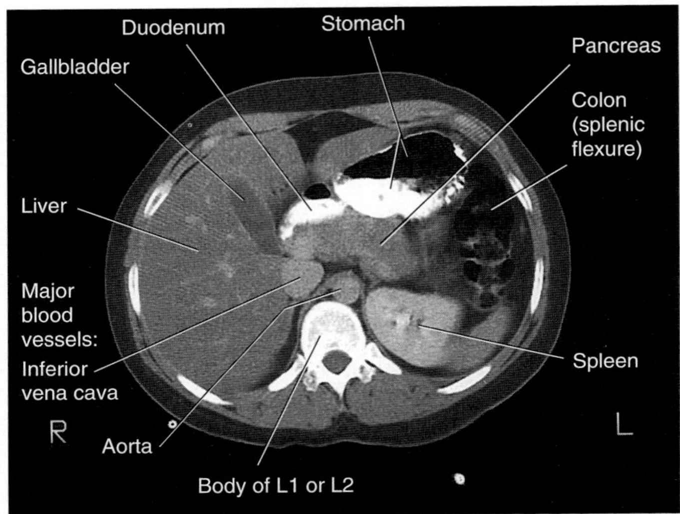

Fig. 3-8. CT image of abdomen, level of stomach, liver, gallbladder, pancreas and spleen.

Spleen

The spleen is not directly associated with the digestive system because it is part of the **lymphatic system**, which, along with the heart and blood vessels, is part of the circulatory system. However, it is an important abdominal organ and occupies a space posterior and to the left of the stomach in the **left upper quadrant**.

The spleen is often visualized on plain abdominal radiographs, particularly if the organ is enlarged. It is a fragile organ and is sometimes lacerated during trauma to the lower left rib cage.

URINARY SYSTEM

In addition to the digestive system, with its accessory organs, the urinary system is also an important abdominal system and will be introduced in this chapter.

The urinary system is composed of:

- two kidneys
- two ureters *(u-re´ter)** or *(yōō-rēt´er)*†
- one urinary bladder
- one urethra *(u-re´thrah)** or *(yōō-rē´thra)*†

Each **kidney** drains by way of its own **ureter** to the single **urinary bladder.** The bladder, situated above and behind the symphysis pubis, serves to store urine. Under voluntary control, the stored urine passes to the exterior via the **urethra.** The two **suprarenal** (adrenal) **glands** of the endocrine system are located at the superomedial portion of each kidney. The bean-shaped kidneys are located on either side of the lumbar vertebral column. The right kidney is usually situated a little lower than the left one, due to the presence of the large liver on the right.

Waste materials and excess water are eliminated from the blood by the kidneys and are transported through the ureters to the urinary bladder.

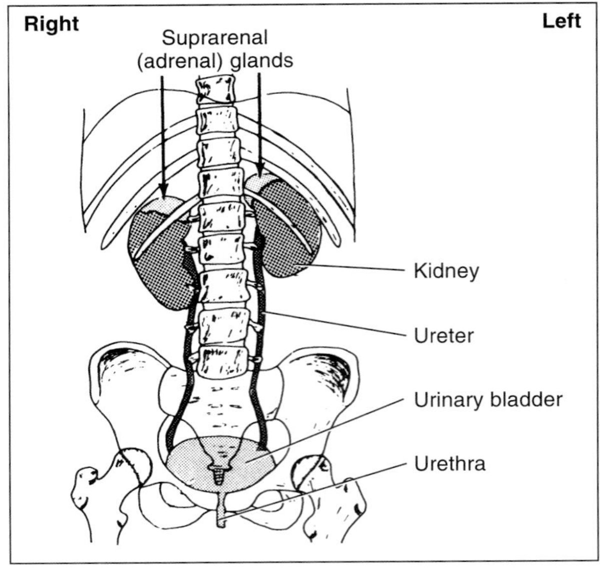

Fig. 3-9. Urinary system.

**Dorland's Illustrated Medical Dictionary*, 27th Edition.
†*Webster's New World Dictionary*, Third College Edition.

Excretory or Intravenous Urogram (IVU)

The kidneys are usually only faintly seen on a plain abdominal radiograph due to a fatty capsule that surrounds each kidney. The contrast medium examination shown in Fig. 3-10 is an **excretory** or **intravenous urogram** (IVU), which is a radiographic examination of the urinary system wherein the contrast media is injected intravenously. During this examination the hollow organs of this system are visualized. The organs as labeled are: (A) **left kidney**, (B) **left ureter**, (C) **urinary bladder**, and (D) **the area of the right suprarenal** (adrenal) **gland**, just above the right kidney. (Additional anatomy and positioning for the urinary system will be covered in Chapter 17.) The four quadrants of the abdomen are included on this IVU radiograph, as will be described on the following page.

Note: The term **Intravenous Pyelogram (IVP)** has often been used for this examination. However, this is **not** an accurate term for this exam because "pyelo" refers to the renal pelvis of the kidney, and the excretory urogram includes a study of the entire urinary tract, which includes the total collecting system. Therefore, throughout this textbook the term **excretory urogram** (EU) or **intravenous urogram** (IVU) will be used.

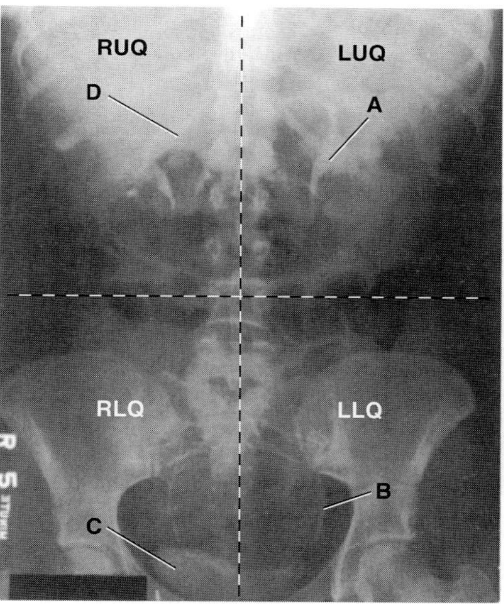

Fig. 3-10. Excretory or intravenous urogram (IVU), (four-quadrant system).

Abdominal Cavity

Peritoneum: The abdominopelvic cavity is lined with a double-walled, saclike membrane called the **peritoneum** *(per″ i-to-ne′ um)*. The outer layer adhering to the abdominal and pelvic cavities is the **parietal** *(pah-ri′ e-tal)* peritoneum, and the inner portion covering certain organs is the **visceral** *(vis′ er-al)* peritoneum. The **peritoneal cavity** is the space inside the peritoneal lining.

Mesentery: Certain portions of the inner visceral peritoneum completely enclose some organs, such as the **small intestine,** to form a double fold called the **mesentery** *(mes′ en-ter″ e),* which stabilizes and supports these structures by connecting them to the posterior abdominal wall. This is seen in the simplified cross-sectional drawing in Fig. 3-11. It is also seen in the midsagittal drawing of Fig. 3-12. Figure 3-12 shows the peritoneal cavity as the large dark gray region making up the peritoneal cavity.

Note: The cross sectional drawing in Fig. 3-11 is simplified to demonstrate peritoneum and mesentery. If all loops of bowel and other organs of the abdominal cavity were drawn in, there would be very little actual space left in the peritoneal cavity, as evident by comparing this drawing to the CT image in Fig. 3-8.

Omentum: **Omentum** *(o-men′ tum)* is a special type of double-fold peritoneum extending from the **stomach to another organ** providing stability and support for these structures. This is shown in Fig. 3-12 as a double fold of peritoneum connecting the stomach to the liver above and also draping down as an apron-like structure in the anterior abdomen region.

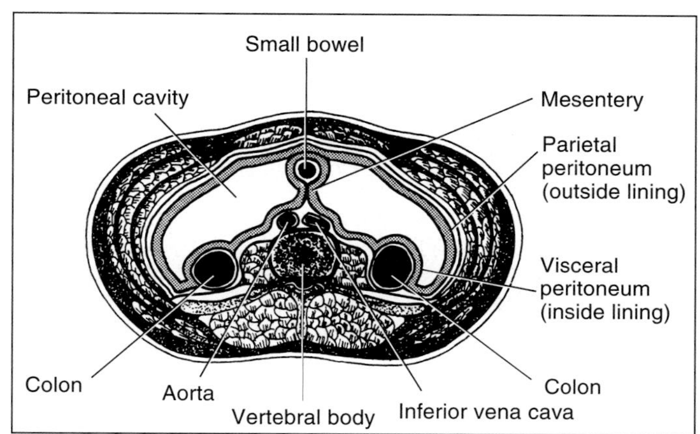

Fig. 3-11. Abdominal cavity (cross-section).

Anatomical Relationships

Abdominal organs that are **not** located within the peritoneal cavity are considered either **retroperitoneal** (behind) or **infraperitoneal** (under) structures. This is an important distinction that should be understood and will be further described in Chapter 19 on the lower GI system.

Summary of Abdominal Organs NOT Located Within the Peritoneal Cavity

Retroperitoneal organs:	Infraperitoneal (pelvic) organs:
–Kidneys	–Lower rectum
–Ureters	–Urinary bladder
–Adrenal glands	–Reproductive organs
–Pancreas	(An exception is the female
–Duodenum	uterus, which extends into the
–Ascending & descending colon	peritoneal cavity)
–Rectum	
–Major abdominal blood vessels	
(aorta and inferior vena cava)	

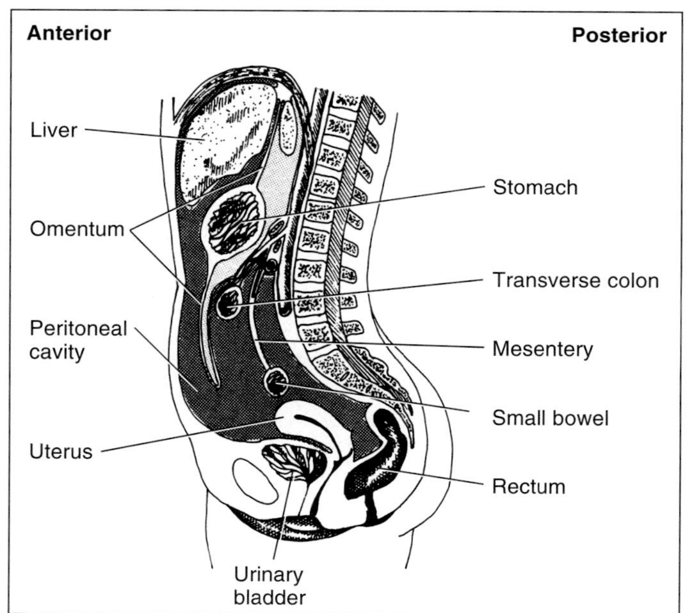

Fig. 3-12. Midsaggital section–Abdominal cavity (female).

QUADRANTS AND REGIONS

To help describe the locations of various organs or other structures within the abdominopelvic cavity, such as the urinary system organs in Fig. 3-10 (on preceding page), the abdomen may be divided into either **four quadrants** or into **nine regions**.

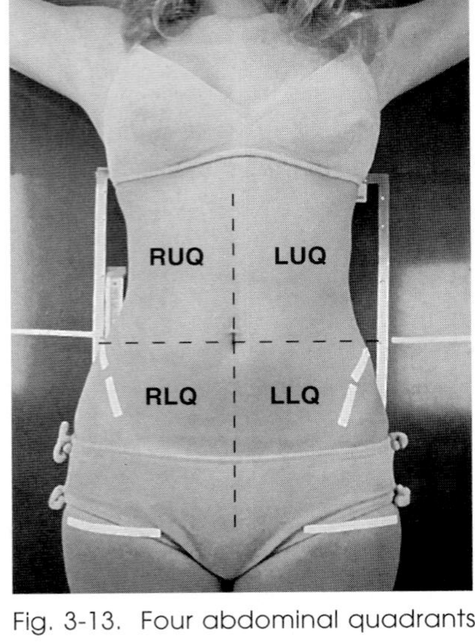

Fig. 3-13. Four abdominal quadrants.

Four Abdominal Quadrants

If two imaginary perpendicular planes (at right angles) were passed through the abdomen at the umbilicus or navel, they would divide the abdomen into four quadrants. One plane would be transverse through the abdomen at the **level of the umbilicus**, which on most people is at the level of the **intervertebral disc between L3 and L4** (3rd and 4th lumbar vertebrae), which is about at the level of the iliac crests on a female.

The vertical plane would coincide with the **midsagittal plane** or midline of the abdomen and would pass through both the umbilicus and the symphysis pubis. These two planes would divide the abdominopelvic cavity into four quadrants: the **right upper quadrant** (RUQ), the **left upper quadrant** (LUQ), the **right lower quadrant** (RLQ), and the **left lower quadrant** (LLQ).

Note: The four-quadrant system is most frequently used in radiographically localizing any particular organ. For example, the liver is located in the RUQ, the stomach is primarily in the LUQ, the spleen in the LUQ, and the right and left kidneys in the RUQ and LUQ respectively.

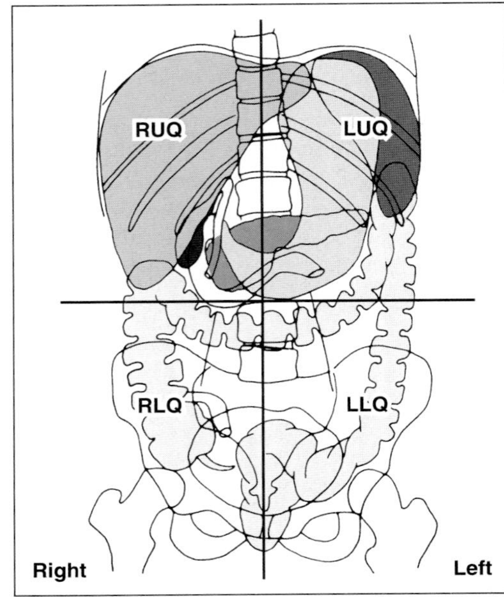

Fig. 3-14. Four quadrants with certain abdominal structures.

Nine Abdominal Regions

The abdominopelvic cavity can also be divided into nine regions by using two horizontal or transverse planes and two vertical planes. The two vertical planes are the **transpyloric plane** and the **transtubercular plane**. The two vertical planes are the **right** and **left lateral planes**. The transpyloric plane is at the level of the lower border of the 1st lumbar vertebra, and the transtubercular plane is at the level of the 5th lumbar vertebra. The right and left lateral planes are parallel to the midsagittal plane and are located midway between it and each anterior superior iliac spine.

Names of Regions: The names of these nine regions are identified below. Radiographers should be familiar with the locations and names of these nine regions. However, generally locating most structures and organs within the four-quadrant system is sufficient for radiographic purposes due to variables that affect specific locations of organs such as body habitus, body position, age, etc., (see organ outlines in Fig. 3-15 for general locations of organs within these nine regions).

1. Right hypochondriac.
2. Epigastric.
3. Left hypochondriac.
4. Right lateral (lumbar).
5. Umbilical.
6. Left lateral (lumbar).
7. Right inguinal (iliac).
8. Pubic (hypogastric).
9. Left inguinal (iliac).

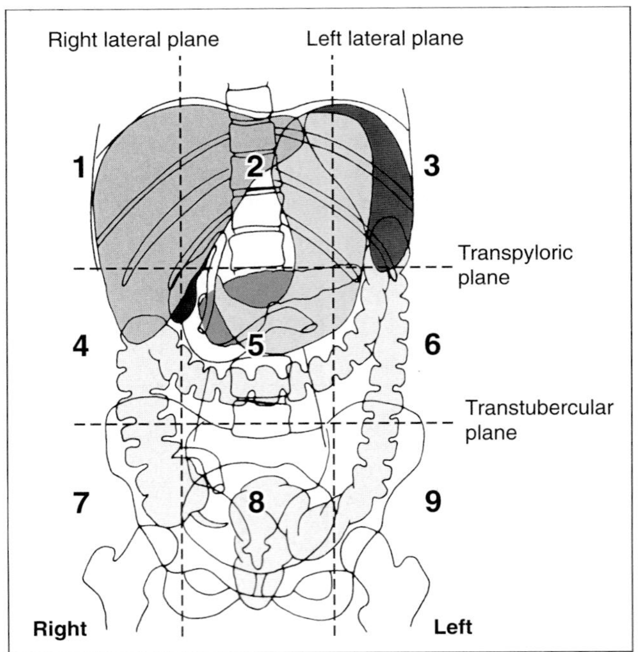

Fig. 3-15. Nine regions with certain abdominal structures.

TOPOGRAPHIC LANDMARKS

Abdominal borders and organs within the abdomen are not visible from the exterior, and because these soft tissue organs cannot be palpated directly, certain bony landmarks are used for this purpose.

Note: Remember that palpation must be done gently because the patient may have painful or sensitive areas within the abdomen and pelvis. Also, be sure that the patient is informed of the purpose of this palpation prior to beginning the palpation.

Seven Landmarks of the Abdomen

The following seven palpable landmarks are important in positioning the abdomen or for locating organs within the abdomen. One may wish to practice finding these bony landmarks on oneself before attempting to locate them on another person or on a patient the first time. Positioning for abdominal radiographs in either AP or PA projections requires a quick but accurate location of these landmarks on all types of patients, the thin as well as the heavy-set or muscular patients that will require more firm palpation.

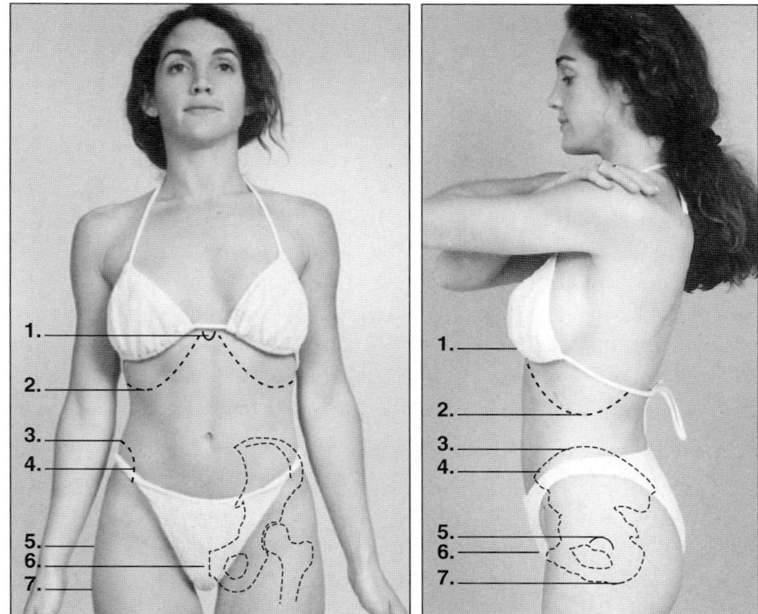

Fig. 3-16. Topographic landmarks. Fig. 3-17.

1. Xiphoid Tip (level of T9-10): The tip of the xiphoid process is the most distal or inferior process of the sternum. This can best be palpated by first gently pressing on the soft abdomen below the distal sternum, then moving upward carefully against the firm distal margin of the xiphoid process.

This landmark approximates the superior anterior portion of the diaphragm, which is also the **superior margin of the abdomen**. This, however, is not a primary landmark for positioning the abdomen because of variations in body types and the importance of including all of the lower abdomen on most abdomen films.

2. Inferior Costal (Rib) Margin (level of L2-3): This landmark is used to locate gallbladder, stomach and other abdominal organs.

3. Iliac Crest (level of L4-5 vertebral interspace): The crest of the ilium is the uppermost portion of the curved border of the ilium. The iliac crest can be easily palpated by pressing inward and downward along the midlateral margin of the abdomen. The uppermost or most superior portion of this crest is the **most commonly used abdominal landmark** and corresponds approximately to level of the **mid abdomen**, which is also at or just slightly below the level of the umbilicus on most persons. If the center of the cassette is centered to this level, the lower abdomen area will generally be included on the lower margin of the film.

Note: To ensure that all of the upper abdomen is included on the film requires centering 1 to 2 inches (3 to 5 cm) above the level of the crest for most patients, which will then usually cut off some of the important lower abdomen. This then would require a second film centered lower to include this lower region.

4. Anterior Superior Iliac Spine (ASIS): The ASIS can be found by locating the iliac crest, then palpating anteriorly and inferiorly until a prominent projection or "bump" is felt (more prominent on females). This is a commonly used landmark for positioning of pelvic and vertebral structures, but can also be a secondary landmark for general abdominal positioning.

5. Greater Trochanter: This landmark is more easily palpated on thin patients. Gentle but very firm palpation is generally required to feel the movement of the trochanter with one hand while rotating the leg internally and externally at the knee area with the other hand. This is not as precise a landmark as other bony landmarks of the pelvis, but the uppermost margin of the trochanter generally lies slightly superior (1 to 1½ in. or 3 to 4 cm) to the level of the symphysis pubis. With practice this can also be used as a secondary landmark for abdomen positioning.

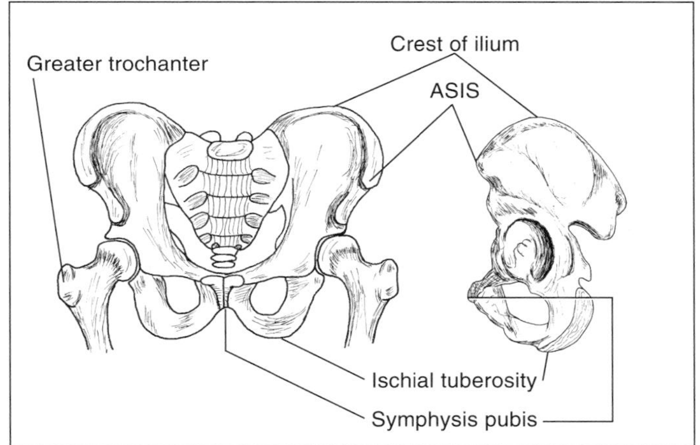

Fig. 3-18. Topographic landmarks of pelvis.

6. Symphysis Pubis: The symphysis pubis is the anterior junction (joint) of the two pelvic bones. The most superior anterior portion of the pubis can be palpated when the patient is in a supine position. This landmark corresponds to the **inferior margin of the abdomen**. Palpation of this area, however, may be embarrassing to some patients. Therefore, with practice one can also determine the level of the symphysis pubis or the lower margin of the abdomen by palpating the greater trochanter, or in reference to the iliac crest as being at the level of the center of the cassette. This then places the lower margin of the film at the symphysis pubis.

7. Ischial Tuberosity: This can be used to determine the lower margin on a PA abdomen with the patient in a **prone position**. These two bony prominences, which can be most easily palpated on thin patients, bear most of the weight of the trunk when one is seated. The lower margins of the ischial tuberosities are about 1 to 1½ inches (4 cm) below or distal to the symphysis pubis. This landmark may be used for positioning a PA projection of the colon when the rectal area is to be included on the film. This, however, may also be uncomfortable and embarrassing for the patient, and other landmarks can and should be used when possible.

Radiographic Positioning

Patient Preparation

Patient preparation for abdominal radiography includes removal of all clothing and any opaque objects in the area to be radiographed. A hospital gown should be put on with the opening and ties in the back, if this type of gown is used. Shoes and socks may remain on the feet.

Some abdominal radiographs, particularly those requiring contrast media, necessitate special instructions to the patient prior to the examination. Instructions may include such things as fasting or a laxative the night before, but the "plain" abdominal radiograph (KUB) or the acute abdominal series are usually taken "as is."

General Positioning Considerations

Make the patient as comfortable as possible on the radiographic table. A pillow under the head and support under the knees will enhance the patient's comfort. Place clean linen on table and cover patient's legs to keep them warm and to protect their modesty.

Breathing Instructions

One of the key factors in good abdominal radiography is the prevention of motion. This may be due to either **voluntary** movements from breathing, or from **involuntary** movements such as peristaltic action of the bowel. The difference between these two types of motion is illustrated in Chapter 1. However, what is important to remember in preventing motion in abdominal radiography is to use **the shortest exposure time possible,** to prevent or minimize the effects of involuntary motion.

A second way to prevent voluntary motion is by **careful breathing instructions** to the patient. Most abdominal radiographs are taken on expiration; the patient is instructed to "take in a deep breath — let it all out and hold it — don't breathe." Before making the exposure, it is important to observe the patient to ensure he (she) is following instructions; and that sufficient time has been allowed for all breathing movements to cease.

Abdominal radiographs are exposed on **expiration**, with the diaphragm in a superior position for better visualization of abdominal structures.

Film Markers

Film markers, such as patient ID information, should be clear and legible. Correctly placed R and L markers and "up side" markers on erect and decubitus projections should be visible without superimposing abdominal structures. On the positioning pages for the abdomen, which follow in this chapter, are suggested locations for all film markers. These are indicated in the small box drawings at the top of the page indicating film size for each projection, as well as the patient ID blocker corner location.

The recommended AEC (Automatic Exposure Control) chambers are also indicated on each positioning page.

Radiation Protection

Patients must be protected from unnecessary radiation for all radiographic examinations. Good radiation protection practices are especially important in abdominal radiography because of the proximity of the radiation-sensitive gonadal organs.

Repeat Exposures: Careful positioning and selection of correct exposure factors are ways of reducing unnecessary exposure from repeat examinations. Following breathing instructions carefully also assists in eliminating repeats due to motion caused by breathing during the exposure.

Collimation: Chapter One states a general collimation rule that **collimation borders should be visible on all four sides if the film is large enough to allow this without "cutting off" essential anatomy.** For abdominal radiographs of small patients, some side collimation smaller than the film size is possible if it does not cut off abdominal anatomy. Extra side collimation can be adjusted manually so the lateral margins of the light field are visible on the outer edges of the patient's abdomen.

Collimation on the top and bottom should be adjusted directly to the margins of the film holder, allowing for divergence of the x-ray beam. Essential anatomy will be cut off on full size adults if extra collimation margins are shown on the top and bottom borders of the abdomen radiograph.

Gonadal Shielding: Chapter One states an important rule that for **all patients of reproductive age gonadal shielding is needed if the gonads lie within or close to** (2 in. or 5 cm) **the primary field, unless such shielding covers an area of primary interest on the image receptor.** Applying this to abdominal radiographs, **gonad shields should be used for males** with the upper edge of the shield carefully placed at the pubic symphysis (Fig. 3-19). For females, gonadal shields may be **used only when such shields do not obscure essential anatomy** in the lower abdominopelvic region. Generally, the decision to shield female gonads on abdomen radiographs should be made by a physician to determine if essential anatomy will be obscured. Top of ovarian shield should be at or slightly above level of ASIS,' and lower border at symphysis pubis (Fig. 3-20).

Exposure Factors

The principal exposure factors for abdominal radiographs are:

1. Medium kVp (70-80).
2. Short exposure time
3. Adequate mAs for sufficient density

Correctly exposed abdominal radiographs on an average-sized patient should visualize the lateral borders of the psoas muscles, lower liver margin, kidney outlines and lumbar vertebrae transverse processes. This requires moderate contrast using medium kVp exposure to allow for visualization of various abdominal structures, including possible small semi-opaque stones in the gall bladder or kidneys.

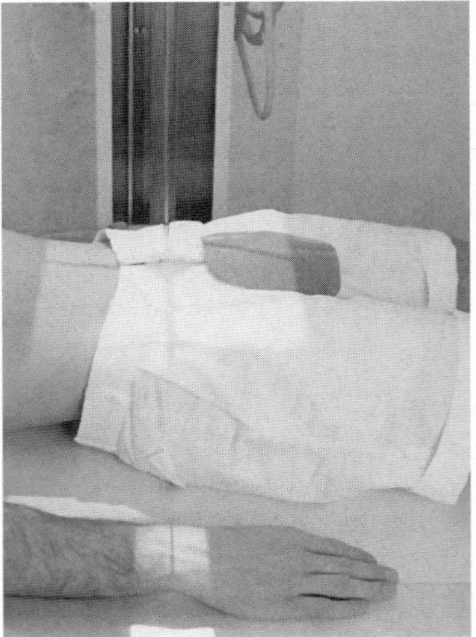

Fig. 3-19. Gonadal shielding-Male.

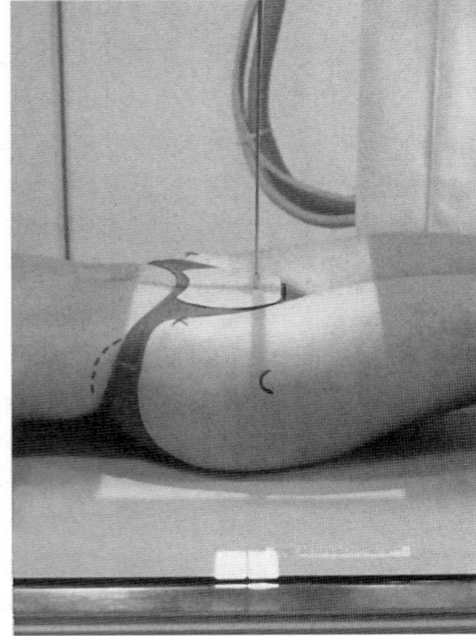

Fig. 3-20. Gonadal shielding-Female (only if shielding does not obscure essential anatomy).

NATIONAL SURVEY

Departmental basic and special procedures for the abdomen are fairly consistent throughout the United States.

Explanations

Abdomen (KUB): Results demonstrate that for the KUB abdomen examination, the **AP supine** is overwhelmingly the basic projection, followed with the **AP erect**. The most common special projections were the **lateral decubitus** and the **dorsal decubitus**.

Acute Abdomen: The acute abdomen series results demonstrate that the **AP supine** and **AP erect** are by far the most frequent basic routines, followed by the **PA chest,** also listed as basic in the acute abdomen series by the majority of respondents.

The **lateral decubitus** is the least common as a basic routine for the acute abdomen series. However, it is much more common as a basic projection in 1995, as compared to 1989 when it was primarily a special projection. (It is known to be common practice to replace the erect abdomen with a lateral decubitus when the patient is unable to assume an erect position.)

In 1995 the centering for the erect abdomen to include the diaphragm was much more common than centering to the crest, even if a PA chest to include the diaphragm is done. This question was not included in the 1989 survey. The PA chest as part of the routine acute abdominal series is more common in the West (82%) as compared to the Mid-U.S. (70%) and the East (61%). (See appendix.)

Because of these differences, this text will list and demonstrate two possible routines for the acute abdomen series. First will be the "three-way" acute abdomen routine, which includes the PA chest, and second, as an alternative, is the "two-way" routine without the PA chest.

One reason the PA chest is included in the three-way acute abdomen series is that the erect chest best visualizes free air under the diaphragm. The erect abdomen will also visualize free air if the film is centered high enough to include the diaphragm; however, the exposure technique for the chest best visualizes this air if present. Also, certain chest diseases, such as basal pneumonia, are frequently associated with abdominal pain, also suggesting the need for a PA chest as part of the acute abdomen routine.

Abdomen Routine

Abdomen	U.S. Average	
	Basic 1995 (1989)	Special 1995 (1989)
• AP supine	98% (98%)	
• AP erect	75% –	12% (21%)
• Lat. decub.		37% (30%)
• Dorsal decub.		34% (5%)
Acute Abdomen Series		
• AP supine	98% –	
• AP erect		
–Center at crest	27% –	
–Center to include diaphragm	73% –	
• PA chest	68% (60%)	
• Lat. decub	51% (23%)	

STANDARD AND SPECIAL OPERATING PROCEDURES

Certain basic and special projections for the abdomen are demonstrated and described on the following pages.

Abdominal Radiographic Routines

Radiographic examinations of the abdomen are done for a wide variety of symptoms and for various purposes as described at the beginning of this chapter. The most common radiographic exam of the abdomen is the "plain" abdomen often called a **KUB** (kidneys, ureters, bladder).

More acute conditions require an **acute abdomen series**, which includes abdominal radiographs taken in various patient positions, such as erect or lateral decubitus using a horizontal x-ray beam. The routines for the acute abdomen series may vary depending on physician preference and what is customary or common in different institutions or different parts of the country as shown in the above survey results.

Basic and Special Projections

Abdomen (KUB)
Basic
• AP supine **94**
Special
• PA prone **95**
• Lat. decub. (AP) **96**
• AP erect **97**
• Dorsal decub. (lat.) **98**

Acute abdomen
(three-way, with PA chest)
Basic
• AP supine **99**
• AP erect **99**
• PA chest erect **99**
Special
• Left lat. decub. (AP) **99**

or

Acute abdomen
(two-way, without PA chest)
Basic
• AP supine **99**
• AP erect (or decub.) **99**

AP Projection–Supine Position

KUB

Abdomen
Basic
• **AP supine (KUB)**

Structures Best Shown

Liver, spleen, kidneys, abnormal masses, calcifications or accumulations of gas. Pelvis, lumbar spine and lower ribs are also well shown.

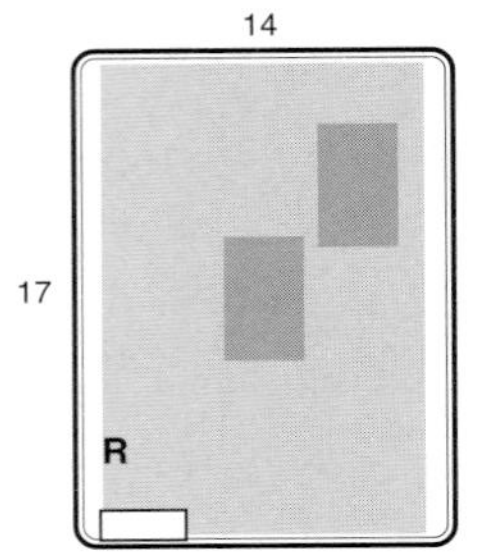

Technical Factors

- Film size–14 x 17 in. (35 x 43 cm), lengthwise.
- Moving or stationary grid.
- 70-80 kVp range.
- Technique and dose:

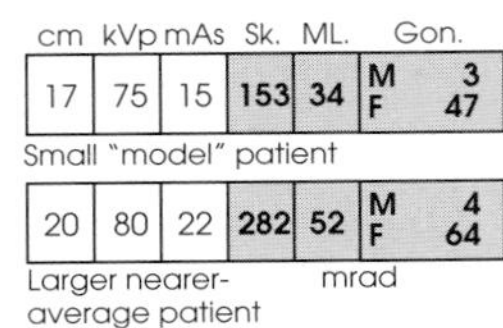

cm	kVp	mAs	Sk.	ML.	Gon.
17	75	15	153	34	M 3 F 47
Small "model" patient					
20	80	22	282	52	M 4 F 64
Larger nearer-average patient			mrad		

Shielding

- Use gonadal shields on males (also on females of reproductive age, only if such shielding does not obscure essential anatomy as determined by a physician).

Patient Position

- Supine with midsagittal plane centered to midline of table and/or cassette. Place arms at patient's sides, away from body.
- Legs extended with support under knees if this is more comfortable.

Part Position

- Center of cassette to **level of iliac crests**, with bottom margin at symphysis pubis (see Notes).
- **No rotation** of pelvis or shoulders (check that both ASISs are the same distance from table-top or film holder).

Central Ray

- CR perpendicular to and directed to **center of film** (to level of iliac crest).
- Minimum 40 in. (102 cm) SID.

Collimation: Collimate closely on sides to skin margins and on top and bottom to film borders.

Respiration: Exposure made at end of **expiration**.

Notes: A tall hyposthenic or asthenic type patient may require **two films lengthwise**, one centered lower to include the symphysis pubis, and the second centered high to include the upper abdomen and diaphragm.

A broad hypersthenic type patient may also require two 14 x 17 films placed **crosswise**, one centered lower to include the symphysis pubis and the second for the upper abdomen, with a minimum of 1 to 2 in. (3 to 5 cm) overlap.

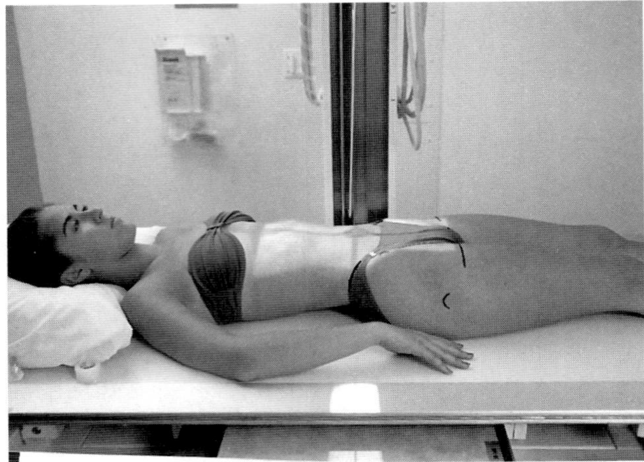

Fig. 3-21. AP abdomen.

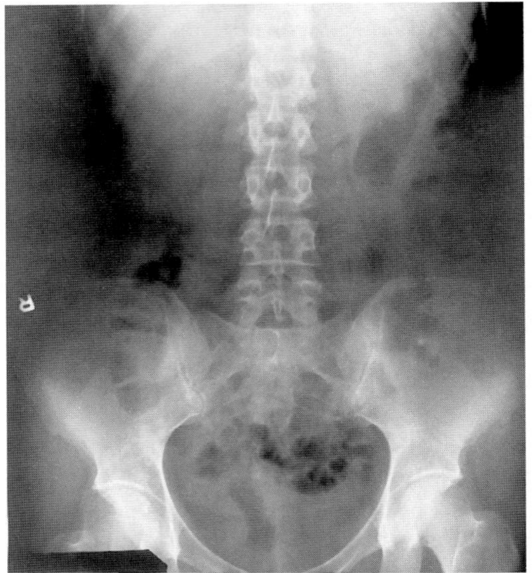

Fig. 3-22. AP abdomen.

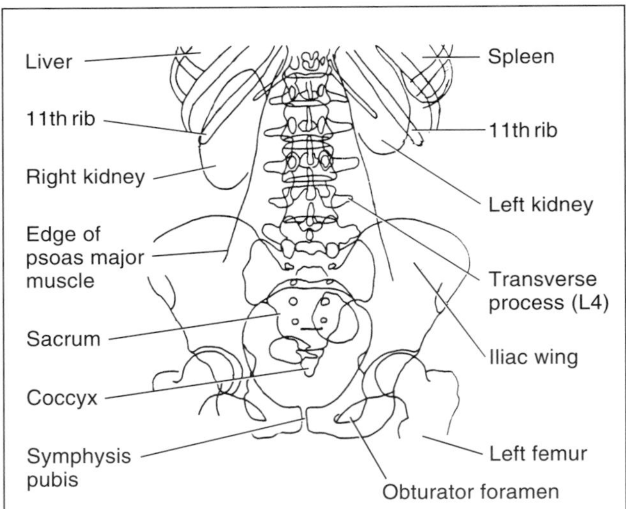

Fig. 3-23. AP abdomen.

Evaluation Criteria

- Lower margin of radiograph should include at least the superior portion of the arch of the symphysis pubis.
- Upper abdomen should be included, visualizing the upper margins of the kidneys as well as the lower portion of the dense liver and the area of the spleen. (See Notes above for possible two radiographs.)
- Vertebral column should be aligned to center of radiograph.
- **No rotation**: Lower rib cage, pelvis and lumbar vertebrae should appear symmetrical. The **outer margins of ribs** should be same distance from the spine; and R and L **iliac wings** should appear equal in size and shape. Elongation of an iliac wing indicates rotation in that direction.
- Lateral collimation margins should be visible for most patients unless such would cut off essential abdominal anatomy.
- **No motion**: Ribs and gas bubble margins appear sharp.
- Should have sufficient exposure (mAs) and long scale contrast (kVp) to visualize psoas muscle outlines, lumbar transverse processes and ribs. Margins of liver and kidneys should be visible on smaller to average size patients.

PA Projection–Prone Position

Abdomen
Special
- **PA prone**
- Lat. decub. (AP)
- AP erect
- Dorsal decub. (lat.)

Structures Best Shown

Liver, spleen, kidneys, abnormal masses, calcifications or accumulations of gas. Pelvis, lumbar spine and lower ribs are also shown.

Note: This projection is **less desirable** if the kidneys are of primary interest **due to the increased OID**.

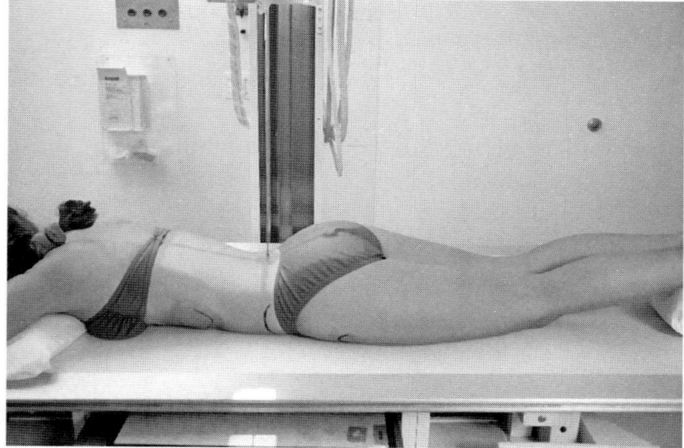

Fig. 3-24. PA abdomen.

Technical Factors

- Film size–14 x 17 in. (35 x 43 cm), lengthwise.
- Moving or stationary grid.
- 70-80 kVp range.
- Technique and dose:

cm	kVp	mAs	Sk.	ML.	Gon.
20	80	22	282	52	M 2 F 47
average size			mrad		

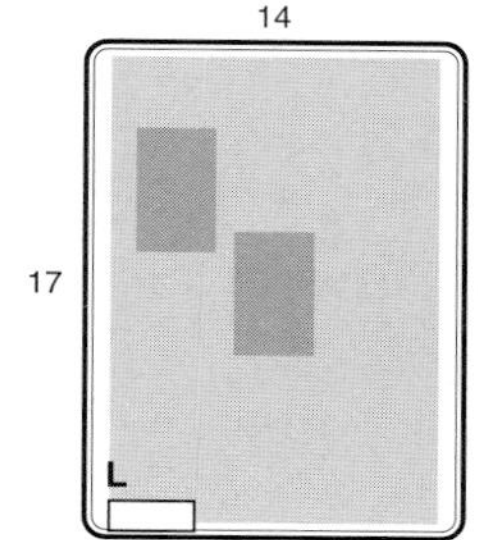

Shielding

- Use gonadal shields on males (also on females of reproductive age, only if such shielding does not obscure essential anatomy as determined by a physician).

Patient Position

- Prone with midsagittal plane of body centered to midline of table and/or film holder.
- Legs extended with support under ankles.
- Arms up beside head, provide clean pillow.

Part Position

- No rotation of pelvis or shoulders and chest.
- Center of cassette to **iliac crest** (see Note above).

Central Ray

- CR perpendicular to and directed to **center of film** (to level of iliac crest).
- Minimum 40 in. (102 cm) SID.

Collimation: Collimate closely on all sides to skin margins and on top and bottom to film borders.

Respiration: Exposure made at end of **expiration**.

Note: Tall asthenic-type patients may require two films lengthwise; broad hypersthenic types may also require two films, but placed crosswise.

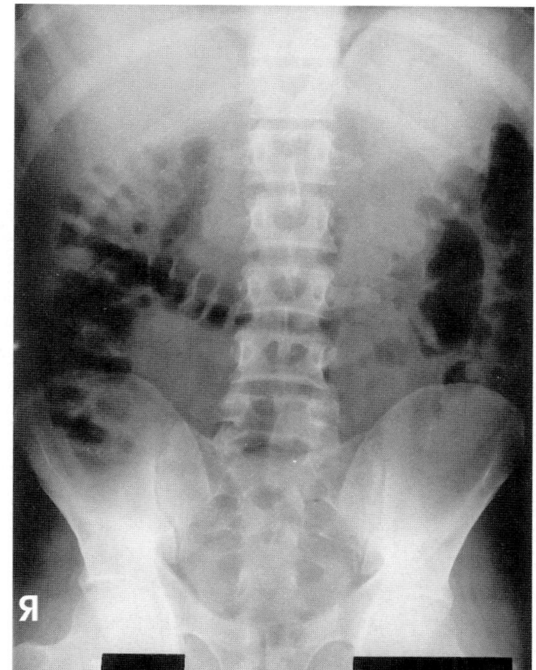

Fig. 3-25. PA abdomen.

Evaluation Criteria

- Lower margin of radiograph should include at least the superior portion of the arch of the symphysis pubis.
- Upper abdomen should be included, visualizing the upper margins of the kidneys as well as the lower portion of the dense liver and the area of the spleen. (See Note above for possible two radiographs.)
- Vertebral column should be aligned to center of radiograph.
- **No rotation**: Pelvis and lumbar vertebrae should appear symmetrical (R and L iliac wings appear equal in size and shape, and spinous processes should appear in center of vertebrae).
- Lateral collimation margins should be visible for most patients unless they cut off essential abdominal anatomy.
- **No motion**: Ribs and gas bubble margins should appear sharp and clear.
- Should have sufficient exposure (mAs) and long-scale contrast (kVp) to visualize psoas muscle outlines, lumbar transverse processes and ribs. Margins of liver and kidneys should be visible on smaller to average size patients.

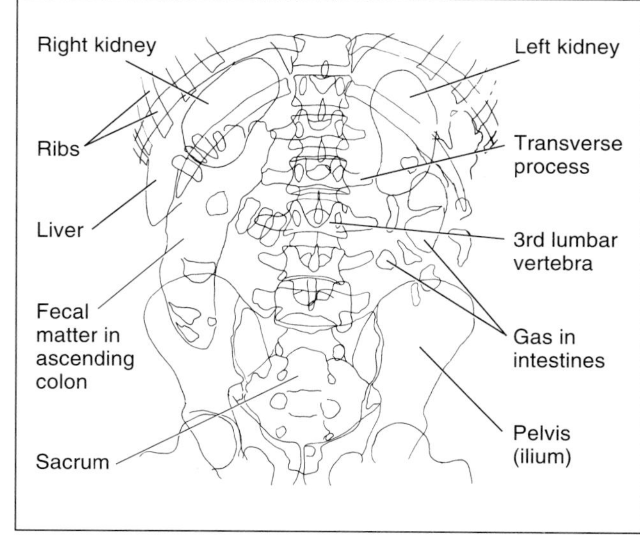

Fig. 3-26. PA abdomen.

Lateral Decubitus Position (AP Projection)

Abdomen
Special
- PA prone
- **Lat. decub. (AP)**
- AP erect
- Dorsal decub. (lat.)

Structures Best Shown

Liver, spleen, kidneys, abdominal masses, air-fluid levels and accumulations of gas or free intra-abdominal air. (Free intra-abdominal air, however, is best demonstrated with chest technique on erect PA chest in three-way acute abdominal series.)

Important: Patient should be on side a minimum of **5 minutes** before exposure (to allow possible free intra-abdominal air to rise or abnormal fluids to accumulate).

Left lateral decubitus best demonstrates free air within abdominal cavity in the area of the liver in the right upper abdomen.

Technical Factors

- Film size–14 x 17 in. (35 x 43 cm), crosswise to the table (lengthwise with the patient).
- Moving or stationary grid.
- 70-80 kVp range.
- Technique and dose:

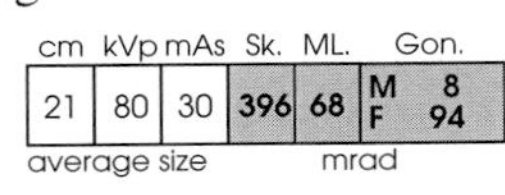

cm	kVp	mAs	Sk.	ML.	Gon.
21	80	30	396	68	M 8 F 94

average size — mrad

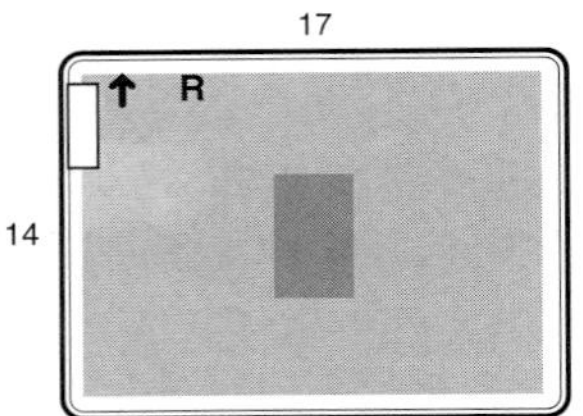

Shielding

- Use gonadal shield on males.

Patient Position

- Lateral recumbent on radiolucent pad, back firmly against table or vertical grid device. (Lock wheels on cart so as not to move away from table or grid.)
- Place patient on firm surface such as a cardiac or back board positioned under the sheet to prevent sagging and anatomy cutoff.
- Knees partially flexed, one on top of the other to stabilize patient.
- Arms up near head, provide clean pillow.

Part Position

- Adjust patient and cart so center of film and CR are about **1 to 2 in. or 3 to 5 cm above level of iliac crests** (to include diaphragm). Top of film will be approximately at level of axilla.
- Ensure **no rotation** of pelvis or shoulders.
- Adjust height of cassette to center midsagittal plane of patient to center of film, but ensure that **up side of abdomen is clearly included on the film.**

Central Ray

- CR **horizontal**, directed to **center of film**, at 1 to 2 in. (3 to 5 cm) above level of iliac crest. (A horizontal beam must be used to show air-fluid levels and free intra-abdominal air.)
- Minimum 40 in. (102 cm) SID.

Collimation: Collimate on four sides.

Respiration: Exposure made at end of **expiration.**

Note: Place arrow or other appropriate marker to indicate the up-side.

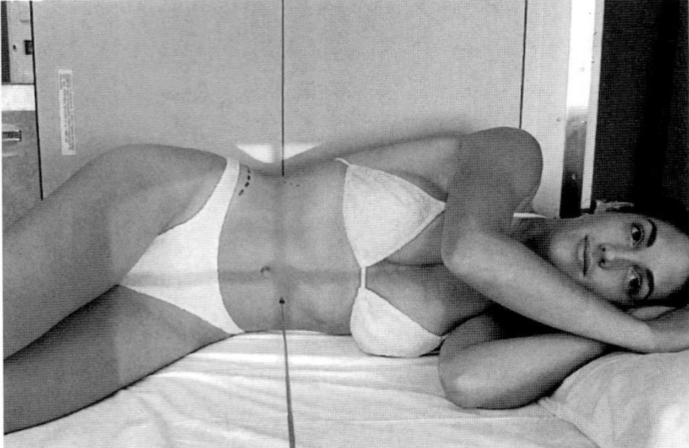

Fig. 3-27. Left lateral decubitus position (AP).

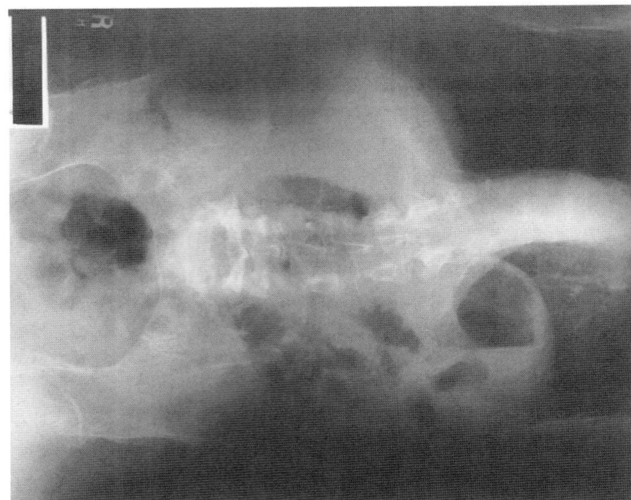

Fig. 3-28. Left lateral decubitus (AP).

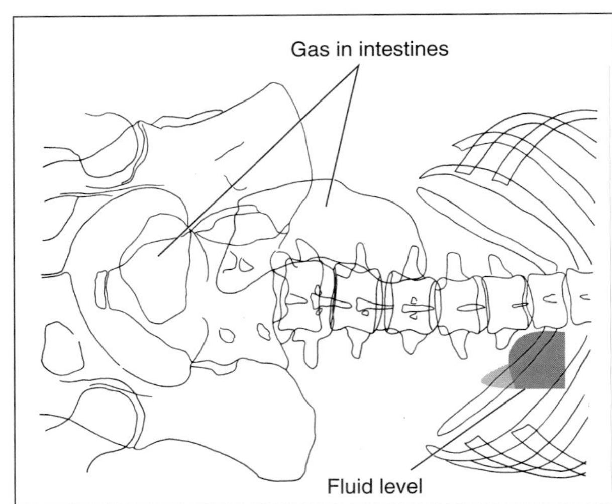

Fig. 3-29. Left lateral decubitus (AP).

Evaluation Criteria

- Upper margin of radiograph should include the diaphragm.
- **No rotation**: Pelvis should appear symmetrical with right and left iliac wings appearing equal in size and shape, and the outer margins of the ribs should be the same distance from the vertebral column.
- If both sides cannot be included, **the upper side must be included.**
- **No motion**: Diaphragm, ribs and gas shadow margins appear sharp.
- Overall exposure and density should appear slightly less than supine abdomen to better visualize air-fluid levels and free intra-abdominal air if present.

AP Projection–Erect Position

Abdomen
Special
- PA prone
- Lat. decub. (AP)
- **AP erect**
- Dorsal decub. (lat.)

Structures Best Shown

Liver, spleen, kidneys, abnormal masses, air-fluid levels, accumulations of gas or free intra-abdominal air.

Technical Factors

- Film size–14 x 17 in. (35 x 43 cm) lengthwise.
- Moving or stationary grid (use erect marker).
- 70-80 kVp range.
- Technique and dose:

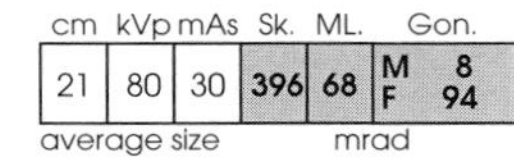
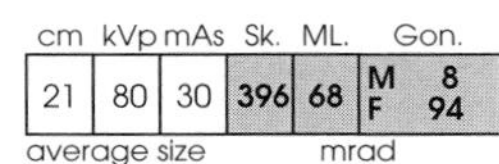

cm	kVp	mAs	Sk.	ML.	Gon.
21	80	30	396	68	M 8 F 94

average size | mrad

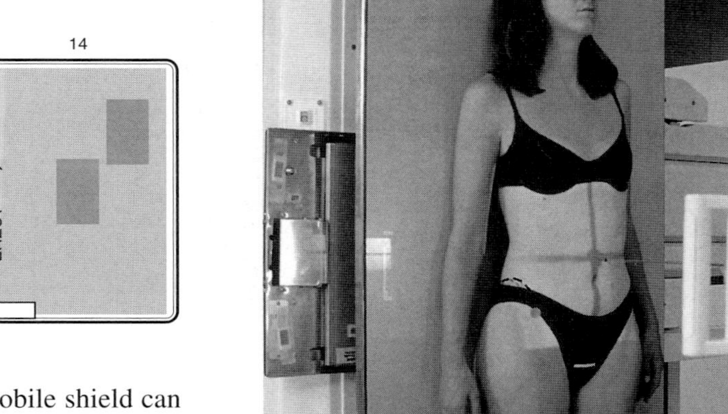

Fig. 3-30. Erect AP–To include diaphragm.

Shielding

- Use gonadal shields on males. An adjustable freestanding mobile shield can be used as for chests.

Patient Position

- Upright, legs slightly spread, back against table or grid device (see Note 1 for weak or unsteady patients).
- Arms at sides away from body.
- Midsagittal plane of body centered to midline of table.

Part Position

- No rotation of pelvis or shoulders.
- Adjust height of film holder so center of film is **1 to 2 in. (3 to 5 cm) above iliac crest,** (to include diaphragm), which for the average patient will place the **top of the film approximately at the level of the axilla** (see Note 2).

Central Ray

- CR **horizontal**, to **center of film**.
- Minimum 40 in. (102 cm) SID.

Collimation: Collimate closely on all four sides–do **NOT** cut off upper abdomen.

Respiration: Exposure made at end of **expiration.**

Note 1: Patient should be upright a minimum of **5 minutes** before exposure. If a patient is too weak to maintain an erect position, a lateral decubitus (AP) should be taken.

Note 2: Generally, centering should be high enough to include diaphragm; however, some routines may include centering to the iliac crests to include all of the lower abdomen **only if** an erect PA chest is also taken to include the diaphragm (see three-way abdomen series); or two radiographs may be taken, especially on a tall asthenic type patient. One centered high to include the diaphragm, and the second centered lower to include the symphysis pubis. Broad hypersthenic type patients may also require two films placed crosswise.

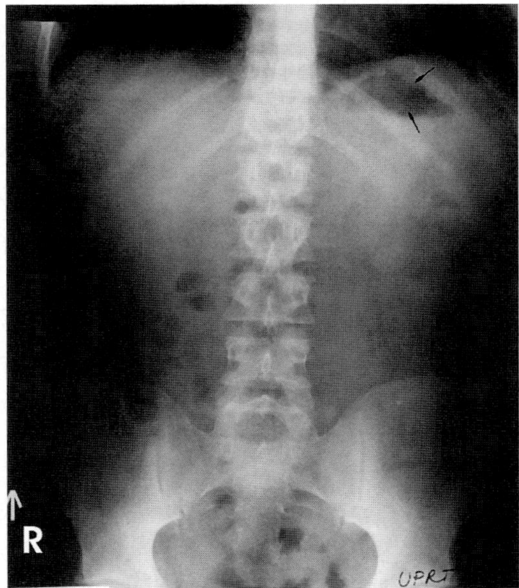

Fig. 3-31. Erect AP–To include diaphragm.

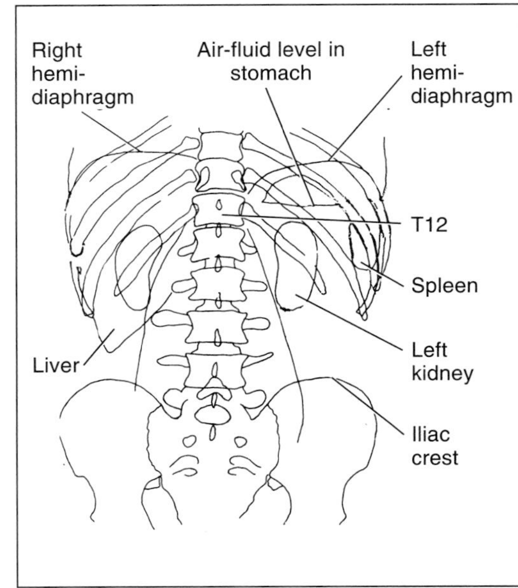

Fig. 3-32. Erect AP.

Evaluation Criteria

- Vertebral column should be aligned to center of radiograph.
- Diaphragm **must** be included, **unless PA erect chest** is also taken.
- **No rotation**: pelvis and lumbar vertebrae should appear symmetrical (R and L iliac wings appear equal in size and shape, and spinous processes should appear in center of vertebrae).
- Lateral collimation margins should be visible for most patients unless such would cut off essential abdominal anatomy.
- **No motion**: ribs, diaphragm and gas bubble margins should appear sharp.
- Should have sufficient exposure (mAs) and long-scale contrast (kVp) to visualize margins of liver and kidneys as well as psoas muscle outline, lumbar transverse processes and ribs on small to average-sized patients, unless these areas are obscured by gas in bowel.
- Free intra-abdominal air should be seen under diaphragm if present.

Dorsal Decubitus Position (Right or Left Lateral)

Abdomen
Special
• PA prone
• Lat. decub. (AP)
• AP erect
• **Dorsal decub. (lat.)**

Structures Best Shown

Abnormal masses, accumulations of gas, air-fluid levels, **aneurysms** (a widening or dilation of the wall of an artery, vein or the heart), **calcification of aorta or other vessels** and **umbilical hernias**.

17

↑ R

14

Technical Factors

- Film size–14 x 17 in. (35 x 43 cm) crosswise.
- Moving or stationary grid.
- 70-80 kVp range.
- Technique and dose:

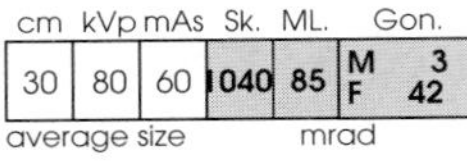

cm	kVp	mAs	Sk.	ML.	Gon.
30	80	60	1040	85	M 3 F 42

average size — mrad

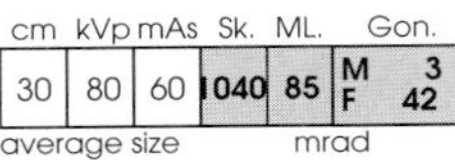

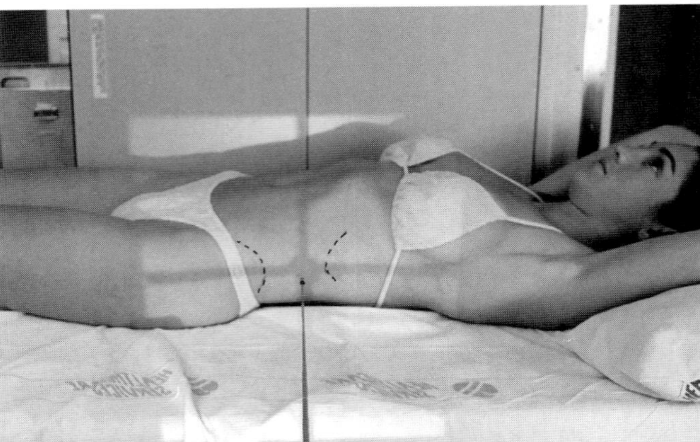

Fig. 3-33. Dorsal decubitus–Right lateral position.

Shielding

- Use gonadal shields on males.

Patient Position

- Supine on radiolucent pad, side against table or vertical grid device. (Secure cart so as not to move away from table or grid device.)
- Pillow under head, arms up beside head, support under partially flexed knees may be more comfortable for the patient.

Part Position

- Adjust patient and cart so center of film and CR is **1 to 2 in. (3 to 5 cm) above level of iliac crest** (to include diaphragm).
- Ensure **no rotation** of pelvis or shoulders. (Ensure that both ASISs' are the same distance from table-top.)
- Adjust height of film holder to align midcoronal plane to centerline of film holder.

Central Ray

- CR **horizontal,** to **center of film** (1 to 2 in. or 3 to 5 cm above iliac crest, and to midcoronal plane).
- Minimum 40 in. (102 cm) SID.

Collimation: Collimate to upper and lower abdomen soft tissue borders.

Respiration: Exposure made at end of **expiration**.

Note: May be taken as a right or left lateral; appropriate R or L lateral marker should be used, indicating which side is against film. An arrow or other marker indicating up side should also be used.

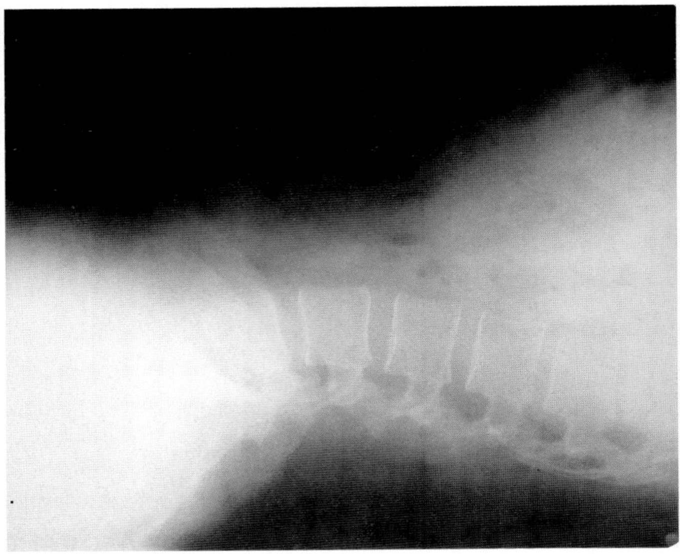

Fig. 3-34. Dorsal decubitus–Right lateral position.

Evaluation Criteria

- The entire diaphragm should be well visualized.
- Collimation borders should be seen on long sides of radiograph on average or small patients without cutting off anterior or posterior aspects of abdomen.
- **No rotation**: Posterior ribs should be superimposed as well as R and L iliac wings and ASISs of pelvis.
- **No motion**: Diaphragm and gas bubble margins should appear sharp.
- Overall density and contrast scale should visualize soft tissue structures within abdomen, especially the ante-vertebral space for possible calcification of aorta and other vessels. Vertebral outlines should be clearly visible below diaphragm.

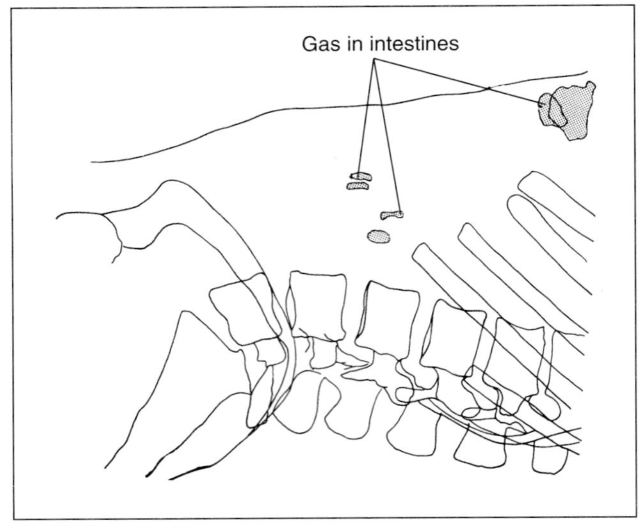

Fig. 3-35. Dorsal decubitus–Right lateral position.

Acute Abdominal Series

• Three-way Abdomen: (1) AP Supine (2) Erect (or Lateral Decub.) Abdomen (3) PA Chest

• Two-way Abdomen: (1) AP Supine (2) Erect (or Lateral Decub.) Abdomen

Acute abdomen
(three-way)
Basic
• **AP supine**
• **AP erect**
• **PA chest**
Special
• **Left lat. decub.**

or

Acute abdomen
(two-way)
Basic
• **AP recumbent**
• **AP erect** (or decub.)
(to include diaphragm)

Clinical Indications for Acute Abdominal Series

1. **Ileus** (small bowel obstruction) or **mechanical ileus** (obstruction of bowel from hernia, adhesions, etc.)
2. **Ascites** *(ah-si'tēz)* (abnormal fluid accumulation in abdomen)
3. **Perforated hollow viscus** (such as bowel or stomach, possible free intraabdominal air)
4. **Intra-abdominal mass**
5. **Post-op** (abdominal surgery)

Remember to **take erect radiographs first** if patient comes to the department in an erect position.

Film Holder, Collimation and Shielding

• 14 x 17 in. (35 x 43 cm), moving or stationary grids. Collimation and shielding the same as described on preceding pages.

Patient and Part Positioning

• Note that on the AP erect abdomen as described on a previous page, some routines may include centering to the iliac crest to include the lower abdomen, **if** the erect PA chest is included to demonstrate possible free intra-abdominal air under the diaphragm.

Most departmental routines, however, include centering higher to include the diaphragm on erect abdomen radiographs even if a PA chest is included in the series. (See survey information, page 93.)

Breathing Instructions

• Chest taken on full inspiration, and abdomen on expiration.

Central Ray

• Same as described on preceding pages.

Notes:

• **Left lateral decubitus** replaces erect position–if the patient is too ill to stand.

• **Horizontal beam** is necessary to visualize air-fluid levels.

• Erect PA chest or AP erect abdomen best visualizes **free air under diaphragm**.

• Patient should be upright or on the side for decubitus, for a minimum of **five minutes** before exposure.

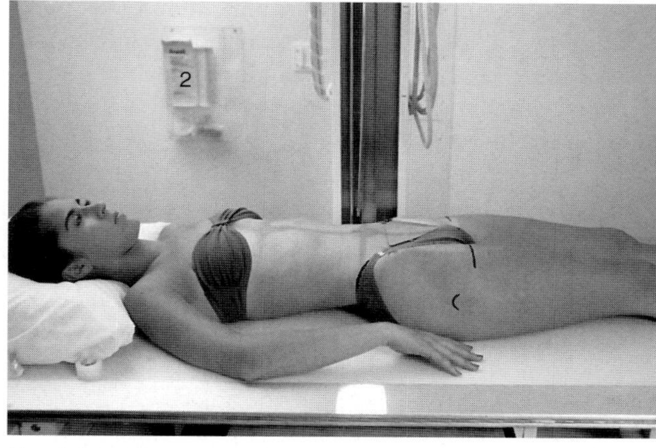

Fig. 3-36. AP supine.

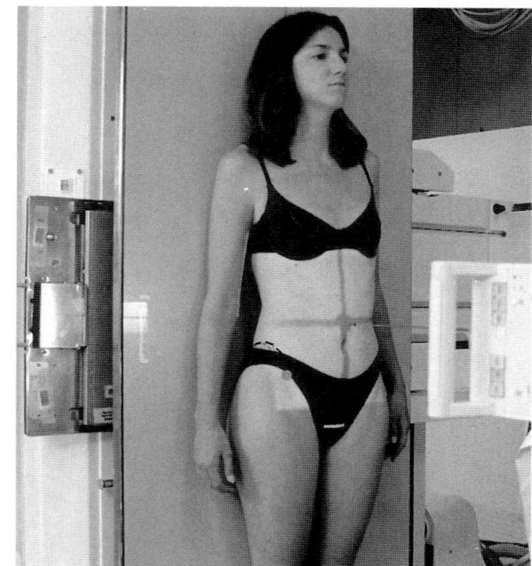

Fig. 3-37. AP erect.

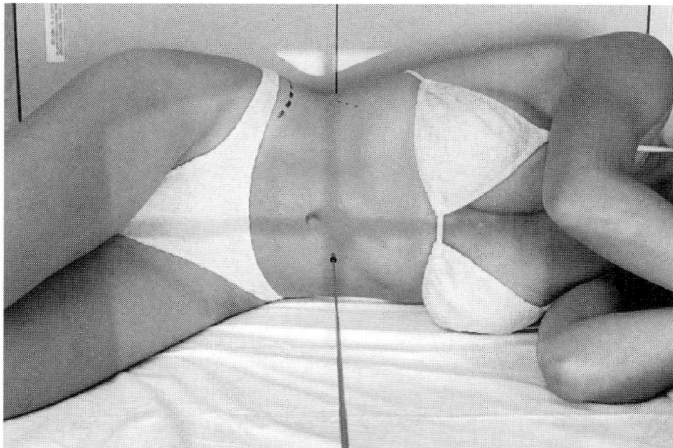

Fig. 3-38. Left lateral decubitus (special projection, if patient cannot stand for AP erect abdomen).

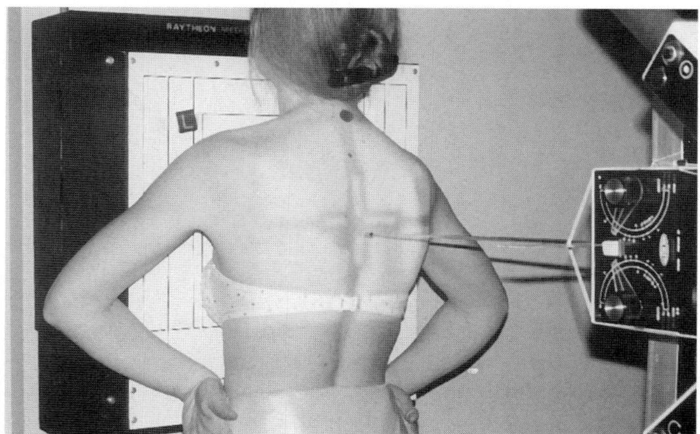

Fig. 3-39. PA chest erect.

Radiographs for Critique

Each of these abdomen radiographs demonstrates some error in positioning which requires a repeat. These, along with accompanying lecture slides of these and other radiographs, will provide a basis for classroom and/or positioning lab discussion. Questions with answers based on these specific critique radiographs are provided in the accompanying student workbook/lab manuals to help prepare students for classroom and/or lab discussions on film critique.

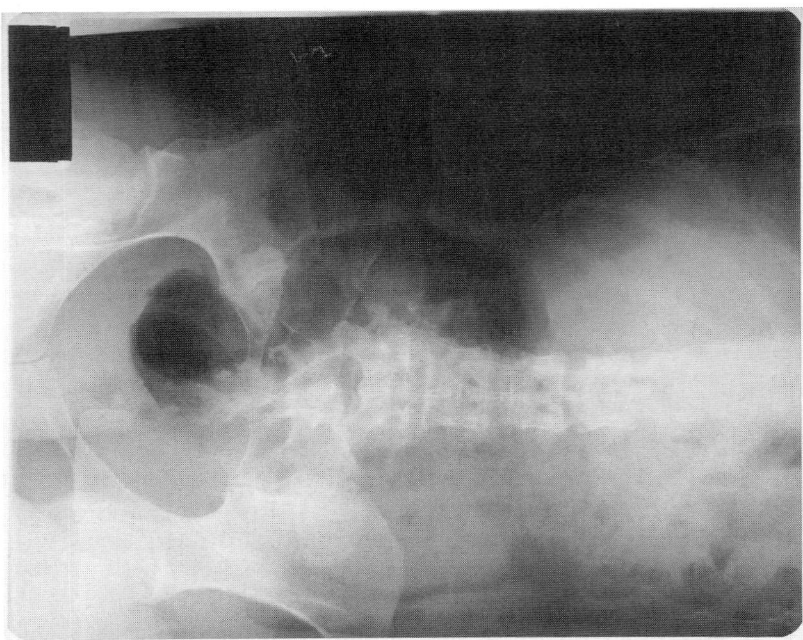

Fig. C3-40. Left lateral decubitus abdomen.

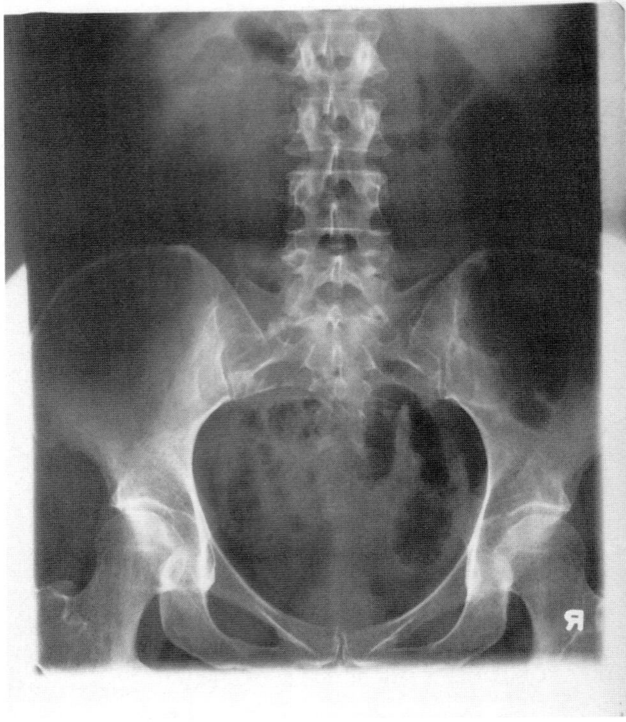

Fig. C3-41. AP supine abdomen – KUB.

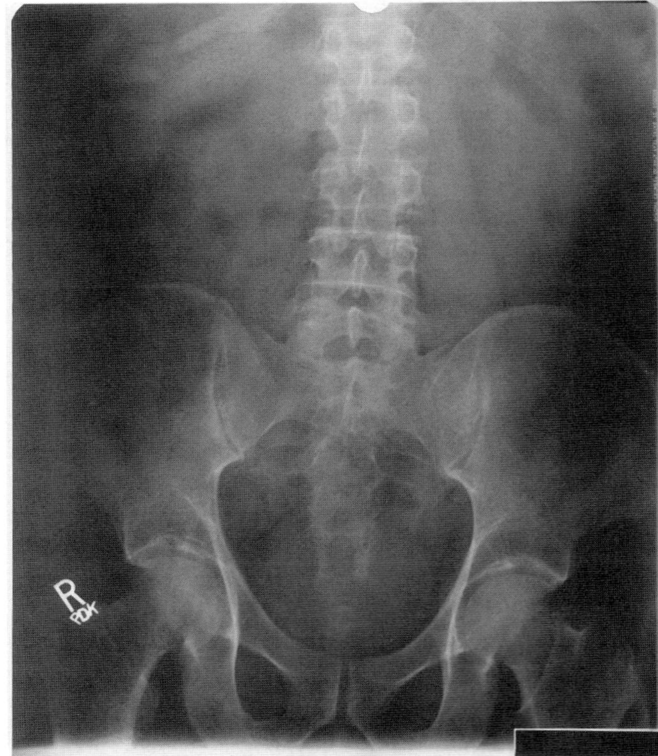

Fig. C3-42. AP supine abdomen.

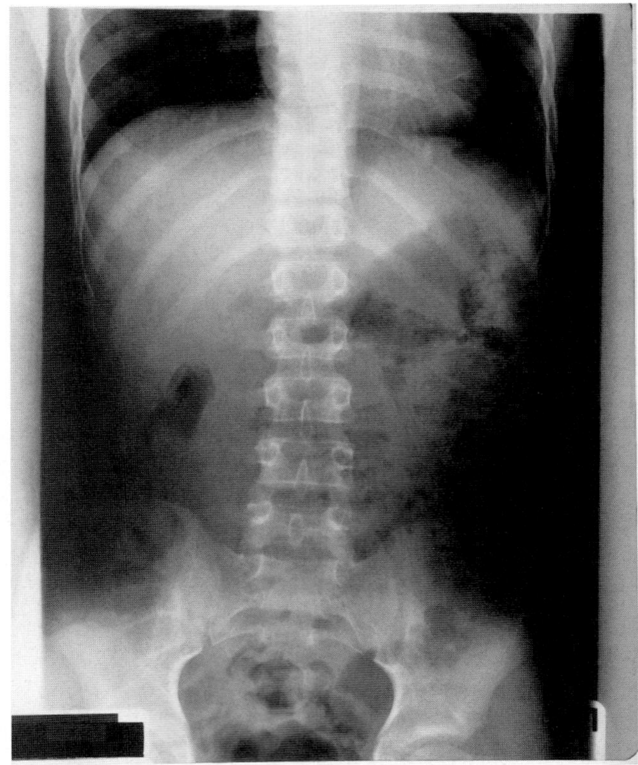

Fig. C3-43. AP abdomen.

CHAPTER 4

Upper Limb

CONTRIBUTIONS BY:
John P. Lampignano, M Ed, RT (R)
Kathy Martensen, BS, RT (R)

4

CONTENTS

Radiographic Anatomy

Hand and wrist **102**

Joints of hand **103**

Carpals **104**

Anatomy review with radiographs **103, 105, 108**

Forearm–Radius and ulna **106**

Distal humerus **107**

Classification of joints **108**

Wrist, forearm and elbow movements **110**

Visualizing fat pads **111**

Radiographic Positioning

Positioning considerations **112**
- Cast conversion chart **112**

Survey information **113**

Basic and special projections **114**

Fingers:
- PA **115**
- PA oblique **116**
- Lateral **117**

Thumb:
- AP **118**
- PA oblique **119**
- Lateral **120**

Hand:
- PA **121**
- PA oblique **122**
- Lateral (fan) **123**
- Lateral (extension and flexion) **124**

Radiographic Positioning cont.

Wrist:
- PA (AP) **125**
- PA oblique **126**
- Lateral **127**
- PA scaphoid views
  - –CR angle, ulnar flexion **128**
  - –Modified Stecher method **129**
- Radial flexion **130**
- Carpal canal
  - –Inferosuperior (Gaynor-Hart method) **131**
  - –Alternate superoinferior **132**
- Carpal bridge **133**

Forearm:
- AP **134**
- Lateral **135**

Elbow:
- AP **136**
- AP oblique
  - –Lateral (external) rotation **137**
  - –Medial (internal) rotation **138**
- Lateral **139**
- Acute flexion (Jones method) **140**
- Trauma axial laterals (Coyle method) **141**
- Radial head laterals **142**

Humerus:
- AP **143**
- Rotational lateral **144**
- Horizontal beam lateral **145**

Proximal humerus–See Shoulder, Chapter 5

Radiographs for critique **146**

Radiographic Anatomy

Upper Limb (Extremity)

The bones of the upper limb can be divided into four main groups: (1) **hand and wrist**, (2) **forearm**, (3) **humerus**, and (4) **shoulder girdle**. The first three groups will be studied in this chapter on the upper limb. The important wrist and elbow joints will be included, but the shoulder joint along with the proximal humerus will be studied in Chapter 5 with the shoulder girdle.

The shape and structure of each of the bones and the articulates or joints of the upper limb must be thoroughly understood by radiographers so that each part can be identified and demonstrated on radiographs.

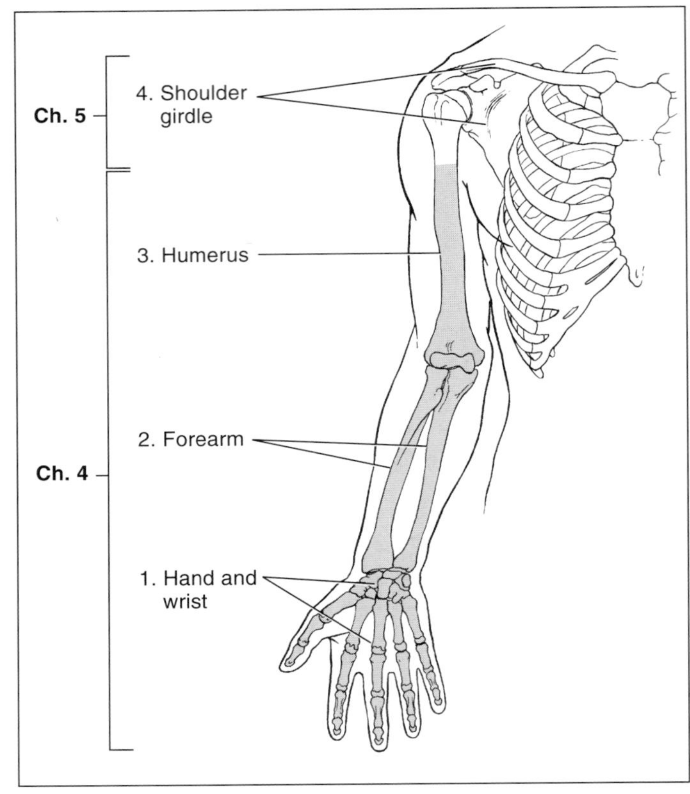

Fig. 4-1. Right upper limb (anterior view).

HAND AND WRIST

The 27 bones on one hand and wrist are divided into three groups:

1. Phalanges (fingers and thumb)	14
2. Metacarpals (palm)	5
3. Carpals (wrist)	8
Total	27

The most distal bones of the hand are the **phalanges** *(fa-lan′jez)*, which make up the digits (fingers and thumb). The second group of bones are the **metacarpals** *(met′ah-kar′pals)*, which make up the palm of each hand. The third group of bones, the **carpals,** *(kar′pals)* comprise the bones of the wrist.

Phalanges–Fingers and Thumb (Digits)

Each finger and thumb is called a **digit**, and each digit consists of two or three separate small bones called **phalanges** [singular is **phalanx** *(fa′lanks)*]. The digits are numbered starting with the thumb as (1) one, and ending with the little finger as (5) five.

Each of the four fingers (digits two, three, four and five) are made up of three phalanges: the **proximal**, **middle** and **distal.** The thumb, or first digit, has just two phalanges, the **proximal** and **distal**.

Each phalanx consists of three parts, a distal rounded **head**, a **body** (shaft), and an expanded **base**, similar to that of the metacarpals

Metacarpals (Palm)

The second group of bones of the hand, making up the palm, are the five **metacarpals**. These bones are numbered the same as the digits, with the first metacarpal being on the thumb or lateral side when the hand is in the anatomical position.

Each metacarpal is made up of three parts similar to the phalanges. Distally, the rounded portion is the **head**. The **body** (shaft) is the long curved portion with the anterior part being concave in shape, and the posterior or dorsal portion convex. The **base** is the expanded proximal end, which articulates with associated carpals.

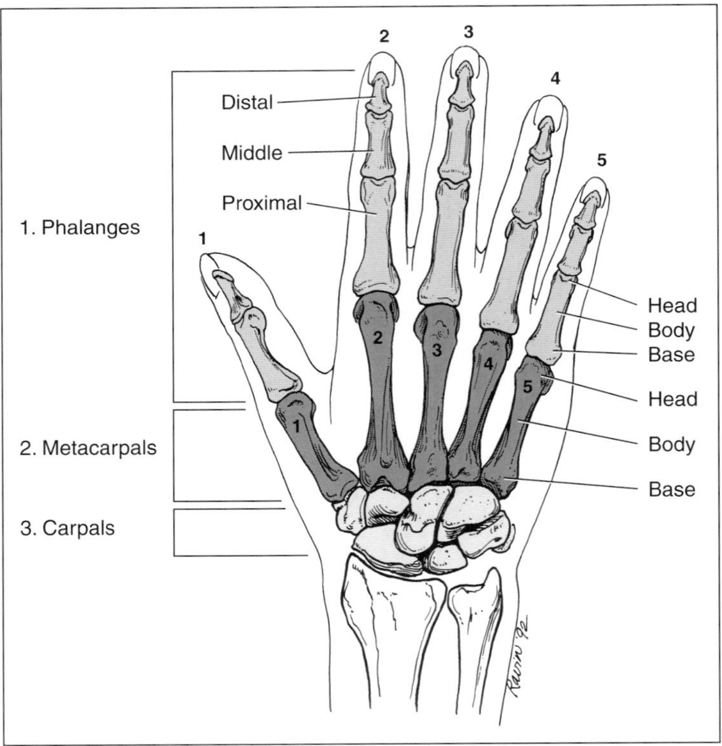

Fig. 4-2. Right hand and wrist (posterior view).

Joints of the Hand

The joints or articulations between the individual bones of the upper limb are important in radiology because small chip fractures may occur near the joint spaces. Therefore, accurate identification of all joints of the phalanges and metacarpals of the hand is required.

Thumb (first digit): The thumb has only two phalanges, so the joint between them is called the **interphalangeal** or **IP joint.** The joint between the first metacarpal and the proximal phalanx of the thumb is called the **first metacarpophalangeal** or **MP joint.** Note that the name of this joint consists of the names of the two bones making up this joint. The proximal bone is named first, followed by the name of the distal bone.

For radiographic purposes, the first metacarpal is considered to be part of the thumb and must be included in its entirety when radiographing the thumb, **from the distal phalanx to the base of the first metacarpal**. This is not the case with the fingers, which for positioning purposes only include the three phalanges: the distal, middle and proximal.

Fingers (second through fifth digits): The second through fifth digits have three phalanges; therefore, they would also have three joints each. Starting from the most distal portion of each digit, the joints are the **distal interphalangeal** or **DIP joint,** followed by the **proximal interphalangeal** or **PIP joint** and, most proximally, the **metacarpophalangeal** or **MP joint.**

Metacarpals: The metacarpals articulate with the phalanges at their distal ends and are called **metacarpophalangeal** or **MP joints.** At the proximal end, the metacarpals articulate with the respective carpals and are called **carpometacarpal** or **CM joints.**

The five metacarpals articulate with specific carpals as follows: (the carpal bones are further identified and described in Figs. 4-5 and 4-6 on the following page)

–1st MC with trapezium –3rd MC with capitate
–2nd MC with trapezoid –4th and 5th MC with hamate

Review Exercise with Radiograph

In identifying joints and phalanges of the hand, it is important to remember that the specific digit and hand must be included in descriptions. A radiograph of a hand (Fig. 4-4) demonstrates the phalanges and metacarpals as well as the joints that have been described above. A good review exercise includes covering up the answers below while identifying each part labeled A-R on this radiograph.

A. Carpometacarpal joint of first digit of right hand.
B. First metacarpal of right hand.
C. Metacarpophalangeal joint of first digit of right hand.
D. Proximal phalanx of the first digit (or thumb) of right hand.
E. Interphalangeal joint of first digit (or thumb) of right hand.
F. Distal phalanx of first digit (or thumb) of right hand.
G. Second metacarpophalangeal joint of right hand.
H. Proximal phalanx of second digit of right hand.
I. Proximal interphalangeal joint of second digit of right hand.
J. Middle phalanx of second digit of right hand.
K. Distal interphalangeal joint of second digit of right hand.
L. Distal phalanx of second digit of right hand.
M. Middle phalanx of fourth digit of right hand.
N. Distal interphalangeal joint of fifth digit of right hand.
O. Proximal phalanx of third digit of right hand.
P. Fifth metacarpophalangeal joint of right hand.
Q. Fourth metacarpal of right hand.
R. Fifth carpometacarpal joint of right hand.

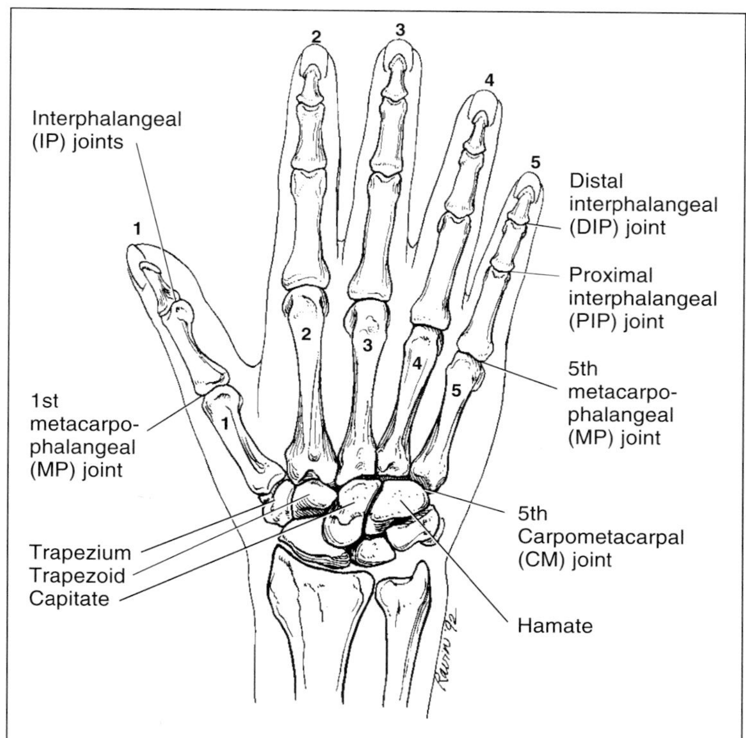

Fig. 4-3. Joints of right hand and wrist.

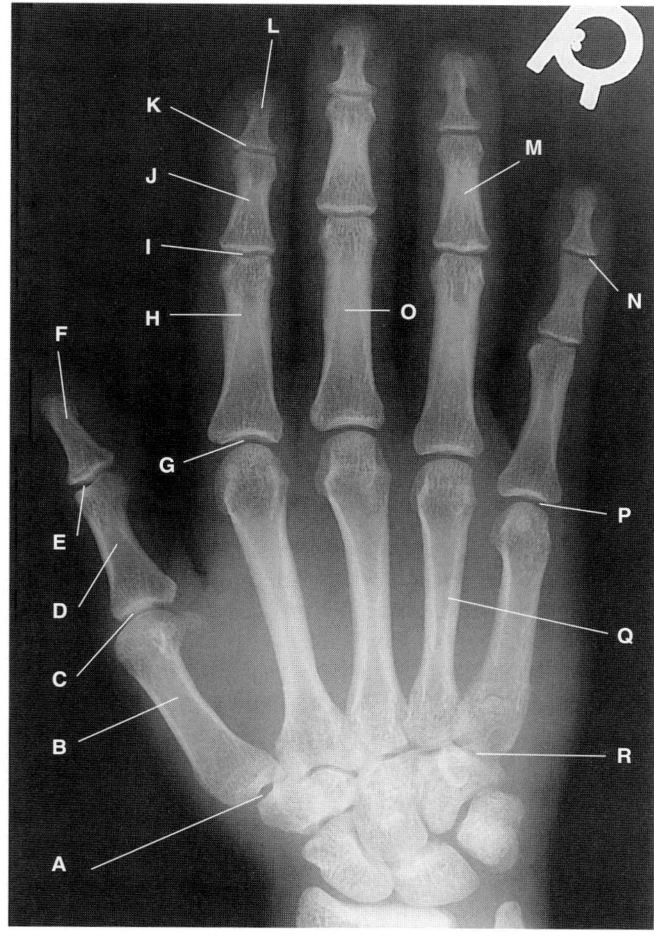

Fig. 4-4. PA radiograph of the right hand.

Carpals (Wrist)

The third group of bones of the hand and wrist are the **carpals** or bones of the wrist. It is easiest to learn the names of the eight carpals by dividing them into two rows of four each.

Proximal row: Beginning on the lateral or thumb side is the **scaphoid**, *(skaf′ oid)* sometimes referred to as the navicular. It should be noted that one of the tarsal bones of the foot is also sometimes called the navicular or scaphoid. However, the correct term for the tarsal bone of the **foot** is **navicular** and the carpal bone of the **wrist** is **scaphoid.**

The **scaphoid**, a boat-shaped bone, is the largest bone in the proximal row and **articulates with the radius proximally.** Its location and articulation with the forearm make it important radiographically because it is **the most frequently fractured carpal bone**.

The **lunate** (moon-shaped) is the second carpal in the proximal row and **also articulates with the radius.** It is distinguished by the deep concavity on its distal surface where it articulates with the capitate of the distal row of carpals (best seen on anterior view, Fig. 4-6).

The **third** carpal is the **triquetrum** *(tri-kwe′ trum),* which has three articular surfaces and is distinguished by its pyramidal shape and its anterior articulation with the small pisiform.

The **pisiform** *(pi′ si-form)* (pea-shaped) is the smallest of the carpal bones and is located anteriorly to the triquetrum as most evident in the anterior view (Fig. 4-6) and the carpal sulcus view in Fig. 4-7.

Distal Row: The second, more distal, row of four carpals articulate with the five metacarpal bones. Starting again on the lateral or thumb side is the **trapezium** *(trah-pe′ ze-um),* a four-sided somewhat irregularly shaped bone located between the scaphoid medially and the first metacarpal distally. Next, the wedge-shaped **trapezoid** *(trap′ e-zoid)*, also four-sided, is the smallest bone in the distal row. This is followed by the largest of the carpal bones, the **capitate** *(kap′ i-tat)* or os magnum, meaning large bone. It can also be remembered by its large rounded head that fits proximally into a concavity formed by the scaphoid and lunate bones.

The last carpal in the distal row is the **hamate** *(ham′ ate),* which is easily distinguished by the hook-like process called the **hamulus** *(ham′ u-lus)*, or hamular process, projecting from its palmar surface (see Fig. 4-7).

Carpal Sulcus (Canal or Tunnel View)

Figure 4-7 is a drawing of the carpals as they would appear looking tangentially down the wrist and arm from the palm or volar side of a hyperextended wrist. This view demonstrates the carpal sulcus formed by the concave anterior or palmar aspect of the carpals. The anteriorly located pisiform and the hamulus process of the hamate are best visualized on this view. This concave area or groove is called the carpal sulcus (carpal tunnel or canal) through which major nerves and tendons pass.

The term "hamate" means hooked, describing the shape of the hamate as seen in the drawing. The trapezium and its relationship to the thumb and trapezoid is well demonstrated.

Summary Chart of Carpal Terminology

The preferred terms as listed will be used throughout this text. Secondary terms listed as synonyms in this chart are terms commonly used in earlier literature.

The names of these eight carpals may be more easily remembered by using a mnemonic like the one in the box on the right.

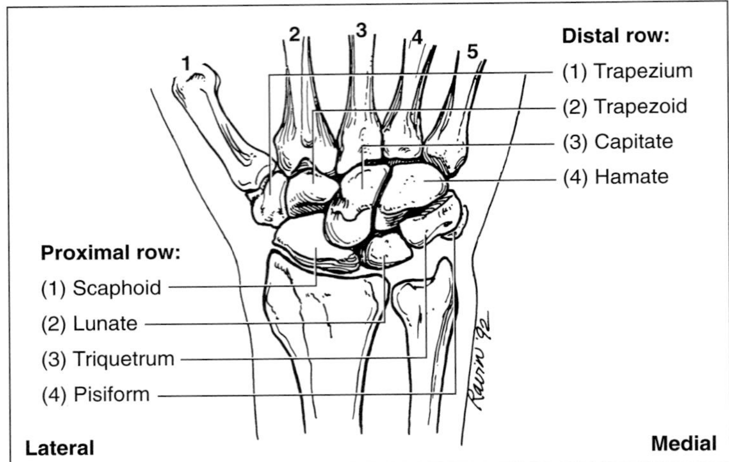

Fig. 4-5. Right carpals (dorsal or posterior view).

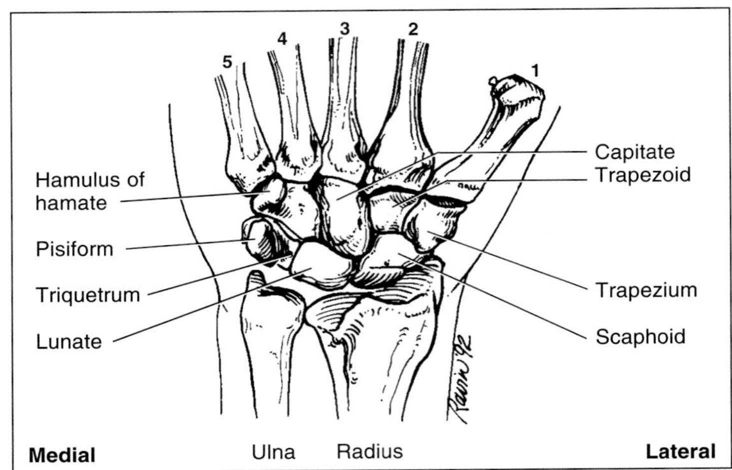

Fig. 4-6. Right carpals (palmar or anterior view).

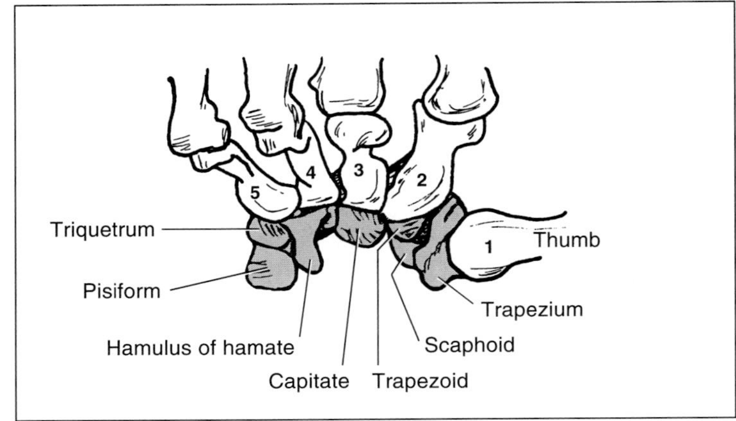

Fig. 4-7. Carpal sulcus (canal or tunnel view).

Mnemonics, Preferred Terms, and Synonyms

Mnemonics	Preferred Term	Synonyms
Send	Scaphoid	(Navicular)
Letter	Lunate	(Semilunar)
To	Triquetrum	(Triangular or Cuneiform)
Peter	Pisiform	
To	Trapezium	(Greater Multangular)
Tell'm (to)	Trapezoid	(Lesser Multangular)
Come	Capitate	(Os Magnum)
Home	Hamate	(Unciform)

REVIEW EXERCISE WITH RADIOGRAPHS

Five projections for the wrist are shown in Fig. 4-8 through 4-12. A good review exercise is to cover up the answers below and identify each of the carpal bones as labeled. Check your answers with those listed below.

Note in the lateral position (Fig. 4-12) that the trapezium (E) and the scaphoid (A) are located more anteriorly. Note also that the ulnar flexion (Fig. 4-10) best demonstrates the scaphoid without the foreshortening and overlapping as seen on the PA (Fig. 4-8). The radial flexion (Fig. 4-9) best demonstrates the interspaces and the carpals on the ulnar (lateral) side of the wrist, namely the hamate (H), the triquetrum (C), pisiform (D) and the lunate (B). The outline of the end-on view of the hamulus process of the hamate (h), can also be seen on this radial flexion radiograph. This hamulus process is also demonstrated well on the carpal canal projection of Fig. 4-11, as is the hook-like process of D the pisiform.

A. Scaphoid
B. Lunate
C. Triquetrum
D. Pisiform
E. Trapezium
F. Trapezoid
G. Capitate
H. Hamate
h. Hamulus (hamular process of hamate)

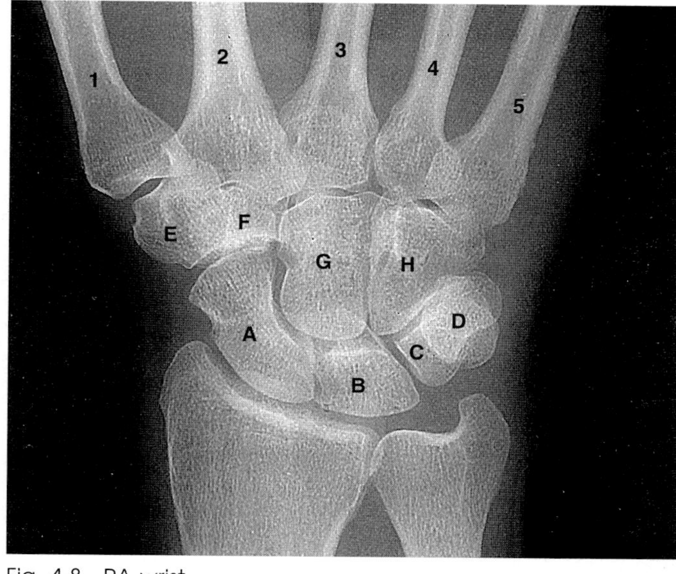

Fig. 4-8. PA wrist.

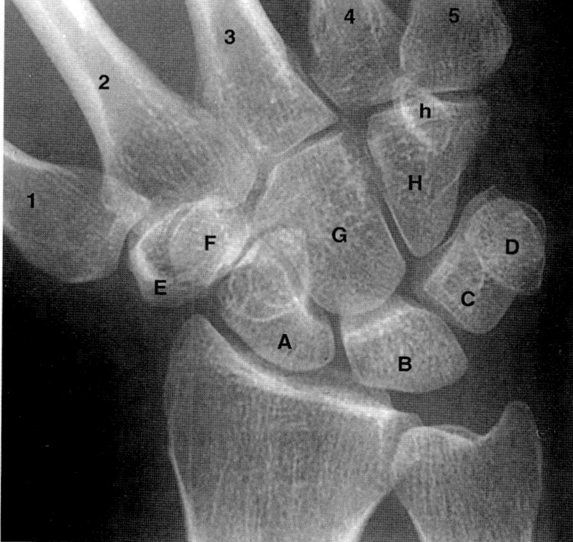

Fig. 4-9. Radial flexion.

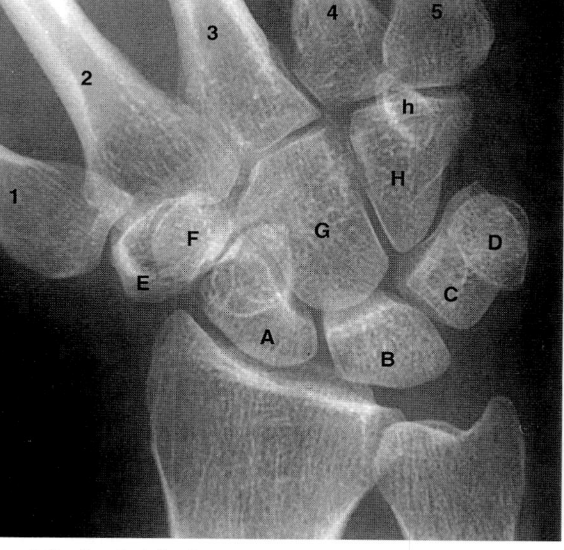

Fig. 4-10. Ulnar flexion.

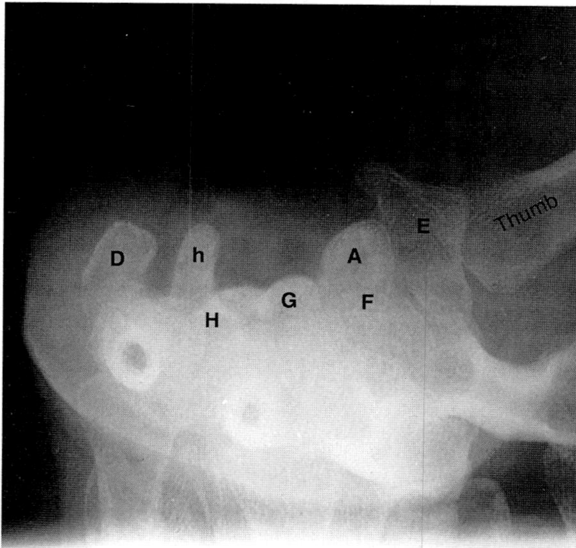

Fig. 4-11. Carpal canal.
The scaphoid (A) is partially superimposed with the trapezoid (F) on this projection.

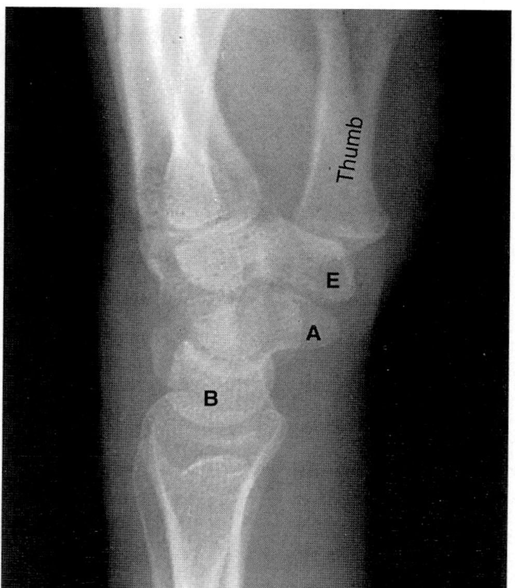

Fig. 4-12. Lateral.

FOREARM–RADIUS AND ULNA

The second group of upper limb bones are those of the forearm, namely, the **radius** on the lateral or thumb side, and the **ulna** on the medial side (Fig. 4-13).

The radius and ulna articulate with each other at the **proximal radioulnar joint** and at the **distal radioulnar joint** as shown in Fig. 4-14. These two joints allow for the rotational movement of the wrist and hand, as will be described later in this chapter.

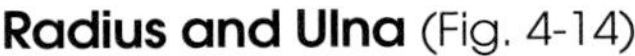

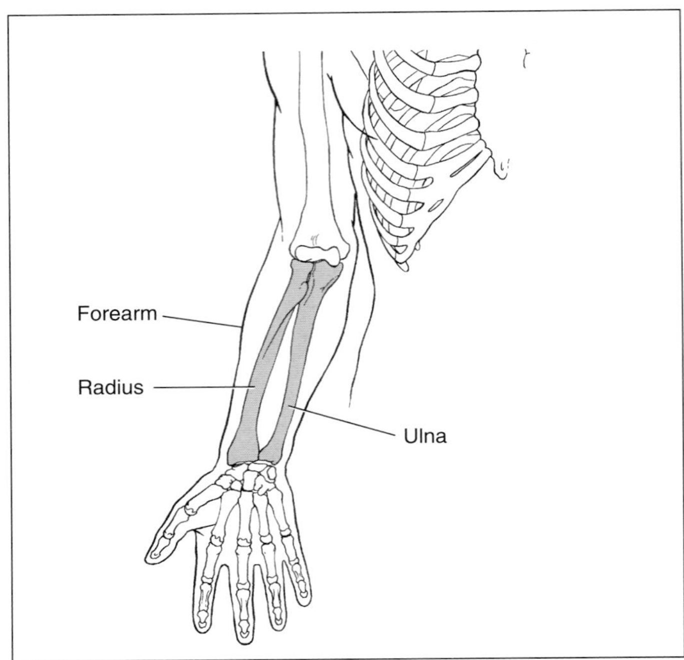

Fig. 4-13. Right upper limb (anterior view).

Radius and Ulna (Fig. 4-14)

Starting at the distal forearm or wrist joint are small conical projections called **styloid processes**, located at the extreme distal ends of both the radius and the ulna. The radial styloid process can be palpated on the thumb side of the wrist joint. The radial styloid process extends more distally than does the ulnar styloid process.

The **ulnar notch** is a small depression on the medial aspect of the distal radius. The head of the ulna fits into the ulnar notch.

The **head of the ulna** is located near the wrist at the **distal** end of the ulna. When the hand is pronated, the ulnar head and styloid process are easily felt and seen on the little finger side of the distal forearm.

The **head of the radius** is located at the **proximal** end of the radius near the elbow joint. The long midportion of both the radius and the ulna is called the **body** (shaft).

The radius is the shorter of the two bones of the forearm and is the only one of the two directly involved in the wrist joint. During the act of pronation, the radius is the bone that rotates around the more stationary ulna.

The proximal radius demonstrates the round disc-like **head** and the **neck** of the radius, a tapered constricted area directly below the head. The rough oval process on the medial and anterior side of the radius, just distal to the neck, is the **radial tuberosity**.

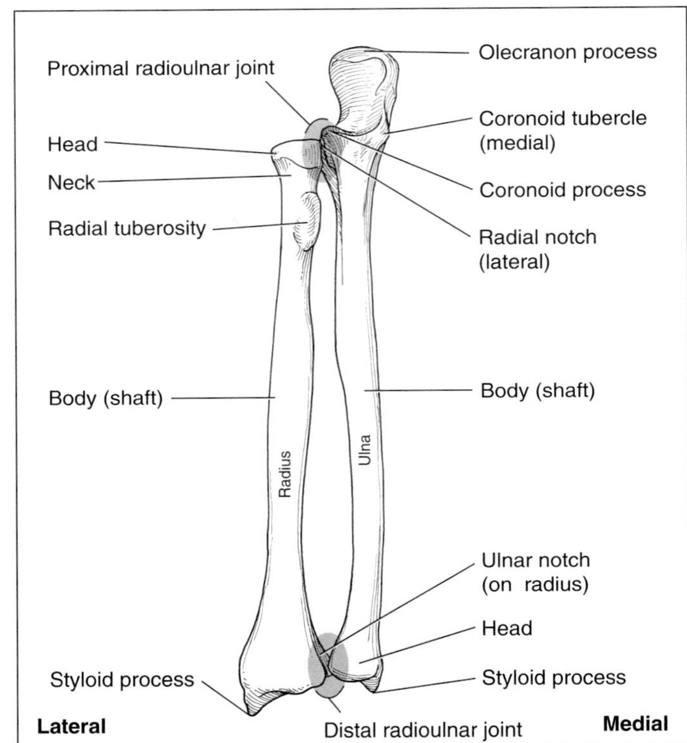

Fig. 4-14. Right radius and ulna (anterior view).

Proximal Ulna (Fig. 4-14 and 4-15)

The ulna is the longer of the two bones of the forearm and is primarily involved in the formation of the elbow joint. The two beak-like processes of the proximal ulna are called the **olecranon** and **coronoid processes**. The olecranon process can be easily palpated on the posterior aspect of the elbow joint.

The medial margin of the coronoid process opposite the radial notch (lateral) is commonly referred to as the **coronoid tubercle** (see Fig. 4-14 and AP elbow radiograph in Fig. 4-19).

The large concave depression or notch articulating with the distal humerus is the **trochlear** *(trok′ le-ar)* **notch** (semilunar notch). The small shallow depression located on the lateral aspect of the proximal ulna is the **radial** *(ra′ de-al)* **notch.** The head of the radius articulates with the ulna at the radial notch. This joint or articulation is the proximal radioulnar joint that combines with the distal radioulnar joint to allow rotation of the forearm during pronation. During the act of pronation the radius crosses over the ulna near the upper third of the forearm (see page 110).

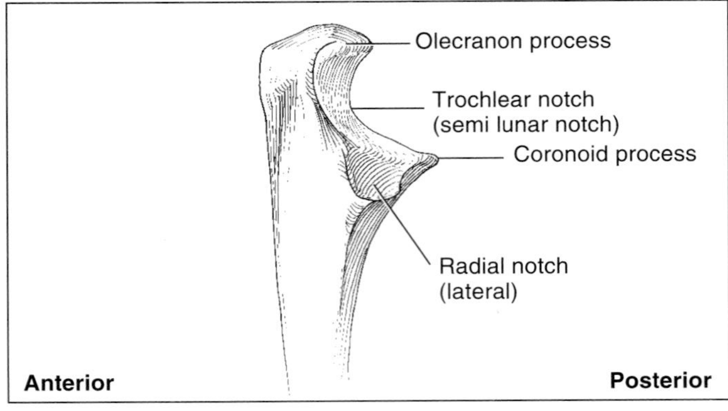

Fig. 4-15. Left proximal ulna (lateral view).

Distal Humerus

The parts of the proximal humerus are covered in Chapter 5 with the shoulder girdle. However, the mid and distal humerus are included in this chapter as part of the elbow joint.

The **body** (shaft) of the humerus is the long center section, and the expanded distal end of the humerus is the **humeral condyle**. The articular portion of the humeral condyle is divided into two parts, the **trochlea** *(trok′ le-ah)* and the **capitulum** *(kah-pit′ u-lum)*.

The **trochlea** (meaning pulley) is shaped like a pulley or spool with two rim-like outer margins, and a smooth depressed center portion called the **trochlear sulcus** or groove. This depression of the trochlea, which continues inferiorly and posteriorly, appears circular on a lateral end-on view and, on a lateral elbow radiograph, appears as a less dense (more radiolucent) area as seen in Figs. 4-17 and 4-20. The **trochlea** is located more medially and articulates with the **ulna**.

The **capitulum**, meaning "little head," which in earlier literature was called **capitellum** *(kap″ i-tel′ um)*, is located on the lateral aspect articulating with the head of the **radius.** (A memory aid is to associate the **cap**itulum, "cap", with the "head" of the radius.)

The articular surface making up the rounded articular margin of the capitulum is just slightly smaller than that of the trochlea, as seen in Fig. 4-18. This becomes significant in evaluating for a true lateral position of the elbow, as does the direct superimposition of the two **epicondyles** *(ep″ e-kon′ dils)*.

The **lateral epicondyle** is the small projection on the lateral aspect of the distal humerus above the capitulum. The **medial epicondyle** is larger and more prominent than the lateral and is located on the medial edge of the distal humerus proximal to the trochlea. In a true lateral position, the directly superimposed epicondyles (which are difficult to recognize) are seen to be proximal to the circular appearance of the trochlear sulcus (Figs. 4-17 and 4-20).

The distal humerus has specific **depressions** on both the anterior and posterior surfaces. The two shallow **anterior depressions** are the **coronoid fossa** and the **radial fossa** (Figs. 4-16 and 4-17). As the elbow is completely flexed, the coronoid process and the radial head are received by these respective fossa, as the names indicate.

The deep **posterior depression** is the **olecranon fossa** (not specifically shown on these drawings). The olecranon process of the ulna fits into this depression when the arm is fully extended. Soft tissue detail by way of specific fat pads located within the deep olecranon fossa is important in trauma diagnosis of the elbow joint.

The lateral view of the elbow (Fig. 4-17) clearly demonstrates specific parts of the proximal radius and ulna. The **head** and **neck** of the radius are well demonstrated, as are the **radial tuberosity** (partially seen on the proximal radius) and the large concave **trochlear (semilunar) notch.**

True Lateral Elbow: Specific positions such as an **accurate lateral** with **90° flexion** with possible associated visualization of fat pads are essential for evaluation of joint pathology for the elbow (see page 111). A good criteria or a good means of evaluating for a true lateral position of the elbow when flexed 90° is the appearance of the three concentric arcs, as labelled in Fig. 4-18. The first and smallest arc is the **trochlear sulcus**. The second intermediate arc appears double-lined as the outer ridges or rounded edges of the **capitulum** and **trochlea.*** (The smaller is the capitulum and the larger is the medial ridge of the trochlea.) The **trochlear notch of the ulna** appears as a third arc of a true lateral elbow. If the elbow is even slightly rotated from a **true** lateral, these arcs will not appear symmetrically aligned in this way, and the elbow joint space will not be as open.

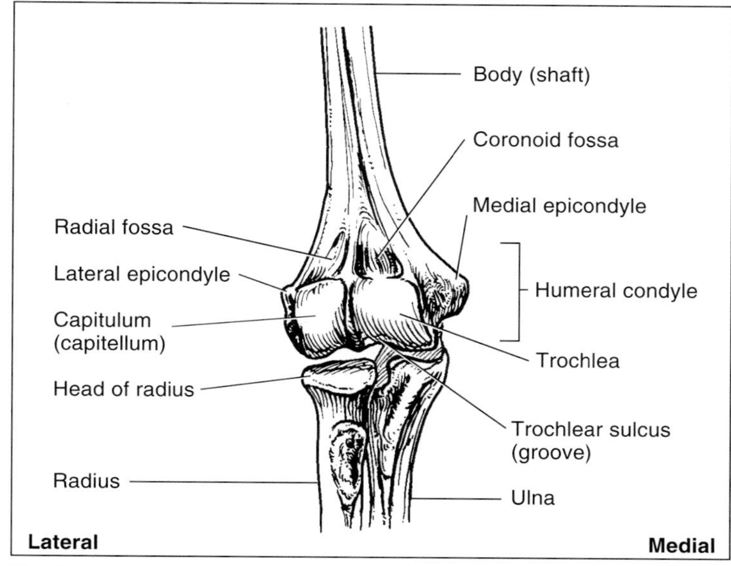

Fig. 4-16. Distal humerus (anterior view).

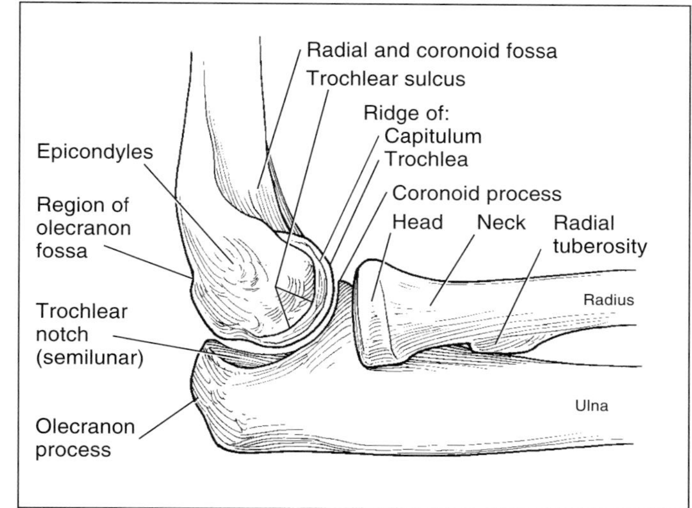

Fig. 4-17. Lateral elbow.

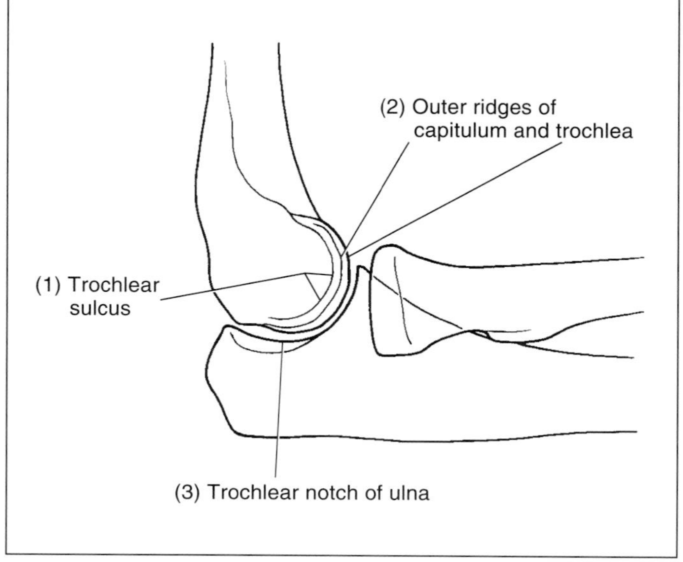

Fig. 4-18. True lateral elbow–3 concentric arcs.*

*Berquist, TH; *Imaging of Orthopedic Trauma and Surgery*; Philadelphia: WB Saunders; 1986 (pp. 583-584).

REVIEW EXERCISE WITH RADIOGRAPHS

These AP and lateral radiographs of the elbow provide a review of anatomy and demonstrate the three concentric arcs as evidence of a true lateral position.

A. Medial epicondyle.
B. Trochlea (medial aspect).
C. Coronoid tubercle.
D. Radial head.
E. Capitulum.
F. Lateral epicondyle.
G. Superimposed epicondyles of humerus.
H. Olecranon process.
I. Trochlear sulcus.
J. Trochlear notch.
K. Double outer ridges of capitulum and trochlea (capitulum is the smaller of the two areas and trochlea the larger).
L. Coronoid process of ulna.
M. Radial head.
N. Radial neck.
O. Radial tuberosity.

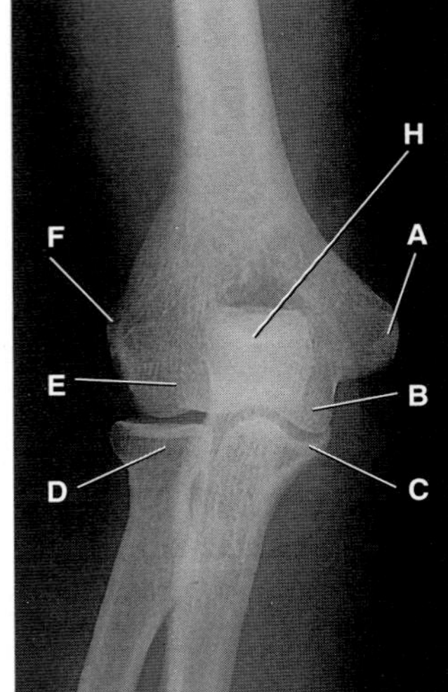

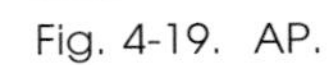
Fig. 4-19. AP.

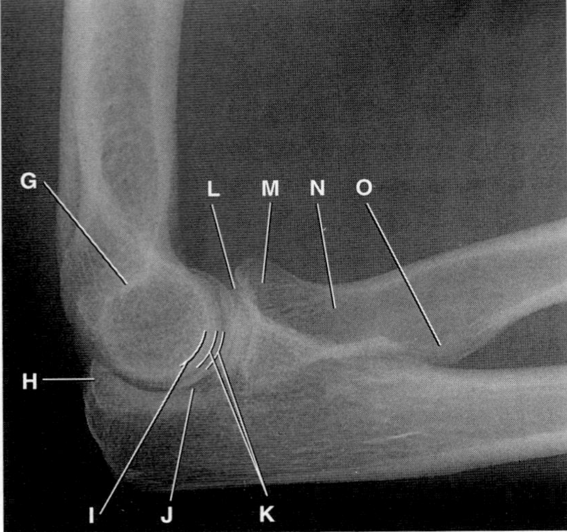

Fig. 4-20. Lateral.

CLASSIFICATION OF JOINTS

A general description of joints or articulations with the various classifications and movement types is described in Chapter One. These will be reviewed and described more specifically for each joint of the hand, wrist, forearm and elbow.

All joints of the upper limb as described in this chapter are classified as **synovial** and therefore are freely movable or **diarthrodial**. Only the movement types differ as follows:

Hand and Wrist

Interphalangeal (IP) Joints: Beginning distally with the phalanges, all interphalangeal joints are **ginglymus** or **hinge type** joints with movements in two directions only, **flexion** and **extension**. This movement is in one plane only, around the transverse axis. This includes the single interphalangeal joint of the thumb (1st digit), and the distal and proximal interphalangeal joints of the fingers (2nd to 5th digits).

Metacarpophalangeal (MP) Joints: The second through fifth metacarpophalangeal joints (the base of the fingers) are **ellipsoidal** or **condyloid type** joints that allow movement in four directions: **flexion**, **extension**, **abduction** and **adduction**. **Circumduction** movement also occurs at these joints, which is a cone-like sequential movement of these four directions.

Both the first metacarpophalangeal and the first carpometacarpal (MP) joints of the thumb are **sellar** or **saddle type** joints. The best example of the saddle joint is the first carpometacarpal joint, as this best demonstrates the shape and the movements of a saddle joint. The first metacarpophalangeal joint is also classified as a saddle joint, although it is not as good an example.

The second through fifth carpometacarpal joints are **plane** or **gliding type** joints, which allow the least amount of movement of the synovial class joints. The joint surfaces are flat or slightly curved with movement limited by a tight fibrous capsule. The intercarpal joints between the various carpals also only have a **plane** or **gliding type** movement.

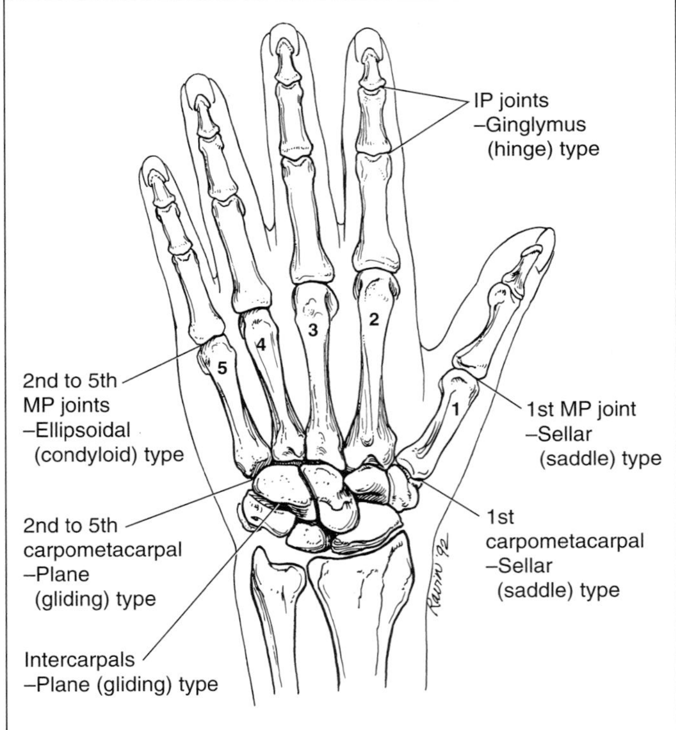

Fig. 4-21. Joints of left hand and wrist (posterior view).

Wrist Joint

The wrist joint is an **ellipsoidal** or **condyloid-type** joint, and is freely movable or **diarthrodial**, of the **synovial classification**. Of the two bones of the forearm, only the radius articulates directly with two carpal bones, the **scaphoid** and the **lunate**. This wrist joint is called the **radiocarpal joint**.

The **triquetral** bone, however, is also part of the wrist joint in that it is opposite the **articular disk**. The articular disk is part of the total wrist articulation, including a joint between the distal radius and ulna of the forearm, called the **distal radioulnar joint**.

The articular surface of the distal radius, along with the total articular disk, forms a smooth concave-shaped articulation with the three carpals to form the complete wrist joint.

The total wrist joint is enclosed by an articular synovial capsule strengthened by four radiocarpal ligaments that allow movements in four directions plus circumduction.

The four ligaments of the wrist are as follows: The **ulnar collateral ligament**, which is attached to the styloid process of the ulna and fans out to attach to the triquetrum and the pisiform. The **radial collateral ligament** extends from the tip of the styloid process of the radius to primarily the lateral side of the scaphoid but also has attachments to the trapezium. The remaining two wrist ligaments are not shown on this posterior view drawing. The first of these is the **dorsal radiocarpal ligament**, a somewhat weaker ligament attaching the posterior border of the distal radius to the adjoining carpals. The **palmar radiocarpal ligament**, also not visualized, is a strong and broad ligament attaching to the anterior aspects of both the radius and ulna to the anterior aspects of the three adjoining carpals, the scaphoid, lunate and triquetrum.

The synovial membrane lines the inner surfaces of these four wrist ligaments in addition to lining the distal end of the radius and the articular surfaces of the adjoining carpal bones.

Visualization of Fat Pads or Stripes: Certain fat pads and fat stripes associated with the wrist joint are important to visualize radiographically. One of these, the scaphoid fat pad or stripe, is located between the radial collateral ligament and the adjoining muscle tendons and can be visualized lateral to the scaphoid. It should be visualized as a soft tissue structure on all PA and oblique wrist radiographs. The absence or displacement of this fat stripe may be the only indication of a fracture of the radial aspect of the wrist (see page 111).

Elbow Joint

The elbow joint is also of the **synovial classification** and is thus freely movable or **diarthrodial**. The elbow joint is generally considered a **ginglymus** (hinge) type joint with flexion and extension movements between the humerus and the ulna and radius. The complete elbow joint, however, includes three joints enclosed in one articular capsule. In addition to the hinge joints between the humerus and ulna and the humerus and radius, the **proximal radioulnar joint** (trochoidal or pivot type) is also considered part of the elbow joint.

See the following pages in this chapter for a discussion of the importance of accurate lateral positioning of the elbow for visualizing certain fat pads within the elbow joint.

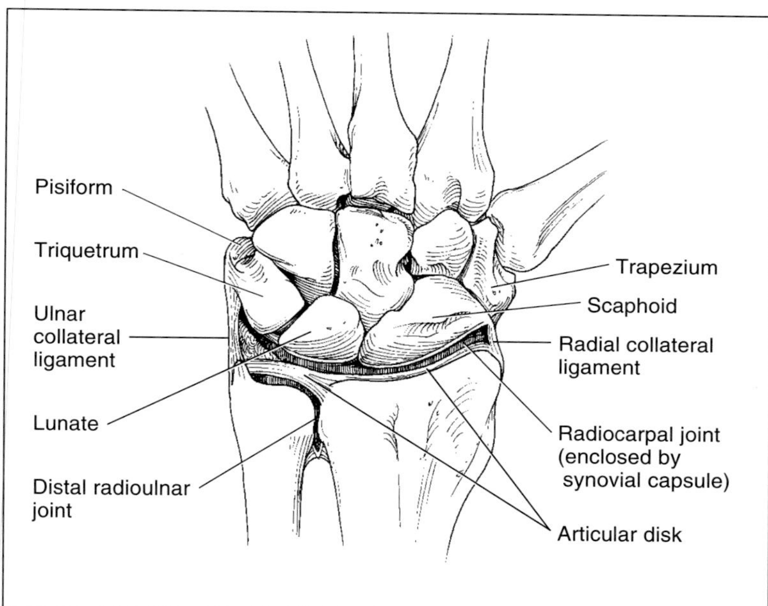

Fig. 4-22. Left wrist joint with articular disk (posterior view).

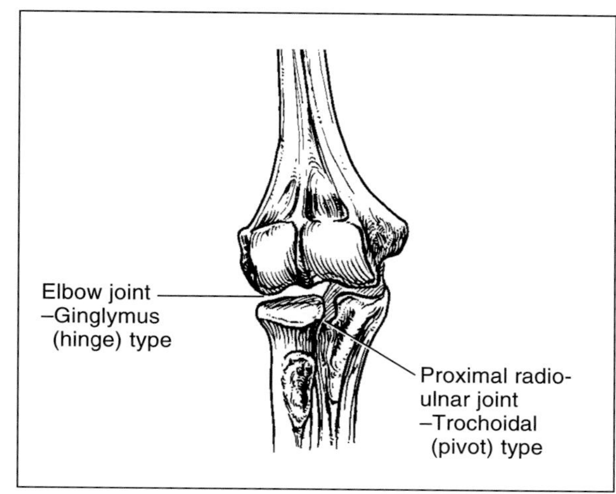

Fig. 4-23. Elbow joint.

Summary of Hand, Wrist, Forearm and Elbow Joints

Classification: ***Synovial*** (Articular capsule containing synovial fluid)

Mobility Type: ***Diarthrodial*** (freely movable)

Movement Type:

1. Interphalangeal joints	–***Ginglymus*** (hinge)
2. Metacarpophalangeal joints:	
First digit (thumb)	–***Sellar*** (saddle)
Second-fifth digits	–***Ellipsoidal*** (condyloid)
3. Carpometacarpal joints:	
First digit (thumb)	–***Sellar*** (saddle)
Second-fifth digits	–***Plane*** (gliding)
4. Intercarpal joints	–***Plane*** (gliding)
5. Wrist (radiocarpal) joint	–***Ellipsoidal*** (condyloid)
6. Proximal and distal: Radioulnar joints	–***Trochoidal*** (pivot)
7. Elbow joint:	
Humeroulnar and Humeroradial	–***Ginglymus*** (hinge)
Proximal radioulnar	–***Trochoidal*** (pivot)

WRIST JOINT MOVEMENT TERMINOLOGY

Certain terminology involving movements of the wrist joint may be confusing but need to be understood by radiographers because special projections of the wrist are described by these movements. These terms are **ulnar flexion** and **radial flexion**.

The term flexion is described in Chapter 1 under Terminology as a "bending of a joint wherein the angle between the parts is decreased." Usual flexion of the wrist joint involves the anterior surface of the wrist and is a forward bending wherein the angle between the anterior hand and forearm is decreased.

Ulnar or radial flexion involves a **lateral bending** at the wrist joint. If the hand is moved toward the ulnar side of the forearm with the hand pronated, the wrist joint near the distal ulna is flexed, and the angle between the lateral aspect of the hand and forearm is decreased. This movement, termed **ulnar flexion**, serves to open up the carpal joints on the opposite side of the wrist. The carpals best demonstrated in this position are those located most medially when the hand is pronated, namely the scaphoid, trapezium and trapezoid. This motion is most often used to obtain a better view of the **scaphoid** (the most commonly fractured carpal bone).

If the hand is forced toward the radial or thumb side of the forearm with the hand pronated, the wrist joint near the distal radius will be flexed laterally. This motion, termed **radial flexion**, serves to open up the carpal joints on the lateral or little finger side of the wrist. The carpals best demonstrated are the lunate, triquetrum, pisiform and hamate. This motion is used most often to better demonstrate the **lunate**.

Note: See Chapter 1, page 24, for an explanation of the terms **ulnar** and **radial deviation**, which in practice are sometimes used as being synonymous with ulnar and radial flexion wrist movements.

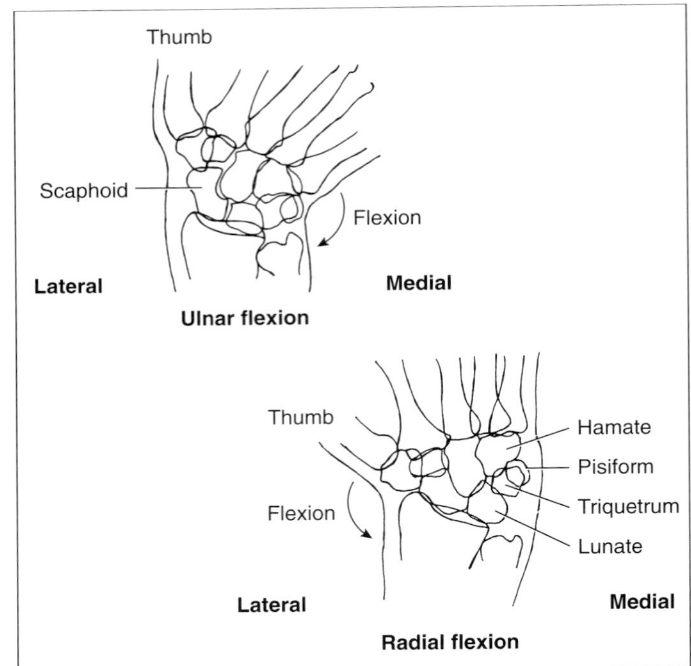

Fig. 4-24. Wrist movements.

FOREARM ROTATIONAL MOVEMENTS

The radioulnar joints of the forearm also involve some special rotational movements which need to be understood in radiographing the forearm. For example, the **forearm generally should not be radiographed in a pronated position (a PA projection)** which may appear to be the most natural position for the forearm and hand. The forearm should routinely be radiographed in an **AP projection** with the hand **supinated**, or palm up. The reason becomes clear in studying the "cross over" position of the radius and ulna when the hand is pronated (Fig. 4-25). This results from the unique pivot-type rotational movements of the forearm involving both the proximal and distal radioulnar joints.

Summary: To prevent superimposition of the radius and ulna resulting from these pivot-type rotational movements, the forearm is radiographed with the **hand supinated** for an **AP projection**.

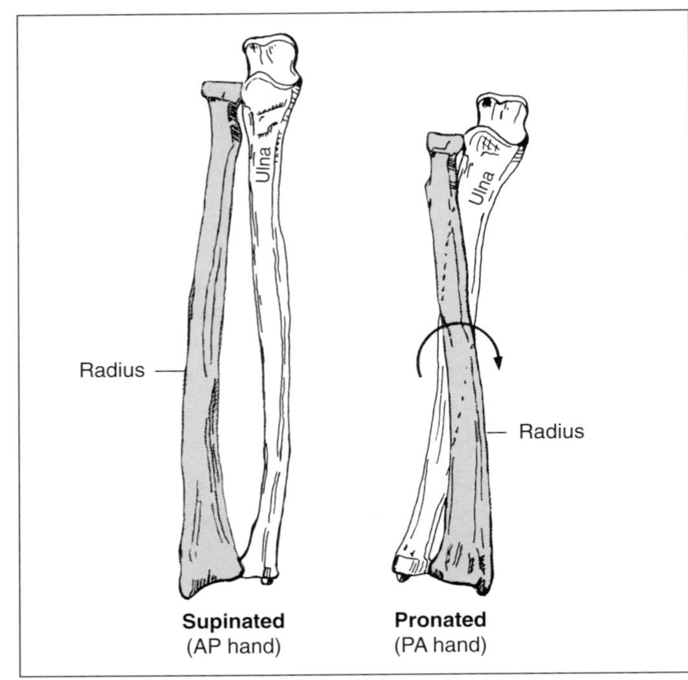

Fig. 4-25. Forearm rotational movements.

ELBOW ROTATIONAL MOVEMENTS

The appearance of the proximal radius and ulna changes as the elbow and distal humerus is rotated either medially or laterally as shown with these radiographs. Note that on the AP radiograph with no rotation, the proximal radius is only slightly superimposed by the ulna (Fig. 4-25a). The radius and ulna can be separated with lateral rotation of the elbow, as shown on the center radiograph; while medial rotation completely superimposes them, as seen on the radiograph on the right. This relationship is crucial in critiquing AP projections of the elbow, and it is important to remember that **lateral rotation separates** the radius and ulna and **medial rotation superimposes**. (This is further demonstrated with the oblique elbow projections on pages 137 and 138.)

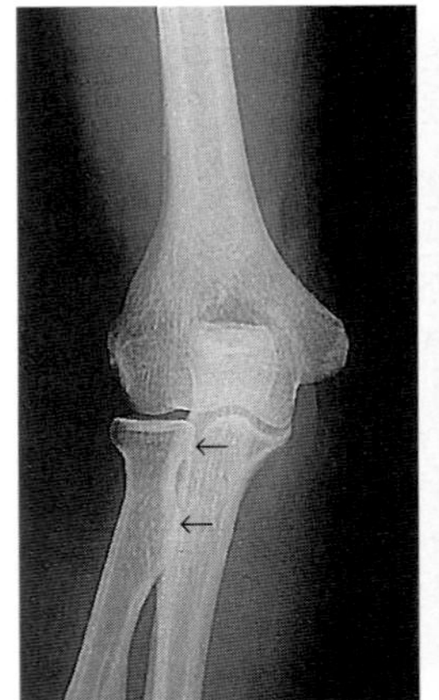

Fig. 4-25a. AP, **no rotation**–Radius and ulna partially superimposed.

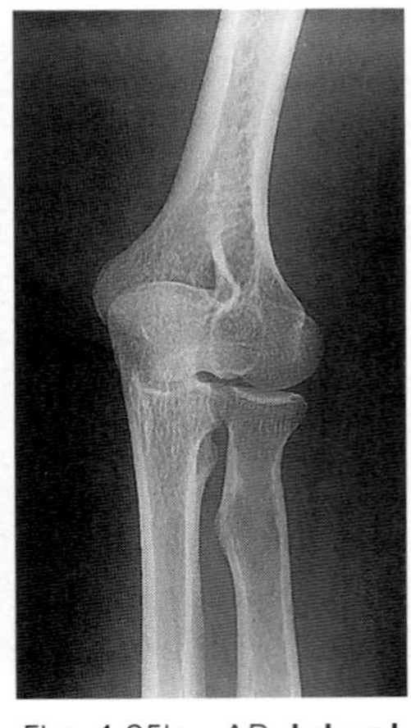

Fig. 4-25b. AP, **lateral rotation**–Separates radius and ulna.

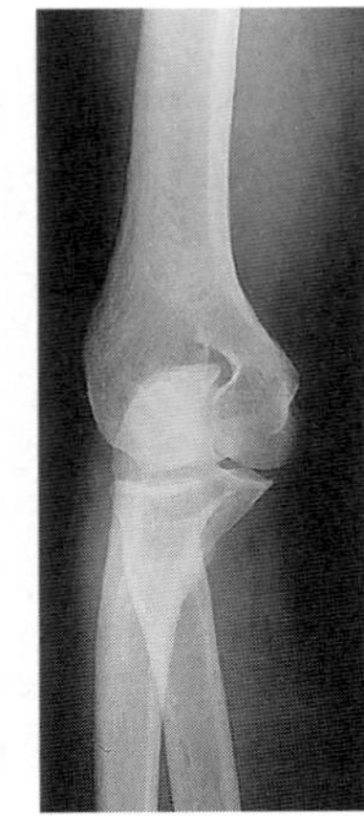

Fig. 4-25c. AP, **medial rotation**–Superimposes radius and ulna.

IMPORTANCE OF VISUALIZING FAT PADS

Radiographs of the upper and lower limbs are taken not only to evaluate for disease or trauma to bony structures, but also to evaluate associated soft tissues such as certain accumulations of fat called **fat pads, fat bands** or **stripes**. In some cases the displacement of an adjoining fat pad or band may be the only indication of disease or significant injury or fracture within a joint region.

For diagnostic purposes the most important fat pads or bands are those located around certain joints of the upper and lower limbs. These fat pads are extra-synovial (outside the synovial sac) but are located within the joint capsule. Therefore, any changes within the capsule itself will alter the normal position and shape of the fat pads. Most often, this change is a result of fluid accumulation (effusion) within the joint, indicating the presence of an injury involving that joint.

When visualized, the radiolucent fat pads are seen as densities which are slightly more lucent than surrounding structures. Fat pads and their surrounding soft tissue are of only slightly different density, making them difficult to visualize on radiographs. This requires long-scale contrast techniques with optimum exposure or density to visualize these soft tissue structures. (They generally will not be visible on printed radiographs without enhancement as shown on this page).

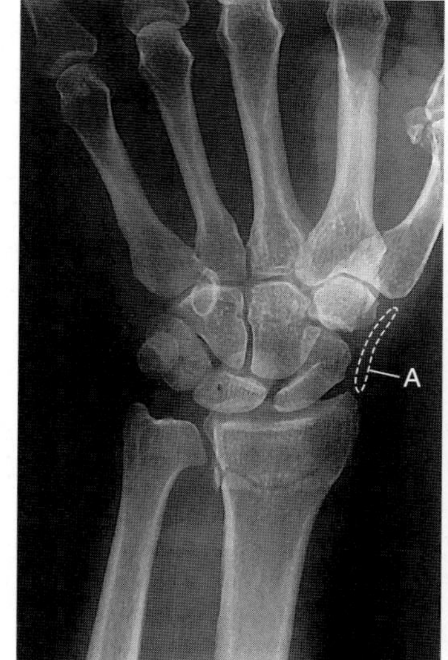

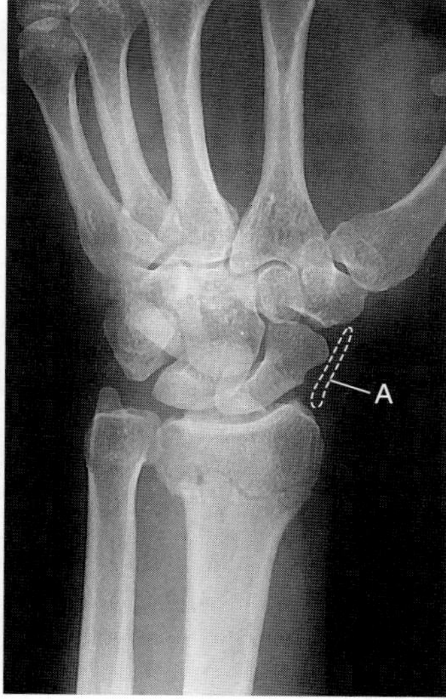

Fig. 4-26. PA and oblique wrist–**Scaphoid fat band (A)**.

Wrist Joint*

The wrist joint includes two important fat stripes. First, a **scaphoid fat stripe (A)** is visualized on the PA and the oblique views. It is elongated and slightly convex in shape and is located between the radial collateral ligament and adjoining muscle tendons immediately lateral to the scaphoid (Fig. 4-26). The absence or displacement of this fat stripe may be the only indicator of a fracture on the radial aspect of the wrist.

A second fat stripe is visualized on the lateral view of the wrist. This **pronator fat stripe (B)** is normally visualized approximately 1 cm (4/10 in.) from the anterior surface of the radius (Fig. 4-27). Subtle fractures of the distal radius can be indicated by the displacement or obliteration of the plane of this fat stripe.

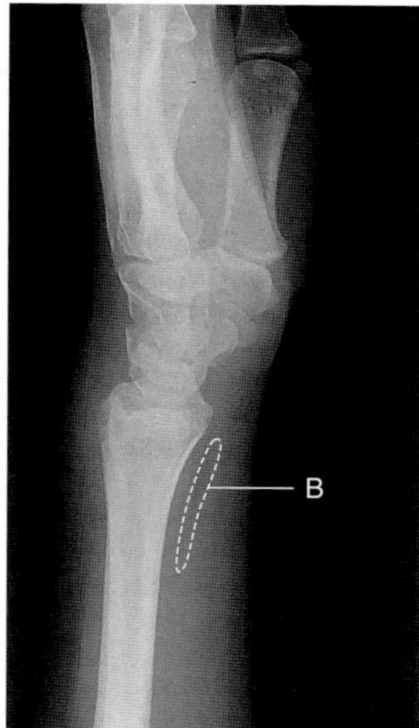

Fig. 4-27. Lateral wrist–**Pronator fat stripe (B)**.

Elbow Joint*†

The three significant fat pads or stripes of the elbow are visualized only on the lateral projection. They are not seen on the AP due to their superimposition over the bony structures. On the lateral view the **anterior fat pad (C)**, which is formed by the superimposed coronoid and radial pads, is seen as slightly radiolucent "teardrop" shapes located just anterior to the distal humerus (Fig. 4-28). Trauma or infection can cause the anterior fat pad to be elevated and more visible and distorted in shape. This is visible only on a lateral elbow flexed 90°.

The **posterior fat pad (D)** is located deep within the olecranon fossa and is normally **not visible** on a negative elbow exam. The visualization of this fat pad, on a 90° flexed lateral elbow radiograph, indicates that a change within the joint has caused its position to be changed, suggesting the presence of joint pathology.

To ensure an accurate diagnosis, it is essential that the elbow **be flexed 90° on** the lateral view. If the elbow is extended beyond the 90° flexed position, the olecranon slides into the olecranon fossa, elevates the posterior fat pad and causes it to visualize. In this situation, the pad will visualize whether the exam is negative or positive. Generally, visualization of the posterior fat pads is considered to be more reliable than the anterior fat pads.

The **supinator fat stripe (E)** is a long thin stripe just anterior to the proximal radius. This can be used as an indicator for diagnosing non-obvious radial head or neck fractures.

In summary, for the anterior and posterior fat pads to be useful diagnostic indicators on the lateral elbow, the elbow must be (1) **flexed 90°**, (2) in a **true lateral position**, and (3) **optimum exposure techniques must be used**.

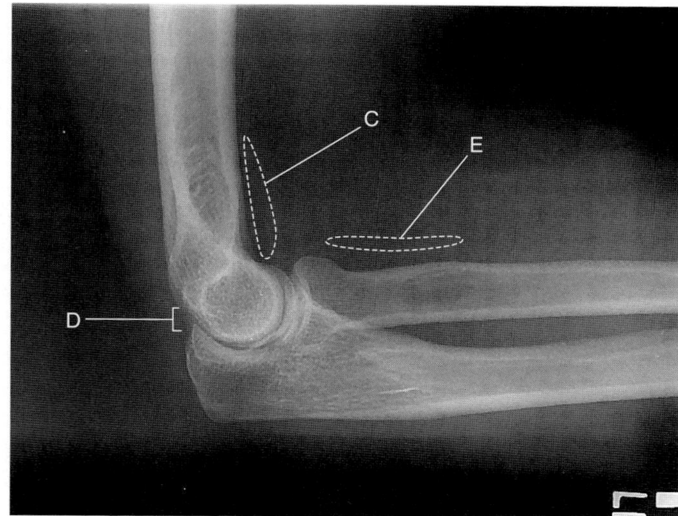

Fig. 4-28. Lateral elbow (anterior and posterior fat pads).
–**Anterior fat pad (C)**.
–**Posterior fat pad (D)**, not visible.
–**Supinator fat stripe (E)**.

*McQuillen-Martensen, K. *Radiographic Critique*, Philadelphia; WB Saunders, 1996.
†Griswold, R. Elbow Fat Pads: A Radiography Perspective, *Radiologic Technology* 1982; 53:303-307.

Radiographic Positioning

General Positioning Considerations

Radiographic examinations involving the upper limb on ambulatory patients are generally done with the patient seated sideways at the end of the table in a position that is not strained or uncomfortable (Fig. 4-29). An extended table-top may make this a little more comfortable, especially if the patient is in a wheelchair. The patient should also be moved away from the x-ray beam out of the region of scatter radiation as much as possible. The height of the table-top should be near shoulder height so the arm can be fully supported as shown.

Trauma Patients: Trauma patients can be radiographed on the table or taken directly on the cart as shown in Fig. 4-30. The patient should be moved to one side to provide the necessary space on the cart for the cassette.

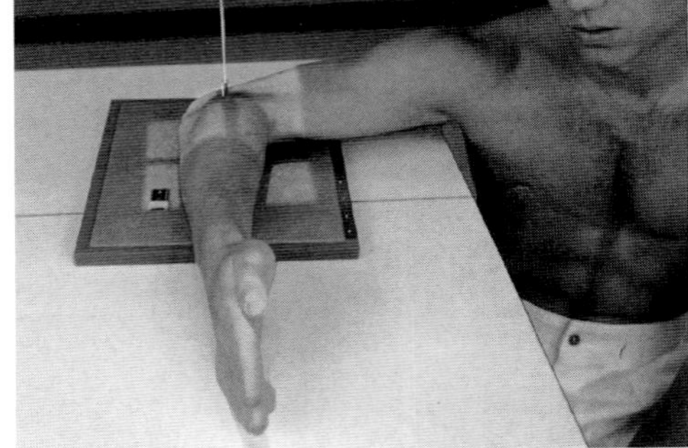

Fig. 4-29. Ambulatory patient–Lateral elbow. (Lead shield should be across lap covering gonads.)

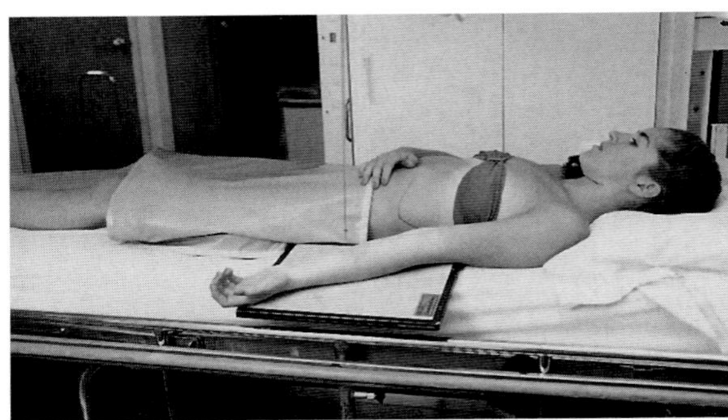

Fig. 4-30. Trauma patient–AP forearm.

Distance

A common minimum SID (source-image receptor distance) is 40 in. or 100 cm. When radiographing with cassettes directly on the table-top, to maintain a constant SID the tube height must be increased as compared with radiographs taken with the cassette in the Bucky tray. This difference is generally 3 to 4 in. (8 to 10 cm) for floating type tabletops.

Gonadal Shielding

Gonadal shielding is important for exams of the upper limb because of the proximity of the gonads to the divergent x-ray beam, as well as scatter radiation. This is true for those patients seated at the end of the table as well as those trauma patients taken on the cart. Therefore a lead vinyl-covered shield should be draped over the patient's lap or gonadal area. Even though the gonadal rule states this should be done on patients of reproductive age when the gonads lie within or close to the primary field, it is a good practice to provide gonadal shielding for all patients.

Collimation, General Positioning and Markers

The collimation rule should again be followed, namely that **collimation borders should be visible on all four sides if the film is large enough to allow this without cutting off essential anatomy**. A general rule concerning film size is to **use the smallest film size possible for the specific part being radiographed**. Four-sided collimation is generally possible, however, even with a minimal size film for most if not all radiographic exams of the upper limb.

Two or more projections may be taken on one film. This requires close collimation.

A general positioning rule especially applicable to the upper limbs is to **always place the long axis of the part being radiographed parallel to the long axis of the film**. Also, **all body parts should be oriented in the same direction** when two or more projections are taken on the same film.

Patient ID information and side markers within the collimation borders must be demonstrated on each radiograph. The patient ID blocker on the cassette should always be placed in **the corner least likely to superimpose essential anatomy.**

Correct Centering

Accurate centering and alignment of the body part to the film and central ray is important for exams of the upper limb where shape and size distortion must be avoided and the narrow joint spaces clearly demonstrated. Therefore the following three positioning principles should be remembered for upper limb exams:

a. Part should be **parallel to plane of film**.
b. CR should be **90° or perpendicular to part and film**.
c. CR should be directed to **correct centering point**.

Fracture Terminology (See Chapter 19 for fracture definitions)

Certain more common fracture terms should be known and understood to determine which projections should be taken to confirm or rule out such fractures. Examples are: Colles,' Smith's, Barton's, Bennett's or scaphoid fractures. These will be noted under "Structures Best Shown" on the positioning pages.

Exposure Factors

The principal exposure factors for radiographs of the upper limbs are:

1. Lower to medium kVp (50-70)
2. Short exposure time
3. Small focal spot
4. Adequate mAs for sufficient density

Correctly exposed radiographs of the upper limbs should visualize soft tissue margins for fat pad visualization and fine trabecular markings of all bones being radiographed.

Cassettes

Cassettes with detail intensifying screens are generally used for adult extremities to achieve optimum recorded detail. Grids are not used for the upper limbs unless the body part, (such as the shoulder) measures more than 10 cm. (Some references suggest a grid for over 13 cm.)

Increase Exposure with Cast

An upper limb with a cast will require an increase in exposure. The thickness of the cast and the body part will affect the increase as follows:

Cast Conversion Chart

Type of cast	Increase in exposure
• Small to medium dry plaster cast:	–increase 5-7 kVp.
• Large or wet plaster cast:	–double mAs **or** –increase 8-10 kVp.
• Fiberglass cast:	–increase 3-4 kVp.

NATIONAL SURVEY

Departmental standard and special operating procedures (departmental routines) for exams of the upper limb were generally consistent throughout the United States.

Finger and Thumb Routine

Fingers	U.S. Average	
	Basic 1995 (1989)	Special 1995 (1989)
• PA (finger only)	70% (57%)	3% (5%)
or		
PA (entire hand)	42% (43%)	6% (11%)
• Lateral	94% (94%)	
• Oblique	84% (87%)	
Thumb		
• AP	91% (93%)	
• Lateral	93% (94%)	
• Oblique (thumb only)	72% (58%)	2% (5%)
or		
Oblique (include PA hand)	25% (35%)	6% (8%)
• PA	20% –	18% –

Hand Routine

Hand	U.S. Average	
	Basic 1995 (1989)	Special 1995 (1989)
• PA	98% (90%)	
• Oblique	98% –	
• Lateral (fan lateral)	83% (62%)	
• Lateral (in extension)		33% –
• Lateral (in flexion)		23% –

Summary

Hand: The routines for the upper limb procedures were generally very consistent throughout the U.S. One exception was the fan lateral for the hand, which was routine for 96% of the Western States, 85% for the Mid U.S., and 77% for the East (see appendix pages). As expected, the lateral in extension also showed a difference with 26% in the East considering it routine, 18% in the Mid U.S., and only 14% in the West.

Wrist: The results for the wrist routine were also very consistent throughout the U.S. The PA, oblique and lateral were routine by 96% to 98%. The most frequent special projections were the carpal canal (52%), the scaphoid ulnar flexion (52%), the carpal bridge (37%), and the radial flexion (35%).

The **Stecher method** for the scaphoid is considered a routine special projection by 40% of the respondents throughout the U.S. in 1995, compared with only 5% in 1989. Therefore this projection has been added in this 4th edition as an alternative to the ulnar flexion, CR angle projection.

Wrist Routine

Wrist	U.S. Average	
	Basic 1995 (1989)	Special 1995 (1989)
• PA	96% (96%)	
• Oblique (45°)	97% (94%)	
• Lateral	98% (98%)	
• Scaphoid (ulnar flexion)		52% (47%)
or		
Scaphoid (Stecher method)		40% (5%)
• Carpal canal		52% (20%)
• Radial flexion		35% (19%)
• Carpal bridge		37% (15%)

Forearm Routine

Forearm	U.S. Average	
	Basic 1995 (1989)	Special 1995 (1989)
• AP	98% (99%)	
• Lateral	98% (99%)	
• Oblique		17% (5%)

Elbow Routine

Elbow	1995–637 (1989–529) U.S. Average	
	Basic 1995 (1989)	Special 1995 (1989)
• AP	98% (99%)	
• Lateral	97% (98%)	
• Oblique (external)	70% –	
• Oblique (internal)	52% –	
• AP (partial flexion)		47% (20%)
• Acute flexion (Jones method)		37% –
• Axial trauma (Coyle method)		20% (3%)

Elbow: The survey results for the oblique elbow show that a majority of the U.S. respondents considered **both** obliques of the elbow routine. The external oblique is more common (70%) than the internal oblique (52%).

There were some differences in the three regions with the East indicating the internal oblique routine by 62%, and the external oblique by 73%. The West indicated 47% for the internal oblique, and 73% for the external.

4

4

Humerus Routine

Humerus (Non-trauma routine)	U.S. Average	
	Basic 1995 (1989)	Special 1995 (1989)
• AP	98% (99%)	
• Rotational lateral	97% (98%)	
Humerus (Trauma routine–possible fracture or dislocation)		
• AP (neutral rotation)	96% (98%)	
• Lateral (mid & distal)	57% (59%)	
• Transthoracic lateral (proximal)	64% (60%)	19% (23%)
• Scapular Y (proximal)	43% (17%)	23% (21%)

Summary
The routines for the **non-trauma humerus** were very consistent with a non-trauma routine of an **AP** and a **rotational lateral**. The trauma lateral routine showed a preference for the transthoracic lateral (64%), compared to the scapular Y (43%). However, the use of the scapular Y for a trauma lateral humerus increased from **17% in 1989** to **43% in 1995**.

STANDARD AND SPECIAL OPERATING PROCEDURES

Certain basic and special projections for the hand, wrist, forearm, elbow and humerus are demonstrated and described on the following pages as suggested standard basic and special departmental routines or procedures.

Basic Projections

Standard or basic projections, also sometimes referred to as routine projections or departmental routines are those projections commonly taken on average patients who are helpful and can cooperate in performing the procedure.

Special Projections

Special projections are those more common projections taken as extra or additional projections to better demonstrate certain pathologic conditions or specific body parts.

Basic and Special Projections

Fingers
Basic
• PA **115**
• PA oblique **116**
• Lateral **117**

Thumb
Basic
• AP **118**
• PA oblique **119**
• Lateral **120**

Hand
Basic
• PA **121**
• PA oblique **122**
• Lateral (fan) **123**
• Lateral (extension and flexion) **124**

Wrist
Basic
• PA (AP) **125**
• PA oblique **126**
• Lateral **127**

Wrist
Special
• Scaphoid views
–CR angle, ulnar flex. **128**
–Mod. Stecher method **129**
• Radial flexion **130**
• Carpal canal
–Inferosuperior **131**
–Superoinferior **132**
• Carpal bridge **133**

Forearm
Basic
• AP **134**
• Lateral **135**

Elbow
Basic
• AP **136**
• AP obliques
–Lateral (external) rotation **137**
–Medial (internal) rotation **138**
• Lateral **139**

Elbow
Special
• Acute flexion (Jones method) **140**
• Trauma axial laterals (Coyle method) **141**
• Radial head laterals **142**

Humerus
Basic
• AP **143**
• Rotational lateral **144**
• Horizontal beam lateral **145**

Proximal humerus
–See Shoulder, Ch. 5.

PA Projection

Fingers
Basic
• **PA**
• Oblique
• Lateral

Structures Best Shown

Distal, middle and proximal phalanges, distal metacarpal and associated joints.

10
8
R

Technical Factors

- Film size–8 x 10 in. (18 x 24 cm).
- Divide in thirds crosswise.
- Detail screen, tabletop.
- 50-60 kVp range.
- Technique and dose:

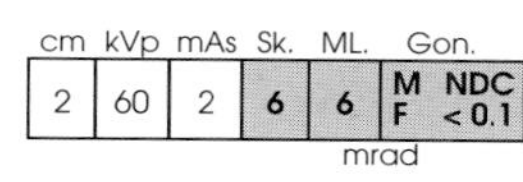

cm	kVp	mAs	Sk.	ML.	Gon.
2	60	2	6	6	M NDC F <0.1

mrad

or

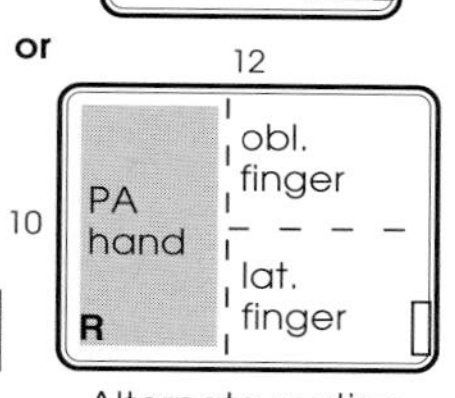

Alternate routine

Alternate Routine

- 10 x 12 in. (24 x 30 cm) crosswise.
- Divide in half to include entire hand.
- An alternate routine includes the entire hand for the PA projection of the finger for possible secondary trauma or pathology to other aspects of the hand and wrist. Oblique and lateral projections would be of affected finger only.

Shielding: Place lead shield over patient's lap.

Patient Position

- Patient seated at end of table with elbow flexed about 90° with hand and forearm resting on table.

Part Position

- Pronate hand with fingers extended.
- Center and align long axis of affected finger to long axis of portion of cassette being exposed.
- Center PIP joint to CR.
- Separate adjoining fingers from affected finger.

Central Ray

- CR perpendicular to film, directed to **proximal interphalangeal (PIP) joint**.
- Minimum 40 in. (102 cm) SID.

Collimation: Collimate on four sides to area of affected finger.

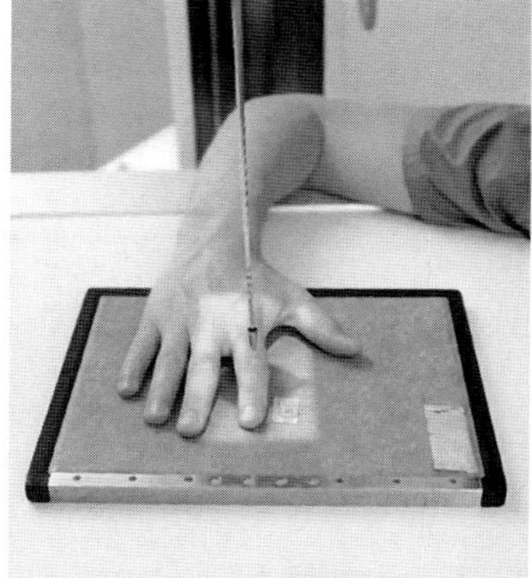

Fig. 4-31. PA–2nd digit.

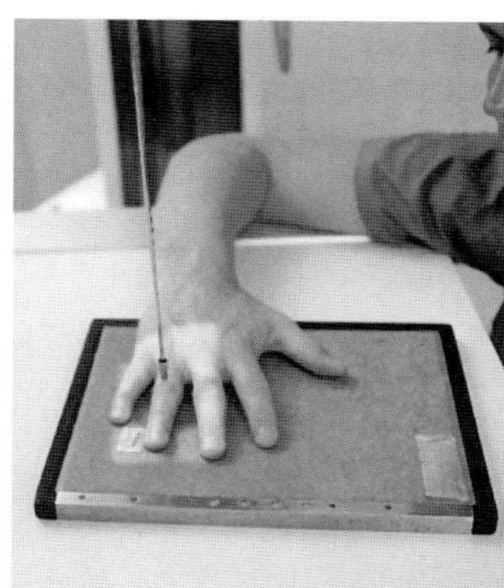

Fig. 4-32. PA–4th digit.

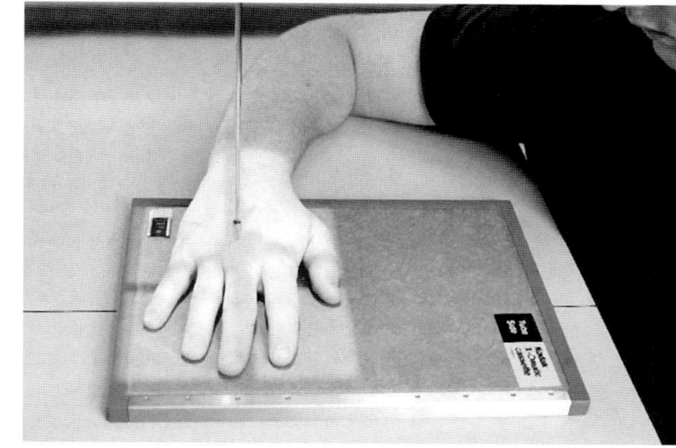

Fig. 4-33. PA hand (alternate routine).

Evaluation Criteria

- Entire finger in question (distal, middle and proximal phalanges) and approximately the distal one-third of metacarpal should be included, with collimation visible on four sides.
- The center of the collimation field should be at the PIP joint.
- Long axis of finger should be aligned to long axis of portion of film being used.
- No rotation of fingers as evidenced by:
  - –The symmetrical appearance of both sides or concavities of the shafts of phalanges and distal metacarpals.
  - –The amount of tissue on each side of the phalanges should appear equal.
- Fingers should be separated from both sides of finger being examined so there is no overlapping of soft tissues.
- Interphalangeal joints should appear open, indicating hand was fully pronated and CR location was correct.

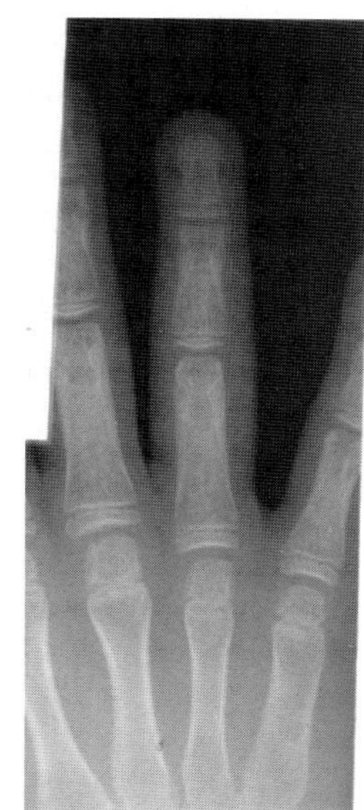

Fig. 4-34. PA–4th digit.

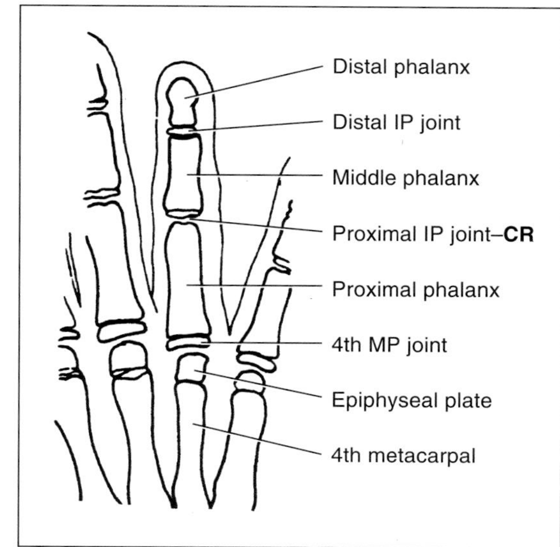

Fig. 4-35. PA–4th digit.

- Optimum exposure and contrast with no motion will demonstrate soft tissue margins and clear, sharp bony trabecular markings.
- **Alternate routine**: See PA hand.

PA Oblique Projection–Medial or Lateral Rotation

Fingers
Basic
• PA
• **Oblique**
• Lateral

Structures Best Shown

Phalanges, interphalangeal and metacarpophalangeal joints in oblique position.

Technical Factors

- Film size–8 x 10 in. (18 x 24 cm).
- Divide in thirds crosswise.
- Detail screen, tabletop.
- 50-60 kVp range.
- **Accessories**: 45° foam wedge block or step wedge.
- Technique and dose:

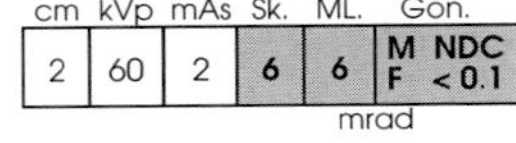

cm	kVp	mAs	Sk.	ML.	Gon.
2	60	2	6	6	M NDC F <0.1

mrad

Shielding: Place lead shield over patient's lap to shield gonads.

Patient Position

- Patient seated at end of table with elbow flexed about 90° with hand and wrist resting on cassette with fingers extended.

Part Position

- Place hand with fingers fully extended against 45° foam wedge block, placing hand in a 45° lateral oblique (thumb side up).
- Position hand on cassette so the long axis of finger is aligned with long axis of the one-third of film being exposed.
- Center PIP joint to CR.
- Separate fingers and carefully place finger being examined against block so it is supported in a 45° oblique and is **parallel to film.**

Central Ray

- CR perpendicular to film, directed to **proximal interphalangeal (PIP) joint.**
- Minimum 40 in. (102 cm) SID.

Collimation: Collimate on four sides to finger being examined.

Optional medial oblique: Second digit may also be taken in a 45° medial oblique (thumb side down) with thumb and other fingers flexed to prevent superimposition. This places part closer to film for improved definition but may also be more painful for patient.

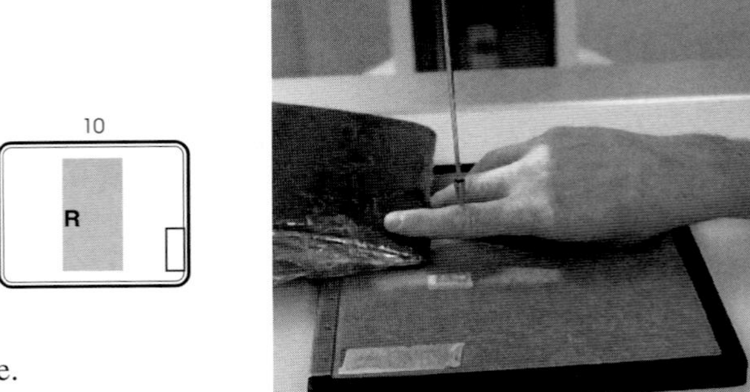

Fig. 4-36. 2nd digit (medial rotation).

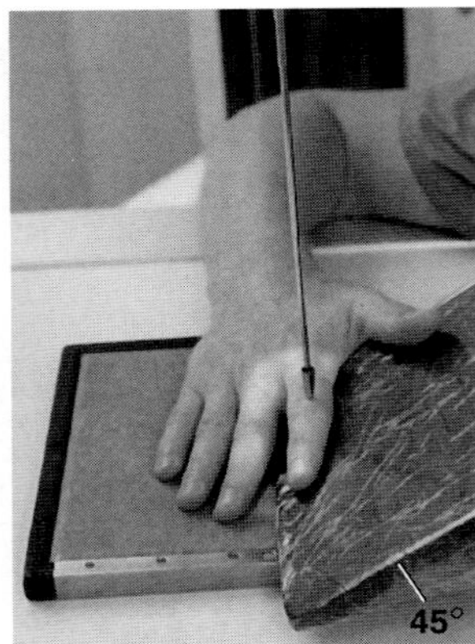

Fig. 4-37. 2nd digit (optional lateral rotation).

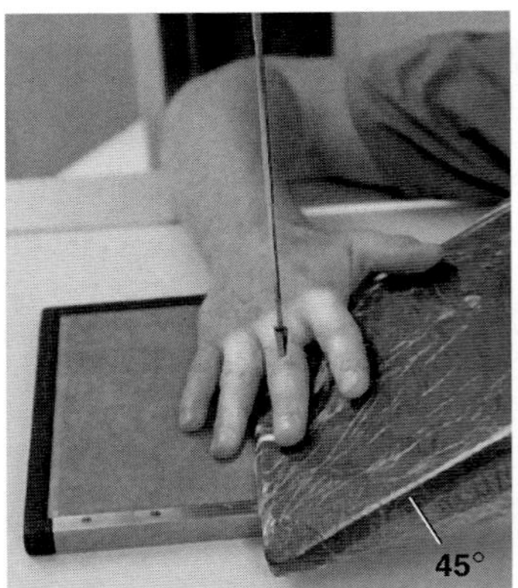

Fig. 4-38. 3rd digit (lateral rotation).

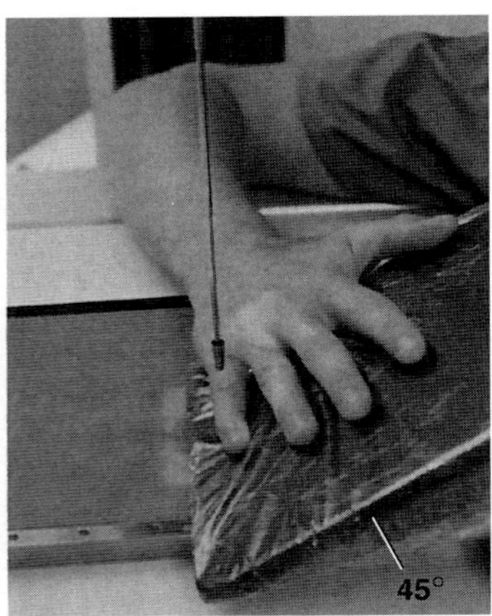

Fig. 4-39. 5th digit (lateral rotation).

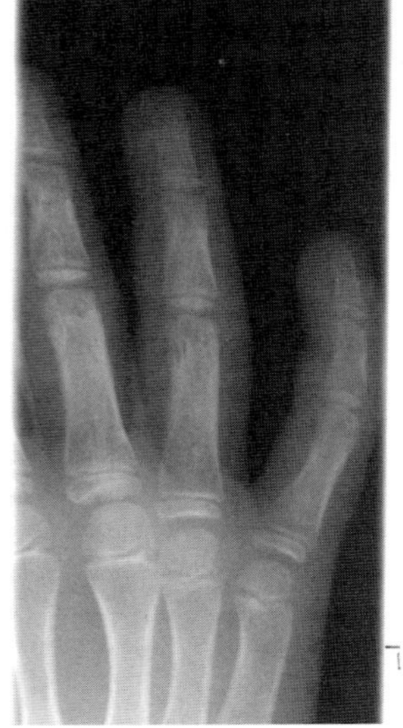

Fig. 4-40. 4th digit.

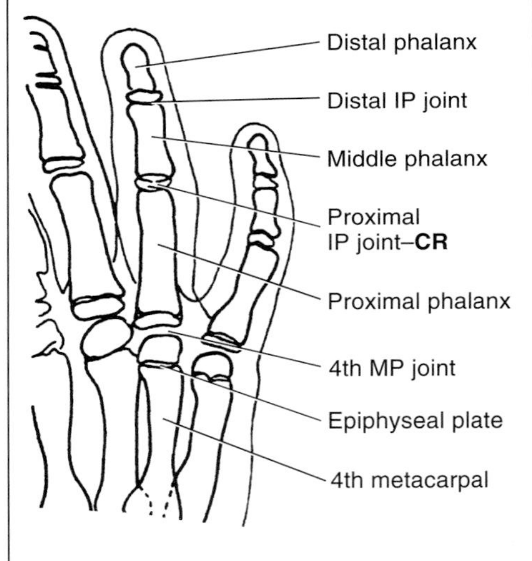

Fig. 4-41. 4th digit.

Evaluation Criteria

- Entire finger in question (distal, medial and proximal phalanges) and the metacarpophalangeal joint should be included, positioned in a 45° oblique with collimation on four sides.
- Long axis of finger should be aligned to long axis of portion of film being used.
- Center of collimation field should be to the PIP joint.
- Interphalangeal and metacarpophalangeal joint spaces should be open, indicating correct central ray location and that the phalanges are parallel to the film.
- Optimum exposure and contrast with no motion will demonstrate soft tissue margins and clear, sharp bony trabecular markings.

Lateral–Lateromedial or Mediolateral Projections

Fingers
Basic
• PA
• Oblique
• **Lateral**

Structures Best Shown

Phalanges, interphalangeal and metacarpophalangeal joints in lateral position.

Technical Factors

10
8
R

- Film size–8 x 10 in. (18 x 24 cm).
- Divide in thirds crosswise.
- Detail screen, tabletop.
- 50-60 kVp range.
- **Accessories**: Sponge support block.
- Technique and dose:

cm	kVp	mAs	Sk.	ML.	Gon.
2	60	2	6	6	M NDC F <0.1

mrad

Shielding: Place lead shield over patient's lap to shield gonads.

Patient Position

- Patient seated at end of table with elbow flexed about 90° with hand and wrist resting on cassette with fingers extended.

Part Position

- Place hand in lateral position (thumb side up) with finger to be examined fully extended centered to portion of film (see Note for 2nd digit lateral).
- Align and center finger to long axis of portion of film being exposed, and to CR.
- Use sponge block or other radiolucent device to support finger and prevent motion. Flex unaffected fingers.
- Center PIP joint to CR.
- Ensure that long axis of finger is **parallel to film**.

Central Ray

- CR perpendicular to film, to **proximal interphalangeal (PIP) joint**.
- Minimum 40 in. (102 cm) SID.

Collimation: Collimate on four sides to finger being examined.

Note: For 2nd digit, a thumb-side-down lateral is advised if patient can assume this position, placing the second digit in contact with cassette. (Definition is improved with less OID).

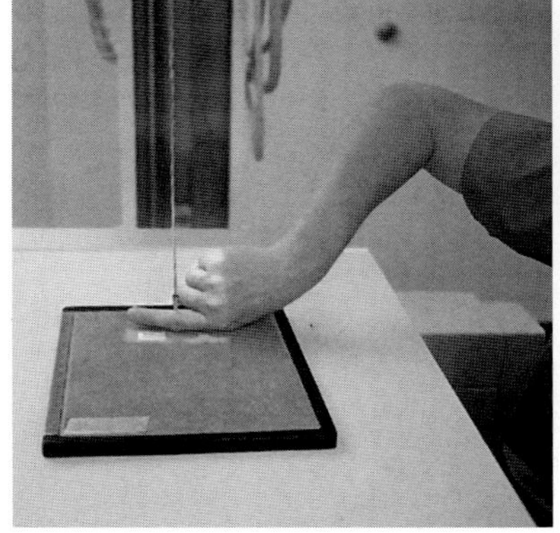

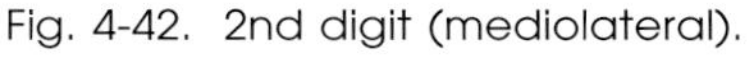

Fig. 4-42. 2nd digit (mediolateral).

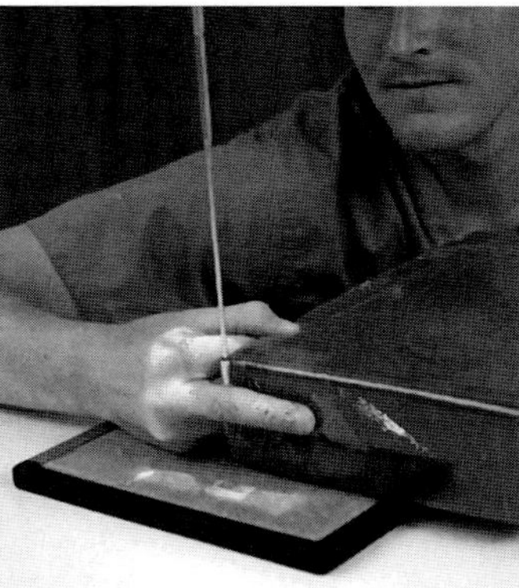

Fig. 4-43. 3rd digit (lateromedial).

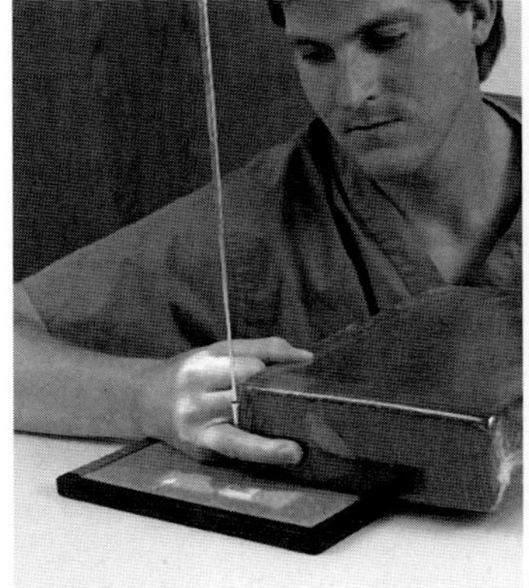

Fig. 4-44. 4th digit (lateromedial).

Fig. 4-45. 5th digit (lateromedial).

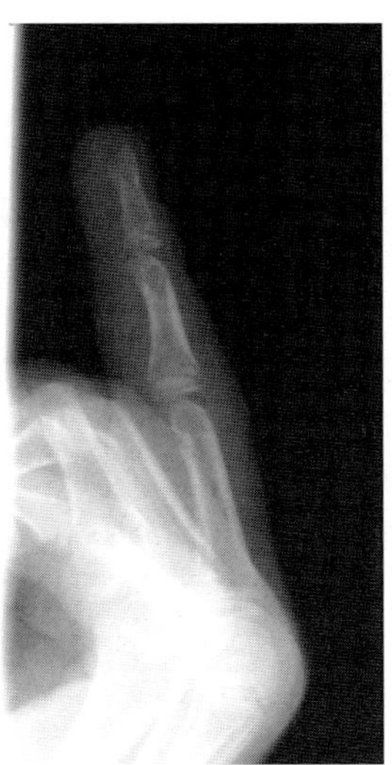

Fig. 4-46. 4th digit.

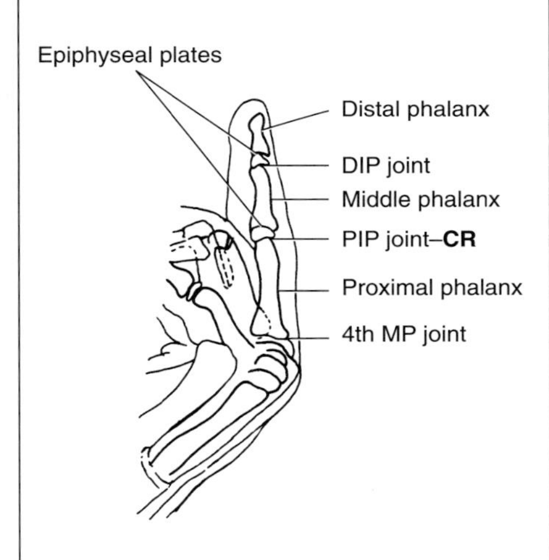

Fig. 4-47. 4th digit.

Evaluation Criteria

- Entire finger in question (distal, middle and proximal phalanges) and the metacarpophalangeal joint should be included with collimation on four sides.
- The center of the collimation field should be at the PIP joint.
- Long axis of finger should be aligned to long axis of portion of film being used.
- Interphalangeal joint spaces should be open, indicating correct central ray location and that the phalanges are parallel to film.
- Finger should be in true lateral position, as indicated by the concave appearance of anterior surface of the shaft of phalanges and by the anterior projecting rounded ends of proximal and middle phalanges.
- Optimum exposure and contrast with no motion will demonstrate soft tissue margins and clear, sharp bony trabecular markings.

AP Projection

Thumb
Basic
• **AP**
• Oblique
• Lateral

Structures Best Shown

Distal and proximal phalanges, first metacarpal and associated joints.

Base of first metacarpal for ruling out a **Bennett's type fracture.**

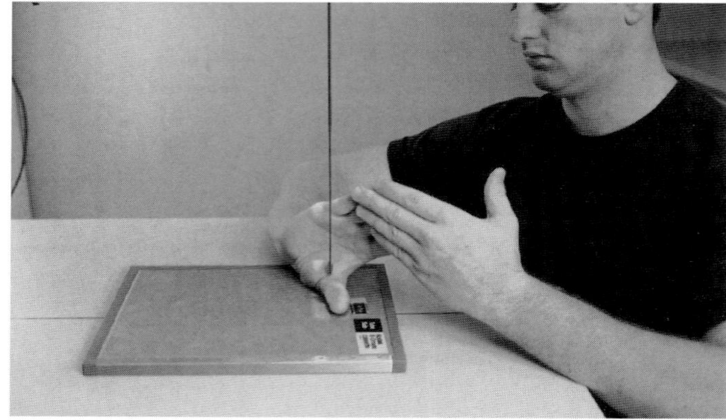

Fig 4-48. AP thumb–CR to 1st MP joint.

Technical Factors

• Film size–8 x 10 in. (18 x 24 cm).
• Divide in thirds crosswise.
• Detail screen, tabletop.
• 50-60 kVp range.
• Technique and dose:

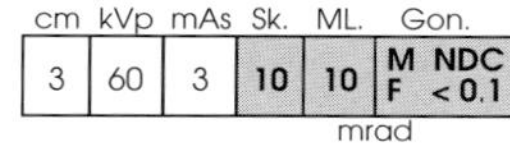

cm	kVp	mAs	Sk.	ML.	Gon.
3	60	3	10	10	M NDC F <0.1

mrad

Shielding: Place lead shield over patient's lap to shield gonads.

Patient Position–AP

• Patient seated facing table, arms extended in front with hand rotated internally to supinate thumb for AP projection (Fig. 4-48).

Part Position–AP

(It is suggested you first demonstrate this awkward position on yourself for the patient to see so they will better understand what is expected of them.)

• Internally rotate hand with fingers extended until posterior surface of thumb is in contact with film (may need to hold fingers back with other hand as shown).
• Align thumb to long axis of portion of film being exposed.
• Center **1st MP joint** to CR and to center of portion of film being exposed. (Remember 1st metacarpal is considered part of thumb.)

Exception–PA (only if patient cannot position for above AP):

• Place hand in a near lateral position and rest thumb on a sponge support block which is high enough so thumb is not obliqued but in position for a **true PA projection**.
• Align thumb to long axis of portion of film being exposed.

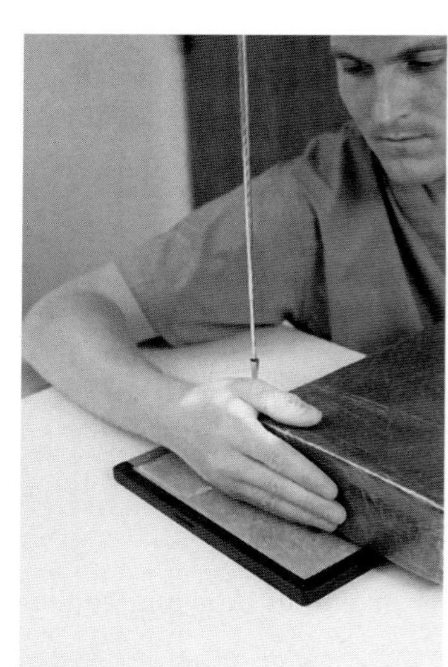

Fig. 4-49. PA (exception).

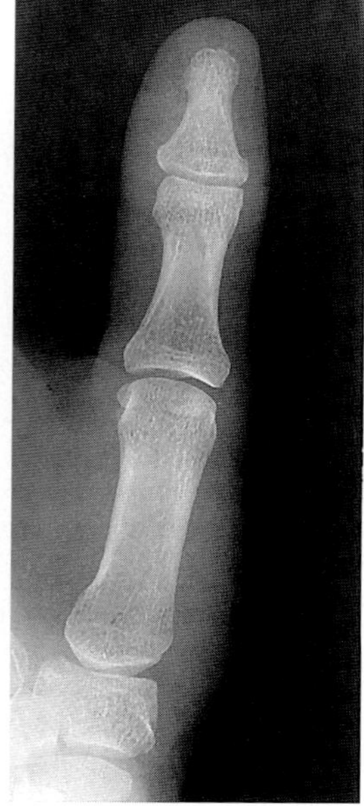

Fig. 4-50. AP thumb.

Note: The PA is not advisable as a routine because of loss of definition due to increased object-image receptor distance (OID).

Central Ray

• CR perpendicular to film, to **1st MP joint**.
• Minimum 40 in. (102 cm) SID.

Collimation: Collimate on four sides to area of thumb remembering the **thumb includes the entire first metacarpal**.

Evaluation Criteria

• Entire thumb (from distal tip of thumb to 1st carpometacarpal joint) should be centered to film, with trapezium included, and well-visualized.
• Collimation on four sides.
• Long axis of thumb should be aligned to long axis of portion of film being used.
• The center of the collimation field should be at the 1st MP joint.
• No rotation as evidenced by symmetrical appearance of both concave sides of phalanges and by the equal amounts of soft tissue appearing on each side of phalanges.
• Interphalangeal and metacarpophalangeal joints should appear open.
• Optimum exposure and contrast with no motion will demonstrate soft tissue margins and clear, sharp bony trabecular markings for the 1st metacarpal and the phalanges.

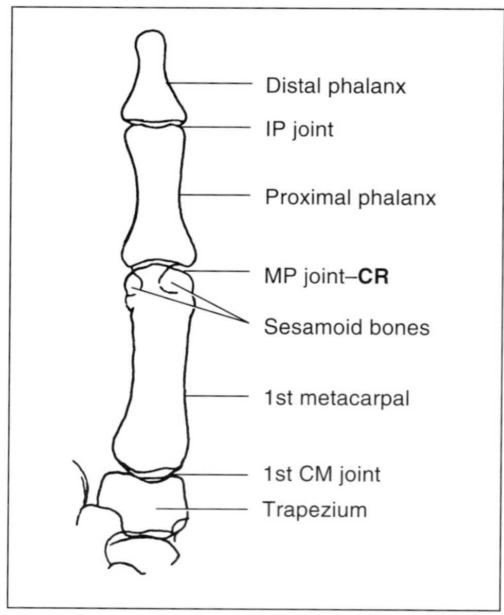

Fig. 4-51. AP thumb.

PA Oblique Projection–Medial Rotation

Thumb
Basic
• AP
• **Oblique**
• Lateral

Structures Best Shown

Distal and proximal phalanges and metacarpal of first digit and associated joints all in oblique position and sesamoid bones if present.

Base of first metacarpal for ruling out a **Bennett's type fracture.**

Technical Factors

- Film size–8 x 10 in. (18 x 24 cm).
- Divide in thirds crosswise.
- Detail screen, tabletop.
- 50-60 kVp range.
- Technique and dose:

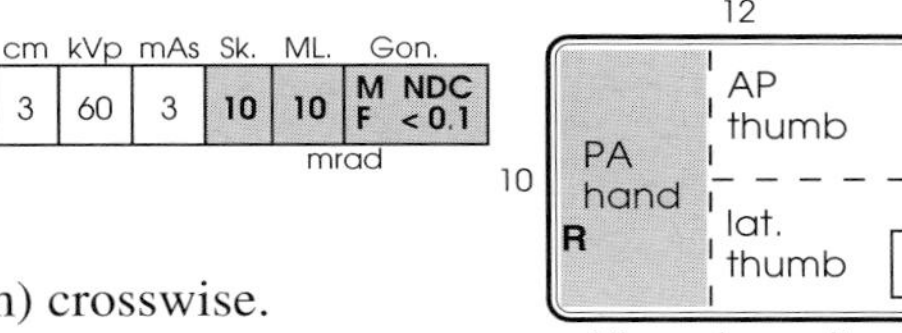

cm	kVp	mAs	Sk.	ML.	Gon.
3	60	3	10	10	M NDC F <0.1
					mrad

Alternate Routine

- 10 x 12 in. (24 x 30 cm) crosswise.
- Divide in half to include entire hand.
- An alternate routine includes the entire hand for the oblique thumb for possible secondary trauma or pathology on other aspects of hand. AP and lateral would be of thumb only.

Shielding: Place lead shield over patient's lap to shield gonads.

Patient Position

- Patient seated at end of table with elbow flexed about 90° with hand resting on cassette.

Part Position 

- Abduct thumb slightly with palmar surface of hand in contact with cassette (this will naturally place thumb into a 45° oblique position).
- Align long axis of thumb to long axis of third of cassette being exposed.
- Center **1st MP joint** to CR and to center of portion of film being exposed.

Central Ray

- CR perpendicular to film, directed to **1st MP joint**.
- Minimum 40 in. (102 cm) SID.

Collimation: Collimate on four sides to thumb, ensure that **all of first metacarpal is included**.

Evaluation Criteria (Oblique thumb only)

- Entire thumb (from distal tip of thumb to 1st carpometacarpal joint) and the carpal bone, trapezium, should be visualized in a 45° oblique position and be centered to portion of film being used, with collimation on four sides.
- The center of the collimation field should be at the 1st MP joint.
- Long axis of thumb should be aligned to long axis of portion of film being used.
- Interphalangeal and metacarpophalangeal joints should appear open.
- Optimum exposure and contrast with no motion will demonstrate soft tissue margins and clear sharp bony trabecular markings for the 1st metacarpal and the phalanges.
- **Alternate routine**: See PA hand.

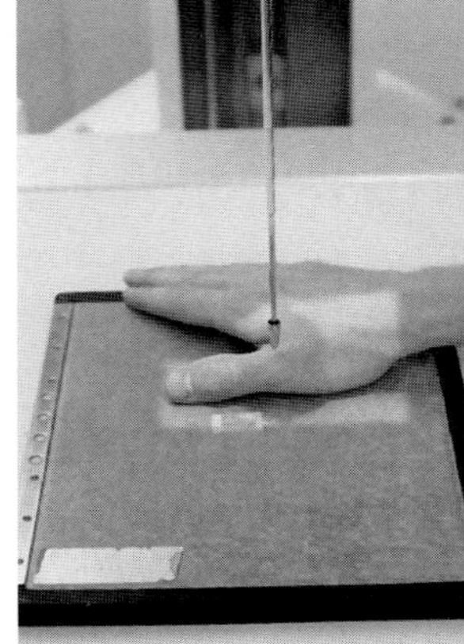

Fig 4-52. Oblique thumb. –CR to 1st MP joint.

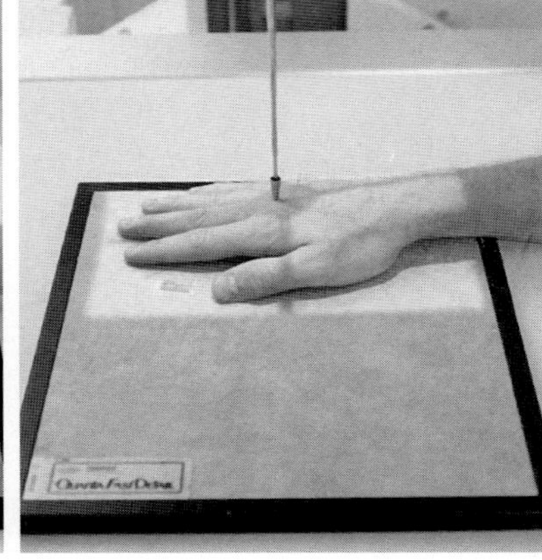

Fig. 4-53. Oblique thumb with PA hand (alternate routine).

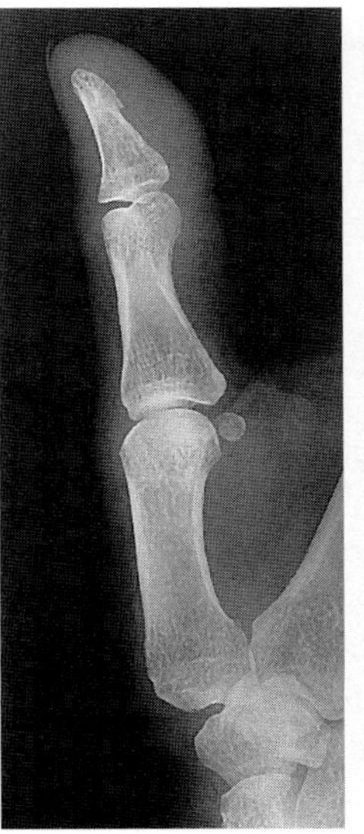

Fig. 4-54. Oblique thumb.

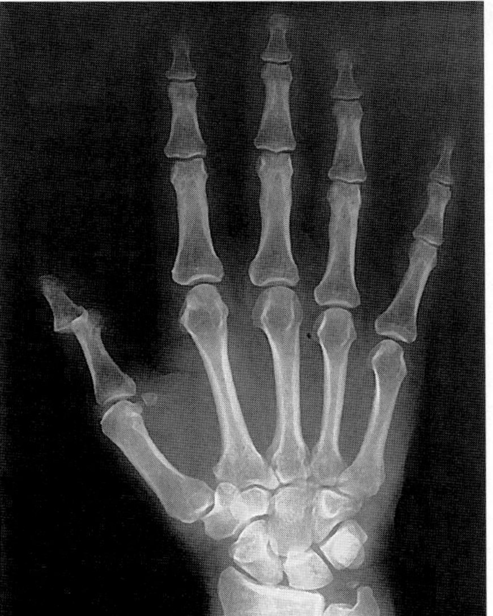

Fig. 4-55. Oblique thumb with PA hand (note dislocated distal phalanx of thumb).

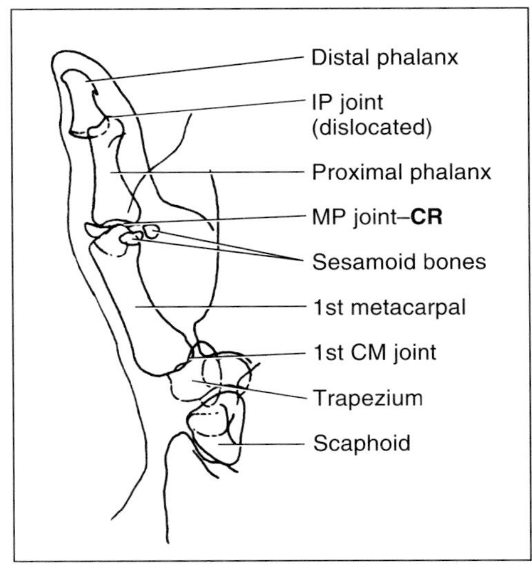

Fig. 4-56. Oblique thumb.

4

Lateral Position

Thumb
Basic
• AP
• Oblique
• **Lateral**

Structures Best Shown

Distal and proximal phalanges and metacarpal of first digit in lateral position along with associated opened joints and sesamoid bones if present.

Base of first metacarpal for ruling out a **Bennett's type fracture.**

Technical Factors

- Film size–8 x 10 in. (18 x 24 cm).
- Divide in thirds crosswise.
- Detail screen, tabletop.
- 50-60 kVp range.
- Technique and dose:

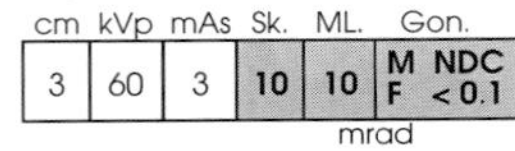

cm	kVp	mAs	Sk.	ML.	Gon.
3	60	3	10	10	M NDC F <0.1

mrad

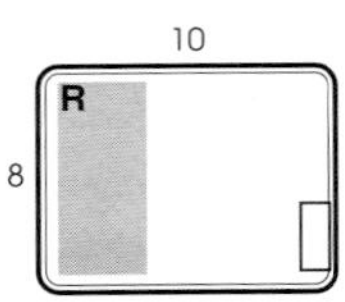

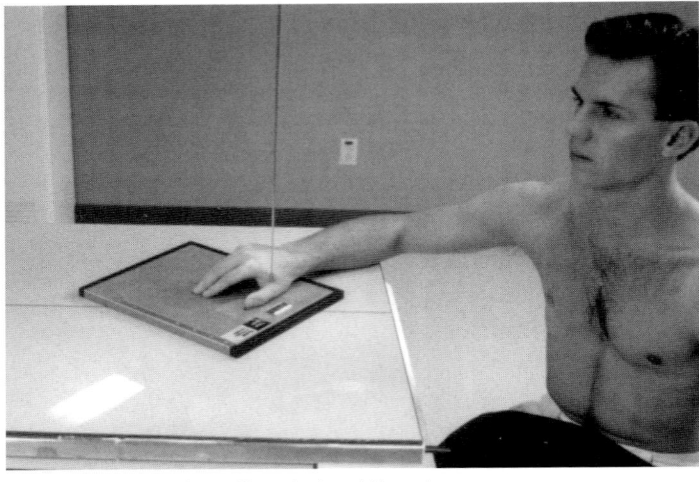

Fig. 4-57. Patient position–Lateral thumb.

Shielding: Place lead shield over patient's lap to shield gonads.

Patient Position

- Patient seated at end of table with elbow flexed about 90° with hand resting on cassette, palm down.

Part Position 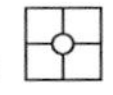

- Start with hand pronated and thumb abducted, with fingers and hand slightly arched, then rotate hand medially slightly until thumb is in a true lateral position. (May need to provide sponge or other support under lateral portion of hand.)
- Align long axis of thumb to long axis of portion of film being exposed.
- Center **1st MP joint** to CR and to center of portion of film being exposed.
- Entire lateral aspect of thumb should be in direct contact with cassette.

Central Ray

- CR perpendicular to film, directed to **1st MP joint**.
- Minimum 40 in. (102 cm) SID.

Collimation: Collimate on four sides to thumb area. (Remember the thumb includes the **entire first metacarpal**.)

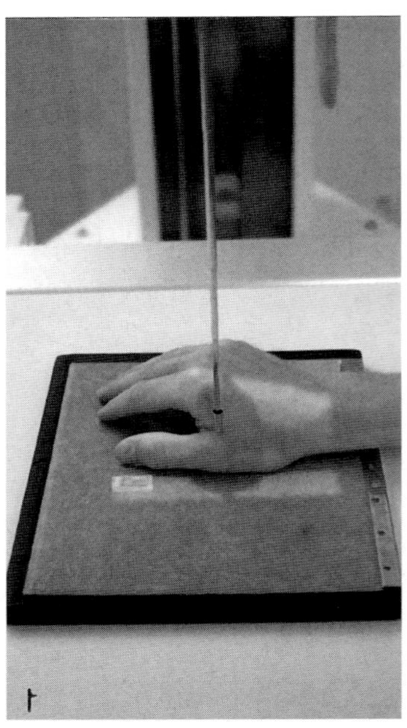

Fig. 4-58. Part position–lateral thumb.
–CR to 1st MP joint.

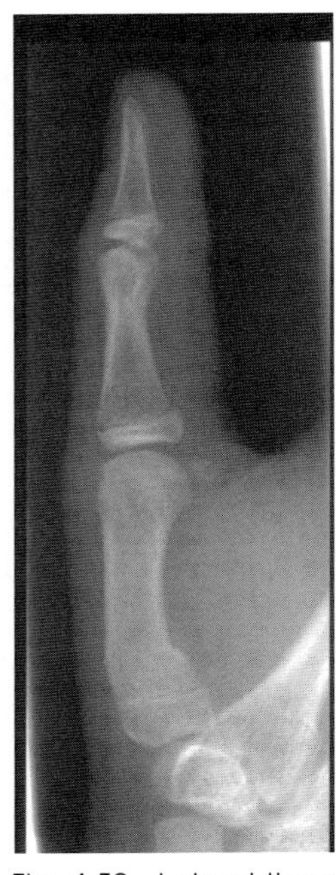

Fig. 4-59. Lateral thumb.

Evaluation Criteria

- Entire thumb (from distal tip of thumb to 1st carpometacarpal joint) and the carpal, trapezium, should be visualized and centered to the film.
- Collimation on four sides.
- The center of the collimation field should be at the 1st MP joint.
- Thumb should be in true lateral position evidenced by the concave shaped anterior surface of proximal phalange and 1st metacarpal, and the relatively straight posterior surfaces.
- Interphalangeal and metacarpophalangeal joints should appear open.
- Optimum exposure and contrast with no motion will demonstrate soft tissue margins and clear sharp bony trabecular markings for the first metacarpal and the phalanges.

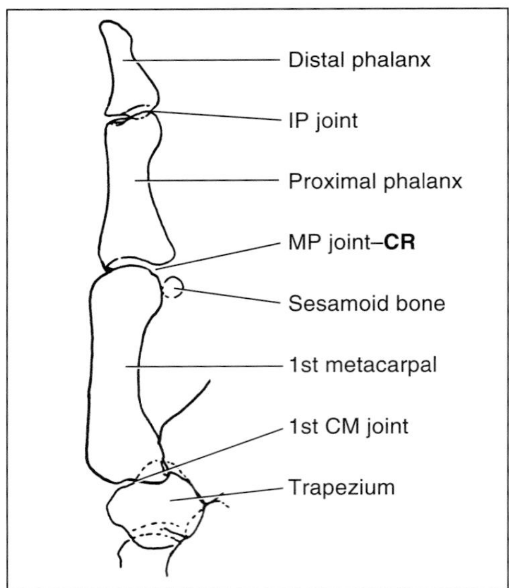

Fig. 4-60. Lateral thumb.

PA Projection

Hand
Basic
• **PA**
• Oblique
• Lateral

Structures Best Shown

Phalanges, metacarpals, carpals and all joints of hand. Results in an oblique view of thumb.

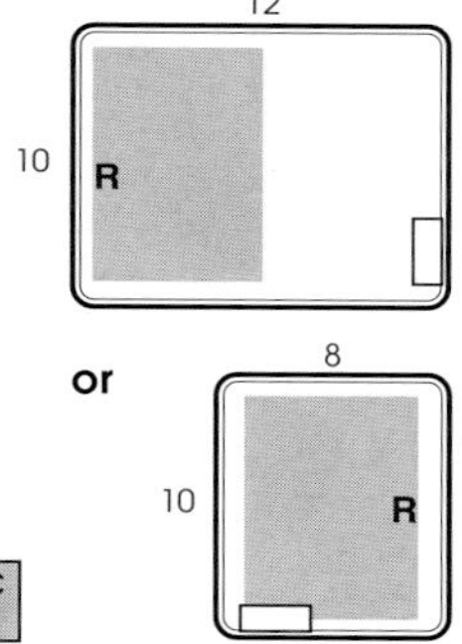

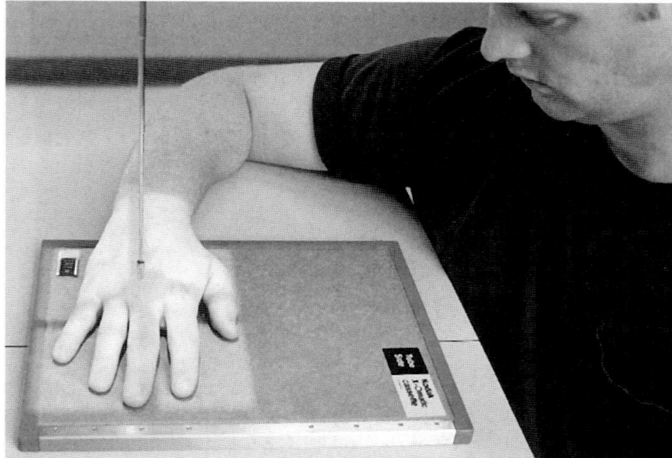

Fig. 4-61. Patient position–PA hand.

Technical Factors

- Film size–10 x 12 in. (24 x 30 cm).
- Divide film in half crosswise or (for large hand)–8 x 10 in. (18 x 24 cm) lengthwise.
- Detail screen, tabletop.
- 50-60 kVp range.
- Technique and dose:

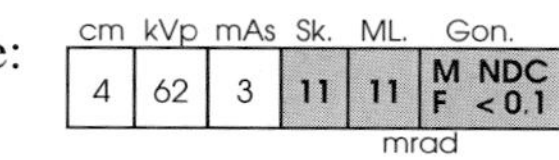

cm	kVp	mAs	Sk.	ML.	Gon.
4	62	3	11	11	M NDC F <0.1
				mrad	

Shielding: Place lead shield over patient's lap to shield gonads.

Patient Position

- Patient seated at end of table with elbow flexed about 90° with hand and forearm resting on table.

Part Position 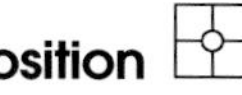

- Pronate hand with palmar surface in contact with cassette; spread fingers slightly.
- Align long axis of hand and forearm with long axis of portion of film being exposed.
- Center hand and wrist to unmasked half of film.
- Center 3rd MP joint of hand to CR.

Central Ray

- CR perpendicular to film, directed to the **3rd MP joint**.
- Minimum 40 in. (102 cm) SID.

Collimation: Collimate on four sides to outer margins of hand and wrist.

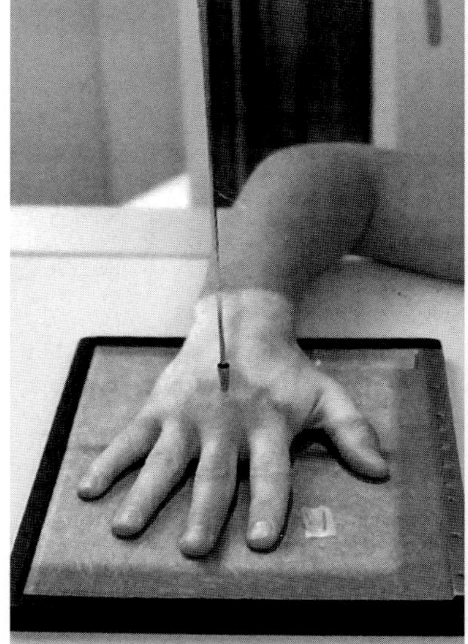

Fig. 4-62. Part position. –CR to 3rd MP joint.

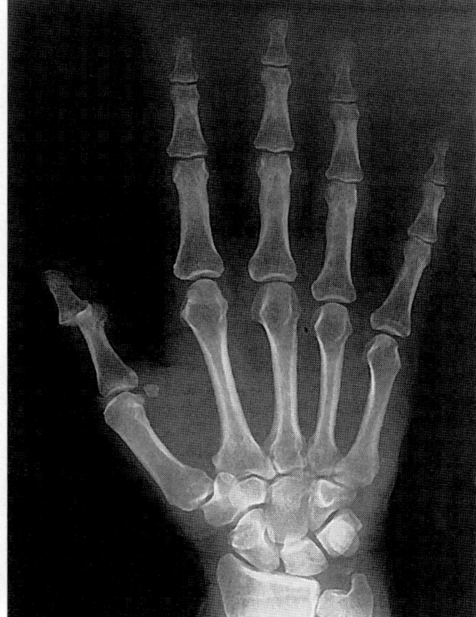

Fig. 4-63. PA hand.

Note: If exams of both hands and/or wrists are requested, generally they should be positioned and exposed separately for correct CR placement.

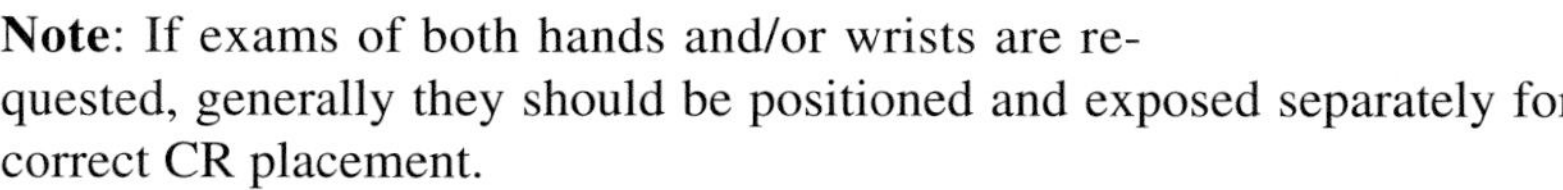

Evaluation Criteria

- Entire hand, wrist and about 1 in. (2.5 cm) of distal forearm should be included with collimation margins visible on four sides.
- Center of collimation field should be to 3rd MP joint, indicating correct CR placement.
- Long axis of hand and wrist should be aligned to long axis of film.
- **No rotation** of hand as evidenced by:
  - –The symmetrical appearance of both sides or concavities of the shafts of the metacarpals and phalanges (except for the first metacarpal and phalanges of the obliqued thumb).
  - –The amount of soft tissue on each side of the phalanges should appear equal.
- Digits should be slightly separated with soft tissues not overlapping.
- Metacarpophalangeal and interphalangeal joints should appear open, indicating correct CR location and that hand was fully pronated.
- Optimum exposure and contrast with no motion will be evidenced by soft tissue margins and fine trabecular markings of the bones appearing sharp.

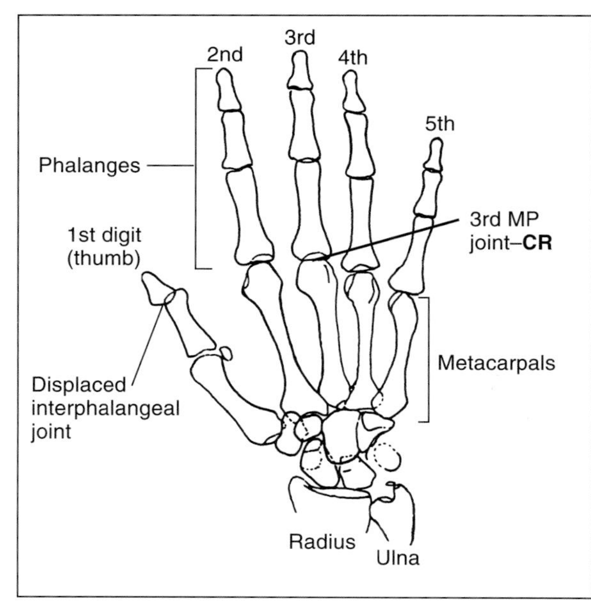

Fig. 4-64. PA hand.

PA Oblique Projection–Lateral Rotation

Hand
Basic
• PA
• **Oblique**
• Lateral

Structures Best Shown

Phalanges, metacarpals, carpals and all joints in oblique position.

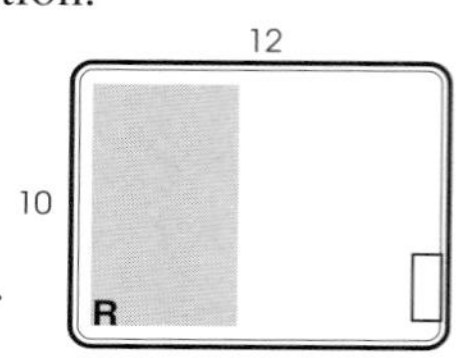

or

Technical Factors

- Film size–10 x 12 in. (24 x 30 cm).
- Divide film in half crosswise or (for large hand)–8 x 10 in. (18 x 24 cm), lengthwise.
- Detail screen, tabletop.
- 50-60 kVp range.
- Technique and dose:

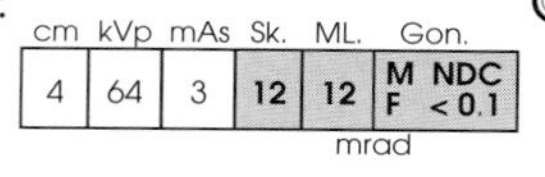

cm	kVp	mAs	Sk.	ML.	Gon.
4	64	3	12	12	M NDC F <0.1

mrad

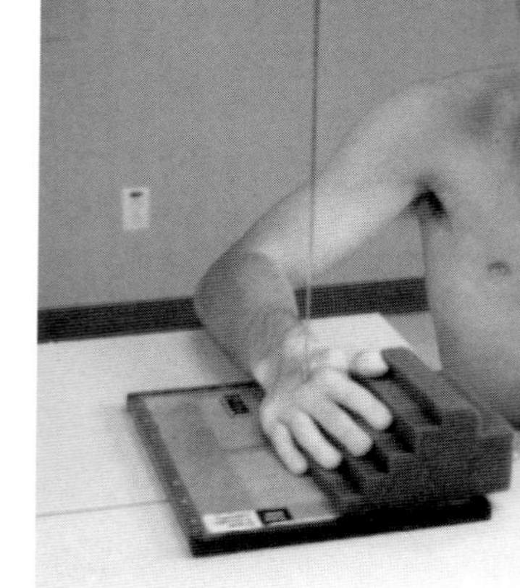

Fig. 4-65. Routine oblique hand (digits parallel).

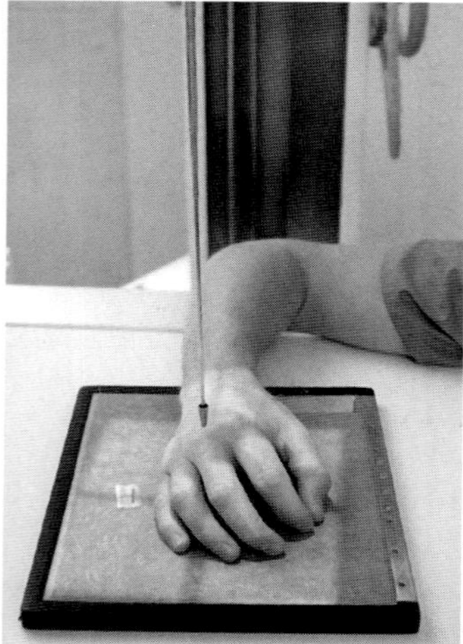

Fig. 4-66. **Exception:** Oblique hand for metacarpals (digits not parallel)–Not recommended for digits.

Shielding: Place lead shield over patient's lap to shield gonads.

Patient Position

- Patient seated at end of table with elbow flexed about 90° with hand and forearm resting on table.

Part Position 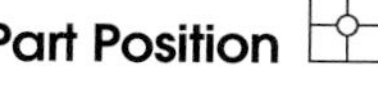

- Pronate hand on cassette; center and align long axis of hand to long axis of portion of film being exposed.
- Center 3rd MP joint of hand to CR.
- Rotate entire hand and wrist laterally 45° and support with radiolucent wedge or step block as shown so all digits are separated and **parallel to film**. (See exception below.)

Central Ray

- CR perpendicular to film, directed to the **3rd MP joint**.
- Minimum 40 in. (102 cm) SID.

Collimation: Collimate on four sides to outer margins of hand and wrist.

Exception: It is advisable for a routine oblique hand to use a support block as shown to place digits parallel to film (Fig. 4-65). This prevents foreshortening of phalanges and obscuring of interphalangeal joints. Only if the phalanges are not in the area of interest, should the oblique position for metacarpals be taken with thumb and finger tips touching cassette (Fig. 4-66).

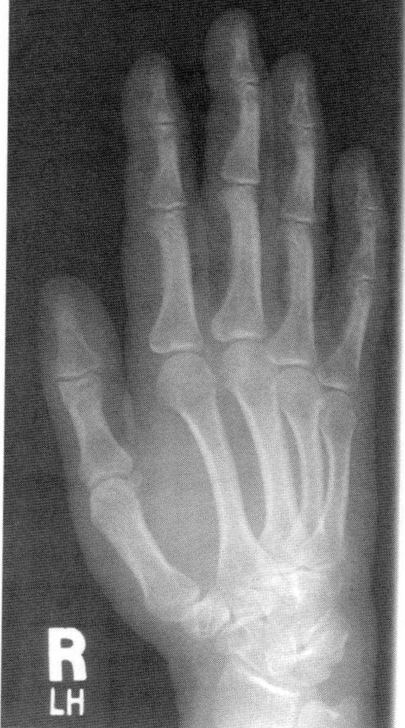

Fig. 4-67. Oblique hand (digits parallel).

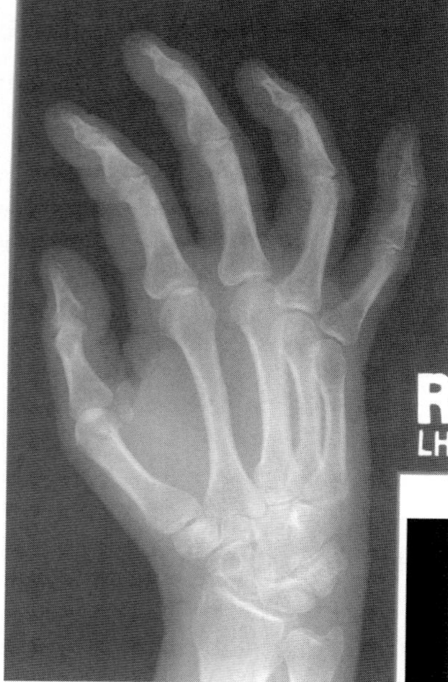

Fig. 4-68. Oblique hand (digits not parallel) –Joint spaces not open.

Evaluation Criteria

- Entire hand, wrist and about 1 inch (2.5 cm) of distal forearm should be visualized with collimation margins on four sides.
- The center of the collimation field should be at the 3rd MP joint.
- Long axis of hand and wrist should be aligned to long axis of film.
- 45° oblique is evidenced by:
  - –Mid-shafts of 3rd, 4th and 5th metacarpals should not overlap.
  - –Some overlap of distal heads of 3rd, 4th and 5th metacarpals but no overlap of distal 2nd and 3rd metacarpals.

  (Excessive overlap of metacarpals indicates excessive rotation, and too much separation indicates insufficient rotation.)
- Metacarpophalangeal and interphalangeal joints should be open without foreshortening of mid and distal phalanges indicating fingers were parallel to film.
- Optimum exposure and contrast with no motion will be evidenced by clear and sharp fine trabecular markings of the bones. Soft tissue margins will also be visualized.

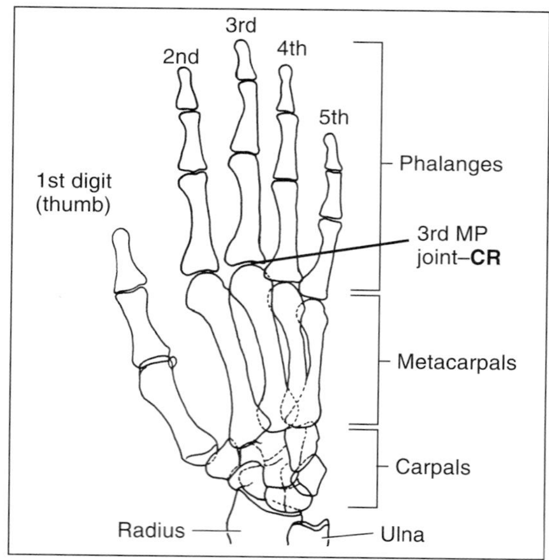

Fig. 4-69. Oblique hand (digits parallel).

"Fan" Lateral–Lateromedial Projection

Hand
Basic
• PA
• Oblique
• **Lateral**

Structures Best Shown

Phalanges separated; metacarpals and carpals superimposed in a lateral position, except for thumb, which is shown in a true PA projection (with some magnification).

Technical Factors

• Film size–8 x 10 in. (18 x 24 cm) lengthwise.
• Detail screen, tabletop.
• 54-64 kVp range. (Increase 4 or 5 kVp from PA.)
• Technique and dose:

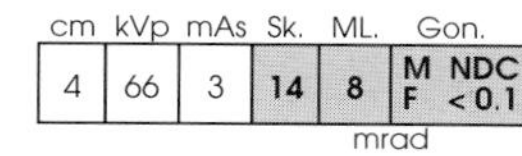

cm	kVp	mAs	Sk.	ML.	Gon.
4	66	3	14	8	M NDC F <0.1
				mrad	

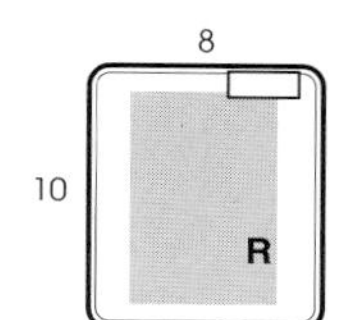

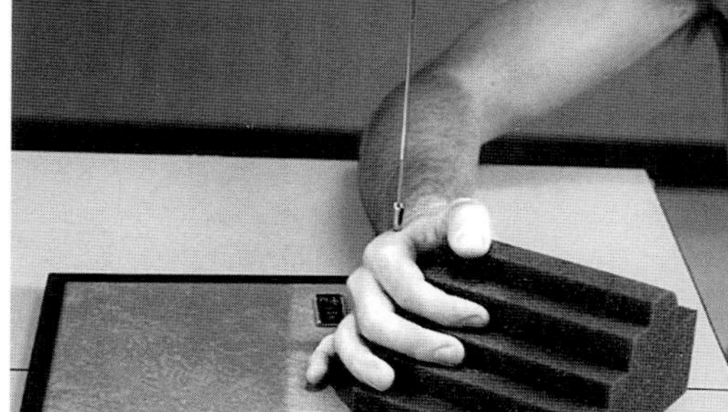
Fig. 4-70. Patient position–Fan lateral hand (keep digits separated and parallel to film).

Shielding: Place lead shield over patient's lap to shield gonads.

Patient Position

• Patient seated at end of table with elbow flexed about 90° with hand and forearm resting on table.

Part Position

• Align long axis of hand to long axis of film.
• Rotate hand and wrist into a lateral position with thumb side up.
• Spread fingers and thumb into a "fan" position and support each digit on radiolucent step block as shown. Ensure that all digits, including the thumb, are separated and are **parallel to film** and that the metacarpals are **not** obliqued but remain in a true lateral position.
• Center 2nd to 5th MP joints to CR.

Central Ray

• CR perpendicular to film, directed to **the 2nd MP joint**.
• Minimum 40 in. (102 cm) SID.

Collimation: Collimate on four sides to outer margins of hand and wrist.

Note: The "fan" lateral position as demonstrated is the preferred lateral for the hand–See following page for alternate projections.

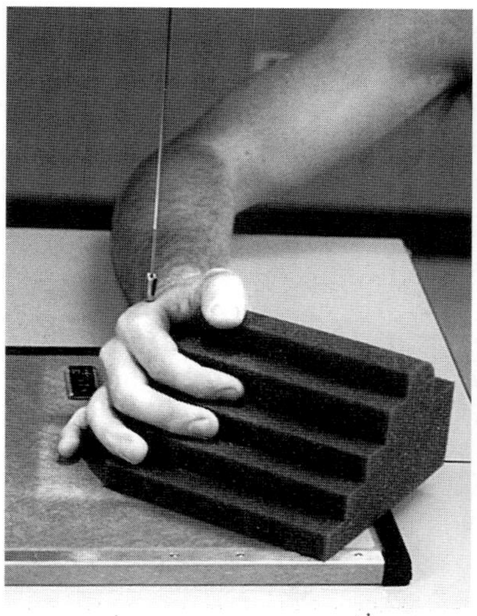
Fig. 4-71. Part position–Fan lateral –CR to 2nd MP joint.

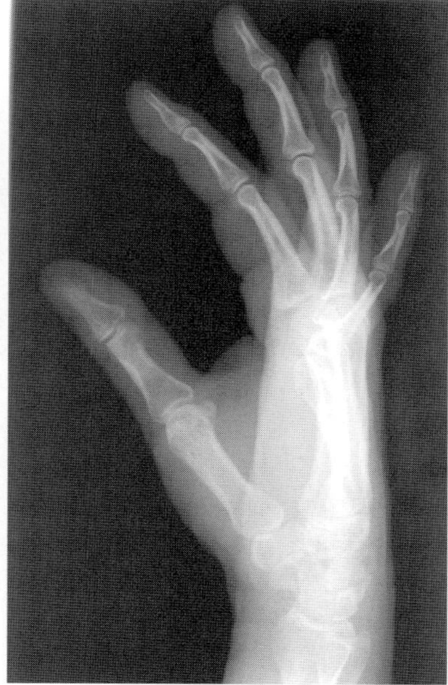
Fig. 4-72. Fan lateral.

Evaluation Criteria

• Entire hand, wrist and about 1 in. (2.5 cm) of the distal forearm should be included with collimation margins visible on four sides.
• The center of the collimation field should be to 2nd MP joint.
• Long axis of hand and wrist should be aligned to long axis of film.
• Hand and wrist should be in a true lateral position evidenced by:
–Distal radius and ulna directly superimposed.
–Metacarpals directly superimposed.
• Fingers should appear equally separated with phalanges in lateral position with joint spaces open, indicating fingers were parallel to film.
• Thumb should appear, as in a near PA projection, completely free of superimposition with joint spaces open.
• Optimum exposure and contrast with no motion will demonstrate outlines of individual metacarpals through shadows of superimposing metacarpals. Mid and distal phalanges of both thumb and fingers should appear sharp and should be visible, but will appear slightly overexposed.

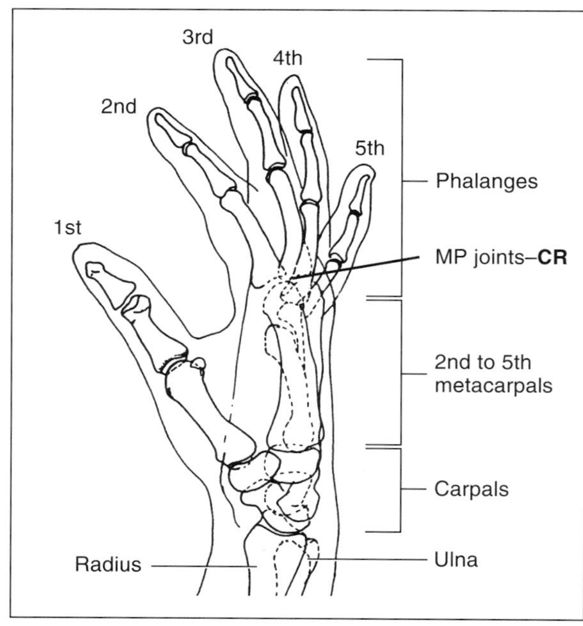

Fig. 4-73. Fan lateral.

Lateral in Extension and Flexion–Lateromedial Projections

(Alternates to Fan Lateral–See Note)

Hand
Basic
• PA
• Oblique
• **Lateral**

Structures Best Shown

Phalanges, metacarpals and carpals superimposed in a lateral position, except for thumb, which is shown in a true PA projection. (With some magnification.)

Technical Factors

- Film size–8 x 10 in. (18 x 24 cm) lengthwise.
- Detail screen, tabletop.
- 54-64 kVp range. (Increase 4 kVp from PA and oblique.)
- Technique and dose:

cm	kVp	mAs	Sk.	ML.	Gon.
4	66	3	14	8	M NDC F <0.1
			mrad		

Shielding: Place lead shield over patient's lap to shield gonads.

Patient Position

- Patient seated at end of table with elbow flexed about 90° with hand and forearm resting on table.

Part Position 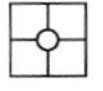

- Rotate hand and wrist 90° to cassette, thumb side up, into a true lateral position, with 2nd to 5th MP joints centered to film and to CR.

Lateral in Extension:

- Extend fingers and thumb and support against a radiolucent support block. Ensure that all fingers are directly superimposed for a true lateral position.

Lateral in Flexion:

- Flex fingers into a natural flexed position with thumb lightly touching the first finger.
- Thumb should be parallel to film.
- Ensure that fingers are directly superimposed with the entire hand in a true lateral position.

Central Ray

- CR perpendicular to film directed to the **2nd to 5th MP joints**.
- Minimum 40 in. (102 cm) SID.

Collimation: Collimate to outer margins of hand and wrist.

Note: These two positions are alternate positions to the recommended fan lateral. The lateral position in extension may be taken for localization of foreign bodies and fractures of metacarpals. The lateral in flexion will demonstrate anteroposterior displacement of fractures of metacarpals. These, however, should **not** be replacements for the fan lateral with possible trauma to the digits due to their superimposition.

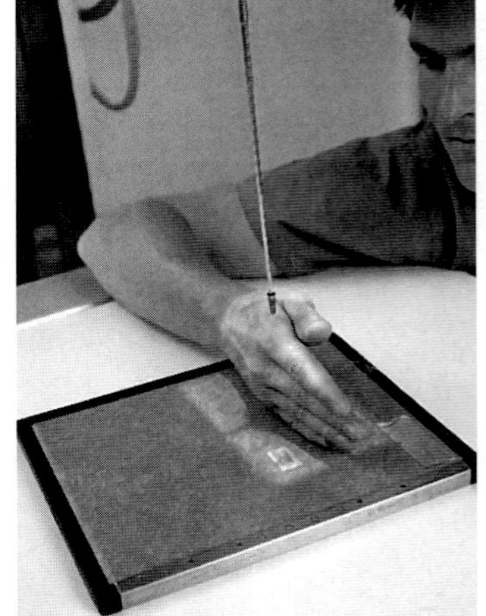

Fig. 4-74. Lateral in extension.

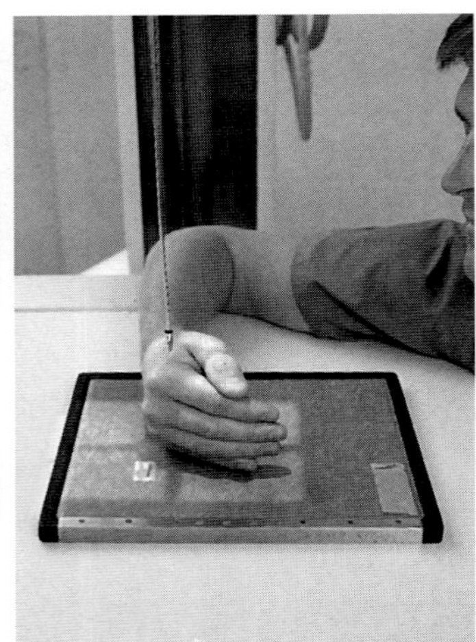

Fig. 4-75. Lateral in flexion.

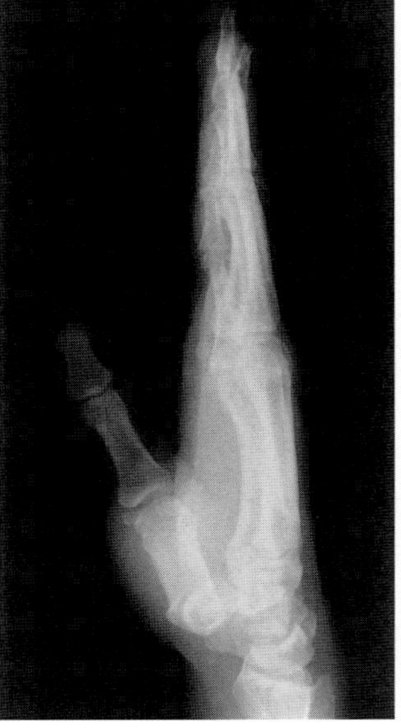

Fig. 4-76. Lateral in extension.

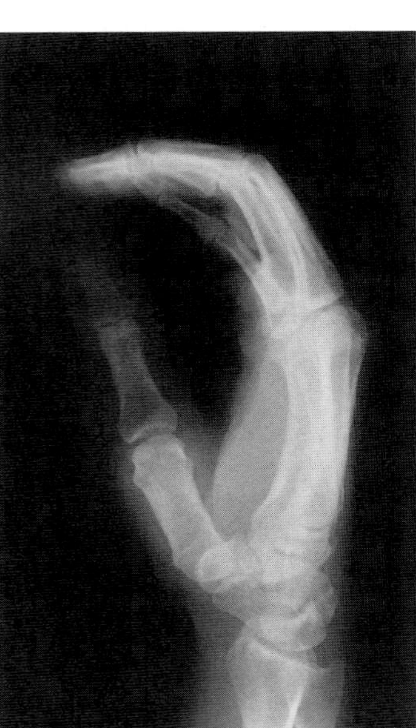

Fig. 4-77. Lateral in flexion.

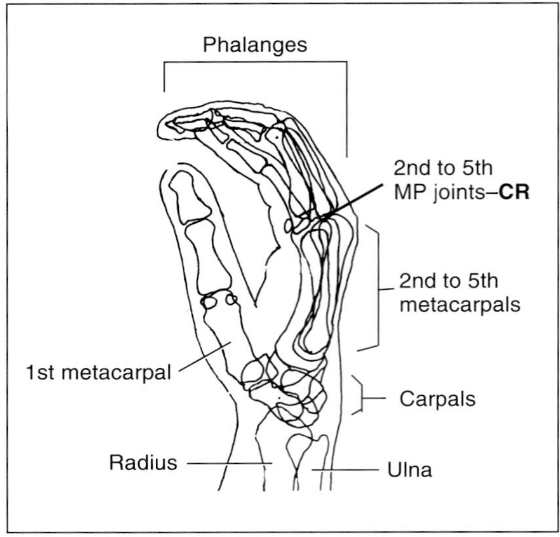

Fig. 4-78. Lateral in flexion.

Evaluation Criteria

- Entire hand, wrist and about 1 inch (2.5 cm) of the distal forearm should be included with collimation margins visible on four sides.
- The center of the collimation field should be at the MP joints.
- Long axis of hand and wrist should be aligned to long axis of film.
- Hand and wrist should be in a true lateral position evidenced by:
  –Distal radius and ulna directly superimposed.
  –Metacarpals and phalanges directly superimposed.
- Thumb should appear, as in a PA projection, free of superimposition with joint spaces open.
- Optimum exposure and contrast without motion will visualize outlines of individual metacarpals and phalanges through shadows of superimposing structures. Trabecular markings of thumb should appear clear and sharp.

PA (AP) Projection

Wrist
Basic
• PA
• Oblique
• Lateral

Structures Best Shown

Mid and proximal metacarpals, carpals, distal radius and ulna and associated joints, and pertinent soft tissues such as fat pads and fat stripes of the wrist joint.

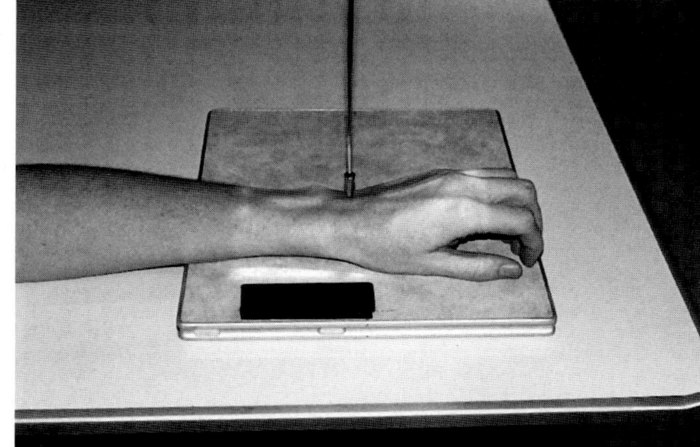

Fig. 4-79. PA wrist.

Technical Factors

- Film size–8 x 10 in. (18 x 24 cm).
- Divide in half, crosswise.
- Detail screen, tabletop.
- 60±6 kVp range.
- Technique and dose:

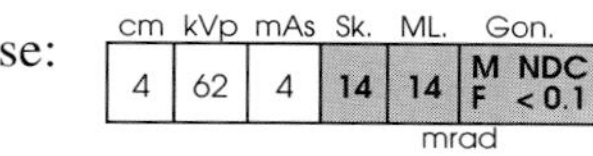

cm	kVp	mAs	Sk.	ML.	Gon.
4	62	4	14	14	M NDC F <0.1

mrad

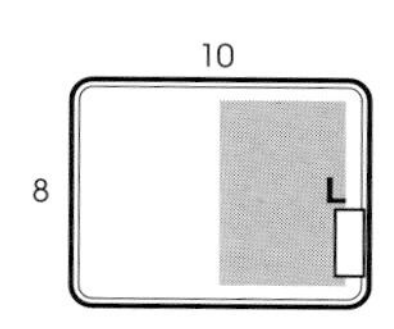

Shielding: Place lead shield over patient's lap to shield gonads.

Patient Position

- Patient seated at end of table with elbow flexed about 90° with hand and wrist resting on cassette, palm down.
- Drop shoulder so shoulder, elbow and wrist are on same horizontal plane.

Part Position

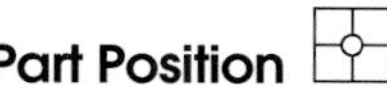

- Align and center long axis of hand and wrist to portion of film being exposed, with carpal area centered to CR.
- With hand pronated, arch hand slightly **to place wrist and carpal area in close contact with cassette** (reduce OID).

Central Ray

- CR perpendicular to film, directed to **midcarpal area**.
- Minimum 40 in. (102 cm) SID.

Collimation: Collimate to wrist on all four sides; include distal radius and ulna and mid metacarpal area.

Alternate AP: To better demonstrate intercarpal spaces and the distal radius and ulna, an AP wrist may be taken with hand slightly arched to place **wrist and carpals in close contact with cassette** (Fig. 4-80). This is a good wrist projection if the patient can assume this position easily.

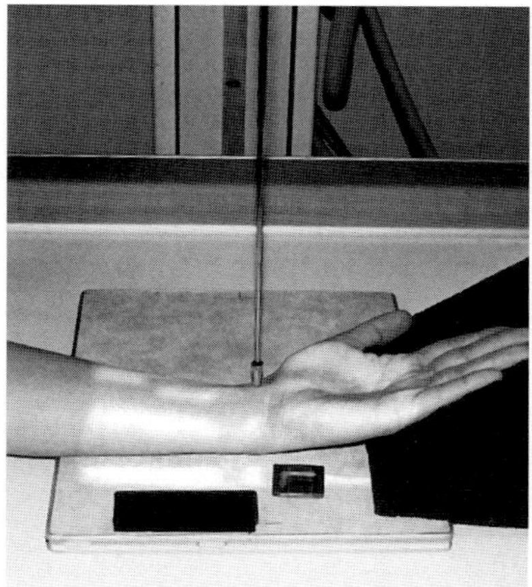

Fig. 4-80. Alternate AP wrist.

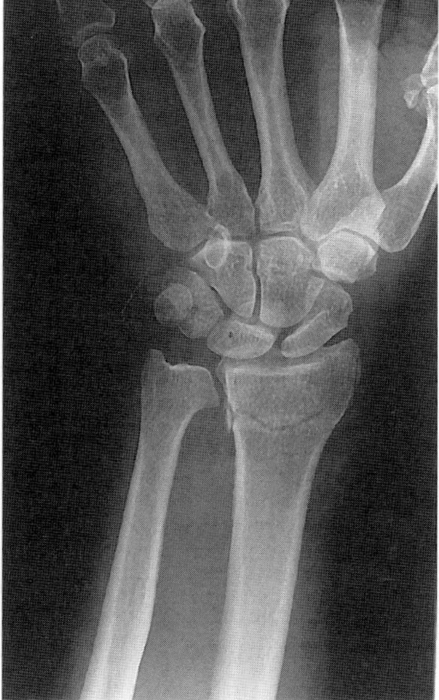

Fig. 4-81. PA wrist.

Evaluation Criteria

- Distal radius, ulna, and all carpals at least to mid-metacarpal area should be visualized, centered to the mid portion and to the long axis of that part of film being used with collimation margins on four sides.
- The center of collimation field should be to midcarpal area.
- **True PA** as evidenced by:
  - –Equal concavity shapes on each side of shafts of proximal metacarpals.
  - –Near equal distances between proximal metacarpals; and separation of distal radius and ulna except for possible minimal superimposition at distal radioulnar joint.
- Optimum exposure and contrast with no motion should visualize soft tissues such as pertinent fat pads, as well as the bony margins of the carpals with sharp borders and clear trabecular markings. (The intercarpal spaces will not all appear open because of irregular shapes and resultant overlapping).

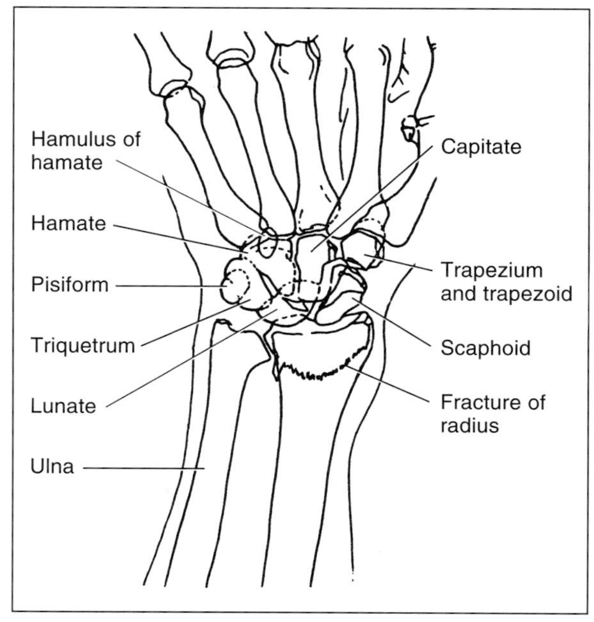

Fig. 4-82. PA wrist.

PA Oblique Projection–Lateral Rotation

Wrist
Basic
• PA
• **Oblique**
• Lateral

Structures Best Shown

Mid and distal metacarpals, carpals (especially trapezium and scaphoid), distal radius and ulna and associated joints and pertinent fat pads and fat stripes of the wrist joint.

10

8 R

Technical Factors

- Film size–8 x 10 in. (18 x 24 cm).
- Divide in half, crosswise.
- Detail screen, tabletop.
- 60±6 kVp range.
- Technique and dose:

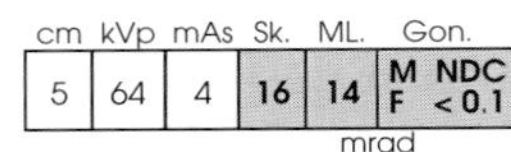

cm	kVp	mAs	Sk.	ML.	Gon.
5	64	4	16	14	M NDC F <0.1

mrad

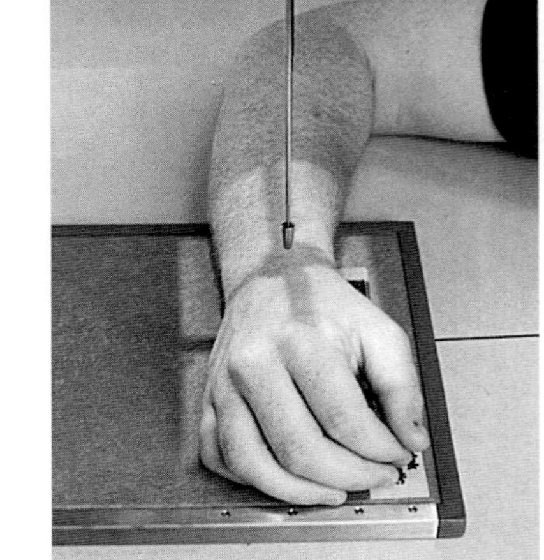

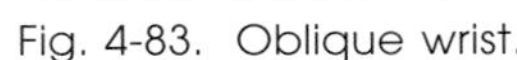

Fig. 4-83. Oblique wrist.

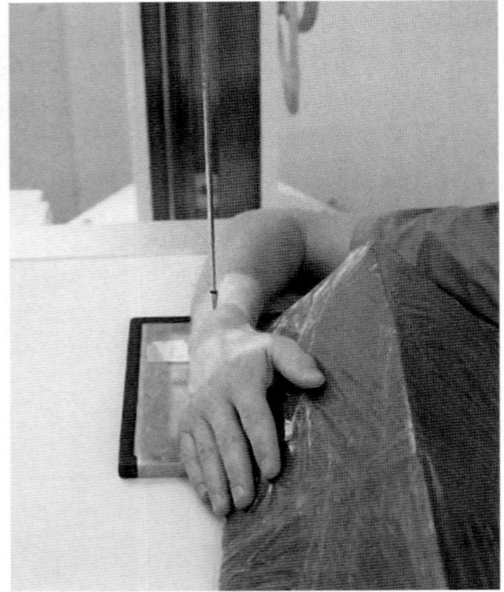

Fig. 4-84. Oblique wrist (with 45° support).

Shielding: Place lead shield over patient's lap to shield gonads.

Patient Position

- Patient seated at end of table with elbow flexed about 90° with hand and wrist resting on cassette, palm down.

Part Position 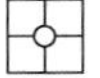

- Align and center hand and wrist to the portion of film being exposed.
- From pronated position, rotate wrist and hand laterally 45°.
- For stability place a 45° support under thumb side of hand to support hand and wrist in a 45° oblique position (Fig. 4-84), or partially flex fingers to arch hand to lightly rest fingertips on cassette (Fig. 4-83).
- Center midcarpal area to CR.

Central Ray

- CR perpendicular to film, directed to the **midcarpal area**.
- Minimum 40 in. (102 cm) SID.

Collimation: Collimate to wrist on four sides, include distal radius and ulna, and at least to the mid-metacarpal area.

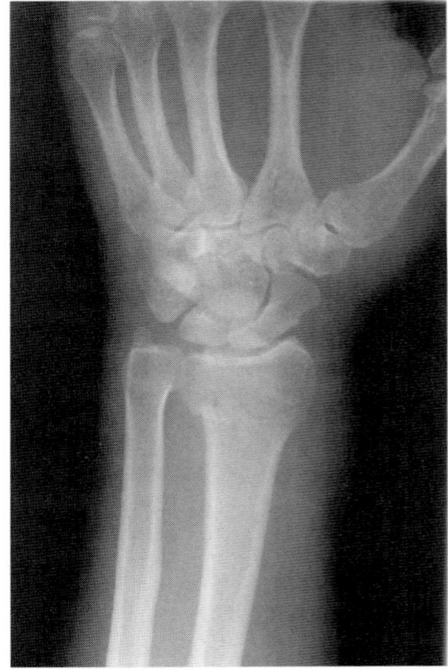

Fig. 4-85. Oblique wrist.

Evaluation Criteria

- Distal radius, ulna, carpals and at least to mid-metacarpal area should be visualized, centered to the mid portion and to the long axis of that part of film being used, with collimation margins on four sides.
- The center of collimation field should be to midcarpal area.
- The trapezium in its entirety should be well visualized, as well as the scaphoid, which has only slight superimposition of other carpals on its medial aspects.
- The proximal 3rd, 4th, 5th metacarpals, as well as the distal radius and ulna, should appear with some superimposition.
- Correct exposure with sufficient contrast and no motion will demonstrate the carpals and their overlapping borders. The trabecular markings of all bones visualized will be sharp and clear. Soft tissue margins such as pertinent fat pads should be visible.

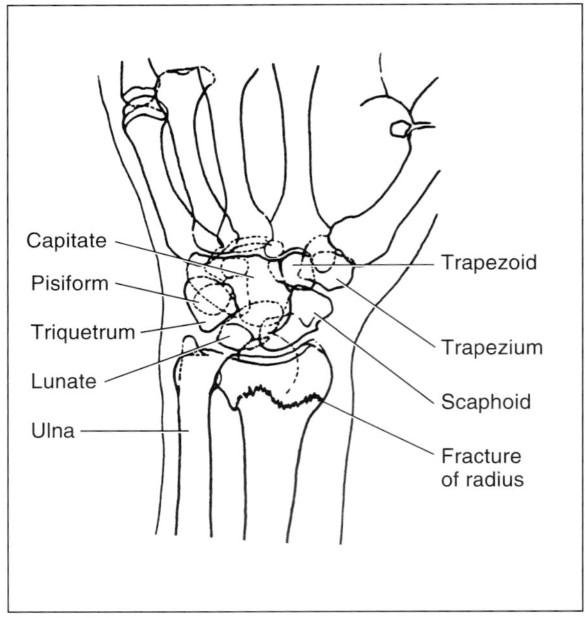

Fig. 4-86. Oblique wrist.

Lateral–Lateromedial Projection

Wrist
Basic
• PA
• Oblique
• **Lateral**

Structures Best Shown

Superimposed proximal metacarpals, carpals, distal radius and ulna and wrist joint, and pertinent fat pads and stripes of the wrist joint.

Posterior lip of distal radius to rule out a **Barton's type fracture**; or distal portion of radius for possible **Colles' fracture** with posterior displacement of distal fragment; or **Smith's fracture** with anterior displacement of distal fragment.

Technical Factors

- Film size–8 x 10 in. (18 x 24 cm), lengthwise.
- Detail screen, tabletop.
- 64±6 kVp range. (Increase 4 kVp from PA and oblique.)
- Technique and dose:

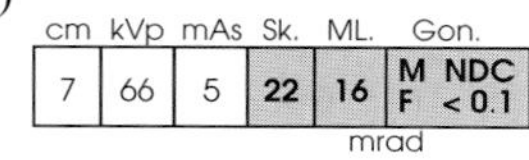

cm	kVp	mAs	Sk.	ML.	Gon.
7	66	5	22	16	M NDC F <0.1
			mrad		

Shielding: Place lead shield over patient's lap to shield gonads.

Patient Position

- Patient seated at end of table with both arm and forearm resting on the table with elbow flexed about 90°. Wrist and hand are placed on cassette in thumb-up lateral position. Shoulder, elbow and wrist should be on same horizontal plane.

Part Position

- Align hand and wrist to the center of and to the long axis of the cassette; center midcarpal area to CR.
- Adjust the hand and wrist into a **true lateral** position with fingers comfortably flexed; or if support is needed to prevent motion, use a radiolucent support block and sandbag and place block against extended hand and fingers as shown.

Central Ray

- CR perpendicular to film, directed to **midcarpal area**.
- Minimum 40 in. (102 cm) SID.

Collimation: Collimate on four sides, including distal radius and ulna, and the metacarpal area.

Evaluation Criteria

- Distal radius and ulna, carpals and at least the mid metacarpal area should be visualized, centered to the mid portion and to the long axis of that part of film being used.
- Collimation margins should be visible on four sides.
- The center of the collimation field should be to the mid carpal region.
- **True lateral** position as evidenced by:
  –Ulnar head of distal ulna should be centered and directly superimposed over radius.
  –Proximal metacarpals should all appear aligned and superimposed.
- Optimum exposure and contrast with no motion will visualize soft tissue such as margins of pertinent fat pads, as well as the borders of the distal ulna through the superimposed radius. The fine trabecular markings of all bones should appear clear and sharp.

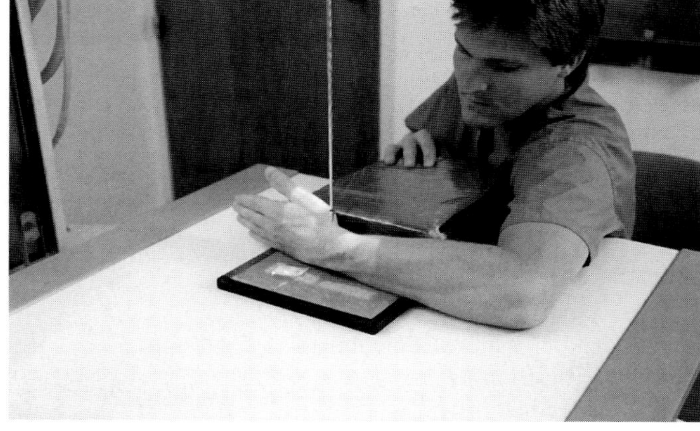

Fig. 4-87. Patient position–Lateral wrist.

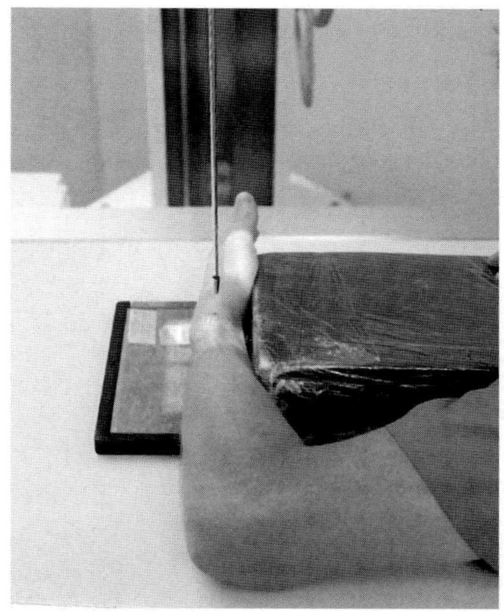

Fig. 4-88. Part position–Lateral wrist.

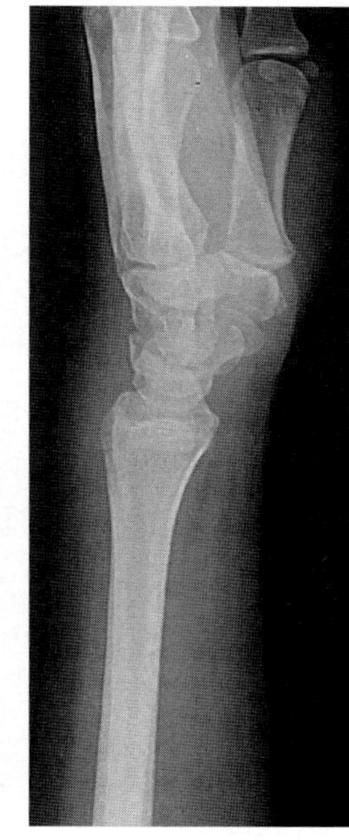

Fig. 4-89. Lateral wrist.

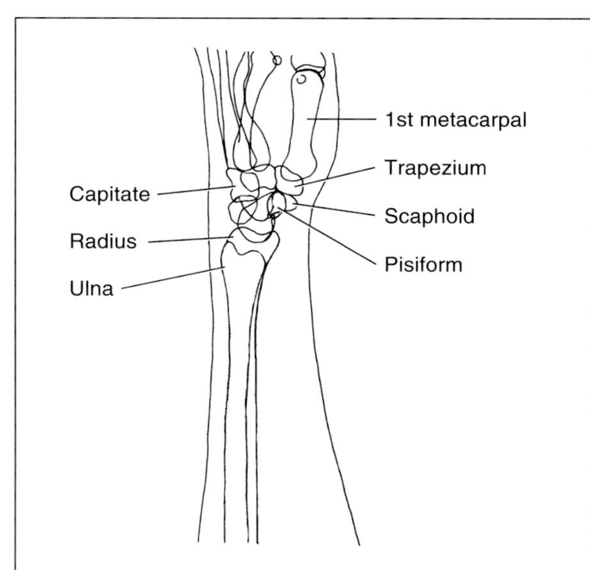

Fig. 4-90. Lateral wrist.

PA Scaphoid–with CR Angle and Ulnar Flexion

Warning: Do **not** attempt this position with possible wrist trauma before routine wrist series has been completed to evaluate for possible fractures of distal forearm and/or wrist.

Wrist
Special
- **Scaphoid views: CR angle, ulnar flex.** Mod. Stecher method
- Radial flexion
- Carpal canal
- Carpal bridge

Structures Best Shown

Scaphoid without foreshortening with opened spaces between adjacent carpals.

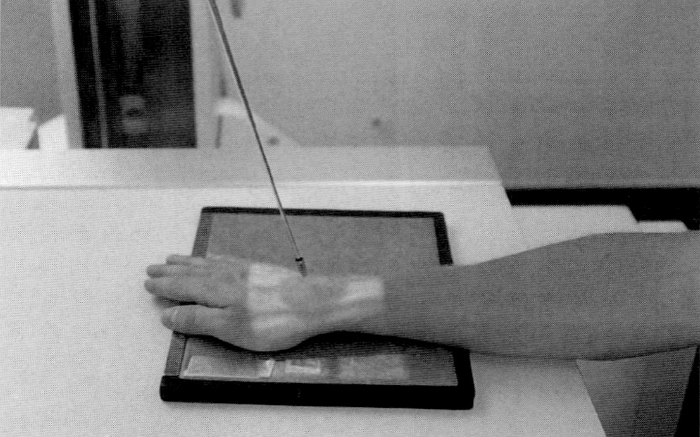

Fig. 4-91. PA wrist (scaphoid)–Ulnar flexion with 15° CR angle.

Technical Factors

- Film size–8 x 10 in. (18 x 24 cm).
- Divide in half, crosswise (if combined with other projections).
- Detail screen, tabletop.
- 60±6 kVp range.
- Technique and dose:

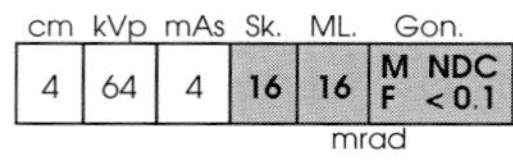

cm	kVp	mAs	Sk.	ML.	Gon.
4	64	4	16	16	M NDC F <0.1
			mrad		

Shielding: Place lead shield over patient's lap to shield gonads.

Patient Position

- Patient seated at end of table with wrist and hand on cassette, palm down with shoulder, elbow and wrist on same horizontal plane.

Part Position 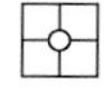

- Position wrist as for a PA projection, palm down with hand and wrist aligned to center of long axis of portion of film being exposed, scaphoid centered to CR.
- Without moving forearm, gently evert the hand (move toward ulnar side) as far as patient can tolerate without lifting or obliquing distal forearm.

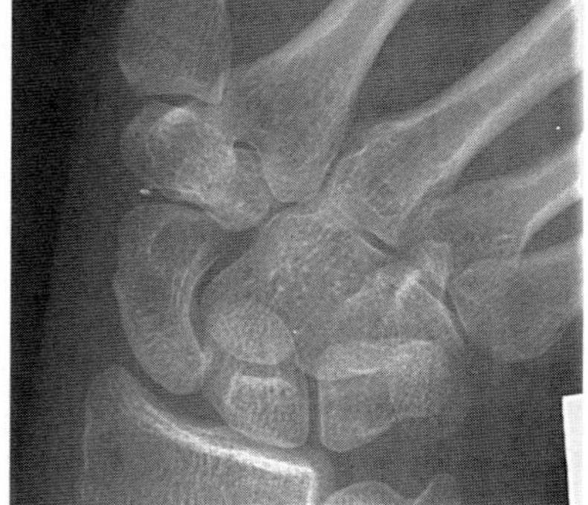

Fig. 4-92. 15° angle.

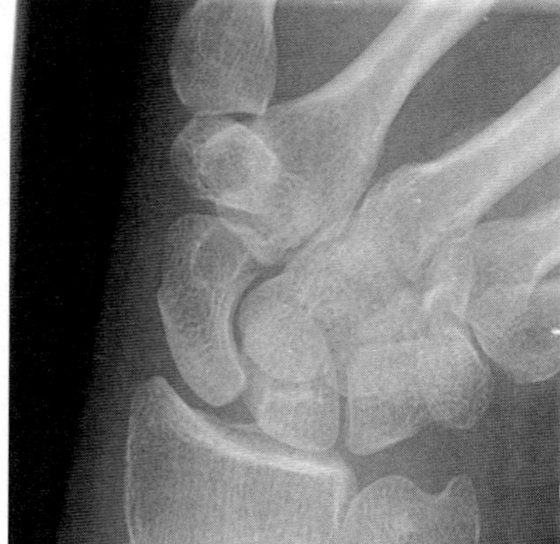

Fig. 4-93. 25° angle.

Central Ray

- Angle CR **10 to 15° proximally** (along long axis of forearm, toward elbow). Direct the CR perpendicular to the scaphoid.
- Center CR to **scaphoid**. (Locate scaphoid at a point ¾ in. or 2 cm distal to radial styloid process.)
- Minimum 40 in. (102 cm) SID.

Collimation: Collimate on four sides to carpal region.

Note: Obscure fractures of the scaphoid may require several projections taken with different CR angles, such as a four-projection series with the CR angled proximally 0°, 10°, 20° and 30°.*

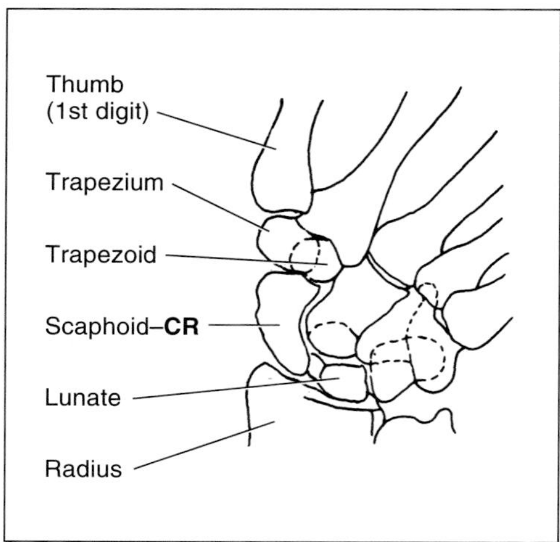

Fig. 4-94. 15° angle.

Evaluation Criteria

- Scaphoid should be clearly demonstrated without distortion (foreshortening), with adjacent carpal interspaces open.
- The distal radius and ulna, the carpals and proximal metacarpals should be visualized. The long axis of forearm should be aligned to long axis of the portion of exposed film with collimation margins evident on four sides.
- The center of collimation field (CR location) should be to the scaphoid.
- No rotation of wrist as evidenced by appearance of distal radius and ulna with only minimal superimposition of distal radioulnar joint.
- Ulnar flexion should be evident by the angle of the long axis of the metacarpals to that of the radius and ulna.
- Correct exposure and contrast with no motion will visualize the scaphoid borders and trabecular markings clearly and sharply.

*Rafert, JA, Long, BW. Technique for diagnosis of scaphoid fractures. *Radiologic Technology* 1991; 63(1):16-21.

PA Scaphoid–Hand Elevated and Ulnar Flexion

Modified Stecher Method*†

Warning: Do **not** attempt ulnar flexion with possible wrist trauma before routine series has been completed to evaluate for possible fractures of distal forearm and/or wrist.

Wrist
Special
- **Scaphoid views:**
  CR angle, ulnar flex.
  Mod. Stecher method
- Radial flexion
- Carpal canal
- Carpal bridge

Structures Best Shown

Scaphoid without foreshortening or superimposition of adjoining carpals.

This is an alternative projection to the CR angle ulnar flexion method demonstrated on the preceding page.

Technical Factors

- Film size–8 x 10 in. (18 x 24 cm).
- Divide in half, crosswise.
- Detail screen, tabletop.
- 60±6 kVp range.
- Technique and dose:

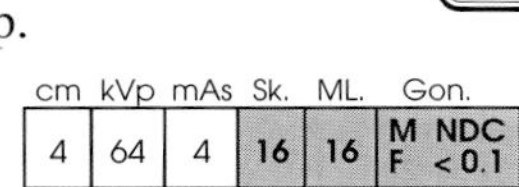

cm	kVp	mAs	Sk.	ML.	Gon.
4	64	4	16	16	M NDC F < 0.1

mrad

Shielding: Place lead shield to shield gonads.

Patient Position

- Patient seated at end of table with elbow flexed resting on table with wrist and hand on cassette, palm down with shoulder, elbow and wrist on same horizontal plane.

Part Position

- Place hand and wrist palm down on cassette with **hand elevated on 20° angle sponge**.
- Ensure that wrist is in direct contact with cassette.
- Gently ulnarflex hand (flex hand toward ulnar side) unless contraindicated due to severity of injury (see Fig. 4-96).
- Center scaphoid to CR.

Alternate method: Clenching the fist along with ulnar flexion results in a similar position of the scaphoid.

Central Ray

- CR **perpendicular to film**, directed to **scaphoid** (¾ in. or 2 cm proximal, and ¾ in. or 2 cm lateral to 1st MP joint).
- Minimum 40 in. (102 cm) SID.

Collimation: Collimate on four sides to carpal region.

Note: Stecher indicated that elevating the hand 20° places the scaphoid parallel to the film. Stecher also suggested that clenching the fist can be an alternative to elevating the hand or angling the CR.* Bridgman recommended ulnar flexion in addition to the hand elevation for less scaphoid superimposition.†

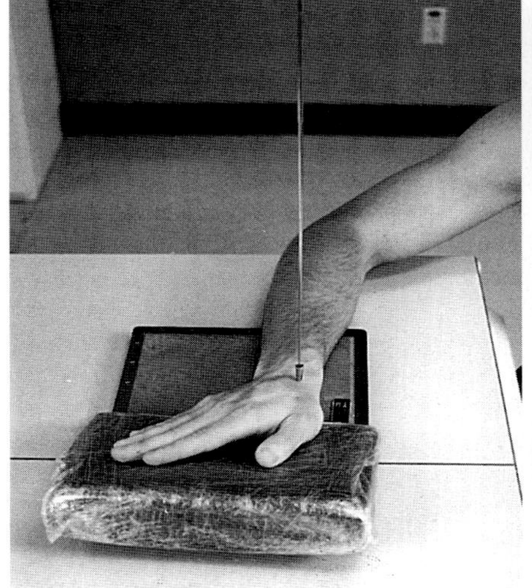

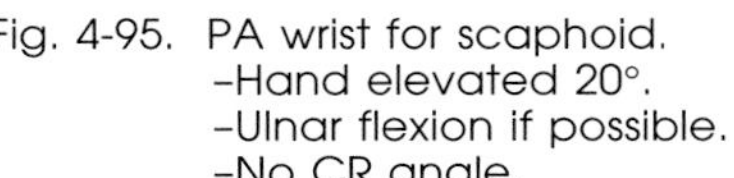

Fig. 4-95. PA wrist for scaphoid.
-Hand elevated 20°.
-Ulnar flexion if possible.
-No CR angle.

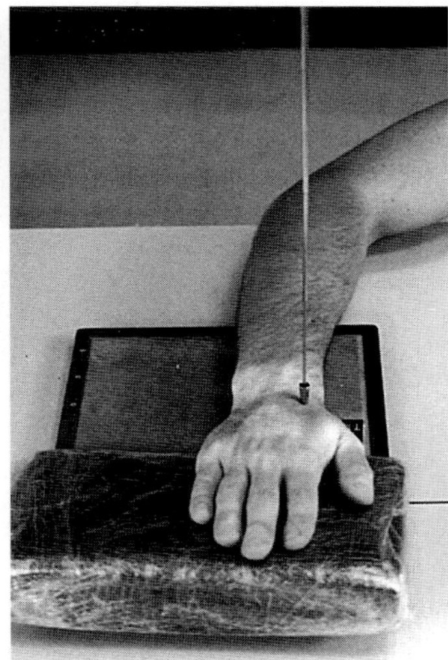

Fig. 4-96. Possible trauma.
-Hand elevated 20°.
-**No** ulnar flexion.
-No CR angle.

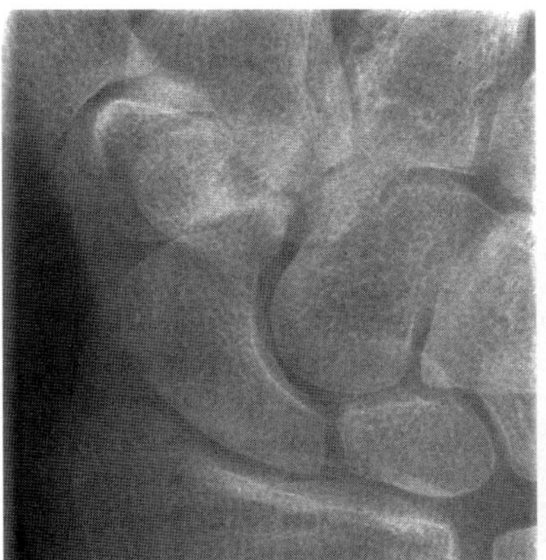

Fig. 4-97. Hand elevated, ulnar flexion.

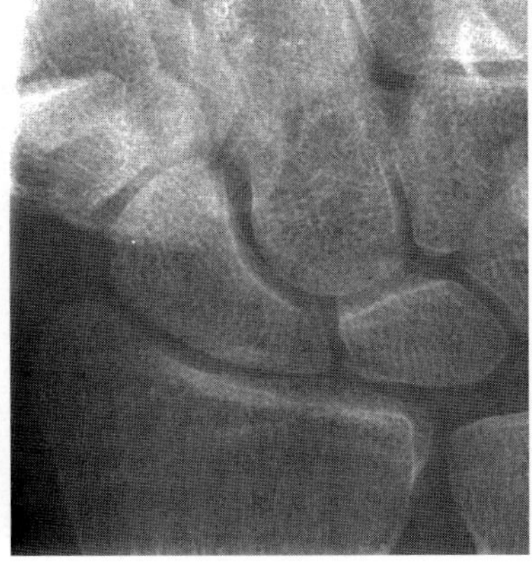

Fig. 4-98. Hand elevated, no ulnar flexion or CR angle.

Evaluation Criteria

- The carpals with adjacent interspaces more open should be best visualized on the lateral (ulnar) side of the wrist.
- The distal radius and ulna, the carpals and proximal metacarpals should be visualized. The long axis of forearm should be aligned to long axis of the portion of exposed film with collimation margins on all four sides.
- The center of collimation field should be to the midcarpal area.
- No rotation of wrist as evidenced by appearance of distal radius and ulna (should be similar to a PA wrist projection).
- Extreme radial flexion should be evident by the angle of the long axis of the metacarpals to that of the radius and ulna.
- Correct exposure and adequate penetration with no motion will visualize the scaphoid borders and trabecular markings clearly and sharply.

*Stecher, WR. Roentgenography of the carpal navicular bone, *AJR* 1937; 37:704-705.
†Bridgman, CF. Radiography of the Carpal Navicular Bone, *Medical Radiography Photography* 1949; 25:104-105.

PA Projection–Radial Flexion

Warning: Do **not** attempt this position with possible wrist trauma before routine series has been completed to evaluate for possible fractures of distal forearm and/or wrist.

Wrist
Special
- Scaphoid views: CR angle, ulnar flex. Mod. Stecher method
- **Radial flexion**
- Carpal canal
- Carpal bridge

Structures Best Shown

Carpals with more **opened interspaces on ulnar (lateral) side of wrist**, especially the **lunate**, **triquetrum**, **pisiform** and **hamate**.

Technical Factors

- Film size–8 x 10 in. (18 x 24 cm).
- Divide in half, crosswise.
- Detail screen, tabletop.
- 64±6 kVp range.
- Technique and dose:

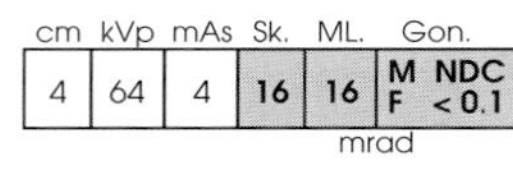

cm	kVp	mAs	Sk.	ML.	Gon.
4	64	4	16	16	M NDC F <0.1

mrad

Shielding: Place lead shield over patient's lap to shield gonads.

Patient Position

- Patient seated at end of table with elbow flexed at 90° resting on table with wrist and hand on cassette, palm down with shoulder, elbow and wrist on same horizontal plane.

Part Position

- Position wrist as for a PA projection, palm down with wrist and hand aligned to center of long axis of portion of film being exposed.
- Without moving forearm, gently invert the hand (move medially toward thumb side) as far as patient can tolerate without lifting or obliquing distal forearm.
- Center midcarpal area to CR.

Central Ray

- CR **perpendicular to film**, directed to **midcarpal area**.
- Minimum 40 in. (102 cm) SID.

Collimation: Collimate on four sides to carpal region.

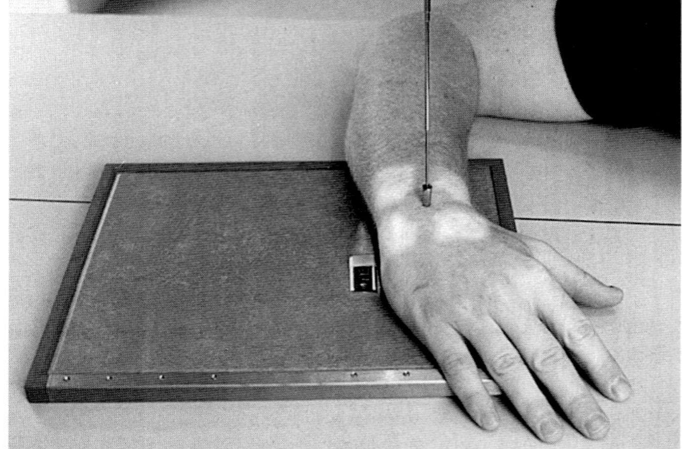

Fig. 4-99. PA wrist–Radial flexion.

Fig. 4-100. Radial flexion.

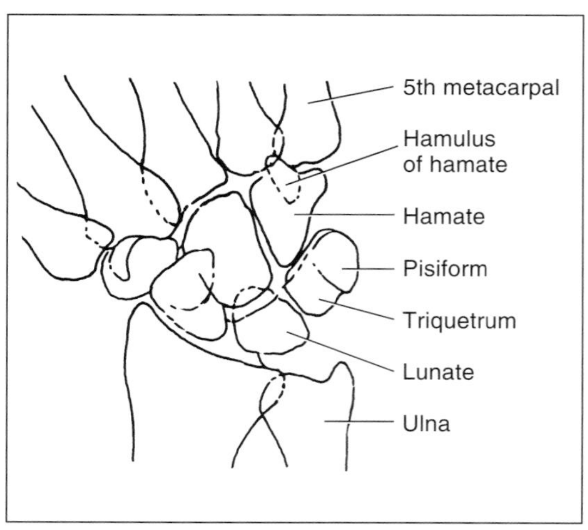

Fig. 4-101. Radial flexion.

Evaluation Criteria

- The carpals with more open adjacent interspaces should be best visualized on the lateral (ulnar) side of the wrist.
- The distal radius and ulna, the carpals and proximal metacarpals should be visualized with collimation margins on all four sides.
- The center of collimation field should be to the midcarpal area.
- No rotation of wrist, as evidenced by appearance of distal radius and ulna (should be similar to a PA wrist projection).
- Extreme radial flexion should be evident by the angle of the long axis of the metacarpals to that of the radius and ulna, and the proximity of the trapezium to the styloid process of the radius.
- Correct exposure and contrast with no motion will visualize the carpal borders and trabecular markings clearly and sharply.

Carpal Canal (Tunnel)–Tangential, Inferosuperior Projection

Gaynor-Hart Method

Warning: Do **not** attempt this position with possible wrist trauma before routine series has been completed to evaluate for possible fractures of distal forearm and/or wrist.

Wrist
Special
- Scaphoid views: CR angle, ulnar flex. Mod. Stecher method
- Radial flexion
- **Carpal canal**
- Carpal bridge

Structures Best Shown

Carpal tunnel or canal (sulcus) made up of the palmar aspect of the trapezium, tuberosity of scaphoid, palmar aspects of trapezoid and capitate, the hamulus process of the hamate, the triquetrum (which is mostly superimposed), and the pisiform.

To rule out abnormal calcification in the carpal sulcus, which may create impingement on the **median nerve** as seen with **carpal tunnel syndrome**.

Technical Factors

- Film size–8 x 10 in. (18 x 24 cm).
- Divide in half, crosswise.
- Detail screen, tabletop.
- 64±6 kVp range.
- Technique and dose:

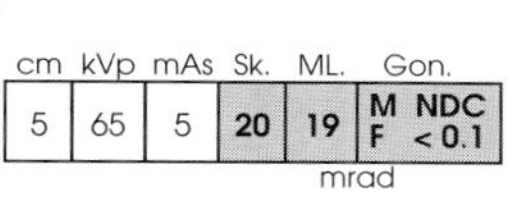

cm	kVp	mAs	Sk.	ML.	Gon.
5	65	5	20	19	M NDC F <0.1

mrad

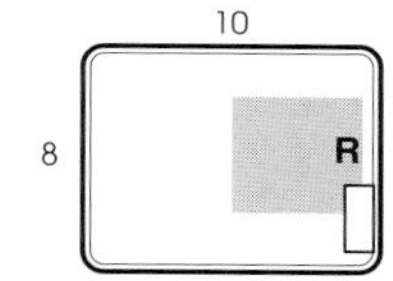

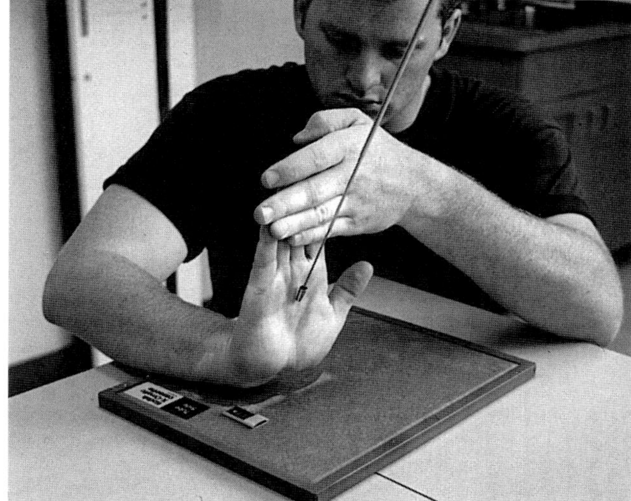

Fig. 4-102. Tangential projection.
–CR 25 to 30° to long axis of hand.

Shielding: Place lead shield over patient's lap to shield gonads.

Patient Position

- Patient seated at end of table with wrist and hand on cassette, palm down, (pronated).

Part Position

- Align hand and wrist to long axis of portion of film being exposed.
- Ask patient to hyperextend wrist (dorsiflex) as far as possible by grasping the fingers with other hand and gently but firmly hyperextending the wrist until the long axis of the metacarpals and fingers are as near vertical as possible (without lifting the wrist and forearm from the cassette). May also have patient pull fingers back, using gauze or tape.
- Rotate entire hand and wrist about **10° internally** (toward radial side) to prevent superimposition of pisiform and hamate.
- Center carpal canal to CR.

Central Ray

- Angle CR **25 to 30° to the long axis of the hand**. (The total CR angle in relationship to the film will have to be increased if patient cannot hyperextend wrist as far as indicated above.)
- Direct CR to a point **≈1½ inches (3 cm) distal to the base of 3rd metacarpal** (center of palm of hand).
- Minimum 40 in. (102 cm) SID.

Collimation: Collimate on four sides to area of interest.

Note: If patient cannot assume this hyperextended position, see alternate superoinferior projection on following page.

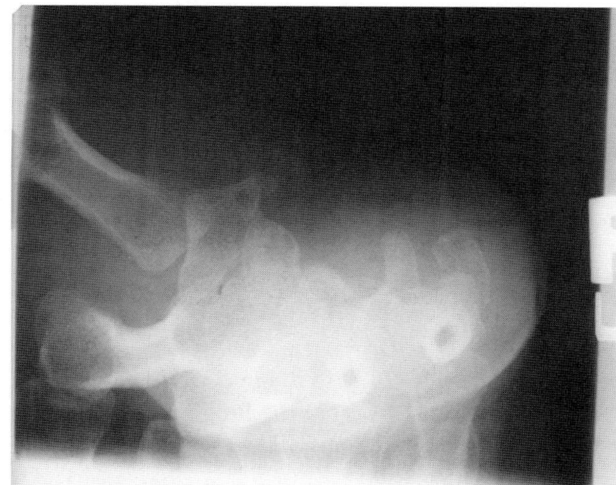

Fig. 4-103. Tangential projection.

Evaluation Criteria

- The carpals should be demonstrated in a tunnel-like "arched" arrangement on the inferosuperior projection.
- The center of the collimation field should be to the midpoint of the carpal canal.
- The pisiform and the hamulus process should be separated and clearly visualized in profile without superimposition.
- The rounded palmar aspect of the scaphoid should be visualized in profile; as well as that aspect of the trapezium articulating with the 1st metacarpal.
- Correct exposure and adequate contrast without motion should visualize the carpals in profile with trabecular markings appearing clear and sharp.

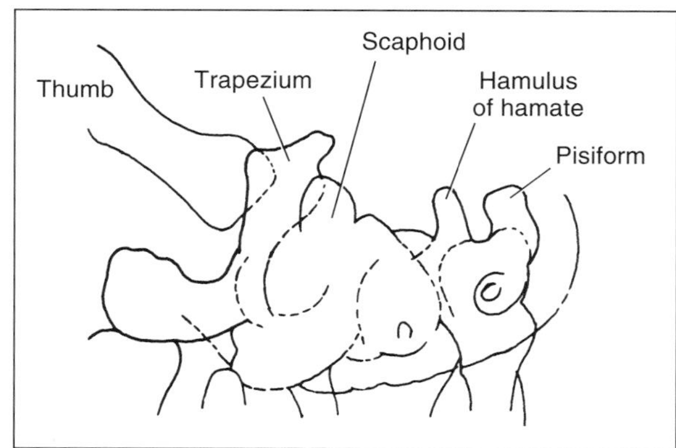

Fig. 4-104. Tangential projection.

Carpal Canal–Alternate Superoinferior Projection

Warning: Do **not** attempt this position with possible wrist trauma before routine series has been completed to evaluate for possible fractures of distal forearm and/or wrist.

Wrist
Special
- Scaphoid views:
  CR angle, ulnar flex.
  Mod. Stecher method
- Radial flexion
- **Carpal canal**
- Carpal bridge

Structures Best Shown

Carpal tunnel or canal made up of the palmar aspect of the trapezium, tuberosity of scaphoid, palmar aspects of trapezoid and capitate, the hamulus process of the hamate, the triquetrum (which is mostly superimposed), and the pisiform.

Technical Factors

10
8 R

- Film size–8 x 10 in. (18 x 24 cm).
- Divide in half, crosswise.
- Detail screen, tabletop.
- 64±6 kVp range.
- Technique and dose:

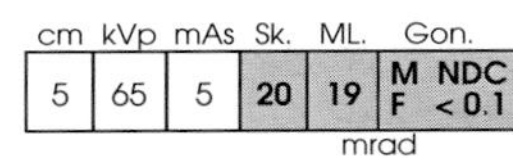

cm	kVp	mAs	Sk.	ML.	Gon. (mrad)
5	65	5	20	19	M NDC F <0.1

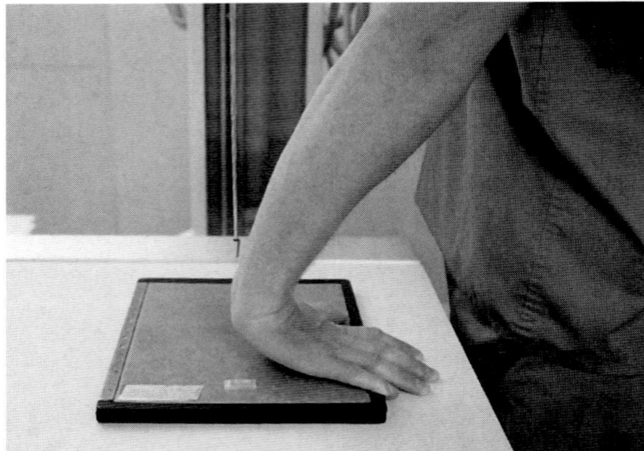

Fig. 4-105. Tangential superoinferior projection. –CR 25 to 30° to forearm.

Alternate Projection: If patient cannot hyperflex wrist sufficiently as shown on preceding page, then this alternate superoinferior projection may be taken. This, however, will not result in the same tunnel view of the arched carpals, and the carpal canal may not be as well visualized in profile as on the inferosuperior projection.

Shielding: Secure a lead shield around patient's waist to shield gonads.

Patient and Part Position 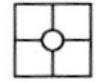

- Have patient stand at end of the table and place the palmar surface of the hand flat on the cassette. Then hyperextend the wrist by slowly leaning forward as far as can be tolerated, allowing the palmar surface of the hand to raise off the cassette 1 to 1½ inches (3 to 4 cm) as shown.
- The long axis of the forearm should be about 25 to 35° from the perpendicular CR.
- Center carpal canal to CR.

Central Ray

- Direct CR **tangentially to the mid carpal canal**, perpendicular to the film or **25 to 30° from the long axis of the forearm**.
- Minimum 40 in. (102 cm) SID.

Collimation: Collimate on four sides to area of interest.

Evaluation Criteria

- The carpals in general should be demonstrated in a tunnel-like "arched" arrangement.
- The center of the collimation field should be to the midpoint of the carpal canal.
- The pisiform and the hamulus process should be clearly visualized in profile without superimposition.
- The rounded palmar aspect of the scaphoid, and the adjacent and mostly superimposed trapezium should be visualized in profile.
- Correct exposure and adequate contrast without motion should visualize the carpals in profile with trabecular markings appearing clear and sharp.

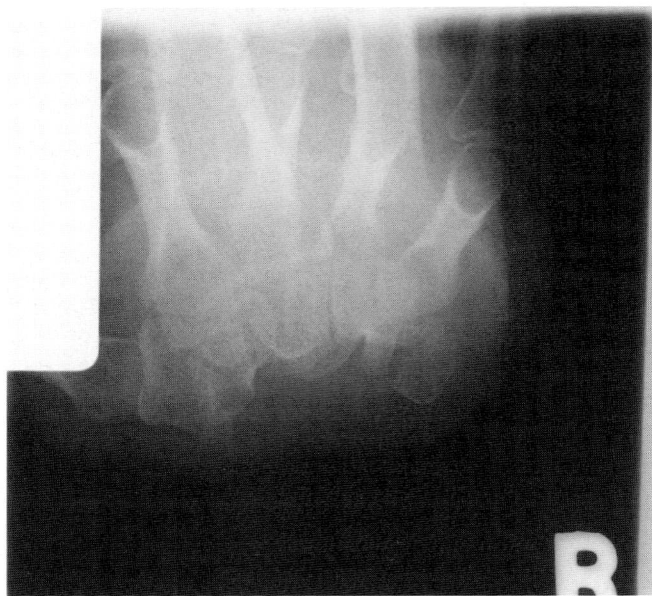

Fig. 4-106. Tangential superoinferior projection.

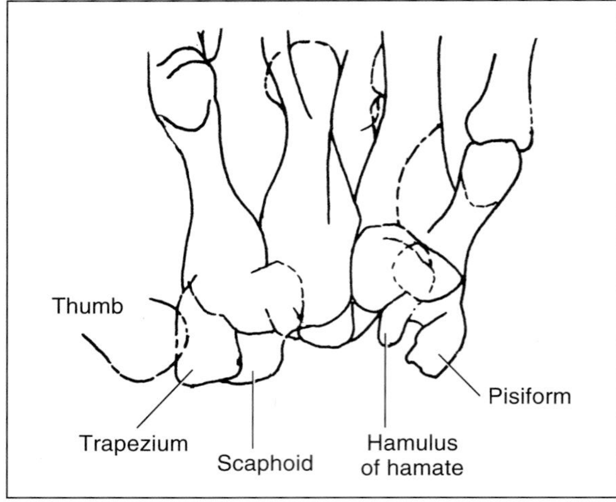

Fig. 4-107. Tangential superoinferior projection.

Carpal Bridge–Tangential Projection

Warning: Do **not** attempt this position with possible wrist trauma before routine series has been completed to evaluate for possible fractures of distal forearm and/or wrist.

Wrist
Special
- Scaphoid views: CR angle, ulnar flex. Mod. Stecher method
- Radial flexion
- Carpal canal
- **Carpal bridge**

Structures Best Shown

Tangential view of carpals, especially for demonstration of possible calcifications or pathology of the dorsal aspect of the carpals.

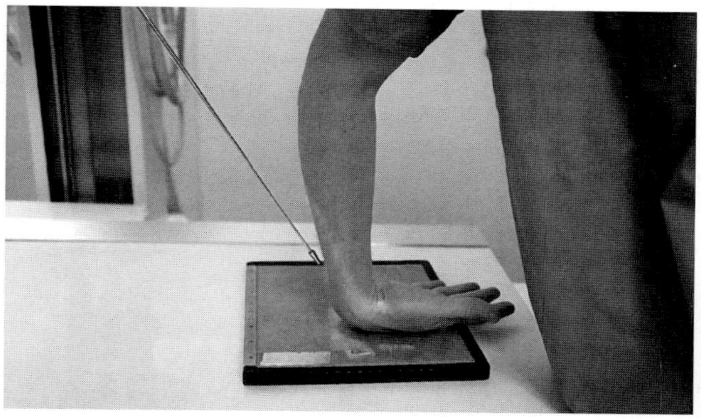

Fig. 4-108. Carpal bridge–Tangential projection. –CR 45° to forearm.

Technical Factors

- Film size–8 x 10 in. (18 x 24 cm).
- Divide in half, crosswise.
- Detail screen, tabletop.
- 64±6 kVp range.
- Technique and dose:

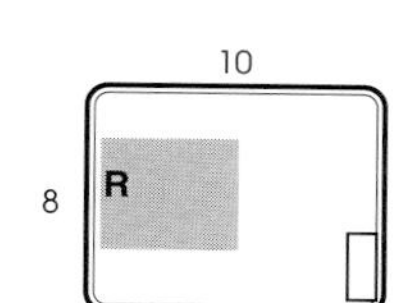

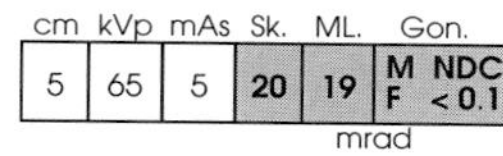

cm	kVp	mAs	Sk.	ML.	Gon.
5	65	5	20	19	M NDC F <0.1
					mrad

Shielding: Secure lead shield around waist to shield gonads.

Patient Position

- With patient standing or seated at end of the table, ask them to lean over and place dorsal surface of hand, **palm upward**, on cassette.

Part Position

- Gently flex wrist as far as can be tolerated, or until the hand and forearm form as near a 90° or right angle as possible.
- Center dorsal aspect of carpals to CR.

Central Ray

- Angle the CR **45° to the large axis of the forearm**.
- Direct the CR to a **midpoint of the distal forearm about 1½ inches proximal to the wrist joint**.
- Minimum 40 in. (102 cm) SID.

Collimation: Collimate on all four sides to area of interest.

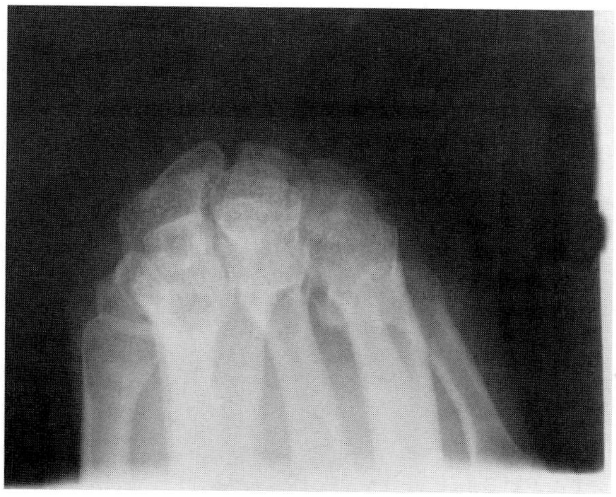

Fig. 4-109. Carpal bridge .

Evaluation Criteria

- Should demonstrate a tangential view of the dorsal aspect of the scaphoid, lunate and triquetrum. An outline of the superimposed capitate and trapezium should also be visible.
- The center of the collimation field should be to the area of the proximal 3rd metacarpal.
- Correct exposure with adequate contrast without motion should visualize sharp borders and trabecular markings of the more posterior carpals as described above. Outlines of the proximal metacarpals should be visualized through other superimposed structures.

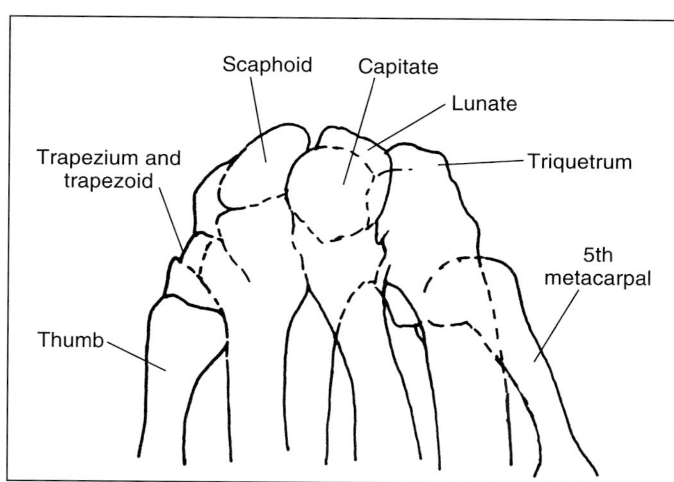

Fig. 4-110. Carpal bridge.

AP Projection

Forearm
Basic
• **AP**
• Lateral

Structures Best Shown

Entire radius and ulna, proximal row of carpals, elbow and distal end of humerus.

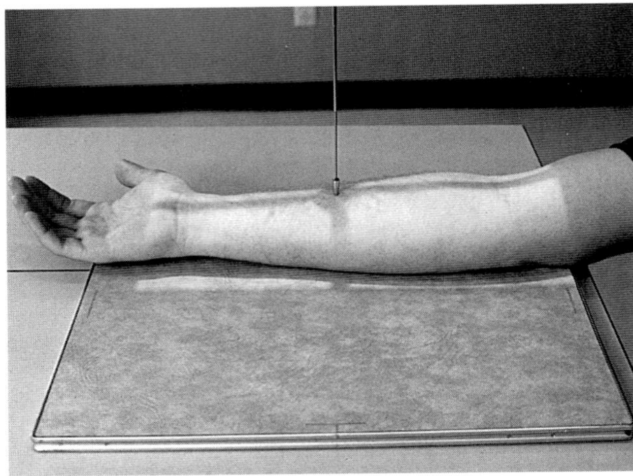

Fig. 4-111. AP forearm (include both joints).

Technical Factors

- Film size–11 x 14 in. (30 x 35 cm, smaller patients)
  –14 x 17 in. (35 x 43 cm, large patients).
- Divide in half, lengthwise.
- Detail screen, tabletop.
- 60±6 kVp range.
- Technique and dose:

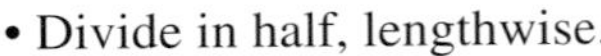

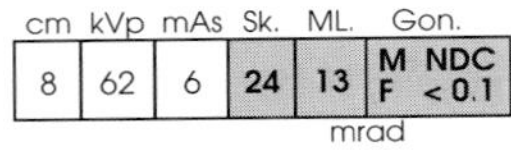

cm	kVp	mAs	Sk.	ML.	Gon.
8	62	6	24	13	M NDC F <0.1

mrad

11 (14)
14 (17)
R

Shielding: Place lead shield over patient's lap to shield gonads.

Patient Position

- Patient seated at end of table with hand and arm fully extended **palm up (supinated)**.

Part Position

- Drop shoulder to place entire upper limb on same horizontal plane.
- Align and center forearm to the long axis of film, ensure that both wrist and elbow joints are included (use as large a film as necessary).
- Have patient lean laterally as necessary to place entire wrist, forearm and elbow in as near a true frontal position as possible. (Medial and lateral epicondyles the same distance from film.)

Central Ray

- CR perpendicular to film, directed to **mid-forearm**.
- Minimum 40 in. (102 cm) SID.

Collimation: Collimate lateral borders to the actual forearm area with minimal collimation at both ends to avoid cutting off anatomy at either joint. Considering divergence of the x-ray beam, ensure that a **minimum** of 1 to 1½ in. (3 to 4 cm) distal to wrist and elbow joints will be included on the film.

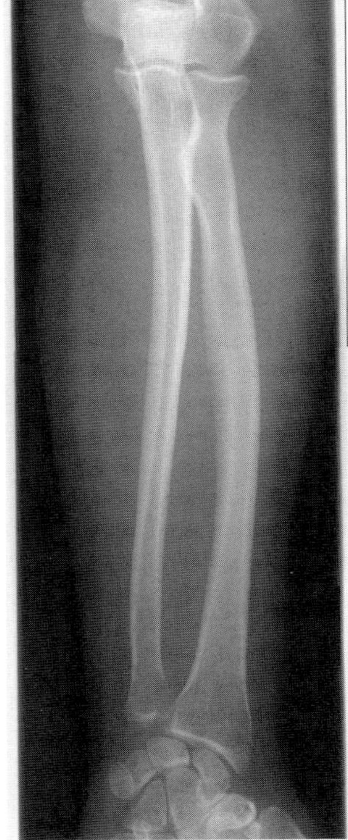

Fig. 4-112. AP (both joints).

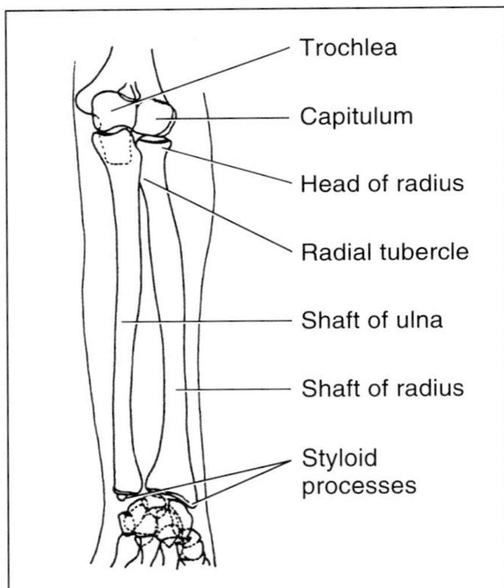

Fig. 4-113. AP (both joints).

Evaluation Criteria

- The long axis of the forearm should be aligned to the long axis of the half of exposed film.
- The carpals should be included distally, and the distal humerus proximally.
- Humeral epicondyles should be visible in profile with radial head, neck and tuberosity slightly superimposed by ulna. There should only be slight superimposition at the distal radioulnar joint.
- Wrist and elbow joint spaces will be only partially opened because of beam divergence.
- Lateral collimation borders should be visible on each side of forearm and borders at both ends should include essential anatomy of joints.
- Optimum exposure with no motion should visualize sharp bone margins and clear trabecular markings throughout.

Lateral-Lateromedial Projection

Forearm
Basic
• AP
• **Lateral**

Structures Best Shown

Lateral view of entire radius and ulna, proximal row of carpals, elbow and distal end of humerus, and pertinent soft tissue such as fat pads or stripes of the wrist and elbow joints.

Technical Factors

- Film size–11 x 14 in. (30 x 35 cm) or –14 x 17 in. (35 x 43 cm).
- Divide in half, lengthwise.
- Detail screen, tabletop.
- 64±6 kVp range (+4 kVp from AP).
- To make best use of the anode-heel effect, place elbow at cathode end of x-ray beam.
- Technique and dose:

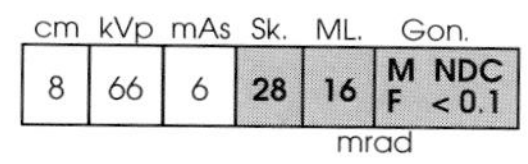

cm	kVp	mAs	Sk.	ML.	Gon.
8	66	6	28	16	M NDC F <0.1

mrad

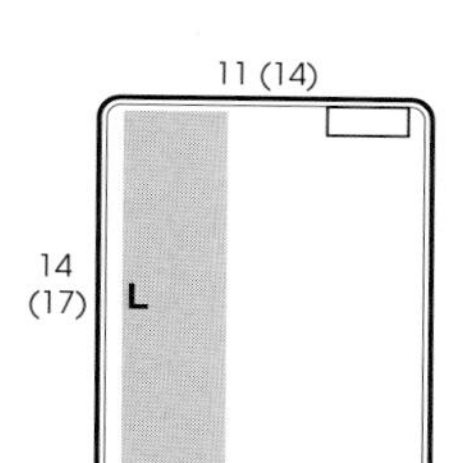

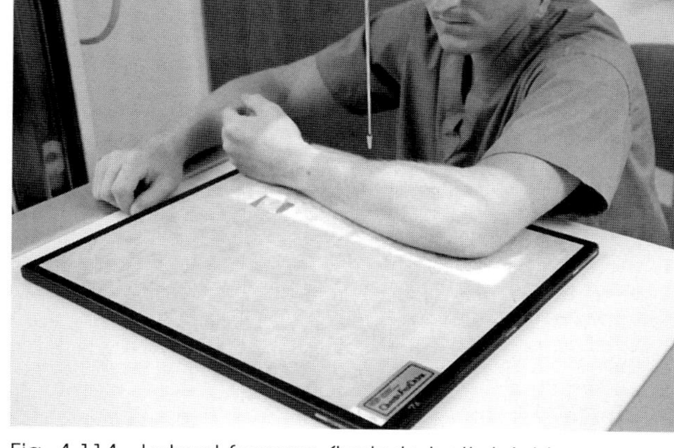

Fig. 4-114. Lateral forearm (include both joints).

Shielding: Place lead shield over patient's lap to shield gonads.

Patient Position

- Patient seated at end of table with elbow flexed 90°.
- Drop shoulder to place entire upper limb on same horizontal plane.

Part Position

- Align and center forearm to the long axis of film; ensure that both wrist and elbow joints are included on film.
- Rotate hand and wrist into **true lateral position** and support hand to prevent motion. (Ensure that distal radius and ulna are directly superimposed.)
- For heavy muscular forearm, place support under hand and wrist as needed to place radius and ulna parallel to film.

Central Ray

- CR perpendicular to film, directed to **mid-forearm**.
- Minimum 40 in. (102 cm) SID.

Collimation: Collimate both lateral borders to the actual forearm area. Also, use less collimation at both ends to avoid cutting off anatomy at either joint. Considering divergence of the x-ray beam, ensure that a **minimum** of 1 to 1½ in. (3 to 4 cm) distal to wrist and elbow joints will be included on the film.

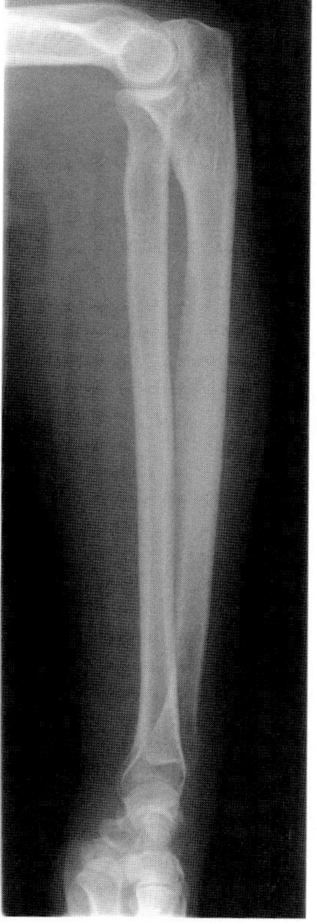

Fig. 4-115. Lateral (both joints).

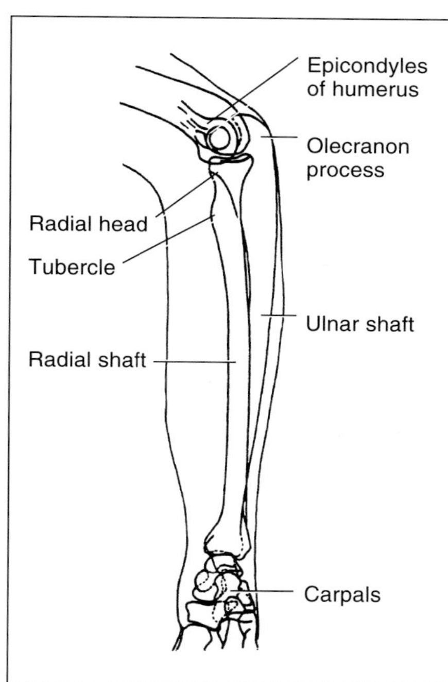

Fig. 4-116. Lateral (both joints).

Evaluation Criteria

- The elbow should be flexed 90° and the forearm should be aligned to the long axis of the half of exposed film.
- The carpals should be visible distally, and the distal humerus proximally.
- **No rotation**: Head of distal ulna should be directly superimposed and centered over radius, and humeral epicondyles should be directly superimposed.
- Radial head should superimpose coronoid process, and radial tuberosity should not be seen in profile.
- Wrist and elbow joints will be only partially open due to beam divergence.
- Lateral collimation borders should be visible, but borders at both ends should be minimal so as not to cut off essential anatomy of joints.
- Optimum exposure with no motion should visualize sharp bone margins and clear trabecular markings throughout, and demonstrate fat pads and stripes at the wrist and elbow joints. Densities should be similar at distal and proximal ends of forearm.

AP Projection

Elbow
Basic
• **AP**
• Oblique:
Lateral (ext.)
Medial (int.)
• Lateral

Structures Best Shown

Distal humerus, elbow joint space and proximal radius and ulna.

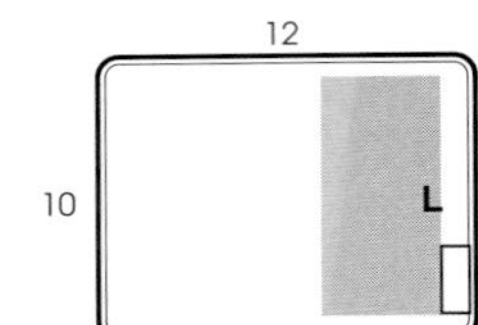

Technical Factors

- Film size–10 x 12 in. (24 x 30 cm).
- Divide in half, crosswise.
- Detail screen, tabletop.
- 64±6 kVp range.
- Technique and dose:

cm	kVp	mAs	Sk.	ML.	Gon.
7	64	6	25	17	M NDC F < 0.1
					mrad

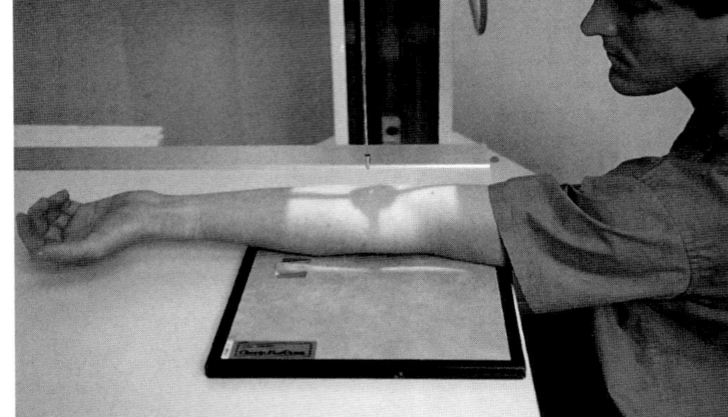

Fig. 4-117. AP elbow (fully extended).

Shielding: Place lead shield over pelvic area.

Patient Position

- Patient seated at end of table with elbow fully extended if possible.

Part Position

Fully Extended:

- Extend elbow, supinate hand and align arm and forearm to long axis of portion of film being exposed.
- Center elbow joint to CR, and to center of portion of film being exposed.
- Have patient lean laterally as necessary for **true AP projection**. (Palpate epicondyles to ensure that they are parallel to the film.)
- Support hand as needed to prevent motion.

Partially Flexed *(if patient cannot fully extend elbow):*

- **Two** AP projections required; one with **forearm parallel** to film, and one with **humerus parallel** to film.
- Place support under wrist and forearm for projection with humerus parallel to film.
- Increase exposure 4 to 6 kVp, because of increased part thickness due to partial flexion.

Central Ray

- CR perpendicular to film, directed to **mid elbow joint**, which is approximately ¾ in. (2 cm) distal to mid point of a line between epicondyles.
- Minimum 40 in. (102 cm) SID.

Collimation: Collimate on four sides to area of interest.

Note: If patient cannot even partially extend elbow, and elbow remains **flexed near 90°,** take the two AP projections as described above under "Partially Flexed," but **angle the CR 10 to 15°** into elbow joint, or if flexed **more than 90°,** take the **Jones positions** (page 140).

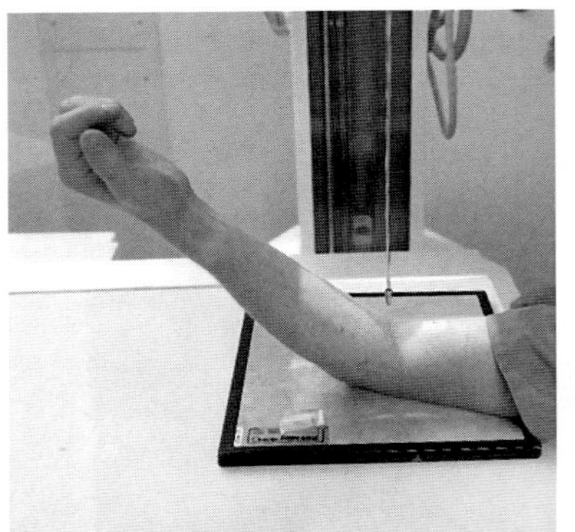

Fig. 4-118. AP elbow (partially flexed). Fig. 4-119.
–Humerus parallel to film. –Forearm parallel to film.

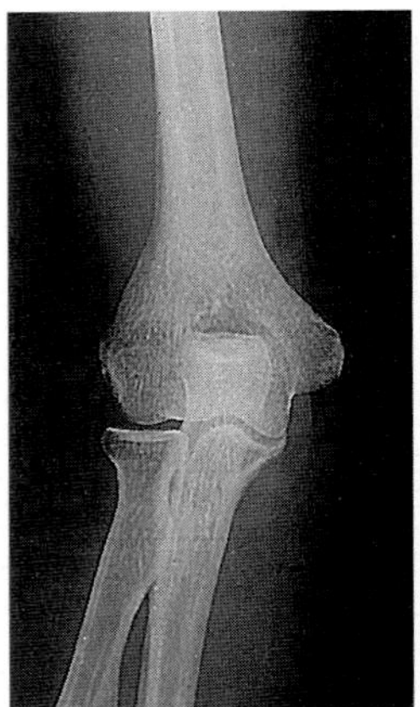

Fig. 4-120. AP (extended).

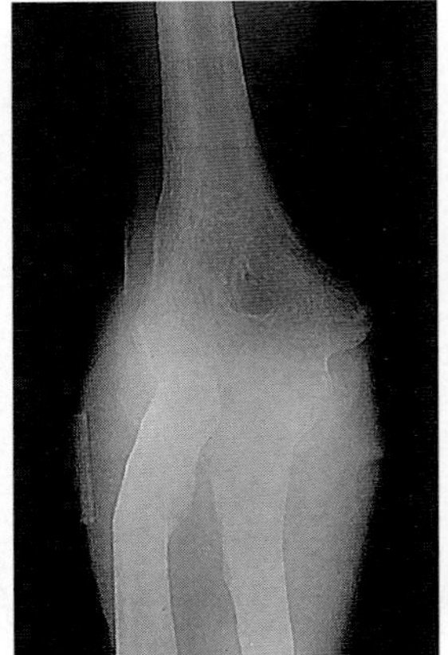

Fig. 4-121. Humerus parallel.

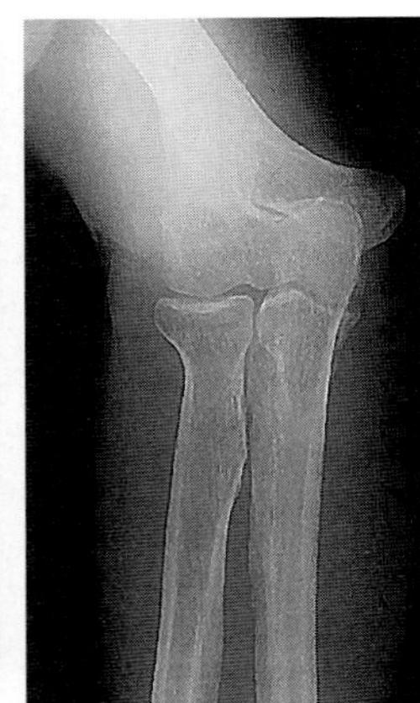

Fig. 4-122. Forearm parallel.

Evaluation Criteria

- Long axis of arm should be aligned to long axis of the portion of the film being exposed.
- Elbow joint space should be open and centered to exposed area of film.
- Collimation borders should be visible on four sides with mid elbow joint to center of collimation field.
- Epicondyles should both be in profile with the medial most prominent.
- A portion of the radial head and about half of neck should be superimposed by ulna.
- Optimum exposure and contrast with no motion should visualize sharp bone margins. Trabecular marking should appear clear and sharp.

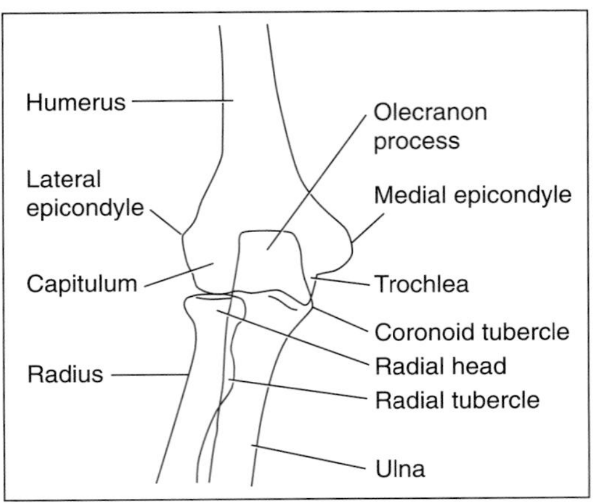

Fig. 4-123. AP (extended).

AP Oblique Projection–Lateral (External) Rotation

Elbow
Basic
- AP
- **Oblique:**
  Lateral (ext.)
  Medial (int.)
- Lateral

Structures Best Shown

Oblique view of distal humerus and proximal radius and ulna.
External oblique: Radial head and neck.

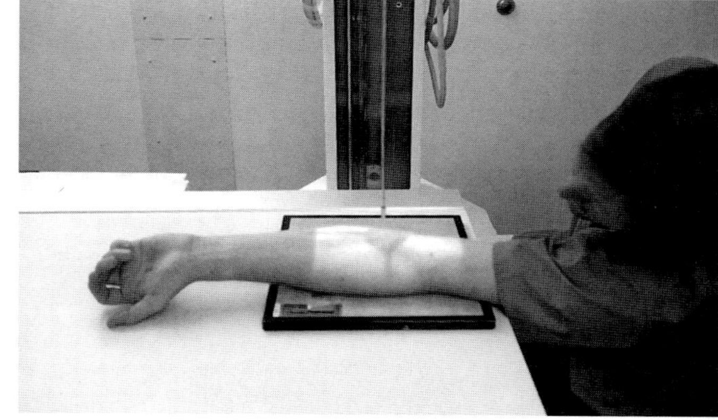

Fig. 4-124. Lateral–External oblique.

Note: Choice of internal and/or external oblique should be determined by departmental routines or by area of interest, coronoid process or radial head and neck.

Technical Factors

12
10
L

- Film size–10 x 12 in. (24 x 30 cm).
- Divide in half, crosswise.
- Detail screen, tabletop.
- 64±6 kVp range.
- Technique and dose:

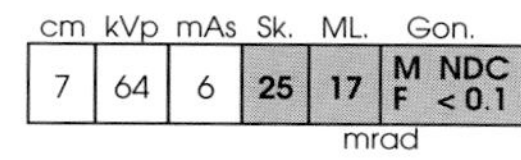

cm	kVp	mAs	Sk.	ML.	Gon.
7	64	6	25	17	M NDC F <0.1

mrad

Shielding: Place lead shield over patient's lap to protect gonads.

Patient Position

- Patient seated at end of table with arm fully extended with shoulder and elbow on same horizontal plane (lower shoulder as needed).

Part Position

- Align arm and forearm to long axis of portion of film being exposed.
- Center elbow joint to CR and to portion of film being exposed.
- Supinate hand and rotate laterally the entire arm so the distal humerus and the anterior surface of elbow joint is ≈45° to cassette. (Will need to lean laterally for sufficient lateral rotation). Palpate epicondyles to determine ≈45° rotation of distal humerus.

Central Ray

- CR perpendicular to film, directed to **mid elbow joint**, (a point approximately ¾ in. (2 cm) distal to midpoint of line between epicondyles as viewed from the x-ray tube).
- Minimum 40 in. (102 cm) SID.

Collimation: Collimate on four sides to area of interest.

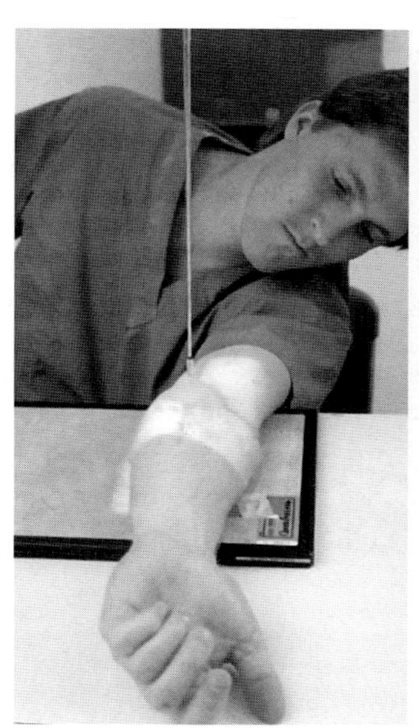

Fig. 4-125. Close-up, showing 45° lateral rotation.

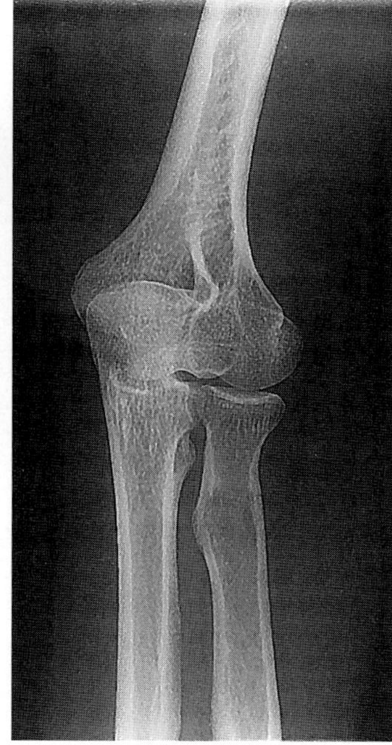

Fig. 4-126. Lateral rotation. -External oblique.

Evaluation Criteria

- Long axis of arm should be aligned to long axis of the half of exposed film with elbow joint centered to center of four-sided collimation.
- The lateral epicondyle and the capitulum should appear elongated and in profile.
- **Radial head, neck and tuberosity** should be visualized entirely free of superimposition.
- Elbow joint space should appear open.
- Optimum exposure and penetration with no motion should visualize sharp bone margins. Trabecular markings should be visible and appear sharp on those parts of humerus, radius and ulna that are not superimposed.

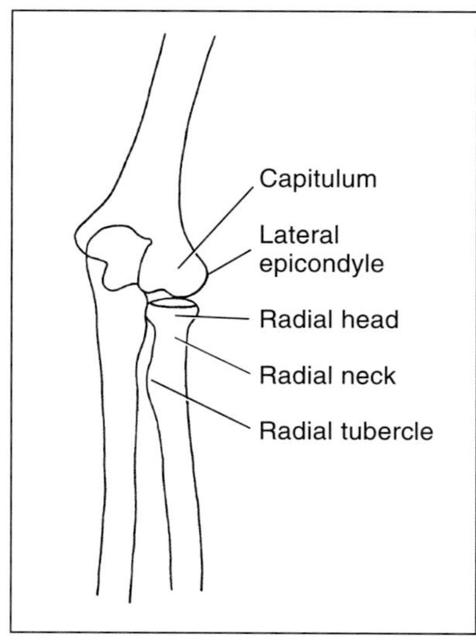

Fig. 4-127. Lateral–External oblique.

AP Oblique Projection–Medial (Internal) Rotation

Elbow
Basic
• AP
• Oblique:
Lateral (ext.)
Medial (int.)
• Lateral

Structures Best Shown

Oblique view of distal humerus and proximal radius and ulna and **olecranon process** seated in olecranon fossa.

Internal oblique: **Coronoid process** of ulna in profile.

Note: Choice of internal and/or external oblique may be determined by departmental routines or by area of interest, either the coronoid process or the radial head and neck. A common routine, however, is to include **both** internal and external obliques (see page 113).

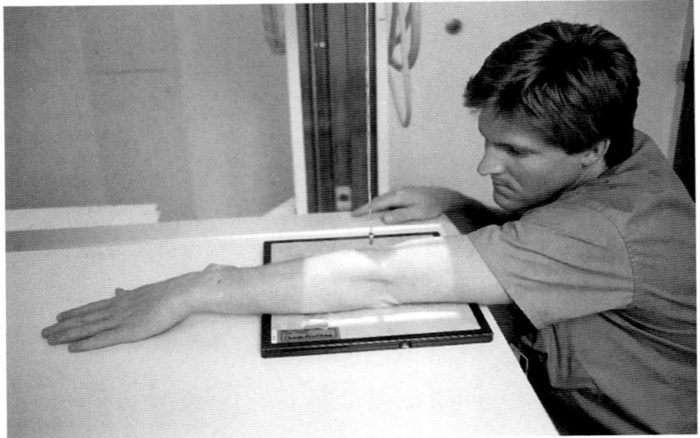

Fig. 4-128. Medial–Internal oblique.

Technical Factors

- Film size–10 x 12 in. (24 x 30 cm).
- Divide in half, crosswise.
- Detail screen, tabletop.
- 66±6 kVp range.
- Technique and dose:

cm	kVp	mAs	Sk.	ML.	Gon.
7	64	6	25	17	M NDC F <0.1
					mrad

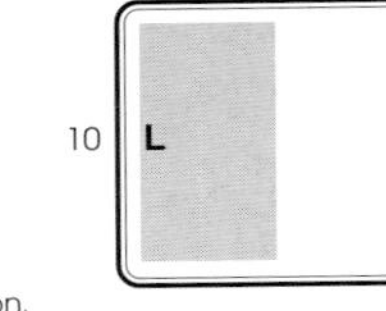

Shielding: Place lead shield over patient's lap to protect gonads.

Patient Position

- Patient seated at end of table with arm fully extended with shoulder and elbow on same horizontal plane (lower shoulder as needed).

Part Position

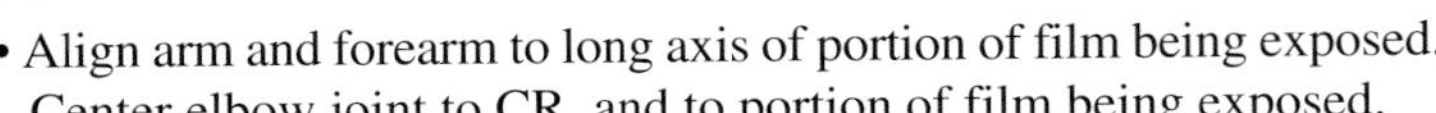

- Align arm and forearm to long axis of portion of film being exposed. Center elbow joint to CR, and to portion of film being exposed.
- Pronate hand into a natural palm down position and rotate arm as needed until distal humerus and anterior surface of elbow is rotated **45°** (palpate epicondyles to determine a 45° rotation of distal humerus.)

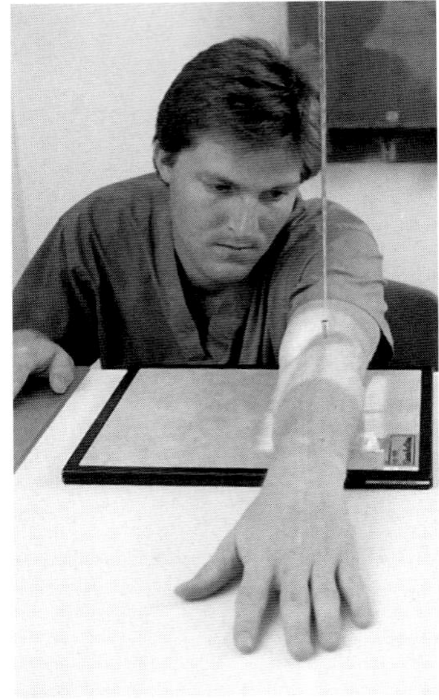

Fig. 4-129. End view, showing 45° internal oblique.

Central Ray

- CR perpendicular to film, directed to **mid elbow joint** (approximately ¾ in. or 2 cm distal to midpoint of line between epicondyles as viewed from the x-ray tube).
- Minimum 40 in. (102 cm) SID.

Collimation: Collimate on four sides to area of interest.

Evaluation Criteria

- Long axis of arm should be aligned to long axis of the half of exposed film with elbow joint centered to center of four-sided collimation.
- The medial epicondyle and the trochlea should appear elongated and in partial profile.
- **Olecranon process** of ulna should appear seated in olecranon fossa, and trochlear notch should be visible in obliqued position.
- **Coronoid process** should be well demonstrated in profile with associated joint space open.
- Radial head and neck should be superimposed and centered over proximal ulna.
- Optimum exposure and contrast with no motion should visualize sharp bone margins. Trabecular markings should be visible and appear sharp on those parts of humerus, radius and ulna that are not superimposed.

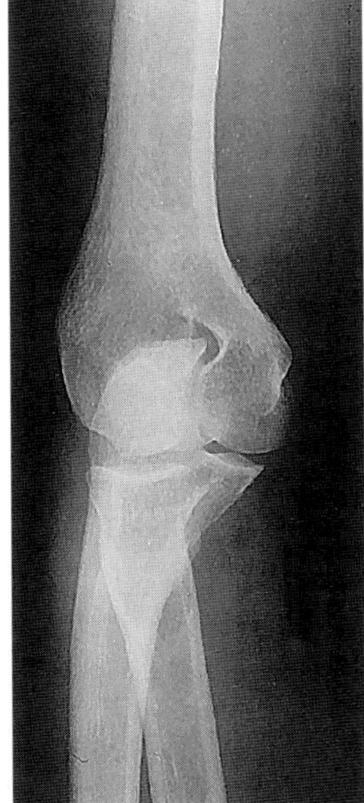

Fig. 4-130. Medial–Internal oblique.

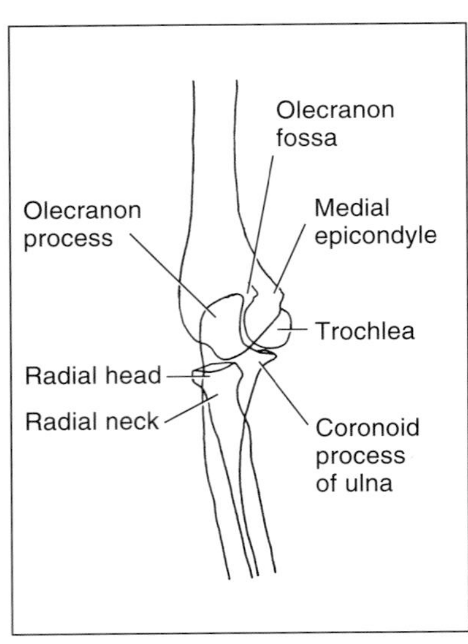

Fig. 4-131. Medial–Internal oblique.

Lateral–Lateromedial Projection

Elbow
Basic
- AP
- Oblique:
  Lateral (ext.)
  Medial (int.)
- **Lateral**

Structures Best Shown

Lateral view of distal humerus and proximal forearm. Clearly visualizes olecranon process with epicondyles superimposed. Also visualizes associated soft tissues including possible elevated or displaced fat pads of the elbow joint.

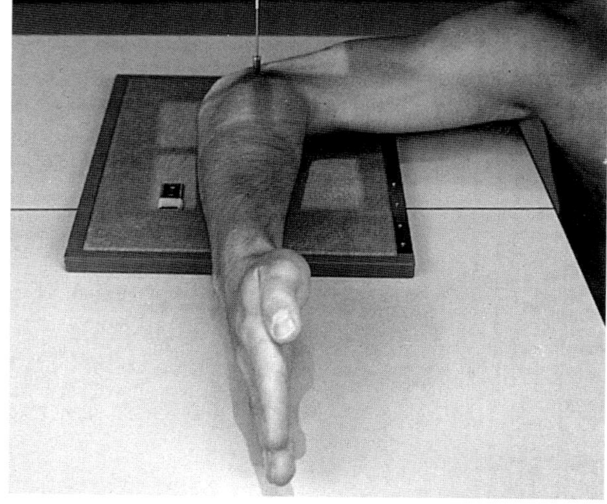

Fig. 4-132. Lateral–Elbow flexed 90° (forearm parallel to film).

Technical Factors

10
8
R

- Film size–8 x 10 in. (18 x 24 cm), crosswise.
- Detail screen, tabletop.
- 66±6 kVp range.
- Technique and dose:

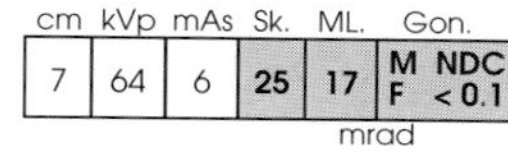

cm	kVp	mAs	Sk.	ML.	Gon.
7	64	6	25	17	M NDC F < 0.1

mrad

Shielding: Place lead shield over patient's lap to protect gonads.

Patient Position

- Patient seated at end of table with elbow **flexed 90°** (see Note).

Part Position

- Align long axis of forearm to long axis of cassette.
- Center elbow joint to CR and to center of film.
- Drop shoulder so humerus and forearm are on same horizontal plane.
- Rotate hand and wrist into true lateral position, thumb side up.
- Place support under hand and wrist to elevate hand and distal forearm as needed for heavy muscular forearm to place forearm parallel to film for true lateral elbow.

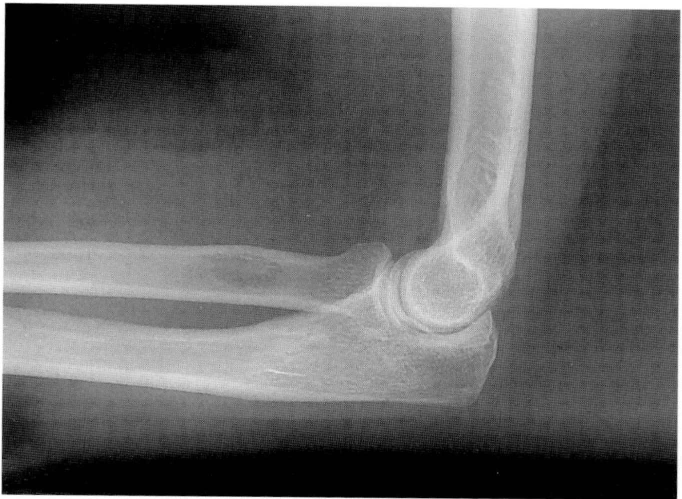

Fig. 4-133. Lateral elbow.

Central Ray

- CR perpendicular to film, directed to **mid elbow joint** (a point approximately 1½ in. or 4 cm medial to easily palpated posterior surface of olecranon process).
- Minimum 40 in. (102 cm) SID.

Collimation: Collimate on four sides to area of interest.

Note: Diagnosis of certain important joint pathology (such as possible visualization of the posterior fat pad) is dependent on 90° flexion of the elbow joint.* Therefore, unless there are counter indications such as severe trauma and/or dislocation, the lower arm should be flexed **90°** or at **a right angle** to the humerus. Also, a second reason for the full 90° flexion is that the olecranon process will not be seen in full profile with less than 90°.

Exception: Certain soft tissue diagnoses require less flexion of only 30 to 35°, but these should be taken only when specifically indicated.

Evaluation Criteria

- Long axis of arm should be aligned to long axis of film with elbow joint flexed 90° and centered to center of film and to four-sided collimation field.
- **True lateral**, best indicated by the three concentric arcs of (1) the trochlear sulcus, (2) double ridges of capitulum and trochlea and (3) trochlear notch of ulna (see Figs. 4-141 and 4-142 and page 101). Also, the humeral epicondyles should be superimposed.
- Olecranon process should be visualized in profile.
- About one-half of the radial head will be superimposed by the coronoid process.
- Optimum exposure with no motion should visualize sharp bone margins and clear trabecular markings throughout, and soft tissue margins, such as possible visualization of the anterior and posterior fat pads.

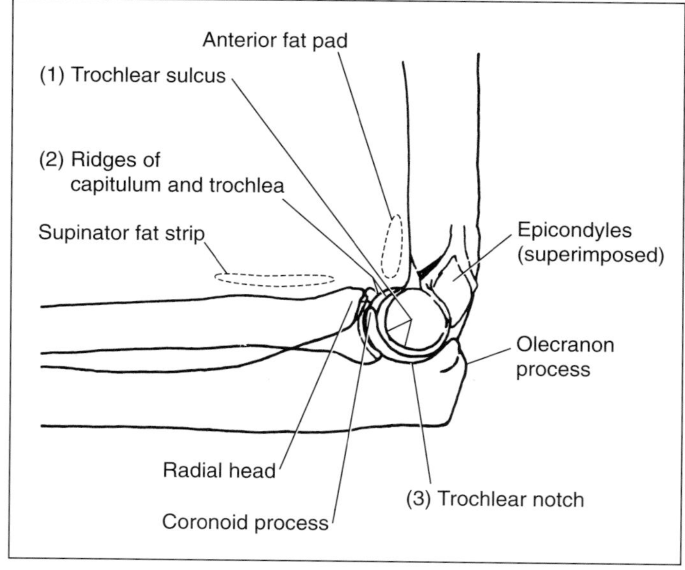

Fig. 4-134. Lateral elbow.

*Griswold, R. Elbow Fat Pads: A Radiography Perspective, *Radiologic Technology* 1982; 53:303-307.

Acute Flexion Projections
Jones Method
(AP projections of elbow when arm cannot be extended)

Elbow
Special
- **Acute flexion (Jones method)**
- Trauma axial (Coyle method)
- Radial head projections

Structures Best Shown
Olecranon process in profile, and superimposed outlines of bones of forearm and arm.

Note: To visualize both the distal humerus and the proximal radius and ulna, **two** projections are required, one with **CR perpendicular to humerus** and one with CR angled to be **perpendicular to forearm**.

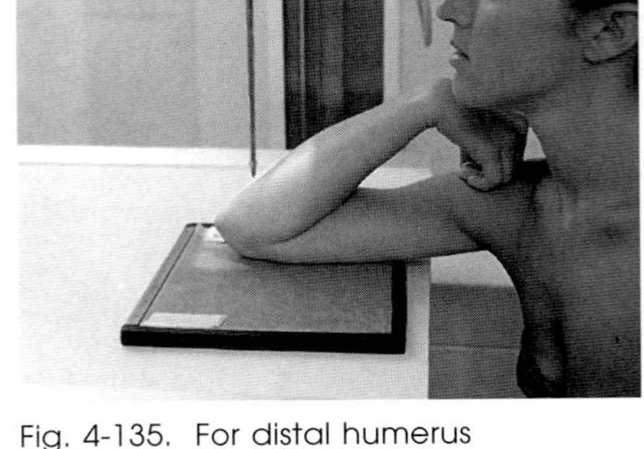
Fig. 4-135. For distal humerus –CR perpendicular to **humerus**.

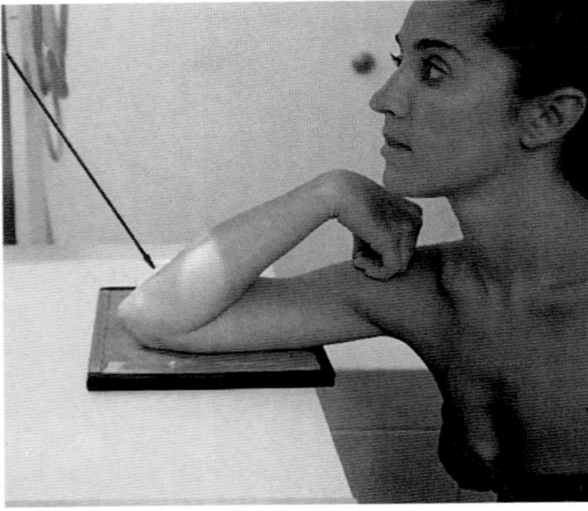
Fig. 4-136. For proximal forearm –CR perpendicular to **forearm**.

Technical Factors
- Film size–8 x 10 in. (18 x 24 cm) lengthwise (or divide in half, crosswise for two projections).
- Detail screen, tabletop.
- 66 ± 6 kVp range. (Increase 4-6 kVp for proximal forearm.)

Shielding: Place lead shield over patient's lap.

Patient Position
- Patient seated at end of table with acutely flexed arm resting on cassette.

Part Position 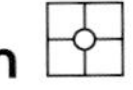
- Align and center humerus to long axis of film with forearm acutely flexed, with fingertips resting on shoulder.
- Adjust cassette to center elbow joint region to center of film.
- Palpate epicondyles and ensure they are the same distances from cassette for **no rotation**.

Central Ray
Distal Humerus:
- CR **perpendicular to film, and humerus**, directed to **a point midway between epicondyles**.
- Minimum 40 in. (102 cm) SID.

Proximal Forearm:
- CR **perpendicular to forearm**, (angle CR as needed) directed to a point approximately **2 in. (5 cm) proximal or superior to olecranon process**.
- Minimum 40 in. (102 cm) SID.

Collimation: Collimate on four sides to area of interest.

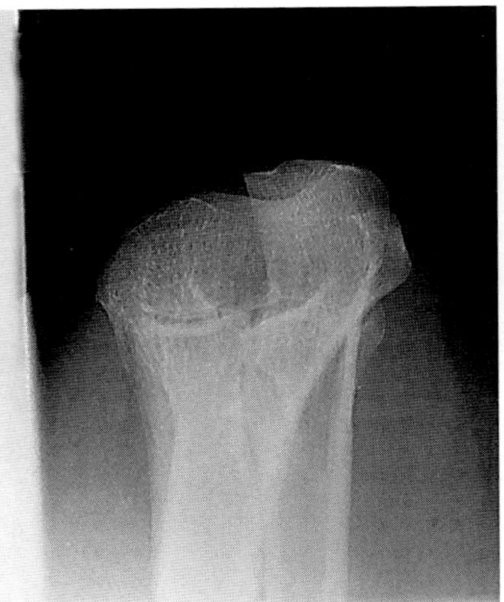
Fig. 4-137. Distal humerus.

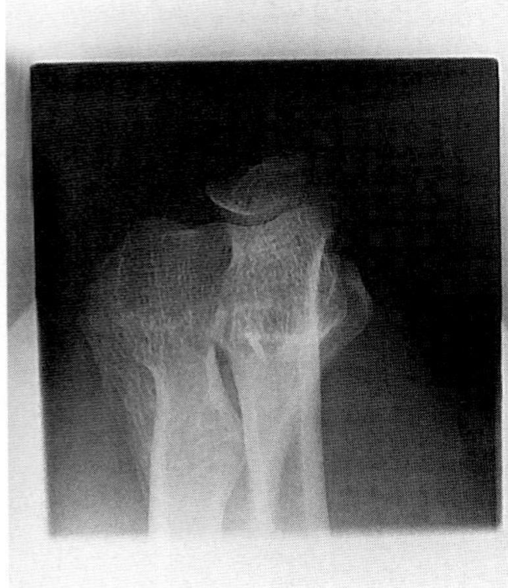
Fig. 4-138. Proximal forearm.

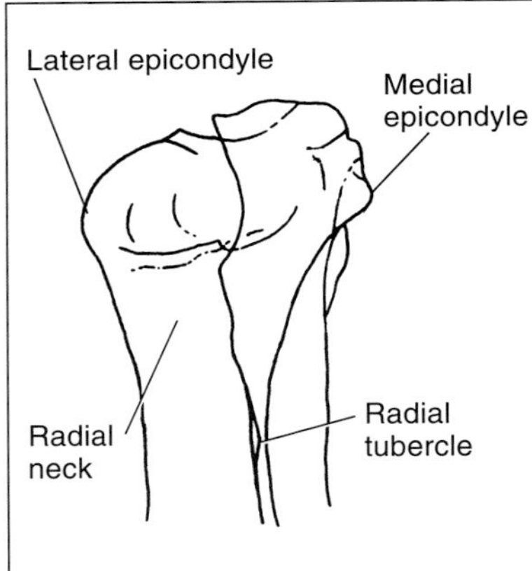

Fig. 4-139. Distal humerus.

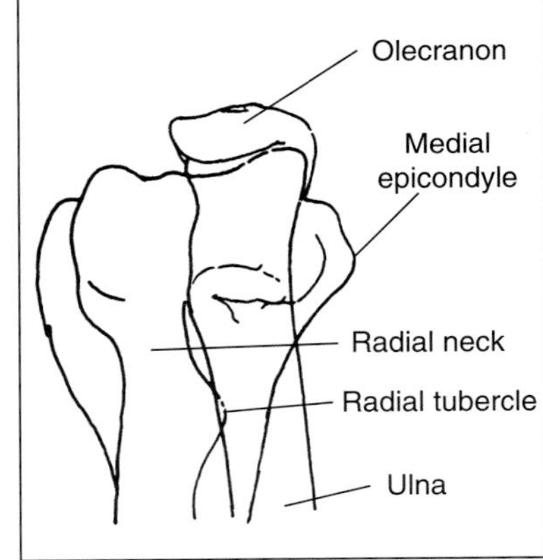

Fig. 4-140. Proximal forearm.

Evaluation Criteria
- Four-sided collimation borders should be visible.

Distal Humerus:
- Forearm and humerus should be directly superimposed.
- Medial and lateral epicondyles, distal margins of trochlea and capitulum and olecranon process all should be seen in profile.
- Joint space and articular surfaces of olecranon process and trochlea should be visualized.
- Optimum exposure will visualize (without overexposure) soft tissues and the olecranon process and other structures of distal humerus in profile. Other parts of humerus and proximal forearm will appear underexposed.

Proximal Forearm:
- Proximal ulna and radius will be superimposed by distal humerus.
- Outline of radial head and neck should be clearly visible through distal humerus.
- Optimum exposure will clearly visualize outlines of proximal ulna and radius superimposed over humerus. Soft tissues will not be readily visible and certain structures in profile will appear dark and overexposed.

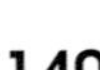

Trauma Axial Laterals–Axial Lateromedial Projections

Coyle Method*

Special projections taken for pathology or trauma to the area of the radial head and/or the coronoid process of ulna. Effective projections when patient cannot extend elbow fully for medial or lateral obliques of the elbow.

Elbow
Special
- Acute flexion (Jones method)
- **Trauma axial (Coyle method)**
- Radial head projections

Structures Best Shown

1. Radial head, neck and tuberosity and articular margin of capitulum.
2. Coronoid process and articular margin of trochlea.

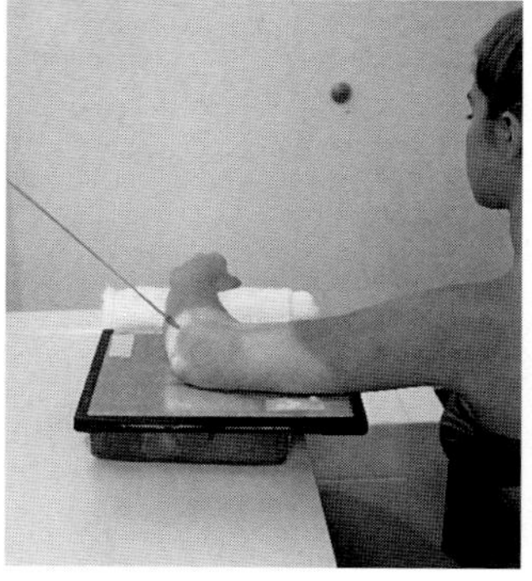

Fig. 4-141. Erect.

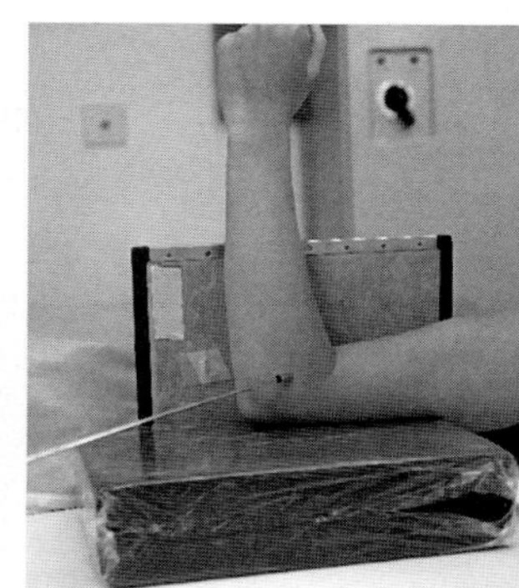

Fig. 4-142. Supine.

1. Angled for radial head–Flexed **90°**.

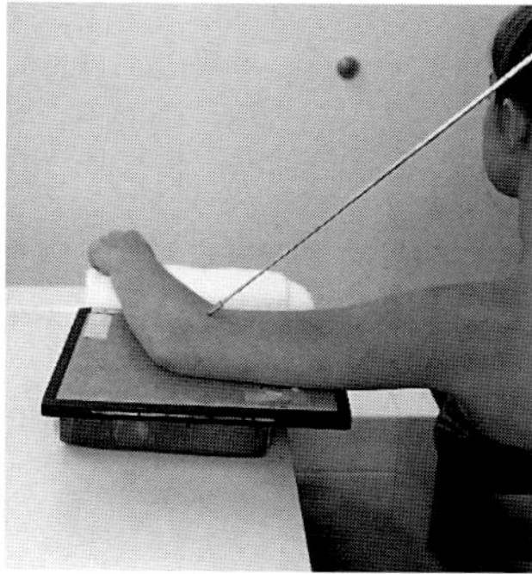

Fig. 4-143. Erect.

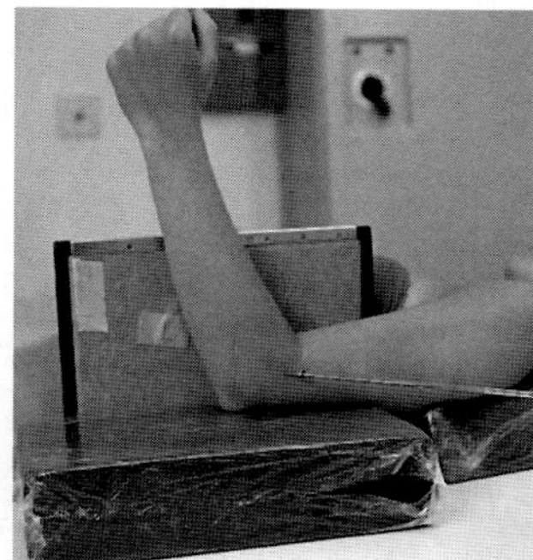

Fig. 4-144. Supine.

2. Angled for coronoid process–Flexed **80°**.

Technical Factors

- Film size–8 x 10 in. (18 x 24 cm) crosswise.
- Detail screen, tabletop.
- 70±6 kVp range. (See Note below.)
- Technique and dose:

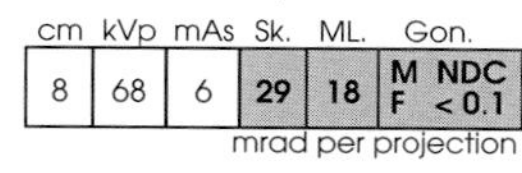

cm	kVp	mAs	Sk.	ML.	Gon.
8	68	6	29	18	M NDC F <0.1

mrad per projection

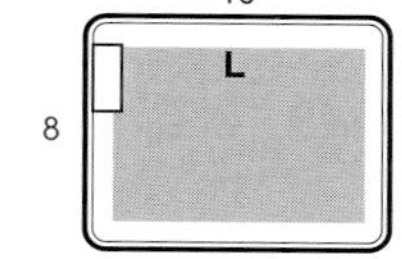

Shielding: Place lead shield over gonadal area.

Patient Position

- Supine or erect seated at end of table.

1. Part Position–Radial Head

- Flex elbow 90° if possible, **pronate hand**.
- CR–Angle **45° toward shoulder**, centered to radial head (mid elbow joint).
- Minimum 40 in. (102 cm) SID.

2. Part Position–Coronoid Process

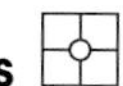

- Elbow flexed **only 80°** from extended position (more than 80° will obscure coronoid process), pronate hand.
- CR–Angle **45° away from shoulder**, into mid elbow joint.
- Minimum 40 in. (102 cm) SID.

Collimation: Collimate on four sides to area of interest.

Note: Increase exposure factors by 4 to 6 kVp from lateral elbow because of angled CR. These projections are effective with or without a splint.

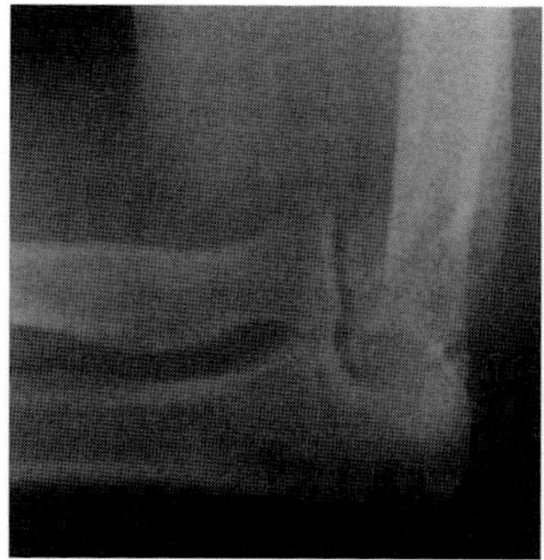

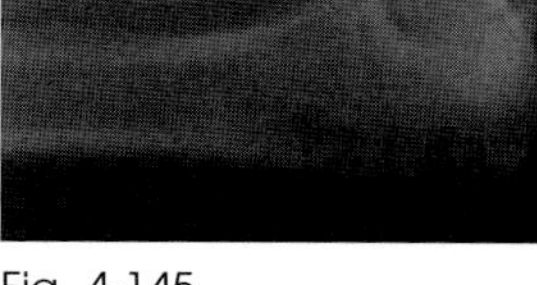

Fig. 4-145.
1. For radial head.

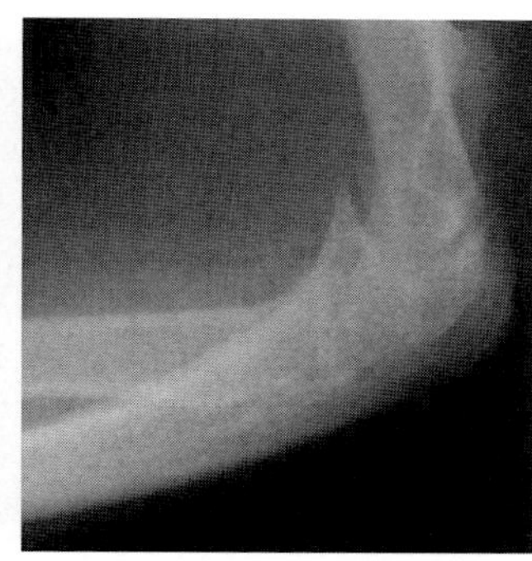

Fig. 4-146.
2. For coronoid process.

Evaluation Criteria for Specific Anatomy

1. Radial Head:

- The joint space between radial head and capitulum should be open and clear.
- The radial head, neck and tuberosity should be in profile free of superimposition except for a small part of the coronoid process.
- The distal humerus and epicondyles will appear distorted due to the 45° angle.

2. Coronoid Process:

- The distal portion of the coronoid will appear elongated but in profile.
- The joint space between coronoid process and trochlea should be open and clear.
- The radial head and neck will be superimposed by ulna.
- Optimum exposure factors should clearly visualize the coronoid process in profile. Bony margins of superimposed radial head and neck will be faintly visualized through the proximal ulna.

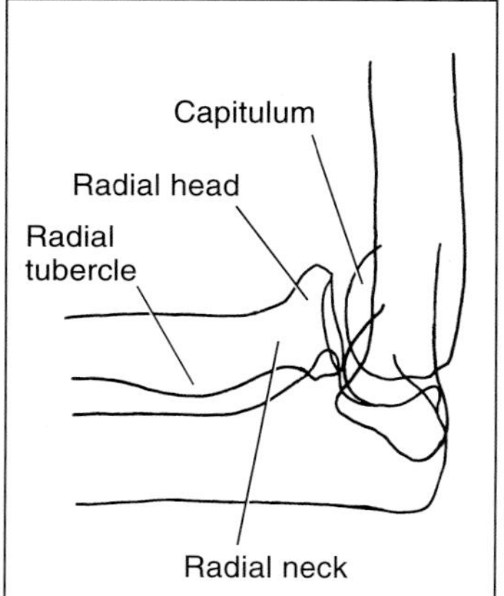

Fig. 4-147.
1. For radial head.

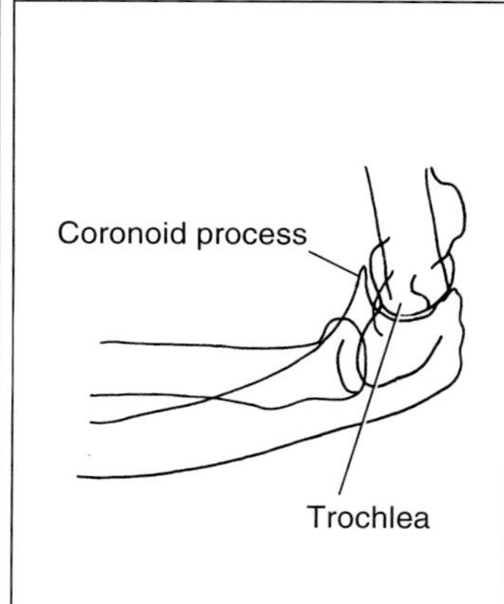

Fig. 4-148.
2. For coronoid process.

*Coyle, George F. *Radiographing Immobile Trauma Patients, Unit 7, Special Angled Views of Joints–Elbow, Knee, Ankle*. Denver: Multi-Media Publishing, Inc.; 1980.

Radial Head Laterals–Lateromedial Projections

Elbow
Special
- Acute flexion (Jones method)
- Trauma axial (Coyle method)
- **Radial head projections**

Structures Best Shown

Series of projections of the radial head and neck projected in profile, with entire head and neck demonstrated without superimposition with varying degrees of rotation.

Technical Factors

- Film size–8 x 10 in. (18 x 24 cm).
  Divide in half.
  or
  –10 x 12 in. (24 x 30 cm).
  Divide in fourths.
- Detail screen, tabletop.
- 66±6 kVp range.
- Technique and dose:

cm	kVp	mAs	Sk.	ML.	Gon.
7	64	6	25	17	M NDC F <0.1

mrad per projection

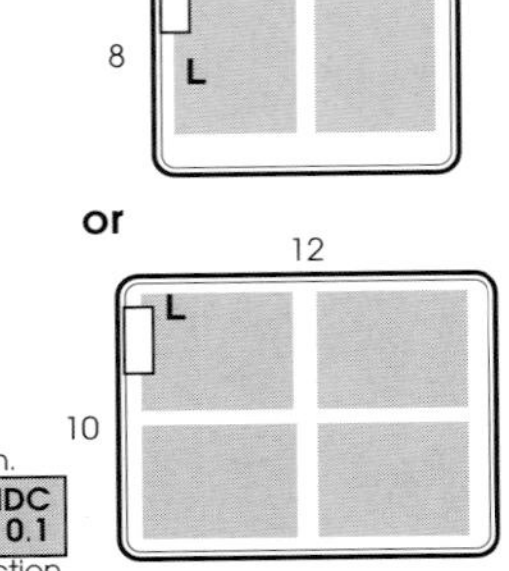

Shielding: Place lead shield over gonadal area.

Patient Position

- Patient seated at end of table, arm **flexed 90°** resting on cassette with humerus, forearm and hand on same horizontal plane.

Part Position

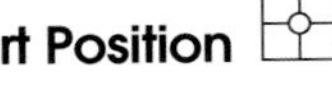

- Center radial head area to center of the portion of film being exposed, positioned so that distal humerus and proximal forearm are placed "square" with, or parallel with, the borders of cassette.
- Center radial head region to CR.
- **Four projections** are taken with the only difference being the rotation of the hand and wrist from (1) maximum external rotation to (4) maximum internal rotation, demonstrating different parts of the radial head projected clear of the coronoid process. (Near complete rotation of radial head occurs in these four projections.)
  1. Supinate hand (palm up), externally rotate as far as can be tolerated.
  2. Place hand in true lateral position (thumb up).
  3. Pronate hand (palm down).
  4. Internally rotate hand (thumb down) as far as can be tolerated.

Central Ray

- CR perpendicular to film, directed to **radial head** (approximately 1 in. or 2 to 3 cm distal to lateral epicondyle).
- Minimum 40 in. (102 cm) SID.

Collimation: Collimate on four sides to area of interest (include at least 3 to 4 in. (10 cm) of proximal forearm as well as distal portion of humerus).

Evaluation Criteria

- Elbow should be flexed 90° in true lateral position evidenced by direct superimposition of epicondyles.
- Radial head and neck will be partially superimposed by ulna but should be completely visualized in profile in the various projections.
- Radial tuberosity should be seen in partial profile adjacent to ulna when hand and wrist are at maximum internal rotation (Fig. 4-155).
- Optimum exposure with no motion should clearly visualize sharp bony margins and clear trabecular markings of the radial head and neck area.

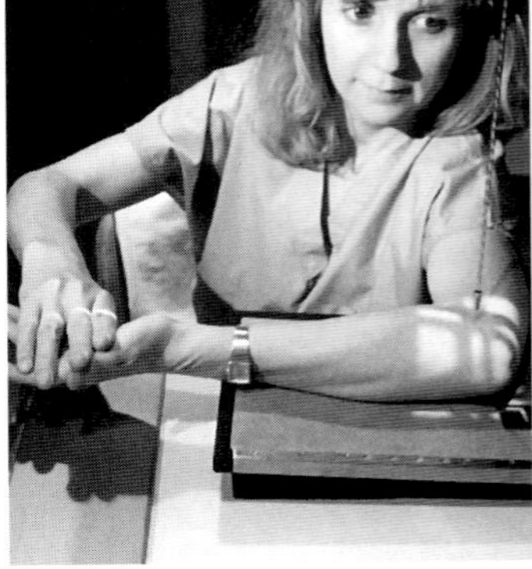
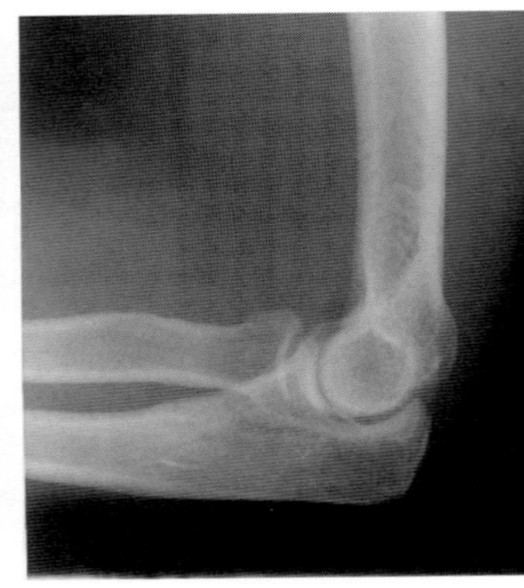

Fig. 4-149. 1. Hand supinated (external rotation). Fig. 4-150.

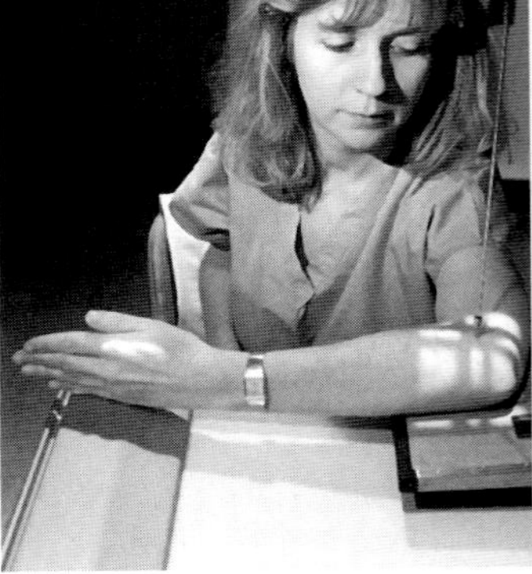

Fig. 4-151. 2. Hand lateral. Fig. 4-152.

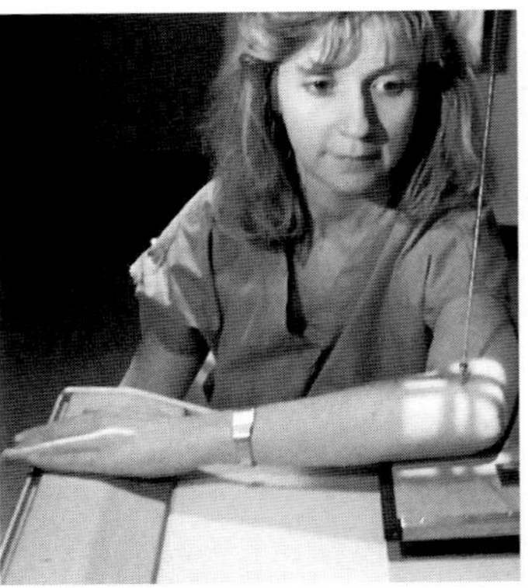
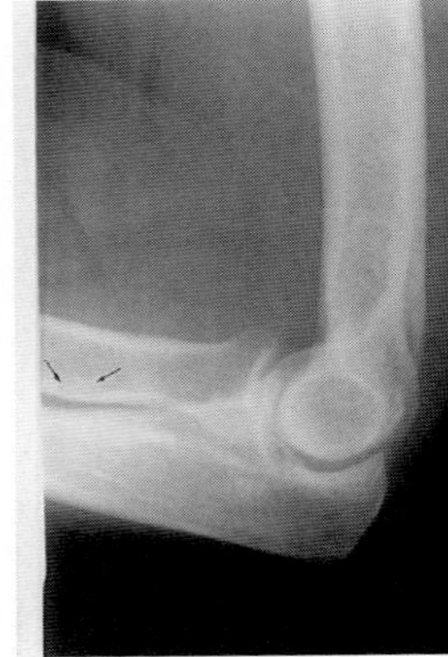

Fig. 4-153. 3. Hand pronated. Fig. 4-154.

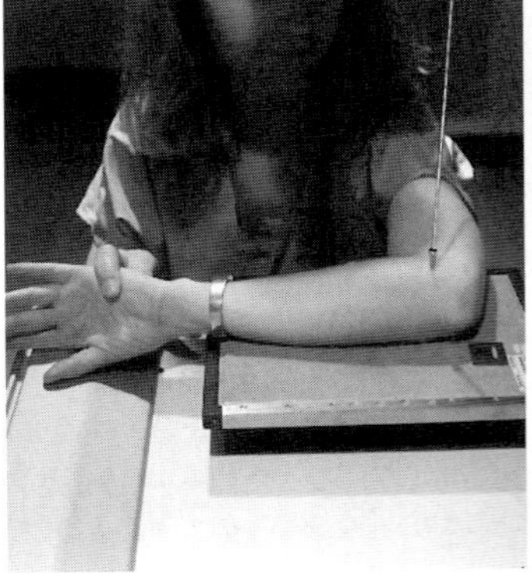
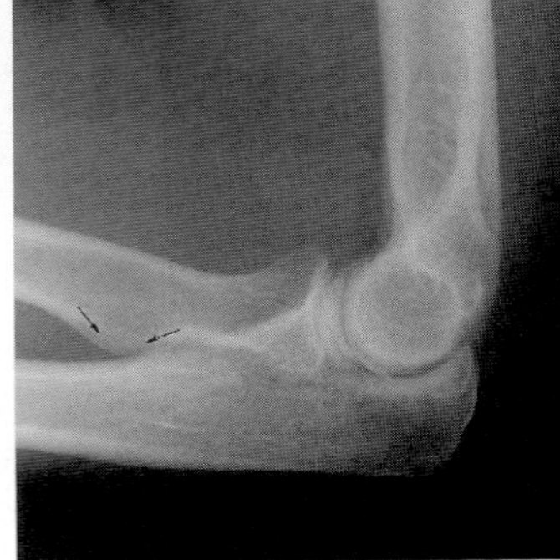

Fig. 4-155. 4. Hand internally rotated. Fig. 4-156.

AP Projection

Warning: Do **NOT** attempt to rotate arm if fracture or dislocation is suspected.

Humerus
Basic
• **AP**
• Rotational lateral
• Cross table lateral

Structures Best Shown

Frontal view of entire humerus.

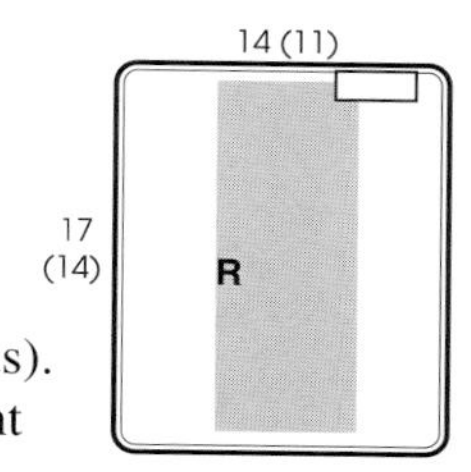

Technical Factors

- Film size–lengthwise (large enough to include entire humerus).
  - –14 x 17 in. (35 x 43 cm), larger patient or
  - –11 x 14 in. (28 x 35 cm), smaller patient.
  (May need to place film diagonally to include both joints on large patients.)
- Moving or stationary grid (non-grid, detail screen may be used for smaller patient).
- 70±6 kVp range.
- Utilize anode-heel effect if possible; shoulder at cathode end of x-ray beam.
- Technique and dose:

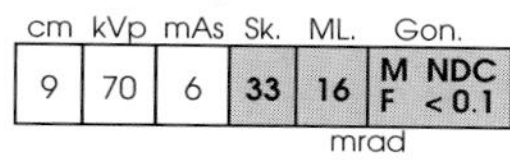

cm	kVp	mAs	Sk.	ML.	Gon.
9	70	6	33	16	M NDC F <0.1
			mrad		

Shielding: Secure or place lead shield over pelvic area.

Patient Position

- May be taken erect or supine.
- Adjust height of cassette so that shoulder and elbow joints are the same distance from ends of film.
- Rotate body toward affected side as needed to bring the shoulder and proximal humerus in contact with cassette.

Part Position

- Align humerus to long axis of film, unless diagonal placement is needed to include both shoulder and elbow joints.
- Extend hand and forearm as far as can be tolerated.
- Abduct arm slightly and gently supinate hand so that **epicondyles of elbow are parallel to** the film.

Central Ray

- CR perpendicular to film, directed to **midpoint of humerus**.
- Minimum 40 in. (102 cm) SID.

Collimation: Collimate on sides to soft tissue borders of humerus and shoulder. (Lower margin of collimation field should include the elbow joint and up to 1 in. or 2.5 cm minimum of proximal forearm.)

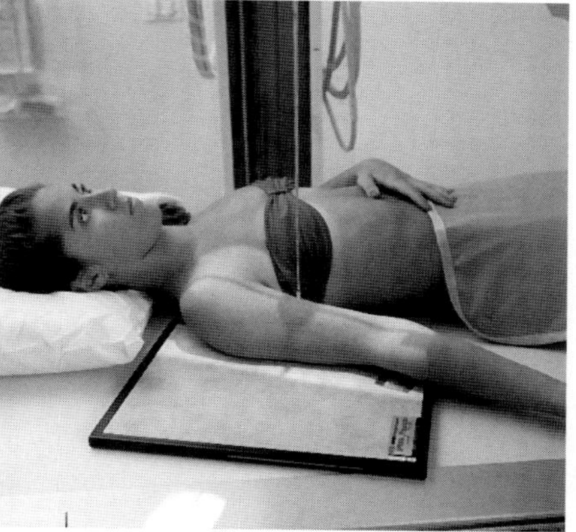

Fig. 4-157. AP supine.

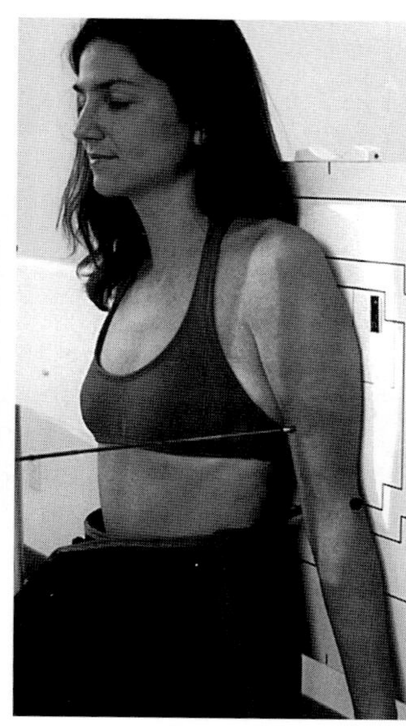

Fig. 4-158. AP erect.

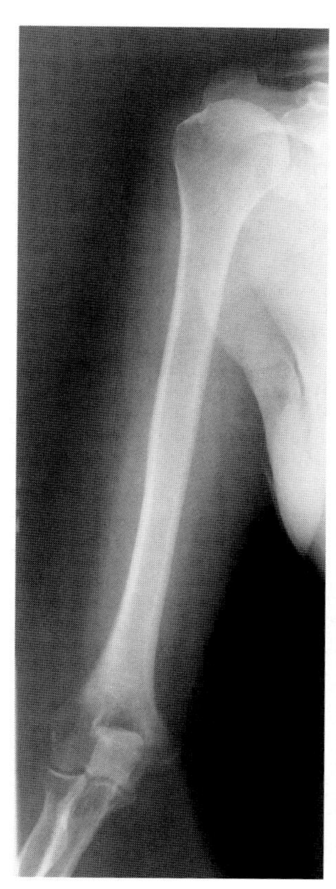

Fig. 4-159. AP.

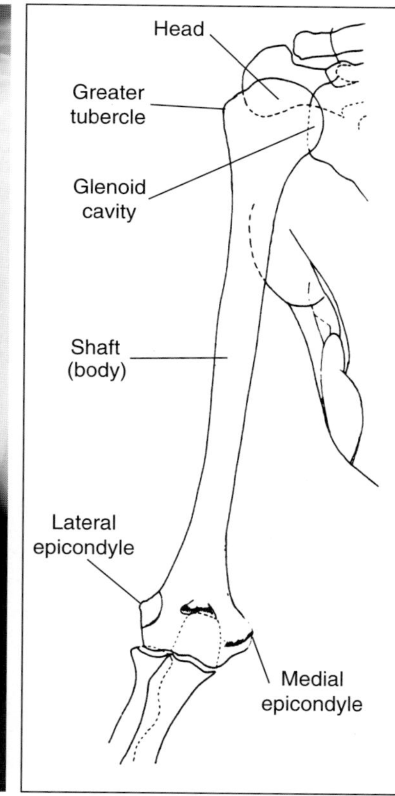

Fig. 4-160. AP.

Evaluation Criteria

- Entire humerus including shoulder and elbow joints and about 1 in. or 3 cm of proximal forearm should be visualized, with collimation margins on all four sides.
- True AP projection as evidenced by:
  - –Greater tubercle seen in profile laterally.
  - –Humeral head seen in profile medially with only minimal superimposition of glenoid cavity.
  - –Outline of lesser tubercle seen just medially to greater tubercle.
  - –Lateral and medial epicondyles of distal humerus seen in profile.
- Optimum exposure with no motion will visualize sharp borders and fine trabecular markings of the entire humerus. The proximal and distal portions of the humerus should appear near equal in exposure density. (Correct utilization of anode-heel effect will facilitate this.)

Rotational Lateral–Lateromedial or Mediolateral Projections

Warning: Do **NOT** attempt to rotate arm if fracture or dislocation is suspected–see trauma routine.

Humerus
Basic
- AP
- **Rotational lateral**
- Horizontal beam lateral

Structures Best Shown

Lateral view of entire humerus.

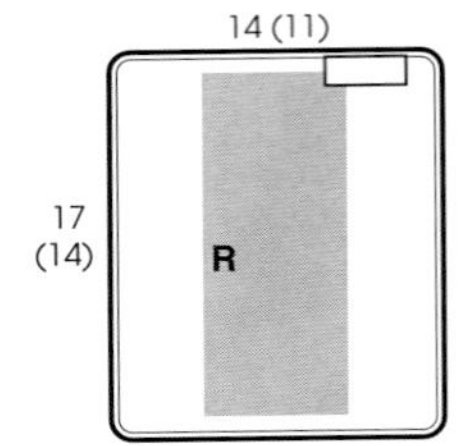

Technical Factors

- Film size–lengthwise, (large enough to include entire humerus)
  - –14 x 17 in. (35 x 43 cm), larger patient
  - or
  - –11 x 14 in. (28 x 35 cm), smaller patient.
- Moving or stationary grid (non-grid, detail screen may be used for smaller patient).
- 70±6 kVp range.
- Utilize anode-heel effect if possible for supine position; shoulder at cathode end of x-ray beam.
- Technique and dose:

cm	kVp	mAs	Sk.	ML.	Gon.
9	70	6	33	16	M NDC F <0.1

mrad

Shielding: Secure or place lead shield over pelvic area.

Patient and Part Position

- May be taken erect or supine.
- Erect with back to film and elbow partially flexed, with body rotated toward affected side as needed to bring humerus and shoulder in contact with cassette. Internally rotate arm as needed for lateral position; **epicondyles are perpendicular** to film.
- The erect position with patient facing film (Fig. 4-162) may be preferred if interest is primarily of mid and distal humerus. The patient is obliqued as needed (20 to 30°) to allow close contact of humerus to film holder; flex elbow 90° as shown.
- If taken supine, extend elbow; internally rotate arm into true lateral. (Fig. 4-163).
- Adjust cassette so shoulders and elbow joints are the same distance from the ends of cassette.
- Epicondyles should be directly superimposed as viewed from the x-ray tube for a true lateral.

Central Ray

- CR perpendicular to film, centered to **midpoint of humerus**.
- Minimum 40 in. (102 cm) SID.

Collimation: Collimate on four sides to soft tissue border of humerus, ensuring that all of shoulder and elbow joints are included.

Respiration: Suspend respiration during exposure.

Evaluation Criteria

- Entire humerus, including elbow and shoulder joints, should be included with collimation margins on all four sides.
- True lateral projection as evidenced by:
  - –Epicondyles directly superimposed.
  - –Lesser tubercle shown in profile medially, partially superimposed by the lower portion of the glenoid cavity.
- Optimum exposure with no motion will visualize sharp borders and fine trabecular markings of the entire humerus. The proximal and distal parts of the humerus should appear near equal in exposure density. (Correct utilization of anode-heel effect will facilitate this.)

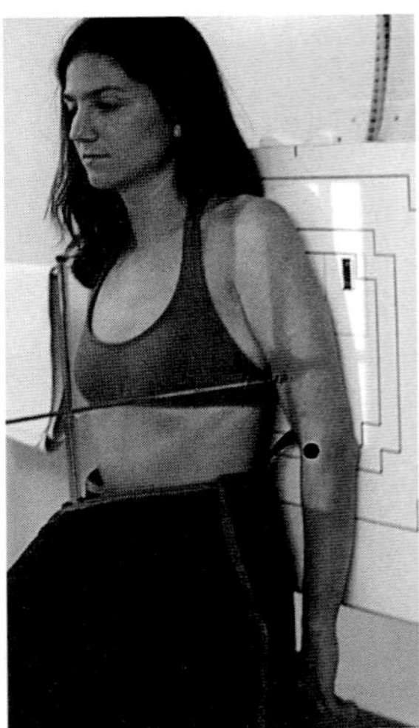

Fig. 4-161. Erect lateral. –Lateromedial, back to film. –Best visualizes entire humerus.

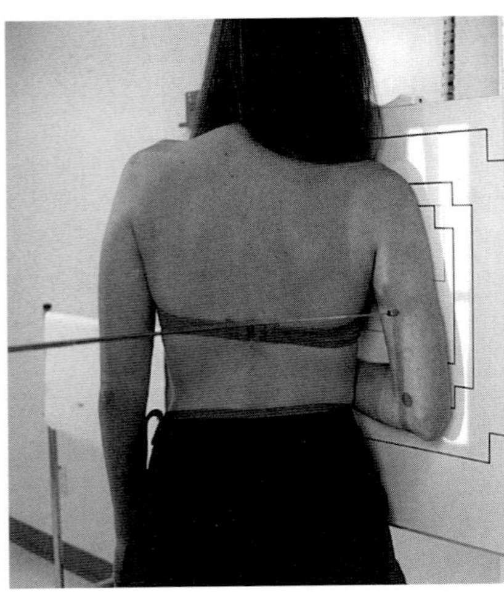

Fig. 4-162. Erect lateral. –Mediolateral, facing film. –Best visualizes mid and distal humerus.

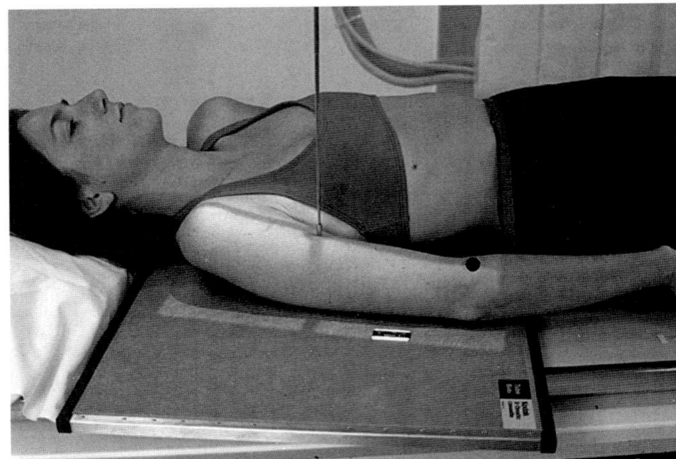

Fig. 4-163. Supine lateromedial projection.

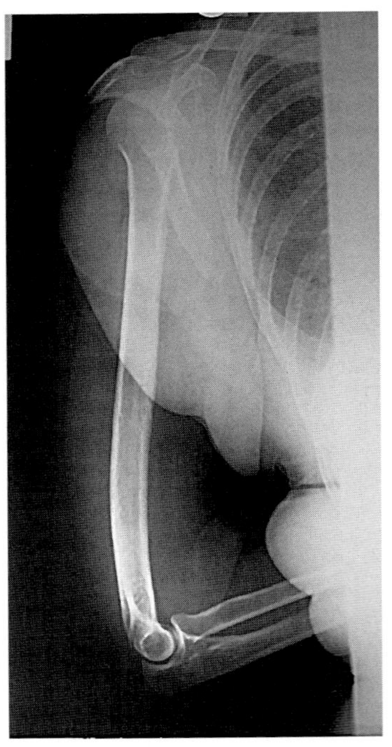

Fig. 4-164. Erect mediolateral.

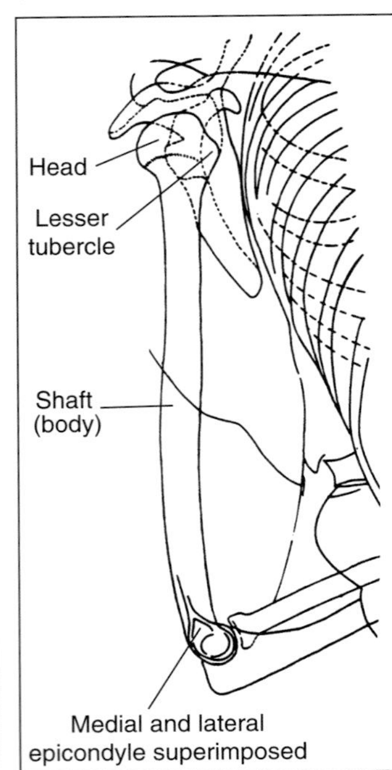

Fig. 4-165. Lateral.

Trauma Horizontal Beam Lateral–Lateromedial Projection

Warning: Do **NOT** attempt to rotate arm if fracture or dislocation is suspected.
Proximal Humerus: See transthoracic lateral, or Scapular Y in Chapter 5.

Humerus
Basic
- AP
- Rotational lateral
- **Horizontal beam lateral**

Structures Best Shown

Lateral view of mid and distal humerus, including elbow joint.

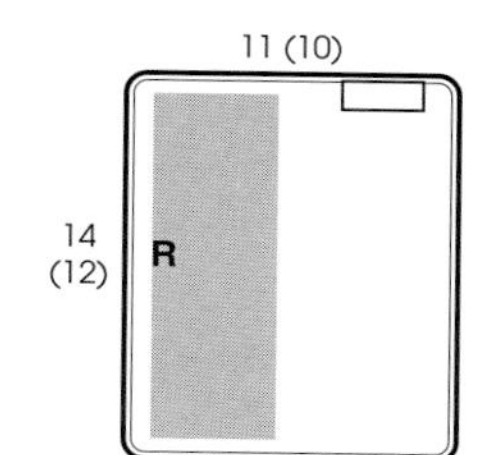

Technical Factors

- Film size–11 x 14 in. (28 x 35 cm)
  or
  –10 x 12 in. (24 x 30 cm), smaller patient.
- Detail screen, non-grid.
- 64±6 kVp range.
- Technique and dose:

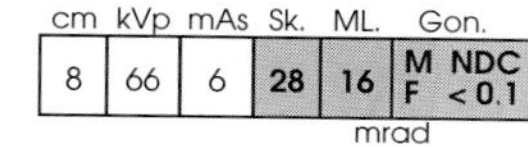

cm	kVp	mAs	Sk.	ML.	Gon.
8	66	6	28	16	M NDC F <0.1

mrad

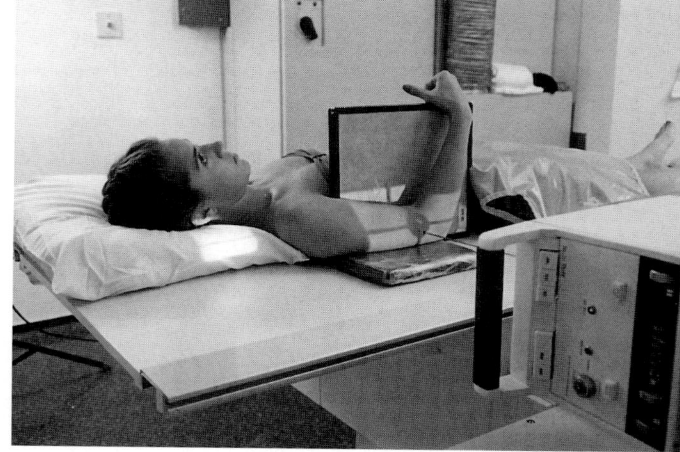

Fig. 4-166. Horizontal beam lateral (mid and distal humerus).

Shielding: Place lead shield **over thorax and pelvis**, between the cassette and patient.

Patient and Part Position

- With patient recumbent, may be taken as a horizontal beam lateral, place support under arm.
- Flex elbow if possible, but do not attempt to rotate arm; projection should be 90° from AP.
- Gently place cassette between arm and thorax (top of film to the axilla).

Central Ray

- CR perpendicular to the **midpoint of distal two-thirds of humerus**.
- Minimum 40 in. (102 cm) SID.

Collimation: Collimate to soft tissue margins.

Respiration: **Suspend respiration** during exposure. (This is important to prevent movement of cassette during the exposure.)

Evaluation Criteria

- Distal two-thirds of humerus and elbow joint should be well-visualized with collimation visible on lateral borders.
- This lateral view should be 90° or at a right angle to an AP trauma projection.
- Optimum exposure with no motion should visualize sharp bony borders and fine trabecular markings of humerus and proximal forearm.

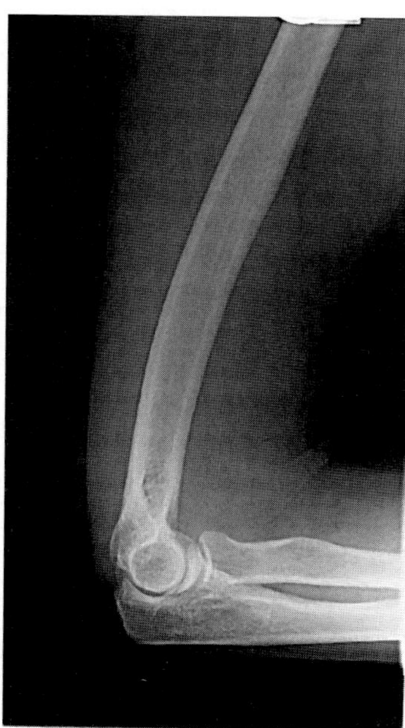

Fig. 4-167. Lateral (mid and distal humerus).

4

Radiographs for Critique

Each of these upper limb radiographs demonstrates some error in positioning which requires a repeat. These, along with accompanying lecture slides of these and other radiographs, will provide a basis for classroom and/or positioning lab discussion. Questions with answers based on these specific critique radiographs are provided in the accompanying student workbook/lab manuals to help prepare students for classroom and/or lab discussions on film critique.

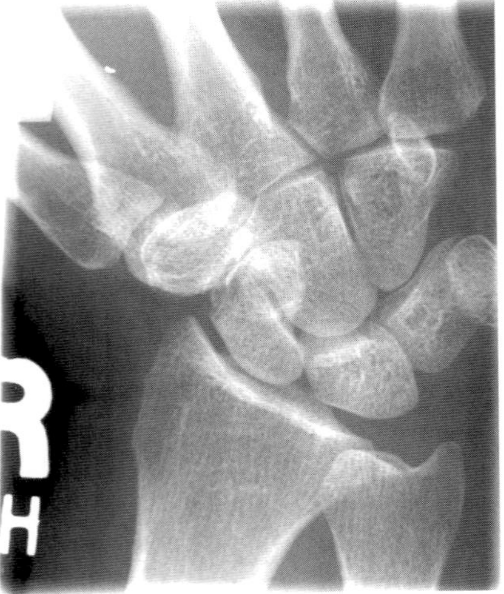

Fig. C4-168. Wrist.

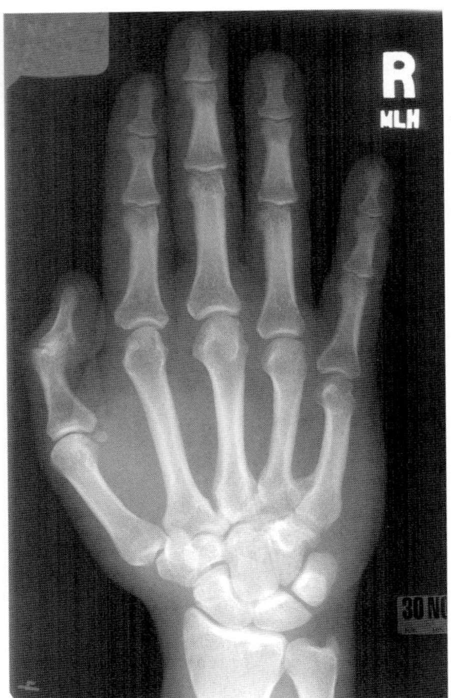

Fig. C4-169. Hand.

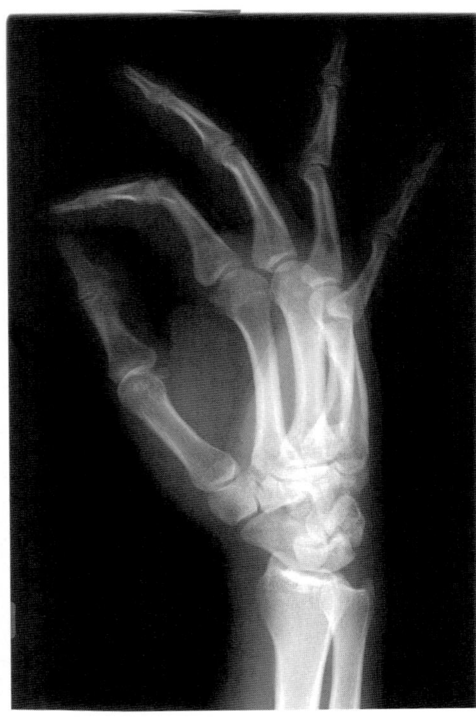

Fig. C4-170. Hand.

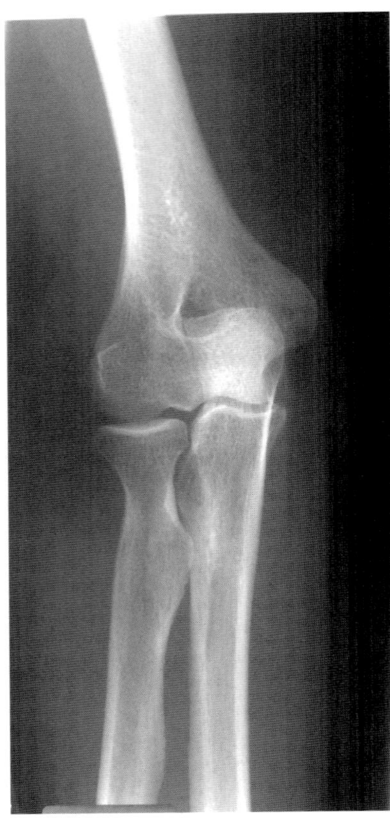

Fig. C4-171. Elbow.

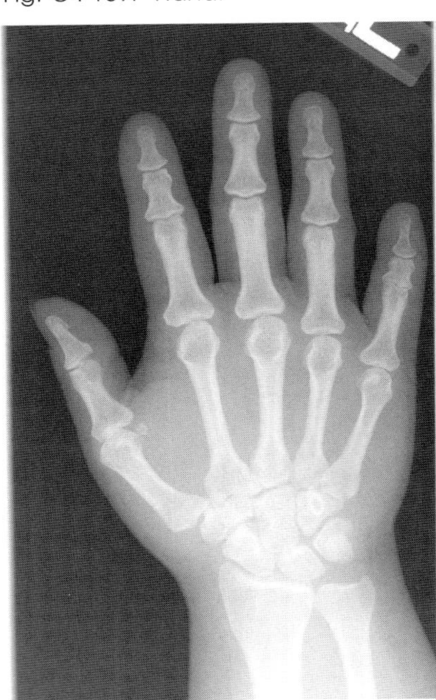

Fig. C4-172. Hand.

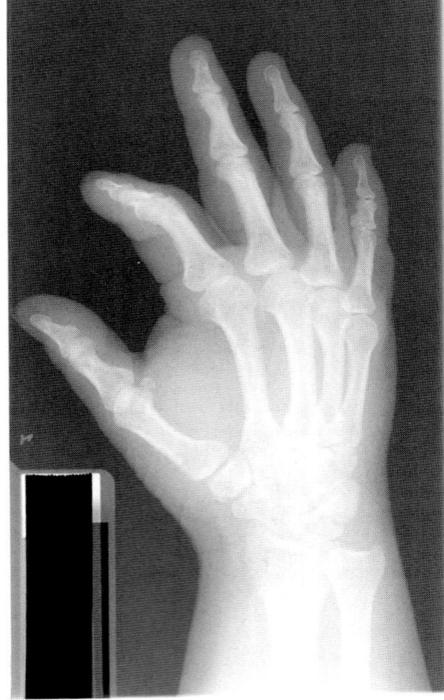

Fig. C4-173. Hand.

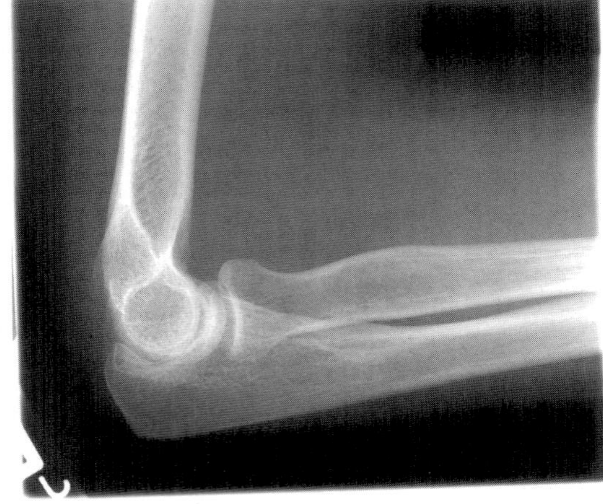

Fig. C4-174. Elbow.

CHAPTER 5

Proximal Humerus and Shoulder Girdle

5

CONTENTS

Radiographic Anatomy

Proximal humerus **148**

Shoulder girdle **149**

Clavicle **149**

Scapula **150**

Anatomy review with radiographs **151**

Classification of joints **152**

Radiographic Positioning

Proximal humerus rotation and related anatomy **153**

Survey information **154**

Basic and special projections **155**

Shoulder (non-trauma routine):
- AP (external rotation) **156**
- AP (internal rotation) **157**
- Inferosuperior axiolateral (Lawrence method) **158**
- Glenoid cavity oblique (Grashey method) **159**
- Intertubercular (bicipital) groove (Fisk method) **160**

Shoulder (trauma routine):
- AP (neutral rotation) **161**
- Scapular Y lateral and Neer method **162**
- Transthoracic lateral (Lawrence method) **163**
- Apical oblique projection (Garth method) **164**

Clavicle:
- AP and AP axial **165**

Acromioclavicular (AC) joints:
- AP bilateral with and without weights **166**

Sternoclavicular joints:
(see Chapter 10–Bony Thorax)

Scapula:
- AP **168**
- Lateral **169**

Radiographs for critique **170**

Radiographic Anatomy

Upper Limb (Extremity)

The hand, wrist and mid and distal humerus of the upper limb were described in Chapter 4. The **proximal humerus** is covered in this chapter along with the shoulder girdle, which includes the **clavicle** and **scapula**.

HUMERUS

The **humerus** is the largest and the longest bone of the upper limb. Its length on an adult equals approximately one-fifth of the body height. The humerus articulates with the **scapula** (shoulder blade) at the shoulder joint.

Proximal Humerus

The proximal humerus is that part of the upper arm which articulates with the scapula, making up the shoulder joint. The most proximal part is the rounded **head** of the humerus. The slightly constricted area directly below and lateral to the head is the **anatomical neck**, which appears as a line of demarcation between the rounded head and the adjoining greater and lesser tubercles.

The process directly below the anatomical neck on the anterior surface is the **lesser tubercle**, *(tu′ber- k′l)* (tuberosity in earlier literature), and the larger lateral process is the **greater tubercle.** The deep groove between these two tubercles is the **intertubercular** *(in″ter-tu-ber′ ku-lar)* **groove** (bicipital groove). The tapered area below the head and tubercles is the **surgical neck**, and distal to the surgical neck is the long **body** (shaft) of the humerus.

The surgical neck is so named because it is the site of frequent fractures requiring surgery of the proximal humerus. Fractures at the thick anatomical neck are more rare.

Anatomy of Proximal Humerus on Radiograph

Figure 5-3 is an AP radiograph of the shoulder taken with **external rotation**, which places the humerus in a **true AP** or frontal position. Note that the drawing in Fig. 5-2 represents a neutral rotation (natural position of arm without internal or external rotation). This places the humerus in an oblique position midway between an AP (external rotation) and a lateral (internal rotation).

Some of the parts are more difficult to clearly visualize on radiographs than on drawings, but a good understanding of locations and relationships between various anatomical parts aids in this identification.

A. Head of humerus
B. Greater tubercle
C. Intertubercular groove
D. Lesser tubercle
E. Anatomical neck
F. Surgical neck
G. Body

The relative location of the greater and lesser tubercles is significant as a way of determining a true frontal view or a true AP projection of the proximal humerus. Note that the **lesser tubercle is located anteriorly, and the greater tubercle is located laterally** in a true AP projection.

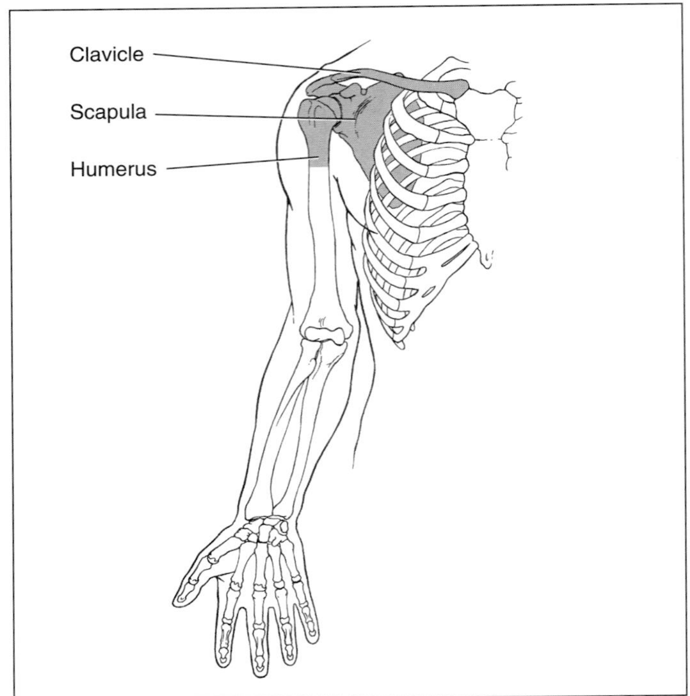

Fig. 5-1. Shoulder girdle.

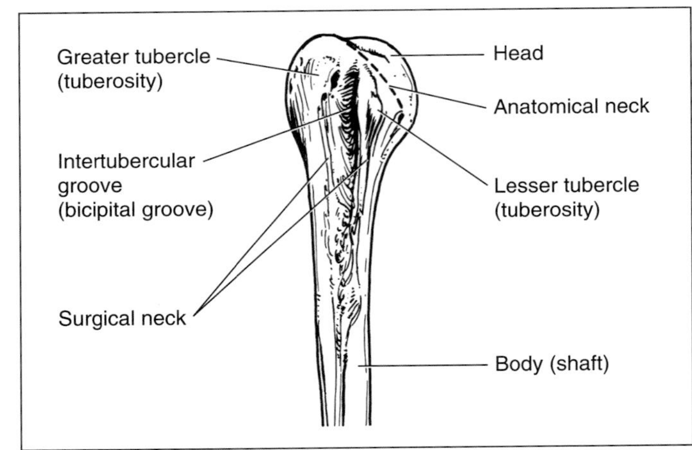

Fig. 5-2. Frontal view of proximal humerus.
-Neutral rotation (oblique position).

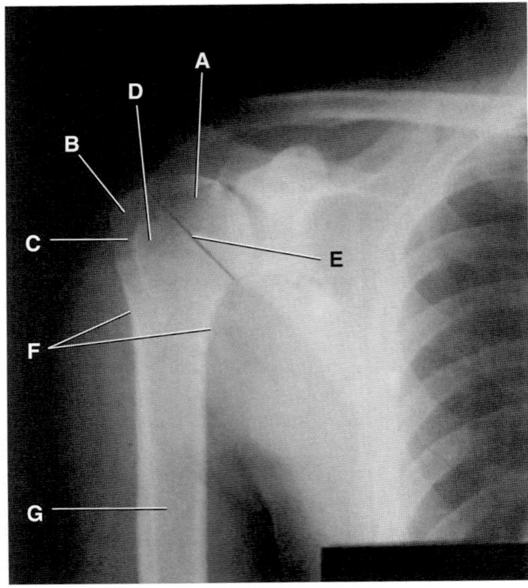

Fig. 5-3. AP shoulder-External rotation.

SHOULDER GIRDLE

The shoulder girdle consists of two bones, the **clavicle** and the **scapula**. The function of the clavicle and scapula is to connect each upper limb to the trunk or axial skeleton. Anteriorly the shoulder girdle connects to the trunk at the upper sternum, but posteriorly the connection to the trunk is incomplete in that the scapula is connected to the trunk by muscles only. Each shoulder girdle and upper limb connect at the shoulder joint between the scapula and the humerus. Each clavicle is located over the upper, anterior rib cage. Each scapula is situated over the upper, posterior rib cage.

The upper margin of the scapula is at the level of the **second posterior rib**, and the lower margin is at the level of the **seventh posterior rib** (T7). Note that the lower margin of the scapula corresponds to T7, also used as a landmark for location of the central ray for chest positioning as described in Chapter 2.

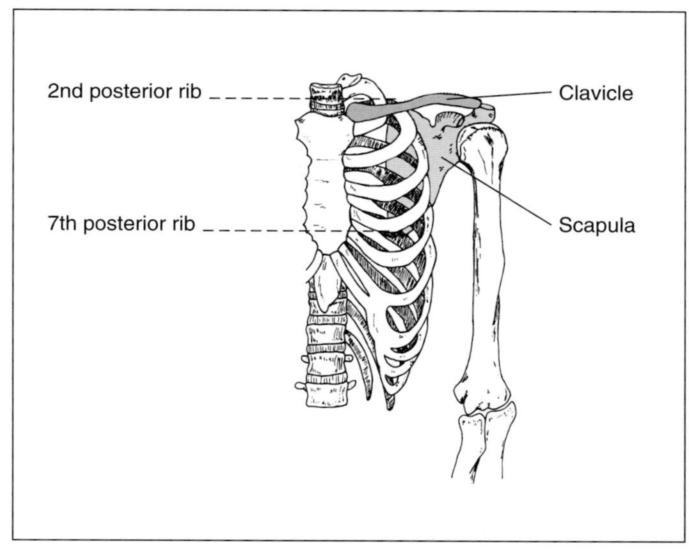

Fig. 5-4. Shoulder girdle.

Clavicle

The clavicle (collar bone) is a long bone with a double curvature having three main parts, the two ends and the long central portion. The lateral or **acromial** *(ah-kro′me-al)* **extremity** (end) of the clavicle articulates with the acromion of the scapula. This joint or articulation is termed the **acromioclavicular** *(ah-kro″me-o-klah-vik′u-lar)* **joint** and can generally be readily palpated.

The medial or **sternal extremity** (end) articulates with the manubrium, which is the upper part of the sternum. This articulation is termed the **sternoclavicular** *(ster″no-klah-vik′u-lar)* **joint.** This joint is also easily palpated and the combination of the sternoclavicular joints on either side of the manubrium help form an important positioning landmark called the **jugular** *(jug′u-lar)* **notch**, also called the suprasternal or manubrial notch in earlier literature.

The **body** (shaft) of the clavicle is the elongated portion between the two extremities.

The acromial end of the clavicle is flattened and has a downward curvature at its attachment with the acromion. The sternal end is more triangular in shape and is also directed downward to articulate with the sternum.

In general, there is a difference in size and shape of the clavicle between male and female. The **female clavicle** is usually **shorter** and **less curved** than is the male clavicle. The clavicle in the male tends to be thicker and more curved in shape, usually being most curved in heavily muscled males.

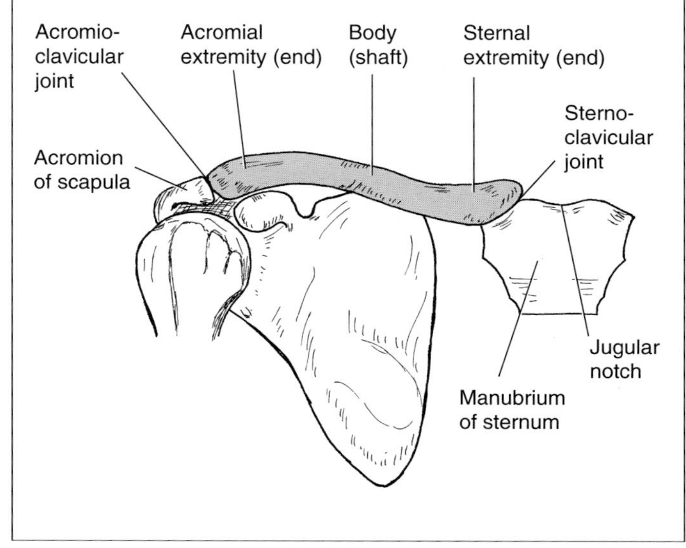

Fig. 5-5. Clavicle.

Radiograph of the Clavicle

The AP radiograph of the clavicle in Fig. 5-6 identifies the two joints and the three parts of the clavicle.

A. Sternoclavicular joint
B. Sternal extremity
C. Body
D. Acromial extremity
E. Acromioclavicular joint

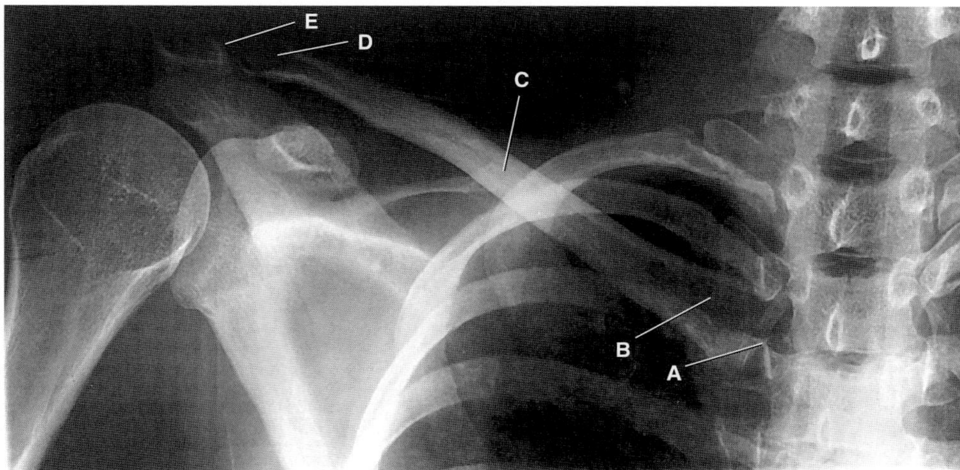

Fig. 5-6. AP radiograph of clavicle.

Scapula

The scapula (shoulder blade), which forms the posterior part of the shoulder girdle, is a flat triangular bone with three borders, three angles and two surfaces. The three borders include the **medial** (vertebral) **border,** which is the long edge or border near the vertebrae, the **superior border**, the uppermost margin of the scapula, and the **lateral** (axillary) **border,** the border nearest the axilla *(ak-sil′ ah).* Axilla is the medical term for the armpit.

Anterior View: The three corners of the triangular-shaped scapula are called angles. The **lateral angle**, sometimes called the head of the scapula, is the thickest part of the scapula and ends laterally in a shallow depression called the **glenoid cavity** (fossa).

The humeral head articulates with the glenoid cavity of the scapula to form the **scapulohumeral** *(skap′ u-lo-hu′ mer-al)* **joint**, also known as the glenohumeral or shoulder joint.

The constricted area between the head and the body of the scapula is the **neck.** The **superior** and **inferior angles** refer to the upper and lower ends of the medial or vertebral border. The **body** (blade) of the scapula is arched for greater strength. The thin, flat, lower part of the body is sometimes referred to as the "wing" or ala of the scapula, although these are not preferred anatomical terms.

The anterior surface of the scapula is termed the **costal** *(kos′ tal)* **surface** because of the proximity to the ribs (*costa*, literally meaning rib). The mid area of the costal surface presents a large concavity or depression, the **subscapular fossa**.

The **acromion** is a long, curved process extending laterally over the head of the humerus. The **coracoid process** is a thick, beak-like process projecting anteriorly beneath the clavicle. The **scapular notch** is a notch on the superior border partially formed by the base of the coracoid process.

Posterior View: Fig. 5-9 shows a prominent structure on the dorsal or posterior surface of the scapula, called the **spine**. The elevated spine of the scapula starts at the vertebral border as a smooth triangular area and continues laterally to end at the **acromion.** The acromion overhangs the shoulder joint posteriorly.

The posterior border or ridge of the spine is somewhat thickened and is termed the **crest** of the spine. The spine separates the posterior surface into an **infraspinous** *(in″frah-spi′ nus)* **fossa** and **a supraspinous fossa**. (Older terms for these fossae are infraspinatus and supraspinatus, respectively.) Both of these fossae serve as surfaces of attachment for shoulder muscles. The names of these muscles are associated with the respective fossae, namely the infraspinous and supraspinous muscles.

Lateral View: The lateral view of the scapula (Fig. 5-10) demonstrates relative positions of the various parts of the scapula. The thin scapula looks like the letter Y in this position. The upper parts of the Y are the acromion and coracoid process. The **acromion** is the expanded distal end of the spine extending superiorly and posteriorly to the **glenoid cavity** (fossa). The **coracoid process** is located more anteriorly in relationship to the glenoid cavity or shoulder joint.

The bottom leg of the Y is the body of the scapula. The posterior surface or back portion of the thin body portion of the scapula is called the **dorsal surface**. The **spine** extends from the dorsal surface at its upper margin. The anterior surface of the body is called the **ventral** (costal) **surface**. The **lateral** (axillary) **border** is a thicker edge or border extending from the **glenoid cavity** to the **inferior angle,** as shown on this lateral view.

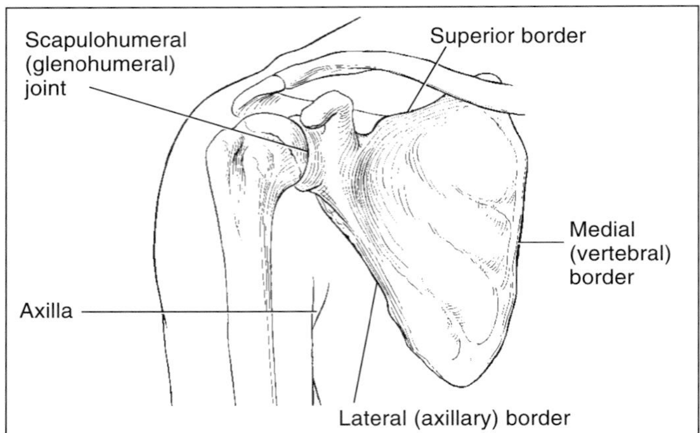

Fig. 5-7. Scapula–Three borders and scapulohumeral (glenohumeral) joint.

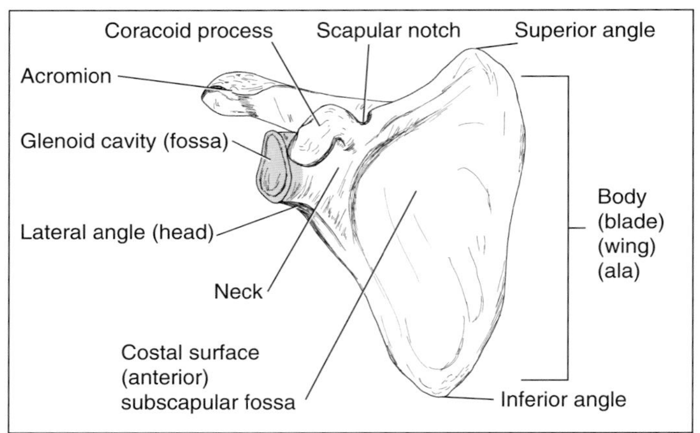

Fig. 5-8. Scapula–Anterior view.

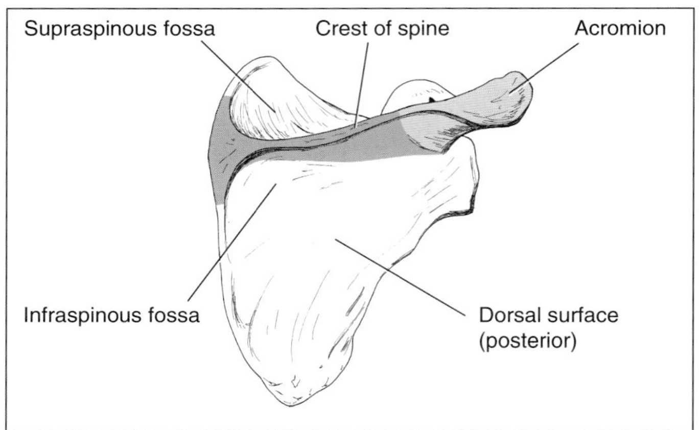

Fig. 5-9. Scapula–Posterior view.

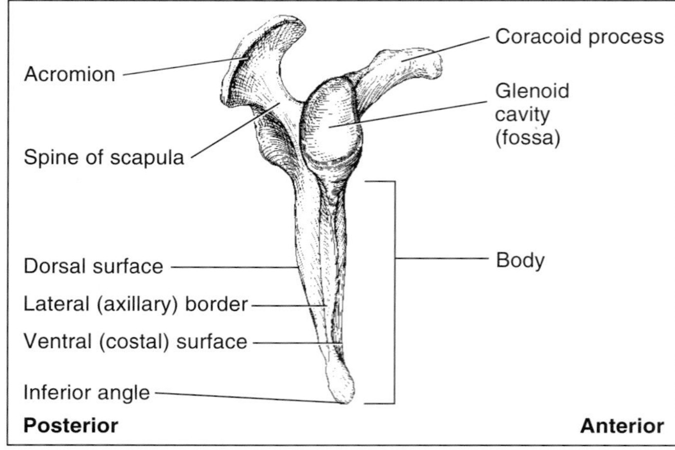

Fig. 5-10. Scapula–Lateral view.

Review Exercise with Radiographs of Scapula

AP Projection: Fig. 5-11 is an AP projection of the scapula taken with the arm abducted so as not to superimpose the scapula. Knowing shapes and relationships of anatomical parts should help in identifying each of these parts.

A. Acromion
B. Neck of scapula (about one inch below the coracoid process)
C. Scapular notch
D. Superior angle
E. Medial (vertebral) border
F. Inferior angle
G. Lateral (axillary) border
H. Glenoid cavity (fossa) or scapulohumeral joint

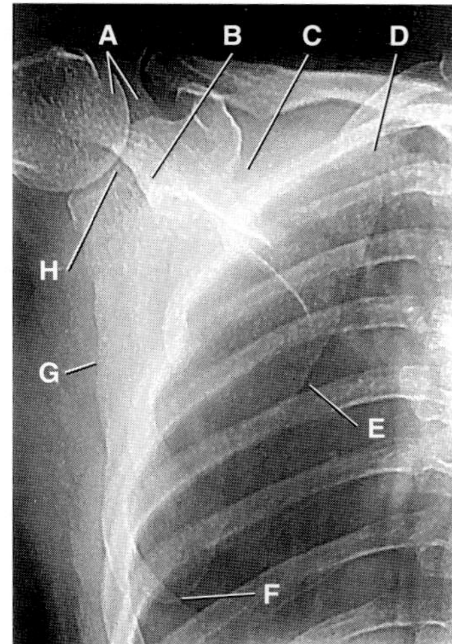

Fig. 5-11. AP projection.

Lateral Projection: This lateral projection of the scapula is taken with the patient in an anterior oblique position with the upper body rotated until the scapula is separated from the rib cage in a true end-on or lateral projection.

A. Acromion
B. Coracoid process
C. Inferior angle
D. Spine of scapula
E. Body of scapula

Note that this lateral view of the scapula results in a Y shape wherein the acromion and the coracoid process make up the upper legs of the Y, and the body makes up the long lower leg.

The scapular Y position is named for this Y shape resulting from a true lateral view of the scapula.

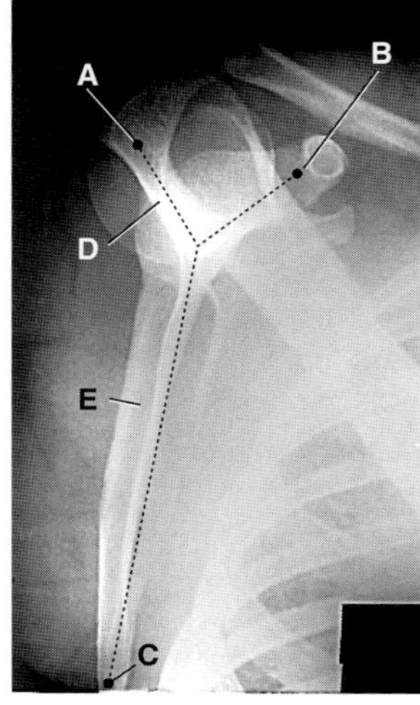

Fig. 5-12. Lateral (scapular Y) position.

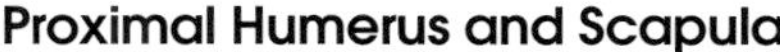

Proximal Humerus and Scapula

Inferosuperior (Axiolateral) Projection: This projection (as illustrated in Fig. 5-14), results in a lateral view of the head and neck of the humerus. It also demonstrates the relationship of the humerus to the glenoid cavity, which makes up the scapulohumeral (shoulder) joint.

The anatomy of the scapula may appear confusing in this position, but knowing and understanding relationships of various parts of the scapula well will enable one to identify those labelled parts on this projection. This will also allow one to place this radiograph correctly on the illuminator (viewbox) for viewing with the correct side up.

Part **A** of Fig. 5-13 is the tip of the **coracoid process**, which is located anterior to the shoulder joint and would therefore be uppermost on the radiograph if the film is placed on the viewbox as the x-ray tube sees it, with the anterior shoulder to the top.

Part **B** is the **glenoid cavity,** which is the articulating surface of the **lateral angle** or **head** of the scapula.

Part **C** is the **spine** of the scapula, which would be located posteriorly with the patient lying on her back as shown in Fig. 5-14.

Part **D** is the **acromion,** which is the extended portion of the spine superimposed over the humerus in this position.

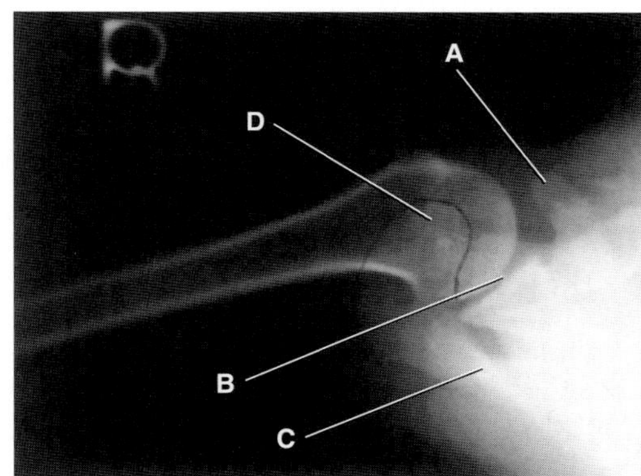

Fig. 5-13. Inferosuperior axial projection.

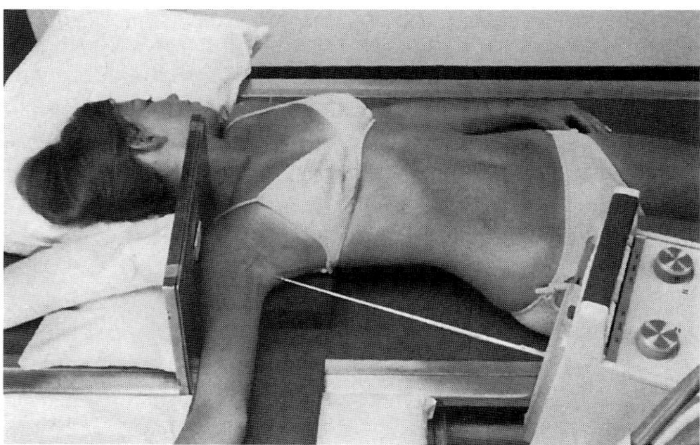

Fig. 5-14. Inferosuperior axial projection.

CLASSIFICATION OF JOINTS

There are only three types of joints or articulations of the shoulder girdle; the **sternoclavicular joint** and the **acromioclavicular joints** of the sternum, and the **scapulohumeral joint** (glenohumeral or shoulder). The classification, mobility type and movement type of these joints are as follows:

Classification

All three joints of the shoulder girdle are classified as **synovial joints**, characterized by a fibrous capsule containing synovial fluid.

Mobility Type

The mobility type of all three of these joints is **freely moveable** or **diarthrodial**. All synovial joints are by nature of their structure freely movable. Therefore, the only difference between these three joints is the movement type.

Movement Type

The **scapulohumeral** (glenohumeral) or shoulder joint involves articulation between the head of the humerus and the glenoid cavity of the scapula. The movement type is a **spheroidal** or **ball and socket** joint, which allows great freedom of movement. These movements are **flexion, extension, abduction, adduction, circumduction, medial** (internal) and **lateral** (external) **rotation.**

The glenoid cavity is very shallow, allowing the greatest freedom in mobility of any joint in the human body, but at some expense to its strength and stability. Even though the strong ligaments, tendons and muscles surrounding the joint provide stability, some stretching of the muscles and tendons can occur causing separation or dislocation of the humeral head from the glenoid cavity. Dislocations at the shoulder joint occur more frequently than at any other joint in the body, requiring the need for frequent radiographic shoulder exams to evaluate for structural damage.

The shoulder girdle also includes two joints involving both ends of the clavicle. These are the sternoclavicular and acromioclavicular joints.

The **sternoclavicular joint** is a **double plane** or **gliding joint** in that the sternal end of the clavicle articulates with both the manubrium or upper portion of the sternum, as well as with the cartilage of the first rib. This allows a limited amount of gliding motion in nearly every direction.

The **acromioclavicular joint** is also a small synovial joint of the **plane** or **gliding movement type**, between the acromial end of the clavicle and the medial aspect of the acromion of the scapula. There are actually two types of movement at this joint. The primary movement is a gliding action between the end of the clavicle and the acromion. There is also some secondary rotary movement as the scapula moves forward and backward with the clavicle. This allows the scapula to adjust its position as it remains in close contact with the posterior chest wall. The rotary type movement, however, is limited, and this joint is generally termed a plane or gliding-type joint.

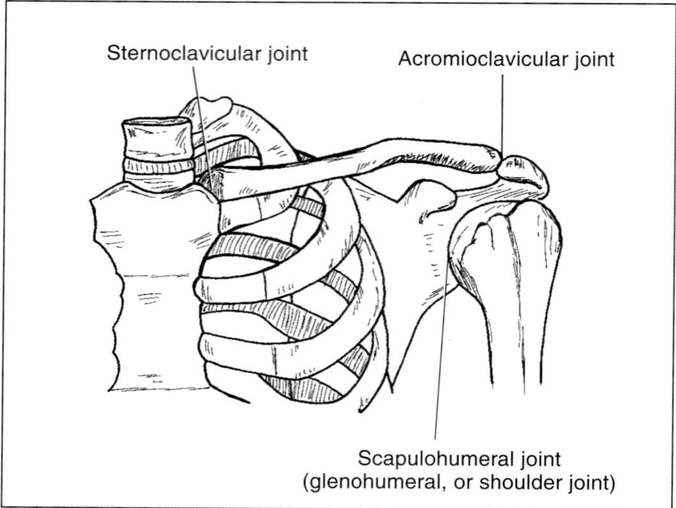

Fig. 5-15. Joints of shoulder girdle.

Summary of Shoulder Girdle Joints	
Classification:	***Synovial*** (articular capsule containing synovial fluid)
Mobility type:	***Diarthrodial*** (freely movable)
Movement types:	
1. Scapulohumeral (glenohumeral) joint	***Spheroidal** or **ball and socket***
2. Sternoclavicular joint	***Plane** or **gliding***
3. Acromioclavicular joint	***Plane** or **gliding***

Radiographic Positioning

PROXIMAL HUMERUS ROTATION

Radiographs of Proximal Humerus

Rotational views of the proximal humerus or shoulder girdle are commonly taken on non-trauma patients when gross fractures or dislocations of the humerus have been ruled out. These AP rotational projections demonstrate the scapulohumeral joint (shoulder joint) well for possible calcium deposits or other pathology. Note specifically the location and shapes of the **greater tubercle (A)** and the **lesser tubercle (B)** on these external, internal and neutral rotation radiographs.

By studying the position and relationships of the greater and lesser tubercles on a radiograph of the shoulder, one can determine the rotational position of the arm. This understanding enables one to know which rotational view is necessary to visualize specific parts of the proximal humerus.

External Rotation: The external rotation position represents a true **AP projection** or frontal view of the humerus in the anatomical position, as determined by the epicondyles of the distal humerus. The arm and elbow are rotated externally until the palm of the hand is forward. This places an imaginary line between the medial and lateral epicondyles **parallel to the film**.

Note: You can check this on yourself by dropping your arm at your side and externally rotating your hand and arm while palpating the epicondyles of your distal humerus.

With this external rotation view the **greater tubercle (A)**, which is located anteriorly in a neutral position, is now positioned in **profile laterally.** The **lesser tubercle (B)** is now located **anteriorly,** just medial to the greater tubercle.

Internal Rotation: The internal rotation results when the hand and arm are rotated internally until the epicondyles of the distal humerus are **perpendicular to the film**, thus placing the humerus in a **true lateral position.** The palm of the hand is turned back or as far posteriorly as needed to place the epicondyles **perpendicular to the film**.

The AP projection of the shoulder taken in the internal rotation position is therefore a lateral position of the humerus in which the **greater tubercle (A)** is now rotated around to the anterior and medial aspect of the proximal humerus. The **lesser tubercle (B)** is seen in profile medially.

Neutral Rotation: The neutral rotation AP projection of the shoulder, as taken on a trauma patient when rotation views cannot be accomplished, generally places the epicondyles of the distal humerus at an **approximate 45° angle to the film**. This results in a 45° oblique position of the humerus when the **palm of the hand is facing inward** against the thigh. The neutral position then is about midway between the external and internal positions and places the greater tubercle anteriorly but still lateral to the lesser tubercle, as seen on the radiograph in Fig. 5-21.

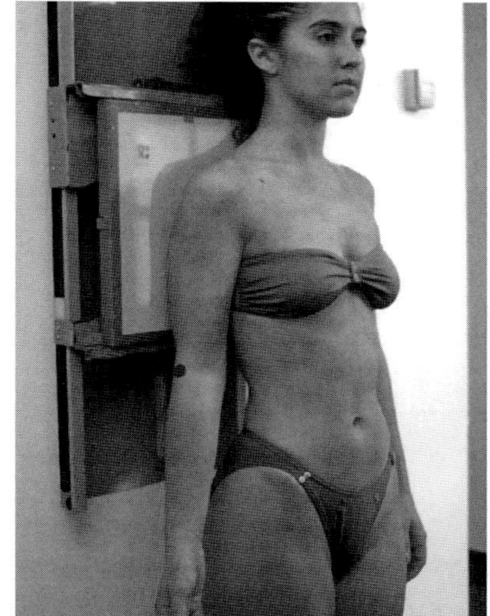

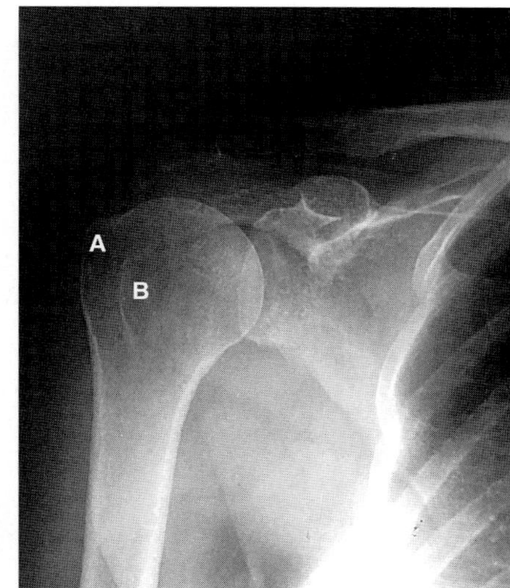

Fig. 5-16. External rotation (AP projection of humerus). Fig. 5-17.

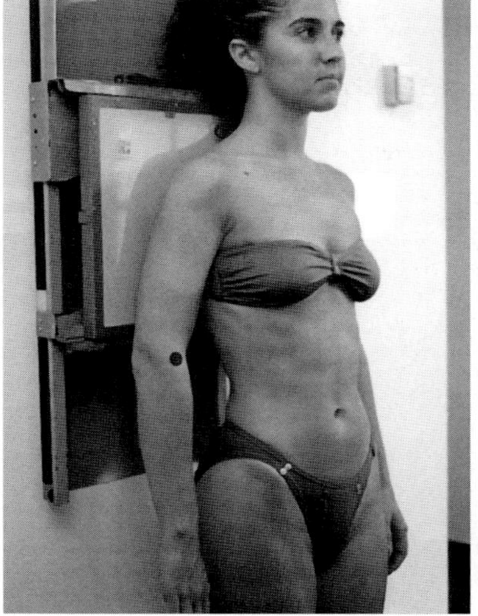

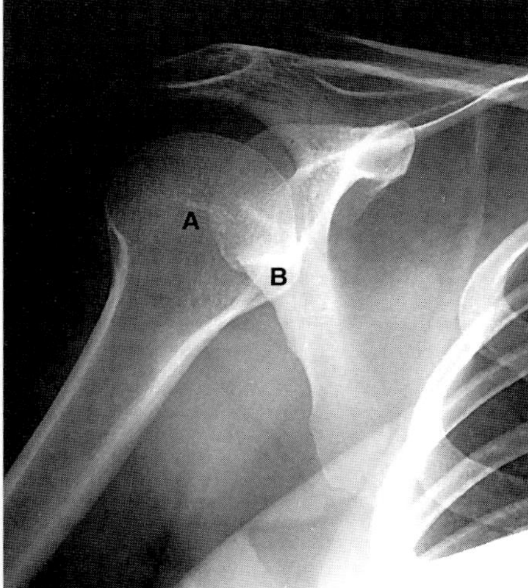

Fig. 5-18. Internal rotation (lateral projection of humerus). Fig. 5-19.

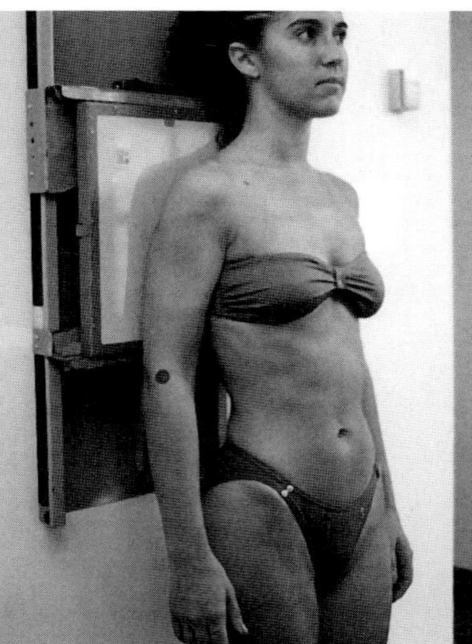

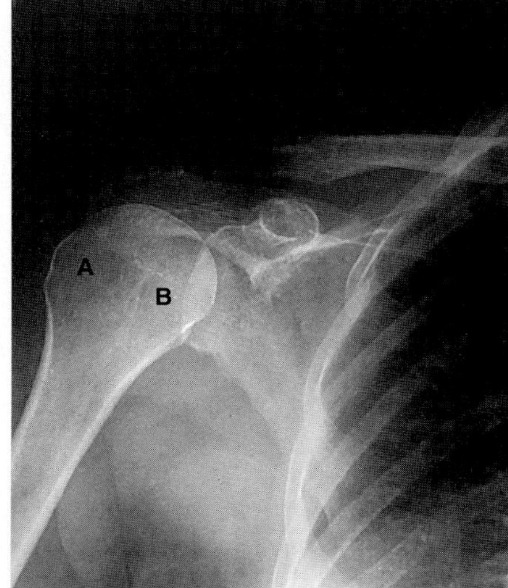

Fig. 5-20. Neutral rotation (oblique projection of humerus). Fig. 5-21.

Positioning, Technique and Shielding Considerations

General positioning considerations for the proximal humerus and shoulder girdle (clavicle and scapula) are similar to other upper and lower limb procedures.

Technique Considerations

Adult shoulders generally measure from 10 to 15 cm, which requires the use of a grid and other technical consideration as listed below. Children and thin, asthenic type adults, may measure less than 10 cm, requiring exposure factor adjustments without the use of grids. AC joints also generally measure less than 10 cm, thus requiring less kVp (67-70) and detail (100) speed screen/films without grids.

Average Adult Shoulder:

1. Medium kVp, 70-80 with grids if over 10 cm (less than 10 cm, 65-70 kVp without grids).
2. Higher mA with short exposure times.
3. Small focal spot.
4. Center cell for AEC if used (manual techniques may be recommended with certain projections).
5. Adequate mAs for sufficient density (to visualize soft tissues as well as bone margins and trabecular markings of all bones).
6. 400 (high) speed screen/film combination recommended with grid techniques.
7. 40 to 44 in. (102 to 112 cm) SID; except for AC joints, which require a 72 in. (180 cm) SID for less beam divergence.

Shielding

Gonads: Generally, gonadal shielding is important for upper limb radiography because of the proximity of parts of the upper limb to the gonads when taken in a supine position. The relationship of the divergent x-ray beam to the pelvic region in an erect seated position also necessitates gonadal protection.

However, for a proximal humerus and/or clavicle, scapula or AC joints, the gonads are of sufficient distance from the primary x-ray beam to result in a gonadal dose of less than 0.1 mrad for females, and NDC (no detectable contribution) for males as shown in patient exposure boxes on each positioning page. However, it is a good practice, and also provides assurance to the patient, to cover the pelvic region whenever possible on all procedures, including the shoulder region.

Thyroid, Lungs and Female Breasts: Radiography of the shoulder region may provide potentially significant doses to the thyroid and lung regions as well as to the female breasts, which are all weighted radiosensitive organs having relative risk of becoming cancerous as compared to whole body effective doses (see Chapter 1, page 39). Therefore **close collimation** to the area of interest is very important, in addition to providing **contact shields** over that portion of the lungs, breast and thyroid regions that do not obscure the area of interest.

NATIONAL SURVEY

Departmental standard and optional operating procedures (departmental routines) for the proximal humerus and shoulder girdle were with a few exceptions similar throughout all regions of the United States.

Shoulder Routine

Shoulder (non-trauma routine)	**U.S. Average** Basic 1995 (1989)	Special 1995 (1989)
• AP (int. and ext. rotation)	96% (92%)	
• Inferosuperior, axial	35% (20%)	34% (15%)
• Post. oblique for glenoid cavity (Grashey method)	24% (20%)	35% (9%)
• Tangential for intertubercular groove	7% –	44% –
Shoulder (trauma routine–possible fracture or dislocation)		
• AP (neutral rotation)	93% (93%)	
• Transthoracic lateral	52% (54%)	26% (19%)
• Scapular Y	62% (41%)	23% (19%)
• Apical oblique, 45° post. obl. 45° caudad	6% (7%)	12% (10%)

Clavicle Routine

Clavicle	**U.S. Average** Basic 1995 (1989)	Special 1995 (1989)
• AP, CR perpendicular	90% (88%)	
• AP, CR 15 to 30° cephalad	94% (86%)	
• PA, CR 15 to 30° caudad	11% (5.5%)	22% (9%)

Scapula Routine

Scapula	**U.S. Average** Basic 1995 (1989)	Special 1995 (1989)
• AP	94% (99%)	
• Lateral (ant. obl.)	76% (93%)	
or		
Lateral (post obl.)	52% –	– (6%)

AC Joints Routine

AC Joints	**U.S. Average** Basic 1995 (1989)	Special 1995 (1989)
• AP, bilateral with and without weights	95% (96%)	

Summary of National Survey Results

Shoulder Routine: The non-trauma shoulder routine was very consistent throughout the United States except for the **posterior oblique (Grashey method)**, which was more common in the West (28%) and Mid U.S. (27%) as compared to the East (19%). The **inferosuperior axial projection** was also more common in 1995 as both a basic routine (35% in 1995 and 20% in 1989), and as a special projection (34% in 1995 and 15% in 1989).

The major change in trauma shoulder routines over the past six years was the lateral projection wherein the **scapular Y** was indicated as the most common basic routine in 1995 (62%) as compared to 1989 (41%).

The **apical oblique** as a special projection in 1995 was twice as common in the West (20%) and Mid U.S. (19%), as compared to the East (10%). (See appendix pages.)

Clavicle Routine: The clavicle routine included both an AP perpendicular (90%) and an AP with 15 to 30° cephalad angle (94%) throughout the United States, with very little regional differences. The PA with caudad angle continues to be a much less common projection (11%), as compared to the AP with cephalad angle (94%).

Scapula Routine: The lateral scapula is more common as an anterior oblique in all regions of the United States (76%), as compared to the posterior oblique (52%). It is known that the posterior obliques are most common for trauma patients in a supine position, as described in Chapter 19 on Mobile and Trauma Radiography. This question was not included in the 1989 survey; therefore, no trend or change can be determined for this lateral scapula projection.

STANDARD AND SPECIAL OPERATING PROCEDURES

Certain basic and special projections for the shoulder, clavicle, AC joints and scapula are demonstrated and described on the following pages as suggested standard basic and special departmental routines or procedures.

Basic Projections

Standard or basic projections, also sometimes referred to as routine projections or departmental routines, are those projections commonly taken on average patients who are helpful and can cooperate in performing the procedure.

Special Projections

Special projections are those more common projections taken as extra or additional projections to better demonstrate certain pathologic conditions or specific body parts.

Basic and Special Projections

Shoulder
(Non-trauma routine)
Basic
- AP external rotation (AP) **156**
- AP internal rotation (lateral) **157**

Special
- Inferosuperior axial **158** (Lawrence method)
- Glenoid cavity post. obl. **159** (Grashey method)
- Tangential projection for intertubercular groove **160** (Fisk method)

Shoulder
(Trauma routine)
Basic
- AP neutral rotation (AP) **161**
- Scapular Y lateral **162**

or
- Transthoracic lateral **163** (Lawrence method)

Special
- Apical oblique **164** (Garth method)

Clavicle
Basic
- AP and AP axial **165**

AC joints
Basic
- AP bilateral with weights and AP bilateral without weights **166**

Scapula
Basic
- AP **168**
- Lateral **169**

AP Projection–External Rotation

AP Proximal Humerus

Warning: Do **NOT** attempt to rotate arm if fracture or dislocation is suspected (see trauma routine).

Shoulder (non-trauma)
Basic
- **AP ext. rotation (AP)**
- AP int. rotation (lateral)

Structures Best Shown

Frontal view of proximal humerus and lateral two-thirds of clavicle and upper scapula, including relationship of humeral head to glenoid cavity. Also demonstrates possible calcium deposits in muscles, tendons or bursal structures of shoulder.

Technical Factors

- Film size–10 x 12 in. (24 x 30 cm), crosswise (or lengthwise to show more of humerus if injury includes proximal half of humerus).
- Moving or stationary grid.
- 70±5 kVp range.
- Technique and dose:

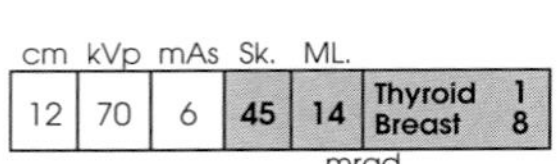

cm	kVp	mAs	Sk.	ML.	Thyroid / Breast (mrad)
12	70	6	45	14	Thyroid 1 Breast 8

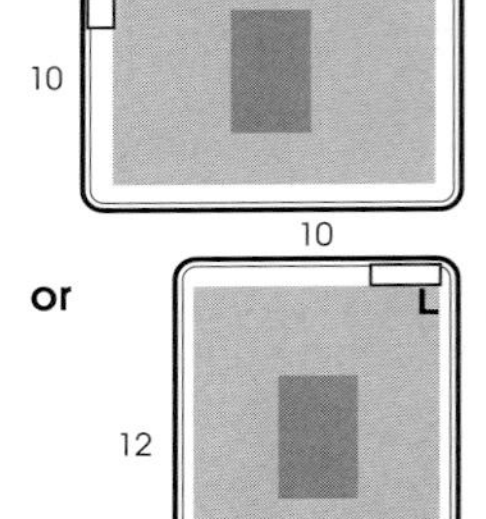

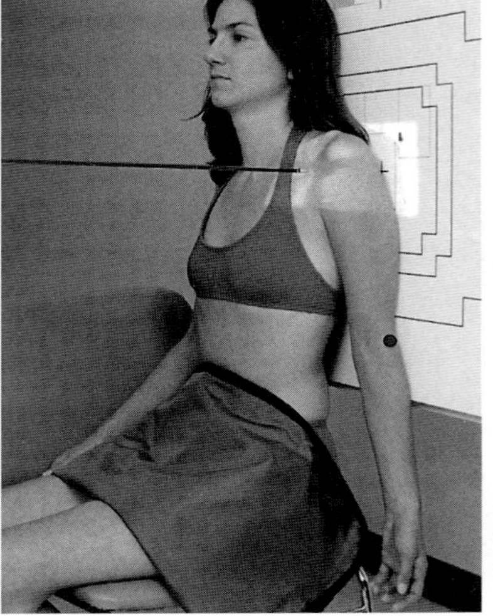

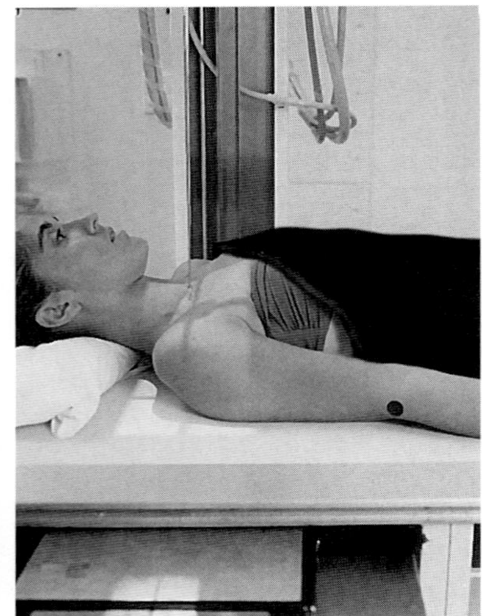

Fig. 5-22. Patient and part position: External rotation–AP. Fig. 5-23.

Shielding: Shield chest and female breast (not over scapula) and pelvis.

Patient Position

- May be taken erect or supine. (Erect is usually less painful for patient if condition allows.)
- Rotate body slightly toward affected side if necessary to place shoulder in contact with film holder or table-top.

Part Position

- Position patient and CR so that the scapulohumeral joint is centered to CR.
- Abduct extended arm slightly, then **externally rotate arm** (supinate hand) until epicondyles of distal humerus are **parallel** to film.

Central Ray

- CR **perpendicular** to film, directed to **mid scapulohumeral joint**, which is ≈¾ in. (2 cm) inferior and slightly lateral to the coracoid process. (See Note.)
- Minimum 40 in. (102 cm) SID.

Collimation: Collimate on four sides, with lateral and upper borders adjusted to soft tissue margins.

Respiration: Suspend respiration during exposure.

Note: The coracoid process may be difficult to palpate directly on most patients, but it can be approximated by knowing that it is about ¾ in. (2 cm) inferior to the lateral portion of the readily palpated clavicle. Also the scapulohumeral joint is found at the base or pit of the concave-like depression just medial to the humeral head.

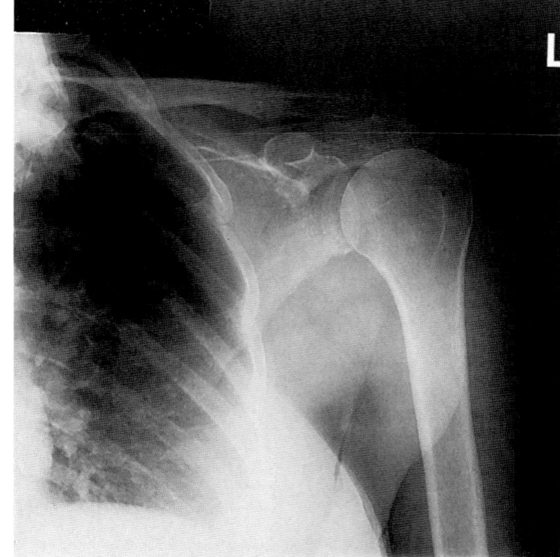

Fig. 5-24. External rotation.

Evaluation Criteria

- Proximal one-third of humerus, upper scapula and lateral two-thirds of clavicle should be included with collimation visible on four sides.
- Center of collimation field should be to scapulohumeral joint, indicating correct CR placement.
- Frontal view of proximal humerus evidenced by the **greater tubercle** being visualized in profile **laterally**. An outline of the lesser tubercle should be seen superimposed over the humeral head.
- Optimum exposure with no motion as evidenced by sharp borders and fine trabecular markings. Correct exposure will visualize the outline of the medial aspect of humeral head through the glenoid cavity and demonstrate soft tissue detail for possible calcium deposits.

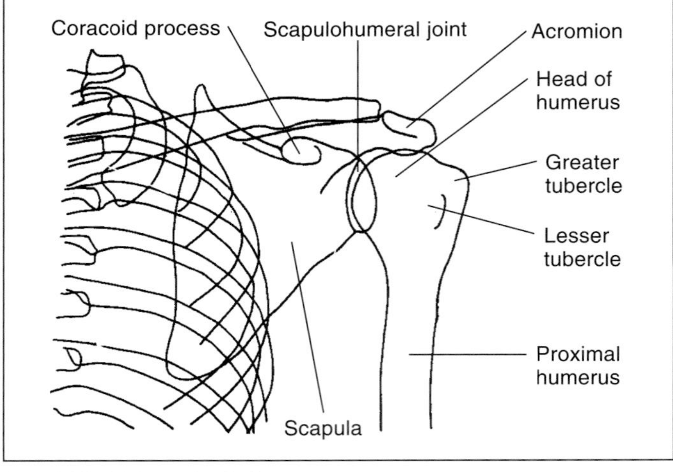

Fig. 5-25. External rotation.

AP Projection–Internal Rotation

Lateral Proximal Humerus

Warning: Do **NOT** attempt to rotate arm if fracture or dislocation is suspected (see trauma routine).

Shoulder (non-trauma)
Basic
- AP ext. rotation (AP)
- **AP int. rotation (lateral)**

Structures Best Shown

Lateral view of proximal humerus and lateral two-thirds of clavicle and upper scapula, including relationship of humeral head to glenoid cavity. Also demonstrates possible calcium deposits in muscles, tendons or bursal structures of shoulder.

Technical Factors

- Film size–10 x 12 in. (24 x 30 cm), crosswise (or lengthwise to show more of humerus if injury includes proximal 1/2 of humerus).
- Moving or stationary grid.
- 80±5 kVp range.
- Technique and dose:

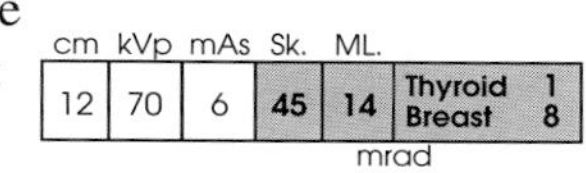

cm	kVp	mAs	Sk.	ML.	mrad
12	70	6	45	14	Thyroid 1, Breast 8

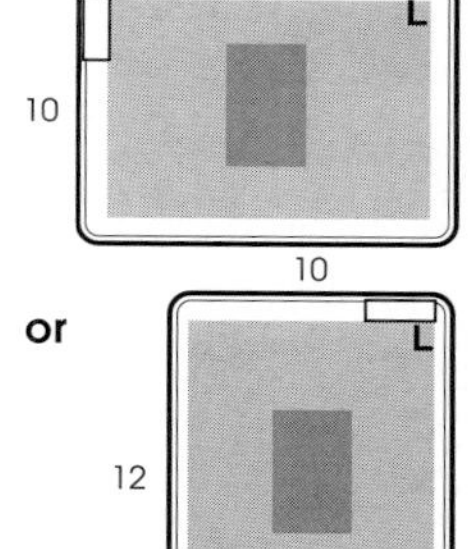

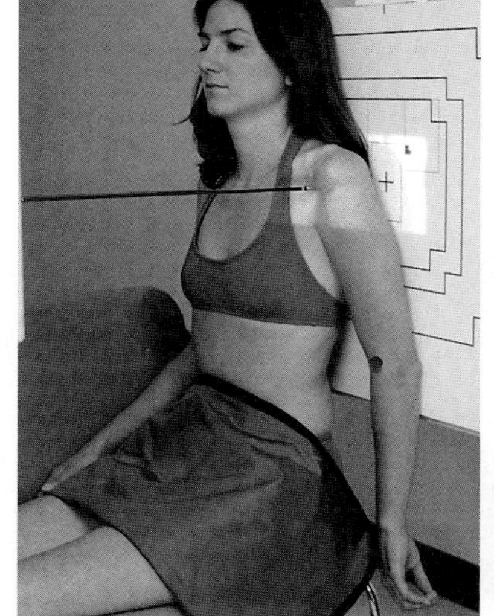

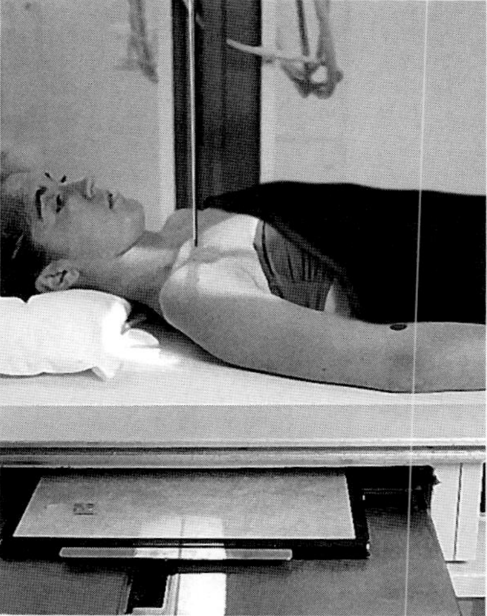

Fig. 5-26. Patient and part position: Internal rotation–Lateral. Fig. 5-27.

Shielding: Shield thyroid, lungs (not over scapula) and pelvic area.

Patient Position

- May be taken erect or supine. (Erect is usually less painful for patient if condition allows.)
- Rotate body slightly toward affected side if necessary to place shoulder in contact with film holder or table-top.

Part Position

- Position patient and CR so that the scapulohumeral joint is centered to CR (see Note).
- Abduct extended arm slightly, then **internally rotate arm** (pronate hand) until epicondyles of distal humerus are **perpendicular** to film.

Central Ray

- CR perpendicular to film, directed to mid scapulohumeral joint, which is ≈¾ in. (2 cm) inferior and slightly lateral to the coracoid process. (See Note.)
- Minimum 40 in. (102 cm) SID.

Collimation: Collimate on four sides, with lateral and upper borders adjusted to soft tissue margins.

Respiration: Suspend respiration during exposure.

Note: The coracoid process may be difficult to palpate directly on most patients, but it can be approximated by knowing that it is about ¾ in. (2 cm) inferior to the lateral portion of the readily palpated clavicle. Also the scapulohumeral joint is generally found at the base or pit of the concave-like depression just medial to the humeral head (which is also about 2 to 3 in. or 5 to 7 cm) inferior and medial to the superolateral borders of shoulder).

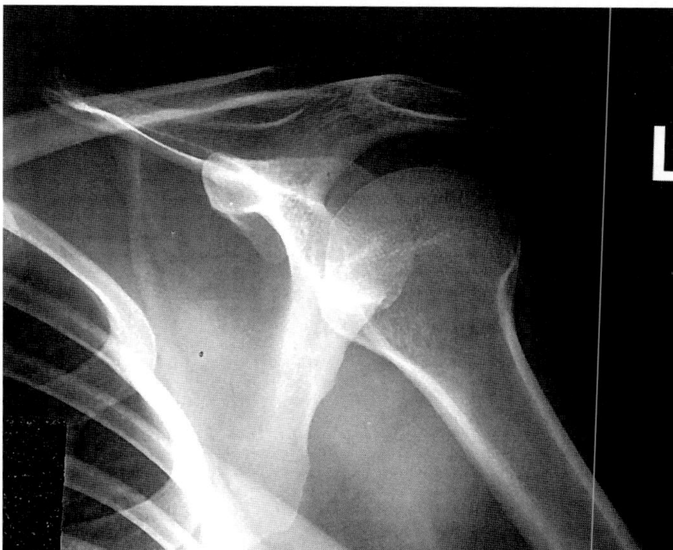

Fig. 5-28. Internal rotation–Lateral.

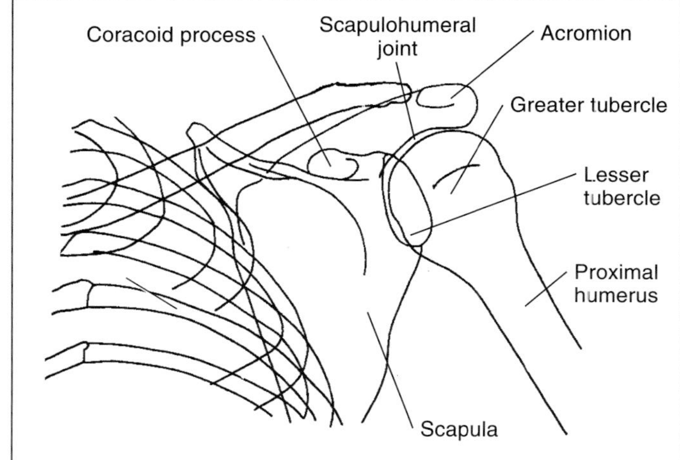

Fig. 5-29. Internal rotation–Lateral.

Evaluation Criteria

- Proximal one-third of humerus, upper scapula and lateral two-thirds of clavicle should be included with collimation visible on four sides.
- Center of collimation field should be to scapulohumeral joint, indicating correct CR placement.
- Lateral view of proximal humerus evidenced by the **lesser tubercle** being visualized in profile **medially** partially superimposed by the lower portion of the glenoid cavity. An outline of the greater tubercle may be seen superimposed over the humeral head.
- Optimum exposure with no motion as evidenced by sharp borders and fine trabecular markings. Correct exposure will visualize the outline of the medial aspect of humeral head through the glenoid cavity, and demonstrate soft tissue detail for possible calcium deposits.

Inferosuperior Axiolateral Projection

Lawrence Method

Warning: Do **NOT** attempt to rotate arm if fracture or dislocation is suspected.

Shoulder (non-trauma)
Special
- **Inferosuperior axial (Lawrence method)**
- Glenoid cavity AP obl. (Grashey method)
- Tangential projection (Fisk method)

Structures Best Shown

Lateral view of proximal humerus and relationship to glenoid cavity. With exaggerated rotation, the Hill-Sachs defect is demonstrated.

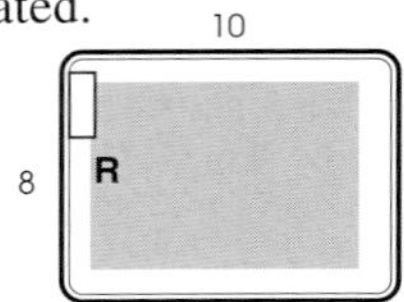

Technical Factors

- Film size–8 x 10 in. (18 x 24 cm) crosswise.
- Stationary grid. (CR to centerline of grid. Crosswise to prevent grid cutoff due to CR angle.)
  No AEC due to small body part and to table-top screen.
- 70±5 kVp range.
- Technique and dose:

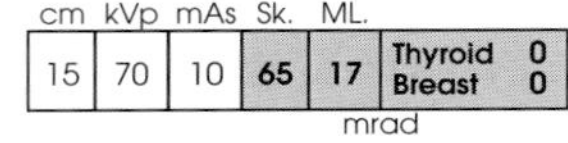

cm	kVp	mAs	Sk.	ML.	
15	70	10	65	17	Thyroid 0 Breast 0

mrad

Shielding: Place lead shield over pelvis and radiosensitive regions.

Patient Position

- Patient supine with shoulder raised about 2 in. (5 cm) from table-top by placing support under arm and shoulder to place body part near center of film.
- Move patient toward the front edge of table-top and place a cart or other arm support against front edge of table to support abducted arm.

Part Position

- Rotate head toward opposite side, and place vertical cassette on table as close to neck as possible, support with sand bags.
- Abduct arm 90° from body if possible; keep in **external rotation**, palm up with support under arm and hand extended over the edge of table.

Central Ray

- Direct CR **medially 25 to 30°**, centered **horizontally to axilla and humeral head.** If abduction of arm is less than 90°, the CR medial angle should also be decreased to 15-20° if possible.
- Minimum 40 in. (102 cm) SID.

Collimation: Collimate closely on four sides.

Respiration: Suspend respiration during exposure.

Alternate position: Exaggerated **external** rotation.* An anterior dislocation of the humeral head may result in a compression fracture of the articular surface of the humeral head, termed the Hills-Sachs defect. This is best demonstrated with this exaggerated external rotation wherein the thumb is pointed down and posteriorly about 45°.

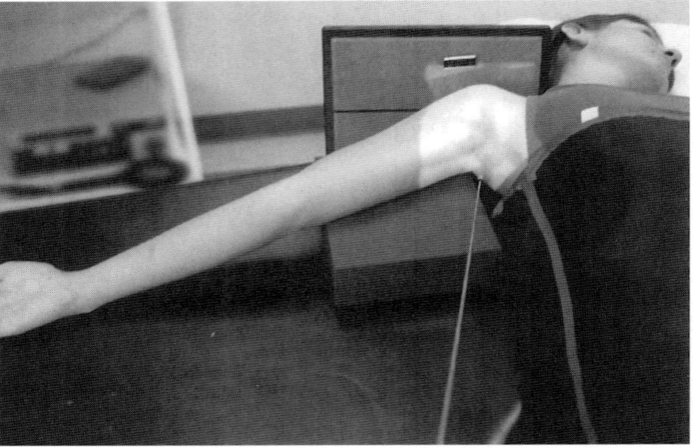

Fig. 5-30. Inferosuperior axial.

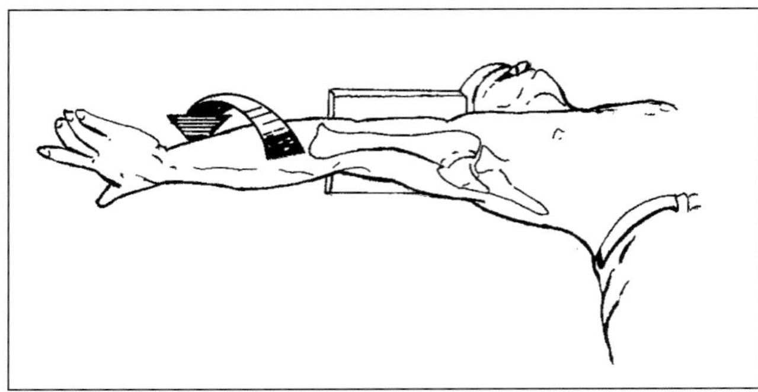

Fig. 5-31. Alternate position–Exaggerated rotation.

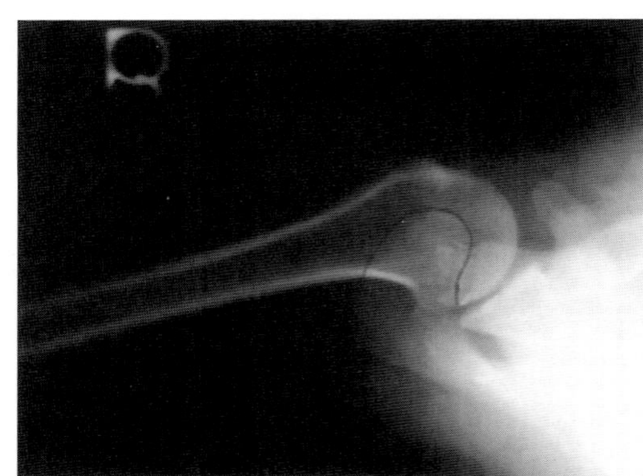

Fig. 5-32. Inferosuperior axiolateral.

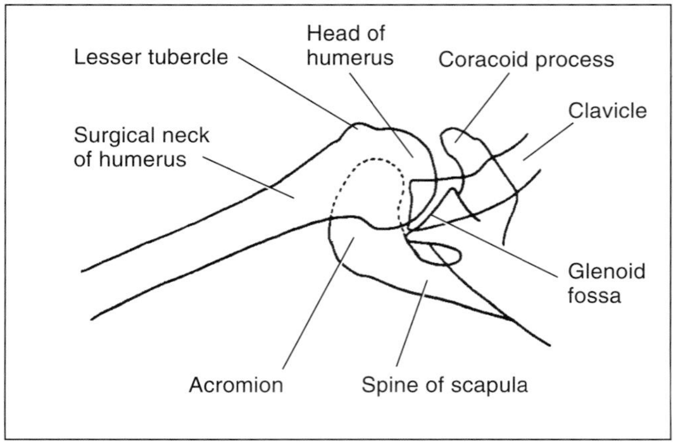

Fig. 5-33. Inferosuperior axiolateral.

Evaluation Criteria

- The neck and head of humerus should be well visualized in a lateral position, evidenced by the **lesser tubercle in profile anteriorly**.
- The relationship of the humeral head and glenoid cavity should be clearly visualized. The spine of the scapula should be seen on edge below the scapulohumeral joint.
- The superior and inferior borders of the glenoid cavity should be directly superimposed, indicating correct CR angle.
- Optimum exposure without motion should visualize sharp borders and fine trabecular markings of the proximal humerus and lateral aspects of scapula. The bony margins of the acromion and distal clavicle should be visible as well as the AC joint through the humeral head. Soft tissue should be visualized.
- Collimation borders should be visible on all four sides.

*Rafert, JA, et al. Axillary Shoulder with Exaggerated Rotation: The Hill-Sachs Defect, *Radiologic Technology* Sept/Oct 1990; 62:18-21.

AP Oblique Projection–LPO or RPO Position

Glenoid Cavity, Grashey Method

Shoulder (non-trauma)
Special
- Inferosuperior axial (Lawrence method)
- **Glenoid cavity AP obl. (Grashey method)**
- Tangential projection (Fisk method)

Structures Best Shown

Glenoid cavity in profile and open scapulohumeral joint space.

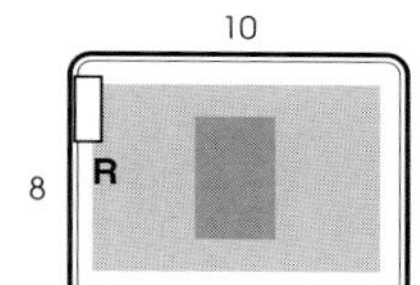

Technical Factors

- Film size–8 x 10 in. (18 x 24 cm), crosswise.
- Moving or stationary grid.
- 75±5 kVp range.
- Technique and dose:

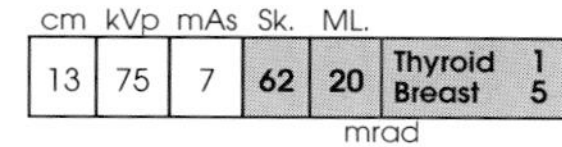

cm	kVp	mAs	Sk.	ML.	mrad	
13	75	7	62	20	Thyroid	1
					Breast	5

Shielding: Place gonadal shielding over thyroid, lungs and pelvic area.

Patient Position

- Erect or supine. (Erect is usually less painful for patient if condition allows.)
- Rotate body **35 to 45°** toward affected side. (See Note.) If done supine, place supports under elevated shoulder and hip to maintain this position.

Part Position

- Center mid scapulohumeral joint to CR.
- Adjust cassette so top of film is about 2 in. (5 cm) above shoulder, and side of film is about 2 in. (5 cm) from lateral border of humerus.
- Abduct arm slightly with arm in neutral rotation.

Central Ray

- CR **perpendicular** to film, **centered to scapulohumeral joint**, which is approximately **2 in. or 5 cm inferior and medial to superolateral border** of shoulder.
- Minimum 40 in. (102 cm) SID.

Collimation: Collimate so upper and lateral borders of the light field are to the soft tissue margins.

Respiration: Suspend respiration during exposure.

Note: The degree of rotation will vary depending on how flat or round shouldered the patient is. Rounded or curved shoulder and back requires more rotation to place body of scapula parallel to film.

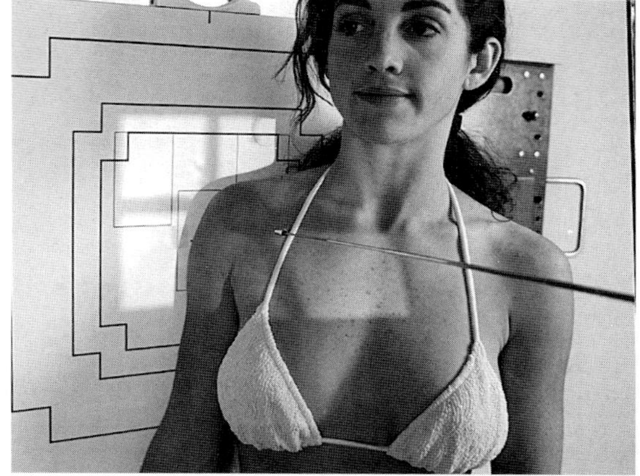

Fig. 5-34. Glenoid cavity posterior oblique–40° RPO.

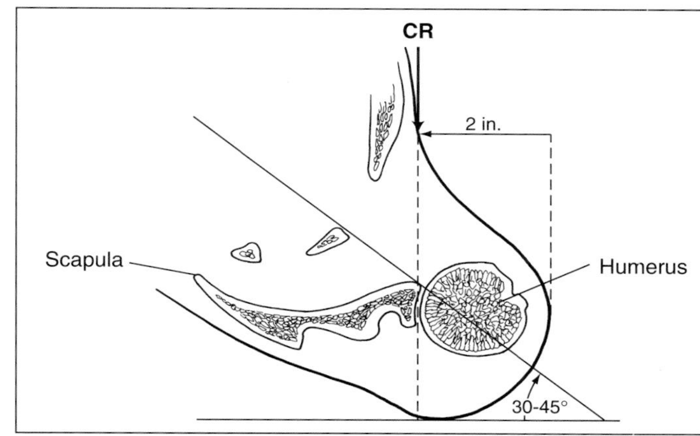

Fig. 5-35. Glenoid cavity posterior oblique.

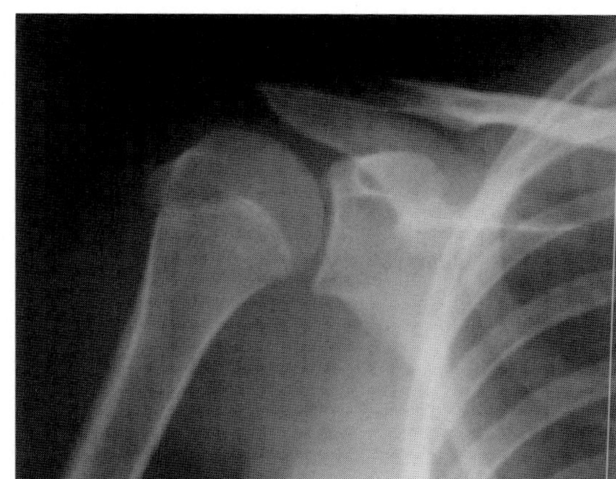

Fig. 5-36. Glenoid cavity posterior oblique.

Evaluation Criteria

- Glenoid cavity should be seen in profile without superimposition of humeral head (joint space should appear open).
  Note: Under-rotation is most common for this projection as evidenced when anterior and posterior glenoid rims are not superimposed.
- Optimum exposure without motion should visualize sharp bony borders and fine trabecular markings of humeral head and the lateral angle or head of scapula. Soft tissue detail in the area of joint space and axilla should be visualized.
- Collimation borders should be visible on four sides to area of soft tissue outer margins. The center of the collimation field should be to the area of the scapulohumeral joint.

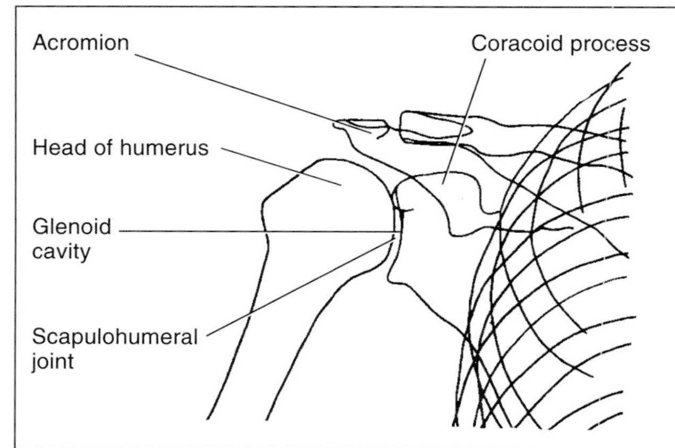

Fig. 5-37. Glenoid cavity posterior oblique.

Tangential Projection–Intertubercular (Bicipital) Groove

Fisk Method

Shoulder (non-trauma)
Special
- Inferosuperior axial (Lawrence method)
- Glenoid cavity AP obl. (Grashey method)
- **Tangential projection (Fisk method)**

Structures Best Shown

Demonstrates humeral tubercles and intertubercular groove in profile unobscured by other structures.

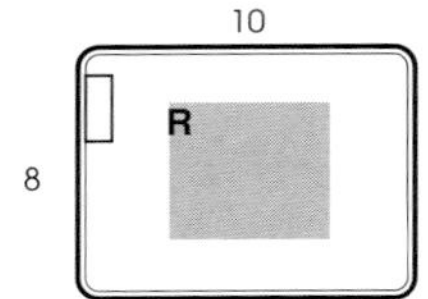

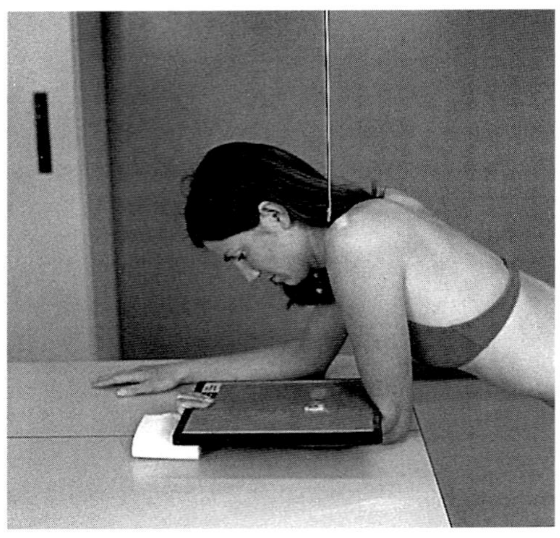

Fig. 5-38. Erect superoinferior tangential projection.

Technical Factors

- Film size–8 x 10 in. (18 x 24 cm), crosswise.
- Detail screen cassette, non grid.
- No AEC due to small body part and tabletop screen.
- 60±5 kVp range.
- Technique and dose:

	cm	kVp	mAs	Sk.	ML.	
Erect	-	65	4	31	10	Thyroid 0 Breast 0
Supine	-	65	3	14	5	Thyroid 0 Breast 0

mrad

Shielding: Place lead shield over pelvis and thorax.

Patient Position and Central Ray

Erect (Fisk method):

- Patient standing, leaning over end of table with elbow flexed and posterior surface of forearm resting on table, hand supinated holding cassette, head turned away from affected side (lead shield placed between back of cassette and forearm reduces backscatter to film).
- Patient leans forward slightly to place humerus **15 to 20°** from vertical.
- CR perpendicular to film, directed to groove area at mid anterior margin of humeral head (groove can be located by careful palpation).

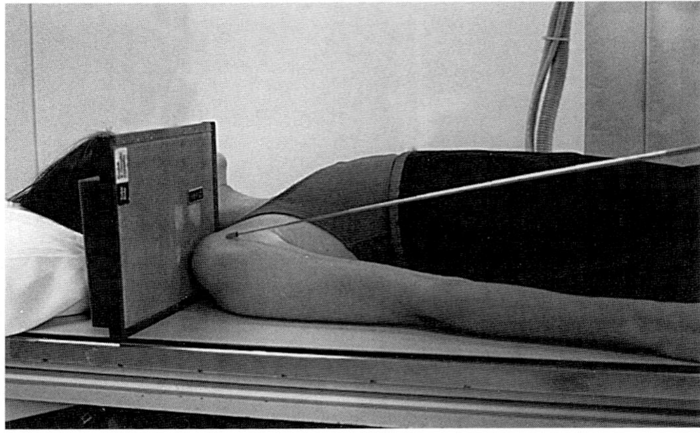

Fig. 5-39. Supine superoinferior tangential projection.

Supine:

- Patient supine, arm at side, hand supinated.
- Vertical cassette placed on table against top of shoulder and against neck (head turned away from affected side).
- CR **10 to 15° posterior from horizontal**, directed to groove at mid anterior margin of humeral head.

Collimation: Collimate closely on four sides to area of anterior humeral head.

Respiration: Suspend respiration during exposure.

Note: Erect is the preferred method if the patient is able, due to the magnification factor combined with the air-gap to absorb scatter.

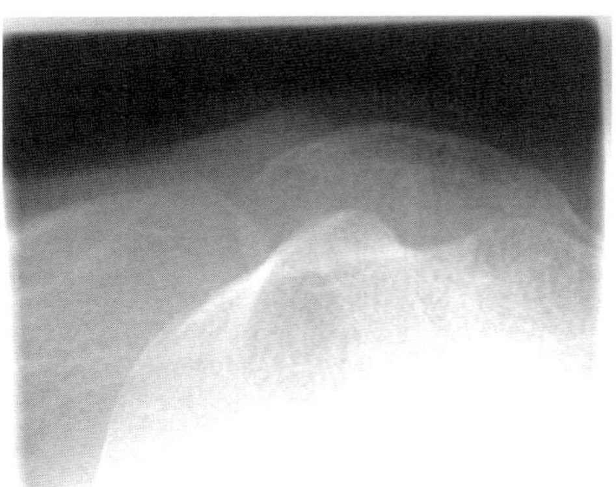

Fig. 5-40. Erect tangential.

Evaluation Criteria

- The anterior margin of the humeral head should be seen in profile, demonstrating the intertubercular groove between the greater and lesser tubercles.
- Collimation field should be limited to the area of anterior humeral head, and the center of the field should be to the intertubercular groove, indicating correct CR location.
- Optimum exposure and contrast without motion should visualize sharp borders and demonstrate the complete borders of the groove seen through soft tissue.

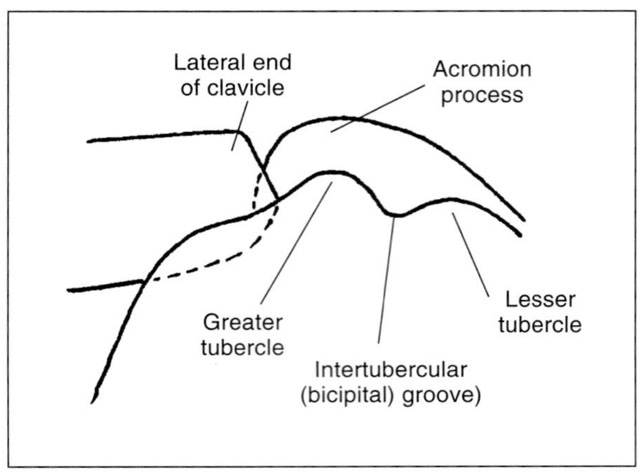

Fig. 5-41. Tangential.

AP Projection–Neutral (NO) Rotation

Warning: Do **NOT** attempt to rotate arm if fracture or dislocation is suspected; take as is in neutral rotation, which generally places humerus in an oblique position.

> **Shoulder** (trauma)
> Basic
> • **AP (neutral rotation)**
> • Scapular Y lateral and Neer method
> or
> • Transthoracic lateral
> Special
> • Apical oblique (Garth method)

Structures Best Shown

Frontal oblique view of proximal humerus; lateral two-thirds of clavicle and upper scapula, including relationship of humeral head to glenoid cavity.

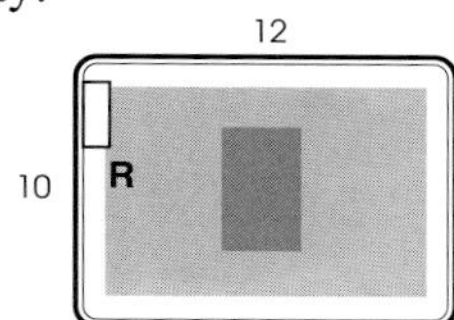

or

10
R
12

Technical Factors

- Film size–10 x 12 in. (24 x 30 cm), crosswise (or lengthwise to show more of humerus if injury includes proximal half of humerus).
- Moving or stationary grid.
- 70±5 kVp range.
- Technique and dose:

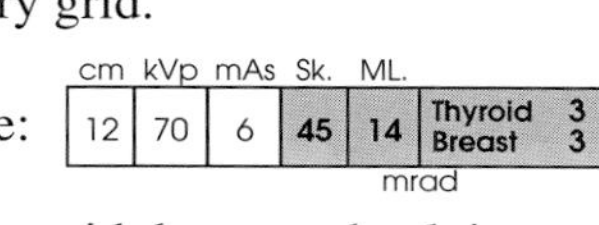

cm	kVp	mAs	Sk.	ML.	mrad
12	70	6	45	14	Thyroid 3 Breast 3

Shielding: Shield thyroid, lungs and pelvic area.

Patient Position

- May be taken erect or supine. (Erect is usually less painful for patient if condition allows.)
- Rotate body slightly toward affected side if necessary to place shoulder in contact with film holder or table-top.

Part Position

- Position patient and CR so that the scapulohumeral joint is centered to CR.
- Place patient's arm at side in "as is" neutral rotation. (Epicondyles are generally approximately 45° to plane of film.)

Central Ray

- CR **perpendicular** to film, directed to **mid scapulohumeral joint**, which is ≈¾ in. (2 cm) inferior and slightly lateral to the coracoid process. (See Note.)
- Minimum 40 in. (102 cm) SID.

Collimation: Collimate on four sides, with lateral and upper borders adjusted to soft tissue margins.

Respiration: Suspend respiration during exposure.

Note: The coracoid process may be difficult to palpate directly on most patients, but it can be approximated by knowing that it is about ¾ in. (2 cm) inferior to the lateral portion of the readily palpated clavicle. Also, the scapulohumeral joint is generally found at the base or pit of the concave-like depression just medial to the humeral head.

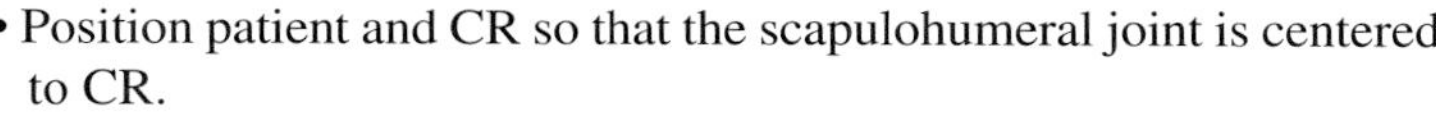

Evaluation Criteria

- Proximal one-third of the humerus, upper scapula and a minimum of lateral two-thirds of clavicle should be included with collimation visible on four sides.
- Center of collimation field should be to scapulohumeral joint, indicating correct CR placement.
- With neutral rotation, greater tubercle will be primarily superimposed over humeral head.
- Optimum exposure with no motion as evidenced by sharp borders and fine trabecular markings. Correct exposure will visualize the outline of the medial aspect of humeral head through the glenoid cavity, and visualize soft tissue detail to show possible calcium deposits.

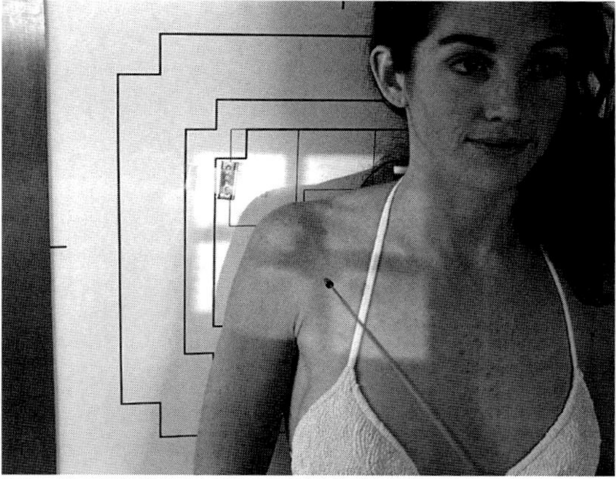

Fig. 5-43. AP erect.

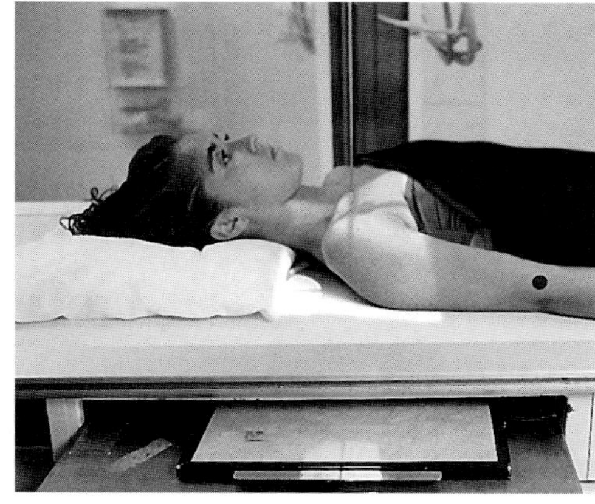

Fig. 5-44. AP supine.

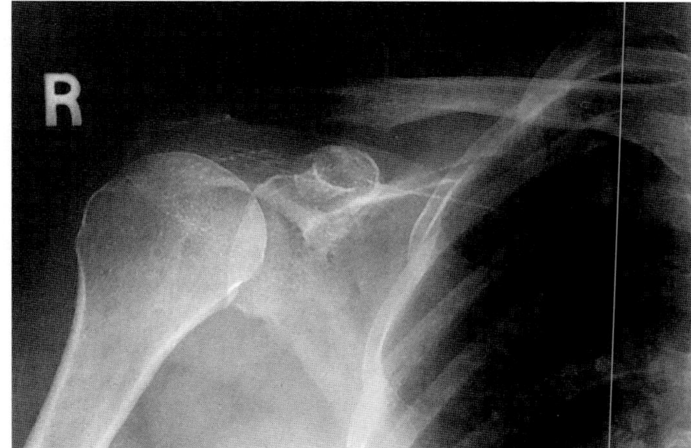

Fig. 5-45. AP projection.

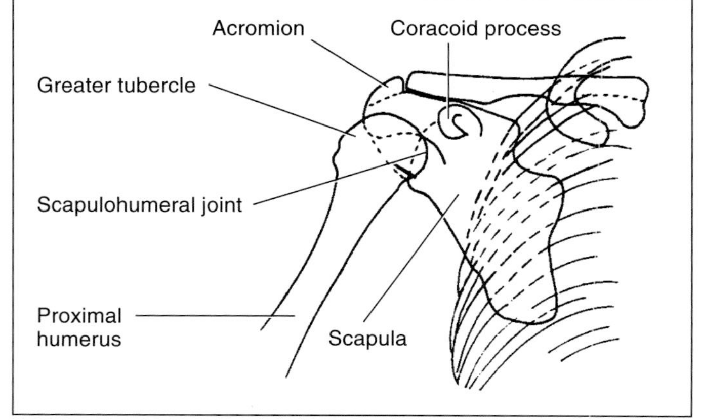

Fig. 5-46. AP projection.

5

Scapular Y Lateral–PA Oblique Projection (RAO or LAO)

and Neer Method (Supraspinatus Outlet Tangential Projection)

Warning: Do **NOT** attempt to rotate arm if fracture or dislocation is suspected.

Shoulder (trauma)
Basic
- AP (neutral rotation)
- **Scapular Y lateral and Neer method**

or
- Transthoracic lateral

Special
- Apical oblique (Garth method)

Structures Best Shown

Proximal humerus superimposed over a lateral view of the scapula. Demonstrates relationship of humeral head to glenoid cavity; and to rule out dislocation or fractures of proximal humerus.

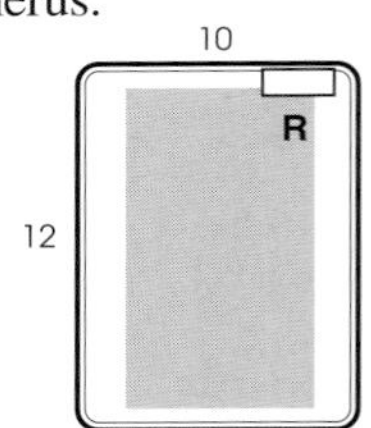

Technical Factors

- Film size–10 x 12 in. (24 x 30 cm), lengthwise.
- Moving or stationary grid.
- AEC not recommended.
- 75±5 kVp range.
- Technique and dose:

cm	kVp	mAs	Sk.	ML.	mrad
16	75	13	126	30	Thyroid 1 Breast 1

Fig. 5-47. Scapular Y lateral. -CR perpendicular.

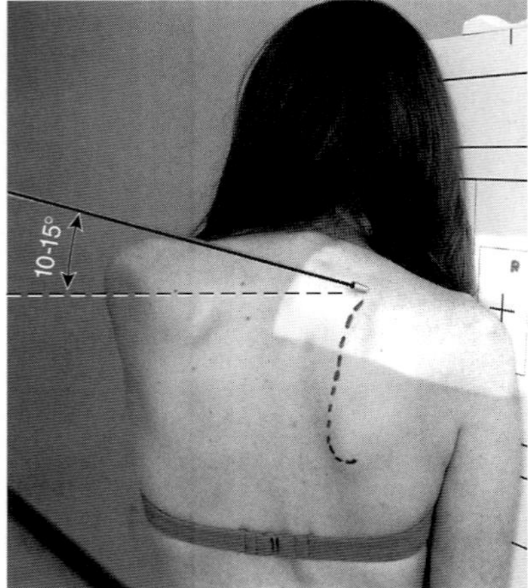

Fig. 5-48. Outlet projection, Neer method–CR 10 to 15° caudad.

Shielding: Shield pelvic area.

Patient Position

- May be taken erect or recumbent, but erect is usually more comfortable for patient.
- With patient facing the cassette, rotate into an anterior oblique position as for a lateral scapula. Average patient will be in a 45 to 60° anterior oblique position. Palpate scapular borders to determine correct location. (See lateral scapula, page 169.)

Part Position

- Center scapulohumeral joint to CR, and to center of film.
- Abduct arm slightly so as not to superimpose proximal humerus over ribs; do not attempt to rotate arm.

Central Ray (Scapular Y lateral)

- CR perpendicular to film, directed to the **scapulohumeral joint** (2 or 2½ in. (5 or 6 cm) below top of shoulder).
- Minimum 40 in. (102 cm) SID.

Fig. 5-49. Scapular Y lateral. -No dislocation.

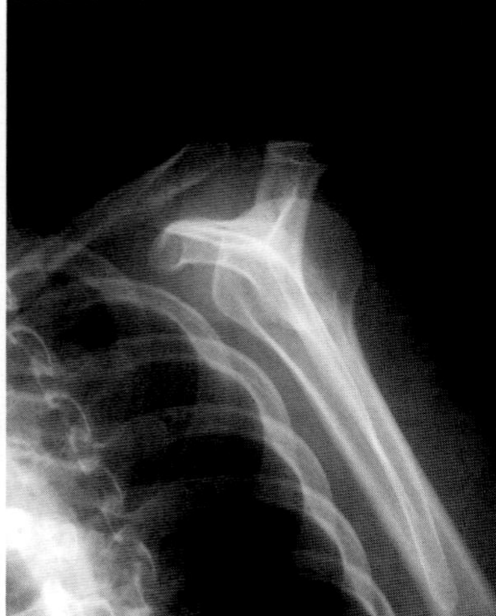

Fig. 5-50. Outlet projection -Neer method.

Neer Method (Supraspinatus Outlet Tangential Projection)*†

This requires a **10 to 15° CR caudal angle centered to the superior margin of humeral head**. Some **reduction in exposure** is needed. This best demonstrates the acromiohumeral space (supraspinatus outlet) for possible subacromial spurs or other abnormalities such as rotator cuff injuries creating shoulder impingement symptoms.

Collimation: Collimate on four sides, to area of interest.

Respiration: Suspend respiration during exposure.

Note: If patient's condition requires, this scapular Y lateral may be taken recumbent in the opposite posterior oblique position with injured shoulder elevated. See Chapter 19: Trauma and Mobile Radiography.

Evaluation Criteria

- The thin body of the scapula should be seen on end, **not** superimposed by ribs.
- The acromion and coracoid processes should appear as nearly symmetrical upper limbs of the Y.
- The humeral head should appear superimposed over the base of the Y **if** the humerus is not dislocated. The proximal humerus will appear medial and inferior to the scapula on an anterior dislocation. (Fig. 5-51.)
- Optimum exposure without motion should visualize well the Y appearance of the lateral scapula, including the outline of the body of the scapula. Bony borders of ribs, scapula and humerus should appear clear and sharp.

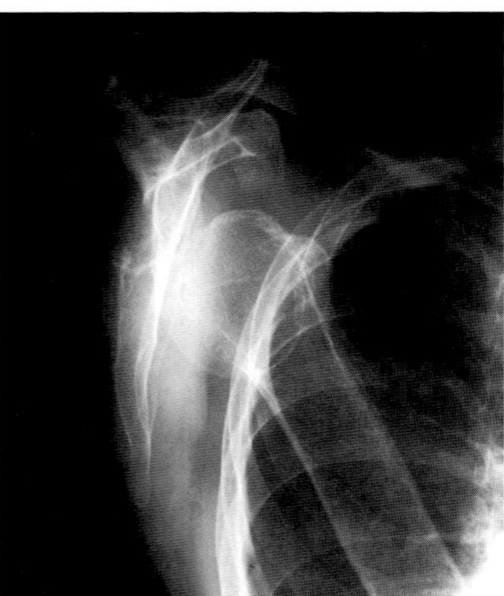

Fig. 5-51. Scapular Y lateral -With anterior dislocation.

*Neer, CS II: Acromioplasty for the Chronic Impingement Syndrome in the Shoulder: A Preliminary Report. *J. Bone Surgery* 1972; 54-A: 41-50.
†Neer, CS II: Supraspinatus Outlet. *Orthrop Trans.* 1987; 11:234.

Transthoracic Lateral Projection–R or L Lateral Position

Lawrence Method

Shoulder (trauma)
Basic
- AP (neutral rotation)
- Scapular Y lateral and Neer method
  or
- **Transthoracic lateral**

Special
- Apical oblique (Garth method)

Structures Best Shown

Lateral view of proximal humerus and relationship of scapulohumeral joint to rule out dislocation or fracture of proximal humerus.

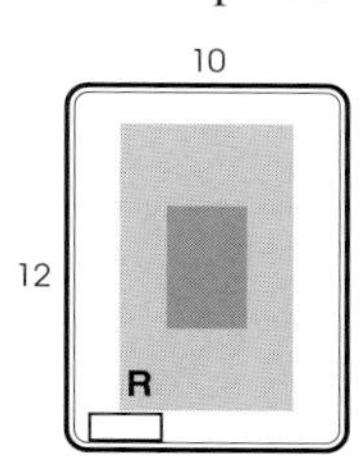

Technical Factors

- Film size–10 x 12 in. (24 x 30 cm), lengthwise.
- Moving or stationary grid, vertical, CR to centerline.
- 75±5 kVp range.
- Minimum of 3 sec. exposure time with breathing technique (4 or 5 sec. is desirable).
- Technique and dose:

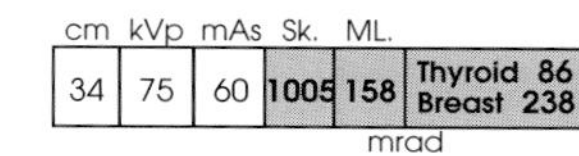

cm	kVp	mAs	Sk.	ML.	
34	75	60	1005	158	Thyroid 86 Breast 238

mrad

Shielding: Secure gonadal shield at waist to cover pelvic area.

Patient Position

- May be taken erect or supine. (Erect preferred, which also may be more comfortable for patient.)
- Place patient in lateral position with side of interest against cassette. With patient supine, place grid lines vertically, and center CR to centerline to prevent grid cutoff.

Part Position

- Affected arm at patient's side in **neutral rotation**; drop shoulder if possible (see Note 1).
- Raise opposite arm and place hand over top of head, elevate shoulder as much as possible to prevent superimposing affected shoulder.
- Center surgical neck and center of film to CR as projected through thorax.
- Ensure that thorax is in a true lateral position or with slight anterior rotation of unaffected shoulder so humerus is not superimposed by thoracic vertebrae.

Central Ray

- CR perpendicular to film directed through thorax to **surgical neck** (see Note 2).
- Minimum 40 in. (102 cm) SID.

Collimation: Collimate on four sides to area of interest, remembering the divergence of x-ray beam.

Respiration: Breathing technique is preferred if patient can cooperate. Patient should be asked to gently breathe short shallow breaths without moving affected arm or shoulder. (This will best visualize proximal humerus by blurring out ribs and lung structures.)

Note 1: With possible fracture or dislocation, **arm should not be rotated** but taken as is, which will result in a 90° or right angle view of proximal humerus, compared to the AP projection also taken without arm rotation. (Forced rotation of arm with a fracture may result in displacement of fractured humeral head or neck.)

Note 2: If patient is in too much pain to drop injured shoulder sufficiently and elevate uninjured arm and shoulder high enough to prevent superimposition of shoulders, **then angle CR 10 to 15° cephalad**.

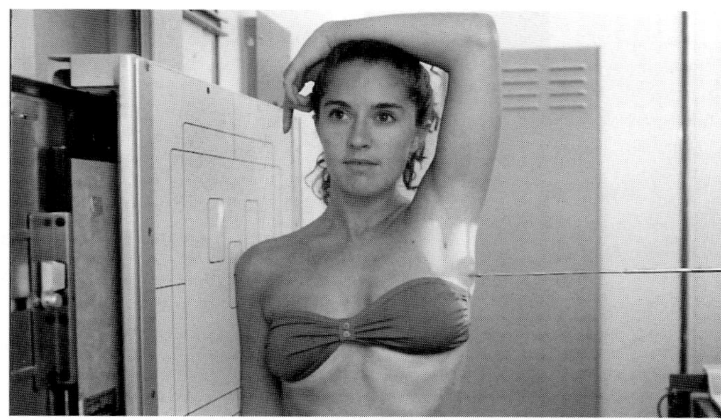

Fig. 5-52. Erect transthoracic lateral projection (R lateral).

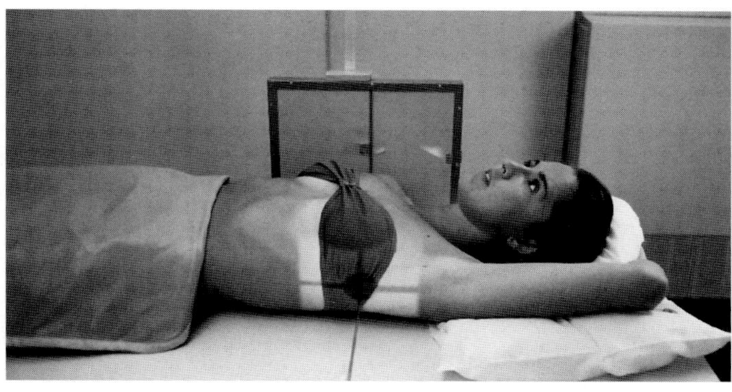

Fig. 5-53. Supine transthoracic lateral projection (R lateral).

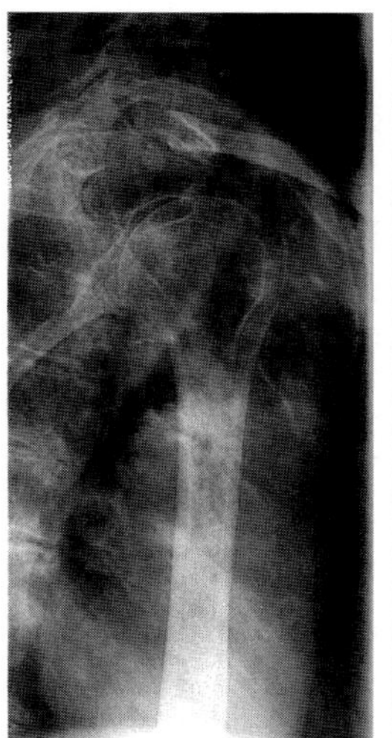

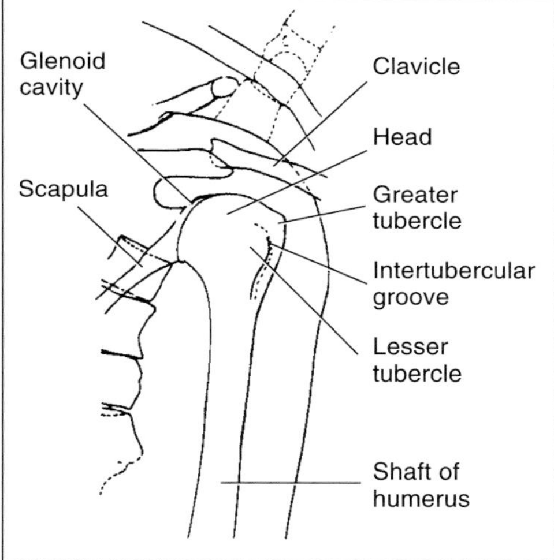

Fig. 5-54. Transthoracic lateral. Fig. 5-55.

Evaluation Criteria

- Proximal half of humerus and scapulohumeral joint should be visualized without superimposition by opposite shoulder.
- The outline of proximal humerus should be clearly visualized anterior to the thoracic vertebrae. Ribs and lung structures should appear blurred if breathing technique was used correctly.
- The relationship of the humeral head and glenoid cavity of scapula should be demonstrated.
- Optimum exposure should visualize the entire border outlines of the humeral head and the proximal half of the humerus.
- Neutral rotation should present a view which is 90° to the AP projection also taken without forced rotation of humerus. (The anterior location of the greater tubercle in the above radiograph indicates some internal rotation of humerus.)

AP Apical Oblique Axial Projection (RPO or LPO Positions)

Garth Method

Shoulder (trauma)
Basic
- AP (neutral rotation)
- Scapular Y lateral and Neer method
  or
  Transthoracic lateral

Special
- **Apical oblique (Garth method)**

Structures Best Shown

The humeral head, glenoid cavity and scapular head and neck are well demonstrated. A good projection for possible scapulohumeral dislocations (especially posterior dislocations), glenoid fractures, Hill-Sachs lesions and soft tissue calcifications. This is a recommended projection for acute shoulder trauma radiography.* This view was also described by Garth et. al. in 1984 to demonstrate scapulohumeral instability.†

Technical Factors

- Film size–8 x 10 in. (18 x 24 cm), lengthwise.
- Moving or stationary grid.
- 75±5 kVp range.
- Technique and dose:

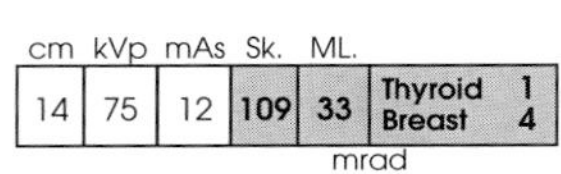

cm	kVp	mAs	Sk.	ML.	mrad	
14	75	12	109	33	Thyroid	1
					Breast	4

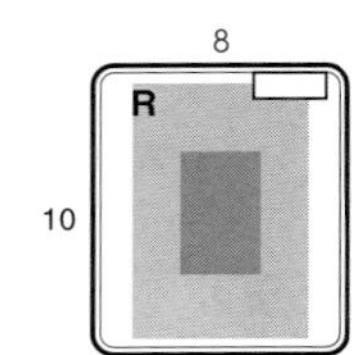

Shielding: Shield lungs and pelvic area.

Patient Position

- Erect or supine. (Erect is usually less painful if patient's condition allows.)
- Rotate body **45° toward affected side**. (Posterior surface of affected shoulder against cassette.)

Part Position

- Center scapulohumeral joint to CR.
- Adjust cassette so the 45° angled CR will direct the scapulohumeral joint to the center of the film.
- Flex elbow and place arm across chest, or with trauma, arm at side as is.

Central Ray

- CR **45° caudad**, centered **to the scapulohumeral joint.**
- Minimum 40 in. (102 cm) SID.

Collimation: Collimate closely to area of interest.

Respiration: Suspend respiration during exposure.

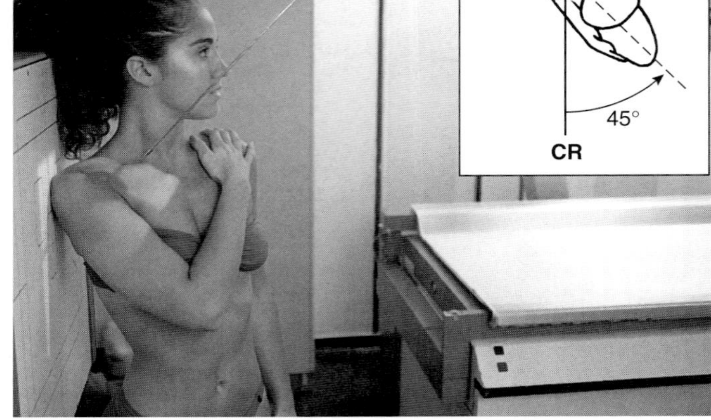

Fig. 5-56. Erect apical oblique axial projection –45° posterior oblique, CR 45° caudad.

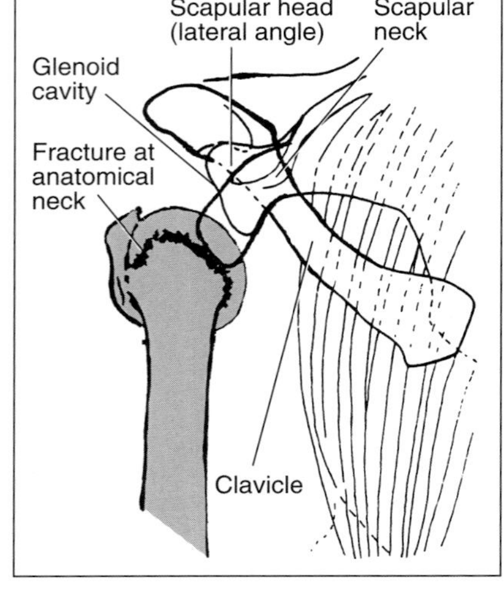

Fig. 5-57. Apical oblique projection. Fig. 5-58.
(Note impacted fracture of humeral head but no scapulohumeral dislocation.)

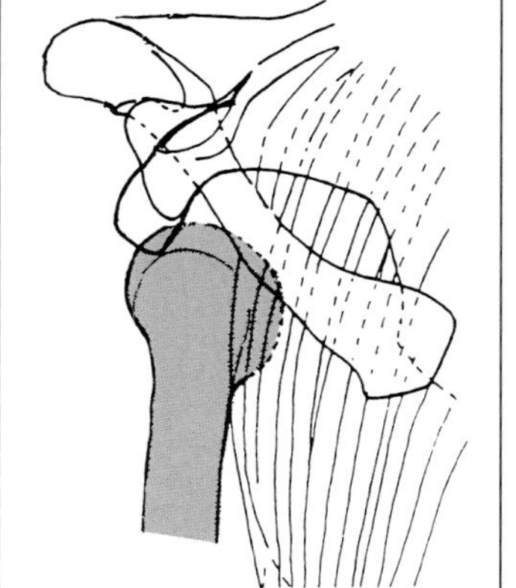

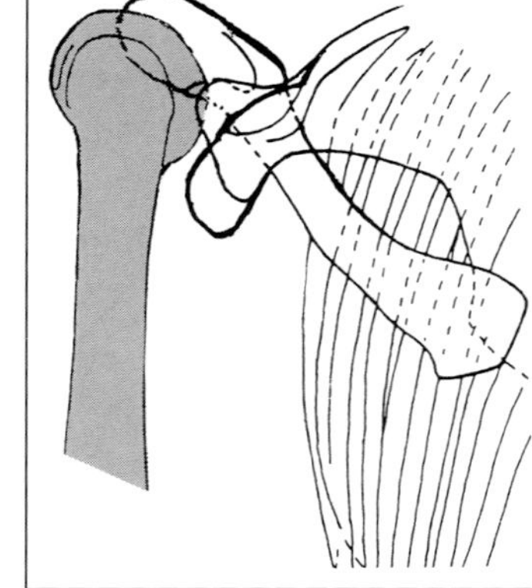

Fig. 5-59. Appearance of humerus if there were a dislocation. Fig. 5-60.
–Anterior dislocation (most common), humerus projected inferiorly. –Posterior dislocation, humerus projected superiorly.

Evaluation Criteria

- The humeral head, glenoid cavity and neck and head of the scapula are well demonstrated free of superimposition except for the coracoid process, which should be visible as projected over the mid scapulohumeral joint region. The clavicle will appear curved and distorted and the acromion and AC joint should be projected superior to the humeral head.
- **Dislocations**: A posterior dislocation of the humerus will project the humeral head superior or cephalic to the glenoid cavity; an anterior dislocation will project the humeral head inferiorly or caudally.
- The center of the collimation field should be to the lateral angle (head) of the scapula.
- Optimum exposure with no motion will be evidenced by sharp borders and fine trabecular markings. Correct exposure will visualize the outline of the scapular spine and coracoid process and soft tissue detail to show possible calcifications.

*Sloth C, Lundgren, JS. The Apical Oblique Radiograph in Examination of Acute Shoulder Trauma. *Europ. J. Radiol.* 1989; 9:147-151.
†Garth Jr., WP, Slappey, CE, Ochs, CW. Roentgenographic Demonstration of Instability of the Shoulder: The Apical Oblique Projection. *Bone Joint Surg.* 1984; 66-A:1450-1453.

AP and AP Axial Projections

Clavicle
Basic
• AP and AP axial

Structures Best Shown

Clavicle, including acromioclavicular and sternoclavicular joints.

Departmental routines most frequently include both the AP 0° and AP axial projections.

Technical Factors

- Film size–10 x 12 in. (24 x 30 cm) crosswise.
- Moving or stationary grid.
- AEC not recommended.
- 70±5 kVp range.
- Technique and dose:

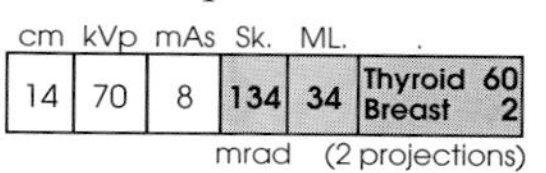

cm	kVp	mAs	Sk.	ML.	
14	70	8	134	34	Thyroid 60 Breast 2

mrad (2 projections)

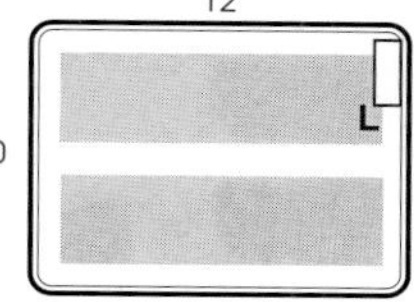
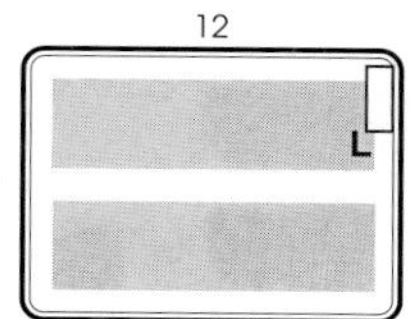

Shielding: Shield female breast and pelvic area.

Patient Position

- Erect or supine with arms at sides, chin raised, looking straight ahead.
- Posterior shoulder should be in contact with cassette or table-top, without rotation of body.

Part Position

- Center clavicle and film holder to CR. (Clavicle can readily be palpated with medial aspect at jugular notch and lateral portion at AC joint above shoulder.)

Central Ray

AP:

- CR **perpendicular,** to **mid clavicle**

AP Axial:

- CR **15 to 30° cephalad,** to **mid clavicle** (see Note).
- Minimum 40 in. (102 cm) SID.

Collimation: Collimate to area of clavicle. (Ensure that both acromioclavicular and sternoclavicular joints are included.)

Respiration: Suspend respiration at end of exhalation.

Alternate PA: May also be taken as a PA projection and/ or a PA axial with 15 to 20° caudal angle.

Note: Thin shoulders (asthenic) require 10 to 15° more angle than thick shoulders and chest (hypersthenic).

Fig. 5-61. AP–CR 0°.

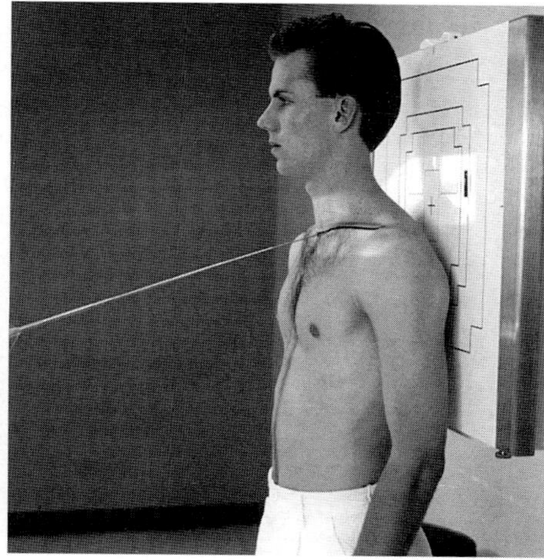

Fig. 5-62. AP axial–CR 15 to 30° cephalad.

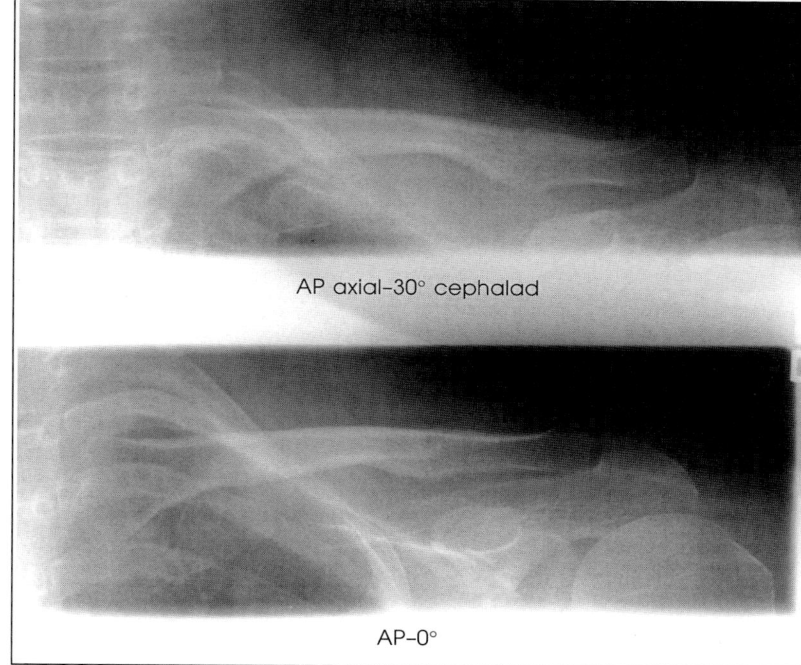

Fig. 5-63. AP axial and AP clavicle–female with thick shoulders.

Evaluation Criteria

AP 0°:

- Collimation borders should be visible with entire clavicle visualized, including both AC and sternoclavicular joints.

AP Axial:

- Correct angulation of CR will project most of the clavicle above the scapula and ribs. Only the medial portion of clavicle will be superimposed by the first and second ribs.
- Optimum exposure will visualize the distal clavicle and AC joint without excessive density. The bony margins of the medial clavicle and sternoclavicular joint should also be visualized through the thorax.

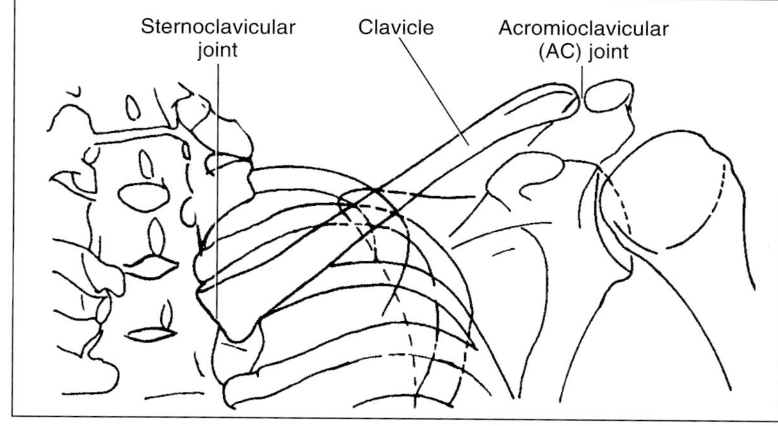

Fig. 5-64. AP clavicle–CR 0°, male.

5

AP Projection

Bilateral With and Without Weights

Warning: Shoulder and/or clavicle projections should be completed first to rule out fractures.

AC joints
Basic
- **AP bilateral with weights and AP bilateral without weights**

Structures Best Shown:

Both AC joint spaces for comparison with and without stress. Demonstrates possible separation of joint spaces.

A widening of one joint space as compared with the other during the weight-bearing projection usually indicates an AC joint separation.

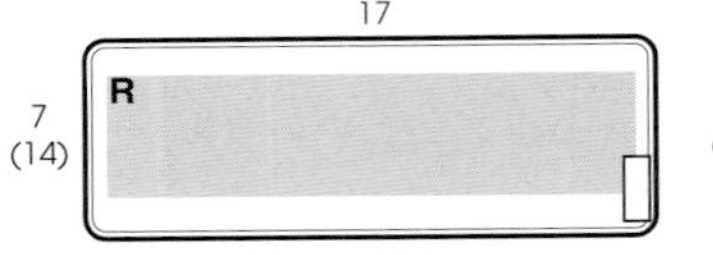

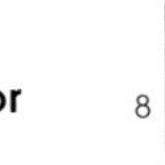

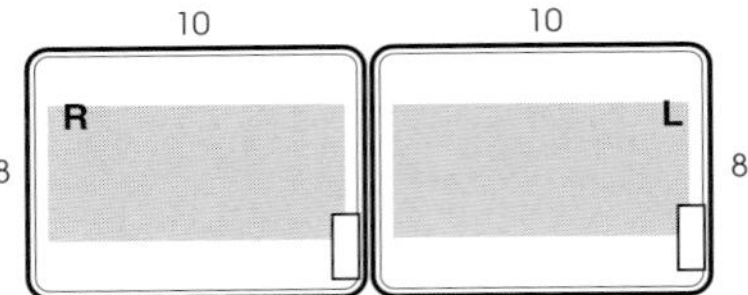

Technical Factors

- Film size–One 7 x 17 in. (18 x 43 cm) crosswise (or 14 x 17 in. if 7 x 17 in. is not available).
- Use "with weight" and "without weight" markers.
- Detail screen, non-grid.
- AEC not recommended.
- 65±5 kVp with screen; 65-70 kVp with grid on larger patients.
- For broad-shouldered patients, use two 8 x 10 in. (18 x 24 cm) cassettes crosswise placed side by side and exposed simultaneously to include both AC joints on one exposure.
- Technique and dose:

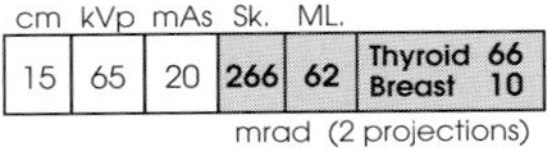

cm	kVp	mAs	Sk.	ML.	
15	65	20	266	62	Thyroid 66 Breast 10

mrad (2 projections)

Shielding: Secure gonadal shield around waist.

Patient Position

- Erect, posterior shoulders against cassette with equal weight on both feet, arms at side, no rotation of shoulders or pelvis, looking straight ahead. (May be taken seated if patient's condition requires.)
- **Two sets** of bilateral AC joints are taken in the same position, one **without weights** and one **stress view with weights.**

Part Position

- Position patient to direct CR to midway between AC joints.
- Center midline of film holder(s) to CR (top of film should be ≈2 in. or 5 cm above shoulders).

Central Ray

- CR perpendicular, to a **midpoint between AC joints**, 1 in. or 2.5 cm above jugular notch.
- Minimum 72 in. (180 cm) SID.

Collimation: Collimate with a long narrow light field to area of interest; upper light border should be to upper shoulder soft tissue margins.

Respiration: Suspend respiration during exposure.

Weights: After the first exposure is made without weights and the cassette(s) has (have) been changed, for large adult patients strap 10 to 15 lb. weights to each wrist and with shoulders relaxed, **gently** allow weights to hang from wrists pulling down on each arm and shoulder. The same amount of weight must be used on each wrist. Less weight (8 to 10 lbs. per limb) may be used for smaller or asthenic patients, and more weight for larger or hypersthenic patients.

Note: Patients should **NOT** be asked to hold on to the weights with their hands, rather the **weights must be attached to the wrists so the hands, arms and shoulders are relaxed**, to determine possible AC joint separation. Holding on to weights may result in false negative radiographs because they will tend to pull on the weights, resulting in contraction rather than relaxation of the shoulder muscles.*

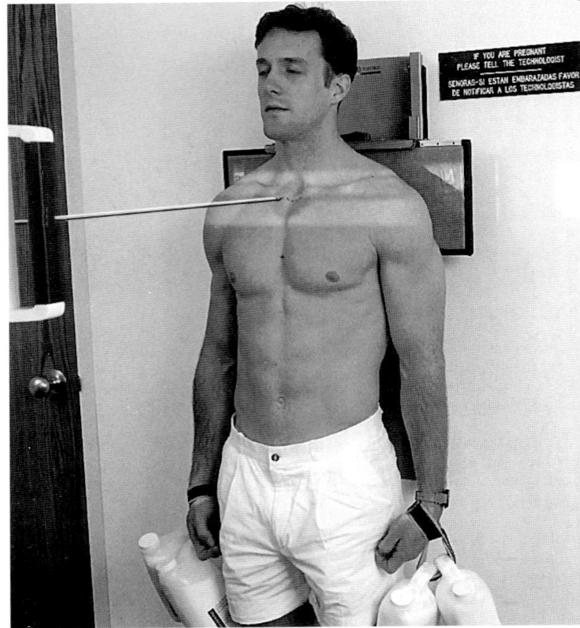

Fig. 5-66. Stress view with weights (weights **tied** to wrists). Male, 10 to 15 lbs, **two** films side-by-side.

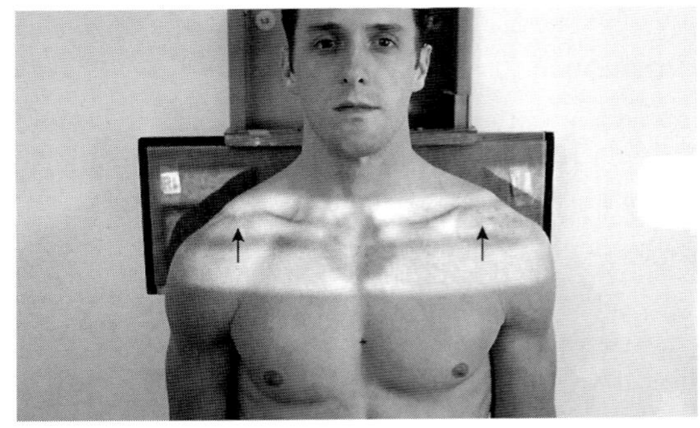

Fig. 5-67. AC joints marked by arrows.

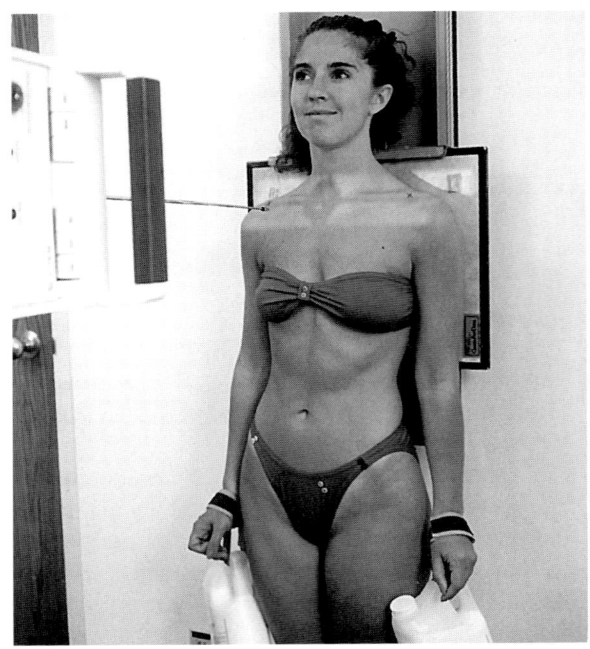

Fig. 5-68. Stress view with weights (weights **tied** to wrists). Female, 8 to 10 lbs, **one** film crosswise.

* James A. Rand, M.D.; Mayo Clinic, Rochester, MN; 1990.

AP Projection continued

Bilateral With and Without Weights

Alternate supine position: If patient's condition requires, may be done supine by tying both ends of a long strip of gauze to patient's wrists and placing around patient's feet with knees partially flexed, then **slowly** and **gently** straighten legs pulling down on shoulders. May also be done by an assistant **gently** pulling down on arms and shoulders.

Warning: This method should only be done by experienced and qualified personnel to prevent additional injury.

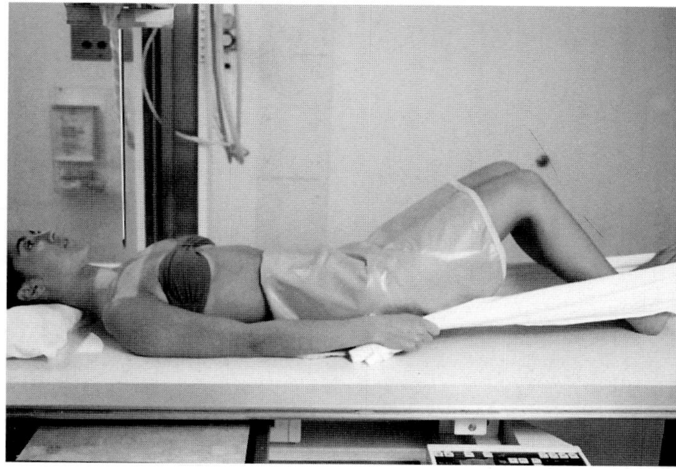

Fig. 5-69. Alternate supine position.

Evaluation Criteria

- Long narrow collimation field should visualize both AC joints as well as the entire clavicles and sternoclavicular joints on one or two separate radiographs exposed simultaneously.
- No rotation, as evidenced by symmetrical appearance of sternoclavicular joints on each side of vertebral column.
- Both AC joints should be on the same horizontal plane.
- Optimum exposure without motion should clearly visualize AC joints and soft tissue without excessive density.
- R and L markers as well as markers indicating stress (with weights) and non stress (without weights) should be visible without superimposing essential anatomy.

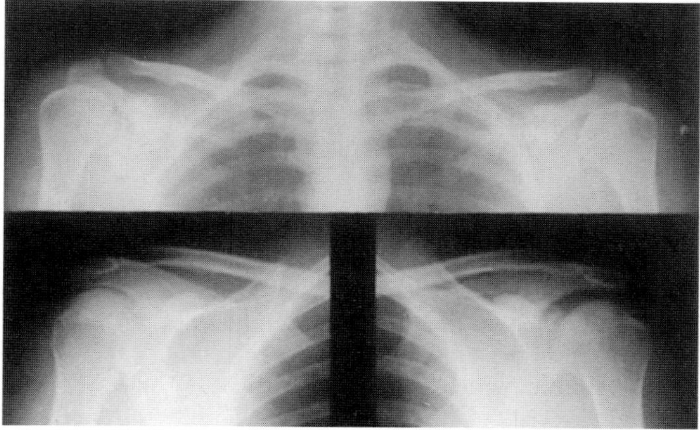

Fig. 5-70. AP acromioclavicular joints (single film and two films exposed simultaneously).

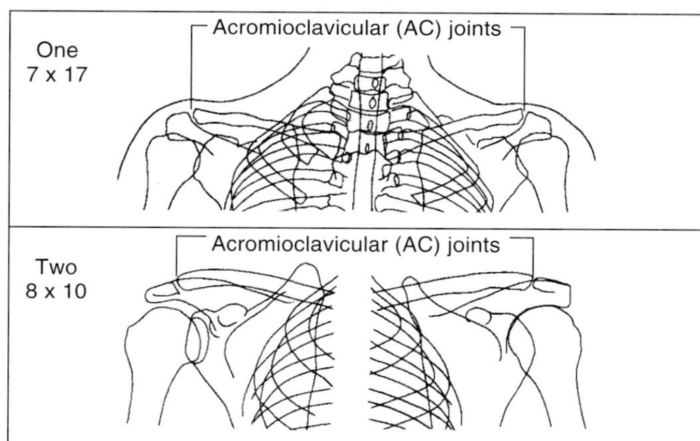

Fig. 5-71. AC joints.

AP Projection

Scapula
Basic
• **AP**
• Lateral

Structures Best Shown

Frontal view of scapula with lateral border free from rib superimposition.

Technical Factors

- Film size–10 x 12 in. (24 x 30 cm) lengthwise.
- Moving or stationary grid.
- 75±5 kVp range.
- Minimum of 3 sec. exposure time with breathing technique. (4 or 5 sec. is desirable).
- Technique and dose:

cm	kVp	mAs	Sk.	ML.	mrad
15	75	7	66	17	Thyroid 1, Breast 25

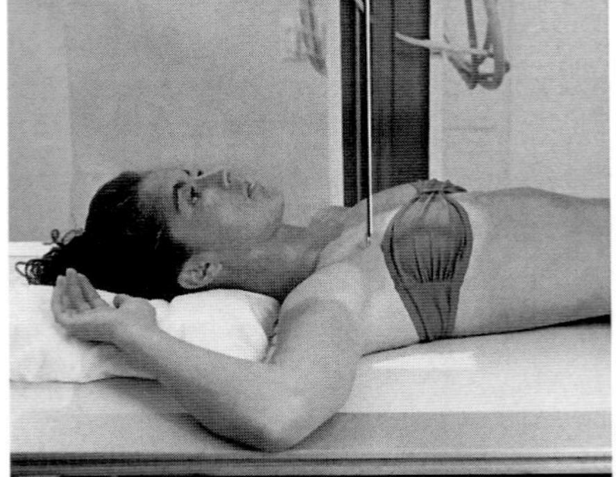

Fig. 5-72. AP supine.

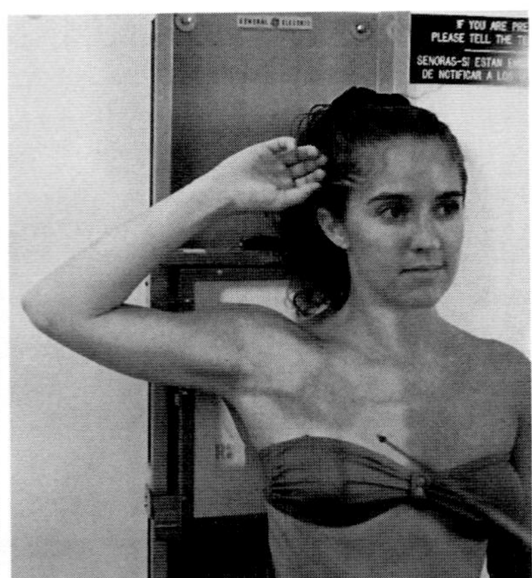

Fig. 5-73. AP erect.

Shielding: Place gonadal shield over pelvic area.

Patient Position

- May be taken erect or supine. (Erect may be more comfortable for patient.)
- Posterior surface of shoulder in direct contact with table-top or cassette without rotation of thorax. (Rotation toward affected side will place scapula into a truer frontal position, but it will also result in greater superimposition of rib cage.)

Part Position

- Position patient so mid scapula area is centered to CR.
- Adjust film holder to center to CR. Top of film should be about 2 in. or 5 cm above shoulder, and lateral border of film about 2 in. or 5 cm from lateral margin of rib cage.
- Gently **abduct arm 90°** and supinate hand. (Abduction will move scapula laterally to clear more of thoracic structures.)

Central Ray

- CR perpendicular, **to mid scapula, 2 in. (5 cm) inferior to coracoid process**, or to **level of axilla and ≈2 in. (5 cm) medial from lateral border of patient**.
- Minimum 40 in. (102 cm) SID.

Collimation: Collimate on four sides to area of scapula.

Respiration: Breathing technique is preferred if patient can cooperate. Ask patient to breathe gently without moving affected shoulder or arm.

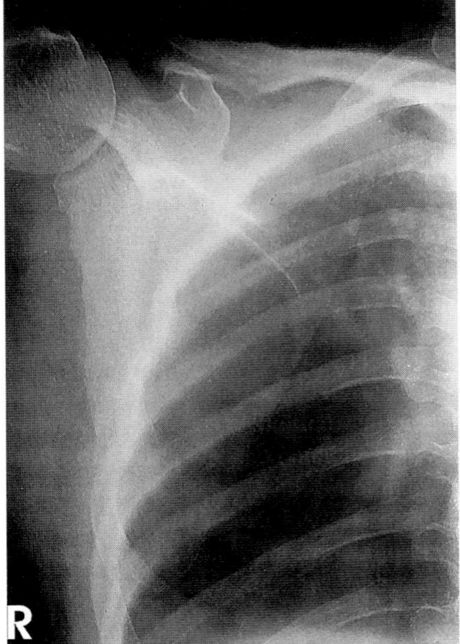

Fig. 5-74. AP scapula.

Evaluation Criteria

- The entire scapula should be visualized. (Approximately half of scapula will be seen through blurred thoracic structures with breathing technique.)
- Collimation borders should be visible on four sides with center of collimation field to mid-scapula area.
- Entire lateral portion of scapula should be visible without superimposition of ribs and lung. (Indicates correct abduction of arm and no rotation or obliquity of thorax.)
- Optimum exposure will visualize bony margins and trabecular markings of lateral portion of scapula. The medial aspect of the scapula should be visualized without excessive density wherein the bony margins of the vertebral border should be visible through the lung field along its entirety. Ribs and lung structures will appear blurred with proper breathing technique.

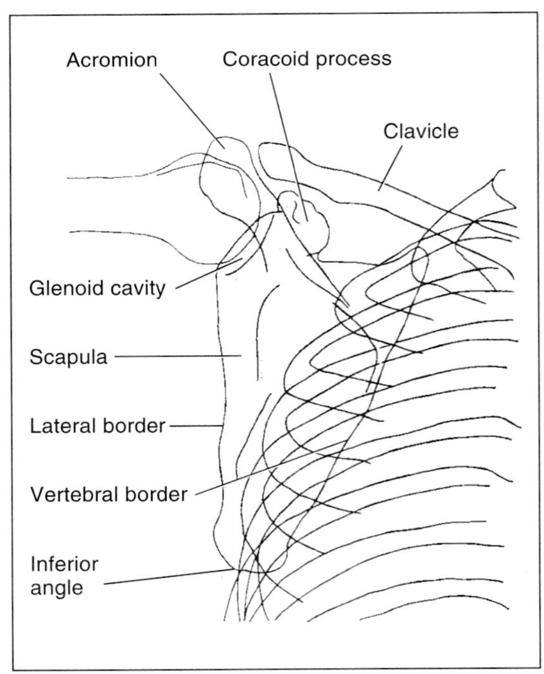

Fig. 5-75. AP scapula.

Lateral Projection–RAO or LAO Body Position

Scapula
Basic
• AP
• **Lateral**

Structures Best Shown

Lateral scapula projected clear of the rib cage. Arm placement should be determined by scapular area of interest to result in the least superimposition of scapula by humerus

Technical Factors

- Film size–10 x 12 in. (24 x 30 cm) lengthwise.
- Moving or stationary grid.
- AEC not recommended.
- 75±5 kVp range.
- Technique and dose:

cm	kVp	mAs	Sk.	ML.	
16	75	13	131	38	Thyroid 0 Breast 0

mrad

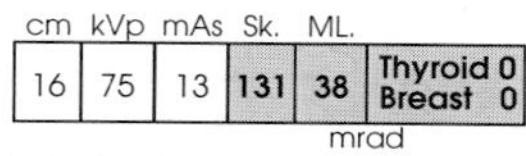

Shielding: Secure gonadal shield around waist.

Patient Position

- Erect or recumbent position. Erect position is preferred.
- Patient facing cassette in an anterior oblique position.

Part Position

- Have patient reach across front of chest and grasp opposite shoulder. This best demonstrates the **body** of the scapula (Figs. 5-76 and 5-77).

or

- Have patient drop affected arm, flex elbow and place arm behind lower back with arm partially abducted, or just let arm hang down at patient's side. This best demonstrates **acromion and coracoid processes** (Figs. 5-78 and 5-79).
- **Palpate borders of scapula** and rotate patient until the scapula is in a **true lateral position**. The average patient will be rotated 30 to 45° from the lateral position. (Results in a 45 to 60° anterior oblique position.) The position of humerus (down at side or up across anterior chest) has an effect on the amount of body rotation required. Less rotation is required with arm up across anterior chest. (The flat posterior surface of scapula should be perpendicular to film.)
- Align patient so as to center mid vertebral border to CR, and to center of film.

Central Ray

- CR to **mid vertebral border of scapula**.
- Minimum 40 in. (102 cm) SID.

Collimation: Collimate to area of scapula.

Respiration: Suspend respiration during exposure.

Recumbent trauma posterior oblique: May also be taken recumbent in the opposite posterior oblique if patient's condition requires. The affected side would then be "up side" away from the film with the body again rotated until the scapula is in a true lateral position. See Chapter 19 for trauma lateral scapula.

Evaluation Criteria

- Entire scapula should be visualized within collimation field in a lateral position, as evidenced by direct superimposition of vertebral and lateral borders.
- Body of scapula should be seen in profile, free of superimposition by ribs.
- As much as possible, the humerus should not superimpose area of interest of the scapula.
- Optimum exposure should visualize the entire scapula without excessive density in area of inferior angle. Bony borders of both the acromion and coracoid processes should be seen through the head of the humerus.

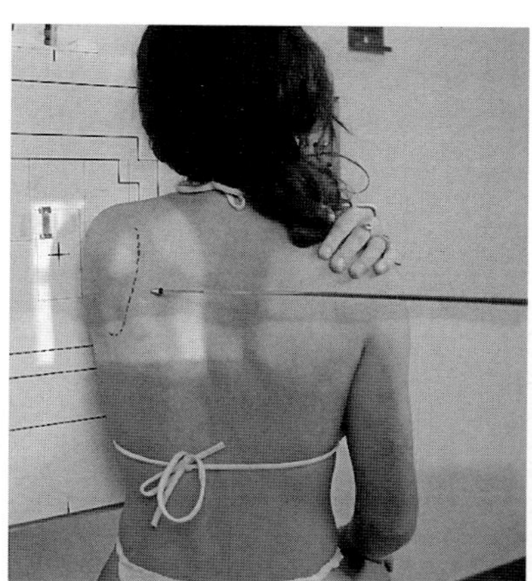

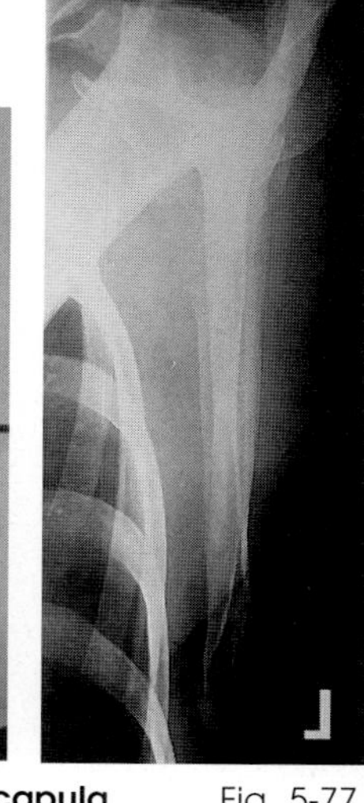

Fig. 5-76. Lateral for **body of scapula**. (≈45° LAO) Fig. 5-77.

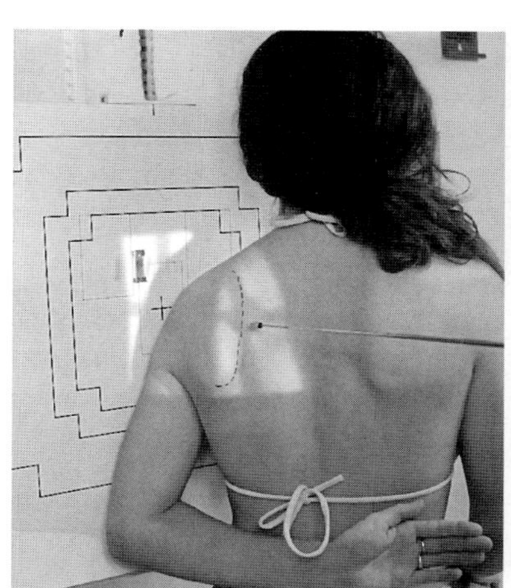

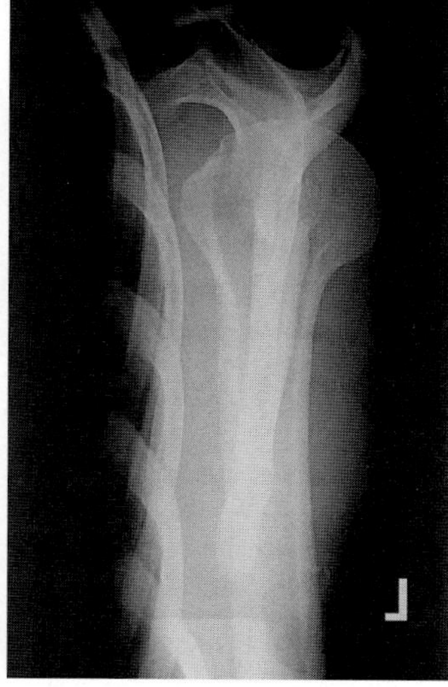

Fig. 5-78. Lateral for **acromion or coracoid process**. (≈60° LAO) Fig. 5-79.

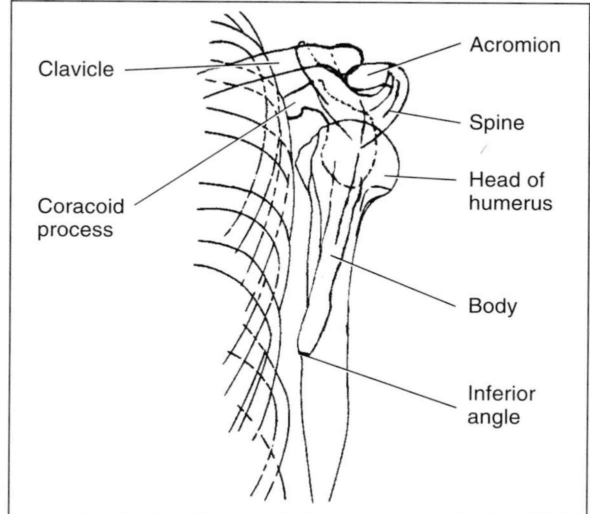

Fig. 5-80. Lateral scapula.

Radiographs for Critique

Each of these proximal humerus and shoulder girdle radiographs demonstrates some error in positioning which requires a repeat. These along with accompanying lecture slides of these and other radiographs will provide a basis for classroom and/or positioning lab discussion. Questions with answers based on these specific critique radiographs are provided in the accompanying student workbook/lab manuals to help prepare students for classroom and/or lab discussions on film critique.

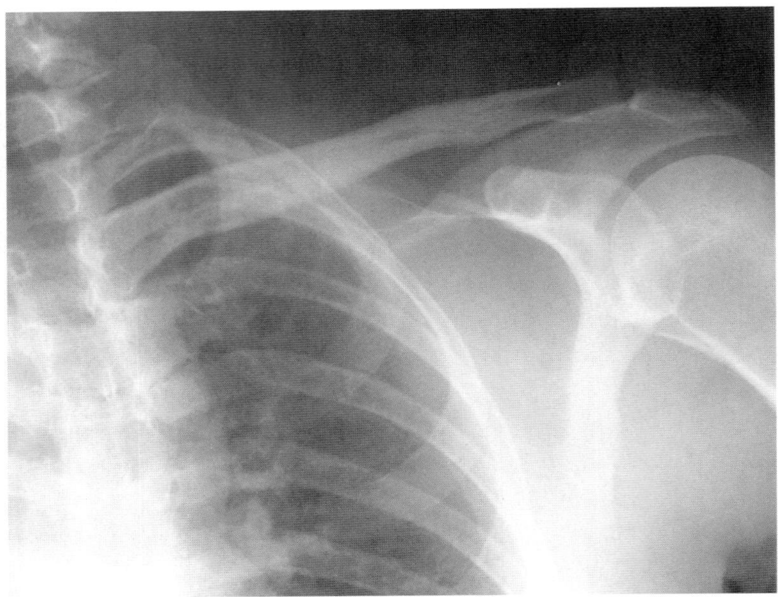

Fig. C5-81. AP clavicle.

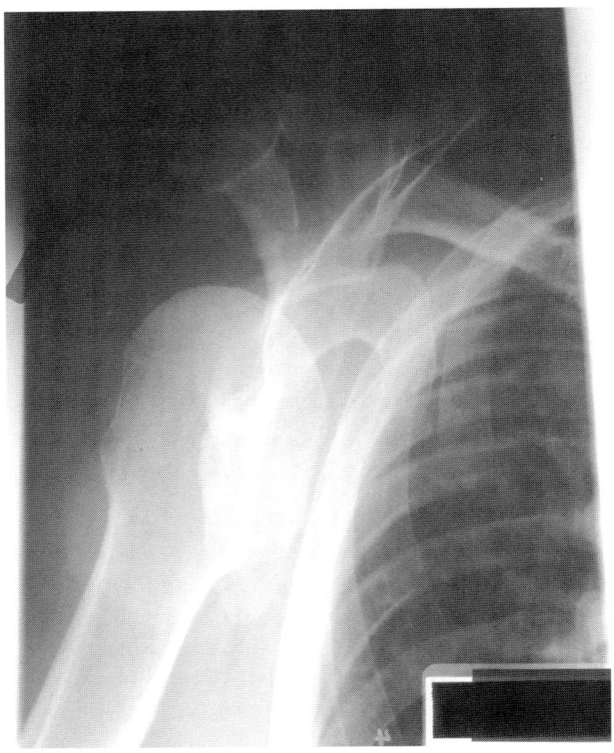

Fig. C5-82. AP apical oblique axial shoulder (Garth method)

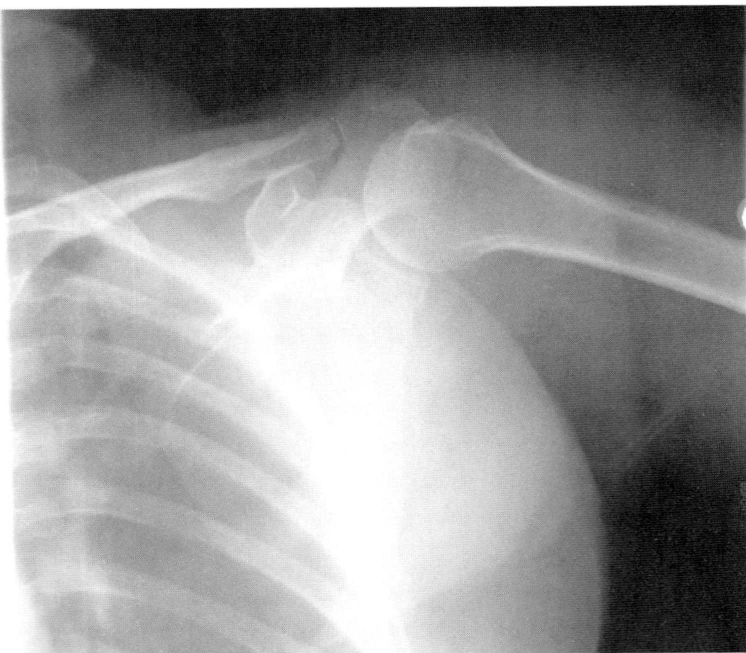

Fig. C5-83. AP scapula.

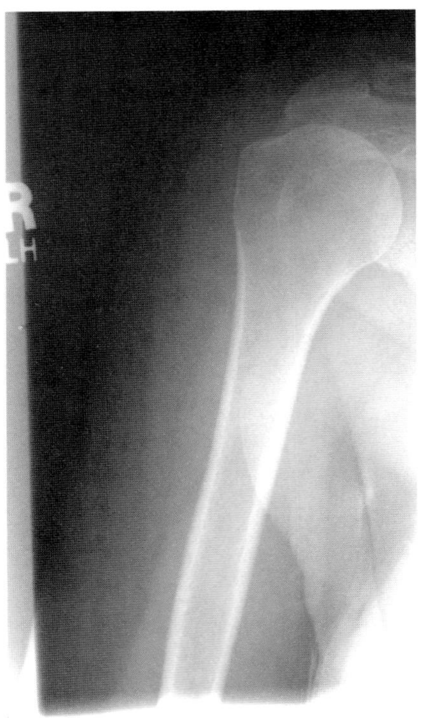

Fig. C5-84. AP shoulder and proximal humerus.

CHAPTER 6

Lower Limb

CONTRIBUTIONS BY:
Eugene D. Frank, MA, RT (R), FASRT
J. Fred Price, MS, RT (R), FASRT

CONTENTS

Radiographic Anatomy

Foot–Phalanges and metatarsals **172**

Joints and sesamoid bones **173**

Tarsals **174**

Arches of foot **175**

Ankle joint **176**

Anatomy review with radiographs **177**

Leg–Tibia and fibula **178**

Distal femur **179**

Knee joint **180**

Anatomy review with radiographs **182**

Classification of joints **183**

Surfaces, projections, and motions of foot and ankle **184**

Radiographic Positioning

Positioning considerations **185**

Survey information **186**

Basic and special projections **188**

Toes:
- AP **189**
- Oblique **190**
- Lateral **191**
- Sesamoids **192**

Foot:
- AP **193**
- Oblique **194**
- Lateral **195**
- AP and lateral (weight-bearing) **196**

Calcaneus:
- Plantodorsal (axial) **197**
- Lateral **198**

Radiographic Positioning cont.

Ankle:
- AP **199**
- AP mortise (15° oblique) **200**
- AP oblique (45°) **201**
- Lateral **202**
- AP stress **203**

Leg–Tibia and fibula:
- AP **204**
- Lateral **205**

Knee:
- AP **206**
- Oblique **207**
- Lateral **208**
- AP (PA) (weight-bearing) **209**

Knee–Intercondylar fossa:
- PA axial (Camp Coventry and Holmblad methods) **210**
- AP axial **211**

Patella and patellofemoral joint:
- PA **212**
- Lateral **213**
- Tangential (Merchant method) **214**
- Tangential (inferosuperior, Hughston and Settegast methods) **215**
- PA oblique and axial oblique (Kuchendorf method) **216**

Mid and distal femur:
- AP **217**
- Lateral **218**

Mid and proximal femur:
- AP (see AP hip, Chapter 7)
- Lateral **219**

Radiographs for critique **220**

Radiographic Anatomy

Lower Limb

The bones of the lower limb are divided into four main groups, the foot, leg, femur and hip. This chapter includes a thorough study of the anatomy and positioning for the three groups, the **foot**, **leg**, and **mid** and **distal femur**. The **ankle** and **knee joints** are also included in this study.

FOOT

The bones of the foot are fundamentally very similar to the bones of the hand and wrist studied in Chapter 4.

The 26 bones of one foot are divided into three groups:

Phalanges (toes/or digits)	14
Metatarsals (instep)	5
Tarsals	7
Total	26

Phalanges–Toes (Digits)

The most distal bones of the foot are the **phalanges**, which make up the toes or digits. The five digits of each foot are numbered one through five starting on the medial or big toe side of the foot. Note that the large toe or first digit has only two phalanges, similar to that of the thumb. These are the **proximal phalanx** and the **distal phalanx**. Each of the second, third, fourth and fifth digits has a **middle phalanx** in addition to a proximal and a distal phalanx. Since the first digit has two phalanges, and digits two through five have three apiece, there are **14 phalanges** in each foot.

The similarities to the hand are obvious in that there are also 14 phalanges in each hand. However, there are two noticeable differences in that the phalanges of the foot are smaller, and their movements are more limited than those of the hand.

When describing any of the bones or joints of the foot, the specific digit and foot should also be identified. For example, the distal phalanx of the first digit of the right foot would leave no doubt as to which bone is in question.

It should be noted that the distal phalanges of the second through fifth toes are very small and may be difficult to identify as separate bones on a radiograph.

Metatarsals

The five bones of the instep are the **metatarsal** bones. These are numbered along with the digits with number one on the medial side and number five on the lateral side.

Each of the metatarsals is composed of three parts. The small, rounded, distal part of each metatarsal is the **head.** The centrally located, long, slender portion is termed the **body** (shaft). The expanded, proximal end of each metatarsal is the **base.**

The **base of the fifth metatarsal** is expanded laterally into a prominent rough **tuberosity**, which provides for the attachment of a tendon. The proximal portion of the fifth metacarpal, including this tuberosity, is readily visible on radiographs and is **a common trauma site** for the foot, therefore, this area must be well visualized on radiographs.

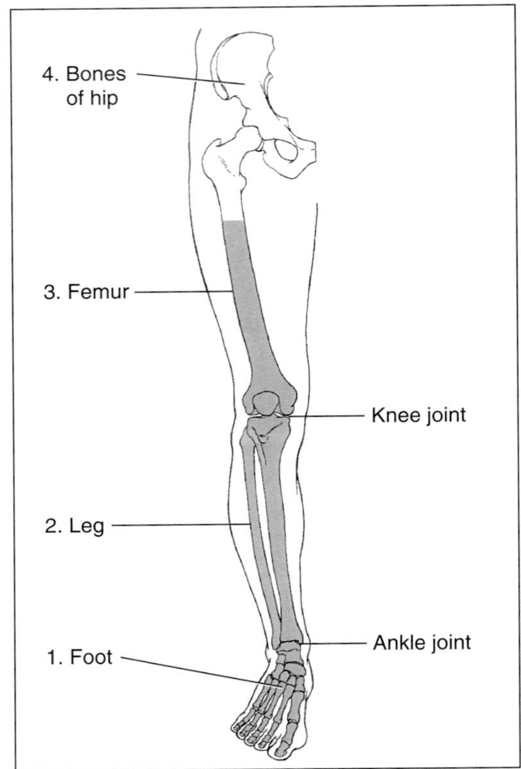

Fig. 6-1. Lower limb.

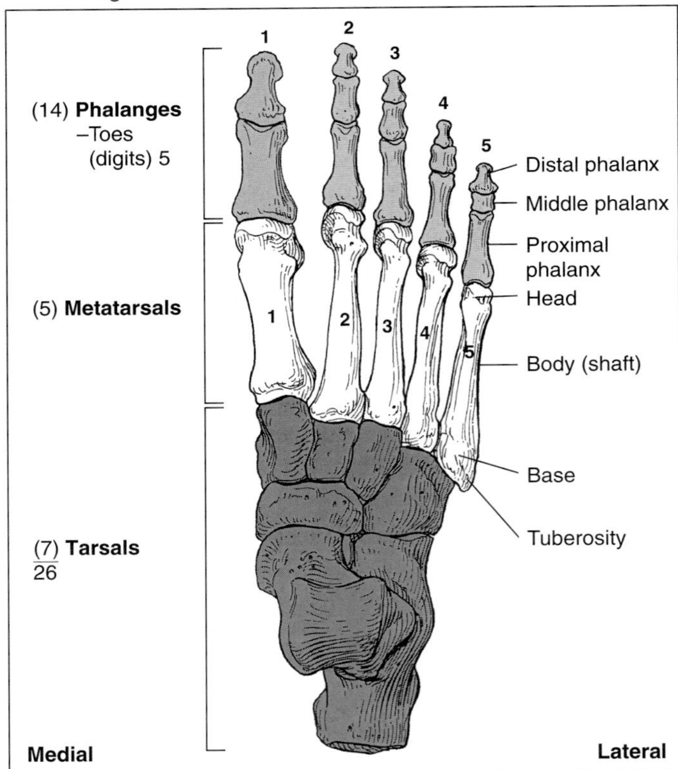

Fig. 6-2. Bones of foot.

Joints of Phalanges (Digits) and Metatarsals

Joints of Digits: The joints or articulations of the digits of the foot are important to identify since fractures may involve the joint surfaces. Each joint of the foot has a name derived from the two bones on either side of that joint. Between the proximal and distal phalanges of the first digit is the **interphalangeal** or **IP joint**.

Since digits two through five are comprised of three bones each, these digits also each have two joints. Between the middle and distal phalanges is the **distal interphalangeal joint** or **DIP** joint. Between the proximal and middle phalanges is the **proximal interphalangeal joint** or **PIP joint.**

Joints of Metatarsals: Each of the joints at the head of the metatarsal is a **metatarsophalangeal** or **MP joint,** while each of the joints at the base of the metatarsal is a **tarsometatarsal joint** or **TM joint.** The base of the third metatarsal or the third tarsometatarsal joint is important because this is the centering point or the central ray (CR) location for an AP and oblique foot.

When describing joints of the foot, it is important to state the name of the joint first, then include which digit or metatarsal as well as which foot. For example, an injury or fracture may be described as near the distal interphalangeal joint of the fifth digit of the left foot.

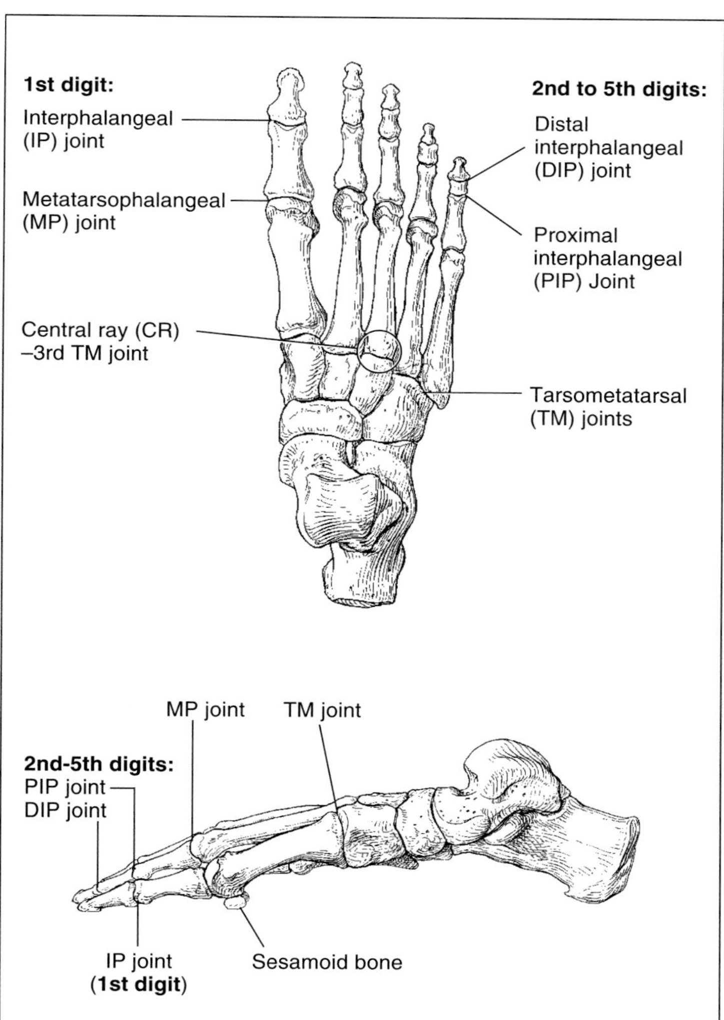

Fig. 6-3. Joints of right foot.

Sesamoid Bones

Several small detached bones, called **sesamoid** bones, are often found in the feet and hands. These extra bones, which are embedded in certain tendons, are often present near various joints. In the upper limbs sesamoid bones are quite small and most often found on the palmar surface near the metacarpophalangeal joints, or occasionally at the interphalangeal joint of the thumb.

In the **lower limbs**, sesamoid bones tend to be larger and more significant radiographically. The largest sesamoid bone in the body is the patella or knee cap, as described later in this chapter. Also, the sesamoid bones illustrated in Fig. 6-3 and 6-4 are almost always present on the posterior or **plantar surface at the head of the first metatarsal** near the first metatarsophalangeal joint. Sesamoid bones may also be found near other joints of the foot. Sesamoid bones are important radiographically, because it is possible to fracture these small bones. Due to their plantar location, they can be quite painful and cause discomfort when placing weight on that foot. Special tangential projections may be necessary to demonstrate a fracture of a sesamoid bone, as will be demonstrated later in this chapter (page 192).

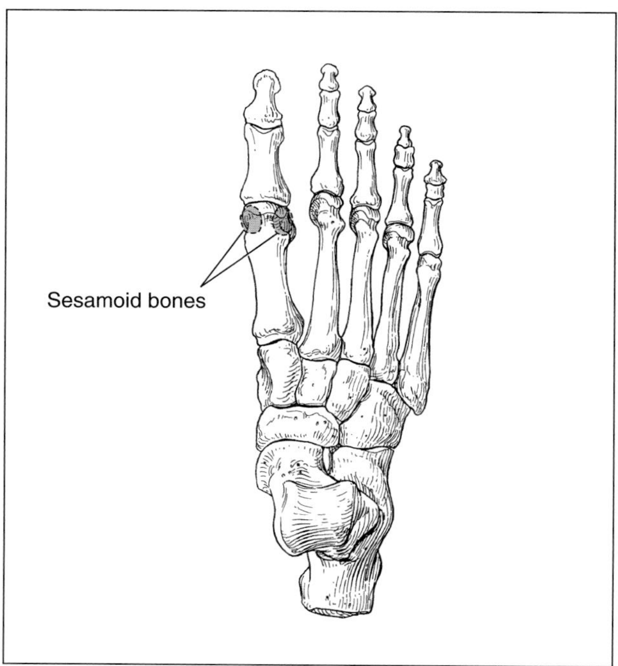

Fig. 6-4. Sesamoid bones.

TARSALS

The seven large bones of the proximal foot are termed tarsal bones. The names of the tarsals can be remembered with the aid of a mnemonic: **C**ome **T**o **C**olorado (the) **N**ext **3 C**hristmases.

(1) **C**ome –**C**alcaneus (Os Calcis)
(2) **T**o –**T**alus (Astragalus)
(3) **C**olorado –**C**uboid
(4) **N**ext –**N**avicular (Scaphoid)
(5-6-7) **3 C**hristmases –**1st, 2nd, 3rd C**uneiforms

Note above that the calcaneus, talus, and navicular bones are also sometimes known by alternative names, the os calcis, astragalus, and scaphoid, respectively. Correct usage, however, dictates that the tarsal bone of the foot should be called the navicular, while the carpal bone of the wrist, which has a similar shape, should be called the scaphoid. (The carpal bone, unfortunately, has more often been called the navicular rather than the preferred scaphoid.)

Similarities to the upper limb are less obvious with the tarsals in that there are only **seven tarsal bones** compared with the **eight carpal bones** of the wrist. Also, the tarsals are larger and less mobile because they provide a basis of support for the body in an erect position, compared with the more mobile carpals of the hand and wrist.

The seven tarsal bones are sometimes referred to as the ankle bones, although only one of the tarsals, the talus, is directly involved in the ankle joint. Each of these tarsals will be studied individually along with a list of the bones with which they articulate.

Calcaneus

The largest and strongest bone of the foot is the calcaneus *(kal-ka′ ne-us)*. The posterior portion is often called the heel bone. The most posterior-inferior part of the calcaneus contains a process called the **tuberosity**. Certain large tendons are attached to this rough and striated proces, which at its widest points has two small rounded processes. The largest of these is labeled as the **lateral process**. The **medial process** is smaller and less pronounced.

Another ridge of bone that varies in size and shape and is visualized laterally on an axial projection is the **peroneal trochlea** *(per″ o-ne′ al trok′ le-ah)*. Sometimes in general this is also called the **trochlear process.** On the medial proximal aspect is a larger more prominent bony process called the **sustentaculum tali** *(sus″ ten-tak′ u-lum)*, literally meaning a support for the talus.

Articulations: The calcaneus articulates with **two** bones; anteriorly with the **cuboid** and superiorly with the **talus.** The superior articulation with the talus forms the important **subtalar** (talocalcaneal) **joint**. There are three specific articular facets at this joint with the talus through which the weight of the body is transmitted to the ground in an erect position. These are the larger **posterior articular facet** and the smaller **anterior** and **middle articular facets.**

Note that the middle articular facet is the upper portion of the prominent sustentaculum tali, which provides the medial support for this important weight-bearing joint.

The deep depression between posterior and middle articular facets is called the **calcaneal sulcus** (Fig. 6-6). This, combined with a similar groove or depression of the talus, forms an opening for certain ligaments to pass through. This opening or space, found in the middle of the subtalar joint, is called the **sinus tarsi** or tarsal sinus (Fig. 6-7).

Talus

The talus is the second largest tarsal bone and is located between the lower leg and the calcaneus. Therefore, the weight of the body is transmitted by this bone through the important ankle and talocalcaneal joints.

Articulations: The talus articulates with **four** bones; superiorly with the **tibia** and **fibula**, inferiorly with the **calcaneus** and anteriorly with the **navicular.**

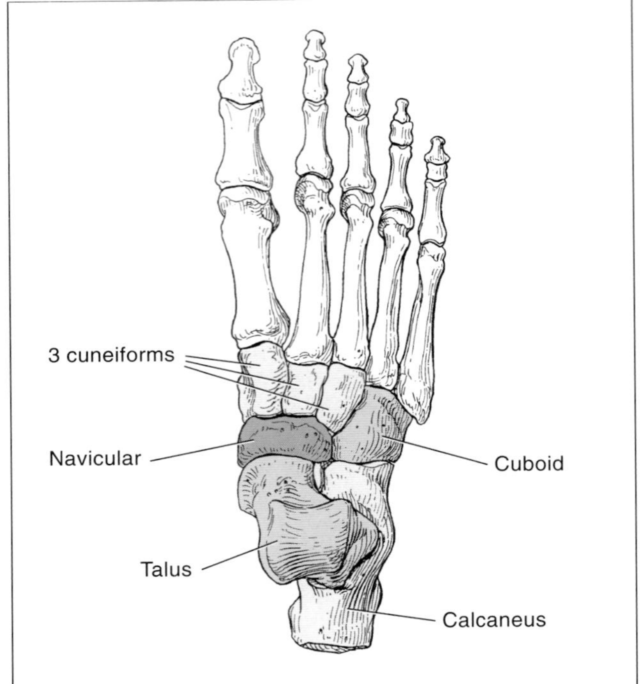

Fig. 6-5. Tarsals (7).

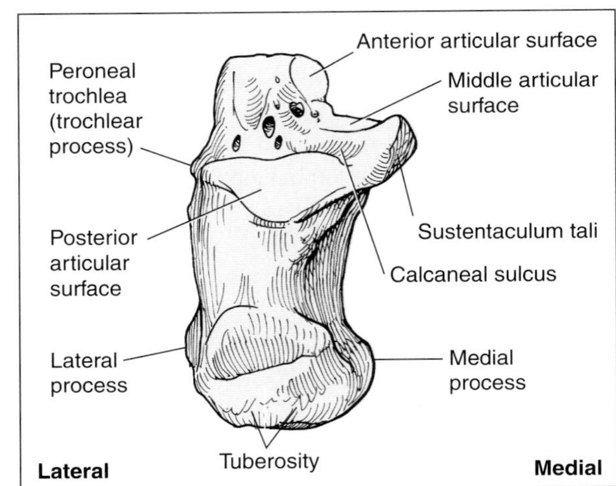

Fig. 6-6. Left calcaneus (superior or proximal surface).

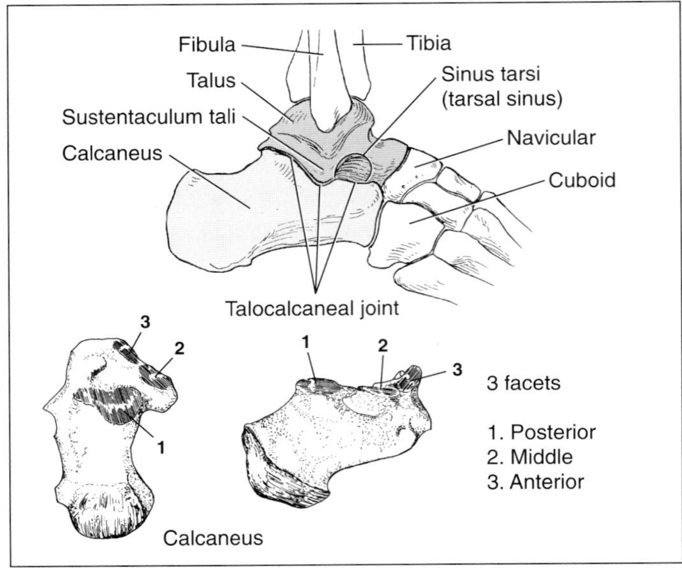

Fig. 6-7. Calcaneus and talus (with ankle and subtalar joints).

Navicular

The navicular is a flattened, oval-shaped bone located on the medial side of the foot between the talus and the three cuneiforms.

Articulations: The navicular articulates with **four** bones, posteriorly with the **talus** and anteriorly with the **three cuneiforms.**

Cuneiforms (3)

The three cuneiforms (meaning wedge shaped) are located on the medial and mid aspects of the foot between the first three metatarsals distally and the navicular proximally. The largest cuneiform, articulating with the first metatarsal, is the **medial** (first or internal) cuneiform. The **intermediate** (second or middle) cuneiform, which articulates with the second metatarsal, is the smallest of the cuneiforms. The **lateral** (third or external) cuneiform articulates with the third metatarsal distally and with the cuboid laterally. All three cuneiforms articulate with the navicular proximally.

Articulations: The **medial cuneiform** articulates with **four** bones: the **navicular** proximally, the **first** and **second metatarsals** distally and the **intermediate** laterally.

The **intermediate cuneiform** also articulates with **four** bones: the **navicular** proximally, the **second metatarsal** distally and the **medial** and **lateral cuneiforms** on each side.

The **lateral cuneiform** articulates with **six** bones: the **navicular** proximally, the **second, third,** and **fourth metatarsals** distally, the **intermediate cuneiform** medially and the **cuboid** laterally.

Cuboid

The cuboid is located on the lateral aspect of the foot, distal to the calcaneus and proximal to the fourth and fifth metatarsals.

Articulations: The **cuboid** articulates with **four** bones: the **calcaneus** proximally, the **lateral cuneiform** medially, and the **fourth** and **fifth metatarsals** distally. (Occasionally, it will also articulate with a fifth bone, the navicular.)

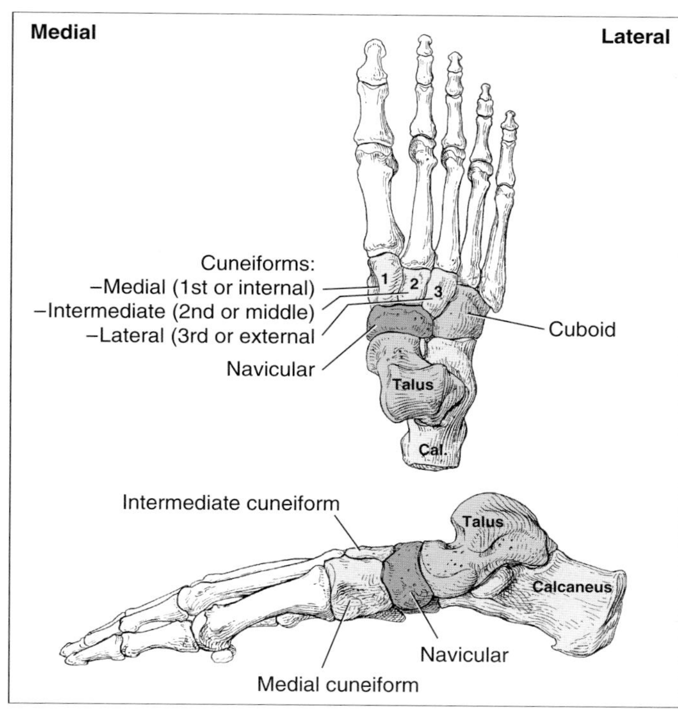

Fig. 6-8. Navicular, cuneiforms (3) and cuboid.

Summary of 7 Tarsals and Articulating Bones of Each

1. Calcaneus (2) –Cuboid –Talus	**5. Intermediate cuneiform (4)** –Navicular –2nd metatarsal –Medial and lateral cuneiforms
2. Talus (4) –Tibia and fibula –Calcaneus –Navicular	**6. Lateral cuneiform (6)** –Navicular –2nd, 3rd, 4th metatarsals –Intermediate cuneiform –Cuboid
3. Navicular (4) –Talus –Three cuneiforms	**7. Cuboid (4)** –Calcaneus –Lateral cuneiform –4th and 5th metatarsals
4. Medial cuneiform (4) –Navicular –1st and 2nd metatarsals –Intermediate cuneiform	

Note: The number in parentheses indicates the total number of bones with which each of these tarsals articulates.

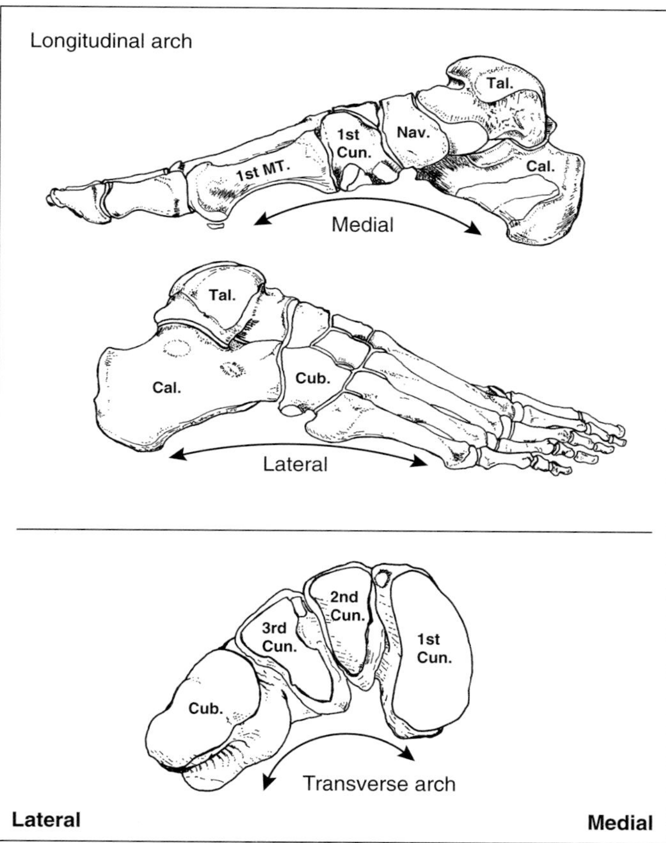

Fig. 6-9. Arches and tarsal relationships.

Arches

Longitudinal Arch: The bones of the foot are arranged in **longitudinal** and **transverse arches** providing a strong, shock-absorbing type support for the weight of the body. The springy, longitudinal arch is composed of a medial and a lateral component with most of the arch on the medial and mid aspects of the foot.

Transverse Arch: The transverse arch is located primarily along the plantar surface of the distal tarsals and the tarsometatarsal joints. The transverse arch is primarily made up by the wedge-shaped cuneiforms, especially the smaller second and third cuneiforms (Fig. 6-9) in combination with the larger first cuneiform and the cuboid.

ANKLE JOINT*

Frontal View

The **ankle joint** is formed by three bones, the two long bones of the lower leg, the **tibia** and **fibula**, and one tarsal bone, the **talus**. The expanded distal end of the slender fibula, which extends well down alongside the talus, is termed the **lateral malleolus**.

The distal end of the larger and stronger tibia has a broad articular surface for articulation with the similarly shaped broad upper surface of the talus. The medial elongated process of the tibia which extends down alongside the medial talus, is termed the **medial malleolus**.

The inferior portions of the tibia and fibula form a deep "socket" or three-sided opening called a **mortise** into which the upper talus fits. The entire three-part joint space of the ankle mortise, however, is **not seen** on a true frontal view (AP projection) due to overlapping of portions of the distal fibula and tibia by the talus. This is caused by the more posterior position of the distal fibula, as shown on these drawings. A 15° internally rotated AP projection, called the **mortise position**, will be demonstrated later (Fig. 6-15) to visualize this entire mortise joint.

The **anterior tubercle** is an expanded process at the distal anterior and lateral tibia, shown to articulate with the inferior talus anteriorly on a lateral view (Fig. 6-11).

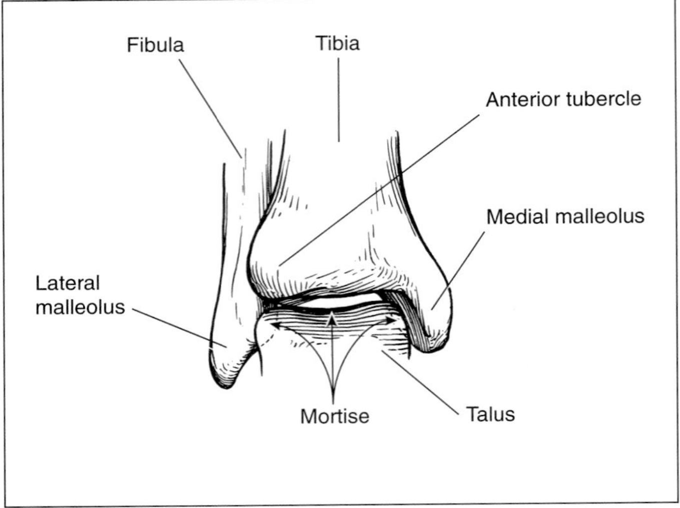

Fig. 6-10. Right ankle joint–Frontal view.

Lateral View

The ankle joint, seen in a true lateral position in Fig. 6-11, demonstrates that the **distal fibula is located about 1 cm or near ½ inch posterior in relationship to the distal tibia**. This relationship becomes important in evaluation for a **true lateral** radiograph of the leg, ankle or foot. A common misconception is to position and rotate the ankle so the medial and lateral malleoli are directly superimposed. However, this will result in a slightly oblique ankle as these drawings illustrate. Therefore, a true lateral requires the lateral malleolus to be about 1 cm posterior to the medial malleolus.

Note also that the more slender lateral malleolus generally extends about 1 cm or near ½ inch more distal than its counterpart, the medial malleolus (best seen on frontal view, Fig. 6-10).

Posterior malleolus is a term not found in general anatomy and physiology texts but is used in orthopedic and radiology references for the **posterior tip of the distal tibia.** It is used in describing a trimalleolar fracture of the ankle, involving the lateral and medial malleoli, and this "posterior" malleolus.

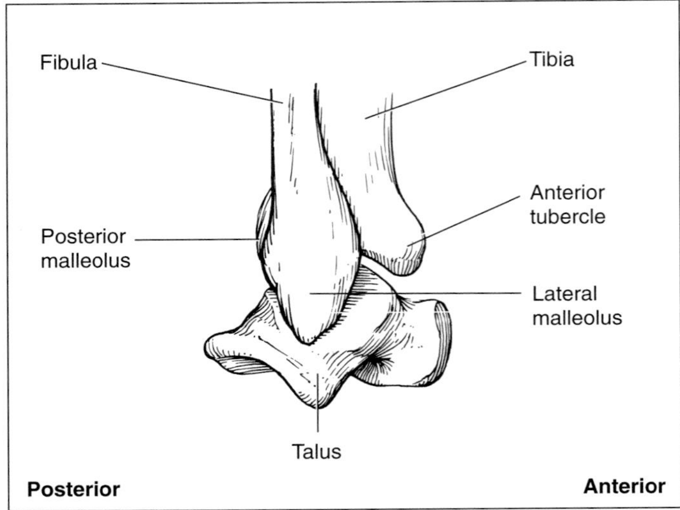

Fig. 6-11. Right ankle joint–True lateral view.

Axial View

An axial view of the inferior margin of the distal tibia and fibula is shown in Fig. 6-12. This axial view visualizes an "end on" view of the ankle joint looking from the bottom up, demonstrating the concave inferior surface of the tibia. Also demonstrated are the relative positions of the **lateral** and **medial malleoli** of the fibula and tibia, respectively. The smaller **fibula** is again shown to be **more posterior.** A line drawn through the midportions of the two malleoli will be approximately **15° to 20°** from the coronal plane (the true side-to-side plane of the body). Therefore, the lower leg and ankle must be rotated 15° to 20° to bring the intermalleolar line parallel to the coronal plane. This relationship of the distal tibia and fibula becomes important in positioning for various views of the ankle joint or ankle mortise as described in the positioning pages of this chapter.

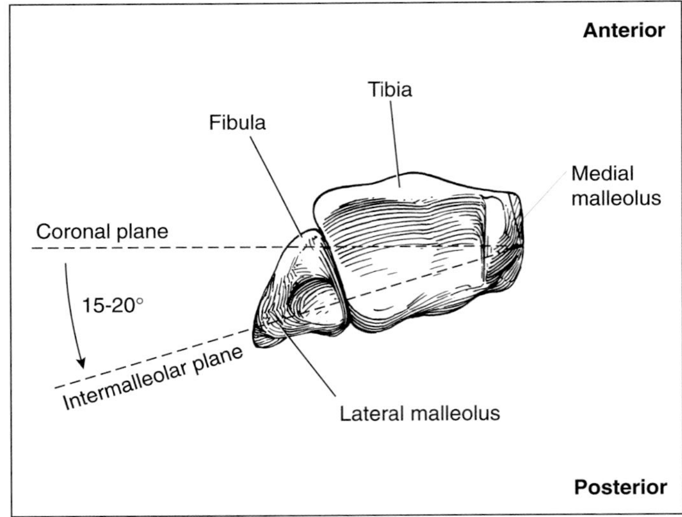

Fig. 6-12. Ankle joint–Axial view.
(Figs. 6-10, 11, 12 Courtesy of Mayo Foundation)

Ankle Joint

The ankle joint is a **synovial joint** of the **ginglymus** or **hinge type** with flexion and extension (dorsiflexion and plantar flexion) movements only. This requires strong collateral ligaments extending from the medial and lateral malleoli to the calcaneus and talus. Lateral stress can result in a "sprained" ankle with stretched or torn collateral ligaments as well as torn muscle tendons.

*Frank, E.D., et. al: Radiography of the Ankle Mortise, *Radiologic Technology* 1991; 62-5: 354-359.

REVIEW EXERCISE WITH RADIOGRAPHS

Three common projections of the foot and ankle are shown with labels for an anatomy review of the bones and joints. A good review exercise is to cover up the answers below and identify or write out all the parts as labelled before checking the answers as listed below.

Lateral Left Foot (Fig. 6-13)

A. Tibia
B. "Posterior malleolus" of tibia
C. Calcaneus
D. Tuberosity of calcaneus
E. Tuberosity at the base of 5th metatarsal
F. Superimposed cuneiforms
G. Navicular
H. Subtalar joint
I. Talus

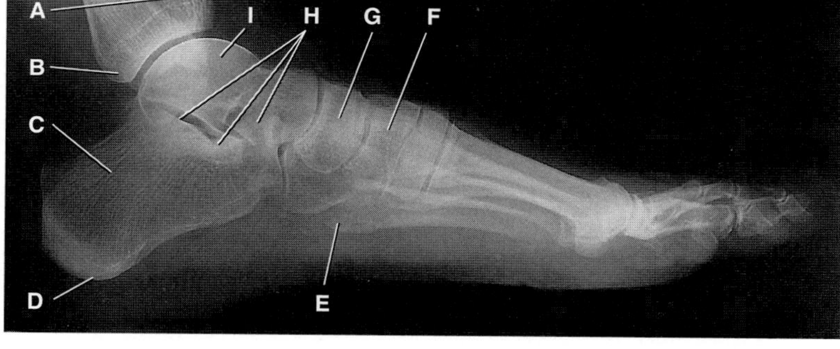

Fig. 6-13. Lateral left foot.

Oblique Right Foot (Fig. 6-14)

A. Interphalangeal joint of 1st digit of right foot
B. Proximal phalanx of 1st digit of right foot
C. Metatarsophalangeal (MP) joint of 1st digit of right foot
D. Head of first metatarsal
E. Body of first metatarsal
F. Base of first metatarsal
G. 2nd or intermediate cuneiform (partially superimposed over 1st or medial cuneiform)
H. Navicular
I. Talus
J. Tuberosity of calcaneus
K. Cuboid
L. Tuberosity of the base of the 5th metatarsal
M. Fifth metatarsophalangeal (MP) joint of right foot
N. Proximal phalanx of 5th digit of right foot

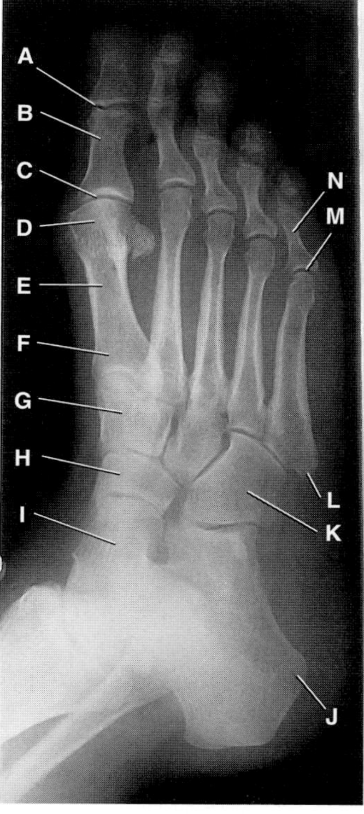

Fig. 6-14. Oblique right foot.

AP Mortise View Right Ankle (Fig. 6-15)

A. Fibula
B. Lateral malleolus
C. "Open" mortise joint of ankle
D. Talus
E. Medial malleolus
F. Tibia

Lateral Ankle (Fig. 6-16)

A. Fibula
B. Posterior malleolus
C. Calcaneus
D. Cuboid
E. Tuberosity at base of 5th metatarsal
F. Navicular
G. Talus
H. Sinus tarsi
I. Anterior tubercle
J. Tibia

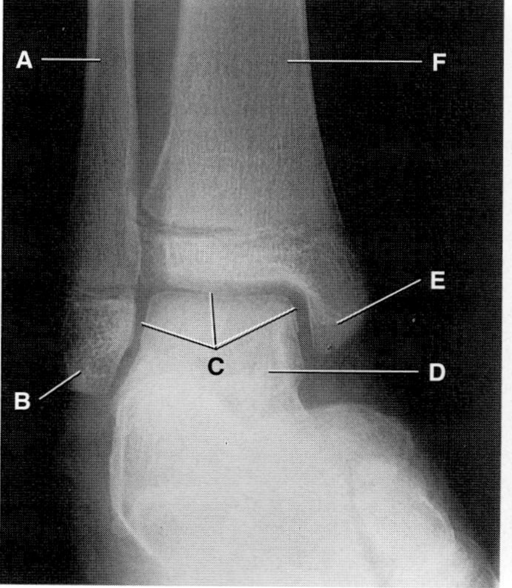

Fig. 6-15. AP right ankle (mortise view–15° medial oblique).

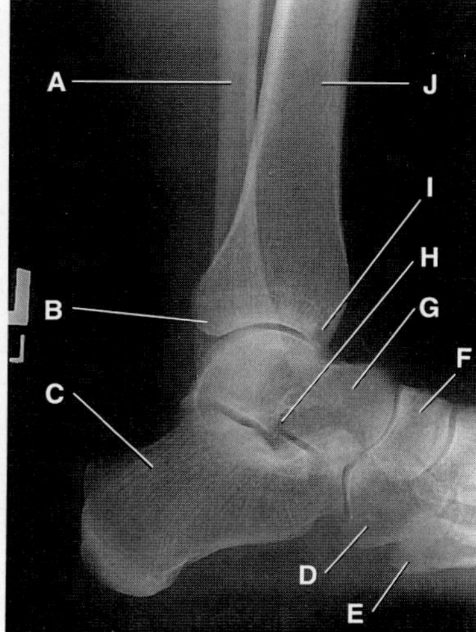

Fig. 6-16. Lateral ankle.

LEG–TIBIA AND FIBULA

The second group of bones of the lower limb to be studied in this chapter are the two bones of the lower leg, the **tibia** and **fibula.**

Tibia

The tibia, as one of the larger bones of the body, is the weight-bearing bone of the lower leg. The tibia can easily be felt through the skin in the anteromedial part of the leg. It is made up of three parts, the central **body** (shaft) and **two extremities.**

Proximal Extremity: The **medial** and **lateral condyles** are the two large processes making up the medial and lateral aspects of the proximal tibia.

The **intercondylar eminence**, sometimes called the tibial spine, includes two small pointed prominences, called the **medial and lateral intercondylar tubercles**, located on the superior surface of the tibial head between the two condyles.

The upper articular surface of the condyles includes two smooth concave **articular facets**, commonly called the **tibial plateau,** which articulate with the femur. As seen on the lateral view (Fig. 6-18) **the articular facets making up the tibial plateau slope posteriorly from 10 to 20°** in relationship to the long axis of the tibia.* This is an important anatomical consideration because in positioning for an AP knee, the central ray must be angled as needed in relationship to the film and tabletop to be parallel to the tibial plateau. This CR angle is essential to demonstrate an "open" joint space on an AP knee projection.

The **tibial tuberosity** on the proximal extremity of the tibia is a rough-textured prominence located on the midanterior surface of the tibia just distal to the condyles. This tuberosity is the distal attachment of the patellar tendon, which connects to the large muscle of the anterior thigh. Sometimes in young persons, the tibial tuberosity separates from the body of the tibia, a condition known as Osgood-Schlatter disease.

The **body** (shaft) is the long portion of the tibia between the two extremities. Along the anterior surface of the body, extending from the tibial tuberosity to the medial malleolus, is a sharp ridge called the **anterior crest** or **border.** This sharp anterior crest is just under the skin surface and is often referred to as the shin or shin bone.

Distal extremity: The distal extremity of the tibia is smaller than the proximal and ends in a short pyramid-shaped process called the **medial malleolus,** which is easily palpated on the medial aspect of the ankle.

The lateral aspect of the distal extremity of the tibia forms a flattened, triangular shaped **fibular notch** for articulation with the distal fibula. The inferior smooth, concave-shaped articular surface is continuous with the articular surface of the medial malleolus for articulation with the talus. This articulation makes up the ankle joint or ankle mortise, as described on a previous page.

Fibula

The smaller fibula can be seen to be located **laterally** and **posteriorly** to the larger tibia. The fibula articulates with the tibia proximally and the tibia and talus distally. The proximal extremity of the fibula is expanded into a **head,** which articulates with the lateral aspect of the posteroinferior surface of the lateral condyle of the tibia. The extreme proximal aspect of the head is pointed and is known as the **apex** (styloid process) of the head of the fibula. The tapered area just below the head is the **neck** of the fibula.

The **body** (shaft) is the long, slender portion of the fibula between the two extremities. The enlarged distal end of the fibula can be felt as a distinct bump on the lateral aspect of the ankle joint and as described earlier is called the **lateral malleolus.**

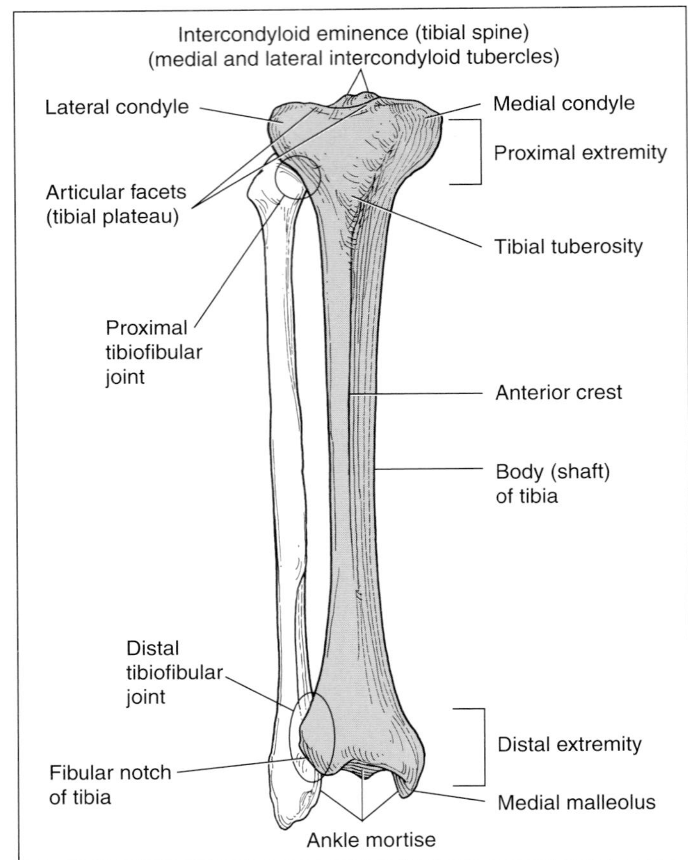

Fig. 6-17. Tibia–Anterior view.

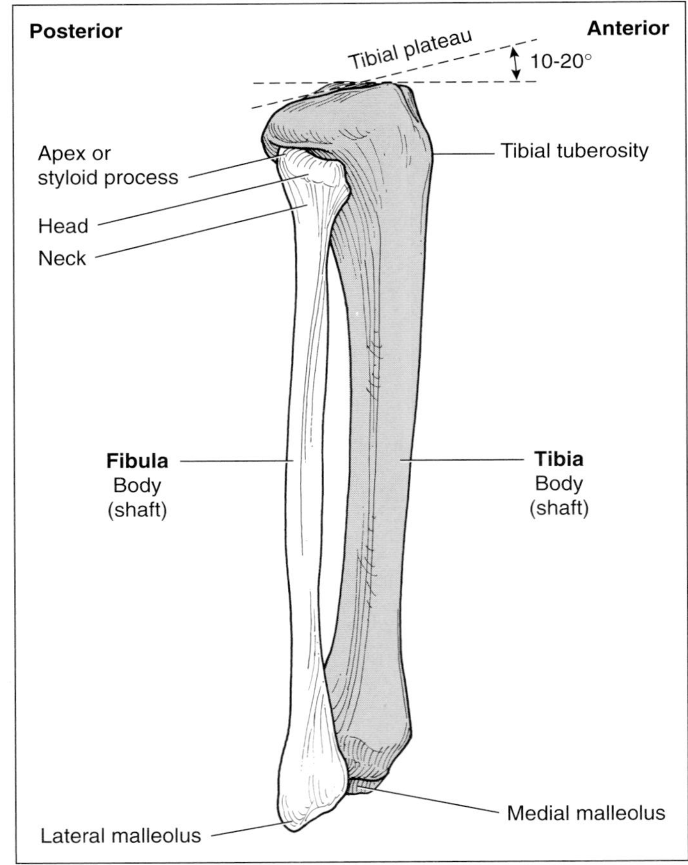

Fig. 6-18. Tibia and fibula–Lateral view.

*Manaster, BJ. *Handbooks in Radiology*. Chicago: Year Book Medical Publishers, Inc; 1989.

FEMUR

The **femur** or thigh bone is the longest and strongest bone in the entire body. The femur is the only long bone between the **hip joint** and the **knee joint.** The proximal femur will be described in Chapter 7 with the hip and pelvis.

Mid and Distal Femur–Anterior View (Fig. 6-19)

Similar to all long bones, the **body** or shaft of the femur is the slender, elongated portion of the bone. The distal femur viewed anteriorly demonstrates the position of the patella or knee cap. The **patella,** which is the largest sesamoid bone in the body, is located anteriorly to the distal femur. Note that the most distal part of the patella is **above** or **proximal** to the actual knee joint by approximately ½ in. (1.25 cm) in this position with the lower leg fully extended. This relationship becomes important in positioning for the knee joint.

The **patellar surface** is the smooth and shallow, triangular-shaped depression at the distal portion of the anterior femur extending up under the lower part of the patella as seen on this drawing. This depression is also sometimes termed the **intercondylar sulcus.** (Sulcus means a groove or depression.) Some literature also refers to this depression as the **trochlear groove.** (Trochlea means pulley or pulley-shaped structure in reference to the medial and lateral condyles.) All three of these terms should be recognized as referring to this smooth, shallow depression.

Note that the patella itself is mostly superior to the patellar surface with the leg fully extended. However, as the leg is flexed, the patella, which is attached to large muscle tendons, moves distally or downward over the patellar surface. This is best shown on the lateral knee drawing (Fig. 6-21) on the following page.

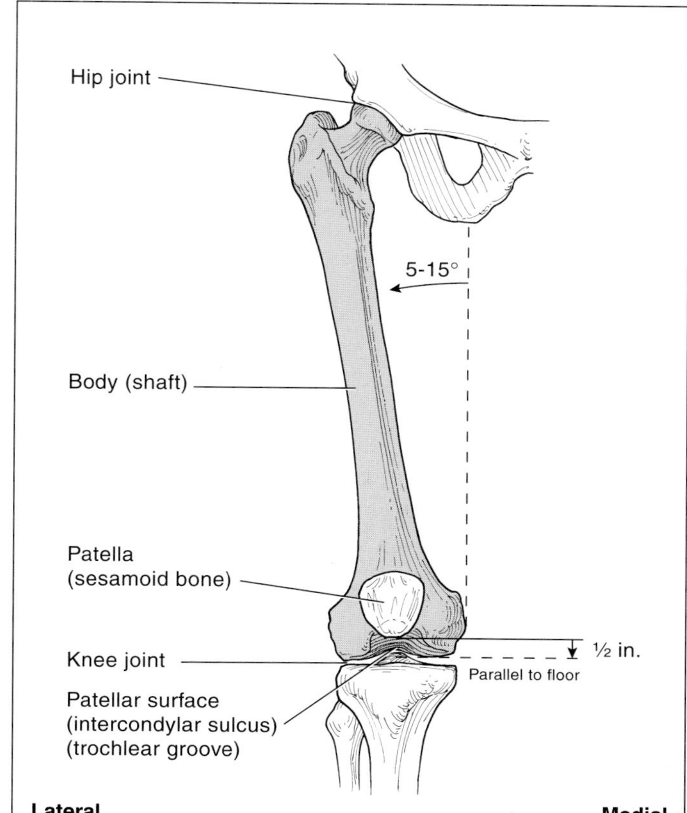

Fig. 6-19. Femur–**Anterior** view.

Mid and Distal Femur–Posterior View (Fig. 6-20)

The posterior view of the distal femur best demonstrates the two large rounded condyles that are joined anteriorly but are separated distally and posteriorly by the deep **intercondylar fossa** or notch. This posterior view demonstrates that the intercondylar fossa is primarily on the distal and posterior aspects of the femur.

The rounded distal portions of the **medial** and **lateral condyles** contain smooth articular surfaces for articulation with the tibia. The **medial condyle extends lower or more distally** than the lateral when the femoral shaft is vertical, as on this drawing. This explains why the **CR must be angled 5 to 7° cephalad for a lateral knee** to cause the two condyles to be directly superimposed when the femur is parallel to the film. The explanation for this is also seen in Fig. 6-20, which demonstrates that in an erect anatomical position, wherein the distal femoral condyles are parallel to the floor at the knee joint, the femoral shaft is at an angle of approximately 10° from vertical for an average adult. The range is 5 to 15°.* This angle would be greater on a short person with a wider pelvis and less on a tall person with a narrow pelvis. Therefore, in general this angle is greater on a female than on a male.

A distinguishing difference between the medial and lateral condyles is the presence of the **adductor tubercle**, a slightly raised area that receives the tendon of an adductor muscle. This tubercle is present on the **lateral and posterior aspects of the medial condyle**. It is best seen on a slightly rotated lateral view of the distal femur and knee. The presence of this adductor tubercle on the medial condyle is important in critiquing a lateral knee for rotation in that it allows the viewer to determine if the knee is under-rotated or over-rotated to correct a positioning error when the knee is not in a true lateral position. This is shown on the radiograph in Fig. 6-33 (page 182) and also will be demonstrated on critique radiographs at the end of the chapter.

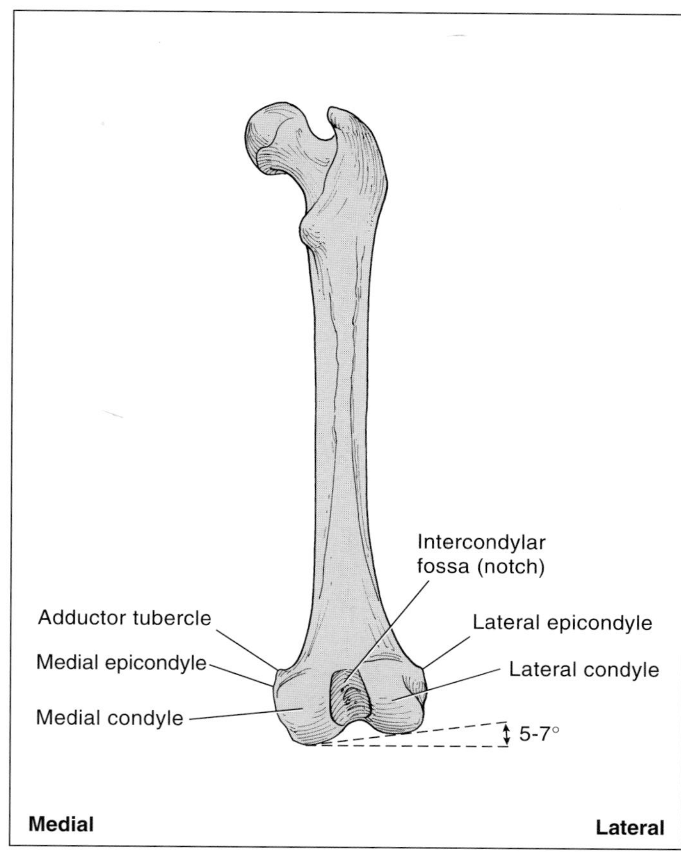

Fig. 6-20. Femur–**Posterior** view.

The **medial** and **lateral epicondyles**, which can be palpated, are rough prominences for attachments of ligaments and are located on the outermost portions of the condyles. The medial epicondyle, along with adductor tubercles, is the more prominent of the two.

*Keats, TE, et al. *Radiology* 1966; 87:904.

Distal Femur and Patella (Lateral View)

The lateral view in Fig. 6-21 demonstrates the relationship of the patella to the **patellar surface** of the distal femur. The patella, as a large sesamoid bone, is embedded in the tendon of the large quadriceps femoris muscle. Therefore, as the lower leg is flexed, the patella moves downward and is drawn inward into the intercondylar groove or sulcus. A partial flexion of near 45°, as shown in this drawing, shows the patella being pulled only partially downward, but with 90° flexion, the patella would move down farther over the distal portion of the femur. This movement and the relationship of the patella to the distal femur becomes important in positioning for the knee joint and for the tangential projection of the patellofemoral joint. (Articulation between patella and distal femur.)

The posterior surface of the knee joint in general is called the **popliteal region.**

The region of the **adductor tubercle** of the medial condyle is identified on this lateral drawing.

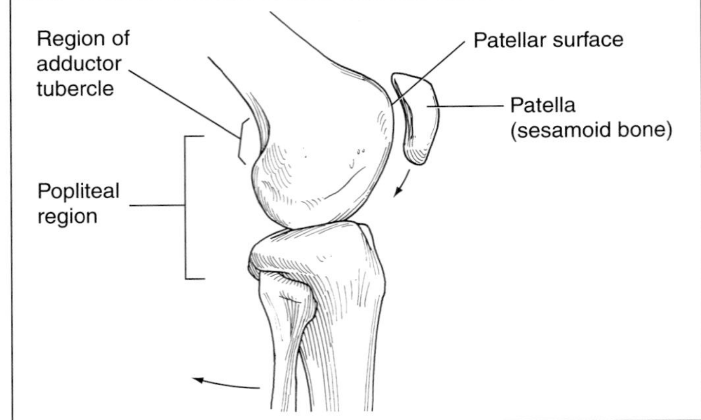

Fig. 6-21. Distal femur and patella–Lateral view.

Distal Femur and Patella (Axial View)

The axial or end on view of the distal femur again demonstrates the relationship of the patella to the **patellar surface** (intercondylar sulcus or trochlear groove) of the distal femur. The patellofemoral joint space is visualized in this axial view (Fig. 6-22). Other parts of the distal femur are also well visualized.

The **intercondylar fossa** (notch) is shown to be very deep on the posterior aspect of the femur. The **epicondyles** are seen as rough prominences on the outermost tips of the large **medial** and **lateral condyles.**

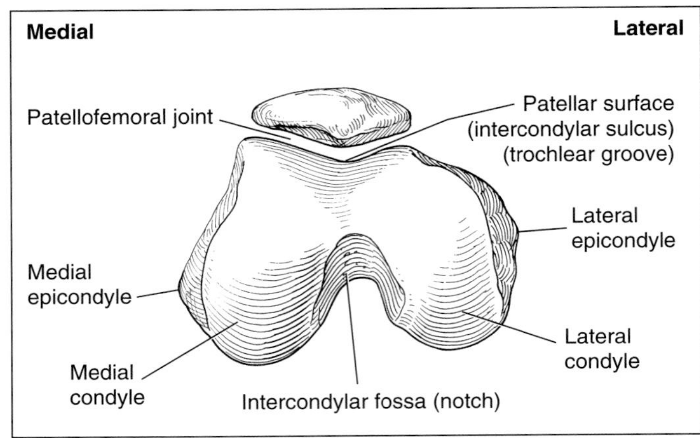

Fig. 6-22. Distal femur and patella–Axial view.

Patella

The **patella** (knee cap) is a flat triangular bone about 2 in. or 5 cm in diameter. The patella appears to be upside down in that its pointed **apex** is located along the **inferior border**, and its **base** is the **superior** or **upper border.** The outer or **anterior surface** is convex and roughened, while the inner **posterior surface** is smooth and oval shaped for articulation with the femur. The patella serves to protect the anterior aspect of the knee joint and acts as a pivot to increase the leverage of the large quadriceps femoris muscle, the tendon of which attaches to the tibial tuberosity of the lower leg. The patella is somewhat loose and movable in its more superior position when the leg is extended and the quadriceps muscles relaxed. However, as the leg is flexed and the muscles tighten, it moves distally and becomes locked into position. It should be noted that the patella articulates only with the femur, not with the tibia.

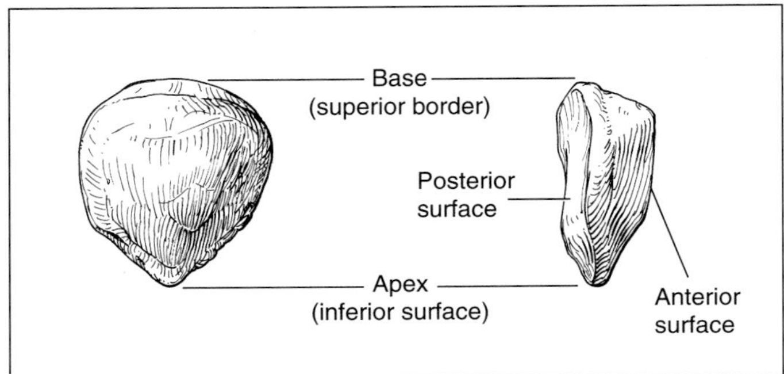

Fig. 6-23. Patella.

KNEE JOINT

The knee joint proper is a large complex joint primarily involving the **femorotibial joint** between the two condyles of the **femur** and the corresponding condyles of the **tibia**. The **patellofemoral joint** is also part of the knee joint wherein the patella articulates with the anterior surface of the distal femur.

Proximal Tibiofibular Joint and Major Knee Ligaments

The proximal fibula is not part of the knee joint in that it does not articulate with any aspect of the femur, even though the **fibular collateral ligament** extends from the femur to the lateral proximal fibula as shown in Fig. 6-24. The head of the fibula, however, does articulate with the lateral condyle of the tibia to which it is attached by this ligament.

Additional major knee ligaments shown on this posterior view are the **tibial collateral ligament** located medially, and the major **posterior** and **anterior cruciate** *(kroo′she-at)* **ligaments** located within the knee joint capsule. The knee joint is highly dependent on these two important pairs of major ligaments for stability.

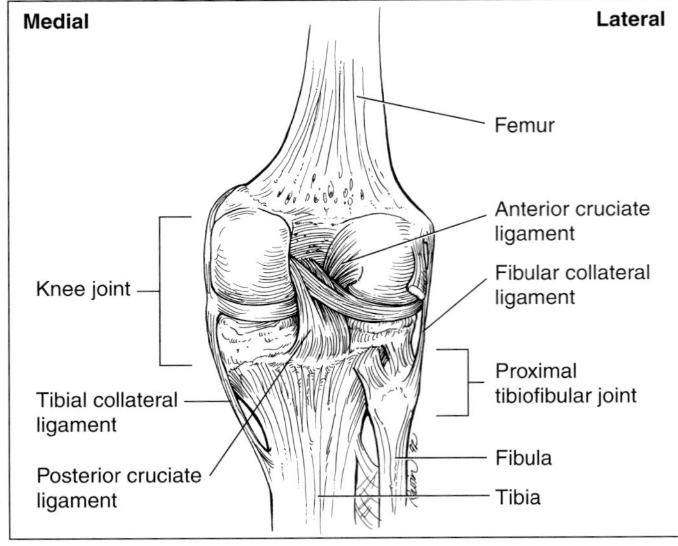

Fig. 6-24. Knee joint and proximal tibiofibular joint–Posterior view.

Knee Joint continued

The two **collateral ligaments** are strong bands at the sides of the knee that **prevent adduction and abduction** movements at the knee. The two **cruciate ligaments** are strong, rounded cords that cross each other as they attach to the respective anterior and posterior aspects of the intercondylar eminence of the tibia. They stabilize the knee joint by **preventing anterior or posterior movement** within the knee joint.

In addition to these two major pair of ligaments, there is also an anteriorly located **patellar ligament** as well as various minor ligaments that help in maintaining the integrity of the knee joint (Fig. 6-26). The patellar ligament is shown as part of the tendon of insertion of the large quadriceps femoris muscle extending over the patella to the tibial tuberosity. The **infrapatellar fat pad** is posterior to this ligament, which aids in protecting the anterior aspect of the knee joint.

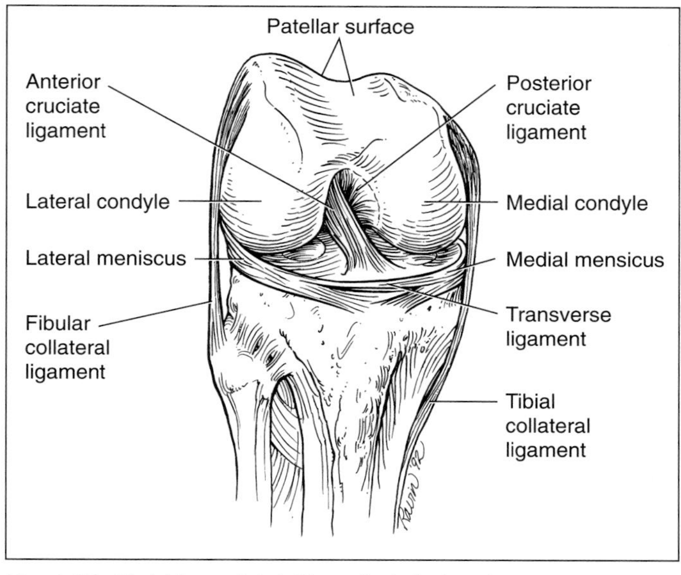

Fig. 6-25. Right knee joint (flexed)–Anterior view.

Synovial Membrane and Cavity

The articular cavity of the knee joint is the largest joint space of the human body. The total knee joint is a synovial type enclosed in an **articular capsule** or **bursa**, a complex multifaceted saclike structure filled with a lubricating-type synovial fluid and lined with synovial membrane closely integrated with certain fibrocartilage and ligaments best demonstrated on a lateral view as seen in Fig. 6-26. This is also demonstrated in the arthrogram radiograph (Fig. 6-28) wherein a combination of negative and positive contrast media has been injected into the articular capsule or bursa.

The articular cavity or bursa of the knee joint extends upwards under and superior to the patella, identified as the **suprapatellar bursa** (Fig. 6-26). Distal to the patella, the **infrapatellar bursa** is separated by a large **infrapatellar fat pad**, which can be identified on radiographs. Posteriorly the bursae continue as various subdivisions or recesses interspaced between certain ligaments and muscle tendons. These spaces posterior and distal to the femur can also be seen filled with negative contrast media on the lateral arthrogram radiograph.

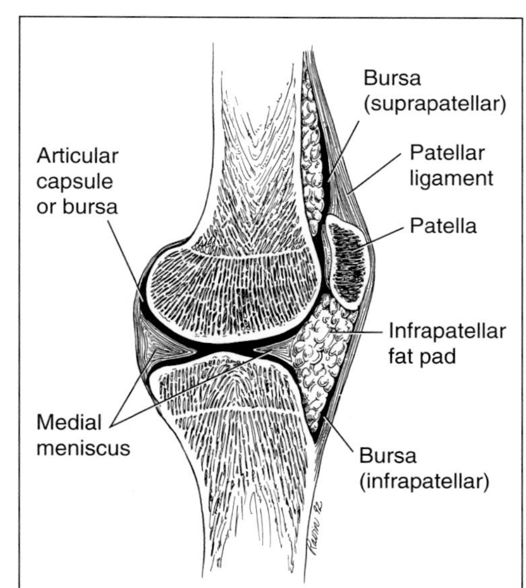

Fig. 6-26. Sagittal section of knee joint.

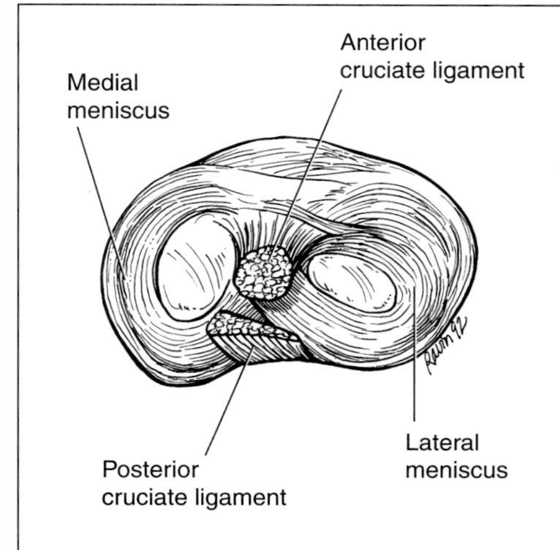

Fig. 6-27. Superior view of articular surface of tibia (shows menisci and cruciate ligament attachments).

Menisci (Articular Disks)

The **medial** and **lateral menisci** *(me-nis′ ci)* are fibrocartilage disks between the articular facets of the tibia (tibial plateau) and the femoral condyles (Fig. 6-27). They are crescent-shaped and are thicker at their external margins and taper to a very thin center portion. They act as shock absorbers to reduce some of the direct impact and stress occurring at the knee joint. Along with the synovial membrane, they are also believed to function in producing synovial fluid, which acts as a lubricant for the articulating ends of the femur and tibia, which are also covered with a tough, slick hyaline membrane.

Knee Trauma

The knee has the greatest potential for trauma injury of any joint in the human body, especially in contact sports such as football or basketball. For example, the most common type of knee injury in football from a blow to the lateral side of the knee is a rupture of the tibial collateral ligament. This injury is also often associated with a tearing of the anterior cruciate ligament and the medial meniscus (torn cartilage). These injuries typically come to the radiology department for either an MRI (magnetic resonance imaging) exam to visualize these soft tissue structures of the knee or for a knee arthrogram.

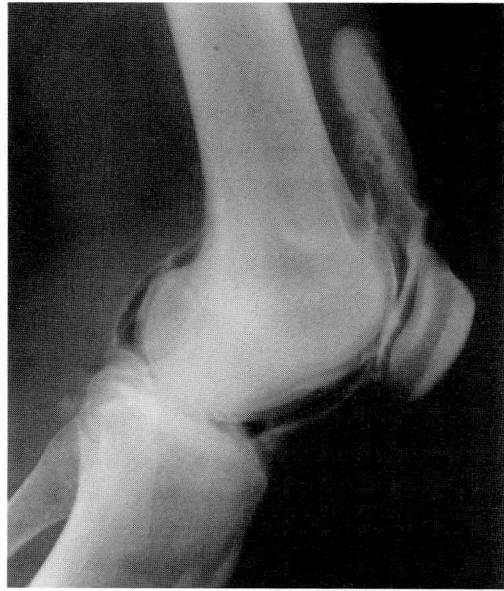

Fig. 6-28. Lateral knee arthrogram radiograph (demonstrates articular capsule or bursa as outlined by a combination of negative and positive contrast media).

REVIEW EXERCISE WITH RADIOGRAPHS

Common projections of the leg, knee and patella are shown with labels for an anatomy review.

AP Leg (Fig. 6-29)

A. Medial condyle of the tibia
B. Body or shaft of tibia
C. Medial malleolus
D. Lateral malleolus
E. Body or shaft of the fibula
F. Neck of fibula
G. Head of fibula
H. Apex (styloid process) of head of fibula
I. Lateral condyle of tibia
J. Intercondylar eminence (tibial spine)

Lateral Leg (Fig. 6-30)

A. Intercondylar eminence (tibial spine)
B. Tibial tuberosity
C. Body or shaft of tibia
D. Body or shaft of fibula
E. Medial malleolus
F. Lateral malleolus
G. Posterior lip of distal tibia (posterior malleolus)

AP Knee (Fig. 6-31)

A. Medial and lateral intercondylar tubercles; extensions of the intercondylar eminence (tibial spine)
B. Lateral epicondyle of femur
C. Lateral condyle of femur
D. Lateral condyle of tibia
E. Articular facets of tibia (tibial plateau)
F. Medial condyle of tibia
G. Medial condyle of femur
H. Medial epicondyle of femur
I. Patella (seen through femur)

Lateral Knee (Fig. 6-32)

A. Base of patella
B. Apex of patella
C. Tibial tuberosity
D. Neck of fibula
E. Head of fibula
F. Apex (styloid process) of head of fibula
G. Superimposed medial and lateral condyles
H. Patellar surface (intercondylar sulcus or trochlear groove)

Lateral Knee (Fig. 6-33)

(Demonstrating some rotation)
I. Adductor tubercle
J. Lateral condyle
K. Medial condyle

Tangential Projection (Patellofemoral Joint) (Fig. 6-34)

A. Patella
B. Patellofemoral joint
C. Lateral condyle
D. Patellar surface (intercondylar sulcus, trochlear groove)
E. Medial condyle

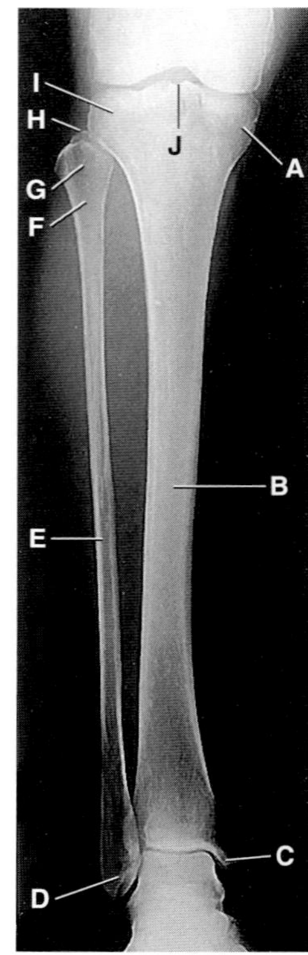

Fig. 6-29. AP leg.

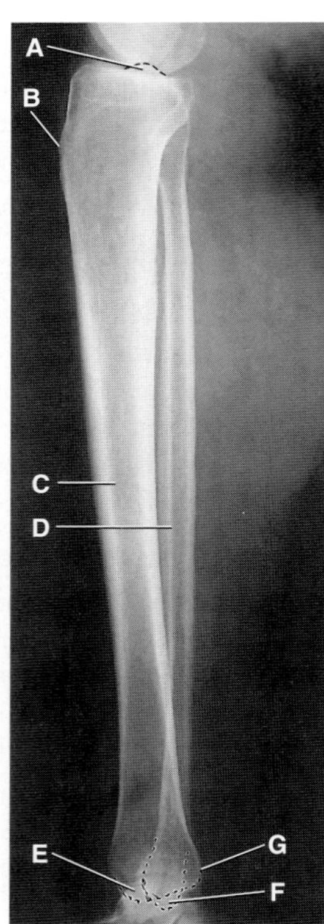

Fig. 6-30. Lateral leg.

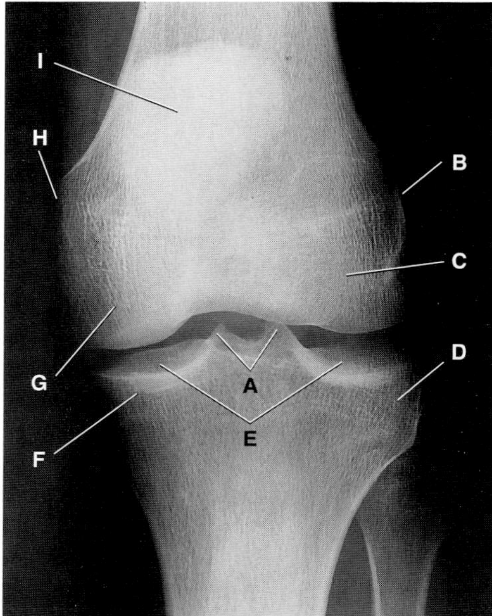

Fig. 6-31. AP knee.

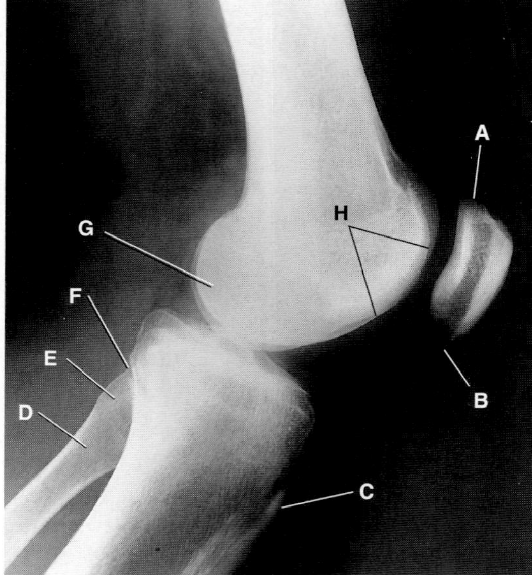

Fig. 6-32. Lateral knee–True lateral.

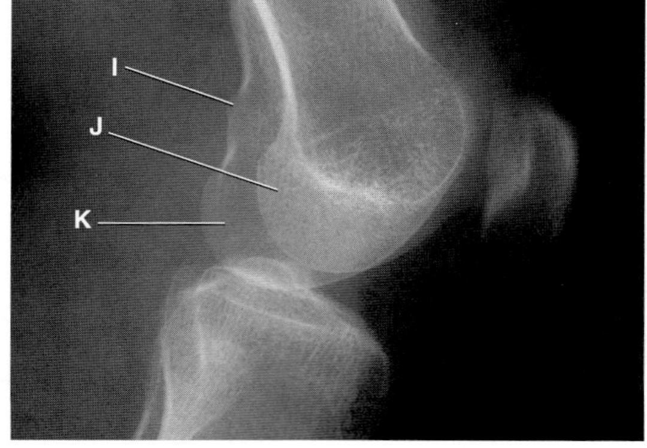

Fig. 6-33. Slightly rotated lateral knee. (medial condyle more posterior)

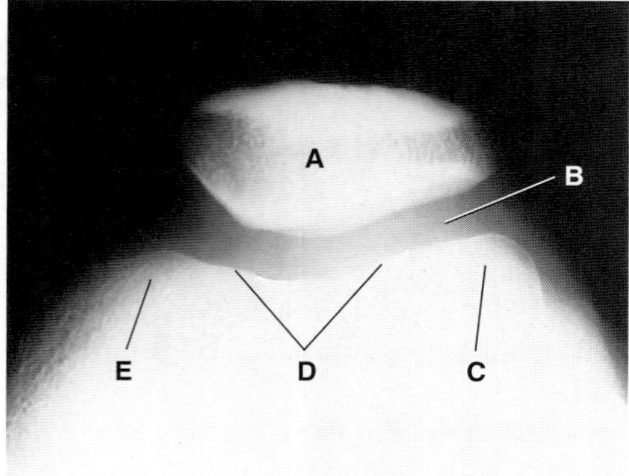

Fig. 6-34. Tangential projection. (patellofemoral joint)

CLASSIFICATION OF JOINTS

The joints or articulations of the lower limb are (with one exception) all classified as **synovial joints** characterized by a fibrous type capsule containing synovial fluid. Therefore, they also are (with the one exception) **diarthrodial** or freely movable.

The one exception to the synovial joint is the **distal tibiofibular joint**, which is classified as a **fibrous joint** with fibrous interconnections between the surfaces of the tibia and fibula. It is of the **syndesmosis type** and is only **slightly movable**, or **amphiarthrodial**. The most distal part of this joint, however, is smooth and lined with a synovial membrane that is continuous with the ankle joint.

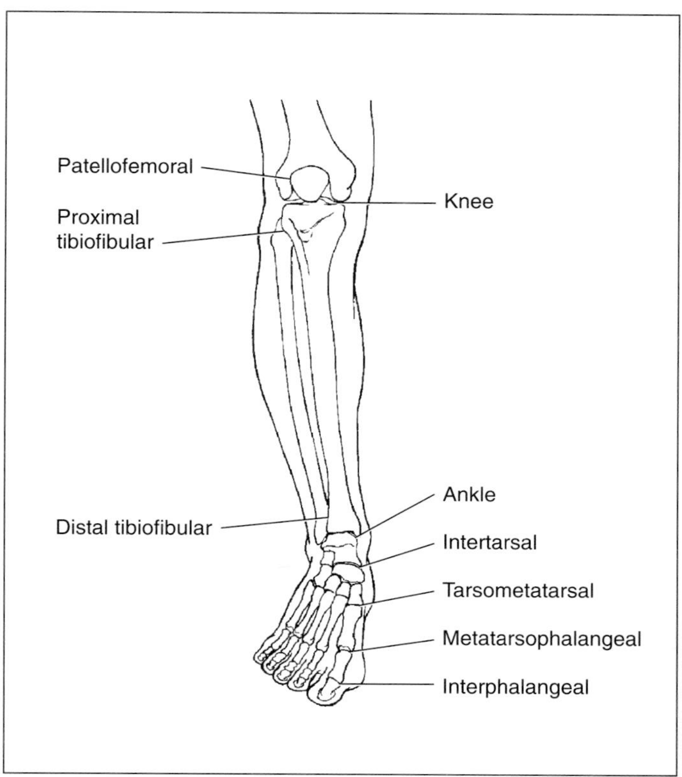

Fig. 6-35. Joints of lower limb.

Summary of Foot, Ankle, Leg and Knee Joints	
All joints of lower limb except distal tibiofibular	
Classification:	***Synovial*** *(articular capsule containing synovial fluid).*
Mobility Type:	***Diarthrodial*** *(freely movable).*
Movement Type:	
1. Interphalangeal joints	***Ginglymus or Hinge:*** Flexion and extension movements.
2. Metatarsophalangeal joints	***Modified Ellipsoidal or Condyloid:*** Flexion, extension, abduction and adduction. (Circumduction like that of the metacarpophalangeal joints of the hand are generally not possible.)
3. Tarsometatarsal joints	***Plane or Gliding:*** Limited gliding movement.
4. Intertarsal joints	***Plane or Gliding:*** Subtalar in combination with some other intertarsal joints provides for gliding and rotation, results in **inversion** and **eversion** of the foot.
5. Ankle joint	***Ginglymus or Hinge:*** Dorsiflexion and plantar flexion only (side-to-side movements only occur with stretched or torn ligaments).
6. Knee joint(s):	
Femorotibial	***Special Type–Ginglymus or Hinge:*** Flexion and extension and some gliding and rotational movements when knee is partially flexed.
Patellofemoral	***Sellar or Saddle:*** Considered a saddle type because of its shape and relationship of the patella to the distal femur.
7. Tibiofibular joint(s):	
Proximal tibiofibular	***Plane or Gliding:*** Limited gliding movement between lateral condyle and head of fibula.
Distal tibiofibular	
Classification:	***Fibrous.***
Mobility Type:	***Amphiarthrodial*** *(slightly movable) of the* ***syndesmosis*** *type.*

SURFACES AND PROJECTIONS OF THE FOOT

Surfaces: The surfaces of the foot are sometimes confusing in that the top or **anterior surface** of the foot is called **dorsum**. Dorsal is usually the posterior part of the body. Dorsum, in this case, comes from the term **dorsum pedis** which refers to the upper surface, or the surface opposite the sole of the foot.

The sole of the foot is the **posterior** surface or **plantar surface**. Using these terms one can describe the common projections of the foot.

Projections: The **anteroposterior** or **AP projection** of the foot is the same as a **dorsoplantar projection.** The less common **posteroanterior** or **PA projection** can also be called a **plantodorsal projection.**

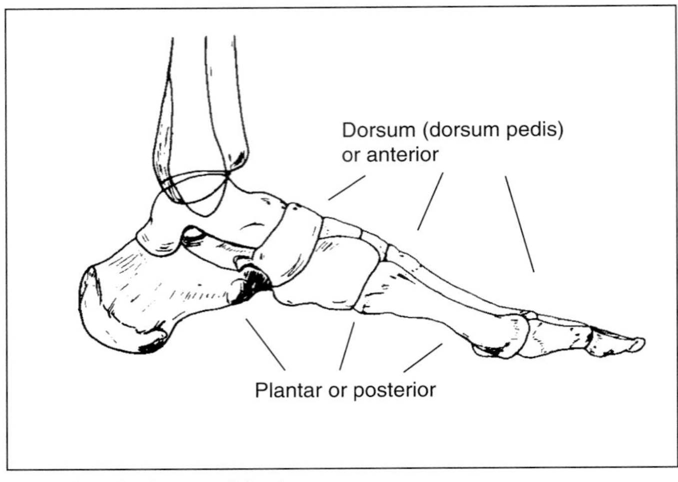

Fig. 6-36. Surfaces of foot.

MOTIONS OF FOOT AND ANKLE

Other confusing terminology involving the ankle and intertarsal joints are: **dorsiflexion, plantar flexion, inversion,** and **eversion.** To decrease the angle (flex) between the dorsum pedis and the anterior part of the lower leg is to dorsiflex at the ankle joint. Extending the ankle joint or pointing the foot and toe downward with respect to the normal position is termed plantar flexion.

Inversion is an inward turning of the ankle and subtalar (talocalcaneal) joints, while eversion is an outward turning. The lower leg does not rotate during inversion or eversion. Most sprained ankles result from an accidental and forced inversion or eversion.

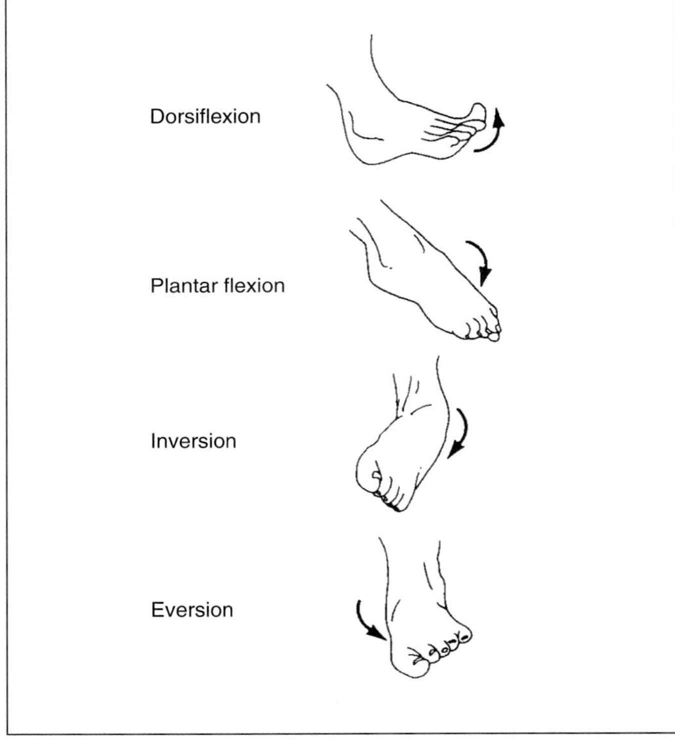

Fig. 6-37. Motions of foot and ankle.

Radiographic Positioning

POSITIONING CONSIDERATIONS

Radiographic examinations involving the lower limb below the knee are generally done table-top as shown in Fig. 6-38. Severe trauma cases or patients who are difficult to move can also be radiographed directly on the cart.

Distance

A common minimum SID (source-image receptor distance) is 40 in. or 102 cm. When radiographing with cassettes directly on the table-top, to maintain a constant SID the tube height must be increased as compared to radiographs taken with the cassette in the Bucky tray. This difference is generally 3 to 4 in. (8 to 10 cm) for floating type table-tops. The same minimum 40 in. (102 cm) SID should also be used when radiographing directly on the cart, unless exposure factors are adjusted to compensate for a change in SID.

Gonadal Shielding

Gonadal shielding is important for exams of the lower limb because of the proximity of the gonads to the divergent x-ray beam as well as scatter radiation. Therefore, a lead vinyl-covered shield should be draped over the patient's gonadal area as shown. Even though the gonadal rule states this should be done on patients of reproductive age when the gonads lie within or close to the primary field, it is a good practice to provide gonadal shielding for all patients.

Bucky Tray Out of Exposure Field: A good practice for all table-top exams of the lower limb is to move the Bucky tray, which is not being used, up under the pelvic region and out from under the exposure field to reduce possible scatter and secondary rays from these structures when they are in the x-ray field under the table-top.

Collimation

The collimation rule should again be followed, namely that **collimation borders should be visible on all four sides if the film is large enough to allow this without cutting off essential anatomy**. A general rule, concerning film size, is to **use the smallest film size possible for the specific part being radiographed.** Four-sided collimation is generally possible, however, even with a minimal size film for most if not all radiographic exams of the lower limb.

Two or more projections may be taken on one film for some exams such as for the toes, foot, ankle or lower leg. This requires close collimation of the part being radiographed.

Four-sided collimation allows for checking radiographs for accuracy of centering and positioning by placing a large imaginary "X" from the four corners of the collimation field. The center point of the "X" indicates the CR location.

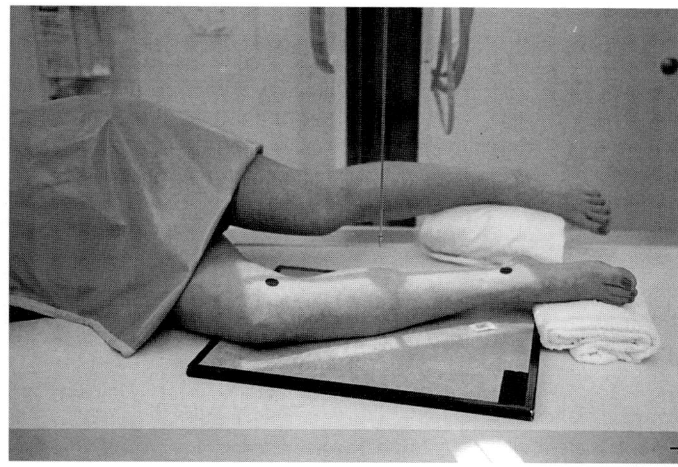

Fig. 6-38. Table-top of lower limb demonstrating:
-correct CR location.
-good collimation.
-gonadal shielding.
-diagonal placement of the film to include both knee and ankle joints.

General Positioning

A general positioning rule especially applicable to both the upper and lower limbs is to **always place the long axis of the part being radiographed parallel to the long axis of the film.** If more than one projection is taken on the same film, the part should be parallel to the long axis of the part of the film being used. Also **all body parts should be oriented in the same direction,** when two or more projections are taken on the same film.

An exception to this rule is the lower leg of an adult. This limb generally has to be placed diagonally to include both the knee and the ankle joints as shown in Fig. 6-38.

Correct Centering

Accurate centering and alignment of the body part to the film and correct central ray location is especially important for exams of the upper and lower limbs where shape and size distortion must be avoided and the narrow joint spaces clearly demonstrated. Therefore, in general, the part being radiographed should **be parallel to the plane of the film holder, the central ray should be 90° or perpendicular** and should be **directed to the correct centering point,** as indicated on each positioning page. (Exceptions to the 90° or perpendicular CR do occur as indicated in the following pages.)

Exposure Factors

The principal exposure factors for radiographs of the lower limbs are:

1. Lower to medium kVp (50-70).
2. Short exposure time.
3. Small focal spot.
4. Adequate mAs for sufficient density.

Correctly exposed radiographs of the lower limbs should generally visualize both soft tissue margins and fine bony trabecular markings of bones being radiographed.

Optional Technique for Foot: An increase to 70 or 75 kVp with accompanying decrease in mAs will increase exposure latitude to result in a more uniform exposure density between the phalanges and the tarsals.

Film Holders

For exams distal to the knee, detail extremity screens are used without grids. Detail (extremity) screens are commonly used for adult extremities for better detail.

A general rule states that grids should be used with body parts measuring over 10 cm. (Some references suggest a grid over 13 cm.) This places the average knee (measuring 9 to 13 cm) at a size where either a screen or grid may be used depending on patient size and departmental preferences. This text recommends a screen on smaller patients measuring 10 cm or less and a grid for larger patients measuring over 10 cm, especially on the AP knee. Anything proximal to the knee such as the mid or distal femur requires the use of a grid. When grids are used, either the moving Bucky grid under the table-top may be used, or fine-lined portable grids.

Placement of Film Markers and Patient ID Information

At the top of each of the following positioning pages is a box drawing demonstrating the correct film holder size and placement (lengthwise or crosswise). A suggested corner placement for the patient ID blocker is shown for each film. However, this is only a suggested location because the location of the blocker changes from manufacturer to manufacturer. The important consideration is to **always place it in the location least likely to superimpose anatomy of interest** for that projection.

The size and location of multiple projections on one film are also shown.

When evaluating final radiographs as part of the evaluation criteria, the patient ID information should always be checked to see if it is legible and not superimposing essential anatomy. Right (R) and left (L) markers should always be visible on the lateral margin of the collimation field **on at least one projection on each film** without superimposing any anatomy of interest.

Increase Exposure with Cast

A lower limb with a cast will require an increase in exposure. The thickness of the cast and the body part, as well as the type of cast, will affect the increase in exposure required. A recommended conversion guide for casts is as follows:

Cast Conversion Guide	
Small to medium dry plaster cast:	–Increase 5-7 kVp
Large or wet plaster cast:	–Double mAs **<u>or</u>** increase 8-10 kVp
Fiberglass cast:	–Increase 3-4 kVp

NATIONAL SURVEY

Departmental standard (basic) and special routines for exams of the lower limbs were very consistent throughout the United States except for the patella routines, which showed some regional differences. The results of this survey determined national norms for routines presented in the positioning pages of this text, which follow. Approximately 530 responses to this survey were received.

Toe Routine

Toe	U.S. Average Basic 1995 (1989)	U.S. Average Special 1995 (1989)
• AP (toes only)	68% (60%)	
• AP (entire foot)	37% (40%)	
• Oblique toes	91% (94%)	
• Lateral toes	87% (85%)	

Foot Routine

Foot	U.S. Average Basic 1995 (1989)	U.S. Average Special 1995 (1989)
• AP, 10-15° toward heel	94% (91%)	
• Medial oblique	95% –	
• Lateral oblique	12% –	18% –
• Lateral:		
–Mediolateral	70% (80%)	
–Lateromedial	22% (16%)	16% (5%)
• Lateral, weight bearing	14% –	51% –
• AP, weight bearing	13% –	41% –
• Club foot (Kite method)		24% –
• Sesamoids (tangential)		29% –

National Survey Continued

Calcaneus Routine

Calcaneus	U.S. Average	
	Basic 1995 (1989)	Special 1995 (1989)
• Lateral	96% (98%)	
• Plantodorsal (axial)	90% (90%)	
• Dorsoplantar (axial)	14% (12%)	19% (11%)

Ankle Routine

Ankle	U.S. Average	
	Basic 1995 (1989)	Special 1995 (1989)
• AP (true AP, no rotation)	95% (60%)	
• AP mortise (15-20° internal rotation)	40% (40%)	29% (14%)
• Oblique (45° internal)	72% (94%)	
• Lateral:		
–Mediolateral	73% (85%)	5% (2%)
–Lateromedial	22% (40%)	14% (5%)
• AP stress views		49% –

Lower Leg Routine

Leg	U.S. Average	
	Basic 1995 (1989)	Special 1995 (1989)
• AP	96% (99%)	
• Lateral	96% (99%)	
• Oblique		16% –

Knee Routine

Knee	U.S. Average	
	Basic 1995 (1989)	Special 1995 (1989)
• AP	92% (91%)	
• PA	10% –	
• AP oblique:		
–45° medial oblique	53% (45%)	21% –
–45° lateral oblique	34% (5%)	26% –
• AP, weight bearing		48% –
• PA, weight bearing		20% –
Intercondylar fossa		
• PA axial:		
–Camp Coventry method	52% (61%)	18% –
–kneeling, Holmblad method	34% (38%)	23% (10%)
• AP axial (Béclere method) (curved cassette)	19% –	21% –

Patella Routine

Patella	U.S. Average	
	Basic 1995 (1989)	Special 1995 (1989)
• PA	65% (65%)	
• Lateral	78% (81%)	
• Tangential		
–Settegast (prone flexed 90°)	64% (68)	13% –
–Hughston (prone flexed 55°)	16% –	21% –
–Merchant (supine flexed 45°)	27% (13%)	26% (18%)
• PA obliques	8% 9%	13% (9%)
• Axial oblique (Kuchendorf)	2% (38%)	15% (3%)

Summary

Toes: The survey indicates that the **"affected toes only"** is routine by about two-thirds (68%) of the U.S. average, and only about one-third (37%) consider taking the **entire AP foot** as routine for the AP toes. This is fairly consistent in all regions of the U.S.

Foot: The **AP**, **medial oblique** and **mediolateral** are the basic routines for the foot throughout the U.S. A regional difference was the **lateromedial,** which was twice as common in the West (40%) as compared to the Mid U.S. (19%) and East (18%). (See Appendix.)

Ankle: The routines for the ankle were fairly consistent throughout the U.S. as an **AP** (true AP), **45° medial oblique** and **lateral** (mediolateral). The **AP mortise 15° oblique** as routine was more common in the West (56%) as compared with the Mid U.S. (36%) and East (39%). This indicates that in 1995 only in the Western States is it considered a routine rather than a special projection by a majority of responding institutions.

Knee: The routine for the knee was consistent throughout the U.S., as an **AP, oblique** and **lateral**. The **medial oblique** was most common (53%) as compared with the **lateral oblique** (34%). This suggests that even though the medial oblique is most common, many institutions in 1995 also include the lateral oblique as part of their routine. This was not evaluated in 1989.

Patella: The survey indicates three basic projections for the patella: **PA**, **lateral** and a **tangential**. The **Settegast method** (patient prone, knee flexed 90°) was the most common tangential projection (60 to 67%) throughout all regions of the United States. The **Hughston method** (patient prone, knees flexed 55%) was considered basic by 24% in the West and only by 13% and 17% in the East and Mid U.S. respectively. The **Merchant method** (patient supine, knees flexed 45°) was basic in the West by 49%, but only 29% in the Mid U.S., and only 18% in the East.

Note: Even though the Settegast method was indicated to be the most common tangential projection throughout the U.S., studies indicate a major disadvantage to this method is the +90° flexion of the knee, which draws the patella into the intercondylar sulcus, thus limiting its diagnostic value (see page 215).

STANDARD AND SPECIAL OPERATING PROCEDURES

Certain basic and special projections for the toes, foot, ankle, leg, knee and mid and distal femur are demonstrated and described on the following pages as suggested standard and special departmental procedures.

Basic Projections

Standard or basic projections, at times referred to as routine projections or departmental routines, are those projections commonly taken on average patients who are helpful and can cooperate in performing the procedure.

Special Projections

Special projections are those more common projections taken as extra or additional projections to better demonstrate certain pathologic conditions or specific body parts.

Basic and Special Projections

Toes
Basic
- AP **189**
- Oblique **190**
- Lateral **191**

Special
- Sesamoids **192** (tangential)

Foot
Basic
- AP **193**
- Oblique **194**
- Lateral **195**

Special
- AP and lateral weight-bearing **196**

Calcaneus
Basic
- Plantodorsal **197** (axial)
- Lateral **198**

Ankle
Basic
- AP **199**
- AP mortise **200**
- Oblique (45°) **201**
- Lateral **202**

Special
- AP stress **203**

Leg
Basic
- AP **204**
- Lateral **205**

Knee
Basic
- AP **206**
- Oblique **207**
- Lateral **208**

Special
- AP (PA) weight-bearing **209**

Knee–Intercondylar fossa
Basic
- PA axial (Camp Coventry and Holmblad methods) **210**

Special
- AP axial **211**

Patella and patellofemoral joint
Basic
- PA **212**
- Lateral **213**
- Tangential (Merchant method) **214**
- Tangential (inferosuperior projection, Hughston and Settegast methods) **215**

Special
- Oblique or axial oblique (Kuchendorf method) **216**

Femur –Mid and distal
Basic
- AP **217**
- Lateral **218**
- Lateral –cross table **218**

Femur –Mid and proximal
Basic
- AP (see AP hip, Ch. 7)
- Lateral **219**

AP Projection

Toes
Basic
- **AP**
- Oblique
- Lateral

Structures Best Shown

Phalanges of digit(s) in question to include distal metatarsal(s) and associated joints.

Technical Factors

- Film size–8 x 10 in. (18 x 24 cm) crosswise.
- Divide in thirds, crosswise.
- Detail screen, table-top.
- 50-60 kVp range.
- Technique and dose:

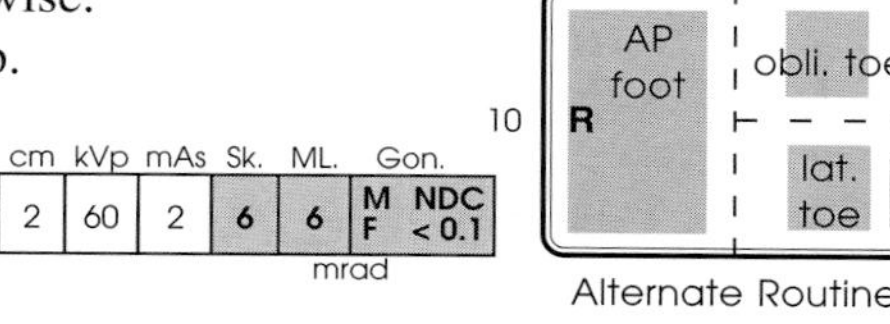

cm	kVp	mAs	Sk.	ML.	Gon.
2	60	2	6	6	M NDC F < 0.1

mrad

Alternate Routine (AP of Entire Foot)

- 10 x 12 in. (24 x 30 cm) crosswise, divide in half.
  Note: Some departments require the entire foot to be included for this AP projection for possible secondary trauma to other parts of the foot. (CR and collimation would be changed accordingly as for an AP foot, see page 193.)

Shielding: Place shield over pelvic region to shield gonads.

Patient Position

- Patient supine or seated on table, knee flexed with plantar surface of foot resting on cassette.

Part Position

- Center and align long axis of digit(s) to CR and long axis of portion of film being exposed.
- Ensure that MP joint(s) of digit(s) in question is (are) centered to CR.

Central Ray

- Angle CR **10 to 15° toward calcaneus** (CR perpendicular to phalanges).
- If a **15° wedge** is placed under foot for parallel part-film alignment, then the CR is **perpendicular** to film, Fig. 6-41.
- CR to **metatarsophalangeal (MP) joint(s)** in question.
- Minimum 40 in. (102 cm) SID.

Collimation: Collimate on four sides to area of interest. On side margins include a minimum of one digit on each side of digit(s) in question.

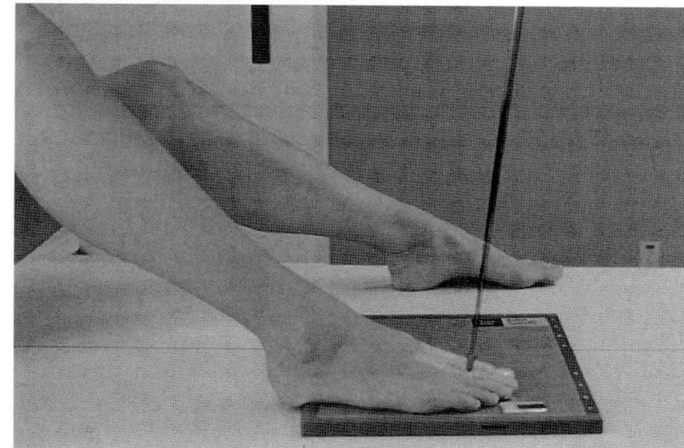

Fig. 6-39. 2nd digit (CR 10 to 15°).

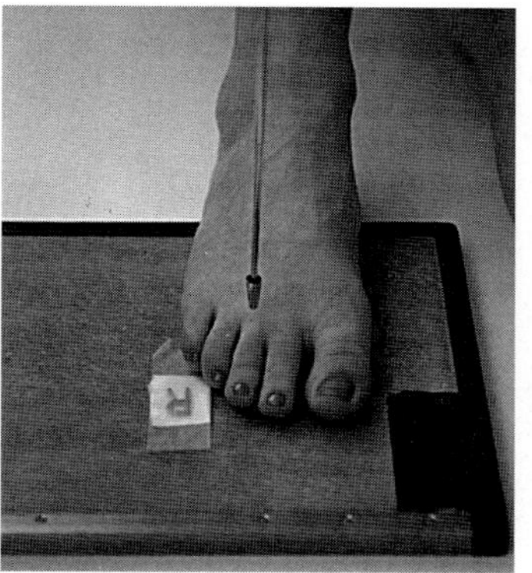

Fig. 6-40. AP 3rd digit (CR 10 to 15°).

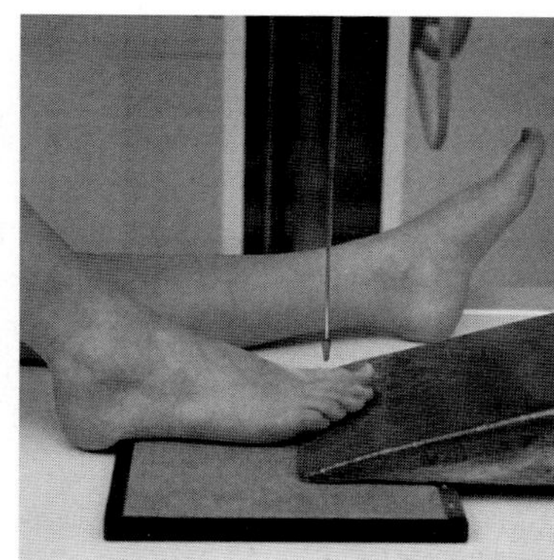

Fig. 6-41. AP 1st digit with wedge (CR perpendicular).

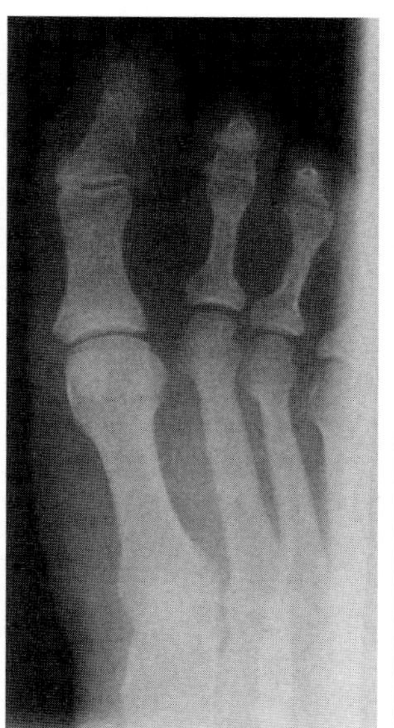

Fig. 6-42. AP 1st digit.

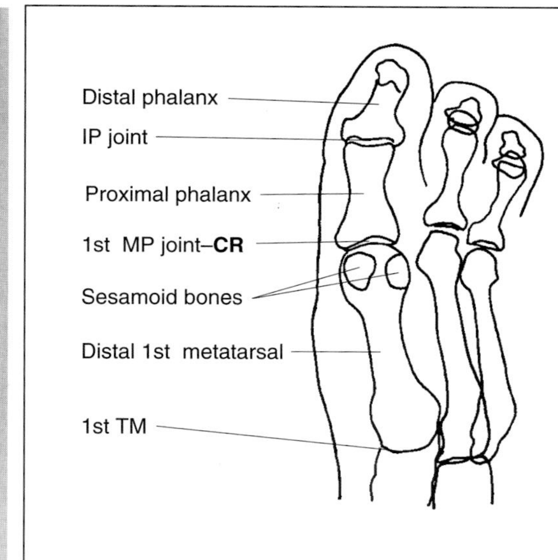

Fig. 6-43. AP 1st digit.

Evaluation Criteria

- Digit(s) in question and a minimum of the distal half of metatarsals should be included.
- Individual digits should be separated with no overlapping of soft tissues.
- Collimation borders should be visible on all four sides with the center at the MP joint(s) in question.
- No rotation as evidenced by symmetrical appearance of concavities on each side of shafts of phalanges and distal metatarsals.
- Interphalangeal and MP joints in question should appear open, indicating correct CR centering and angle.
- Optimum exposure and contrast with no motion will visualize sharp borders and fine trabecular markings. Soft tissue margins and detail should be visible.
- **Alternate routine**: See AP foot.

AP Oblique Projection–Medial or Lateral Rotation

Toes
Basic
- AP
- **Oblique**
- Lateral

Structures Best Shown

Phalanges of digit(s) in question to include distal metatarsal(s) and associated joints.

Technical Factors

- Film size–8 x 10 in. (18 x 24 cm) crosswise.
- Divide in thirds, crosswise.
- Detail screen, table-top.
- 50-60 kVp range.
- Technique and dose:

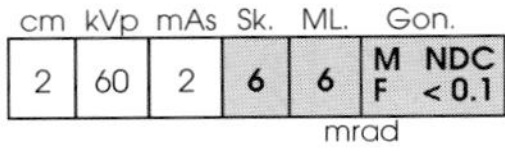

cm	kVp	mAs	Sk.	ML.	Gon.
2	60	2	6	6	M NDC F <0.1

mrad

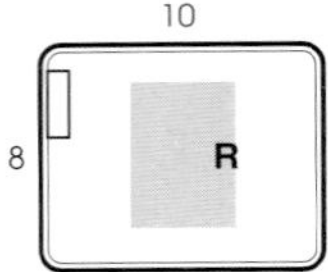

Shielding: Place lead shield over pelvic area to shield gonads.

Patient Position

- Patient supine or seated on table, knee flexed with plantar surface of foot resting on cassette.

Part Position 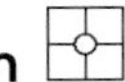

- Center and align long axis of digit(s) to CR and long axis of portion of film being exposed.
- Ensure that MP joint(s) of digit(s) in question is (are) centered to CR.
- Rotate the leg and foot 30 to 45° medially for the 1st, 2nd and 3rd digits, and laterally for the 4th and 5th digits.
- Use 45° radiolucent support under elevated portion of foot to prevent motion.

Central Ray

- CR **perpendicular** to film, directed to MP joint(s) in question.
- Minimum 40 in. (102 cm) SID.

Collimation: Collimate on four sides to include phalanges and a minimum of distal two-thirds of metatarsals. On side margins include a minimum of one digit on each side of digit(s) in question.

Evaluation Criteria

- Digit(s) in question and distal half of metatarsals should be included without overlap (superimposition).
- Collimation borders should be visible on all four sides with the center at the MP joint(s) in question.
- Interphalangeal and MP joint spaces in question should appear open.
- Correct obliquity should be evident by increased concavity on one side of shafts and by overlapping of soft tissues of digits. Heads of metatarsals should appear directly side by side with no (or only minimal) overlapping.
- Optimum exposure and contrast with no motion will visualize sharp borders and fine trabecular markings. Soft tissue margins and detail should be visible.

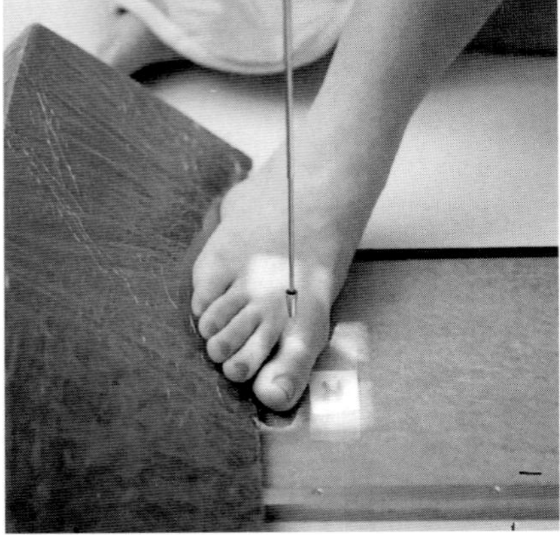

Fig. 6-44. Medial rotation–1st digit.

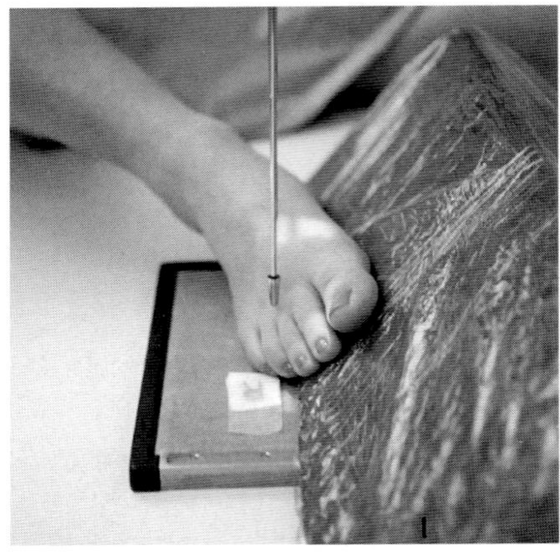

Fig. 6-45. Lateral rotation–4th digit.

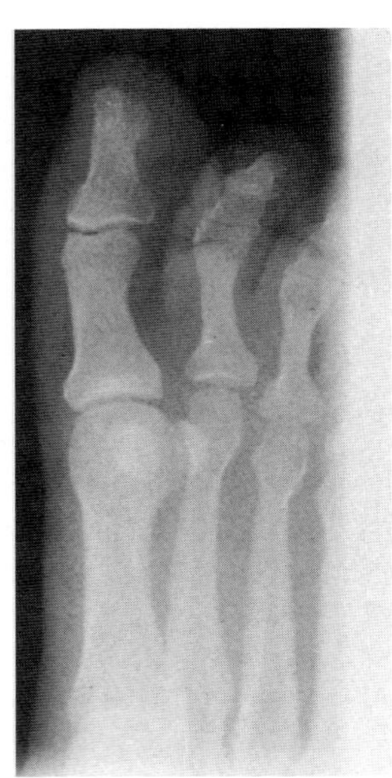

Fig. 6-46. Oblique–1st digit

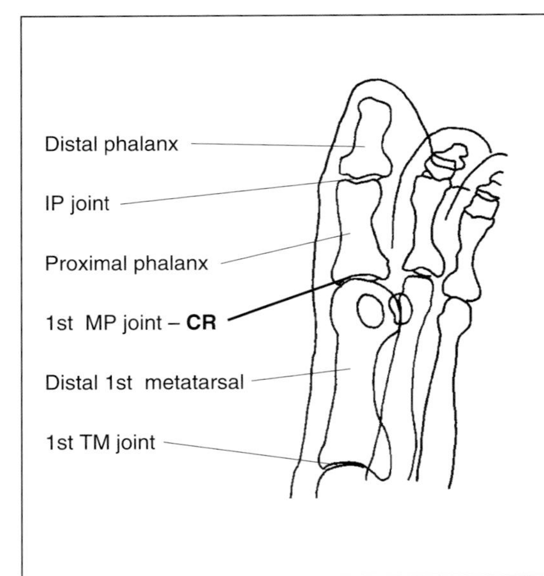

Fig. 6-47. Oblique–1st digit.

Lateral–Mediolateral or Lateromedial Projections

Toes
Basic
• AP
• Oblique
• **Lateral**

Structures Best Shown

Phalanges of digit in question free of superimposition.

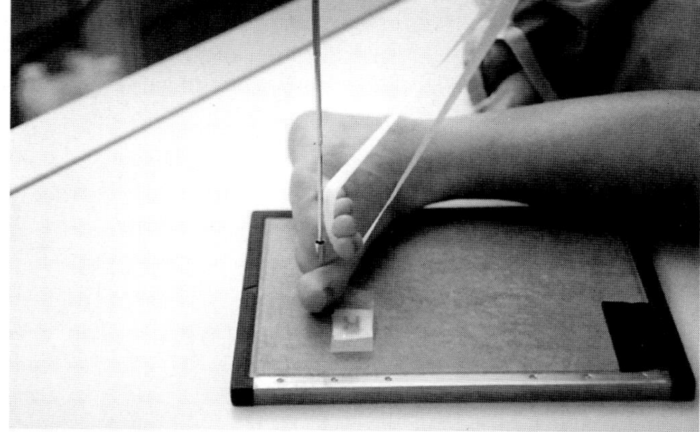

Fig. 6-48. Lateromedial–1st digit.

Technical Factors

- Film size–8 x 10 in. (18 x 24 cm) crosswise.
- Divide in thirds, crosswise.
- Detail screen, table-top.
- 50-60 kVp range.
- Technique and dose:

cm	kVp	mAs	Sk.	ML.	Gon.
2	60	2	6	6	M NDC F < 0.1

mrad

Shielding: Place lead shield over pelvic area to shield gonads.

Patient and Part Position

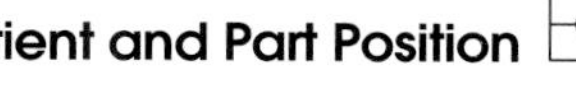

- Rotate affected leg and foot medially (lateromedial) for 1st, 2nd and 3rd digits and laterally (mediolateral) for 4th and 5th digits.
- Adjust cassette to center and align long axis of toe in question to CR and to long axis of portion of film being exposed.
- Ensure that IP joint or PIP joint in question is centered to CR.
- Use tape, gauze or tongue blade to flex and separate unaffected toes to prevent superimposition.

Central Ray

- CR **perpendicular** to film.
- CR directed to **interphalangeal joint for 1st digit**, and to **PIP joint for 2nd to 5th digits**.
- Minimum 40 in. (102 cm) SID.

Collimation: Collimate closely on four sides to affected digit.

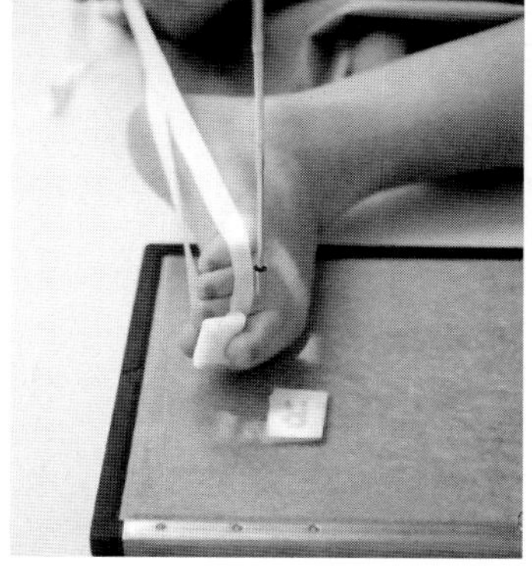

Fig. 6-49. Lateromedial –2nd digit.

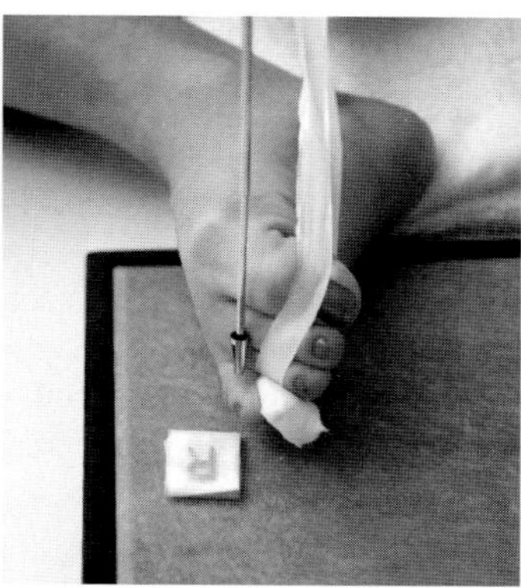

Fig. 6-50. Mediolateral –4th digit.

Evaluation Criteria

- Phalanges of digit in question should be seen in lateral position free of superimposition by other digits. Toenail should be seen on edge in profile. (When total separation of toes is not possible, especially 3rd to 5th digits, the proximal phalanx should be included and visualized through superimposed structures.)
- Interphalangeal joints should appear open and unobstructed. The MP joint should be visualized even if superimposed.
- Optimum exposure and contrast with no motion will visualize sharp borders and fine trabecular markings. Soft tissue margins and detail should be visible.

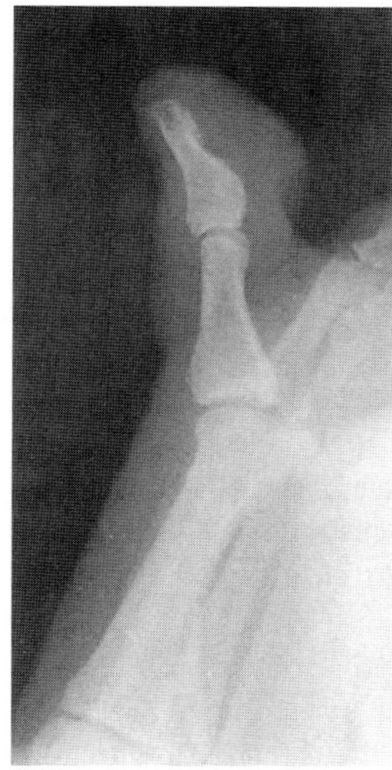

Distal phalanx
Interphalangeal joint
Proximal phalanx
1st metatarso-phalangeal joint

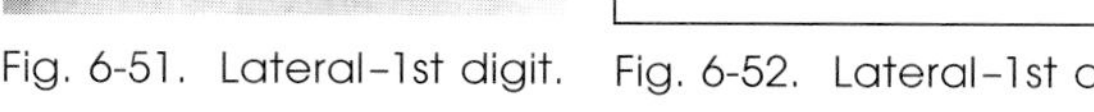

Fig. 6-51. Lateral–1st digit. Fig. 6-52. Lateral–1st digit.

Tangential Projection

Toes
Special
• **Sesamoids (tangential)**

Structures Best Shown

Sesamoids and head of 1st metatarsal in profile.

Note: A lateral of 1st digit in dorsiflexion may also be taken to visualize these sesamoids.

Technical Factors

- Film size–8 x 10 in. (18 x 24 cm) crosswise. (Divide in half if combined with another projection.)
- Detail screen, table-top.
- 50-60 kVp range.
- Technique and dose:

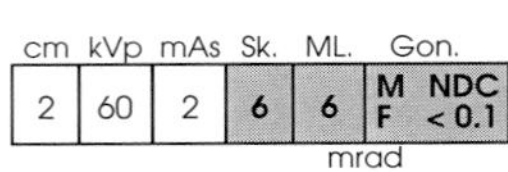

cm	kVp	mAs	Sk.	ML.	Gon.
2	60	2	6	6	M NDC F <0.1
					mrad

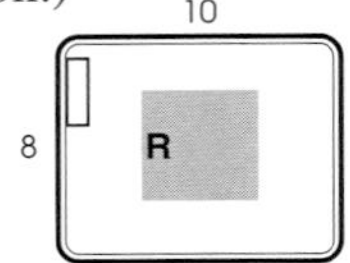

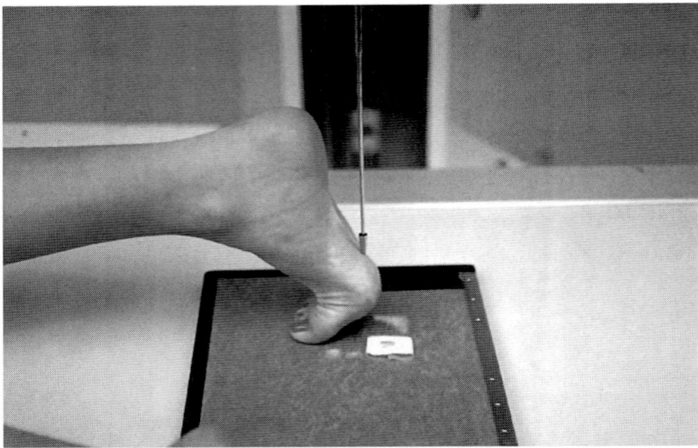

Fig. 6-53. Tangential projection–Patient prone.

Shielding: Place lead shield over pelvic area to shield gonads.

Patient Position

- Patient prone, provide pillow for head and small sponge or folded towel under lower leg for patient comfort.

Part Position

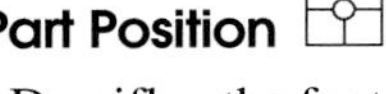

- Dorsiflex the foot so that the plantar surface of the foot forms about a **15 to 20° angle** from vertical.
- Dorsiflex the 1st digit (great toe), and rest on cassette to maintain position.
- Ensure that long axis of foot is not rotated; place sandbags or other support on both sides of foot to prevent movement.

  Note: This is an uncomfortable and often painful position; do not keep patient in this position longer than necessary.

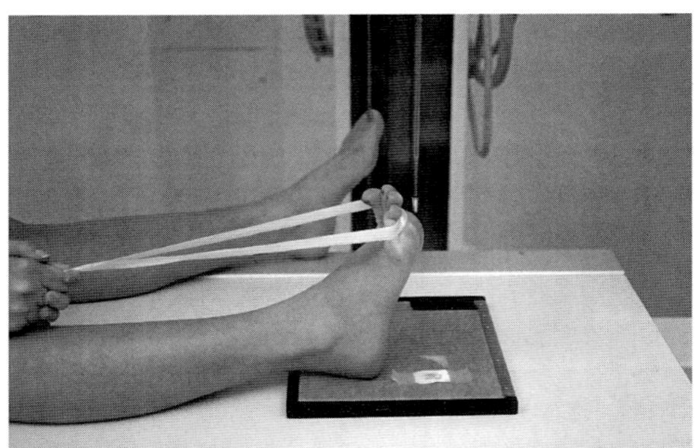

Fig. 6-54. Alternate projection–Patient supine.

Central Ray

- CR **perpendicular** to film, directed tangentially to posterior aspect of **head of 1st metatarsal**. (Depending on the amount of dorsiflexion of foot, may need to angle CR slightly for a true tangential projection.)
- Minimum 40 in. (102 cm) SID.

Collimation: Collimate closely to area of interest. Include at least the 1st, 2nd and 3rd distal metatarsals for possible sesamoids but with CR at 1st MP joint.

Alternate projection: If patient cannot tolerate the above prone position, this may be taken in a reverse projection with patient supine by using a long strip of gauze for patient to hold the toes as shown. CR would again be directed tangential to head of 1st metatarsal. Use support to prevent motion. This, however, is not a desirable projection because of the increased OID with accompanying magnification and loss of definition and should only be done if patient cannot tolerate prone position.

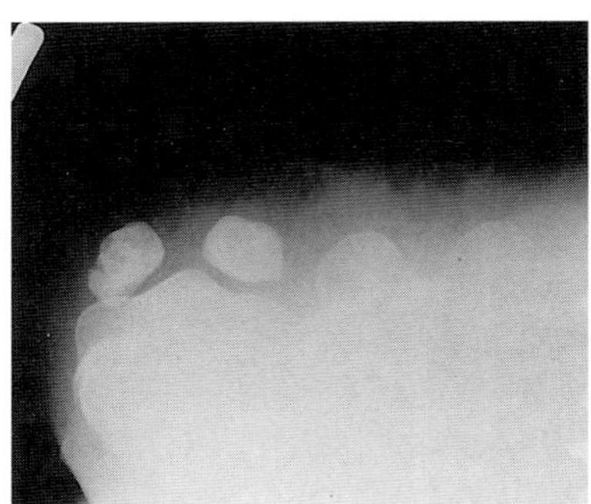

Fig. 6-55. Tangential projection.

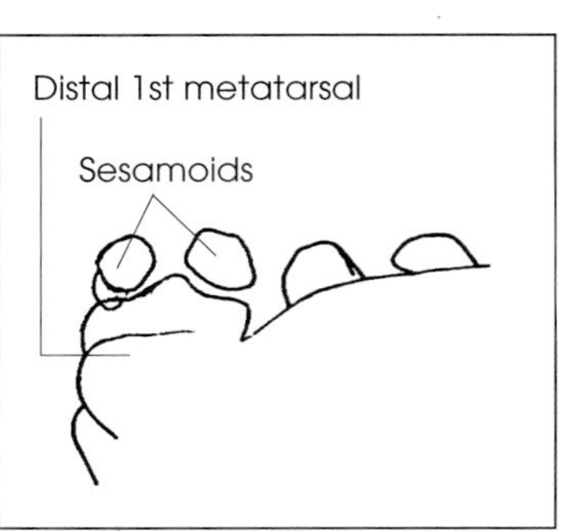

Fig. 6-56. Tangential projection.

Evaluation Criteria

- Sesamoids should be seen in profile free of superimposition.
- A minimum of the first three distal metatarsals should be included in collimation field for possible sesamoids, with the center of the four-sided collimation field at the distal portion of the head of 1st metatarsal.
- Optimum exposure without motion should visualize sharp borders and trabecular markings of sesamoid bones and distal portions of the heads of the metatarsals, without the sesamoids appearing overexposed.

AP Projection

Dorsoplantar Projection

Foot
Basic
• **AP**
• Oblique
• Lateral

Structures Best Shown

Phalanges, metatarsals, cuneiforms, cuboid and navicular.

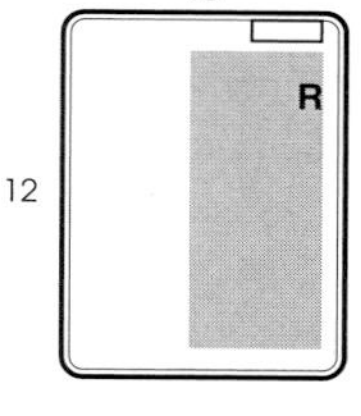

Technical Factors

- Film size–10 x 12 in. (24 x 30 cm), lengthwise. (Divide in half for AP and oblique.)
- Detail screen, table-top.
- 60±5 kVp range; or 70-75 kVp for increased exposure latitude for more uniform density of phalanges and tarsals.
- Technique and dose @ 70 kVp:

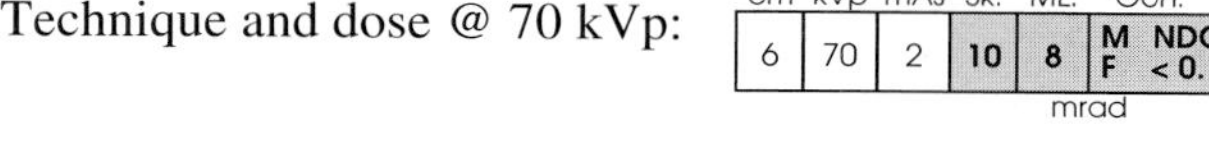

cm	kVp	mAs	Sk.	ML.	Gon.
6	70	2	10	8	M NDC F <0.1
			mrad		

Shielding: Place lead shield over pelvic area to shield gonads.

Patient Position

- Patient supine, pillow for head, flex knee and place plantar surface (sole) of affected foot flat on cassette.

Part Position

- Extend (plantar flex) foot but maintain plantar surface resting flat and firmly on cassette.
- Align and center long axis of foot to CR and to long axis of portion of film being exposed. (Use sandbags if necessary to prevent cassette from slipping on table-top.)
- If immobilization is needed, flex opposite knee also and rest against affected knee for support.

Central Ray

- CR angled **10° posteriorly** (toward heel), CR perpendicular to metatarsals.
- Direct CR to **base of 3rd metatarsal.**
- Minimum 40 in. (102 cm) SID.

Collimation: Collimate to outer margins of foot on four sides.

Fig. 6-57. AP foot–CR 10°.

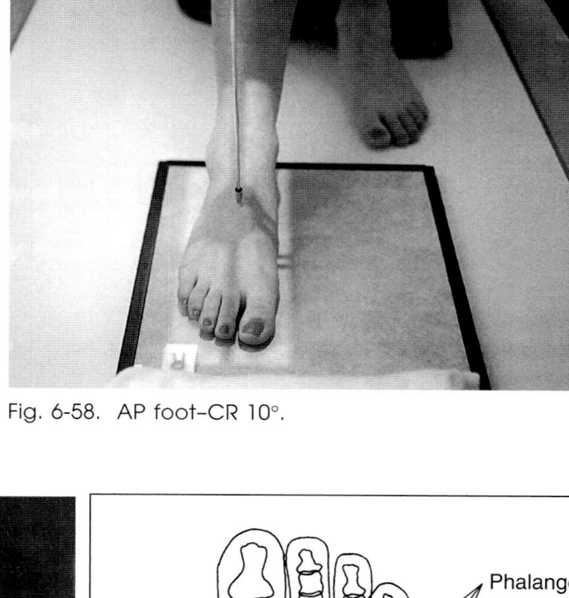

Fig. 6-58. AP foot–CR 10°.

Evaluation Criteria

- Entire foot should be visualized including all phalanges and metatarsals, as well as the navicular, cuneiforms and cuboids.
- Center of four-sided collimation field should be at the base of 3rd metatarsal.
- No rotation as evidenced by near equal distance between 2nd through 5th metatarsals. Bases of 1st and 2nd metatarsals are generally separated but bases of 2nd to 5th metatarsals will appear to be overlapped.
- Sesamoid bones (if present) should be seen through head of 1st metatarsal.
- MP joints should generally appear open. IP joints however, may appear partially closed due to divergent rays.
- Optimum density and contrast with no motion should visualize sharp borders and trabecular markings of distal phalanges as well as tarsals distal to talus. (See optional technique for more uniform densities between phalanges and tarsals.)

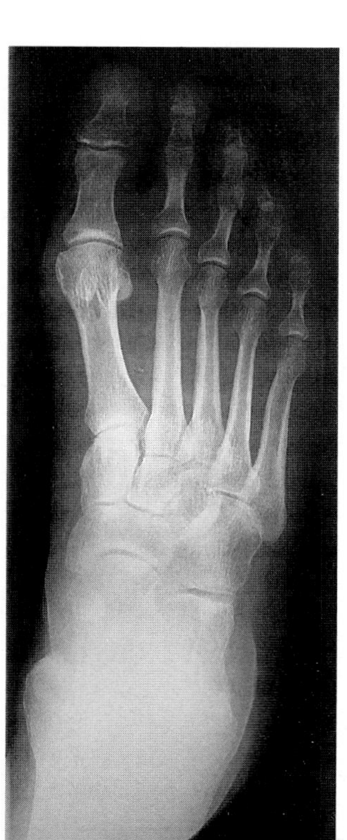

Fig. 6-59. AP foot.

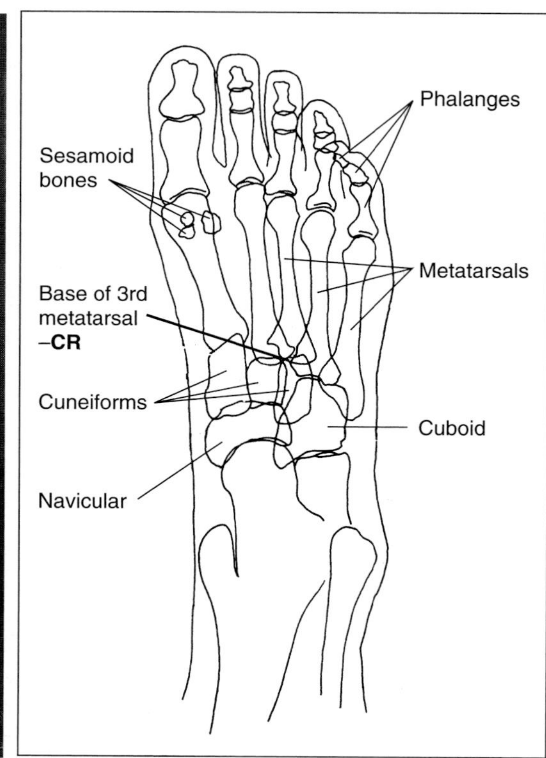

Fig. 6-60. AP foot.

AP Oblique Projection–Medial Rotation

Foot
Basic
• AP
• **Oblique**
• Lateral

Structures Best Shown

Phalanges, metatarsals, cuboid, 3rd cuneiform, navicular and distal calcaneus with associated intertarsal spaces.
Note: An alternate lateral rotation may be requested as an additional oblique for specific anatomy.

Technical Factors

- Film size–10 x 12 in. (24 x 30 cm), lengthwise. (Divide in half for AP and oblique.)
- Detail screen, table-top.
- 60±5 kVp range; or 70-75 kVp for increased exposure latitude for more uniform density between phalanges and tarsals.
- Technique and dose @ 70 kVp:

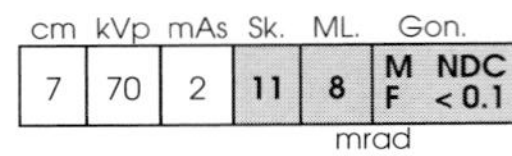

cm	kVp	mAs	Sk.	ML.	Gon.
7	70	2	11	8	M NDC F <0.1
			mrad		

Shielding: Place lead shield over pelvic area to shield gonads.

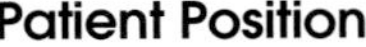

Patient Position

- Patient supine, pillow for head. Flex knee, with plantar surface of foot on table.
- Body turned slightly away from side in question.

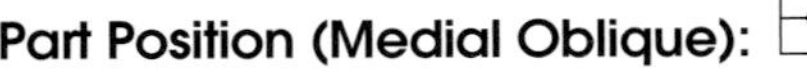

Part Position (Medial Oblique):

- Extend foot but maintain plantar surface resting flat and firmly on cassette.
- Align and center long axis of foot to CR and to long axis of portion of film being exposed.
- Rotate foot **medially** to place **plantar surface 30 to 45° to plane of film.** (See Note.)
- Use 45° radiolucent support block to prevent motion. Use sandbags if necessary to prevent cassette from slipping on table-top.

Central Ray

- CR **perpendicular** to film, directed to **base of 3rd metatarsal.**
- Minimum 40 in. (102 cm) SID.

Collimation: Collimate to outer margins of skin on four sides.

Note: Some department routines call for a 40 to 45° medial oblique and others prefer only 30°. This text recommends 40 to 45° for the medial oblique, which results in better separation at the bases of 2nd to 5th metatarsals and between individual tarsals due to the natural transverse arch of the foot.

Alternate Lateral Oblique:

- Rotate the foot laterally 30° (less oblique required because of the natural arch of the foot).
- A lateral oblique will best demonstrate the space between 1st and 2nd metatarsals and between 1st and 2nd cuneiforms. The navicular will also be best visualized on the lateral oblique.

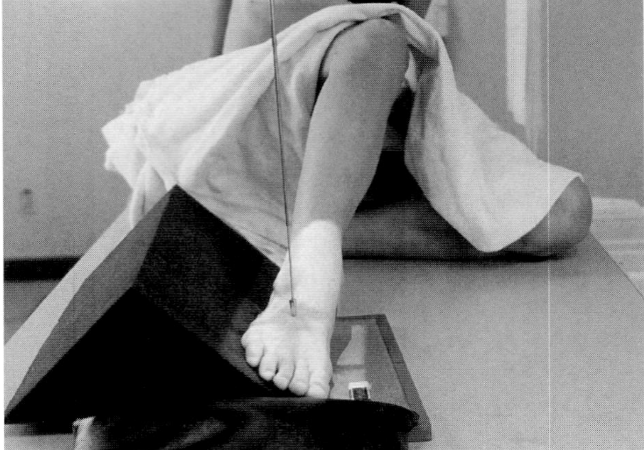

Fig. 6-61. 30 to 45° medial oblique.

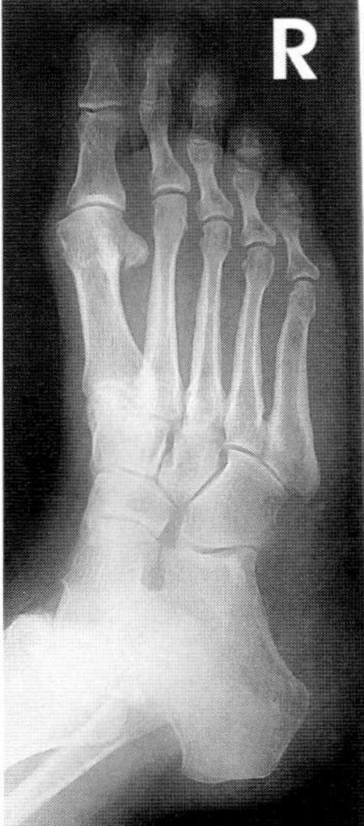

Fig. 6-62. 45° medial oblique.

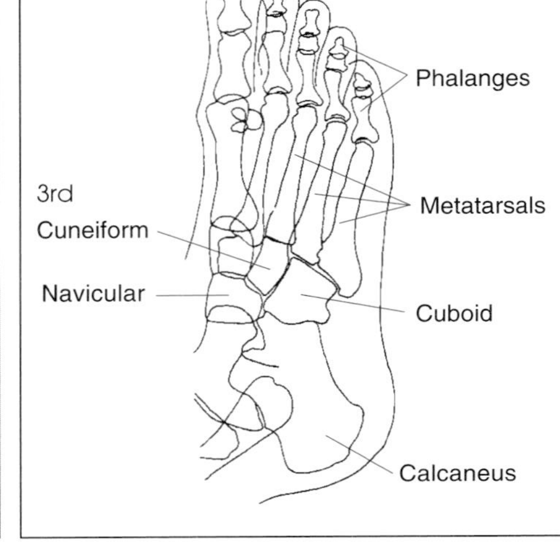

Fig. 6-63. 45° medial oblique.

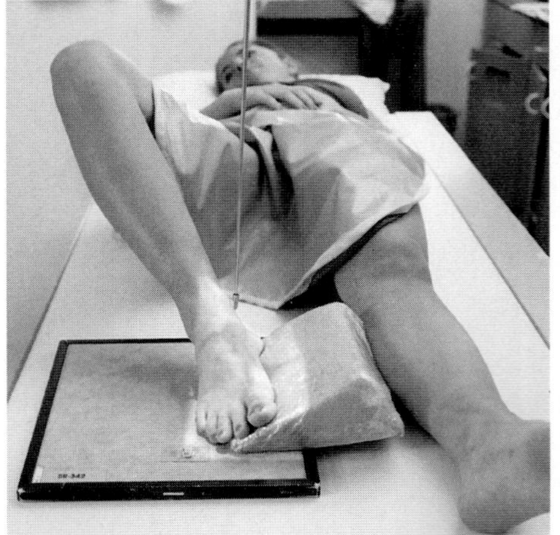

Fig. 6-64. Alternate 30° lateral oblique.

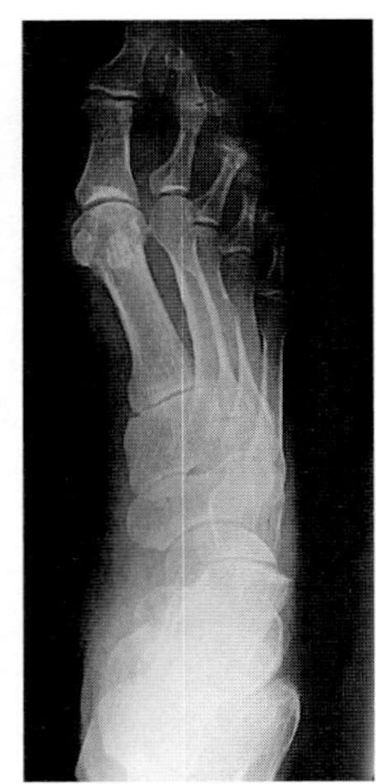

Fig. 6-65. Lateral oblique.

Evaluation Criteria

Medial Oblique (45°):

- Entire foot should be visualized from distal phalanges to posterior calcaneus and proximal talus.
- Center of four-sided collimation should be to base of 3rd metatarsal.
- Third through 5th metatarsals should be completely free of superimposition. First and 2nd metatarsals should also be free of superimposition except for base area.
- Tuberosity at base of 5th metatarsal should be well visualized.
- Optimum density and contrast with no motion should visualize sharp borders and trabecular markings of phalanges, metatarsals and tarsals.

Alternate Lateral Oblique (30°):

- Bases of 1st and 2nd metatarsals should not overlap, and space between 1st and 2nd cuneiform should be open. Outline of the navicular should be seen in its entirety.

Lateral–Mediolateral or Lateromedial Projections

Foot
Basic
- AP
- Oblique
- **Lateral**

Structures Best Shown

Tarsals are partially superimposed. Ankle joint and subtalar joint are seen partially superimposed, metatarsals and phalanges are superimposed.

Technical Factors

- Film size–8 x 10 in. (18 x 24 cm)–smaller foot.
  or
  –10 x 12 in. (24 x 30 cm)–larger foot.
- Detail screen, table-top.
- 60±5 kVp range.
- Technique and dose:

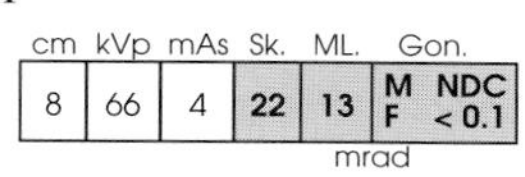

cm	kVp	mAs	Sk.	ML.	Gon.
8	66	4	22	13	M NDC F < 0.1

mrad

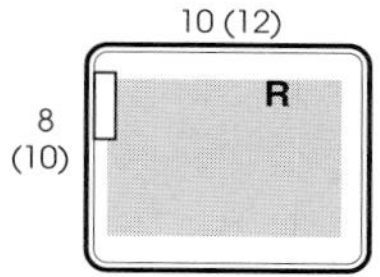

Shielding: Place lead shield over pelvic area to shield gonads.

Patient Position

Note: **Mediolateral** projection recommended because this is more comfortable for trauma patient.

- Patient in lateral recumbent position, affected side down.
- Provide pillow for head.
- Flex knee of affected limb about 45°; place opposite leg **behind** the injured limb to prevent over-rotation of affected leg.

Part Position 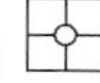

- Carefully dorsiflex the foot if possible to assist in positioning for a true lateral foot and ankle.
- Place support under leg and knee as needed so that **plantar surface is perpendicular to film.**
- Align long axis of foot to long axis of film (unless diagonal placement is needed to include entire foot).
- Center mid area of base of metatarsals to CR.

Central Ray

- CR **perpendicular** to film, directed to **medial cuneiform** (base of 3rd metatarsal).
- Minimum 40 in. (102 cm) SID.

Collimation: Collimate to the outer skin margins of the foot, to include about 1 in. or 2 to 3 cm proximal to ankle joint.

Alternate lateromedial projection: May be taken as an alternate lateral. Is usually more uncomfortable or painful for patient, even though it may be easier to achieve a true lateral in this position.

Evaluation Criteria

- Entire foot should be visualized and a minimum of 1 in. or 2 cm of distal tibia-fibula.
- Center of four-sided collimation field should be at medial cuneiform (base of 3rd metatarsal).
- Distal fibula should be seen superimposed over posterior portion of tibia.
- Tibiotalar joint space should be clearly visualized.
- Metatarsals should generally be superimposed with only a portion of the tuberosity at base of 5th metatarsal seen in profile distally.
- Optimum density and contrast should visualize borders of superimposed tarsals and metatarsals. Borders and trabecular markings of calcaneus and non-superimposed parts of other tarsals should appear sharp and visible.

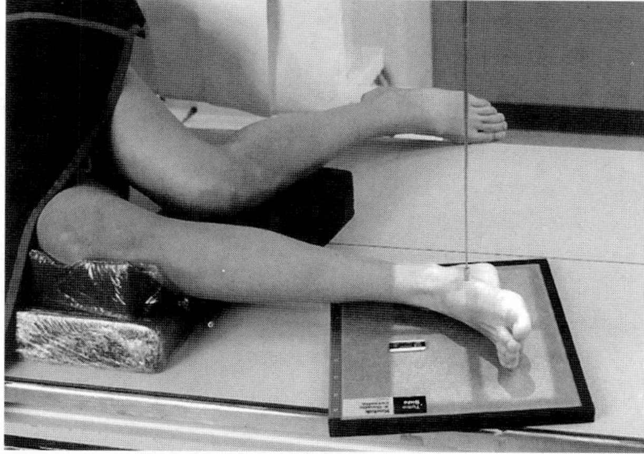

Fig. 6-66. **Mediolateral** projection.

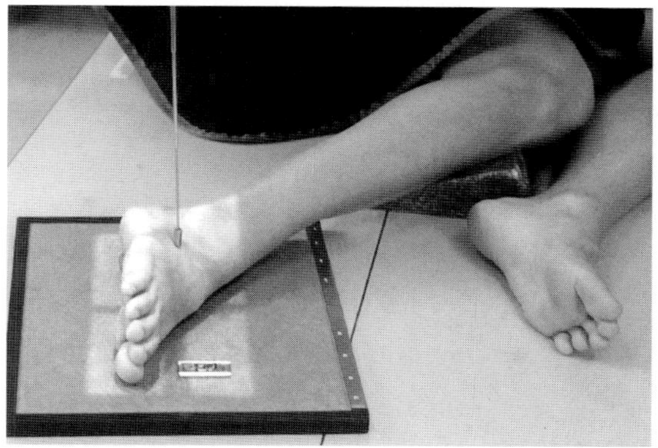

Fig. 6-67. Alternate **lateromedial.**

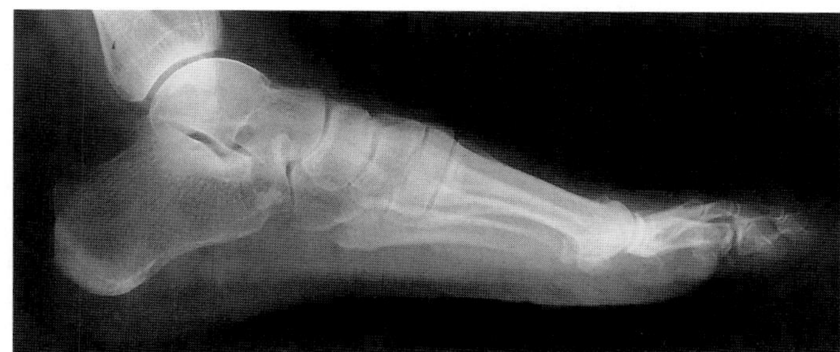

Fig. 6-68. Mediolateral foot.

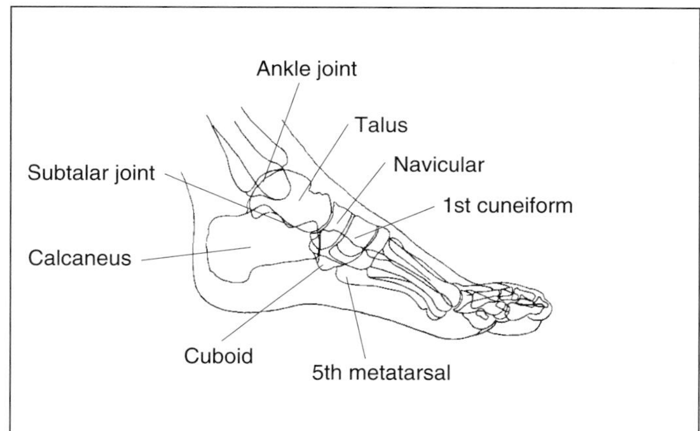

Fig. 6-69. Lateral foot.

AP and Lateral Weight-Bearing Projections

Foot
Special
• **AP and lateral (weight-bearing)**

Structures Best Shown

AP and lateral view of bones of the feet to show the condition of arches with full weight of body.

Note: Laterals of both feet are usually taken for comparison.

Technical Factors

- Film size–8 x 10 in. (18 x 24 cm) and –10 x 12 in. (24 x 30 cm).
- Detail screen.
- 65±5 kVp range.

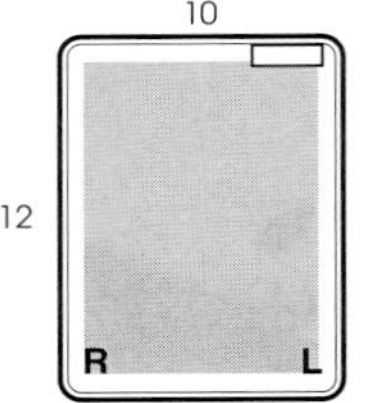

AP both feet

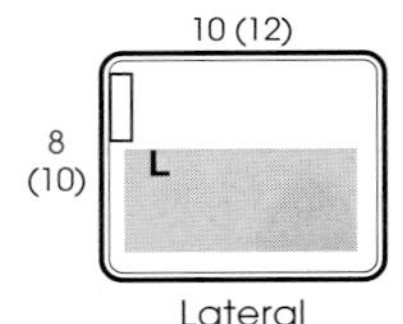

Lateral

Shielding: Shield gonadal area.

Part Position and CR

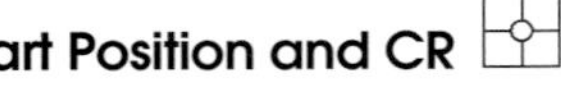

Note: Some AP routines include separate projections of each foot taken with CR centered to individual foot.

AP:

- Patient standing erect, full weight evenly distributed on both feet, standing lateral. Feet directed straight ahead, parallel to each other.
- **CR 15° posteriorly** to **midpoint between feet** at level of **base of metatarsals.**

Lateral:

- Patient standing erect, weight evenly distributed on **both** feet.
- Standing on wood blocks on a step stool, or on the footrest attached to the table as shown. Can also use a special wood box with a film slot for cassette. (Needs to be high enough from floor to get x-ray tube down into a horizontal beam position.)
- Provide some support for patient onto hold to for security.
- Support vertical cassette between feet, with long axis of foot to long axis of film.
- After first lateral is taken, cassettes are changed and patient is turned for lateral of other foot for comparison.
- **CR** directed **horizontally**, to **level of base of 3rd metatarsal.**
- Minimum 40 in. (102 cm) SID.

Collimation: Collimate to margins of feet (foot).

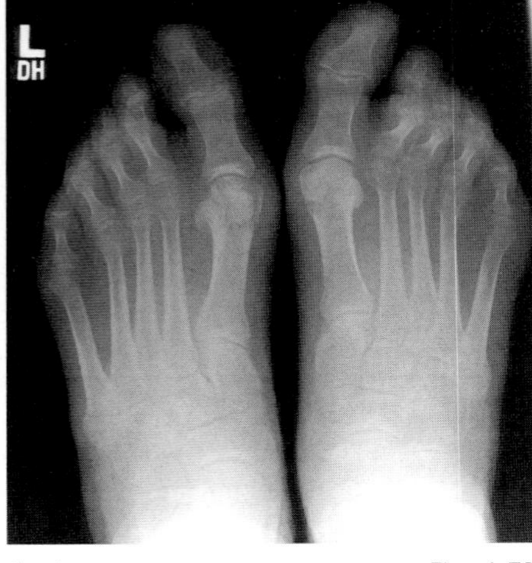

Fig. 6-70. AP–Both feet. Fig. 6-71.

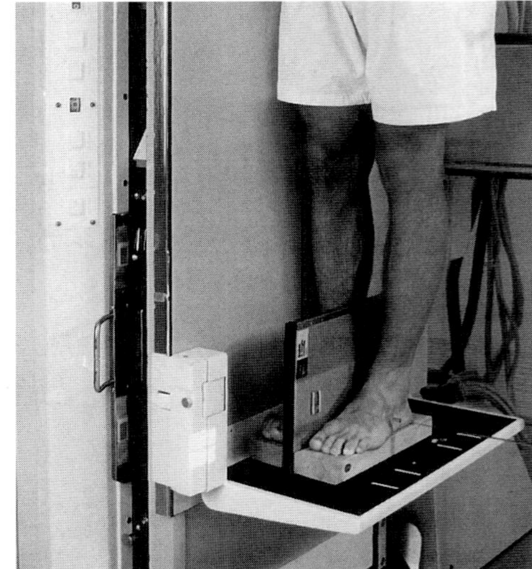

Fig. 6-72. Lateral–Left foot.

Evaluation Criteria

AP:

- Frontal view of bilateral feet with parallel phalanges and metatarsals without rotation.

Lateral:

- Entire foot should be visualized and a minimum of 1 in. or 2 cm of distal tibia-fibula.
- Center of collimation field should be to level of base of 3rd metatarsal.
- Distal fibula should seem superimposed over posterior half of the tibia.
- Plantar surfaces of heads of metatarsals should appear directly superimposed.
- Optimum density and contrast should visualize borders of superimposed tarsals and metatarsals.

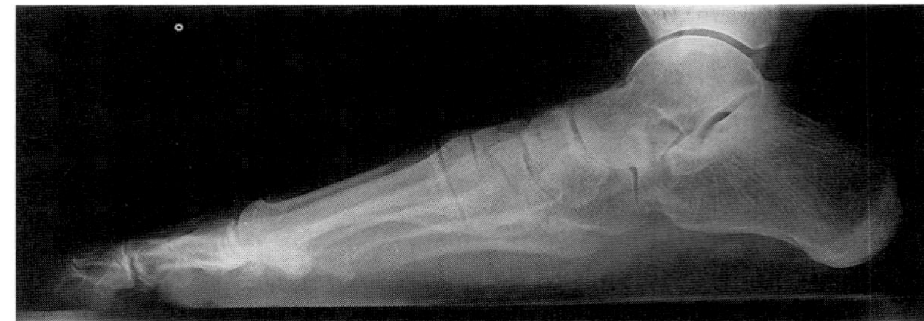

Fig. 6-73. Weight-bearing lateral.

Plantodorsal (Axial) Projection

Calcaneus
Basic
- **Plantodorsal (axial)**
- Lateral

Structures Best Shown

An axial view of the calcaneus (os calcis), with the sustentaculum tali and the tuberosity shown in profile.

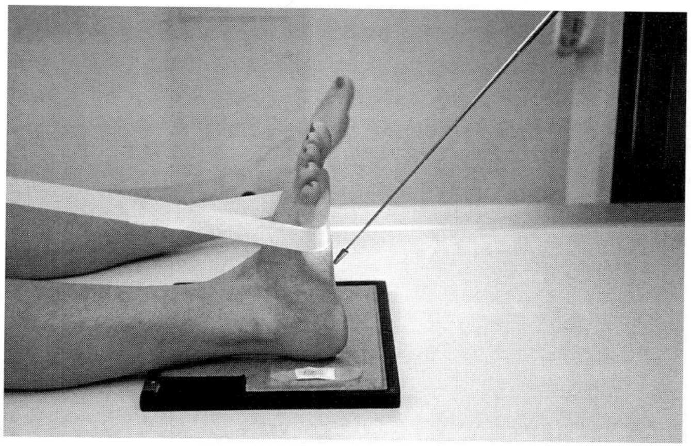

Fig. 6-74. Plantodorsal (axial) projection of calcaneus.

Technical Factors

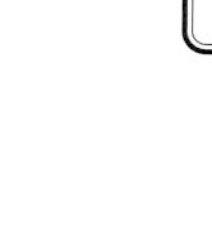

- Film size–8 x 10 in. (18 x 24 cm)
- Divide in half, crosswise.
- Detail screen, table-top.
- 70±5 kVp range.
  (Increase 8-10 kVp from other foot projections to best visualize proximal calcaneus and/or calcanes-talus relationship.)
- Technique and dose:

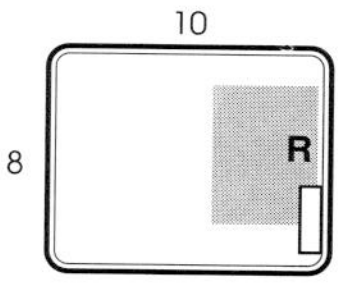

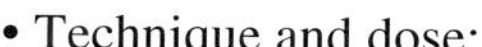

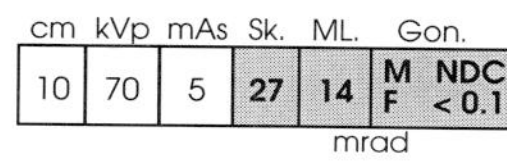

cm	kVp	mAs	Sk.	ML.	Gon.
10	70	5	27	14	M NDC F < 0.1

mrad

Shielding: Place lead shield over pelvic area to shield gonads.

Patient Position

- Patient supine or seated on table.
- Leg fully extended.

Part Position

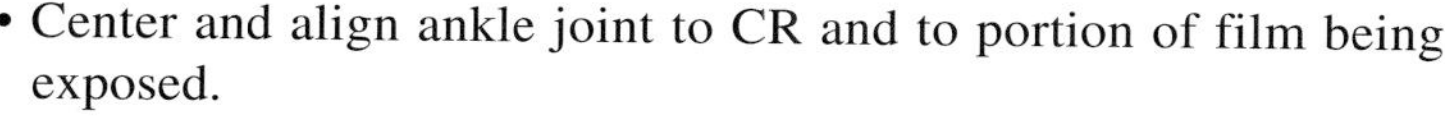

- Center and align ankle joint to CR and to portion of film being exposed.
- Dorsiflex foot so that plantar surface is near perpendicular to film.
- Loop gauze around foot and ask patient to pull gently but firmly and hold the plantar surface of foot as near perpendicular to film as possible. (Do **not** keep in this position any longer than necessary as this may be very uncomfortable for patient.)

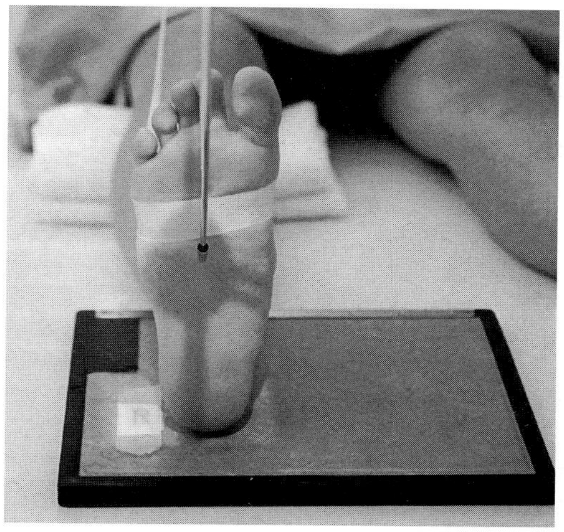

Fig. 6-75. Plantodorsal (axial) projection.

Central Ray

- Direct CR to the **base of 3rd metatarsal** to emerge just distal and inferior to lateral malleolus.
- Angle CR **40° cephalad from long axis of foot** (which would also be 40° from vertical **if** long axis of foot is perpendicular to film).
- Minimum 40 in. (102 cm) SID.

Collimation: Collimate closely to area of calcaneus.

Evaluation Criteria

- Entire calcaneus should be visualized, from the tuberosity posteriorly, to the talocalcaneal joint anteriorly.
- No rotation. The bases of the 1st and 5th metatarsals should **not** be visible on either side. A portion of the sustentaculum tali should appear in profile medially.
- Optimum density and contrast will at least faintly visualize the talocalcaneal joint without overexposing the distal tuberosity area.

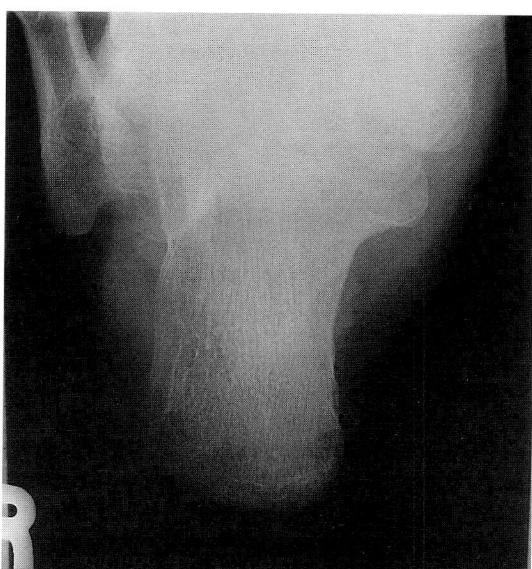

Fig. 6-76. Plantodorsal projection.

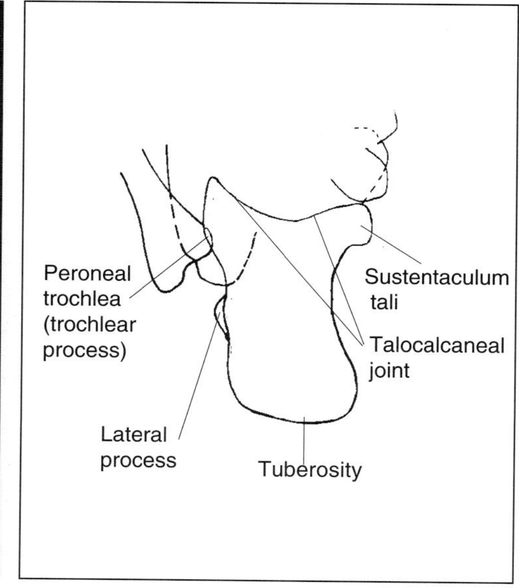

Fig. 6-77. Plantodorsal projection.

Lateral–Mediolateral Projection

Calcaneus
Basic
• Plantodorsal
• **Lateral**

Structures Best Shown

Lateral view of the calcaneus, talus and talocalcaneal joint.

Technical Factors

- Film size–8 x 10 in. (18 x 24 cm)
- Divide in half, crosswise.
- Detail screen, table-top.
- 60±5 kVp range.
- Technique and dose:

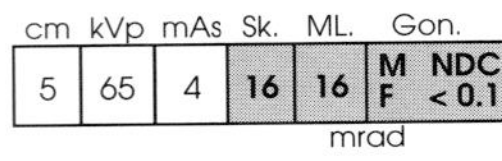

cm	kVp	mAs	Sk.	ML.	Gon.
5	65	4	16	16	M NDC F <0.1
			mrad		

Shielding: Place lead shield over pelvic area to shield gonads.

Patient Position

- Lateral recumbent position, affected side down, pillow for head.
- Flex knee of affected limb about 45°; place opposite leg behind the injured limb.

Part Position

- Adjust cassette to center calcaneus to CR and to unmasked portion of cassette, with long axis of foot parallel to long axis of film.
- Place support under knee and leg as needed to place plantar surface perpendicular to film.
- Position ankle and foot for a **true lateral,** which places the lateral malleolus about 1 cm posterior to the medial malleolus.
- Dorsiflex foot so plantar surface is at right angle to leg and place support against ball of foot if needed to immobilize or to maintain this position.

Central Ray

- CR **perpendicular** to film, directed to a point **1½ in. (3.5 cm) inferior to medial malleolus.**
- Minimum 40 in. (102 cm) SID.

Collimation: Collimate to outer skin margins to include the ankle joint proximally.

Evaluation Criteria

- Calcaneus and talus should be visualized without rotation as evidenced by lateral malleolus superimposed over the posterior half of the tibia and talus. Tarsal sinus and calcaneocuboid joint space should appear open.
- Four-sided collimation should include ankle joint proximally and talonavicular joint and base of 5th metatarsal anteriorly.
- Optimum exposure will visualize some soft tissue as well as more dense portions of calcaneus and talus. The outline of the distal fibula should be faintly visible through the talus. Trabecular markings will appear clear and sharp.

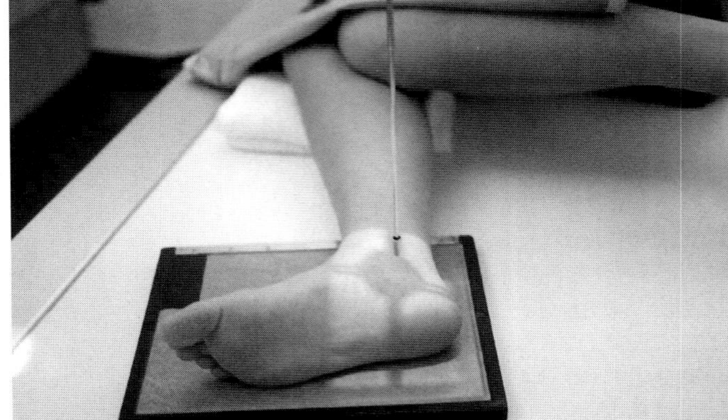

Fig. 6-78. Mediolateral calcaneus.

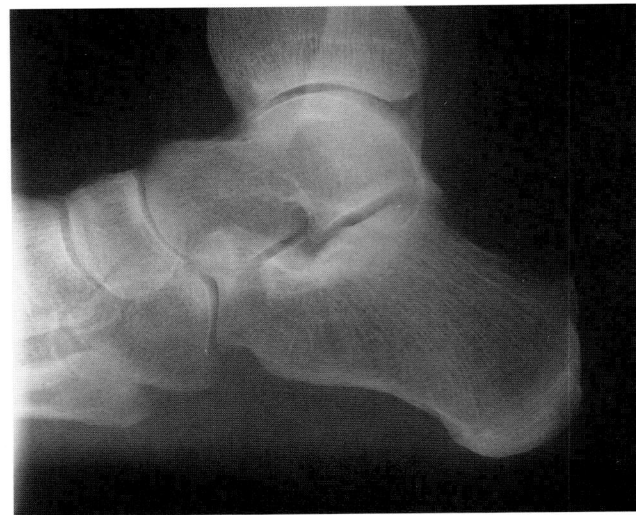

Fig. 6-79. Mediolateral calcaneus.

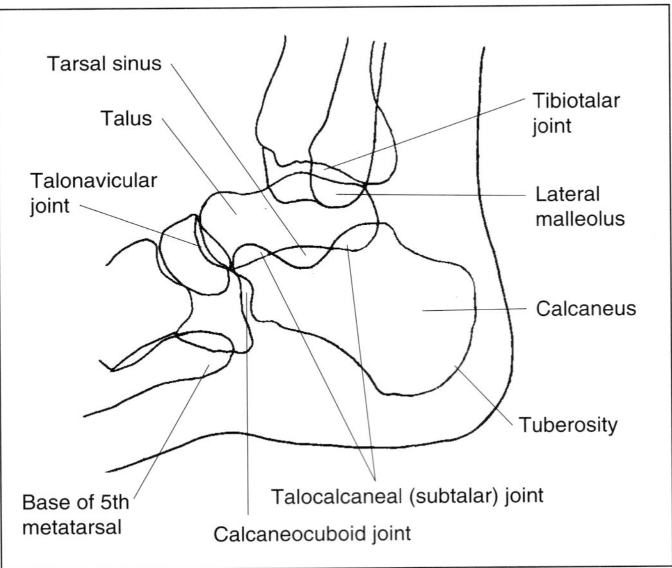

Fig. 6-80. Mediolateral calcaneus.

AP Projection

Ankle
Basic
• **AP**
• AP mortise (15°)
• Oblique (45°)
• Lateral

Structures Best Shown

Frontal view of ankle joint, distal tibia and fibula and proximal talus and proximal 5th metatarsal. (The lateral portion of the ankle joint space will not appear open on this projection–See mortise projection on following page.)

12

10

R

Technical Factors

- Film size–10 x 12 in. (24 x 30 cm).
- Divide in half, crosswise.
- Detail screen, table-top.
- 60±5 kVp range.
- Technique and dose:

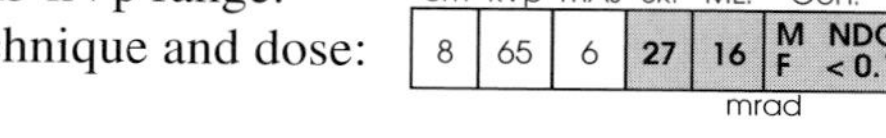

cm	kVp	mAs	Sk.	ML.	Gon.
8	65	6	27	16	M NDC F < 0.1

mrad

Shielding: Place lead shield over pelvic area to shield gonads.

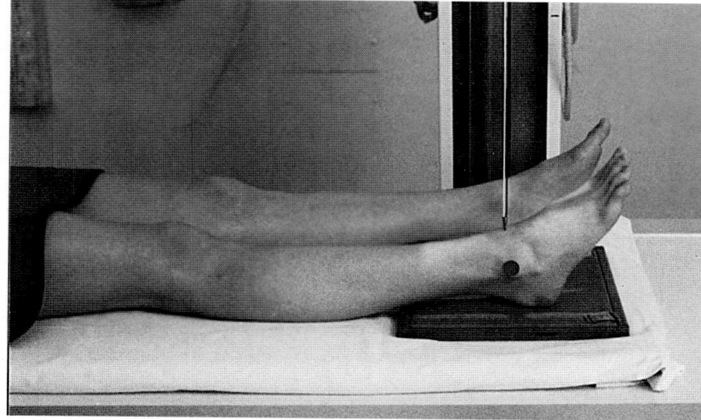

Fig. 6-81. AP ankle.

Patient Position

- Patient supine, pillow under head.
- Legs fully extended (small sand bag or other support under knee may increase comfort for some patients).

Part Position

- Center and align ankle joint to CR and to long axis of portion of film being exposed.
- Do not force dorsiflexion of the foot but allow it to remain in its natural position as shown in Fig. 6-81. (See Note 1.)
- Adjust the **foot and ankle** for a **true AP projection**. Ensure that the entire lower leg is not rotated. The intermalleolar line will **not** be parallel to film. (See Note 2.)

Central Ray

- CR **perpendicular** to film, directed to **a point midway between malleoli.**
- Minimum 40 in. (102 cm) SID.

Collimation: Collimate to lateral skin margins, include proximal one-half of metatarsals and distal tibia-fibula.

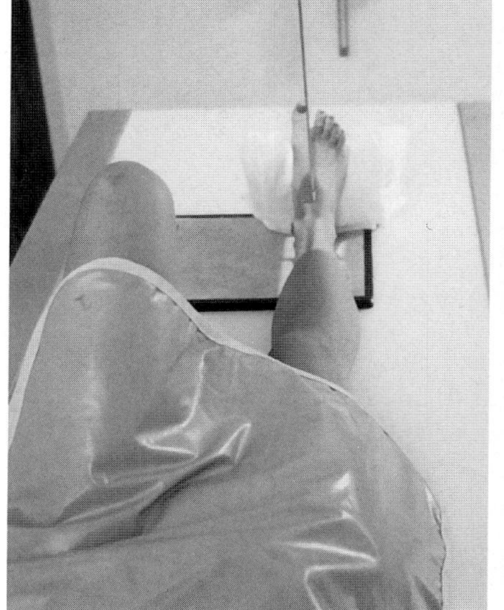

Fig. 6-82. AP ankle.

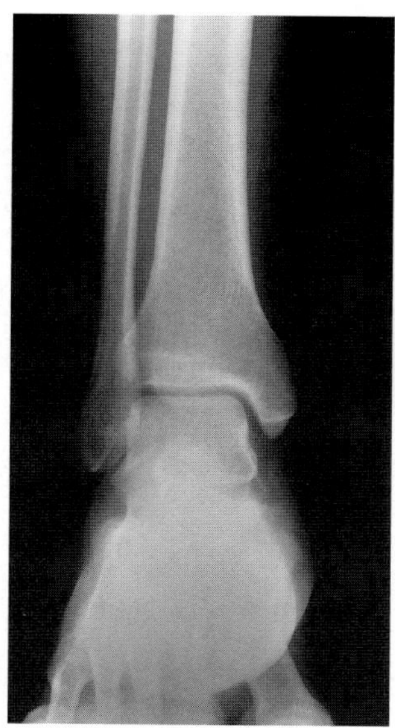

Fig. 6-83. AP ankle. (Courtesy of E. Frank R.T.)

Note 1: Forced dorsiflexion of the foot can be painful and may cause additional injury, also some extension or plantar flexion of the foot allows for visualization of base of 5th metatarsal, a common fracture site with trauma to ankle and/or foot.

Note 2: The malleoli will **not** be the same distance from the film in the anatomical position with a true AP projection. (The lateral malleolus will be about 15° more posterior.) The lateral portion of the mortise joint therefore should **not** appear open. If this portion of the ankle joint did appear open on a true AP, it may suggest a spread of the ankle mortise from ruptured ligaments.*

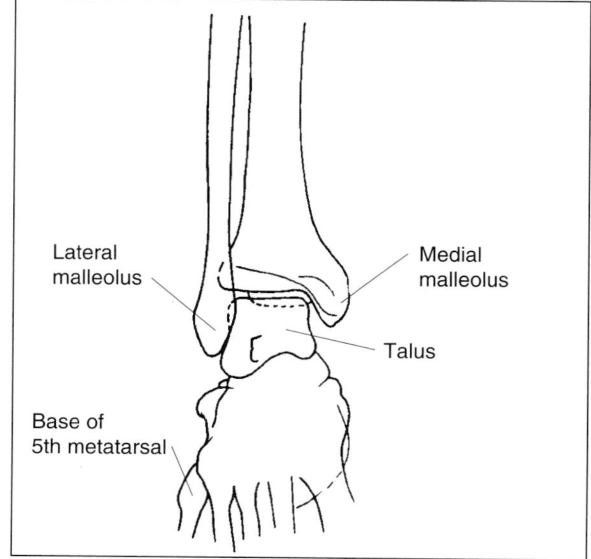

Fig. 6-84. AP ankle.

Evaluation Criteria

- The center of four-sided collimation should be to mid ankle joint. The area from the **distal third of the tibia-fibula** to the **proximal half of the metatarsals** should be included.
- The medial and upper portion of the ankle joint mortise should appear open, but the lateral portion will appear closed due to overlap of the distal fibula and a corner of the talus.
- Up to half the thickness of the distal fibula will overlap that of the medial tibia.
- Optimum exposure should visualize soft tissue, the lateral and medial malleoli, the talus and the distal tibia-fibula.
- With no motion and good exposure technique, trabecular markings and bony margins should appear sharp and clear.

*Frank, E.D. et al, Mayo Clinic: Radiography of the Ankle Mortise, *Radiologic Technology* 1991; 62-5: 354-359.

AP Mortise Projection–15 to 20° Medial Rotation

Ankle
Basic
- AP
- **AP mortise (15°)**
- Oblique (45°)
- Lateral

Structures Best Shown

Frontal view of entire ankle mortise, and frontal oblique view of proximal metatarsals (especially base of 5th metatarsal, a common fracture site).

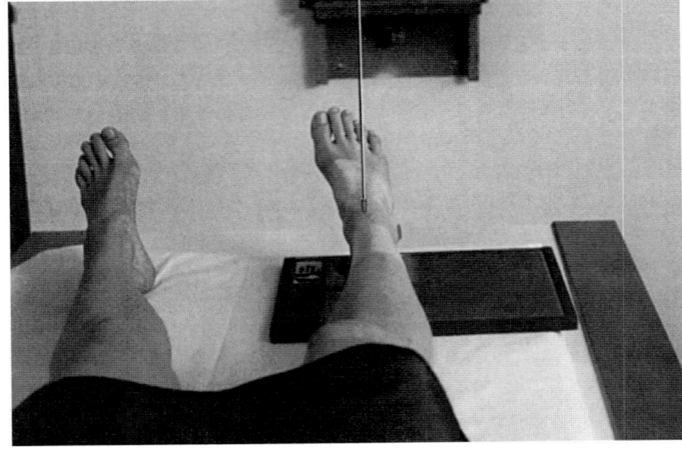

Fig. 6-85. AP mortise projection –15 to 20° AP medial rotation.

Technical Factors

- Film size–10 x 12 in. (24 x 30 cm).
- Divide in half, crosswise.
- Detail screen, table-top.
- 60±5 kVp range.
- Technique and dose:

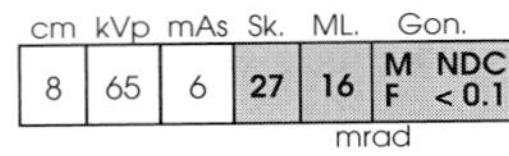

cm	kVp	mAs	Sk.	ML.	Gon.
8	65	6	27	16	M NDC F < 0.1
			mrad		

Shielding: Place lead shield over pelvic area.

Patient Position

- Patient supine, pillow under head.
- Legs fully extended (small sandbag or other support under knee increases comfort of patient).

Part Position

- Center and align ankle joint to CR and to long axis of portion of film being exposed.
- Do not dorsiflex foot but allow to remain in natural extended (plantar flexed) position. (Allows for visualization of base of 5th metatarsal, a common fracture site with trauma to ankle and/or foot.)
- Internally rotate **entire leg and foot** about **15 to 20°** until the **intermalleolar line is parallel to film.**
- Place support against foot if needed to prevent motion.

Central Ray

- CR **perpendicular** to film, directed to **a point midway between malleoli.**
- Minimum 40 in. (102 cm) SID.

Collimation: Collimate to lateral skin margins, include proximal metatarsals and distal tibia-fibula.

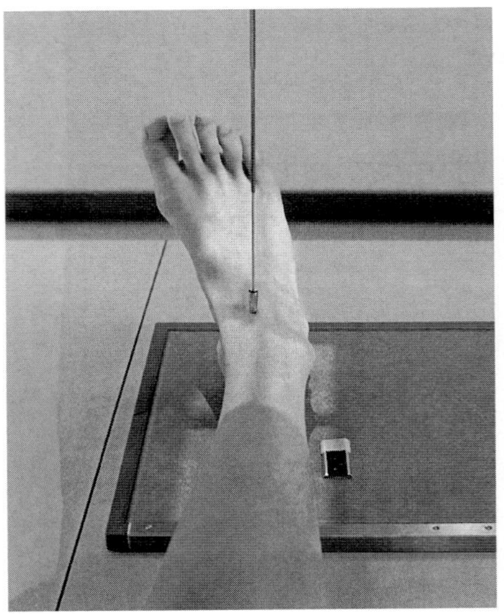

Fig. 6-86. Mortise projection, demonstrating 15° medial rotation of foot.

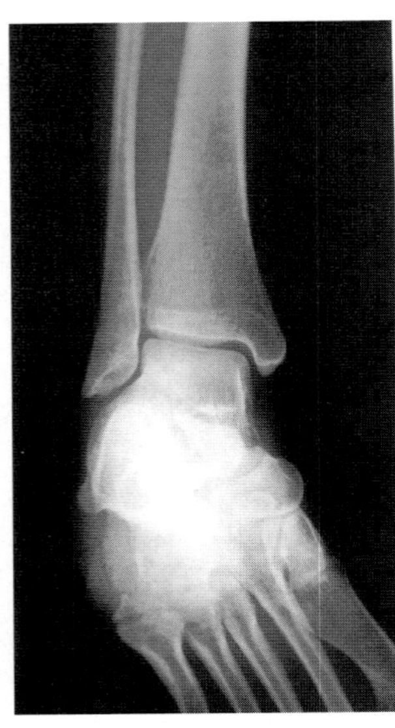

Fig. 6-87. Mortise projection. (Courtesy of John Garner R.T.)

Notes: This position should not be a substitute for either the AP projection or the oblique ankle position, but rather should be a separate projection of the ankle taken routinely when potential trauma or sprains of the ankle joint are involved.*

This is also a common projection taken during open reduction surgery of the ankle.

Evaluation Criteria

- Center of four-sided collimation should be to mid ankle joint. The area from the **distal third of the tibia-fibula** to the **proximal half of metatarsals** should be included. (Note fracture at base of 5th metatarsal, which in this case was not demonstrated on routine AP and oblique projections of the foot.)
- The **entire ankle mortise should appear open** with no overlap between distal fibula and talus, or between tibia and talus (3 to 4 mm space over entire talar surface is normal; an extra 2 mm widening is abnormal).†
- There should only be minimal overlap at the distal tibiofibular joint space.
- Optimum exposure should visualize some soft tissue with sufficient density for the talus and distal tibia and fibula.
- With no motion and good exposure technique, trabecular markings and bony margins should appear sharp and clear.

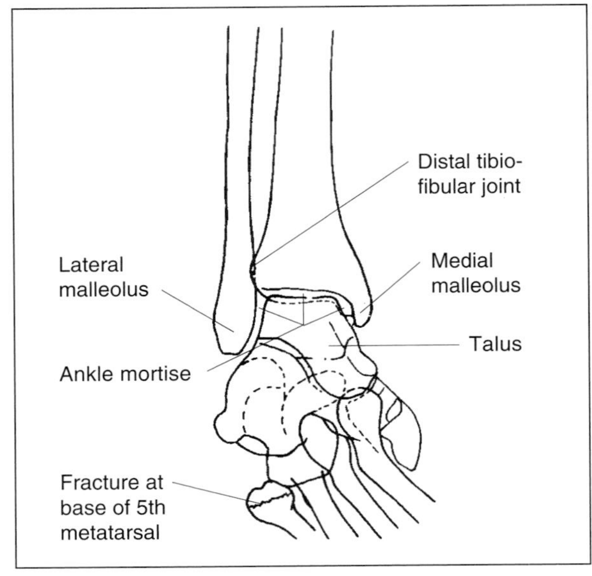

Fig. 6-88. Mortise projection.

*Frank, E.D. et al, Mayo Clinic: Radiography of the Ankle Mortise, *Radiologic Technology*, 62-5: 354-359, 1991.
†Manaster, BJ. *Handbooks in Radiology, Skeletal Radiology*. St. Louis: Year Book; 1989.

AP Oblique Projection–45° Medial Rotation

Ankle
Basic
• AP
• AP mortise (15°)
• **Oblique (45°)**
• Lateral

Structures Best Shown

Distal tibiofibular joint and a more complete view of the distal fibula and lateral malleolus. Also demonstrates the base of 5th metatarsal.

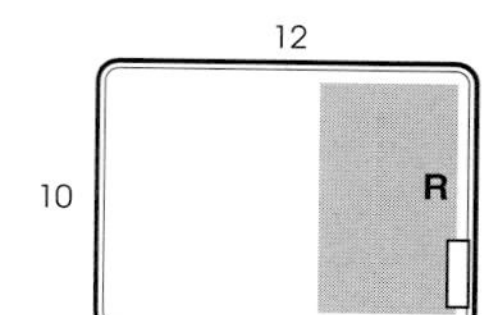

Technical Factors

- Film size–10 x 12 in. (24 x 30 cm).
- Divide in half, crosswise.
- Detail screen, table-top.
- 60±5 kVp range.
- Technique and dose:

cm	kVp	mAs	Sk.	ML.	Gon.
8	65	6	27	16	M NDC F <0.1

mrad

Shielding: Place lead shield over pelvic area to shield gonads.

Patient Position

- Patient supine, pillow under head.
- Legs fully extended (small sand bag or other support under knee increases comfort of patient).

Part Position 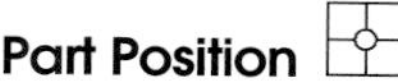

- Center and align ankle joint to CR and to long axis of portion of film being exposed.
- If patient's condition allows, dorsiflex the foot if needed so the plantar surface is at least 80 to 85° from the film (10-15° from vertical). See Note.
- Similar to mortise position except **rotate leg & foot** internally **45°**.

Central Ray

- CR **perpendicular** to film, directed to **a point midway between malleoli.**
- Minimum 40 in. (102 cm) SID.

Collimation: Collimate to lateral skin margins; include distal tibia-fibula and proximal metatarsals (see Note).

Alternate lateral oblique: Sometimes a lateral or external oblique is requested to rule out subtle fractures and/or to visualize parts of the talocalcaneal joint. The entire leg and foot would be rotated **externally 45°**.

Note: If the foot is extended or plantar flexed more than 10 or 15° from vertical, the calcaneus will be superimposed over the lateral malleolus on this 45° oblique, thus obscuring an important area of interest. The base of the 5th metatarsal will still be demonstrated in this position.

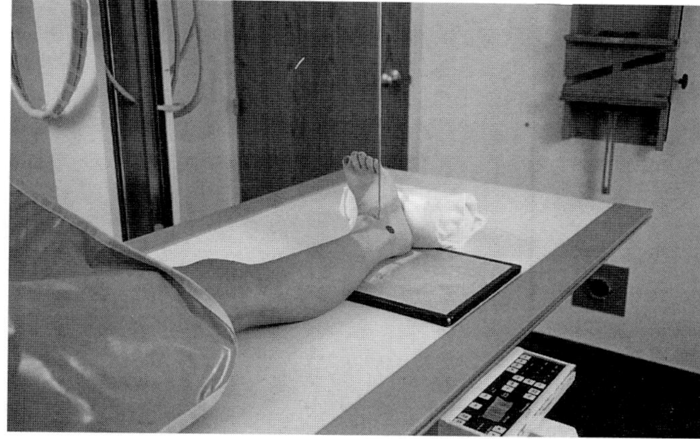

Fig. 6-89. AP 45° medial oblique projection –45° medial rotation of long axis of foot.

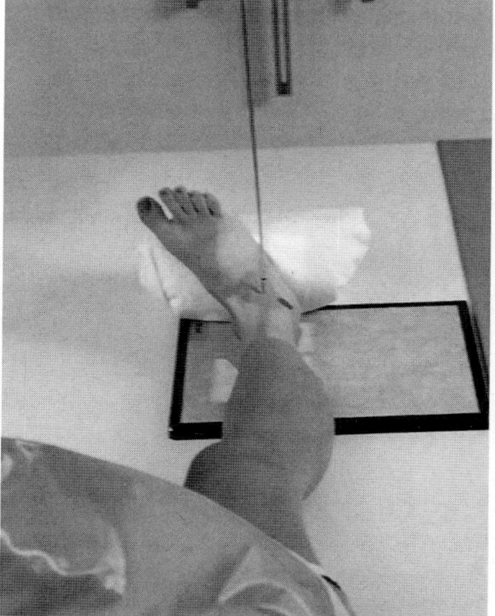

Fig. 6-90. 45° medial oblique (top view).

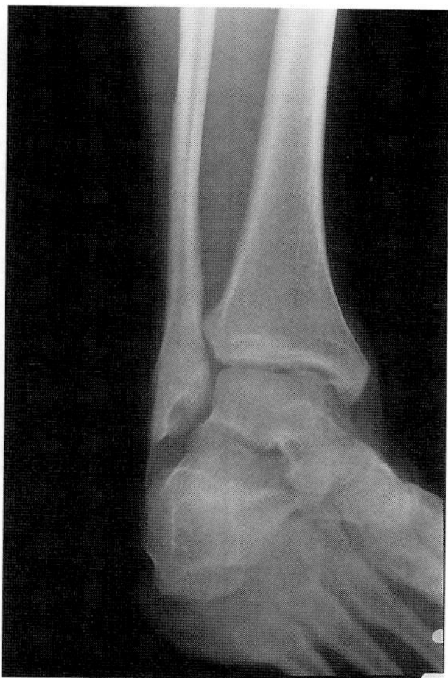

Fig. 6-91. 45° internal oblique.
(Courtesy of E. Frank, R.T.)

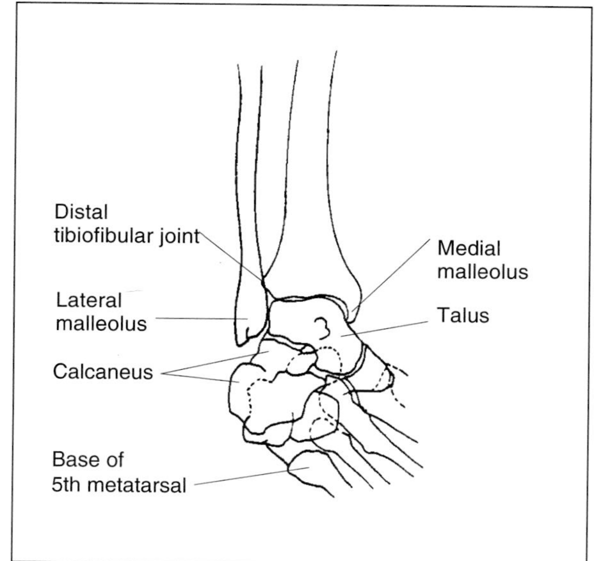

Fig. 6-92. 45° internal oblique.

Evaluation Criteria

- The center of four-sided collimation should be to mid ankle joint. The area from the **distal third of the tibia-fibula** to the **proximal half of the metatarsals** should be included.
- The calcaneus will not superimpose the lateral malleolus with correct dorsiflexion of the foot.
- The distal tibiofibular joint space should be primarily open with only minimal "touching" on an average ankle.
- Both the distal fibula and tibia may have some overlap with the talus.
- Optimum exposure should visualize soft tissue, the lateral and medial malleoli, the talus and proximal metatarsals, and the distal tibia and fibula.
- With no motion and good exposure technique, trabecular markings and bony margins should appear sharp and clear.

Lateral–Mediolateral (or Lateromedial) Projection

Ankle
Basic
- AP
- AP mortise (15°)
- Oblique (45°)
- **Lateral**

Structures Best Shown

Lateral view of distal tibia and fibula, ankle joint, talus and calcaneus, and adjoining tarsals to include base of 5th metatarsal.

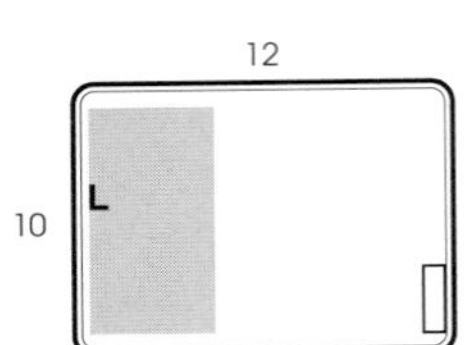

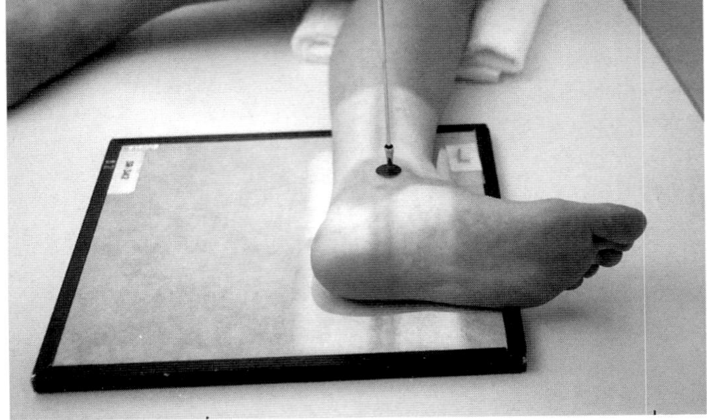

Fig. 6-93. Mediolateral ankle.

Technical Factors

- Film size–10 x 12 in. (24 x 30 cm)
- Divide in half, crosswise.
- Detail screen, table-top.
- 60±5 kVp range.
- Technique and dose:

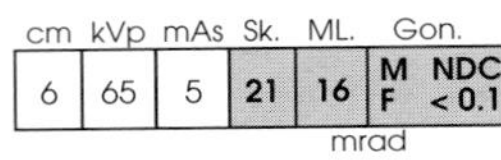

cm	kVp	mAs	Sk.	ML.	Gon.
6	65	5	21	16	M NDC F < 0.1
			mrad		

Shielding: Place lead shield over pelvic area.

Patient Position

- Lateral recumbent position, affected side down, pillow for head.
- Flex knee of affected limb about 45°; place opposite leg behind the injured limb.

Part Position (Mediolateral Projection)

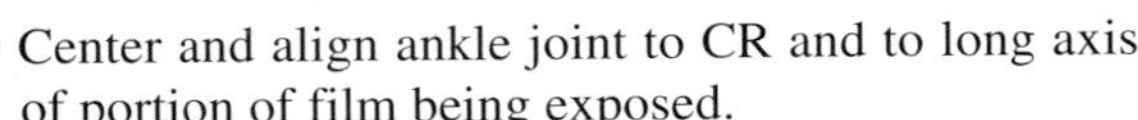

- Center and align ankle joint to CR and to long axis of portion of film being exposed.
- Place support under knee as needed to place leg and foot in a **true lateral position.** The distal fibula and lateral malleolus will be about 15 to 20° **posterior** to distal tibia and medial malleolus. (See p. 178.)
- Dorsiflex foot so plantar surface is at a right angle to leg or as far as patient can tolerate; do **not** force. (This will help maintain a true lateral position.)

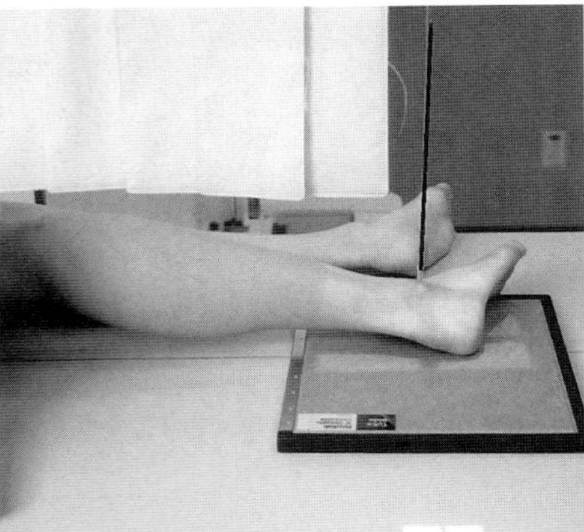

Fig. 6-94. Alternate lateromedial ankle.

Fig. 6-95. Mediolateral ankle.

Central Ray

- CR **perpendicular** to film, directed to **medial malleolus.**
- Minimum 40 in. (102 cm) SID.

Collimation: Collimate to skin margins to include distal tibia and fibula and to mid metatarsal area of foot.

Alternate lateromedial projection: This lateral may be taken rather than the more commonly preferred mediolateral. (This position is more uncomfortable for patient.) It would be positioned similarly to the mediolateral projection except patient is turned on opposite side (affected side up, see Fig. 6-94).

Evaluation Criteria

- Center of four-sided collimation should be to mid ankle joint.
- The talus and calcaneus should be seen in their entirety, as well as portions of the adjoining tarsal bones and the base of the 5th metatarsal.
- The upper arch of the tibiotalar joint should appear open with a uniform joint space.
- The lateral malleolus and distal fibula will appear superimposed over the posterior half of the talus, and the posterior half or two-thirds of the tibia.
- Optimum exposure should visualize the outline of the distal fibula as well as some soft tissue detail. Trabecular markings and borders of all bones visualized should appear clear and sharp.

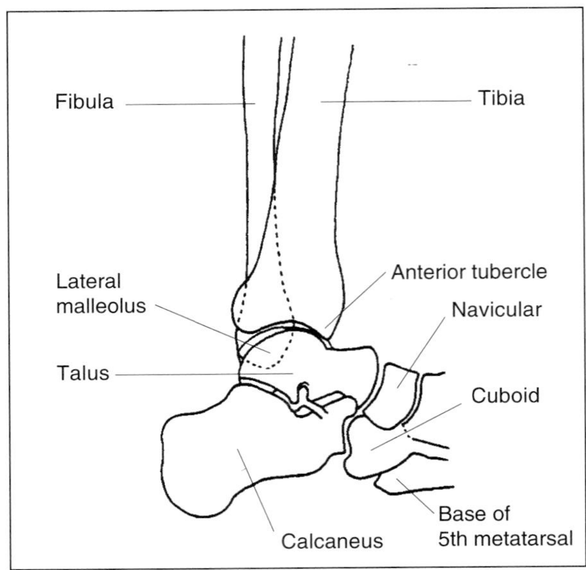

Fig. 6-96. Lateral ankle.

AP Stress Projections

Inversion and Eversion Positions

Warning: Proceed with utmost care with injured patient.

Ankle
Basic
- AP
- AP mortise (15°)
- Oblique (45°)
- Lateral

Special
- **AP stress**

Structures Best Shown

Ankle joint for evaluation of joint separation and ligament tear or rupture.

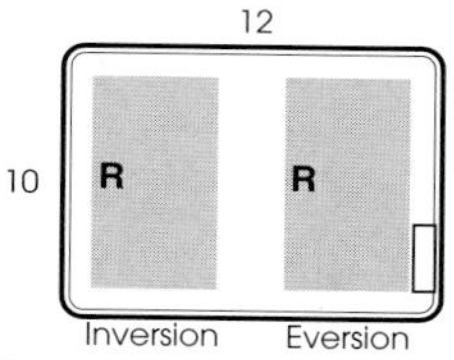

Technical Factors

- Film size–10 x 12 in. (24 x 30 cm).
- Divide in half, crosswise.
- Detail screen, table-top.
- 60±5 kVp range.
- Technique and dose:

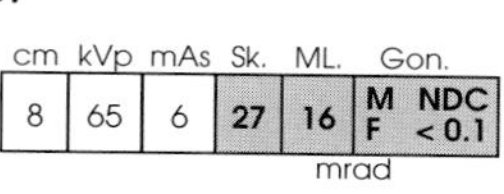

cm	kVp	mAs	Sk.	ML.	Gon.
8	65	6	27	16	M NDC F <0.1
				mrad	

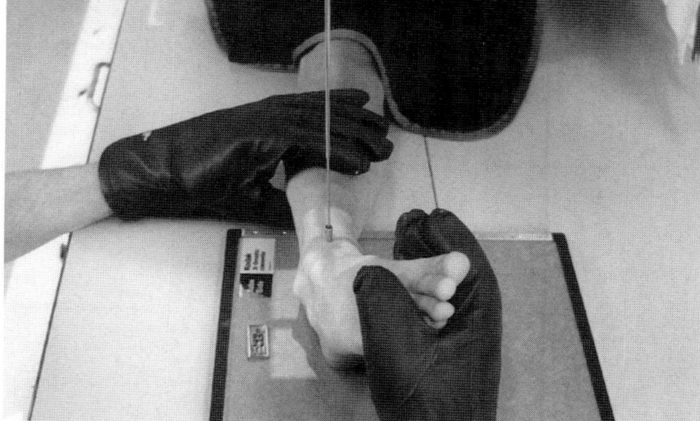

Fig. 6-97. Inversion stress.

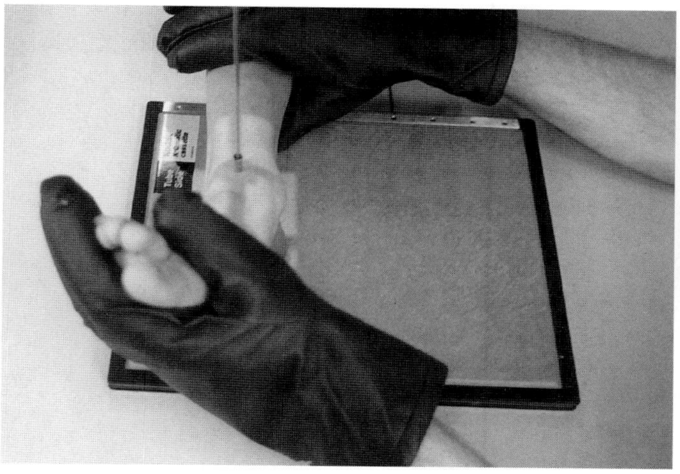

Shielding: Place shielding over gonadal area of patient. Supply lead gloves and a lead apron for physician if stress positions are hand held during exposures.

Patient Position

- Patient supine, pillow under head.
- Leg fully extended, support under knee.

Fig. 6-98. Eversion stress.

Part Position

- Center and align ankle joint to CR and to long axis of portion of film being exposed.
- Dorsiflex the foot to as near right angle to the leg as possible.
- With leg and ankle in position for a **true AP** with no rotation, stress is applied wherein the entire plantar surface is turned medially for inversion and laterally for eversion. (See Note.)

Central Ray

- CR **perpendicular** to film, directed to a point **midway between malleoli**.
- Minimum 40 in. (102 cm) SID.

Collimation: Collimate to lateral skin margins, include proximal metatarsals and distal tibia-fibula.

Note: A physician or another health professional must be present to either hold the foot and ankle in these stress views, or to strap into position with weights, or to have patient hold this position with long gauze looped around ball of foot. If this is too painful for patient, local anesthesia may be injected by the physician.

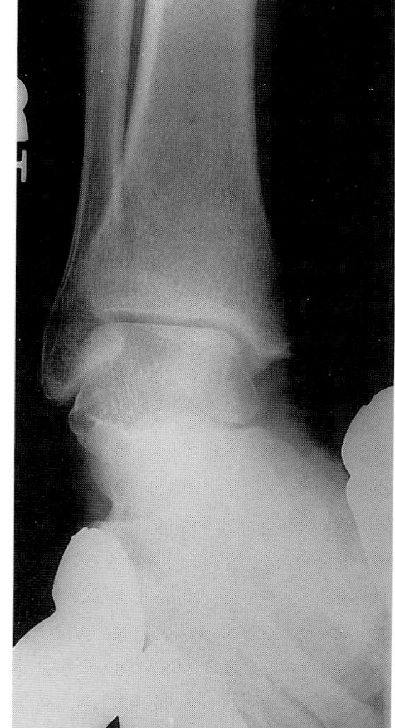

Fig. 6-99. Inversion.

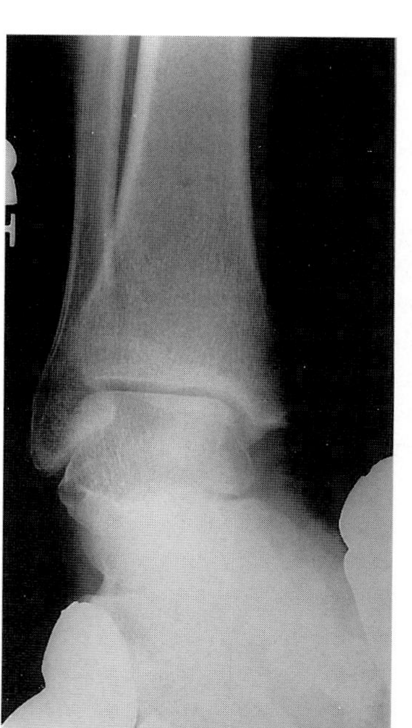

Fig. 6-100. Eversion.

Evaluation Criteria

- The center of four-sided collimation should be to mid ankle joint. The area from the distal tibia-fibula to the proximal metatarsals should be included.
- The appearance of the joint space may vary greatly depending on the severity of ligament damage.
- With no motion and good exposure technique, trabecular markings and bony margins should appear sharp and clear.
- Optimum exposure should visualize soft tissue, the lateral and medial malleoli, the talus and the distal tibia and fibula.

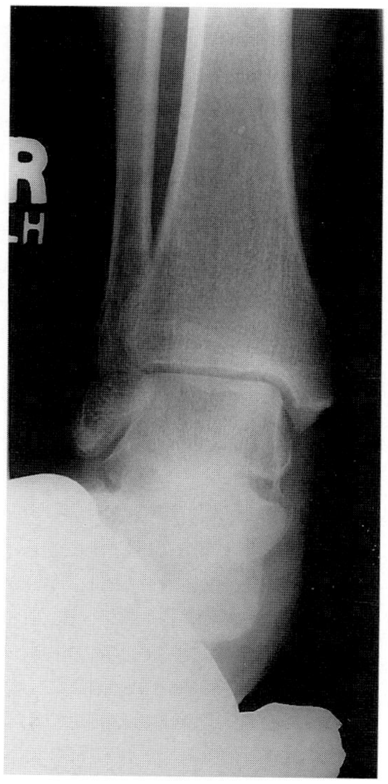

AP Projection

Leg
• **AP**
• Lateral

Structures Best Shown

Tibia and fibula and knee and/or ankle joints.

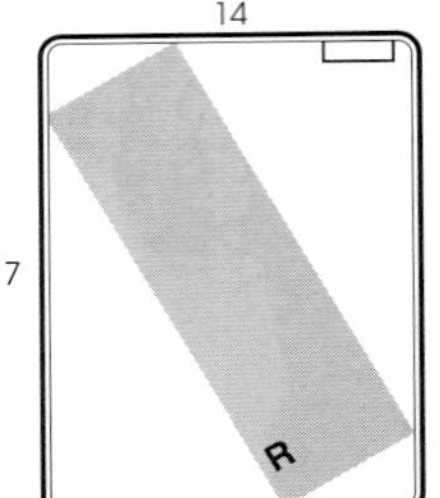

Diagonal placement

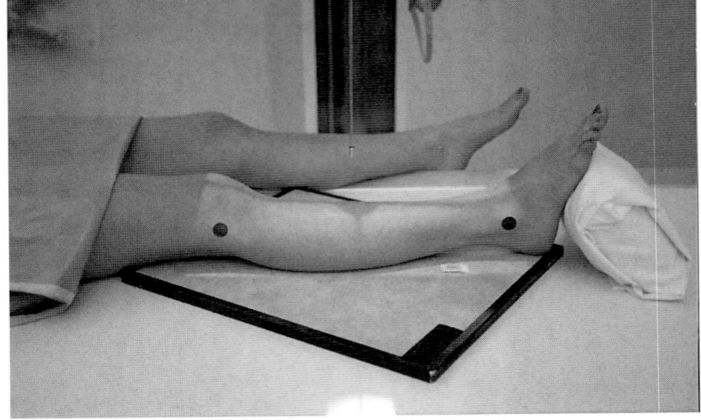
Fig. 6-101. AP leg–Include both joints.

Technical Factors

- Film size–14 x 17 in. (35 x 43 cm) divided in half lengthwise (or diagonal which requires 44 in. or 112 cm minimum SID).
- Detail screen, table-top.
- 70±5 kVp range.
- To make best use of anode-heel effect, place knee at cathode end of x-ray beam.
- Technique and dose:

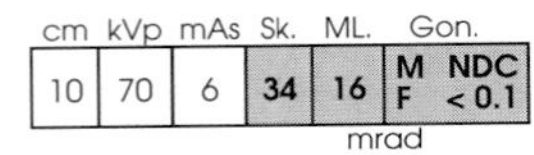

cm	kVp	mAs	Sk.	ML.	Gon.
10	70	6	34	16	M NDC F < 0.1

mrad

Shielding: Place lead shielding over gonadal area.

Patient Position

- Patient supine, pillow for head.
- Leg fully extended.

Part Position

- Adjust pelvis, knee and leg into a true AP with no rotation.
- Place sand bag against foot if needed for stabilization, dorsiflex foot to 90° to leg if possible.
- Ensure that both ankle and knee joints are 1 to 2 in. (3 to 5 cm) from ends of film (so that divergent rays will not project either joint off film).
- For most adults the leg must be placed diagonally (corner to corner) on one 14 x 17 film to ensure that both joints are included. (Also, if needed, a second smaller film may be taken of the joint nearest the injury site.)

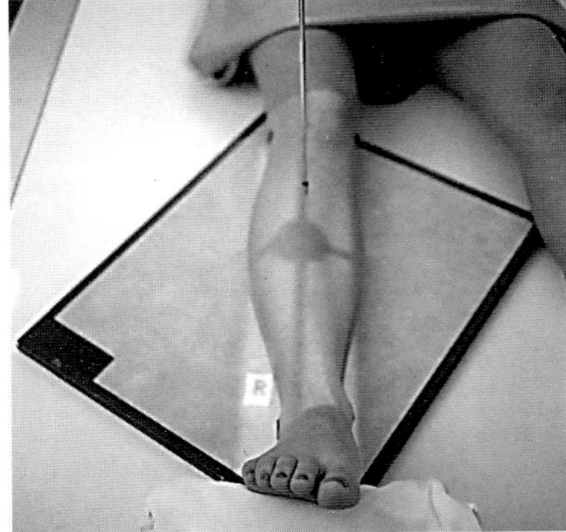
Fig. 6-102. AP leg–Include both joints.

Central Ray

- CR **perpendicular** to film, directed to **midpoint of leg.**
- Minimum 40 in. (102 cm) SID. May increase to 44 or 48 in. (112 to 122 cm) to reduce divergence of x-ray beam to include more of body part.

Collimation: Collimate on both sides to skin margins, with full collimation at ends of film borders to include maximum knee and ankle joints.

Alternate follow-up exam routine: The routine for follow-up exams of long bones in some departments is to include only the one joint nearest the site of injury and to place this joint a minimum of 2 in. (5 cm) from the end of the film for better demonstration of this joint. However, for initial exams it is **especially important when the injury site is at the distal leg to also include the proximal tibiofibular joint area** because it is common to have a second fracture at this site. For an extra-large patient a second AP projection of the knee and proximal leg may be needed on a smaller film.

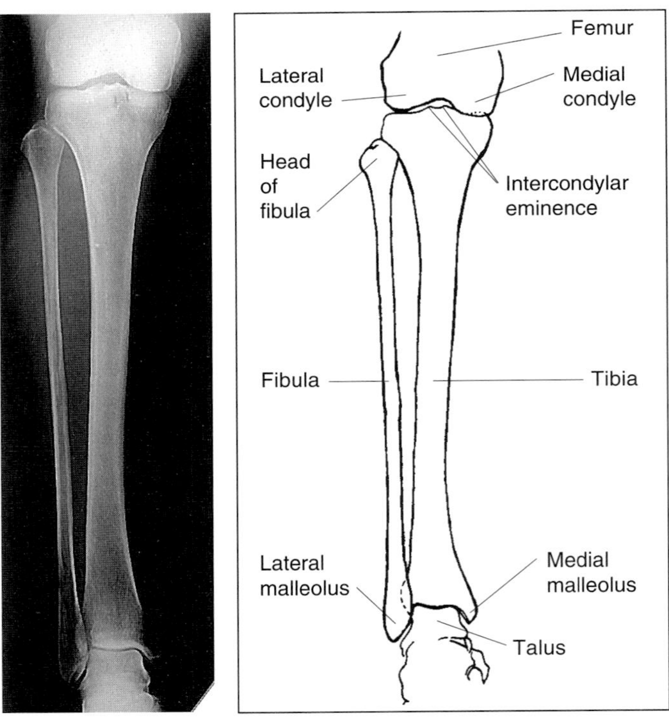

Fig. 6-103. AP leg–Both joints. Fig. 6-104.
(Courtesy of Jim Sanderson, RT)

Evaluation Criteria

- The entire tibia and fibula should be included with both the ankle and knee joints included on one (or two if needed) film(s). (Exception is alternate routine on follow-up exams.)
- Close side collimation border but any end collimation border visibility should be minimal, to maximize visualization of both joints.
- Overlap of the fibula and tibia will be visible at both the proximal and distal ends.
- Optimum exposure with correct use of the anode-heel effect will result in near equal density at both ends of the film.
- Good exposure density without motion will result in visualization of sharp trabecular markings and sharp borders of entire tibia and fibula.

Lateral–Mediolateral Projection

Leg
- AP
- **Lateral**

Structures Best Shown

Tibia, fibula, knee and/or ankle joints.

Technical Factors

- Film size–14 x 17 in. (35 x 43 cm) divide in half lengthwise (or diagonal which requires 44 in. or 112 cm minimum SID).
- Detail screen, table-top.
- 70±5 kVp range.
- To make best use of anode-heel effect, place knee at cathode end of x-ray beam.
- Technique and dose:

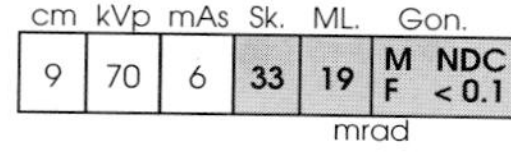

cm	kVp	mAs	Sk.	ML.	Gon.
9	70	6	33	19	M NDC F <0.1
				mrad	

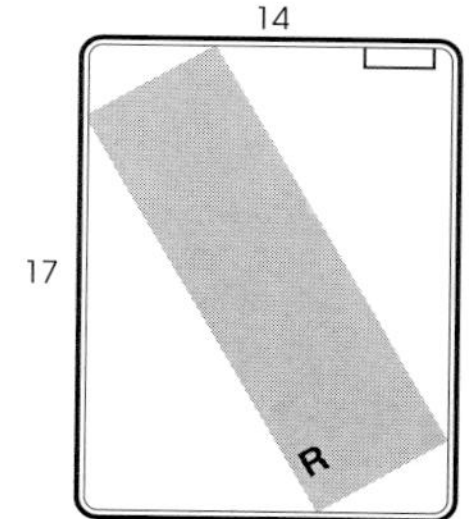

Diagonal placement

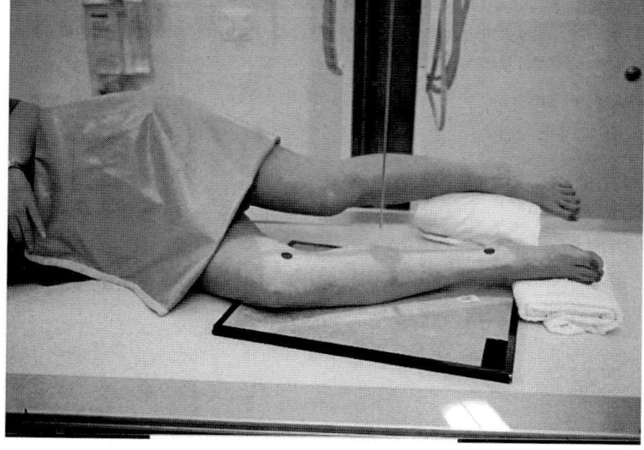

Fig. 6-105. Mediolateral leg–Include both joints.

Shielding: Place shield over pelvic and gonadal area.

Patient Position

- Patient in lateral recumbent position, injured side down, pillow for head.
- Generally the opposite leg may be placed behind the affected leg and supported with a pillow or sand bags.

Part Position

- Flex knee about 45° and ensure that leg is in a true lateral position. (Plane of patella should be perpendicular to film.)
- Ensure that both ankle and knee joints are 1 to 2 in. (3 to 5 cm) from ends of film so that divergent rays will not project either joint off film.
- For most adults the leg must be placed diagonally (corner to corner) on one 14 x 17 film to ensure that both joints are included. (Also if needed a second smaller film may be taken of the joint nearest the injury site.)

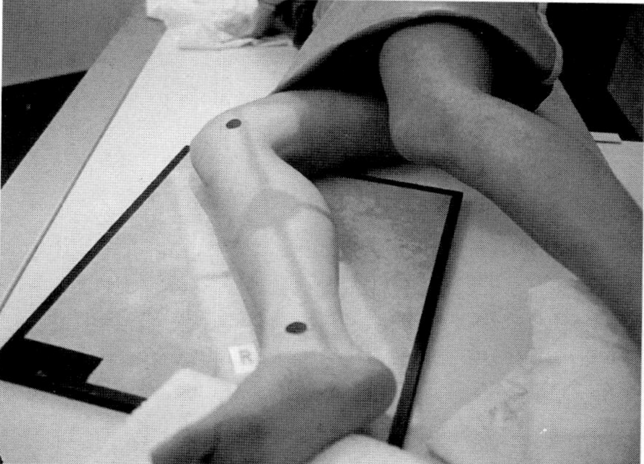

Fig. 6-106. Mediolateral leg–Include both joints.

Central Ray

- CR **perpendicular** to film, directed to **mid leg.**
- Minimum 40 in. (102 cm) SID. May increase to 44 or 48 in. (112 to 122 cm) to reduce divergence of x-ray beam to include more of body part.

Collimation: Collimate on both sides to skin margins, with full collimation at ends of film borders to include maximum knee and ankle joints.

Alternate follow-up exam routine: The routine for follow-up exams of long bones in some departments is to include only the one joint nearest the site of injury and to place this joint a minimum of 2 in. (5 cm) from the end of the film for better demonstration of this joint. However, for initial exams it is especially important when the injury site is at the distal leg to also include the proximal tibiofibular joint area because it is common to have a second fracture at this site. For an extra-large patient, a second AP projection of the knee and proximal leg may be needed on a smaller film.

Cross-table lateral: If patient cannot be turned, this can be taken cross table with cassette placed on edge between legs. Place a support under injured leg to center leg to film, and direct horizontal beam from lateral side of patient.

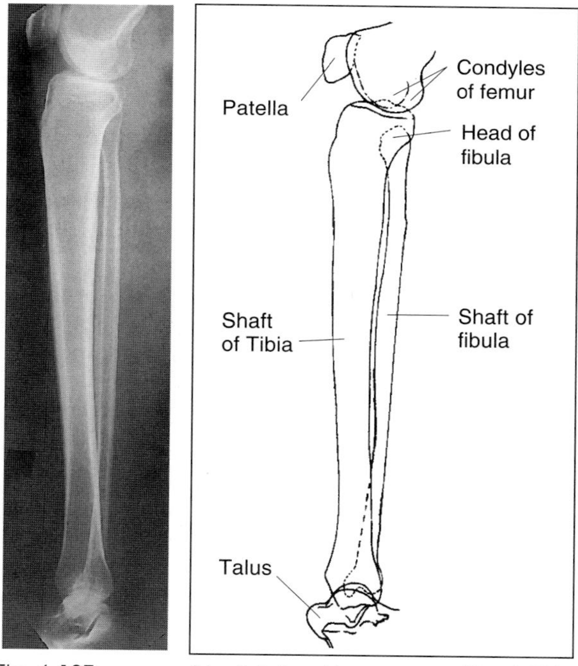

Fig. 6-107. Mediolateral leg. Fig. 6-108.
(Courtesy of Jim Sanderson, RT.)

Evaluation Criteria

- The entire tibia and fibula should be included with both the ankle and knee joints included on one (or two if needed) film(s). (Exception is alternate routine on follow-up exams.)
- Close side collimation borders should be visible but only minimal if any border should be visible at the ends to maximize visualization of both joints.
- A portion of the proximal head of the fibula will be superimposed by the tibia, and outlines of the distal fibula will be seen through the posterior half or two-thirds of the tibia. The majority of the shaft or body areas of the tibia and fibula will lie parallel to each other, not superimposed.
- Optimum exposure with correct use of the anode-heel effect will result in near equal density at both ends of the film.
- Good exposure density without motion will result in visualization of sharp trabecular markings and sharp borders of entire tibia and fibula.

AP Projection

Knee
Basic
• **AP**
• Oblique
• Lateral

Structures Best Shown

Distal femur, proximal tibia and fibula, patella and knee joint.

Technical Factors

- Film size–8 x 10 in. (18 x 24 cm), lengthwise.
- Grid or Bucky, >10 cm (70±5 kVp).
- Screen, table-top, <10 cm (65±5 kVp).
- Technique and dose:

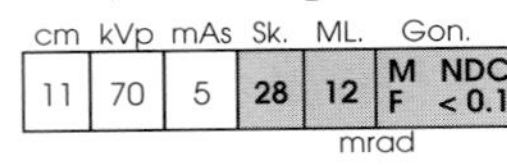

cm	kVp	mAs	Sk.	ML.	Gon.
11	70	5	28	12	M NDC F <0.1

mrad

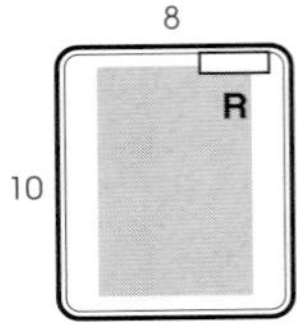

Shielding: Place shield over gonadal area.

Patient Position

- Patient supine with no rotation of pelvis, pillow for head.
- Leg fully extended.

Part Position 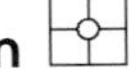

- Align and center leg and knee to CR and to midline of table or cassette.
- Rotate leg internally 3 to 5° for a true AP knee (or until **interepicondylar line is parallel** to plane of film).
- Place sandbags by foot and ankle to stabilize if needed.

Central Ray

- CR **parallel to tibial plateau**, average-size patient CR perpendicular to film (see Note).
- Direct CR to a point **¾ in. or 2 cm** distal to apex of patella.
- Minimum 40 in. (102 cm) SID.

Collimation: Collimate on both sides to skin margins, at ends to film borders.

Note: A suggested guideline for determining that CR is parallel to tibial plateau for open joint space is to measure distance from ASIS to table-top to determine CR angle as follows:*

- < 19 cm, **3 to 5° caudad** (thin thighs and buttocks)
- < 19-24 cm, **0° angle** (average thighs and buttocks)
- > 24 cm, **3 to 5° cephalad** (thick thighs and buttocks)

Evaluation Criteria

- The center of the collimation field should be to the mid knee joint space.
- The femorotibial joint space should be open with the articular facets of the tibia seen on end with only minimal surface area visualized.
- No rotation will be evidenced by the symmetrical appearance of the femoral and tibial condyles and the joint space. The approximate medial half of the fibular head should be superimposed by the tibia.
- Optimum exposure will visualize the outline of the patella through the distal femur and the fibular head and neck will not appear overexposed.
- Trabecular markings of all bones should be visible and appear sharp. Soft tissue detail should be visible.

*Martensen, KM. Alternate AP Knee Method Assures Open Joint Space. *Radiologic Technology* 1992; 64:1, 19-23.

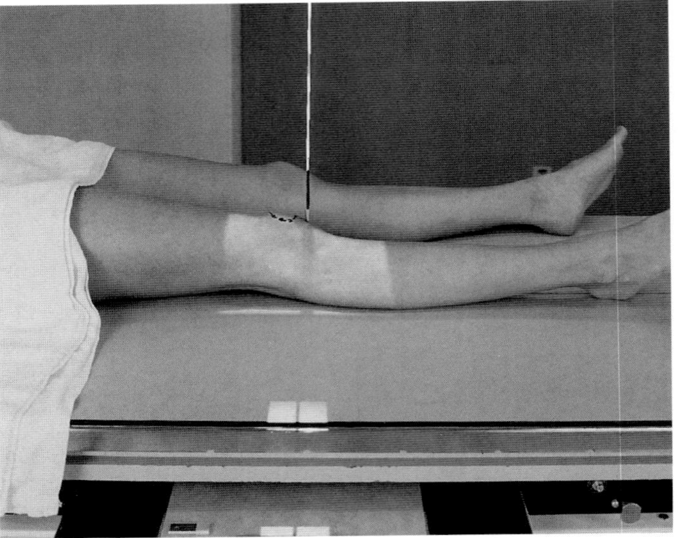

Fig. 6-109. AP knee
-CR perpendicular to film (average patient).

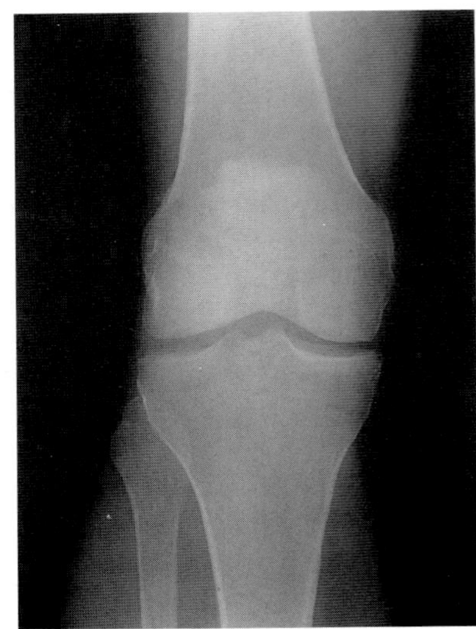

Fig. 6-110. AP knee-0° CR.

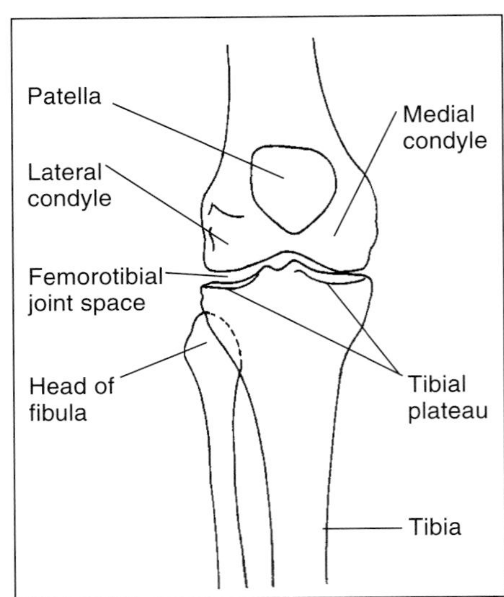

Fig. 6-111. AP knee-0° CR.

AP Oblique Projection–Medial or Lateral Rotation

Knee
Basic
• AP
• **Oblique**
• Lateral

Structures Best Shown (Medial Oblique)

Distal femur, proximal tibia, fibular head and neck and lateral condyles of femur and tibia without superimposition. Proximal tibiofibular joint and tibiofemoral (knee) joint.

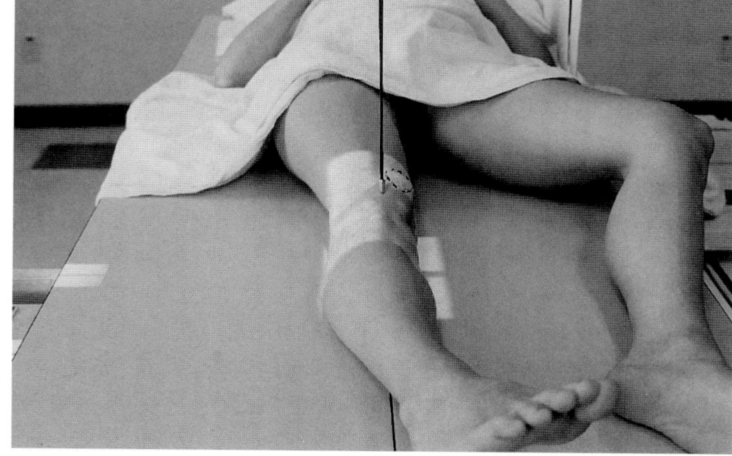

Fig. 6-112. AP medial oblique.

Technical Factors

- Film size–8 x 10 in. (18 x 24 cm), lengthwise.
- Grid or Bucky, > 10 cm (70±5 kVp).
- Screen, table-top, < 10 cm (65±5 kVp).
- Technique and dose:

cm	kVp	mAs	Sk.	ML.	Gon.
10	70	5	28	13	M NDC F < 0.1

mrad

(Film: 8 x 10, R)

Shielding: Place shield over gonadal area.

Patient Position

- Patient semi-supine with entire body and leg rotated partially away from side of interest.
- Place support under elevated hip, pillow for head.

Part Position (Medial Oblique) 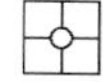

- Align and center leg and knee to CR and to midline of table or cassette.
- Rotate entire leg **internally 45°**. (Interepicondylar line should be 45° to plane of film.)
- If needed, stabilize foot and ankle in this position with sandbags.

Central Ray

- Angle CR 0° on average patient (see AP knee)
- Direct CR to **midpoint of the knee** at a level **¾ in. (2 cm) distal to apex of patella.**.
- Minimum 40 in. (102 cm) SID.

Collimation: Collimate on both sides to skin margins, with full collimation at ends to film borders to include maximum femur and tibia/fibula.

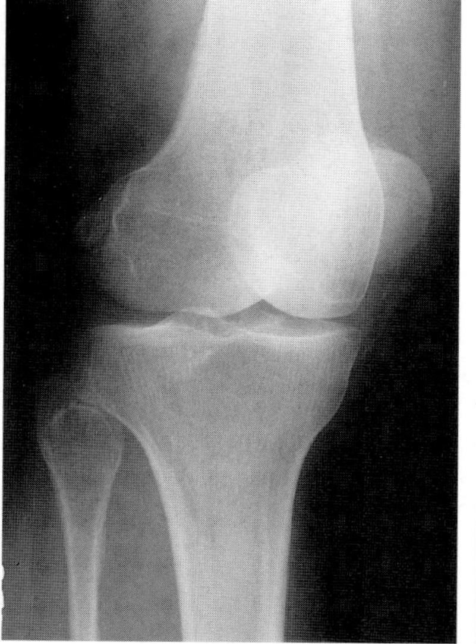

Fig. 6-113. AP medial oblique.

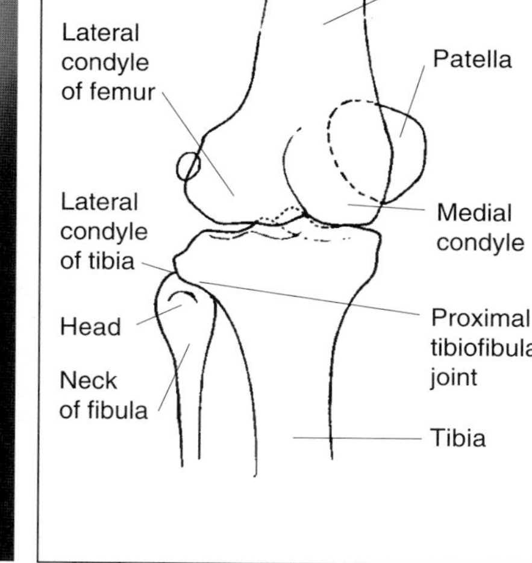

Fig. 6-114. AP medial oblique.

Optional Lateral Oblique: A 45° lateral (external) rotation oblique may be taken as an optional projection if a second oblique view of the knee area is desired. Positioning would be similar but with the entire leg **rotated laterally 45°**. Some departmental routines include **both** medial and lateral obliques.

Note: The terms medial (internal) oblique or lateral (external) oblique positions refer to the direction of rotation of the anterior or patella surface of the knee. This is true for descriptions of either AP and PA oblique projections.

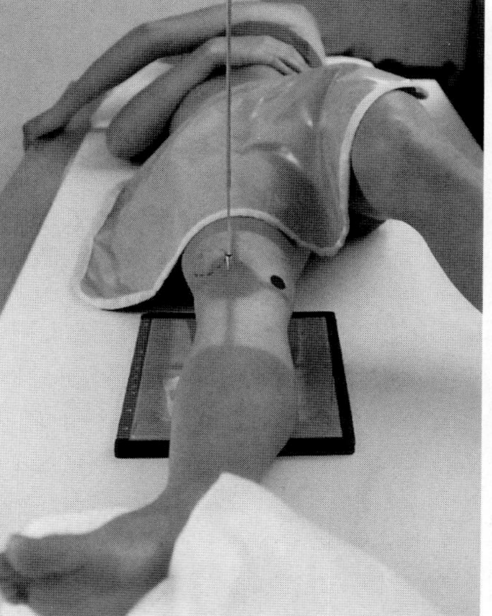

Fig. 6-115.

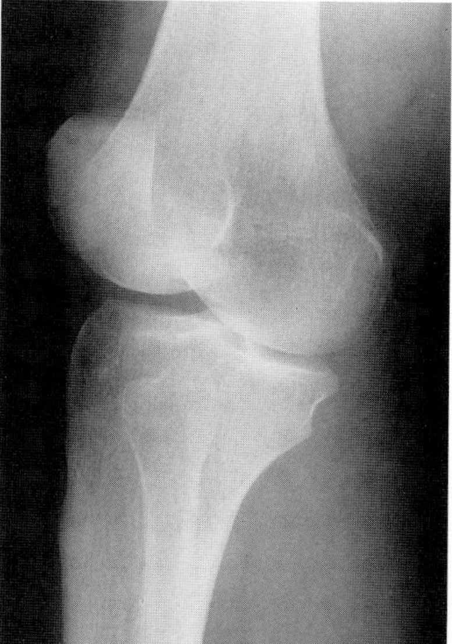

Fig. 6-116.

Optional AP lateral oblique.

Evaluation Criteria

AP Medial (Internal) Oblique:

- The proximal tibiofibular articulation should appear open, and the lateral condyles of femur and tibia are seen in profile with head and neck of fibula visualized without superimposition.
- Approximately half of the patella should be seen free of superimposition by the femur.
- Optimum exposure should visualize soft tissue in knee joint area and trabecular markings of all bones should appear clear and sharp. Head and neck area of fibula should not appear overexposed.

AP Lateral (External) Oblique:

- Medial condyles of femur and tibia are visualized in profile, and proximal fibula is seen superimposed over mid portion of proximal tibia.

Lateral-Mediolateral Projection

Knee
Basic
• AP
• Oblique
• **Lateral**

Structures Best Shown

Distal femur, proximal tibia, fibula, patella and tibiofemoral joint and patellofemoral joints.

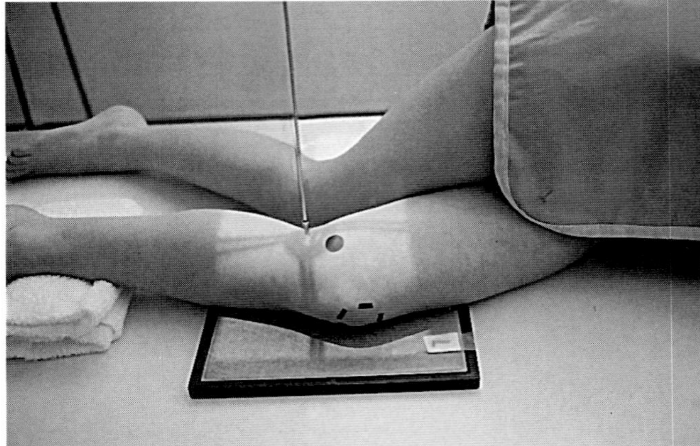

Fig. 6-117. Mediolateral–5 to 7° cephalad.

Technical Factors

8

10

L

- Film size–8 x 10 in. (18 x 24 cm), lengthwise.
- Grid or Bucky, > 10 cm (70±5 kVp).
- Screen, table-top, < 10 cm (65±5 kVp).
- Technique and dose:

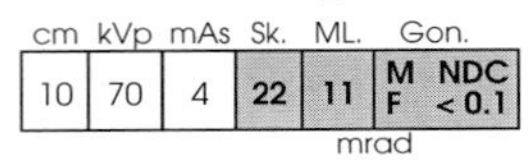

cm	kVp	mAs	Sk.	ML.	Gon.
10	70	4	22	11	M NDC F < 0.1

mrad

Shielding: Place shield over gonadal area.

Patient Position

- Patient in lateral recumbent position, affected side down, pillow for head.
- Provide support for knee of opposite limb placed behind knee being examined.

Part Position

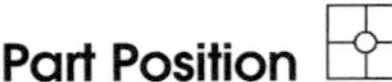

- Adjust rotation of body and leg until knee is in a **true lateral** position (femoral epicondyles directly superimposed and plane of patella perpendicular to plane of film).
- Flex knee **15 to 20°**. (see Note 1.)
- Align and center leg and knee to CR and to midline of table or cassette.

Central Ray

- Angle CR **5 to 7° cephalad**. (See Note 2.)
- Direct CR to a point **¾ in. (2 cm) distal to** medial epicondyle.
- Minimum 40 in. (102 cm) SID.

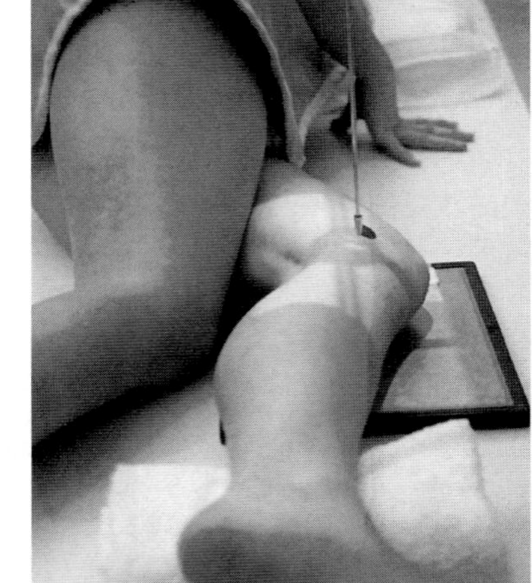

Fig. 6-118. Demonstrates front-to-back centering to CR.

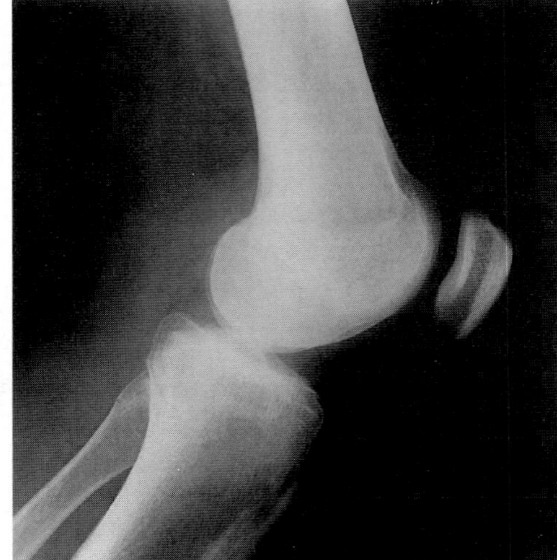

Fig. 6-119. Mediolateral knee.

Collimation: Collimate on both sides to skin margins, with full collimation at ends to film borders to include maximum femur and tibia/fibula.

Cross table lateral: If patient cannot be turned, this can also be taken cross table with cassette placed on edge between legs. Place support under knee to center knee to film and direct horizontal beam from lateral side of patient.

Note 1: Additional flexion will tighten muscles and tendons which may obscure important diagnostic information in the joint space. The patella will be drawn into the intercondylar sulcus also obscuring soft tissue information from effusion and/or fat pad displacement. Additional flexion may also result in fragment separation of patellar fractures if present.

Note 2: Angle CR 7 to 10° on short patient with wide pelvis, and only about 5° on tall, male patient with narrow pelvis. (See p. 179.)

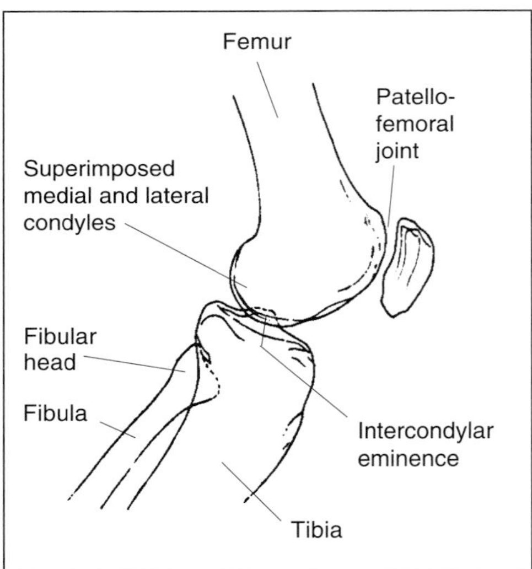

Fig. 6-120. Mediolateral projection.

Evaluation Criteria

- **True lateral**: Femoral condyles should be directly superimposed. The 5 to 10° cephalad angle of CR should result in direct superimposition of the **distal borders** of the condyles, and a true lateral without rotation will directly superimpose the **posterior borders**.
- The tibiofemoral joint space should be open with only the pointed intercondylar eminence (tibial spines) superimposed by the femoral condyles.
- The patella should be seen in profile with the patellofemoral joint space open.
- For the average patient about one-half of the fibular head will be superimposed by the tibia.
- Over or under rotation can be determined by identifying the adductor tubercle on medial condyle (p. 182, Fig. 6-33) and by the amount of superimposition of fibular head by tibia. (Over rotation, less superimposition of fibular head; under rotation, more superimposition.)
- Optimum exposure will visualize important soft tissue detail including fat pads anterior to knee joint, and sharp trabecular markings.

AP (PA) Weight-Bearing Bilateral Knee Projection

Knee
Special
• **AP (PA) weight-bearing**

Structures Best Shown

Joint spaces of the knees are demonstrated for possible cartilage degeneration or other knee joint deformities. Both knees included for comparison.

Most commonly taken AP, but may be taken PA as demonstrated if requested.

Technical Factors

- Film size–11 x 14 in. (28 x 35 cm), crosswise.
- Moving or stationary grid.
- 70±5 kVp range.
- Technique and dose:

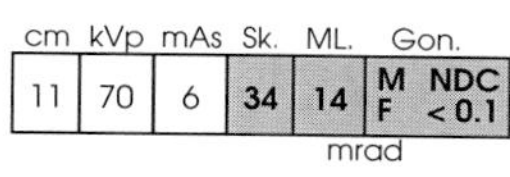

cm	kVp	mAs	Sk.	ML.	Gon.
11	70	6	34	14	M NDC F <0.1

mrad

14

11

R

Shielding: Shield gonadal area.

Part Position (AP) 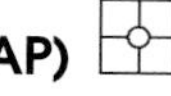

- Patient erect, standing on attached step or on step stool to place patient high enough for horizontal beam x-ray tube.
- Feet straight ahead with weight evenly distributed on both feet, provide support handles for patient stability.
- Bilateral legs and knees aligned and centered to CR and to midline of table and cassette. Cassette height adjusted to CR.

Central Ray

- CR **perpendicular to film** (average-sized patient), or **5-10° caudad** on thin patient, directed to **midpoint between knee joints** at level of **¾ in. (2 cm) below apex of patellae**.
- Minimum 48 in. (122 cm) SID suggested for less divergence of x-ray beam (adjust exposure factors accordingly).

Collimation: Collimate to bilateral knee joint region.

Alternate PA: Patient facing the table or film holder, knees flexed ≈20°, feet straight ahead, thighs against table-top or film holder.

CR directed **10° caudad** (parallel to tibial plateaus) to **level of knee joints**.

Note: The CR angle should be parallel to tibial plateau to best demonstrate "open" knee joint spaces. (See knee anatomy, page 178, to understand correct CR angles on AP or PA projections.)

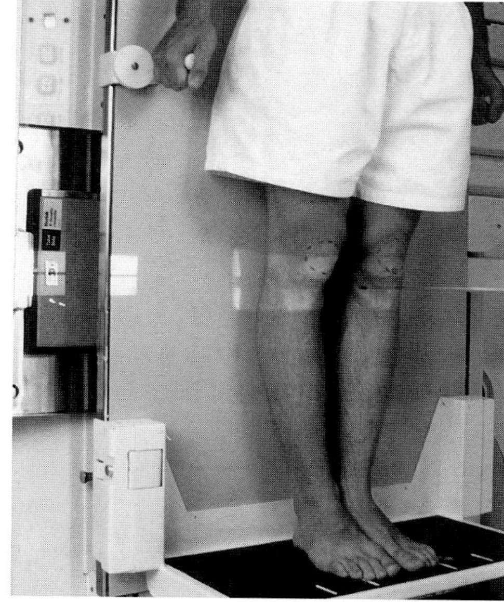

Fig. 6-121. AP bilateral weight-bearing –CR perpendicular to film, or 5-10° caudad on thin patient.

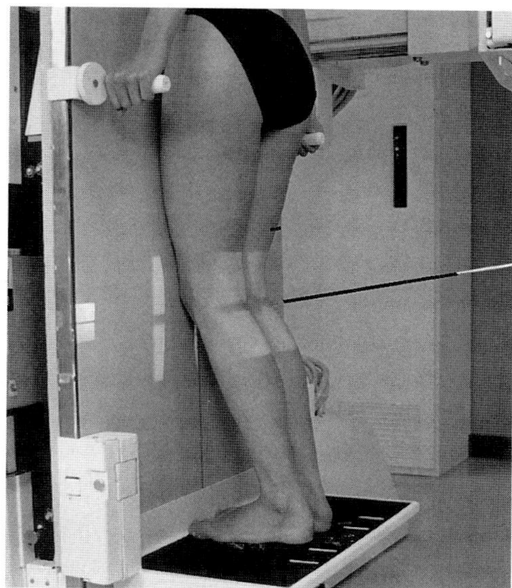

Fig. 6-122. Alternate PA bilateral weight-bearing –CR 10° caudad, if knees are partially flexed as shown.

Evaluation Criteria

- Collimation field should be centered to knee joint spaces, and should include sufficient femur and tibia to determine long axis of these long bones for alignment determinations.
- No rotation of both knees, evident by symmetrical appearance of femoral and tibial condyles.
- Knee joint spaces should appear "open" if CR angle was correct (parallel to tibial plateau).
- Optimum exposure should visualize faint outlines of patellae through femora, soft tissue should be visible and trabecular markings of all bones should appear clear and sharp.

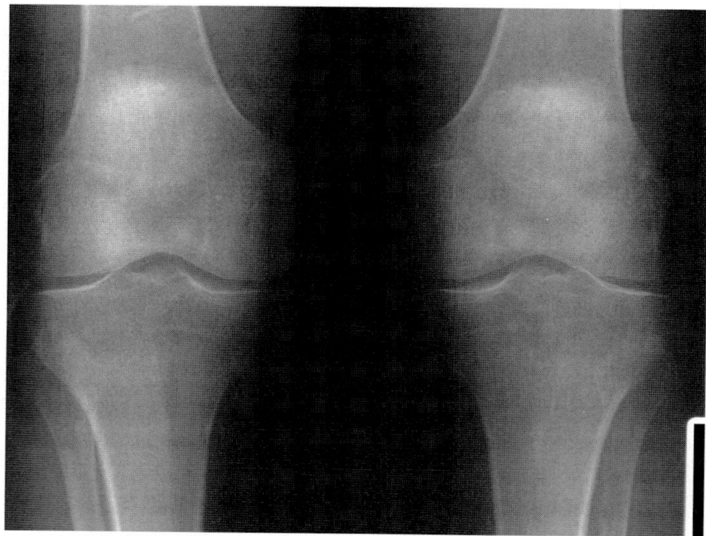

Fig. 6-123. AP bilateral weight-bearing, CR 10° caudad.

PA Axial Projection–Tunnel View

(1) Camp Coventry Method and (2) Holmblad Method

Knee
–Intercondylar fossa
Basic
• **PA axial**

Structures Best Shown

Intercondylar fossa shown in profile, femoral and tibial condyles, intercondylar eminence and articular facets of tibia.

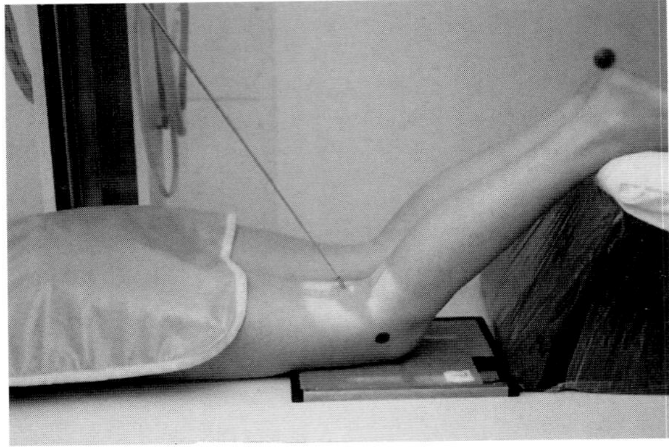

Fig. 6-124. (1) Camp Coventry method –Prone position (40 to 50° flexion).

Note: Two methods are described for demonstrating these structures. The prone position *(*Fig. 6-124*)* is an easier position for the patient. The Holmblad kneeling method provides another option with a slightly different projection of these structures with an increase in the amount of knee flexion.

Technical Factors

- Film size–8 x 10 in. (18 x 24 cm), lengthwise.
- Moving or stationary grid (or screen, <10 cm).
- 75±5 kVp range. (Increase 4-6 kVp from PA knee for increased penetration.)
- Technique and dose: (With 12:1 Bucky grid)

cm	kVp	mAs	Sk.	ML.	Gon.
11	78	5	36	17	M NDC F <0.1
			mrad		

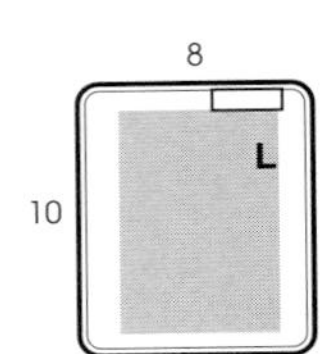

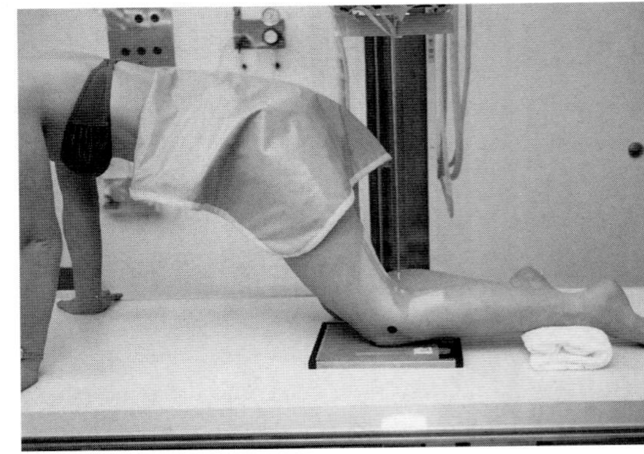

Fig. 6-125. (2) Holmblad method –Kneeling position (60 to 70° flexion).

Shielding: Place lead shield over gonadal area. Secure around waist in kneeling position and extend shield down to at least the mid femur level.

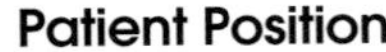

Patient Position

(1): Patient prone, pillow for head.
(2): Patient kneeling on x-ray table.

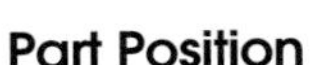
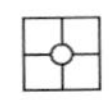

Part Position

(1) Prone:
- Flex knee **40 to 50**°, place support under ankle.
- Center cassette to knee joint considering projection of CR angle.

(2) Kneeling:
- With patient kneeling on "all fours," place cassette under affected knee; film centered to popliteal crease.
- Ask patient to support body weight primarily on opposite knee.
- Place padded support under ankle and leg of affected limb to reduce pressure on injured knee.
- Ask patient to slowly **lean forward 20 to 30**°, and hold that position. (Results in 60 to 70° knee flexion.)

Central Ray

(1) Prone: CR **perpendicular to lower leg** (40 to 50° caudad to match degree of flexion).
(2) Kneeling: CR **perpendicular to film and lower leg.**
- Direct CR to **mid popliteal crease.**
- Minimum 40 in. (102 cm) SID.

Collimation: Collimate on four sides to knee joint area.

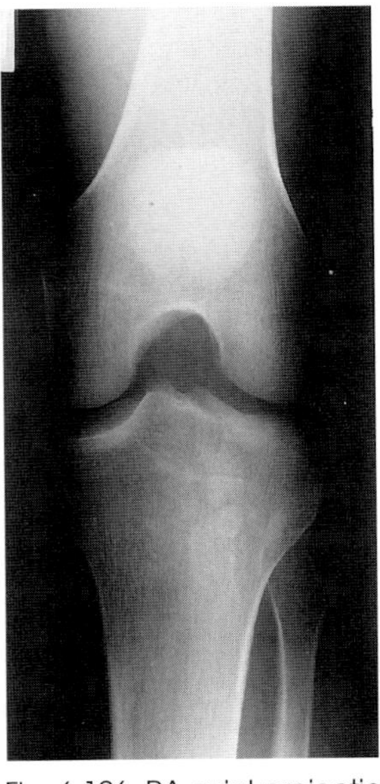

Fig. 6-126. PA axial projection.

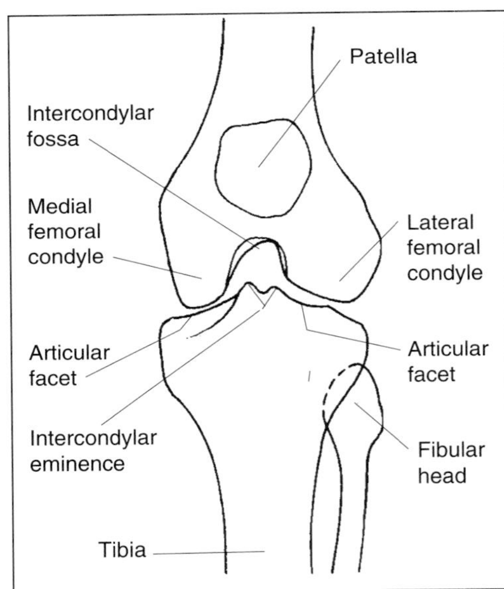

Fig. 6-127. PA axial projection.

Evaluation Criteria

- Center of four-sided collimation field should be to mid knee joint area.
- For this projection it is most important that the intercondylar fossa appear in profile, open without superimposition by patella.
- No rotation will be evidenced by symmetrical appearance of the distal posterior femoral condyles and superimposition of approximately half of fibular head by tibia.
- Articular facets and intercondylar eminence of tibia should be well visualized without superimposition.
- Optimum exposure should visualize soft tissue in the knee joint space and an outline of patella through the femur.
- Trabecular markings of femoral condyles and proximal tibia should appear clear and sharp.

AP Axial Projection

Knee
–Intercondylar fossa
Basic
• PA axial
Special
• **AP axial**

Structures Best Shown

Intercondylar fossa shown in profile, femoral and tibial condyles, intercondylar eminence (tibial spines) and articular facets of tibial (tibia plateau).

Note: This is a reversal of the PA axial projection for those who cannot assume the prone position. This, however, is **not** a preferred projection because of the distortion from the CR angle and increased part-film distance, unless a curved cassette is available. This projection also increases exposure to gonadal region.

Technical Factors

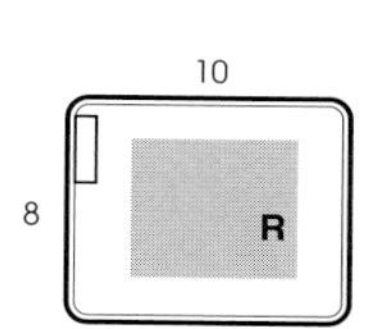

- Film size–8 x 10 in. (18 x 24 cm), crosswise.
- Curved cassette preferred if available to reduce part/film distance.
- Detail screen, small focal spot (65±5 kVp range), (Grid not needed due to air gap.)

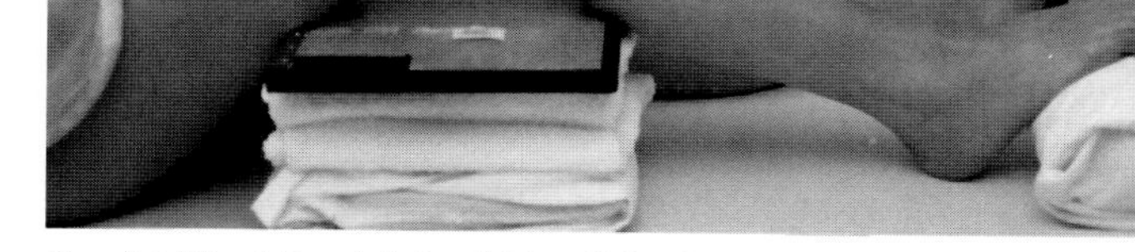

Fig. 6-128. AP axial–8 x 10 in. (18 x 24 cm) cassette crosswise (40° flexion, 40° CR angle).

Shielding: Place lead shield over pelvic area extending to mid femur.

Patient Position

- Patient supine with support under partially flexed knee with entire leg in the anatomical position with **no rotation.**

Part Position

- Flex knee **40 to 45°** and place support under cassette as needed to place cassette firmly against posterior thigh and leg as shown in Fig. 6-129.
- If curved cassette is available, place under knee as shown in Fig. 6-130.
- Adjust cassette as needed to center film to mid knee joint area.

Central Ray

- CR **perpendicular** to lower leg (40 to 45° cephalad).
- Direct CR to a point **¾ in. (2 cm) distal to apex of patella.**
- Minimum 40 in. (102 cm) SID.

Collimation: Collimate on four sides to knee joint area.

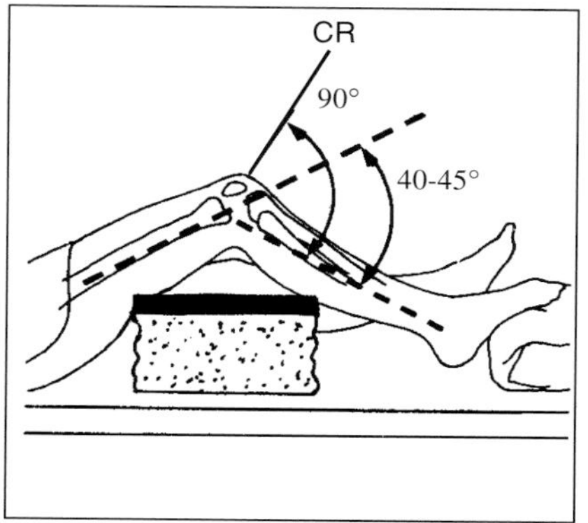

Fig. 6-129. With 8 x 10 in. flat cassette.

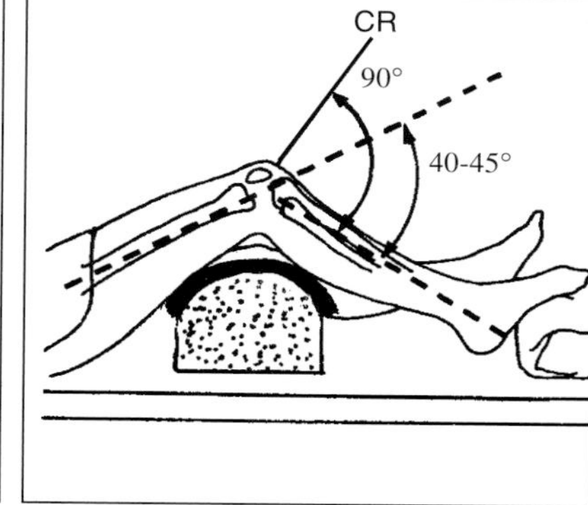

Fig. 6-130. With curved cassette (Béclere method).

Evaluation Criteria

- Center of four-sided collimation field should be to mid knee joint area.
- The intercondylar fossa should appear in profile, open without superimposition by patella. The intercondylar eminence and tibial plateau and distal condyles of femur should be clearly visualized.
- **No rotation**: Will be evidenced by symmetrical appearance of the distal posterior femoral condyles and superimposition of approximately half of fibular head by the tibia.
- Optimum exposure should visualize soft tissue in the knee joint space and an outline of patella through the femur.
- Trabecular markings of femoral condyles and proximal tibia should appear clear and sharp.

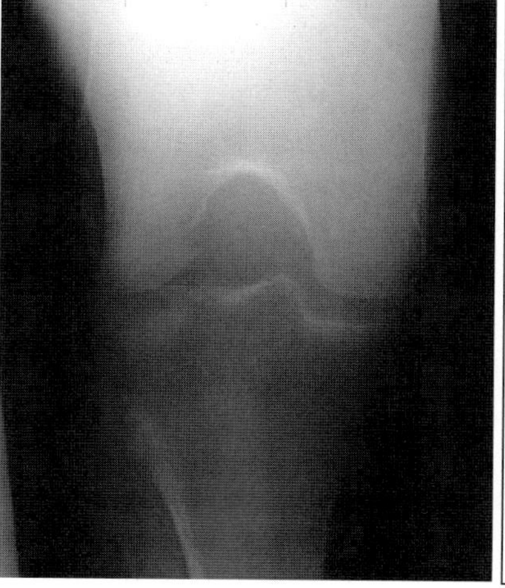

Fig. 6-131. AP axial–40° flexion and CR angle.

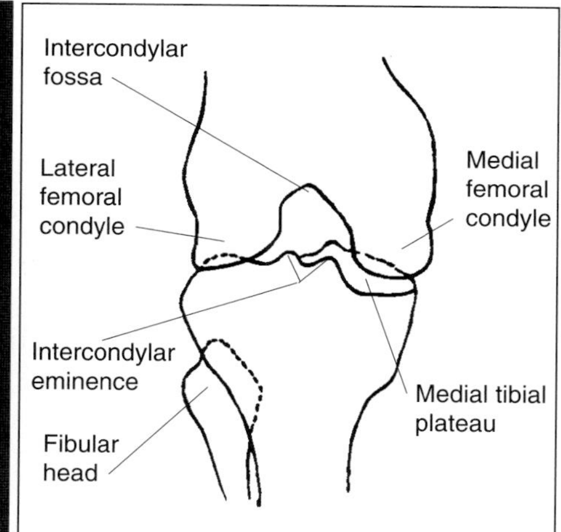

Fig. 6-132. AP axial.

PA Projection

Patella
- **PA**
- Lateral
- Tangential

Structures Best Shown

Knee joint and patella. (PA projection visualizes patella better than AP because of closer part/film distance.)

Technical Factors

- Film size–8 x 10 in. (18 x 24 cm), lengthwise.
- Moving or stationary grid (or screen, <10 cm).
- 75±5 kVp range.
  (Increase 4 to 6 kVp from PA knee technique for better patella visualization.)
- Technique and dose:

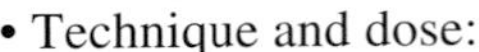

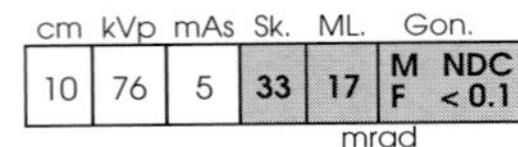

cm	kVp	mAs	Sk.	ML.	Gon.
10	76	5	33	17	M NDC F <0.1
			mrad		

Shielding: Place shield over gonadal area.

Patient Position

- Patient prone, legs extended, pillow for head.
- Place support under ankle and leg with smaller support under femur above knee to prevent direct pressure on patella.

Part Position 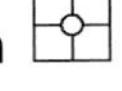

- Align and center long axis of leg and knee to midline of table or grid cassette.
  True PA: Interepicondylar line should be parallel to plane of film. (This usually requires about 5° internal rotation of anterior knee.)

Central Ray

- CR **perpendicular** to film. Direct CR to **mid patella area** (which is usually at approximately the mid popliteal crease).
- Minimum 40 in. (102 cm) SID.

Collimation: Collimate closely on four sides to include just the area of the patella and knee joint.

Notes: With a potential fracture of patella, extra care should be taken to **not flex knee** and **provide support under thigh** (femur) so as not to put direct pressure on patella area.

May also be taken as an AP projection positioned like an AP knee if patient cannot assume a prone position.

Evaluation Criteria

- Four-sided collimation field should include patella and knee joint area with the center at the mid patella area.
- Sufficient exposure will visualize soft tissue in joint area and also clearly visualize the outline of patella as seen through the distal femur.
- No rotation, as evidenced by symmetrical appearance of the condyles. The patella normally will be slightly off center toward the medial aspect of the femur.

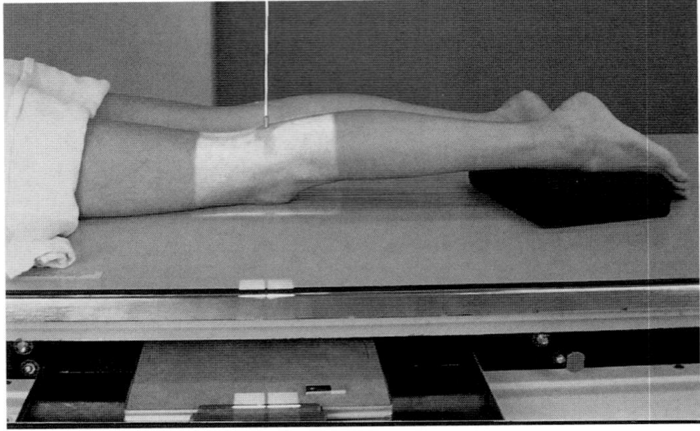

Fig. 6-133. CR 0° to mid patella–PA patella.

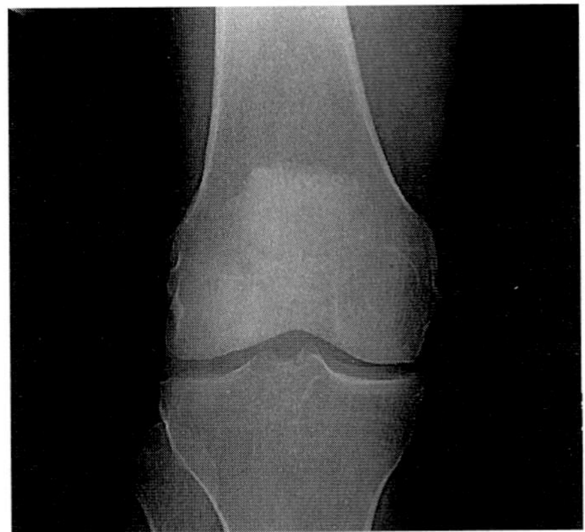

Fig. 6-134. PA patella.

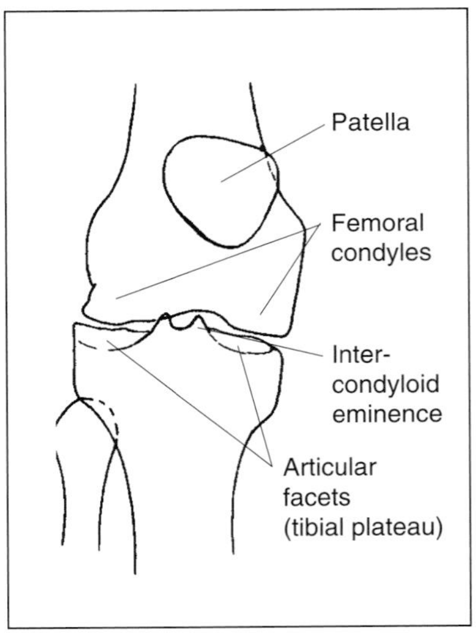

Fig. 6-135. PA patella.

Lateral–Mediolateral Projection

Patella
- PA
- **Lateral**
- Tangential

Structures Best Shown

Patella (in profile), patellofemoral joint and tibiofemoral joint.

Technical Factors

- Film size–8 x 10 in. (18 x 24 cm), lengthwise.
- Moving or stationary grid, 70±6 kVp range or smaller patient (<10 cm), screen table-top, 60±5 kVp range.
  (Decrease 4-6 kVp from lateral knee technique to avoid overexposing the patella.)
- Technique and dose:

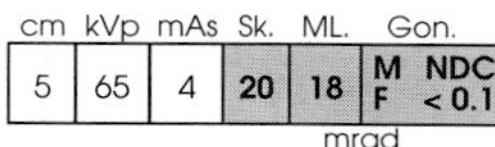

cm	kVp	mAs	Sk.	ML.	Gon.
5	65	4	20	18	M NDC F < 0.1

mrad

Shielding: Place shield over gonadal area.

Patient Position

- Patient in lateral recumbent position, affected side down, pillow for head.
- Provide support for knee of opposite limb placed either behind or in front of affected knee.

Part Position

- Adjust rotation of body and leg until knee is in a **true lateral** position (femoral epicondyles directly superimposed and plane of patella perpendicular to plane of film).
- Flex knee **only 5 or 10°**. (Additional flexion may separate fracture fragments if present.)
- Align and center long axis of patella to CR and to centerline of table or cassette.

Central Ray

- CR **perpendicular** to film. Direct CR to the **distal aspect of the patellofemoral joint.**
- Minimum 40 in. (102 cm) SID.

Collimation: Collimate closely on four sides to include just the area of the patella and knee joint.

Note: This can also be taken as a cross table lateral with no knee flexion on a severe trauma patient.

Evaluation Criteria

- Four-sided collimation should include patella and knee joint with the center to the distal aspect of the patellofemoral joint space.
- **True lateral**: The anterior and posterior borders of the femoral condyles should be directly superimposed. The patellofemoral joint space should appear open.
- Optimum exposure will visualize the patella well without overexposure. Soft tissue detail of the knee joint should also be visible. The trabecular markings of the patella and other bones should appear clear and sharp.

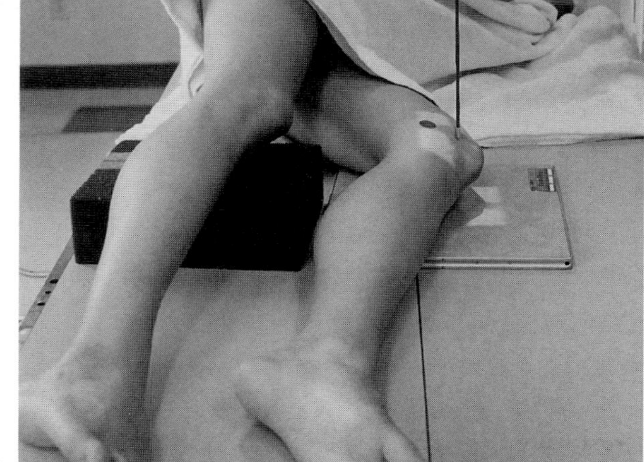

Fig. 6-136. Lateral patella.

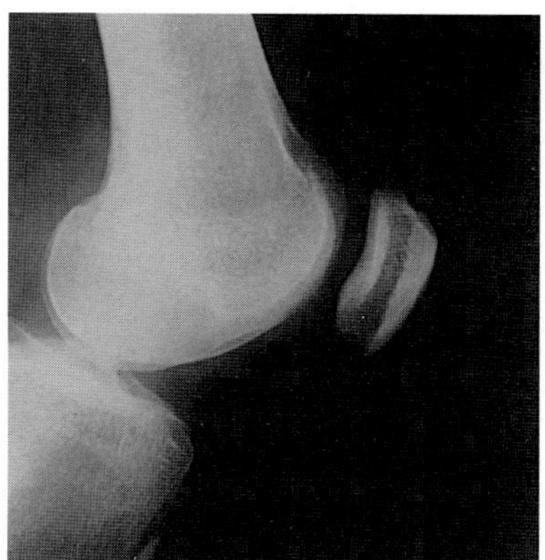

Fig. 6-137. Lateral patella.

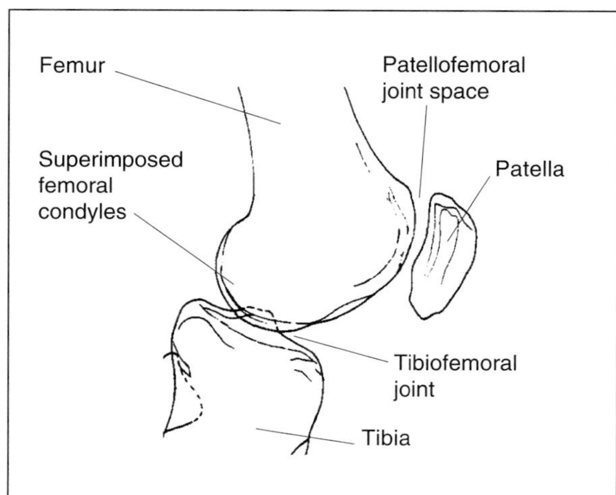

Fig. 6-138. Lateral patella.

Tangential (Axial or Sunrise/Skyline) Projections

Merchant Bilateral Method

Patella
- PA
- Lateral
- **Tangential**

Structures Best Shown

An axial view of patella, intercondylar sulcus, and patellofemoral joint with quadriceps femoris muscle in relaxed state.

12

10 R L

Technical Factors

- Film size–10 x 12 in. (24 x 30 cm), crosswise.
- Detail screen, small focal spot. (Grid is not needed because of air gap due to increased OID.)
- 65±5 kVp range.
- Some type of leg support and cassette holder should be used.
- Technique and dose:

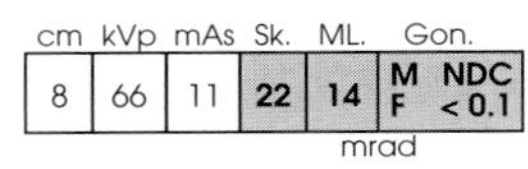

cm	kVp	mAs	Sk.	ML.	Gon.
8	66	11	22	14	M NDC F < 0.1
				mrad	

Shielding: Place lead shield over entire pelvic area.

Patient Position

- Patient supine with knees **flexed 40 to 45°** over the end of the table, resting on a leg support. Patient in general needs to be comfortable and relaxed for quadriceps muscles to be totally relaxed (see Note).

Part Position

- Place support under knees to raise distal femora so they are parallel to table-top.
- Place knees and feet together and secure legs together below the knees to prevent rotation and to allow patient to be totally relaxed.
- Place cassette on edge against legs about 12 in. (30 cm) below the knees, **perpendicular** to x-ray beam.

Central Ray

- Angle CR caudad, **30° from horizontal** (CR 30° to femora). Adjust CR angle if needed for true tangential projection of patellofemoral joint spaces.
- Direct CR to a point **midway between patellae.**
- 48 in. (120 cm) to 72 in. (180 cm) SID (increased SID reduces magnification.)

Collimation: Collimate **tightly** on all sides to patellae.

Note: Patient comfort and total relaxation are essential. The quadriceps femoris muscles must be relaxed to prevent subluxation of patellae, wherein they are pulled into the intercondylar sulcus or groove, which may result in false readings.*

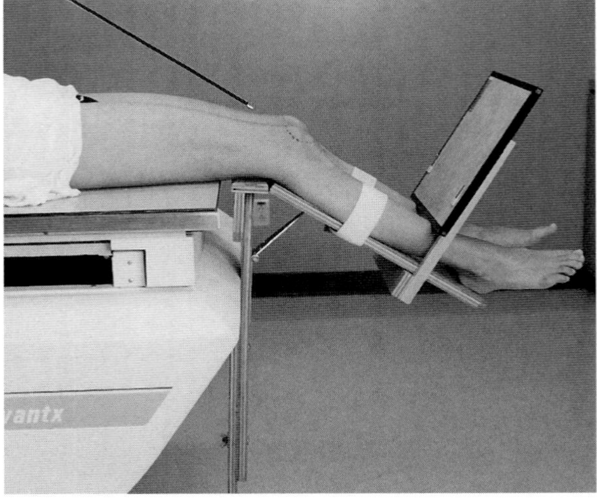

Fig. 6-139a. Patient position–Bilateral tangential, knees flexed 40 to 45°.

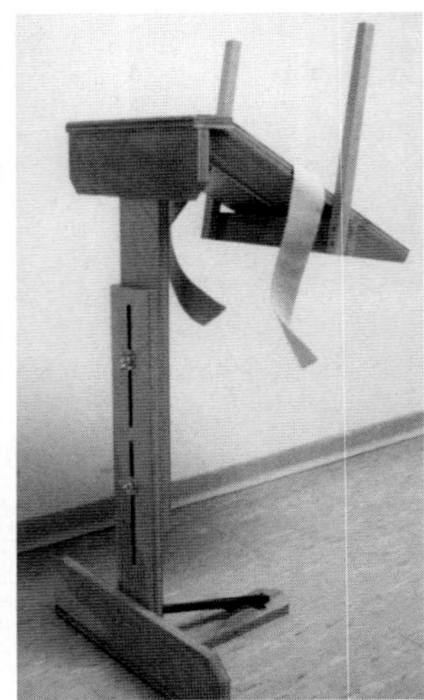

Fig. 6-139b. Adjustable type leg support and film holder. (Courtesy of St. Joseph's Hospital and Medical Center, Phoenix, AZ.)

Fig. 6-140. Bilateral tangential.

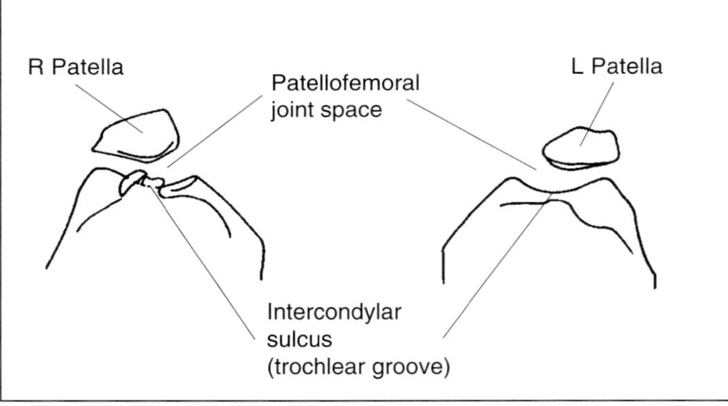

Fig. 6-141. Bilateral tangential.

Evaluation Criteria

- Four-sided rectangular collimation field should be limited to area of patellae and anterior femoral condyles.
- The intercondylar sulcus (trochlear groove) and patella of each distal femur should be visualized in profile.
- Patellofemoral joint space should be open with bony margins of condyles and patellae clearly defined.
- Optimum exposure should clearly visualize soft tissue and joint space margins and trabecular markings of patellae. Femoral condyles will appear underexposed with only the anterior margins clearly defined.

*Merchant, AC, et al. Roentgenographic Analysis of Patellofemoral Congruence, *J. Bone and Joint Surg*. 1974; 56-A:1391-96.

Patella
• PA
• Lateral
• **Tangential**

Tangential (Axial or Sunrise/Skyline) Projections

1. Inferosuperior projection, (patient supine, 45° knee flexion)
2. Hughston Method (Patient prone, 55° knee flexion)
3. Settegast Method (Patient prone, 90° knee flexion)

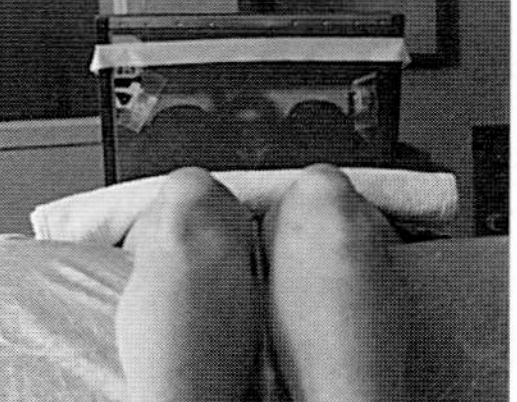

Fig. 6-142. Profile of patellae seen in light field. (Inferosuperior projection)

Summary: Three additional methods for the tangential projections of the patellae and patellofemoral joints are described in a suggested order of preference. Advantages and disadvantages of each are noted. **Both sides** are generally taken for comparison.

Technical Factors

• Film size–10 x 12 in. (24 x 30 cm) or 8 x 10 in. (18 x 24 cm), crosswise.
• Detail screen, small focal spot.
• 65±5 kVp range.

12
10
L R

1. Inferosuperior Projection

(May be taken unilaterally on separate films, or bilaterally on one film placed crosswise as shown.)

• Patient supine, legs together with sufficient size support placed under knees for maximum 45° knee flexion. (Legs relaxed.)
• Ensure no leg rotation, feet up.
• Place cassette on edge, resting on mid thighs, tilted so as to be perpendicular to CR. Use sandbags and tape as shown, or other methods to stabilize cassette in this position. It is **not** recommended that patient be asked to sit up to hold cassette in place because this places patient's head and neck region into path of x-ray beam.

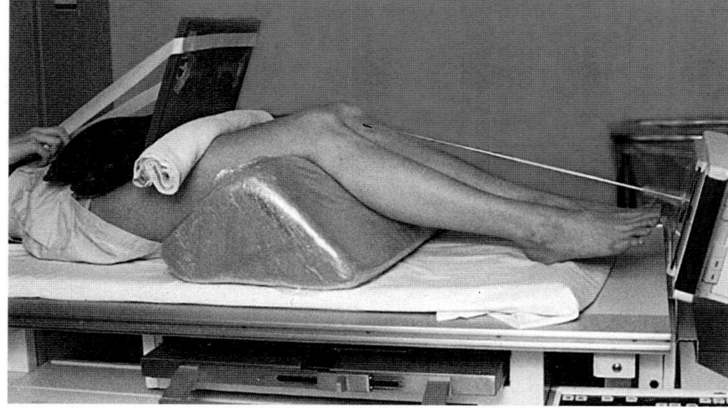

Fig. 6-143. **Inferosuperior projection**–40 to 45° flexion of knees.

Central Ray

• Direct CR inferosuperiorly, ≈10-15° angle from lower legs to be **tangential to patellofemoral joint.** Palpate borders of patella to determine specific CR angle required to pass through infrapatellar joint space.
• 40-48 in. (102-122 cm) SID.

Note 1: The major advantage to this method is it does not require special equipment and it is a relatively comfortable position for patient. Therefore total relaxation can be achieved with 40-45° knee flexion if proper sized support is placed under knees. The only disadvantage is in holding or supporting the cassette in this position if the patient cannot cooperate fully.

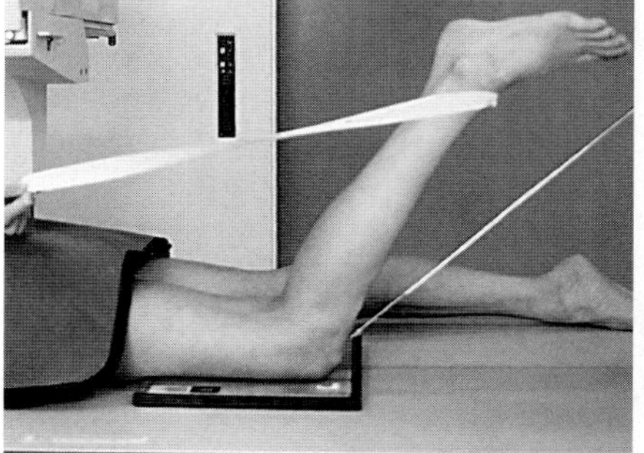

Fig. 6-144. **2. Hughston method*** –45° flexion of knee.

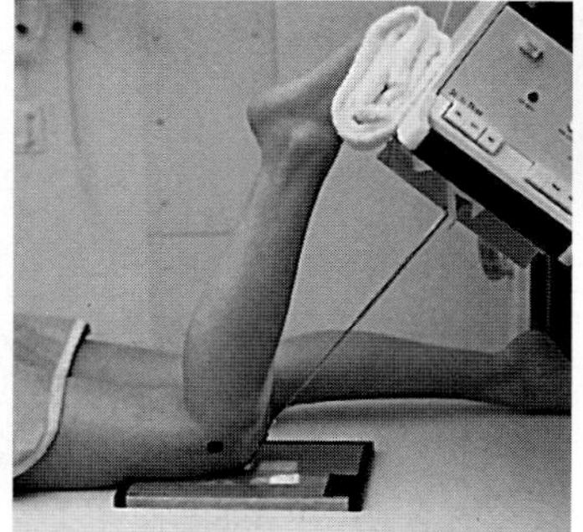

Fig. 6-145. **2. Hughston method*** –55° flexion of knee.

2. Hughston Method* (May be done bilaterally on one film.)

• Patient prone with cassette placed under knee. Slowly flex knee 45 to 55° (see Note 3). Have patient hold foot with gauze, or rest foot against collimator or other support. Place pad between foot and possible **hot** collimation.

Central Ray

• CR ≈**15-20° from long axis of lower leg**. (Tangential to patellofemoral joint.)
• Direct CR to **mid patellofemoral joint**
• Minimum 40 in. (102 cm) SID.

Note 2: This is a relatively comfortable position for patient and relaxation of the quadriceps can be achieved. The major disadvantage is the image distortion caused by the film-body part-beam alignment, and the difficulty of less angle knee flexion due to modern equipment and large collimators.

Note 3: Some authors suggest only 20° of flexion to prevent patella from being drawn into patellofemoral groove, which may prevent detection of subtle abnormalities in alignment.†

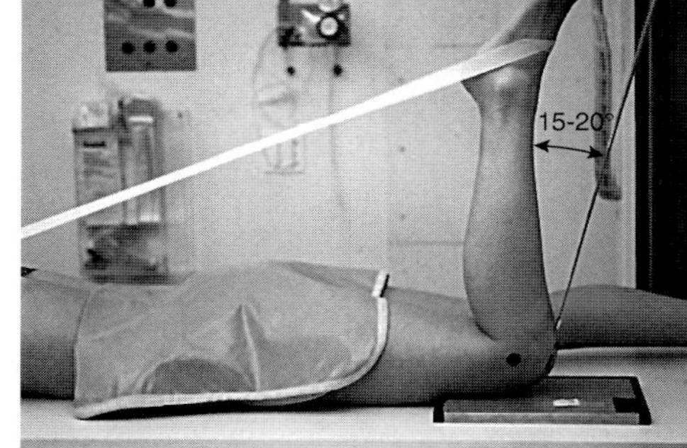

Fig. 6-146. **3. Settegast Method** –90° flexion of knee (see Note 4).

3. Settegast Method

Warning: This acute flexion of knee should **not** be attempted until fracture of patella has been ruled out by other projections.

• Patient prone with cassette under knee. Slowly flex knee to a **minimum of 90°**. Patient holds on to gauze or tape to maintain position.

Central Ray

• CR **tangential to patellofemoral joint space**, (≈15 to 20° from lower leg).
• Minimum 40 in. (102 cm) SID.

Note 4: The major disadvantage to this method is that the acute knee flexion makes this impossible to use with knee trauma. Also the tightened quadriceps tend to center the patella and draw it into the intercondylar sulcus, thus reducing the diagnostic value of this projection.††

*Hughston, AC. Subluxation of the Patella, *J Bone and Joint Surg* 1968; 50-A: 1003-26.
†Manaster, BJ. Handbooks in Radiology. *Skeletal Radiology*. St. Louis: Year Book Pub.; 1989.
††Turner, GW, Burns, CB. Erect Position/Tangential Projection of the Patellofemoral Joint. *Radiologic Technology*. 1982; 54-1: 11-14.

PA Oblique Projections–Internal and External Rotation

Axial Oblique–Kuchendorf Method

Patella
Special
• Oblique

Structures Best Shown

Oblique views of patella free of superimposition. (Each half of patella is shown free of superimposition in these two obliques.)

PA axial obliques (Kuchendorf method): A 25 to 30° CR caudad angle will project more of the patella free of superimposition of the femur.

Technical Factors

12

10

L

- Film size–10 x 12 in. (24 x 30 cm), crosswise.
- Divide in half for each oblique.
- Detail screen, table-top.
- 60±5 kVp range.
- Technique and dose:

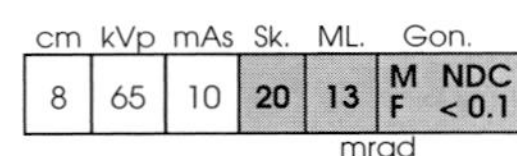

cm	kVp	mAs	Sk.	ML.	Gon.
8	65	10	20	13	M NDC F <0.1
			mrad		

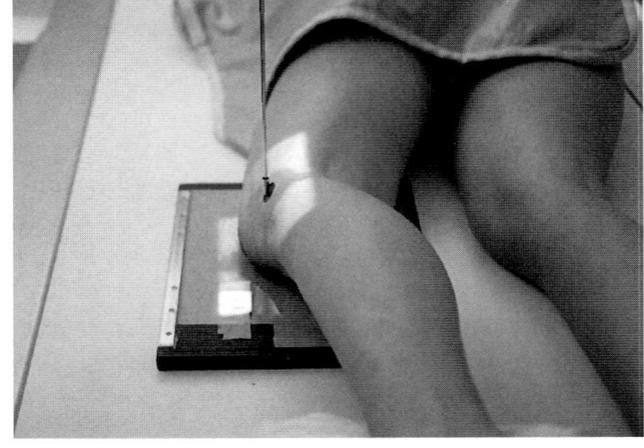

Fig. 6-147. PA external oblique (lateral portion of patella free of superimposition).

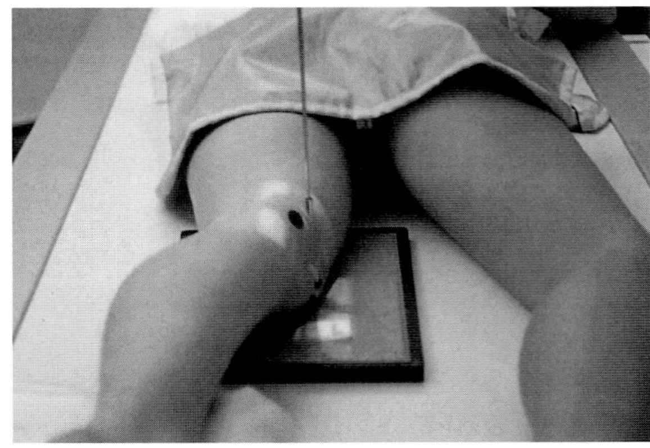

Fig. 6-148. PA internal oblique (medial portion of patella free of superimposition).

Shielding: Place shield over gonadal area.

Patient Position

External Oblique: Patient prone, turned up slightly oblique away from affected side with hand and arm of affected side up by head and opposite arm down by side. Provide pillow for head.

Internal Oblique: Same as above but patient turned into opposite oblique.

Part Position

External Oblique: Rotate the anterior or patella area of the leg externally. Generally a 35 to 40° rotation from a PA is required.

Internal Oblique: Same as above but rotate leg internally to displace the patella medially.

- Flex knee slightly to relax quadriceps muscles, place support under ankle.
- Center patella area to CR and to center of unmasked half of film.

Central Ray

- CR **perpendicular** to film, directed to **mid patella,** or **25-30° caudad** (Kuchendorf method).
- Minimum 40 in. (102 cm) SID.

Collimation: Collimate to region of patella.

Optional PA axial (Kuchendorf method): Positioning is the same as above oblique projections. Central ray is angled **25 to 50° caudad,** directed to **mid patella.**

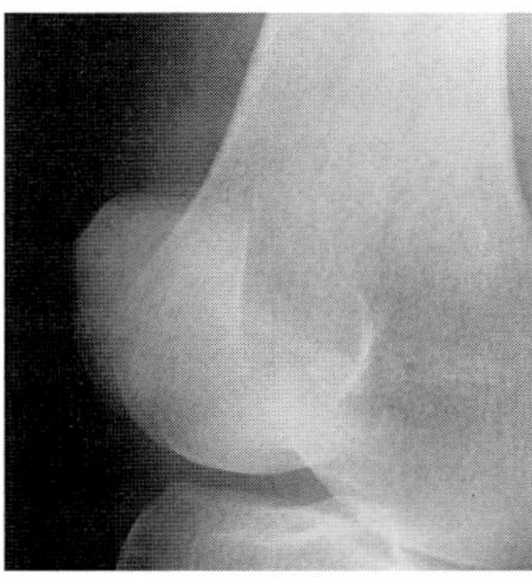

Fig. 6-149. External oblique –CR 0°.

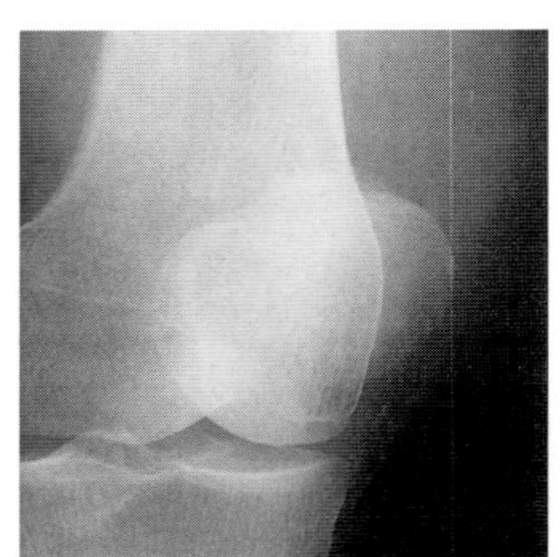

Fig. 6-150. Internal oblique –CR 0°.

Evaluation Criteria

- Four-sided collimation field should include only the patella and knee joint area.
- Half or more of the patella should be seen in profile on each oblique not superimposed by femur.
- PA axial projection projects patella inferiorly with less superimposition by femur.
- Optimum exposure should visualize the border outline of the patella through the femur and also clearly visualize the portion of the patella in profile without overexposure. Trabecular markings of that portion of the patella free of superimposition should be visible and appear clear and sharp.

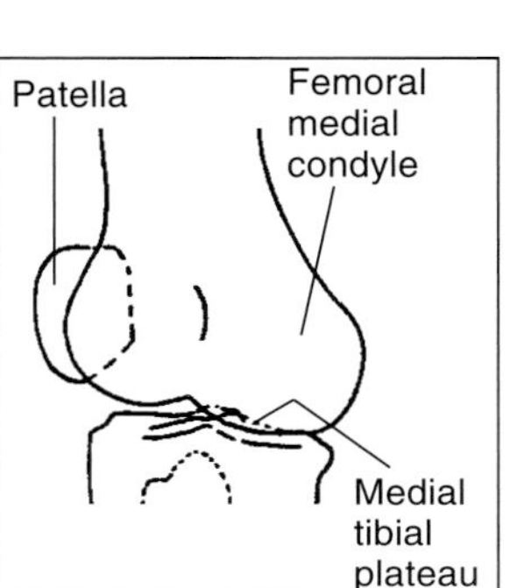

Fig. 6-151. External oblique.

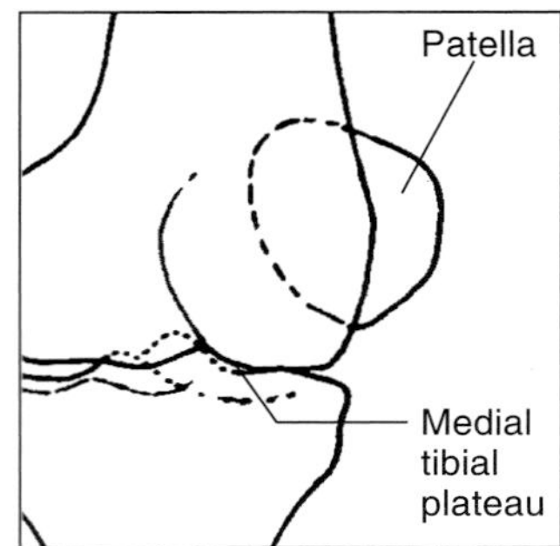

Fig. 6-152. Internal oblique.

AP Projection

Note: If site of interest is in area of proximal femur, a unilateral hip routine or a pelvis is recommended, as described in Chapter 7.

Femur–Mid and distal
Basic
- **AP**
- Lateral

Structures Best Shown

Mid and distal femur, including knee joint.

Technical Factors

- Film size–14 x 17 in. (35 x 43 cm), lengthwise.
- Moving or stationary grid.
- 75±5 kVp range.
- Due to anode-heel effect, place hip or head end of patient at cathode end of x-ray beam.
- Technique and dose:

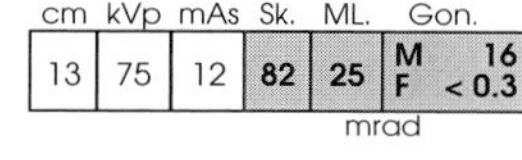

cm	kVp	mAs	Sk.	ML.	Gon.
13	75	12	82	25	M 16 F <0.3
			mrad		

Shielding: Place lead shield over pelvic area to ensure correct gonadal shielding because of proximity to primary beam.

Patient Position

- Patient supine, femur centered to midline of table, pillow for head. (May also be done on stretcher with portable grid placed under femur.)

Part Position

- Align femur to CR and to midline of table or film. (Mid and proximal femur tends to be in lateral part of thigh.)
- Rotate leg internally about 5° for a true AP as for an AP knee.
- Ensure that knee joint is included on film, considering the divergence of the x-ray beam. (Lower cassette margin should be about 2 in. or 5 cm below knee joint.)

Central Ray

- CR **perpendicular** to femur and film, directed to **midpoint of film.**
- Minimum 40 in. (102 cm) SID.

Collimation: Collimate closely on both sides to femur with end collimation to film borders.

Routine to include both joints: Some departmental routines include both joints on at least one projection on all initial femur exams. For a large adult a second smaller film (10 x 12 in.) should then be used for an AP of either the knee or the hip, ensuring that both hip and knee joints are included. If the hip is included, the leg should be rotated 10 to 15° internally to place the femoral neck in profile.

Evaluation Criteria

- Femur should be centered to collimation field with knee joint space a minimum of 1 in. (2.5 cm) from distal film margin. There should only be minimal collimation borders visible on proximal and distal margins of film.
- Knee joint space will not appear fully open due to divergent x-ray beam.
- **No rotation**: Femoral and tibial condyles should appear symmetrical in size and shape with the outline of patella near the center of distal femur (patella usually is slightly toward medial side of femur). The approximate medial half of fibular head should be superimposed by tibia.
- Optimum exposure with correct use of anode-heel effect will result in near uniform density of entire femur. Fine trabecular markings should be clear and sharp throughout length of femur.

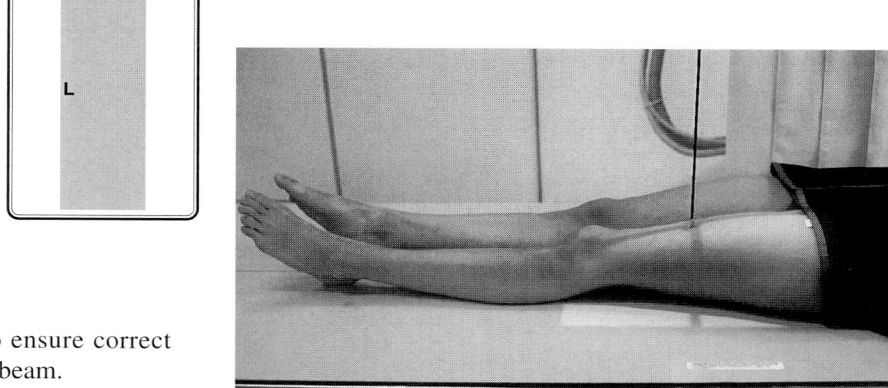

Fig. 6-153. AP–Mid and distal femur (head at cathode end).

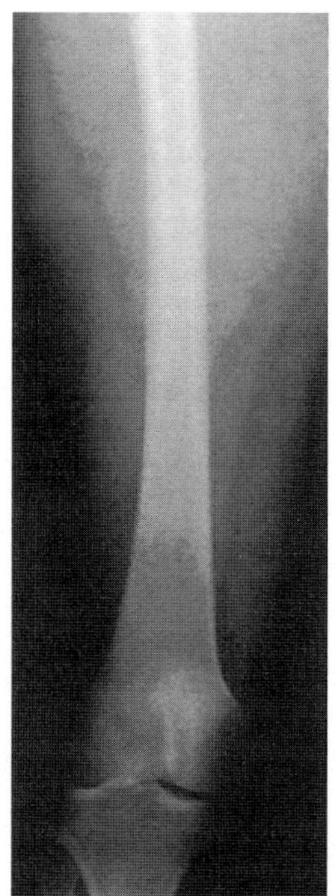

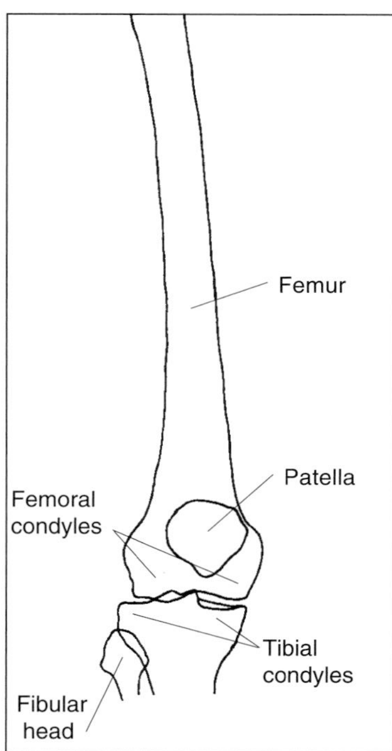

Fig. 6-154. AP–Mid and distal femur. Fig. 6-155.

Lateral–Mediolateral or Lateromedial Projections

Note: For possible trauma if site of interest is in area of proximal femur, a unilateral trauma hip routine is recommended, as described in Chapter 7. For non-trauma lateral of mid and proximal femur, see following page.

Femur–Mid and distal
Basic
• AP
• **Lateral**

Structures Best Shown

Mid and distal femur including knee joint.

Technical Factors

- Film size–14 x 17 in. (35 x 43 cm), lengthwise.
- Moving or stationary grid.
- 75±5 kVp range.
- Due to anode-heel effect, place the hip of patient at cathode end of x-ray beam.
- Technique and dose: (With 12:1 Bucky Grid)

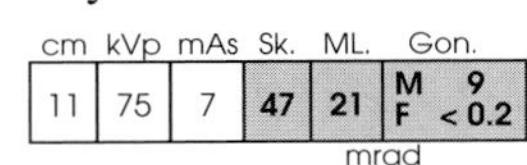

cm	kVp	mAs	Sk.	ML.	Gon.
11	75	7	47	21	M 9 F <0.2
					mrad

Shielding: Place lead shield over pelvic area to shield gonads.

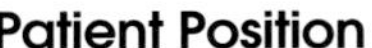

Patient Position

- Lateral recumbent, or supine for trauma patient.

Part Position 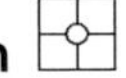

Lateral Recumbent (Fig. 6-156):

Warning: Do not attempt this position with severe trauma.

- With patient on affected side, flex knee approximately 45° and align femur to midline of table or film (remember the femur tends to be in anterior part of thigh).
- Place unaffected leg behind affected leg (or in front of affected leg if this assists in a true lateral position).
- Adjust cassette to include knee joint on film (lower cassette margin should be about 2 in. or 5 cm below knee joint). A second film to include the proximal femur and hip will generally be required on an adult. (See following page.)

Trauma Lateromedial Projection (Fig. 6-157):

- Place support under affected leg and support foot and ankle in true AP position.
- Place cassette on edge against medial aspect of thigh to include knee, with horizontal x-ray beam directed from lateral side.

Trauma Mediolateral Projection (Fig. 6-158):

- Elevate unaffected leg and place a high support under foot and ankle.
- With support under affected leg, place cassette on edge against lateral thigh with horizontal x-ray beam directed from medial side.

Central Ray

- CR **perpendicular** to femur and film, directed to **midpoint of film.**
- Minimum 40 in. (102 cm) SID.

Collimation: Collimate closely on both sides to femur with end collimation to film borders.

Evaluation Criteria

- Femur should be centered to collimation field with knee joint space a minimum of 1 in. (2.5 cm) from distal film margin. There should only be minimal collimation borders visible on proximal and distal margins of film.
- Knee joint will not appear open and distal margins of the femoral condyles will not be superimposed due to divergent x-ray beam.
- **True lateral**: Anterior and posterior margins of femoral condyles should be superimposed and aligned. Patellofemoral joint space should be open.
- Optimum exposure with correct use of anode-heel effect will result in near uniform density of entire femur. Fine trabecular markings should be clear and sharp throughout length of femur.

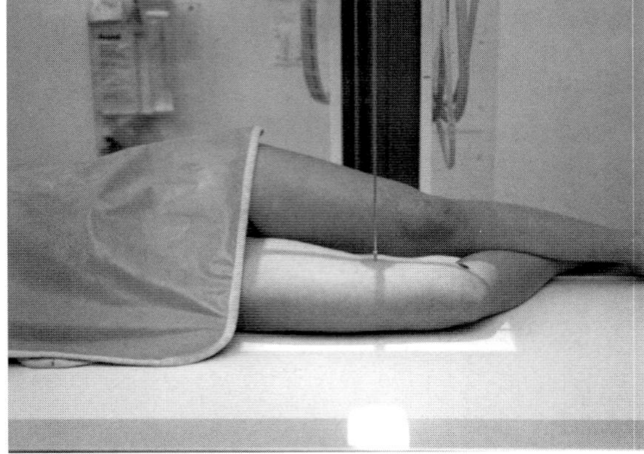

Fig. 6-156. Mediolateral mid and distal femur.

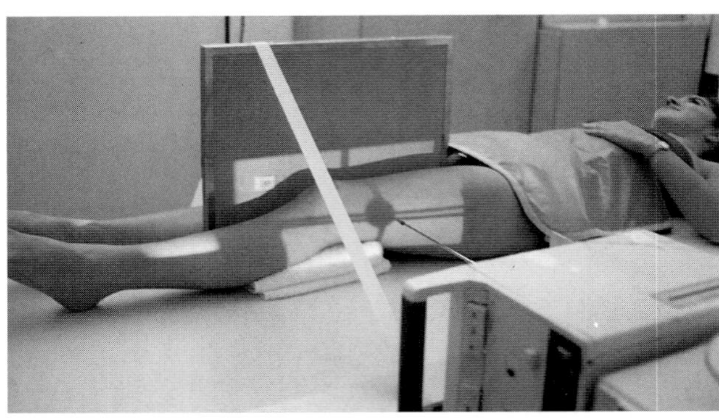

Fig. 6-157. Trauma lateromedial (horizontal beam) projection.

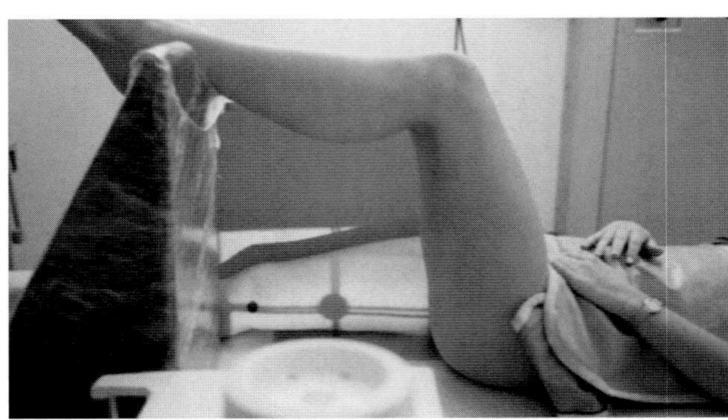

Fig. 1-158. Alternate mediolateral (horizontal beam) projection.

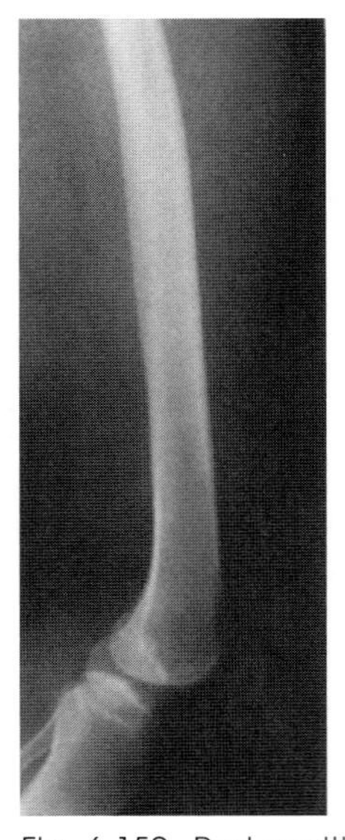

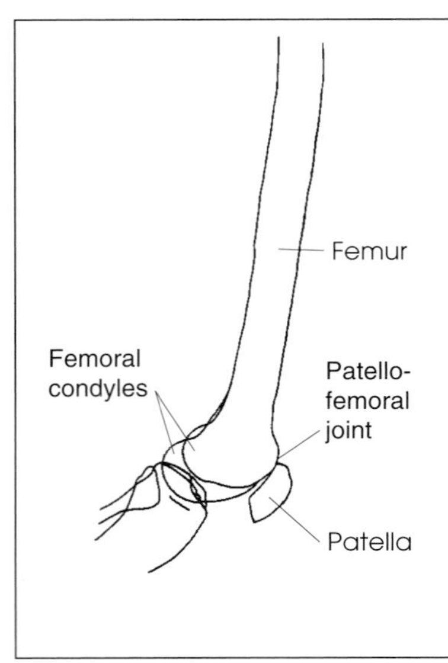

Fig. 6-159. Part position–Mid and distal femur. Fig. 6-160.

Lateral–Mediolateral Projection

Warning: Do not attempt this position for patient with possible fracture of hip or proximal femur. Refer to trauma lateral hip routine in Chapter 7.

Femur–Mid and proximal
Basic
- AP (see AP hip, Ch. 7)
- **Lateral**

Structures Best Shown

Mid and proximal femur including lateral hip.

Technical Factors

- Film size–14 x 17 in. (35 x 43 cm), lengthwise.
- Moving or stationary grid.
- 75±5 kVp range.
- To make best use of the anode-heel effect, place the hip at cathode end of x-ray beam.
- Technique and dose:

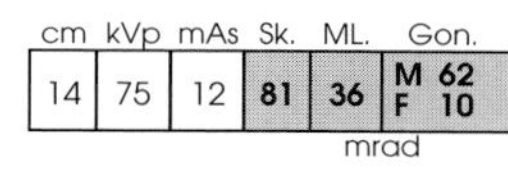

cm	kVp	mAs	Sk.	ML.	Gon.
14	75	12	81	36	M 62 F 10

mrad

Shielding: Generally gonadal shielding is difficult on this projection without obscuring essential anatomy.

Patient Position 

- Patient in lateral recumbent position with affected side down; provide pillow for head.
- Ask patient to grasp the edge of table to maintain this position. (Do not pinch fingers when moving Bucky Tray.)

Part Position

- Flex affected knee about 45° and align femur to midline of table.
- Place folded towel or other support under the affected leg for true lateral.
- With unaffected knee flexed, place leg behind affected leg for support, and have patient roll back (posteriorly) about 15° to prevent superimposition of proximal femur and hip joint.
- Adjust cassette to include hip joint on film considering the divergence of the x-ray beam. (Palpate anterior superior iliac spine and place upper film margin at the level of this landmark.)

Central Ray

- CR **perpendicular** to femur and film, directed to **midpoint of film.**
- Minimum 40 in. (102 cm) SID.

Collimation: Collimate closely on both sides to femur with end collimation to film borders.

Alternate routine to include both joints: Some departmental routines include both joints on all initial femur exams. On a large adult this requires a second smaller film (10 x 12 in. or 24 x 30 cm) of either the hip or knee joint.

Evaluation Criteria

- Femur should be centered to collimation field with hip joint a minimum of 1 in. (2.5 cm) from proximal film margin.
- There should only be minimum collimation borders on proximal and distal margins of film.
- Proximal femur and hip joint should not be superimposed by opposite limb.
- **True lateral**: Evidenced by the superimposition of the greater and lesser trochanters by the femur with only a small part of the lesser trochanter visible on medial side. The greater trochanter should be nearly symmetrically superimposed by the neck of the femur.
- Optimum exposure should result in near uniform density of entire femur. Fine trabecular markings should appear clear and sharp throughout entire femur.

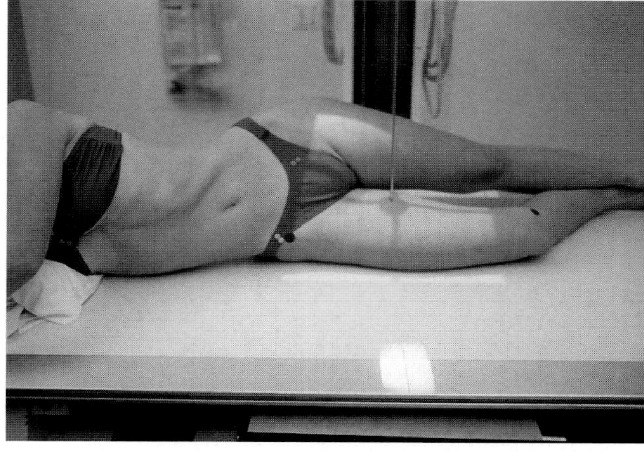

Fig. 6-161. Mediolateral–Mid and proximal femur.

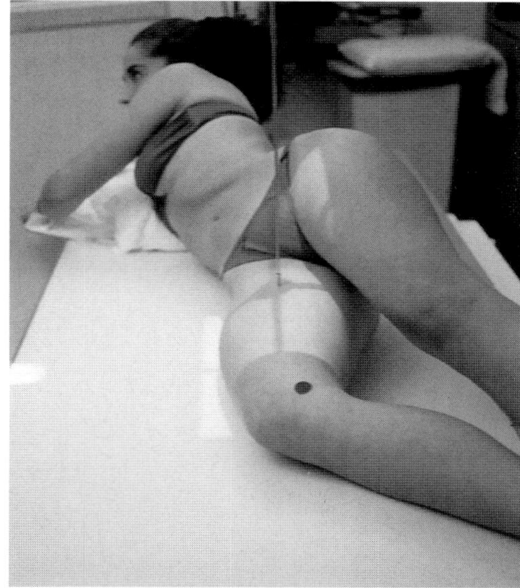

Fig. 6-162. Mediolateral –Mid and proximal femur.

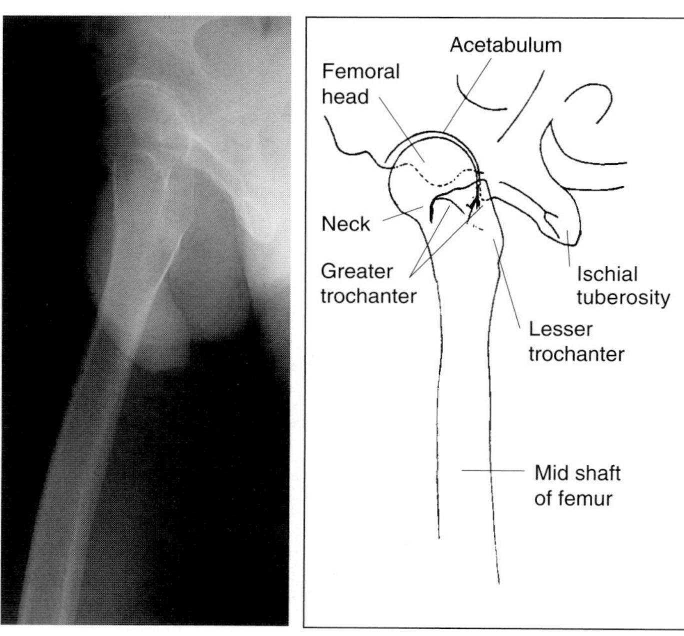

Fig. 6-163. Mediolateral–Mid and proximal femur. Fig. 6-164.

Radiographs for Critique

Each of these lower limb radiographs demonstrates some error in positioning which requires a repeat. These, along with accompanying lecture slides of these and other radiographs, will provide a basis for classroom and/or positioning lab discussion. Questions with answers based on these specific critique radiographs are provided in the accompanying student workbook/lab manuals to help prepare students for classroom and/or lab discussions on film critique.

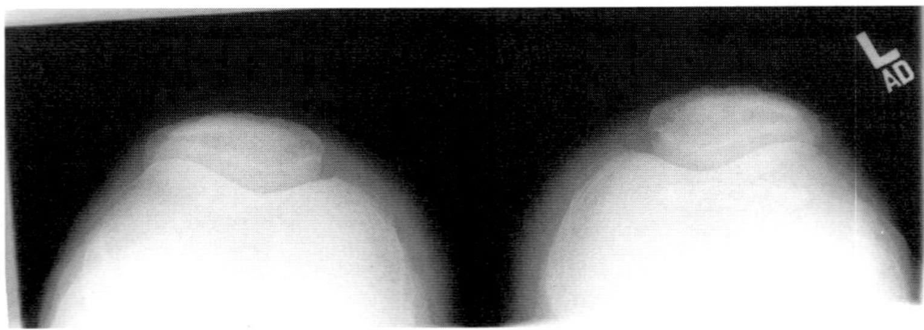

Fig. C6-165. Bilateral tangential patella.

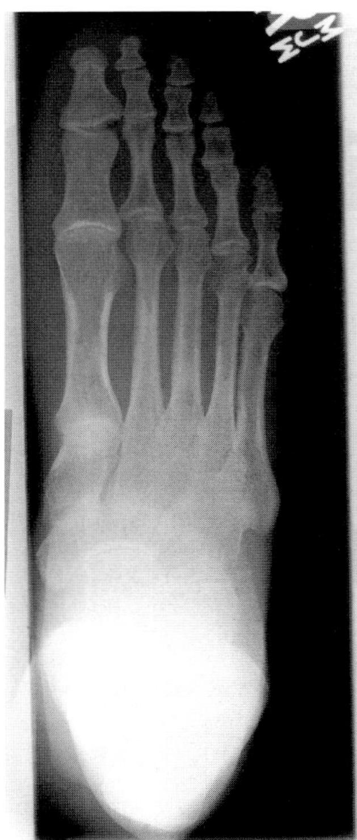

Fig. C6-166. AP foot.

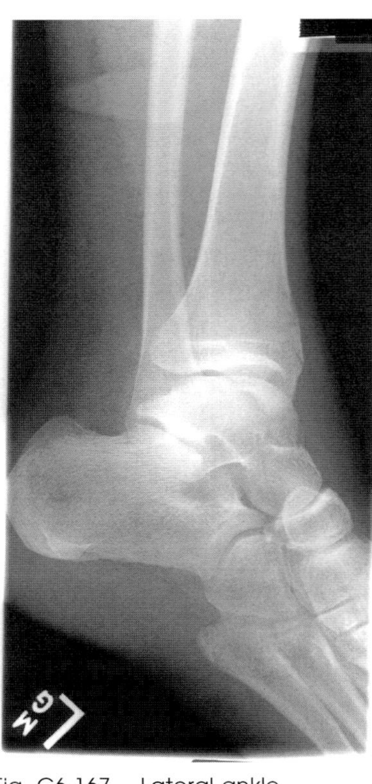

Fig. C6-167. Lateral ankle.

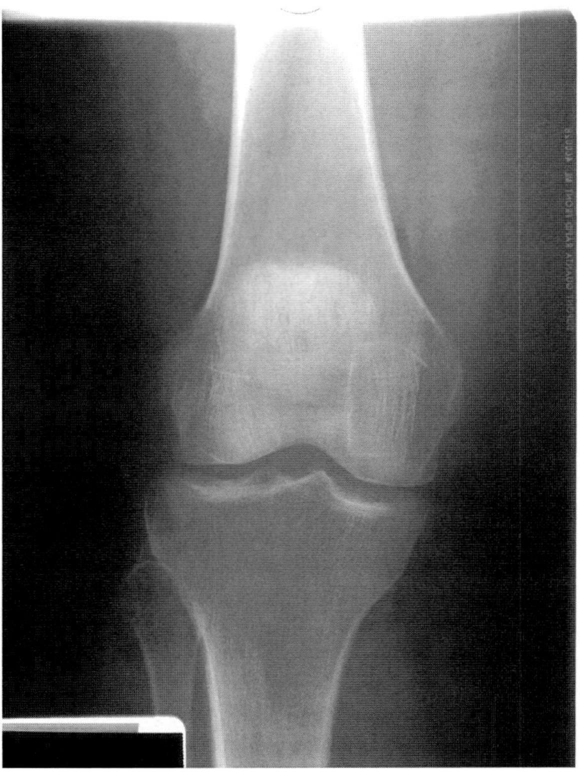

Fig. C6-168. AP knee.

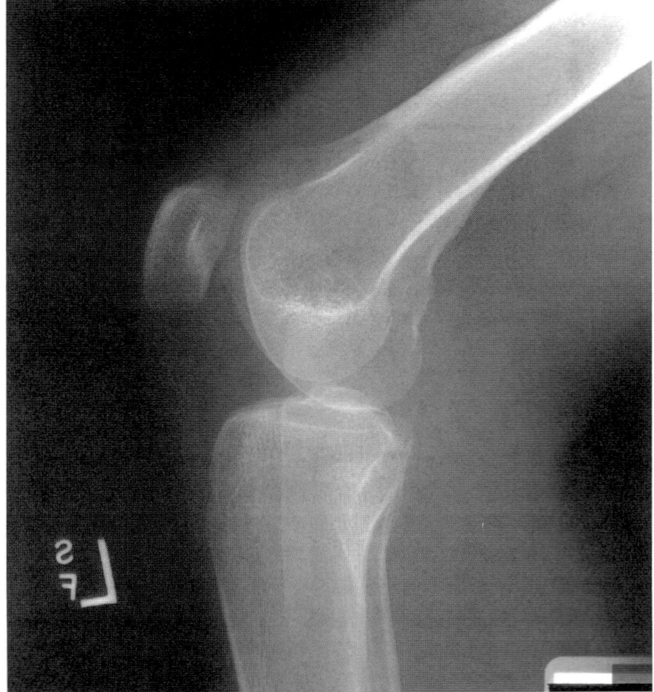

Fig. C6-169. Lateral knee.

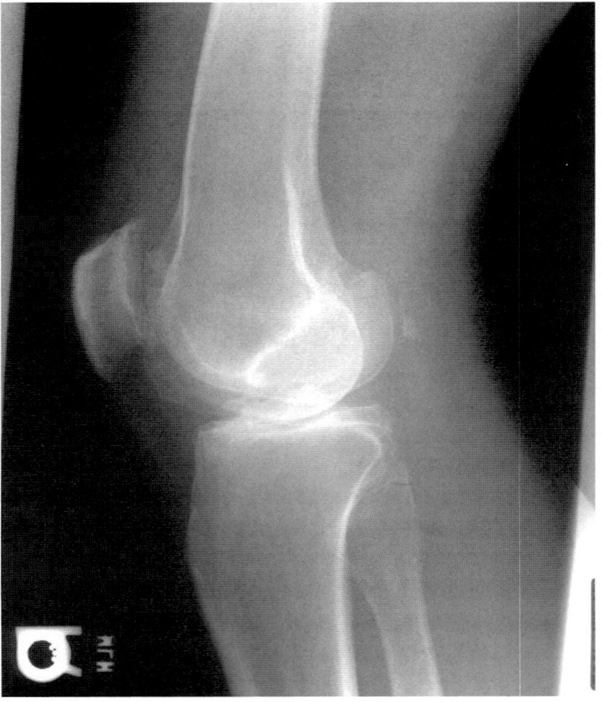

Fig. C6-170. Lateral knee.

CHAPTER 7

Proximal Femur and Pelvic Girdle

CONTENTS

Radiographic Anatomy

Femur **222**

Pelvis **223**

Hip bone **223**

Topographical landmarks **224**

True and false pelvis **225**

Birth canal **225**

Male vs. female pelvis **226**

Review exercise with radiographs **227**

Classification of joints **228**

Radiographic Positioning

Positioning considerations:
- Locating femoral head and neck **229**
- Effect of lower limb rotation **230**
- Gonadal shielding **231**

Survey results and routine and special projections **232**

Pelvis:
- AP **234**
- AP bilateral frog-leg (modified Cleaves method) **235**
- AP axial–Anterior pelvic bones (Taylor method) **236**
- Anterior oblique–Acetabulum (Teufel method) **237**

Hip and proximal femur:
- AP unilateral hip **238**
- Axiolateral (inferosuperior) (Danelius-Miller method) **239**
- Unilateral frog-leg (modified Lauenstein and Hickey method) **240**
- Modified axiolateral (Clements-Nakayama method) **241**

Sacroiliac joints:
- AP axial **242**
- Posterior obliques **243**
- Anterior obliques **244**

Radiographs for critique **245**

Radiographic Anatomy

Lower Limb (Extremity)

The first two groups of bones of the lower limb, the foot and leg, were described in Chapter 6 along with the distal femur and the associated knee and ankle joints.

The third and fourth groups of lower limb bones to be discussed in this chapter are the **proximal femur**, the **pelvic girdle** and the **bones of the hip**. The joints involving these two groups of bones, which will also be included in this chapter, are the important **hip joint** and the **sacroiliac** and **symphysis pubis** joints of the pelvic girdle.

FEMUR

The **femur** is the longest and strongest bone in the entire body. The entire weight of the body is transferred through this bone and the associated joints at each end. Therefore these joints are a frequent source of pathology when trauma occurs.

Proximal Femur

The proximal femur consists of four essential parts, the (1) head, (2) neck, and (3) greater and (4) lesser trochanters *(tro-kan′ ters)*. The **head** of the femur is rounded and smooth for articulation with the hip bones. It contains a depression or pit near its center called the **fovea capitis** *(fo′ ve-ah cap′ i-tis)* wherein a ligament is attached to the head of the femur.

The **neck** of the femur is a strong pyramidal process of bone connecting the head to the body or shaft in the region of the trochanters.

The **greater trochanter** is a large prominence located **superiorly** and **laterally** to the femoral shaft and is palpable as a bony landmark. The **lesser trochanter** is a smaller, blunt, conical eminence that projects **medially** and **posteriorly** from the junction of the neck and shaft of the femur. The trochanters are joined posteriorly by a thick ridge called the **intertrochanteric** *(in″ ter-tro″ kan-ter′ ik)* **crest**. The **body** or **shaft** of the femur is long and almost cylindrical.

Angles of Proximal Femur: The angle of the neck to the shaft on an average adult is approximately **125°**, with a variance of plus or minus 15° depending on the width of the pelvis and the length of the lower limbs. For a long-legged male with a narrow pelvis, the femur would be nearer vertical, which would then change the angle of the neck to about 140°. This angle would be less (110 to 115°) for a shorter female with a wider pelvis.

On an average adult in the anatomical position, the longitudinal plane of the femur is about **10° from vertical**, as shown on the left in Fig. 7-3. This vertical angle is nearer 15° on a female with a wide pelvis and shorter limbs, and only about 5° on a long-legged male. This angle affects positioning and CR angles for a lateral knee, as described in Chapter 6, Figs. 6-20 and 6-21.

Another angle of the neck and head of the femur that is important radiographically is the **15 to 20° anterior angle** of the head and neck in relationship to the body of the femur (right drawing of Fig. 7-3). The head projects somewhat anteriorly or forward as a result of this angle. This becomes important in radiographic positioning wherein the femur and leg must be rotated **15 to 20° internally** to place the femoral neck parallel to the film for a true AP projection of the proximal femur.

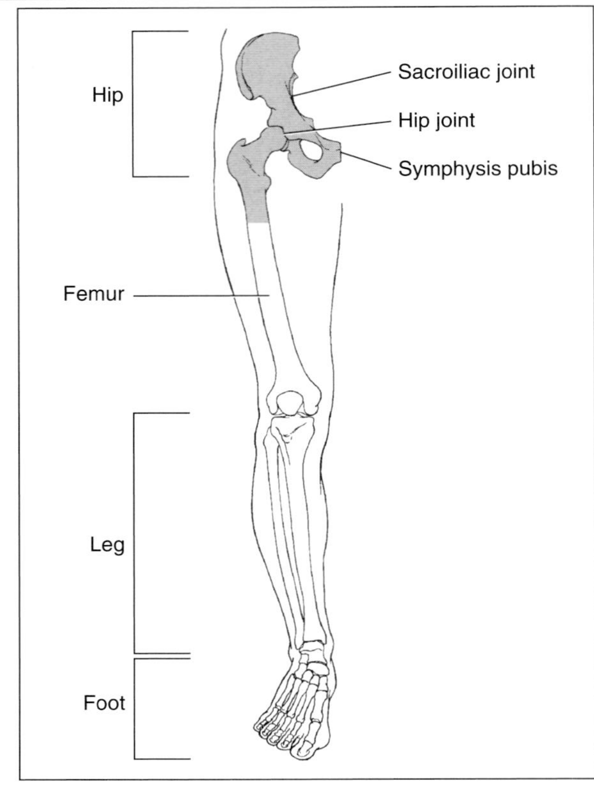

Fig. 7-1. Lower limb.

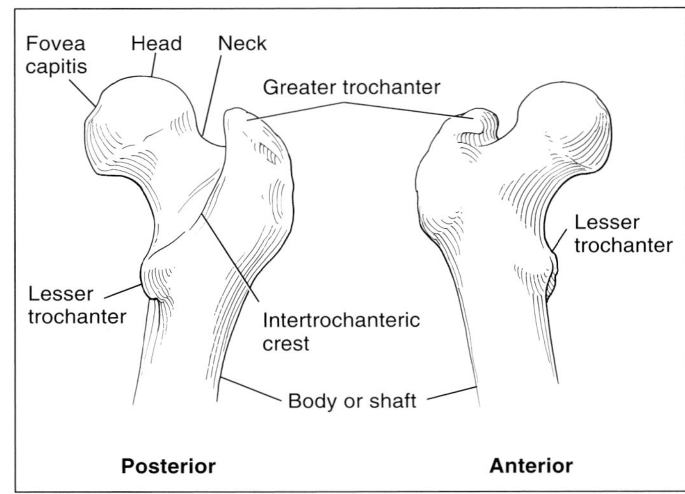

Fig. 7-2. Proximal femur.

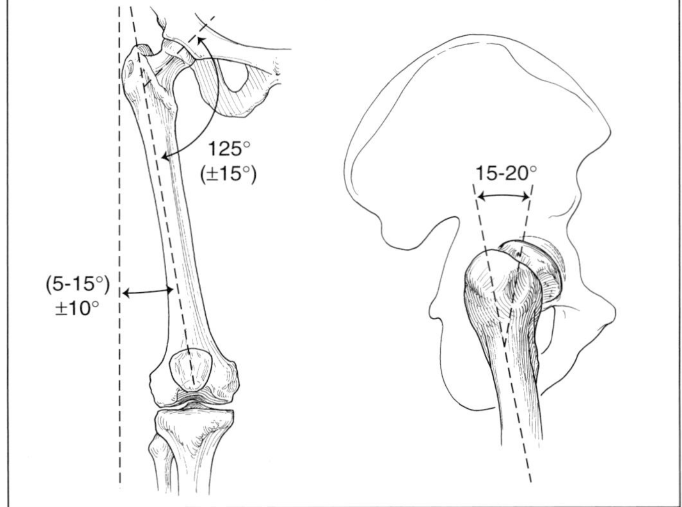

Fig. 7-3. Angles of proximal femur.

Pelvis

The total **pelvis** (meaning a basin) serves as the base of the trunk and forms the connection between the vertebral column and the lower limbs. The pelvis consists of four bones: two **hip bones (ossa coxae**, also called innominate bones), one **sacrum** *(sa′ krum)* and one **coccyx** *(kok′ siks)*.

It should be noted that sometimes the term **pelvic girdle** is used in reference to the total pelvis. This, however, is incorrect in that the **pelvic girdle consists only of the two hip bones**, and the term **pelvis includes the sacrum and coccyx**.*

Note: The sacrum and coccyx are also considered to be part of the distal vertebral column and in this textbook will be covered in Chapter 9 along with the lumbar spine.

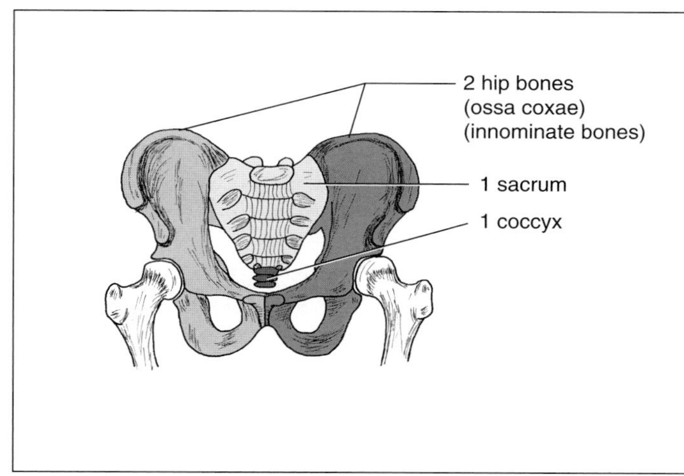

Fig. 7-4. Pelvis–Four bones, two hip bones, sacrum and coccyx.

HIP BONE

Each hip bone is composed of three divisions: (1) **ilium** *(il′ e-um)*, (2) **ischium** *(is′ ke-um)* and (3) **pubis** *(pu′ bis)*. In a child, these three divisions are separate bones, but they fuse into one bone during the middle teens. The fusion occurs in the area of the **acetabulum** *(as″ e-tab′ u-lum)*. The acetabulum is a deep, cup-shaped cavity that accepts the head of the femur to form the hip joint.

The ilium is the largest of the three divisions and is located superior to the acetabulum. The ischium is inferior and posterior to the acetabulum, while the pubis is inferior and anterior. Each of these three parts will be described in detail as follows:

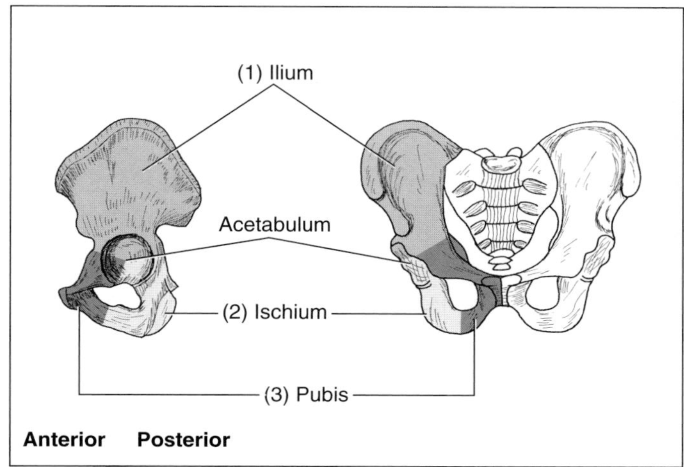

Fig. 7-5. Hip bone–Three parts.

Ilium

Each **ilium** is composed of a **body** and an **ala** or wing. The body of the ilium is the more inferior portion near the acetabulum and includes the upper two-fifths of the acetabulum. The ala or wing portion is the thin and flared upper part of the ilium.

The **crest** of the ilium is the upper margin of the ala and extends from the **anterior superior iliac spine** (ASIS) to the **posterior superior iliac spine** (PSIS). In radiographic positioning, the uppermost peak of the crest is often referred to as the **iliac crest,** but it actually extends between the ASIS and PSIS.

Below the anterior superior iliac spine (ASIS) is a less prominent projection referred to as the **anterior inferior iliac spine**. Similarly, inferior to the posterior superior iliac spine is the **posterior inferior iliac spine**.

Positioning Landmarks: The two most important positioning landmarks of these borders and projections are the **crest of the ilium** (the iliac crest) and the **anterior superior iliac spine** (ASIS).

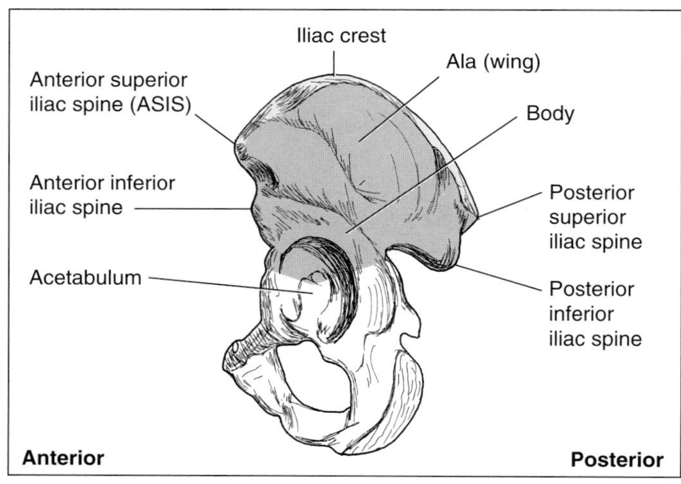

Fig. 7-6. Ilium.

**Gray's Anatomy, 13th ed.*, pp. 261, 270.

Ischium

The **ischium** is that part of the hip bone inferior and posterior to the acetabulum. Each ischium is divided into a **body** and a **ramus**. The upper portion of the body of the ischium makes up the posteroinferior two-fifths of the acetabulum. The lower portion of the body of the ischium (formerly called the superior ramus) projects caudally and medially from the acetabulum ending at the **ischial tuberosity**. Projecting anteriorly from the ischial tuberosity is the **ramus of the ischium**.

The rounded, roughened area near the junction of the lower body and the inferior rami is a landmark termed the **tuberosity** of the ischium, or **ischial** *(is′ ke-al)* **tuberosity**.

Posterior to the acetabulum is a bony projection termed the **ischial spine**. The ischial spine is also shown to be visible on a frontal view of the pelvis as shown in Fig. 7-8. (It is also seen in the anatomy review radiograph, Fig. 7-17.)

Directly above the ischial spine is a deep notch termed the **greater sciatic notch**. Below the ischial spine is a smaller notch termed the **lesser sciatic notch**.

Positioning Landmark: The ischial tuberosities bear most of the weight of the body when one sits, and can be palpated through the soft tissues of each buttock when in a prone position. However, because of discomfort and possible embarrassment to the patient, this landmark is not as commonly used as the already described ASIS and crest of the ilium.

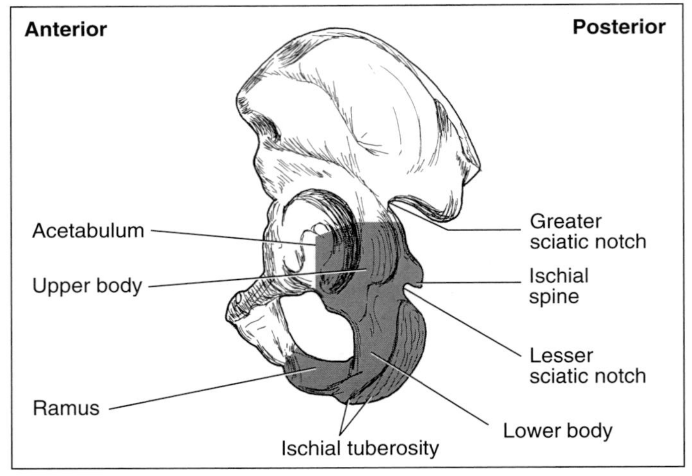

Fig. 7-7. Ischium.

Pubis

The last of the three divisions of one hip bone is the **pubis** or **pubic bone**. The **body** of the pubis is anterior and inferior to the acetabulum and includes the anteroinferior one-fifth of the acetabulum.

Extending anteriorly and medially from the body of each pubis is a **superior ramus**. The two superior rami meet in the midline to form a slightly movable joint, the **symphysis pubis** *(sim′ fi-sis pu′ bis)*. Each **inferior ramus** passes down and posterior from the symphysis pubis to join the inferior ramus of the respective ischium.

The **obturator foramen** *(ob′ tu-ra″ tor fo-ra′ men)* is a large opening formed by the ramus and body of each ischium, and by the pubis. The obturator foramen is the largest foramen in the human skeletal system.

Positioning Landmark: The superior margin of the symphysis pubis is a positioning landmark used in pelvis and hip positioning, as well as positioning for the abdomen since this defines the lowermost margin of the abdomen.

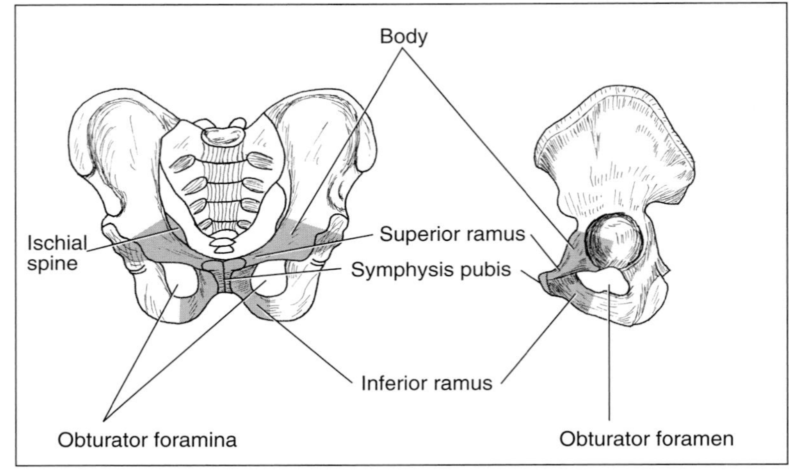

Fig. 7-8. Pubis (pubic bone).

SUMMARY OF TOPOGRAPHICAL LANDMARKS

Important positioning landmarks of the pelvis are reviewed in Fig. 7-9. The most superior aspect of the **iliac crest** and the **ASIS** are easily palpated. The ASIS is one of the more frequently used positioning landmarks of the pelvis. It is also most commonly used to check for rotation of the pelvis and/or lower abdomen by determining if the distance between the ASIS and tabletop is the same on both sides.

The **greater trochanter** of the femur can be located by firm palpation in the soft tissues of the upper thigh. Note that the upper margin of the greater trochanter is about 1 inch (2.5 cm) above the upper border of the **symphysis pubis**, while the **ischial tuberosity** is 1½ to 2 inches (4-5 cm) below the symphysis pubis. These distances will vary between a male and female pelvis because of general differences in shape of the male and female pelvis as will be described later in this chapter.

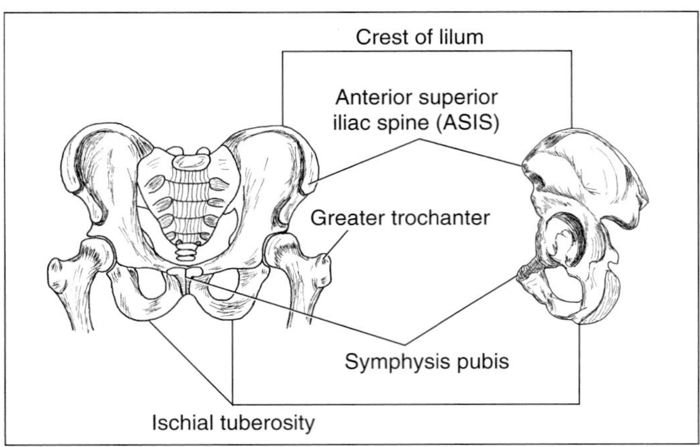

Fig. 7-9. Bony topographical landmarks of the pelvis.

TRUE AND FALSE PELVIS

A plane through the **brim** of the pelvis divides the pelvic area into two cavities. The pelvic brim is defined by the upper part of the symphysis pubis anteriorly and the upper, prominent part of the sacrum posteriorly. The general area above or superior to the oblique plane through the pelvic brim is termed the **greater** or **false pelvis**. The flared portion of the pelvis formed primarily by the alae or wings of the ilia form the lateral and posterior limits of the greater or false pelvis, while the abdominal muscles of the anterior wall define the anterior limits. The lower abdominal organs and a fetus within the pregnant uterus rest on the floor of the greater pelvis.

The area inferior to a plane through the pelvic brim is termed the **lesser** or **true pelvis**. The lesser or true pelvis is a cavity completely surrounded by bony structures. The size and shape of the true pelvis is of greatest importance during the birth process since **the true pelvis forms the actual birth canal**.

True Pelvis

The oblique plane defined by the brim of the pelvis is termed the **inlet** of the true pelvis. The **outlet** of the true pelvis is defined by the two ischial tuberosities and the tip of the coccyx. The three sides of the triangularly shaped outlet are formed by a line between the ischial tuberosities and a line between each ischial tuberosity and the coccyx. The area between the inlet and outlet of the lesser or true pelvis is termed the **cavity** of the true pelvis. During the birth process, the baby must travel through the inlet, cavity and outlet of the true pelvis.

Birth Canal

During a routine delivery, the baby's head first travels through the pelvic inlet, then to the mid cavity, and finally through the outlet to exit in a forward direction as shown in Figs. 7-12 and 7-13.

Because of the sensitivity to radiation by the fetus, radiographs of the pelvis generally are **not** taken during pregnancy. If the size or dimensions of the birth canal of the pelvis is in question, certain ultrasound procedures can be done to evaluate for potential problems during the birthing process.

Note: In the past certain radiographic procedures called **cephalopelvimetry** *(sef″ ah-lo-pel-vim′ e-tre)* **exams** were performed whereby a specific type of metal ruler (Colcher-Sussman ruler) was placed next to the pelvis for AP and lateral projections. In this way the amount of magnification could be determined and actual measurements of the baby's head could be made as well as inlet and outlet measurements of the mother's pelvis. First and second editions of this textbook described and illustrated this procedure in detail but these have been omitted from more recent editions because of the advances in sonography (ultrasound), which now make this the preferred method for achieving this information. (Ultrasound procedures do not use the potentially hazardous ionizing radiation to the fetus as do x-ray exams such as cephalopelvimetry.)

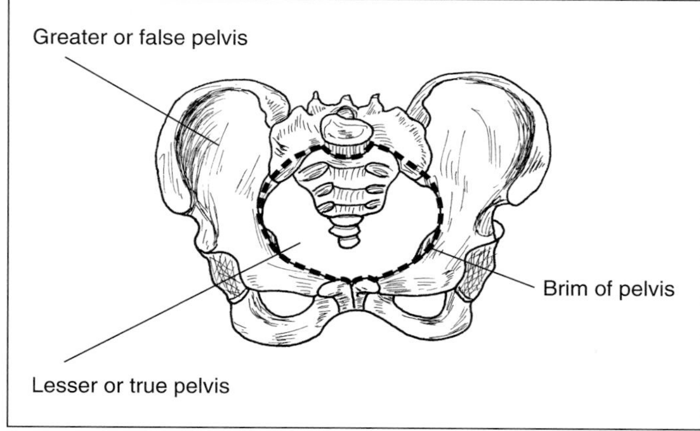

Fig. 7-10. Pelvic cavities.

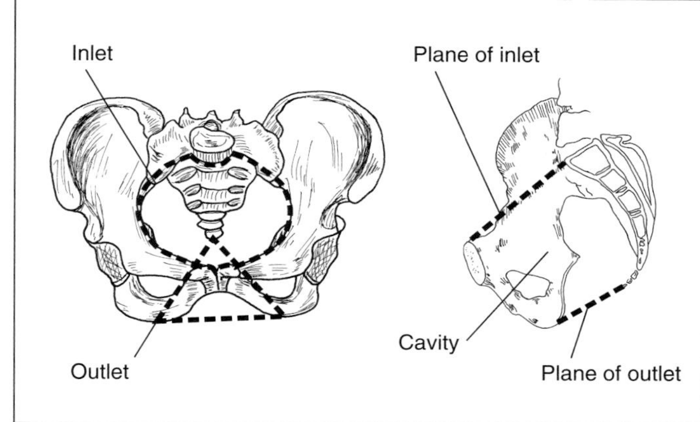

Fig. 7-11. Lesser or true pelvis.

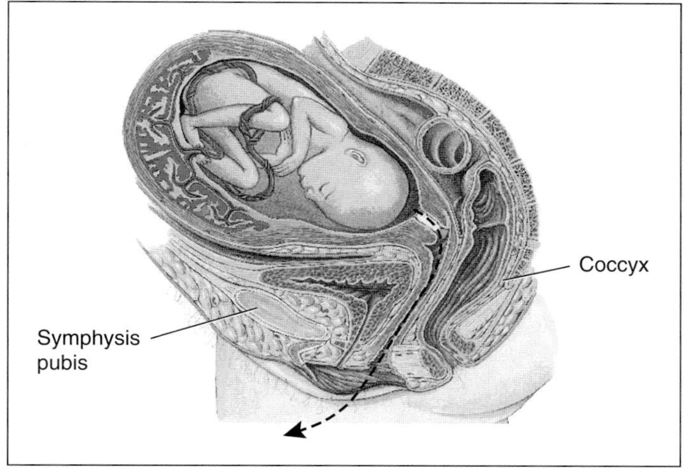

Fig. 7-12. Birth canal–Sagittal sectional view.

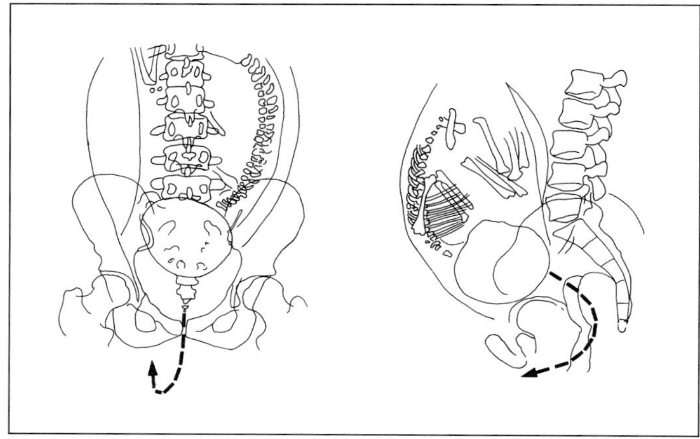

Fig. 7-13. Birth canal.

Male vs. Female Pelvis

The general shape of the female pelvis varies enough from the male pelvis to enable one to discriminate one from the other on pelvis radiographs. In general, the **female pelvis** is wider with the ilia more flared and more shallow from front to back. The **male pelvis** is narrower, deeper and less flared. In overall appearance on a frontal view, the female pelvis is wider. Therefore the first difference between the male and female pelvis is the difference in the **overall general shape** of the entire pelvis.

A second major difference is the **angle of the pubic arch**, formed by the inferior rami of the pubis just below the symphysis pubis. In the female, this angle is usually obtuse or greater than 90°, while in the male the pubic arch usually forms an acute angle, less than 90°.

A third difference is the **shape of the inlet**. The inlet of the female pelvis is usually nearer round, while in the male it is usually more oval or heart-shaped. The general shape of the pelvis does vary considerably from one individual to another, so that the pelvis of a slender female may resemble a male pelvis. In general, however, the differences are usually obvious enough that one can determine the sex of the patient from a radiograph of the pelvis.

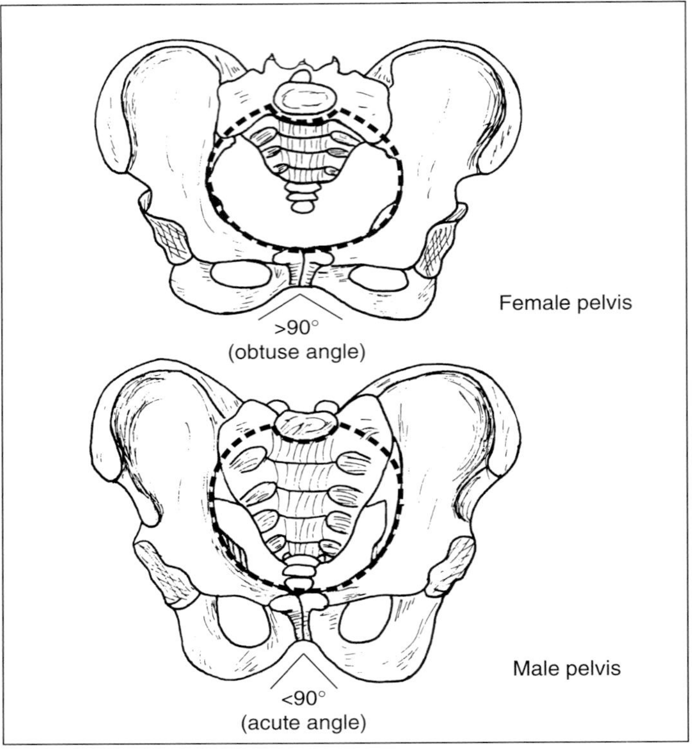

Fig. 7-14. Pelvis–Male vs. female.

Summary of Male and Female Pelvic Characteristics

	Male	*Female*
1. General shape	narrower, deeper, less flared	wider, more shallow, more flared
2. Angle of pubic arch	acute angle (< 90°)	obtuse angle (> 90°)
3. Shape of inlet	more oval	more round

Male vs. Female Pelvis Radiographs

Figs. 7-15 and 7-16 are pelvic radiographs of a female and a male subject, respectively. Note the three differences between this typical female and male pelvis.

First, in overall shape, the male pelvis appears narrower and deeper with a less flared appearance of the ilia.

Second, the acute angle of less than 90° of the pubic arch on the male is obvious, as compared to the greater than 90° angle on the female pelvis below. This is commonly one of the more noticeable differences.

Third, the shape of the inlet on the male pelvis is not as broad or rounded as compared to the female pelvis, even though the inlet on this male pelvis is more rounded and not as oval or heart shaped as on some males.

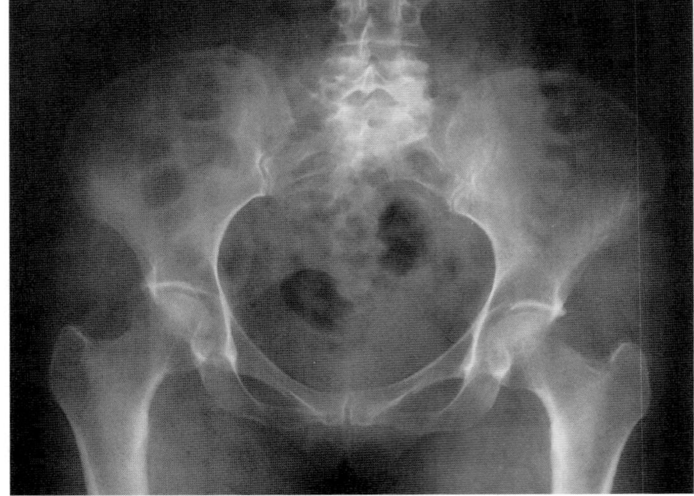
Fig. 7-15. Female pelvis.

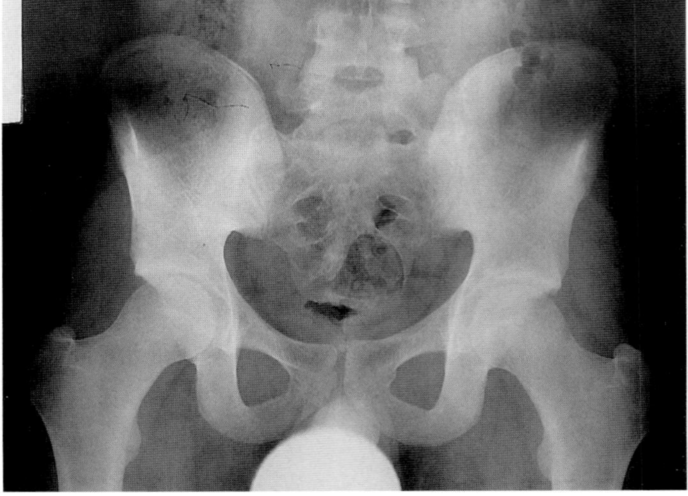
Fig. 7-16. Male pelvis.

REVIEW EXERCISE WITH RADIOGRAPHS

Key pelvic anatomy is labeled on the AP pelvis radiograph of Fig. 7-17. A good review exercise is to first cover up the answers while identifying these parts.

A. Iliac crest
B. ASIS (anterior end of crest)
C. Body of the left ischium
D. Ischial tuberosity
E. Symphysis pubis
F. Inferior ramus of the right pubis
G. Superior ramus of the right pubis
H. Right ischial spine
I. Acetabulum of right hip
J. Neck of right femur
K. Greater trochanter of right femur
L. Head of right femur
M. Ala or wing of right ilium

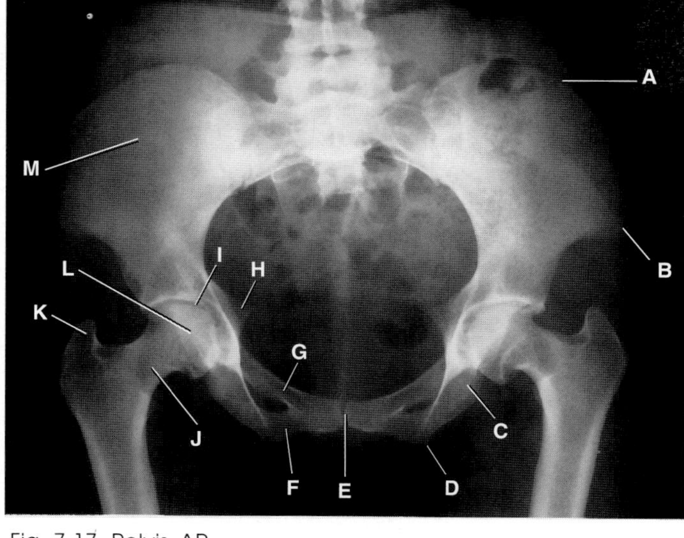

Fig. 7-17. Pelvis–AP.

Lateral Hip

This demonstrates a good lateral radiograph of the proximal femur and hip taken with an inferosuperior projection (horizontal beam lateral) as demonstrated by the positioning drawing of Fig. 7-19.

A. Acetabulum
B. Femoral head
C. Femoral neck
D. Shaft or body
E. Lesser trochanter
F. Greater trochanter
G. Ischial tuberosity

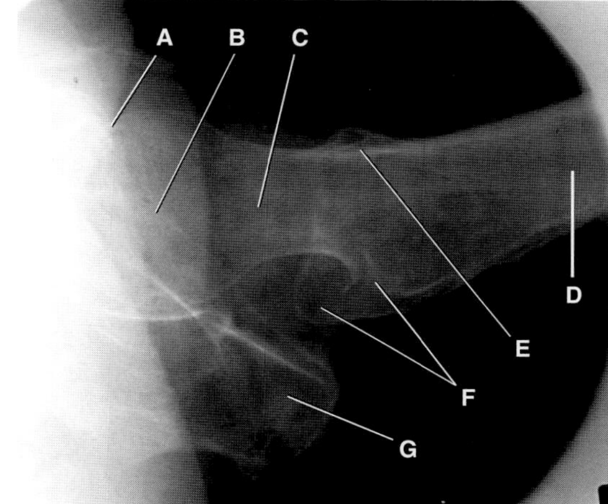

Fig. 7-18. Inferosuperior projection.

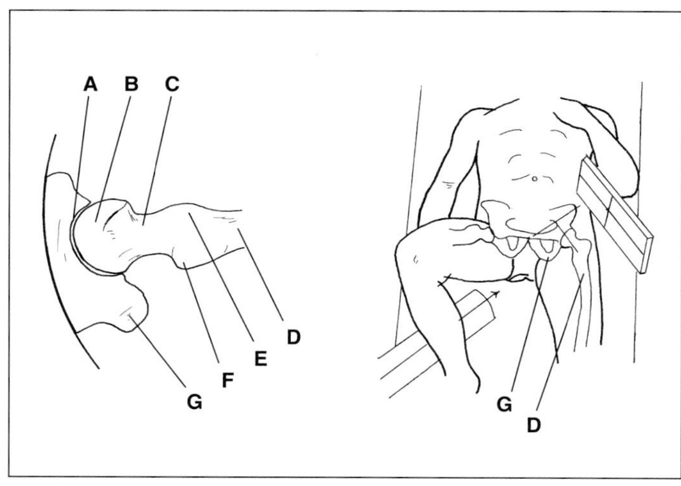

Fig. 7-19. Proximal femur and hip –Lateral (inferosuperior projection).

CLASSIFICATION OF JOINTS

The number of joints or articulations of the proximal femora and the pelvis are limited, with the hip joint being the most obvious. These joints of the pelvic girdle, as listed below, will again be described according to their **classification**, **mobility type** and **movement type**.

Sacroiliac joints–Between sacrum and each ilium.
Symphysis pubis–Between right and left pubic bones.
Union of acetabulum–A temporary growth joint of each acetabulum that solidifies in mid teen years.
Hip joints–Between head of femur and acetabulum of pelvis.

Sacroiliac Joints

The sacroiliac joints are wide, flat joints located on each side obliquely between the sacrum and each ilium. These joints are situated at an unusual oblique angle requiring special positioning to visualize the joint spaces radiographically.

The sacroiliac joint is classified as a **synovial joint** in that it is enclosed in a **fibrous articular capsule** containing synovial fluid. The bones are joined by firm sacroiliac ligaments. Generally, synovial joints by their nature are considered freely movable or diarthrodial joints. However, the sacroiliac joint is a special type of synovial joint which permits little movement and is thus **amphiarthrodial**. The reason for this is the joint surfaces are very irregularly shaped and the interconnecting bones are snugly fitted since they serve a weight-bearing function. This restricts movement and the cavity of the joint or the joint space may be reduced in size or even be nonexistent in older persons, especially in males.

Symphysis Pubis

The symphysis pubic is the articulation of the right and left pubic bones in the midline of the anterior pelvis. The most superior, anterior aspect of this joint is palpable and is an important positioning landmark, as already described.

The symphysis pubis is classified as a **cartilaginous joint** of the **symphysis subtype** in that only limited movement is possible (**amphiarthrodial**). The two articular surfaces are separated by a **fibrocartilaginous disk** and held together by certain ligaments. This **interpubic disk** of fibrocartilage is a relatively thick pad (thicker in females than males), which is capable of being compressed or partially displaced, thereby allowing some limited movement of these bones such as in pelvic trauma, or during the birthing process in females.

Union of Acetabulum

The three divisions of each hip bone are separate bones in a child but come together in the acetabulum by fusing during the middle teens to become completely indistinguishable in an adult. Therefore, this is classified as a **cartilaginous type** joint of the **synchondrosis subtype,** which is **immovable** or **synarthrodial** in an adult. This is considered a temporary type of growth joint similar to the joints between the epiphyses and diaphyses of long bones in growing children.

Hip Joint

The hip joint is classified as a **synovial type**, as truly characterized by a large fibrous capsule containing synovial fluid. It is a **freely movable** or **diarthrodial** joint and is the truest example of a **spheroid** (ball and socket) movement type.

The head of the femur forms more than half of a sphere as it fits into the relatively deep, cup-shaped acetabulum. This makes the hip joint inherently strong as it supports the weight of the body while still permitting a high degree of mobility. The articular capsule surrounding this joint is strong and dense with the thickest part being above, as would be expected since this is in line with the weight-bearing function of the hip joints. A series of strong bands of ligaments surround the articular capsule and joint in general, making this a very strong and stable joint.

Movements of the hip joint include **flexion** and **extension**, **abduction** and **adduction**, **medial** (internal) and **lateral** (external) **rotation** and **circumduction**.

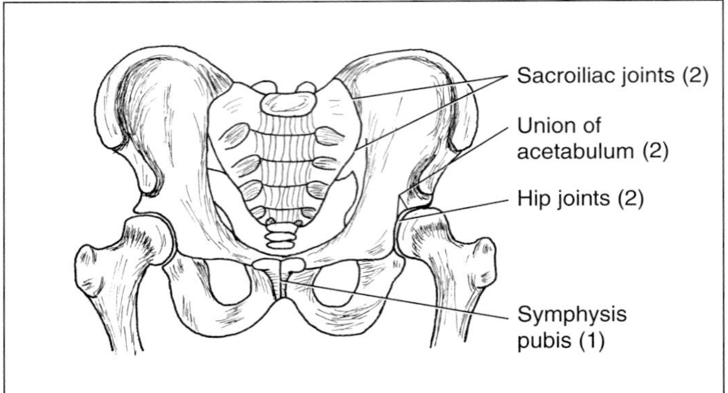

Fig. 7-20. Joints of pelvis.

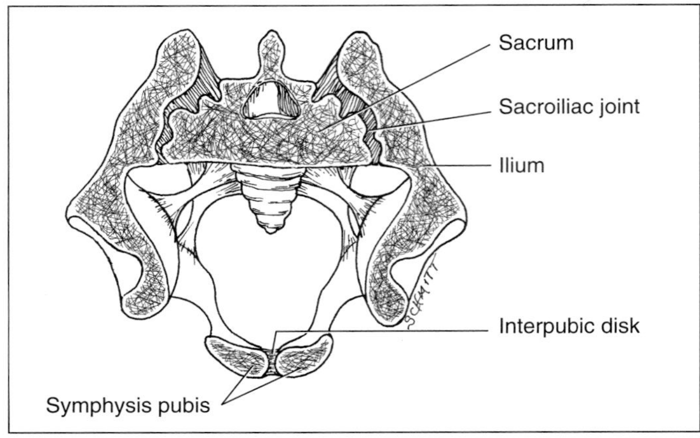

Fig. 7-21. Coronal section showing sacroiliac and symphysis pubis joints.

Summary of Pelvic Joints	
Classification:	
• Sacroiliac joint • Hip joint	***Synovial***
• Symphysis pubis • Union of acetabulum	***Cartilaginous***
Mobility type:	
• Sacroiliac joint • Symphysis pubis	***Amphiarthrodial*** *(limited movement)*
• Hip joint	***Diarthrodial*** *(freely movable)*
Movement type:	
• Hip joint	***Spheroidal*** *(ball and socket)*

Radiographic Positioning

POSITIONING CONSIDERATIONS

Location of Head and Neck

Radiographic positioning of the hip joint is a challenge for radiographers. Interrelationships of the pelvis and the hip joint must be thoroughly understood. One must be able to find the location of the femoral head and femoral neck by two prominent positioning landmarks, which are the **ASIS** and the **upper border of the symphysis pubis.** A primary method of locating either the head or neck of the femur is to first find the midpoint of an imaginary line drawn between the ASIS and the symphysis pubis. The **neck** of the femur is approximately **2½ in.** (6 to 7 cm) or ≈3 to 4 finger widths distal to the midpoint of this line. The **head** of the femur is approximately **1½ in.** (≈4 cm) or ≈2 finger widths below the midpoint of this line (see Figs. 7-22 and 7-23).

A second method of locating the femoral neck is as follows: Approximately 1 inch (2.5 cm) medial to the ASIS at the level of the upper margin of the symphysis pubis.

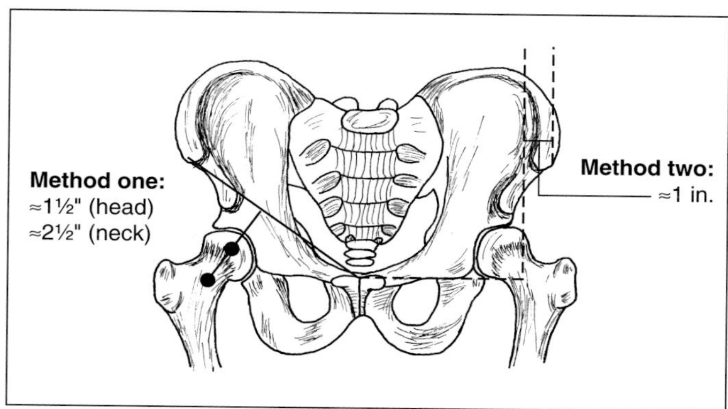

Fig. 7-22. Head or neck localization.

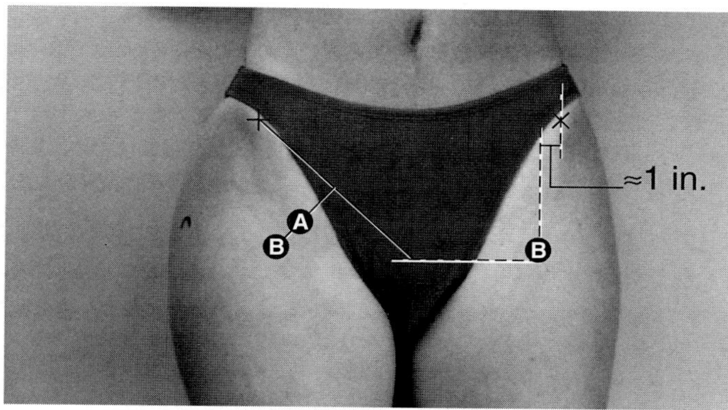

Fig. 7-23. Head (A) or neck (B) localization.

Appearance of Proximal Femur in Anatomical Position

As described earlier in this chapter under anatomy of the proximal femur, the head and neck of the femur project approximately 15 to 20° anteriorly or forward with respect to the rest of the femur and lower leg. Therefore when the leg is in the true anatomical position as for a true AP leg, the proximal femur is actually rotated posteriorly by 15 to 20°. Therefore the femoral neck appears shortened and the **lesser trochanter is visible** when the leg and ankle are truly AP as in a true anatomical position.

Internal Rotation of Leg

By **internally rotating the entire leg**, the proximal femur and hip joint will be projected in a **true AP** projection. The neck of the femur is now parallel to the imaging surface and will not appear foreshortened.

The **lesser trochanter** is key in determining (on a radiograph) the correct leg position. If the entire leg is internally rotated a full 15 to 20°, the outline of the lesser trochanter will generally not be visible at all, or only slightly visible on some patients as it is obscured by the shaft of the femur. If the leg is straight AP, or if externally rotated, then the lesser trochanter is visible. (See illustrations on following page.)

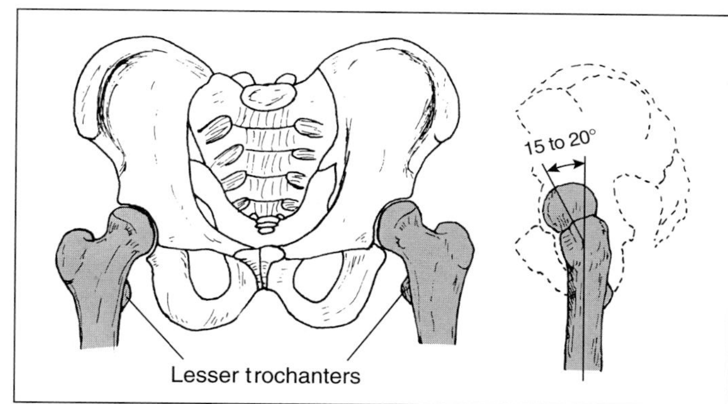

Fig. 7-24. Anatomical position.
(True AP of knee, leg and ankle–But not hip.)

Evidence of Hip Fracture

The femoral neck is a common fracture site for an older patient who has fallen. The typical physical sign for such a fracture is the **external rotation** of the involved foot as shown on the right in Fig. 7-25, and on the lower illustrations of the following page.

Positioning Warning! If such evidence of a hip fracture is present (external foot rotation), a pelvis radiograph should be taken "as is" **without** attempting to internally rotate the leg as would be necessary for a true AP hip projection. This radiograph should then be viewed by a radiologist to rule out a fracture. If this radiograph is negative, then standard hip or pelvis radiographs can be taken with internal leg rotation. Forcing an internal rotation of the leg with a fracture would be very painful, and even more important, may displace the femoral head and/or neck at the fracture site.

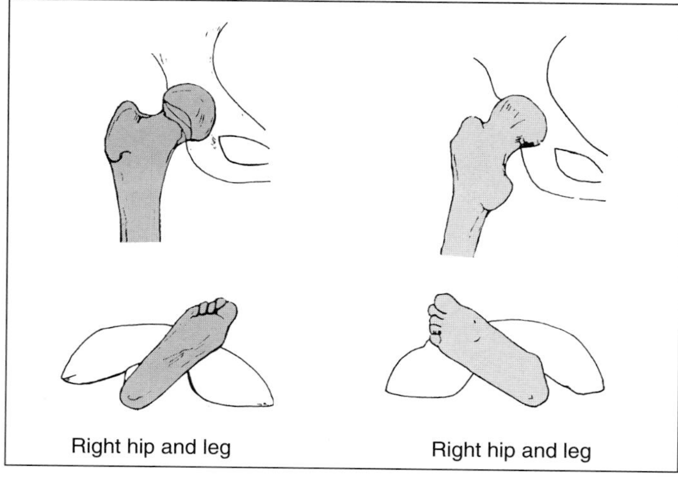

Fig. 7-25. Internal rotation. (True AP of hip.) External rotation. (Typical hip fracture position.)

Positioning considerations continued

Summary: Effect of Lower Limb Rotation

These photos and associated pelvis radiographs demonstrate the effect of lower limb rotation on the appearance of the proximal femora.

1. Anatomical Position:
- –Long axes of feet vertical.
- –Femoral necks partially foreshortened.
- –Lesser trochanters **partially visible**.

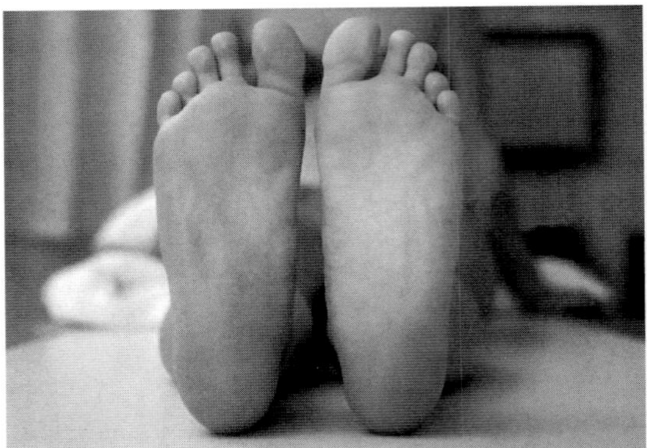

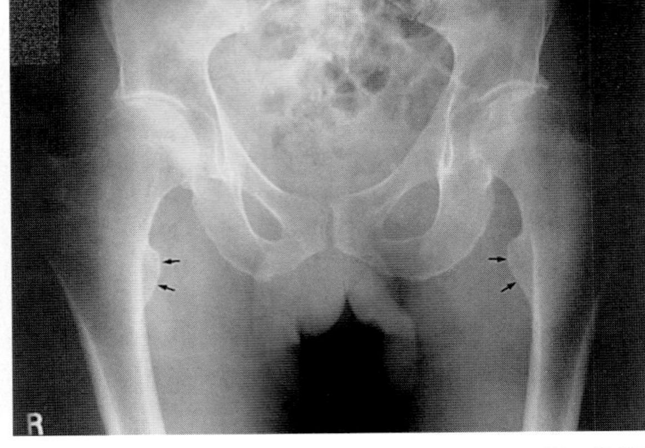

Fig. 7-26. 1. Anatomical position. Fig. 7-27.

2. 15 to 20° Medial Rotation:
(The desired position for visualizing pelvis and hips.)
- –Long axes of feet and lower limbs rotated 15 to 20° internally.
- –Femoral heads and necks in profile.
- –True AP projection of proximal femurs.
- –Lesser trochanters **not visible** or only slightly visible on some patients.

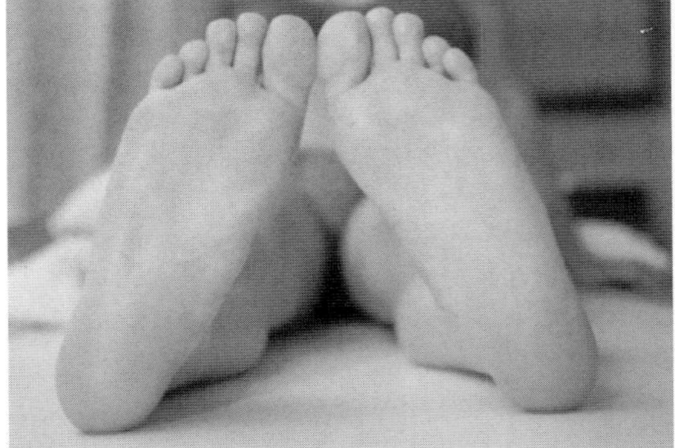

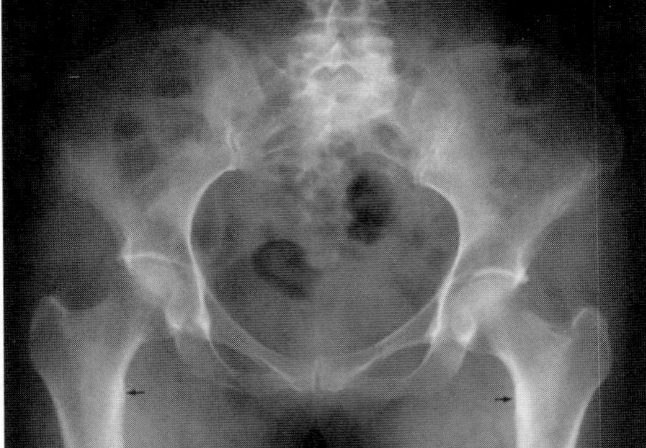

Fig. 7-28. 2. 15 to 20° medial rotation. Fig. 7-29.

3. External Rotation:
- –Long axes of feet and lower limbs equally rotated laterally in a normal relaxed position.
- –Femoral necks greatly foreshortened.
- –Lesser trochanters **visible in profile internally**.

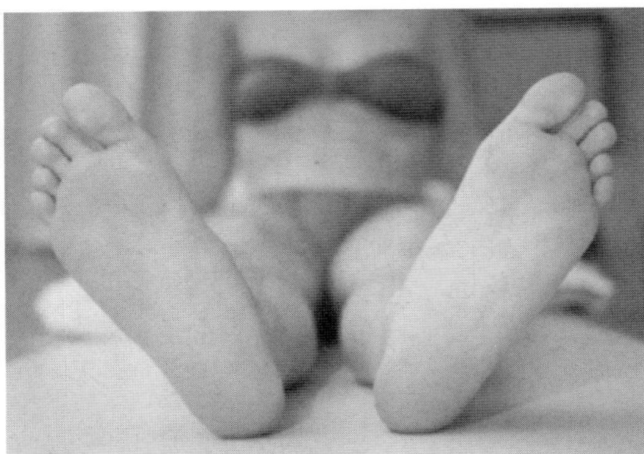

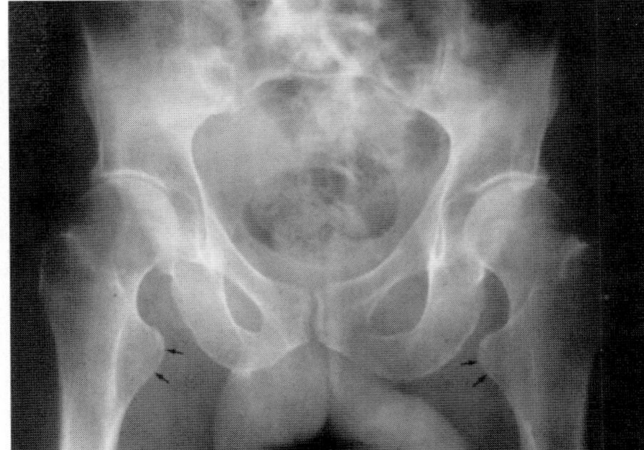

Fig. 7-30. 3. External rotation. Fig. 7-31.

4. Typical Rotation with Hip Fracture:
- –Long axis of foot is externally rotated on side of hip fracture.
- –Unaffected foot and limb in neutral position.
- –Lesser trochanter on externally rotated limb is more visible, and neck area is foreshortened.

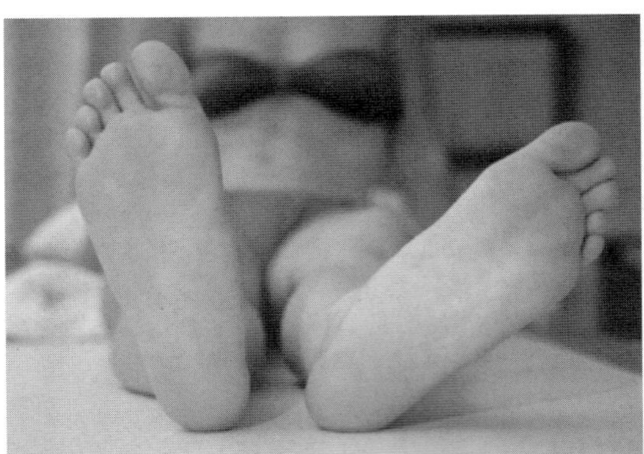

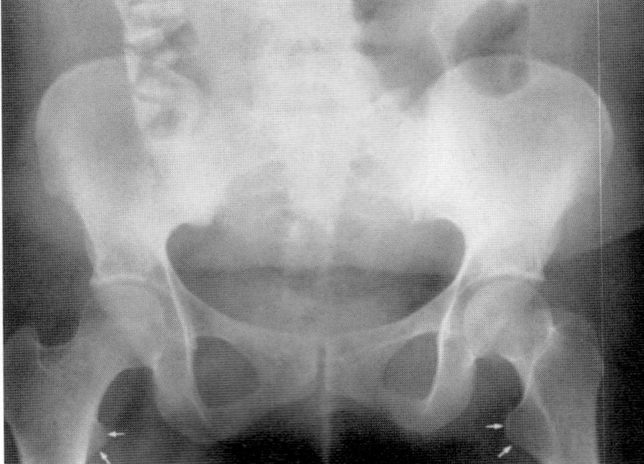

Fig. 7-32. 4. Typical rotation with hip fracture. Fig. 7-33.

Shielding Guidelines

Accurate gonadal shielding for pelvis and hip exams is especially critical because of the proximity of the radiation sensitive gonads to the primary rays.

Male Shielding: This is easier for males in that small contact shields, such as shown in Fig. 7-34, can be used on **all males of reproductive age or younger**. The shields are placed over the area of the testes without covering up essential anatomy of the pelvis or hips. However, care must be taken for pelvis radiographs that the top of the shield be placed at the **inferior margin of the symphysis pubis** to cover the testes adequately without obscuring the pubic and ischial areas of the pelvis.

Female Shielding: Ovarian contact shields for females of childbearing age or younger, however, require more critical placement to shield the area of the ovaries without covering up essential pelvic or hip anatomy. Vinyl-covered lead material cut into various shapes and sizes can be used for this purpose for an AP pelvis or bilateral hip radiograph as shown in Fig. 7-36 and as described in Chapter 1, page 43.

For a unilateral hip or proximal femur, larger contact shields can be used to cover the general pelvic area without covering the specific hip being radiographed, as shown in Fig. 7-35. Accurate location of the femoral head and neck makes this type of gonadal shielding possible.

Gonadal shielding may not be possible for females on certain AP pelvis projections in which the entire pelvis, including the sacrum and coccyx must be demonstrated. Also gonadal shielding may not be possible on certain lateral hip projections for both male and females, such as the lateral inferosuperior projection, in which shielding may obscure essential anatomy. However **gonadal shielding should be used whenever possible for both males and females** along with **close collimation** for all hip and pelvis projections. General pelvic trauma requiring visualization of the entire pelvis may prohibit ovarian shielding for females. Departmental policy regarding gonadal shielding for pelvic procedures on females should be determined by each radiographer.

Exposure Factors and Patient Dosage: In the interest of reducing total radiation dose to the patient, a higher kVp range of 90±5 may be used for hip and pelvis exams. This higher kVp technique, with lower mAs, results in a lower radiation dose to the patient. Higher kVp, however, does decrease contrast and may not be advisable, especially on older patients who may have some loss of bone mass or density due to osteoporosis (see below), thus requiring even lower kVp than average.

Clinical Indicators

1. **Proximal femur (hip) fractures**: Most common with older or geriatric patients with varying degrees of **osteoporosis** (os"te-o-po-ro'sis) or **avascular necrosis** (AVN). Both osteoporosis (loss of bone mass from metabolic or other factors) and avascular (loss of blood circulation) necrosis (cell death) frequently lead to a weakening or collapse of weight-bearing joints such as the hip joint, and fractures will occur with only minimal trauma.

2. **Pelvic ring fractures:** Due to the closed ring structure of the pelvis, a severe blow or trauma to one side of the pelvis may result in a fracture site away from the primary trauma, thus requiring clear radiographic visualization of the entire pelvis.

3. **Congenital hip dislocation** (CHD): Hip dislocations caused by conditions present at birth may require frequent hip radiographs. See Chapter 20, Pediatric Radiography.

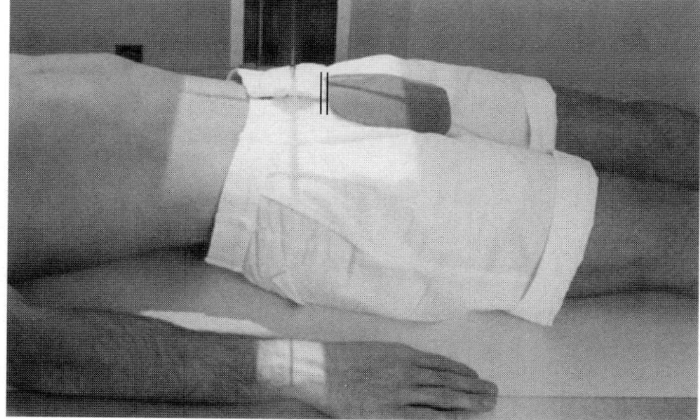

Fig. 7-34. Male gonadal shielding for hips and pelvis.

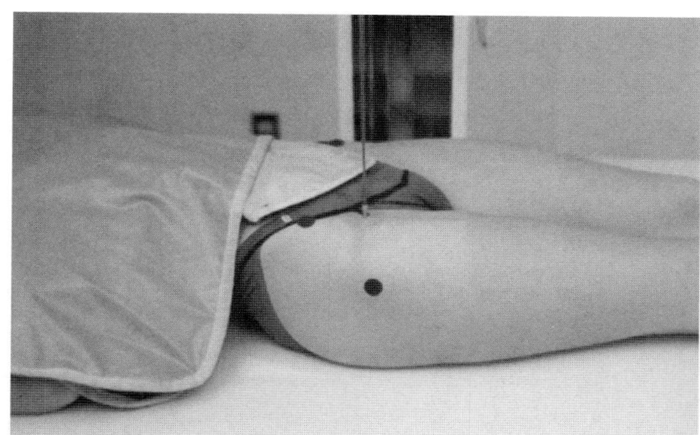

Fig. 7-35. General abdominal and pelvic shielding for proximal femur to include hip.

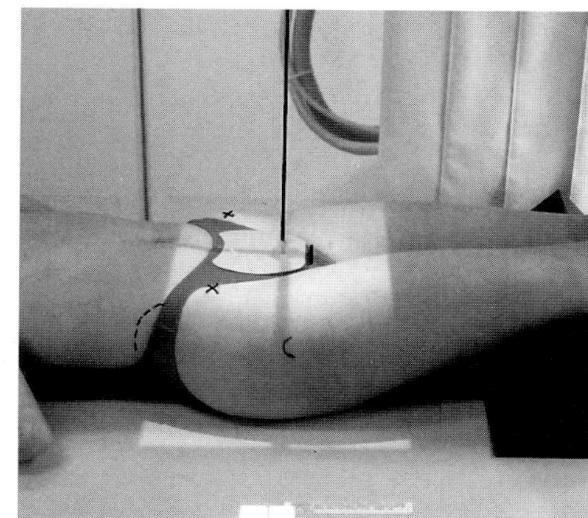

Fig. 7-36. Female gonadal (ovarian) shielding for bilateral hips and proximal femurs.

NATIONAL SURVEY

Departmental standard (basic) and optional routines for exams of the proximal femur and pelvis and the sacroiliac joints were very consistent throughout the United States.

Hip and Proximal Femur Routine

Hip	U.S. Average	
	Basic 1995 (1989)	Special 1995 (1989)
• AP pelvis	92% (82%)	
• AP hip only	71% (43%)	
• Unilateral frog-leg (non-trauma)	71% (82%)	10% –
• Axiolateral (inferosuperior) (trauma) (Danelius-Miller method)	48% (36%)	– (17%)
• Modified axiolateral (Clements-Nakayama method)		26% (11%)

Pelvis Routine

Pelvis	U.S. Average	
	Basic 1995 (1989)	Special 1995 (1989)
• AP pelvis	97% (98%)	
• AP bilateral frog-leg (non-trauma)	42% (28%)	21% (17%)
• AP axial –Anterior pelvic bones	42% –	24% –
• Anterior oblique –Acetabulum		25% –

Sacroiliac Joints Routine

Sacroiliac joints	U.S. Average	
	Basic 1995 (1989)	Special 1995 (1989)
• AP pelvis	57% (41%)	
• Obliques: posterior–25-30°	64% (69%)	8% –
or anterior–25-30°	27% (25%)	12% –
• AP–25-30° cephalad	71% (62%)	

Summary:

Hip and Proximal Femur: The survey supported the routine of taking the **AP pelvis** to include both hips for comparison even when a single hip exam is requested.

For the lateral hip, the results support this text's recommended routine of a **lateral frog-leg for non-trauma**, and an **axiolateral (inferosuperior) for trauma patients**.

Pelvis: The survey supported the **AP pelvis** as the common projection for the pelvis, with 28% in 1989 and 42% in 1995, indicating they also take the **bilateral frog-leg** routinely on non-trauma patients.

The two most common additional projections for the pelvis in 1995 were the AP axial for the anterior pelvic bones (42% basic, 24% special), and the anterior oblique for the acetabulum at 25%.

Sacroiliac Joints: The most common routine for the sacroiliac joints per this survey were **AP with a 25 to 30° cephalad angle** and the **posterior obliques**. The anterior obliques are less frequently included as part of this routine.

STANDARD AND SPECIAL OPERATING PROCEDURES

Certain basic and special projections or positions for the proximal femora and pelvis are demonstrated and described on the following pages as suggested standard and special departmental procedures.

Pelvis Decision Guide

The following guide is provided as **a suggested sequence of possible basic and special projections** of the proximal femur and pelvis, as described and illustrated in this textbook. The basic **AP pelvis** is considered to be the **initial baseline evaluation projection** for either hip or general pelvis pathology or trauma. This is then followed by **additional lateral projections for the hip and proximal femur**, or additional **special projections of the pelvis** for possible trauma to other parts of the pelvis. The entire AP pelvis is considered basic for a possible hip fracture even if the side of injury is known so that both hips can be demonstrated for comparison purposes.

AP Pelvis 234
AP projection of entire pelvis
(Bilateral hips)

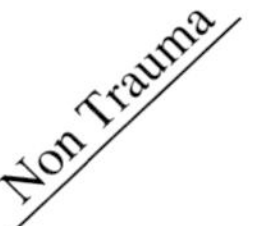

Trauma

Basic – proximal femur and hip
1. AP bilateral frog-leg **235**
   (modified Cleaves)
   or
2. Unilateral frog-leg **240**
3. AP unilateral hip **238**
   (post-op or follow-up exams)

Basic – proximal femur and hip
1. Axiolateral (inferosuperior) **239**
   (Danelius-Miller method)

Special – proximal femur and hip
2. Modified axiolateral hip **241**
   (Clements-Nakayama method)
3. Mediolateral projection (Chapter 19, page **571**)
   (Sanderson method)

Special – pelvis
4. AP axial **236**
   - Anterior pelvic bones
5. Anterior oblique **237**
   - Acetabulum

Basic Projections

Standard or basic projections, at times referred to as routine projections or departmental routines, are those projections commonly taken on average patients who are helpful and can cooperate in performing the procedure.

Special Projections

Special projections are those more common projections taken as extra or additional projections to better demonstrate certain pathologic conditions or specific body parts.

Pelvis
Basic
- AP pelvis **234**
- AP bilateral frog-leg **235**
  (Modified Cleaves method)

Special
- AP axial **236**
  –Anterior pelvic bones
  (Taylor method)
- Anterior oblique **237**
  –Acetabulum
  (Teufel method)

Hip and proximal femur
Basic
- AP unilateral hip **238**

Trauma lateral
- Axiolateral (inferosuperior **239**
  (Danelius-Miller method)

Special non-trauma lateral
- Unilateral frog-leg **240**

Special trauma lateral
- Modified axiolateral **241**
  (Clements-Nakayama method)

Sacroiliac joints
Basic
- AP axial **242**
- Posterior obliques **243**

Special
- Anterior obliques **244**

AP Pelvis Projection (Bilateral Hips)

An AP pelvis serves as a basic projection for unilateral hip trauma for comparison purposes.

Warning: Do **not** attempt to internally rotate legs if a hip fracture or dislocation is suspected. Take with affected leg "as is."

Pelvis
Basic
- **AP**
- AP bilateral frog-leg (modified Cleaves)

Structures Best Shown

Pelvic girdle, L5, sacrum and coccyx, femoral heads, necks and greater trochanters.

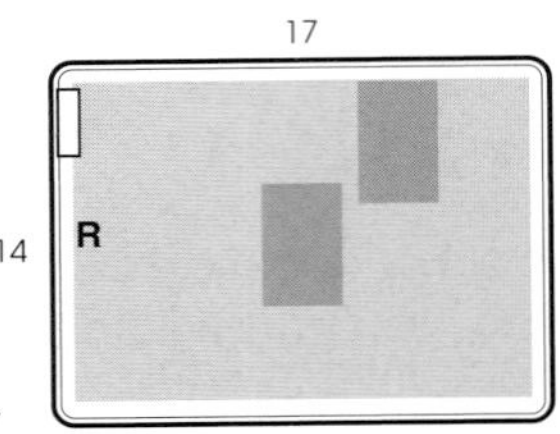

Technical Factors

- Film size–14 x 17 in. (35 x 43 cm), crosswise.
- Moving or stationary grid.
- 80±5 kVp range or 90±5 kVp range.
- Technique and dose @ 80 kVp:

@ 90 kVp:

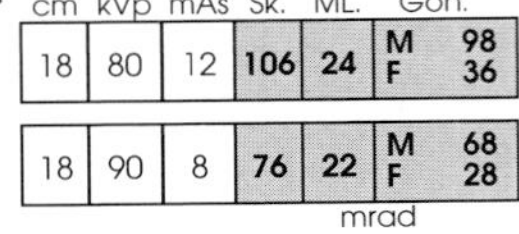

	cm	kVp	mAs	Sk.	ML.	Gon.
@ 80 kVp	18	80	12	106	24	M 98 F 36
@ 90 kVp	18	90	8	76	22	M 68 F 28

mrad

Shielding: Gonadal shielding should be done on all males of reproductive age. Ovarian shielding on females, however, is generally not possible without obscuring essential pelvic anatomy (unless interest is in area of hips only).

Patient Position

- Patient supine, arms at sides or across upper chest; provide pillow for head and support for under knees

Part Position

- Align midsagittal plane of patient to center line of table and to CR.
- Ensure that pelvis is **not rotated**; the distance from tabletop to each ASIS should be equal.
- Separate legs and feet, then **internally rotate** long axes of feet and lower limbs **15 to 20°**. See **warning** above. (May need to place sandbag between heels and tape top of feet together or use additional sandbags against feet to retain this position.)
- Center cassette to CR or midway between the level of the ASIS and the symphysis pubis. Palpate the iliac crest to ensure that the superior border of the pelvis is included on the upper margin of the film, considering the divergent x-ray beam (see Note).

Central Ray

- CR **perpendicular**, directed to **midway between the level of the ASISs and the symphysis pubis** (This will be ≈2 in. or 5 cm inferior to level of ASIS, which is also ≈2 in. or 5 cm superior to symphysis pubis.)
- Minimum 40 in. (102 cm) SID.

Collimation: Collimate to lateral skin margins and to upper and lower film borders.

Respiration: Suspend respiration during exposure.

Note: This centering will ensure that entire pelvis is included on the film, as well as the proximal femora for both the male and female pelvis with the normal variations in shape and size.

The higher kVp range of 90±5 with lower mAs will reduce patient dosage as shown in dose icon boxes above.

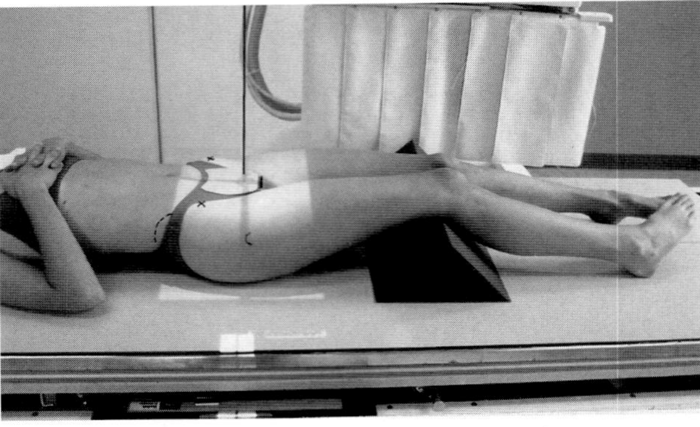

Fig. 7-37. Patient and part position–AP pelvis.

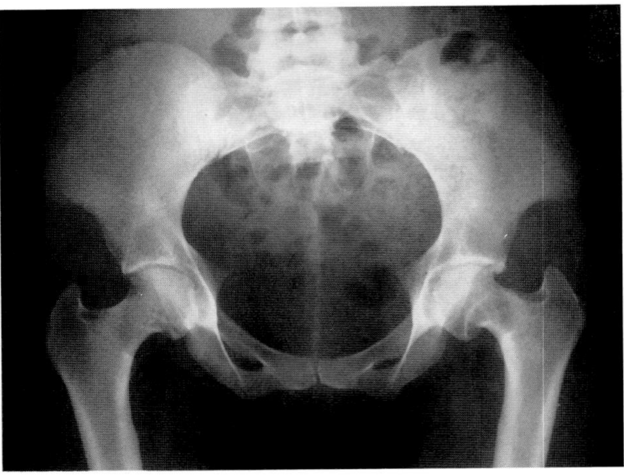

Fig. 7-38. AP pelvis.

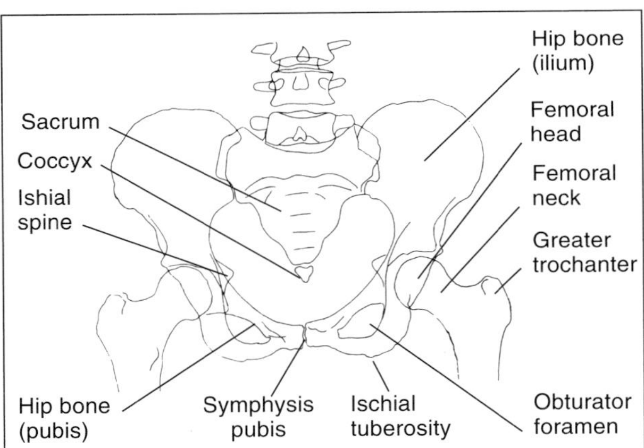

Fig. 7-39. AP pelvis.

Evaluation Criteria

- Entire pelvis and proximal femora should be included and centered on film.
- Collimation borders will be minimal on larger patients. Smaller patients should show equal lateral collimation borders just lateral to greater trochanters.
- **No rotation**: The iliac ala or wings should appear symmetrical and equal in size as well as the two obturator foramina. The right and left ischial spines (if visible) should appear equal in size as well.

Note: An elongated ilium or obturator foramen indicates rotation in that direction (elongation of R ilium indicates rotation towards right).

- Lesser trochanters should not be visible at all, or for many patients only the tips will be visible, and greater trochanters should appear equal in size and shape.
- Optimum exposure will visualize L5 and sacrum area and margins of the femoral heads and acetabula, as seen through overlying pelvic structures without overexposing the ischium and pubic bones. Trabecular markings of proximal femora and pelvic structures will appear clear and sharp.

AP Bilateral "Frog-leg" Projection

Modified Cleaves Method

Warning: Do **not** attempt this position on patient with destructive hip disease or with potential hip fracture or dislocation.

Pelvis
Basic
• AP
• **AP bilateral frog-leg (modified Cleaves)**

Structures Best Shown

Femoral heads, necks, and trochanteric areas on one radiograph for purpose of comparison. Entire pelvis is shown.

For non-trauma hip or congenital hip dislocation (CHD).

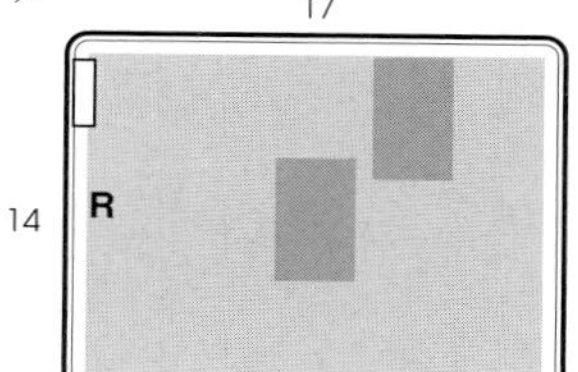

Technical Factors

- Film size–14 x 17 in. (35 x 43 cm), crosswise.
- Moving or stationary grid.
- 80±5 kVp range or 90±5 kVp range.
- Technique and dose:

@ 80 kVp

cm	kVp	mAs	Sk.	ML.	Gon.
18	80	12	**106**	**28**	M **98** F **36**

mrad

Shielding: Shield gonads for both male and female without obscuring essential anatomy (see Note 1).

Patient Position

- Patient supine, pillow for head, arms across upper chest.

Part Position

- Align patient to midline of table and/or cassette and to CR.
- Pelvis must **not be rotated** (equal distance of ASISs to table-top).
- Center cassette to CR, at the level of femoral heads, or 1 in. (2.5 cm) superior to symphysis pubis.
- Flex both hips and knees as demonstrated.
- Place the plantar surfaces of feet together and abduct **both femurs 40 to 45° from vertical**. (See Note 2.) Ensure that **both** femurs are **abducted the same amount** and that there is **no rotation** of pelvis.
- Finalize all positioning, shield placement, tube placement, etc., and be ready to make exposure immediately after patient assumes this final, uncomfortable position.

Central Ray

- CR **perpendicular** to film, directed to a point **1 in. (2.5 cm) superior to symphysis pubis**.
- Minimum 40 in. (102 cm) SID.

Collimation: Collimate to film borders on four sides.

Respiration: Suspend respiration during exposure.

Note 1: This projection is frequently performed for periodic follow-up exams on younger patients, thus the importance of **correctly placed gonadal shielding for ;oth male and female, ensuring that hip joints are not covered**.

Note 2: Less abduction of femurs such as only 20-30° from vertical provides for the least foreshortening of femoral necks, but this foreshortens the entire proximal femora, which may not be desirable.

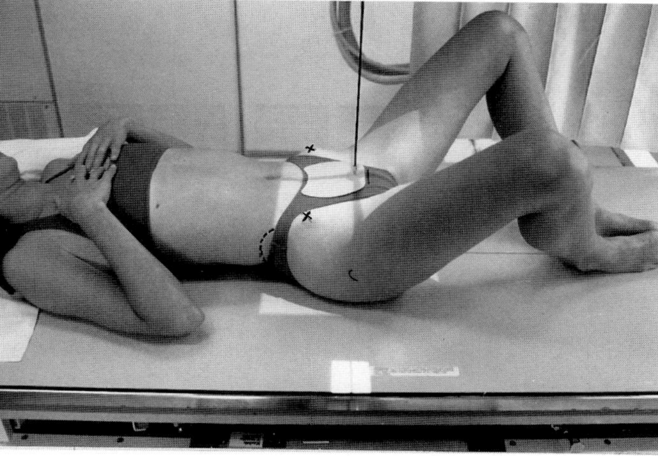

Fig. 7-40. Bilateral "frog-leg"– femora abducted 40-45°.

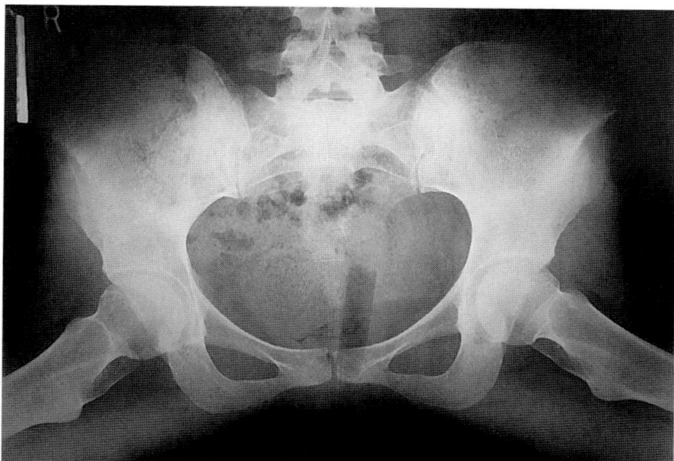

Fig. 7-41. Bilateral "frog-leg."
(Courtesy of Kathy Martensen, R.T.)

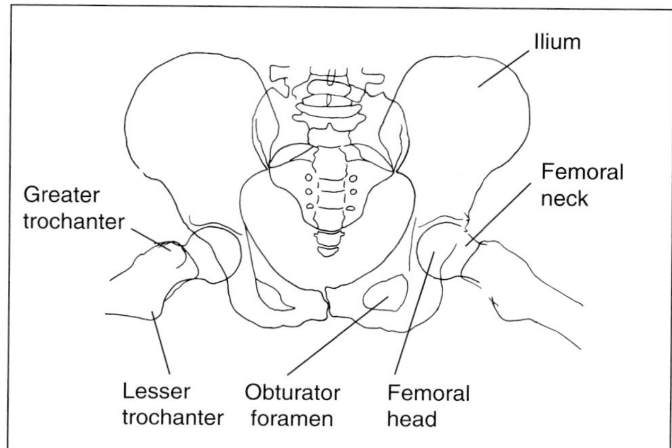

Fig. 7-42. Bilateral "frog-leg."

Evaluation Criteria

- The pelvic girdle should be centered to the film or collimation field from right to left with the mid point being at about 1 in. (2.5 cm) superior to the symphysis pubis.
- **No rotation**, as evidenced by the symmetrical appearance of the pelvic bones, especially the ala of the ilium and the two obturator foramina.
- The lesser trochanters should appear equal in size, as projected beyond the lower or medial margin of the femora.
- The greater trochanters will appear mostly superimposed over the femoral necks, which will appear foreshortened (see note 2 above).
- The femoral heads, necks and greater trochanters should appear symmetrical if both thighs were abducted equally.
- Optimum exposure will visualize the margins of the femoral head and the acetabulum through overlying pelvic structures without overexposing other parts of the proximal femur or pelvic structures. Trabecular markings of greater trochanter and neck areas will appear clear and sharp.

AP Axial Projection

Taylor Method

Pelvis
Special
• **AP axial–Anterior pelvic bones**
• Anterior oblique –Acetabulum

Structures Best Shown

Elongated and/or magnified view of pubic and ischial rami to assess for pelvic trauma or displacement of pubic or ischial structures.

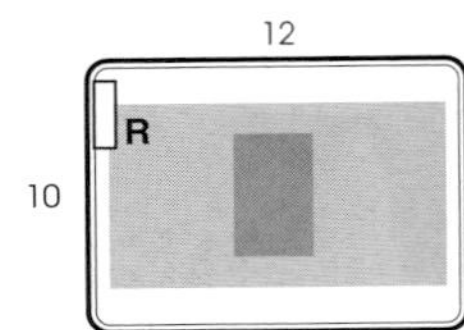

Technical Factors

- Film size–10 x 12 in. (24 x 30 cm), crosswise.
- Moving or stationary grid.
- 80±5 kVp range
  or
- 90±5 kVp range.
- Technique and exposure @ 80 kVp:

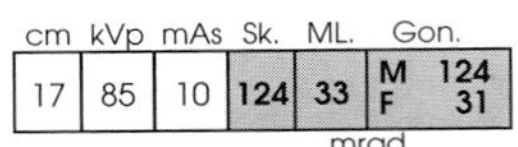

cm	kVp	mAs	Sk.	ML.	Gon.
17	85	10	124	33	M 124 F 31
				mrad	

Shielding: Gonadal shielding may be done only if great care is taken not to obscure essential pelvic anatomy.

Patient Position

- Patient supine, pillow for head, legs extended with support under knees for comfort.

Part Position

- Align midsagittal plane to CR and to midline of table and/or cassette.
- Ensure **no rotation** of pelvis (ASIS to table-top distance the same on both sides).
- Center cassette to projected CR.

Central Ray

- Angle CR **cephalad**, **20 to 35° for males** and **30 to 45° for females**. (These different angles are due to differences in shapes between male and female pelves.)
- Direct CR to a midline point **2 in. (5 cm) distal to** the superior border of the **symphysis pubis**.
- Minimum 40 in. (102 cm) SID.

Collimation: Collimate closely on four sides to area of interest.

Respiration: Suspend respiration during exposure.

Evaluation Criteria

- Elongated and magnified pubic and ischial bones superimposed over the sacrum and coccyx should be centered to film and/or collimation field.
- Lateral margins of collimation field should extend equally on both sides to just lateral to the femoral heads and acetabula.
- **No rotation**: Obturator foramina should appear equal in size and shape.
- Optimum exposure will visualize the femoral head margins and the acetabula through overlying pelvic structures without overexposing other parts of the pubis and ischial bones. With no part motion the trabecular markings of pubic and ischial bones will appear clear and sharp.

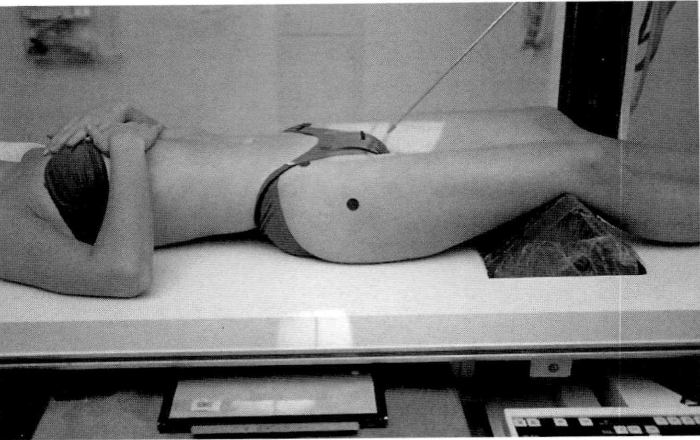

Fig. 7-43. AP axial of anterior pelvic bones – CR 40° cephalad.

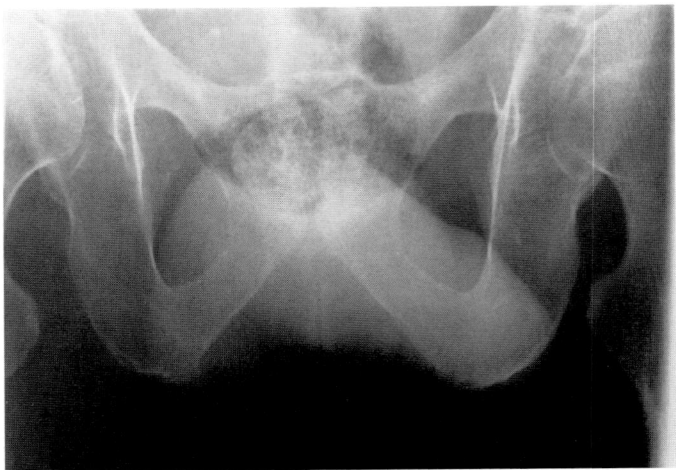

Fig. 7-44. AP axial.

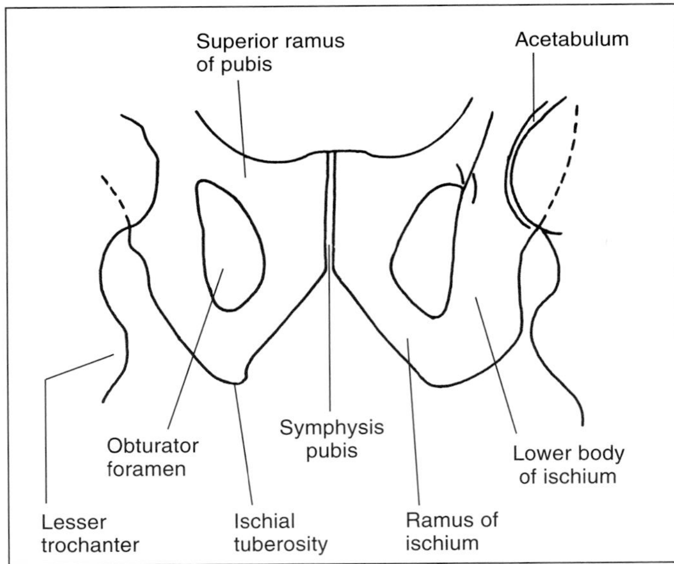

Fig. 7-45. AP axial.

Anterior Oblique Position

Teufel Method

Pelvis
Special
• AP axial–Anterior pelvic bones
• **Anterior oblique –Acetabulum**

Structures Best Shown

Superior and posterior rim of acetabulum, femoral head margin including the fovea capitis.

Both right and left obliques generally taken for comparison.

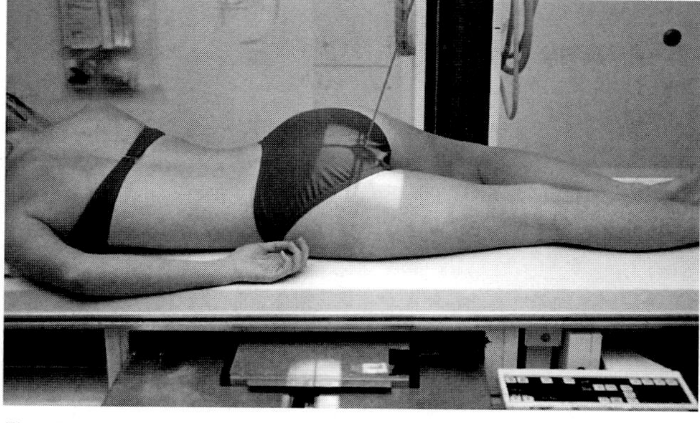

Fig. 7-46. LAO–Left (downside) acetabulum. –CR 12° cephalad.

Technical Factors

- Film size –8 x 10 in. (18 x 24 cm), lengthwise or –10 x 12 in. (24 x 30 cm), lengthwise.
- Moving or stationary grid.
- 80±5 kVp range or 90±5 kVp range.
- Technique and exposure:

8 (10)
10 (12)
L

@ 80 kVp

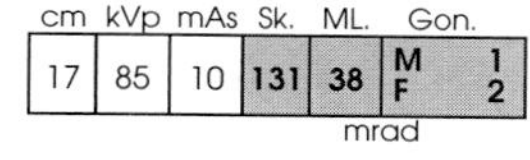

cm	kVp	mAs	Sk.	ML.	Gon.
17	85	10	131	38	M 1 F 2

mrad

Shielding: Shield gonads only if possible without obscuring essential anatomy (use close collimation).

Patient Position–Anterior Oblique Positions

- Patient semiprone, pillow for head, **affected side down**, supported by partially flexed knee and arm of elevated side.

Part Position

- Adjust the patient into a **35 to 40° anterior oblique** (anterior pelvis surface and thorax 35 to 40° from tabletop).
- Align downside femoral head area to midline of table. (Femoral head area is approximately 2 in. or 5 cm lateral of midsagittal plane.)
- Center cassette to CR about 1 in. (2.5 cm) superior to level of greater trochanter, or about 3 in. (8 cm) superior to the level of the ischial tuberosity. (Palpating this may be uncomfortable for patient.)

Central Ray

- CR **12° cephalad**, directed **to acetabulum,** at the level of distal tip of coccyx or about **1 in.** (2.5 cm) **superior to level of greater trochanter, and about 2 in.** (5 cm) **lateral of coccyx at midsagittal plane**.
- Minimum of 40 in (102 cm) SID.

Alternate Posterior Obliques (Judet Oblique Acetabulum Positions): If patient cannot be turned into an anterior oblique position due to trauma or other conditions, a posterior oblique can be done with patient supine. (See Chapter 19, trauma pelvis.)

Collimation: Collimate closely on four sides to area of interest.

Respiration: Suspend respiration during exposure.

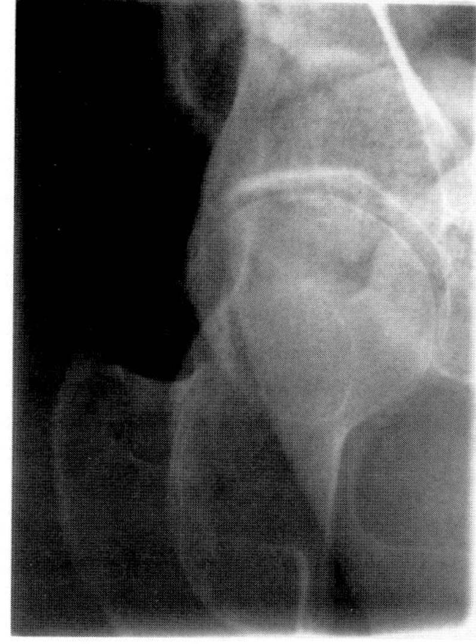

Fig. 7-47. LAO–Left (downside) acetabulum.

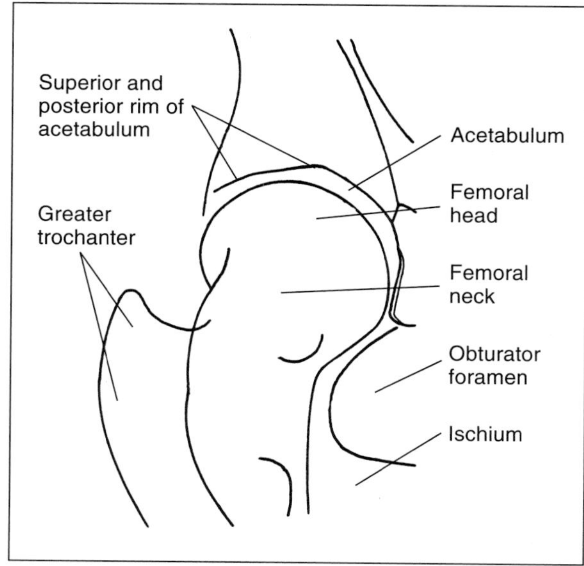

Fig. 7-48. LAO–Left superior and posterior rim of acetabulum.

Evaluation Criteria

- Acetabulum should be centered to film and/or collimation field.
- Femoral head and neck should appear in profile with superior articular margin of head, including the area of the fovea capitis clearly defined, as well as the margins of the acetabulum and the joint space.
- Optimum exposure should clearly demonstrate the acetabulum and femoral head region. Trabecular markings of distal head and the neck area should appear clear and sharp.

AP Unilateral Hip Projection

Warning: Do not attempt to rotate legs if fracture is suspected. A basic AP pelvis to include both hips for comparison should be completed prior to an AP unilateral hip for possible hip or pelvis trauma.

Hip and proximal femur
Basic
- **AP unilateral hip**
- Axiolateral (trauma hip) (inferosuperior)

Structures Best Shown

A post-op or follow-up exam to demonstrate the acetabulum, femoral head, neck and greater trochanter, and the condition and placement of any existing orthopedic appliance.

Technical Factors

- Film size–10 x 12 in. (24 x 30 cm), lengthwise.
- Moving or stationary grid.
- 80±5 kVp range, or 90±5 kVp range.
- Technique and dose: @ 80 kVp

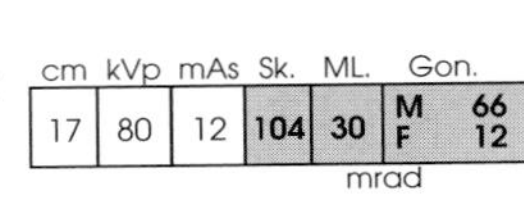

cm	kVp	mAs	Sk.	ML.	Gon.
17	80	12	104	30	M 66 F 12

mrad

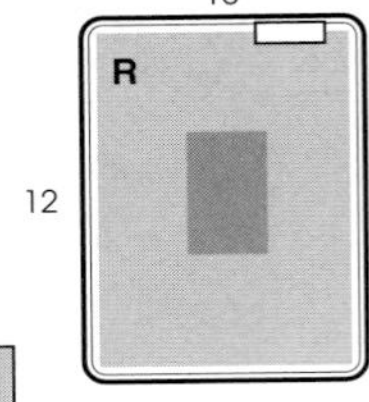

Fig. 7-49. AP right hip.

Shielding: Place shield over gonads and pelvic area, **ensuring affected hip is not obscured**.

Patient Position

- Patient supine, arms at sides or across upper chest.
- Provide pillow for head and support under knees.

Part Position

- Locate **femoral neck** and align to CR and to midline of table and/or film.
- Ensure **no rotation** of pelvis (equal distance from ASIS to table).
- Rotate affected leg **internally 15 to 20°** (see warning above).

Central Ray

- CR **perpendicular** to film, directed to **mid femoral neck**. Femoral neck is 2½ in. or 6 to 7 cm inferior and perpendicular to midpoint of line between ASIS and symphysis pubis. Femoral neck can also be located on a longitudinal line about **1 in. or 2.5 cm medial to ASIS at level of greater trochanter** or ≈1 in. or 2.5 cm above level of symphysis pubis.
- Minimum 40 in. (102 cm) SID.

Collimation: Collimate on four sides to area of interest or to film borders.

Respiration: Suspend respiration during exposure.

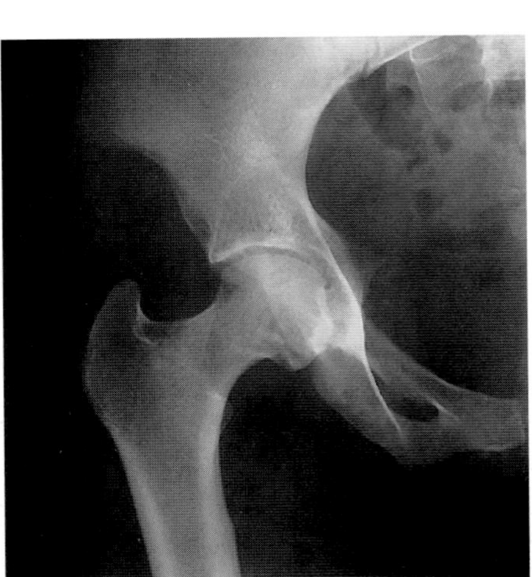

Fig. 7-50. AP hip.

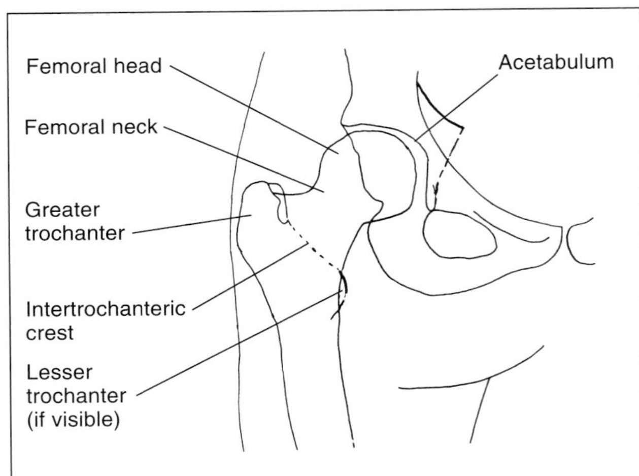

Fig. 7-51. AP hip.

Evaluation Criteria

- The proximal one-third of the femur should be visualized along with the acetabulum and adjacent parts of the pubis, ischium and ilium.
- The hip joint space, including the perimeter borders of the femoral head should be clearly visualized.
- The lesser trochanter should not project beyond the medial border of the femur at all or on some patients only its very tip is seen with sufficient internal rotation of leg, indicating the greater trochanter, femoral head and neck are seen in full profile without foreshortening.
- Any existing orthopedic appliance should be seen in its entirety.
- Optimum exposure will visualize the margins of the femoral head and the acetabulum through overlying pelvic structures without overexposing other parts of the proximal femur or pelvic structures. Trabecular markings of greater trochanter and neck areas will appear clear and sharp.

Axiolateral (Inferosuperior) Projection

Danelius-Miller Method

Warning: Do not attempt to internally rotate leg on initial trauma exam.

Note: This is a common projection for trauma, surgery, post-surgery or other patients who cannot move or rotate legs for frog-leg lateral.

Hip and proximal femur
Basic
• AP unilateral hip
• **Axiolateral (trauma) (inferosuperior)**

Structures Best Shown

Lateral view of acetabulum and femoral head, neck and trochanteric area for **trauma hip** situtations.

10

12

R

Technical Factors

- Film size–10 x 12 in. (24 x 30 cm), crosswise.
- Stationary grid cassette (lead strips in crosswise direction if the patient is raised from the table top sufficiently to center the CR and body part to center line of grid to prevent grid cutoff).
- 80±5 kVp range.
- Technique and dose:

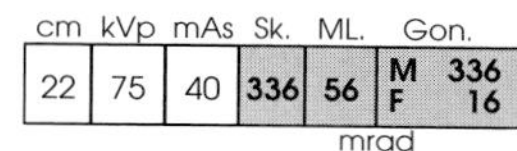

cm	kVp	mAs	Sk.	ML.	Gon. (mrad)
22	75	40	336	56	M 336, F 16

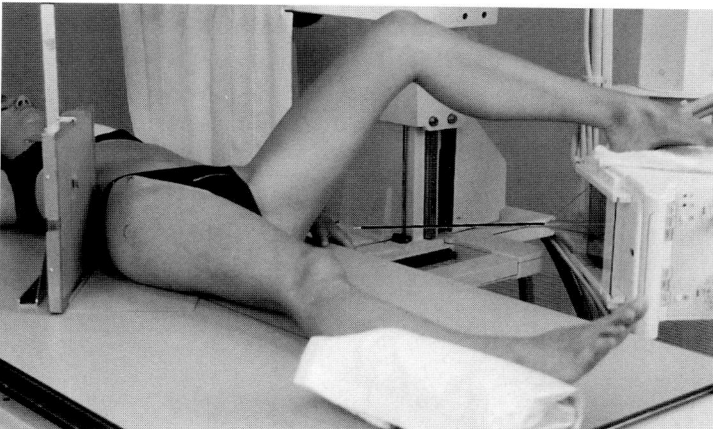

Fig. 7-52. Axiolateral hip.

Shielding: Gonadal shielding is not possible without obscuring essential anatomy; **close collimation is important**.

Patient Position

(May be done on stretcher or bedside if patient cannot be moved, see Chapter 19, Trauma Pelvis.)

- Patient supine, pillow for head.
- Elevate pelvis 1 to 2 in. (3-5 cm) if possible by placing supports under pelvis (more important for thin patient).

Part Position

- Flex and elevate unaffected leg so thigh is in near vertical position and outside of the collimation field. Support in this position. If foot is rested on collimator as shown, provide folded sheets or padding to prevent burning of foot.
- Check to ensure **no rotation** of pelvis (equal ASIS-table distance).
- Place cassette in crease above iliac crest and adjust so it is **parallel to femoral neck** and **perpendicular to CR**. Use cassette holder if available, or use sandbags to hold cassette in place.
- Internally rotate affected leg 15 to 20° **unless contraindicated** by possible fracture or other pathology (see warning above).

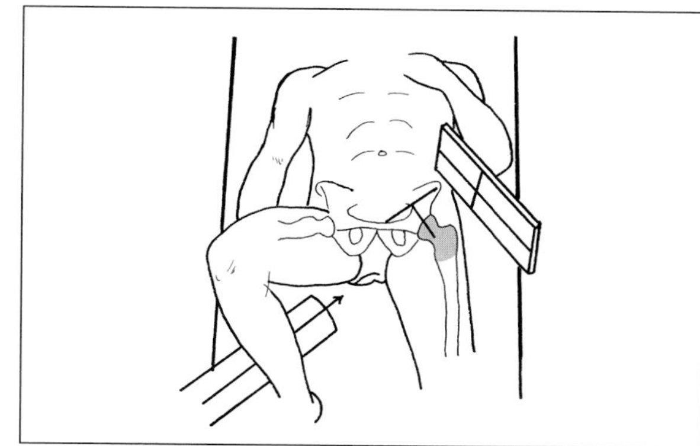

Fig. 7-53. Axiolateral hip.

Central Ray

- CR **perpendicular** to femoral neck and to film.
- Minimum 40 in. (102 cm) SID.

Collimation: Tight collimation on four sides to femoral head and neck region.

Respiration: Suspend respiration during exposure.

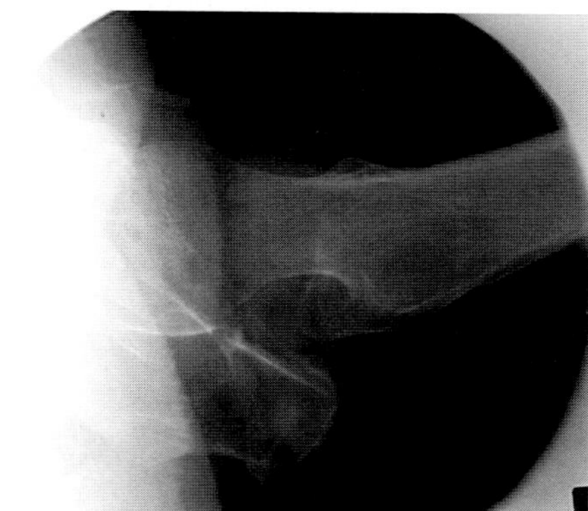

Fig. 7-54. Axiolateral hip.

Evaluation Criteria

- Entire femoral head, neck and trochanter and acetabulum should be seen visualized.
- Only the most distal part of femoral neck should be superimposed by greater trochanter.
- Only a small part if any of lesser trochanter is visualized with inversion of affected leg.
- Soft tissue from raised unaffected leg is not superimposed over affected hip.
- No visible grid lines; grid lines indicate incorrect tube film alignment.
- Optimum exposure will visualize femoral head and neck without overexposing proximal femoral shaft.

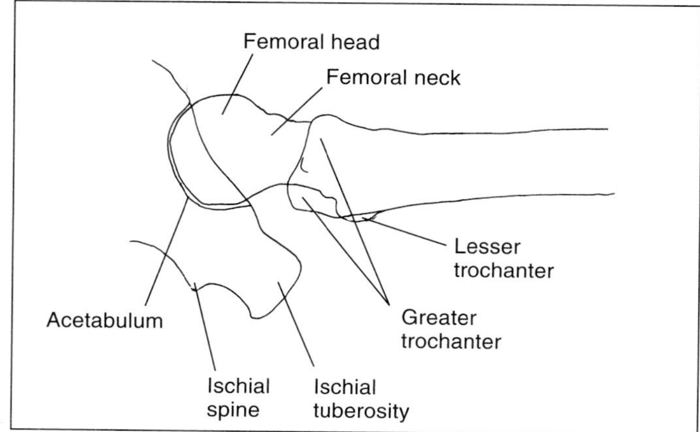

Fig. 7-55. Axiolateral hip.

7

Unilateral "Frog-leg" Projection–Mediolateral

Modified Lauenstein and Hickey Method

Warning: Do **not** attempt this position on patient with destructive hip disease or with potential hip fracture or dislocation. (This could result in significant displacement of fracture fragments. See lateral trauma projections.)

Hip and proximal femur
Special - non-trauma
- **Unilateral frog-leg**

Special - trauma
- Modified axiolateral (Clements-Nakayama method)

Structures Best Shown

Lateral view of acetabulum and femoral head, neck and trochanteric area, for **non-trauma hip** situations.

Technical Factors

- Film size–10 x 12 in. (24 x 30 cm), crosswise.
- Moving or stationary grid.
- 80±5 kVp range, or 90±5 kVp range.
- Technique and dose: @ 80 kVp

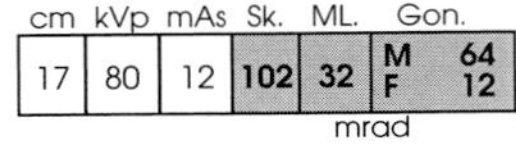

cm	kVp	mAs	Sk.	ML.	Gon.
17	80	12	102	32	M 64 F 12
				mrad	

Shielding: Shield over gonads, ensuring affected hip is not obscured.

Patient Position

- Patient supine with affected hip area aligned to CR and midline of table and/or film.

Part Position

- Flex knee and hip on affected side as shown.
- Abduct femur 40 to 45° from vertical which places femoral neck parallel to film. (See Note 1.)
- Center affected femoral neck to CR and midpoint of film. (Femoral neck is 2½ in. or 6 to 7 cm inferior and perpendicular to mid point of line between ASIS and symphysis pubis.)

Central Ray

- CR **perpendicular** to film (see Note 2), directed to **mid femoral neck** (center of film).
- Minimum 40 in. (102 cm) SID.

Collimation: Collimate closely on four sides to area of interest.

Respiration: Suspend respiration during exposure.

Note 1: The optimum femur abduction for demonstrating the femoral neck without foreshortening is 20 to 30° from vertical on most patients. This does result in some foreshortening of the proximal femur region, which may be objectionable.

Note 2: A 20 to 25° cephalad CR angle is sometimes preferred, in which the greater trochanter will not superimpose as much of the proximal neck area (Fig. 7-58).

Evaluation Criteria

- Proximal one-third of femur should be visualized, along with hip joint and acetabulum.
- The greater trochanter will superimpose most of femoral neck area.
- Lesser trochanter will be only partially seen more distally than the greater trochanter.
- Optimum exposure will visualize the margins of the femoral head and the acetabulum through overlying pelvic structures without overexposing other parts of the proximal femur. Trabecular markings of proximal femur should appear clear and sharp.

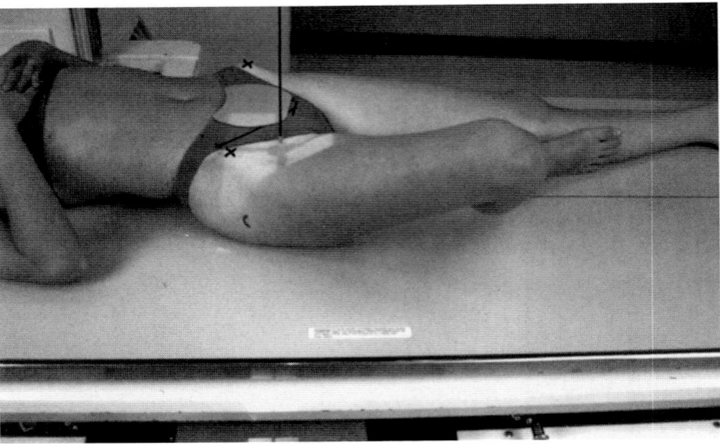

Fig. 7-56. Unilateral frog-leg position (leg abducted 40-45° from vertical, CR 0°.

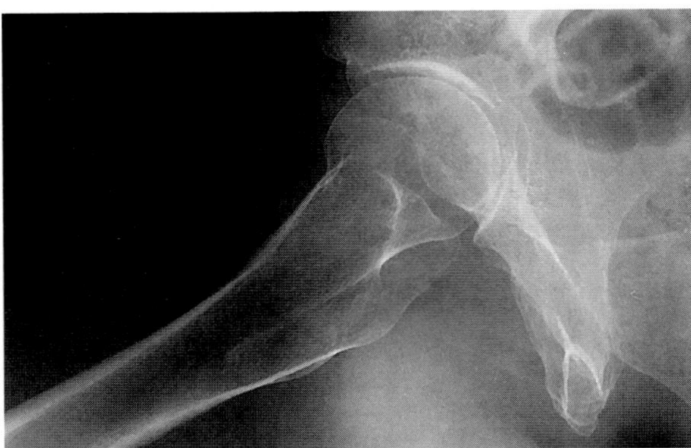

Fig. 7-57. For femoral neck–CR 0°.

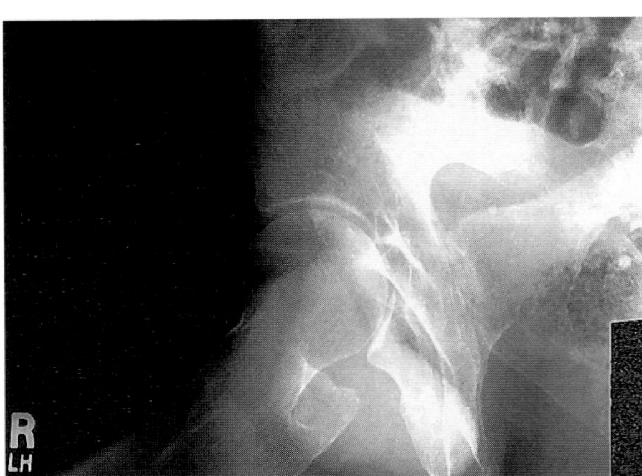

Fig. 7-58. Unilateral frog-leg – CR 20° cephalad.

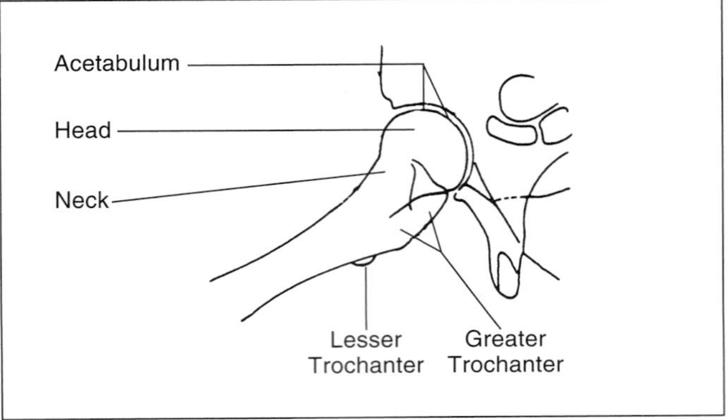

Fig. 7-59. Unilateral frog-leg.

Modified Axiolateral Projection–Possible Trauma

Clements-Nakayama Method*

Hip and proximal femur
Special - non-trauma
• Unilateral frog-leg
Special - trauma
• **Modified axiolateral (Clements-Nakayama method)**

Structures Best Shown

Lateral oblique view of acetabulum and femoral head, neck and trochanteric area.

Note: This can be used with possible bilateral hip fractures or with bilateral arthroplasty (surgery for hip prosthesis) with limited movement possible of both affected and unaffected legs and hips.

Technical Factors

- Film size–8 x 10 in. (18 x 24 cm), lengthwise.
- Stationary grid cassette. (Cassette on edge with 15° tilt, grid lines parallel to table top.)
- 80±5 kVp range.

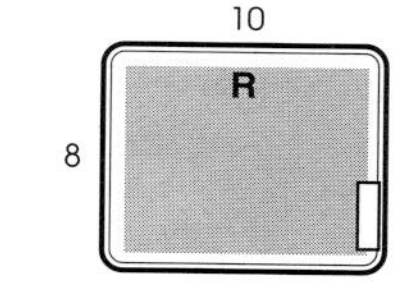

Shielding: Shield gonads as much as possible without obscuring essential anatomy.

Patient Position

- Supine, affected side near edge of table with both legs fully extended.
- Provide pillow for head, arms across upper chest.

Part Position

- Leg remains in neutral (anatomical) position. (15° posterior CR angle compensates for internal leg rotation.)
- Rest cassette on extended Bucky tray, which places the bottom edge of cassette about 2 in. (5 cm) below the level of the tabletop.
- Tilt cassette about 15° from vertical and adjust alignment of cassette to ensure that face of cassette is **perpendicular** to CR to prevent grid cutoff.

Central Ray

- CR angled **30 to 40° mediolateral**, which should be **perpendicular to** and **centered to femoral neck**, angled downward (posteriorly) **15 to 20°** from horizontal.
- Centerline of cassette centered to projected CR.
- Minimum 40 in. (102 cm) SID.

Collimation: Collimate closely on four sides to area of interest.

Respiration: Suspend respiration during exposure.

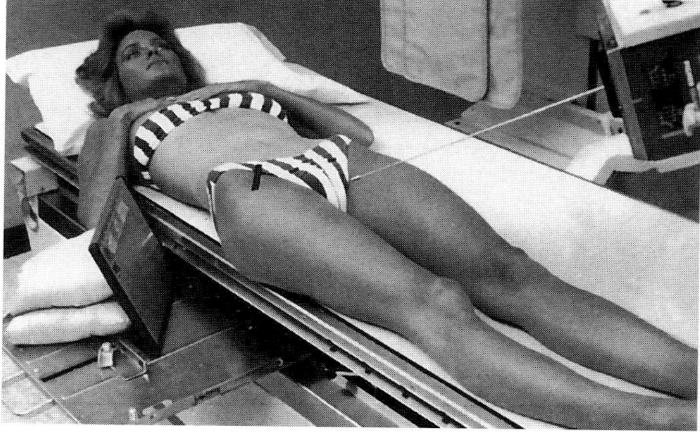

Fig. 7-60. Modified axiolateral–15° tilt.

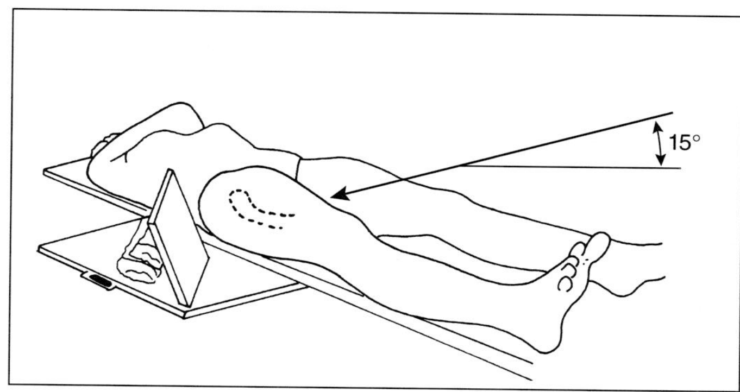

Fig. 7-61. Modified axiolateral.

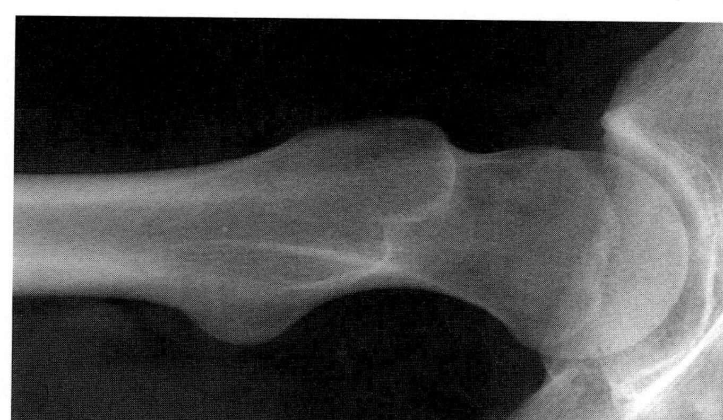

Fig. 7-62. Modified axiolateral.

Evaluation Criteria

- Entire femoral head, neck and trochanters should be seen centered to mid film area.
- Femoral head and neck should be seen in profile with only minimal superimposition by greater trochanter.
- Lesser trochanter is seen projecting below femoral shaft. (With leg in neutral or anatomical position, the amount of lesser trochanter seen will be minimal, and with increased external rotation of leg, this will decrease.)
- Optimum exposure will visualize femoral head and neck without overexposing proximal femoral shaft. No excessive grid lines visible on radiograph.

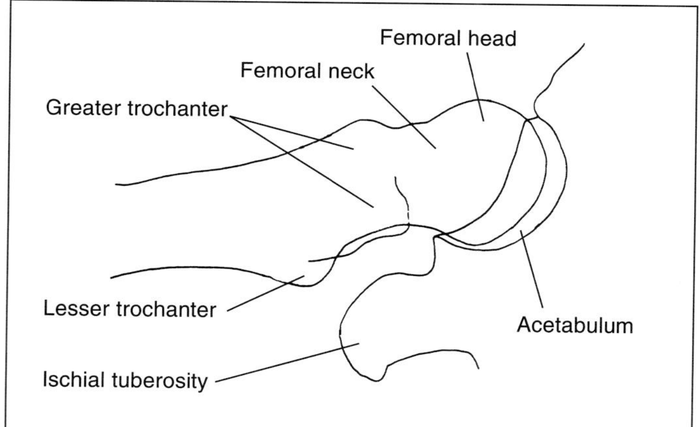

Fig. 7-63. Modified axiolateral.

*Clements, RS, Nakayama, HK. Radiographic Methods in Total Hip Arthroplasty; *Radiologic Technology* 1980; 51:589-600.

AP Axial Projection

Sacroiliac joints
- **AP axial**
- Posterior obliques

Special
- Anterior obliques

Structures Best Shown

Sacroiliac joints, L5-S1 junction, sacrum and coccyx.

Note: The urinary bladder should be emptied before beginning this procedure. It is also desirable to have the lower colon free of gas and fecal material, which may require a cleaning enema as ordered by a physician.

Technical Factors

- Film size–10 x 12 in. (24 x 30 cm), lengthwise.
- Moving or stationary grid.
- 90±5 kVp range.
  (Increase 6-10 kVp due to axial projection.)
- Technique and dose:

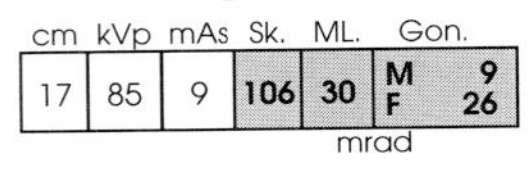

cm	kVp	mAs	Sk.	ML.	Gon.
17	85	9	106	30	M 9 F 26

mrad

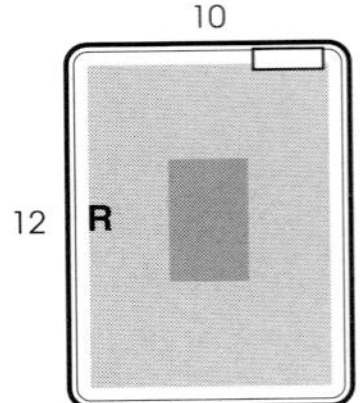

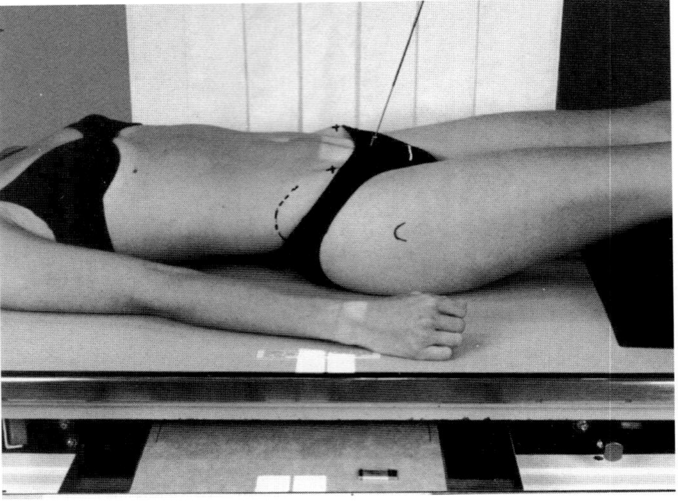

Fig. 7-64. AP axial of SI joints – CR 30 to 35° cephalad.

Shielding: Carefully place gonadal shielding for males. Ovarian shielding on females is not possible because such shielding would directly obscure area of interest.

Patient Position

- Patient supine, pillow for head, legs extended with support under knees for comfort.

Part Position

- Align midsagittal plane to CR and to midline of table and/or cassette.
- Ensure **no rotation** of pelvis (ASIS-table distance the same on both sides).
- Center of cassette to projected CR.

Central Ray

- Angle **CR 30 to 35° cephalad** (generally males require about 30° and females or those with an increase in the lumbosacral curve require nearer 35°).
- Direct CR to a midline point **midway between the level of the ASIS and the symphysis pubis**. This is also about 1½ to 2 in. (4 to 5 cm) below or distal to a bisecting line between the ASISs.
- Minimum 40 in. (102 cm) SID.

Collimation: Collimate to area of interest, but ensure that side margins do not cut off sacroiliac joints.

Respiration: Suspend respiration during exposure.

Alternate AP pelvis: Some departmental routines indicate a full AP pelvis with no CR angle as part of an SI joint routine in addition to or in place of this AP axial.

Alternate PA axial projection: If patient cannot assume the supine position, this can also be taken as a PA with patient prone, using a 30 to 35° **caudad** angle. The CR would be centered to the level of the iliac crest.

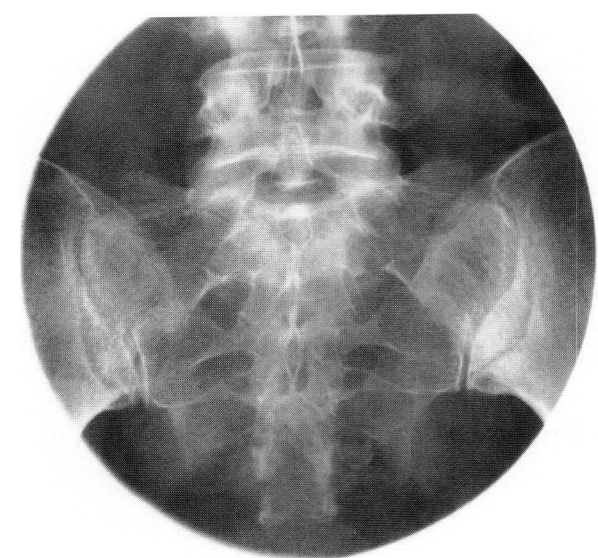

Fig. 7-65. AP axial.

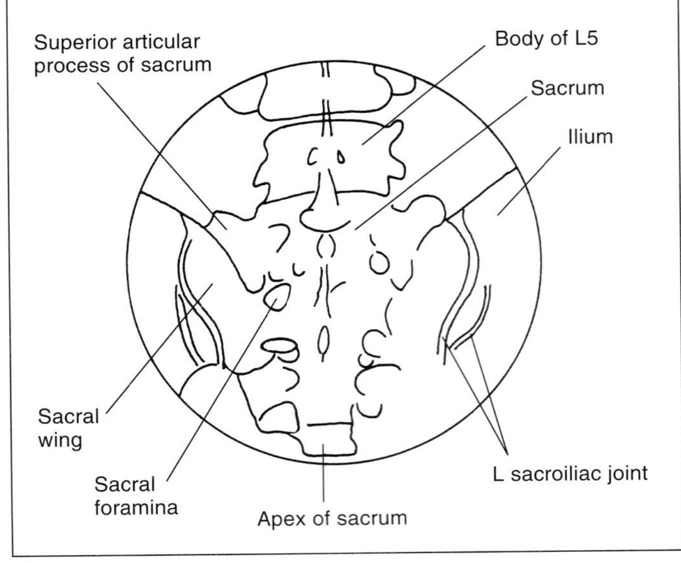

Fig. 7-66. AP axial.

Evaluation Criteria

- The sacroiliac joints and the first two segments of the sacrum should be centered to the collimation field and/or film.
- The sacroiliac joint spaces and the L5-S1 junction should appear open, indicating correct CR angulation.
- Optimum exposure should visualize the margins of the sacroiliac joint spaces.

Posterior Oblique Positions (LPO and RPO)

Sacroiliac joints
- AP axial
- **Posterior obliques**

Special
- Anterior obliques

Structures Best Shown

Sacroiliac joints **farthest from film**. **Both sides** are done for comparison.

Note: May also be taken as anterior obliques, see following page.

Technical Factors

- Film size–10 x 12 in. (24 x 30 cm), lengthwise.
- Moving or stationary grid.
- 85±5 kVp range.
- Technique and dose:

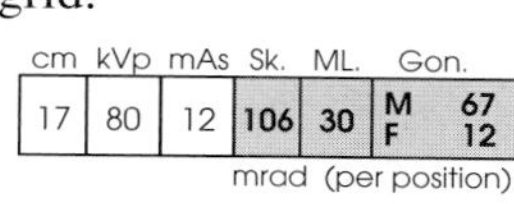

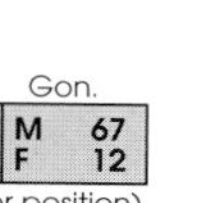

cm	kVp	mAs	Sk.	ML.	Gon.
17	80	12	106	30	M 67 F 12

mrad (per position)

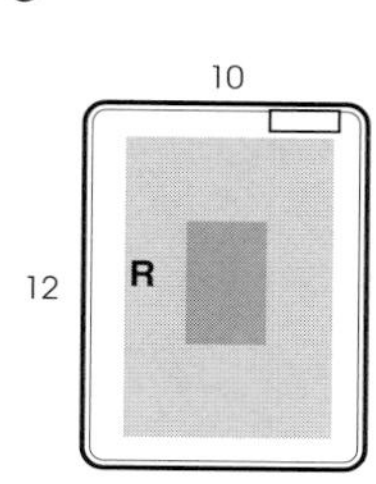

Shielding: Carefully shield gonads without obscuring sacroiliac joint area. (Can readily be done on males but requires more care with females.) Ensure close collimation.

Patient Position

- Patient supine, pillow for head.

Part Position

- Turn into **25 to 30°** posterior oblique, **side of interest is elevated**.
- **LPO** will visualize **right joint**.
- **RPO** will visualize **left joint**.
- Use some angle measuring device to ensure correct and consistent angles on **both** obliques.
- Place support under elevated hip and flex elevated knee. Ask patient to reach across and grasp edge of table to help maintain this position.
- Align joint of interest to CR and to midline of table and/or cassette. (Note CR entrance point as described below.)
- Center film to CR.

Central Ray

- CR **perpendicular**, directed to a point **1 in. (2.5 cm) medial** to upside ASIS. (See Note for optional cephalad angle.)
- Minimum 40 in. (102 cm) SID.

Collimation: Collimate closely on four sides to area of interest.

Respiration: Suspend respiration during exposure.

Note: To demonstrate the inferior or distal part of the joint more clearly, the CR may be angled 15 to 20° **cephalad**.

Fig. 7-67. RPO for left side (upside) SI joints.

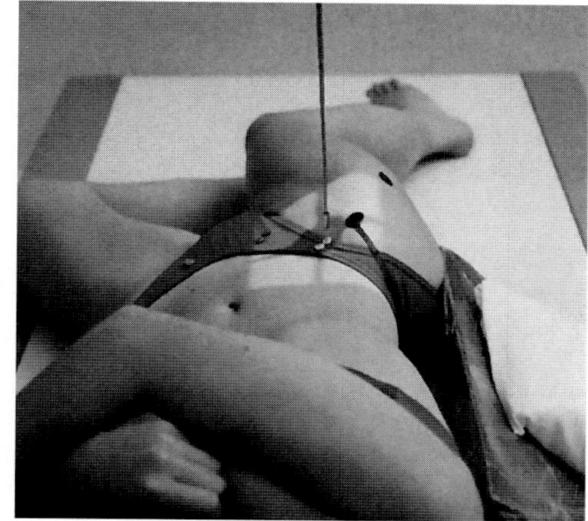

Fig. 7-68. LPO for right side (upside).

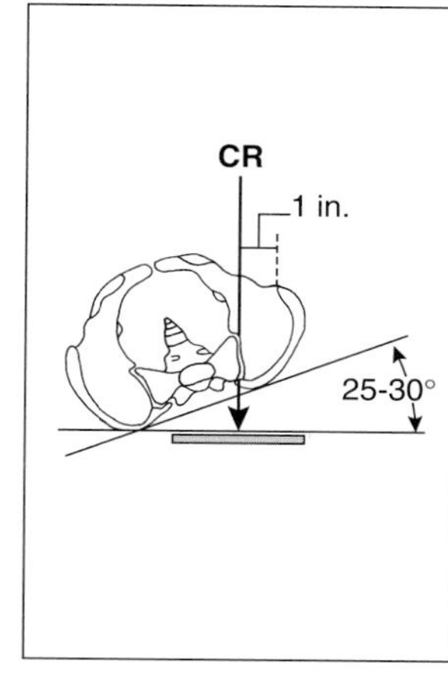

Fig. 7-69. LPO.

Evaluation Criteria

- Joint space on side of interest should appear open.
- The ala of the ilium and the sacrum should have no overlap, indicating the correct obliquity. (Overlap indicates too much obliquity.)
- Optimum exposure will clearly visualize the margins of the joint space along its entirety.

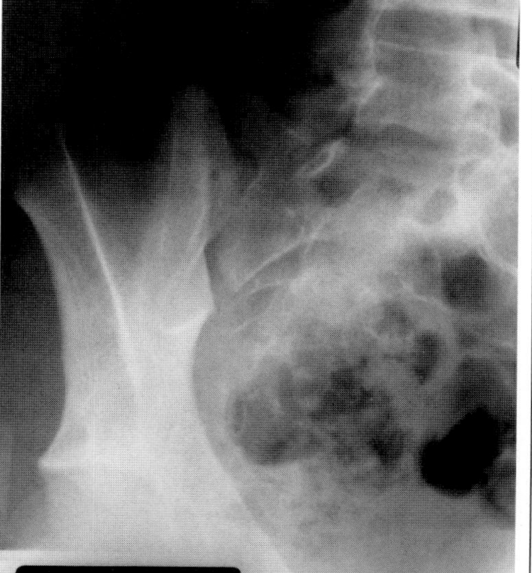

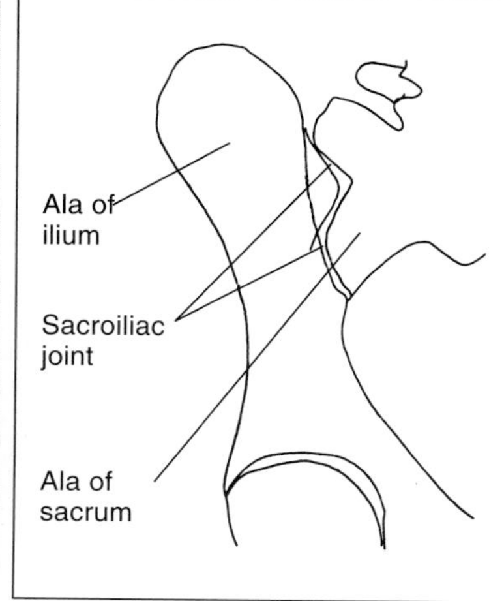

Fig. 7-70. Left posterior oblique projection (upside). Fig. 7-71.
(Courtesy of Kathy Martensen, R.T.)

Anterior Oblique Positions (LAO and RAO)

Sacroiliac joints
- AP axial
- Posterior obliques

Special
- **Anterior obliques**

Structures Best Shown

Profile view of sacroiliac joint **closest to film. Both sides** are done for comparison.

Technical Factors

- Film size–2 each: 10 x 12 in. (24 x 30 cm), lengthwise.
- Moving or stationary grid.
- 85±5 kVp range.
- Technique and dose:

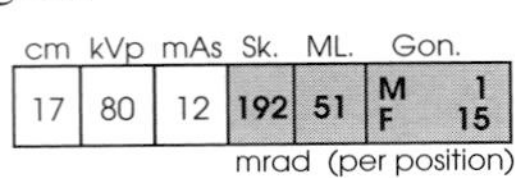

cm	kVp	mAs	Sk.	ML.	Gon.
17	80	12	192	51	M 1 F 15

mrad (per position)

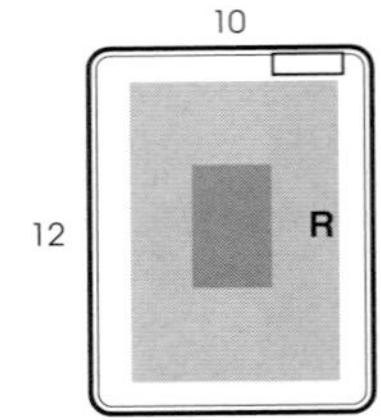

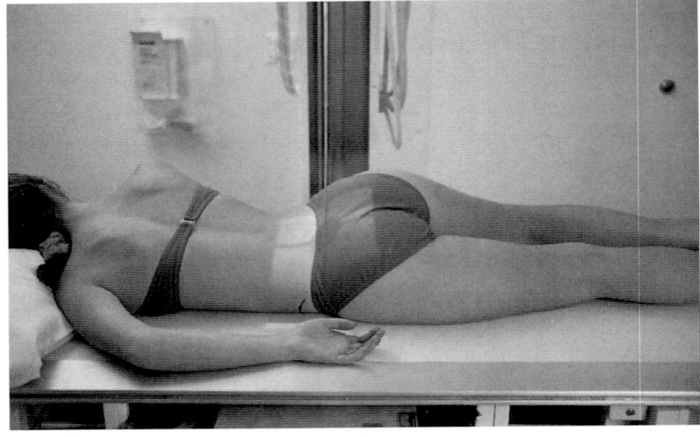

Fig. 7-72. LAO for left side (downside) SI joints.

Shielding: Carefully place gonadal shielding for males. Ovarian shielding on females is more difficult without obscuring area of interest. Ensure close collimation.

Patient Position

- Patient in semiprone position, **affected side down**, pillow for head.
- Flex elevated knee, place elevated arm in front of head with opposite arm down behind back.

Part Position

- Adjust body into 25 to 30° anterior oblique, **side of interest down**.
- **LAO** will visualize **left** joint.
- **RAO** will visualize **right** joint.
- Align joint of interest to CR and to midline of table and/or cassette. (Note CR entrance point as described below.)
- Center film to CR.

Central Ray

- CR **perpendicular**, directed to a point **1 in. (2.5 cm) lateral** (below) the **vertebral spinous processes at level of the ASIS**. This will exit at a point 1 in. (2.5 cm) medial to downside ASIS. (See Note for optional caudad angle.)
- Minimum 40 in. (102 cm) SID.

Collimation: Collimate closely on four sides to area of interest.

Respiration: Suspend respiration during exposure.

Note: To best demonstrate the inferior or distal aspect of the joint, the CR may be angled 15 to 20° **caudad**.

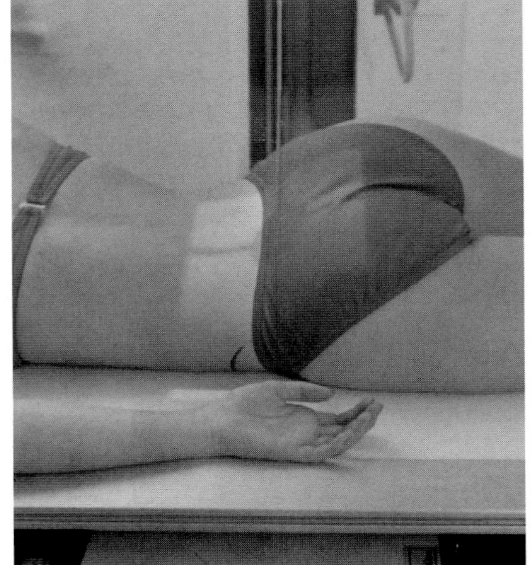

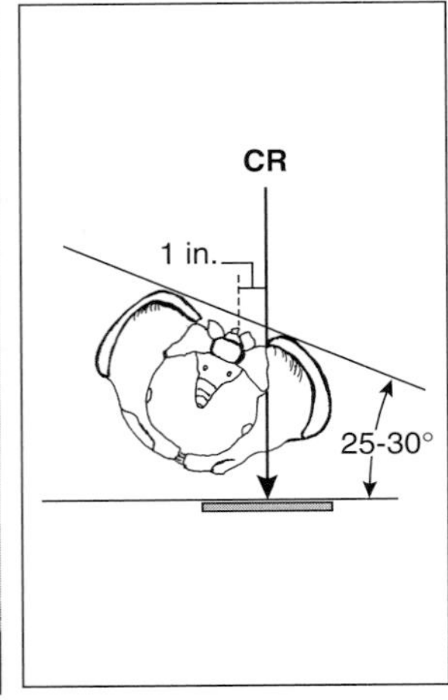

Fig. 7-73. Anterior oblique (LAO) position (downside). Fig. 7-74.

Evaluation Criteria

- Joint space closest to the film should appear open.
- The ala of the ilium and the sacrum should have no overlap, indicating the correct obliquity. (Overlap indicates too much obliquity.)
- Optimum exposure will clearly visualize the margins of the joint space along its entirety.

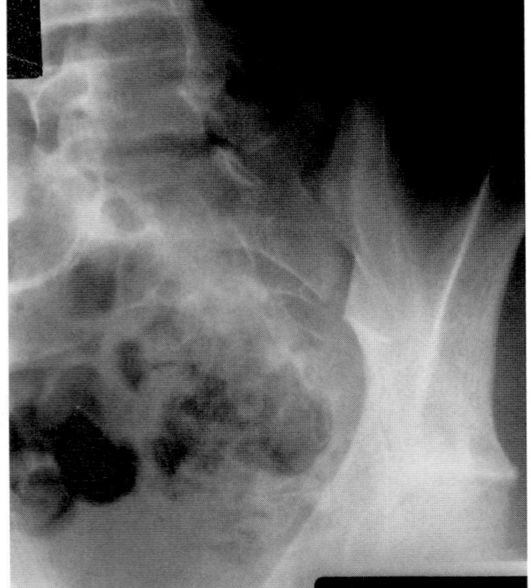

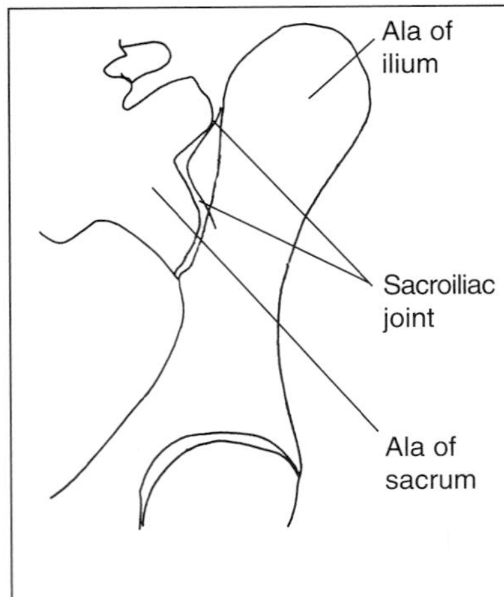

Fig. 7-75. Anterior oblique position. Fig. 7-76.

Radiographs for Critique

Each of these radiographs demonstrates some error in positioning which requires a repeat. These, along with accompanying lecture slides of these and other radiographs, will provide a basis for classroom and/or positioning lab discussion. Questions with answers based on these specific critique radiographs are provided in the accompanying student workbook/lab manuals to help prepare students for classroom and/or lab discussions on film critique.

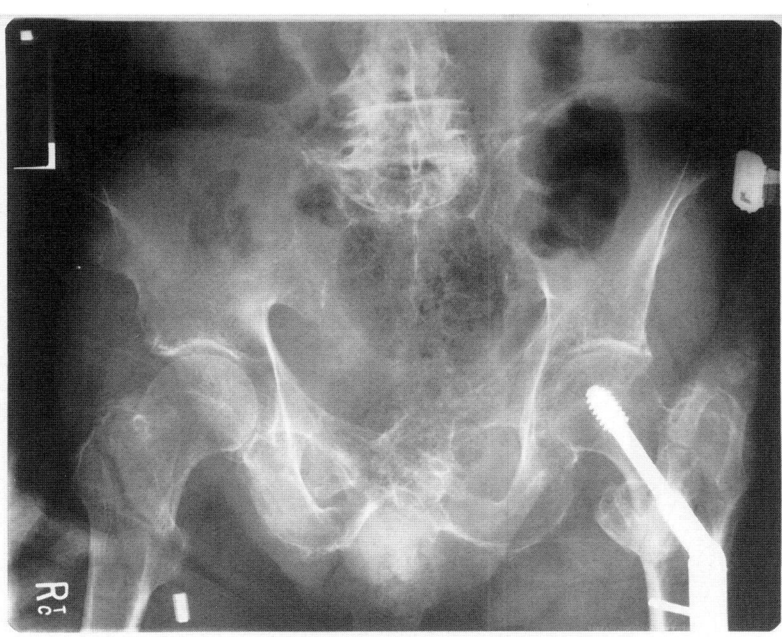

Fig. C7-77. AP pelvis (83-year-old).

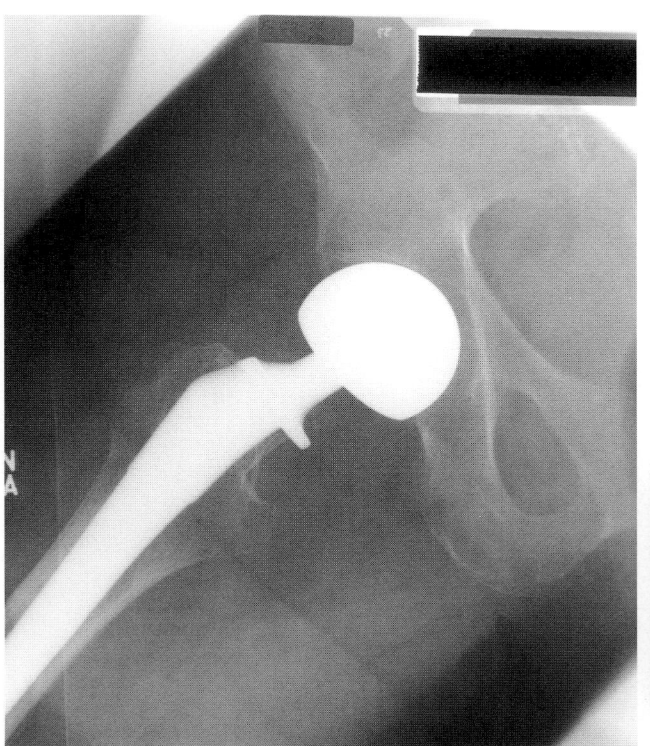

Fig. C7-78. Unilateral frog-leg (84-year-old).

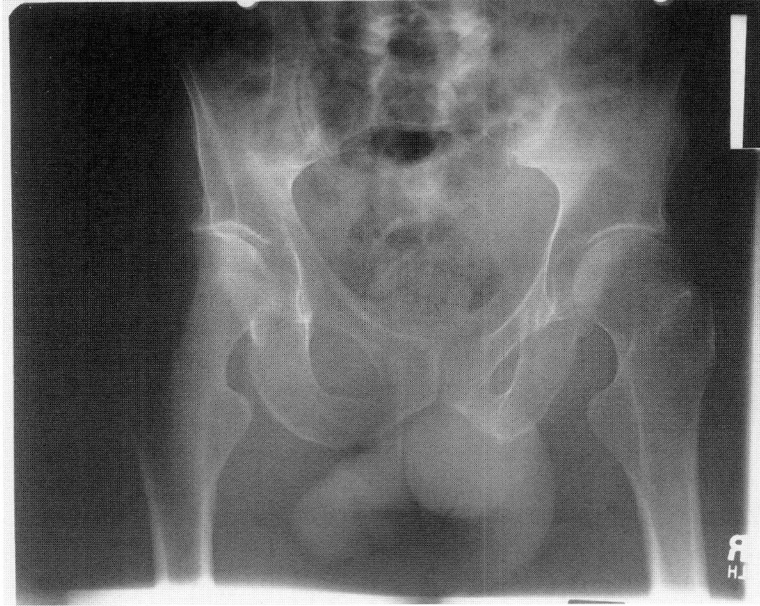

Fig. C7-79. AP pelvis (57-year-old).

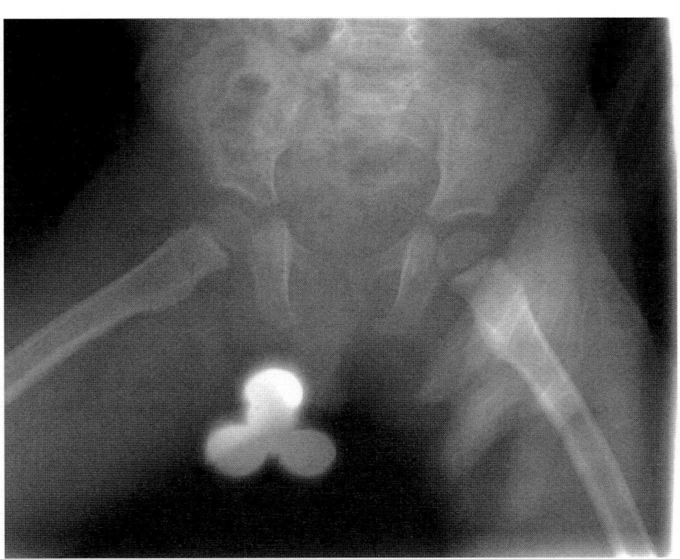

Fig. C7-80. Bilateral frog-leg (2-year-old).

CHAPTER 8

Cervical and Thoracic Spine

CONTRIBUTIONS BY:
Alex Backus, MS, RT (R)

CONTENTS

Radiographic Anatomy

Vertebral column **248**

Vertebral (spinal) curvatures **249**

Typical vertebra **250**

Cervical vertebrae **252**

Atlas (C1) and axis (C2) **253**

Thoracic vertebrae **254**

Anatomy review with radiographs **256**

Intervertebral foramina
vs. zygapophyseal joints **258**

Radiographic Positioning

Topographical landmarks **260**

Positioning considerations **262**

Survey information **263**

Basic and special projections **264**

Cervical spine (basic):
- AP open mouth (C1 and C2) **265**
- AP axial **266**
- Obliques **267**
- Lateral **268**
- Lateral, horizontal beam **269**
- Cervicothoracic lateral (swimmer's) **270**
(For additional cervical trauma projections–see Chapter 19)

Cervical spine (special):
- Alternate method for C7-T1 **271**
- Lateral–Hyperflexion and hyperextension **272**
- AP (Fuch method) or PA (Judd method) **273**
- AP chewing or wagging jaw (Ottonello method) **274**

Thoracic spine (basic):
- AP **275**
- Lateral **276**

Thoracic spine (special):
- Oblique **277**

Radiographs for critique **278**

8

Radiographic Anatomy

VERTEBRAL COLUMN

The vertebral *(ver′ te-bral)* column, commonly called the spine or spinal column, is a complex succession of many bones called **vertebrae** *(ver′ te-bre)*, (singular is **vertebra** *[ver′ te-brah])*. It provides a flexible supporting column for the trunk and head; and also transmits the weight of the trunk and upper body to the lower limbs. This column is located in the midsagittal plane, forming the posterior or dorsal aspect of the bony trunk of the body.

Spinal Canal: The spinal canal, which follows the various curves of the spinal column, begins at the base of the skull and extends distally into the sacrum. This canal contains the spinal cord and is filled with cerebrospinal fluid.

Spinal Cord: The spinal cord, which is enclosed and protected by the spinal canal, begins with the **medulla oblongata** *(me-dul′ ah ob″ long-ga′ tah)* of the brain. It passes through the foramen magnum of the skull and continues through the **first cervical vertebra** all the way down to the **lower border of the first lumbar vertebra** where it tapers off to a point called the **conus medullaris** *(ko′ nus med′ u″ lar-is)*.

Intervertebral Disks: The typical adult vertebrae are separated by tough fibrocartilaginous disks. These cushion-like disks are tightly bound to the vertebrae for spinal stability but also allow for flexibility and movement of the vertebral column.

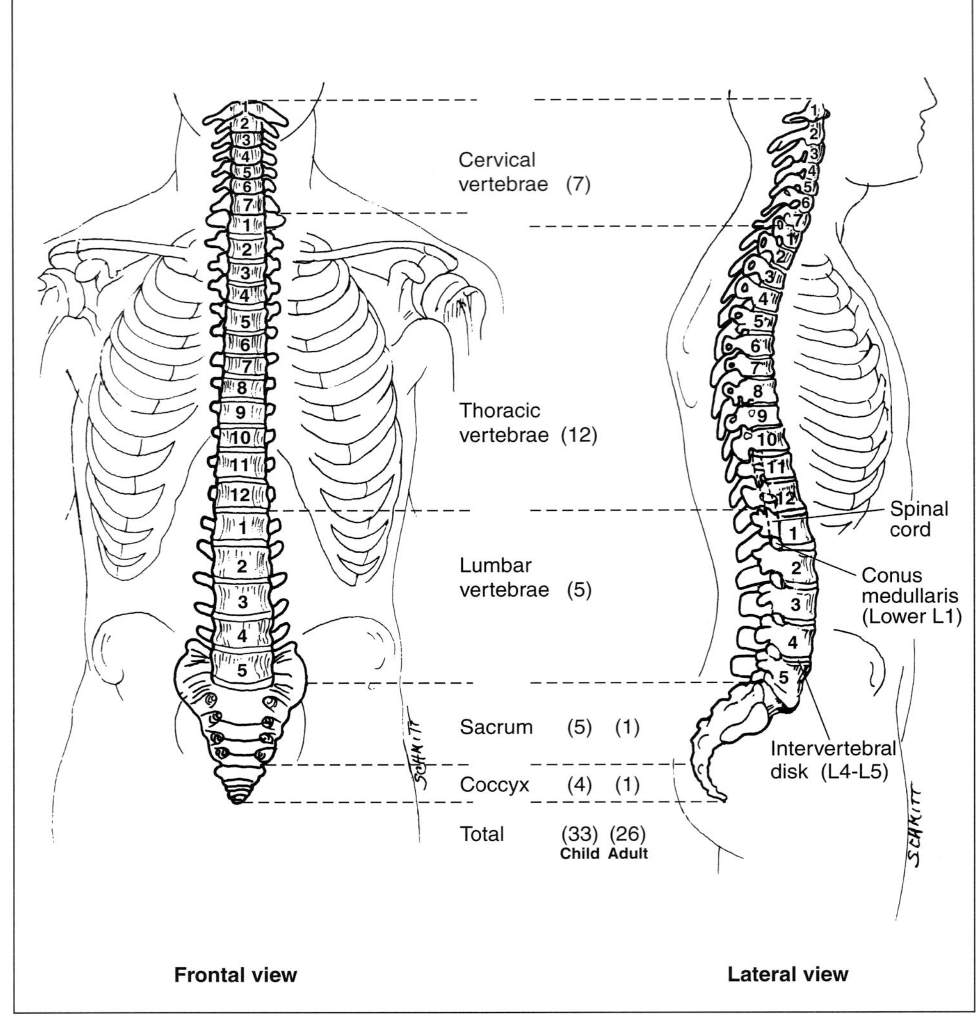

Fig. 8-1. Vertebral column.

Divisions

The entire vertebral column is divided by regions into **five groups** or divisions. Within each of these five regions there are a certain number of vertebrae that have distinctive characteristics of that particular region.

Detailed anatomy and positioning of the first two divisions, the cervical and thoracic vertebrae, will be covered in this chapter. The last three divisions, the lumbar vertebrae (spine), sacrum and coccyx are covered in Chapter 9.

Cervical Vertebrae: The first seven vertebrae have general similarities that group them as **cervical vertebrae**. While there may be a slight variation in the height of each vertebra from one individual to another, the average human has **seven cervical vertebrae**.

Thoracic Vertebrae: The next twelve vertebrae each connect to a pair of ribs. There are twelve pairs of ribs and **twelve thoracic vertebrae**. An older and incorrect term for the thoracic vertebrae is dorsal vertebrae. However, all of the vertebrae, being located on the posterior or dorsal aspect of the body, could correctly be called dorsal vertebrae; therefore, the twelve vertebrae of the upper back should correctly be called thoracic vertebrae.

Lumbar Vertebrae: The largest and most massive individual vertebrae are the **five lumbar vertebrae**. These vertebrae are the largest and strongest in the vertebral column because the entire body weight as supported by the vertebrae increases toward the lower end of the column. For this reason the disks between the lower lumbar vertebrae are common sites for stress and pathology creating pain and back problems, especially for mammals such as humans who walk in an upright position.

Sacrum and Coccyx: Each of the vertebrae in the cervical, thoracic and lumbar regions forms as a separate vertebra in the child, and is retained as a separate bone in the adult. The sacrum *(sa′ krum)* and coccyx *(kok′ siks)*, however, are different. In the newborn there are **five sacral** *(sa′ kral)* **segments**, and from **three** to **five coccygeal** *(kok-sij′ e-al)* **segments**. Some references suggest **four** coccygeal segments as normal, for an average total of **33 separate bones** in the vertebral column of a young child.

In the adult, however, the sacrum and coccyx tend to fuse into two single bones. Counting the sacrum and coccyx as single bones, the adult vertebral column therefore is composed of **26 separate bones**.

VERTEBRAL (SPINAL) CURVATURES

The vertebral column forms a series of anteroposterior curves (Fig. 8-2). Soon after birth the **thoracic** and **sacral** (pelvic) curves begin to develop. These two **posterior convex** curves are called **primary curves.** As a child begins to raise his head and later begins to sit up, the first **compensatory curve** forms in the opposite direction in the cervical region. This **cervical curve** is the least pronounced of the four curves, and is described as a posterior **concave** curve.

The second compensatory curve to form is the **lumbar curvature**, also a **concave** curve. This lumbar curvature develops when the child learns to walk. Both of the lower curves, the lumbar and sacral (pelvic), are usually more pronounced in the female than they are in the male.

Note: The terms **concave** (a rounded inward or depressed surface like a "cave") and **convex** (a rounded outward or elevated surface) are curves in relationship to the **posterior surface**, as viewed from the side. If described in reference to the anterior, these curvatures would be described with opposite terms with the cervical being convex and the thoracic concave. In medicine, however, it is more common to describe these from the back or the posterior, as described in this textbook and as defined in *Dorland's Medical Dictionary*, 27th ed.

These primary and compensatory curvatures are normal and serve an important function by increasing the strength of the vertebral column and by helping maintain balance along a center line of gravity in the upright position.

Certain terms are commonly used to describe these curvatures when they become exaggerated or abnormal. These terms, **lordosis**, **kyphosis**, and **scoliosis**, are described as follows:

Lordosis

The term lordosis *(lor-do′ sis)*, meaning swayback, is a condition in which the **lumbar curvature is exaggerated**. This **abnormal increased concavity** of the lumbar spine may result from pregnancy or extreme obesity by the increased weight of the abdominal contents. It may also be caused by poor posture, rickets or tuberculosis of the spine.

Kyphosis

Kyphosis *(ki-fo′ sis)* is an **abnormal** or **exaggerated thoracic "humpback" curvature** with **increased convexity**, in reference to the posterior. This greater than normal curvature of the thoracic spine may also be caused by poor posture, rickets or tuberculosis of the spine.

Scoliosis

An abnormal or exaggerated sideways or **lateral curvature** is called **scoliosis** *(sko″ le-o′ sis)*. If the spine is viewed from the back (illustrated in Fig. 8-4), the vertebral column is usually near straight with little lateral curvature. Occasionally, there is a slight lateral curvature in the upper thoracic region of a healthy adult. This curvature is usually associated with the dominant extremity, so this curvature may be convex to the right in a right-handed person and convex to the left in a left-handed person.

A more serious type of problem occurs when there is a pronounced S-shaped lateral curvature. This deformity is termed **scoliosis** and may cause severe deformity of the entire thorax. The effect of scoliosis is more obvious if it occurs in the lower vertebral column, where it may create a tilting of the pelvis with a resulting effect on the lower limbs, creating a "limp" or uneven walk.

Summary: **Lordosis** refers to an abnormal or exaggerated lumbar or "swayback" type curvature with **increased concavity**. **Kyphosis** describes an abnormal or exaggerated thoracic or "humpback" type curvature with **increased convexity**, and **scoliosis** refers to an abnormal "sideways" or **lateral curvature**.

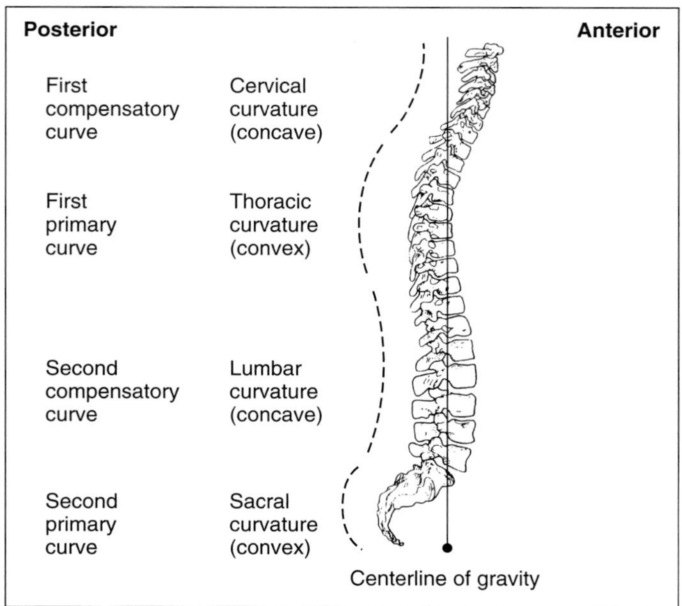

Fig. 8-2. Normal adult curvature (side view).

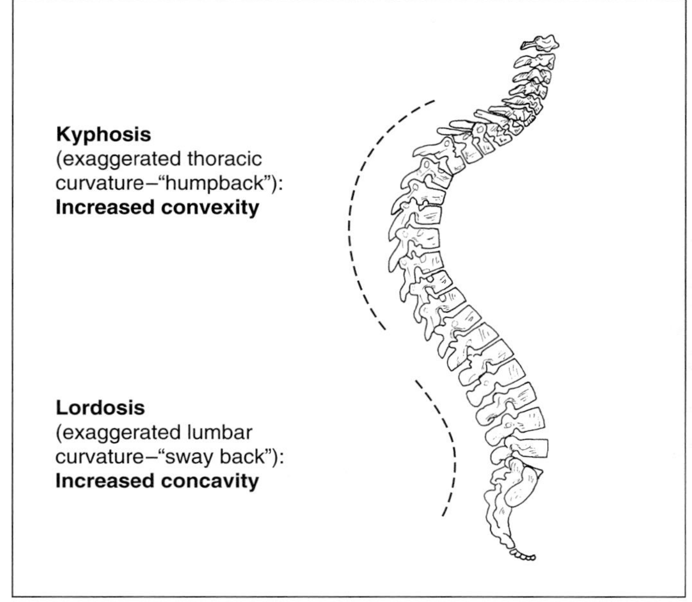

Fig. 8-3. Lordosis–Kyphosis.

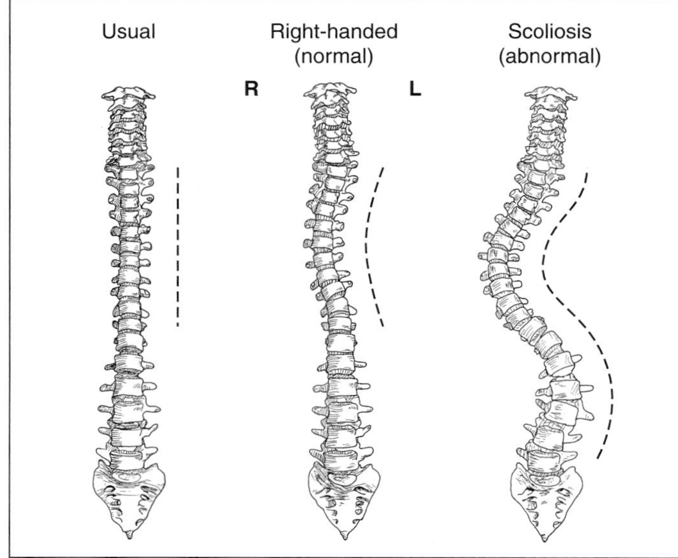

Fig. 8-4. Scoliosis–Lateral curvatures (posterior view).

8

TYPICAL VERTEBRA ANATOMY

Although the vertebrae in the different regions vary in size and shape, all are similar in basic structure. A typical vertebra consists of two main parts as follows:

(1) Body

The body is the thick, weight-bearing anterior part of the vertebra. Its superior and inferior surfaces are flat and rough for attachment of the intervertebral disks.

(2) Vertebral Arch

The second part of a typical vertebra consists of a ring or arch of bone extending posteriorly. With the body extending anteriorly, the vertebral arch forms a circular opening containing the spinal cord. This opening is called the **vertebral foramen**.

When a number of vertebrae are stacked, as they are in the normal articulated vertebral column, the succession of vertebral foramina forms a tubelike opening along the complete length of the spine. This opening, called the **vertebral** (spinal) **canal**, encloses and protects the spinal cord.

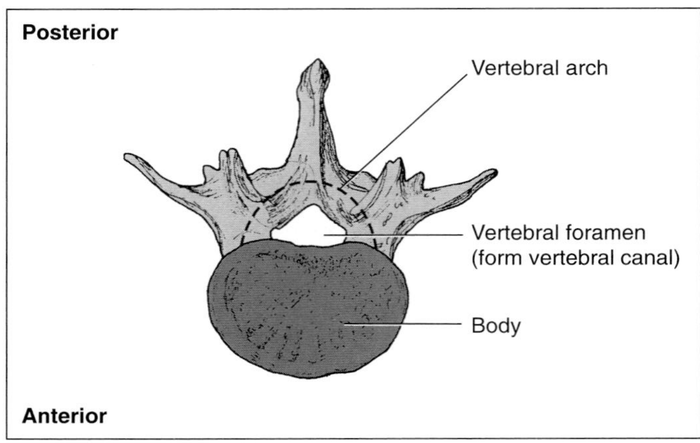

Fig. 8-5. Typical vertebra (demonstrates two main parts).

Superior View: Part of the vertebral arch is formed by two projections, termed **pedicles**, *(ped′i-kuls)* that extend posteriorly from either side of the body. Pedicle is a Latin term meaning "little foot." The pedicles form most of the sides of the vertebral arch.

The posterior part of the vertebral arch is formed by two somewhat flat layers of bone termed laminae. A **lamina** *(lam′i-na)* extends posteriorly from each pedicle to unite in the midline.

Extending laterally from approximately the junction of each pedicle and lamina is a projection termed the **transverse process**. Specific vertebrae, namely the seven cervical vertebrae, contain openings or foramina in each transverse process called transverse foramina, as described and illustrated in a following section.

At the midline junction of the two laminae, extending posteriorly, is another process called the **spinous process**. The spinous processes are the most posterior extensions of the vertebrae and can often be palpated along the dorsal surface of the neck and back.

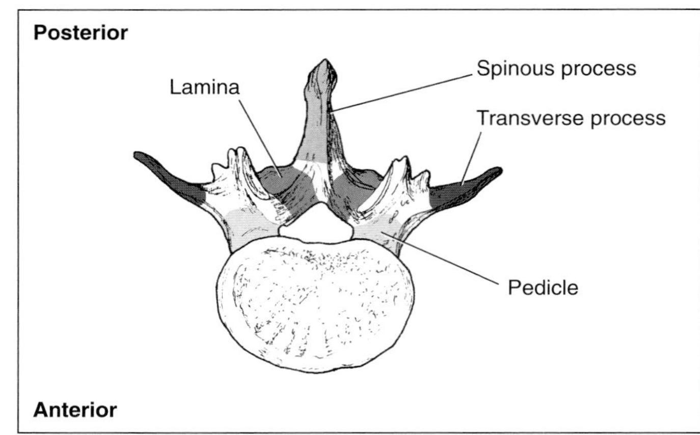

Fig. 8-6. Typical vertebra–Superior view.

Lateral View: A typical vertebra as seen from the side is illustrated in Fig. 8-7. The **body** is the large anterior portion, and the **spinous process** is the posterior portion. Extending posteriorly from the body on each side are the **pedicles**, which terminate in the area of the **transverse process**. Continuing posteriorly from the origin of the transverse process on each side are the two **lamina**, which end at the spinous process.

Along the upper surface of each pedicle is a notch termed the **superior vertebral notch**, and along the lower surface of each pedicle is another deeper notch termed the **inferior vertebral notch**. These notches, along with the floor of the pedicles, help form the important **intervertebral foramina** when vertebrae are stacked to form the vertebral column as described on the following page (see Fig. 8-9).

Summary: The typical vertebra has **two pedicle**s and **two laminae** that form the vertebral arch and the vertebral foramen containing the spinal cord, **two transverse processes** extending laterally, **one spinous process** extending posteriorly, and the large anterior **body**. Each typical vertebrae also has four **articular processes** described and illustrated on the following page.

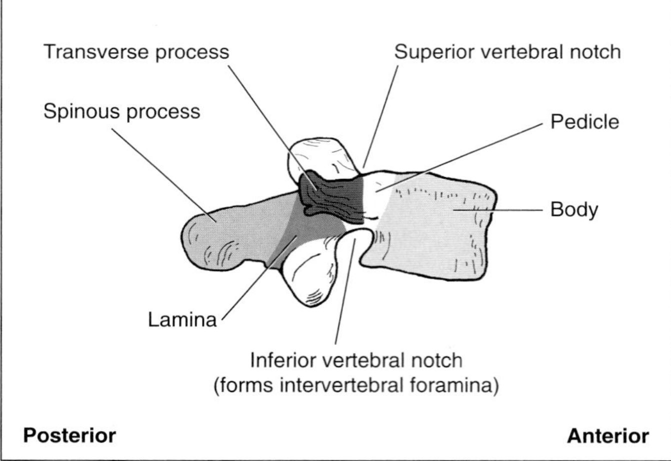

Fig. 8-7. Typical vertebra–Lateral view.

Articular Processes

Each typical vertebra has **four articular processes** projecting from approximately the area of the junction of the pedicles and laminae. As seen from the front (anterior) and side (lateral) in Fig. 8-8, the processes projecting upward are called the **superior articular processes**, and the processes projecting downward are the **inferior articular processes.** The importance of these processes becomes apparent when vertebrae are stacked together to form the vertebral column (Fig. 8-9). The two superior articular processes of one vertebra articulate with the two inferior articular processes of the vertebra above, forming joints called **zygapophyseal** *(zi′ gah-po-fiz′ e-al)* **joints**. In earlier literature these were called apophyseal *(ah″ po-fiz′ e-al)* joints.

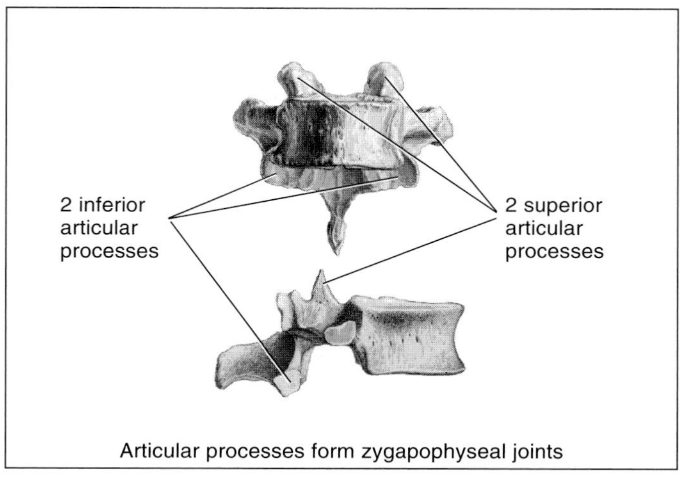

Fig. 8-8. Typical vertebra–Articular processes (anterior and lateral views).

Zygapophyseal (Apophyseal) Joints

Since there are two superior and two inferior articular processes on each vertebra, there are also two zygapophyseal joints between any two vertebrae, one on each side. It is often necessary to demonstrate these joints on certain radiographs of the vertebral column.

The term **facet** *(fas′ et)* is sometimes used interchangeably with the term zygapophyseal joint; however, the facet is actually only the **articulating surface** of the superior and inferior articular processes. The superior facets or articulating surfaces are only seen on either posterior or oblique views. The inferior facets are seen on anterior, oblique and lateral views (Fig. 8-9).

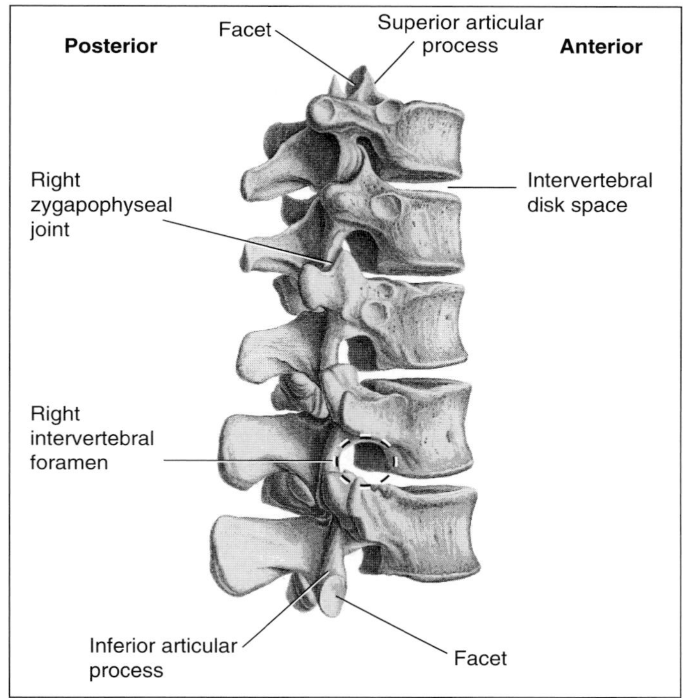

Fig. 8-9. Zygapophyseal joints and intervertebral foramina (lateral oblique view).

Intervertebral Foramina

In the articulated vertebral column, the floor portion of the pedicles of stacked vertebrae along with the inferior vertebral notches of the vertebra above, and the superior vertebral notches of the vertebra below, form the important openings, the **intervertebral foramina.** Therefore, between every two vertebrae there are two intervertebral foramina, one on each side, through which important spinal nerves and blood vessels pass.

The zygapophyseal joints and the intervertebral foramina must be demonstrated radiographically by the appropriate projection in each of the three major portions of the vertebral column as described and illustrated in later sections.

Intervertebral Disk

Intervertebral disks are found between the bodies of any two vertebrae except between the first and second cervical vertebra since the first cervical vertebra has no body. These fibrocartilage disks provide a resilient cushion between the vertebrae, helping to absorb shock such as received from jumping or other types of vigorous exercises. The vertebral column would be rigidly immovable without the intervertebral disks and zygapophyseal joints.

As labeled in Fig. 8-10, each disk consists of an outer fibrous portion termed the **annulus fibrosus** *(an′ u-lus fi-bro′ sis)*, and a soft semi-gelatinous inner part called the **nucleus pulposus** *(nu′ kle-us pul′ po-sus)*. The intervertebral disk is similar to an oblong donut, with the outer part being the annulus fibrosus, and the hole of the donut (when filled), being similar to the nucleus pulposus.

If, due to injury, the soft inner part protrudes into the spinal canal to press on the spinal cord or spinal nerves located in the spinal canal (see small arrows), severe pain and possible numbness radiating into the extremities will occur. This condition is called a "slipped disk" or, more properly, **herniated nucleus pulposus (HNP)**. This is also well demonstrated on an MRI image of the cervical spine region in Fig. 8-30, page 257.

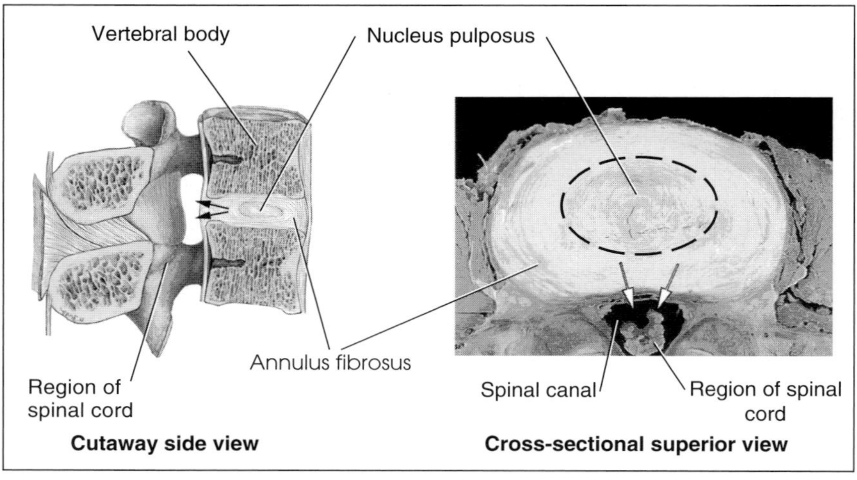

Fig. 8-10. Intervertebral disk.

CERVICAL VERTEBRAE CHARACTERISTICS

The cervical vertebrae show little resemblance to either the lumbar or thoracic vertebrae which are more typical in appearance. In fact, the upper two cervical vertebrae, C1 (the **atlas**) and C2 (the **axis**), are quite unusual as described on the following page.

The third through sixth cervical vertebrae are typical cervical vertebrae. The last or **seventh cervical vertebra** assumes many of the features of the thoracic vertebrae, including an extra long and more horizontal spinous process which can be palpated at the base of the neck. This gives C7 its special name, the **vertebra prominens**, the spinous process of which is long and prominent, making it a useful landmark for locating specific cervical and upper thoracic vertebrae and for locating the center of the lungs for chest positioning.

Superior View: Fig. 8-12 shows a typical cervical vertebra (C3-6) as viewed from above. While the parts forming the vertebral arch are all present, and the vertebra has the usual processes, they are somewhat different from those of either the typical lumbar or thoracic vertebra.

The **transverse processes** are quite small and arise from both the **pedicle** and the **body**, rather than from the pedicle-lamina junction. In addition, there is a hole in each transverse process called a **transverse foramen**. The vertebral artery and vein, and certain nerves pass through these successive transverse foramina. Therefore **one unique characteristic of all cervical vertebrae** is that they **each have three foramina**; the right and left transverse foramina and the single large vertebral foramen.

The **spinous processes** of C2 through C6 are fairly short and usually end in two tips rather than only one. This double or forked tip is called a **bifid tip, a second unique characteristic** of cervical vertebrae, specifically for C2 through C6. The bodies are small and oblong in shape with some overlapping when they are stacked in the cervical vertebral column.

***Lateral View** (Fig. 8-13):* A typical cervical vertebra as viewed from the side illustrates that the **body** is the most anterior structure and the **spinous process** is the most posterior structure. Located behind the transverse process at the junction of the pedicle and the lamina between the superior and inferior articular processes is a short column of bone that is much more supportive than the similar area in the rest of the spinal column. This column of bone is termed the **articular pillar**, sometimes shortened to just **pillar**, or to **lateral mass** if referring to C1. Located on top of each pillar is the **superior articular process**. On the bottom is found the **inferior articular process** for formation of the **zygapophyseal joint**.

Each cervical vertebra and vertebral body continues to get larger, progressing down to the seventh cervical.

Zygapophyseal Joints

The superior and inferior articular processes, as located over and under the articular pillars, are directly lateral to the large vertebral foramen. Therefore, the **zygapophyseal joints of the second through seventh cervical vertebrae are located at right angles or 90°** to the midsagittal plane and would be visualized radiographically in a **true lateral projection**.

The zygapophyseal joints between C1 and C2 are visualized only on a true frontal (AP) view.

Intervertebral Foramina

The intervertebral foramina can be identified by the pedicles which make up the floor of these foramina as shown in Figs. 8-12 and 8-14. The **intervertebral foramina are situated at a 45° angle** to the midsagittal plane, and open anteriorly as shown on this drawing. They are also directed at a 15° inferior angle due to the shape and the overlapping of the cervical vertebrae. Therefore, to "open up" and visualize these foramina radiographically, a **45° oblique position** is required, and a **15° cephalad angle** of the x-ray beam for posterior oblique (AP) projections.

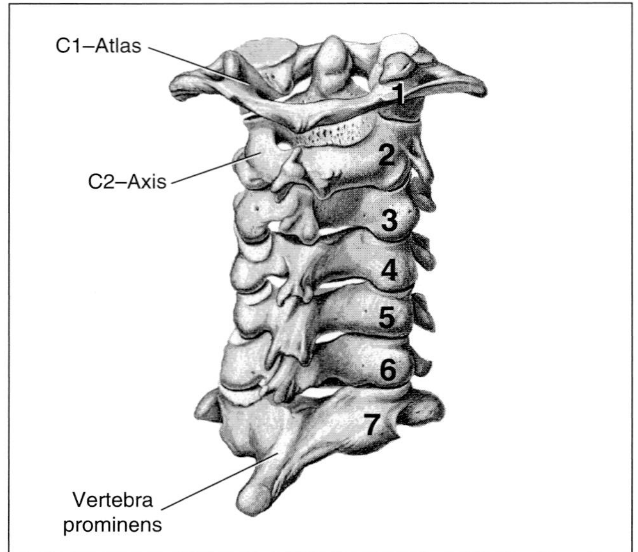

Fig. 8-11. Seven cervical vertebrae–Oblique posterior view.

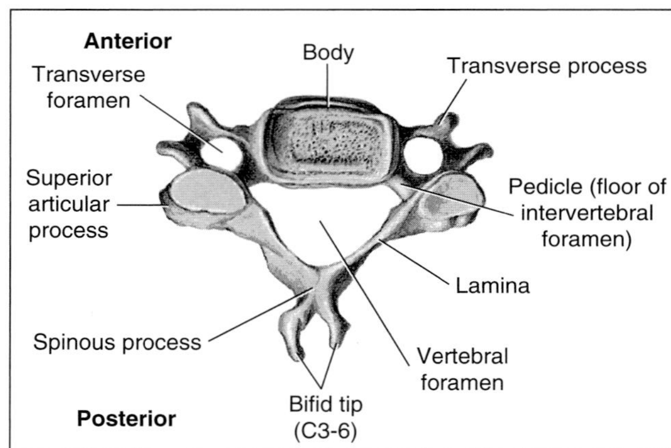

Fig. 8-12. Typical cervical vertebra–Superior view.

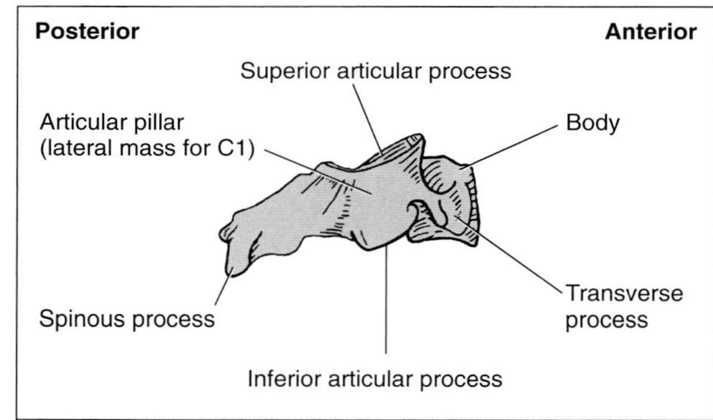

Fig. 8-13. Typical cervical vertebra–Lateral view.

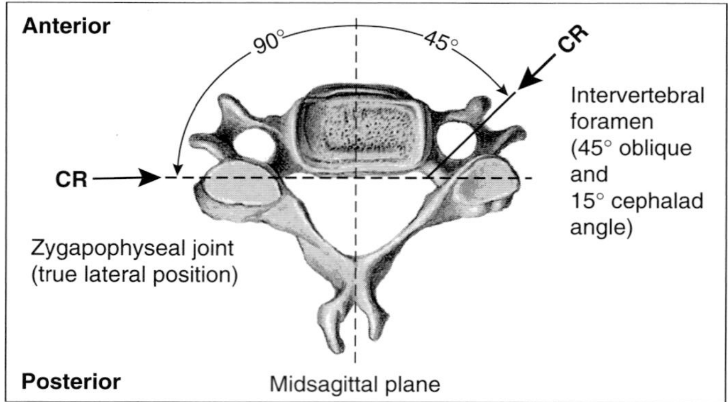

Fig. 8-14. Typical cervical vertebra (superior view).
-Zygapophyseal joints, 90° (true lateral).
-Intervertebral foramina, 45° oblique.

Atlas (C1) (Figs. 8-15 and 8-17)

The first cervical vertebra, the **atlas**, a name derived from the Greek god who bore the world upon his shoulders, least resembles a typical vertebra. Anteriorly, there is no body, but simply a thick arch of bone termed the **anterior arch**, which contains a small anterior tubercle. The **dens** or **odontoid process** is part of the second cervical vertebra (see Fig. 8-16), but is demonstrated in a sectional view of C1 (Fig. 8-15) to show it's location and how it is held in place by the **transverse atlantal ligament**.

The dens is actually the body of C1, because embryologically the C1 body fuses to C2 and becomes the dens. Therefore, in an adult, the dens projects up through the anterior portion of the large central opening of C1. This is well demonstrated on the posterior oblique view of C1-2 (Fig. 8-17) and the frontal open-mouth view radiograph of Fig. 8-18.

Posteriorly, another arch of bone of C1, the **posterior arch**, generally bears a small **posterior tubercle** at the midline (Fig. 8-15). This tubercle is all that remains of a spinous process for the atlas.

Each **superior articular process** presents a large depressed surface called **superior facet** for articulation with the respective occipital condyle of the skull. These articulations between C1, the atlas, and the occipital condyles of the skull are called **atlanto-occipital** articulations.

The **transverse processes** are smaller, but still contain the **transverse foramina** distinctive of all cervical vertebrae.

The **articular pillars**, or **lateral masses** as called for C1, are again shown as that portion of bone between the superior and inferior articular processes. For the atlas these portions are the most bulky and solid part of this vertebra to support the weight of the head, thus the term lateral masses.

Axis (C2) (Figs. 8-16 and 8-17)

The most distinctive feature of the second cervical vertebra, the **axis**, is the radiographically important **dens** or **odontoid process**, the conical process projecting up from the upper surface of the **body.**

Rotation of the head primarily occurs between C1 and C2, with the dens acting as a pivot helping to make this type of motion possible. The superior facets of the superior articular processes articulating with the skull also assist in rotation of the head.

Severe stress as the possible result of a forced flexion-hyperextension "whiplash" type of injury may cause a fracture of the dens. Any fracture of the vertebral column at this level could result in serious damage to the spinal cord as well.

As seen in Fig. 8-16, the **inferior articular process** for articulation with C3 lies inferior to the **lamina.** Below and lateral to the superior articular process is the transverse process with its **transverse foramen.** The blunt **spinous process** extends posteriorly.

Relationship of C1 and C2 (Figs. 8-17 and 8-18)

The relationship of C2, with its dens, to C1, and the relationship of C1 to the base of the skull, are highly important. Fig. 8-18 demonstrates the view as seen on an AP radiograph of the upper cervical spine taken with the mouth wide open. The anterior arch of C1, which lies in front of the dens, is only faintly visible on this frontal view because it is a fairly thin piece of bone compared to the larger, more dense dens.

Normally, articulations between C2 and C1, such as the **zygapophyseal joints**, are **perfectly symmetrical**. Accordingly, **the relationship of the dens to C1 must also be perfectly symmetrical**. Both injury and improper positioning can render these areas asymmetrical. For example, **rotation of the skull** can alter the symmetry of these spaces and joints thus imitating an injury. Therefore accurate positioning for this region is essential. The parts are labeled on the drawing of Fig. 8-17, and the radiograph of Fig. 8-18 as follows:

A. Centrally located dens.
B. Left transverse process of C1.
C. Left lateral mass of C1.
D. Inferior articular surface of C1.
E. Left zygapophyseal joint.
F. Body of C2.
G. Right superior articular surface of C2.

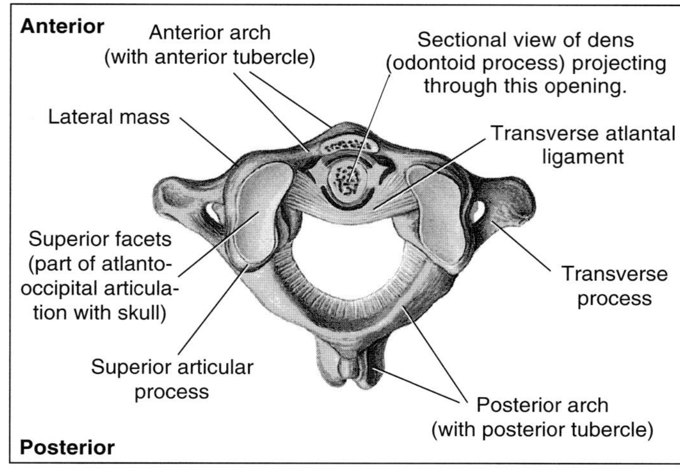

Fig. 8-15. Atlas (C1)–Superior view.

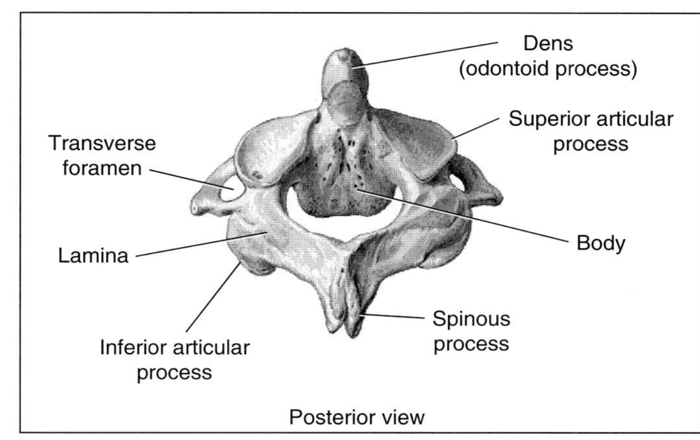

Fig. 8-16. Axis (C2)–Posterior superior view.

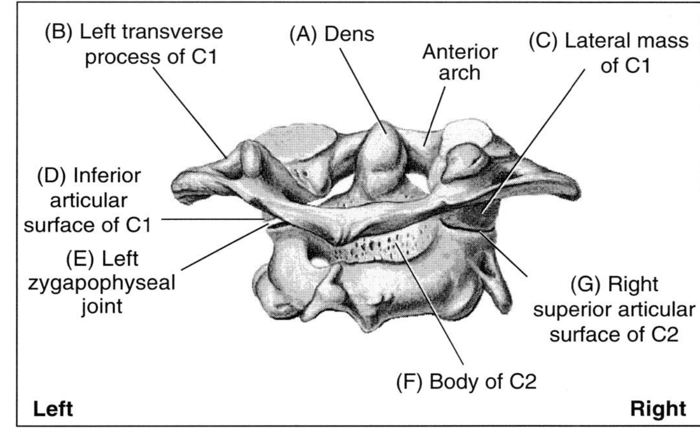

Fig. 8-17. C1 and C2–Posterior oblique view.

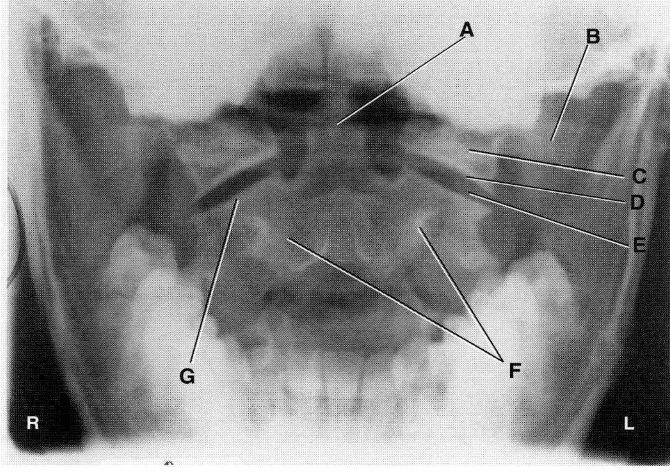

Fig. 8-18. AP open mouth radiograph.

THORACIC VERTEBRAE CHARACTERISTICS

An overview of the twelve thoracic vertebrae reveals a marked difference in size and appearance of upper vertebrae as compared to lower ones as demonstrated in Fig. 8-19.

The middle four thoracic vertebrae, 5, 6, 7 and 8, are considered typical thoracic vertebrae. The lower four are larger and assume some of the characteristics of the lumbar vertebrae, while the upper four gradually get smaller and assume features of the cervical region. This difference in size contributes to density of these vertebrae as seen on an AP radiograph wherein the upper unequal thoracic vertebrae appear dark and overexposed compared to the lower larger vertebrae.

Rib Articulations

The one important feature of all thoracic vertebrae that serves to distinguish them from all others is that **all thoracic vertebrae have facets for articulation with ribs.** Each thoracic vertebra is closely associated with one pair of ribs. Since there are 12 pairs of ribs, there are also 12 thoracic vertebrae. Note in Fig. 8-20 that the two lumbar vertebrae, L1 and L2 do not show facets for rib articulations.

Costovertebral Joints: A unique characteristic of thoracic vertebrae is that all 12 vertebrae have either **a full facet** *(fas′ et)* or **two partial facets**, called **demifacets** *(dem″ e-fas′ et)*, on each side of the body. Each facet or combination of two demifacets accepts the head of a rib to form a **costovertebral joint** (Figs. 8-19, 8-20 and 8-21).

Those vertebrae with two demifacets share the heads of two ribs, one on the right and one on the left. The demifacet on the bottom of one vertebra articulates with the superior portion of the head of a particular rib, while the demifacet near the top of the next vertebra articulates with the inferior part of the same head.

The first thoracic vertebra (T1) has on each side of its body a superior whole facet and an inferior demifacet. This indicates that the heads of the **first pair of ribs** articulate with the **upper part of T1** vertebra, (top of Fig. 8-19). This fact becomes important when identifying T1 vertebrae by association with the posterior first pair of ribs, which are readily seen on radiographs of the cervical and thoracic spine.

Thoracic vertebrae 10, 11 and 12 (T10-12) have a **single costal facet on each side** indicating the heads of the 10th, 11th & 12th ribs articulate with the respective vertebrae at these facets. This again provides a means of identifying these specific vertebrae.

Costotransverse Joints: In addition to the costovertebral joint, each of the **first ten thoracic vertebrae** also have facets (one on each transverse process) that articulate with the tubercles of ribs 1 through 10. These articulations are termed **costotransverse joints**. Note in Figs. 8-19 and 8-20 that T11 and T12 do not show facets at the ends of the transverse process for rib articulations. Thus as the first ten pairs of ribs flare out away from the upper ten vertebrae, the tubercle of each rib articulates with one transverse process to form a costotransverse joint, **while ribs 11 and 12 only articulate at the costovertebral joints**.

The superior cross-sectional view of the rib articulations (Fig. 8-21) demonstrates that the ribs 1 to 10 do articulate with the thoracic vertebrae at both the body and transverse process. However, these are not always clearly separated joints but tend to blend together as a **single extended articulation enclosed in synovial capsules** lined by synovial membrane. Thus these are **synovial joints,** which are **diarthrodial** or slightly movable of the **plane** or gliding **movement type**. This allows for slight gliding movements at these two sites of articulation. This is further demonstrated and described in Chapter 10 on the bony thorax.

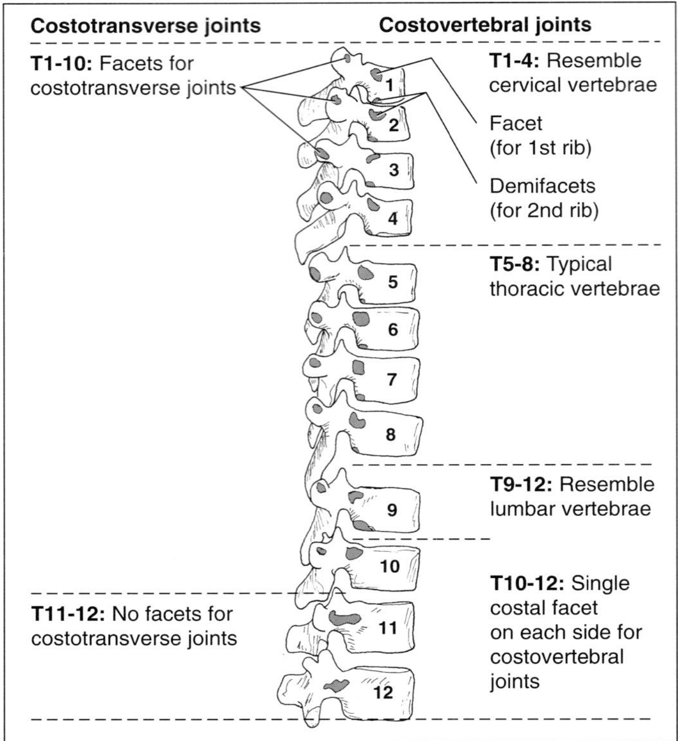

Fig. 8-19. Thoracic vertebrae (rib articulations).

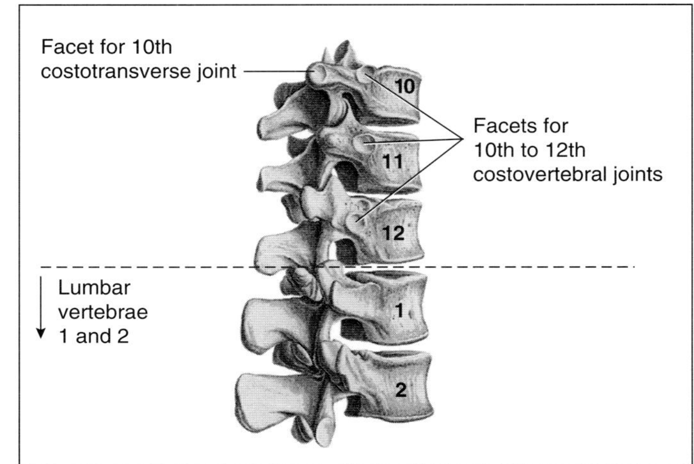

Fig. 8-20. T10-L2 (rib articulations on T10-12 only).

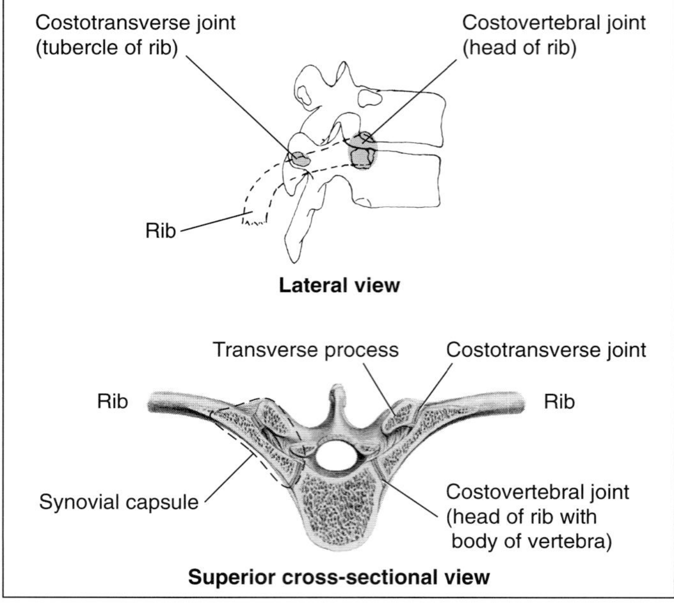

Fig. 8-21. Costovertebral and costotransverse joints–Ribs 1 to 10.

Typical Thoracic Vertebrae

Superior and Lateral Views *(Fig. 8-22)***:** A typical thoracic vertebra as seen from above and from the side is illustrated. The **body** is the most anterior structure, while the **spinous process** is the most posterior structure. The spinous process seems fairly short when viewed in this direction, but remember that it is projected primarily downward.

The vertebral arch is composed of the two **pedicles** projecting from the body and the two **laminae**. Each **transverse process** projects from the junction of the pedicle and the lamina on each side.

The articular **facet of the inferior articular process** is shown which articulates with the superior process of the adjoining vertebrae below it to form the **zygapophyseal joint**. This is best illustrated in the lateral oblique view of Fig. 8-23.

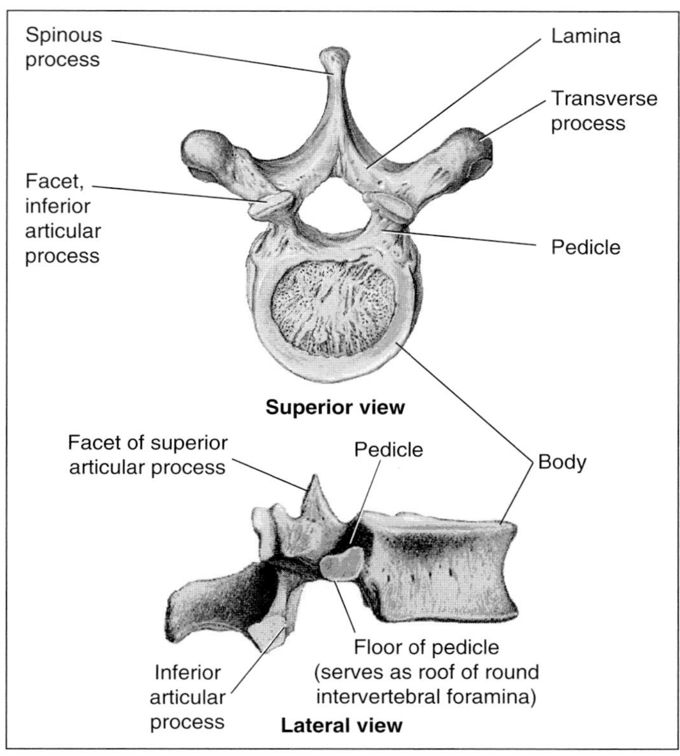

Fig. 8-22. Typical thoracic vertebrae.

Lateral Oblique View *(Fig. 8-23)***:** The two **transverse processes** of thoracic vertebra T1 through T10 are shown to be unique in that each of these has a facet near its end for articulation with ribs as described on the preceding page.

The **superior articular processes** (facing primarily posteriorly) and the **inferior articular processes** (facing more anteriorly) are again shown to connect the successive thoracic vertebrae to form the **zygapophyseal** (apophyseal) joints.

On each side, between any two thoracic vertebrae, are **intervertebral foramina**. The main distinguishing characteristic of the thoracic vertebrae, however, is the fact that each thoracic vertebra possess facets for rib articulation.

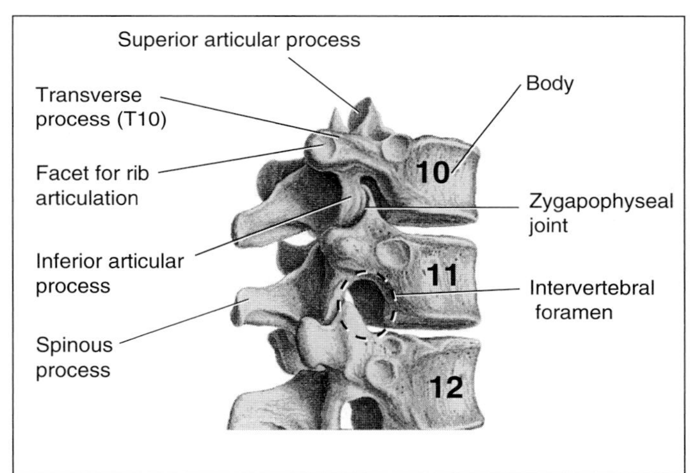

Fig. 8-23. Typical thoracic vertebrae (lateral oblique view).

Zygapophyseal Joints

The structure and angles of the facets of the inferior and superior articular processes making up the zygapophyseal joints differ markedly from that of the cervical vertebrae. These joints on the cervical vertebrae form an angle of 90°, but on the thoracic vertebrae, this angle is from **70° to 75° from the midsagittal plane**. Therefore, to demonstrate these joints radiographically on the thoracic spine requires a **70° to 75° oblique**, which is 15° to 20° from the lateral position.

Intervertebral Foramina

The location of the intervertebral foramina can be identified on these drawings by the pedicles which make up the roof and floor of these foramina or openings. As demonstrated in Fig. 8-24, the openings of the intervertebral foramina on the thoracic vertebra are located at right angles or **90° to the midsagittal plane** as compared to 45° on the cervical. Therefore, to demonstrate these foramina radiographically, **a true lateral position** is required for thoracic vertebrae rather than the 45° oblique for cervical vertebrae.

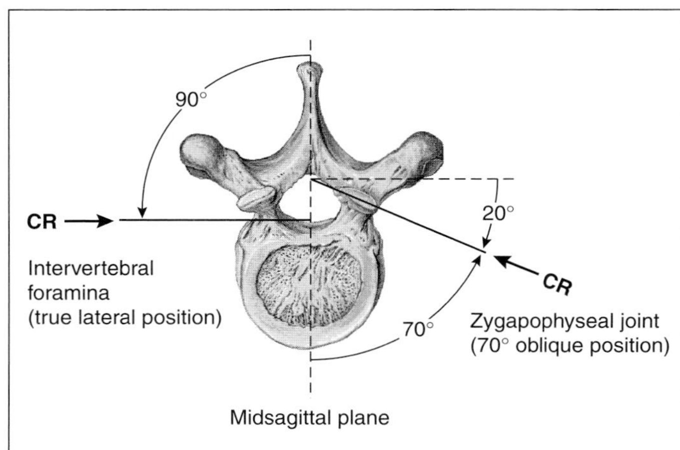

Fig. 8-24. Typical thoracic vertebrae.
- Intervertebral foramina, 90° (true lateral).
- Zygapophyseal joints, 70 to 75° (oblique).

ANATOMY REVIEW WITH RADIOGRAPHS

AP Cervical Spine (Fig. 8-25)

A conventional AP radiograph of the cervical spine is illustrated. Usually, the first two or three thoracic vertebrae, as well as C7 up to C3, are seen well on this projection. Identifying specific cervical vertebrae is possible by starting with T1, which can be identified by the attachment of the first pair of ribs. Therefore, to localize T1, locate the most superior ribs and find the vertebra to which they appear to connect. After locating T1, the visible cervical vertebrae can be identified by starting at C7 and counting upward.

Part **A** on this radiograph is the first thoracic vertebra, determined by discovering that part **B** is the first rib on the patient's right side.
Part **C** is the fourth cervical vertebra (count up from T1 and C7).
Part **D** is the articular pillar or lateral mass region of C3.

Note: The white area at the top of the radiograph is created by the combined shadows of the base of the skull and the mandible. These structures effectively cover up the first two cervical vertebrae on this type of radiograph.

Part **E** is the spinous process of C3 seen on end.

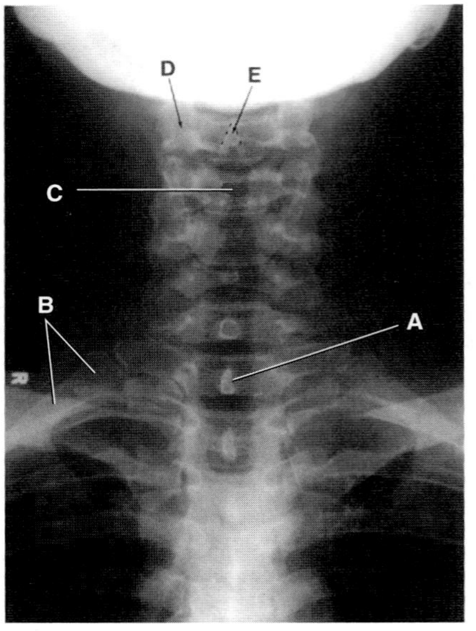

Fig. 8-25. AP C spine.

8

AP and Lateral Thoracic Spine

Individual thoracic vertebrae can best be identified on the AP projection because of rib associations. The posterior ribs 1 to 12 can be readily seen and counted thus identifying specific thoracic vertebra. This is more difficult on the lateral thoracic spine unless the sternum can also be seen.

***AP T Spine** (Fig. 8-26):*

A. 1st posterior rib
B. 10th posterior rib
C. Spinous process of T11, faintly seen on edge through body.
D. Body of T12
E. Intervertebral disk space between T8 and T9
F. Body of T7 (center of T spine and of average chest)
G. Body of T1 (remember heads of 1st ribs articulate with upper portion of T1)

***Lateral T spine** (Fig. 8-27):*

A. Body of T3. Count up from T12, assuming the top edge of T12 is at the level of costophrenic angle (posterior tip) of diaphragm.
B. Body of T7 (center of T spine and of chest)
C. Intervertebral foramina between T11 and T12 (best demonstrated on a lateral projection for the T spine).

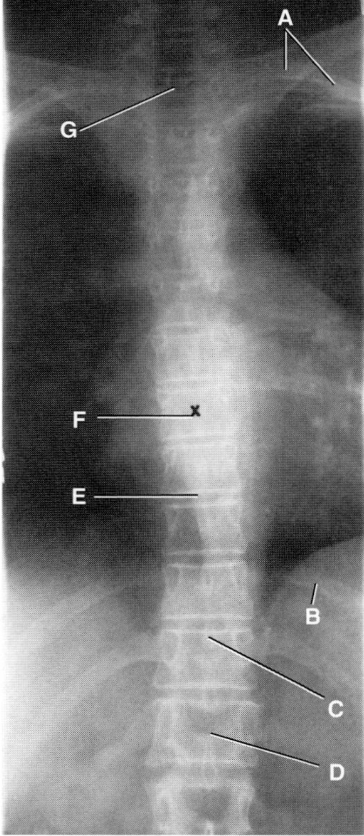

Fig. 8-26. AP T spine.

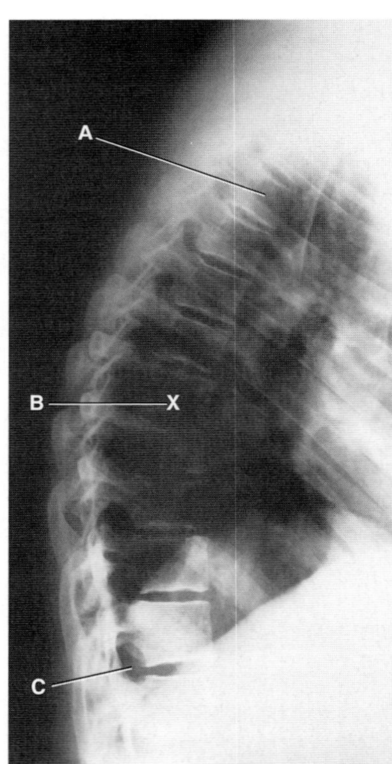

Fig. 8-27. Lateral T spine.

Lateral Cervical Spine (Fig. 8-28)

The single most important radiograph in any cervical spine series is a good lateral. A good lateral cervical spine radiograph is demonstrated in Fig. 8-28. Radiographers should always try to show all seven cervical vertebrae on any lateral cervical spine radiograph if this is possible. At times this is difficult on those patients with thick shoulders and a short neck, and a special "swimmer's" lateral may need to be taken to include C7. This radiograph is an exceptional lateral cervical, visualizing even the body of T1. Most patients have shorter necks and thicker shoulders making visualization of C7 and T1 more difficult. In order to determine if all seven cervical vertebrae are being shown, locate the atlas, or C1, and count downward. Remember that C1 has a posterior arch with a small tubercle resembling a small spinous process which can be readily identified on a lateral view. Therefore counting this as the 1st spinous process, (labeled as B), one can count down to C7, the body of which is marked with an X.

The lower anterior margins of the last four or five cervical vertebral bodies have a slight lipped appearance which, along with the general shape of the bodies, requires that the central ray (CR) be angled approximately **20° cephalad** (toward the head) to "open up" these lower **intervertebral spaces**. This is demonstrated by the CR arrow angled 20° cephalad to pass through these intervertebral spaces.

A. Dens (odontoid process) enhanced with dotted lines on this visual, seen extending up through C1.
B. Posterior arch and tubercle of the atlas, C1 (also see A in Fig. 8-29)
C. Body of C3
D. Zygapophyseal joint between C4 and C5 (Best shown on a lateral projection for the cervical spine)
E. Spinous process of C6
F. Body of C7
G. Spinous process of C7, vertebral prominens (a positioning landmark)

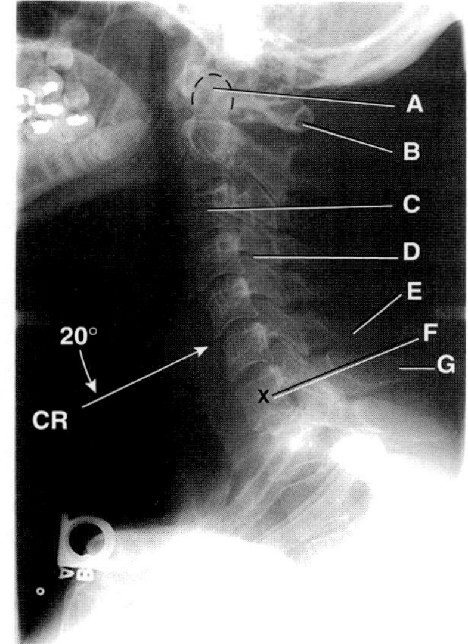

Fig. 8-28. Lateral C spine.

Oblique Cervical Spine (Fig. 8-29)

A good **oblique cervical spine** radiograph is shown in Fig. 8-29. An important purpose of the oblique position is to show the **intervertebral foramina.** Spinal nerves to and from the spinal cord are transmitted through these intervertebral foramina. Remember this is taken in a **45° oblique position** with the central ray angled **15° cephalad**, if taken as posterior obliques.

A. Posterior arch and tubercle of Cl
B. Intervertebral foramen between C4 and C5 (count down from C1)
C. Pedicle of C6
D. Body of C7

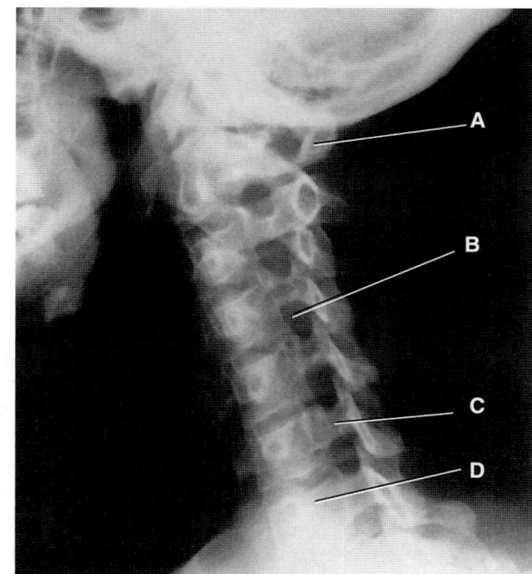

Fig. 8-29. Oblique C spine.

MRI Image, Sagittal Section of Lateral Cervical Spine (Fig. 8-29)

The MRI sagittal section image of a cervical spine clearly demonstrates not only bony structure but soft tissue as well.

The vertebral canal containing the **spinal cord** (A) is seen as the tubelike column directly posterior to the cervical vertebrae. The spinal cord is a continuation of the **medulla oblongata** (B) of the brain. A herniation of the disk between C5 and C6 is demonstrated with a slight posterior displacement, causing mild spinal cord displacement (see arrows).

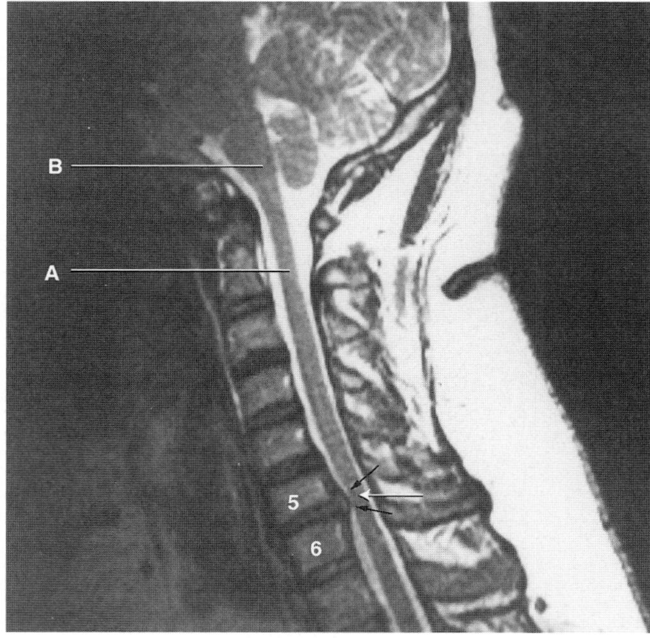

Fig. 8-30. MRI sagittal section, C spine. (Demonstrates herniated disk between C5 and C6.)

INTERVERTEBRAL FORAMINA VS. ZYGAPOPHYSEAL JOINTS

Two anatomical areas of the spine that generally need to be demonstrated by the proper radiographs are the **intervertebral foramina** and the **zygapophyseal joints**. This is especially important for the cervical spine. The physician gains important information concerning the relationship of consecutive vertebrae by studying these two areas on the appropriate radiograph. To complicate matters, however, depending on the part of the spine to be radiographed (cervical, thoracic, or lumbar), a different body position is required to best show each anatomical area.

Cervical Spine Skeleton (Figs. 8-31 and 8-32)

Two photographs of the cervical vertebrae are shown in position to visualize these areas on the cervical vertebrae. On the left is a cervical section of the vertebral column in a left lateral position, while to the right is a 45° left posterior oblique position (LPO). The **zygapophyseal joints** visualize well on the **lateral position** (see arrows).

On the right, the posterior oblique with a 45° rotation shows that the intervertebral foramina are clearly opened (see arrows). It is important to know that the **left posterior oblique** position opens up the foramina on the **right side**, and a 15° CR **cephalad angle** is needed. Therefore, on a **posterior oblique** cervical spine radiograph, the upside is the side on which the intervertebral foramina are opened well.

If this were taken in an **anterior** oblique position, the foramina **closest** to the film, the downside would be open, and a 15° **caudad angle** would be required.

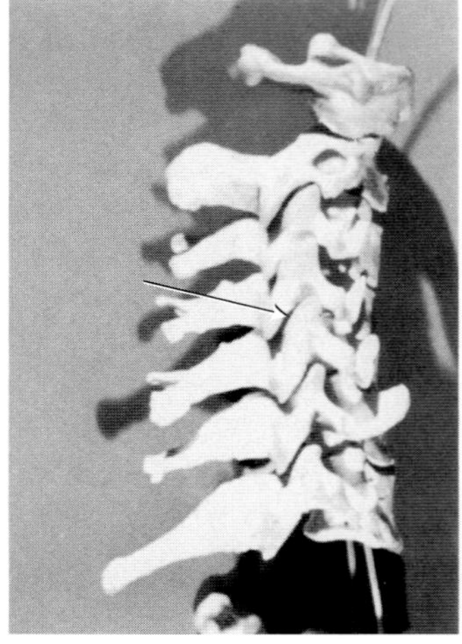

Fig. 8-31. Left lateral.
-Zygapophyseal joints.

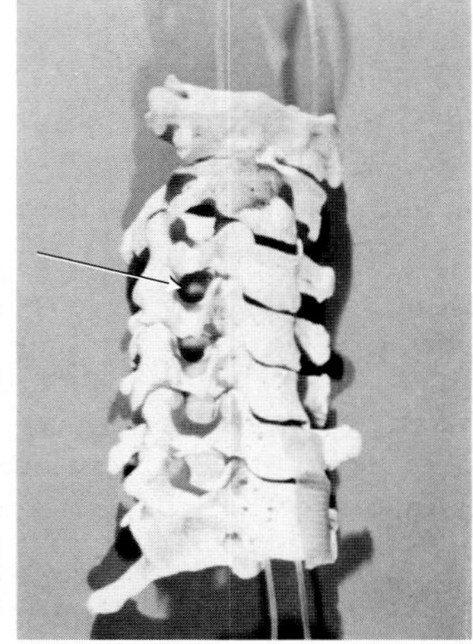

Fig. 8-32. Oblique (LPO).
-Right Intervertebral foramina (upside).

Cervical Spine Radiographs (Figs. 8-33 and 8-34)

The two radiographs of the cervical spine illustrate the same anatomy in the same two positions as shown on the skeleton above. The lateral position on the left best shows the zygapophyseal joints. The joint on each side is superimposed upon the joint on the opposite side. One should remember that the zygapophyseal joints are located between the articular pillars of each vertebra.

The oblique cervical spine radiograph on the right shows the circular intervertebral foramina opened. In each oblique radiograph only one set of foramina are opened, while the ones on the opposite side are closed. Since this position is a **left posterior** oblique, the **right intervertebral foramina** or those on the **upside** are being shown.

It is important to remember that the LPO will show the same anatomy as the RAO. Therefore, if the patient were placed in an **anterior** oblique position, the **downside** foramina to the film will be shown. Thus in either case, LPO or RAO, the right intervertebral foramina will be visualized.

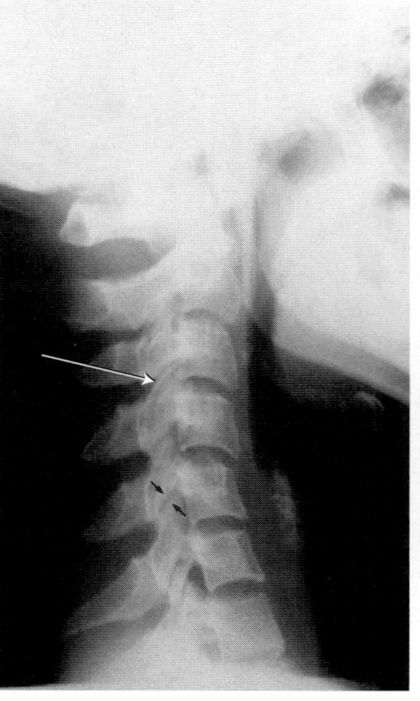

Fig. 8-33. Lateral (left)
-Zygapophyseal joints demonstrated.

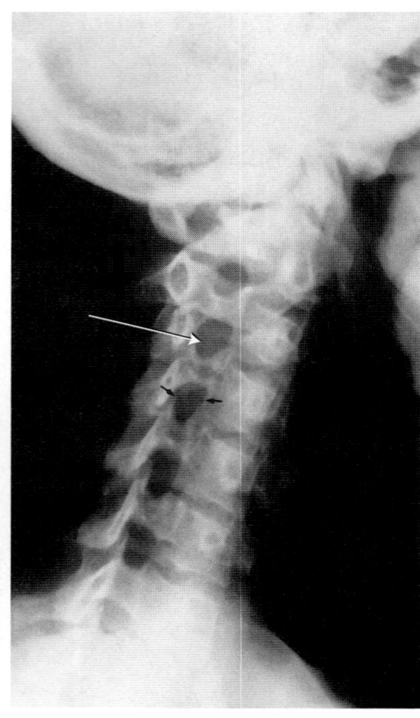

Fig. 8-34. Oblique (LPO)
-Right intervertebral foramina (upside).

Summary Chart

Cervical Spine	
Intervertebral foramina – 45° oblique	*Zygapophyseal joints – 90° lateral*
CR 15° cephalad - upside visualized LPO – Right foramina RPO – Left foramina **CR 15° caudad - downside visualized** LAO – Left foramina RAO - Right foramina	R or L Lateral

Thoracic Spine Skeleton (Figs. 8-35 and 8-36)

Two photographs of the thoracic vertebrae are shown. The thoracic vertebrae on the left are in a lateral position, and on the right, an oblique position. The **lateral position** of the thoracic spine best shows the **intervertebral foramina**. A **70° oblique** is necessary to open up the **zygapophyseal joints** on the thoracic spine.

The **posterior** oblique position on the right shows the zygapophyseal joint on the **upside**. **Anterior** obliques would demonstrate the **downside** joints.

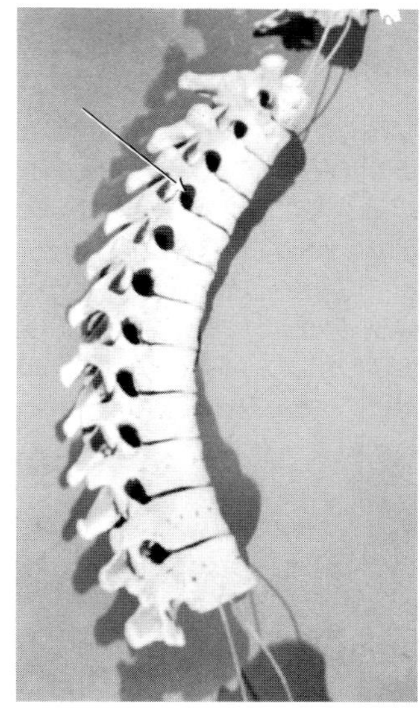

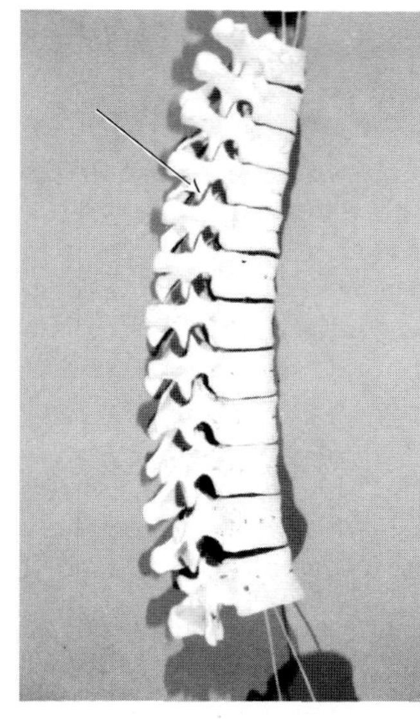

Fig. 8-35. Thoracic spine. Left lateral -Intervertebral foramina.

Fig. 8-36. Thoracic spine. Oblique (LPO) -Upside zygapophyseal joints.

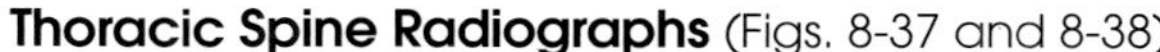

Thoracic Spine Radiographs (Figs. 8-37 and 8-38)

Radiographs of the thoracic spine in the lateral position, and in the 70° oblique position correspond to the position of the thoracic skeleton directly above. Observe that the round openings of the superimposed **intervertebral foramina** are best visualized on the **lateral** radiograph on the left (see arrows).

The **zygapophyseal joints** are best visualized on the **oblique** radiograph on the right. The oblique radiograph is in a 70° LPO position, which should best visualize the zygapophyseal joints on the **upside,** or those farthest away from the film. The LPO position best shows the **right zygapophyseal** joints.

If the obliques were taken as **anterior** obliques, the opposite would be true, the **downside** joints would be demonstrated. An **LAO** would demonstrate the **left** zygapophyseal joints. Therefore, an LAO would demonstrate the same side joints as an RPO, as seen in the chart below.

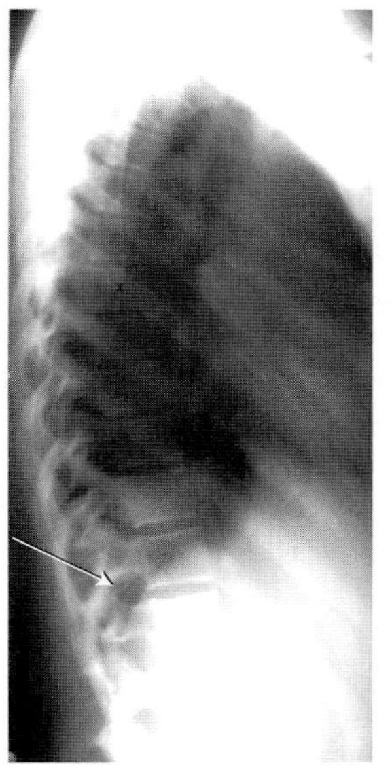

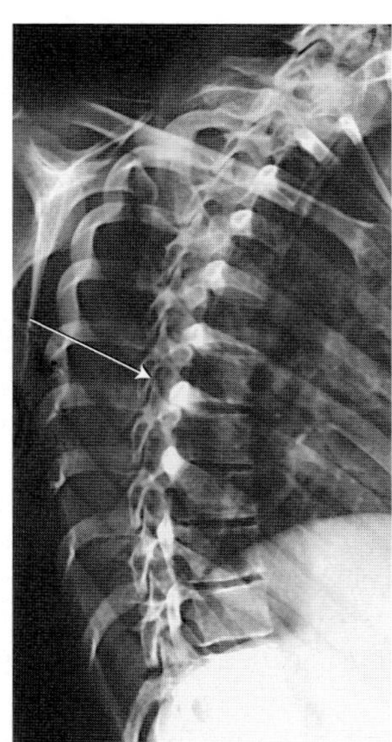

Fig. 8-37. Thoracic spine. Left lateral -Intervertebral foramina.

Fig. 8-38. Thoracic spine. Oblique (LPO) -Right (upside) zygapophyseal joints.

Summary Chart

Thoracic Spine

Intervertebral foramina – 90° lateral	*Zygapophyseal joints – 70° oblique*
R or L Lateral	**Posterior Obliques – Upside** LPO – Right zygapophyseal RPO – Left zygapophyseal **Anterior Oblique –Downside** LAO – Left zygapophyseal RAO – Right zygapophyseal

Summary of Intervertebral Foramina and Zygapophyseal Joints

The chart on the right summarizes which position of each region of the spine best visualizes either the intervertebral foramina or the zygapophyseal joints. The **intervertebral foramina** are best shown on the **oblique cervical**, and on the **lateral thoracic or lumbar**.

The zygapophyseal joints are best seen on the **lateral cervical**, the near **lateral thoracic (70°)** and the **45° oblique lumbar** (as will be described in Chapter 9).

The **upper body**, the cervical and thoracic regions, shows the **upside** best, while the **lower body** shows the **downside** best when radiographed anterior to posterior as posterior obliques.

Total Vertebrae Summary

	Intervertebral foramina	*Zygapophyseal joints*
Cervical:	Oblique 45° Upside (LPO or RPO)	Lateral
Thoracic:	Lateral	Posterior oblique – 70° Upside (LPO or RPO)
Lumbar: (Chapter 9)	Lateral	Posterior oblique – 45° Downside (LPO or RPO)

Radiographic Positioning

TOPOGRAPHICAL LANDMARKS

Sternum

The sternum provides some useful landmarks for locating various levels of the thoracic spine. The sternum is divided into three basic sections. The upper section is called the **manubrium.** The very top part of the manubrium, the **jugular** (suprasternal) **notch**, can be easily felt. The central portion of the sternum is called the **body.** The manubrium and body connect at a slight, easily located angle termed the **sternal angle.** The most inferior end of the sternum is called the **xiphoid process.** It takes some pressure to locate the xiphoid process on a patient.

With careful palpation or probing of these topographic landmarks, certain anatomical structures and relationships between structures can be determined. For example, the level of specific thoracic vertebrae can be determined from these three sternal landmarks—the jugular notch, the sternal angle and the xiphoid process. Both the sternal angle and the xiphoid process can be palpated, although they are not as easy to locate as the jugular notch.

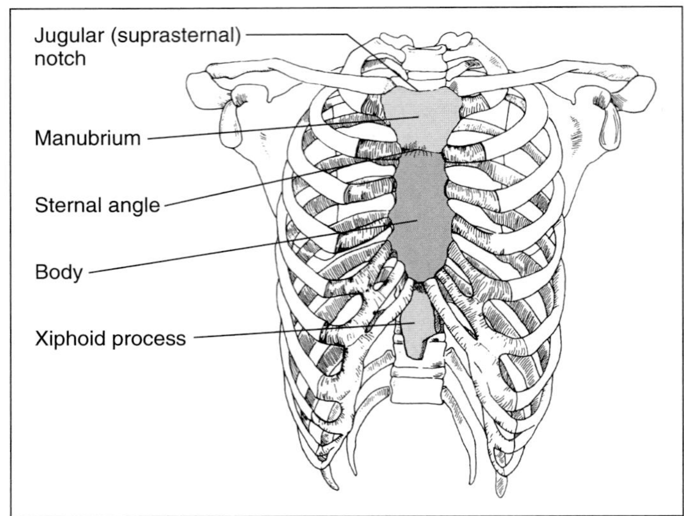

Fig. 8-39. Sternum.

Thoracic Spine

The bottom part of the xiphoid process, the **xiphoid tip,** is at the level of **T10** as indicated by line **A**. The **sternal angle** (line **C**) locates the **junction of T4 and T5**. The sternal angle is most easily located if one first locates the jugular notch and then follows the manubrium down about 2 in. or 5 cm until a slight bump is felt. The slight bump on the surface of the sternum should be the sternal angle. The second pair of ribs attach just lateral to the sternal angle.

One of the most important centering points for the thoracic spine is line **B** which locates **T7** at a level of **3 to 4 in.** (8 to 10 cm) **below the jugular notch**. The approximate center of the thoracic portion of the vertebral column is at the level of T7. The mid seventh thoracic vertebra is the center of the 12 thoracic vertebrae since the lower thoracic vertebrae are larger in size than the upper thoracic vertebrae.

The jugular notch is identified by line **D**, which is at the same level as the **disk space between T2 and T3.** Often, on a prepared skeleton, the jugular notch is closer to T 1, but this is not true on a person standing upright. On an average, standing adult, T1 is located 1½ in. or (3.75 cm) above the jugular notch, marked as line **E**.

The first thoracic vertebra can also be located by palpating posteriorly at the base of the neck for the prominent spinous process of C7, the **vertebra prominens**. Note that the long sloping vertebra prominens extends downward with its tip at the level of the body of T1.

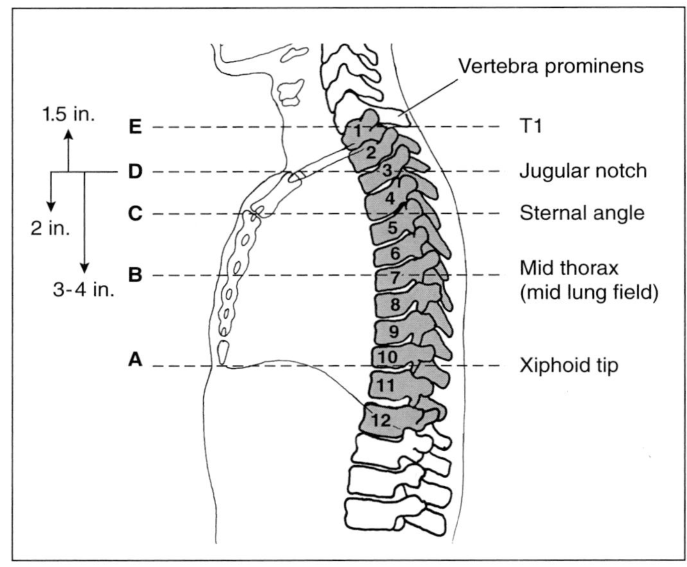

Fig. 8-40. T spine landmarks.

Cervical Spine

The prominent topographical landmarks of the cervical region are illustrated. The prominent spinous process of the last cervical vertebra, **C7** (vertebra prominens), is at about the same level as the **body of T1**. On an average patient this is slightly above the level of the shoulders as shown on the model on the following page. The shoulders occasionally superimpose the last cervical vertebra on a lateral cervical spine radiograph. When this problem occurs, the shoulders must be depressed as much as possible.

The most prominent part of the **thyroid cartilage,** or "Adam's apple" **(B)**, is at an approximate level of C5. This is not a reliable bony landmark, however, and varies between the level of C4 to C6. With the head in a neutral position, the angle of the jaw, or **gonion (C),** is at the same level as **C3.** The **mastoid tip (D)** corresponds to the level of **C1**. The **EAM** (external acoustic meatus) **(E)** is easy to locate on any person and is about **1 inch or 2.5 cm above the level of C1.**

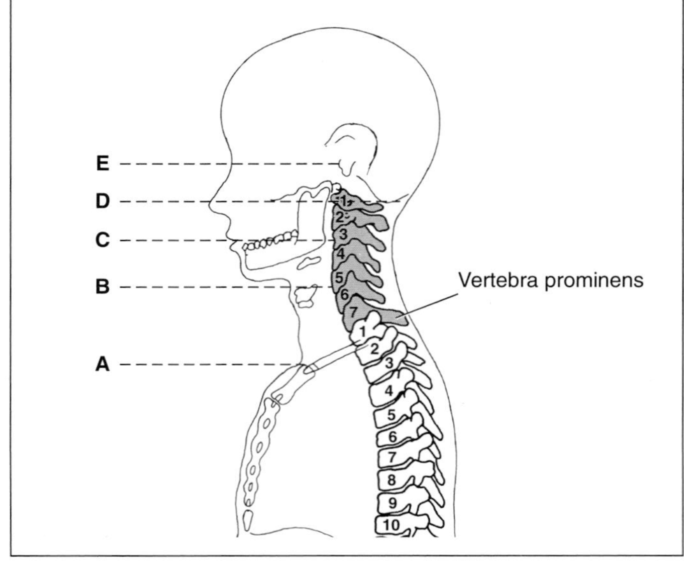

Fig. 8-41. C spine landmarks.

Sternum and T Spine Landmarks

The standard landmarks for the sternum and thoracic spine, which are illustrated on the model below, are as follows:

A. Line **A** is at the level of the **xiphoid tip**, which locates **T10**.
B. An important centering point is represented by line **B**, which anteriorly is 3 to 4 inches (8 to 10 cm) **below the jugular notch** at the level of **T7**. This is the center of the thoracic spine as well as the center of the lungs. Posteriorly this is about a handspread, 7 to 8 inches (18 to 20 cm), **below the vertebra prominens**. On a well developed male such as this model, anteriorly this would be 4 to 5 in. (8 to 10 cm) below the jugular notch, and posteriorly 8 inches (20 cm) below the vertebra prominens as described in Chapter 2 on chest positioning. For a smaller male and for the average female these would be 3 to 4 in. (8 to 10 cm) anteriorly, and about 7 inches (18 cm) posteriorly.
C. Line **C,** is at the **sternal angle** and corresponds to the disk space between **T4** and **T5**.
D. The **jugular notch** which corresponds to line **D** is at the level of the junction between **T2 and T3**.
E. Line **E** corresponds to **T1**, the vertebra prominens, about 1 to 2 inches or (2.5 to 5 cm) above the jugular notch.

The sternum and the vertebra prominens can be used to locate individual thoracic vertebra. The use of these landmarks becomes necessary when well-collimated radiographs are required of specific thoracic vertebrae.

C Spine Landmarks

These cervical spine landmarks are also identified on the side view of this model (Fig. 8-43).

C7-T1: The tops of the shoulders on an average adult are located slightly below the level of C7-T1. This landmark does vary on different people, however, since on a very thin patient the shoulders may go down to T2 or T3. For a well developed male, such as this model, the shoulders slope and vary in such a way that they do **not** present a reliable positioning landmark. Since the spinous process of C7 (at level of T1), the **vertebra prominens**, is very prominent (especially with head tipped forward), it should be used to help locate C7 and T1 rather than the top of the shoulders. This is an important landmark for the radiographer due to the importance of including all of C7 on a lateral cervical radiograph.

C4-C5: The **thyroid cartilage** of the larynx or "Adam's apple" localizes the **approximate** level of **C4** or **C5**. On most patients the upper margin of the thyroid cartilage corresponds nearer to the level of C4.

C3: The **angle** or **gonion** of the mandible is at the level of **C3** when the head is in a neutral position.

C1: The top of the cervical spine, or **C1**, is at the level of the **mastoid tip**. The mastoid tip can also be used to find the most inferior level of the base of the skull. The occipital condyles and foramen magnum are basal skull structures in line with the mastoid tip.

EAM: The **EAM** (external auditory meatus) is about 1 inch (2.5 cm) above the level of C1.

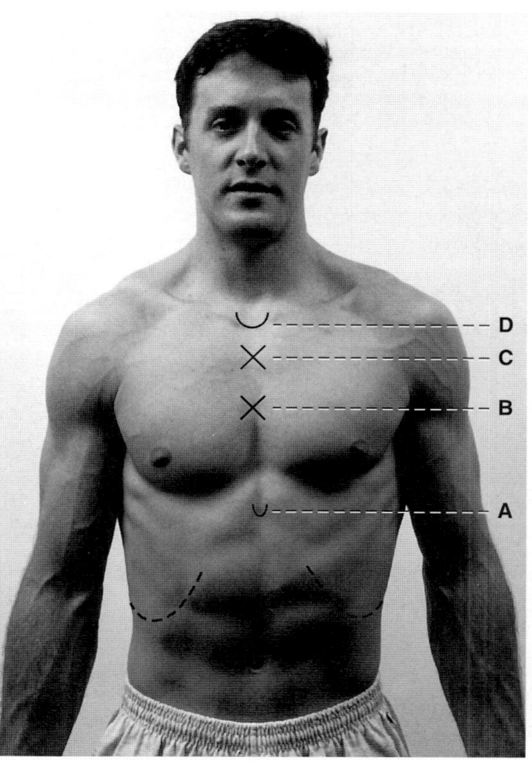

Fig. 8-42.

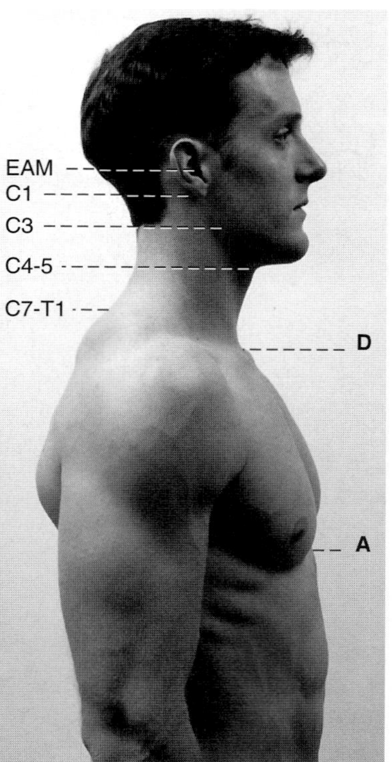

Fig. 8-43.

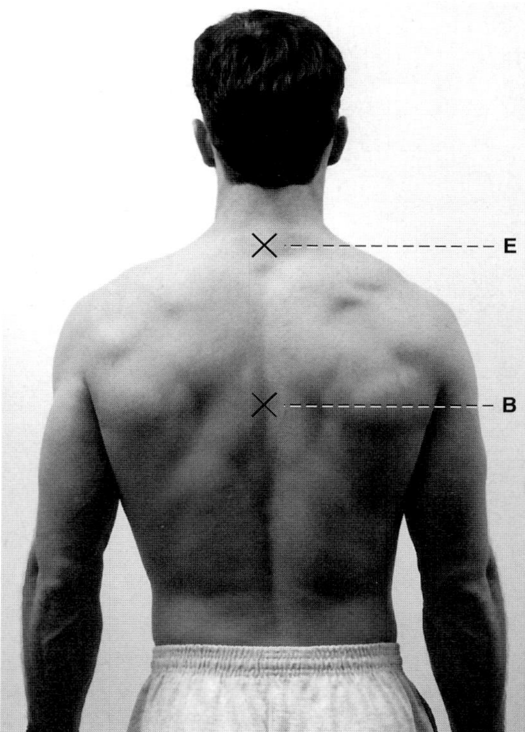

Fig. 8-44.

Sternum, T spine and C spine landmarks.

POSITIONING CONSIDERATIONS

Radiographic examinations of the cervical spine are generally taken erect, either seated or standing in front of a chest-board type film holder with a moving or stationary grid, or with the table in an erect position. They can also be taken recumbent on the table if the patient's condition requires this.

Generally all spine exams are done using a grid except possibly for the cervical spine on small patients, which can be done with screens and no grid. The lateral cervical is also frequently taken with screens and no grid due to the object image distance (OID), which provides for an air gap that reduces the amount of scatter reaching the film.

Thoracic and lumbosacral spines are taken on the table with Bucky grids, except for certain special scoliosis exams with flexion and extension, and right and left bending positions, which need to be taken erect as described in Chapter 9.

Distance and Focal Spot

Certain cervical spine projections, such as the lateral and obliques, are generally taken with an **increased SID** of 60 to 72 inches (150-172 cm) to compensate for the increased OID, resulting in less magnification and better detail.

The **small focal spot** should also always be used for cervical spines, especially the lateral and obliques due to the loss of detail occurring with the increase in OID. The lateral thoracic and lumbar spine also results in a greater OID. However, one must be aware of tube-rating limitations, and the small focal spot may not be able to be used for lateral thoracic, lumbar or sacrum and coccyx imaging on large adult patients.

Patient Protection

Optimum radiation protection practices are important in spine radiography. This is due to the proximity of the exposure field to radiosensitive tissues such as the **gonads** for thoracic and lumbar spines. Additional radiosensitive areas include the **thyroid and parathyroid glands**, **lungs** and **female breasts** for the cervical and thoracic spine. The exposure to each of these radiosensitive areas can be minimized by close collimation and the use of correctly-placed contact shields. Also, the thyroid dose can be reduced significantly on cervical obliques with anterior obliques rather than posterior obliques (see comparative patient dose icon boxes on page 267).

Exposure Factors

The principal exposure factors for radiographs of the spine include:

1. Medium to Higher kVp:
C spine–70-80 kVp, T and L spine–80-95 kVp.

Note: The use of **higher kVp increases exposure latitude**, especially on the AP thoracic spine due to the smaller size upper thoracic vertebra bodies as compared to the lower vertebrae, and also the thickness difference of the upper thorax and mediastinum as compared to the lower thorax. Sometimes compensation "wedge" type filters are used to achieve a more uniform density for the entire AP thoracic spine.

Higher kVp with corresponding mAs reductions also **reduces patient doses** as seen in the patient dose icon boxes on page 276 describing positioning for the lateral T spine.

2. Exposure Time:
The lateral thoracic spine is most commonly taken with a **breathing technique** requiring a minimum of 3 or 4 seconds exposure time to blur out structures overlying the thoracic vertebrae.

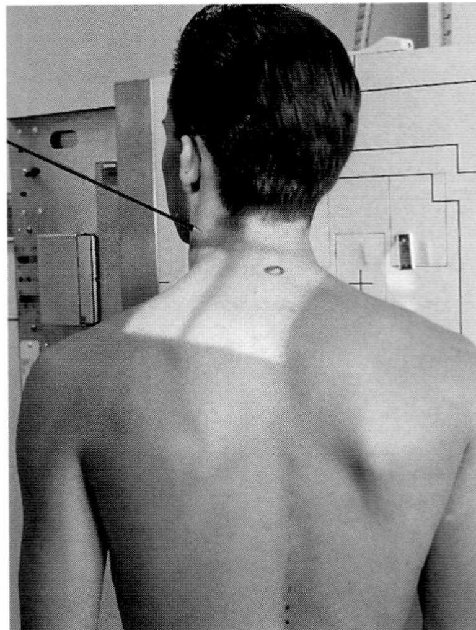

Fig. 8-45. Anterior cervical oblique.

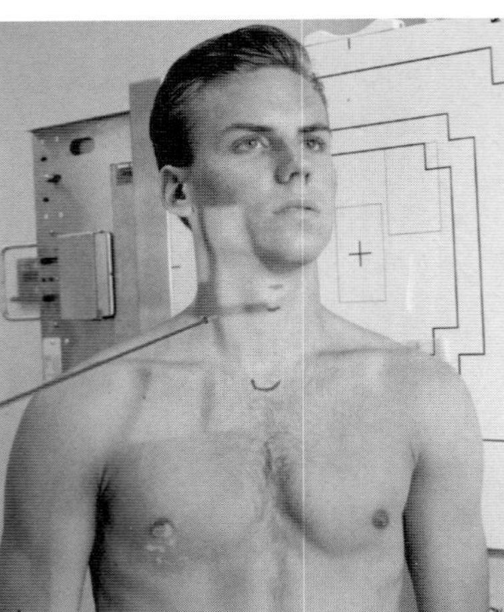

Fig. 8-46. Posterior cervical oblique.
-60 in. SID.
-Small focal spot.
-Anterior obliques reduce thyroid doses.

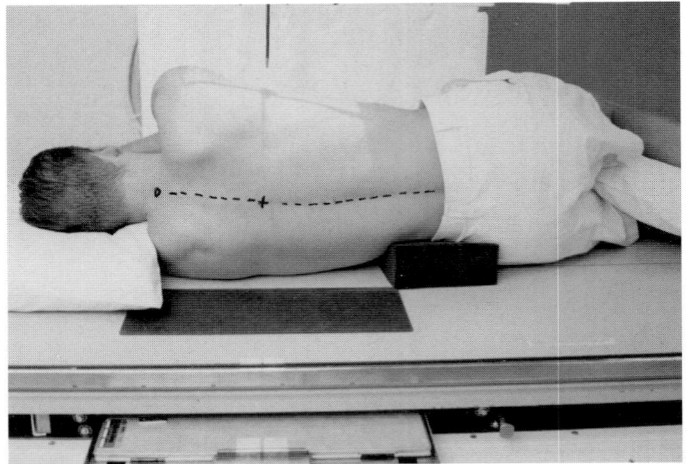

Fig. 8-47. Lateral T spine–With lead blocker behind patient.
-Vertebral column near parallel to table top.

3. Wide-latitude, Higher Speed, Screens and Films:
Special high-latitude film-screen combinations such as the Kodak Insight™ system or other wide-latitude thoracic screen-film systems have been developed to provide a **wider latitude** of visible densities along with requiring some lower patient exposures.

Minimize Effect of Scatter Radiation: Higher kVp and penetration of thick dense tissue both result in the production of significant scatter radiation from body tissues which degrade the radiographic image. This is most evident on the lateral thoracic and lumbar spine and the lateral sacrum and coccyx. This can be minimized two ways, first with **close collimation**; and second with a **lead blocker** placed on the table-top next to the patient (Fig. 8-47).

Part/Film Alignment: Correct part/film alignment is especially important for lateral projections of the vertebral column wherein the primary beam including the divergent rays must pass through "open" intervertebral spaces. This requires close attention to placing the right amount of support under the patient in the waist region to result in the entire **vertebral column being near parallel or equal distance from the table-top** (Fig. 8-47).

Optimum object-film-CR alignment is a challenge for lateral thoracic and lumbar spines due to the wide range of body builds among male and female patients. This is illustrated in the positioning pages for these projections.

NATIONAL SURVEY

Departmental standard (basic) and special routines of the cervical or thoracic spine did not show a significant difference in the different regions of the U.S.

Cervical Spine Routine

Cervical spine	U.S. Average	
	Basic 1995 (1989)	Special 1995 (1989)
• AP–20° cephalad	97% (88%)	
• AP–open mouth (C 1 and C 2)	97% (86%)	
• Lateral	94% (93%)	
• Obliques–Anterior	65%	
–Posterior	60%	
• Swimmer's lateral (cervicothoracic–C7-T1)	50% (59%)	43% (26%)
• Lateral –Flexion and extension		63% (31%)
• AP "chewing" or "wagging jaw" (Ottonello method)		31% (10%)
• AP dens (Fuch method)		33% –
• PA dens (Judd method)		25% –

Thoracic Spine Routine

Thoracic spine	U.S. Average	
	Basic 1995 (1989)	Special 1995 (1989)
• AP	95% (98%)	
• Lateral		
–Breathing	83% –	
–Expiration	13% –	
–Inspiration	19% –	
• Obliques		28% (13%)

Summary

Cervical Spine: Some significant results in cervical spine projections were the **anterior obliques** (65%) vs. **posterior obliques** (60%). Thus it appears that it is slightly more common to do these as anterior obliques which is also recommended in this text due to the lower doses to the thyroid (see page 267). The same holds true for the special projection for the dens with the **Fuch method (AP)** as compared to the **Judd method (PA)** (see page 273). Other considerations, however, such as OID and patient comfort may be reasons why the AP dens (33%) is a more frequent special projection than the PA dens (25%).

The survey also indicates that the **AP "chewing"** (Ottonello method) for C1-2 vertebra is three times more common as a special projection in 1995 (31%) as compared to 1989 (10%). The frequency of two other special cervical projections also increased by about two fold in 1995 as compared to 1989. These are **swimmer's lateral** and the **laterals in flexion and extension**.

Thoracic Spine: The survey demonstrated that for the lateral thoracic, the **breathing technique** is by far the most common routine (83%) followed with inspiration (19%) and the least frequent, expiration (13%). (A trend for this cannot be determined because the same question was not included in the 1989 survey.)

The percent of institutions doing oblique thoracic spine as special projections increased to 28% in 1995 from only 13% in 1989.

STANDARD AND SPECIAL OPERATING PROCEDURES

Certain basic and special projections for the thoracic and cervical spine are demonstrated and described on the following pages as suggested standard (basic) and special departmental procedures.

Basic Projections

Standard or basic projections, also sometimes referred to as routine projections or departmental routines, are **those projections taken on average patients who are helpful and can cooperate in performing the procedure.**

Special Projections

Optional projections are **those more common projections or positions taken as extra or additional projections to better demonstrate certain pathologic conditions or specific body parts.**

Basic and Special Projections

Cervical spine
Basic
- AP open mouth (C1 and C2) **265**
- AP axial **266**
- Obliques **267**
- Lateral **268**
- Lateral, horizontal beam **269**
- Swimmer's lateral (cervicothoracic) **270**

Cervical spine
Special
- Alternate method for C7-T1 **271**
- Lateral
  –Hyperflexion and hyperextension **272**
- AP (Fuch method) **273** and PA (Judd method) **273**
- AP chewing or wagging jaw (Ottonello method) **274**

Thoracic spine
Basic
- AP **275**
- Lateral **276**

Special
- Obliques **277**

Warning! Trauma to head and/or neck area with **possible fracture** or **subluxation** (partial dislocation) requires a horizontal beam cervical lateral taken first **without** moving patient's head and neck. Cervical collar, if present, should **NOT** be removed. This radiograph should be viewed by physician **before** attempting to move patient's head or neck for other cervical and/or skull trauma projections.

Additional C spine trauma projections are included in Chapter 19, Mobile and Trauma Radiography.

8

AP "Open Mouth" Projection-C1 and C2

Warning: Do not attempt any head or neck movement with potential cervical trauma without first reviewing a horizontal beam lateral radiograph (see page 269).

Cervical spine
Basic
- **AP open mouth (C1 & C2)**
- AP
- Obliques – PA or AP
- Lateral
- Swimmer's lateral

Structures Best Shown

Dens (odontoid process) and vertebral body of C2, lateral masses of C1 and zygapophyseal joints between C1 and C2.

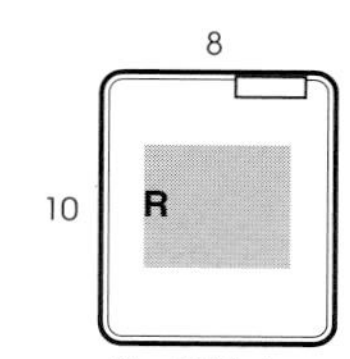

Technical Factors

- Film size–8 x 10 in. (18 x 24 cm), lengthwise.
- Moving or stationary grid.
- 75±5 kVp range.
- Technique and dose:

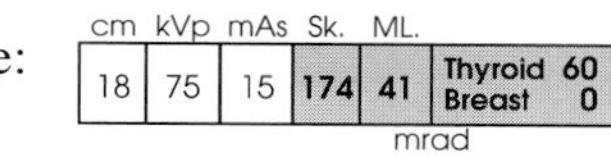

cm	kVp	mAs	Sk.	ML.	mrad
18	75	15	174	41	Thyroid 60 Breast 0

Shielding: Place lead shield over chest and neck to shield thyroid and breast region.

Patient Position

- Supine (or erect) with arms by sides.
- Head on table surface, provide immobilization if needed.

Part Position

- Align midsagittal plane to CR and midline of table.
- Adjust head so that with mouth open a line from **lower margin of upper incisors to the base of the skull** (mastoid tips) **is perpendicular** to table and/or film.
- Assure there is **no rotation** of the head or thorax.
- Assure that **mouth is wide open** during exposure. (Do this as the last step and work quickly as it is difficult to maintain this position.)

Central Ray

- CR **perpendicular to film**, directed through **center of open mouth.**
- Center cassette to CR.
- Minimum 40 in. (102 cm) SID.

Collimation: Close four-sided collimation to area of interest.

Respiration: Suspend respiration during exposure.

Notes: Make sure that when patient is instructed to open mouth that only the lower jaw moves.

Instruct the patient to keep the tongue in the lower jaw to prevent its shadow from superimposing the atlas and axis.

If unable to demonstrate the upper dens, see Fuchs or Judd method (page 273).

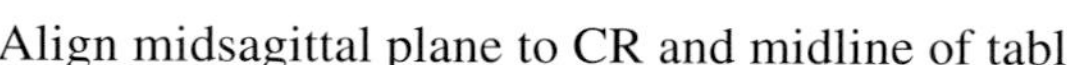

Evaluation Criteria

- The atlas and axis including the dens in its entirety, and the C1-2 zygapophyseal joint space should be clearly demonstrated through the open mouth.
- Optimum head position, indicated by the lower margin of the **upper incisors** superimposing the **base of the skull**.
- **No rotation**: Evidenced by equal distances from lateral masses and/or transverse processes of C1 to condyles of mandible, and by center alignment of spinous process of C2. Rotation can imitate pathology by causing unequal spaces between lateral masses and dens.
- Optimum exposure should demonstrate both bone and soft tissue density.

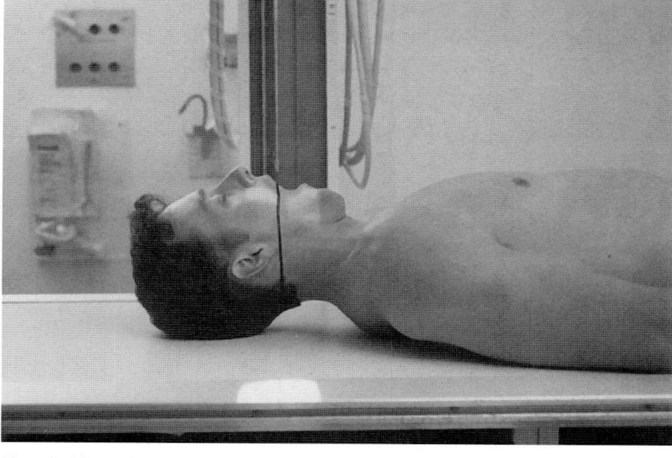

Fig. 8-48. AP open mouth–C1-2.

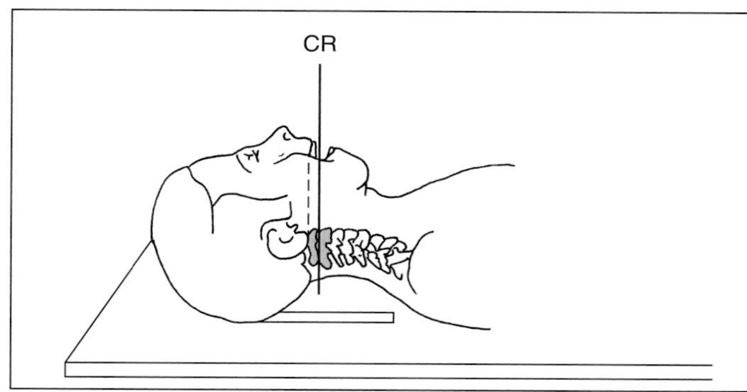

Fig. 8-49. AP open mouth–C1-2.

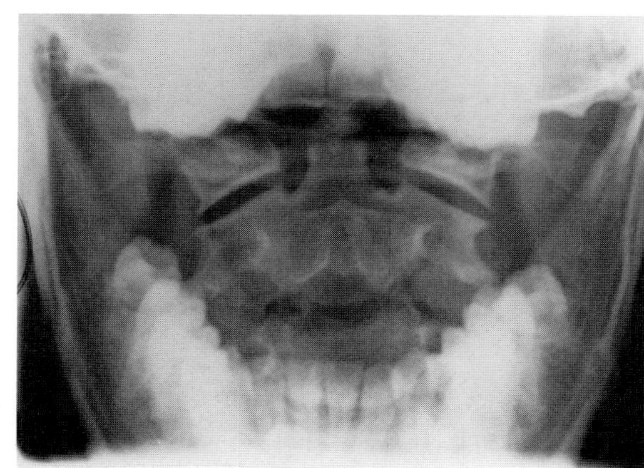

Fig. 8-50. AP open mouth–C1-2.

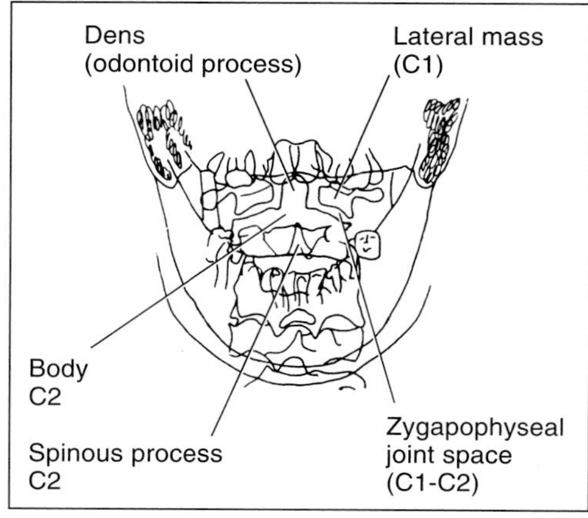

Fig. 8-51. AP open mouth–C1-2.

AP Axial Projection

Cervical spine
Basic
- AP open mouth (C1 & C2)
- **AP**
- Obliques – PA or AP
- Lateral
- Swimmer's lateral

Structures Best Shown

Vertebra from C3 through T2 or T3 to include vertebral bodies, space between pedicles, intervertebral disk spaces and spinous processes.

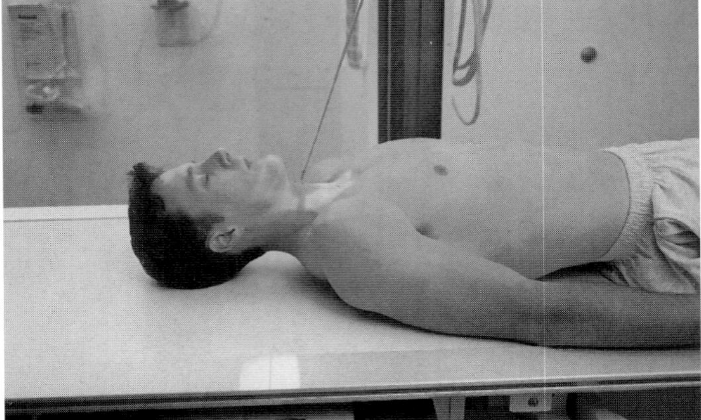

Fig. 8-52. AP supine, 15 to 20° cephalad angle.

Technical Factors

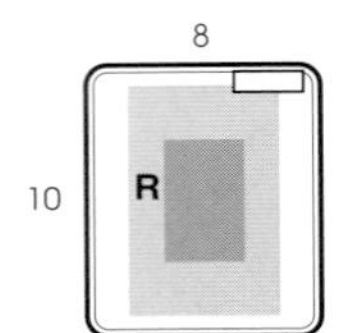

- Film size–8 x 10 in. (18 x 24 cm), lengthwise.
- Moving or stationary grid.
- 75±5 kVp range.
- Technique and dose:

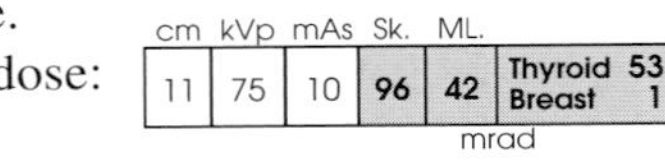

cm	kVp	mAs	Sk.	ML.	
11	75	10	96	42	Thyroid 53 Breast 1
				mrad	

Shielding: Place lead shield over chest region for thyroid and breast shielding.

Patient Position

- Supine or erect, with arms by sides.
- Head on table surface, provide immobilization if needed.

Part Position 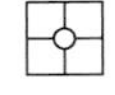

- Align **midsagittal plane to CR and midline of table** and/or film.
- Adjust head so that a line from the occlusal plane (chewing surface of teeth) to the base of the skull (mastoid tips) is **perpendicular to table** and/or film. Line from tip of mandible to base of skull should be **parallel to angled CR**.
- Ensure there is **no rotation** of the head or thorax.

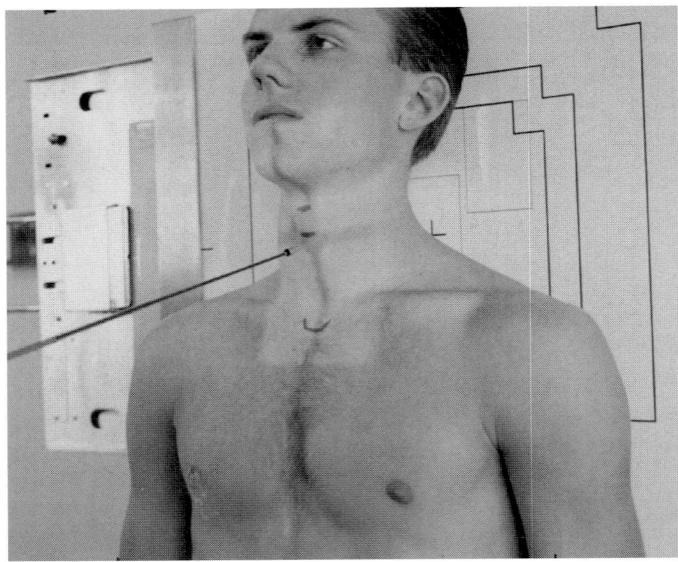

Fig. 8-53. AP erect, 15 to 20° cephalad angle.

Central Ray

- CR angled **15 to 20° cephalad**, to enter at the level of the lower margin of thyroid cartilage **(C5-6)**.
- Center cassette to CR (top of cassette will be 1 to 2 in. (3 to 5 cm) above level of EAM).
- Minimum 40 in. (102 cm) SID.

Collimation: Close four-sided collimation to area of interest.

Respiration: Suspend respiration during exposure.

Notes: Patient should not swallow during exposure.

Cephalad angulation will open up intervertebral disk spaces.

Evaluation Criteria

- C3 to T1 should be clearly seen.
- **No rotation**; spinous processes and sternoclavicular joints should be equidistant from the spinal borders.
- **Intervertebral disk spaces should be open** indicating correct CR angle.
- The mandible and base of the skull will be superimposed over the first two cervical vertebra.
- Optimum exposure should demonstrate both bone and soft tissue density.

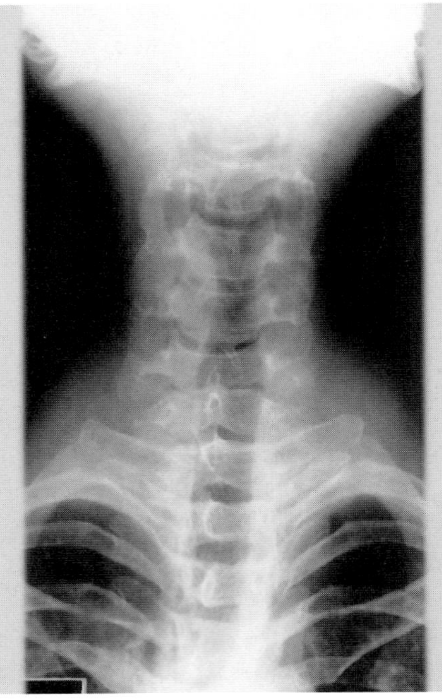

Fig. 8-54. AP, 15 to 20° cephalad angle.

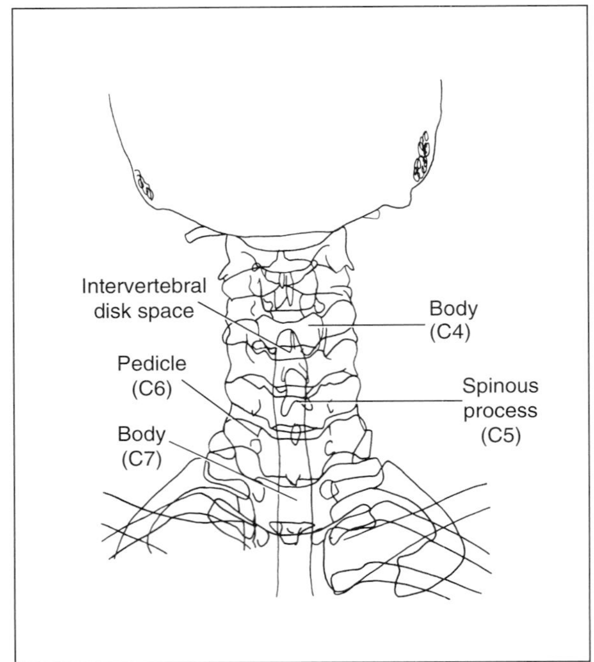

Fig. 8-55. AP, 15 to 20° cephalad angle.

PA or AP Oblique Projections–LAO, RAO or LPO, RPO Positions

Cervical spine
Basic
- AP open mouth (C1 & C2)
- AP
- **Obliques – PA or AP**
- Lateral
- Swimmer's lateral

Structures Best Shown

PA obliques: Intervertebral foramina and pedicles closest to film.
AP obliques: Intervertebral foramina and pedicles farthest from the film.

Both right and left obliques must be taken as either PA or AP obliques. **PA obliques** are preferred due to reduced thyroid doses.

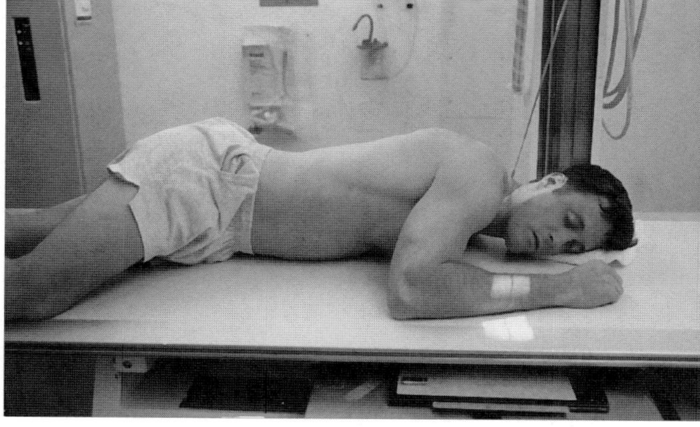

Fig. 8-56. PA oblique–Recumbent LAO position.
–CR 15 to 20° **caudad.**

Technical Factors

- Film size–8 x 10 in. (18 x 24 cm), lengthwise.
- Moving or stationary grid.
- 75±5 kVp range.
- Technique and dose–

	cm	kVp	mAs	Sk.	ML.	mrad
Ant. obl.	11	75	10	129	50	Thyroid 5, Breast 0
–Post. obl.	11	75	10	129	50	Thyroid 69, Breast 4

Patient Position

- Erect position preferred (sitting or standing), or may be taken recumbent if patient's condition requires.

Part Position 

- Center spine to **CR** and **midline** of table and/or film.
- Arms at side; if recumbent, place arms as needed to help maintain position.
- Rotate body and head 45°. (Use protractor or other angle gauge to assure 45°.) See Note about head rotation.
- Extend chin to prevent mandible from superimposing vertebrae. Do not elevate chin too much to cause base of skull to superimpose C1.

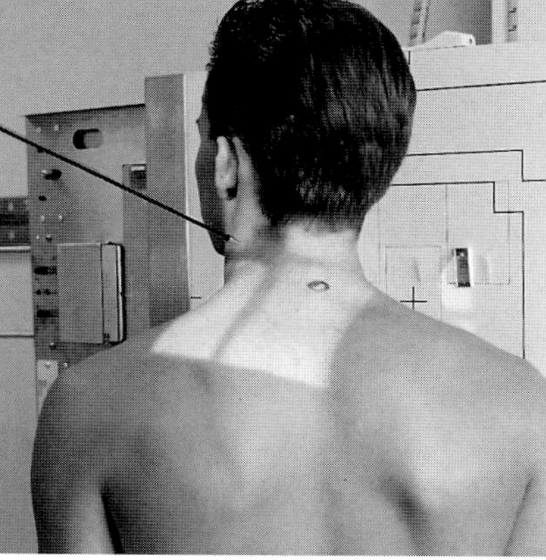

Fig. 8-57. Erect RAO position.
–CR 15 to 20° **caudad** (less thyroid dose).

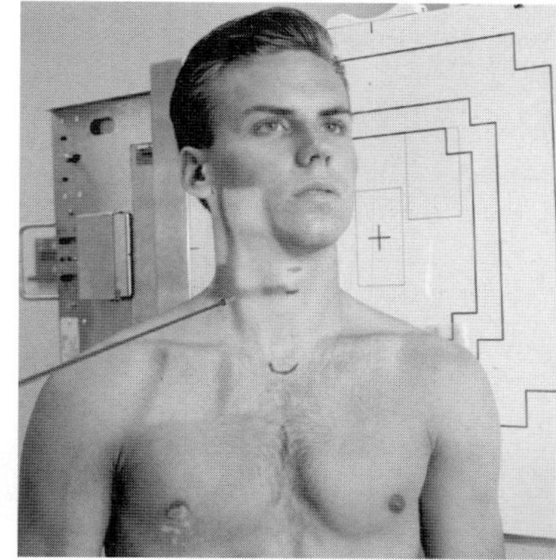

Fig. 8-58. Optional AP obliques, LPO.
–CR 15 to 20° **cephalad**.

Central Ray

PA Obliques:
- **15° to 20° caudad** to **C4** (level of upper margin of thyroid cartilage).

AP Obliques:
- **15° to 20° cephalad** to **C4** (to lower thyroid cartilage).
- Center cassette to projected CR.
- 60 to 72 in. (152 to 183 cm) SID.

Collimation: Four-sided collimation to area of interest (to near upper and lower film borders).

Respiration: Suspend respiration.

Note: Departmental option: The head may be turned toward film to a near lateral position. (This results in some rotation of upper vertebrae but prevents superimposition of vertebra by mandible.)

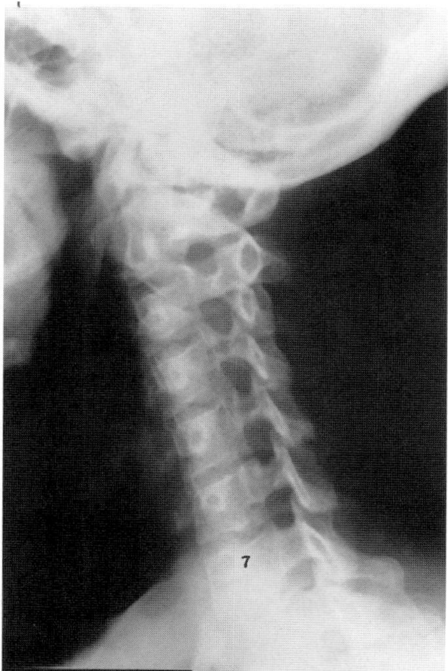

Fig. 8-59. Oblique.

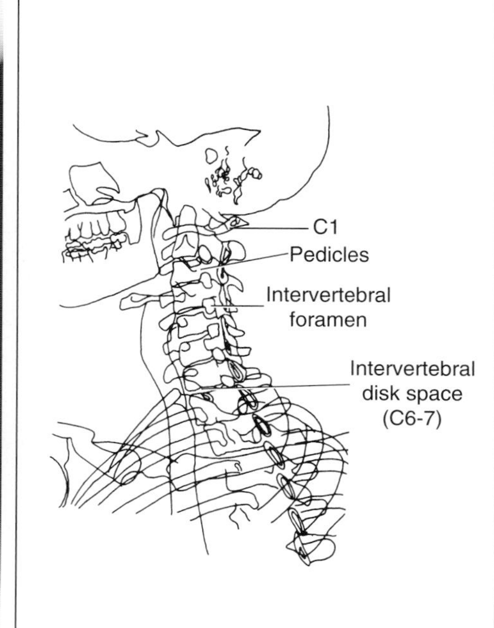

Fig. 8-60. Oblique.

Evaluation Criteria

- C1 through C7 should be clearly seen with open intervertebral foramina and open intervertebral disk spaces.
- Incorrect CR angle will close and obscure intervertebral disk spaces.
- Over or under rotation will narrow and partially obscure the intervertebral foramina.
- The rami of the mandible should not superimpose the upper cervical vertebra.
- The base of the skull should not superimpose C1.
- Cervical pedicles should be demonstrated.
- Optimum exposure should demonstrate soft tissue including margins of the air column, as well as proper bone density of the entire cervical vertebrae.

Lateral Position

Cervical spine
Basic
• AP open mouth (C1 & C2)
• AP
• Obliques – PA or AP
• **Lateral**
• Swimmer's lateral

Structures Best Shown

Cervical vertebral bodies, intervertebral joint spaces, articular pillars, spinous processes and zygapophyseal joints. **Trauma patients**: Lateral horizontal beam, page 269.

Technical Factors

- Film size–10 x 12 in. (24 x 30 cm), lengthwise. or for smaller patient–8 x 10 in. (18 x 24 cm).
- Moving or stationary grid (optional).
- 75±5 kVp range.
- Technique and dose: @ 72"

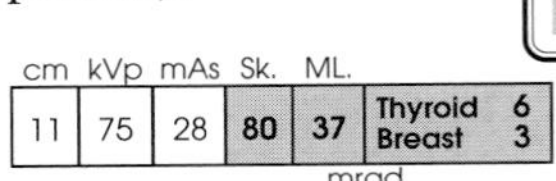

cm	kVp	mAs	Sk.	ML.	
11	75	28	**80**	**37**	Thyroid 6 Breast 3

mrad

Patient Position

- Erect lateral, either sitting or standing with shoulder against vertical film holder.

Fig. 8-61. Erect L lateral.

Part Position

- Align midcoronal plane to CR and midline of table and/or cassette holder.
- Centering cassette to CR should place top of cassette about 1 to 2 in. (3 to 5 cm) above EAM.
- Depress shoulders (for equal weights to both arms, see Note 1).
- Ask patient to **relax** and **drop shoulders down and forward as far as possible**. (Do this as the last step before exposure as this is a difficult position to maintain.)
- Extend chin forward (to prevent superimposition of upper cervical by mandible).

Fig. 8-62. Erect L lateral (front-to-back centering).

Central Ray

- CR **perpendicular** to film, directed horizontally to **C4-5** (level of upper margin of thyroid cartilage).
- Center cassette to CR.
- 60 to 72 in. (152 to 183 cm) SID. (See Note 2).

Respiration: Suspend respiration on **full expiration** (for maximum shoulder depression).

Collimation: Four-sided collimation to area of interest. (With smaller film, collimate to near upper and lower film borders.)

Note 1: Adding 5 to 10 lb. weights to each arm may help in pulling down shoulders.

Note 2: Long (72 in.) SID compensates for increased OID, and provides for less divergence of useful x-ray beam to reduce shoulder superimposition of C7.

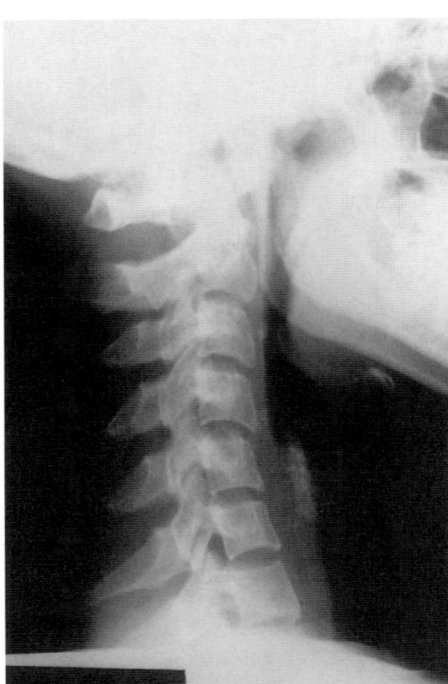

Fig. 8-63. Lateral.

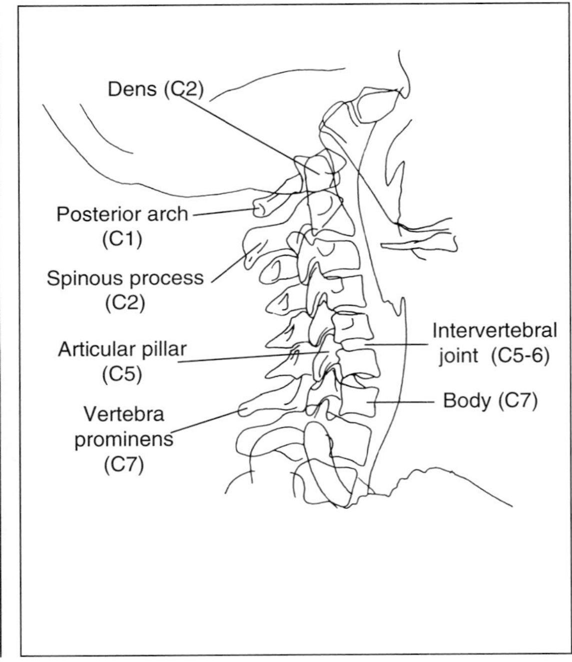

Fig. 8-64. Lateral.

Evaluation Criteria

- C1 through C7 should be clearly seen. If C7 is not seen, a special view (Swimmer's) should be done of the cervicothoracic region.
- Center of collimation field should be to C4-5 region.
- The rami of the mandible should not be superimposed over C1-C2.
- No rotation of head is indicated by superimposition of both rami of the mandible. Lower cervical rotation is evidenced by lack of superimposition of R and L side apophyseal joints.
- Optimum exposure with no rotation should demonstrate soft tissue including margins of the air column, as well as proper bone density of the entire cervical vertebrae.

Lateral Position, Horizontal Beam

Warning: Do not remove cervical collar and do not move head or neck until this lateral radiograph has ruled out cervical fracture or subluxation.

Cervical spine
(trauma patient)
Basic
• Lateral (horizontal beam)

Structures Best Shown

Cervical vertebral bodies, intervertebral joint spaces, articular pillars, spinous processes and zygapophyseal joints.

Technical Factors

- Film size –8 x 10 in. (18 x 24 cm)
  or –10 x 12 in. (24 x 30 cm), lengthwise.
- Non-grid cassette or grid (see Note 1).
- 70±5 kVp range.
- Technique and dose:
  @72"

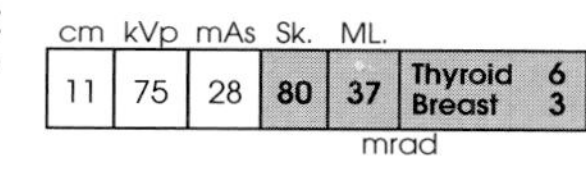

cm	kVp	mAs	Sk.	ML.	
11	75	28	80	37	Thyroid 6 Breast 3
				mrad	

10 (8)
L
12 (10)

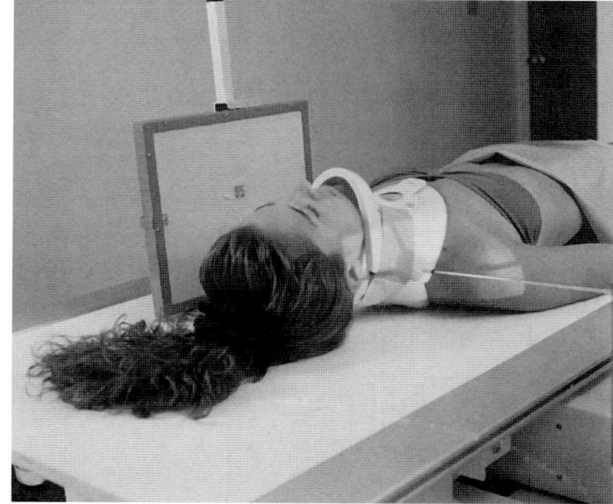

Fig. 8-65. R lateral–Horizontal beam.

Shielding: Place lead shield over pelvic area to shield gonads.

Patient Position

- Supine on stretcher or table.

Part Position

- Do **not** manipulate or move head or neck.
- Support cassette vertically against shoulder, or place stretcher next to vertical grid device.
- Center cassette to CR, which should place top of cassette about 1 to 2 in. (3 to 5 cm) above EAM.
- Depress shoulders. (See Note 2.)

Central Ray

- CR **perpendicular** to film, directed horizontally to **C4** (level of upper margin of thyroid cartilage).
- 60 to 72 in. (158 to 183 cm) SID. (See Note 3.)

Collimation: Four-sided collimation to area of interest.

Respiration: Suspend respiration on full **expiration** (this will help to depress shoulders).

Note 1: Generally a non-grid cassette can be used for smaller or average patients due to the increased OID and the resultant air-gap effect.

Note 2: Traction on arms will help depress shoulders but should only be done by a qualified assistant and/or with the consent or assistance of a physician.

Note 3: Long SID compensates for increased magnification caused by an increase in OID with resultant loss of image sharpness, also results in less diveregence of useful x-ray beam to reduce shoulder superimposition of C7.

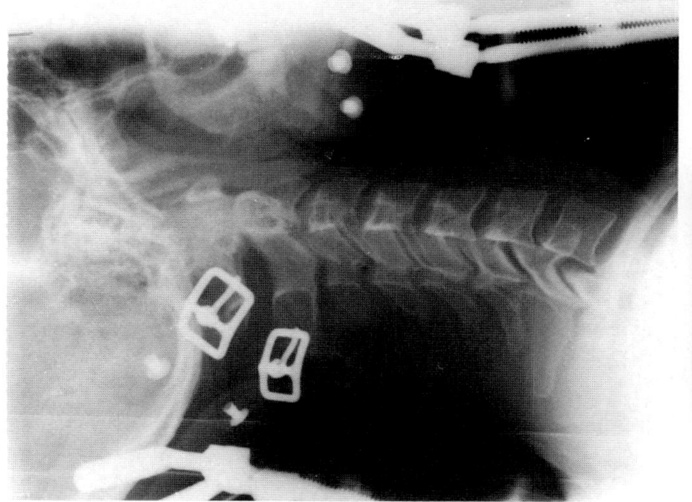

Fig. 8-66. Lateral–Horizontal beam.

Evaluation Criteria

- C1 through C7 should be clearly seen. If C7 is not seen, the horizontal beam swimmer's lateral may be taken to visualize C7, or the physician must review the film and grant permission before any additional (or special) views are obtained involving patient movement.
- Optimum exposure should demonstrate soft tissue as well as proper bone density of all aspects of the cervical vertebrae.

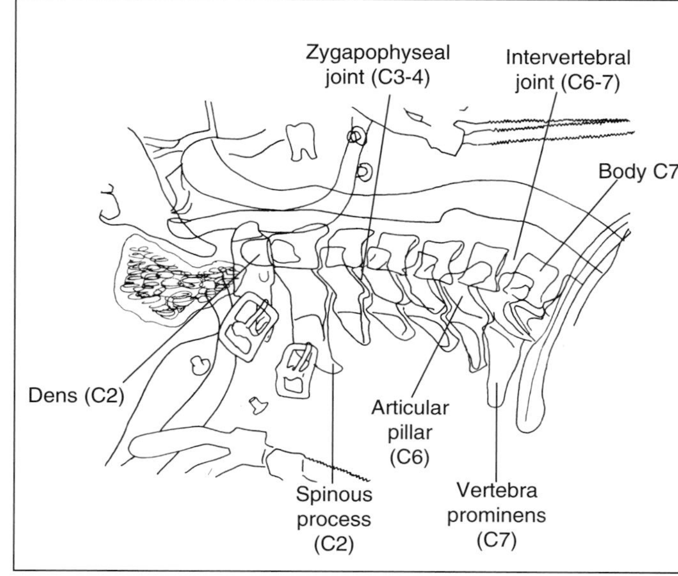

Fig. 8-67. Lateral–Horizontal beam.

8

Cervicothoracic (Swimmer's) Lateral Position

Twining Method, for C4-T3 region

Cervical spine
Basic
- AP open mouth (C1 & C2)
- AP
- Obliques
- Lateral
- **Swimmer's lateral**

Structures Best Shown

Cervical and thoracic vertebral bodies, intervertebral disk spaces, and zygapophyseal joints of C4 to T3.

Good projection when C7 is not visualized on lateral cervical.

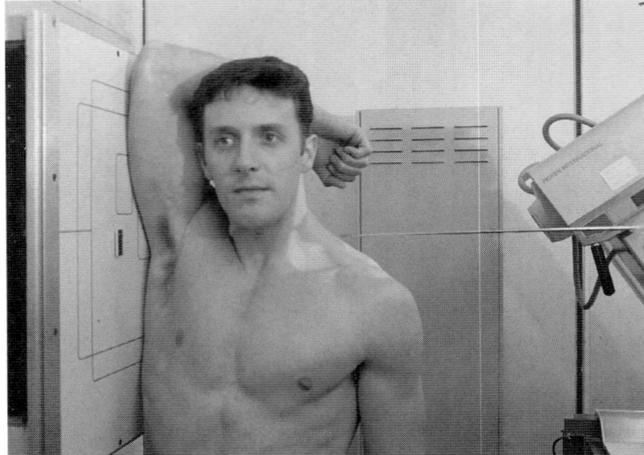

Fig. 8-68. Swimmer's lateral.

Technical Factors

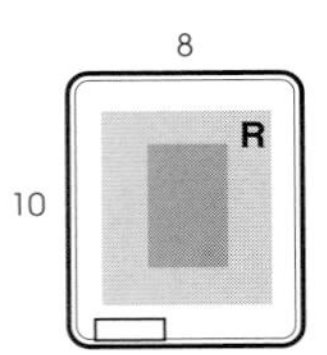

- Film size–8 x 10 in. (18 x 24 cm), lengthwise.
- Use moving or stationary grid.
- 80±5 kVp range. (Increase 5-10 kVp from lateral cervical.)
- Technique and dose: @ 72"

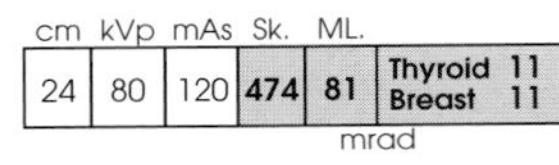

cm	kVp	mAs	Sk.	ML.	
24	80	120	474	81	Thyroid 11 Breast 11
			mrad		

Patient Position

- Erect position preferred (sitting or standing), or may be done recumbent if patient's condition requires.

Part Position 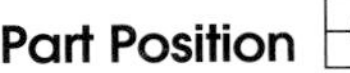

- Align mid coronal plane to CR and midline of table or cassette holder.
- Place arm and shoulder nearest film up, flex elbow and rest forearm on head for support.
- Position arm and shoulder away from film down and slightly anterior to place humeral head anterior to vertebrae.
- Maintain thorax and head in as true a lateral position as possible.

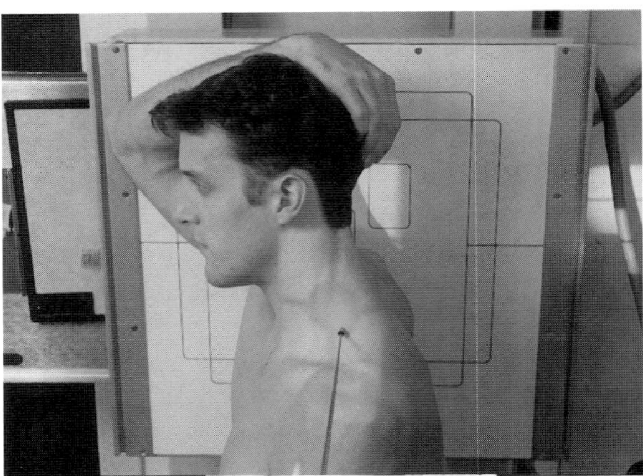

Fig. 8-69. Swimmer's lateral.

Central Ray

- CR **perpendicular** to film. (See Note.)
- Center to **T1**, which is approximately 1 in. (2.5 cm) above level of jugular notch anteriorly, and at level of vertebra prominens posteriorly.
- Center cassette to CR.
- 60 to 72 in. (152 to 183 cm) SID.

Collimation: Close four-sided collimation to area of interest (about 4 x 6 in.). Close collimation improves contrast and the visibility of anatomy.

Respiration: Suspend breathing on full **expiration**.

Note: A slight caudad angulation of 3 to 5° may be necessary to help separate the two shoulders, especially on a heavily muscled patient or one who cannot sufficiently depress the shoulder away from the film.

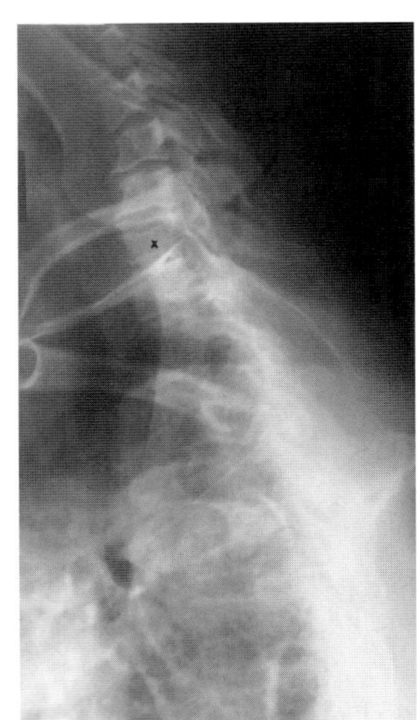

Fig. 8-70. Swimmer's lateral.

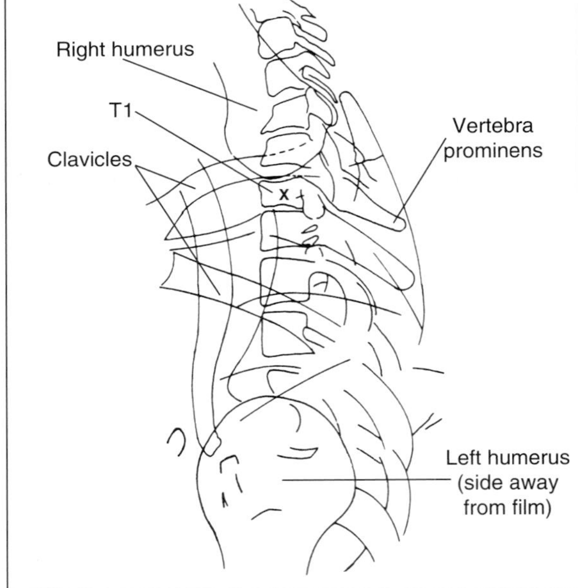

Fig. 8-71. Swimmer's lateral.

Evaluation Criteria

- The center of collimation field should be to T1 region.
- Vertebral rotation should appear to be minimal.
- C4 to T3 should be clearly seen in outline when properly exposed.
- The humeral heads should be separated vertically. The humeral head and arm closest to the film superimposes the lower cervical to provide a more uniform density of the lower cervical and upper thoracic vertebrae.
- The magnified humeral head which was depressed and farthest from the film should appear distal to T4 or T5 area.
- Optimum exposure should clearly visualize outlines of vertebrae including intervertebral spaces of C4 to T3 through shoulder structures without overpenetrating upper cervicals.

Alternate Method of Visualizing C7-T1

Modified Swimmer's*

Cervical spine
Special
- **Alternate method for C7-T1**
- Lateral–Hyperflexion and hyperextension
- AP (Fuch method) PA (Judd method)
- AP chewing or wagging jaw (Ottonello method)

Structures Best Shown

Lower cervical and upper thoracic vertebral bodies, intervertebral disk spaces, and zygapophyseal joints.

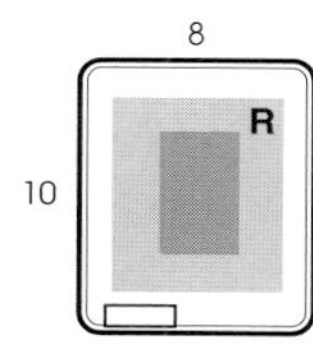

Technical Factors

- Film size–8 x 10 in. (18 x 24 cm), lengthwise.
- Use moving or stationary grid.
- 80±5 kVp range.
  (Increase 5-10 kVp from lateral cervical.)
- Technique and dose:
  @72"

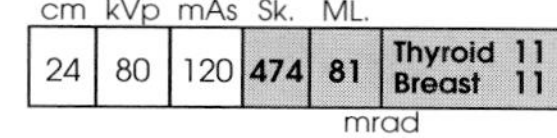

cm	kVp	mAs	Sk.	ML.	
24	80	120	474	81	Thyroid 11 Breast 11

mrad

Patient Position

- Erect position preferred (sitting or standing), or may be done recumbent if patient's condition requires.

Part Position 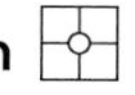

- Align **mid coronal plane to CR and midline** of table or cassette holder.

Modified Swimmer's Method:

- **Elevate hand and arm closest to film** and rest hand on head. This placement of arm tends to pull the shoulder superiorly and anteriorly to separate humeral heads.
- Pull arm and shoulder away from film **down and forward or anteriorly** as far as possible while maintaining a lateral position of the head, neck and thorax. (This places humeral head anterior to vertebrae.)

Central Ray

- CR **perpendicular**, centered to T1 at level of vertebra prominens posteriorly and about 1 in. (2.5 cm) superior to jugular notch.
- Center cassette to CR.
- 40 to 60 in. (102 to 152 cm) SID.

Collimation: Collimate closely to area of interest.

Respiration: Suspend breathing on **full expiration**.

Note: Consistent visualization of C7-T1 region on all types of patients is a challenge and each radiographer will develop a method which works best for him/her. The positions demonstrated and described on this page and the preceding page provide several options for different types of patients which can be used successfully.

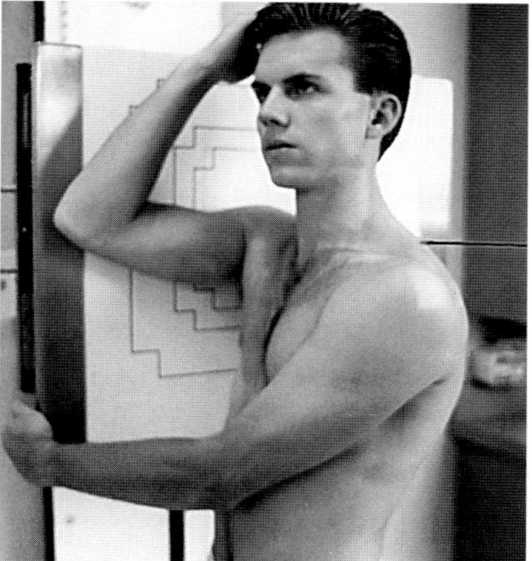

Fig. 8-72. Modified swimmer's method.
-Right shoulder raised and forward.
-Left shoulder down and forward.

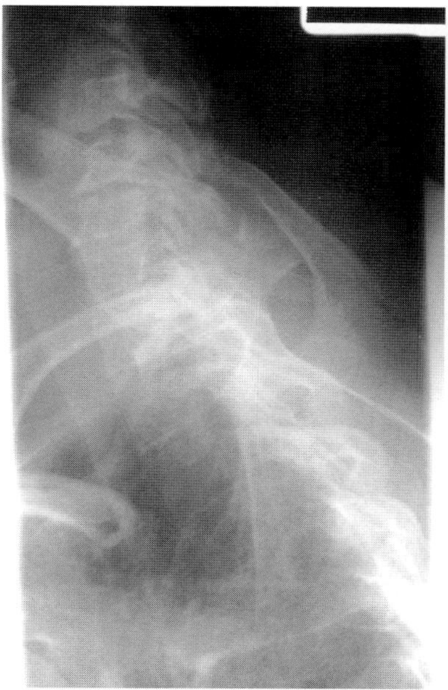

Fig. 8-73. Modified swimmer's. (Female, short neck, thick shoulders)

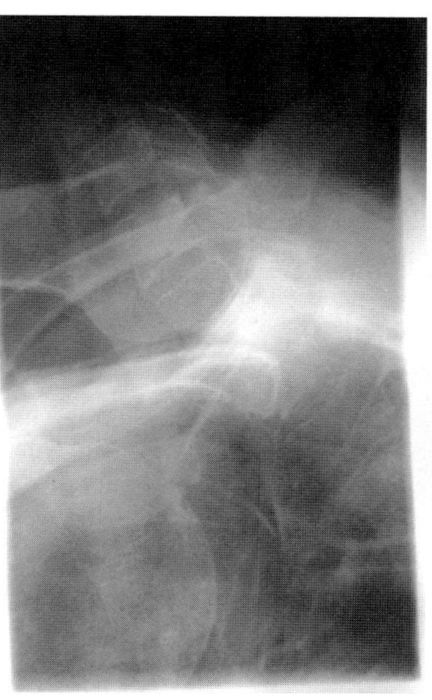

Fig. 8-74. Modified swimmer's. (Male, short neck, thin shoulders)

Evaluation Criteria

- The center of collimation field should be to T1 region.
- Vertebral rotation should appear to be minimal.
- C4 to T3 should be clearly seen in outline when properly exposed.
- The humeral heads should be **separated vertically** with the magnified humeral head away from the film placed **anterior to the T vertebrae**. The humeral head closest to the film superimposes C7 and T1 to provide a more uniform density of the lower C vertebrae with that of the upper T vertebrae.
- Optimum exposure should clearly visualize outlines of vertebrae including intervertebral spaces of C4-T3 through shoulder structures without overpenetrating upper cervicals.

*Described by Karen Brown, RT (R).

Lateral Positions–Hyperflexion and Hyperextension

Warning: **Never** attempt these positions on trauma patient before cervical fractures have been ruled out.

Cervical spine
Special
- Alternate methods for C7-T1
- **Lateral–Hyperflexion and hyperextension**
- AP (Fuch method) PA (Judd method)
- AP chewing or wagging jaw (Ottonello method)

Structures Best Shown

Functional study to demonstrate motion or lack of motion of cervical vertebra. Performed to rule out "whiplash" type injuries.

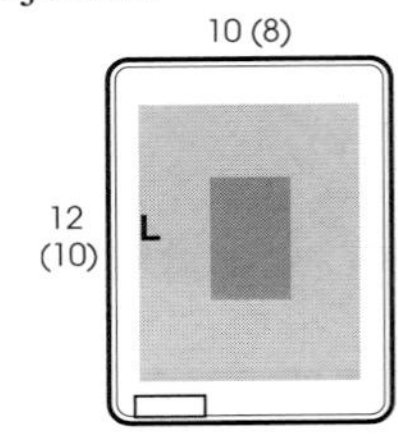

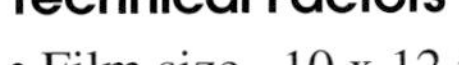

Technical Factors

- Film size –10 x 12 in. (24 x 30 cm), lengthwise. or – 8 x 10 in. (18 x 24 cm), lengthwise.
- Moving or stationary grid (optional).
- 75±5 kVp range.
- Technique and dose (per projection): @ 72"

cm	kVp	mAs	Sk.	ML.	mrad
11	75	28	80	37	Thyroid 6, Breast 3

Patient Position

- Erect lateral, either sitting or standing, arms at sides.

Part Position

- Align mid coronal plane of vertebrae to CR and midline of film.
- Ensure a **true lateral position**, no rotation of pelvis, shoulders or head.
- Relax and **depress shoulders** as far as possible (weights on each arm may be used).
- For **hyperflexion**: Chin should be depressed until it touches the chest or as much as patient can tolerate (do not allow patient to move forward to ensure that entire cervical is included on film).
- For **hyperextension**: Chin should be raised and head leaned back as much as possible (do not allow patient to move backward to ensure that entire cervical is included on film).

Central Ray

- CR **perpendicular** to film, directed horizontally to area of **C4-5** (level of upper margin of thyroid cartilage with head in neutral position).
- 60 to 72 in. (158 to 183 cm) SID.
- Center height of cassette to level of CR. (Top of cassette should be about 2 in. or 5 cm above level of EAM.)

Collimation: Four-sided collimation to area of interest. Ensure that both upper and lower cervical vertebrae are included, especially on hyperflexion projection.

Respiration: Suspend respiration on full expiration.

Note: These are uncomfortable for patient; do not keep in these positions longer than necessary.

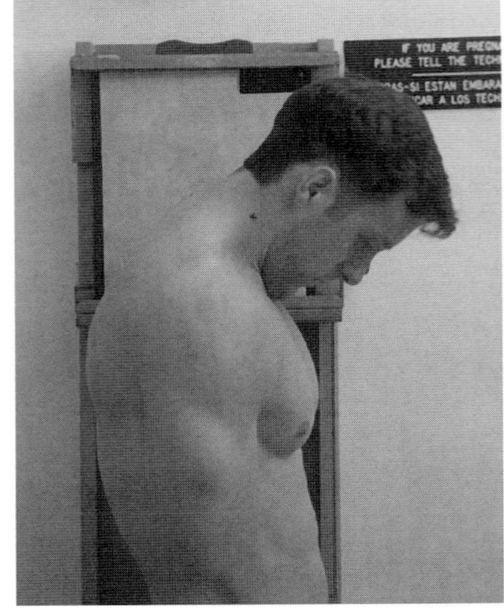

Fig. 8-76. Hyperflexion.

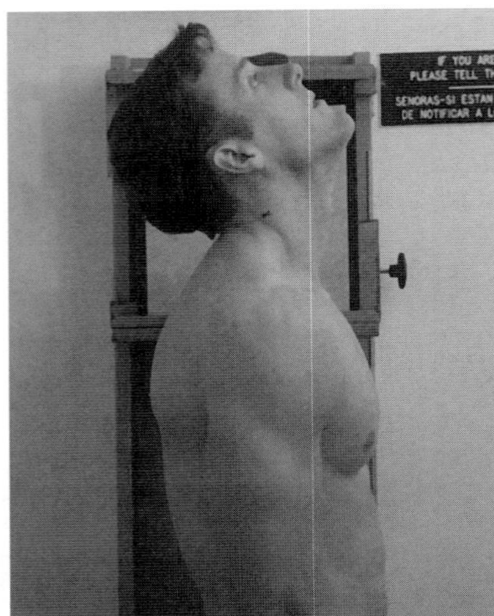

Fig. 8-77. Hyperextension.

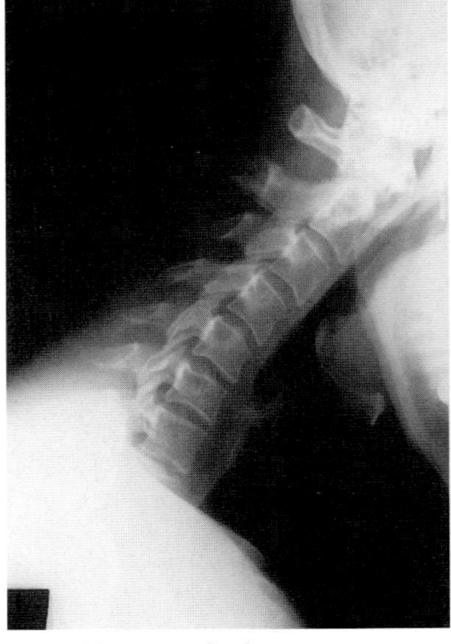

Fig. 8-78. Hyperflexion.

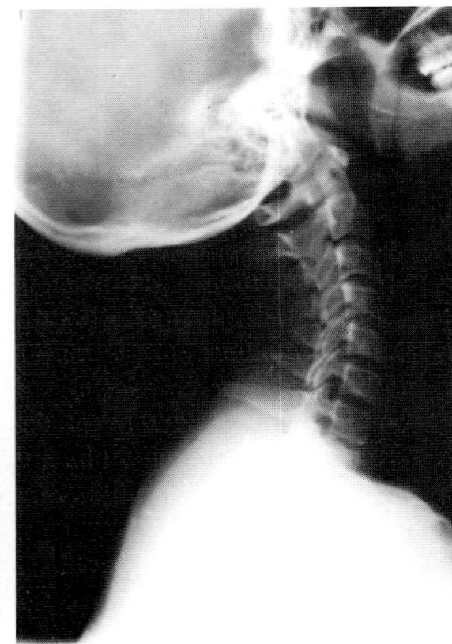

Fig. 8-79. Hyperextension.

Evaluation Criteria

- C1 through C7 should be included on film. (C7 however, may not be completely visualized on some patients.)
- Center of collimation field should be to region of C4-5.
- No rotation of head is indicated by superimposition of rami of mandible.
- For **hyperflexion**: Spinous processes should be well separated.
- For **hyperextension**: Spinous processes should be in close proximity.
- Optimum exposure should demonstrate soft tissue as well as proper bone density of entire cervical vertebrae.

AP or PA Projection for C1-2 (Dens)

Fuch Method (AP) or Judd Method (PA)

Warning: Do not attempt on trauma patients without first ruling out C spine fracture or subluxation.

This is an alternate projection to the AP open-mouth of C1-2, especially to demonstrate the upper portion of dens.

Cervical spine
Special
- Alternate methods for C7-T1
- Lateral–Hyperflexion and hyperextension
- **AP (Fuch method) PA (Judd method)**
- AP chewing or wagging jaw (Ottonello method)

Structures Best Shown

Visualizes the dens (odontoid process) and other structures of C1-C2 within the foramen magnum.

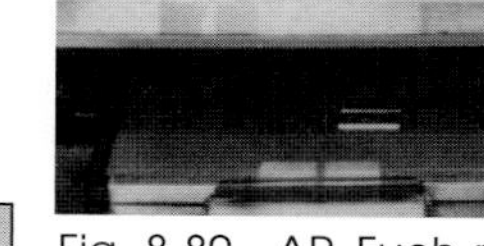

Fig. 8-80. AP–Fuch method.

Fig. 8-81. PA–Judd method (less thyroid dose).

Technical Factors

- Film size–8 x 10 in. (18 x 24 cm) crosswise
- Moving or stationary grid.
- 75±5 kVp range.

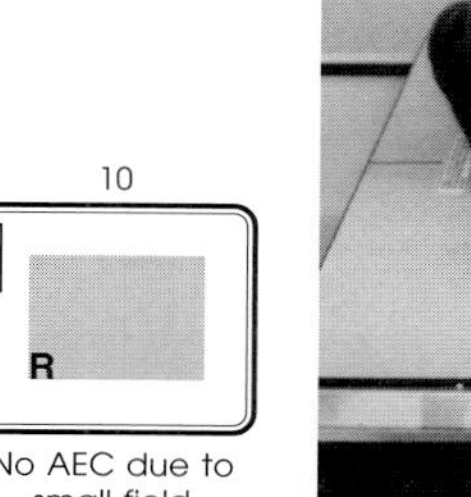

No AEC due to small field

	cm	kVp	mAs	Sk.	ML.		
Technique and dose–AP:	11	75	15	237	51	Thyroid / Breast	6 / 0
Technique and dose–PA:	11	75	15	173	40	Thyroid / Breast	3 / 0

mrad

Shielding: Shield chest area for thyroid and female breasts (best shielding is close collimation).

Patient and Part Position 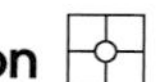

- Supine (AP), or prone (PA) with midsagittal plane aligned to CR and midline of table.

AP:

- Elevate chin as needed to bring **MML** (mentomeatal line) **near perpendicular to tabletop** (adjust CR angle as needed to be parallel to MML).
- Ensure that there is **no rotation** of head. (Angles of mandible equidistant to table-top).
- Center film to projected CR.
- CR **parallel to MML**, directed to **inferior tip of mandible.**

PA:

- This is a reverse position to the AP. Chin is resting on table-top and is extended to bring MML near perpendicular to table (may adjust CR as needed to be parallel to MML).
- Ensure **no rotation of head**, film centered to projected CR.
- CR **parallel to MML**, through mid-occipital bone, about 1 in (2.5 cm) inferoposterior to mastoid tips and angles of mandible.

Collimation: Close four-sided collimation to C1-2 region.

Respiration: Suspend respiration on full expiration.

Note: Positioning for these two projections is similar to Waters and reverse-Waters except for the CR location.

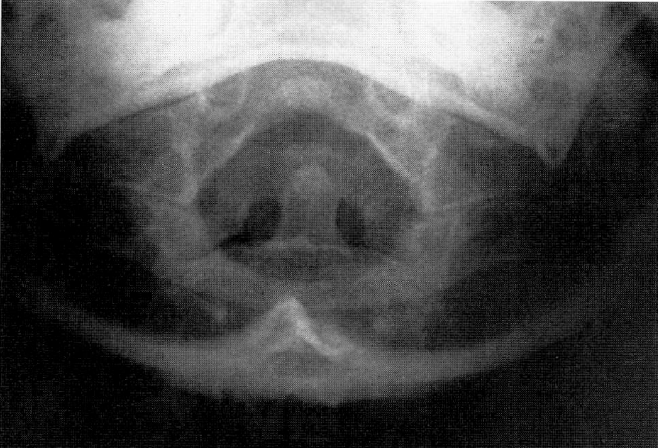

Fig. 8-82. AP or PA dens.

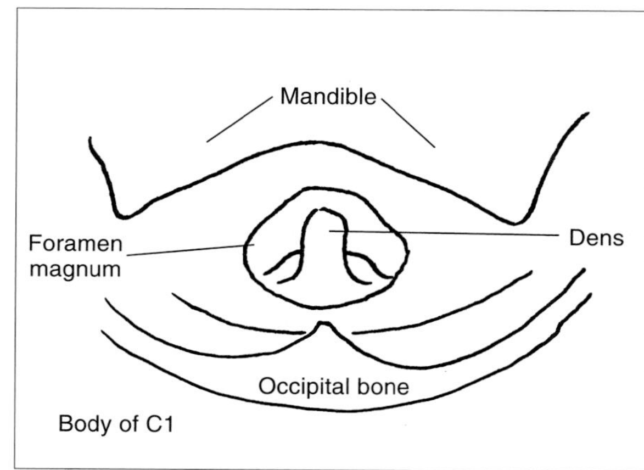

Fig. 8-83. AP or PA for C1-C2, dens.

Evaluation Criteria

- Dens process should be centered with foramen magnum.
- **No rotation**: Can be evaluated by the symmetrical appearance of the mandible arched over the foramen magnum.
- **Correct extension** of head and neck can be evaluated by the tip of the mandible clearing the superior portion of the dens and the foramen magnum.
- Optimum exposure with no motion will demonstrate clear and sharp outline of dens and other structures of C1 and C2 within foramen magnum.

AP "Chewing" or "Wagging Jaw" Projection

Ottonello Method

Cervical spine
Special
- Alternate methods for C7-T1
- Lateral–Hyperflexion and hyperextension
- AP (Fuch method) PA (Judd method)
- **AP chewing or wagging jaw (Ottonello method)**

Structures Best Shown

Entire cervical spine with mandible blurred.

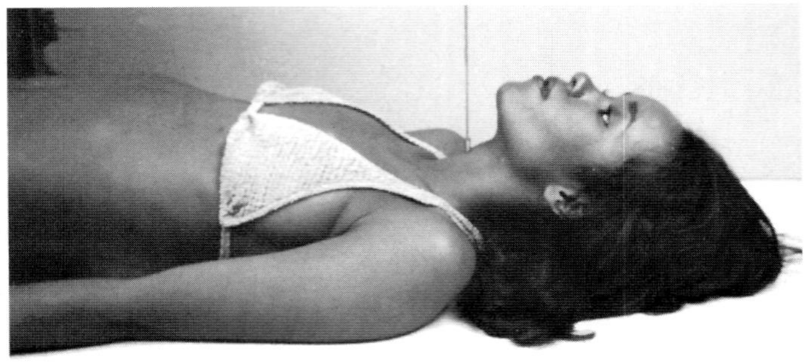

Technical Factors

- Film size–8 x 10 in. (18 x 24 cm), lengthwise.
- Moving or stationary grid.
- Use low mA and long (> 3 sec) exposure time.
- 75±5 kVp range.
- Technique and dose:

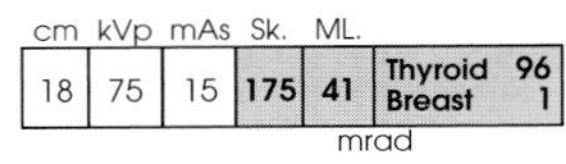

cm	kVp	mAs	Sk.	ML.	
18	75	15	175	41	Thyroid 96 / Breast 1
				mrad	

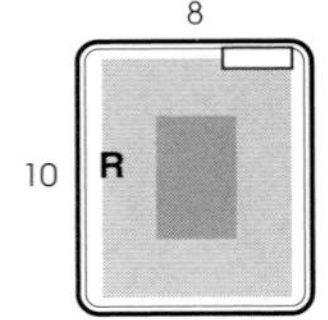

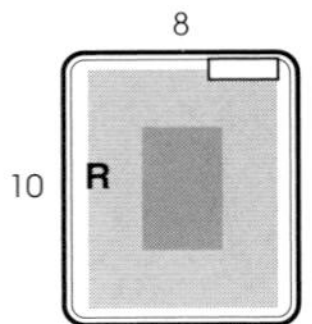

Fig. 8-85. Position for AP "chewing."

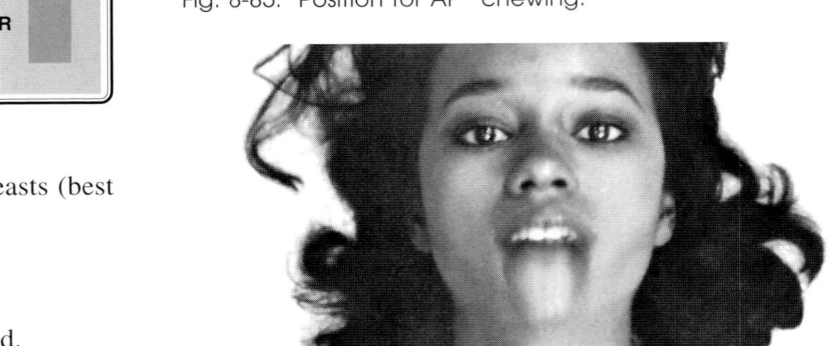

Fig. 8-86. AP "chewing" during exposure.

Shielding: Shield thyroid and chest area for female breasts (best shielding is close collimation).

Patient Position

- Supine with arms at side.
- Head on table surface, provide immobilization, if needed.

Part Position 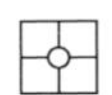

- Align midsagittal plane to CR and midline of table.
- Adjust head so that a line drawn from **lower margin of upper incisors to the base of the skull is perpendicular** to table.
- Immobilize head if needed to ensure no movement.
- Ensure there is **no rotation** of the head or thorax.
- Mandible must be in **continuous motion** during exposure.
- Ensure that **only the mandible moves**. The head must not move, and the **teeth must not make contact**.

Central Ray

- CR **perpendicular** to film, centered to **C4-5** (upper margin of thyroid cartilage).
- Center cassette to CR.
- Minimum 40 in. (102 cm) SID.

Collimation: Four-sided collimation to area of interest.

Respiration: May be suspended, or fully exhaled while saying "AHHH."

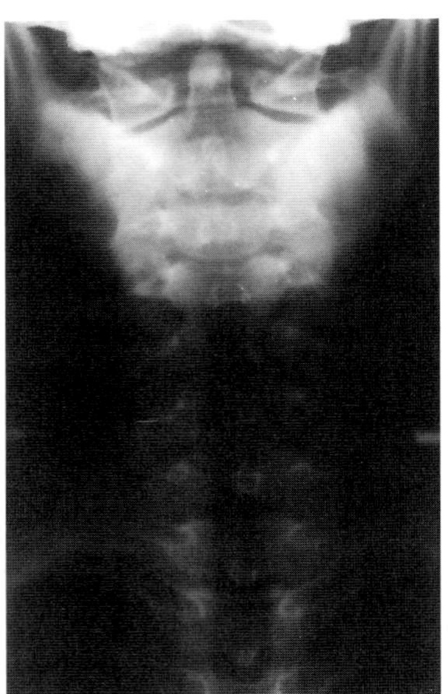

Fig. 8-87. AP "chewing."

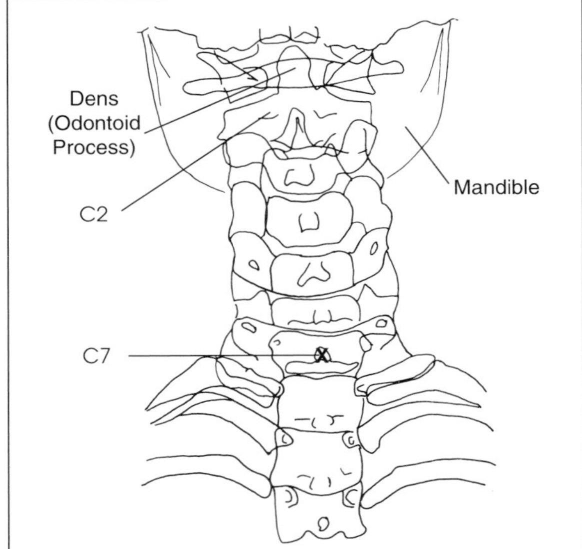

Fig. 8-88. AP "chewing."

Notes: Practice with patient prior to exposure. Having the patient say "AHHHH" during exposure prevents the tongue from moving.

Increase 2-4 kVp from AP to compensate for mandibular and tongue shadow.

Evaluation Criteria

- All seven vertebrae should be clearly seen with mandibular blurring.
- The C1-2 area should be lighter but still well visualized.
- There should be no motion of the cranium or the cervical spine.
- Optimum exposure should demonstrate both the upper and lower cervical regions even though lower vertebrae will appear somewhat darker.

AP Projection

Thoracic spine
Basic
• **AP**
• Lateral
Special
• Obliques

Structures Best Shown

Thoracic vertebral bodies, intervertebral joint spaces, distance between pedicles, spinous and transverse processes, posterior ribs and costovertebral articulations.

14

17

R

Technical Factors

- Film size–14 x 17 in. (35 x 43 cm), lengthwise.
- Moving or stationary grid.
- 80±5 or 90±5 kVp range.
- May use wedge compensation filter with thicker part of filter at head end for more uniform density (especially for thick or heavily-muscled chests with greater difference in thickness between superior and mid T spine region.

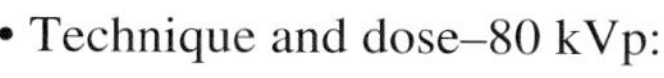

- Technique and dose–80 kVp:
- Technique and dose–90 kVp:

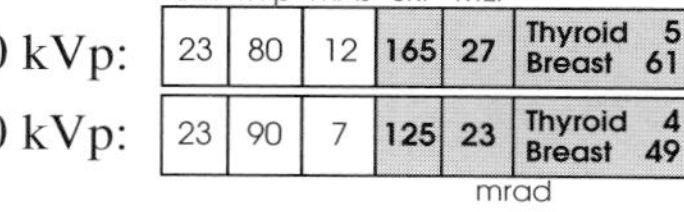

	cm	kVp	mAs	Sk.	ML.	
80 kVp	23	80	12	165	27	Thyroid 5 Breast 61
90 kVp	23	90	7	125	23	Thyroid 4 Breast 49

mrad

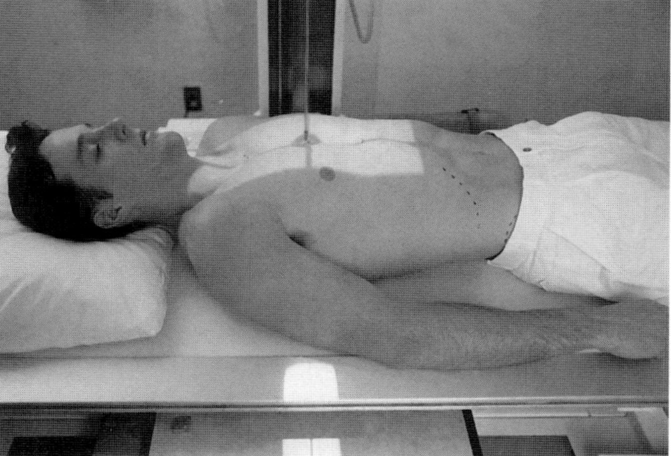

Fig. 8-89. AP T spine.

Shielding: Shield pelvic area and abdominal region. Also, use close collimation and/or breast shields for young females without obscuring vertebrae column region.

Patient Position

- Supine with **head at anode end of table**. This orientation will utilize the **anode-heel effect** to result in a more uniform density from T1 to T12.
- Arms at side, head on table or on a thin pillow, **knees up** (straighten spine).

Part Position 

- Align midsagittal plane to CR and midline of table.
- **Flex knees and hips** to reduce thoracic curvature.
- Assure there is **no rotation** of the pelvis or thorax.

Central Ray

- CR **perpendicular** to film.
- Center to **T7**, which is 3 to 4 in. (8 to 10 cm) below jugular notch, or 1 to 2 in. (3 to 5 cm) below sternal angle. (Centering is similar to AP chest.)
- Center cassette to CR (top of cassette should be about 1 to 1½ in. or 3 to 5 cm. above level of shoulder).
- Minimum 40 in. (102 cm) SID.

Collimation: Collimate on lateral margins to expose a field 4 or 5 in. (10 or 12 cm) wide, with upper and lower borders to film margins.

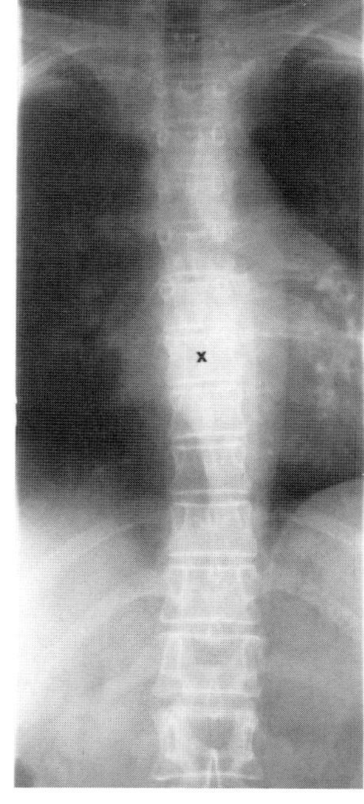

Fig. 8-90. AP.

Respiration: Suspend respiration on **expiration** (expiration reduces air volume in thorax for more uniform density of complete T spine.

Notes: T7 rather than the T6-7 interspace is the center of the 12 vertebrae thoracic spine since lower vertebrae are larger.

Higher kVp with lower mAs decreases patient dose and also decreases overall contrast which may not be preferred by some radiologists. However, it does **increase exposure latitude** (less difference in density between upper and lower T spine regions).

Evaluation Criteria

- The spinal column from C7 to L1 should be seen centered to the midline of the film.
- Good collimation will include side collimation borders medial to female breast shadows.
- Sternoclavicular joints should be seen equidistant from the spine indicating no rotation.
- Vertebral bodies should be well penetrated from T1 to T12.
- Optimum exposure and the use of a wedge filter in addition to correct use of the anode-heel effect should clearly visualize the lower thoracic vertebral body margins and intervertebral joint spaces without overexposing the upper thoracic vertebrae.

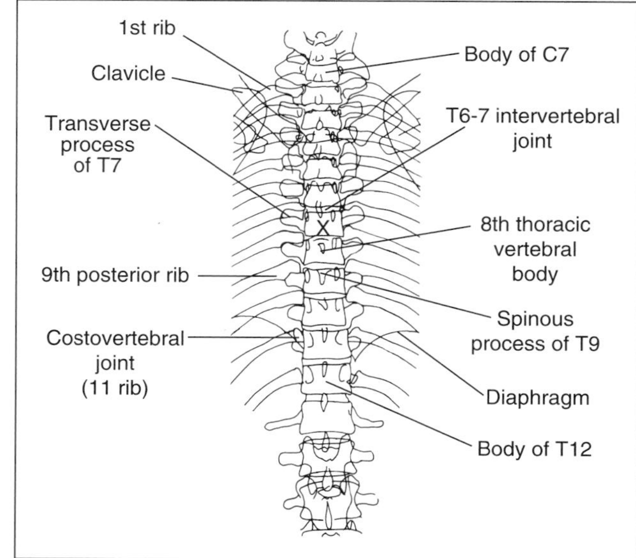

Fig. 8-91. AP.

8

Lateral Position

Thoracic spine
Basic
• AP
• **Lateral**
Special
• Obliques

Structures Best Shown

Thoracic vertebral bodies, intervertebral joint spaces and intervertebral foramina. Upper 2 or 3 vertebrae are not well visualized.

Take (swimmer's) lateral (page 271) if upper thoracic vertebrae are of special interest.

Technical Factors

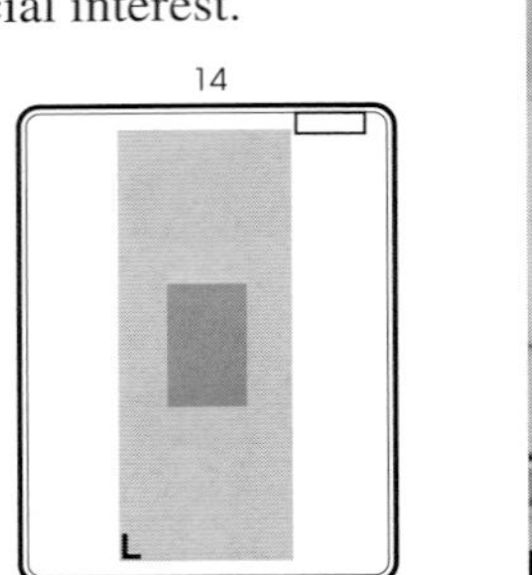

- Film size–14 x 17 in. (35 x 43 cm), lengthwise.
- Moving or stationary grid.
- 85±5 kVp range.
- With breathing technique use low mA and 3 to 4 sec. exposure.
- Place lead blocker on table behind patient to reduce scatter to film.
- Technique and dose:

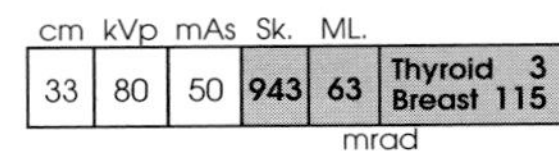

cm	kVp	mAs	Sk.	ML.	mrad
33	80	50	943	63	Thyroid 3 Breast 115

Fig. 8-92. Left lateral T spine, with proper waist support and lead blocker on table-top behind patient.

Shielding: Shield pelvic and abdominal areas to shield gonads. Use close collimation to reduce exposure to thyroid and female breasts.

Patient Position

- Lateral recumbent, head on pillow, knees flexed.

Part Position

- Align midcoronal plane to CR and midline of table.
- Raise arms to right angles to body with elbows flexed.
- Support waist so entire spine is near parallel to table (palpate spinous processes to determine this). See Note.
- Flex hips and knees for stability with support between knees.

Central Ray

- CR **perpendicular** to film and thoracic spine.
- Center to **T7**, which is 3 to 4 in. (8 to 10 cm) below jugular notch or 7 to 8 in. (18 to 21 cm) below the vertebra prominens (see chest positioning).
- Center cassette to CR (top of cassette should be about 2 in. or 5 cm above level of shoulders).
- Minimum 40 in. (102 cm) SID.

Collimation: Collimate on lateral margins to expose a field 5 or 6 in. (13 to 15 cm) wide, with upper and lower borders to film margins.

Respiration: Use breathing technique or suspend respiration after full expiration. Breathing technique blurs out unwanted rib and lung markings overlying the T vertebrae.

Note: The correct amount of support under the waist will cause the lower T vertebra to be the same distance from the table-top as upper T vertebrae. A female with wide hips and a narrow waist will require substantially more support under waist, or an alternate way to achieve open disk space without sufficient support under the waist is to angle the CR 3 to 5° cephalad to be perpendicular to the long axis of the T spine.

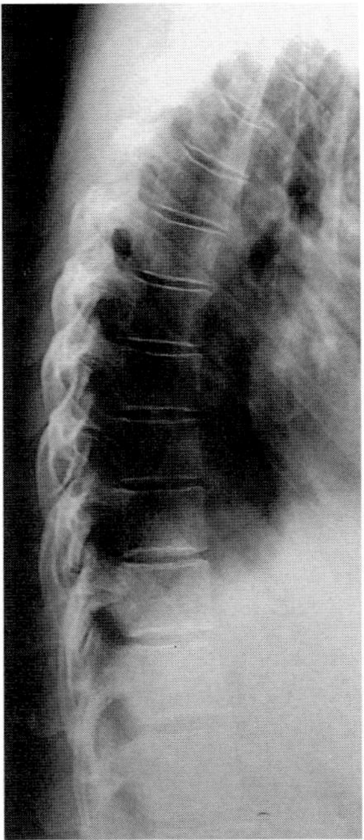

Fig. 8-93. Lateral with breathing.

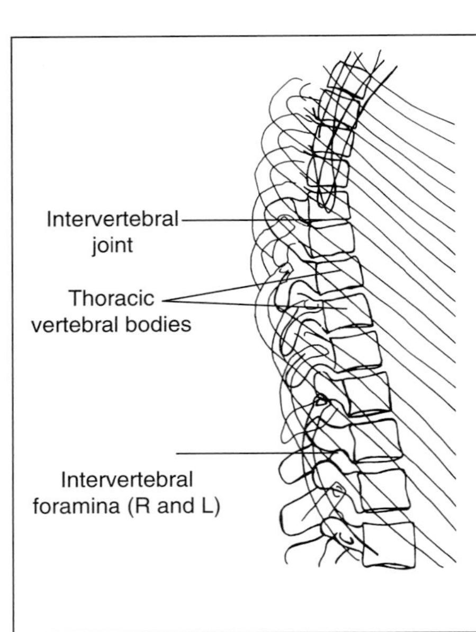

Fig. 8-94. Lateral.

Evaluation Criteria

- The spinal column from C7 to L1 should be seen centered to the midline of the film. For most patients the upper vertebra will be underexposed due to superimposition of shoulders.
- Intervertebral disk spaces should be open. (Insufficient waist support will cause the lower T disk spaces to appear closed.)
- Vertebral bodies should be in lateral profile without rotation as indicated by superimposed posterior ribs.
- Optimum exposure should demonstrate the lower two-thirds of the thoracic spine with blurring of the ribs and lung markings if breathing technique is used.

Oblique Position–Anterior (PA) or Posterior (AP) Obliques

Thoracic spine
Basic
• AP
• Lateral
Special
• **Obliques**

Structures Best Shown

Zygapophyseal joints: RPO and LPO demonstrate upside joints (farther from film). RAO and LAO demonstrate downside joints (closest to film).

Both right and left obliques are take for comparison.

14

17

R

Technical Factors

- Film size–14 x 17 in. (35 x 43 cm), lengthwise.
- Moving or stationary grid.
- 80±5 kVp range.
- Technique and dose:

	cm	kVp	mAs	Sk.	ML.	mrad
Post. obli.	32	80	20	365	27	Thyroid 1 Breast 72
Ant. obli.	32	80	20	365	27	Thyroid 1 Breast 17

Shielding: Shield pelvic and abdominal regions.

Patient Position

- Lateral recumbent, head on pillow (or erect if patient's condition requires this).

Part Position

- Align **midaxillary plane to CR and midline of table.**
- Rotate the body 20° from true lateral to create a **70° oblique** from plane of table.
- Flex hips, knees, and arms for stability as needed:

Posterior Oblique:

- (LPO or RPO), arm nearest table should be up and forward; arm nearest tube should be down and posterior.

Anterior Oblique:

- (LAO or RAO), arm nearest table should be down and posterior; arm nearest tube should be up and forward.

Central Ray

- CR **perpendicular** to film.
- Center to **T7**, which is 3 to 4 in. (8 to 10 cm) below jugular notch or 2 in. (5 cm) below sternal angle.
- Center cassette to CR (top of cassette should be about 1½ in. or 3 cm above level of shoulders).
- Minimum 40 in. (102 cm) SID.

Collimation: Close four-sided collimation to area of interest.

Respiration: Suspend breathing on full expiration.

Notes: Patient's thorax is 20° from lateral for each oblique, some type of angle guide may be used to determine correct rotation (Figs. 8-95 and 8-96).

May take as posterior or anterior obliques.

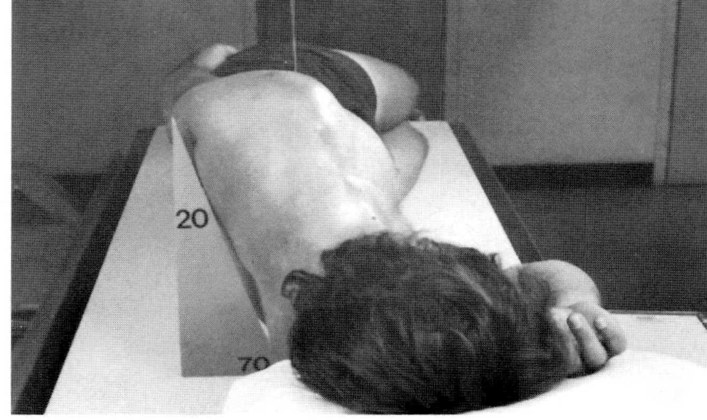

Fig. 8-95. Posterior oblique (RPO).

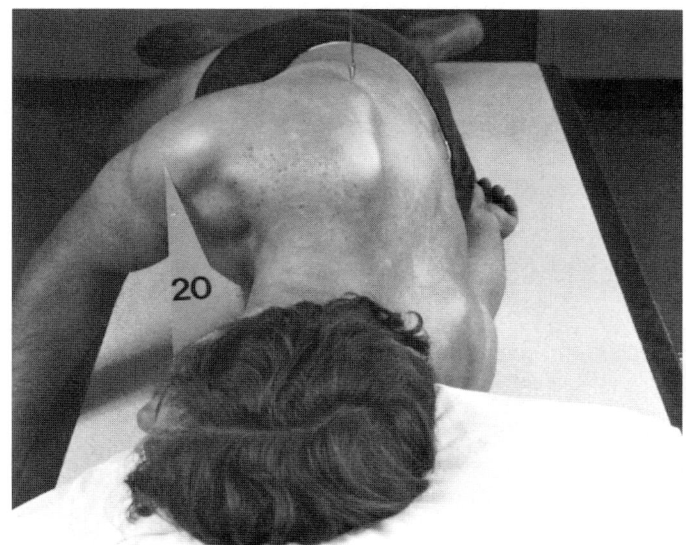

Fig. 8-96. Anterior oblique (LAO).

Evaluation Criteria

- All twelve thoracic vertebra should be seen and centered to the midline of the film.
- The zygapophyseal joints should be open and well demonstrated, but the amount of kyphosis will determine how many apophyseal joints will be seen.
- Optimum exposure should demonstrate wide exposure latitude to visualize all parts of the 12 thoracic vertebrae.

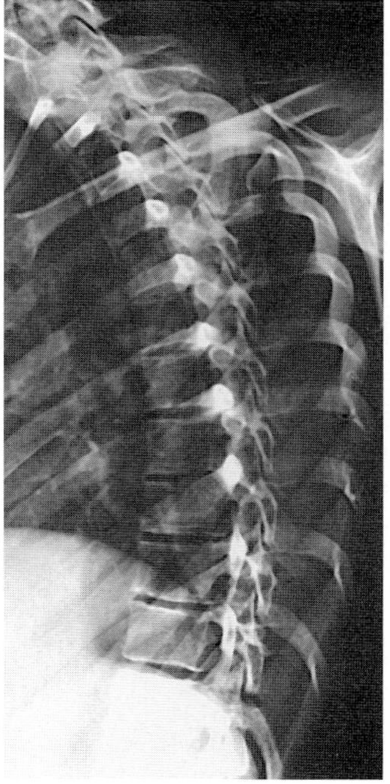

Fig. 8-97. Oblique.

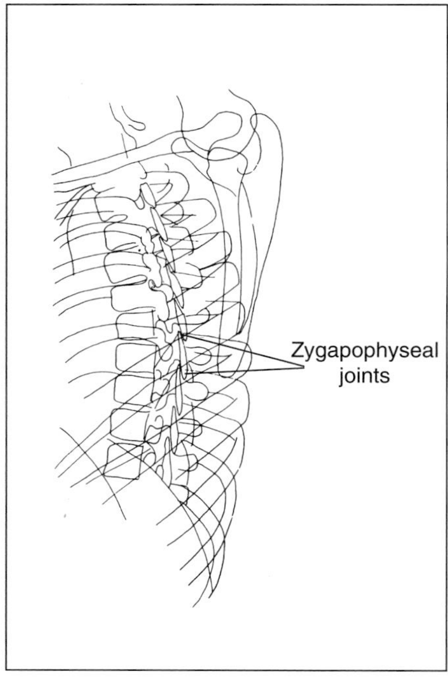

Fig. 8-98. Oblique.

Radiographs for Critique

Each of these radiographs demonstrates some error in positioning which requires a repeat. These, along with accompanying lecture slides of these and other radiographs, will provide a basis for classroom and/or positioning lab discussion. Questions with answers based on these specific critique radiographs are provided in the accompanying student workbook/lab manuals to help prepare students for classroom and/or lab discussions on film critique.

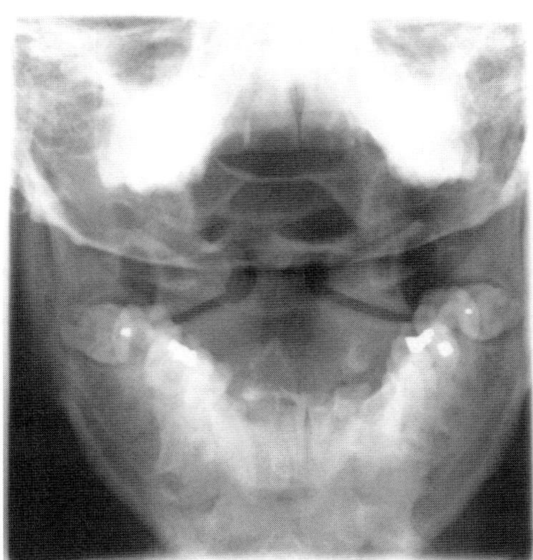

Fig. C8-99. AP open mouth (C1-C2)

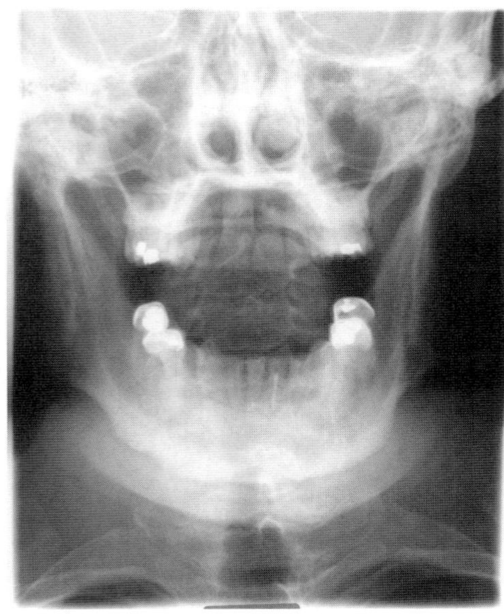

Fig. C8-100. AP open mouth (C1-C2)

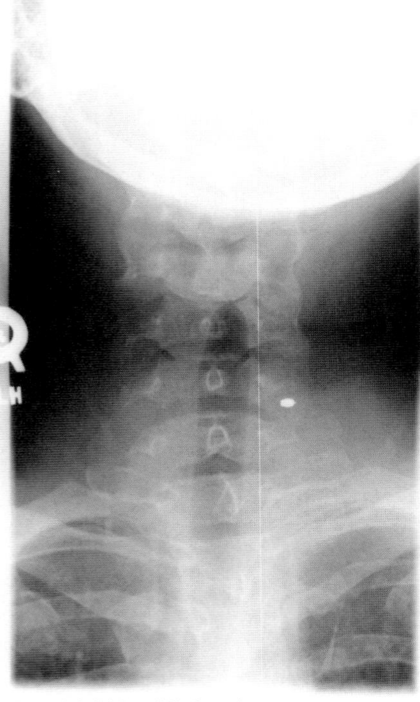

Fig. C8-101. AP C spine

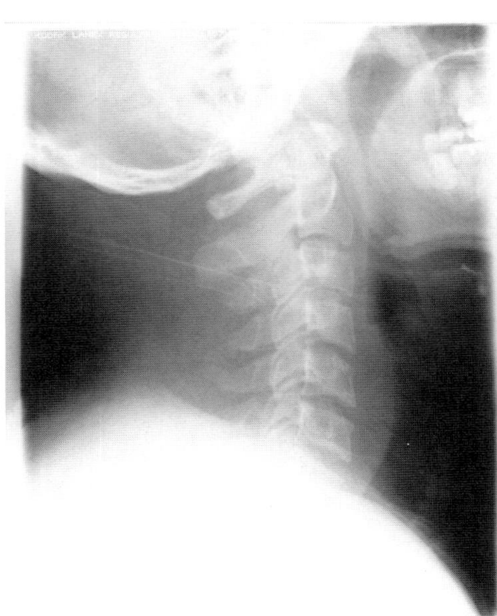

Fig. C8-102. Lateral C spine

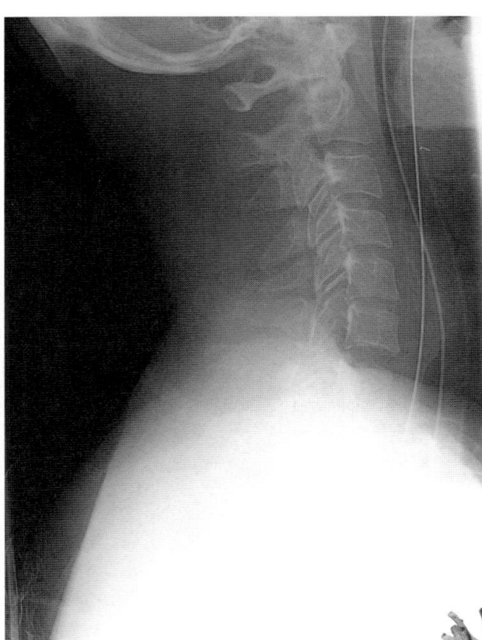

Fig. C8-103. Horizontal beam lateral C spine (with cervical collar).

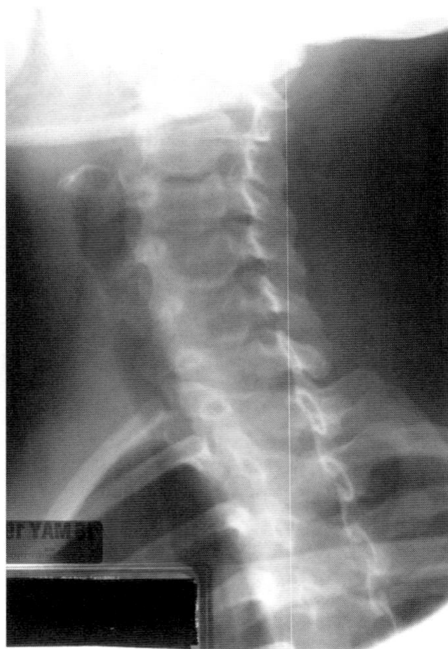

Fig. C8-104. Oblique C spine

CHAPTER 9

Lumbar Spine, Sacrum and Coccyx

CONTRIBUTIONS BY:
Alex Backus, MS, RT (R)

CONTENTS

Radiographic Anatomy

Lumbar vertebrae **280**

Sacrum **281**

Coccyx **282**

Anatomy review with radiographs **283**

Classification of joints **284**

Radiographic Positioning

Topographical landmarks **286**

Positioning considerations **287**

Survey results and basic and special projections **288**

Lumbar spine:
- AP (or PA) **289**
- Obliques **290**
- Lateral **291**
- Lateral L5-S1 **292**
- AP axial L5-S1 **293**

Scoliosis series:
- PA (AP) **294**
- Erect lateral **295**
- AP (Ferguson method) **296**
- AP (PA) R and L bending **297**

Spinal fusion series:

- AP (PA) R and L bending **297**
- Lateral–Hyperextension and hyperflexion **298**

Sacrum and coccyx:
- AP axial sacrum **299**
- AP axial coccyx **300**
- Lateral sacrum **301**
- Lateral coccyx **302**

Radiographs for critique **303**

9

LUMBAR VERTEBRAE

The third, fourth and fifth divisions of the vertebral column to be described in this chapter are the **lumbar**, **sacrum**, and **coccyx**, respectively. The anatomy and positioning of these will be studied beginning with the **lumbar vertebrae**.

Lateral and Superior Views

Joining the thoracic vertebrae distally are the five large **lumbar vertebrae**. A typical lumbar vertebra as seen from the side is illustrated in Fig. 9-1. The **bodies** of the lumbar vertebrae are large in comparison to the vertebral bodies in the thoracic and cervical regions, with the last body, L5, being largest of all. The **transverse processes** are fairly small, while the posteriorly projecting **spinous process** is quite large and blunt. The palpable lower tip of each lumbar spinous process lies at the level of the intervertebral disk space inferior to each vertebral body.

Intervertebral Foramina: The **intervertebral foramina** are well seen from the side and are best visualized on a **true lateral** of the lumbar spine. This is demonstrated on the superior view of Fig. 9-2 which shows the 90° orientation of the intervertebral foramen in relationship to the midsagittal plane. The intervertebral foramen would be the spaces or openings on each side of the central vertebral foramen formed by the roof and floor of the right and left pedicles when two vertebrae are stacked on each other. These appear as rounded openings or foramina on a lateral projection of the lumbar spine.

Zygapophyseal Joints: The **superior** and the **inferior articular processes** are best shown on a lateral view (Fig. 9-1). These processes form the **zygapophyseal** (apophyseal) **joints** when several vertebrae are stacked on top of each other. The articular facets making up this joint form an angle of from **30° to 50°** to the midsagittal plane as shown in Fig. 9-2. The upper lumbar are nearer the 50° angle, and the lower or distal lumbar are nearer the 30°. The average angle for the lumbar spine is 45°.

The **laminae** are large sturdy structures in a lumbar vertebra as demonstrated on superior and posterior views. The portion of each lamina lying between the two articular processes has a special name, the **pars interarticularis**. Occasionally the pars interarticularis fails to unite the front and back of an individual vertebra (usually at L4 or L5). This congenital (developmental) condition allows the front part of one vertebra to slip forward on the vertebral body below it, a condition known as **spondylolisthesis** *(spon′ di-lo-lis′ the-sis)*.

Posterior and Anterior Views

The posterior view in Fig. 9-3 demonstrates the general appearance of a lumbar vertebra as seen on an AP radiograph of the lumbar spine. Since the **spinous process** is being seen on end, just the outline of this process shows through the body on an AP radiograph.

The **transverse processes** extending to each side are clearly shown on these views. The **superior and inferior articular processes** are also visualized; however, the actual zygapophyseal joint is best seen on an oblique radiograph of the lumbar vertebral column because of the angle of the articular facets as described above.

A common defect, most often seen in the fifth lumbar vertebra, is the failure of two lamina to unite at the center line, leaving a space or opening where the spinous process is usually found. This congenital condition, termed **spina bifida** *(spi′ nah bif′ i-da)*, generally causes no problems as long as the structures within the vertebral canal remain in place. However, sometimes the soft tissues of the spinal cord coverings herniate posteriorly through this opening.

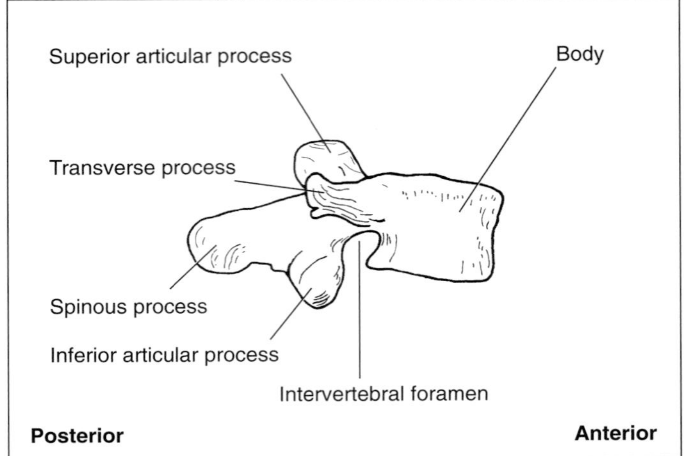

Fig. 9-1. Lumbar vertebra–Lateral view.

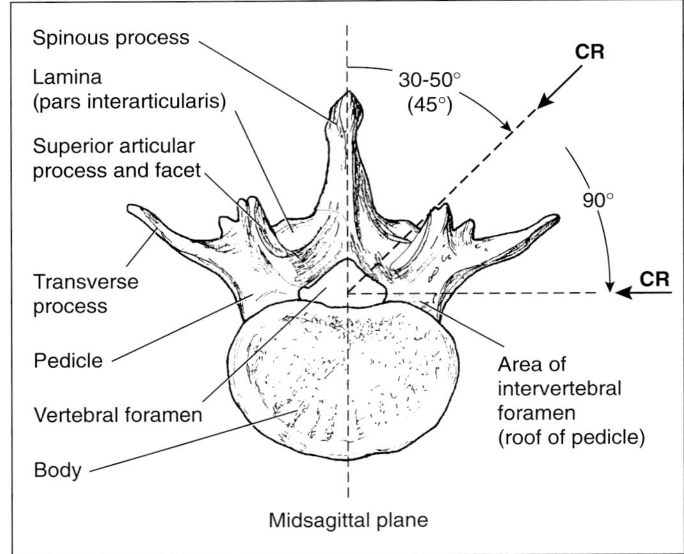

Fig. 9-2. Lumbar vertebra–Superior view.

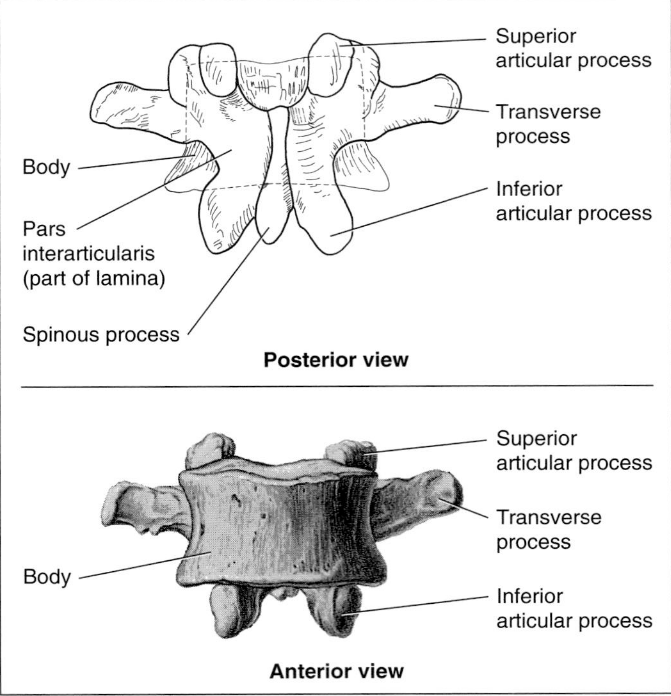

Fig. 9-3. Lumbar vertebra–Posterior and anterior views.

SACRUM

Anterior Sacrum

Immediately distal to the lumbar vertebrae is the **sacrum.** The anterior surface of a sacrum is illustrated in Fig. 9-4. The bodies of the original five segments can be seen, but they have fused into a single bone in the adult. The sacrum is shaped somewhat like a shovel, with the **apex** the most inferior portion. The anterior or pelvic surface is concave, thereby adding to the capacity of the pelvic cavity.

Four sets of foramina are shown on the anterior surface. These foramina are remnants of the intervertebral foramen (openings between vertebrae) which serve to transmit nerves and blood vessels. In the sacrum they are called the **pelvic** (anterior) **sacral foramina**.

The large masses of bone lateral to the central body of the first sacral segment are called the **alae** or wings of the sacrum. The upper surface of the sacrum closely resembles the last lumbar vertebra with which it articulates. Each **superior articular process** of the sacrum forms a zygapophyseal (apophyseal) joint with the inferior articular process of the fifth lumbar vertebra.

The anterior ridge of the body of the first sacral segment helps to form the posterior wall of the **inlet of the true pelvis**, and is termed the **promontory** of the sacrum, best demonstrated on a lateral view (Fig. 9-5).

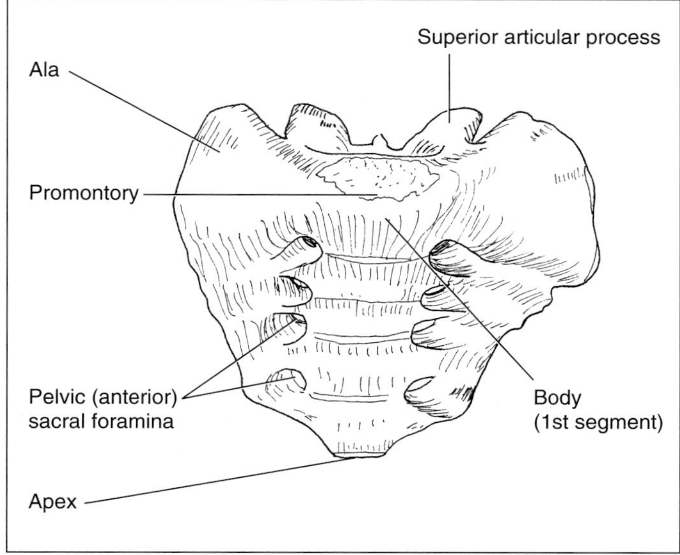

Fig. 9-4. Sacrum–Anterior view.

Lateral Sacrum and Coccyx

A lateral drawing of both the sacrum and the coccyx in Fig. 9-5 clearly illustrates the dominant curve of the sacrum and the forward projection of the coccyx. These curves determine how the central ray must be angled for a true AP projection of the sacrum or the coccyx.

The **sacral promontory** is the anterior projecting ridge portion of the sacrum. Directly posterior to the body of the first segment is the opening to the **sacral canal**, which is a continuation of the vertebral canal and contains certain sacral nerves. The **superior articular processes** (B), which articulate with the inferior articular processes of L5, are demonstrated projecting upward on each side of the opening of the sacral canal (Fig. 9-5 and 9-6). The **median sacral crest** is formed by the fused spinous processes of the sacral vertebrae.

As seen in Figs. 9-5 and 9-6, the posterior surface of the sacrum is much rougher and more irregular than the smooth anterior or pelvic surface.

The sacrum articulates with the ilium of the pelvis at the **auricular surface** (A), called this because of its resemblance in shape to the auricle of the ear. This large auricular surface, which projects **posteriorly,** is best demonstrated on the posterior view of the sacrum (Fig. 9-6).

The **sacral horns** (cornua) (D) are the small tubercles representing the inferior articular processes projecting down on each side of the fifth sacral segment. This is best seen on the lateral view of the sacrum where they are seen to project inferiorly and posteriorly to join the corresponding **horns** (cornua) of the **coccyx.**

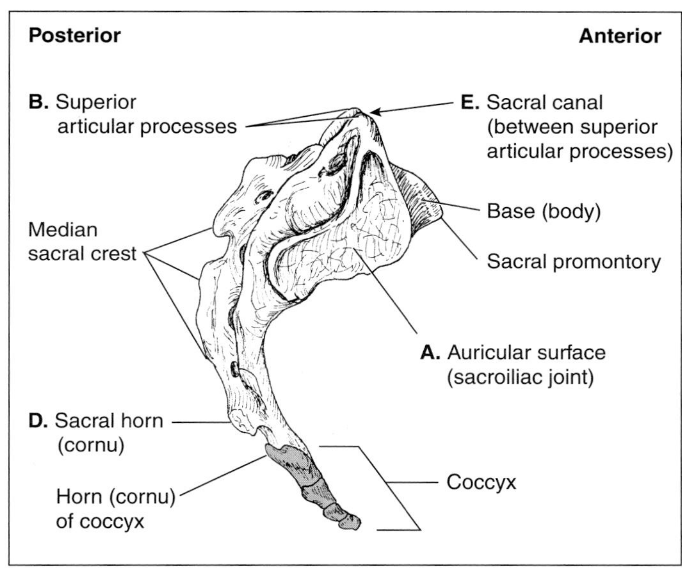

Fig. 9-5. Sacrum and coccyx–Lateral view.

Posterior Sacrum

Fig. 9-6 is a photograph of an actual sacrum as seen from the posterior aspect. Clearly seen is the large, wedge-shaped (A) **auricular surface,** which articulates with a similar surface on the ilium to form the **sacroiliac joint**. Each sacroiliac joint opens **obliquely posteriorly at an angle of 30°**.

The **articulating facets of the superior articular processes** (B), also open to the rear and are shown on this photograph. There are eight, four on each side, **posterior sacral foramina** (C), corresponding to the same number of anterior sacral foramina.

The **sacral horns** (cornua) (D) are seen as small bony projections at the very inferoposterior aspect of the sacrum. Remnants of the enclosed sacral canal (E) can also be seen. (Deteriorating bone structure leaves this canal partially open on this bone specimen.)

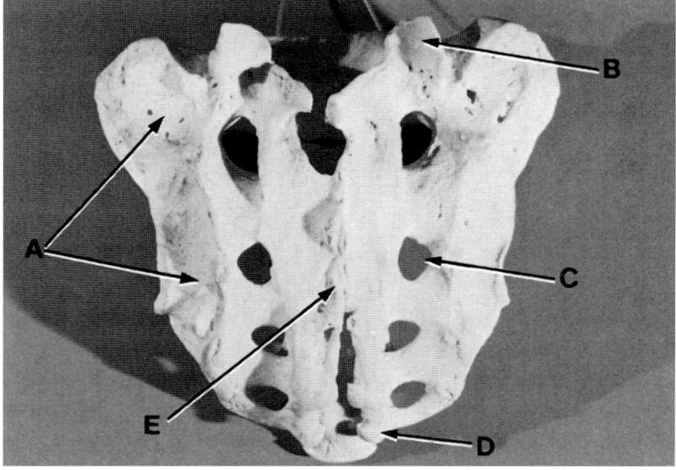

Fig. 9-6. Sacrum–Posterior view.

9

COCCYX

Anterior Coccyx (Fig. 9-7)

The most distal portion of the vertebral column is the **coccyx**. The anterior surface of the "tailbone" or coccyx is illustrated in this figure. This portion of the vertebral column has greatly regressed in the human, so there remains little resemblance to vertebrae. Three to five coccygeal segments (an average of four) have fused in the adult to form the single coccyx. The drawing in Fig. 9-7 demonstrates four formerly separate segments present in a youth, now fused into a single bone as an adult. The photograph of a coccyx in Fig. 9-8 demonstrates five segments now mostly fused in the adult coccyx.

The most superior segment is the largest and broadest of the four sections and even has two lateral projections that are small **transverse processes.** The distal pointed tip of the coccyx is termed the **apex**, while the broader, superior portion is termed the **base.**

Occasionally the second segment does not fuse solidly with the larger first segment (as shown in Fig. 9-8); however, the coccyx usually is one, small, fairly insignificant end of the vertebral column.

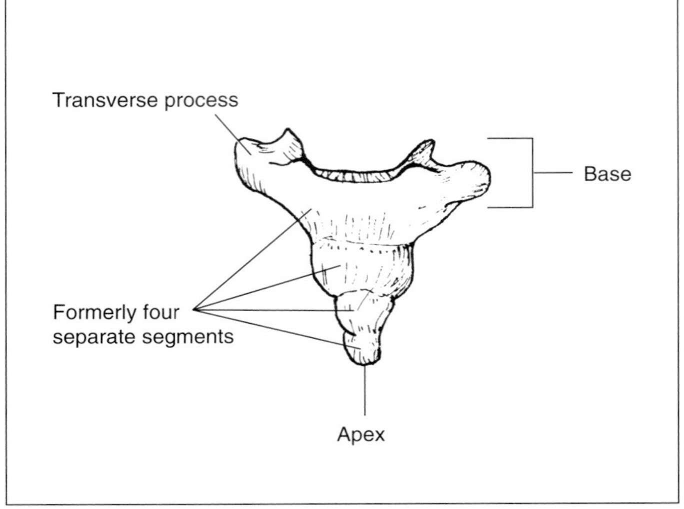

Fig. 9-7. Coccyx–Anterior view.

Posterior Coccyx (Fig. 9-8)

The posterior aspect of an actual coccyx is pictured in Fig. 9-8 along with a common U.S. postage stamp to allow a size comparison of the two. (Note that a portion of the transverse process is missing on the upper right aspect of this specimen.)

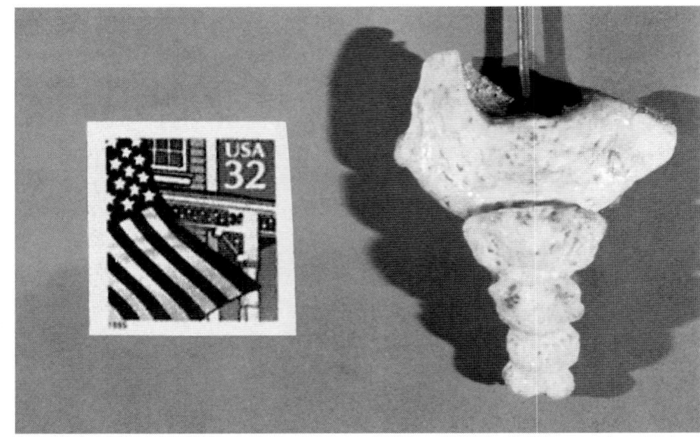

Fig. 9-8. Coccyx–Posterior view (actual size).

Lateral Sacrum and Coccyx Radiograph (Fig. 9-9)

The lateral sacrum on this radiograph is seen as a large solid bone, as compared to the much smaller coccyx. The long axis of the sacrum is shown to be angled posteriorly, requiring a cephalad angle of the CR on an AP projection. This angle is greater on an average female as compared to the average male.

Ordinarily the coccyx curves anteriorly as seen and identified on this lateral radiograph, so the apex points toward the symphysis pubis of the anterior pelvis. This forward curvature is frequently more pronounced in males and less pronounced, with less curvature, in females. The coccyx projects into the birth canal in the female and, if angled excessively forward, it can impede the birth process.

The most common injury associated with the coccyx results from a direct blow to the lower vertebral column when a person is in a sitting position. A wild ride on a toboggan might provide the type of force required to angulate the coccyx more forward than normal and make sitting down an action to be avoided for a period of time.

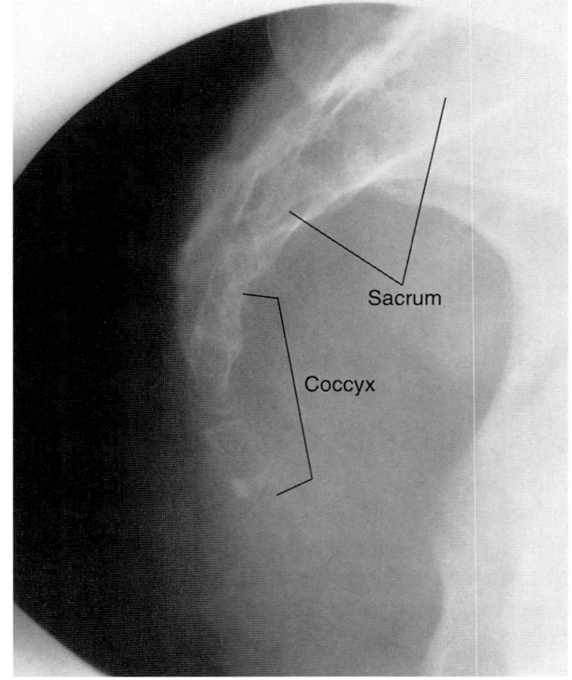

Fig 9-9. Lateral sacrum and coccyx.

ANATOMY REVIEW

Superoinferior Projection (Fig. 9-10)

Certain parts on this radiograph of an individual lumbar vertebra taken from a disarticulated skeleton are labeled as follows:

A. Spinous process.
B. Lamina.
C. Pedicle.
D. Vertebral foramen.
E. Body.
F. Transverse process.

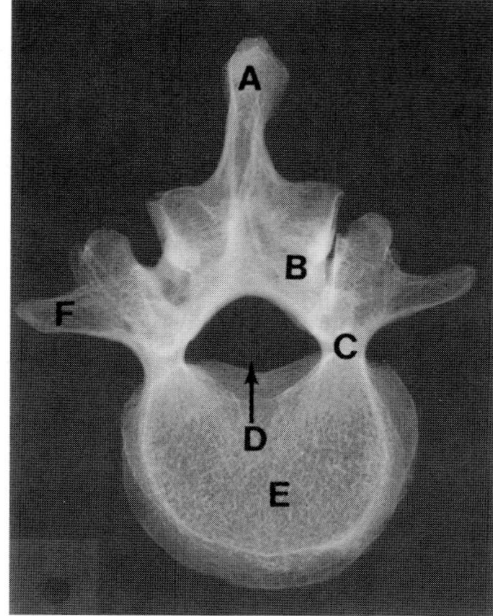

Fig. 9-10. Lumbar vertebra (superoinferior projection).

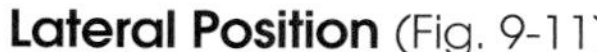

Lateral Position (Fig. 9-11)

Parts labeled A through F on the lateral view of a disarticulated lumbar vertebra are as follows:

A. Body.
B. Inferior vertebral notch, or the floor of the pedicle making up the upper portion of the rounded intervertebral foramen.
C. Area of the articulating facet of the inferior articular process (actual articular facet not shown on this lateral view). When vertebrae are stacked, these make up the zygapophyseal joints.
D. Spinous process.
E. Superior articular process.
F. Pedicle.

Note that this lateral view would "open up" and demonstrate the intervertebral foramina well (the larger round opening directly under B, the inferior vertebral notch). However, it would not demonstrate the zygapophyseal joints. This would require a 45° oblique view.

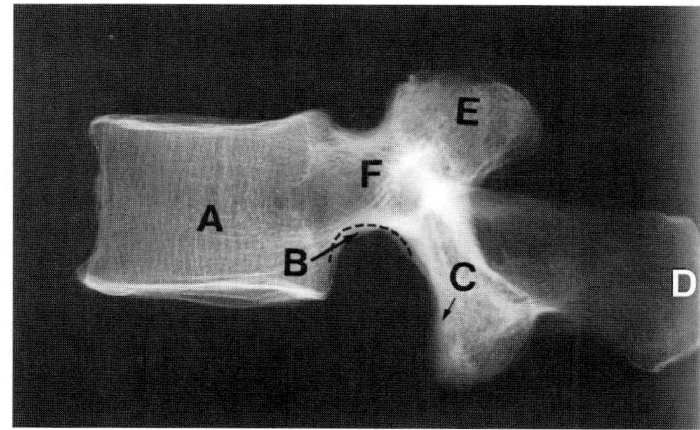

Fig. 9-11. Lumbar vertebra (lateral position).

AP Projection (Fig. 9-12)

Individual structures are more difficult to identify when the vertebrae are superimposed by the soft tissues of the abdomen as demonstrated on this AP lumbar spine radiograph. Those structures labeled A through F are:

A. Transverse process of L5.
B. Lower lateral portion of the body of L4.
C. Lower part of the spinous process of L4 as visualized on end.
D. One inferior articular process of L3.
E. Superior articular process of L4.
F. L1-2 intervertebral disk space.

The facets of the inferior and superior articular processes (D and E) make up one zygapophyseal joint not visualized on this AP projection. It is, however, demonstrated on a 45° oblique projection of lumbar vertebrae (see Fig. 9-16 on following page).

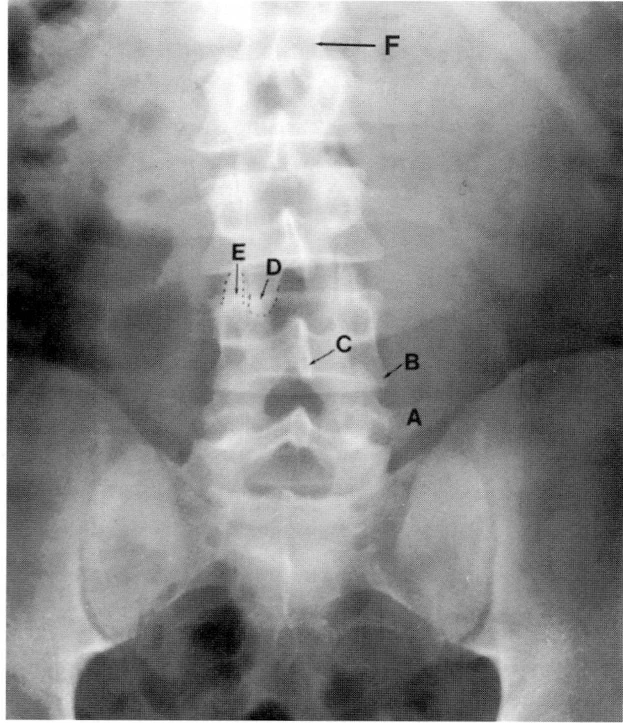

Fig. 9-12. Lumbar spine (AP projection).

Anatomy Review continued

Lateral Lumbosacral Spine (Fig. 9-13)

Radiograph of entire lumbosacral spine in lateral position:

A. Body of L1
B. Body of L3
C. Intervertebral disk space between L4 and L5
D. Body of L5
E. Superimposed intervertebral foramina between L2 and L3.

AP Lumbosacral Spine (Fig. 9-14)

AP projection of entire lumbosacral spine labeled as follows:

A. Last thoracic vertebra (T12)
B. First lumbar vertebra
C. Third lumbar vertebra
D. Fifth lumbar vertebra

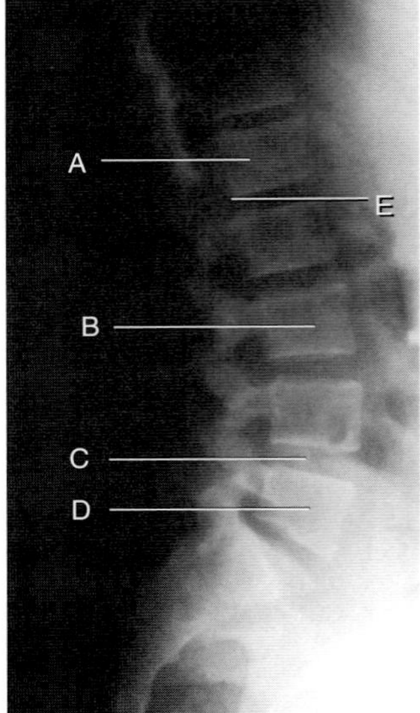

Fig. 9-13. Lumbosacral spine -Lateral.

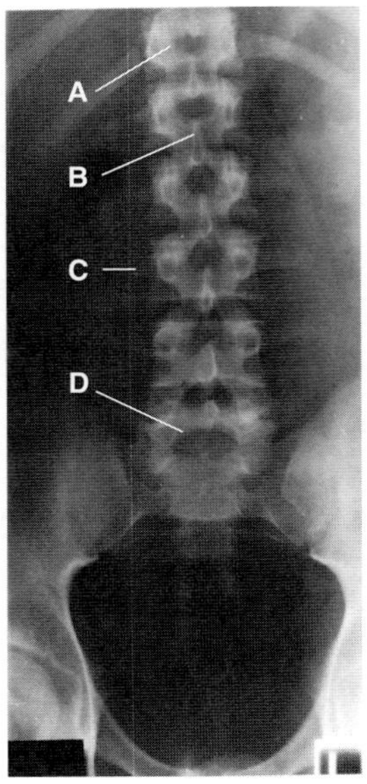

Fig. 9-14. Lumbosacral spine-AP.

OBLIQUE LUMBAR VERTEBRAE

Appearance of "Scotty Dog"

Any bone and its parts, when seen in an oblique position, are more difficult to recognize than the same bone seen in the conventional frontal or lateral view. A vertebra is no exception; however, imagination can help us in the case of the lumbar vertebrae. A good 45° oblique will project the various structures in such a way that a "Scotty dog" seems to appear. The drawing in Fig. 9-15 shows the various components of the "Scotty dog.'' The head and neck of the dog are probably the easiest features to recognize. The neck is one **pars interarticularis** (part of the lamina which primarily makes up the shoulder region of the dog). The **ear** of the dog is one **superior articular process**, while the **eye** is formed by one **pedicle**. One **transverse process** forms the **nose. The front legs** are formed by one **inferior articular process.**

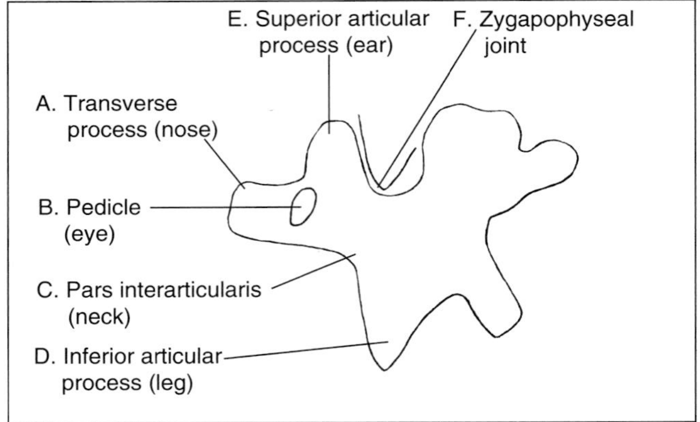

Fig. 9-15. The "Scotty dog."

Oblique Lumbar Radiograph (Fig. 9-16)

The radiograph in Fig. 9-16 shows the "Scotty dog" appearance that should be visible on a good oblique radiograph of the lumbar spine.

A. Nose of the "Scotty dog," formed by one transverse process.
B. Eye is one pedicle seen on end.
C. Collar around the neck of the dog, which is the area of the pars interarticularis.
D. Front leg of the animal, formed by one inferior articular process.
E. Pointed ear, one of the superior articular processes.
F. Zygapophyseal joint, formed by front leg of the "scotty" above and ear of the "scotty" below.

Each of the five lumbar vertebrae should assume a similar "Scotty dog" appearance with zygapophyseal joint spaces open on a correctly obliqued lumbar radiograph.

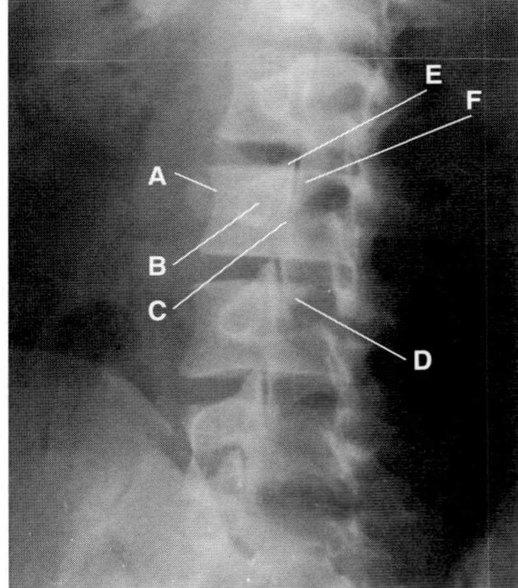

Fig. 9-16. Oblique lumbar spine (the "Scotty dog").

CLASSIFICATION OF JOINTS

There are two types or classifications of joints or articulations involving the vertebral column.

(1) Zygapophyseal (Apophyseal) Joints

The zygapophyseal joints between the superior and inferior articular processes are classified as **synovial joints**, which are **diarthrodial** or freely movable, with a **plane (gliding) type** movement.

(2) Intervertebral Joints

The intervertebral joints between the bodies of any two vertebrae containing intervertebral disks which are made up of fibrocartilage are only slightly movable. These joints which are tightly bound by cartilage are thus classified as **cartilaginous joints**. They are **amphiarthrodial** (slightly movable) of the **symphyses** subclass, similar to the symphysis pubis of the pelvis.

There is not a great deal of motion between any two vertebrae, however the combined effect of all the vertebrae in the column does allow a considerable range of motion. The possible movements are flexion, extension, lateral flexion (bending) and rotation. Certain radiographic exams of the spinal column involving hyperflexion and hyperextension and/or right and left bending routines can measure this range of motion.

INTERVERTEBRAL FORAMINA VS ZYGAPOPHYSEAL JOINTS

Intervertebral Foramina - Lateral Lumbar Spine

The intervertebral foramina for the lumbar spine are visualized on a true lateral projection, as demonstrated in the Fig. 9-13 radiograph on the preceding page.

Zygapophyseal Joints - Oblique Lumbar Spine

Oblique projections commonly taken of the lumbar spine require a good understanding of the anatomy of the vertebrae and the zygapophyseal joints to know how much to oblique, and to know which side is being demonstrated since they can be taken in either anterior or posterior oblique positions.

Posterior Oblique: As the drawing and photographs of the skeleton demonstrate, the **downside** joints are visualized on **posterior** obliques. The downside zygapophyseal joints are not visible on the skeleton since they are "under" the bodies of the vertebrae (Fig. 9-18), but as seen on the inferosuperior sectional drawing, the downside or right joints would be demonstrated on a right posterior oblique (RPO). This is seen on the RPO radiograph in Fig. 9-19, which clearly shows the ears and legs of the "Scotty dogs," or the right zygapophyseal joints (see arrows).

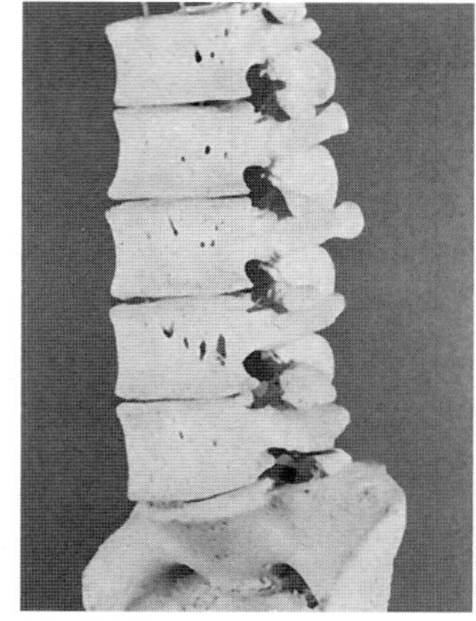

Fig. 9-17

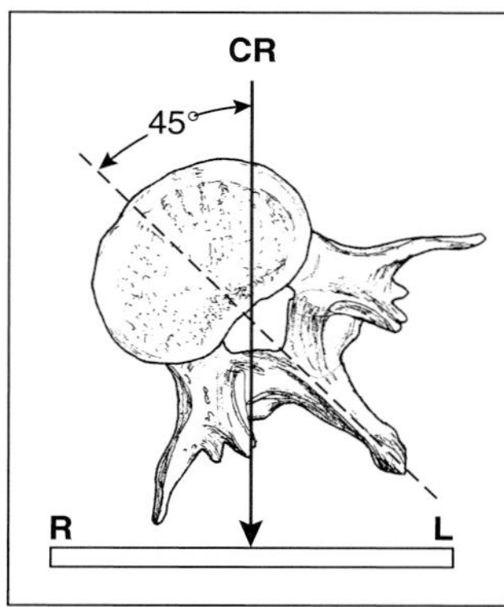

Fig. 9-18.

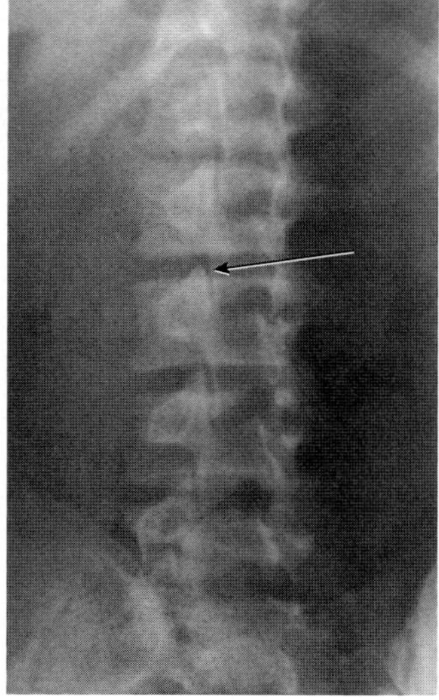

Fig. 9-19.
Posterior oblique lumbar spine.
RPO–Downside or **right** joints.

Anterior Oblique: Anterior obliques of the lumbar spine may be more comfortable for the patient and allow the natural lumbar curvature of the spine to coincide with the divergence angle of the x-ray beam.

As demonstrated, an **anterior** oblique visualizes the **upside** joints. Therefore, a right anterior oblique (RAO) visualizes the upside or left zygapophyseal joints (Figs. 9-21 and 9-22).

The degree of obliquity depends on which area of the lumbar spine is of specific interest. A 45° oblique is for the general lumbar region, but if interest is specifically in **L1 or L2**, the degree of obliquity should be increased to **at least 50°**. If interest is in the **L5-S1** area, the obliquity would be **only about 30°** from an AP or PA. There is some variance among patients, but in general the upper lumbar region requires more degrees of obliquity than the lower regions. The reason for this is the upper lumbar vertebrae take on some shape characteristics of the thoracic vertebrae, which require 70° of obliquity to demonstrate the zygapophyseal joints as described in the preceding chapter.

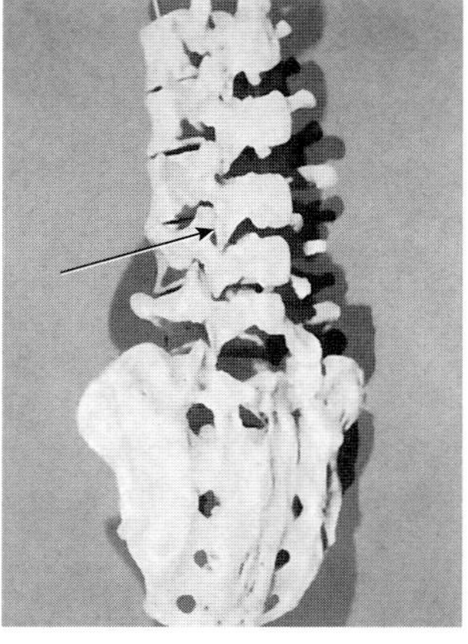

Fig. 9-20

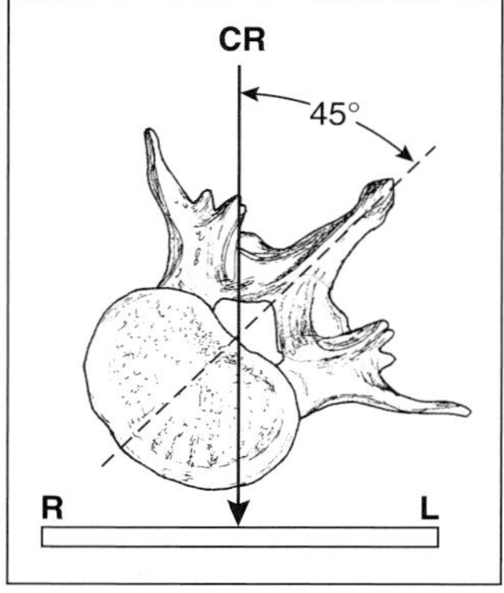

Fig. 9-21.

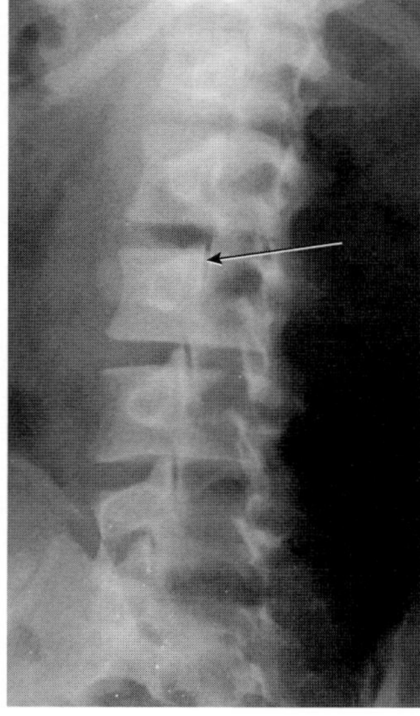

Fig. 9-22.
Anterior oblique lumbar spine.
RAO–Upside or **left** joints.

Summary Chart

Lumbar Spine	
Intervertebral foramina – 90° lateral	***Zygapophyseal joints – 45° obliques***
R or L Lateral	**Posterior obliques - downside** RPO – Right foramina LPO – Left foramina **Anterior oblique - upside** RAO – Left foramina LAO – Right foramina

Radiographic Positioning

TOPOGRAPHICAL LANDMARKS

Correct positioning for the small coccyx and the larger sacrum and lumbar spine require a thorough understanding of certain topographical landmarks which can be easily and accurately palpated.

The most reliable topographical landmarks for the spine are the various palpable bony prominences that are fairly constant from one person to another. However, it should be emphasized that the landmarks as presented refer to an average healthy, erect, normally developed adult male or female. These landmarks will vary in subjects with anatomical and, especially, skeletal anomalies. The very young and the very old will also have slightly different features than the average adult.

Lower Spine Landmarks

The drawings on the right and the photographs below illustrate various landmarks relative to the lower vertebral column.

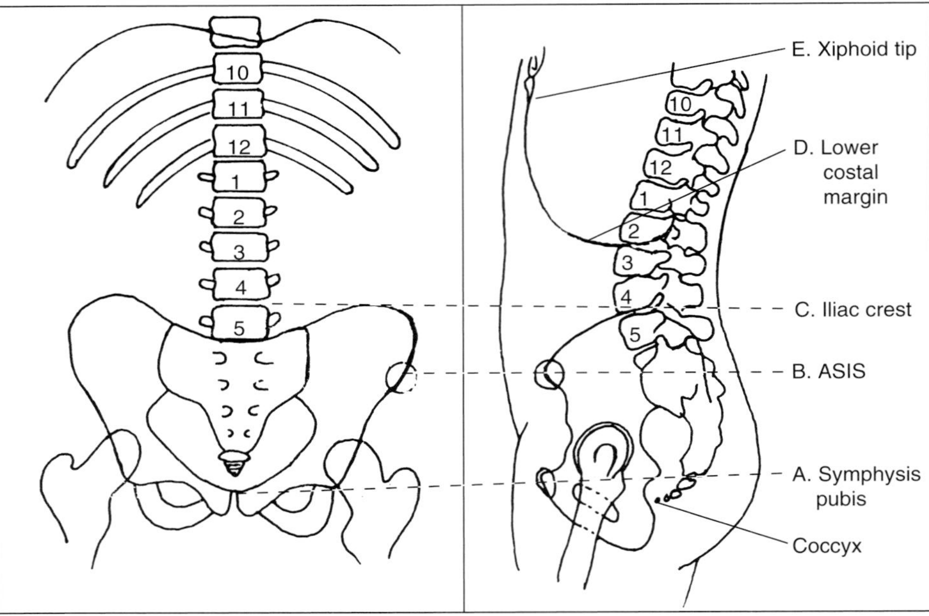

Fig. 9-23. Lower spine landmarks.

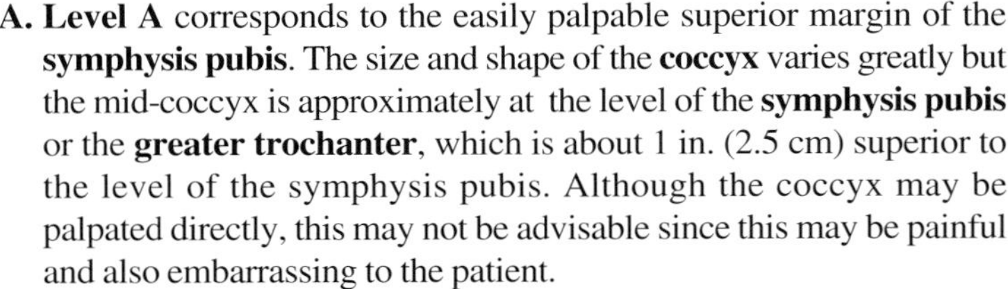

A. Level A corresponds to the easily palpable superior margin of the **symphysis pubis**. The size and shape of the **coccyx** varies greatly but the mid-coccyx is approximately at the level of the **symphysis pubis** or the **greater trochanter**, which is about 1 in. (2.5 cm) superior to the level of the symphysis pubis. Although the coccyx may be palpated directly, this may not be advisable since this may be painful and also embarrassing to the patient.

Note on the photographs below and the drawings above that the greater trochanters are approximately 1 to 1½ in. (3 to 4 cm) above the upper border of the symphysis pubis at the level of the coccyx.

B. The **anterior superior iliac spine** (ASIS) is at about the same **level (B)** as the **second sacral segment.**

C. Level C is the most superior portion of the **iliac crest** and is at approximately the same level as the junction of the **fourth and fifth lumbar vertebrae.**

D. The lowest margin of the ribs or **lower costal margin** (D) is at the approximate level of **L2 or L3**.

E. The **xiphoid tip** is approximately at the level of **T9 or T10**.

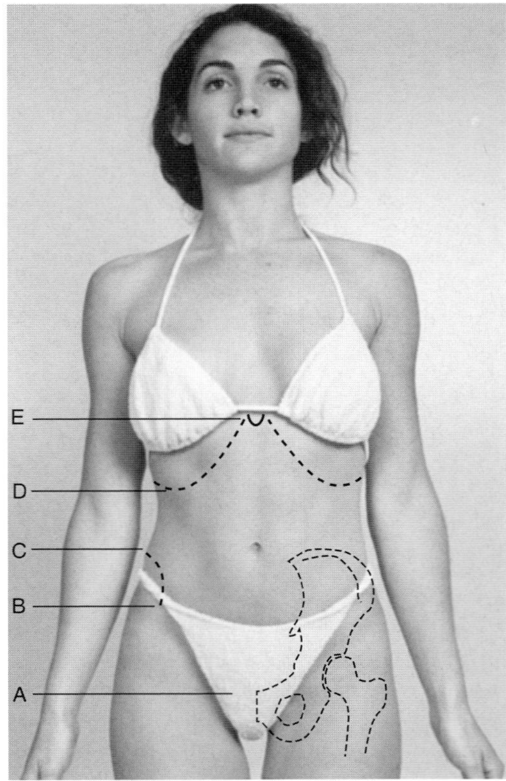

Fig. 9-24.

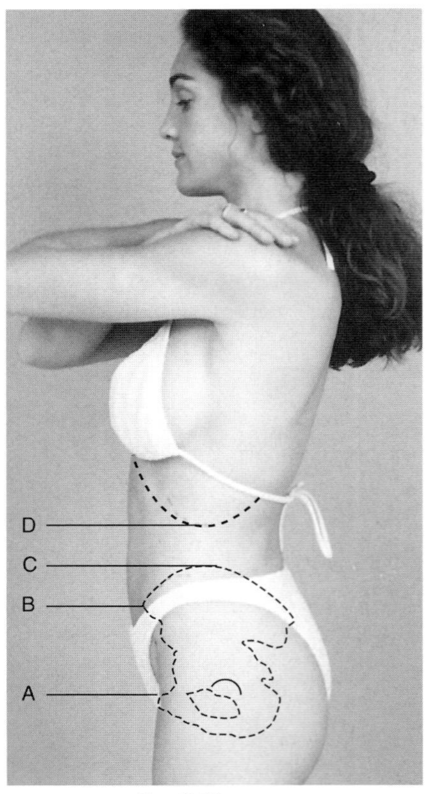

Fig. 9-25.

Lower spine landmarks.

POSITIONING CONSIDERATIONS

Gonadal Shielding

Gonadal shielding and other protection practices such as close collimation are especially important because of the proximity of the lumbar spine, sacrum and coccyx to the gonads. Gonadal shielding can and should **always be used on males** of reproductive age on coccyx, sacrum or lumbar spine radiographs. The gonadal shield should be placed with the top edge of the shield at the lower margin of the symphysis pubis.

If the area of interest includes the sacrum and/or coccyx, gonadal shielding for females may not be possible without obscuring essential anatomy. However, if the area of interest is the lumbar spine, gonadal shields should be used on all children and males and females of reproductive age.

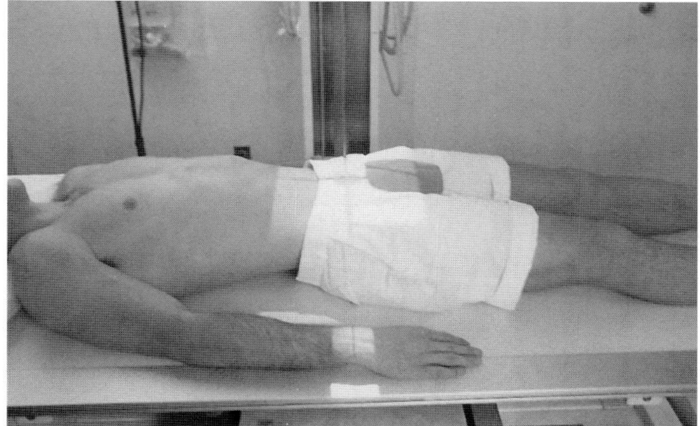

Fig. 9-26. Male gonadal shielding-Lumbar spine.

AP Projection-Lumbar Spine (Knees Up)

Frontal lumbar spine radiographs are commonly taken as AP projections with the **knees and hips flexed** to straighten the spine. Flexing the knees and hips (Fig. 9-28) reduces the lumbar curvature and brings the back in contact with the table, and the lumbar vertebral column nearer parallel to the film. The incorrect position is shown in Fig. 9-27 wherein the pelvis is tipped forward slightly when the lower limbs are extended, which exaggerates the lumbar curvature. The flexing of the knees and hips is a simple positioning step but important because it straightens the spine and opens up the intervertebral spaces on an AP lumbar projection.

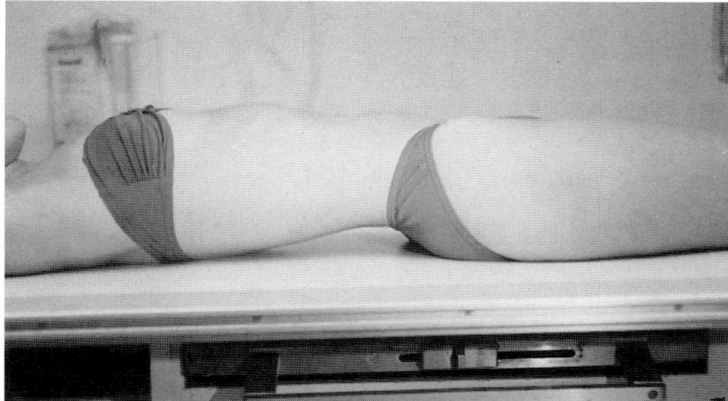

Fig. 9-27. **Incorrect**-Lower limbs extended (AP lumbar spine).

PA vs. AP Projections: Even though the AP projection with knees and hips flexed is a common routine for the lumbar spine, there is a distinct advantage in taking this as a PA projection in a prone position. The prone position places the lumbar spine with its natural lumbar curvature in such a way that the intervertebral disk spaces are nearer parallel to the divergent x-ray beam. This opens up and provides better visualization of the margins of the intervertebral disk spaces. However, the negative factor against the PA is the increased OID with accompanying magnification and loss of detail, especially for a patient with a large abdomen.

The female patient gonadal dose for an AP projection is approximately 35% higher than for a PA due to the slightly anterior to midline placement of female ovarion structures.

The survey results indicate that in 1995, 97% of institutions included the AP lumbar spine as routine, and only 5% the PA.

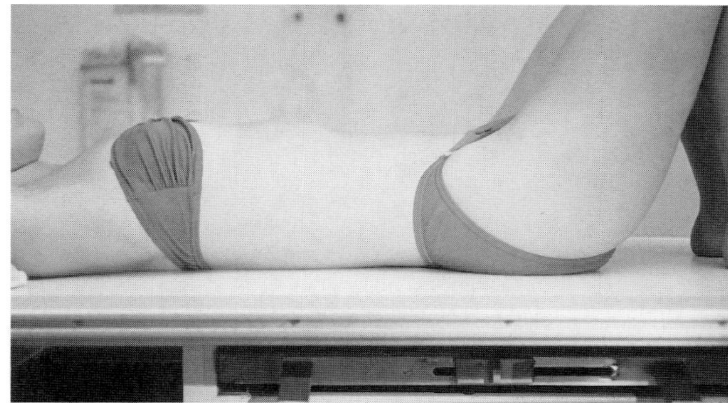

Fig. 9-28. **Correct**-Knees and hips flexed (AP lumbar spine).

kVp Range

Increasing the kVp and decreasing the mAs accordingly reduces patient doses but produces a lower contrast image. Higher kVp increases scatter radiation, which tends to degrade the radiographic image. This can be minimized two ways, with close collimation on all projections, and for the lateral, the use of a lead blocker placed on the table-top next to the patient (Fig. 9-29). Each radiographer should determine the preference of the radiologist and the departmental policies regarding preferred kVp ranges. Comparative patient doses are listed on positioning pages. The lead blocker, however, should be used on all lateral spine projections to absorb scatter and improve image quality.

SID

A common minimum SID is 40 in. (102 cm), but an increased SID of 42, 44, or even 46 in. (107, 112 or 117 cm) not only reduces magnification and increases detail but also results in less skin dose to the patient.

Other advantages of increased SID for radiography of the spine are a decrease in the anode-heel effect and less angle of divergence of the x-ray beam, which facilitates in the "opening up" of intervertebral spaces when the vertebral column is parallel to the film.

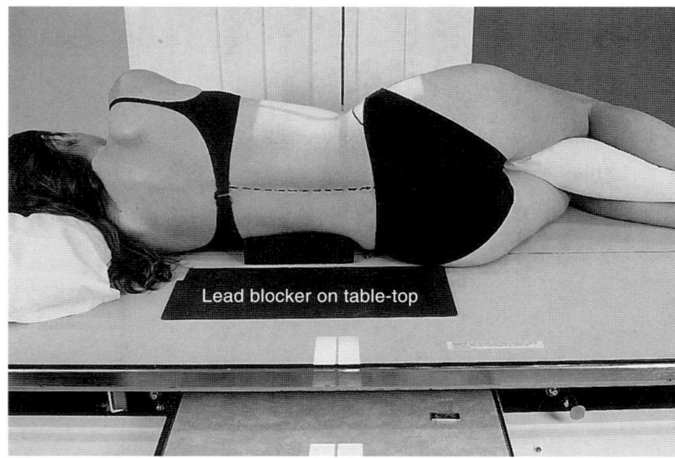

Fig. 9-29. Lateral lumbar spine with lead blocker on table-top.

9

NATIONAL SURVEY

Departmental standard (basic) and special routines of the coccyx, sacrum and lumbar spine were very consistent throughout the United States.

Lumbosacral Spine Routine

L.S. spine	U.S. Average Basic 1995 (1989)	U.S. Average Special 1995 (1989)
• AP	97% (98%)	
or		
PA	5% –	
• Lateral	97% (99%)	
• L5-S1 lateral spot	94% (90%)	
• Posterior obliques (45°)	62% (69%)	20% –
or		
Anterior obliques (45°)	28% –	18% –
• AP L5-S1 (30-35° cephalad)	20% (16%)	20% (8%)
• AP fusion, R and L bending		44% –
• Lateral flexion and extension		60% (2%)
• AP or PA scoliosis series (Ferguson method)		44% –

Sacrum and Coccyx Routine

Sacrum and coccyx	U.S. Average Basic 1995 (1989)	U.S. Average Special 1995 (1989)
• AP sacrum (15-25° cephalad)	98% (98%)	
• AP coccyx (10-20° caudad)	96% (96%)	
• Lateral sacrum and coccyx combined	81% –	
• Separate laterals of sacrum and coccyx	28% –	

Summary

The results reveal the following:

Lumbar Spine: The AP lumbar spine (97%) is much more common as a basic projection than a PA (5%). The posterior obliques also are more common (62%) than anterior obliques (28%) for the lumbar spine. The obliques of the lumbar spine are considered basic or routine rather than special projections by the majority of institutions.

Sacrum and Coccyx: The combined lateral (81%) is much more common than separate laterals of the sacrum and coccyx (28%). This is a recommended routine in this text also due to the relatively high gonadal doses from these projections.

STANDARD AND SPECIAL OPERATING PROCEDURES

Certain basic and special projections or positions for the coccyx, sacrum and lumbar spine are demonstrated and described on the following pages as suggested standard and optional departmental procedures.

Basic Projections

Standard or basic projections, also sometimes referred to as routine projections or departmental routines, are those projections or positions commonly taken on average patients who are helpful and can cooperate in performing the procedure.

Special Projections

Optional projections are those more common projections or positions taken as extra or additional projections to better demonstrate certain pathologic conditions or specific body parts.

Basic and Special Projections

Lumbar spine
Basic
- AP (or PA) **289**
- Obliques–Ant. or post. **290**
- Lateral **291**
- Lateral L5-S1 **292**

Special
- AP axial L5-S1 **293**

Scoliosis series
Basic
- PA (AP)
  –Erect and/or recumbent **294**
- Erect lateral **295**

Special
- AP (Ferguson method) **296**
- AP (PA)
  –R and L bending **297**

Spinal fusion series
Basic
- AP (PA)
  –R and L bending **297**
  (same as for scoliosis series)
- Lateral–hyperextension and hyperflexion **298**

Sacrum and coccyx
Basic
- AP axial sacrum **299**
- AP axial coccyx **300**
- Lateral sacrum **301**
- Lateral coccyx **302**

AP (or PA) Projection

Lumbar spine
Basic
- **AP (or PA)**
- Obliques–Ant. or post.
- Lateral
- Lateral L5-S1

Structures Best Shown

Lumbar vertebral bodies, intervertebral joints, spinous and transverse processes, laminae, SI joints and sacrum.

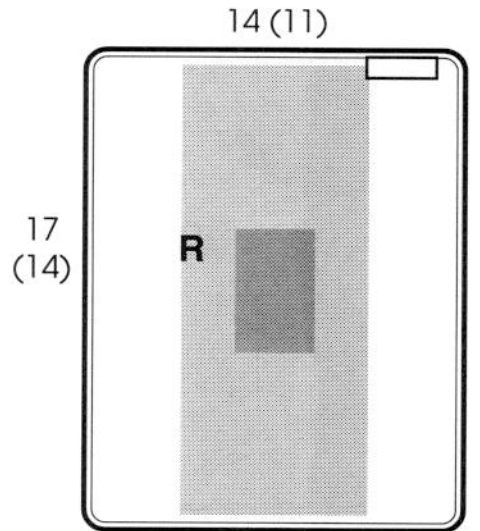

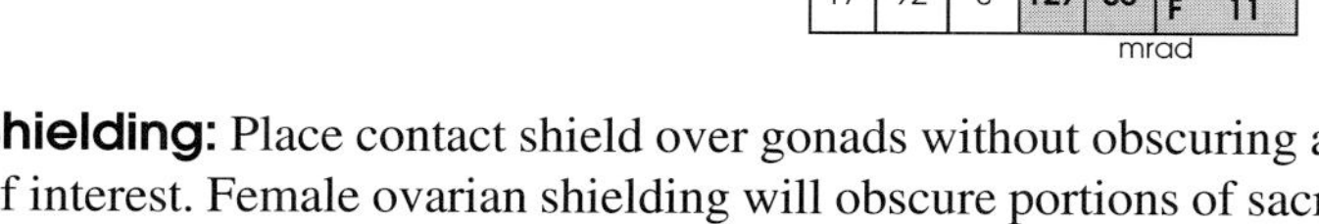

cm	kVp	mAs	Sk.	ML.	Gon.
17	80	15	175	45	M 1 F 19
17	92	8	127	36	M 1 F 15
17	92	8	127	36	M 0 F 11

mrad

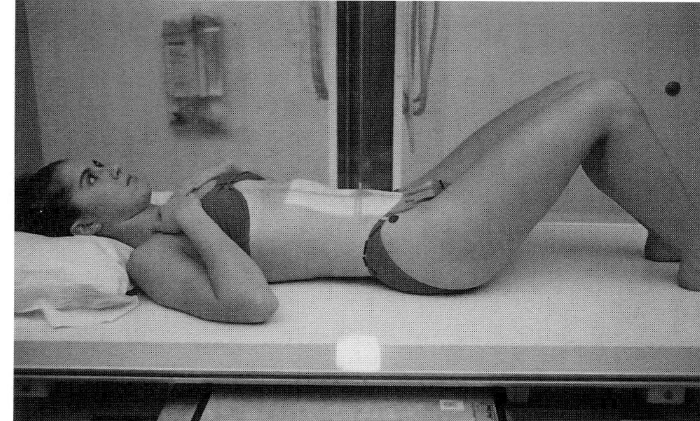

Fig. 9-30. AP projection (centered for 14 x 17 film).

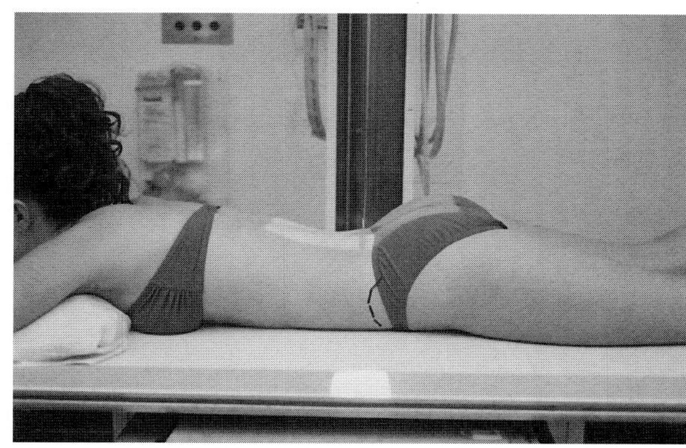

Fig. 9-31. Alternate PA projection.

Shielding: Place contact shield over gonads without obscuring area of interest. Female ovarian shielding will obscure portions of sacrum and coccyx.

Patient Position

- Supine with **knees and hips flexed** and head on pillow. (May also be done PA prone or erect AP or PA, see Notes below.)

Part Position

- Align midsagittal plane to CR and midline of table.
- Place arms at side or up on chest.
- Ensure **no rotation** of torso or pelvis.

Central Ray

- CR perpendicular to film centered to:

  Larger Film (14 x 17): Center to **level of iliac crest** (L4-5 interspace). This will include lumbar vertebrae, sacrum and possibly coccyx. Center cassette to CR.

  Smaller Film (11 x 14): Center to **level of 1 to 1½ in.** (3 to 4 cm) **above iliac crest** (L3). This will include primarily the five lumbar vertebrae. Center cassette to CR.
- Minimum 40 in. (102 cm) SID.

Collimation: Four-sided collimation with superior and inferior borders to near film margins.

Respiration: Suspend breathing on **expiration**.

Notes: Flexion of knees and hips straightens the spine, which helps open up intervertebral spaces.

May be done prone as a PA projection, which may open up interspaces better. This increases OID; therefore, use a small focal spot.

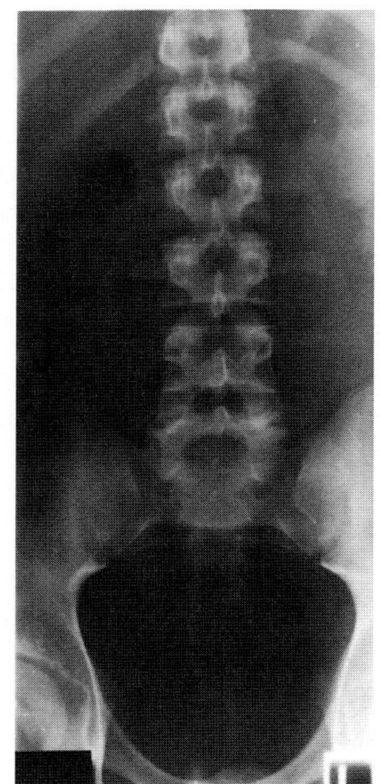

Fig. 9-32. AP projection (centered for 14 x 17 film).

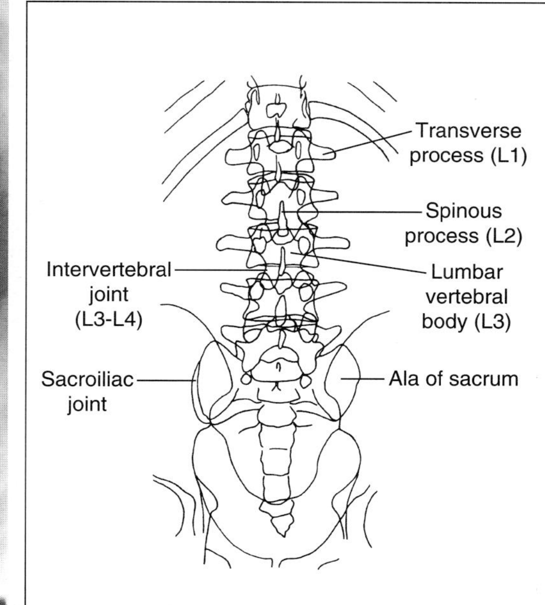

Fig. 9-33. AP projection.

Evaluation Criteria

- The spinal column from approximately T11 to the distal sacrum should be seen if 14 x 17 film is used centered to midline of film and collimation field. (With 11 x 14 film, T12 to S1 should be visible.)
- SI joints should be equidistant from spinous processes indicating no pelvic rotation. Spinous processes should appear in midline of vertebral column and R and L transverse processes should appear equal in length.
- Lateral margins of collimation field should include the SI joints and psoas muscle outlines.
- Optimum exposure should clearly visualize the lumbar vertebral body margins and intervertebral joint spaces without overexposing psoas muscle outlines and/or transverse processes.

Obliques–Anterior and Posterior Oblique Positions

Lumbar spine
Basic
• AP (or PA)
• Obliques–Ant. or post.
• Lateral
• Lateral L5-S1

Structures Best Shown

Zygapophyseal (apophyseal) joints. (RPO and LPO show downside. RAO and LAO show upside.) "Scotty dogs" should be visualized and zygapophyseal joint should appear open on good oblique.

Both right and left obliques are taken.

Technical Factors

- Film size–2 ea. 11 x 14 in. (30 x 35 cm), lengthwise, or 10 x 12 in. (24 x 30 cm)
- Use moving or stationary grid.
- 75-80 kVp range (or 85-92 kVp and reduce mAs and dose).
- Use small focal spot if equipment allows.
- Technique and dose:

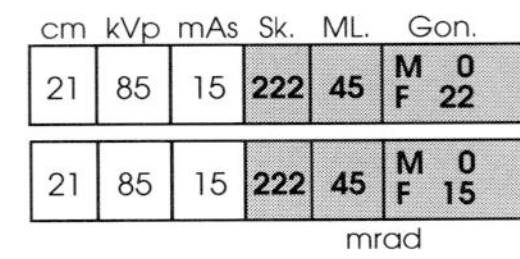

	cm	kVp	mAs	Sk.	ML.	Gon. (mrad)
Post. obli.	21	85	15	222	45	M 0 F 22
Ant. obli.	21	85	15	222	45	M 0 F 15

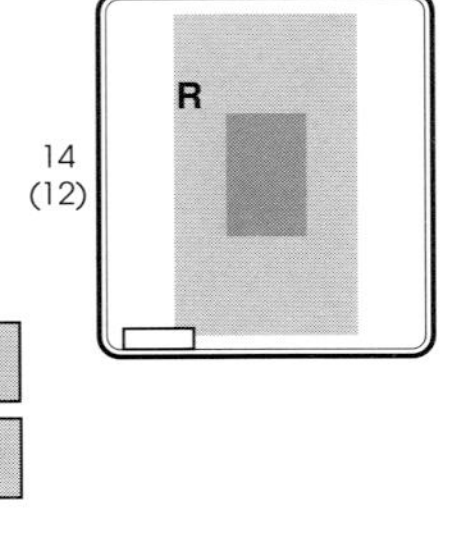

Shielding: Place contact shield over gonads without obscuring area of interest.

Patient Position

- Semisupine (RPO and LPO) or semiprone (RAO and LAO).

Part Position

- Position patient and **rotate body 45°** so as to place spinal column directly over midline of table, aligned to CR.
- Flex knee for stability as shown.
- Support lower back and pelvis with radiolucent sponges to maintain position. (Grasping edge of table may result in pinched fingers.)

Central Ray

- CR perpendicular to film.
- Center to **level of 1 to 1½ in. (3 to 4 cm) above level of iliac crest.**
- Center 1½ in. (4 cm) laterally on upside from midline of patient.
- Center cassette to CR.
- Minimum 40 in. (102 cm) SID.

Collimation: Four-sided collimation to area of interest.

Respiration: Suspend breathing on expiration.

Note: A **50°** oblique from plane of table best visualizes the zygapophyseal joints at **L1-2**, and **30°** for **L5-S1**.

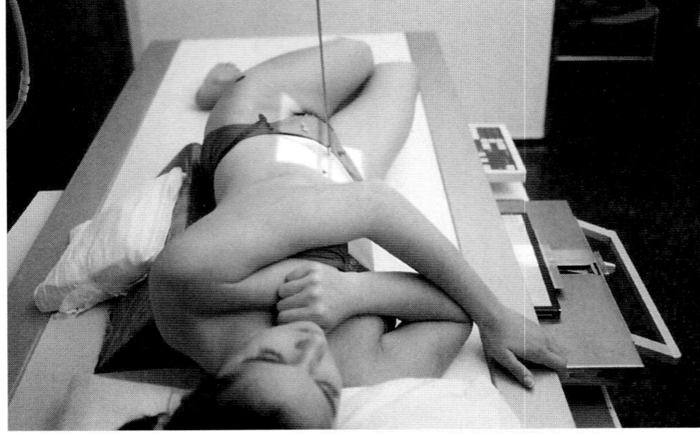

Fig. 9-34. **45° RPO**, visualizes **right** (downside) zygapophyseal joints.

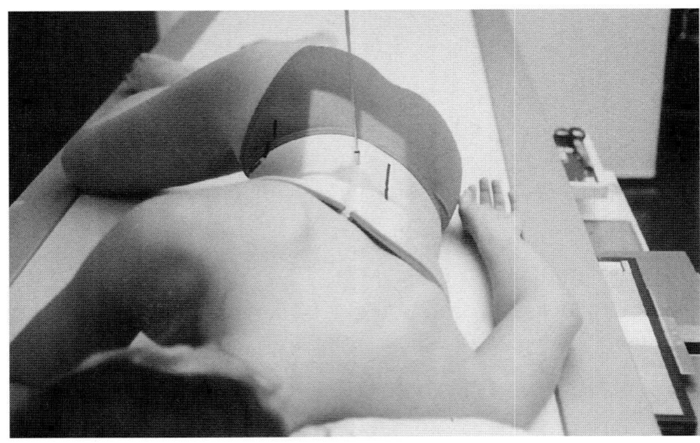

Fig. 9-35. **45° LAO**, visualizes **right** (upside) zygapophyseal joints.

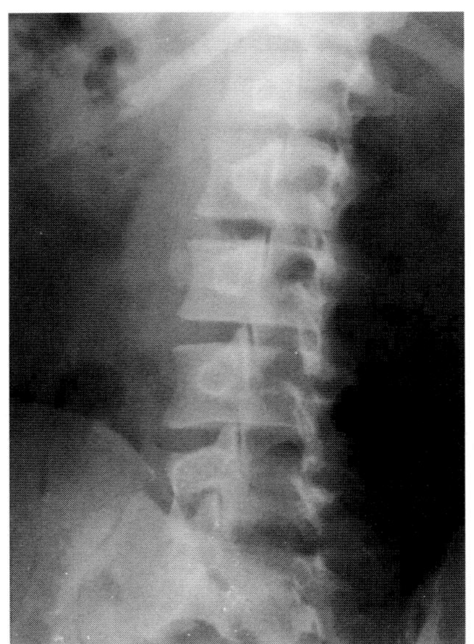

Fig. 9-36. 45° oblique.

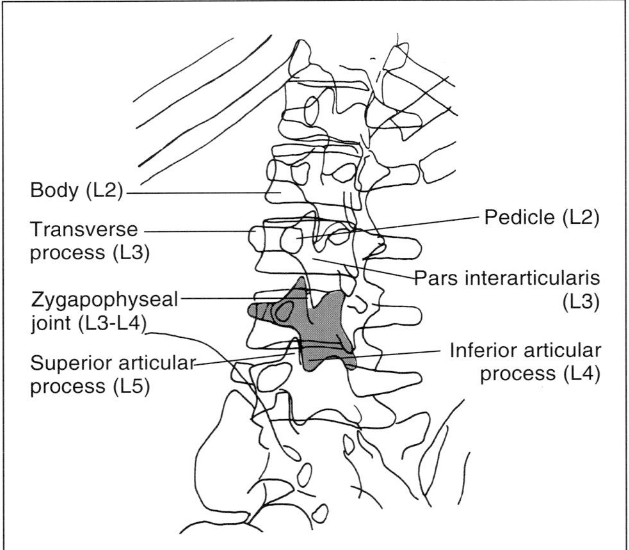

Fig. 9-37. 45° oblique.

Evaluation Criteria

- The spinal column from T11 to S1 should be seen.
- Spinal column should be in midline of collimation field and film.
- "Scotty dogs" and **open zygapophyseal joints** should be visualized on all five vertebral vertebrae.
- A properly 45° obliqued patient puts the pedicle ("eye") of "Scotty dog" near the center of the vertebral body. Posterior displacement of the pedicle ("eye") indicates too much obliquity and anterior displacement indicates not enough obliquity.
- Optimum exposure should clearly visualize the zygapophyseal joints from L1 to L5 without overexposing other vertebral margins.

Lateral Position

Lumbar Spine
Basic
• AP (or PA)
• Obliques–Ant. or post.
• **Lateral**
• Lateral L5-S1

Structures Best Shown

Vertebral bodies, intervertebral joints, spinous processes, L5-S1 junction, sacrum and first four intervertebral foramina.

A good projection for demonstrating **compression fractures** of lumbar vertebrae.

Technical Factors

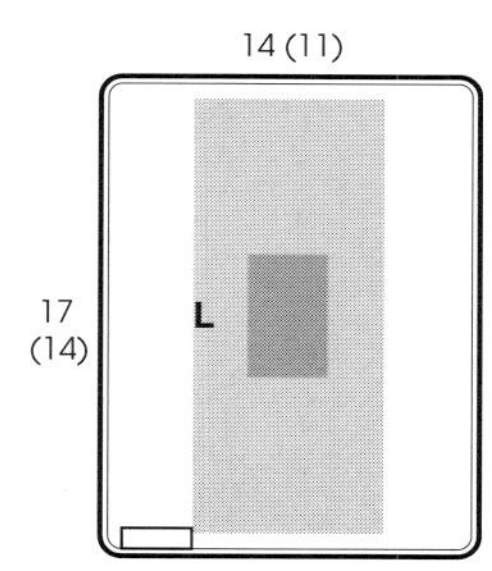

- Film size–2 ea. 14 x 17 in. (35 x 43 cm), lengthwise, or 11 x 14 in. (30 x 35 cm)
- Use moving or stationary grid.
- 85-95 kVp range
- Use small focal spot if equipment allows.
- Place lead blocker on table behind patient.
- Technique and dose:

	cm	kVp	mAs	Sk.	ML.	Gon.
(Female model)	27	90	50	1008	134	M 0 F 29
(Male model)	30	90	65	1310	174	M 0 F 38
						mrad

Shielding: Shield gonads without obscuring area of interest. Ovarian shielding for females may obscure pertinent anatomy.

Patient Position

- Lateral recumbent, pillow for head, knees and hips flexed with support between knees and ankles and under knee resting on table to better maintain a true lateral position.

Part Position 

- Align mid axillary plane to CR and midline of table.
- Place radiolucent support under small of waist, as needed to place the long axis of the spine near parallel to the table (palpate spinous processes to determine this). (See Notes.)
- Place pelvis and torso in **true lateral position.**

Central Ray

- CR **perpendicular to long axis of spine**.
  Larger Film (14 x 17): Center to **level of iliac crest** (L4). This will include lumbar vertebrae, sacrum and possibly coccyx. Center cassette to CR.
  Smaller Film (11 x 14): Center **1½ in. (4 cm) above iliac crest** (L3). This will include primarily the five lumbar vertebrae. Center cassette to CR.
- Minimum 40 in. (102 cm) SID.

Collimation: Closely collimate on lateral borders. (Light field will appear small due to divergent rays and the distance from the upside skin surface to the film.)

Respiration: Suspend breathing on expiration.

Notes: A slight sag of the spine will help open up the intervertebral joints considering the divergence of the x-ray beam **if** both ends of the lumbar spine are the same distance from table. The average male and some females require no CR angle. A person with a wider pelvis and narrow thorax may require a 2 to 5° caudad angle even with support, as shown in Fig. 9-39.

If patient has a natural side curvature (scoliosis) of the lower spine, as determined by viewing the spine from the back with hospital gown open and patient standing evenly on both feet, the patient should be placed in whichever lateral position that **places the sag or convexity of the spine down** to better open the intervertebral spaces.

Another way to prevent too much sag of the spine is to have the patient reach up and extend arm on side away from film overhead, which tends to lift and straighten the spine.

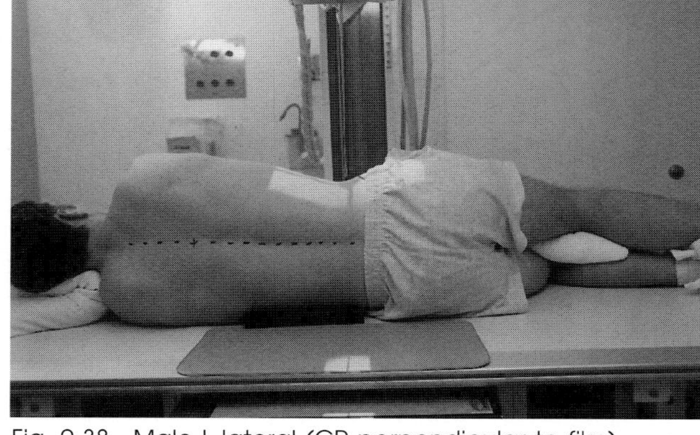

Fig. 9-38. Male L lateral (CR perpendicular to film).

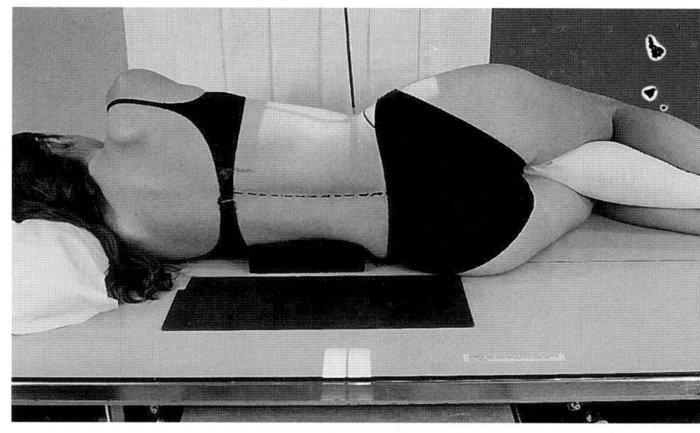

Fig. 9-39. Female R lateral (optional, CR 2 to 5° caudad).

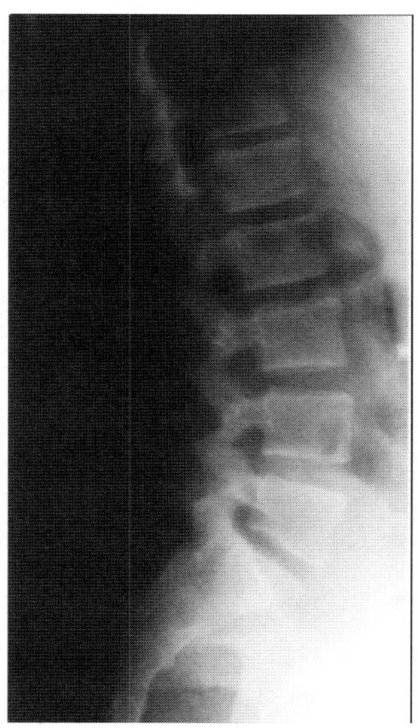

Fig. 9-40. Lateral.

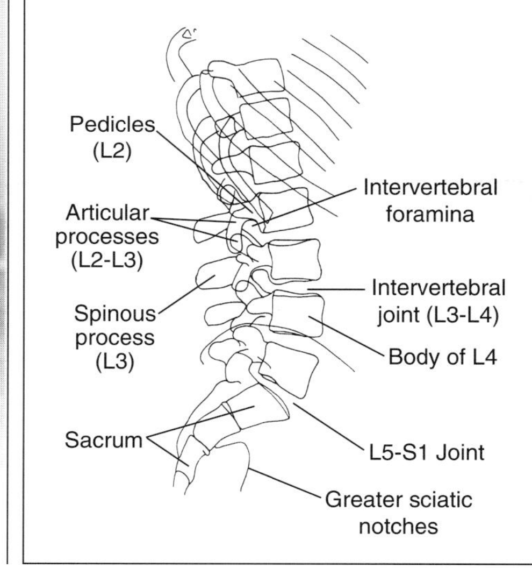

Fig. 9-41. Lateral.

Evaluation Criteria

- Using larger 14 x 17 in. film, vertebra from T12 to the distal sacrum should be seen in lateral profile centered to the film and the collimation field.
- Using smaller 11 x 14 in. film, T12 through S1 should be visualized.
- Intervertebral foramina should appear open.
- Intervertebral joint spaces should appear open from T12 to S1.
- No rotation as evidenced by superimposed greater sciatic notches.
- Optimum exposure should clearly visualize the vertebral bodies and joint spaces without overexposure of other vertebral structures.

Lateral L5-S1 Position

Lumbar spine
Basic
- AP (or PA)
- Obliques–Ant. or post.
- Lateral
- **Lateral L5-S1**

Structures Best Shown

L5-S1 joint space in lateral position.
A good projection for ruling out spondylolisthesis involving L4-L5 or L5-S1.

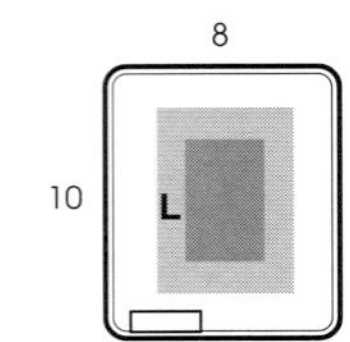

Technical Factors

- Film size–8 x 10 in. (18 x 24 cm), lengthwise.
- Use moving or stationary grid.
- 90-100 kVp range
(increase ≈5 kVp from lateral due to close collimation).
- Place lead blocker on table behind patient to reduce scatter to film.
- Technique and dose:

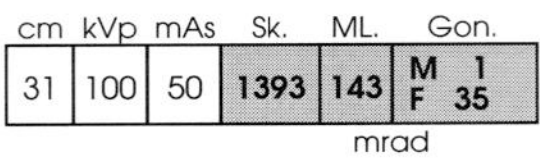

cm	kVp	mAs	Sk.	ML.	Gon.
31	100	50	1393	143	M 1 F 35

mrad

Shielding: Shield gonads without obscuring area of interest. Ovarian shielding for females may obscure a portion of sacrum.

Patient Position

- Lateral recumbent, pillow for head, knees and hips flexed with support between knees and ankles and under knee resting on table to better maintain a true lateral position.

Part Position

- Align mid axillary plane to CR and midline of table.
- Flex knees and hips.
- Place radiolucent support under small of waist. (See Notes.)
- Place pelvis and torso in **true lateral** position.

Central Ray

- CR **perpendicular** to film with sufficient waist support; or **angle 5 to 8° caudad** with less support. (See Notes below.)
- Center CR **1½ in.** (4 cm) **inferior to iliac crest** and **1½ in.** (4 cm) **anterior to posterior surface** of body. Center cassette to CR.
- Minimum 40 in. (102 cm) SID.

Collimation: Close four-sided collimation to area of interest. Use extension cylinder cone if available; if not available, collimate closely.

Respiration: Suspend breathing on expiration.

Notes: If waist is not supported sufficiently, resulting in a sagging of the spinal column, the CR must be angled caudad as needed to be perpendicular to L5-S1 region.

High amounts of secondary/scatter radiation is generated. Use close collimation, higher ratio grids and lead masking.

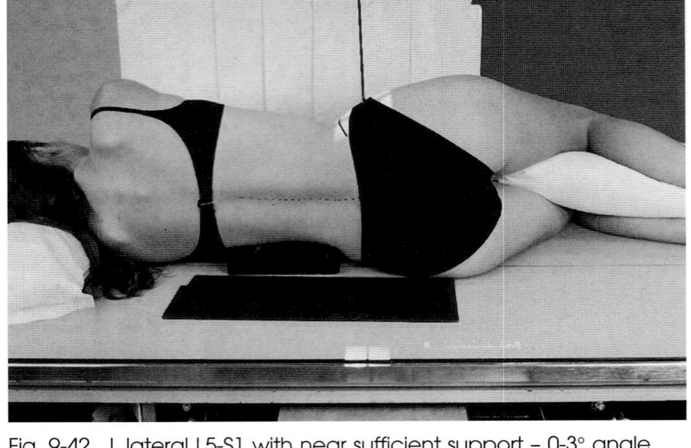

Fig. 9-42. L lateral L5-S1 with near sufficient support - 0-3° angle.

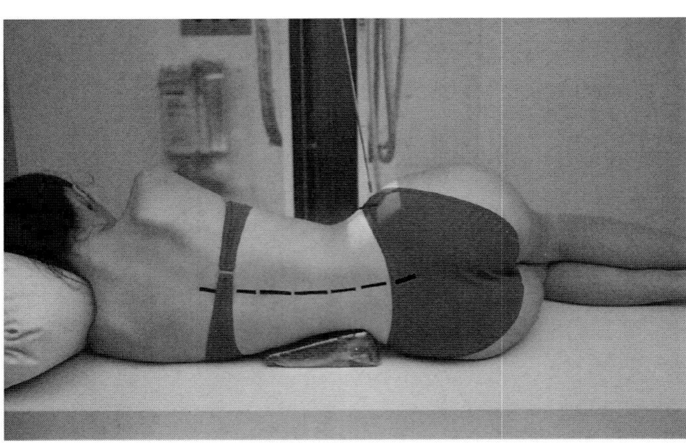

Fig. 9-43. L lateral L5-S1 with less support–CR 5 to 8° caudad.

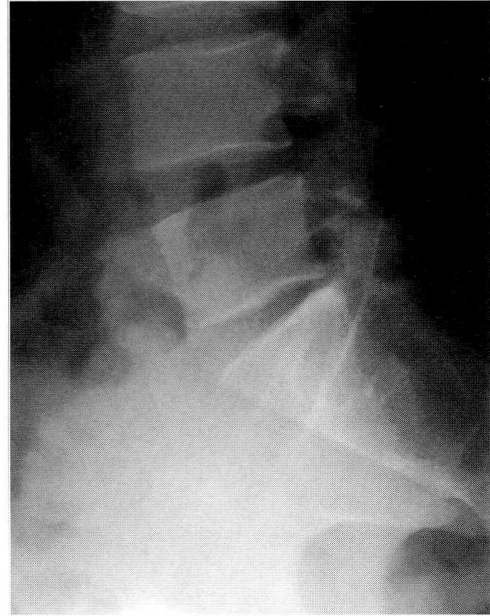

Fig. 9-44. Lateral L5-S1.

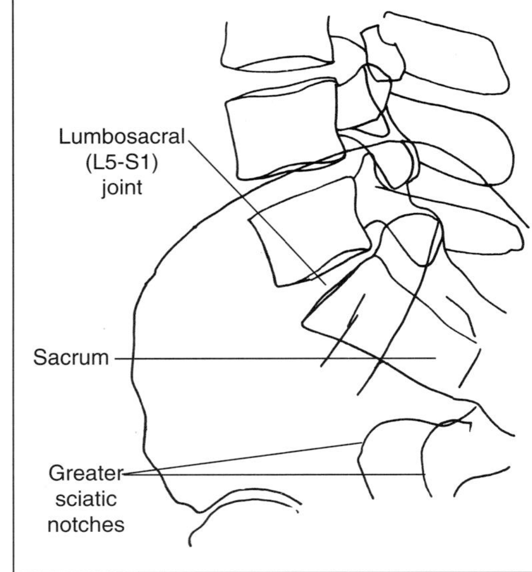

Fig. 9-45. Lateral L5-S1.

Evaluation Criteria

- L5-S1 joint space should be open and in center of exposure field and film.
- There should be no rotation of torso and pelvis as evidenced by superimposed anteroposterior dimensions of greater sciatic notches of posterior pelvis. (The above radiograph demonstrates some rotation.)
- L4, L5 and S1 should be seen in their entirety.
- Optimum exposure should clearly visualize the L5-S1 joint space through the superimposed ilia of the pelvis without excessive burnout of other vertebral structures.

AP Axial L5-S1 Projection

Lumbar spine
Special
• **AP axial L5-S1**

Structures Best Shown

L5-S1 joint space and sacroiliac joints in AP projection.

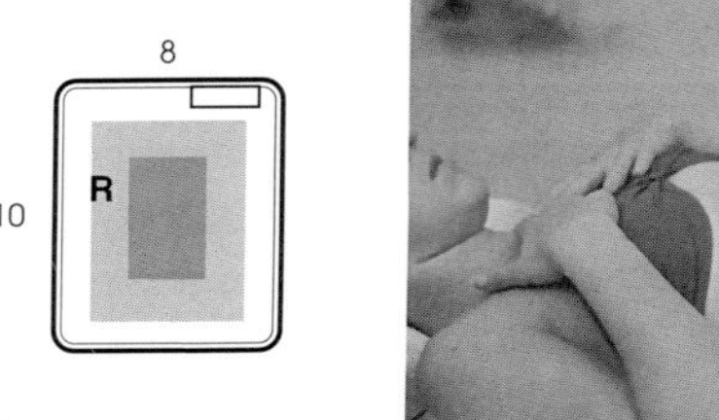

Technical Factors

- Film size–8 x 10 in. (18 x 24 cm), lengthwise.
- Use moving or stationary grid.
- 80-85 kVp range.
  (Increase 8-10 kVp from AP due to axial projection)
- Technique and dose:

cm	kVp	mAs	Sk.	ML.	Gon.
17	85	20	263	75	M 3 F 41

mrad

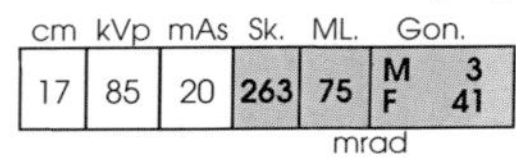

Shielding: Shield gonads without obscuring area of interest. Female ovarian shielding will obscure portion of sacroiliac joints.

Patient Position

- Supine, pillow for head, legs extended with support under knees for comfort.

Part Position

- Place arms at side or up on chest.
- Align midsagittal plane to CR and midline of table.
- Ensure **no rotation** of torso or pelvis.

Central Ray

- Angle CR **cephalad**, **30° (males)** to **35° (females)**.
- CR should enter at the **level of the ASIS** centered to the **midline** of the body.
- Center cassette to projected CR.
- Minimum 40 in. (102 cm) SID.

Collimation: Close four-sided collimation to area of interest.

Respiration: Suspend breathing dur-
ing exposure.

otes: Angled AP projection "opens"
-S1 joint.
Lateral projection of L5-S1 is gen-
ly more informative than this AP
ction.
ay also be done **prone** with **ceph-**
ngle of CR. (Increases OID.)

Fig. 9-46. AP axial L5-S1–30 to 35° cephalad.

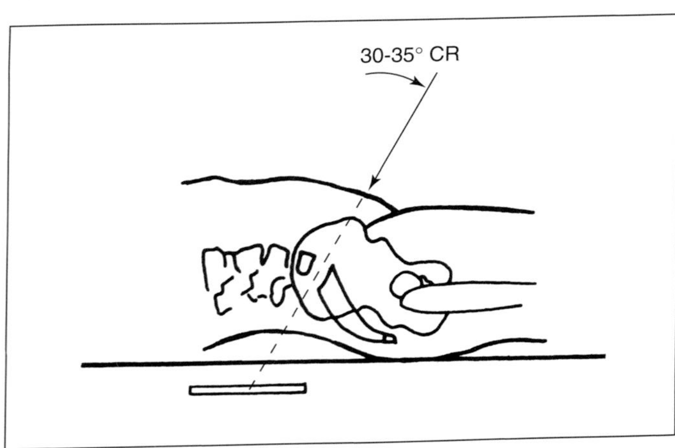

Fig. 9-47. AP axial L5-S1.

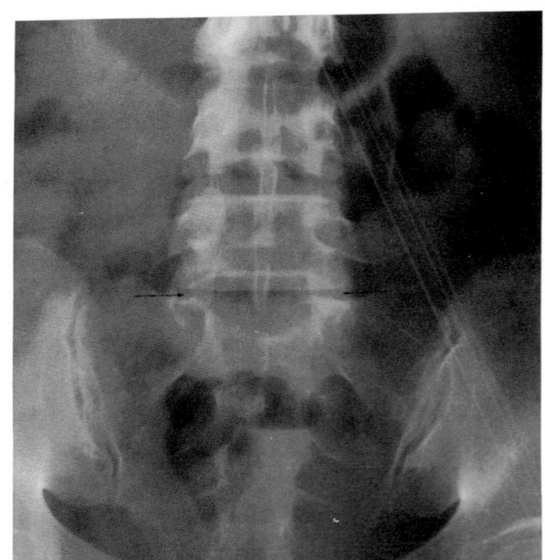

Fig. 9-48. AP axial L5-S1–30° cephalad.

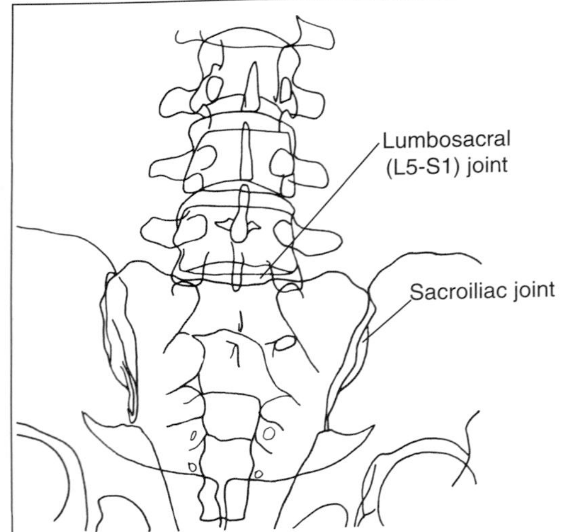

Fig. 9-49. AP axial L5-S1.

Criteria

hould be demonstrated and in center of exposure field

ts should be demonstrated and be equidistant from
no pelvic rotation.
ure should clearly visualize both the L5-S1 joint
roiliac joints.

PA (AP) Projection

Scoliosis series
Basic
- **PA (AP)**
  - **–Erect and/or supine**
- Erect lateral

Special
- AP (Ferguson method)
- AP–R and L bending

Structures Best Shown

Thoracic and lumbar spine in the PA or AP projection to evaluate for abnormal lateral curvature (scoliosis) of the spine.

A scoliosis series frequently includes two AP (or PA) films taken for comparison, one erect and one recumbent.

Technical Factors

- Film size–14 x 17 in. (35 x 43 cm), lengthwise. Larger patients–use 14 x 36 in. if available. (A long cassette with two films placed end to end may also be used.)
- Use moving or stationary grid.
- Use compensating filters for more uniform density.
- Relatively high kVp (80-100) range for long scale contrast and decreased patient dose. (See Notes.)
- Use erect marker for erect position.
- Technique and dose at 60 in. SID:

	cm	kVp	mAs	Sk.	ML.	Breasts	Gon.
PA	23	90	25	447	81	16	M 1 F 43
AP	23	90	25	447	81	164	M 2 F 43

mrad

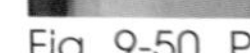
Fig. 9-50. PA erect.

Shielding: Shield gonadal region without obscuring area of interest. Use breast shields for young females. Shadow shields placed on collimator may be used as shown in Fig. 9-51 and as evident in Fig. 9-53.

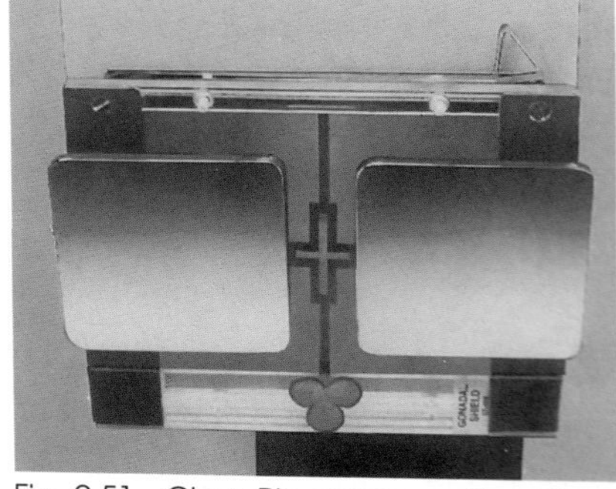
Fig. 9-51. Clear Pb compensating filters with breast and gonadal shields attached to bottom of collimator with magnets. (Courtesy of Nuclear Associates, Carle, NY)

Patient Position

- Erect and recumbent position, weight evenly distributed on both feet.

Part Position

- Align midsagittal plane to CR and midline of film holder. Arms at side.
- **No rotation** of torso or pelvis if possible. (Scoliosis may be accompanied with twisting and rotation of vertebrae making some rotation unavoidable.)

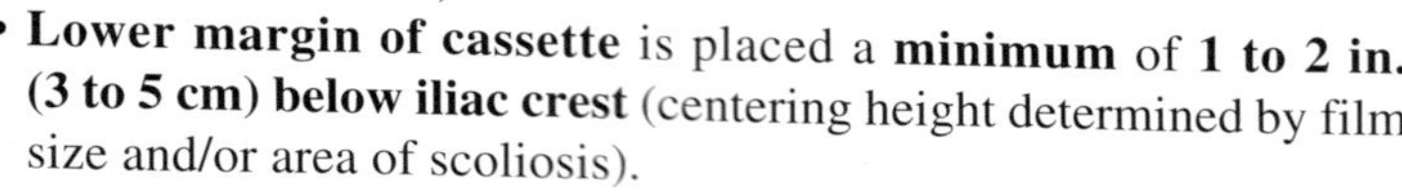

- **Lower margin of cassette** is placed a **minimum** of **1 to 2 in. (3 to 5 cm) below iliac crest** (centering height determined by film size and/or area of scoliosis).

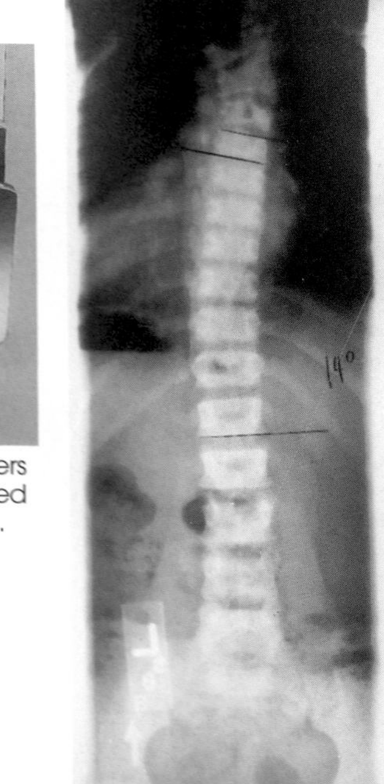
Fig. 9-52. PA erect –14 x 17 in. film

Central Ray

- CR perpendicular, directed to **midpoint of film.**
- 40 to 60 in. (102 to 152 cm) SID (longer SID required with larger film).

Collimation: Collimate on four sides to area of interest. Too narrow side collimation is not recommended on **initial film** since deformities of adjacent areas of ribs and pelvis also need to be evaluated.

Respiration: Suspend breathing on **expiration.**

Notes: A relative high kVp will result in a longer scale contrast and a more uniform density between thoracic and lumbar vertebrae. A second benefit of higher kVp is a reduction in total radiation dose to patient.

A PA rather than AP projection is recommended because of the significantly reduced dosage to radiation sensitive areas such as female breasts and the thyroid gland. Studies have shown this results in approximately 90% reduction in dosage to the breasts.*

Scoliosis generally requires repeat examinations over a period of time on young patients emphasizing the need for careful shielding.

Evaluation Criteria

- Vertebral column should be i…
- Iliac crests should be a m… above bottom edge of f…
- The distal lumbar ve… margin of the film a… (Younger and sma… and thoracic ver…
- Optional 36 i… thoracic and…

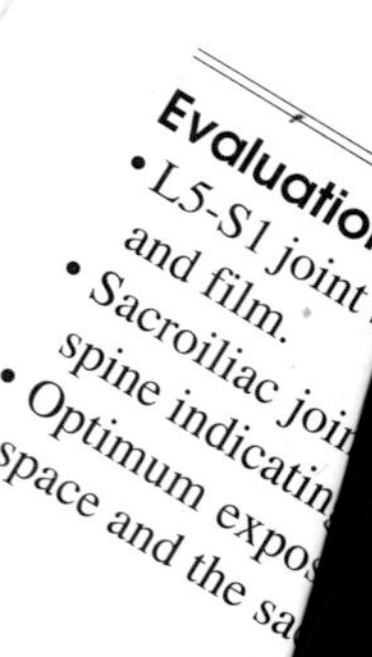

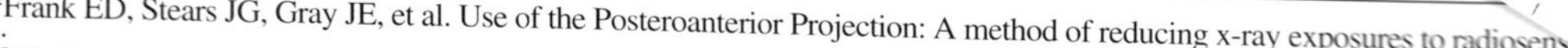
*Frank ED, Stears JG, Gray JE, et al. Use of the Posteroanterior Projection: A method of reducing x-ray exposures to radiosens…

Erect Lateral Position

Scoliosis series
Basic
- PA (AP)
  - Erect and/or supine
- **Erect lateral**

Special
- AP (Ferguson method)
- AP (PA)–R and L bending

Structures Best Shown

Thoracic and lumbar spine in lateral projection to demonstrate possible spondylolisthesis (anterior displacement of one vertebra over another) or degrees of kyphosis or lordosis.

Technical Factors

- Film size–14 x 17 in. (35 x 43 cm), lengthwise, or 14 x 36 in. on larger patients if available. (A long cassette with 2 films placed end to end may also be used.)
- Use stationary or moving grid.
- Use erect marker.
- Use compensating filter for more uniform density.
- 90-100 kVp range. (See Note.)
- Technique and dose at 60 in. SID:

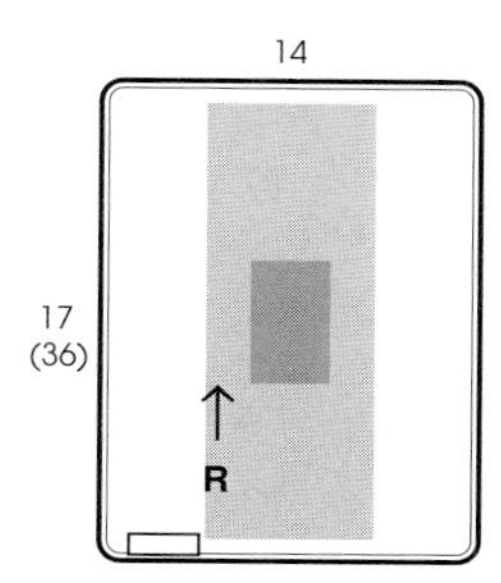

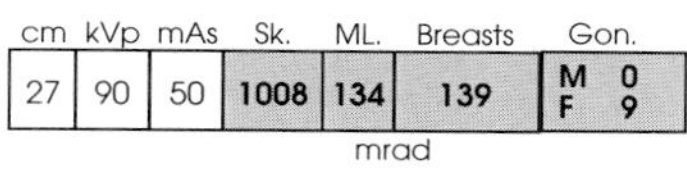

cm	kVp	mAs	Sk.	ML.	Breasts	Gon.
27	90	50	1008	134	139	M 0 F 9
			mrad			

Shielding: Place contact shield or shadow shield over gonads without obscuring area of interest. Use breast shields for young females.

Patient Position

- Patient in erect lateral position with arms folded above head, or if unsteady grasping a support in front of patient.
- The side of the convexity of primary curve should be against film.

Part Position

- Place pelvis and torso in as **true a lateral position** as possible.
- Align midaxillary plane of body to CR and midline of film.
- Lower margin of cassette a **minimum of 1 to 2 in. (3 to 5 cm) below level of iliac crests** (centering height determined by film size and area of scoliosis).

Central Ray

- CR **perpendicular** directed to **midpoint of film**.
- 40 to 60 in. (102 to 152 cm) SID (longer SID required with larger film).

Collimation: Four-sided collimation to area of interest. Use side collimation to area of vertebral column, however, use caution to **not** cut off a portion of vertebral column due to the increase in curvature.

Respiration: Suspend breathing on **expiration.**

Note: A relative high kVp will produce a long scale contrast for a more uniform density of thoracic and lumbar vertebrae.

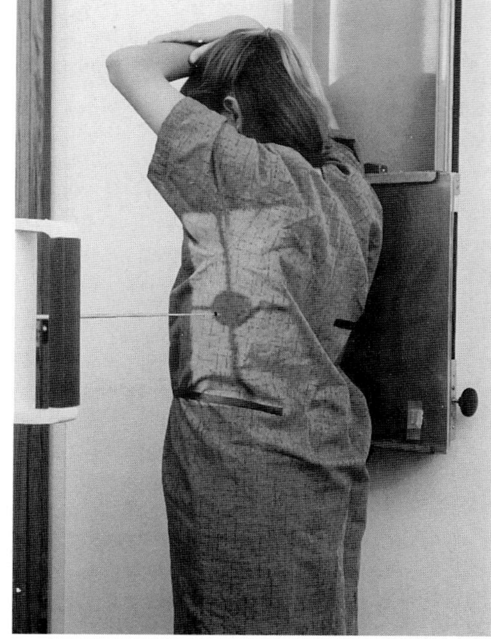

Fig. 9-54. Erect R lateral.

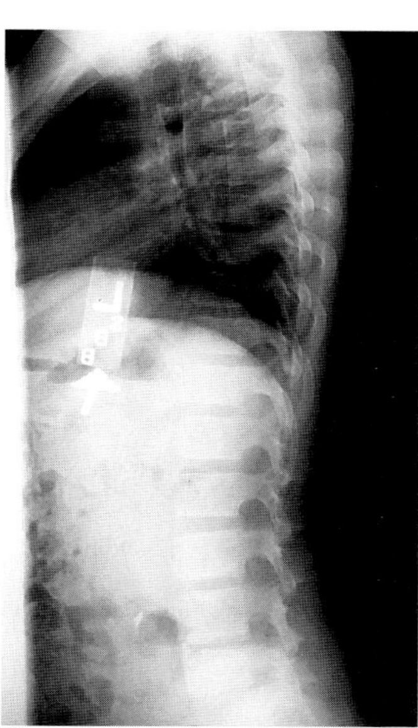

Fig. 9-55. Erect lateral.

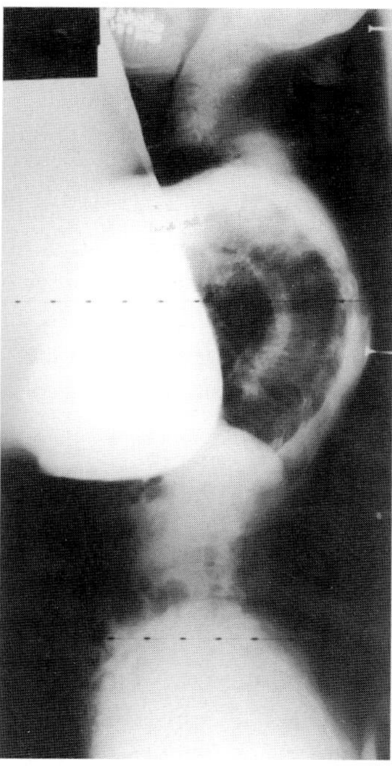

Fig. 9-56. Erect lateral. Clear Pb lateral thoracic compensating filter and breast shadow shield in place.
(Courtesy of Nuclear Associates, Carle, NY)

Evaluation Criteria

- Thoracic and lumbar vertebra should be demonstrated in as true a lateral position as possible. (Some rotation of pelvis and/or thorax may be apparent since scoliosis generally is accompanied by a twisting or rotation of involved vertebrae.)
- One inch (2.5 cm) minimum of the iliac crests should be seen on lower margin of film.
- Vertebral column should be in center of collimation field and film.
- Optimum exposure and long scale contrast will visualize outline of distal lumbar vertebrae without overexposing thoracic vertebrae.
- Right or left and erect markers must be visible without superimposing essential anatomy.

AP Projection–Ferguson* Method

Scoliosis series
Basic
• PA (AP)
–Erect and/or supine
• Erect lateral
Special
• **AP (Ferguson method)**
• AP (PA)–R and L bending

Structures Best Shown

Thoracic and lumbar spine in the AP projection to identify deforming (primary) curve from compensatory curve.

Two films are taken, one standard erect AP and one with the foot or hip on the **convex side** of the curve elevated.

Technical Factors

- Film size–2 ea. 14 x 17 in. (35 x 43 cm), lengthwise.
- Use moving or stationary grid.
- Use erect marker.
- Relatively high kVp (80-100) range for long scale contrast and wider exposure latitude.
- Use compensating filters for more uniform density.
- Technique and dose, per exposure at 60 in. SID:

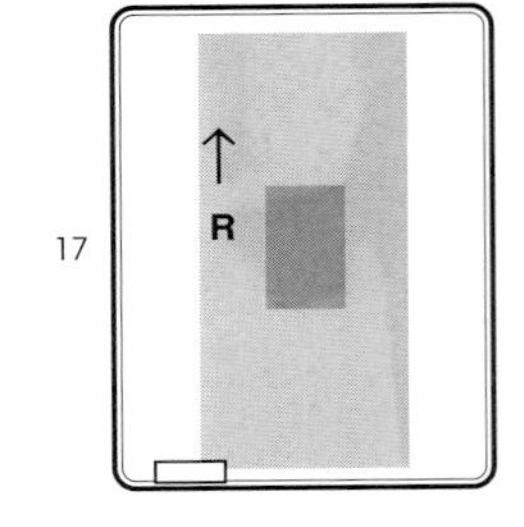

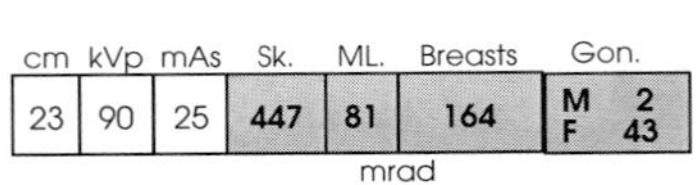

cm	kVp	mAs	Sk.	ML.	Breasts	Gon.
23	90	25	447	81	164	M 2 F 43
			mrad			

Shielding: Place contact shield or shadow shield over gonads without obscuring area of interest. Use breast shields for young females.

Patient Position

- Patient in AP position, either seated or standing with arms at side.
- For second film, place a block under foot (or hip if seated) on **convex side** of curve enough so patient can barely maintain position **without assistance**. A 3 to 4 in. (8 to 10 cm) block of some type may be used under buttock if sitting, or foot if standing (Fig. 9-58).

Part Position

- Align **midsagittal plane to CR and midline of table**. Arms at side.
- **No rotation** of torso or pelvis if possible.
- Bottom edge of cassette is placed a minimum 1 to 2 in. (3 to 5 cm) below level of iliac crest.

Central Ray

- CR **perpendicular**, centered to **mid point of film.**
- 40 to 72 in. (152 to 180 cm) SID; longer SID recommended.

Collimation: Four-sided collimation to area of interest.

Respiration: Suspend breathing on **expiration.**

Notes: No form of support (i.e. compression band) is to be used in this exam. For second film patient should stand or sit with block under one side unassisted.

May be done as PA projections, which reduces dosage to radiation-sensitive areas of chest and neck.

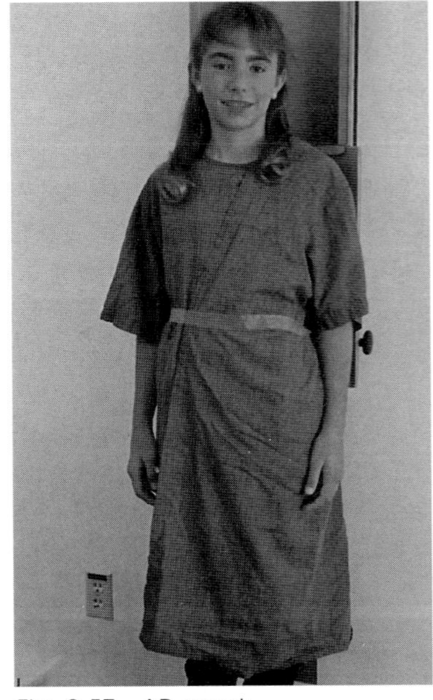

Fig. 9-57. AP erect.

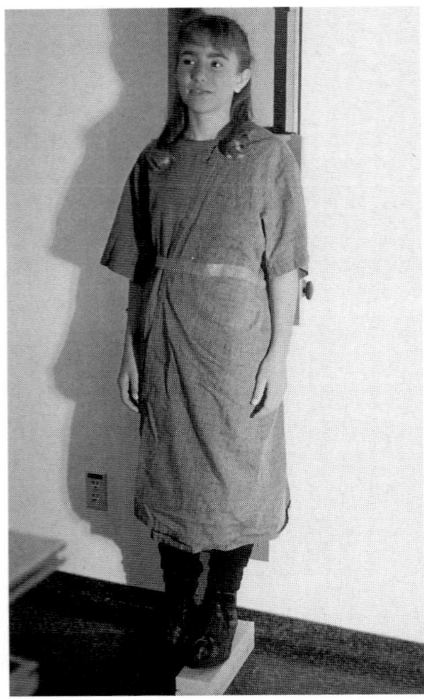

Fig. 9-58. AP with block under foot on **convex side** of curve.

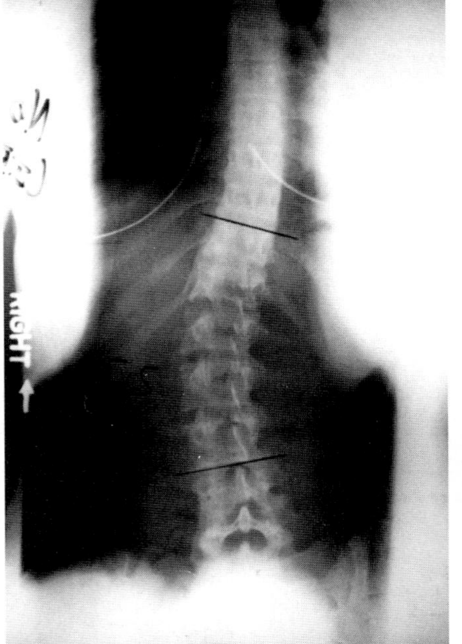

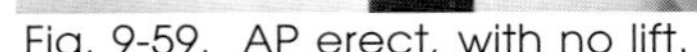

Fig. 9-59. AP erect, with no lift.

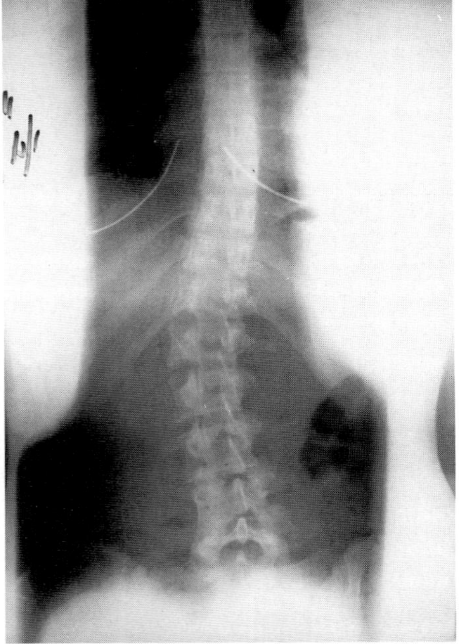

Fig. 9-60. AP erect, with lift.

Note: These radiographs demonstrate convexity to the right which would require elevation of the **right** side.

Evaluation Criteria

- All of thoracic and lumbar vertebra should be demonstrated in AP position.
- A minimum of one inch (2.5 cm) of iliac crest should be seen on lower film margin.
- Vertebral column should be in center of film and/or collimation field.
- Optimum exposure should clearly visualize the distal lumbar region without overexposure of the proximal thoracic region.
- Correct placement of gonad shields (and breast shields on females) should be evident.
- Right or left and erect markers must be visible but not superimposed by essential anatomy.

*Ferguson, AB. *Roentgen Diagnosis of the Extremities and Spine*, New York: Harper & Row Publishers, 1939.

AP (PA) Projection–Right and Left Bending

Scoliosis series
Basic
- PA (AP)
  –Erect and/or supine
- Erect lateral

Special
- AP (Ferguson method)
- **AP (PA)–R and L bending**

Structures Best Shown

Thoracic and lumbar spine in the AP (or PA) projection.

Two films are taken, one bending to right and one bending to left, to determine range of motion of spine

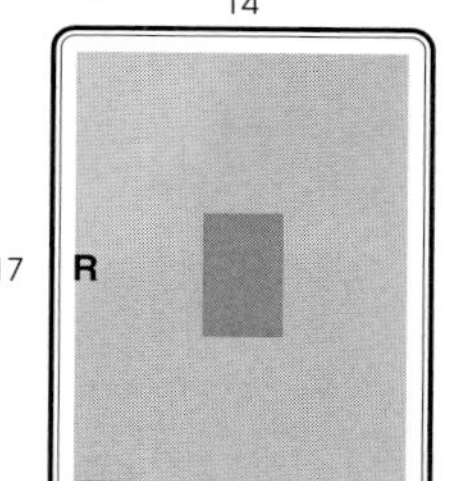

Technical Factors

- Film size–2 each 14 x 17 in. (35 x 43 cm), lengthwise.
- Use moving or stationary grid.
- Use erect marker for erect position.
- Relatively high kVp (80-100) range for long-scale contrast and wider exposure latitude.
- Technique and dose per projection at 44 in. SID:

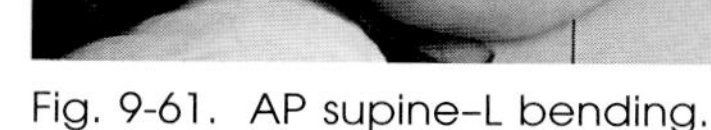

	cm	kVp	mAs	Sk.	ML.	Breasts	Gon.
AP	17	80	15	177	42	6	M 0 F 26

mrad

Shielding: Place contact shield over gonads without obscuring area of interest. Use breast shields for young females if AP.

Patient Position

- May be taken erect or recumbent, AP or PA, arms at side.

Part Position

- Start by aligning midsagittal plane to CR and midline of table.
- **No rotation** of torso or pelvis if possible.
- Bottom edge of cassette is placed **1 to 2 in. (3 to 5 cm) below iliac crest.**
- With the pelvis acting as a fulcrum, have patient bend (lateral flexion) **as far as possible** to either side.
- If recumbent, both the upper torso and the legs may be moved to achieve maximum lateral flexion.
- Repeat above when doing opposite side.

Central Ray

- CR **perpendicular**, directed to **midpoint of film.**
- 40 to 60 in. (102 to 152 cm) SID; longer SID recommended.

Collimation: Four-sided collimation to near borders of film to not cut off any portion of spine.

Respiration: Suspend breathing on **expiration.**

Notes: The pelvis must remain as stationary as possible during positioning.

Pelvis acts as a fulcrum (pivot point) during changes of position.

May be done as PA projections if taken erect, which significantly reduces exposure to radiation sensitive areas.

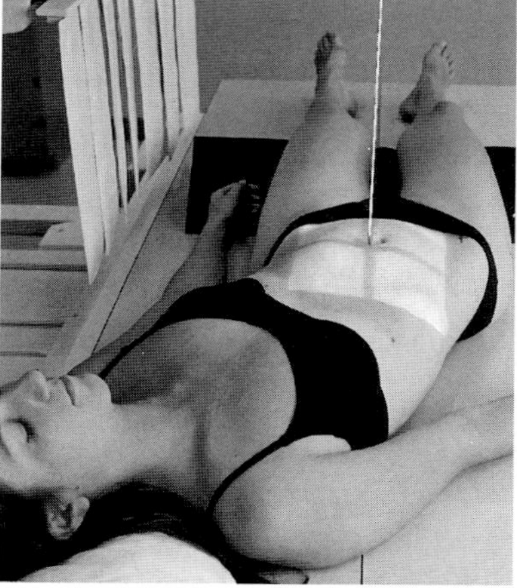

Fig. 9-61. AP supine–L bending.

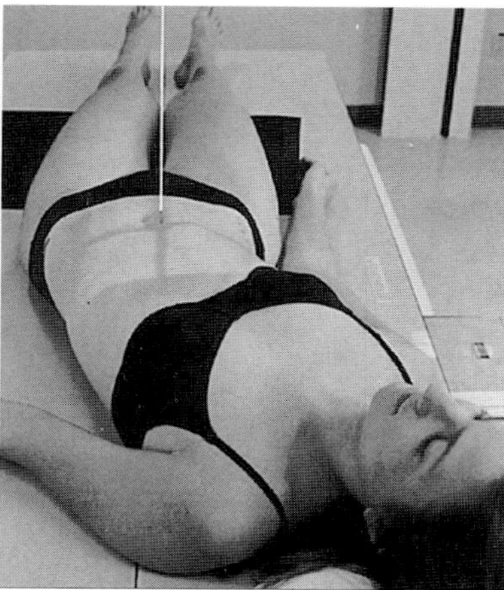

Fig. 9-62. AP supine–R bending.

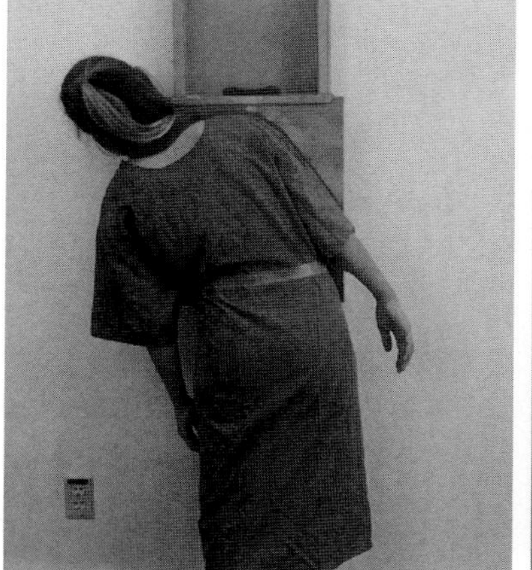

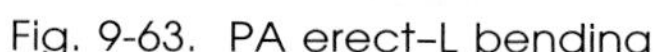

Fig. 9-63. PA erect–L bending.

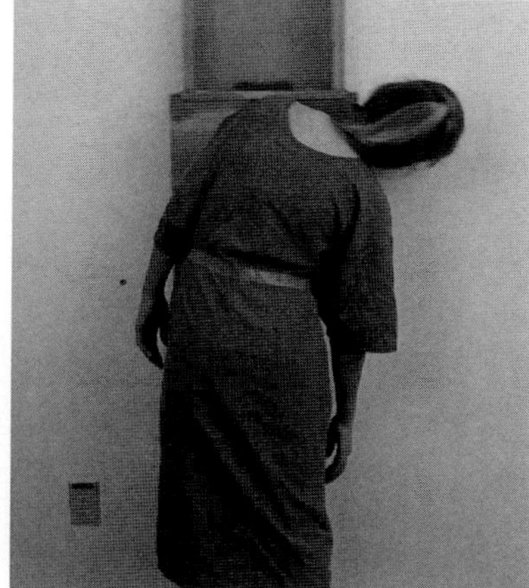

Fig. 9-64. PA erect–R bending.

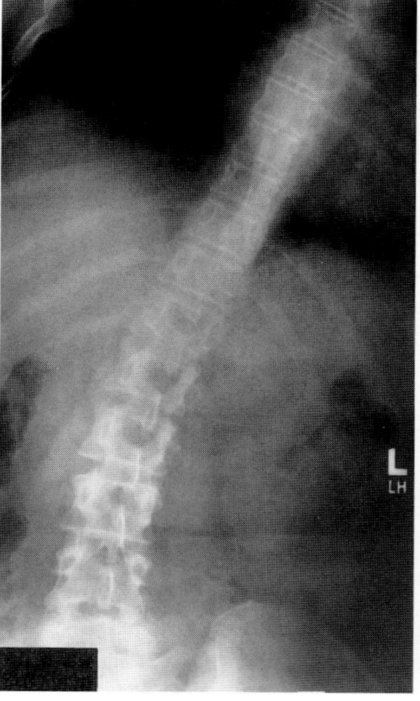

Fig. 9-65. AP–L bending.

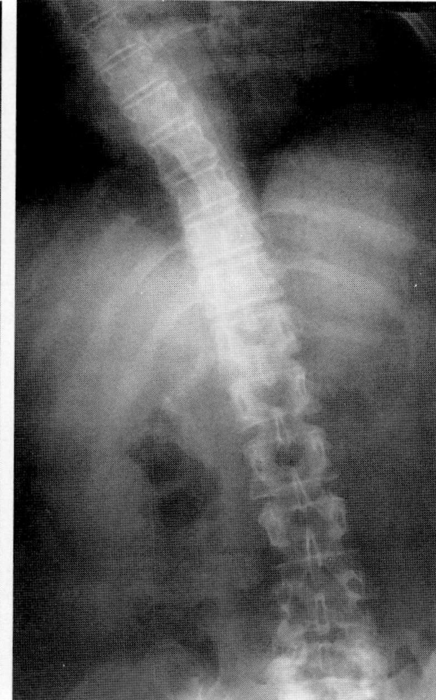

Fig. 9-66. AP–R bending.

Evaluation Criteria

- Thoracic and lumbar vertebra should be demonstrated in extreme lateral flexion (both R and L) on two separate films.
- Iliac crests should be at least 1 inch or 2.5 cm above bottom of radiograph.
- Rotation of pelvis and/or thorax may be apparent since scoliosis generally is accompanied by rotation of involved vertebrae.
- Optimum exposure should clearly visualize the distal lumbar region without overexposure of the proximal thoracic region.
- Right or left markers (and erect marker if erect) must be visible not superimposed by essential anatomy.

Lateral Positions–Hyperextension and Hyperflexion

Spinal fusion series
Basic
- AP (PA)–R and L bending (page 297)
- **Lateral –Hyperextension and hyperflexion**

Structures Best Shown

Two AP (PA) and two lateral projections of the lumbar spine at the site of the fusion.

Purpose: To demonstrate anteroposterior mobility (if any) at fusion site.

Two films are taken (one with hyperflexion and one with hyperextension).

Right and left bending positions are also generally part of a spinal fusion series and are the same as for the scoliosis series on preceding pages.

Technical Factors

- Film size–2 ea. 14 x 17 in. (35 x 43 cm).
- Use stationary or moving grid.
- 85-90 kVp range. Place lead blocker behind patient.
- Use extension and flexion markers.
- Technique and dose, per projection:

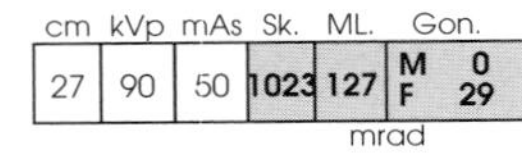

cm	kVp	mAs	Sk.	ML.	Gon.
27	90	50	1023	127	M 0 F 29

mrad

Shielding: Place contact shield over gonads without obscuring area of interest.

Patient Position

- Patient in lateral recumbent position with pillow for head and support between knees. (See Notes for possible erect position.)

Part Position

- Start by aligning mid coronal plane to midline of table.

Hyperflexion:
- Using pelvis as fulcrum, have patient get into fetal position (bend forward) and draw legs up **as far as possible.**

Hyperextension:
- Using pelvis as fulcrum, have patient move torso and legs posteriorly **as far as possible** to hyperextend long axis of body.
- Ensure there is no rotation of thorax or pelvis.

Central Ray

- CR perpendicular to film.
- Center CR to **site of fusion** if known, or to level of **L3**, level of lower costal margin or about 1½ in. or 3 to 4 cm above iliac crest.
- Center cassette to CR.
- Minimum 40 in. (102 cm) SID.

Collimation: Four-sided collimation to near borders of film (if 10 x 12). Larger films require more collimation, especially side collimation.

Respiration: Suspend respiration on expiration.

Notes: May also be done erect sitting on a stool, first leaning forward as far as possible gripping the stool legs; then leaning backwards as far as possible gripping the back of the stool to maintain this position.

Pelvis must remain as stationary as possible during positioning.

Pelvis acts as a fulcrum (pivot point) during changes of position.

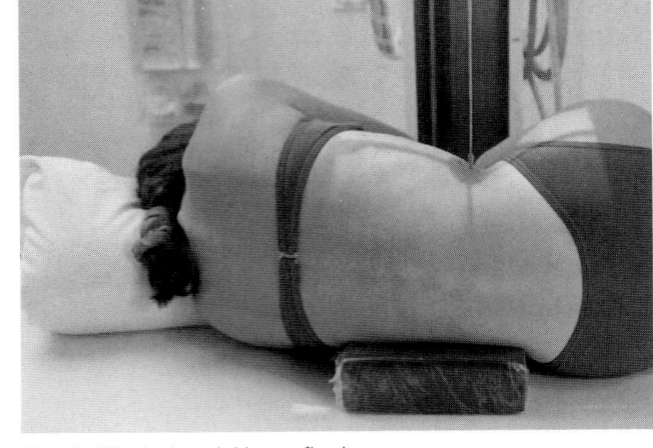

Fig. 9-67. Lateral–Hyperflexion.

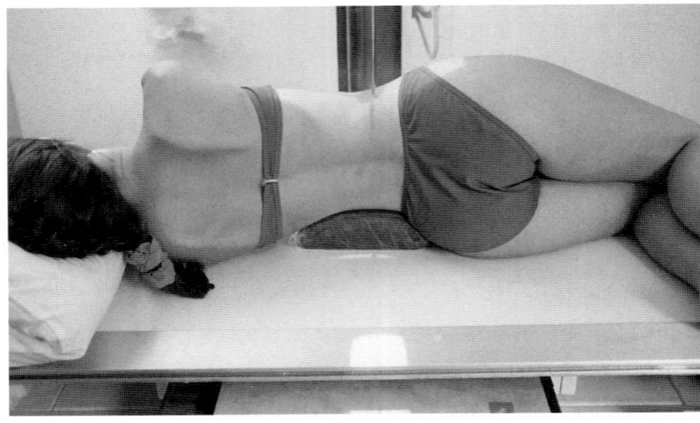

Fig. 9-68. Lateral–Hyperextension.

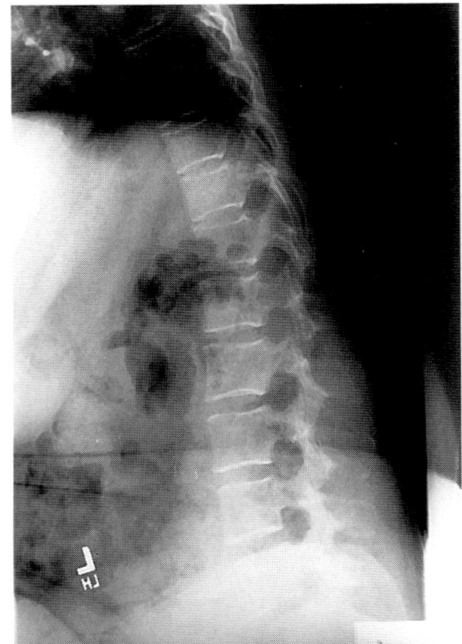

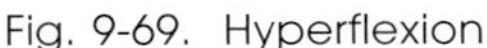

Fig. 9-69. Hyperflexion.

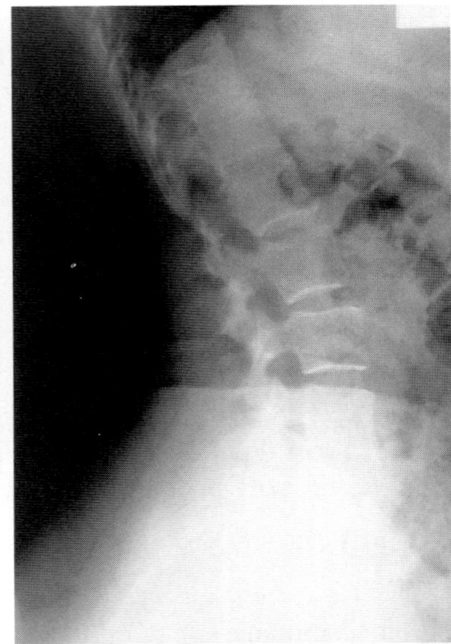

Fig. 9-70. Hyperextension.

Evaluation Criteria

- Site of fusion should be in center of collimation field and film.
- Lower lumbar vertebra should be demonstrated in extreme hyperflexion and hyperextension on two separate films.
- L5 should be in midline of film.
- No rotation of thorax or pelvis; posterior ribs are superimposed.
- Optimum exposure will clearly visualize outlines of lumbar vertebrae and intervertebral joint spaces.
- R or L and hyperextension/hyperflexion markers should be visible without superimposing essential anatomy.

AP Axial Sacrum Projection

Sacrum and coccyx
Basic
- **AP axial sacrum**
- AP axial coccyx
- Lateral

Structures Best Shown

Frontal view of sacrum not foreshortened, SI joints and the L5-S1 junction.

Note: The urinary bladder should be emptied before beginning this procedure. It is also desirable to have the lower colon free of gas and fecal material, which may require a cleaning enema as ordered by a physician.

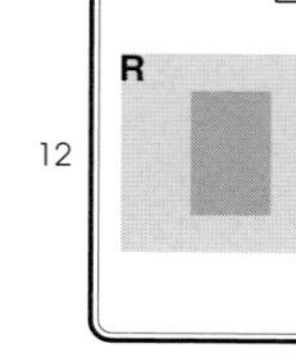

Technical Factors

- Film size–10 x 12 in. (24 x 30 cm), lengthwise.
- Use moving or stationary gird.
- 75-80 kVp range
  (or 85-92 kVp and reduce mAs in half).

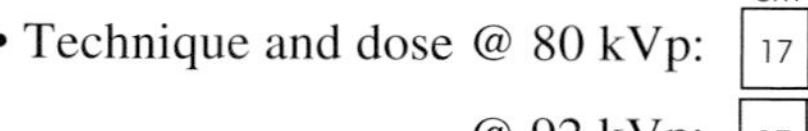

- Technique and dose @ 80 kVp:

@ 92 kVp:

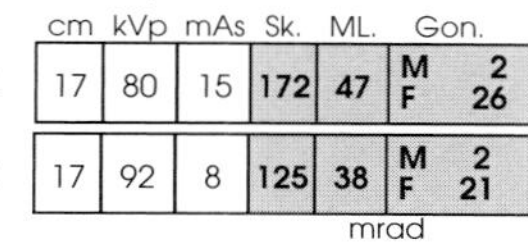

	cm	kVp	mAs	Sk.	ML.	Gon.
@ 80 kVp	17	80	15	172	47	M 2 F 26
@ 92 kVp	17	92	8	125	38	M 2 F 21

mrad

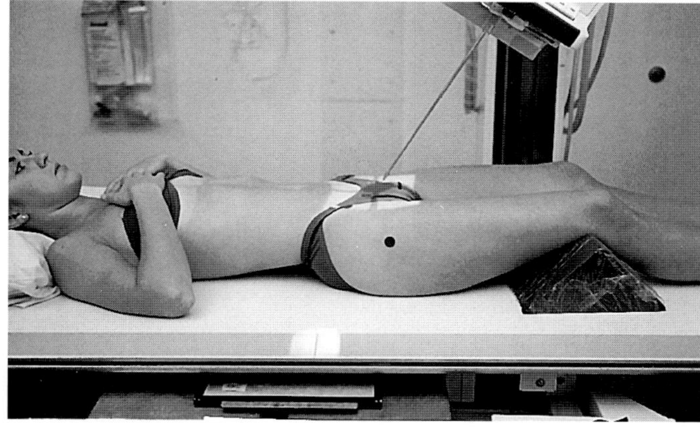

Fig. 9-71. AP–15° cephalad.

Shielding: Use gonadal shielding for males. Ovarian shielding on females is not possible without obscuring area of interest.

Patient Position

- Supine, pillow for head, legs extended with support under knees for comfort.

Part Position

- Align **midsagittal plane to CR and midline of table**.
- Ensure there is **no rotation** of pelvis.

Central Ray

- CR angled **15° cephalad**, to enter at **midsagittal plane midway between level of symphysis pubis and ASIS**.
- Center cassette to projected CR.
- Minimum 40 in. (102 cm) SID.

Collimation: Close four-sided collimation to area of interest.

Respiration: Suspend breathing on expiration.

Notes: May need to increase CR angle to 20° cephalad for females or patients with an apparent greater posterior curvature or tilt of the sacrum and pelvis.

Female sacrum is generally shorter and wider than male sacrum (a consideration in close four-sided collimation).

May be done prone (angle **15° caudad**) if necessary due to patient's condition.

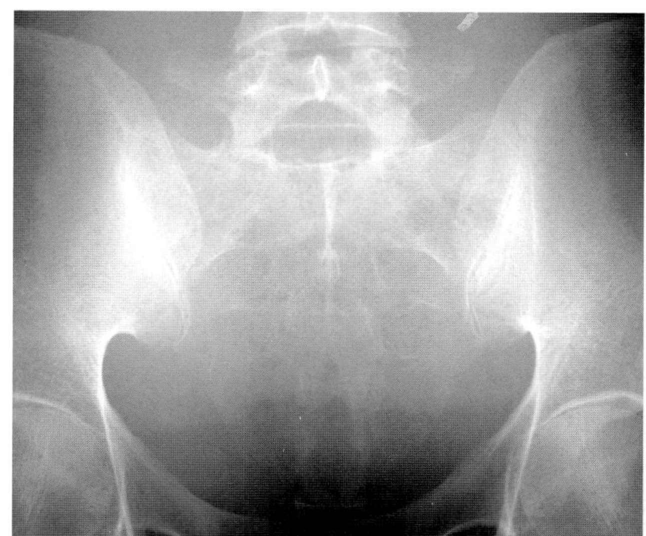

Fig. 9-72. AP sacrum–15° cephalad.

Evaluation Criteria

- Sacrum should be centered to film and collimation field.
- Sacrum should be free of foreshortening and superimposition by pubis and sacral foramina should be visualized.
- Inferior portion of sacrum should be centered in the pelvic opening, indicating no rotation of pelvis.
- Sacral region should be free of excessive gas, fecal matter and a "full" bladder.
- Optimum exposure should demonstrate sufficient contrast and density to clearly visualize the area of the sacrum.

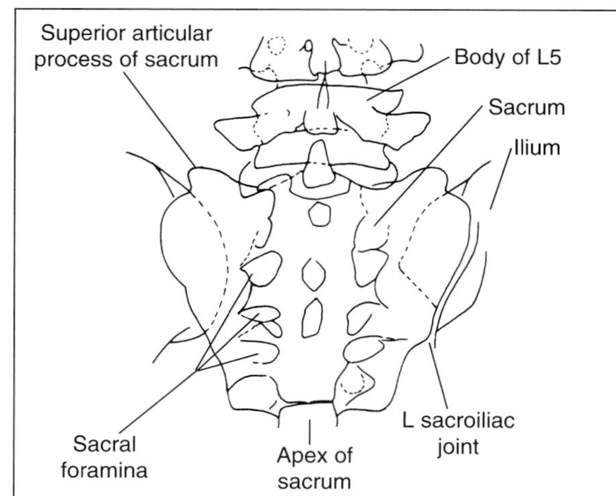

Fig. 9-73. AP sacrum–15° cephalad.

AP Axial Coccyx Projection

Sacrum and coccyx
Basic
• AP axial sacrum
• **AP axial coccyx**
• Lateral

Structures Best Shown

Coccyx free of self-superimposition and superimposition of symphysis pubis.

Note: The urinary bladder should be emptied before beginning this procedure. It is also desirable to have the lower colon free of gas and fecal material which may require a cleaning enema as ordered by a physician.

Technical Factors

8 / 10 / R

- Film size–8 x 10 in. (18 x 24 cm), lengthwise.
- Use moving or stationary gird.
- 70-75kVp range (or 80-85 kVp and reduce mAs and dose in half).
- Technique and dose @ 80 kVp:
- Technique and dose @ 92 kVp:

	cm	kVp	mAs	Sk.	ML.	Gon.
@ 80 kVp	17	80	15	172	47	M 2 F 26
@ 92 kVp	17	92	8	125	38	M 2 F 21
						mrad

Shielding: Use gonadal shielding for males. Ovarian shielding on females is not possible without obscuring area of interest.

Patient Position

- Supine, pillow for head, legs extended with support under knees for comfort.

Part Position

- Align midsagittal plane to midline of table and/or cassette.
- Ensure there is **no rotation** of pelvis.

Central Ray

- CR angled **10° caudad**, to enter **2 in.** (5 cm) **superior to symphysis pubis**.
- Center cassette to projected CR.
- Minimum 40 in. (102 cm) SID.

Collimation: Close four-sided collimation to area of interest. (Close collimation is important for adequate contrast and detail to clearly visualize all segments of the coccyx, and for radiation protection purposes.)

Respiration: Suspend breathing on expiration.

Notes: May need to increase CR angle to 15° caudad with a greater anterior curvature of the coccyx if this is apparent by palpation or as evidenced on the lateral.

May be done **prone** (angle **10° cephalad**) if necessary due to patient's condition, with CR centered to the coccyx, which is easily palpable.

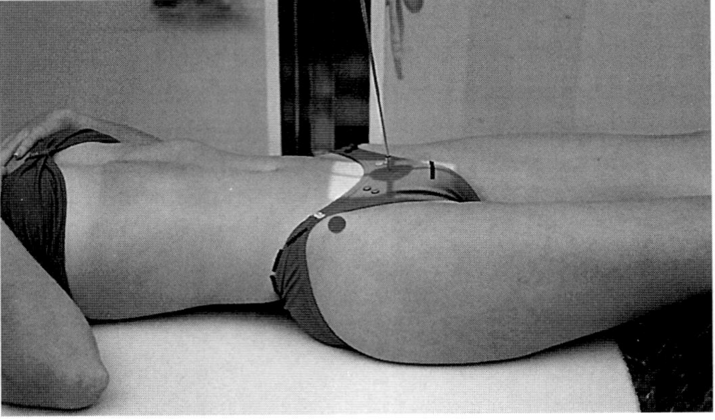

Fig. 9-74. AP coccyx–10° caudad.

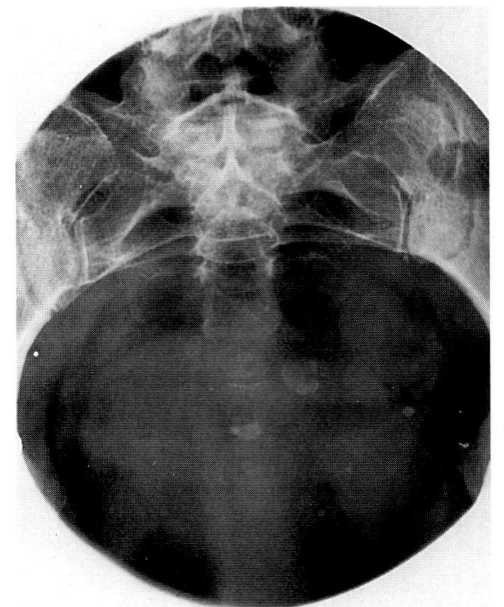

Fig. 9-75. AP coccyx–10° caudad. (Courtesy of Jim Sanderson, RT)

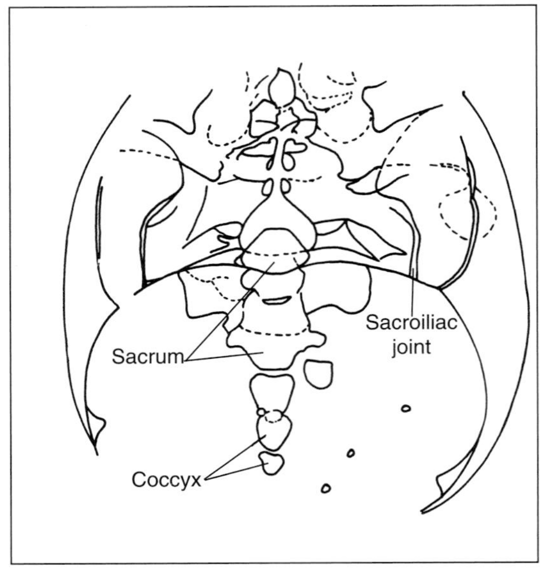

Fig. 9-76. AP coccyx–10° caudad.

Evaluation Criteria

- Coccyx should be seen free of superimposition and projected superior to pubis.
- Coccyx region should be free of excessive gas, fecal matter and a "full" bladder.
- Coccygeal segments should be open. If not, they may be fused or CR angle may need to be increased. (The greater the curvature of the coccyx, the greater the degree of angulation needed.)
- Coccyx should be equidistant from the lateral walls of the pelvic opening, indicating no rotation.
- Coccyx should be in center of collimation field and film.
- Optimum exposure with relatively high (short scale) contrast should clearly visualize all segments of the coccyx without overexposing the most distal segment.

Lateral Sacrum Position–R or L

Sacrum and coccyx
Basic
- AP axial sacrum
- AP axial coccyx
- **Lateral**

Structures Best Shown

Sacrum and L5-S1 joint.

Note: The sacrum and coccyx are commonly ordered together. Separate AP projections are required with different CR angles, **but the lateral can be taken as one projection** with centering to include both the sacrum and coccyx. This is recommended to decrease gonadal doses.

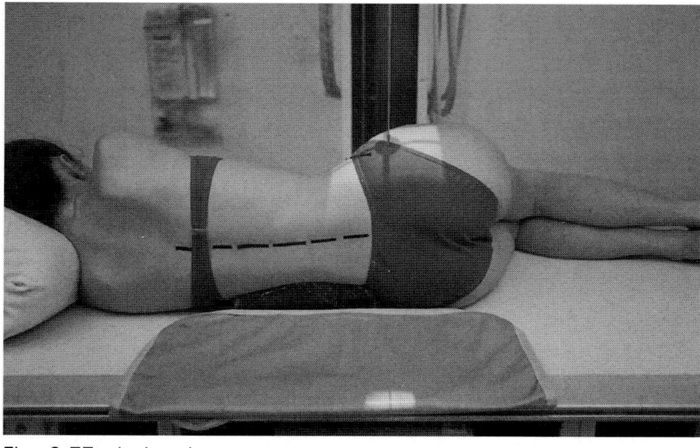

Fig. 9-77. Lateral sacrum.

Technical Factors

- Film size–10 x 12 in. (24 x 30 cm), lengthwise.
- Use moving or stationary grid.
- 90±5 kVp range.
- Place lead blocker on table behind patient to reduce scatter to film.
- AEC not recommended due to size and location of body part and collimation field.
- Technique and dose:

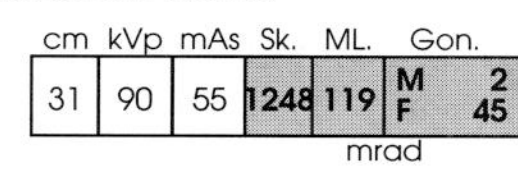

cm	kVp	mAs	Sk.	ML.	Gon.
31	90	55	1248	119	M 2 F 45

mrad

Shielding: Shield gonads without obscuring area of interest. (Complete ovarian shielding on females may obscure a portion of sacrum.)

Patient Position

- Lateral recumbent, pillow for head.

Part Position

- Flex hips and knees.
- Place support under small of waist and between knees and ankles.
- Align **long axis of sacrum to CR and to midline** of table.
- Place pelvis and body in **true lateral position**.

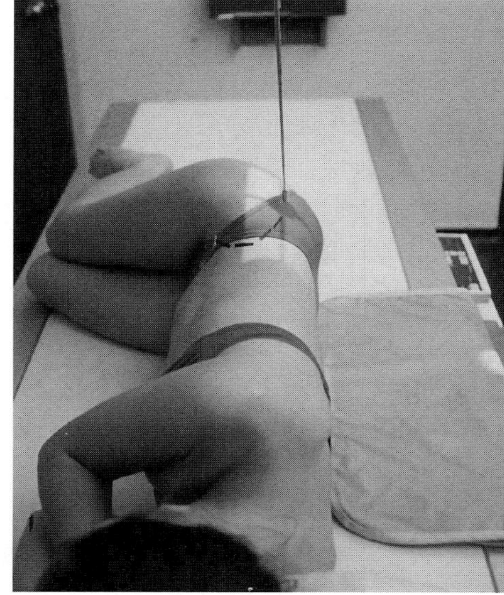

Fig. 9-78. Lateral sacrum.

Central Ray

- CR perpendicular to table and film.
- Center CR **2 in.** (5 cm) **anterior to posterior sacral surface at level of ASIS (S2).**
- Center cassette to CR.
- Minimum 40 in. (102 cm) SID.

Collimation: Close four-sided collimation to area of interest.

Respiration: Suspend breathing on expiration.

Note: High amounts of secondary and scatter radiation are generated. Close collimation and a lead blocker shield placed on table-top directly behind patient reduces scatter to film.

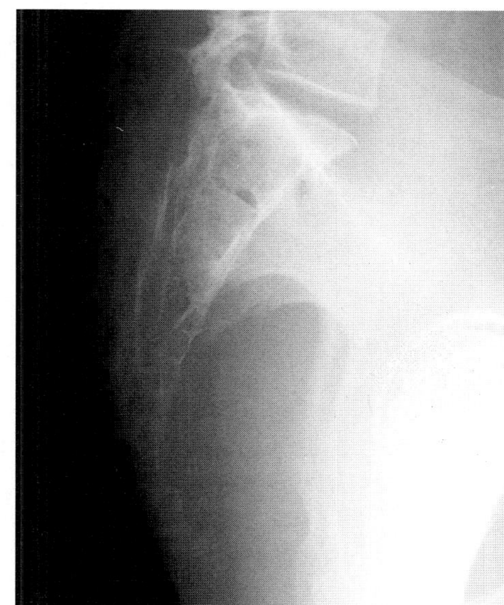

Fig. 9-79. Lateral sacrum and coccyx.

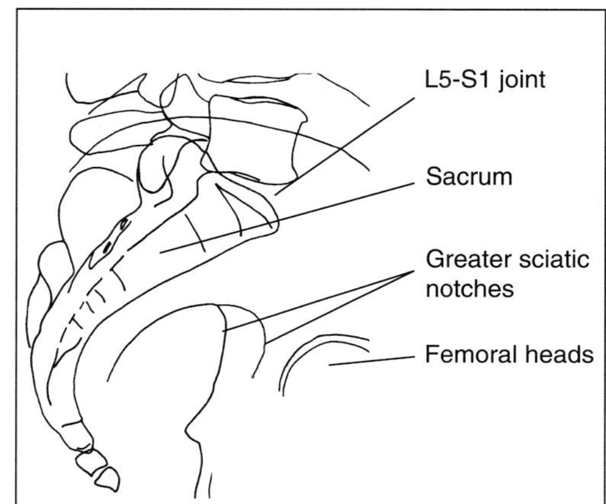

Fig. 9-80. Lateral sacrum.

Evaluation Criteria

- Sacrum and coccyx should be seen in lateral profile in center of film and center of four-sided collimation field, (if lateral sacrum and coccyx are combined as in Fig. 9-79).
- Posterior margins of pelvis including greater sciatic notches and femoral heads are aligned anteroposteriorly, indicating no rotation of pelvis.
- Optimum exposure should clearly visualize the entire sacrum. (The distal coccyx segments may appear slightly overexposed.)

Lateral Coccyx Position

Sacrum and coccyx
Basic
- AP axial sacrum
- AP axial coccyx
- **Lateral**

Structures Best Shown

Coccyx (anterior angulation is best demonstrated in this position).

Note: The sacrum and coccyx are commonly ordered together, and a single lateral can be taken centered to **include both the sacrum and coccyx**. This is recommended to decrease gonadal doses.

Technical Factors

- Film size–8 x 10 in. (18 x 24 cm), lengthwise.
- Use moving or stationary grid.
- 80±5 kVp range.
- Place lead blocker on table behind patient to reduce scatter to the film.
- AEC not recommended due to size and location of body part and collimation field.
- Technique and dose:

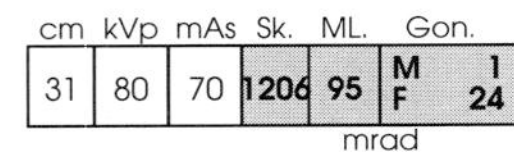

cm	kVp	mAs	Sk.	ML.	Gon.
31	80	70	1206	95	M 1 F 24
					mrad

Shielding: Shield gonads without obscuring area of interest. Complete ovarian shielding on females may obscure a portion of sacrum and/or coccyx.

Patient Position

- Lateral recumbent, pillow for head.

Part Position

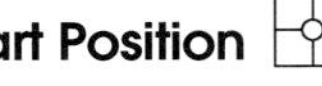

- Flex hips and knees.
- Place support under small of waist, and between knees and ankles.
- Align **long axis of coccyx with CR and midline of table** and/or cassette. (Remember the superficial location of coccyx.)
- Place pelvis and body in **true lateral** position.

Central Ray

- CR perpendicular to table.
- Center CR to **level of about 2 in. (5 cm) distal to level of ASIS, and 1 to 2 in. (3 to 5 cm) anterior to posterior surface of sacrum and coccyx**.
- Center cassette to CR.
- Minimum 40 in. (102 cm) SID.

Collimation: Close four-sided collimation to area of interest.

Respiration: Suspend breathing on expiration.

Note: Do not overexpose. When taken separately, the coccyx requires a lower kVp range and less exposure than the lateral sacrum.

Evaluation Criteria

- Coccyx should be seen in lateral profile in center of collimation field and film. (Close four-sided collimation should be evident.)
- Segment interspaces should be open if not fused.
- Optimum exposure should clearly visualize all segments of the coccyx.
- No rotation of pelvis as indicated by anteroposterior alignment of greater sciatic notches. (Some rotation is evident on the above radiograph.)

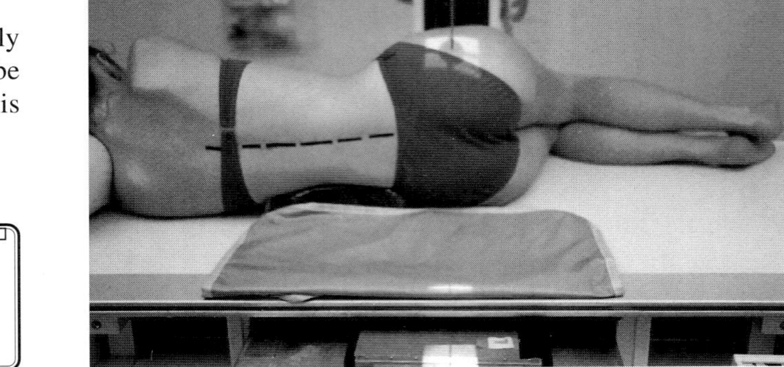

Fig. 9-81. Lateral coccyx.

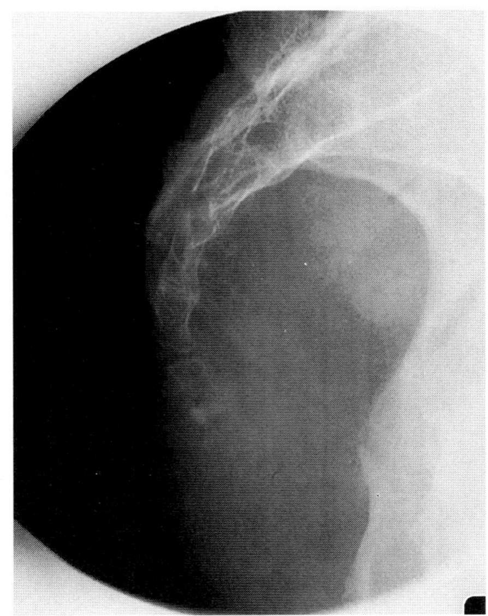

Fig. 9-82. Lateral coccyx.
(Courtesy of Jim Sanderson, RT)

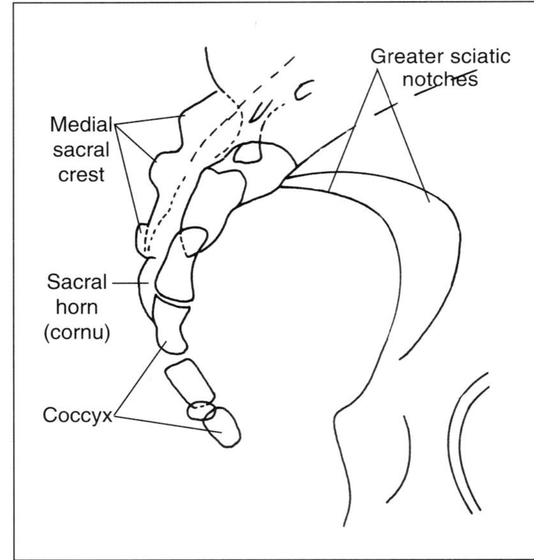

Fig. 9-83. Lateral coccyx.

Radiographs for Critique

Each of these radiographs demonstrates some error in positioning which requires a repeat. These, along with accompanying lecture slides of these and other radiographs, will provide a basis for classroom and/or positioning lab discussion. Questions with answers based on these specific critique radiographs are provided in the accompanying student workbook/lab manuals to help prepare students for classroom and/or lab discussions on film critique.

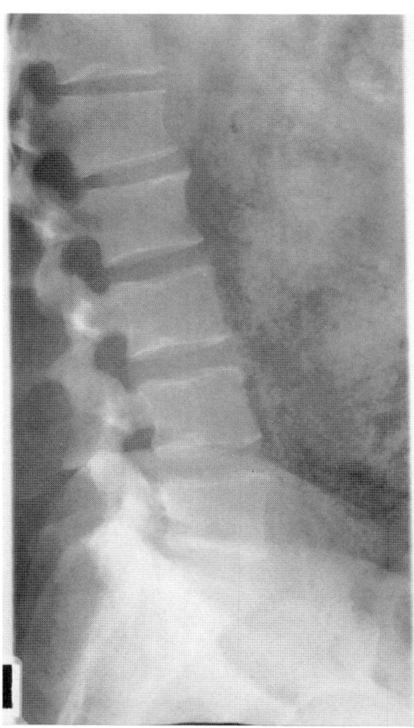

Fig. C9-84. Lateral L spine.

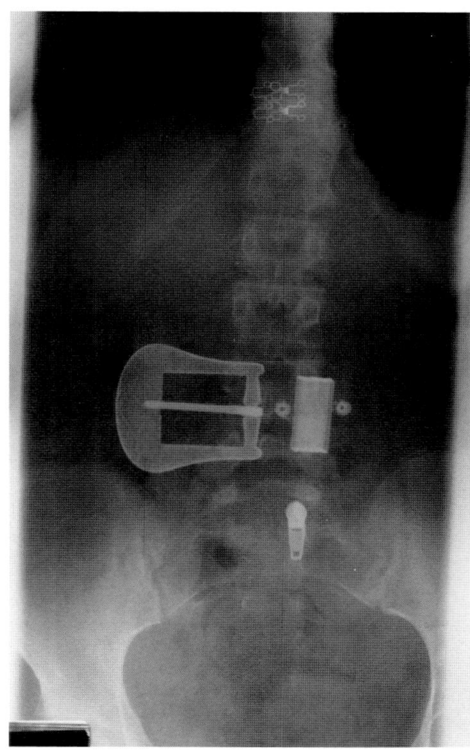

Fig. C9-85. AP lumbar spine.

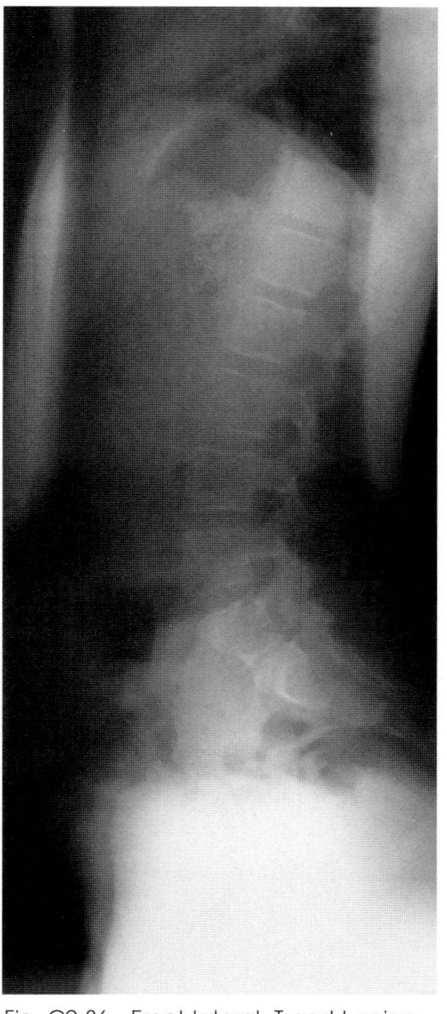

Fig. C9-86. Erect lateral, T and L spine–part of scoliosis series.

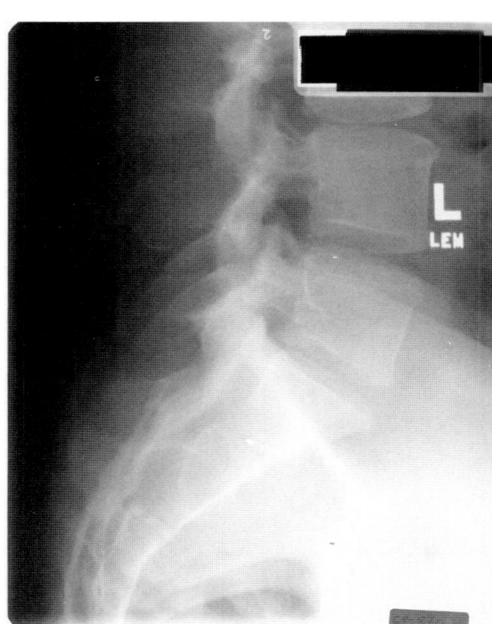

Fig. C9-87. Lateral L5-S1.

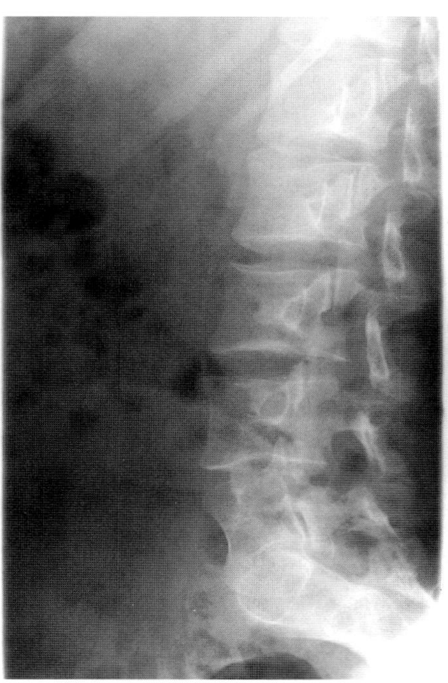

Fig. C9-88. Oblique L spine.

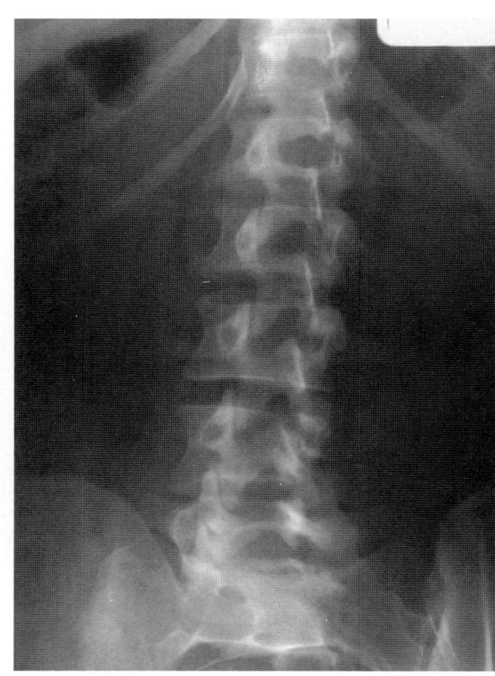

Fig. C9-89. Oblique L spine.

CHAPTER 10

Bony Thorax, Sternum and Ribs

CONTRIBUTIONS BY:
John P. Lampignano, M Ed, RT (R)

CONTENTS

Radiographic Anatomy

Bony thorax, sternum and palpable landmarks **306**

Ribs **307**

Articulations of thorax **308**

Anatomy review with radiographs **309**

Radiographic Positioning

Positioning considerations for sternum **310**

Positioning considerations for ribs **311**

Survey results and basic and special projections **313**

Sternum:
- RAO **314**
- Lateral **315**

Sternoclavicular joints:
- PA **316**
- Anterior obliques **317**

Ribs:
- Posterior ribs (AP) **318**
- Anterior ribs (PA) **319**
- Axillary ribs (oblique) **320**

Radiographs for critique **322**

Radiographic Anatomy

Bony Thorax

The main function of the bony thorax is to serve as an expandable bellows-like chamber wherein the interior capacity expands and contracts during inspiration and expiration respectively. This is caused by alternate action of muscles attached to the rib cage and atmospheric pressure causing the air to move in and out of the lungs during respiration.

The bony thorax consists of the **sternum** anteriorly, the **thoracic vertebrae** posteriorly (Fig.10-3), and the **12 pairs of ribs** connecting the sternum to the vertebral column. The bony thorax serves to protect important organs of the respiratory system and vital structures within the mediastinum, such as the heart and great vessels.

The red marrow of the ribs and sternum are primary sites of red blood cell formation. Therefore, it is important to shield the sternum, thyroid gland, lungs and female breasts whenever possible while radiographing upper body parts.

The sternum is also a common site for marrow biopsy in which, under a local anesthetic, a needle is inserted into the marrow cavity of the sternum to withdraw a sample of red bone marrow.

The drawing in Fig. 10-3 shows the relationship of the sternum to the 12 pairs of ribs and 12 thoracic vertebrae. As demonstrated in these drawings, the thin sternum superimposes the structures within the mediastinum as well as the dense thoracic spine in a direct frontal position. Therefore an AP or PA projection radiograph would show the thoracic spine well, but would show the sternum only faintly, if at all.

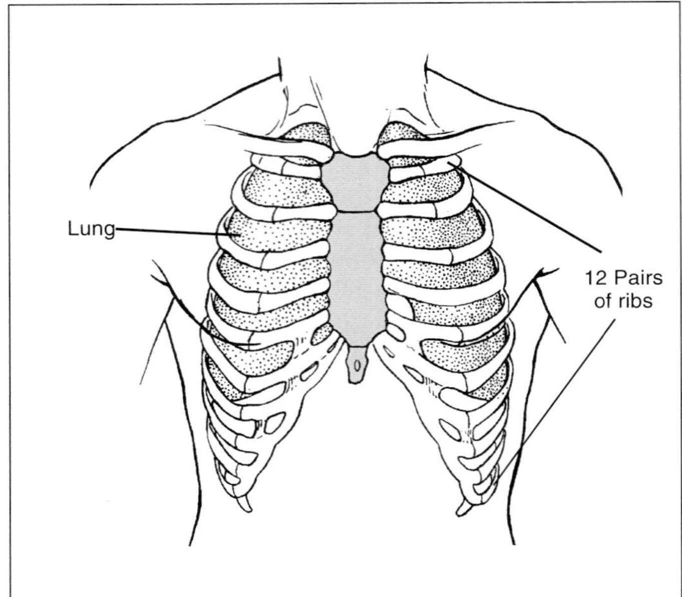

Fig. 10-1. Bony thorax, expandable enclosure for lungs.

STERNUM

The adult sternum is a thin, narrow, flat bone with three divisions. The upper portion is termed the **manubrium** *(mah-nu′ bre-um)*, which is from the Latin, meaning *handle*. The adult manubrium averages 2 inches or 5 centimeters in length.

The longest part of the sternum is the **body,** which is about 4 inches or 10 centimeters long. The Latin word for body is *corpus*. Another, but older, term for the body is *gladiolus*, which means *sword*. The union of the four segments of the body begins during puberty and is not completed until about the age of 25.

The most inferior portion of the sternum is the **xiphoid** *(zi′foid)* **process**, which consists of cartilage during infancy and youth and usually does not become totally ossified until about age 40. The xiphoid process is generally rather small; however, it can be quite variable in size, shape, and degree of ossification.

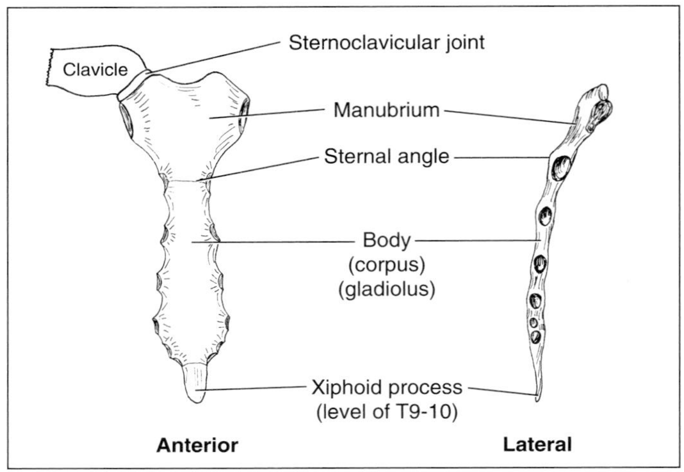

Fig. 10-2. Sternum.

Palpable Landmarks (Fig. 10-2)

The uppermost border of the manubrium is easy to palpate and is called the **jugular notch.** Other secondary names for this area are **suprasternal** or **manubrial notch,** all of which describe the slightly notched area between the two clavicles along the upper border of the sternum. The jugular notch is at the level of T2-3.

The lower end of the manubrium joins the body of the sternum to form a palpable prominence, the **sternal angle.** This is also an easily palpated landmark used for location of other structures of the bony thorax. The sternal angle is at the level of the disc space between **T4 and T5** in an average-shaped, upright adult.

The **xiphoid tip** corresponds to the level of **T9-T10**. The **inferior rib angle** (lowest costal margin) corresponds to the level of **L2** or **L3**.

Sternoclavicular Articulation: Each **clavicle** joins the manubrium lateral to the jugular notch on each side and is called the **sternoclavicular joint**, which is the only bony connection between each upper limb and the bony thorax.

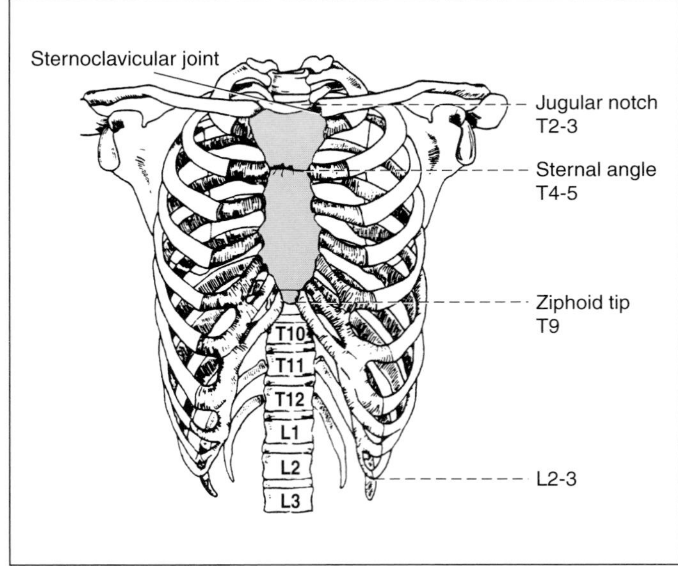

Fig. 10-3. Bony thorax–Sternum, ribs, thoracic vertebrae (landmarks and associated vertebrae).

Sternal Rib Articulations: The **clavicles** and the **cartilages** of the **first seven pairs of ribs** connect directly to the sternum. Below each clavicular notch and sternoclavicular joint is a depression or **facet** for articulation with the cartilage of the first rib.

The drawing in Fig. 10-4 illustrates that the anterior ribs do not unite directly with the sternum, but do so with a short piece of cartilage termed **costocartilage.** The costocartilages and ribs have been added to one side of this drawing to show this relationship.

The second costocartilage connects to the sternum at the level of the sternal angle. An easy way to locate the anterior end of the second rib is to locate the sternal angle first, then feel laterally along the cartilage and the bone of the rib.

The third through the seventh costocartilages connect directly to the body of the sternum.

Ribs #8, #9 and #10 also possess costocartilage, but these connect to the number 7 costocartilages, which then connect to the sternum.

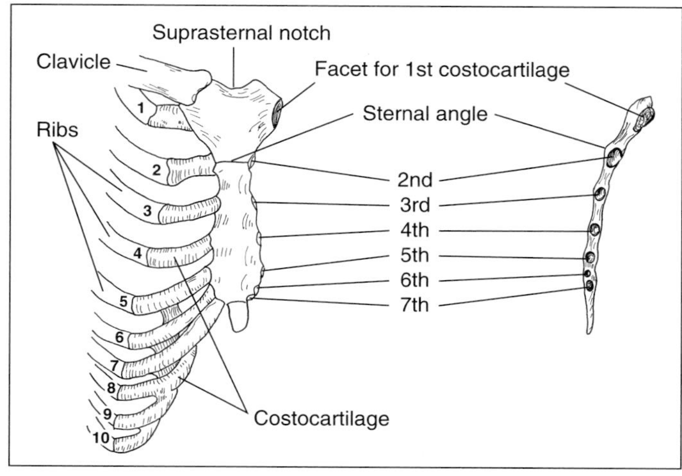

Fig. 10-4. Sternal rib articulations.

RIBS

Each rib is numbered according to the thoracic vertebra to which it attaches; therefore the ribs are numbered from the top down. The first seven pairs of ribs are considered **true ribs.** Each true rib attaches directly to the sternum by its own costocartilage. The term **false ribs** applies to the last five pairs of ribs, numbered 8, 9, 10, 11 and 12.

The drawing in Fig. 10-5 again clearly shows that, although ribs 8 through 10 have costocartilages, they connect to the costocartilage of the seventh rib.

The last two pairs of false ribs are unique in that they do not possess costocartilage. The term **floating ribs** can be used to designate these two pairs of ribs.

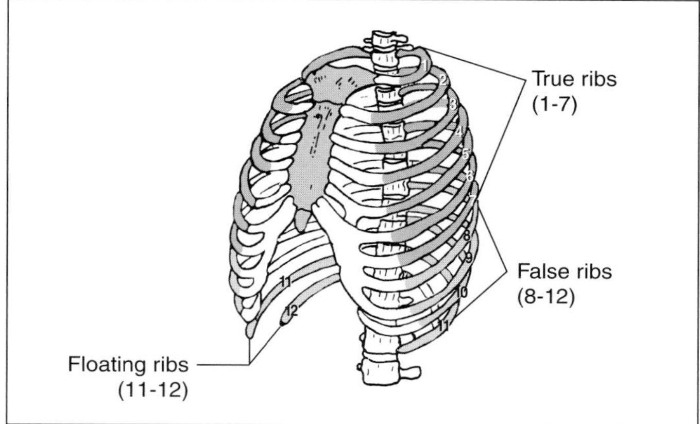

Fig. 10-5. Ribs.

Summary: Ribs **1 to 7** are termed **true ribs** and connect directly to the sternum. The last five pair of ribs, **8 to 12** are termed **false ribs**. The last two pair of ribs, **11 and 12** which are also false ribs, are termed **floating ribs** because they are not connected anteriorly.

Typical Rib

Inferior View: A typical rib viewed from its inferior surface is illustrated in Fig. 10-6. A central rib is used to show the common characteristics of a typical rib. Each rib has two ends, a posterior or **vertebral end,** and an anterior or **sternal end.** Between the two ends is the **shaft** or body of the rib.

The vertebral end consists of a **head,** which articulates with one or two thoracic vertebral bodies, and a flattened **neck.** Lateral to the neck is an elevated **tubercle** that articulates with the transverse process of a vertebra and allows for attachment of a ligament. The shaft extends laterally from the tubercle, then angles forward and downward. The area of forward angulation is termed the **angle** of the rib.

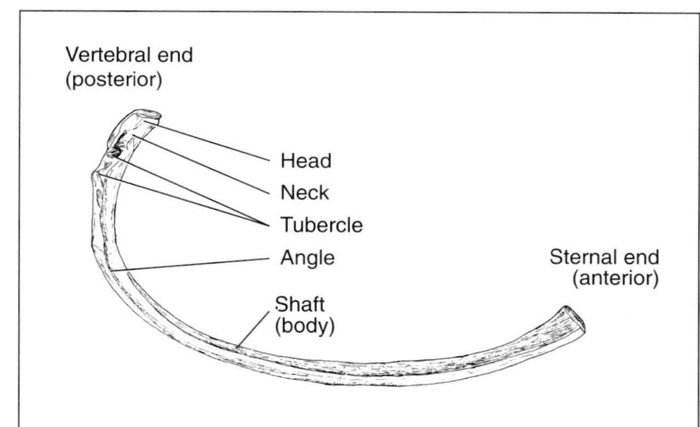

Fig. 10-6. Typical rib–Inferior view.

Posterior View: Seen on this posterior view are the **head, neck** and **tubercles** at the vertebral end of the rib. Progressing laterally, the angle of the rib is where the shaft bends forward and downward toward the sternal end. As seen in Fig. 10-7, the posterior or vertebral end of a typical rib is 3 to 5 inches (7.5 to 12.5 cm) **higher** than the anterior or sternal end. Therefore, when viewing a radiograph of a chest or ribs, one must remember that the part of a rib most superior is the posterior end, or the end nearest the vertebrae. The anterior end is more inferior.

The lower inside margin of each rib protects an **artery**, a **vein** and a **nerve**; therefore, rib injuries are very painful and may be associated with substantial hemorrhage. This inside margin, containing the blood vessels and nerves, is termed the **costal groove.**

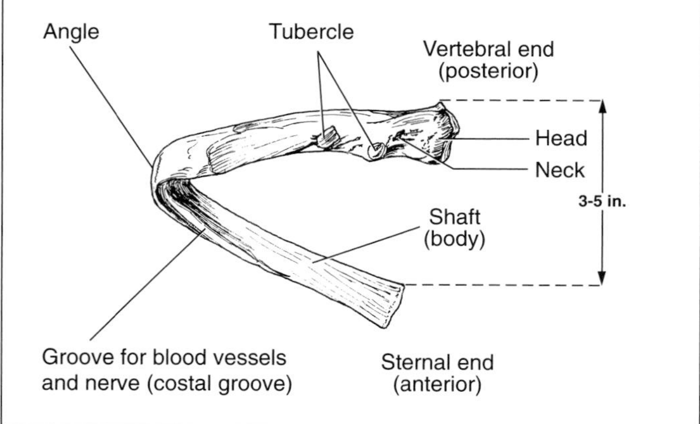

Fig. 10-7. Typical rib–Posterior view.

Rib Cage (Fig. 10-8)

The drawing in Fig. 10-8 illustrates the bony thorax with the sternum and costocartilages removed. The fifth ribs have been shaded to better illustrate the downward angulation of the ribs.

Not all ribs have the same appearance. The first ribs are short and broad, and are the most vertical of all the ribs. Counting downward from the short first pair, the ribs get longer and longer down to the seventh ribs. From the seventh ribs down they get shorter and shorter through the fairly short twelfth or last pair of ribs. The first ribs are the most sharply curved. The bony thorax is **widest** at the lateral margins of the **eighth or ninth ribs.**

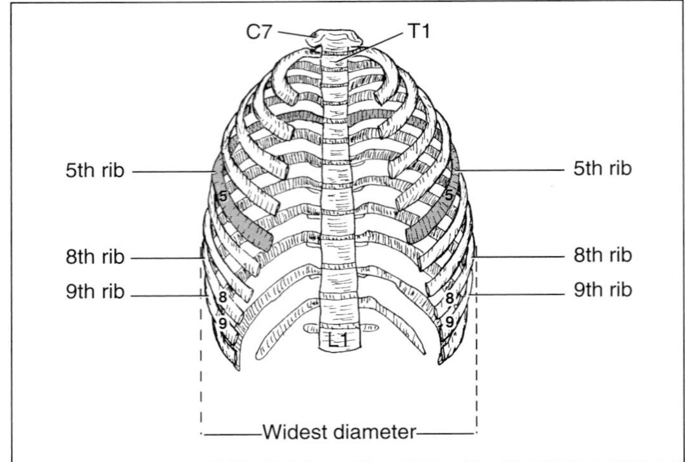

Fig. 10-8. Rib cage.

ARTICULATIONS OF THORAX

Anterior Articulations (Fig. 10-9)

A frontal view of an articulated thorax is illustrated in Fig. 10-9. The joints or articulations of the anterior bony thorax are identified on this photograph. The joints along with the classification and the types of motion allowed are as follows:

Part A (shown on left side at 4th rib) is the joint between costocartilage and the sternal end of the fourth rib, and is called a **costochondral union** or **junction**. These (ribs 1-10) are a unique type of union wherein the cartilage and bone are bound together by the periosteum of the bone itself. This permits **no motion**, therefore, they are **synarthrodial.**

Part B is one **sternoclavicular joint.** The sternoclavicular joints are **synovial** joints, containing articular capsules that permit **a gliding motion** and are therefore **diarthrodial** joints.

Part C is the **sternocostal joint** of the first rib. The cartilage of the first rib attaches directly to the manubrium with no synovial capsule and allows **no motion (synarthrodial)**. Therefore, this is a **cartilaginous** class joint of the **synchondrosis** type.

Part D is the fourth sternocostal joint, typical of the second through the seventh joints between costocartilage and sternum. These are **synovial** joints, which allow a slight **plane (gliding) motion**, making them **diarthrodial** joints.

Part E represents the continuous borders of the **interchondral joint** between the costal cartilage of the anterior sixth through tenth ribs. These are all interconnected by a **synovial** type joint with a long thin articular capsule lined by synovial membrane. These allow a slight **plane (gliding) type movement (diarthrodial)**, facilitating movement of the bony thorax during the breathing process.

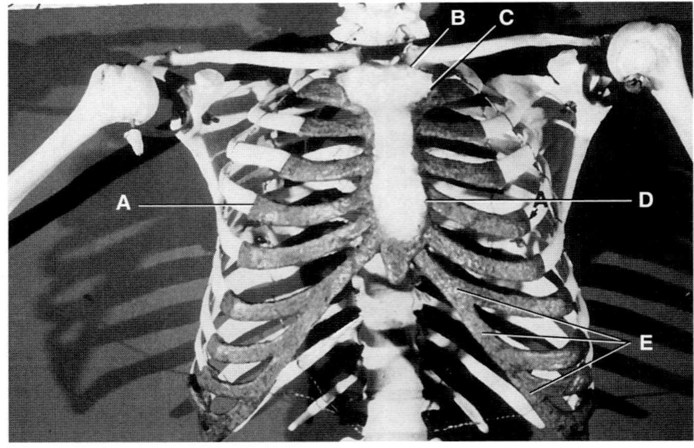

Fig. 10-9. Articulated thorax.

Posterior Articulations (Fig. 10-10)

The remaining posterior types of joints in the bony thorax, **parts F** and **G**, are illustrated in Fig. 10-10. The joints between the ribs and the vertebral column, the **costotransverse joints (F)** and the **costovertebral joints (G),** are **synovial** joints with articular capsules lined by synovial membrane which allow a **gliding motion,** and are therefore **diarthrodial**.

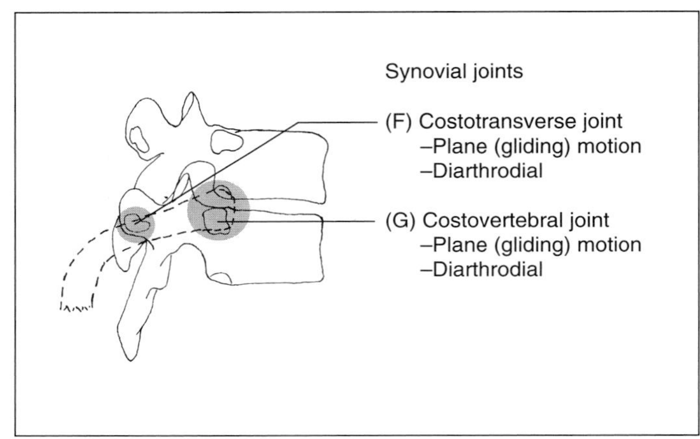

Fig. 10-10. Posterior articulations.

Summary of Thorax Articulations

	Joints	Classification	Movement type
(A)	1st-10th Costochondral unions (between costocartilage and ribs)	Unique type of union	Immovable–synarthrodial
(B)	Sternoclavicular joints (between clavicles and sternum)	Synovial	Plane (gliding)–diarthrodial
(C)	1st Sternocostal joint (between 1st rib and sternum)	Cartilaginous–synchondrosis	Immovable–synarthrodial
(D)	2nd-7th Sternocostal joints (between 2nd-7th ribs and sternum)	Synovial	Plane (gliding)–diarthrodial
(E)	6th-10th Interchondral joints (between anterior 6-10th costal cartilages)	Synovial	Plane (gliding)–diarthrodial
(F)	1st-12th Costotransverse joints (between ribs and transverse processes of T vertebrae)	Synovial	Plane (gliding)–diarthrodial
(G)	1st-12th Costovertebral joints (between heads of ribs and T vertebrae)	Synovial	Plane (gliding)–diarthrodial

ANATOMY REVIEW

Sternum (Fig. 10-11)

The sternum is both difficult to radiograph successfully and difficult to study anatomically on the finished radiograph. The parts of the sternum listed A through G on the photograph of an actual sternum in Fig. 10-11 are:

A. Jugular (suprasternal) notch.
B. Clavicular notch.
C. Facet for the costocartilage of the first rib.
D. Manubrium.
E. Sternal angle.
F. Body or corpus.
G. Area of the xiphoid process.

Part **B** is the area of articulation of the clavicle to the sternum. Remember that the clavicle articulates just lateral to the jugular notch and just above the articulation of the cartilage of the first rib.

Also, on this particular sternum the xiphoid process has not ossified, but the lower bracket **(G)** indicates the area where it would normally be found if it were cartilaginous or osseous.

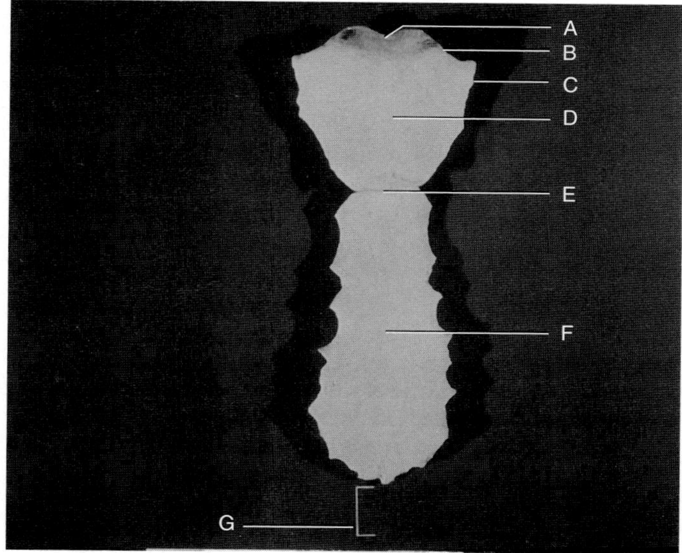

Fig. 10-11. Sternum.

Sternum Radiographs (Figs. 10-12 and 10-13)

RAO: Radiographs of the sternum in an anterior oblique position are illustrated in Figs. 10-12 and 10-13. These are conventional frontal radiographs of the sternum taken in a 15 to 20° anterior oblique position. The slight degree of obliquity tends to project the thoracic vertebrae to one side of the sternum.

The various parts of the sternum are difficult to visualize on radiographs of the sternum, so parts of the radiograph in Fig. 10-12 have been enhanced. The labeled parts are:

A. Sternal end of one clavicle.
B. Jugular notch.
C. Manubrium.
D. Sternal angle.
E. Body.
F. Area of xiphoid process.

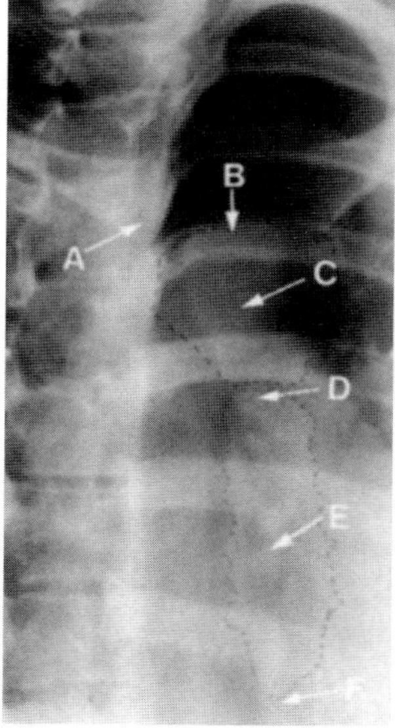

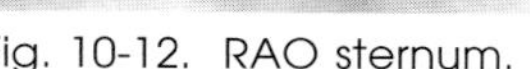
Fig. 10-12. RAO sternum.

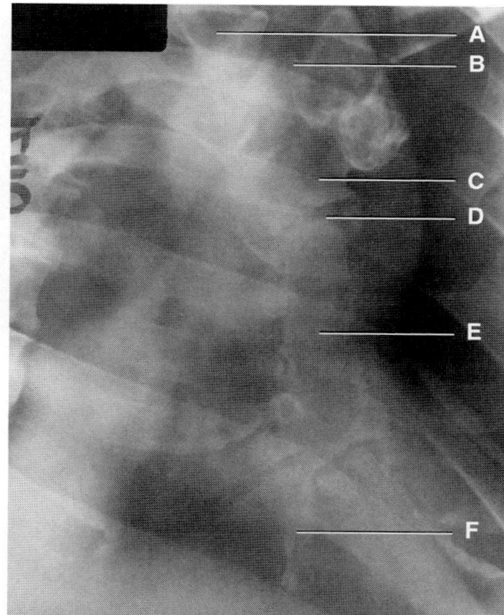

Fig. 10-13. RAO sternum.

Typical Rib (Fig. 10-14)

A photograph of a typical rib as viewed from the undersurface is illustrated in Fig. 10-14. **A**, **B** and **C** are structures at the posterior or vertebral end of the rib.

A. Head.
B. Neck.
C. Tubercle of this rib.
D. Angle of the rib.
E. Portion of the costal groove.
F. Shaft (body)
G. Sternal end (anterior)

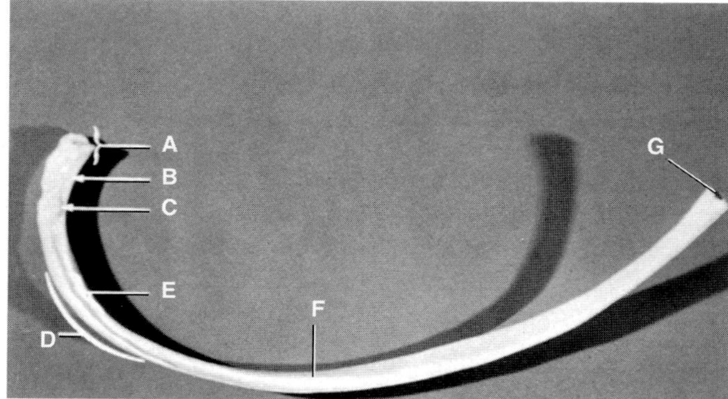

Fig. 10-14. Typical rib.

Radiographic Positioning

POSITIONING CONSIDERATIONS FOR THE STERNUM

The sternum is difficult to radiograph because of its bony composition and position within the thorax. The sternum is made up primarily of spongy bone with a thin layer of hard, compact bone surrounding it. Therefore, it is easy to overexpose.

Also the sternum is an anterior midline structure that is in the same plane as the thoracic spine. Since the thoracic spine is much more dense, it is virtually impossible to see the sternum in a true AP or PA projection. Therefore, a frontal view is obtained in a 15 to 20° RAO position to shift the sternum just to the left of the thoracic vertebrae and into the homogenous heart shadow. (See Fig. 10-15.)

The degree of obliquity is dependent on the size of the thoracic cavity. A shallow or thin chest requires more obliquity than a deep one to cast the sternum away from the thoracic spine. For example, a patient with a large, barrel-chested thorax with a greater anteroposterior measurement requires **less** rotation (≈15°). A thin-chested patient requires **more** rotation (≈20°). This principle is illustrated by the drawings in Figs. 10-16 and 10-17.

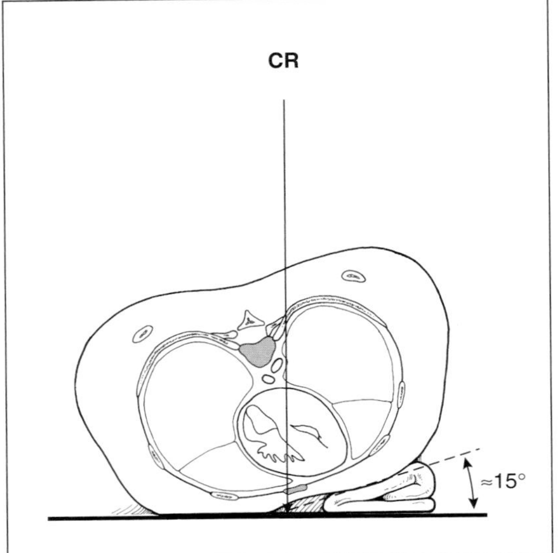

Fig. 10-15. Large, barrel-chested thorax, ≈15°.

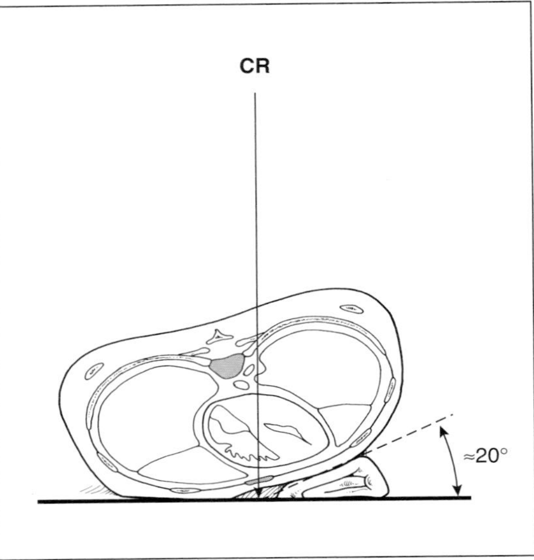

Fig. 10-16. Thin-chested thorax, ≈20°.

Breathing Technique

A breathing technique involves the patient taking short, shallow breaths during the exposure. If performed properly, the lung markings overlying the sternum will become obscured, while the image of the sternum remains sharp and well defined. This requires a low kVp range, low mA, and a long exposure time of 3 or 4 seconds. The radiographer must be sure the thorax in general isn't moving during the exposure other than from the gentle breathing motion.

Because of the low bony density of the sternum, even if the breathing technique is not used, a relatively low kVp and adequate mAs technique are required.

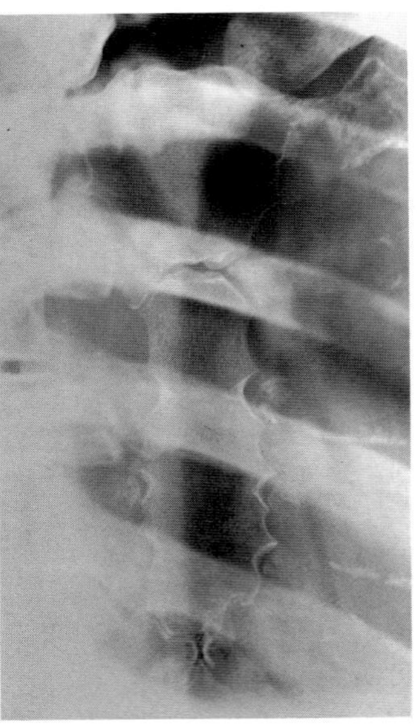
Fig. 10-17. RAO sternum, breathing technique.

Use a Safe SID

It has been a common practice to lower the source-image-receptor distance (SID) to a minimal range to create magnification with resultant blurring of overlying posterior ribs. While this produces visible images of the sternum, it also results in an increase in the radiation exposure to the patient. A safe and practical SID of no less than 30 inches should be used, remembering the radiation safety rule described in Chapter 1, (a **minimum of 12 inches** or [30 cm] **SOD** [source object distance], the distance between the target of the x-ray tube and the closest skin surface of the patient).

Tomography

Tomography, if such equipment is available, is a common method for radiographing the sternum in a frontal view without loss of detail from overlying structures.

POSITIONING CONSIDERATIONS FOR RIBS

Specific projections performed in a rib series are generally determined by the patient's clinical history and the department protocol.

The radiographer must obtain a complete clinical history that includes (a) the nature of the trauma or pathology, (b) the location of the rib pain or injury, (c) whether the patient has been coughing up blood or fluid, and (d) whether the patient is able to stand.

The following positioning tips are provided to assist the radiographer in producing a diagnostic study of the ribs:

Above or Below Diaphragm

The location of the trauma determines which region of the ribs are radiographed. Ribs above the diaphragm require a different technique, different breathing instructions, and generally different body positions than ribs located below the diaphragm.

The upper ten or eleven posterior ribs are generally the minimum ribs above the dome or central portion of the diaphragm on a full inspiration as described in Chapter 2 on the chest. However, with painful rib injuries the patient may not be able to take as full an inspiration and only nine, or even eight posterior ribs may be seen above the diaphragm on inspiration.

Above Diaphragm: To best demonstrate the above-diaphragm ribs, the radiographer should:

(a) Take the radiographs **erect**, if patient is able to stand or sit. This allows better inspiration of the lungs with the diaphragm dropping to its lowest position. Also, most rib injuries are very painful and body movement creating pressure against the rib cage, such as from movements on the x-ray table, can cause severe pain and discomfort.

(b) Suspend respiration and expose upon **inspiration**. This should project the diaphragm below the eighth or ninth, or even tenth ribs on full inspiration.

(c) Select a relatively **low kVp** technique (65-75 range). Since the upper ribs are surrounded by lung tissue, a lower kVp will preserve radiographic contrast and visualize the ribs through the air-filled lungs. However, if the site of injury is over the heart area, a higher kVp may be used to obtain a longer scale contrast to visualize ribs both through the heart shadow and through the lung fields.

Below Diaphragm: To best demonstrate these ribs below the diaphragm, the radiographer should:

(a) Take the radiographs with patient **recumbent** (supine). This will allow the diaphragm to rise to the highest position, and also results in a "less thick" abdomen (especially on heavy patients as the abdomen flattens out when recumbent). This provides better visualization of the lower ribs through abdominal structures.

(b) Suspend respiration and expose upon **expiration.** This should allow the diaphragm to rise to the level of the sixth or seventh ribs, again providing a uniform background density for below-diaphragm ribs.

(c) Select a **medium kVp** technique (75-85). Since the lower ribs are surrounded by the muscular diaphragm and must be demonstrated through dense abdominal structures, a medium kVp will ensure proper penetration of these tissues.

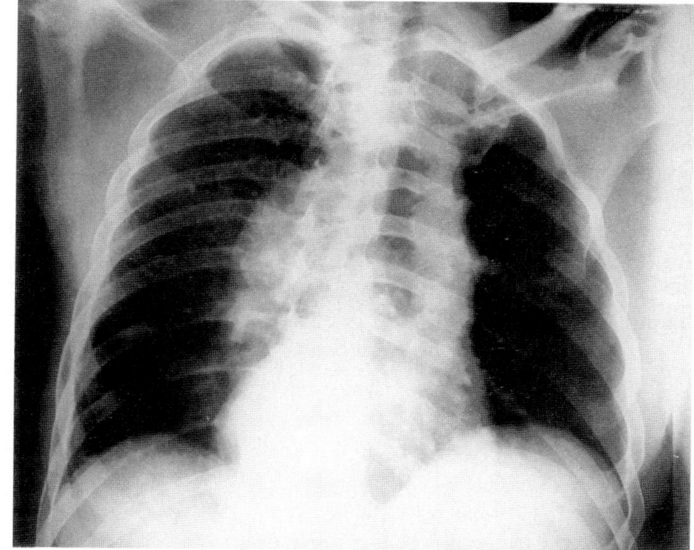

Fig. 10-18. Ribs above diaphragm (slightly oblique).
-Erect if possible.
-Inspiration.
-Low kVp (65-75).

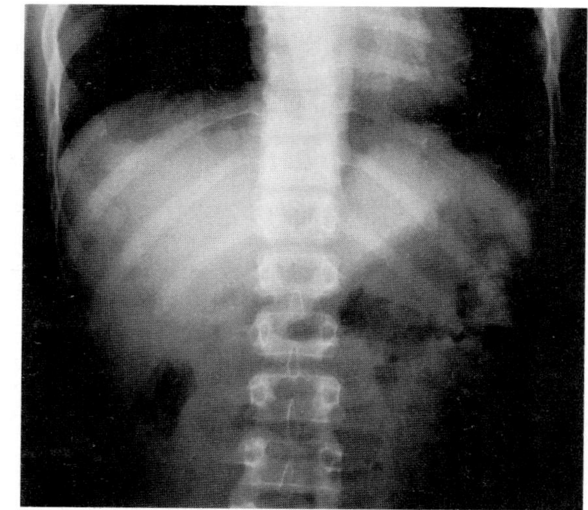

Fig. 10-19. Ribs below diaphragm.
-Recumbent.
-Expiration.
-Medium kVp (75-85).

Positioning Considerations For Ribs continued

Recommended Projections

Departmental routines for ribs may vary depending on the preference of radiologists. One recommended routine is as follows:

Select the projections that will place the **area of interest closest to the film,** and **rotate the spine away from the area of interest.**

For example, if a patient has a history of trauma to the **left posterior ribs**, the two preferred projections with this routine are a straight **AP** and a **left posterior oblique.** (Above or below diaphragm technique would be determined by the level of injured ribs.) The LPO will move the spinous processes **away from** the left side. The left posterior ribs are closest to the film and also placed nearer parallel to the film to reduce foreshortening of these ribs.

A second example is a patient who has trauma to the **right anterior ribs**. Two preferred projections are a straight **PA** and a **left anterior oblique.** The **PA** will place the site of injury closest to the film and the **LAO** will rotate the spinous process **away from** the site of trauma.

Marking the Site of Injury

Some departments prefer that the radiographer tape a small, metallic "BB" or some other **small** type of marker over the site of injury. This will give the radiologist the general location of the trauma or pathology. This policy varies in different departments, and each radiographer should know departmental policy regarding this.

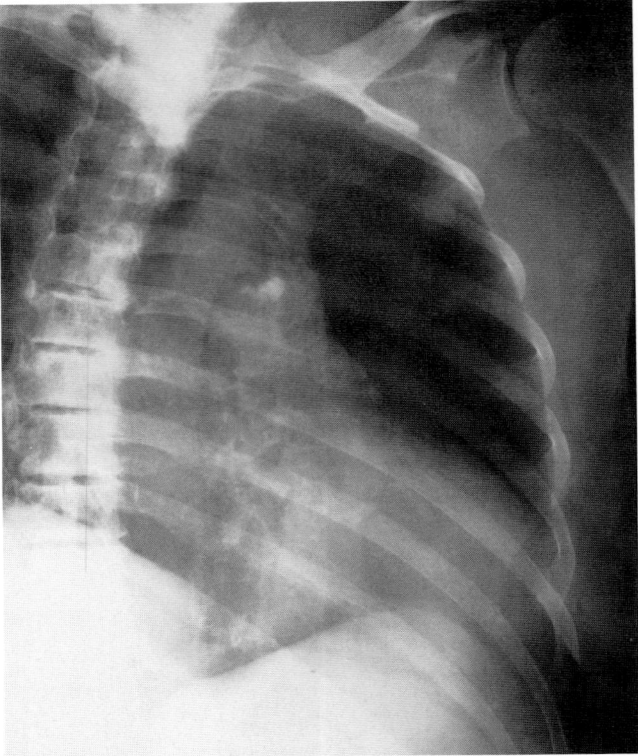

Fig. 10-20. LPO ribs.
-Injury to right posterior ribs.
-Metallic marker to site of injury (optional).

Chest Radiographs

Departmental policy and routines also differ concerning the inclusion of chest x-rays as part of a rib exam routine. However, injury to the thorax often creates respiratory dysfunctions, and patients with a history of rib injuries should have an **erect PA and lateral** projection of the chest taken with lung technique to rule out a possible pneumothorax and hemothorax. If the patient cannot assume an erect position for this, a **decubitus position** using a horizontal beam should be included if possible to determine air-fluid levels. This is described in Chapter 2 on the chest.

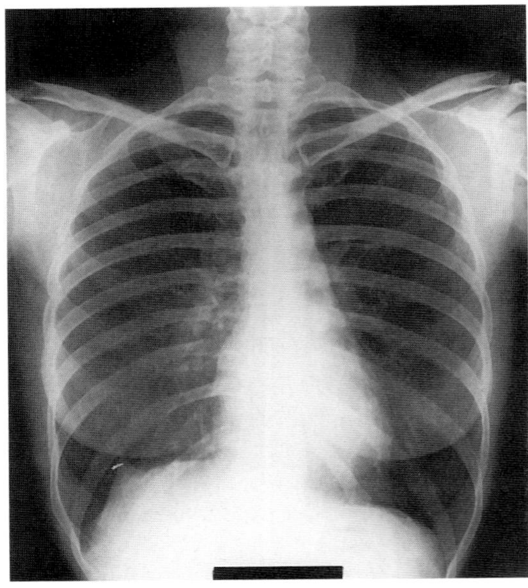

Fig. 10-21. PA chest, to rule out a possible pneumothorax and/or hemothorax.

NATIONAL SURVEY

A survey of the operating procedures (department routines) was conducted throughout the United States. The following information was compiled from the survey indicating the national norm for basic and optional projections of the sternum and ribs. In regard to ribs, specific projections / positions are often determined by the location of the trauma.

Sternum Routine

Sternum	U.S. Average	
	Basic 1995 (1989)	Special 1995 (1989)
• Lateral	92% (97%)	
• RAO (15-20°) (breathing) or	78% (95%)	
RAO (inspiration)	24% –	
• LAO	15% –	18% (5%*)
• Tomograms	5% –	21% (2%*)

*Write-ins by survey respondents.

Sternoclavicular Joints Routine

Sternoclavicular joints	U.S. Average	
	Basic 1995 (1989)	Special 1995 (1989)
• PA	81% –	
• Anterior oblique (10-15°)	74% –	
• PA axial	5% –	12% –

Ribs Routine

Ribs	U.S. Average	
	Basic 1995 (1989)	Special 1995 (1989)
• AP or PA (above or below diaphragm)	92% (89%)	
• Two obliques (R and L anterior or posterior)	55% (27%)	
• Single oblique (anterior or posterior)	45% (66%)	
• PA chest* (to rule out pneumothorax or hemothorax)	59% (66%)	

*Unless chest is ordered as a separate exam.

Summary

Sternum: For the sternum routine, the **lateral** is the most common basic projection, and the **RAO with breathing technique** is much more common (78%), as compared to an RAO with inspiration (24%). The LAO is not common as either a basic or special projection, but tomograms were indicated as special projections by 21% in 1995. This question was not included in the 1989 survey.

Sternoclavicular Joints: The straight **PA** and the **right and left anterior obliques** were the common basic projections in 1995, as expected. This also was not included in the 1989 survey.

Ribs: The 1995 survey indicated that **two obliques** (right and left) are more common (55%) as basic projections than single obliques (45%). This was a major change from 1989, when the single oblique was indicated to be more common (66% vs. 27%). The **PA chest** continues to be a basic projection for rib exams by a majority of survey respondents (59% in 1995 and 66% in 1989).

STANDARD AND SPECIAL OPERATING PROCEDURES

Certain basic and special projections or positions for the sternum and ribs are demonstrated and described on the following pages as suggested standard and special departmental procedures.

Basic Projections

Standard or basic projections, also sometimes referred to as routine projections or departmental routines, are those projections or positions commonly taken on average patients who are helpful and can cooperate in performing the procedure.

Special Projections

Special projections are those more common projections or positions taken as extra or additional projections to better demonstrate certain pathologic conditions or specific body parts.

Basic and Special Projections

Sternum
Basic
• RAO **314**
• Lateral **315**

Sternoclavicular joints
Basic
• PA **316**
• Obliques **317**

Ribs
• Posterior ribs (AP) **318**
or
• Anterior ribs (PA) **319**
• Axillary ribs
(anterior or posterior obliques) **320**
• PA chest (Chapter 2, page 72)

RAO Position

Sternum
Basic
• **RAO**
• Lateral

Structures Best Shown

Entire sternum superimposed over homogenous heart shadow.

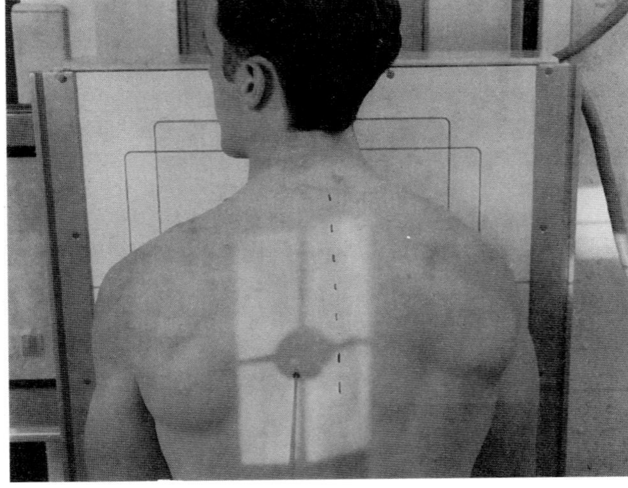

Fig. 10-22. Erect-RAO sternum.

Technical Factors

- Film size–10 x 12 in. (24 x 30 cm), lengthwise.
- Moving or stationary grid.
- Minimum 3 sec. exposure with breathing technique.
- 65±5 kVp range.
- Technique and dose:

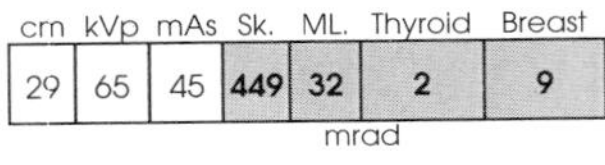

cm	kVp	mAs	Sk.	ML.	Thyroid	Breast
29	65	45	**449**	**32**	2	9
			mrad			

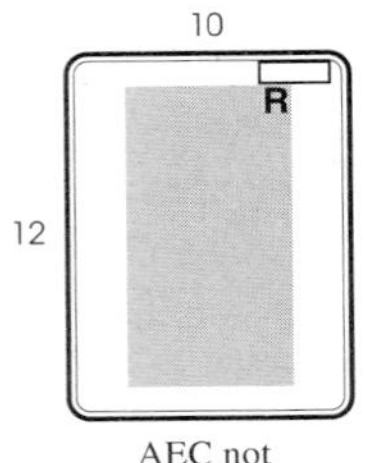

Shielding: Shield gonadal region.

Patient Position

- Erect (preferred), or semiprone position slightly obliqued, right arm down by side, left arm up.

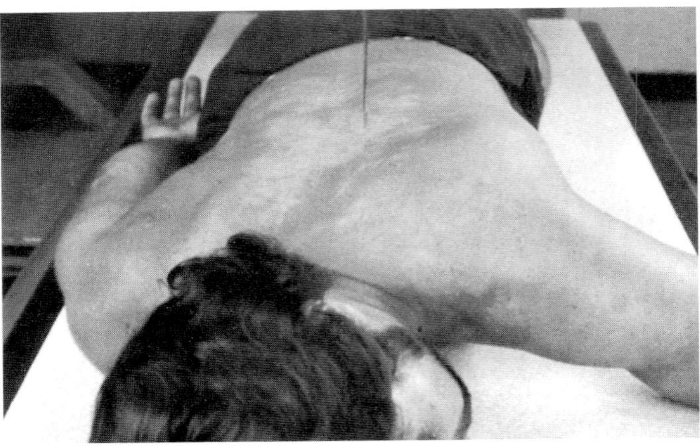

Fig. 10-23. Recumbent-RAO sternum.

Part Position

- Oblique patient **15 to 20°** to the right side, RAO (See Note 1).
- Align long axis of sternum to CR and to midline of x-ray table and/or film.
- Place top of cassette about 1½ in. (4 cm) above the jugular notch.

Central Ray

- CR perpendicular to film holder.
- CR directed to **center of sternum** (to left of midline and midway between the jugular notch and xiphoid process).
- 30 to 40 in. (77 to 102 cm) SID. (See Note 2).

Collimation: Collimate to area of sternum (should result in about a 5 in. or 13 cm wide collimation field).

Respiration: Breathing technique preferred if patient can cooperate (for blurring of overlying lung markings).

Note 1: A large deep-chested thorax requires less rotation than a thin-chested thorax to shift the sternum just to the left of vertebral column superimposed over the homogenous heart shadow. The amount of required rotation can also be determined by placing one hand on the sternum and the other on the spinous processes and determining that these two points are not superimposed as viewed from the position of the x-ray tube.

Note 2: Shorter SID causes magnification and loss of recorded detail of overlying posterior thoracic structures, resulting in better visibility of the sternum. However, a shorter SID results in increased skin dosage and a **minimum of 12 in. (30 cm) SOD** (source object distance) should be maintained as stated earlier in this chapter.

Severe trauma: Can be taken in **LPO position** if patient cannot turn in a semiprone position.
(See Chapter 19, page 559).

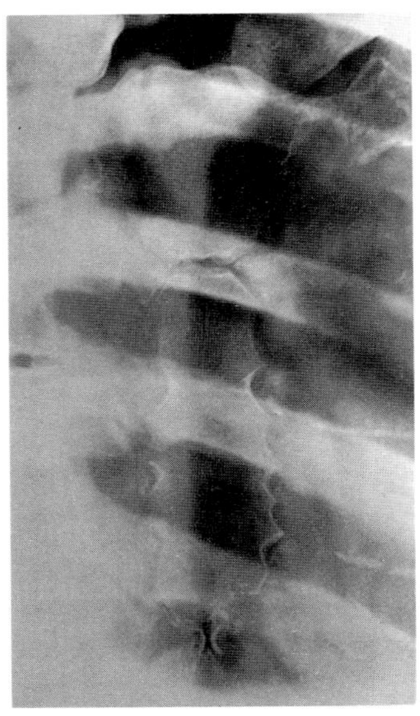

Fig 10-24. RAO.

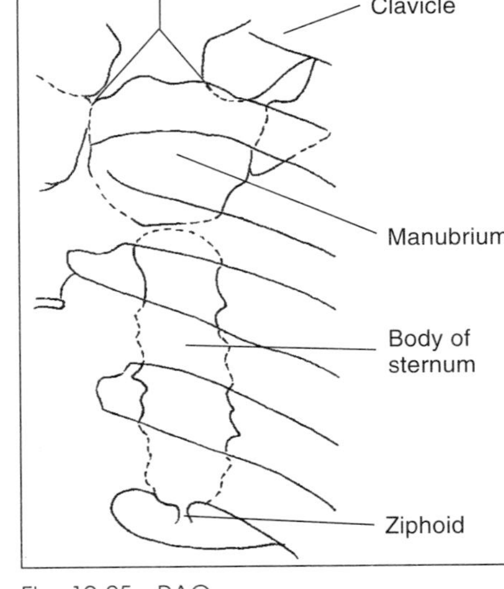

Fig. 10-25. RAO.

Evaluation Criteria

- Entire sternum visualized, superimposed over the heart shadow.
- Correct rotation places entire sternum alongside vertebral column without superimposition of any part of sternum by vertebrae.
- Optimum exposure visualizes outline of sternum through overlying ribs. Lung markings should appear blurred with breathing technique.

Lateral Position - R or L Lateral

Sternum
Basic
• RAO
• **Lateral**

Structures Best Shown

Entire sternum with minimal overlap of soft tissues.

Technical Factors

• Film size–10 x 12 in. (24 x 30 cm), lengthwise.
• Moving or stationary grid.
• 70 - 75 kVp range.
• Technique and dose:

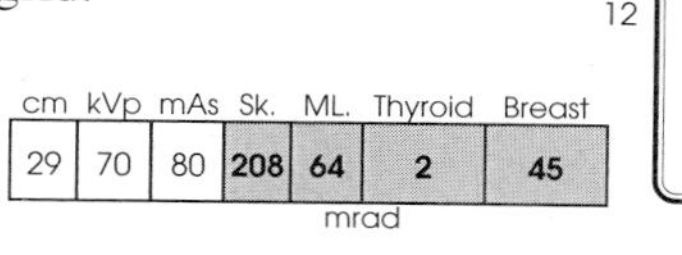

cm	kVp	mAs	Sk.	ML.	Thyroid	Breast
29	70	80	**208**	**64**	**2**	**45**

mrad

10
12
R

AEC not recommended

Shielding: Shield gonadal region.

Patient Position

• Erect (preferred), or lateral recumbent.

Part Position

Erect:
• Standing or seated with shoulders and arms **drawn back**.

Lateral Recumbent:
• Lying on side with arms up above head, keep shoulders back.
• Place top of cassette 1½ in. (4 cm) above the jugular notch.
• Align long axis of sternum to CR and midline of table and/or film.
• Ensure a true lateral, **no rotation.**

Central Ray

• CR perpendicular to film holder.
• CR directed to **center of sternum** (midway between the jugular notch and xiphoid process).
• 60 to 72 in. (152-183 cm) SID recommended to reduce magnification of sternum caused by increased OID.
• Center cassette to CR.

Collimation: Close four-sided collimation to area of sternum.

Respiration: Suspend and expose upon **inspiration**.

Note: Large pendulous breasts of female patients may be drawn to the sides and held in position with a wide bandage.

Severe trauma: Can be taken as a horizontal beam lateral with patient supine on stretcher, as a lateral dorsal decubitus position (Fig. 10-28).

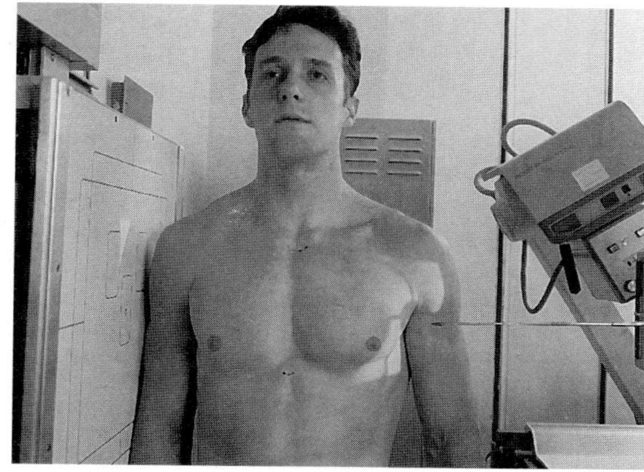

Fig. 10-26. Lateral–Erect.

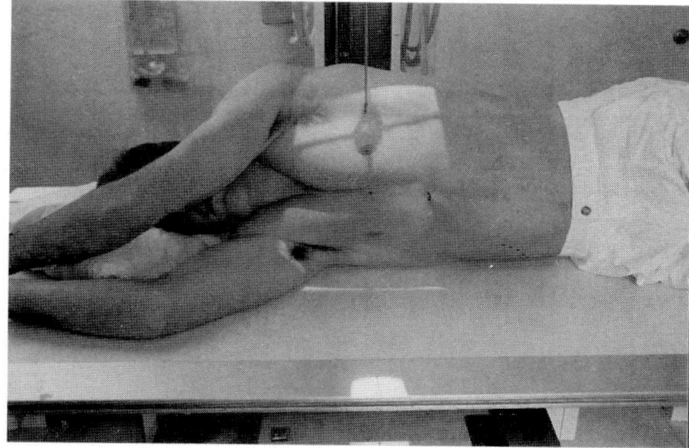

Fig. 10-27. Lateral–Recumbent.

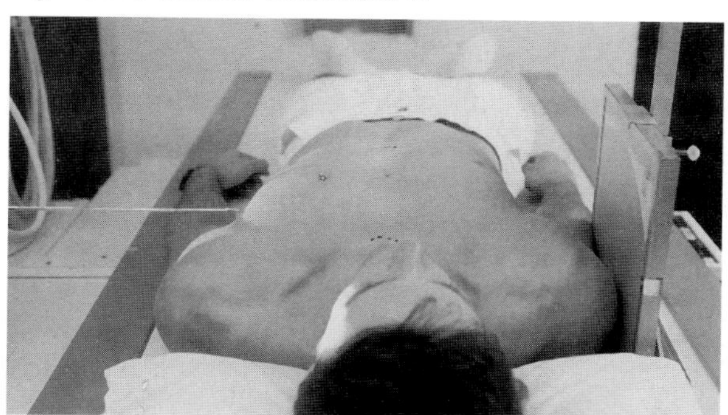

Fig. 10-28. Horizontal beam lateral (Dorsal decubitus).

Evaluation Criteria

• Entire sternum is visualized without superimposition by ribs or soft tissue of arms or shoulders.
• No rotation of the sternum. (Rotation leads to superimposition of ribs over sternum.)
• Optimum exposure and contrast to visualize sternum, from proximal manubrium to distal xiphoid.

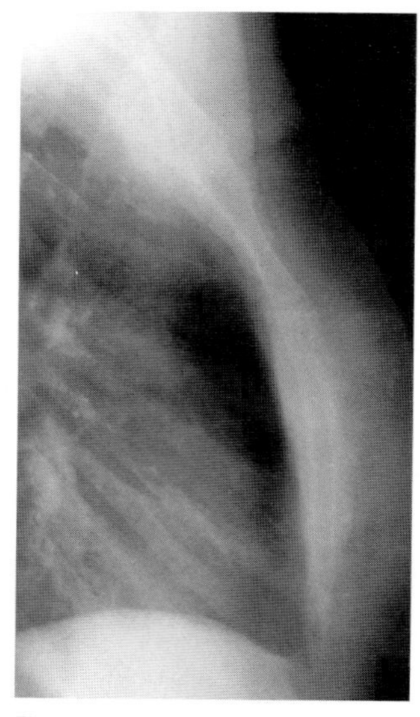

Fig. 10-29. Lateral.

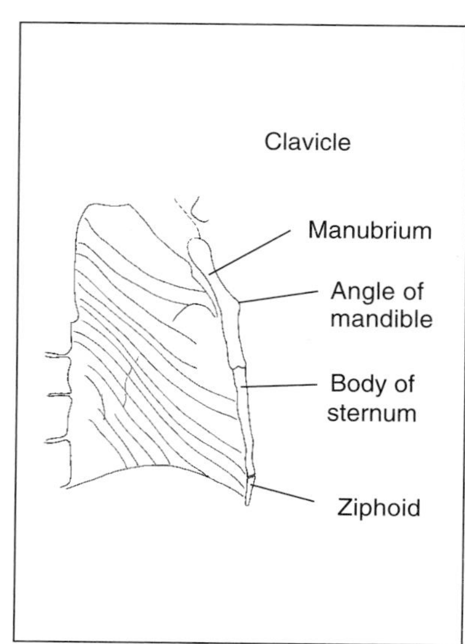

Fig. 10-30. Lateral.

10

PA Projection

Sternoclavicular joints
Basic
• PA
• Anterior obliques

Structures Best Shown

A frontal view of medial aspects of both clavicles and the sternoclavicular joints for possible joint separation or other pathology.

Technical Factors

- Film size–8 x 10 in. (18 x 24 cm), crosswise.
- Moving or stationary grid.
- 65±5 kVp range.
- Technique and dose:

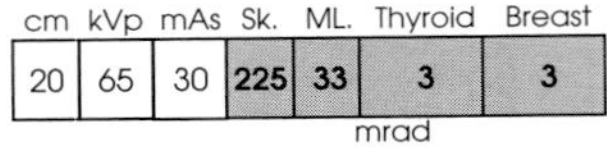

cm	kVp	mAs	Sk.	ML.	Thyroid	Breast
20	65	30	225	33	3	3
			mrad			

Shielding: Shield gonadal region.

Patient Position

- Patient prone, pillow for head turned to one side, arms up beside head, or down by side (may also be taken PA erect if patient prefers).

Part Position

- Align midsagittal plane to CR and to midline of table.
- No rotation of thorax or shoulders.
- Center cassette to CR (3 in. or 7 cm distal to vertebral prominens at level of T2-3).

Central Ray

- CR **perpendicular**, centered to **level of T2-3**, or ≈3 in. (7 cm) distal to vertebral prominens.
- Minimum 40 in. (102 cm) SID.

Collimation: Close collimation to area of interest.

Respiration: Suspend and expose upon **inspiration**.

Note: Tomographic study of the SC joints may improve visibility of the joints.

Evaluation Criteria

- Medial aspects of clavicles are visualized through ribs on each side of vertebrae, centered to film and to collimation field.
- **No rotation**: Evident by equal distances of sternoclavicular joints on each side of vertebrae, or midline.
- Optimum exposure and contrast will visualize outlines of portions of manubrium and the medial aspects of the clavicles making up the sternoclavicular joints, as seen through superimposing ribs and lung structures.

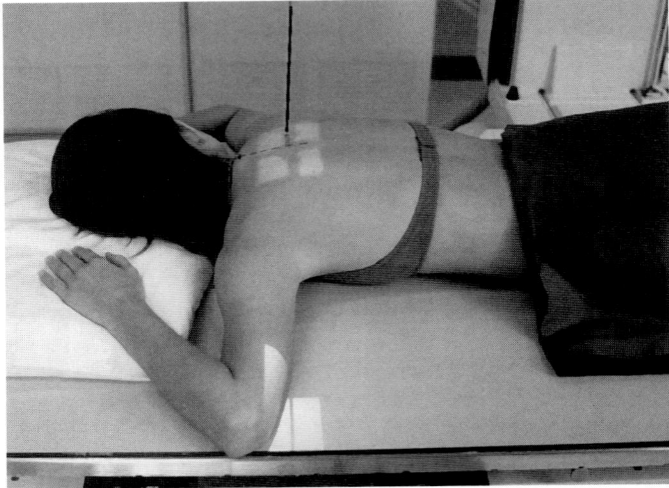

Fig. 10-31. PA bilateral, S-C joints.

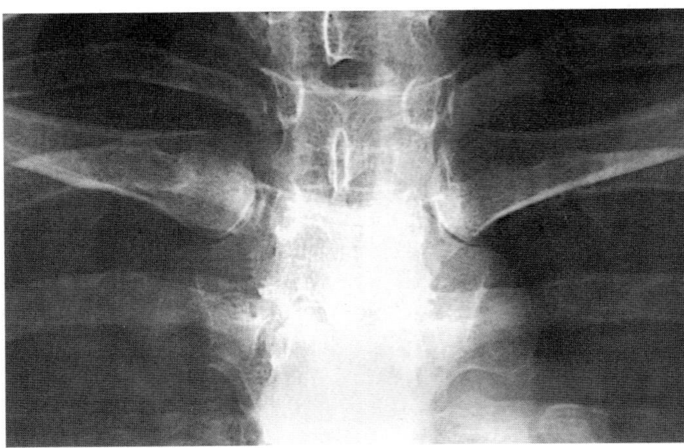

Fig. 10-32. PA bilateral, S-C joints.

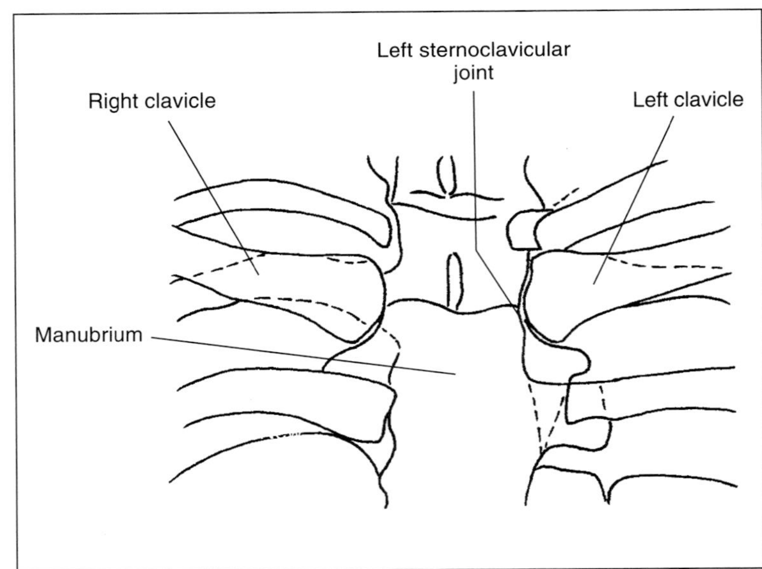

Fig. 10-33. PA bilateral, S-C joints.

Anterior Oblique Positions - RAO and LAO

Right and left obliques commonly taken for comparison.

Sternoclavicular joints
Basic
- PA
- **Anterior obliques**

Structures Best Shown

An obliqued frontal view of sternoclavicular joints shifted away from the vertebral column.

Best visualizes the sternoclavicular joint on **downside**, the side closest to the film.

Fig. 10-34. 15 to 20° RAO, for right S-C joints.

Technical Factors

- Film size–8 x 10 in. (18 x 24 cm), crosswise.
- Moving or stationary grid.
- 65±5 kVp range.
- Technique and dose:

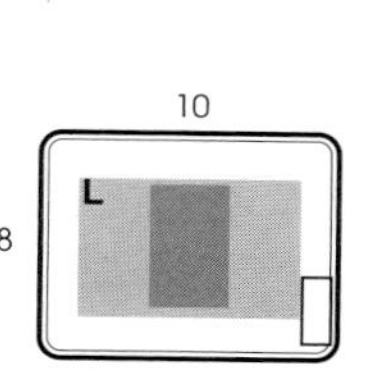

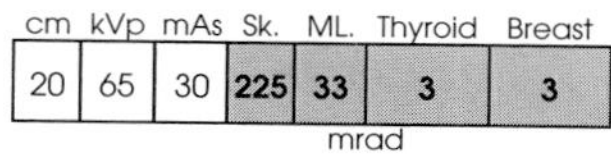

cm	kVp	mAs	Sk.	ML.	Thyroid	Breast
20	65	30	225	33	3	3

mrad

Shielding: Shield gonadal region.

Patient Position

- Prone, with slight rotation (15 to 20°) of thorax with upside arm in front of face and opposite arm down behind patient.

Part Position 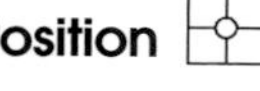

- With patient obliqued 15 to 20°, align and center spinous process 1 to 2 in. (3 to 5 cm) lateral (toward upside) to CR and midline of table and/or film.
- Center cassette to CR.

Central Ray

- CR perpendicular, to **level of T2-3**, or ≈3 in. (7.5 cm) distal to vertebra prominens, and 1 to 2 in. (3 to 5 cm) lateral (toward upside) to midsagittal plane.
- Minimum 40 in. (102 cm) SID.

Collimation: Close collimation to area of interest.

Respiration: Suspend and expose upon **inspiration**.

Alternate projections: (1) AP posterior obliques can be taken as 15 to 20° posterior obliques with patient supine if patient's condition requires. (2) AP or PA with cross-angle CR can also be achieved with patient in supine or prone position without rotation, wherein the CR is angled 10 to 15° laterally to project joints away from vertebrae. A portable grid placed crosswise on tabletop is needed to prevent grid cutoff.

Note: With less obliquity (10-15°) the opposite S-C joint would be best visualized next to the vertebral column.

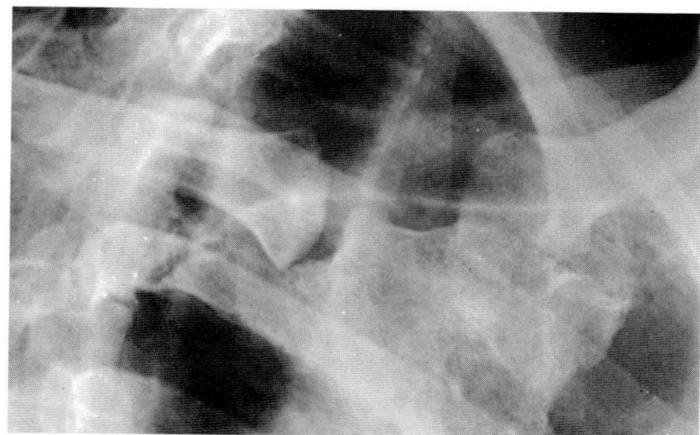

Fig. 10-35. 15 to 20° RAO, best demonstrates right (downside S-C joint.

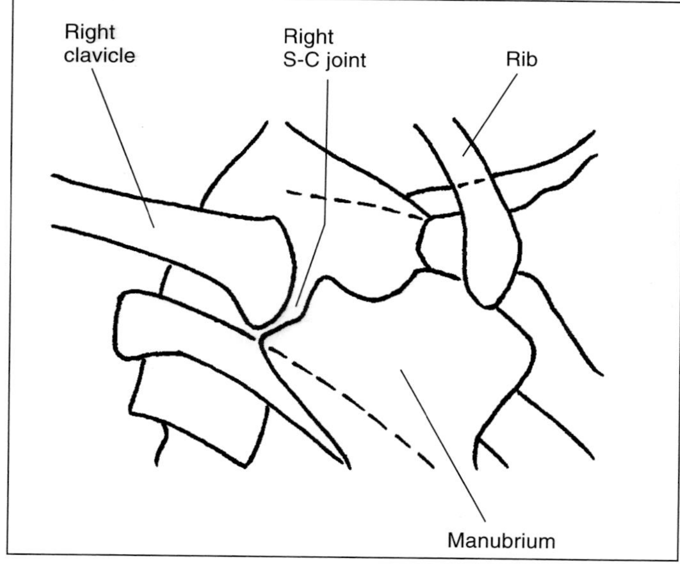

Fig. 10-36. 15 to 20° RAO.

Evaluation Criteria

- Visualization of manubrium and medial portions of clavicles, and sternoclavicular joint in question **shifted away from vertebral column**.
- Optimum exposure and contrast to visualize sternum, from proximal manubrium to distal xiphoid.

AP Projection

Above or Below Diaphragm

Ribs
Basic
- **Posterior ribs (AP)**
  or
  Anterior ribs (PA)
- Axillary ribs (anterior or posterior obliques)
- PA chest (page 72)

Structures Best Shown

Posterior ribs, above or below the diaphragm.

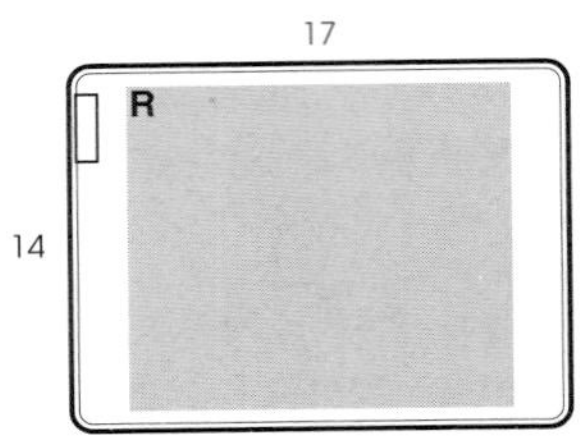

AEC not recommended

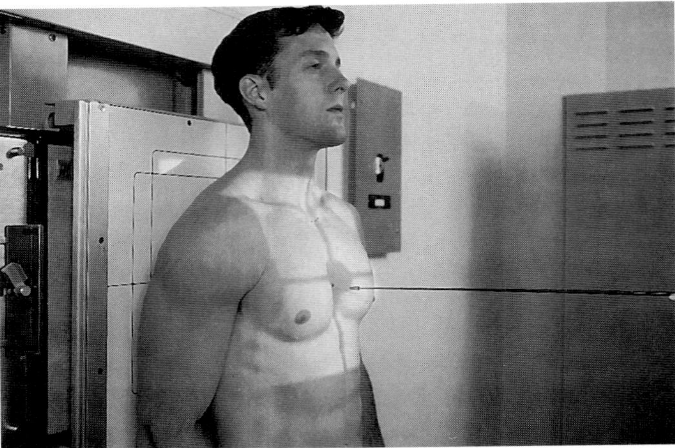

Fig. 10-37. AP erect–Above diaphragm.

Technical Factors

- Film size - 14 x 17 in. (35 x 43 cm).
- Film crosswise (see Note).
- Moving or stationary grid.
- Above diaphragm: 65-75 kVp.
- Below diaphragm: 75-85 kVp.
- Technique and dose:

@ 72" (above dia.)

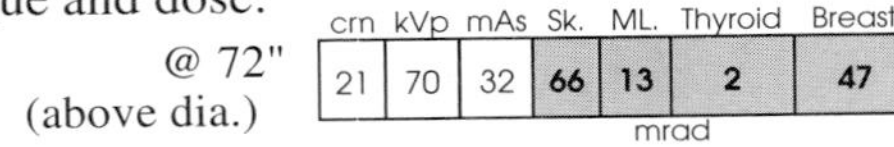

cm	kVp	mAs	Sk.	ML.	Thyroid	Breast
21	70	32	66	13	2	47

mrad

Shielding: Place lead shield over pelvic region, with top of shield at iliac crest.

Patient Position

- Erect preferred for above diaphragm if patient's condition allows; and supine for below diaphragm.

Part Position

- Align midsagittal plane to CR and to midline of table and/or film holder.
- Rotate shoulders anteriorly to remove scapulae from lung fields.
- **Raise chin** to prevent superimposing upper ribs, look straight ahead.
- **No rotation** of thorax or pelvis.

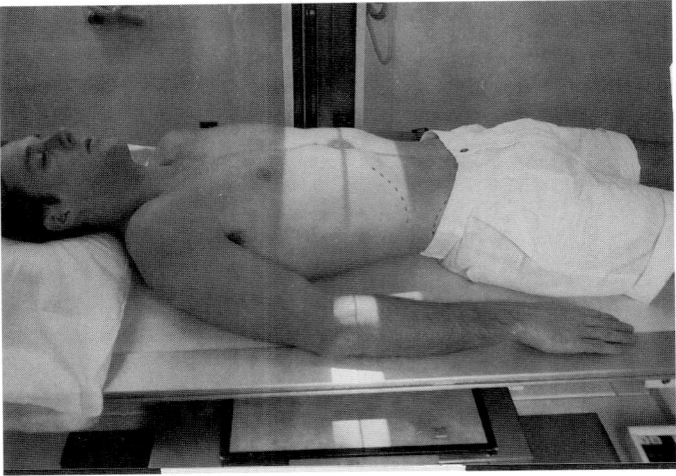

Fig. 10-38. AP supine–Below diaphragm.

Central Ray

Above Diaphragm:

- CR **perpendicular** to film holder, centered to **3 or 4 in.** (8 to 10 cm) **below jugular notch** (level of T7).
- Center cassette to level of CR (top of cassette should be about 1½ in. or 4 cm above shoulders).

Below Diaphragm:

- CR **perpendicular, centered to midway between xiphoid and lower rib cage**.
- Center cassette to level of CR (bottom of cassette should be at the level of iliac crest).
- Minimum 40 in. (102 cm) SID.

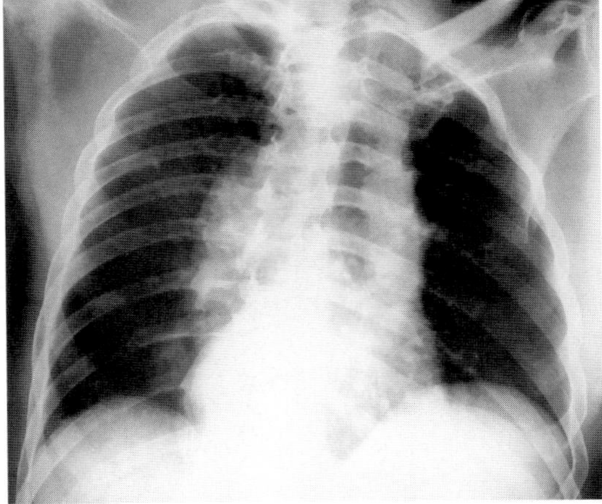

Fig 10-39. AP (slight oblique)–Above diaphragm. (Some rotation is evident on this radiograph.)

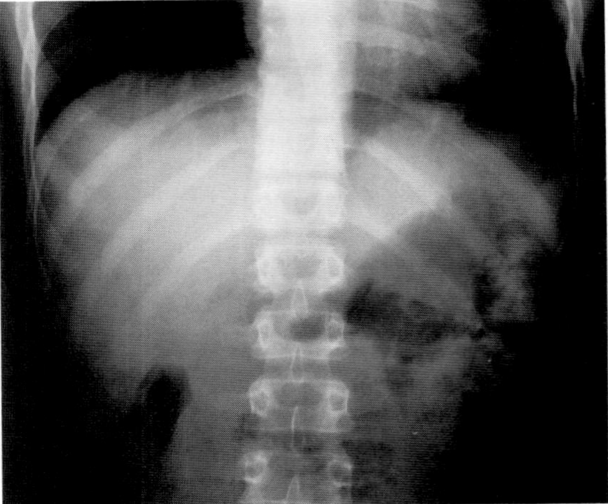

Fig. 10-40. AP–Below diaphragm.

Collimation: Collimate to outer margins of thorax.

Respiration: Suspend and expose upon **inspiration** for **above** diaphragm, and **expiration** for **below** diaphragm.

Note: Place film crosswise for both above and below diaphragm ribs except for small patients because average width of thorax is greater than height as discussed in Chapter 2. (This is more important at shorter SID with greater magnification than at a 72 in. [183 cm] SID as for chests.)

Evaluation Criteria

- ***Above Diaphragm:*** The first through eighth or ninth posterior ribs should be visualized above the diaphragm.
- No motion is seen on the radiograph.
- Rotation of the thorax should not be evident.
- Optimum exposure and penetration should visualize ribs through the heart shadow without overexposing midposterior ribs through the lung fields.
- ***Below Diaphragm:*** The ribs below the diaphragm should be visualized through dense abdominal organs.

PA Projection
Above Diaphragm

> **Ribs**
> Basic
> • Posterior ribs (AP)
> or
> **Anterior ribs (PA)**
> • Axillary ribs (anterior or posterior obliques)
> • PA chest (page 72)

Structures Best Shown

Anterior ribs, above the diaphragm. (Below diaphragm rib injuries are generally to posterior ribs and AP projections are taken.)

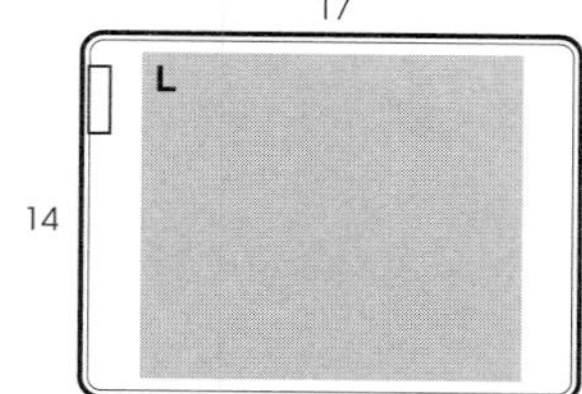

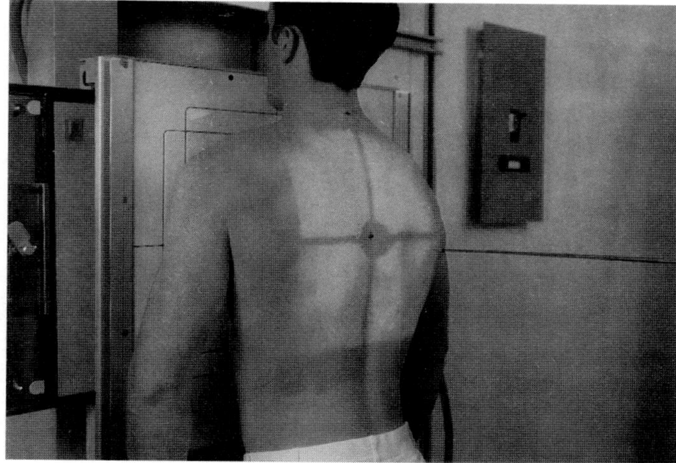

Fig. 10-41. PA ribs–Above diaphragm.

Technical Factors

- Film size–14 x 17 in. (35 x 43 cm), crosswise.
- Moving or stationary grid.
- 65-75 kVp range (above diaphragm).
- Technique and dose:

cm	kVp	mAs	Sk.	ML.	Thyroid	Breast
21	70	32	66	13	0	2
			mrad			

Shielding: Place lead shield over gonadal region.

Patient Position

- Erect preferred, or prone if necessary, with arms down to the side.

Part Position

- Align midsagittal plane to CR and to midline of table and/or film holder.
- Rotate shoulders anteriorly to remove scapulae from lung fields.
- **No rotation** of thorax or pelvis.

Central Ray

- CR **perpendicular** to film holder, centered to **T7** (7 to 8 in. or 18 to 20 cm below vertebra prominens as for PA chest).
- Center cassette to level of CR. (Top of cassette should be about 1½ in. or 4 cm above shoulders.)
- Minimum 40 in. (102 cm) SID or 72 in (180 cm), SID as per chest projections.

Collimation: Collimate along lateral margins of thorax, and to upper and lower margins of film.

Respiration: Suspend and expose upon **inspiration.**

PA erect chest: It is common departmental policy to include an erect PA chest projection with lung exposure techniques to rule out respiratory dysfunctions such as a pneumothorax or hemothorax, which may accompany rib injuries (Fig. 10-43). Positioning is similar to that for PA ribs, above diaphragm, as shown in Fig. 10-41 and described above. Chest exposure factors should be used.

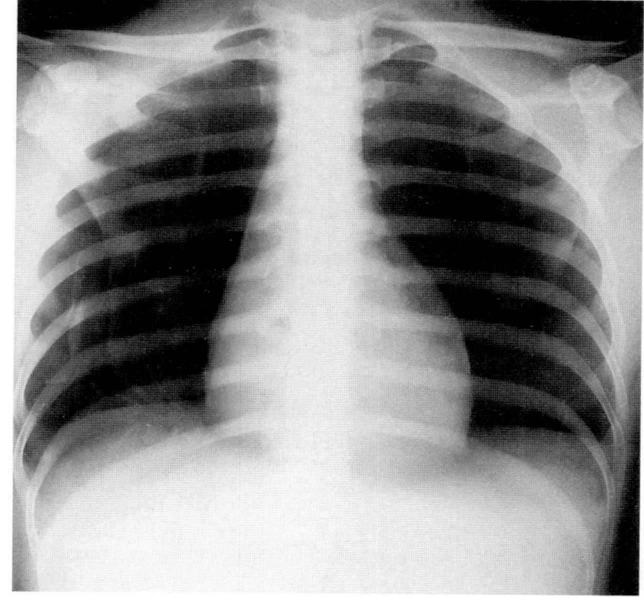

Fig. 10-42. PA ribs.

Evaluation Criteria

- The first through eighth or ninth posterior ribs should be visualized above the diaphragm.
- No motion of the ribs as seen on the radiograph.
- No rotation of the thorax.
- Optimum exposure and penetration should visualize outlines of all ribs above the diaphragm, including ribs through the heart shadow without excessive burnout of other ribs.

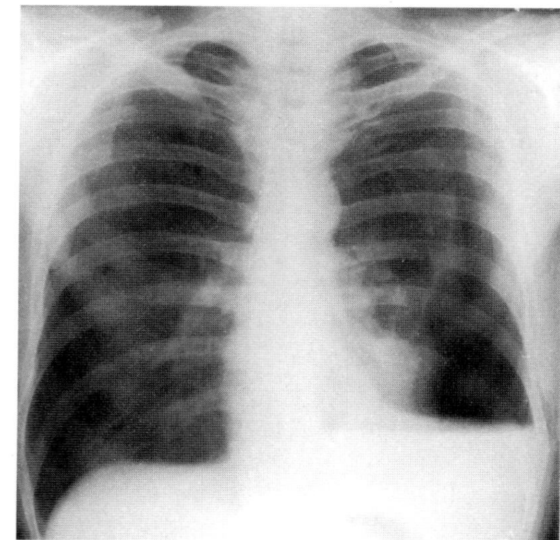

Fig. 10-43. PA erect chest. (Demonstrates a combination hemo- and pneumothorax on left side).

Posterior or Anterior Oblique Positions

Above or Below Diaphragm

Ribs
Basic
- Posterior ribs (AP)
  or
  Anterior ribs (PA)
- **Axillary ribs (anterior or posterior obliques)**
- PA chest (page 72)

Structures Best Shown

Axillary margin of ribs on the side of interest projected without self-superimposition.
Posterior/lateral injury: Posterior obliques, affected side toward film.
Anterior/lateral injury: Anterior obliques, affected side away from film. (See Note 1.)

Technical Factors

- Film size–14 x 17 in. (35 x 43 cm) crosswise
  or –11 x 14 in. (28 x 35 cm) crosswise.
- Moving or stationary grid.
- 70-75 kVp range above diaphragm, or 80-85 kVp below diaphragm.
- Attach metallic marker to area of injury if this is part of departmental routine (Note 2).
- Technique and dose:

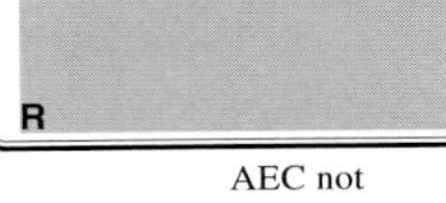

AEC not recommended

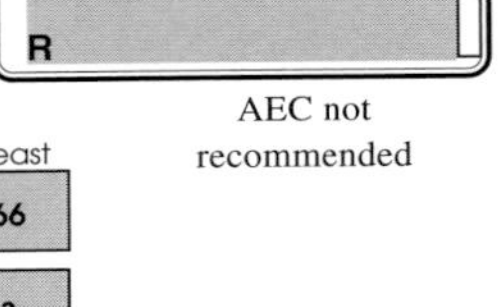

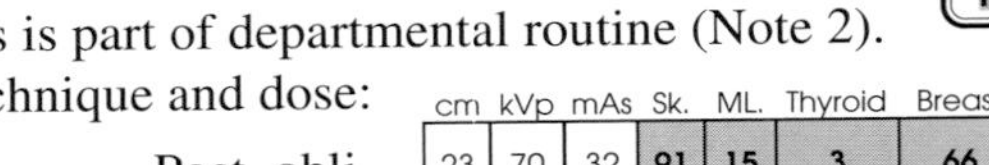

	cm	kVp	mAs	Sk.	ML.	Thyroid	Breast
Post. obli.	23	70	32	91	15	3	66
Ant. obli.	23	70	32	91	15	1	3

mrad

Shielding: Place lead shield over gonadal region.

Patient Position

- Erect preferred for above diaphragm if patient's condition allows; or supine for below diaphragm.

Part Position

- Rotate patient into 45° posterior or anterior oblique, **affected side closest to film** on **posterior** oblique; and **affected side away from film** on **anterior** oblique. (Rotate spine **away** from site of injury.)
- Raise elevated side arm above head; extend opposite arm down and behind patient away from thorax.
- If recumbent, flex knee of elevated side to help maintain this position.
- Support body with positioning blocks if needed.
- Align a plane of the thorax midway between the spine and the lateral margin of thorax on side of interest to CR and to midline of the table and/or film (ensure that side of interest is **not** cut off).

Central Ray

- CR **perpendicular** to film holder, centered midway between lateral margin of ribs and spine.

Above Diaphragm:

- CR to level 3 or 4 in. (8 to 10 cm) below jugular notch **(T7)**. (Top of cassette about 1½ in. or 4 cm above shoulders.)

Below Diaphragm:

- CR to level midway between xiphoid and lower rib cage. (Bottom of cassette should be about at level of iliac crest.)
- 72 in. (183 cm), or minimum 40 in. (102 cm) SID.

Collimation: Collimate to near film borders on all four sides to not cut off rib cage for possible primary and secondary sites of rib injuries.

Respiration: Suspend and expose on **inspiration** for above diaphragm ribs, and on **expiration** for below diaphragm ribs.

Note 1: For this recommended routine, an injury to the **right** side would require an **RPO** or an **LAO**.
Injury to the **left** side would require an **LPO** or an **RAO**.

Note 2: Some departmental routines include taping a small metallic "BB" directly on the patient at the injury site to assist in locating possible rib

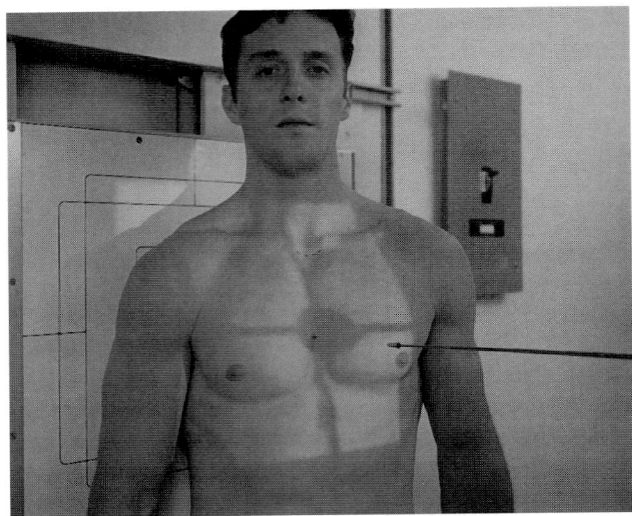

Fig. 10-44. RPO (injury to the **right posterior** ribs, above diaphragm).

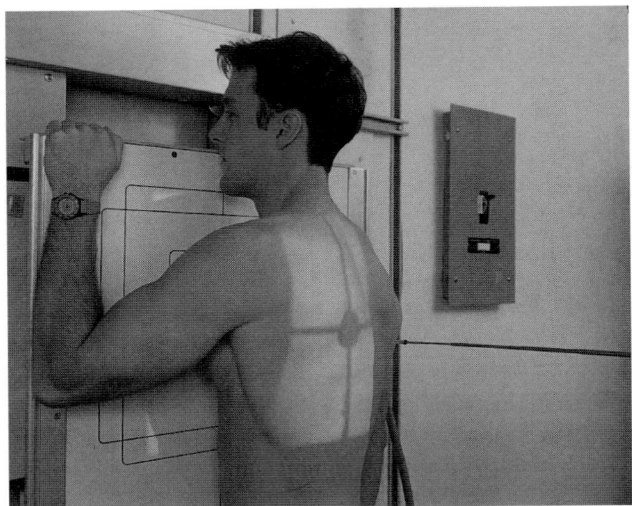

Fig. 10-45. RAO (injury to **left anterior** ribs, above diaphragm).

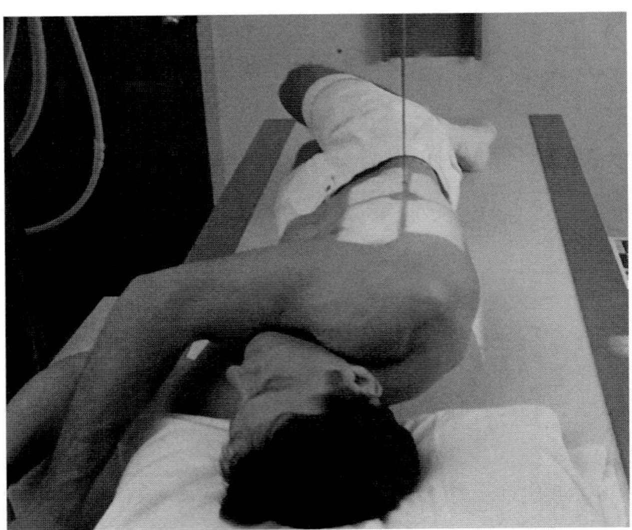

Fig. 10-46. LPO (injury to **right anterior** ribs, below diaphragm).

Posterior or Anterior Oblique Position continued

Alternate routine (additional collimated projection): Some departmental routines include one well-collimated oblique position of the region of injury in profile taken on a smaller film (10 x 12 or 11 x 14).

Evaluation Criteria

- A 45° oblique should be evident in that the distance between the vertebral column and the lateral rib margin on the affected side should be about twice the distance on the unaffected side.
- No motion of the rib margins should be evident on the radiograph.
- The axillary portion of the ribs, involving the site of injury (above or below diaphragm), should be elongated, clearly seen and included in the collimation field.

Above Diaphragm Ribs:

- Upper nine or ten pairs of ribs should be included and seen above the diaphragm.
- Optimum exposure and contrast should visualize the ribs through the heart shadow and lateral rib margins without overexposing ribs through the mid lung fields.

Below Diaphragm Ribs:

- Lower ribs, the eighth through twelfth, should be included and seen below the diaphragm.
- Optimum exposure and contrast should clearly visualize the ribs below the diaphragm as seen through the dense abdominal structures. (Ribs above the diaphragm in the mid lung field area will appear dark and overexposed.)

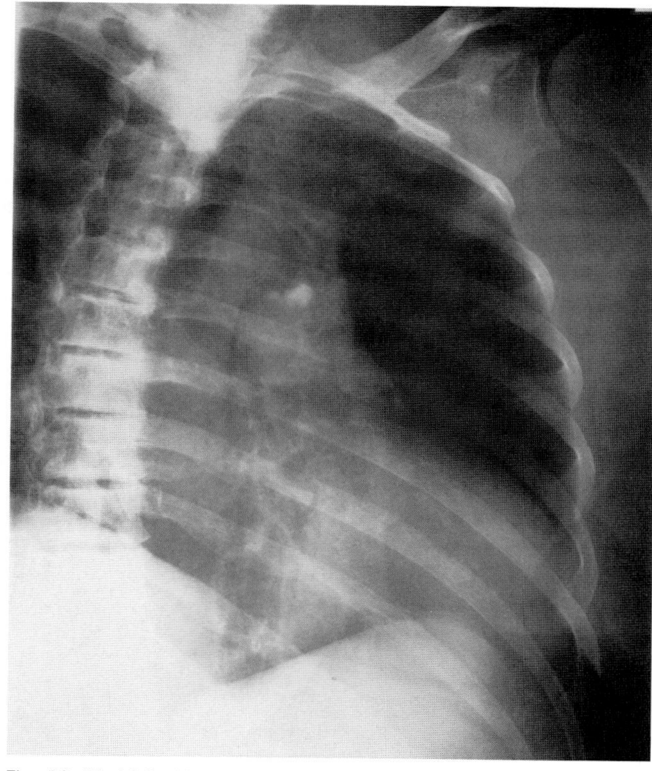

Fig. 10-47. LPO–Above diaphragm.

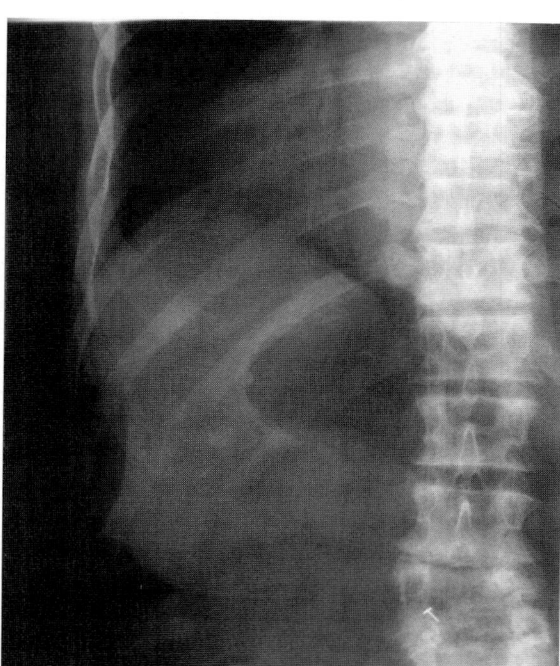

Fig. 10-48. AP below diaphragm centered for right ribs.

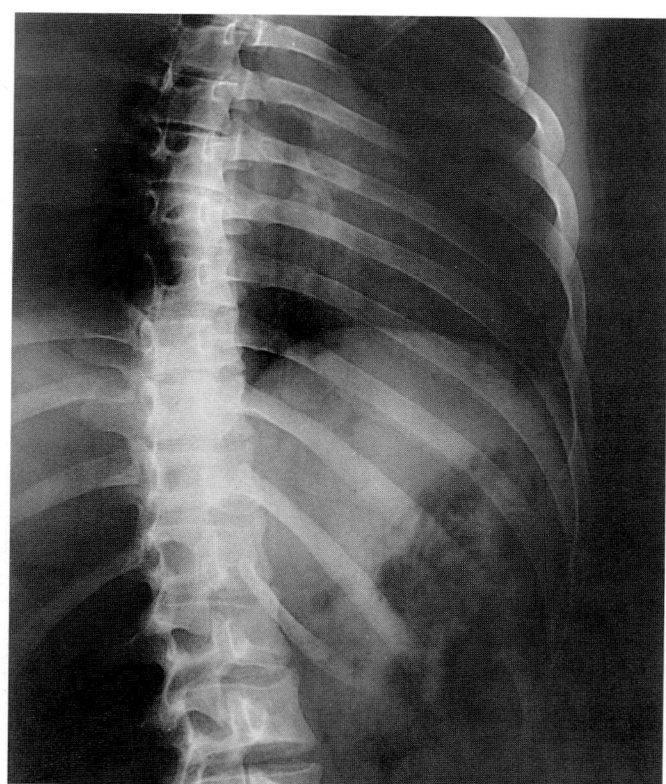

Fig. 10-49. LPO–Below diaphragm, left ribs.
Note: Centering should be a little lower.

Radiographs for Critique

Each of these radiographs demonstrate some error in positioning which requires a repeat. These along with accompanying lecture slides of these and other radiographs will provide a basis for classroom and/or positioning lab discussion. Questions with answers based on these specific critique radiographs are provided in the accompanying student workbook/lab manuals to help prepare students for classroom and/or lab discussions on film critique.

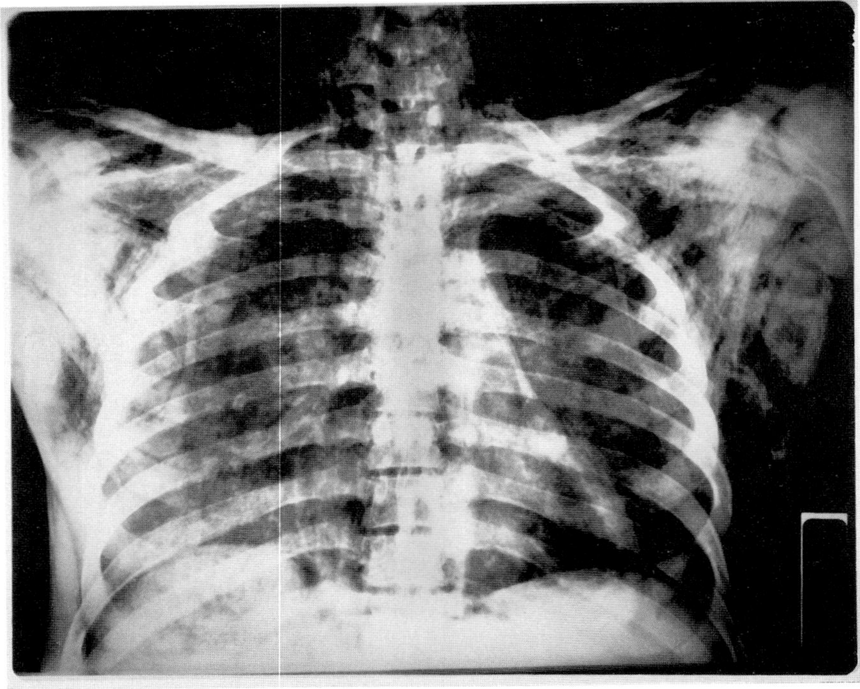

Fig. C10-50. Ribs–Above diaphragm.
(Courtesy of Bill Collins, RT)

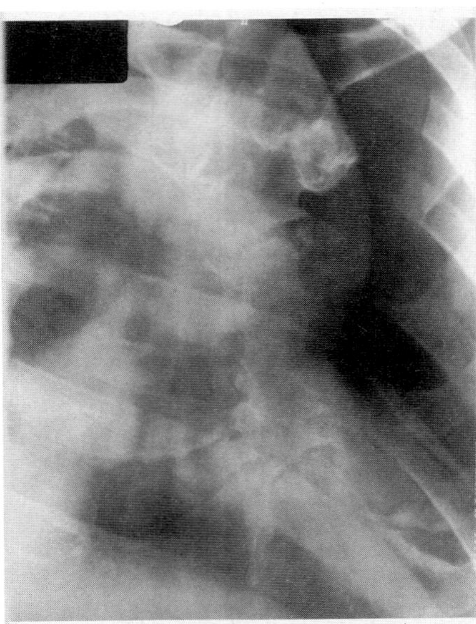

Fig. C10-51. Oblique sternum.

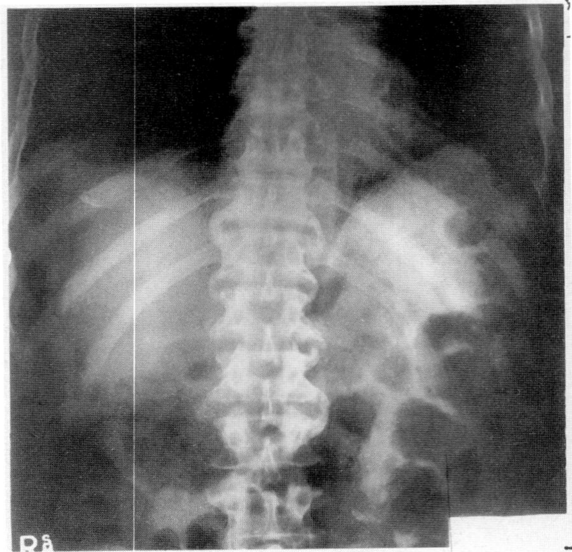

Fig. C10-52. Ribs–Below diaphragm.

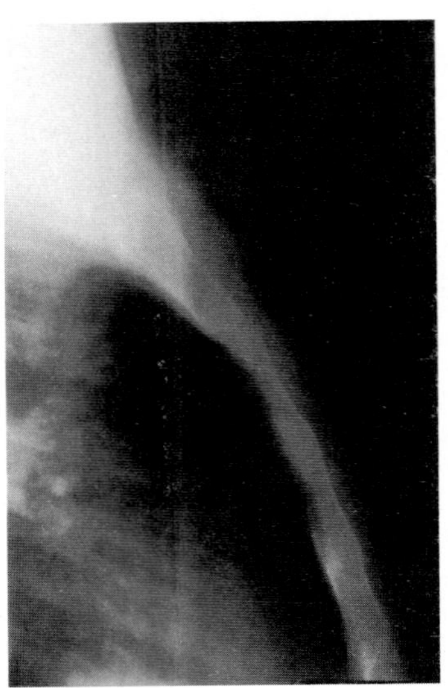

Fig. C10-53. Lateral sternum.

CHAPTER 11

Skull and Cranial Bones

CONTRIBUTIONS BY:
Kathy Martensen, BS, RT (R)
Barry T. Anthony, RT (R)

CONTENTS

Radiographic Anatomy

Skull–Cranial and facial bones **324**

Cranial bones:
- Frontal bone **325**
- Parietal bones **326**
- Occipital bone **326**
- Temporal bones **327**
- Sphenoid bone **328**
- Ethmoid bone **329**

Joints of the cranium (sutures) **330**

Anatomy review with radiographs **331**

Facial bones:
- Maxillary bones **332**
- Zygomatic bones **334**
- Nasal and lacrimal bones **334**
- Inferior nasal conchae **335**
- Palatine bones **335**
- Mandible **336**

Joint classifications **337**

Orbits **338**

Anatomy review **340**

Radiographic Positioning

Skull morphology **343**

Cranial topography (landmarks) **344**

Skull positioning lines **345**

Positioning considerations **346**

Survey results **347**

Basic and special projections **348**

Cranium (skull series):
- AP axial (Towne method) **349**
  or PA axial (Haas method) **350**
- Lateral **351**
- PA axial 15° (Caldwell method) **352**
  or PA axial 25 to 30° **352**
- PA 0° **353**
- Submentovertex (SMV) **354**
  (basilar position)

Sella turcica:
- Lateral **355**
- AP axial (Towne method) **356**
- PA axial 0°
  or PA axial 25° cephalad (Haas method) **357**

Radiographs for critique **358**

Skull trauma series–**Chapter 19**

Radiographic Anatomy

Skull

As with other body parts, radiography of the skull requires a good understanding of all related anatomy. The anatomy of the skull is very complex and extensive, and requires careful and detailed study as covered in this chapter.

The **skull** or bony skeleton of the head rests on the superior end of the vertebral column and is divided into two main sets of bones; the cranium, which consists of eight **cranial bones**, and the fourteen **facial bones**.

The cranium is that part of the skull that surrounds and protects the brain, while that portion anterior and inferior to the brain case is termed the facial skeleton or the facial bones.

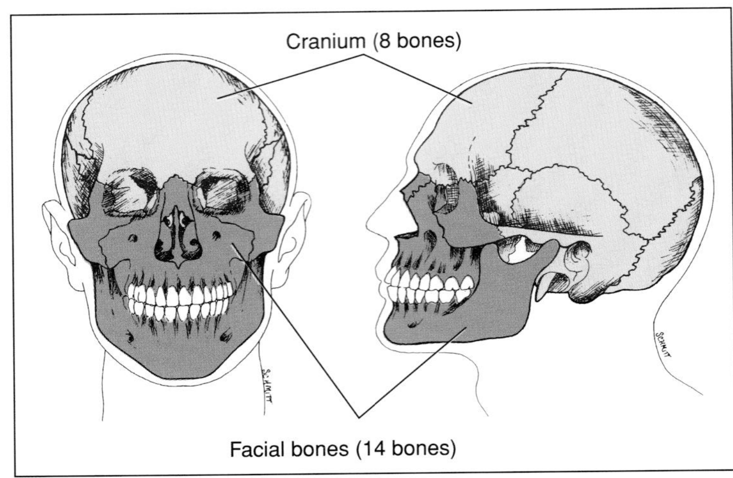

Fig. 11-1. Skull–Bony skeleton of head (cranial and facial bones).

CRANIAL BONES (8)

The eight bones of the cranium are divided into calvarium (skull cap), and floor. Each of these two areas more or less consists of four bones:

Calvarium (skull cap)

1. Frontal
2. Right parietal *(pah-ri′ĕ-tal)*
3. Left parietal
4. Occipital *(ok-sip′i-tal)*

Floor

5. Right temporal
6. Left temporal
7. Sphenoid *(sfe′noid)*
8. Ethmoid *(eth′moid)*

The eight bones making up the calvarium (skull cap) and floor or base of the cranium are demonstrated on these frontal, lateral and superior cutaway view drawings. These eight cranial bones are fused in an adult to form a protective enclosure for the brain. Each of these cranial bones will be demonstrated and described individually in the pages that follow.

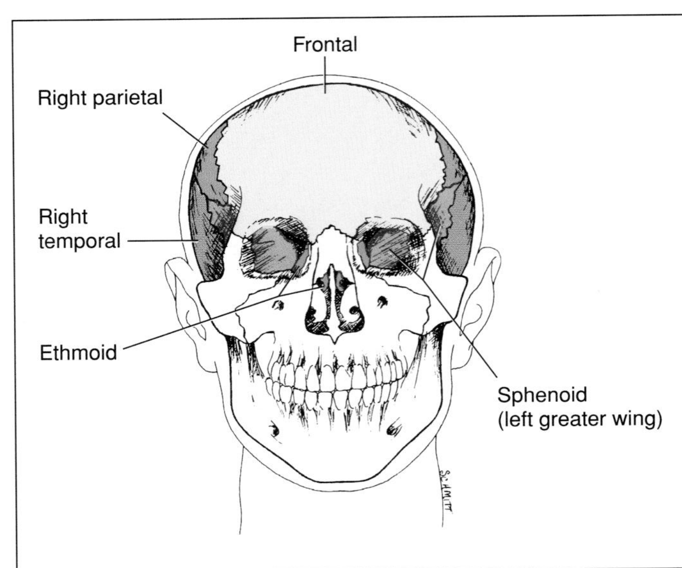

Fig. 11-2. Cranium–Frontal view.

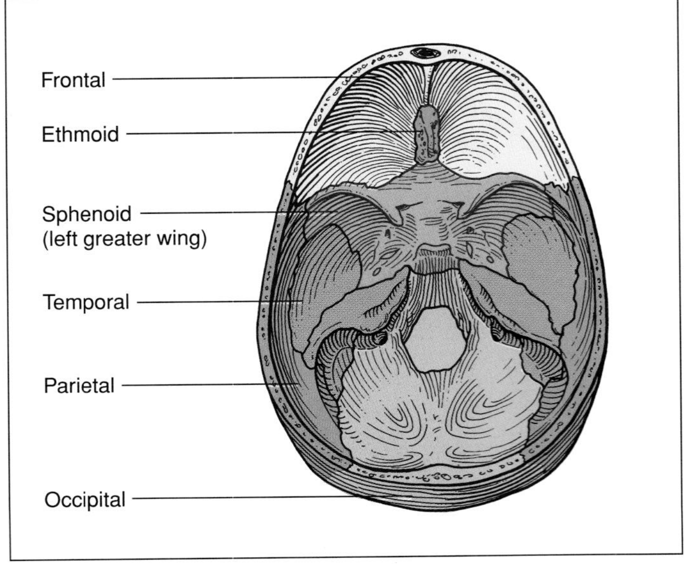

Fig. 11-3. Cranium–Superior cutaway view.

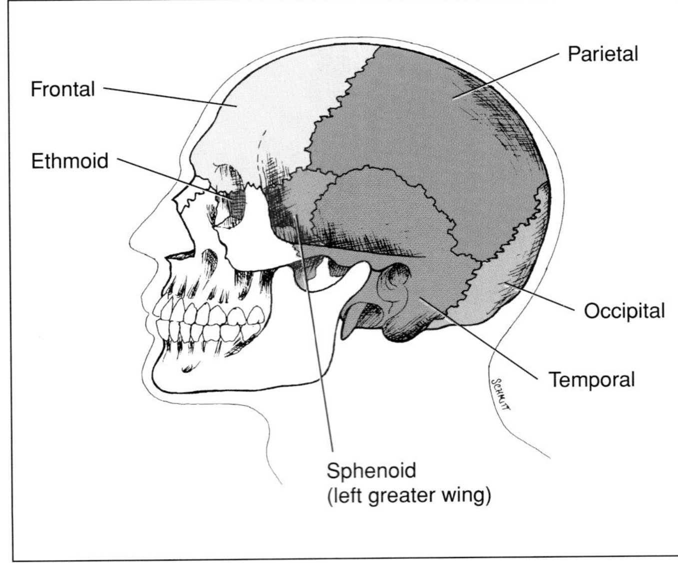

Fig. 11-4. Cranium–Lateral view.

CRANIAL BONES

After the description of each of these eight bones will be a listing of those specific adjoining bones with which they articulate, or with which they are joined since in an adult they are all fused or immovable. Some of the bones with which the cranial bones articulate are facial bones, which are described later in this chapter. Knowing all of these "articulations" helps in learning the specific locations and relationships of each of these bones beginning with the frontal bone.

Frontal Bone

As viewed from the front, the bone of the calvarium most readily visible is the **frontal bone**. This bone, which forms the forehead and the superior part of each orbit, consists of two main parts, each of which is labeled on these drawings. The **squamous** or **vertical portion** forms the forehead, while the **orbital** or **horizontal portion** forms the superior part of the orbit.

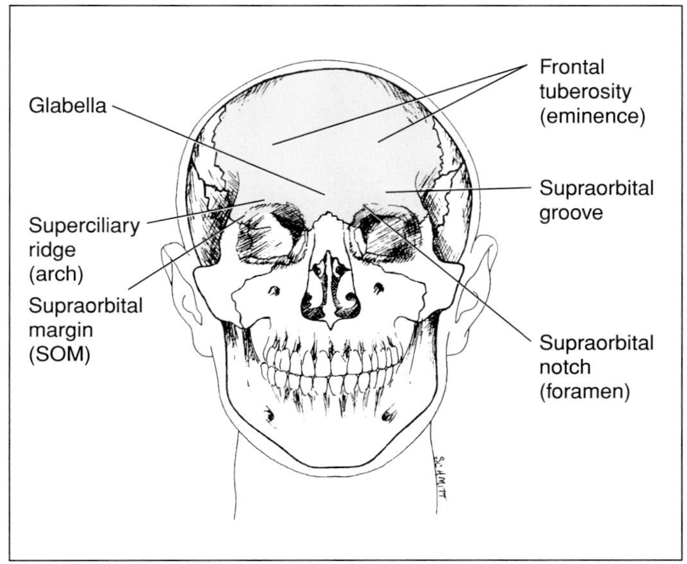

Fig. 11-5. Frontal bone–Frontal view.

Squamous or Vertical Portion (Frontal and Lateral Views): The **glabella** is the smooth raised prominence between the eyebrows just above the bridge of the nose.

The **supraorbital groove (SOG)** is the slight depression above each eyebrow. This becomes an important landmark because it corresponds to the floor of the anterior fossa of the cranial vault, which is also at the level of the orbital plate or the highest level of the facial bone mass (Fig. 11-7).

Note: This SOG can be located on yourself by placing your finger against the length of your eyebrow and feeling the raised arch of bone, then allowing your finger to slide upward and drop slightly into the SOG.

The superior rim of each orbit is the **supraorbital margin** or **SOM**. The **supraorbital notch** (foramen) is a small hole or opening within the supraorbital margin slightly medial to its mid point. A nerve and an artery pass through this small opening.

That ridge of bone beneath each eyebrow is termed the **superciliary ridge** (arch). Between the superciliary arches is the glabella.

On each side of the squamous portion of the frontal bones above the supraorbital grooves, is a larger rounded prominence termed the **frontal tuberosity** (eminence).

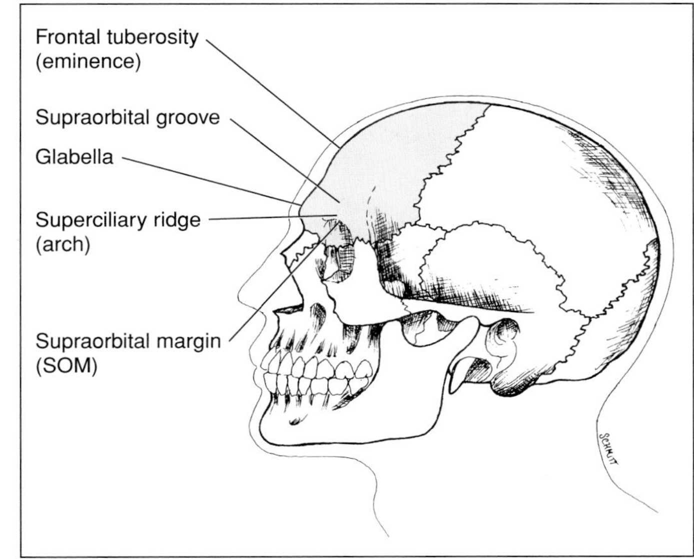

Fig. 11-6. Frontal bone–Lateral view.

Orbital or Horizontal Portion (Inferior View): As seen from the inferior aspect, the frontal bone shows primarily the **horizontal or orbital portion**. The **supraorbital margins**, the **superciliary ridges**, the **glabella** and the **frontal tuberosities** can all be seen.

The **orbital plate** on each side forms the superior part of each orbit. Below the orbital plates lie facial bones, and above the orbital plates is the anterior part of the floor of the brain case.

Each orbital plate is separated from the other by the **ethmoidal notch**. The ethmoid bone, one of the bones of the floor of the cranium, fits into this notch. The **nasal** (frontal) **spine** is found at the anterior end of the ethmoidal notch.

Articulations: The frontal bone articulates with **four** cranial bones; right and left parietals, the sphenoid and the ethmoid. These can be identified on frontal, lateral and superior cutaway drawings on the preceding page. (The frontal bone also articulates with eight facial bones to be described later.)

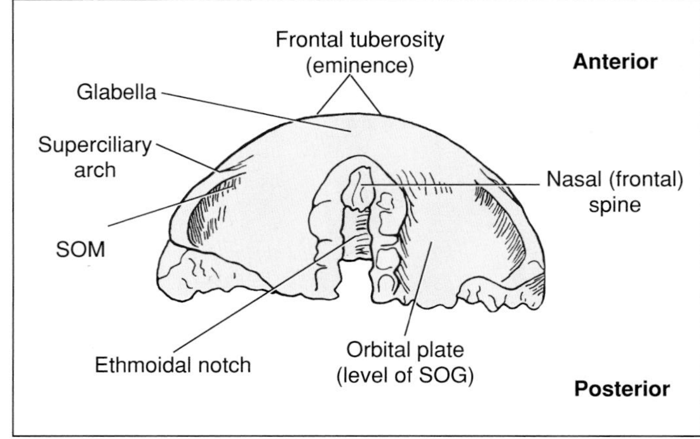

Fig. 11-7. Orbital portion of frontal bone–Inferior view.

Parietal Bones

The paired **right** and **left parietal bones** are well demonstrated on the side and top view drawings of Fig. 11-8 and 11-9. The lateral walls of the cranium and part of the roof are formed by the two parietal bones. Each of the parietals is roughly square in shape and has a concave internal surface.

The widest portion of the entire skull is located between the **parietal tubercles (eminences)** of the two parietal bones. The frontal bone is primarily anterior to the parietals, the occipital is posterior, the temporals inferior and the greater wings of the sphenoid inferior and anterior.

Articulations: Each parietal articulates with **five** cranial bones; the frontal, the occipital, a temporal, the sphenoid and the opposite parietal.

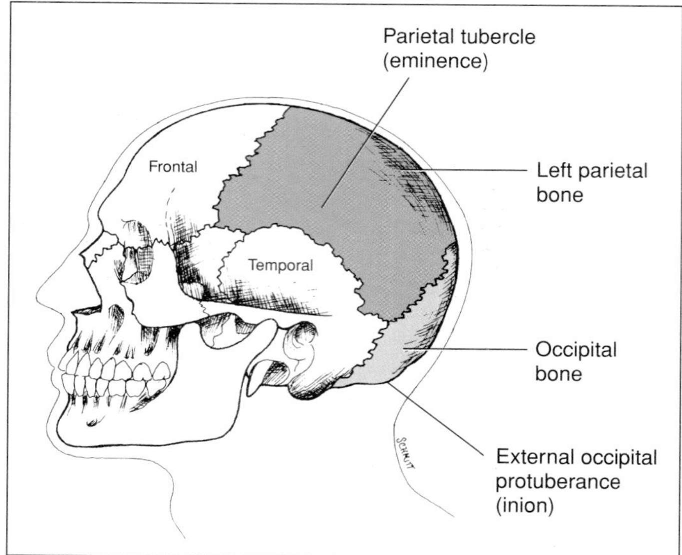

Fig. 11-8. Parietal and occipital bones–Side view.

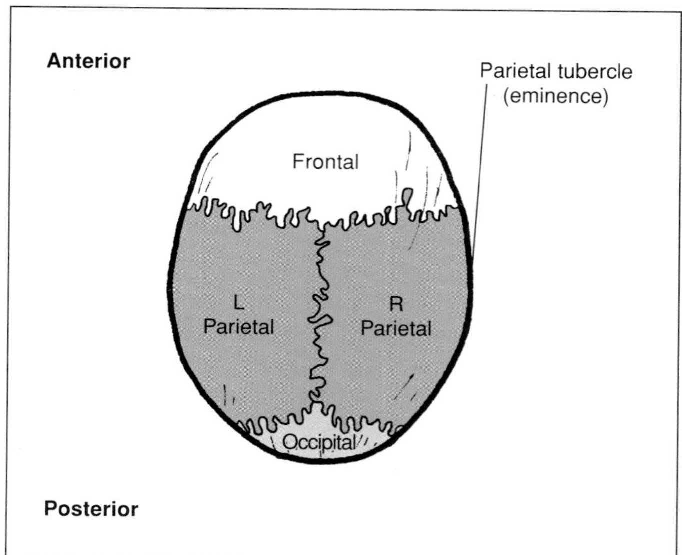

Fig. 11-9. Parietal and occipital bones–Top view.

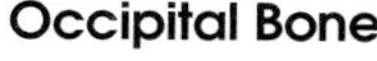

Occipital Bone

The inferoposterior portion of the calvarium or skull cap is formed by the single occipital bone. The external surface of the occipital bone presents a rounded part termed the **squamous portion**. The squamous portion forms most of the back of the head and is that part of the occipital bone superior to the **external occipital protuberance**, or **inion**, the prominent "bump" or protuberance at the inferoposterior portion of the skull.

The large opening at the base of the occipital bone through which the spinal cord passes as it leaves the brain is termed the **foramen magnum**, literally meaning "great hole".

The two **lateral condylar portions (occipital condyles)** are oval processes with convex surfaces, one on each side of the foramen magnum. These articulate with depressions on the first cervical vertebra, the atlas. This two-part articulation between the skull and the cervical spine is called the **occipito-atlantal joint(s)**.

Articulations: The occipital articulates with **six** bones; the two parietals, the two temporals, the sphenoid and the atlas (first cervical vertebra).

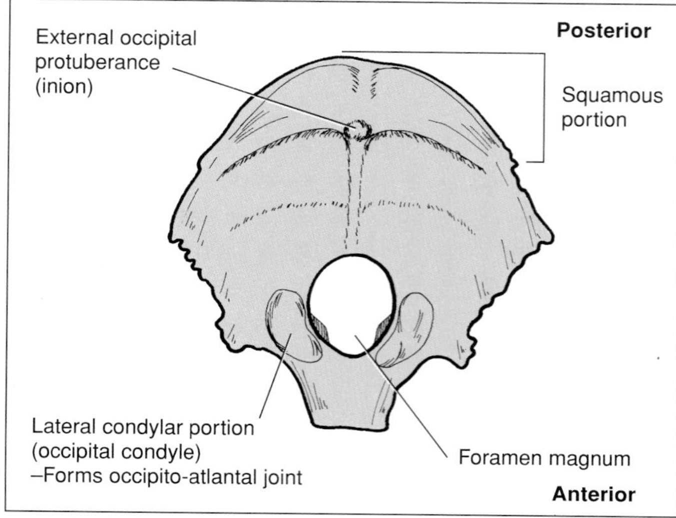

Fig. 11-10. Occipital bone-Inferior view.

Temporal Bones

Lateral view (Fig. 11-11): The paired **right** and **left temporal bones** are complex structures housing the delicate organs of hearing and balance. As seen from the side in this lateral view drawing, the left temporal bone is situated between the greater wing of the sphenoid bone anteriorly, and the occipital bone posteriorly.

Extending anteriorly from the squamous portion of the temporal bone is an arch of bone termed the **zygomatic** *(zi′ go-mat′ ik)* **process.** This process meets the temporal process of the zygomatic bone (one of the facial bones) to form the easily palpated **zygomatic arch**.

Inferior to the zygomatic process and just anterior to the **EAM,** external acoustic (auditory) meatus, is the **temporomandibular fossa**, into which the mandible fits to form the **TMJ** or **temporomandibular joint**.

Inferiorly between the mandible and the EAM is a slender bony projection called the **styloid process**.

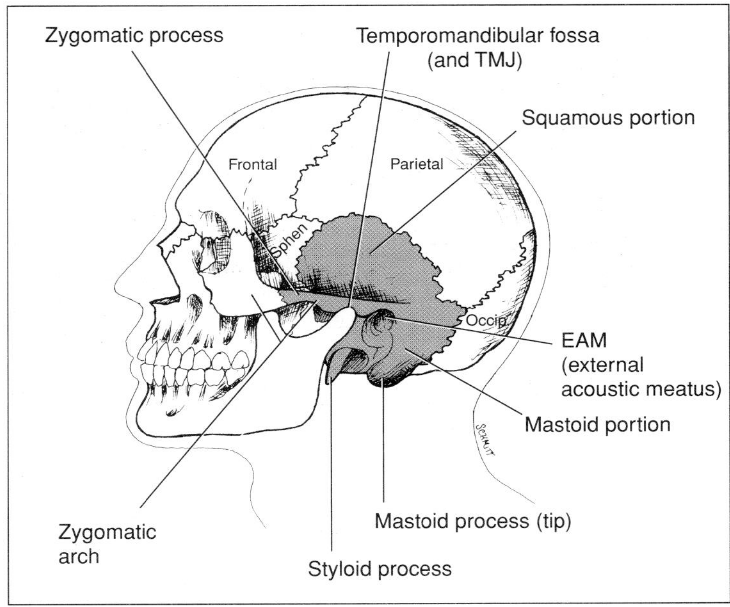

Fig. 11-11. Temporal bone–Lateral view.

Frontal Cutaway View (Fig. 11-12): Each temporal bone is divided into **three primary parts.** First is the thin upper portion forming part of the wall of the skull, the **squamous portion**. This part of the skull is quite thin and is therefore the most vulnerable portion of the entire skull to fracture, which may result in hemorrhage beneath the bony surface.

The second portion is the area posterior to the EAM, the **mastoid portion**, with its prominent **mastoid process** or **tip**. Many air cells of the mastoid sinuses are located within the mastoid process.

The third main portion is the dense **petrous portion**, also called the **petrous pyramid** or **pars petrosa**. Sometimes this is also called the **petromastoid portion** of the temporal bone since internally this includes the petrous portion. The upper border or ridge of the petrous pyramids are commonly called the **petrous ridges**.

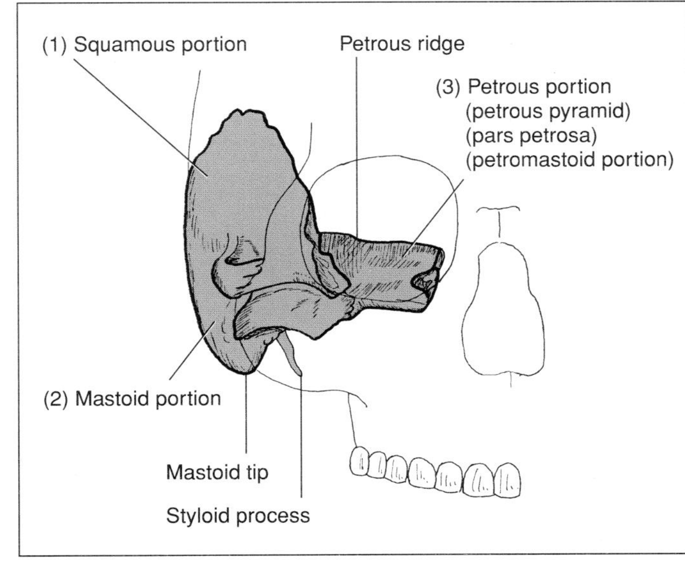

Fig. 11-12. Temporal bone, 3 primary parts – Frontal cutaway view.

Superior View (Fig. 11-13): The entire floor of the cranium is well visualized in this drawing. The single occipital bone resides between the paired temporal bones. The third main portion of each temporal bone is the **petrous** *(pet′ rus)* **portion**, is again shown in this top view. This pyramid-shaped portion of the temporal bone is the thickest and densest bone in the cranium. The petrous pyramids project anteriorly and toward the midline from the area of the **EAM**.

The delicate organs of hearing and balance are housed in and protected by the dense petrous pyramids. The **petrous ridge** of these pyramids **corresponds to the level of an external landmark,** the **TEA** (top of the ear attachment). Near the center of the petrous pyramid on the posterior surface just superior to the **jugular foramen** is an opening or orifice termed the **internal acoustic meatus**, which serves to transmit the nerves of hearing and equilibrium.

Note: The specific openings of both the external and internal acoustic meatus are not visualized on this superior view drawing because they are under a portion of the petrous pyramid structure on this view.

Detailed anatomy of the organs of hearing and equilibrium is included in Chapter 13 along with conventional radiography of the mastoids and special projections for the temporal bone. CT and MRI however, have largely replaced conventional radiography of this region.

Articulations: Each temporal articulates with **three** cranial bones; a parietal, the occipital and the sphenoid. (Each temporal also articulates with two facial bones.)

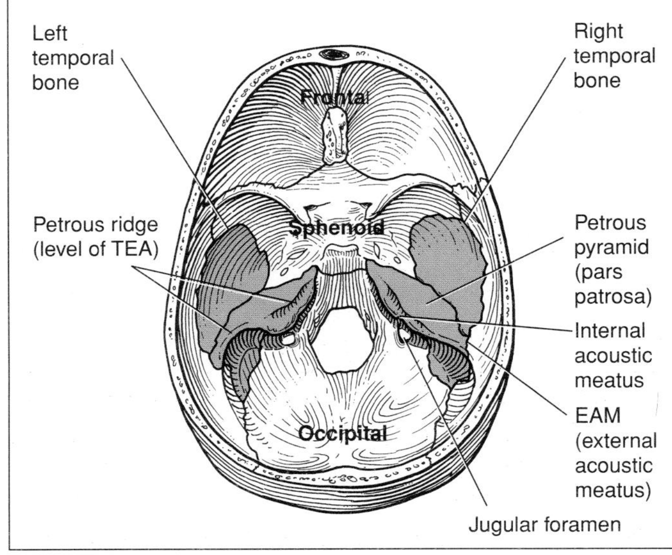

Fig. 11-13. Temporal bones–Superior view.

Sphenoid Bone

Superior View: The single centrally located **sphenoid bone** forms the anchor for all eight cranial bones. The central portion of the sphenoid is the body, which lies in the midline of the floor of the cranium and contains the sphenoid sinuses as best shown on the medial sectional drawing of Fig. 11-18 on the following page.

The central depression on the body is termed the **sella turcica** *(sel' a-tur' si-ka)*. This depression looks like a saddle from the side as shown in Fig. 11-16 on the following page and derives its name from words meaning Turkish saddle. The sella turcica partially surrounds and protects a major gland of the body, the **hypophysis** or **pituitary gland**. Posterior to the sella turcica is the back of the saddle, the **dorsum sellae** *(dor' sum sel' e)*, also best seen on the lateral drawing of Fig. 11-16.

The **clivus** *(kli' vus)* is a shallow depression just posterior to the base of the dorsum sellae (Fig. 11-14). This depression is continuous with a similar groove at the base of the occipital bone sloping upward from the foramen magnum to where it joins the sphenoid. This area forms a base of support for the pons portion of the brain. Thus a portion of the clivus is formed by the base of the occipital bone and a portion by the posterior surface of the body of the sphenoid.

Extending laterally from the body to either side are two pairs of wings. The smaller pair, termed the **lesser wings**, are triangular in shape and are nearly horizontal, ending in the two **anterior clinoid processes.** They project laterally from the upper, anterior portion of the body and extend to about the middle of each orbit. The **greater wings** extend laterally from the sides of the body and form a portion of the floor of the cranium, as well as a portion of the sides of the cranium as shown on lateral external surface drawings such as Fig. 11-4 on a preceding page.

There are **three pairs** of small openings or foramina in the greater wings for passage of certain nerves and blood vessels. Lesions that can cause erosion of these foramina can be detected radiographically. The **foramen rotundum** *(ro-tun' dum)* and the **foramen ovale** *(o-va' le)* are seen as small openings on the both the superior and oblique view drawings. The location of the pair of small rounded **foramen spinosum** *(spi-no' sum)* are also seen on the superior view drawing (Fig. 11-14).

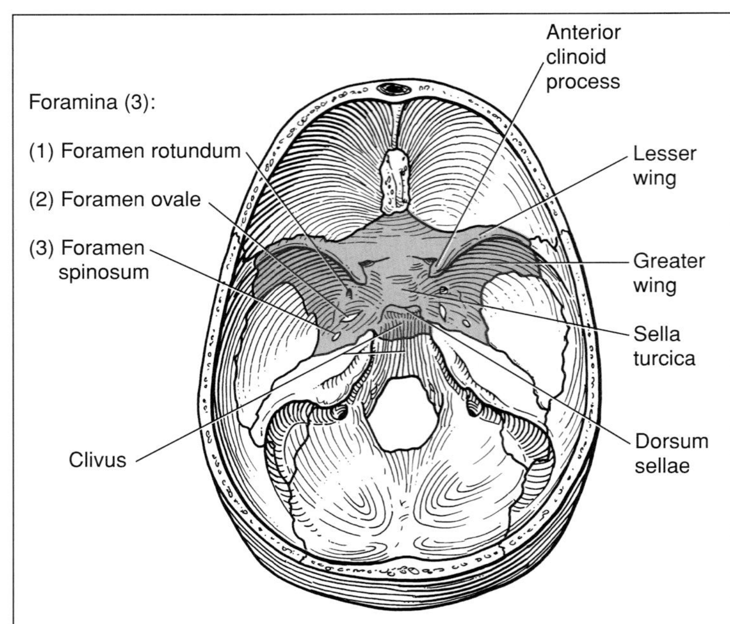

Fig. 11-14. Sphenoid bone–Superior view.

Oblique View: An oblique drawing of the sphenoid bone demonstrates the complexity of this bone. Using one's imagination, the shape of the sphenoid has been compared to a bat with its wings and legs extended as in flight. The centrally located depression, the **sella turcica**, is again seen on this view.

Arising from the most posterior aspect of the **lesser wings** are two bony projections termed **anterior clinoid processes.** The anterior clinoids are somewhat larger and are spread farther apart than are the **posterior clinoid processes**, which extend superiorly from the **dorsum sellae**, best seen on the lateral drawing in Fig. 11-16.

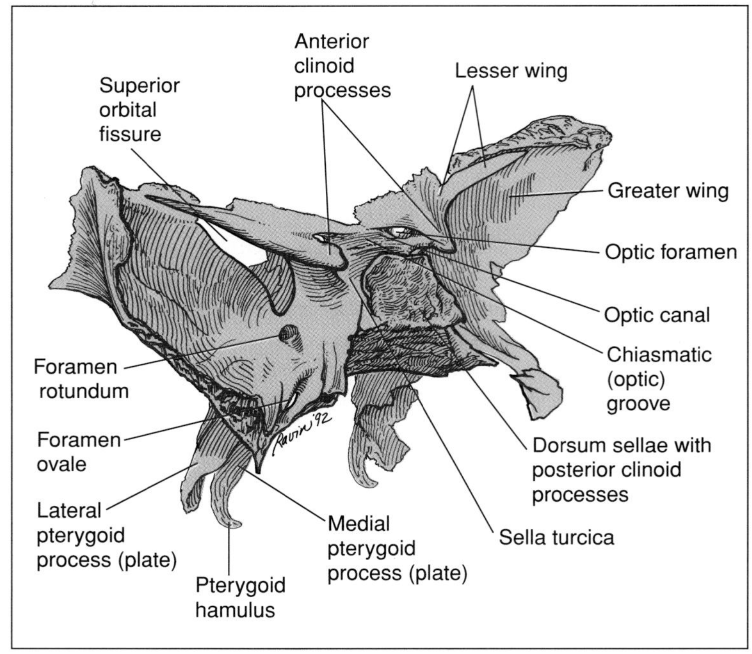

Fig. 11-15. Sphenoid bone–Oblique view.

Between the anterior body and the lesser wings on each side are groove-like canals through which the optic nerve and certain arteries pass into the orbital cavity. This begins in the center as the **chiasmatic** *(ki-az-mat' ik)* or **optic groove**, which leads on each side to an **optic canal**, which ends at the **optic foramen** or opening into the orbit. The optic foramina can be demonstrated radiographically with frontal oblique projections of the orbits.

Slightly lateral and posterior to the optic foramina on each side are irregular shaped openings, seen best on this oblique view, called **superior orbital fissures**. These openings provide additional communication with the orbits for numerous nerves and blood vessels. The foramen rotundum and the foramen ovale are seen again on this oblique view.

Projecting downward from the inferior surface of the body are four processes that correspond to the legs of the imaginary bat. The more lateral, somewhat flat extensions are termed the **lateral pterygoid** *(ter' i-goyd)* **processes**, sometimes called plates. Directly medial to these are the two **medial pterygoid processes** or plates which end inferiorly in small hook-like processes called **pterygoid hamuli**. The pterygoid processes or plates form part of the lateral walls of the nasal cavities.

Sella Turcica–Lateral View: In a true lateral position, the sella turcica would look similar to this drawing. Deformity of the sella turcica is often the only clue that a lesion exists intracranially; therefore, radiography of the sella turcica may be very important.

The depression of the **sella turcica** and the **dorsum sellae** are best seen from the side. The **anterior clinoid processes** are anterior and superior to the sella turcica, while the **posterior clinoid processes** are seen as small extensions located superior to the dorsum sellae.

Articulations: Because of its central location the sphenoid articulates with **all seven** of the other cranial bones. (The sphenoid also articulates with five facial bones.)

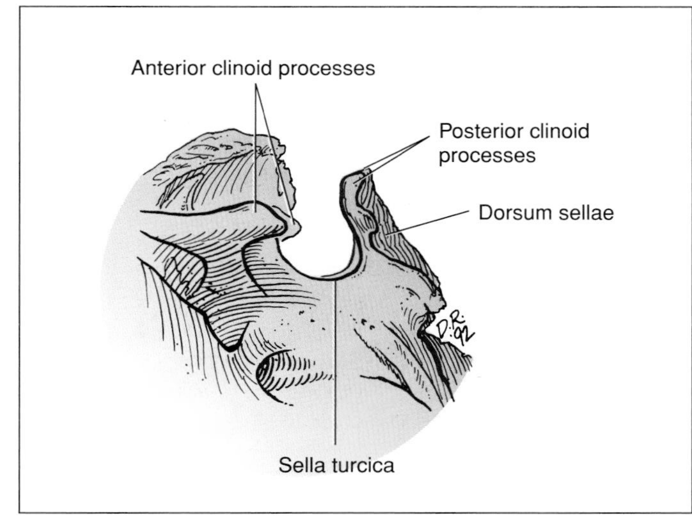

Fig. 11-16. Sella turcica of sphenoid bone–Lateral view.

Ethmoid Bone

The eighth and last cranial bone to be studied is the **ethmoid bone**. The single ethmoid bone lies primarily below the floor of the cranium. Only the top of the ethmoid is shown on a superior view (left drawing in Fig. 11-17), situated in the ethmoidal notch of the frontal bone.

A magnified coronal sectional view of the entire ethmoid is shown on the right. The small upper horizontal portion of the bone is termed the **cribriform plate** and contains many small openings or foramina through which pass the olfactory nerves, the nerves of smell. Projecting superiorly from the cribriform plate, similar to a rooster's comb, is the **crista galli** *(kris′ ta gal′ le)*.

The major portion of the ethmoid lies beneath the floor of the cranium. Projecting downward in the midline is the **perpendicular plate** which helps to form the bony nasal septum. The two **lateral labyrinths** (masses) are suspended from the under surface of the cribriform plate on each side of the perpendicular plate. The lateral masses contain the ethmoid air cells or sinuses and help form the medial walls of the orbits and the lateral walls of the nasal cavity. Extending medially and downward from the medial wall of each labyrinth are thin scroll-shaped projections of bone. These projections are termed the **superior** and **middle nasal conchae** *(kong′ ha)* or **turbinates**, best shown on facial bone drawings, page 335.

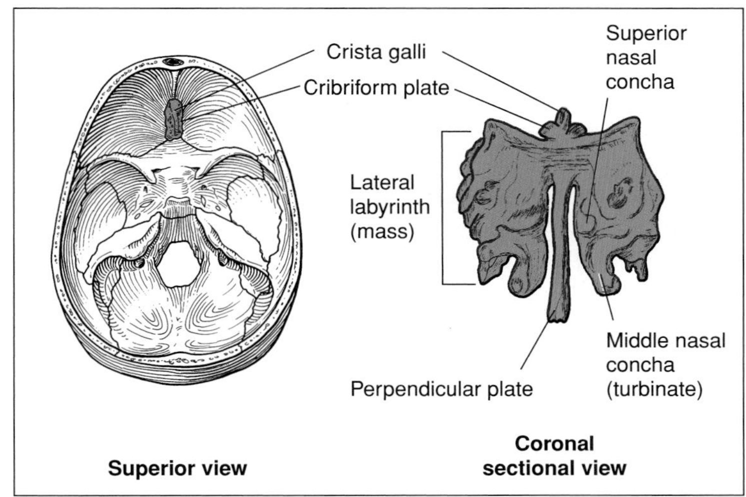

Fig. 11-17. Ethmoid bone.

Articulations: The ethmoid articulates with **two** cranial bones, the frontal and the sphenoid. (It also articulates with 11 facial bones.)

Cranium–Medial Sectional View (Fig. 11-18)

This drawing represents the right half of the skull, sectioned near the midsagittal plane. The centrally located **sphenoid** and **ethmoid** bones are well demonstrated showing their relationship to each other and to the other cranial bones.

The ethmoid bone is seen to be located anterior to the sphenoid bone. The smaller **crista galli** and **cribriform plate** project superiorly, and the larger **perpendicular plate** extends inferiorly. The perpendicular plate forms the upper portion of the bony nasal septum.

The sphenoid bone, containing the saddle-shaped sella turcica, is located directly posterior to the ethmoid bone. Shown again is one of the two long slender shaped **pterygoid processes** or plates extending down and forward ending with the small pointed process called the **pterygoid hamulus**. The center body portion of the sphenoid bone in this sectional view demonstrates a hollow-like area containing the **sphenoid sinus**.

The larger **frontal bone** also demonstrates a cavity in this sectional view directly posterior to the glabella containing the **frontal sinus**.

An interior view of the large rounded **parietal bone** is shown making up most of the lateral and superior portion of the calvarium.

The vomer (a facial bone) is shown as a midline structure between parts of the sphenoid and ethmoid (see page 335).

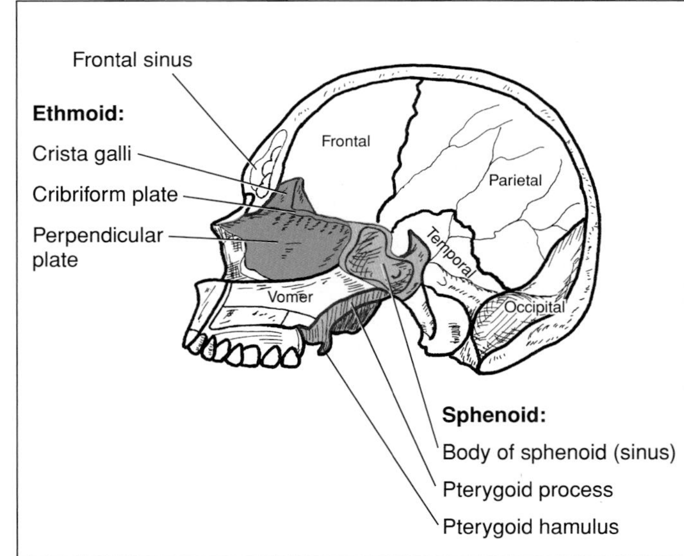

Fig. 11-18. Cranium–Medial section, sphenoid and ethmoid bones.

The **squamous portion** of the **temporal bone** is demonstrated just inferior to the parietal bone, where it also forms part of the lower wall of the cranium. The large **occipital bone** is shown to make up the lower posterior/inferior wall and floor of the cranium.

JOINTS OF THE CRANIUM–SUTURES

Adult Cranium

The articulations or joints of the cranium are called **sutures** and belong in the class of joints termed **fibrous joints**. Since in an adult they are **immovable**, they are called **synarthrodial**. These are demonstrated in Fig. 11-19 in lateral, top and posterior views.

The **coronal** *(ko-ro′ nal)* **suture** separates the frontal bone from the two parietals. Separating the two parietal bones in the midline is the **sagittal suture**.

Posteriorly, the **lambdoidal** *(lam′ doy-dal)* **suture** separates the two parietals from the occipital bone.

The **squamosal** *(skwa-mo′ sal)* **suture** is formed by the inferior junction of each parietal bone with the respective temporal bone.

Each end of the sagittal suture is identified as a point or area with a specific name as labeled. The anterior end of the sagittal suture is termed the **bregma** *(breg′ mah)*, while the posterior end is the **lambda** *(lam′ dah)*. The right and left **pterions** *(ter′ re-ons)* are points at the junction of the parietals, temporals and the greater wings of the sphenoid (**posterior** end of sphenoparietal suture per *Gray's Anatomy*).

The right and left **asterions** *(as-te′ re-ons)* are points posterior to the ear where the squamosal and lambdoidal sutures meet. These six recognizable bony points are used in surgery or other cases where specific reference points for cranial measurements are necessary.

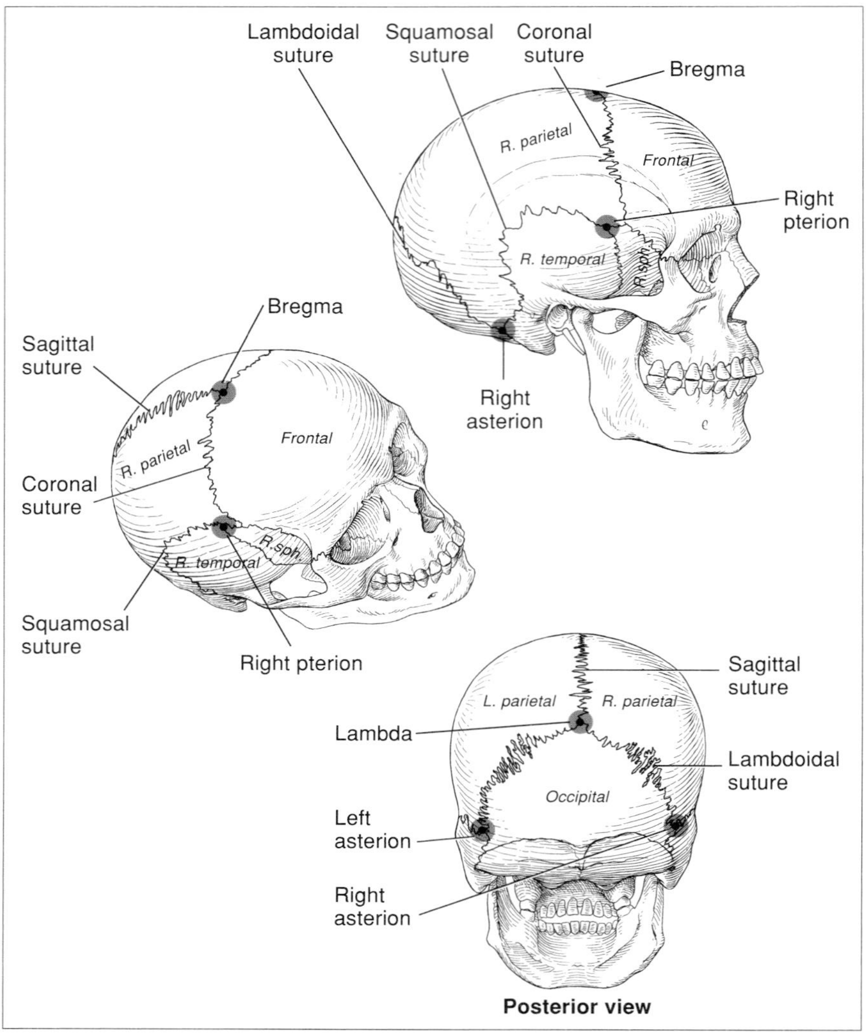

Fig. 11-19. Adult cranial sutures–**Fibrous joints, synarthrodial** (immovable).

Infant Cranium

The calvarium or skull cap on an infant is very large in proportion to the rest of the body, but the facial bones are quite small as seen on these drawings (Fig. 11-20). Ossification of the individual cranial bones is incomplete at birth and the sutures are membranous-covered spaces that fill in soon after birth. However certain regions where sutures join are slower in their ossification and these are called **fontanels**. The cranial sutures themselves generally do not completely close until about the 12th or 13th year, and some may not completely close until adulthood.

Fontanels: Early in life, the bregma and lambda are not bony, but are membrane-covered openings or "soft spots." These "soft spots" are termed the **anterior** and **posterior fontanels** *(fon″ tah-nels′)* in an infant. The anterior fontanel is the largest and at birth is about 2.5 cm wide and 4 cm in length. It doesn't completely close until about 18 months of age.

Two smaller lateral fontanels which close soon after birth are the **sphenoid** (pterion in an adult) and **mastoid** (asterion in an adult) **fontanels**, located respectively at the sphenoid and mastoid angles of the parietal bones on each side of the head. Thus there are a total of **six fontanels** in an infant as follows:

Infant	**Adult**
1. Anterior fontanel	–Bregma
2. Posterior fontanel	–Lambda
3. Right sphenoid fontanel	–Right pterion
4. Left sphenoid fontanel	–Left pterion
5. Right mastoid fontanel	–Right asterion
6. Left mastoid fontanel	–Left asterion

Sutural or Wormian Bones

Certain small irregular bones called sutural or Wormian bones sometimes develop in the adult skull sutures. These small, irregular-shaped, isolated bones are most often found in the lambdoid suture, but occasionally are also found in the region of the fontanels, especially the posterior fontanel. In the adult skull these are completely ossified and are only visible by the sutural lines around their borders.

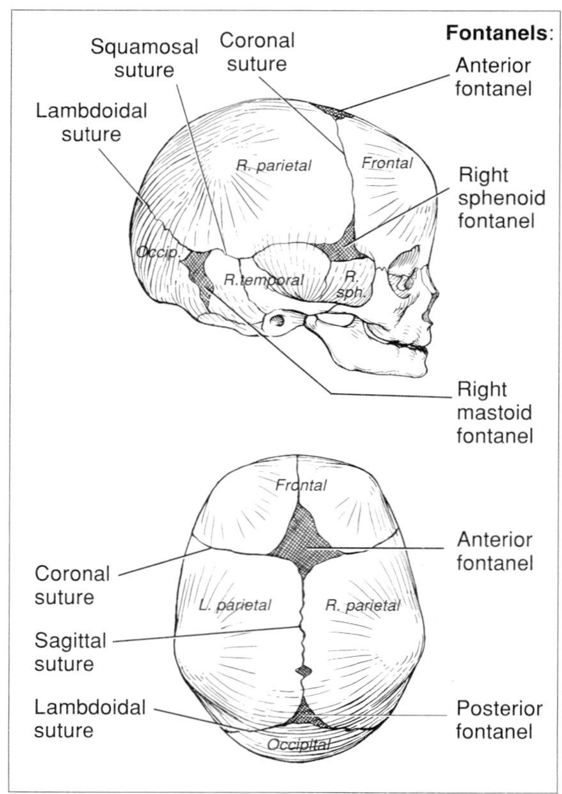

Fig. 11-20. Infant cranial sutures and **fontanels**.

ANATOMY REVIEW WITH RADIOGRAPHS

Following are review exercises for anatomy of the eight cranial bones as labelled on radiographs.

A recommended method of review and reinforcement is to cover up the answers below and first attempt to identify each of the labelled parts from memory. Specific anatomical parts may be more difficult to recognize on radiographs as compared to drawings but knowing locations as well as relationships to surrounding structures and bones should aid in identifying these parts.

Cranial Bones–PA Caldwell Projection

A. Supraorbital margin of R. orbit
B. Crista galli of ethmoid
C. Sagittal suture (posterior skull)
D. Lambdoidal suture (posterior skull)
E. Petrous ridge

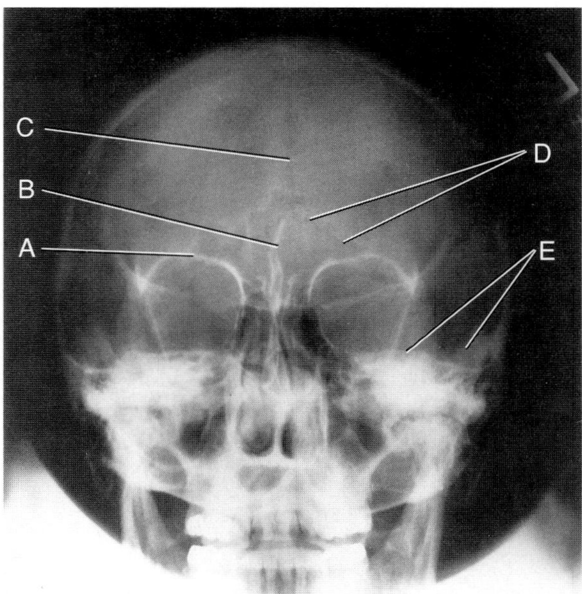

Fig. 11-21. PA Caldwell projection.

Cranial Bones–AP Axial Projection

A. Dorsum sella of sphenoid
B. Posterior clinoid processes
C. Petrous ridge or petrous pyramid
D. Parietal bone
E. Occipital bone
F. Foramen magnum

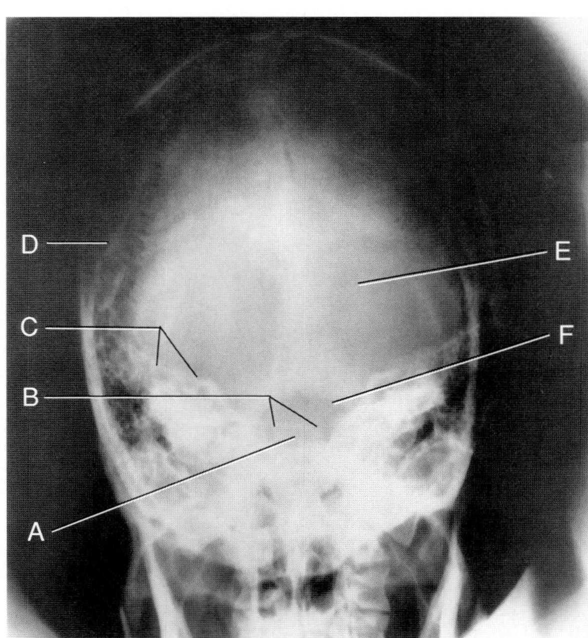

Fig. 11-22. AP axial projection.

Cranial Bones–Lateral Projection

A. External acoustic meatus (EAM)
B. Mastoid portion of temporal bone
C. Occipital bone
D. Lambdoidal suture
E. Clivus
F. Dorsum sellae
G. Posterior clinoid processes
H. Anterior clinoid processes
I. Vertex of cranium
J. Coronal suture
K. Frontal bone
L. Sella turcica
M. Body of sphenoid (sphenoid sinus)

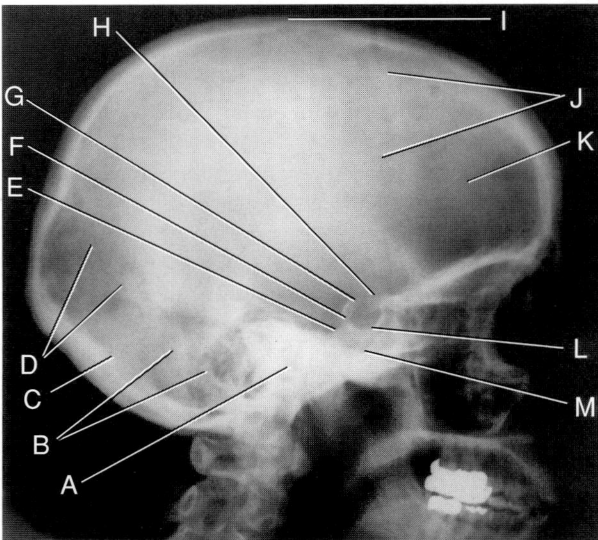

Fig. 11-23. Lateral projection.

FACIAL BONES (14)

In addition to the eight cranial bones, there are also **14 facial bones** making up the skull or bony skeleton of the head. The anatomy of the facial bones is included in this chapter due to their close relationship to the adjoining cranial bones. The positioning, however, for all the procedures involving the facial bones is included in Chapter 12 which follows.

Each of the facial bones are identified on the frontal and lateral drawings of Figs. 11-24 and 11-25, except for the two palatine bones and the vomer which are located internally and not visible on a dry skeleton from the exterior. These are identified on sectional drawings later in this chapter.

The 14 facial bones contribute to the shape and form of a person's face. In addition, the cavities of the orbits, nose and mouth are largely constructed from the bones of the face. Of the 14 bones making up the facial skeleton, only two are single bones. The remaining 12 consist of six pairs of bones with similar bones on each side of the face.

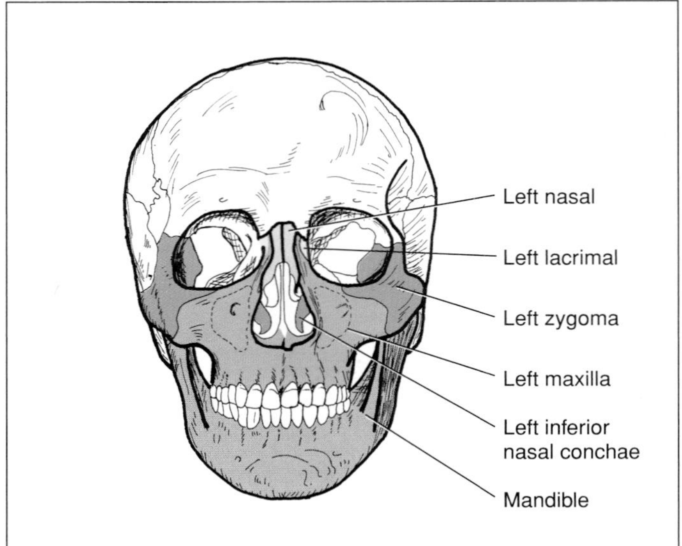

Fig. 11-24. Facial bones–Frontal view.

Facial Bones

2 –Maxillae *(mak-sil′ e)* (upper jaw) or maxillary bones
2 –Zygoma or zygomatic bones *(zi′ go-mat′ ik)*
2 –Lacrimal bones *(lak′ ri-mal)*
2 –Nasal bones
2 –Inferior nasal conchae *(kong′ ke)*
2 –Palatine bones *(pal′ ah-tin)* } Not visible on exterior skeletal drawings
1 –Vomer *(vo′ mer)* }
1 –Mandible (lower jaw)

14 Total

Each of the facial bones will be separated and studied individually, or as pairs for those six paired bones. After the description of each of these facial bones will be a listing of those specific adjoining bones with which they articulate, or with which they are joined since in an adult they are all fused and immovable except for the mandible. Knowing these anatomical relationships helps in understanding the structure of the total skull or bony skeleton of the head.

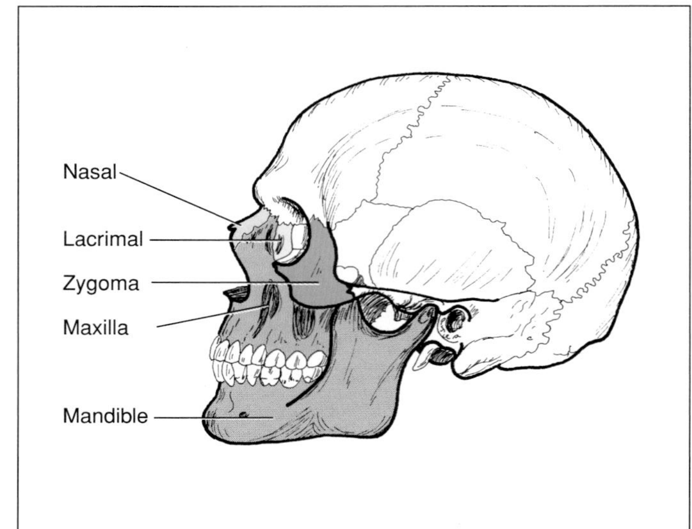

Fig. 11-25. Facial bones–Lateral view.

Right and Left Maxillary Bones

The first pair of facial bones to be studied are the two **maxillae or maxillary bones,** which are the **largest immovable bones of the face**. The only facial bone that is larger than the maxilla is the movable lower jaw or mandible. All of the other bones of the upper facial area are closely associated with the two maxillae, thus they are structurally the most important bones of the upper face. The right and left maxillary bones are solidly united at the midline below the nasal septum. Each maxilla assists in the formation of three cavities of the face: (1) the mouth, (2) the nasal cavity, and (3) one orbit.

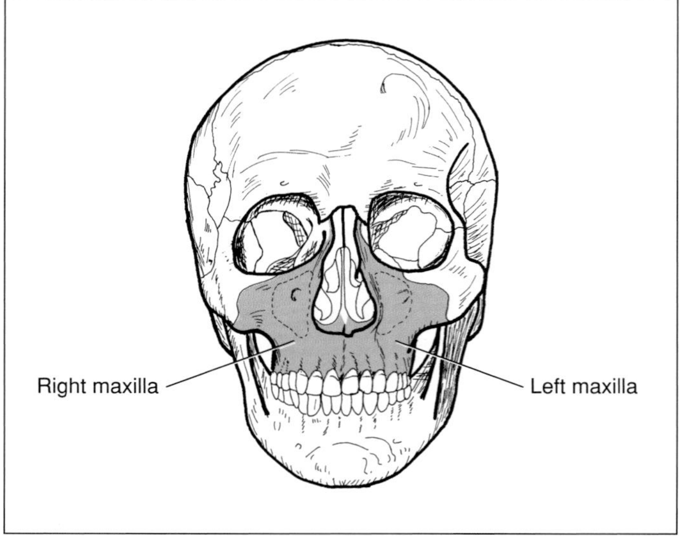

Fig. 11-26. Right and left maxillae.

Lateral View of Left Maxilla: Each maxilla consists of a centrally located **body** and **four processes** projecting from that body. Three of these processes are more obvious and are seen on these lateral and frontal drawings. The fourth process, the palatine process, is described below as part of the hard palate.

The **body** of each maxilla is the centrally located portion that lies lateral to the nose. One of the three processes is the **frontal process**, which projects upward along the lateral border of the nose toward the frontal bone. The **zygomatic process** projects laterally to unite with the zygomatic bone. The third process, the **alveolar process**, is the inferior or lower aspect of the body of each maxilla. The eight upper teeth on each side are embedded in cavities along the inferior margin of the alveolar process.

The two maxillae are solidly united in the midline anteriorly. At the upper part of this midline union is the **anterior nasal spine**. A blow to the nose sometimes results in this nasal spine being separated from the maxillae.

A point at the base of the anterior nasal spine is called the **acanthion**, described later in this chapter as a surface landmark at the midline point where the nose and upper lip meet.

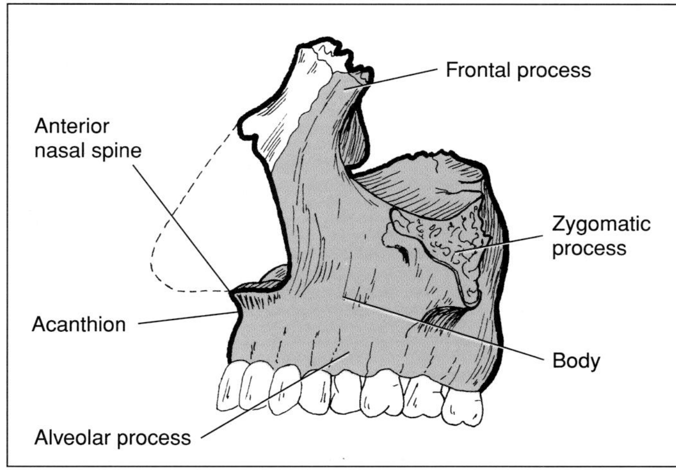

Fig. 11-27. Left maxilla–Lateral view.

Frontal View: The relationship of the two maxillary bones to the remainder of the bones of the skull is well demonstrated in this frontal view (Fig. 11-28). Note again **three processes** as seen in the frontal view of the skull. Extending upward toward the frontal bone is the **frontal process**. Extending laterally toward the zygomatic bone is the **zygomatic process**, and supporting the upper teeth is the **alveolar process**.

The body of each maxillary bone contains a large air-filled cavity known as a **maxillary sinus**. There are several of these air-filled cavities found in certain bones of the skull. These sinuses communicate with the nasal cavity and are collectively termed paranasal sinuses and will be described further in the chapter which follows.

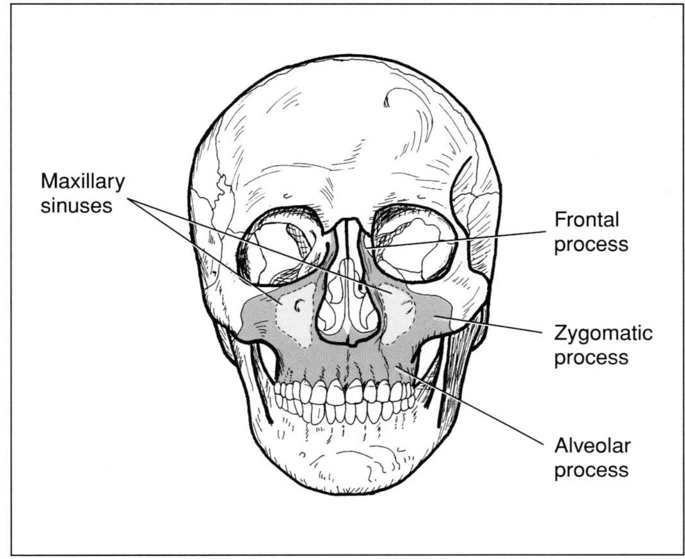

Fig. 11-28. Maxillae–Frontal view.

Hard Palate (Inferior Surface): The **fourth process** of each maxillary bone is the **palatine process**, which can only be demonstrated on an inferior view of the two maxillae (Fig. 11-29). The two palatine processes form the anterior portion of the roof of the mouth, called the hard or bony palate. The two palatine processes are solidly united in the midline to form a synarthrodial or immovable joint. A common congenital defect called a cleft palate is an opening between the palatine processes, caused by an incomplete joining of the two bones.

The posterior part of the hard palate is formed by the horizontal portions of two other facial bones, the **palatine bones**. Note that the posterior part of the hard palate is formed by the two palatine bones, while the anterior part of the hard palate is formed by the palatine processes of the two maxillary bones.

Only the horizontal portions of the L-shaped palatine bones are visible on this view. The vertical portion is demonstrated later on a cutaway drawing in Fig. 11-34.

The two small inferior portions of the sphenoid bone of the cranium are also shown on this inferior view of the hard palate. These two processes, the **pterygoid hamuli**, are likened to the outstretched legs of a bat as described in an earlier drawing (Fig. 11-15).

Articulations: Each maxilla articulates with **two cranial bones**, the frontal and the ethmoid; and with **seven facial bones**, a zygomatic, a lacrimal, a nasal, a palatine, an inferior nasal concha, the vomer and the opposite maxilla.

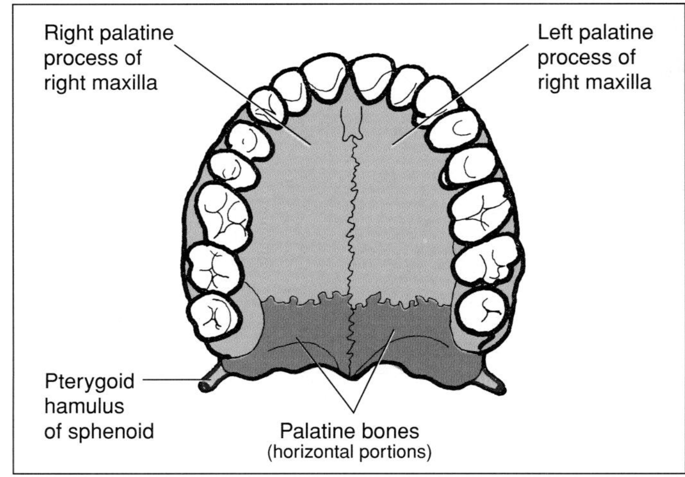

Fig. 11-29. Maxillae and palatine bones–Inferior surface.

Right and Left Zygomatic Bones

One **zygoma** or **zygomatic bone** is located lateral to the zygomatic process of each maxilla. These bones, sometimes termed **malar bones**, form the prominence of the cheek and make up the lower outer portion of each orbit.

Projecting posteriorly from the zygomatic bone is a slender process connecting with the zygomatic process of the temporal bone to form the **zygomatic arch**. The zygomatic arch is a fairly delicate structure and is sometimes fractured or "caved in" by a blow to the cheek. Note that the anterior portion of the zygomatic arch is formed by the zygomatic bone and the posterior portion by the temporal bone. The **zygomatic prominence** is a positioning landmark and refers to this prominent portion of the zygomatic bone.

Articulations: Each zygomatic articulates with **three cranial bones**, the frontal, the sphenoid, and a temporal; and with **one facial bone**, a maxilla.

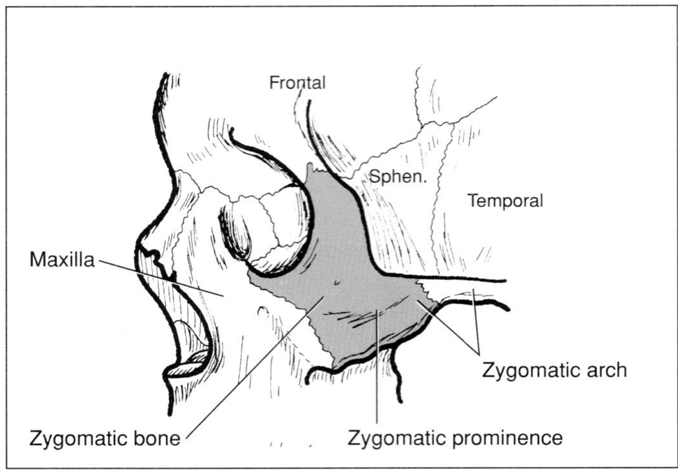

Fig. 11-30. Zygomatic bone–Lateral view.

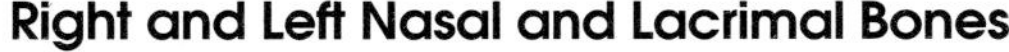

Right and Left Nasal and Lacrimal Bones

The lacrimal and nasal bones are the thinnest and most fragile bones in the entire body.

Lacrimal Bones: The two small and very delicate lacrimal bones (about the size and shape of a fingernail) lie anteriorly on the medial side of each orbit just posterior to the frontal process of the maxilla. Lacrimal, derived from a word meaning tear, is appropriate since the lacrimal bones are closely associated with the tear ducts.

Nasal Bones: The two fused nasal bones form the bridge of the nose and are somewhat variable in size. Some persons have very prominent nasal bones, while others are quite small. Much of the nose is made up of cartilage and only the upper portion at the bridge of the nose is formed by the two nasal bones. The nasal bones lie just anterior and superior to the frontal process of the maxillae and just inferior to the frontal bone. The point of junction of the two nasal bones with the frontal bone is a positioning landmark termed the **nasion**.

Articulations:

Lacrimal–Each lacrimal articulates with **two cranial bones**, the frontal and the ethmoid; and with **two facial bones**, a maxilla and an inferior nasal concha.

Nasal–Each nasal also articulates with **two cranial bones**, the frontal and the ethmoid; and with **two facial bones**, a maxilla and the opposite nasal bone.

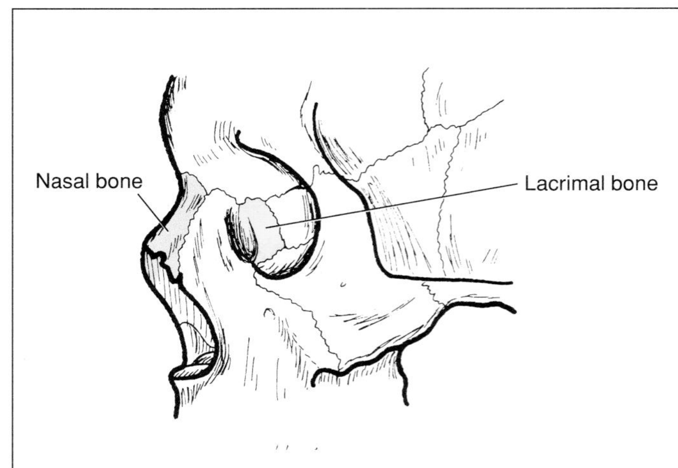

Fig. 11-31. Nasal and lacrimal bones–Lateral view.

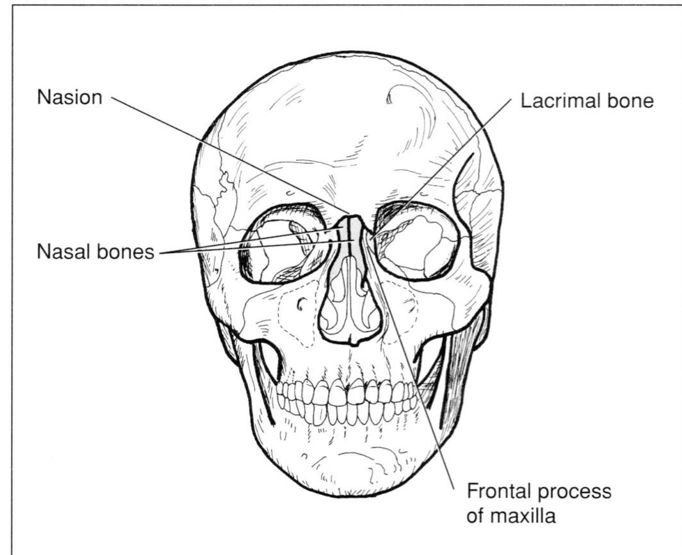

Fig. 11-32. Nasal and lacrimal bones–Frontal view.

Right and Left Inferior Nasal Conchae

Within the nasal cavity are two thin, curved or scroll-shaped facial bones termed the **inferior nasal conchae** (turbinates). These two bones project from the lateral walls of the nasal cavity on each side and extend medially.

The **superior and middle nasal conchae** (turbinates) are similar scroll-like projections that extend from the ethmoid bone into the nasal cavities. (These two pairs are not shown separately on the frontal drawing but are shown in Fig. 11-34.)

In summary, there are three pairs of nasal conchae or turbinates. The **superior and middle pairs are parts of the ethmoid bone**, while the **inferior pair are separate facial bones**.

The effect of the three pairs of turbinates is to divide the nasal cavities into various departments. These irregular compartments tend to break up or mix the flow of air coming into the nasal cavities before it reaches the lungs. In this way the incoming air is somewhat warmed and cleaned as it comes in contact with the mucous membrane covering the conchae, before it reaches the lungs.

Sectional Drawing

Inferior Nasal Conchae: The relationship between the various nasal conchae and the lateral wall of one nasal cavity is illustrated in this sectional drawing (Fig. 11-34). The midline structures making up the nasal septum have been removed so that the lateral portion of the right nasal cavity can be seen. Note that the **superior and middle conchae** are part of the ethmoid bone, and the **inferior nasal conchae** are separate facial bones. The **cribriform plate** and the **crista galli** of the ethmoid bone help to separate the cranium from the facial bone mass.

Right and Left Palatine Bones

The two **palatine bones** are difficult to visualize when studying a dry skeleton because they are located internally and are not visible from the outside. Each palatine bone is roughly "L"-shaped. The vertical portion of the "L" extends upward between one maxilla and one pterygoid plate of the sphenoid bone. The horizontal portion of each "L" helps to make up the posterior portion of the hard palate as shown in an earlier drawing in Fig. 11-29.

Articulations:
Inferior nasal conchae–Each inferior nasal conchae articulates with **one cranial bone**, the ethmoid; and with **three facial bones**, a maxilla, a lacrimal and a palatine.
Palatine–Each palatine articulates with **two cranial bones**, the sphenoid and the ethmoid; and **four facial bones**, a maxilla, an inferior nasal conchae, the vomer and the opposite palatine.

Bony Nasal Septum

The midline structures of the nasal cavity, including the **bony nasal septum**, are shown on this sagittal view drawing. The bony nasal septum is formed by two bones, the **ethmoid** and the **vomer**. It is formed superiorly by the **perpendicular plate** of the ethmoid bone, and inferiorly by the single vomer bone. Anteriorly, the nasal septum is cartilaginous and is termed the **septal cartilage**.

The bony nasal septum, which can be demonstrated radiographically, is thus formed by the perpendicular plate of the ethmoid bone and the vomer bone. In severe trauma to the nasal bone area, the septum may get pushed to one side, away from the midline. This injury would be termed a deviated nasal septum.

Vomer

The single **vomer bone** (meaning plowshare) is a thin triangular-shaped bone that forms the inferoposterior part of the nasal septum.

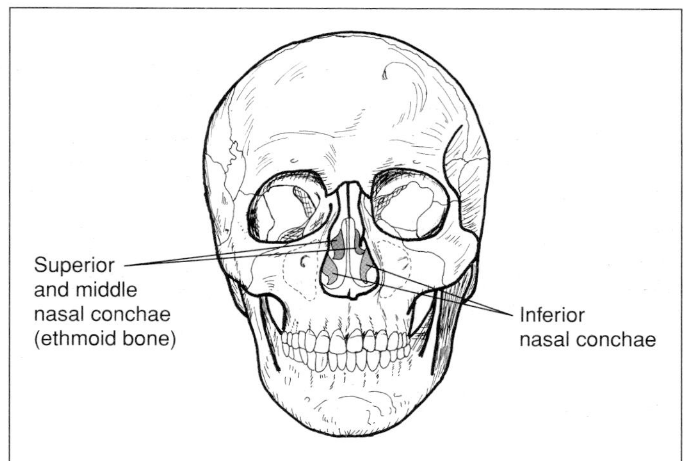

Fig. 11-33. Inferior nasal conchae.

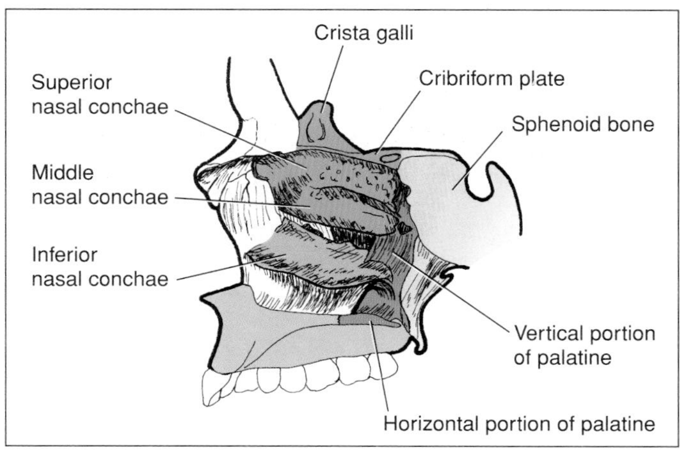

Fig. 11-34. Inferior nasal conchae and palatine bones.

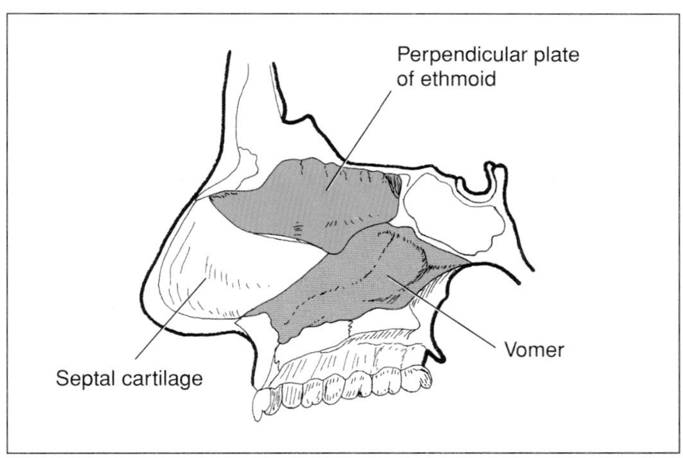

Fig. 11-35. Bony nasal septum and vomer.

The surfaces of the vomer are marked by small furrowlike depressions for blood vessels, a source of nose bleed with trauma to the nasal area. A deviated nasal septum describes the clinical condition wherein the nasal septum is deflected or displaced laterally from the midline of the nose. This deviation usually occurs at the site of junction between the septal cartilage and the vomer. A severe deviation can entirely block the nasal passageway making breathing through the nose impossible.

Articulations: The vomer articulates with **two cranial bones**, the sphenoid and ethmoid; and with **four facial bones**, the right and left palatine and the right and left maxilla. (The vomer also articulates with the septal cartilage.)

Mandible

The last and the largest of the facial bones is the lower jaw or **mandible**. It is the only movable bone in the adult skull. This large facial bone, which is a single bone in the adult, actually originates as two separate bones. The two bones in the infant join to become one bone at approximately 1 year of age.

Lateral View: The **angle** (gonion) of the mandible divides each half of the mandible into two main parts. That area anterior to the angle is termed the **body** of the mandible, while that area superior to each angle is termed the **ramus**. Since the mandible is a single bone, the body actually extends from the left angle around to the right angle.

The lower teeth are rooted in the mandible; therefore, an **alveolar process** or ridge extends along the entire superior portion of the body of the mandible.

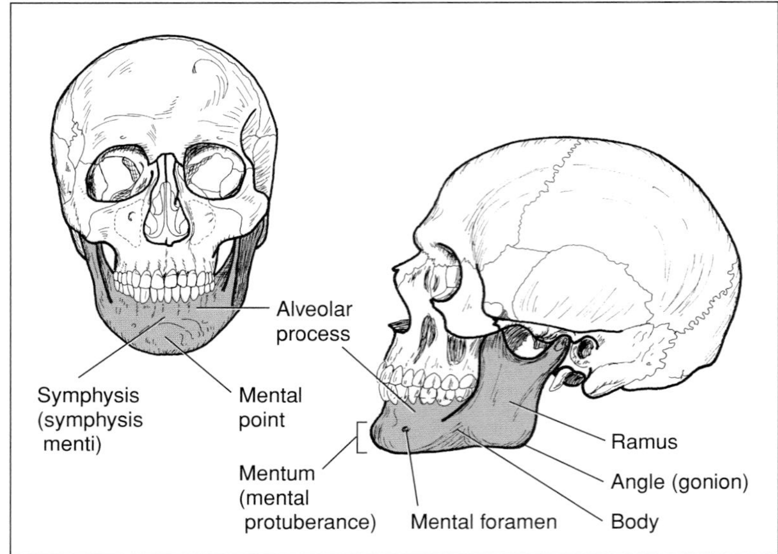

Fig. 11-36. Mandible–Lateral and frontal views.

Frontal View: The anterior aspect of the adult mandible is best seen on a frontal view. The single body forms from each lateral half and unites at the anterior midline. This union is called the **symphysis** of the mandible, or **symphysis menti**. The flat triangular area below the symphysis projecting forward as the chin is called the **mentum** or **mental protuberance**. The center of the mental protuberance is described as the **mental point**. Mentum and mental are Latin words referring to the general area known as the chin. The mental point is a specific point of the chin whereas the mentum is the entire area.

Located on each half of the body of the mandible are the **mental foramina**. These foramina serve as passageways for nerves and blood vessels.

Ramus: The upper portion of each **ramus** terminates in a "U"-shaped notch termed the **mandibular notch**. At each end of the mandibular notch is a process. The process at the anterior end of the mandibular notch is termed the **coronoid process**. The coronoid process does not articulate with another bone and cannot be easily palpated since it lies just inferior to the zygomatic arch. It serves as a site for muscle attachment.

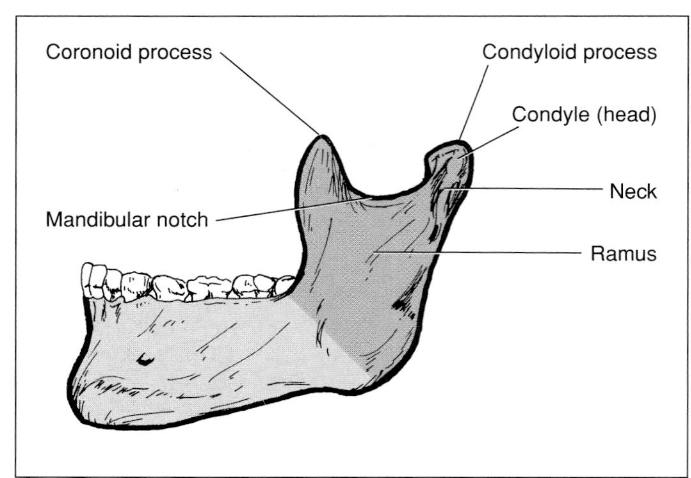

Fig. 11-37. Ramus of mandible–Left side.

Memory aid: The **coronoid process** of the mandible must not be confused with the **coronoid process** of the proximal ulna of the forearm, or the **coracoid process** of the scapula. One way to remember these terms is to associate "n" in coronoid with the "n's" in ulna and in mandible.

The posterior process of the upper ramus is termed the **condyloid process** and consists of two parts. The rounded end of the condyloid process is called the **condyle** or **head**, while the constricted area directly below the condyle is the **neck**. The condyle of the condyloid process fits into the temporomandibular fossa of the temporal bone to form the **temporomandibular joint** or **TMJ**. (See following page.)

Submentovertex Projection: The horseshoe shape of the mandible is well visualized on a **submentovertex** (SMV) projection (Fig. 11-38). Note that the mandible is a fairly thin structure, which explains why it is susceptible to fractures. The area of the chin or **mentum** is well demonstrated, as are the **body** and **rami** of the mandible. The relative positions of the upper ramus and its associated **coronoid process** and **condyle** are also demonstrated with this projection. Note that the condyles project inward and the coronoid processes slightly outward on this view as is demonstrated on radiographs of this projection.

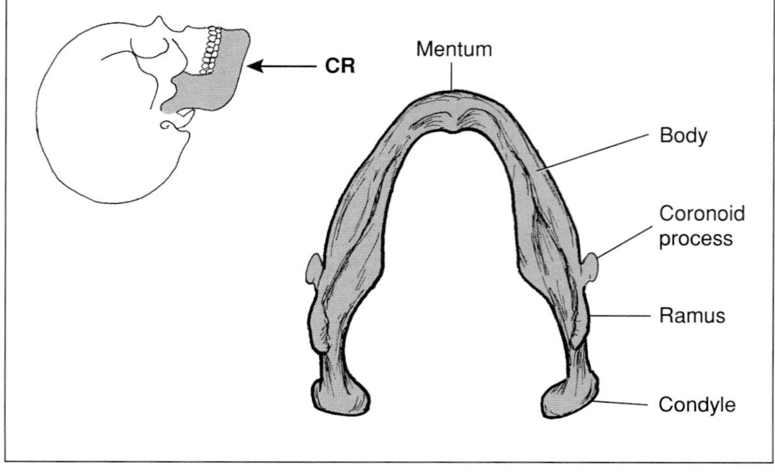

Fig. 11-38. Submentovertex (SMV) projection of mandible.

Temporomandibular Joint (TMJ)

The temporomandibular joint (TMJ), the only movable joint in the skull, is shown on this lateral drawing and on the lateral view photograph of a dry skull (Figs. 11-39 and 11-40). The relationship of the mandible to the temporal bone of the cranium is well demonstrated.

The TMJ is formed by the **condyle** or head of the condyloid process of the mandible fitting into the **temporomandibular fossa** of the temporal bone. The TMJ is located just anterior and slightly superior to the **EAM**.

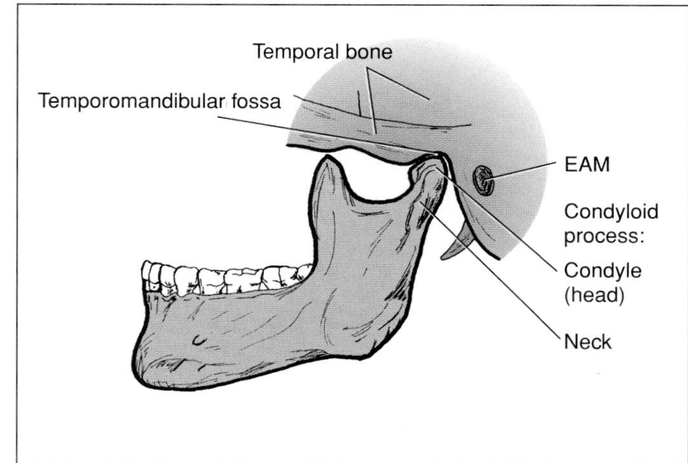

Fig. 11-39. Temporomandibular joint (TMJ).

JOINT CLASSIFICATIONS (SKULL & MANDIBLE)

Synovial Joints (Diarthrodial)

The TMJ is classified as a **synovial type** joint which is **diarthrodial** or freely movable. This synovial joint is divided into upper and lower synovial cavities by a single articular fibrous disc. A series of strong ligaments join the condylar neck of the mandible to the lower borders of the zygomatic process of the temporal bone.

The two-part articular capsule is lined by synovial membrane and divided by the articular disc. This complete two-part synovial joint along with its fibrous articular disc allows for not only a **hinge type motion** but also a **gliding movement** wherein the mandibular condyle glides forward as the mouth is opened. This movement is further facilitated by a shallow temporomandibular fossa of the temporal bone with which the condyle or head of mandible articulates.

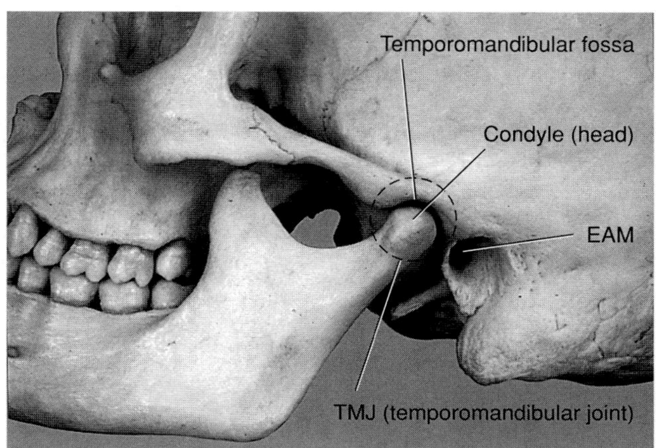

Fig. 11-40. Joints of mandible.

Fibrous Joints (Synarthrodial)

There are two types of **fibrous** joints involving the skull. These are both **synarthrodial** or immovable joints. First are the **sutures** between cranial bones as already described in this chapter. Second is a unique type of fibrous joint involving the teeth and the mandible and the maxillae. This is a **gomphosis** *(gom-fo′ sis)* subclass type fibrous joint between the roots of the teeth and the alveolar processes of both the maxillae and the mandible.

TMJ Motion: The drawings and radiographs below illustrate the TMJ in both an **open** and a **closed mouth** position. When one opens the mouth widely, the condyle moves forward to the front edge of the fossa. If the condyle slips too far anteriorly, the joint may dislocate. If the TMJ dislocates, either by force or by jaw motion, it may be difficult or even impossible to close the mouth, which returns the condyle to its normal position.

Radiographs (Open and Closed Mouth): Two axiolateral projections (Schuller method) of the TMJ are shown below in closed and open mouth positions. The range of anterior movement of the condyle in relationship to the temporomandibular fossa is clearly demonstrated.

Joints of Mandible

Temporomandibular joint	Alveoli and roots of teeth
Classification: ***Synovial*** *(diarthrodial)*	Classification: ***Fibrous*** *(synarthrodial)*
Movement type: ***Ginglymus*** *(hinge)*, ***Plane*** *(gliding)*	Subclass: ***Gomphosis***

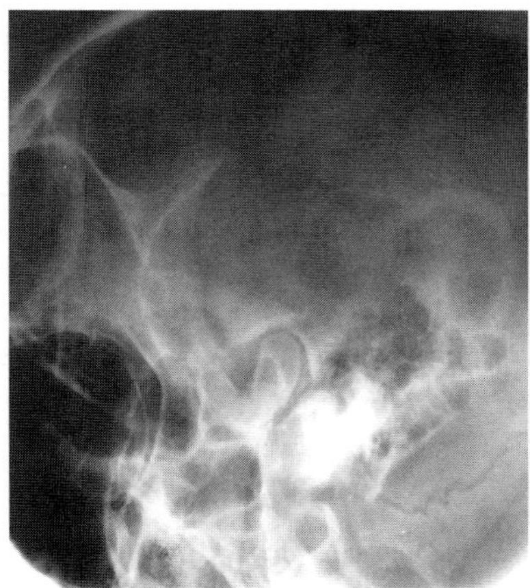

Fig. 11-41. Closed mouth.

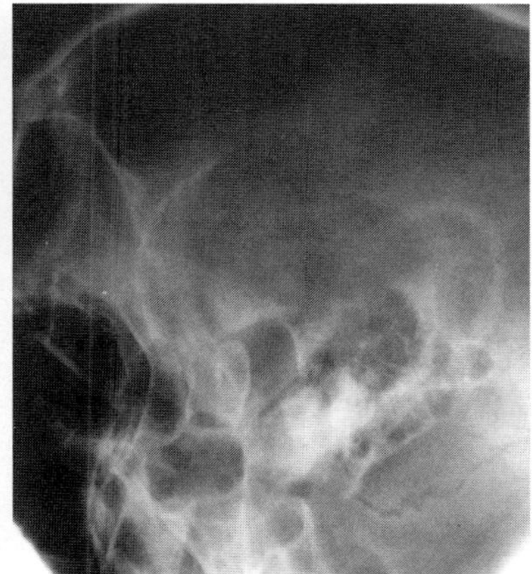

Fig. 11-42. Open mouth.

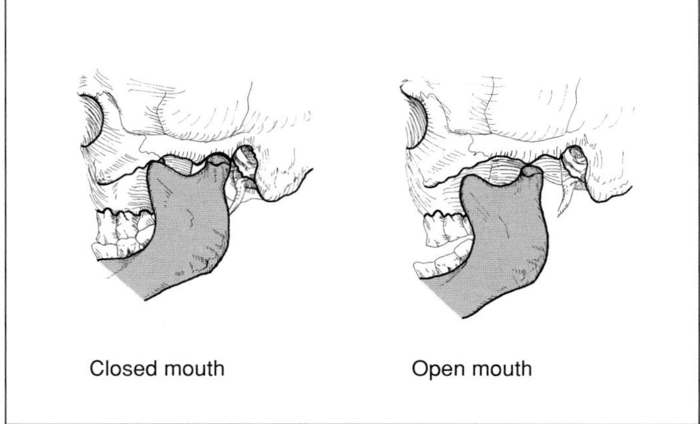

Fig. 11-43. TMJ motion.

ORBITS

The complex anatomy of the 14 facial bones helps to form several facial cavities. Those cavities formed in total or in part by the facial bones are the mouth or oral cavity, the nasal cavities and the bilateral orbits. The mouth and nasal cavities are primarily passageways and, as such, are not often examined specifically by radiographers. The orbits, however, containing the vital organs of sight and associated nerves and blood vessels, are frequently radiographed. The structure and shape of the orbits are illustrated in this simplified drawing. Each orbit is a **cone-shaped**, bony-walled structure composed of parts of **seven bones**.

The rim of the orbit, corresponding to the outer circular portion of the cone, is called the **base**. The base of the orbit is seldom a true circle however, and may even look like a figure with four definite sides. The most posterior portion of the cone, the **apex**, corresponds to the **optic foramen** through which the optic nerve passes.

The long axis of the orbits project both upward and toward the midline. If one's head were placed in an upright AP or lateral position with the orbitomeatal line adjusted parallel to the floor, each orbit would project upward or superiorly at an angle of **30°**, and toward the midsagittal plane at an angle of **37°**. These two important angles are used during radiographic positioning of the optic foramina. Remember that each optic foramen is located at the apex of its respective orbit. In order to radiograph either optic foramen it is necessary to both extend the patient's chin by 30° and rotate the head 37°. The central ray is then projected through the base of the orbit along the long axis of the cone-shaped orbit.

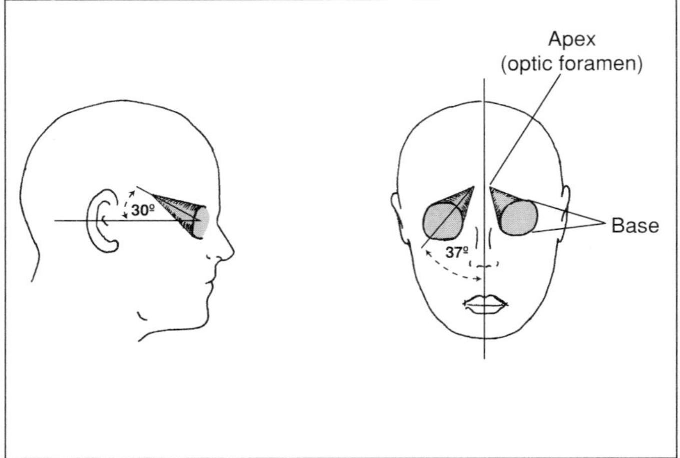

Fig. 11-44. Orbits (cone-shaped).

Bony Composition of Orbits

Each orbit is composed of parts of seven bones. The circumference or circular base of each orbit is composed of parts of **three** bones, the **frontal bone (orbital plate)** from the cranium, and the **maxilla** and **zygoma** from the facial mass. Inside each orbital cavity are a roof, a floor and two walls, parts of which are also formed by these three bones. The orbital plate of the frontal bone forms most of the roof of the orbit. The zygoma forms much of the lateral wall and some of the floor of the orbit, while a portion of the maxilla helps to form the floor.

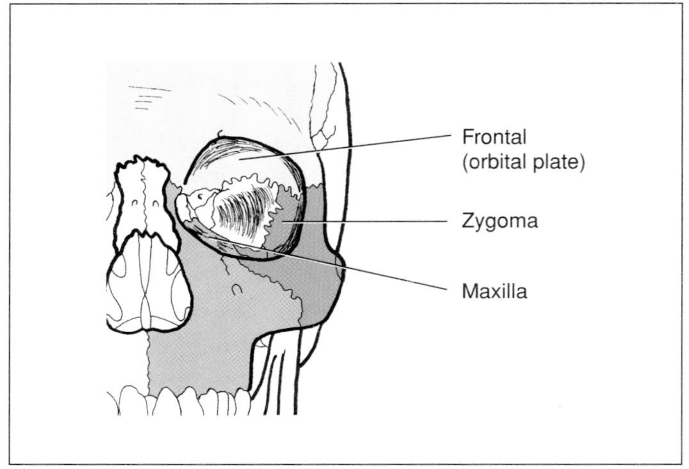

Fig. 11-45. Base of orbit–Three bones (direct frontal view).

All seven bones that form each orbit are shown in Fig. 11-46. The **frontal**, **zygoma** and **maxilla** make up the base of the orbit. Some of the medial wall of the orbit is formed by the thin **lacrimal bone**. The **sphenoid** and **ethmoid** bones make up most of the posterior orbit, while only a small bit of the **palatine** bone contributes to the very innermost posterior portion of the floor of each orbit.

In summary, the **seven** bones making up each orbit include **three cranial bones** and **four facial bones** as follows:

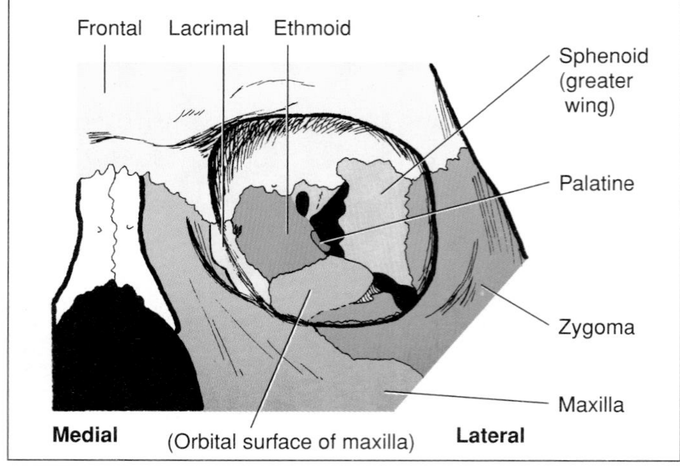

Fig. 11-46. Orbit–Seven bones (slightly oblique frontal view).

Summary Chart – Bones of Orbits

Cranial bones	*Facial bones*
1. Frontal	1. Maxilla
2. Sphenoid	2. Zygoma
3. Ethmoid	3. Lacrimal
	4. Palatine

11

Openings in Posterior Orbit

Each orbit also contains three holes or openings in the posterior portion of the orbit, as demonstrated. The **optic foramen** is a small hole in the sphenoid bone, located posteriorly at the apex of the cone-shaped orbit. The **superior orbital fissure** is a cleft or opening between the greater and lesser wings of the sphenoid bone, located lateral to the optic foramen. A third opening is the **inferior orbital fissure**, located between the maxilla, zygomatic bone and greater wing of the sphenoid.

The small root of bone separating the superior orbital fissure and the optic canal is known as the **sphenoid strut**. The optic canal is a small canal into which the optic foramen opens. Therefore, any abnormal enlargement of the optic nerve could cause erosion of the sphenoid strut, which is actually a portion of the lateral wall of the optic canal.

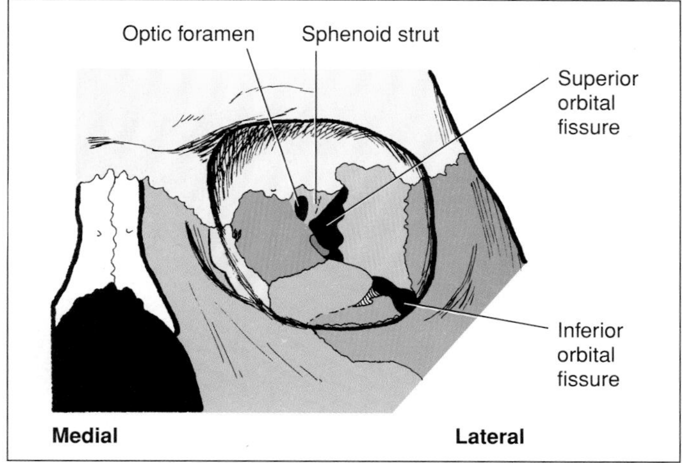

Fig. 11-47. Orbits–Posterior openings (slightly oblique frontal view).

Orbital Fractures

"Blowout" Fracture: Due to the unique construction of the orbit (a closed cone) and to the fact that the orbit is filled with structures containing large amounts of water (water does not compress), certain fractures are common to the orbit. One type of fracture is called a **"blowout" fracture**. If the front of the orbit is struck solidly, such as with a ball or a fist, the contents of the cavity have no place to go. Since the bone along the floor of the orbit is quite thin, the orbital contents "blowout" in that direction. Since the orbital contents involve vision, diagnosis of this type of fracture must be made early in treatment.

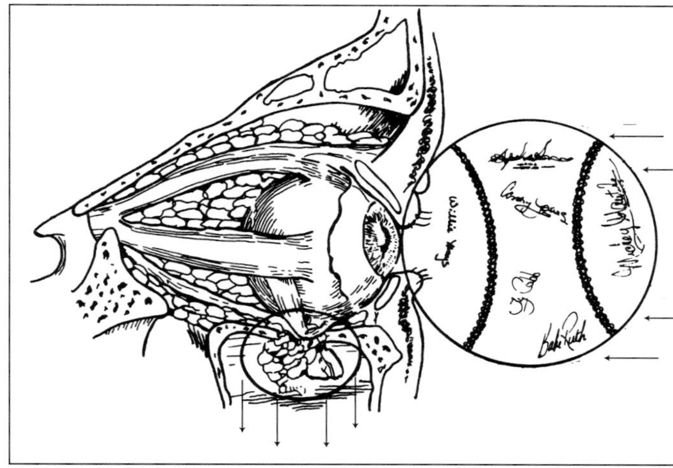

Fig. 11-48. "Blowout" fracture.

"Tripod" Fracture: Another unique fracture of the facial bone area is called the **"tripod" fracture**. This fracture essentially involves the zygomatic bone and its three connections. If fractures were to occur at the three points of attachment with the maxilla, temporal and frontal bones, as might result from a direct blow to the cheek, then the result is a free-floating zygomatic bone or a "tripod" fracture. The bones in this area of the body are highly vascular. Healing is quite rapid, which can be both good and bad. If either a "blowout" or "tripod" fracture is not diagnosed early, the fracture may heal out of place and cause additional problems. The fracture might even have to be rebroken to be set properly.

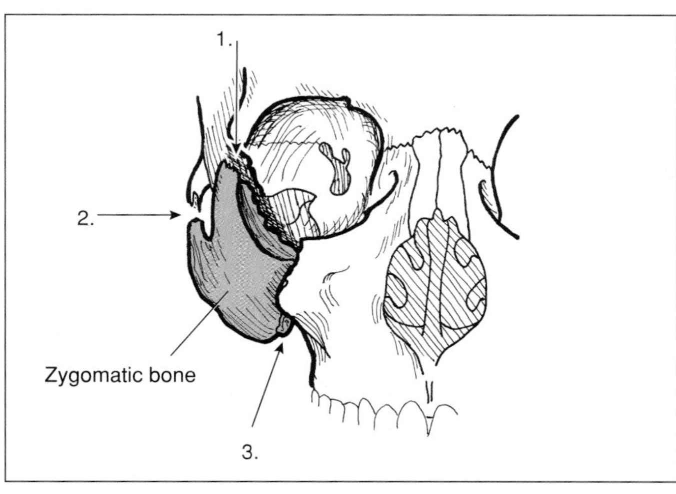

Fig. 11-49. "Tripod" fracture.

ANATOMY REVIEW

Review exercises for anatomy of the cranial and facial bones follow as demonstrated on both a dry skull and on radiographs. Not all specific anatomy shown on the dry skull can be identified on these radiographs but those parts that are identifiable are labeled as such. A good learning and/or review exercise is to carefully study both the dry skull illustrations and the radiographs, and identify each part before looking at the answers below.

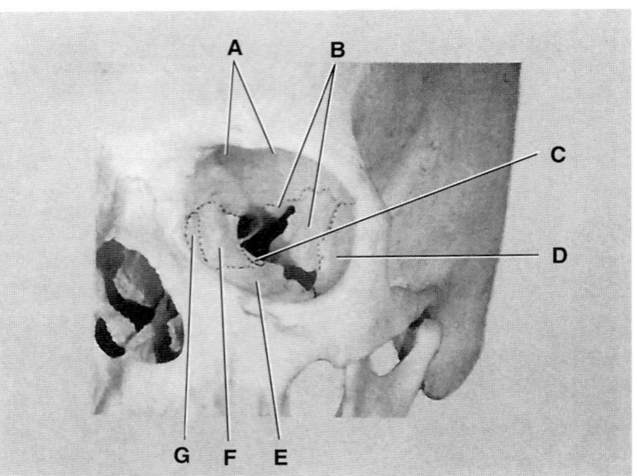

Fig. 11-50. A. Seven bones of left orbit.

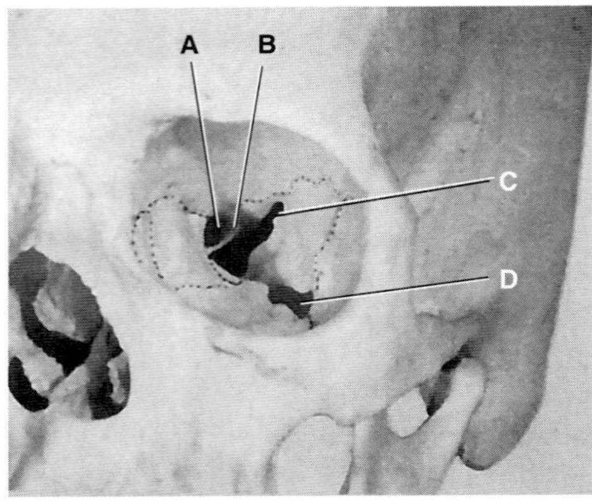

Fig. 11-51. B. Openings of left orbit.

Orbital Structures and Openings

A. Seven Bones of Left Orbit *(Fig. 11-50):*

A. Frontal bone (orbital plate)
B. Sphenoid bone
C. Small portion of palatine bone
D. Zygomatic bone
E. Maxillary bone
F. Ethmoid
G. Lacrimal

B. Openings of Left Orbit *(Fig. 11-51):*

A. Optic foramen
B. Sphenoid strut
C. Superior orbital fissure
D. Inferior orbital fissure

C. Parieto-orbital Projection of Orbits *(Fig. 11-52):*

A. Orbital plate of frontal bone
B. Sphenoid bone
C. Optic foramen and canal
D. Superior orbital fissure
E. Inferior orbital margin
F. Sphenoid strut (part of inferior and lateral wall of optic canal)
G. Lateral orbital margin
H. Superior orbital margin

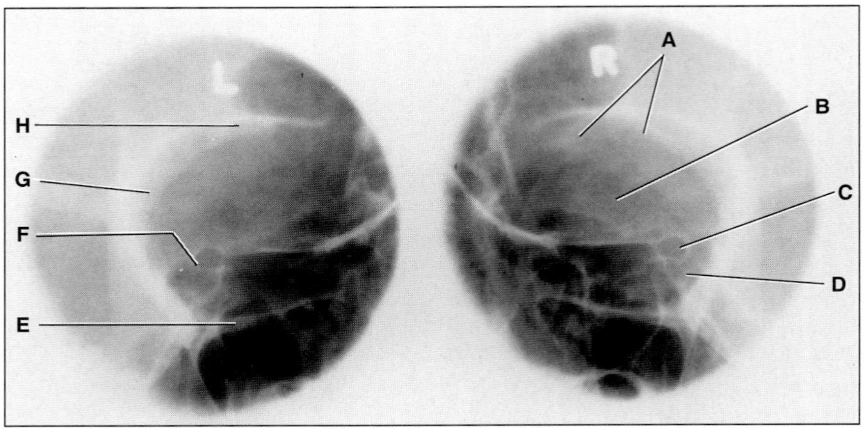

Fig. 11-52. C. Parieto-orbital projection of orbits.

Facial Bones–Frontal View (Fig. 11-53)

A. Left nasal bone
B. Frontal process of left maxilla
C. Optic foramen
D. Superior orbital fissure
E. Inferior orbital fissure
F. Middle nasal conchae of ethmoid bone
G. Vomer facial bone (lower portion of bony nasal septum)
H. Left inferior nasal conchae of facial bone
I. Anterior nasal spine of maxillary bones
J. Alveolar process of left maxilla
K. Alveolar process of left mandible
L. Mental foramen
M. Mentum or mental protuberance
N. Body of right mandible
O. Angle (gonion) of right mandible
P. Ramus of right mandible
Q. Body of right maxilla (contain maxillary sinuses)
R. Zygomatic prominence of right zygomatic bone
S. Outer orbit portion of right zygomatic bone
T. Sphenoid bone (cranial bone)

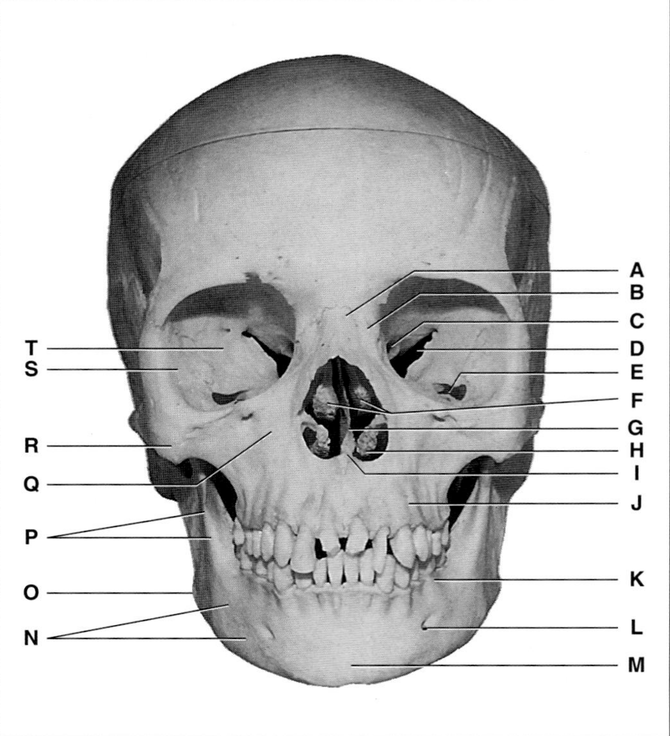

Fig. 11-53. Facial bones–Frontal view.

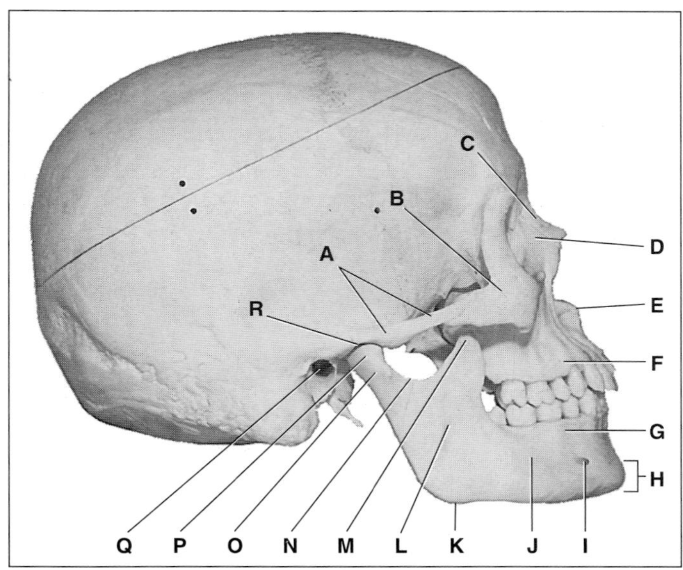

Fig. 11-54. Facial bones–Lateral.

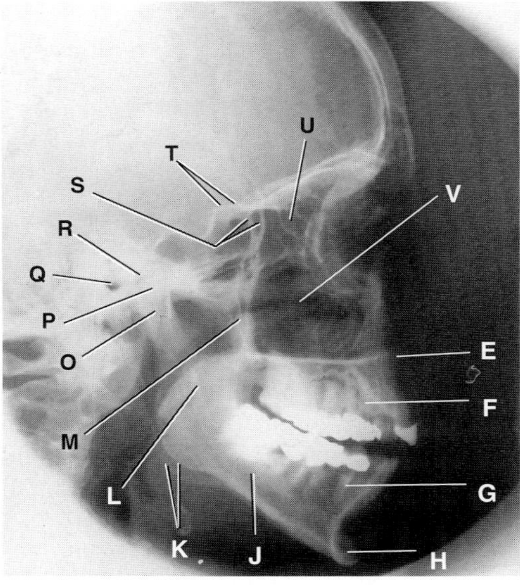

Fig. 11-55. Facial bones–Lateral.

Facial Bones–Lateral

(Figs. 11-54 and 11-55 above)

- *A. Zygomatic arch
- *B. R. zygomatic bone
- *C. R. nasal bone
- *D. Frontal process of R. maxilla
- E. Anterior nasal spine
- F. Alveolar process of maxilla
- G. Alveolar process of mandible
- H. Mentum or mental protuberance
- *I. Mental foramen
- J. Body of mandible
- K. Angle (gonion)
- L. Ramus of mandible
- *M. Coronoid process
- N. Mandibular notch
- O. Neck of mandibular condyle
- P. Condyle or head of mandible
- Q. External acoustic meatus (EAM)
- R. Temporomandibular fossa of temporal bone
- †S. Greater wings of sphenoid
- †T. Lesser wings of sphenoid with anterior clinoid processes
- †U. Ethmoid sinuses between orbits
- †V. Body of maxilla containing maxillary sinuses

* Skeleton only (Fig. 11-54). † Radiograph only (Fig. 11-55).

Facial Bones–Parietoacanthial (Waters)

(Figs. 11-56 and 11-57 below)

The photograph (Fig. 11-56) represents the skull in a parietoacanthial projection (Waters position), with the head tilted back. This results in a parietoacanthial projection, which is one of the more common projections to visualize the facial bones.

A. Zygomatic prominence
B. Body of maxilla (contains maxillary sinuses)
C. Bony nasal septum (perpendicular plate of ethmoid and vomer bone)
D. Anterior nasal spine
E. Zygomatic arch
F. Coronoid process
G. Condyle (head)
H. Mastoid process of temporal bone
I. Angle of mandible
J. Foramen magnum (radiograph demonstrates the dens or odontoid process within foramen magnum)

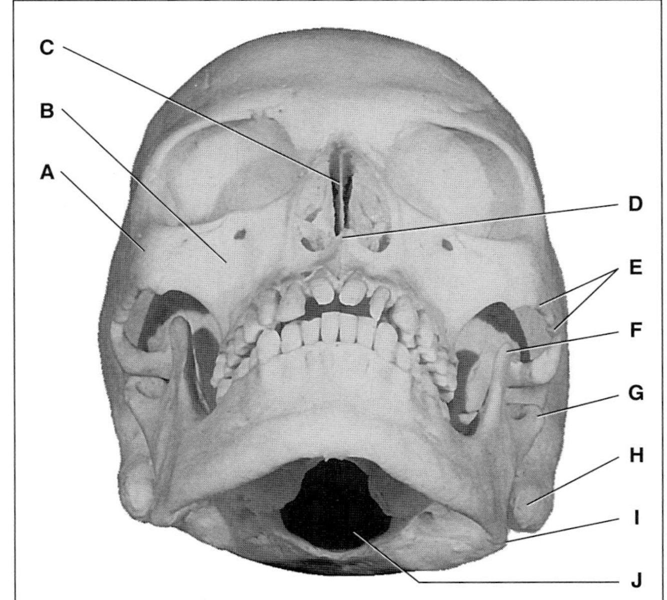

Fig. 11-56. Facial bones–Parietoacanthial projection (Waters). Fig. 11-57.

Anatomy Review continued

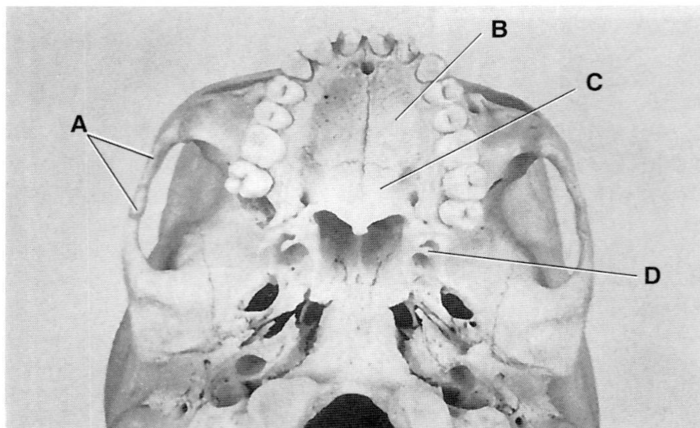

Fig. 11-58. Facial bones–Inferior view.

Facial Bones–SMV (Inferior View)

The photograph above illustrates an inferior view of the dry skull with the mandible removed. The submentovertex projection radiograph on the right is positioned with the top (vertex) of the head against the film with the central ray entering under the chin (mentum).

Skull only *(Fig 11-58):*

A. Zygomatic arch
B. Palatine process of maxilla
C. Horizontal process of palatine
D. Pterygoid hamulus of sphenoid

Radiograph only *(Fig. 11-59):*

E. Foramen ovale of sphenoid
F. Foramen spinosum of sphenoid
G. Foramen magnum
H. Petrous pyramid of temporal bone
I. Mastoid portion of temporal bone
J. Sphenoid sinus in body of sphenoid
K. Condyle (head) of mandible
L. Posterior border (vertical portion) of palatine bone
M. Vomer or bony nasal septum
N. Right maxillary sinuses
O. Ethmoid sinuses

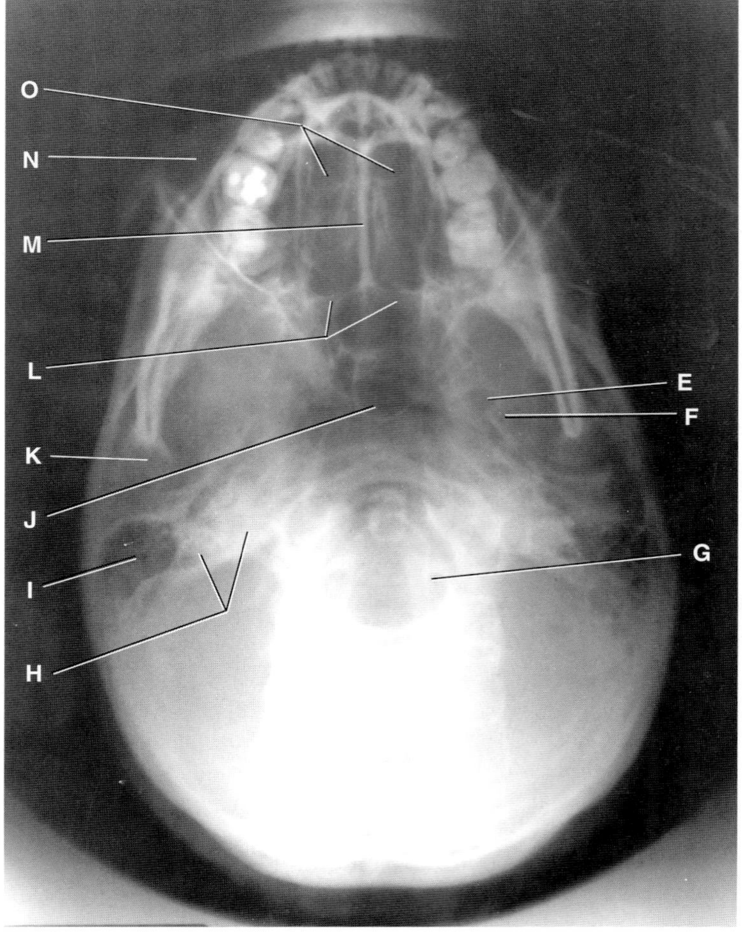

Fig. 11-59. Submentovertex (SMV) projection.

Radiographic Positioning

Skull Radiography

Traditionally skull radiography has been one of the most difficult and challenging parts of the body to radiograph. A good understanding of the anatomy and relationships of bones and structures of the skull as described in this chapter is essential prior to beginning a study of radiographic positioning of the cranium or facial bones. Radiographing certain parts of the skull such as the more obscure internal structures by conventional radiographs is less common today due to advances in other imaging modalities such as computed tomography (CT) and magnetic resonance imaging (MRI). However, in some situations these newer imaging modalities will not be available or practical to use and every radiographer should be able to do conventional film radiography as described in this chapter.

SKULL MORPHOLOGY
(Skull Classifications by Shape & Size)

Mesocephalic Skull

The shape of the average head is termed **mesocephalic** *(mes′ o-se-fal′ ik)*. The average caliper measurements of the adult skull are 15 centimeters between the parietal eminences (lateral), 19 centimeters from frontal eminence to external occipital protuberance (AP or PA), and 23 centimeters from vertex to beneath the chin (SMV projection). While most adults have a skull of the average size and shape, there are exceptions to the rule.

A general basis for describing skull types is by comparing the width of the skull at the parietal eminence to the length measured from the frontal eminence to the external occipital protuberance. For an average mesocephalic skull the **width is between 75 and 80% of the length.***

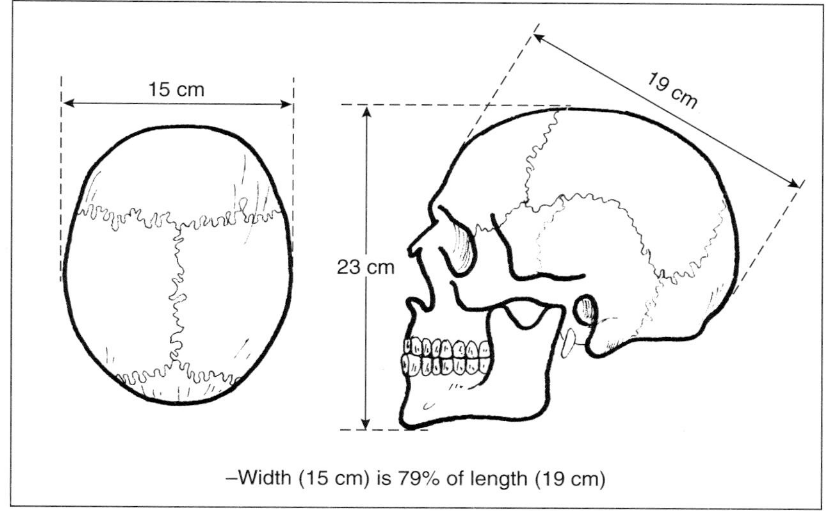

Fig. 11-60. Average skull (mesocephalic).

Brachycephalic and Dolichocephalic Skulls

Variations of the average-shaped or mesocephalic skull include the **brachycephalic** *(brak′ e-se-fal′ ik)* and the **dolichocephalic** *(dol′ i-ko-se-fal′ ik)* designations. The short, broad head is termed brachycephalic; while the long, narrow head is called dolichocephalic.

The width of the brachycephalic type **is 80% or greater** than the length. The width on the long, narrow dolichocephalic is **less than 75%** of the length.*

A second variation to remember is the angle difference between the petrous pyramids and the midsagittal plane. In the average-shaped, mesocephalic head, the petrous pyramids form an angle of **47°**. An angle **greater than 47°** (approximately 54°) is found in the brachycephalic skull; while an angle **less than 47°** (approximately 40°) is found in the dolichocephalic designation.

Positioning Considerations Related to Skull Morphology: The positioning descriptions including CR angles and head rotations as described in this text are based on the average-shaped mesocephalic skull. For example, the axiolateral oblique projection (Law method) for the mastoids or the temporomandibular joints requires 15° of head rotation (Chapter 12). A long, narrow dolichocephalic head would require slightly more than 15° of rotation and a short, broad brachycephalic type would require less than 15°. The 45° oblique Stenvers method projection for the mastoids would also require a slight adjustment for these variations in skull shapes.

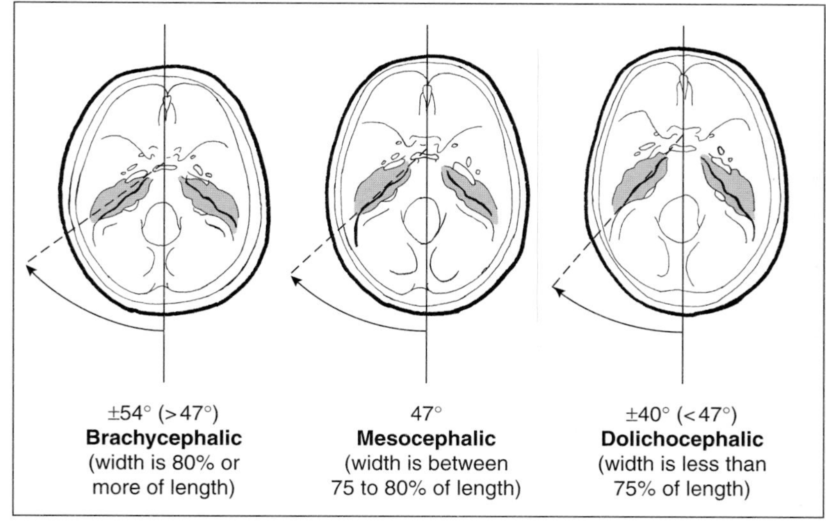

Fig. 11-61. Variable shapes.

*Gray, H. *Gray's Anatomy,* 30th ed. Philadelphia: Lea and Febiger; 1985.

CRANIAL TOPOGRAPHY (SURFACE LANDMARKS)

Certain surface landmarks and localizing lines must be used for accurate positioning of the cranium. Each of the following topographical structures can either be seen or palpated.

Body Planes

The **midsagittal** or **median plane (MSP)** divides the body into left and right halves. This plane is important in accurate positioning of the cranium since, for every frontal or lateral projection, the midsagittal plane is either perpendicular to, or parallel to, the plane of the film.

The **interpupillary (IPL)** or **interorbital line** is a line connecting either the pupils or the outer canthi of the patient's eyes. When the head is placed in a **true lateral** position, the interpupillary line must be exactly perpendicular to the plane of the film.

Frontal and Side View Landmarks

The **superciliary ridge** (arch) is that ridge or arch of bone extending across the forehead directly above each eye.

Slightly above this ridge is a slight groove or depression termed the **supraorbital groove** or SOG.

Note: You should remember that the SOG is important because it corresponds to the highest level of the facial bone mass, which is also the level of the **floor of the anterior fossa** of the cranial vault.

The **glabella** *(glah-bel′ ah)* is the smooth, slightly depressed triangular area between and slightly superior to the eyebrows and above the bridge of the nose.

The **nasion** *(na′ ze-on)* is the depression at the bridge of the nose. Anatomically, the nasion is the junction of the two nasal bones and the frontal bone.

The **acanthion** *(ah-kan′ the-on,* little thorn) is the midline point at the junction of the upper lip and the nasal septum. This is the point where the nose and upper lip meet.

The **angle** or **gonion** *(go′ ne-on)*, refers to the lower posterior angle on each side of the jaw or mandible.

A flat triangular area projects forward as the chin (mentum) in the human. The mid point of this triangular area of the chin as it appears from the front is termed the **mental point**.

Ear: Parts of the ear which may be used as positioning landmarks are the **auricle** or **pinna** (external portion of ear), the large flap of ear made of cartilage, and the **tragus**, the small cartilaginous flap covering the opening of the ear. The **TEA** (Top of Ear Attachment) refers to the superior attachment of the auricle, or that part where the side frames of one's eyeglasses rest. This is an important landmark because it corresponds to the **level of the petrous ridge** on each side.

Eye: The junctions of the upper and lower eyelids are termed **canthi** *(kan′ thi)*. Thus the **inner canthus** *(kan′ thus)* is where the eyelids meet near the nose, while the more lateral junction of the eyelids is termed the **outer canthus**.

The superior rim of bony orbit of the eye is termed the **supraorbital margin** or **SOM**, and the inferior rim is termed the **infraorbital margin** or **IOM**. Another landmark is the **midlateral orbital margin**, that portion of the lateral rim near the outer canthus of the eye.

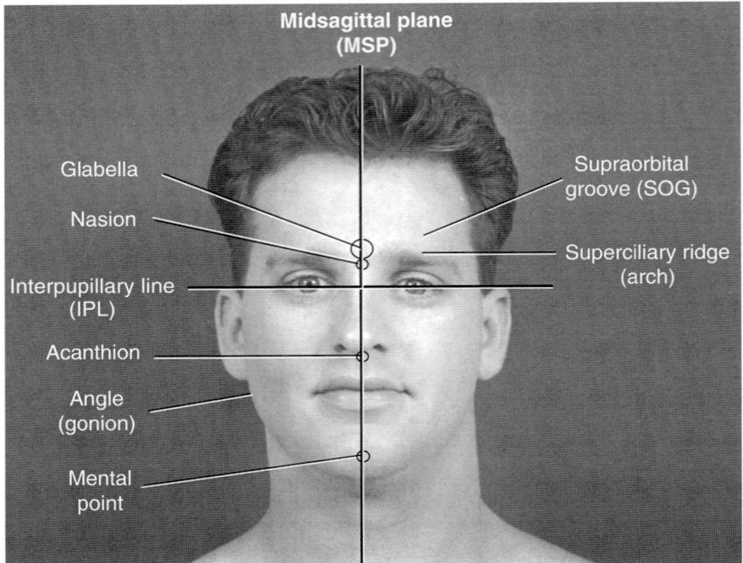

Fig. 11-62. Body planes and landmarks.

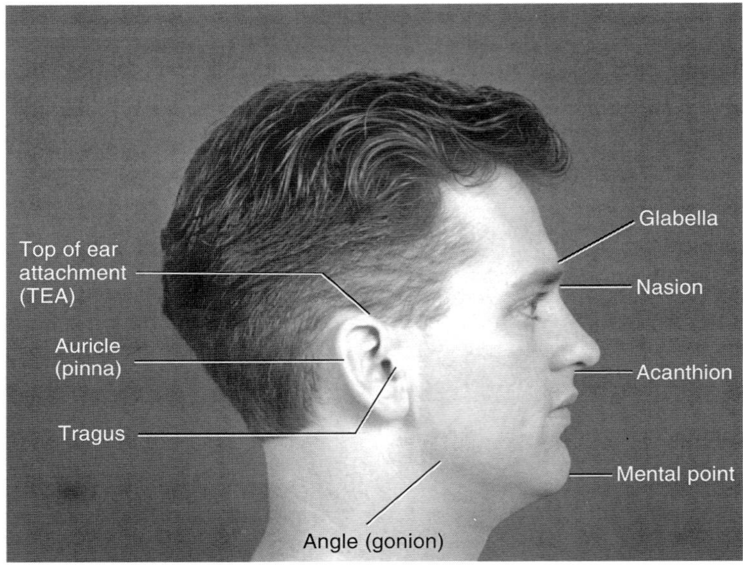

Fig. 11-63. Surface landmarks.

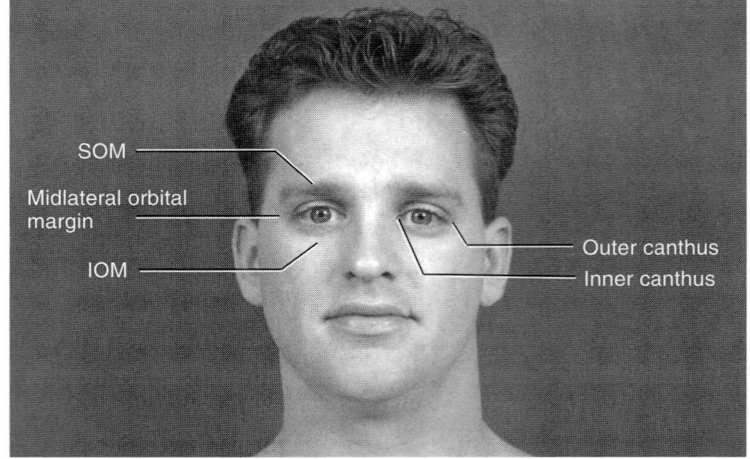

Fig. 11-64. Base of orbit landmarks.

Skull Positioning Lines

Certain positioning lines are important in skull radiography. These lines are formed by connecting certain anterior landmarks to the mid point of the **external acoustic (auditory) meatus (EAM)**. The EAM is the opening of the external ear canal. The center point of this opening is called the **auricular point**.

The most superior of these positioning lines is the **glabellomeatal line (GML)**, which is not as precise as the other lines since the glabella is an area and not a specific point. The GML refers to a line between the glabella and the EAM.

The **orbitomeatal line (OML)** is a frequently used positioning line located between the outer canthus (mid-lateral orbital margin) and the EAM.

The **infraorbitomeatal line (IOML)** is formed by connecting the middle of the infraorbital margin to the EAM. Two older terms identify this same line as **Reid's base line** or **anthropological base line**. Sometimes this is also referred to as just the **base line** of the cranium, although these terms are not used in this text.

There is an average **7 to 8°** angle difference between the orbitomeatal and the infraorbitomeatal lines. There is also an approximate **7 to 8°** average angle difference between the orbitomeatal and glabellomeatal lines. Knowing the angle differences between these three lines is helpful in making positioning adjustments for specific projections of the cranium and facial bones.

The **acanthiomeatal line (AML)** and the **mentomeatal line (MML)** are important in radiography of the facial bones. These lines are formed by connecting the acanthion and the mental point, respectively, to the EAM.

A line from the junction of the lips to the EAM, called the **lips-meatal line (LML)** is a positioning line used in this textbook to position for a specific projection of the facial bones called a modified Water's projection.

The **glabelloalveolar line (GAL)** connects the glabella to a point at the anterior aspect of the alveolar process of the maxilla. This line is used for positioning a tangential projection for the nasal bones.

The **inion** *(in′e-on)* is the most prominent point of the external occipital protuberance, a rise or bump along the midline of the lower back of the head near the junction of the head and neck where posterior muscles attach. An extension of the IOML posteriorly approximates the location of the inion.

Skull Positioning Aids

Various types of positioning aids can be used for determining precise angles required for accurate cranial or facial bones positioning. One common example of such is **a cardboard straightedge** cut at a specific angle, to accurately position the cranium. In Fig. 11-66, a 90° straightedge is shown to determine that the orbitomeatal line has been placed perpendicular to the film plane by depressing the chin as needed, or by placing a support under the back of the head if the chin cannot be depressed far enough. The chin can be raised or lowered to change the perpendicular reference line to be used in relationship to the central ray.

Other types of adjustable devices can be used for determining various degrees of angle in skull positioning. One example is the "angle finder" which indicates the number of degrees from horizontal, or in this example the degrees between the OML and the table-top (film).

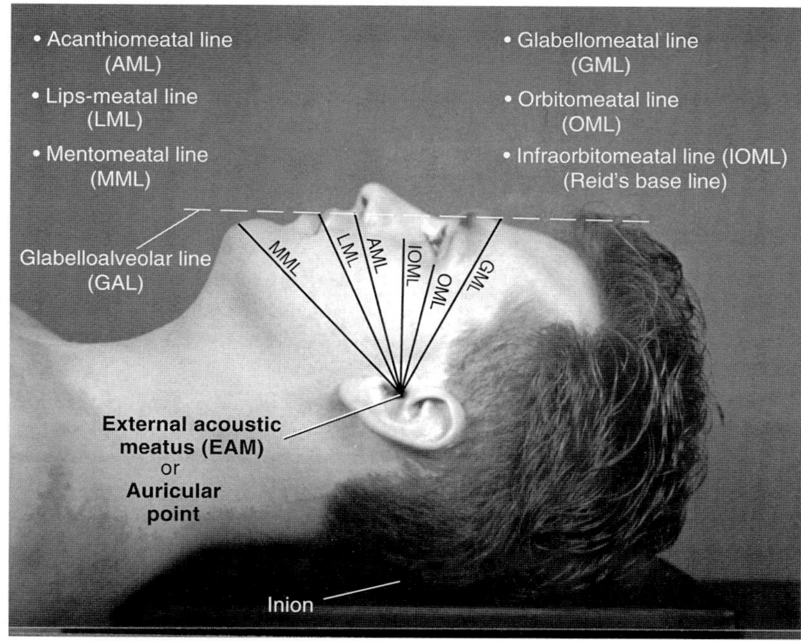

Fig. 11-65. Positioning lines.

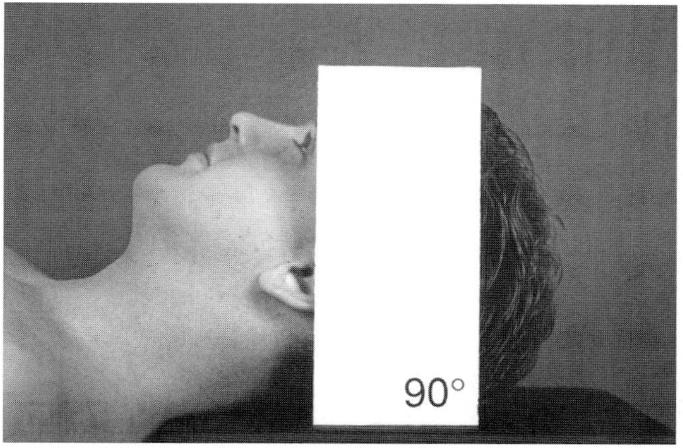

Fig. 11-66. Positioning aid–90° straightedge.

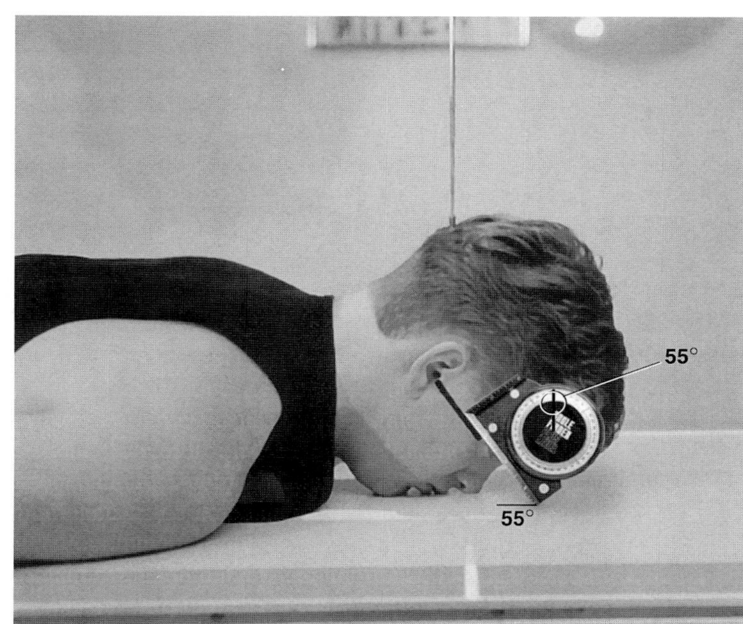

Fig. 11-67. Positioning aid–"Angle finder" demonstrating 55° OML to film (PA modified Waters projection)

(Courtesy of Dasco Pro Inc., Rockford, IL.)

POSITIONING CONSIDERATIONS

Erect vs. Recumbent

Projections of the skull may be taken recumbent or erect if the patient's condition allows. The erect can be accomplished by utilizing an upright head unit, a standard x-ray table in the vertical position or an erect grid-film holder. The erect position allows the patient to be quickly and easily positioned and permits a horizontal beam to be utilized. A horizontal beam is necessary to visualize any existing air fluid levels within the inner cranial or sinus cavities.

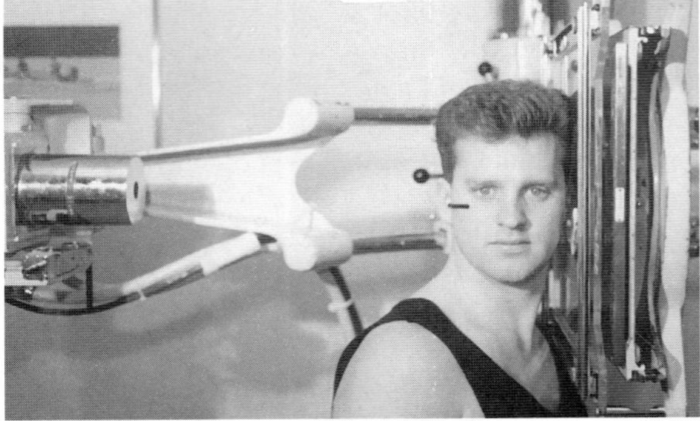

Fig. 11-68. Erect–Head unit.

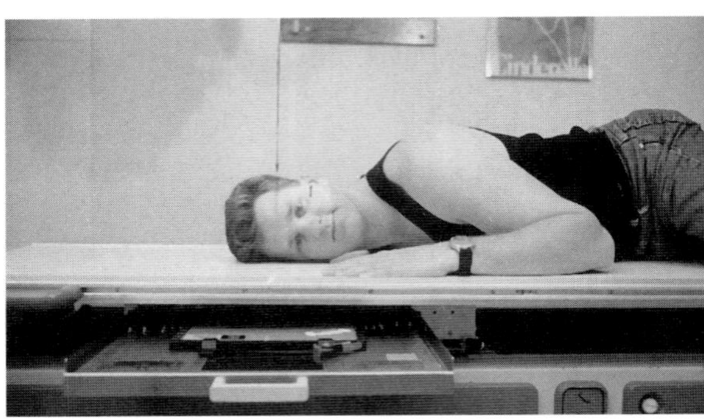

Fig. 11-69. Recumbent–Table-top.

Patient Comfort

Patient motion almost always results in an unsatisfactory radiograph. During skull radiography the head must be placed in precise positions and held there long enough to obtain a motionless exposure. Always remember that there is a patient attached to the other end of the skull being manipulated. Every effort should be made to make the body as comfortable as possible and to utilize positioning aids such as sponges, sandbags and compression devices.

Except for severe trauma patients, patients should be asked to suspend respiration (hold their breath) during the exposure to help in preventing motion of the head from breathing movements of the thorax, especially if the patient is in a prone position. This, however, generally is not necessary for erect skull radiographs.

Personal Hygiene: Cranial and facial radiography may require the patient's face to be in direct contact with the table-top or erect film holders. Therefore, it is important these surfaces be cleaned with disinfectant between patients.

Exposure Factors

The principal exposure factors for radiographs of the skull are:

- Medium kVp, 75-85.
- Short exposure time.
- Small focal spot (if equipment allows).
- Adequate mAs for anatomical area of interest.

SID

Certain types of head unit equipment as demonstrated in this chapter have a fixed SID of 36 in. (91 cm). A common table SID with cassette in bucky is listed as 40 in. (102 cm) **minimum distance.** Some departments increase this to 42 or 44 in. (107 to 112 cm) resulting in a reduction in skin dose and less magnification.

Radiation Protection

The best protection for minimizing radiation exposure to the patient in skull radiography is first, to use **good collimation practices**, and second to **minimize repeats**. The special head units generally utilize a circle or rectangular diaphragm to limit the exposure field to approximately the size of film. Adjustable collimators are used with conventional table units and collimation borders should be adjusted closely to the area of interest.

The exposure factors and patient doses provided in the icon boxes on positioning pages are calculated for an SID of 40 in. or 102 cm, (doses would be about 30% higher at 36 in. (91 cm) with same exposure factors).

Gonadal Shielding: Generally, gonadal shielding does not need to be used in skull radiography. According to publication HEW 76-8031; *Handbook of Selected Organ Doses for Projections Common in Diagnostic Radiology,* with accurate collimation there is no detectable contribution to gonadal exposure when radiographing the skull. However, shields placed over the pelvic region can be used for patient assurance.

Thyroid and Breast Shielding: Frontal views (AP) of the skull and facial bones can result in additional exposure to the radiosensitive thyroid (and breast on females). A contact shield placed over the neck and chest can be used for these projections. When provided a choice, PA rather than AP projections should be selected.

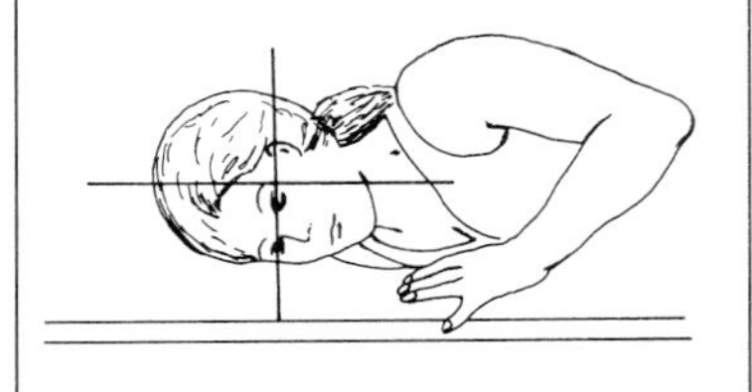

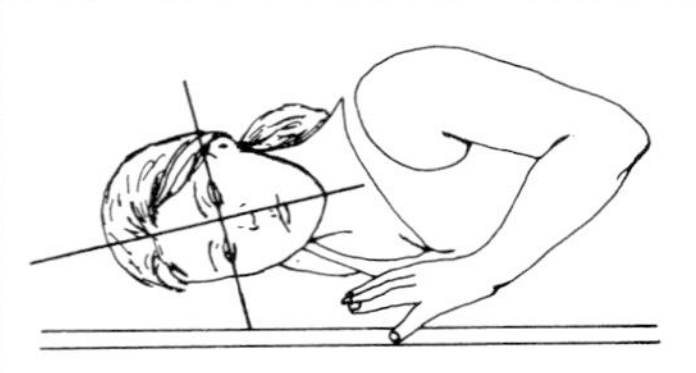

Fig. 11-70. Rotation. Tilt.

Causes of Positioning Errors

When positioning a patient's head, it is necessary to look at various facial features and palpate numerous anatomical landmarks in order to place certain planes precisely in relation to the plane of the film. Although the human body is supposed to be bilaterally symmetrical, (that is, the right half is supposed to be exactly like the left half), this supposition is not always true. The ears, nose and jaw are often asymmetrical. The nose frequently deviates to one side of the midsagittal plane, while the ears are not necessarily in the same place nor of the same size on each side.

The lower jaw or mandible is also often asymmetrical. Bony parts, such as the mastoid tips and the orbital margins, are safer landmarks to use. While you often look at the patient's eyes during positioning, it is best not to look at the nose in between, which is frequently not straight.

Five Common Positioning Errors

Rotation (1) and **tilt** (2) are two very common positioning errors. Rotation of the skull almost always results in a retake, therefore it is important that the head is not turned to one side. Tilt is a tipping or slanting of the midsagittal plane to one side, even though rotation is not present.

Excessive flexion (3) or **excessive extension** (4) of the head (chin elevated or lowered too much) along with an **incorrect CR** (5) angle are 5 potential positioning errors in skull and facial bone positioning that must be avoided.

11

NATIONAL SURVEY

Departmental standards (basic) and optional routines for exams of the cranium and sella turcica were somewhat consistent throughout the United States. The results of this survey determined national norms for routines as presented in the positioning pages which follow.

Skull Series Routine

Cranium (skull) series	U.S. Average	
	Basic 1995 (1989)	Special 1995 (1989)
• AP axial (Towne method)	93% (95%)	
• Lateral	89% (89%)	
• PA axial 15° caudad (Caldwell method)	63% (57%)	
or		
PA 0°	51% (55%)	
or		
PA axial 25 to 30° caudad	11% –	10% –
• Basilar (SMV)	24% (21%)	35% (8%)
• PA axial 25° cephalad (Haas method)		30% –
Trauma skull series (Chapter 19)		
• Lateral (cross table)	79% –	
• AP 15° cephalad	36% (51%)	11% (20%)
or		
AP 0°	55% (43%)	11% –
• AP axial (Towne method)	63% (20%)	7% (13%)

Sella Turcica Routine

Sella turcica	U.S. Average	
	Basic 1995 (1989)	Special 1995 (1989)
• Lateral	80% (96%)	
• AP axial–37°	59% (30%)	
or		
AP axial–30° (Towne method)	– (20%)	
• PA 0° cephalad	– (24%)	
• PA 25° axial (Haas method)	– (13%)	

Summary

Skull Series: The most common projections for the routine skull series continues to be the **AP Towne** (93%), **lateral** (89%) and **PA Caldwell** (63%). This was very consistent throughout all regions of the U.S. and did not change significantly from 1989.

The **PA axial 25° cephalad (Haas method)** was indicated to be a special projection for the skull series by 30% of survey responders. This was a higher frequency than in 1989, but the question previously was asked as part of the sella turcica routine rather than the skull series, which may have affected the results.

Trauma Skull Series: The basic projections most common for the trauma skull series are the **horizontal beam lateral** (79%), **AP axial (Towne)** (63%) and **AP 0°** (55%). This did change some from the 1989 survey which indicated the AP 15° cephalad to be more common than the AP 0°.

Note: The description of these **trauma projections** has been moved from this skull chapter to the new **Chapter 19** on mobile and trauma radiography.

Sella Turcica: The lateral, as expected, was the most common basic projection for the sella turcica, with other less frequent AP or PA projections indicated. Each of these will be included as possible special projections for the sella turcica in this chapter.

STANDARD AND SPECIAL OPERATING PROCEDURES

Certain basic and special projections or positions for the cranium (skull series) and the sella turcica are demonstrated and described on the following pages as suggested standard and special departmental procedures.

Basic Projections

Standard or basic projections, also sometimes referred to as routine projections or departmental routines are those projections or positions commonly taken on average patients who are helpful and can cooperate in performing the procedure.

Special Projections

Special projections are those more common projections taken as extra or additional projections to better demonstrate certain pathologic conditions or specific body parts.

Basic and Special Projections

(For trauma skull series see Chapter 19–Trauma and Mobile Radiography.)

Skull series
Basic
- AP axial (Towne method) **349**
  or PA axial (Haas method) **350**
- Lateral **351**
- PA axial 15° (Caldwell method) **352**
  or PA axial 25 to 30° **352**
  or PA 0° **353**

Special
- Submentovertex (SMV) **354**

Sella turcica
Basic
- Lateral **355**
- AP axial (Towne method) **356**

Special
- PA axial 10°
  or PA axial 25° cephalad **357**
  (Haas method)

AP Axial Projection
Towne Method

Skull series
Basic
• **AP axial (Towne method)** or PA axial (Haas method)
• Lateral
• PA 15° (Caldwell method) or PA 25 to 30°
• PA 0°

Structures Best Shown

Occipital bone, petrous pyramids and foramen magnum with dorsum sellae and posterior clinoids in its shadow.

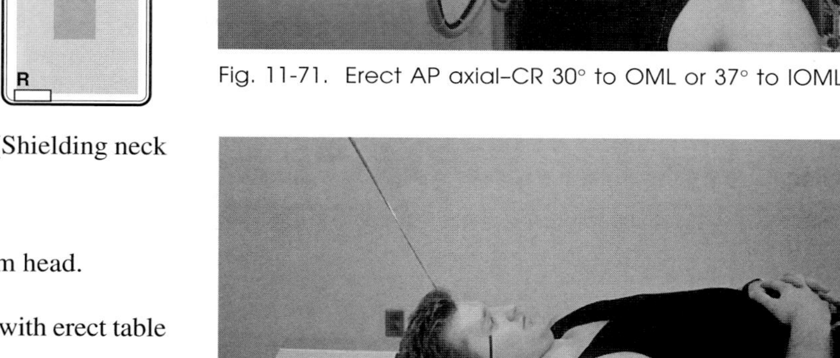

Fig. 11-71. Erect AP axial–CR 30° to OML or 37° to IOML.

Technical Factors

- Film size–10 x 12 in. (24 x 30 cm), lengthwise.
- Moving or stationary grid.
- 70-80 kVp range.
- Use small focal spot.
- Technique and dose:

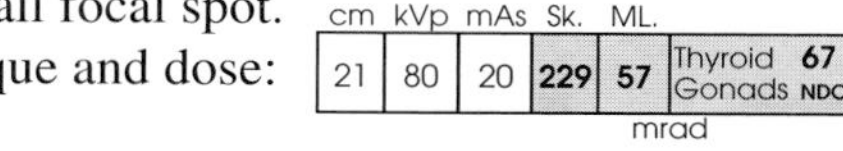

cm	kVp	mAs	Sk.	ML.	
21	80	20	229	57	Thyroid 67 Gonads NDC

mrad

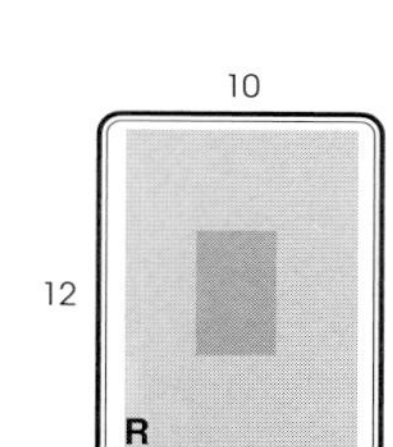

Shielding: Place contact shield over upper thorax region. (Shielding neck and thyroid region may obscure area of interest.)

Patient Position

- Remove all metal, plastic or other removable objects from head.
- Patient erect or supine on table.
- Erect may be done with dedicated head unit if available or with erect table or other erect grid-film holder device.

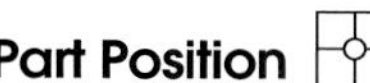

Part Position

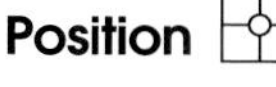

- Depress chin, bringing **OML (or IOML) perpendicular** to film. Add radiolucent support under head if needed. (See Note).
- Align midsagittal plane to CR and to midline of head unit or table-top.
- Ensure **no head rotation and/or tilt**, EAMs same distance from table-top.
- Ensure that vertex of skull is in x-ray field.

Fig. 11-72. Supine–AP axial, CR 30° to OML or 37° to IOML.

Central Ray

- Angle CR **30° caudad to OML** (See Note).
- Center at midsagittal plane, **2½ in.** (6 cm) **above glabella**, or to pass through ≈¾ in. (2 cm) superior to the level of EAMs.
- Center cassette to projected CR.
- SID: Head unit, 36 in. (91 cm). Table, minimum 40 in. (102 cm).

Collimation: Collimate to outer margins of skull on all sides.

Respiration: Suspend respiration.

Note: If patient is unable to depress the chin sufficiently to bring the **OML** perpendicular to the film even with a small sponge under head, the infraorbitomeatal line **(IOML)** can be placed perpendicular instead and the CR angle increased to **37°** caudad. This maintains the **30° angle between OML and CR** and demonstrates the same anatomical relationships. (There is a 7° difference between the OML and IOML.)

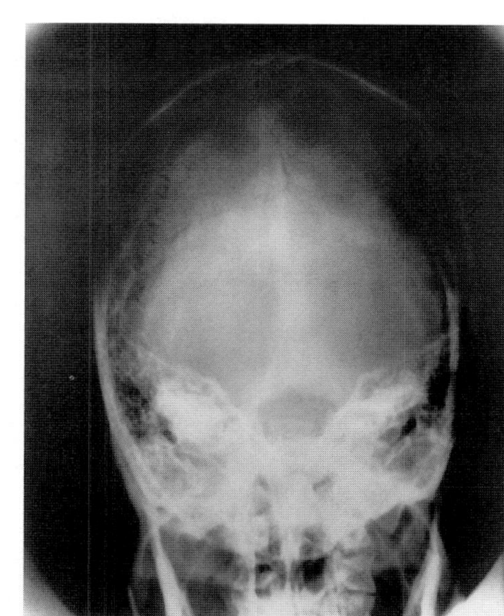

Fig. 11-73. AP axial.

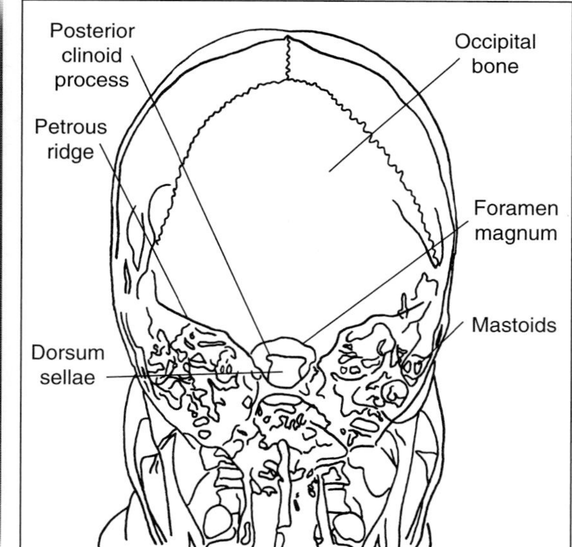

Fig. 11-74. AP axial.

Evaluation Criteria

- Dorsum sella and posterior clinoids are projected into foramen magnum (indicates correct CR angle and proper head flexion/extension).
- Entire skull visualized on radiograph with vertex of skull near top of film.
- Equal distance from foramen magnum to lateral margin of skull on each side (indicates no rotation).
- Petrous ridges are symmetrical and visualized superior to the mastoids.
- Sufficient penetration and exposure, without motion, to visualize occipital bone and sellar structures within foramen magnum.

PA Axial Projection
Haas Method

Skull series
Basic
- AP axial (Towne method) **or PA axial (Haas method)**
- Lateral
- PA 15° (Caldwell method) or PA 25 to 30°
- PA 0°

Structures Best Shown

Occipital bone, petrous pyramids and foramen magnum with dorsum sellae and posterior clinoids in its shadow.

This is an alternate for those patients who cannot flex the neck sufficiently for the reversal position of an AP Towne. Results in magnification of occipital area and sellar structures but results in smaller doses to facial region and thyroid.

Not recommended for occipital bone due to excessive magnification.

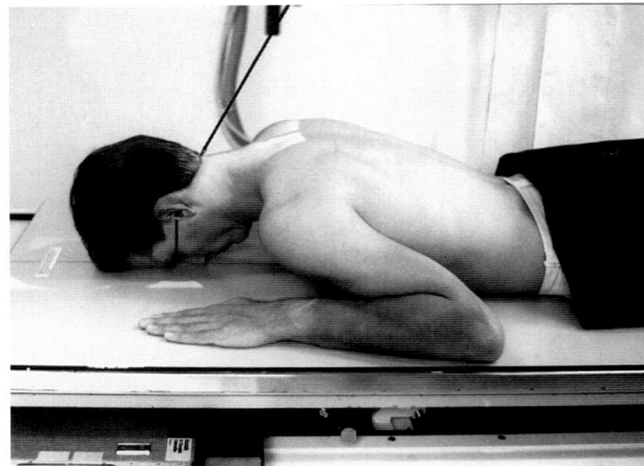
Fig. 11-75. PA axial–CR 25° cephalad to OML.

Technical Factors

- Film size–10 x 12 in. (24 x 30 cm), lengthwise
- Moving or stationary grid.
- 70-80 kVp range.
- Use small focal spot.
- Technique and dose:

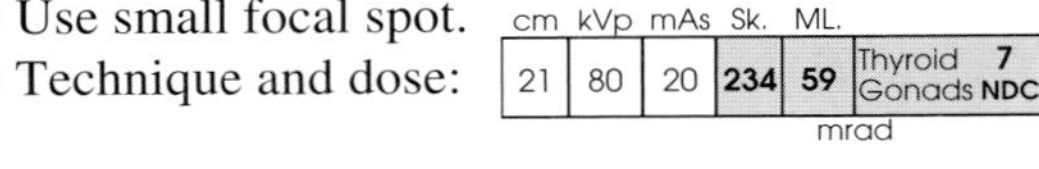

cm	kVp	mAs	Sk.	ML.	
21	80	20	**234**	**59**	Thyroid **7** Gonads **NDC**

mrad

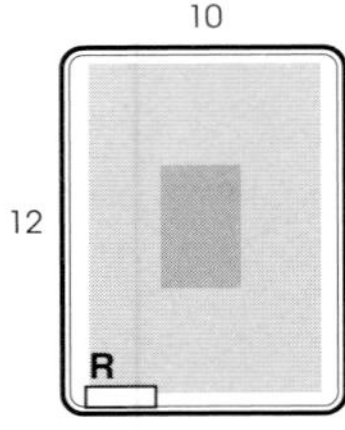

Patient Position

- Remove all metal, plastic or other removable objects from head.
- Patient erect or prone. Start with forehead and nose touching table-top.

Part Position 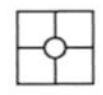

- Flex neck, bringing **OML perpendicular** to film.
- Align midsagittal plane to CR and to midline of film holder and/or table-top.
- Ensure **no rotation or tilt**, EAMs same distance from table-top (midsagittal plane perpendicular to table-top).

Central Ray

- Angle CR **25° cephalad to OML**.
- Center CR at midsagittal plane, **through level of EAMs**.
- Center cassette to projected CR.
- SID: Head unit, 36 in. (91 cm).
  Table, minimum 40 in. (102 cm).

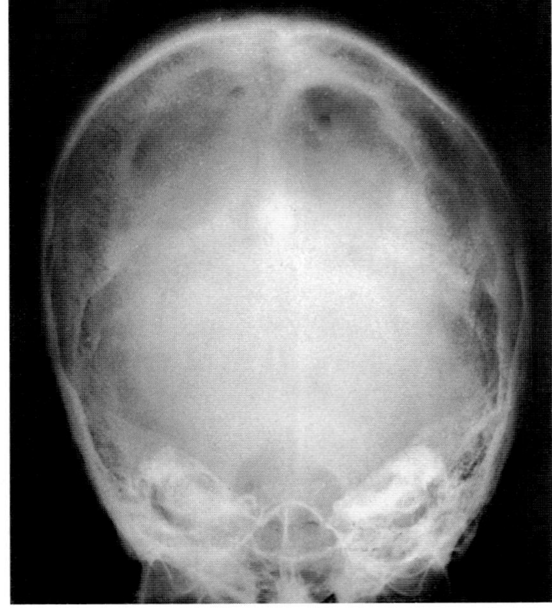
Fig. 11-76. PA axial.

Collimation: Collimate to outer margins of skull on all sides.

Respiration: Suspend respiration.

Evaluation Criteria

- Entire skull visualized on radiograph with vertex of skull near top of film.
- Equal distance from foramen magnum to lateral margin of skull on each side.
- Dorsum sella and posterior clinoids are projected into foramen magnum, which will appear larger due to increased OID.
- Petrous ridges are symmetrical and visualized superior to the mastoids.
- Sufficient penetration and exposure, without motion, to visualize occipital bone and sellar structures within foramen magnum.

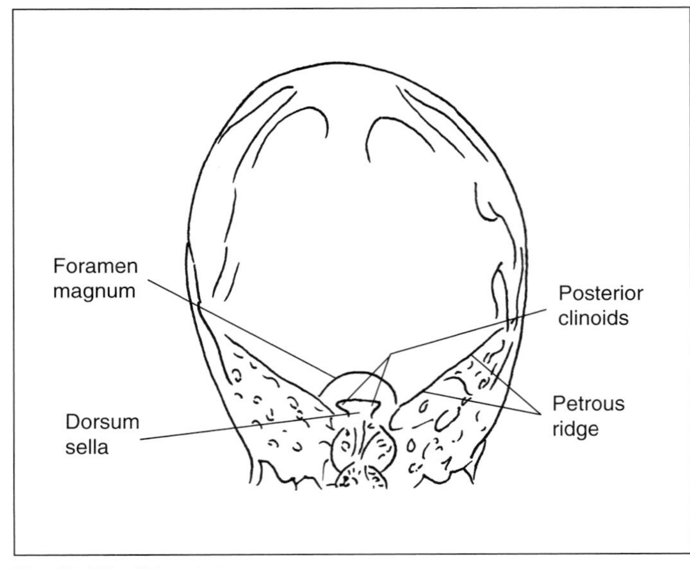

Fig. 11-77. PA axial.

Lateral Position – Right and/or Left Lateral

Skull series
Basic
- AP axial (Towne method) or PA axial (Haas method)
- **Lateral**
- PA 15° (Caldwell method) or PA 25 to 30°
- PA 0°

Structures Best Shown

Best projection for demonstrating the parietal bones. Also demonstrates the total lateral cranium closest to film, sella turcica, anterior and posterior clinoids, dorsum sellae, and greater and lesser wings of sphenoid.

A common general skull routine includes both right and left laterals.

Trauma Routine: A horizontal beam lateral is required to demonstrate air fluid levels. See Chapter 19 for trauma skull positioning.

Technical Factors

- Film size–10 x 12 in. (24 x 30 cm), crosswise.
- Moving or stationary grid.
- 70-80 kVp range.
- Use small focal spot.
- Technique and dose:

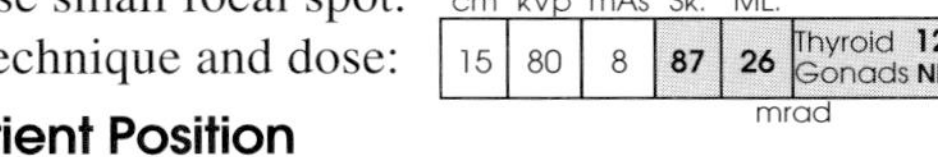

cm	kVp	mAs	Sk.	ML.	
15	80	8	**87**	**26**	Thyroid **12** Gonads **NDC**

mrad

12 10 L

Patient Position

- Remove all metal, plastic or other removable objects from head.
- Patient erect or semi-prone.

Part Position 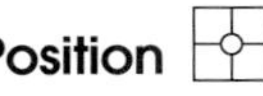

- Place head in a **true lateral position**, with side of interest closest to film, oblique body as needed for patient comfort. (A way to check for rotation is to palpate the external occipital protuberance posteriorly and the nasion or glabella anteriorly and insure that these two points are the same distance from the table-top.)
- Align **midsagittal plane parallel** to film, ensuring **no rotation or tilt**.
- To prevent head tilting, bring **interpupillary line perpendicular** to film. (See Note.)
- Adjust chin to bring **IOML line perpendicular** to front edge of cassette. (GAL will be parallel to front edge of cassette.)

Central Ray

- Align CR **perpendicular** to film.
- Center to a point about **2 in**. (5 cm) **superior to EAM**.
- Center cassette to CR.
- SID: Head unit, 36 in. (91 cm). Table, minimum 40 in. (102 cm).

Collimation: Collimate to outer margins of skull on all sides.

Respiration: Suspend respiration during exposure.

Note: For patients in the recumbent position, a radiolucent support placed under the chin will help in maintaining a true lateral position. A large-chested patient may require a radiolucent sponge under entire head to prevent tilt; and a thin patient may require support under upper thorax.

Evaluation Criteria

- Entire skull visualized on radiograph.
- The cranium is seen without rotation or tilt when:
  - –Mandibular rami, greater and lesser wings of sphenoid and external auditory canals are superimposed.
  - –Sella turcica and clivus are demonstrated in profile without rotation.
- GAL should be parallel to front edge of radiograph, indicating correct flexion/extension.
- Tilt can best be determined by superimposition of orbital roofs (plates).
- Sufficient penetration and exposure, without motion, visualizes sellar structures without overexposing parietal region.

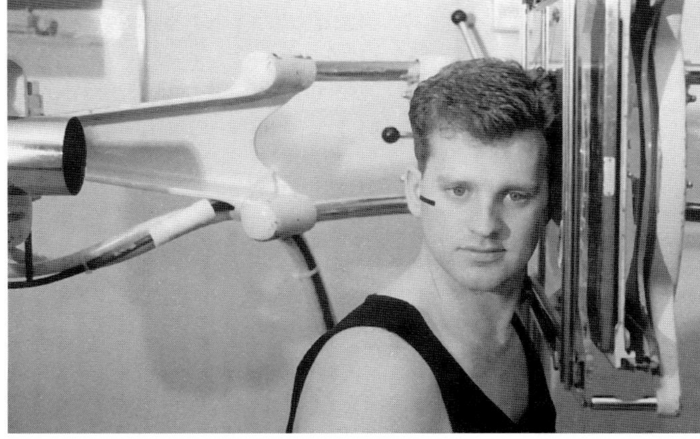

Fig. 11-78. Left lateral–Erect.

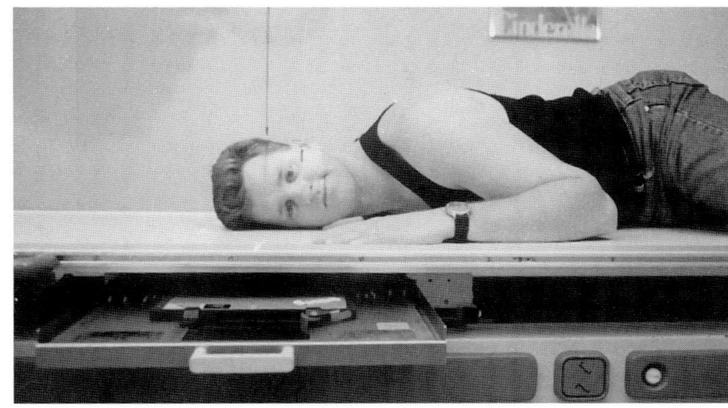

Fig. 11-79. Right lateral–Recumbent.

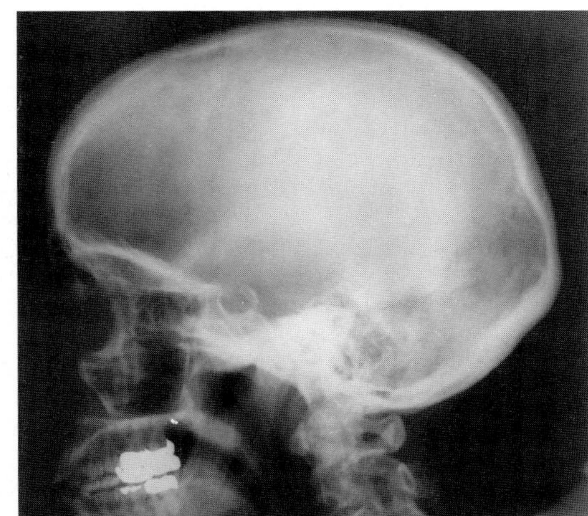

Fig. 11-80. Lateral.

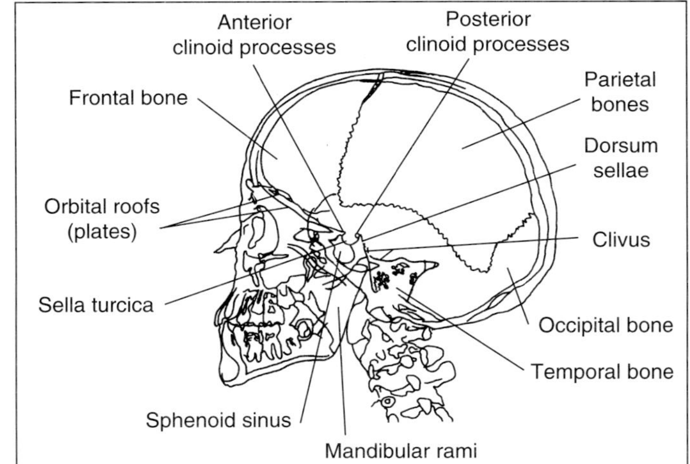

Fig. 11-81. Lateral.

PA Axial Projection

15° CR (Caldwell Method) or 25 to 30° CR

Skull series
Basic
- AP axial (Towne method) or PA axial (Haas method)
- Lateral
- **PA 15° (Caldwell method)** or PA 25 to 30°
- PA 0°

Structures Best Shown

Greater and lesser sphenoid wings, frontal bone, superior orbital fissures, frontal and ethmoid sinuses, foramen rotundum, orbital margin, crista galli, and possibly internal auditory canals.

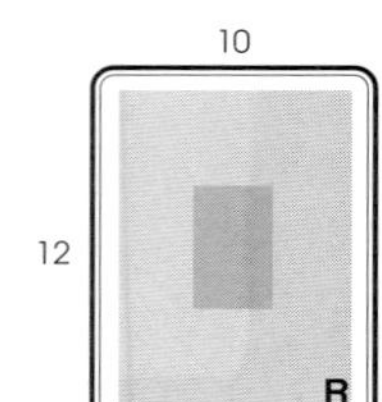

Fig. 11-82. PA–CR 15° caudad, OML perpendicular.

Technical Factors

- Film size–10 x 12 in. (24 x 30 cm), lengthwise.
- Moving or stationary grid.
- 70-80 kVp range.
- Small focal spot.
- Technique and dose:

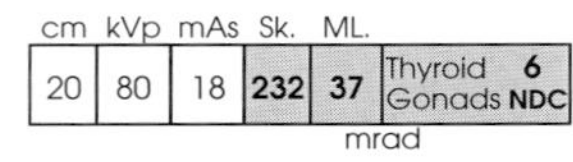

cm	kVp	mAs	Sk.	ML.	
20	80	18	232	37	Thyroid 6 / Gonads NDC
			mrad		

Patient Position

- Remove all metal, plastic or other removable objects from head.
- Patient erect or prone.

Part Position 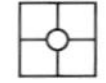

- Rest patient's nose and forehead against head unit or table-top.
- Flex neck as needed to bring **OML perpendicular** to film.
- Align **midsagittal plane perpendicular** to midline of head unit or table-top preventing head rotation and/or tilting.
- Center cassette to CR and to nasion.

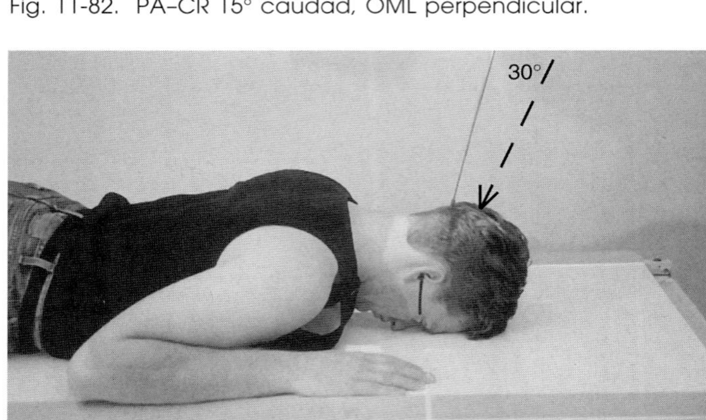

Fig. 11-83. PA–CR 15° caudad, OML perpendicular (and alternate CR 30° caudad-dotted arrow).

Central Ray

- CR angled **15° caudad** and **centered to exit at nasion**.
- Alternate with **CR 25 to 30° caudad** also centered to **exit at nasion**.
- SID: Head unit, 36 in. (91 cm).
  Table, minimum 40 in. (102 cm).

Collimation: Collimate to skull margins.

Respiration: Suspend respiration.

Alternate 25 to 30°: An alternate projection is a **25 to 30° caudad** tube angle to better visualize the superior orbital fissures, the foramen rotundum and the inferior orbital rim region.

Note: A lesser CR caudal angle and/or increased head flexion (chin down) will project the petrous pyramids higher into the orbits.

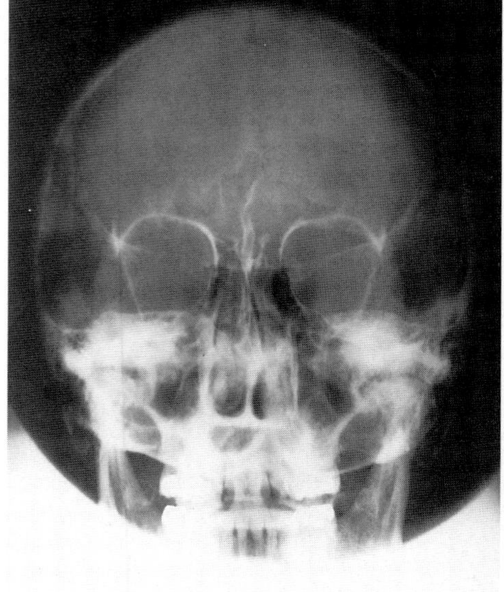

Fig. 11-84. PA–15° caudad (Caldwell).

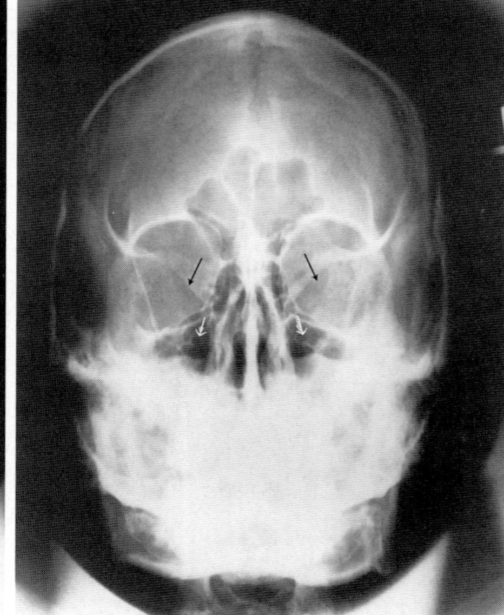

Fig. 11-85. Alternate PA–30° caudad.

Evaluation Criteria

- Entire skull visualized on radiograph.
- **No rotation**: distance from oblique orbital line to lateral margin of skull on each side is equal.
- Superior orbital fissures are symmetrically visualized within orbits.
- Sufficient penetration and exposure, without motion, to visualize frontal bone and sellar structures without overexposing perimeter regions of skull.

PA with 15° caudad angle:
- Petrous pyramids and internal auditory canals (if they can be visualized) are projected into the lower one-third of orbits.
- Superior orbital margin is visualized without superimposition.

PA with 25 to 30° caudad angle:
- Petrous pyramids are projected at the level of, or just below the inferior orbital rim, allowing visualization of the entire orbital margin.
- Foramen rotundum adjacent to each inferior orbital rim is visualized (see white arrows).
- Superior orbital fissures (black arrows) are visualized within orbits.

PA Projection

0° CR

Skull series
Basic
- AP axial (Towne method) or PA axial (Haas method)
- Lateral
- PA 15° (Caldwell method) or PA 25 to 30°
- **PA 0°**

Structures Best Shown

Frontal bone, crista galli, internal auditory canals, frontal and ethmoid sinuses, petrous ridges, greater and lesser wings of sphenoid and dorsum sellae.
A primary projection for frontal bone.

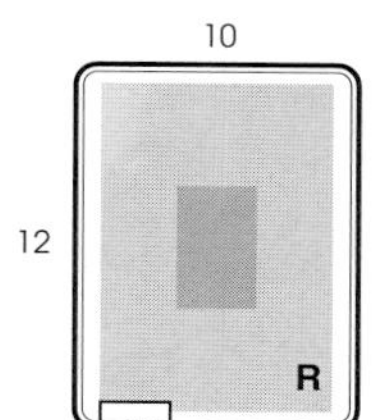

Technical Factors

- Film size–10 x 12 in. (24 x 30 cm), lengthwise.
- Moving or stationary grid.
- 70-80 kVp range.
- Use small focal spot.
- Technique and dose:

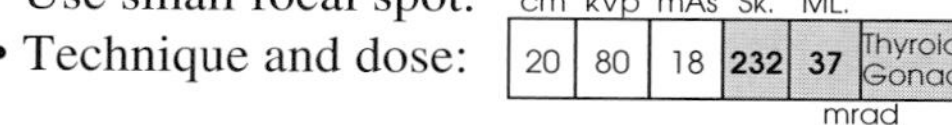

cm	kVp	mAs	Sk.	ML.	
20	80	18	232	37	Thyroid 6 Gonads NDC
			mrad		

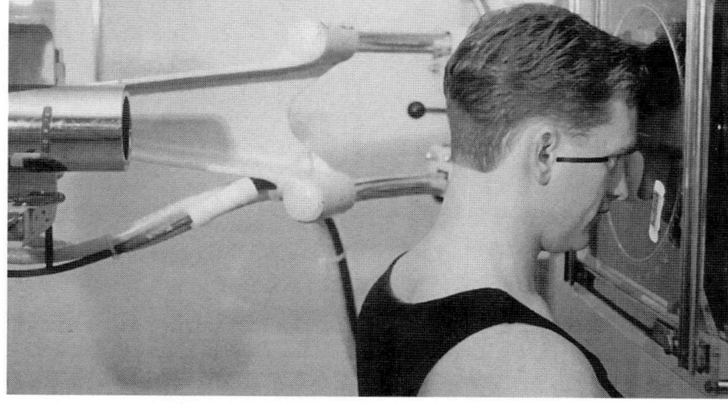

Fig. 11-86. PA–0° CR, OML perpendicular.

Patient Position

- Remove all metal, plastic or other removable objects from head.
- Patient erect or prone.

Part Position

- Rest patient's nose and forehead against head unit or table-top.
- Flex neck bringing **OML perpendicular** to film.
- Align **midsagittal plane perpendicular** to midline of table preventing head rotation and/or tilting (EAMs same distance from table-top).
- Center cassette to CR and to glabella.

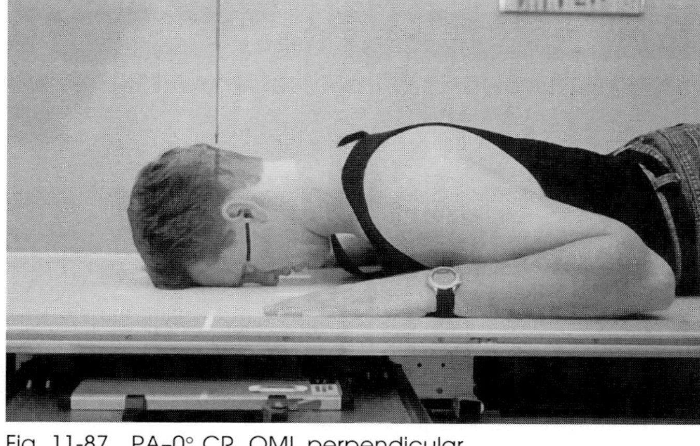

Fig. 11-87. PA–0° CR, OML perpendicular.

Central Ray

- CR **perpendicular** to table and **centered to exit at glabella**.
- SID: Head unit, 36 in. (91 cm).
  Table, minimum 40 in. (102 cm).

Collimation: Use 10 x 12 in. circle diaphragm or collimate to outer margins of skull on all sides.

Respiration: Suspend respiration during exposure.

Evaluation Criteria

- Entire skull visualized on radiograph.
- Petrous ridges superimpose superior orbital region.
- Petrous pyramids fill orbits.
- Distance from oblique orbital line to lateral margin of skull on each side is equal.
- Posterior and anterior clinoids are visualized just superior to ethmoid sinuses.
- Sufficient penetration and exposure, without motion, to visualize frontal bone.

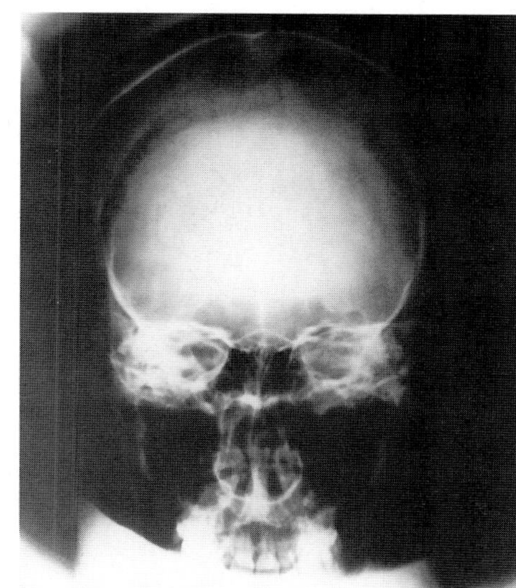

Fig. 11-88. PA–0° CR.

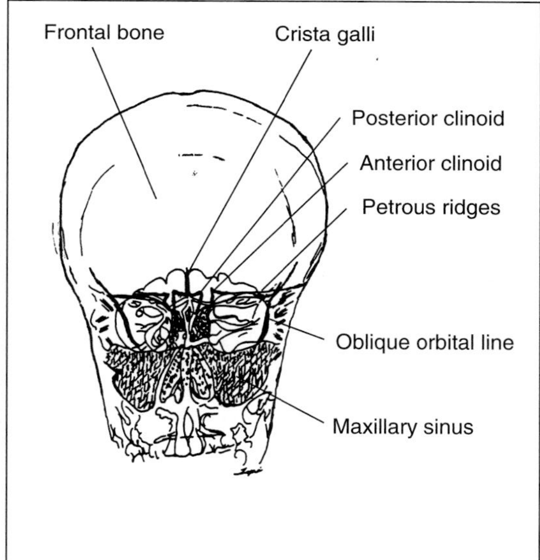

Fig. 11-89. PA–0° CR.

11

Submentovertex (SMV) Projection

Warning: Rule out cervical fracture or subluxation on trauma patient before attempting this projection.

Skull Series
Special
• **Submentovertex (SMV)**

Structures Best Shown

Foramen ovale and spinosum, mandible, sphenoid and ethmoid sinuses, **mastoid processes**, petrous ridges, hard palate, foramen magnum, and occipital bone.

Technical Factors

- Film size–10 x 12 in. (24 x 30 cm), lengthwise.
- Moving or stationary grid.
- 70-80 kVp range.
- Use small focal spot.
- Technique and dose:

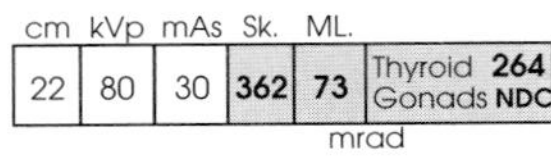

cm	kVp	mAs	Sk.	ML.	
22	80	30	**362**	**73**	Thyroid **264** Gonads **NDC**

mrad

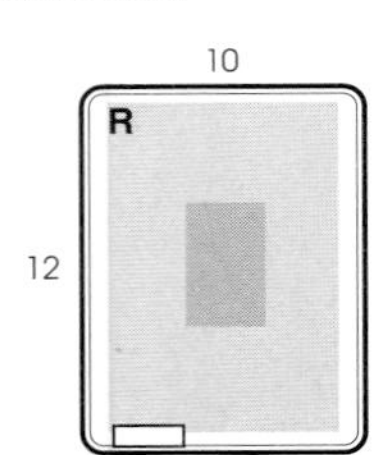

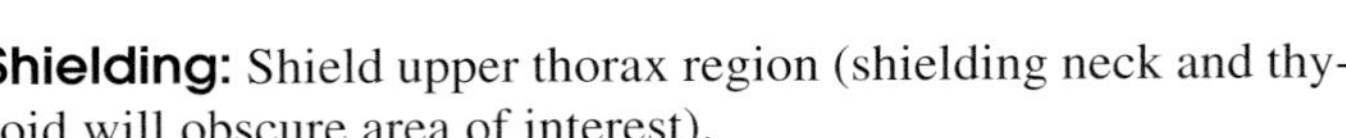

Shielding: Shield upper thorax region (shielding neck and thyroid will obscure area of interest).

Patient Position

- Remove all metal, plastic or other removable objects from head.
- Patient in an erect or supine position.
- Erect, which is easier for patient, may be done with dedicated head unit if available or with erect table or other erect grid-film holder.

Part Position 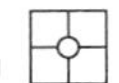

- Raise chin, hyperextending neck if possible until **infraorbitomeatal line (IOML) is parallel to film**. (See Notes.)
- Head rests on vertex.
- Align **midsagittal plane perpendicular** to midline of head unit or table-top, thus **avoiding tilt and/or rotation**.
- If taken supine, extend head over end of table and support cassette and head as shown keeping **IOML parallel to film** and **perpendicular to CR**. (If table will not tilt as shown in Fig. 11-91, build up pillow under patient's back to allow sufficient head extension.

Central Ray

- CR directed **perpendicular to infraorbitomeatal line**.
- Center at ¾ in. (2 cm) anterior to level of EAMs (midway between angles of mandible).
- Center cassette to CR with plane of film parallel to IOML.
- SID: Head unit, 36 in. (91 cm). Table, min. 40 in. (102 cm).

Collimation: Collimate to outer margins of skull on all sides.

Respiration: Suspend respiration.

Notes: If patient is unable to sufficiently extend neck, compensate by angling CR **perpendicular to IOML**. The cassette can also be angled as needed to maintain the film perpendicular to CR.

Position is very uncomfortable for patient; move quickly.

Fig. 11-90. Submentovertex (SMV) erect. –CR perpendicular to IOML.

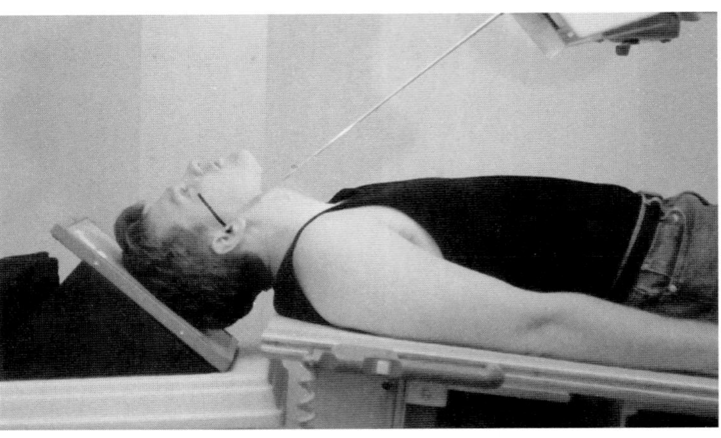

Fig. 11-91. Submentovertex (SMV) table-top with grid cassette. –CR perpendicular to IOML.

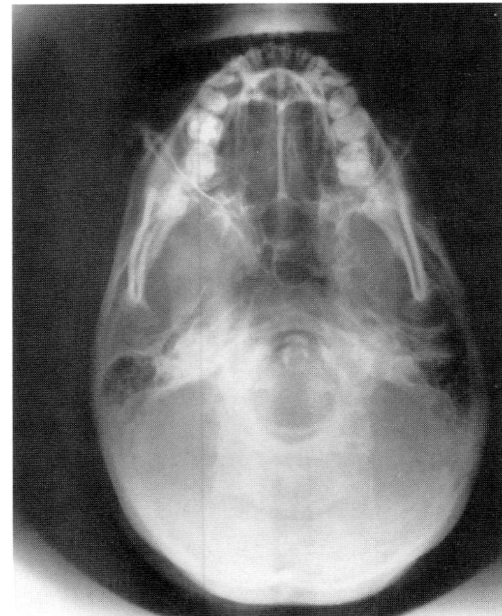

Fig. 11-92. Submentovertex.

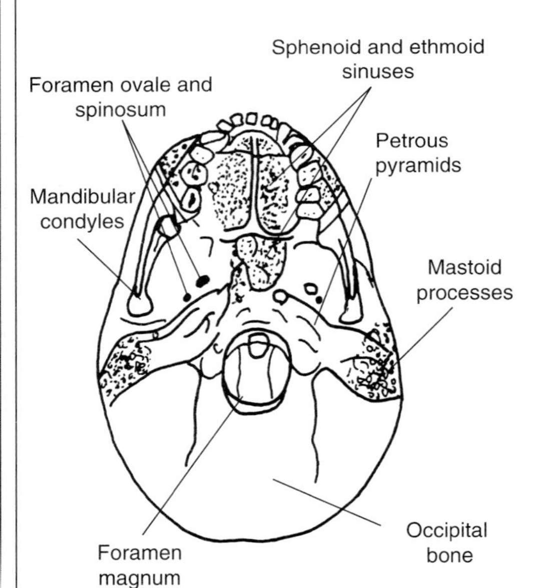

Fig. 11-93. Submentovertex.

Evaluation Criteria

- Entire skull visualized on radiograph.
- **Mandibular condyles are projected anterior to petrous pyramids** (indicates correct skull extension).
- Mandibular symphysis superimposes anterior frontal bone.
- Distance from bilateral mandibular structures to lateral border of skull are equal.
- Foramen ovale and spinosum are visualized.
- Sufficient penetration and exposure to clearly visualize outline of foramen magnum.

Lateral Position - Right or Left Lateral

Sella Turcica
Basic
- **Lateral**
- AP axial (Towne method)

Structures Best Shown

Sella turcica, anterior and posterior clinoid processes, dorsum sellae and clivus.

Technical Factors

- Film size–8 x 10 in. (18 x 24 cm), crosswise.
- Moving or stationary grid.
- 70-80 kVp range.
- AEC not recommended due to small exposure field.
- Use small focal spot.
- Technique and dose:

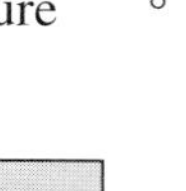

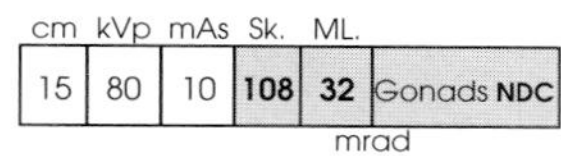

cm	kVp	mAs	Sk.	ML.	
15	80	10	108	32	Gonads NDC
				mrad	

Patient Position

- Remove all metal, plastic or other removable objects from head.
- Patient in an erect or prone position.

Part Position

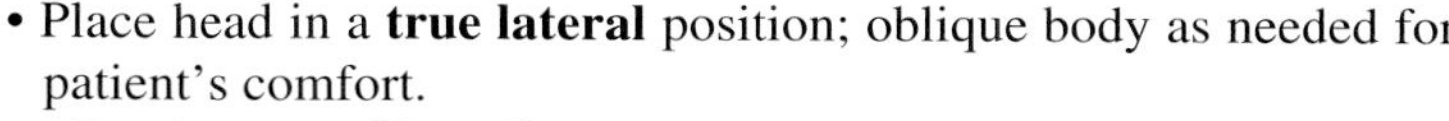

- Place head in a **true lateral** position; oblique body as needed for patient's comfort.
- Align **interpupillary line perpendicular** to head unit or table-top.
- Bring **midsagittal plane parallel** with head unit or table-top.
- Place **infraorbitomeatal line perpendicular** to front edge of cassette.

Central Ray

- Align CR **perpendicular** to film.
- Center to a **point ½ in**. (2 cm) **anterior** and **½ in. superior** to the external auditory meatus (EAM).
- Center cassette to CR.
- SID: Head unit, 36 in. (91 cm).
  Table, minimum 40 in. (102 cm).

Collimation: Use a circle diaphragm or collimate on all sides to yield a field size of approximately 4 in. (10 cm).

Respiration: Suspend respiration during exposure.

Note: To obtain a sharply detailed image of the sella turcica, the utilization of a small focal spot and close collimation is essential.

Evaluation Criteria

- The sella turcica is located in the center of the radiograph, with the body and lesser wings of the sphenoid and the clivus within the collimated field.
- Close four-sided collimation should be evident.
- The cranium is visualized without rotation or tilt:
  - –The sella turcica and clivus are demonstrated in profile without rotation.
  - –The anterior and posterior clinoids are superimposed.
  - –The greater wings and lesser wings of sphenoid are superimposed.
- Sufficient penetration and exposure, without motion, to clearly visualize sella turcica and pituitary fossa.

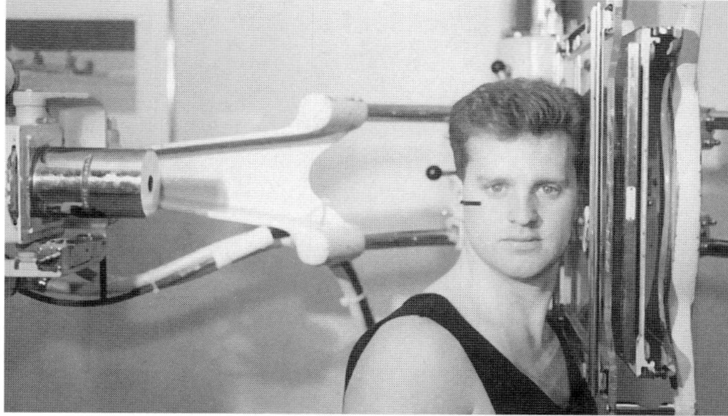

Fig. 11-94. Left lateral sella turcica–Erect.

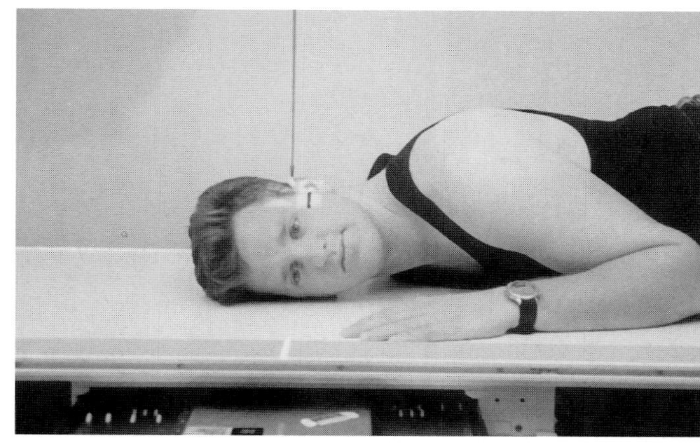

Fig. 11-95. Right lateral sella turcica–Recumbent.

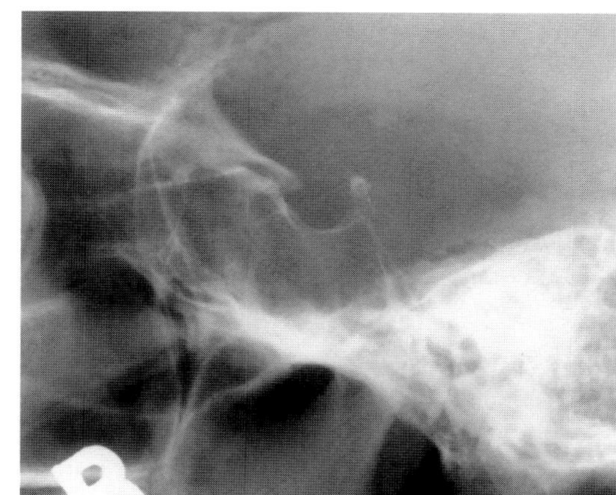

Fig. 11-96. Lateral sella turcica.

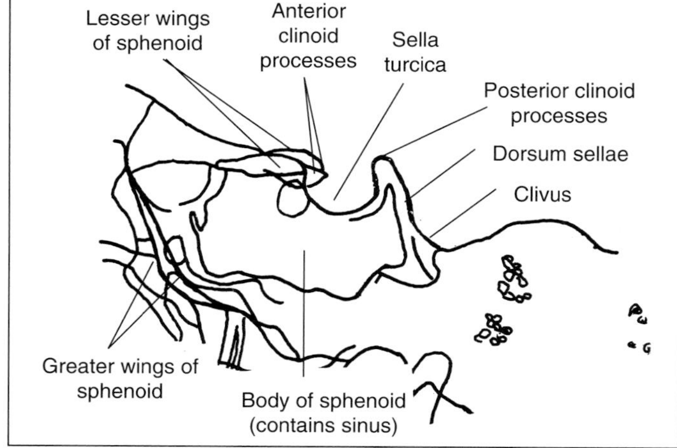

Fig. 11-97. Lateral sella turcica.

AP Axial Projection

Towne Method

Sella Turcica
Basic
• Lateral
• **AP axial (Towne method)**

Structures Best Shown

Dorsum sellae, anterior and posterior clinoids, foramen magnum, petrous ridges and occipital bone.

Technical Factors

- Film size–8 x 10 in. (18 x 24 cm), lengthwise.
- Moving or stationary grid.
- 80±5 kVp range, AEC not recommended.
- Use small focal spot.
- Technique and dose:

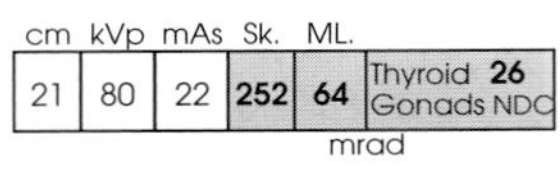

cm	kVp	mAs	Sk.	ML.	
21	80	22	**252**	**64**	Thyroid **26** Gonads NDC

mrad

Shielding: Shield upper thorax region.

Patient Position

- Remove all metal, plastic or other removable objects from head.
- Patient in an erect or supine position.

Part Position

- Rest patient's posterior skull against head unit or table-top.
- Flex neck to bring **IOML perpendicular** to film.
- Align **midsagittal plane perpendicular** to midline of head unit or table.

Central Ray

- Angle CR **37° caudad** if **dorsum sellae** and **posterior clinoids** are of primary interest.
- Angle CR **30° caudad** if the **anterior clinoids** are of primary interest.
- Center at midsagittal plane, **1½ in**. (4 cm) **above superciliary arch**.
- Center cassette to projected CR.
- SID: Head unit, 36 in. (91 cm); Table, minimum 40 in. (102 cm).

Collimation: Use a circle diaphragm or cylinder cone, collimate on all sides to size of approximately 4 in. (10 cm) square.

Respiration: Suspend respiration during exposure.

Note: To obtain a sharply detailed image of the dorsum sellae, a small focal spot and close collimation is essential.

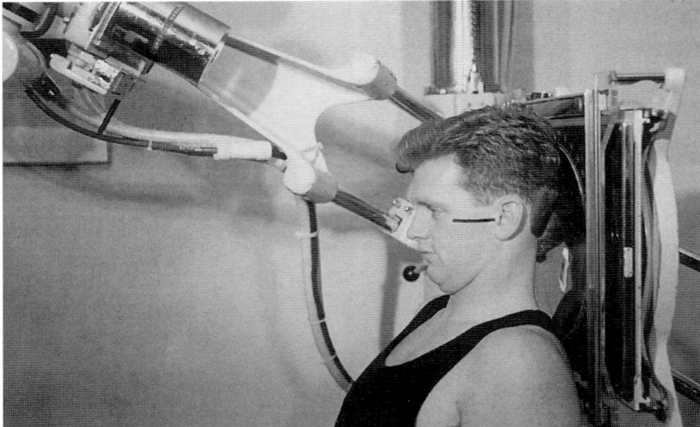

Fig. 11-98. AP axial–CR 30 to 37° caudad, IOML perpendicular.

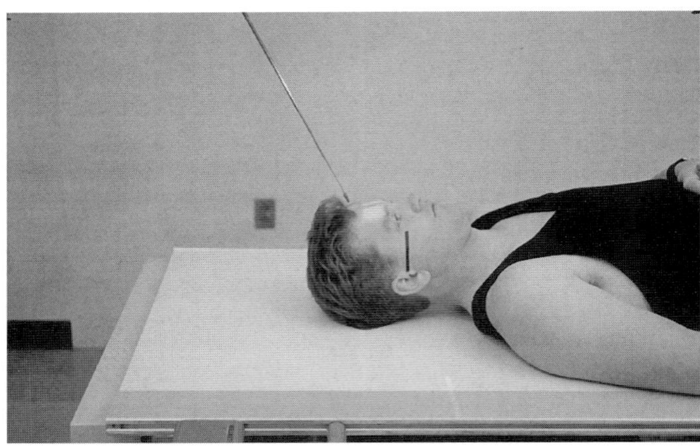

Fig. 11-99. AP axial–CR 30 to 37° caudad, IOML perpendicular.

Evaluation Criteria

- The dorsum sellae is located in center of the radiograph, with petrous ridges and occipital bone within the collimated field.
- Sufficient penetration and exposure, without motion, to visualize dorsum sellae.

37° caudad angle:

- Dorsum sellae and posterior clinoids are projected into foramen magnum.
- Cranium is seen without rotation or tilt:
  - –Petrous ridges are symmetrical.
  - –Equal distance from dorsum sellae to each side of foramen magnum.

30° caudad angle:

- Anterior clinoids are clearly visualized, adjacent to each petrous ridge, directly above the foramen magnum.
- Cranium is seen without rotation or tilt:
  - –Petrous ridges are symmetrical.
  - –Equal distance from midsagittal plane, which can be identified by the perpendicular plate, to each anterior clinoid.
- Dorsum sellae is projected above the foramen magnum superimposing the occipital bone.

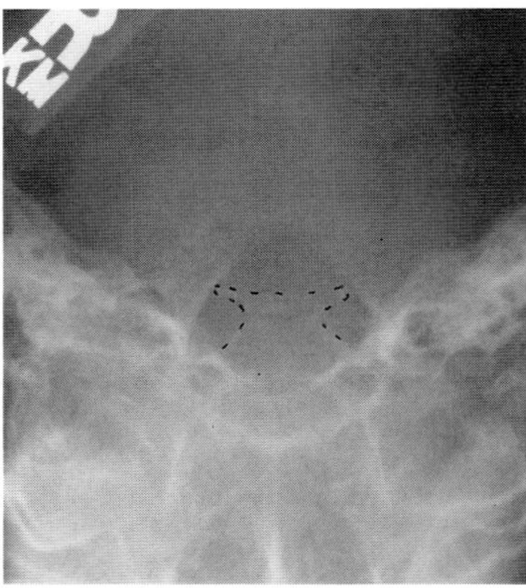

Fig. 11-100. 37° caudad.

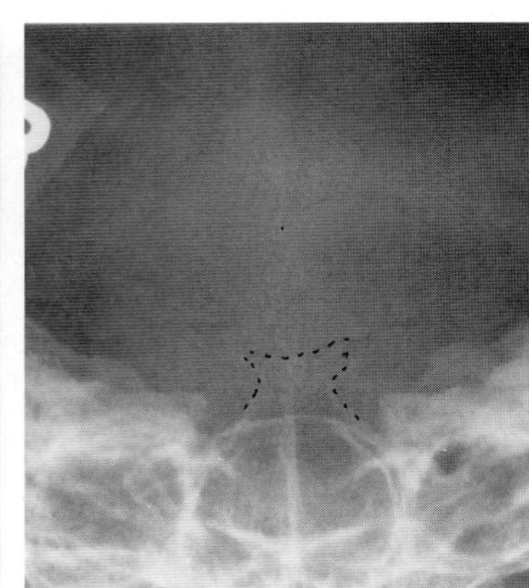

Fig. 11-101. 30° caudad.

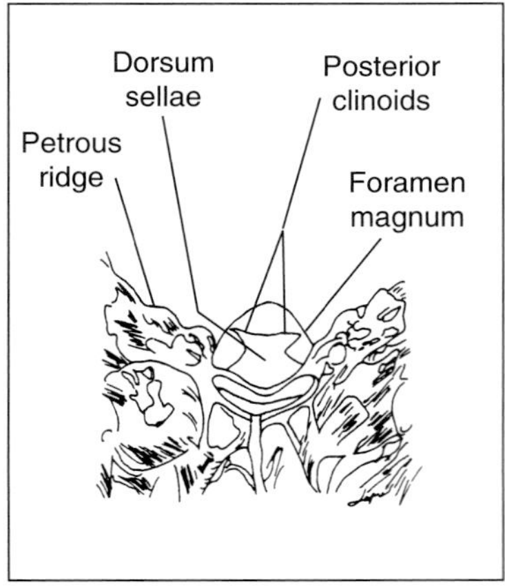

Fig. 11-102. 30° caudad.

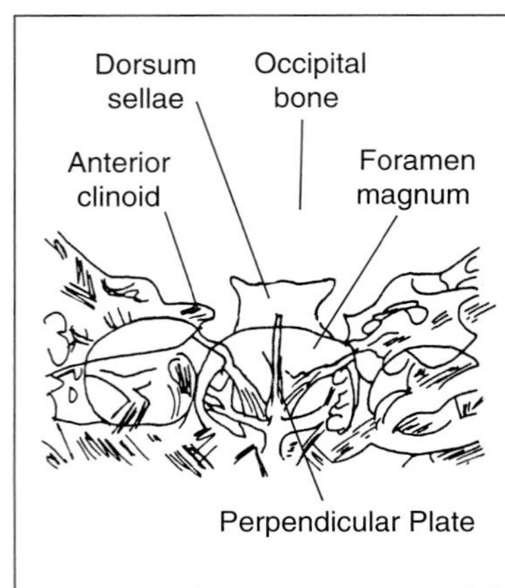

Fig. 11-103. 37° caudad.

PA Axial Projection

10° Cephalad or 25° Cephalad (Haas Method)

Sella Turcica
Special
• **PA axial 10° cephalad or PA axial 25° cephalad (Haas method)**

Structures Best Shown

Dorsum sellae, tuberculum sellae, anterior and posterior clinoids and petrous ridges.

PA 25° cephalad best visualizes dorsum sella and posterior clinoids within foramen magnum.

Technical Factors

- Film size–8 x 10 in. (18 x 24 cm), lengthwise.
- Moving or stationary grid.
- 80±5 kVp range, AEC not recommended.
- Use small focal spot.
- Technique and dose:

cm	kVp	mAs	Sk.	ML.	
20	80	22	**271**	**46**	Thyroid **7** Gonads **NDC**

mrad

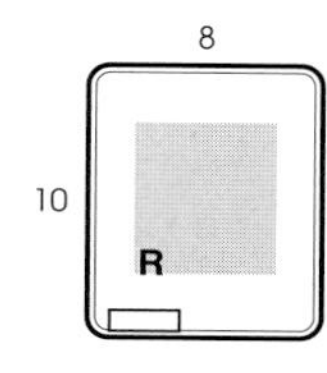

Patient Position

- Remove all metal, plastic or other removable objects from head.
- Patient in an erect or prone position (erect preferred).

Part Position

- Rest patient's nose and forehead against head unit or table.
- Flex chin until **orbitomeatal line is perpendicular** to film.
- Align midsagittal plane perpendicular to midline of table.
- Center cassette to CR and glabella.

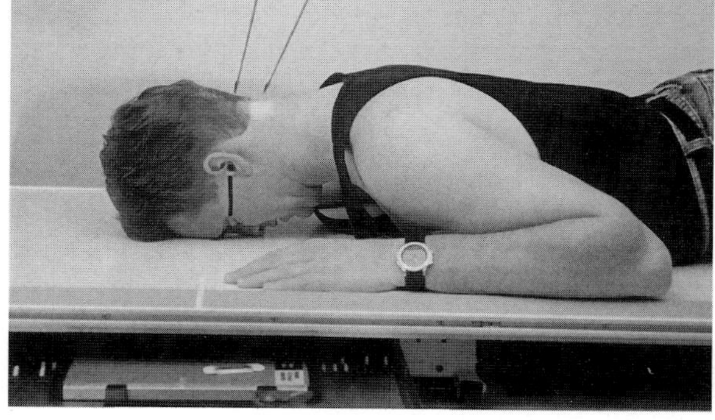

Fig. 11-104. PA axial–CR 10° cephalad, OML perpendicular (25° cephalad – Haas method).

Central Ray

- Angle **CR 10°** and/**or 25° cephalad, to exit at glabella.**
- Center cassette to projected CR.
- SID: Head unit, 36 in. (91 cm).

Table, minimum 40 in. (102 cm).

Collimation: Use a circle diaphragm or cylinder cone, or collimate on all sides to yield a field size of approximately 4 in. (10 cm).

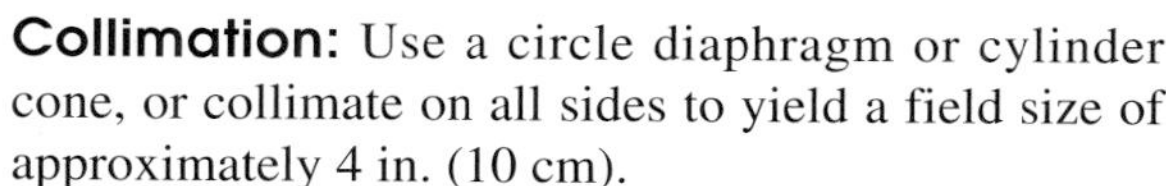

Respiration: Suspend respiration during exposure.

Note: To obtain a sharply detailed image of the dorsum sellae, the utilization of a small focal spot and close collimation is essential.

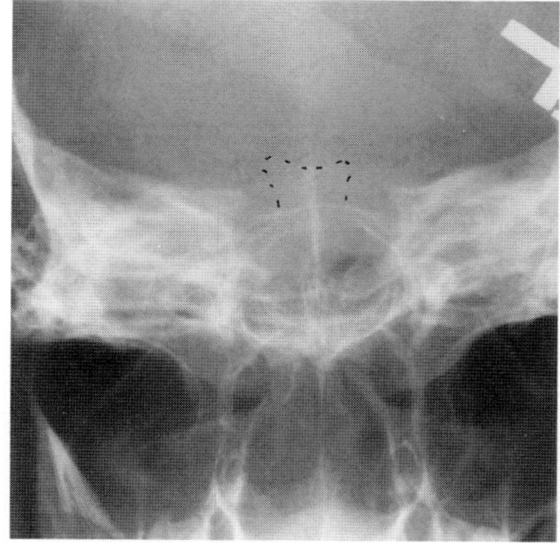

Fig. 11-105. PA axial–10° cephalad.

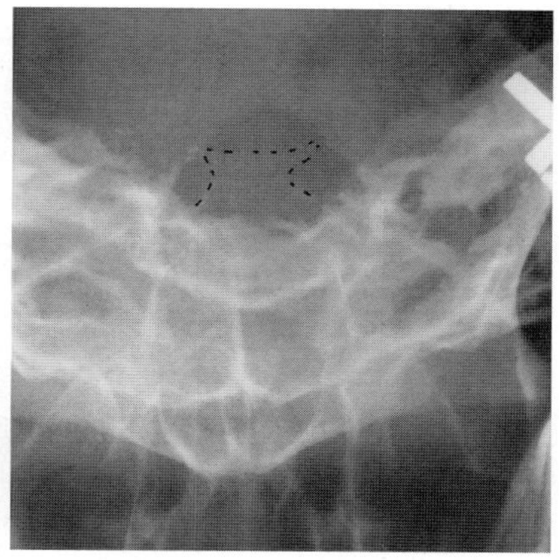

Fig. 11-106. PA axial–25° cephalad.

Evaluation Criteria

- The dorsum sellae is located in the center of the radiograph, with the petrous ridges and foramen magnum within the collimated field.
- Close four-sided collimation should be evident.
- Cranium is seen without rotation or tilt:
  –Petrous ridges are symmetrical.
  –Equal distance from midsagittal plane, which can be identified by the perpendicular plate, to each anterior clinoid.
- Anterior clinoids are clearly visualized adjacent to each petrous ridge, directly above the foramen magnum.
- Sufficient penetration and exposure, without motion, to visualize dorsum sellae.

PA axial–10° cephalad:

- Dorsum sellae is projected above the foramen magnum, superimposing the occipital bone.

PA axial–25° cephalad:

- Dorsum sellae and posterior clinoids are visualized within the outline of the foramen magnum .

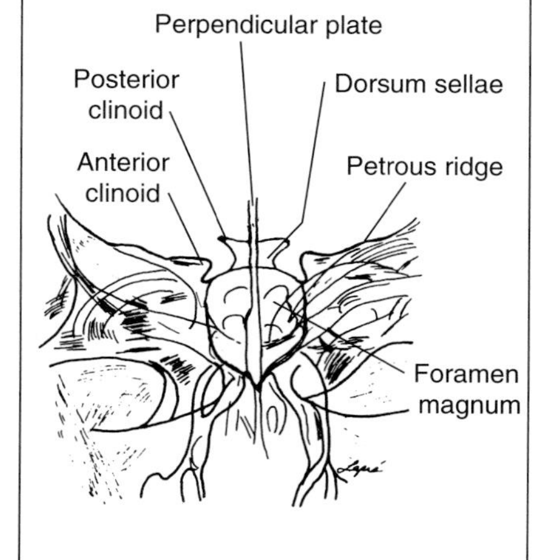

Fig. 11-107. PA axial–10° cephalad.

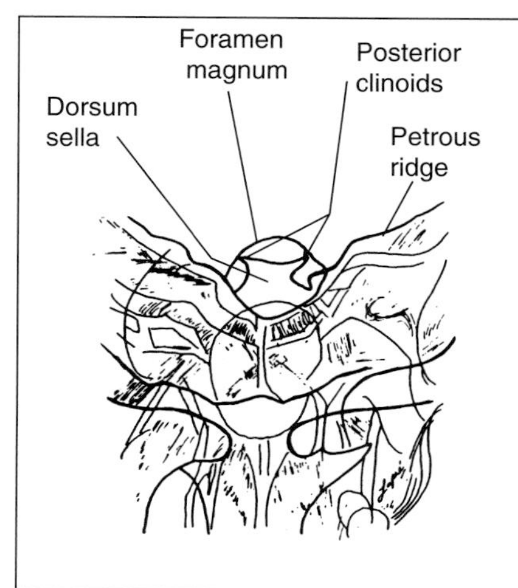

Fig. 11-108. PA axial–25° cephalad.

Radiographs for Critique

Each of these skull radiographs demonstrates some error in positioning which requires a repeat. These, along with accompanying lecture slides of these and other radiographs, will provide a basis for classroom and/or positioning lab discussion. Questions with answers based on these specific critique radiographs are provided in the accompanying student workbook/lab manuals to help prepare students for classroom and/or lab discussions on film critique.

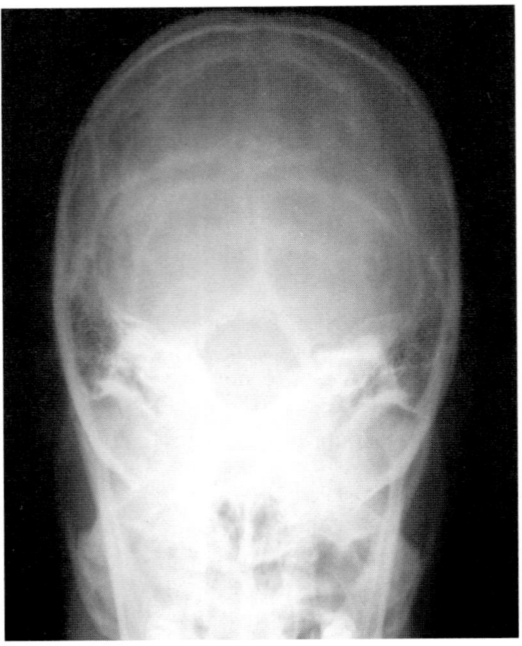

Fig. C11-109. AP Towne

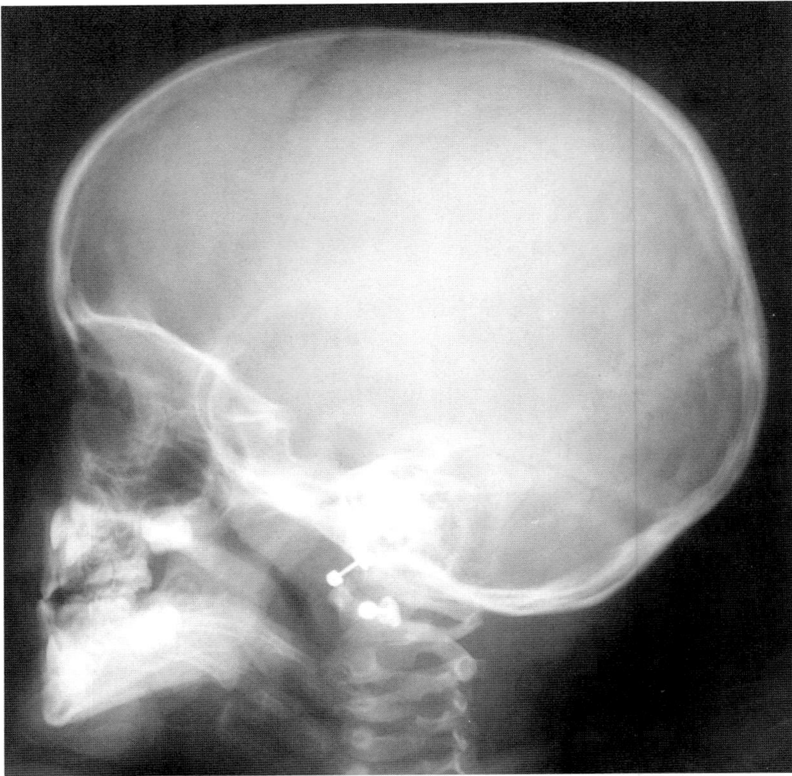

Fig. C11-110. Lateral skull–4-year-old.

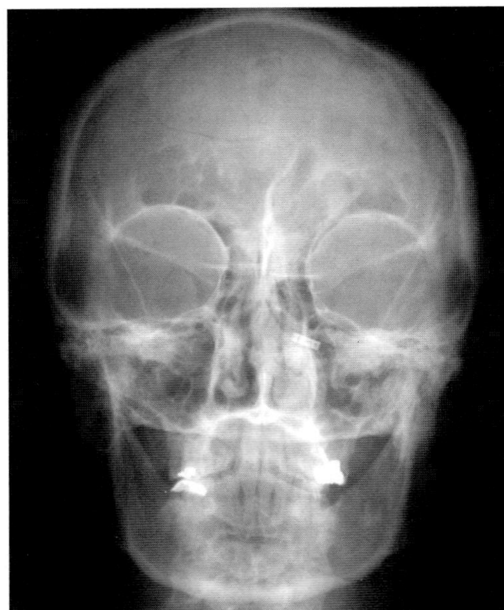

Fig. C11-111. Caldwell, PA or AP?

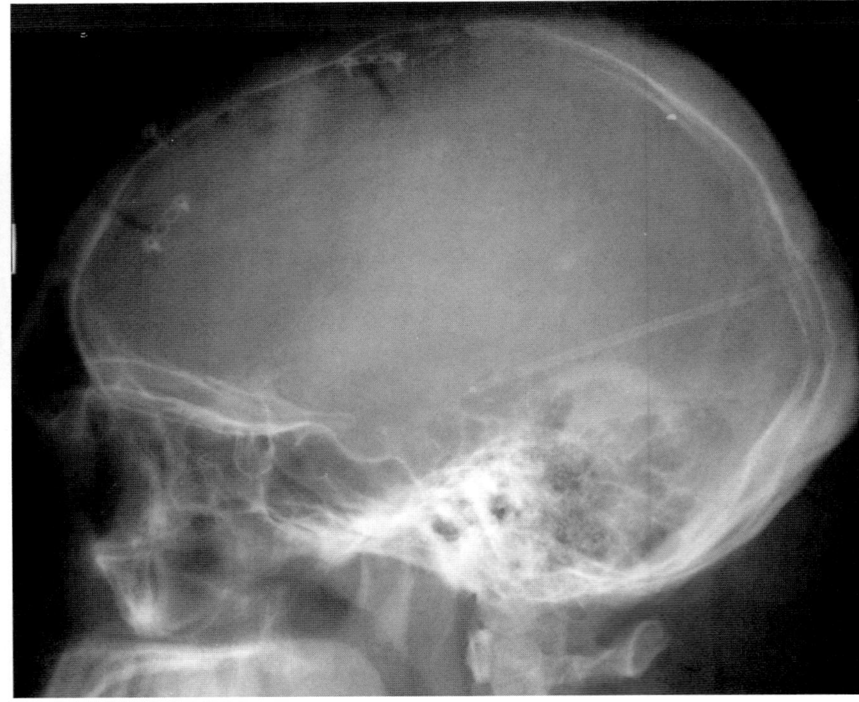

Fig. C11-112. Lateral skull–54-year-old post trauma.

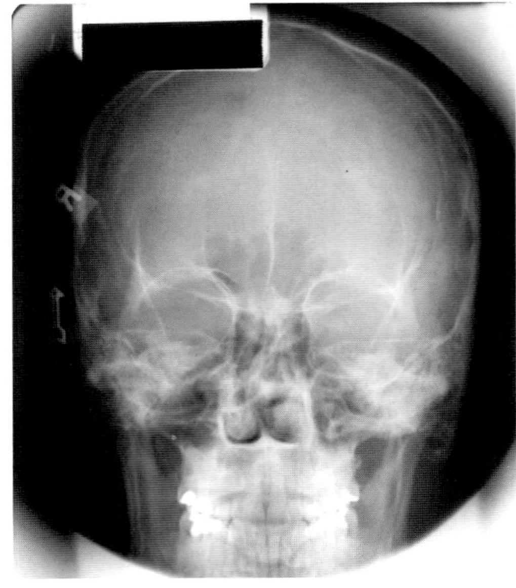

Fig. C11-113. Caldwell, PA or AP?

CHAPTER 12

Facial Bones

CONTRIBUTIONS BY:
Kathy Martensen, BS, RT (R)
Barry T. Anthony, RT (R)

CONTENTS

Radiographic Anatomy

Radiographic anatomy of the facial bones is included in the preceding Chapter 11 on the skull and cranial bones.

Radiographic Positioning

Special projections and anatomical relationships **360**

Positioning considerations **360**

Survey information **361**

Basic and special projections **362**

Facial bones:
- Lateral **363**
- Parietoacanthial (Waters method) **364**
- PA axial (Caldwell method) **365**
- Modified parietoacanthial (modified Waters method) **366**

Radiographic Positioning cont.

Nasal bones:
- Lateral **367**
- Parietoacanthial (Waters method) **364**
- PA axial (Caldwell method) **365**
- Superoinferior (axial) **368**

Zygomatic arches:
- Submentovertex (SMV) **369**
- Oblique inferosuperior (tangential) **370**
- Parietoacanthial (Waters method) **364**
- AP axial (modified Towne method) **371**

Optic foramina:
- Parieto-orbital (Rhese method) **372**
- Parietoacanthial (Waters method) **364**
- PA axial (Caldwell method) **365**

Orbits:
- Modified parietoacanthial (modified Waters) **366**

Mandible:
- Axiolateral **373**
- PA and PA axial **374**
- AP axial (Towne method) **375**
- Submentovertex (SMV) **376**
- Panorex **377**

Temporomandibular joints:
- AP axial (modified Towne method) **379**
- Axiolateral oblique (modified Law method) **380**
- Axiolateral (Schuller method) **381**
- Tomography **382**

Radiographs for critique **384**

12

Radiographic Positioning

SPECIAL PROJECTIONS AND ANATOMICAL RELATIONSHIPS

PA Skull Projection

The PA skull on the right (Fig. 12-2) was taken with no tube angulation and with the OML (dotted line in Fig. 12-1) perpendicular to the plane of the film. The central ray is therefore parallel to the OML (orbitomeatal line). This results in the **petrous pyramids being projected directly into the orbits** so that the orbits appear totally filled by the petrous pyramids. Drawn on both radiographs (Figs. 12-1 and 12-2) is a line through the roof of the orbits and through the petrous ridges. With the orbits superimposed by the petrous pyramids, very little facial bone detail can be demonstrated radiographically. Therefore this PA projection has limited value for visualizing facial bones.

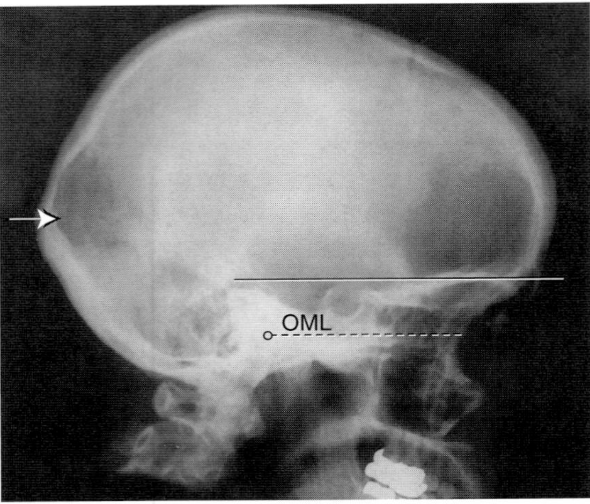

Fig. 12-1. Lateral skull for comparison of bony relationships–CR parallel to OML.

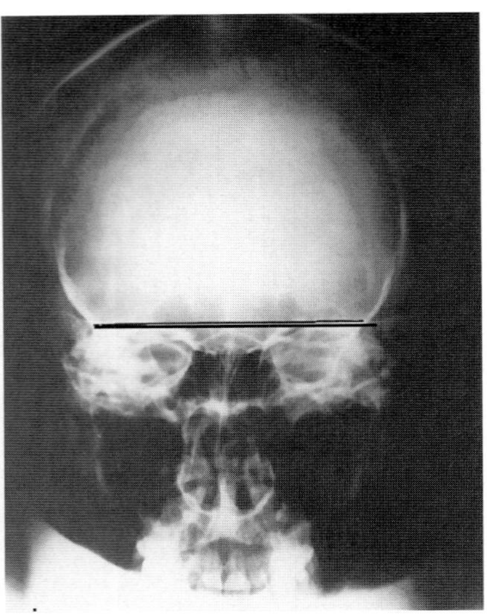
Fig. 12-2. Skull–PA projection.

Parietoacanthial (Waters) Projection

In order to better visualize the facial bone mass, the petrous pyramids must be removed from the facial bone area of interest. This can be done either by tube angulation or by extending the neck. The radiographs to the right (Figs. 12-3 and 12-4) demonstrate how this can be accomplished. The neck is extended by raising the chin so that the **petrous pyramids will be projected just below the maxillary sinuses**. The central ray is now parallel to the mentomeatal line (MML). The radiograph on the right (Waters method, Fig. 12-4), if done correctly as described later in this chapter, demonstrates the petrous ridges (see arrows) projected below the maxillae and maxillary sinuses. Thus, except for the mandible, the **facial bones are now projected superior to** and **not superimposed** over the dense petrous pyramids.

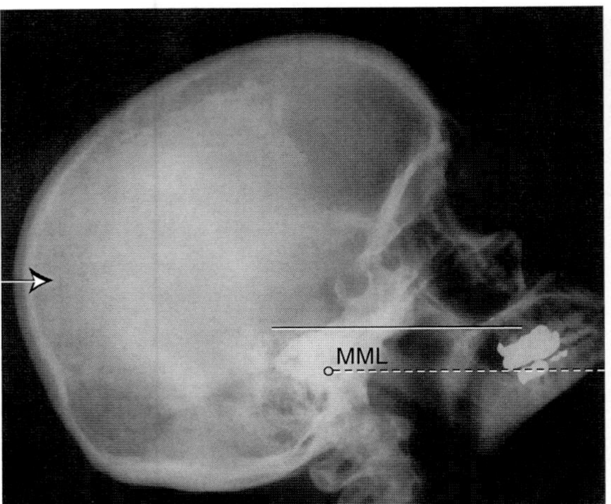

Fig. 12-3. Lateral skull for comparison of bony relationships–CR parallel to MML.

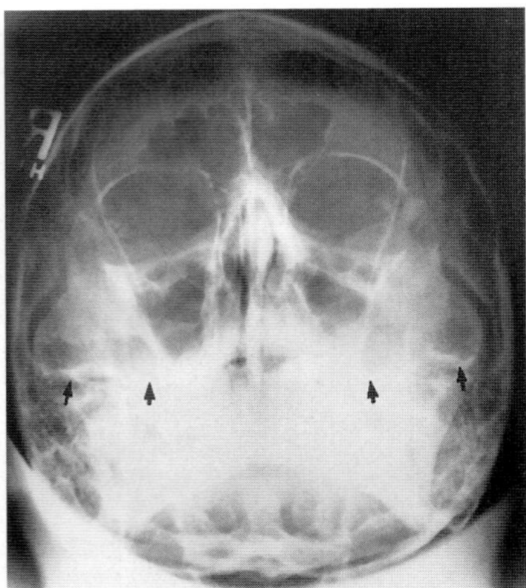
Fig. 12-4. Facial Bones–Parietoacanthial (Waters) projection.

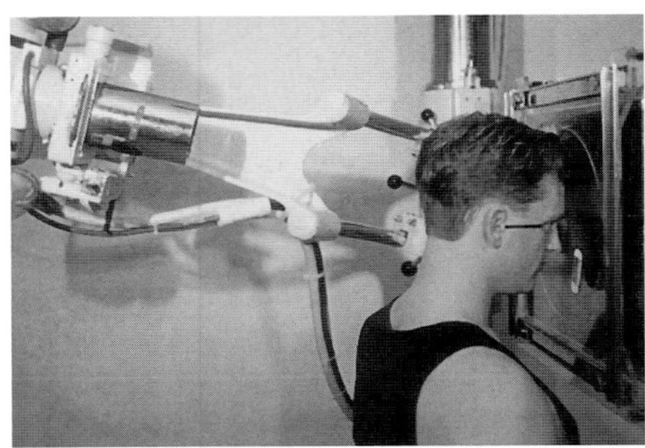
Fig. 12-5. PA, erect–Head unit.

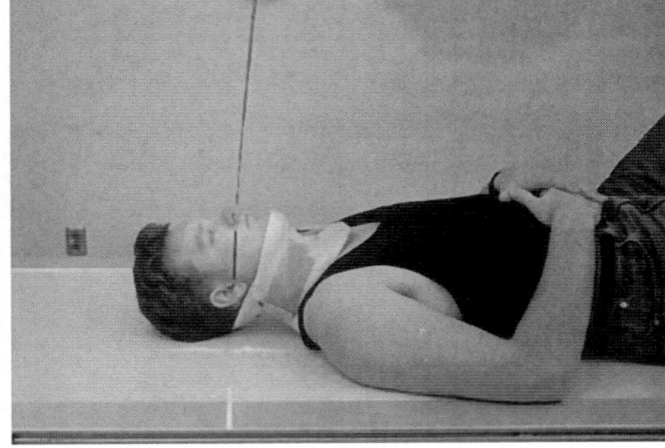
Fig. 12-6. AP, supine–Trauma patient.

POSITIONING CONSIDERATIONS

Erect vs. Recumbent

Positioning considerations for the facial bones are similar to that of the skull as described in the previous chapter.

Facial bone projections may be taken erect if the condition of the patient allows. This can be done with an erect table or erect grid-film holder device, such as the head unit in Fig. 12-5. It is easier to move the patient's entire body as needed in an erect position to accurately adjust the various planes and positioning lines of the head for accurate skull positioning (especially with obese or hypersthenic type patients). Also fluid levels in the sinuses or other cranial cavities may be indicators of cranial trauma, which is only visible in the erect position or with horizontal beam projections.

Trauma patients generally need to be radiographed in a recumbent position, especially with possible neck injuries. Most of these facial bone projections can be taken supine without moving the patient by compensating CR angles and/or CR-part-film alignments as demonstrated in Chapter 19 on mobile and trauma radiography. However, certain AP skull or facial bones are only taken when the patient cannot turn into the prone position because of an increase in OID of the facial bones and since the thyroid and neck structures receive more radiation with an AP projection than with a PA.

NATIONAL SURVEY

Departmental standards (basic) and special routines for exams of the facial bones were somewhat consistent throughout the United States. The results of this survey determined national norms for departmental routines as presented in the positioning pages that follow:

Facial Bones Routine

Facial bones	U.S. Average	
	Basic 1995 (1989)	Special 1995 (1989)
• Lateral	95% (94%)	
• PA Waters (parietoacanthial)	87% (87%)	
• PA Caldwell	73% (35%)	
• PA modified Waters	30% (24%)	28% –

Optic Foramina Routine

Optic foramina	U.S. Average	
	Basic 1995 (1989)	Special 1995 (1989)
• Rhese oblique (bilateral)	78% (97%)	
• PA Waters	53% (14%)	
• PA Caldwell	45% (11%)	10% –
• PA modified Waters	20% –	15% –

Zygomatic Arch Routine

Zygomatic arch	U.S. Average	
	Basic 1995 (1989)	Special 1995 (1989)
• SMV	73% (81%)	
• PA Waters (parietoacanthial)	– (62%)	
• AP Towne	59% (42%)	
• Oblique axial (tangential)	66% (33%)	
• Lateral	– (30%)	

Nasal Bones Routine

Nasal bones	U.S. Average	
	Basic 1995 (1989)	Special 1995 (1989)
• PA Waters	92% (95%)	
• Lateral–both sides	95% (81%)	
or		
Lateral–one side	– (21%)	
• PA Caldwell	16% (20%)	14% –
• Superoinferior (axial)	8% (12%)	18% –

Mandible Routine

Mandible	U.S. Average	
	Basic 1995 (1989)	Special 1995 (1989)
• Axiolateral–oblique	89% (82%)	
• PA 0°	80% (78%)	
• AP Towne	72% (46%)	
• PA semi-axial (20-25° cephalad)	25% (31%)	13% –
• Panorex	– (16%)	
• PA modified Waters	– 13%	
• SMV	14% (12%)	26% –

Temporomandibular Joints Routine

TMJ	U.S. Average	
	Basic 1995 (1989)	Special 1995 (1989)
• Lateral (Law)	37% (57%)	12% –
or		
Lateral (Schuller)	25% (48%)	13% –
• Tomograms	37% (26%)	24% –
• AP Towne	56% (13%)	8% –
• Panorex	– (7%)	

Summary

Facial Bones: The frequency of the **PA Caldwell** as a basic facial bone projection more than doubled in 1995 compared to 1989 (73% vs. 35%).

Optic Foramina: The frequency of both the **PA Waters** and **PA Caldwell** also both increased significantly in 1995.

Mandible: The **AP Towne** is more frequently used as a basic projection in 1995 as compared to 1989 (72% vs. 46%).

TMJ: The **lateral Law** and the **lateral Schuller** decreased significantly while the **AP Towne** increased by more than fourfold.

STANDARD AND OPTIONAL OPERATING PROCEDURES

Certain basic and special projections or positions for exams involving the facial bones are demonstrated and described on the following pages as suggested standard and special departmental procedures.

Basic Projections

Standard or basic projections, also sometimes referred to as routine projections or departmental routines, are those projections commonly taken on average patients who are helpful and can cooperate in performing the procedure.

Special Projections

Special projections are those more common projections taken as extra or additional projections to better demonstrate certain pathologic conditions or specific body parts.

Basic and Special Projections

Trauma facial bone projections are included in Chapter 19 on Trauma and Mobile Radiography.

Facial bones
Basic
- Lateral **363**
- Parietoacanthial **364** (Waters method)
- PA (Caldwell method) **365**

Special
- Modified parietoacanthial **366** (modified Waters method)

Nasal bones
Basic
- Lateral **367**
- Parietoacanthial **364** (Waters method)

Special
- PA (Caldwell method) **365**
- Superoinferior (axial) **368**

Zygomatic arches
Basic
- Submentovertex (SMV) **369**
- Oblique inferosuperior (tangential) **370**
- AP axial **371** (modified Towne method)

Special
- Parietoacanthial **364** (Waters method)
- Lateral **363**

Optic foramina
Basic
- Parieto-orbital **372** (Rhese method)
- Parietoacanthial **364** (Waters method)
- PA (Caldwell method) **365**

Special
- Modified parietoacanthial **366** (modified Waters method)

Orbits (facial bones)
Basic
- Modified parietoacanthial **366** (modified Waters method)

Mandible
Basic
- Axiolateral **373**
- Cross table axiolateral (trauma) (see Chapter 19)
- PA 0° and 20-25° cephalad **374**
- AP axial **375** (Towne method)

Special
- Submentovertex (SMV) **376**
- Panorex **377**

TMJs
Basic
- AP axial **379** (modified Towne method)

Special
- Axiolateral 15° oblique **380** (modified Law method)
- Axiolateral **381** (Schuller method)
- Tomography **382**

Lateral Position–Right or Left Lateral

Facial bones
Basic
• **Lateral**
• Parietoacanthial (Waters method)
• PA axial (Caldwell method)

Structures Best Shown

Superimposed facial bones, greater wings of the sphenoid, orbital roofs, sella turcica, zygoma and mandible.

Technical Factors

- Film size–8 x 10 in. (18 x 24 cm), lengthwise.
- Moving or stationary grid.
- 70-80 kVp range.
- Use small focal spot.
- Technique and dose:

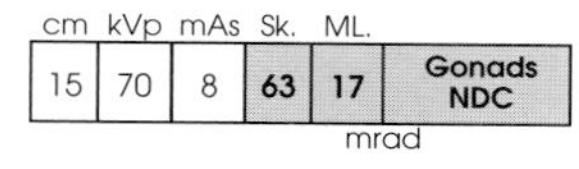

cm	kVp	mAs	Sk.	ML.	Gonads
15	70	8	63	17	NDC

mrad

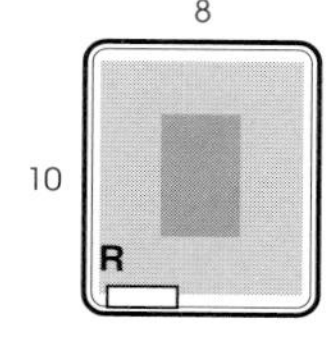

Fig. 12-7. Left lateral–Erect.

Patient Position

- Remove all metal, plastic or other removable objects from head.
- Patient erect or prone.

Part Position

- Rest lateral side of head against head unit or table-top, **with side of interest closest to cassette.**
- Adjust head into a **true lateral position**, oblique body as needed for patient's comfort (palpate the external occipital protuberance posteriorly and the nasion or glabella anteriorly and ensure that these two points are the same distance from the table-top). Place support sponge under chin if needed.
- Align **midsagittal plane parallel** to film.
- Align **interpupillary line perpendicular** to film.
- Adjust chin to bring the **infraorbitomeatal line perpendicular** to front edge of cassette.

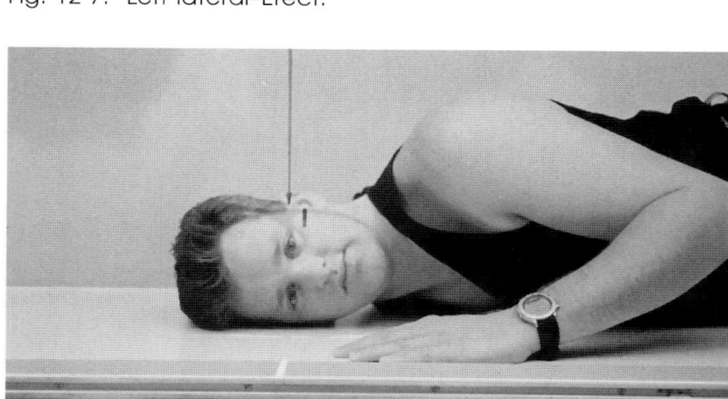

Fig. 12-8. Right lateral–Recumbent.

Central Ray

- Align CR **perpendicular** to head unit or table.
- Center CR to **zygoma**, at a level **halfway between outer canthus and EAM.**
- Center cassette to CR.
- SID: Head unit, 36 in. (91 cm). Table, minimum 40 in. (102 cm).

Collimation: Use an 8 x 10 in. circle diaphragm or collimate on all sides to within 1 in. (2.5 cm) of nearest facial bone.

Respiration: Suspend respiration.

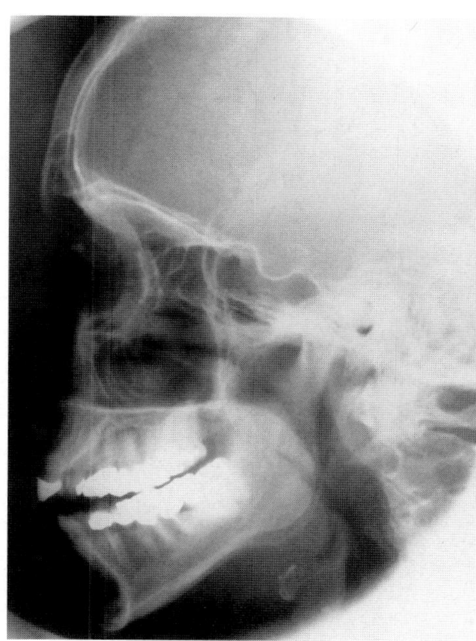

Fig. 12-9. Lateral.

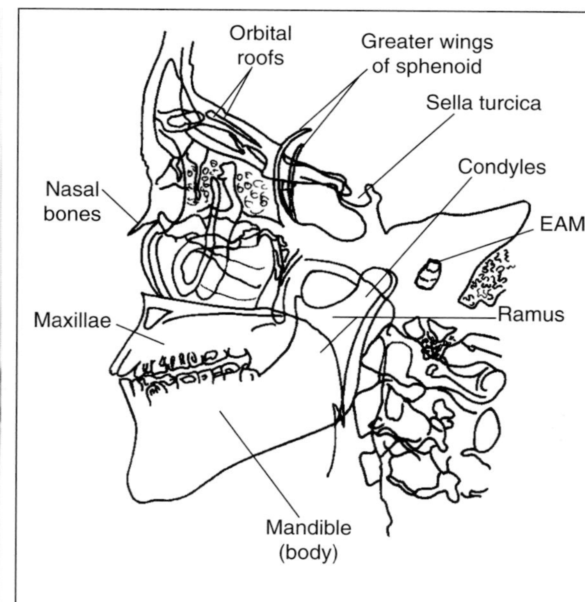

Fig. 12-10. Lateral.

Evaluation Criteria

- The superimposed zygomatic bones are located in the center of the radiograph, with the EAMs and orbital roofs visualized within the collimated field.
- The cranium is not rotated or tilted:
  - –No rotation: mandibular rami are superimposed.
  - –No tilt: orbital roofs and greater wings of sphenoid are superimposed.
- Sufficient penetration and exposure, without motion, to visualize maxillary region.

Parietoacanthial Projection

Waters Method

Facial bones
Basic
- Lateral
- **Parietoacanthial (Waters method)**
- PA axial (Caldwell method)

Structures Best Shown

Inferior orbital rim, maxillae, nasal septum, zygomatic bones, zygomatic arches and anterior nasal spine.

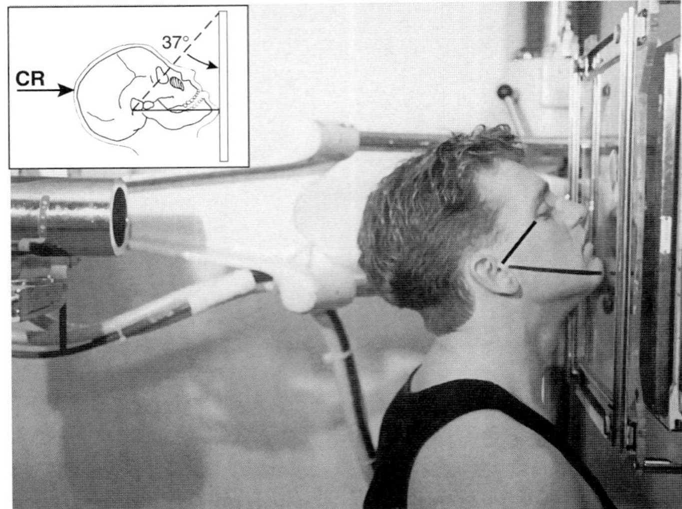

Fig. 12-11. Parietoacanthial (Waters)–**MML perpendicular** (OML 37°).

Technical Factors

- Film size –10 x 12 in. (24 x 30 cm), lengthwise.
  or –8 x 10 in. (18 x 24 cm)
- Moving or stationary grid.
- 70-80 kVp range.
- Use small focal spot.
- Technique and dose:

cm	kVp	mAs	Sk.	ML.	
24	80	18	251	38	Gonads NDC

mrad

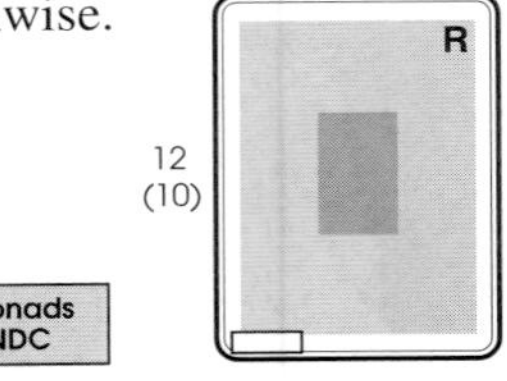

Patient Position

- Remove all metal, plastic or other removable objects from head.
- Patient erect or prone. (Erect preferred if patient's condition allows.)

Part Position 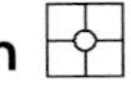

- Extend neck, resting chin against table-top.
- Adjust head until **mentomeatal line (MML) is perpendicular.** OML will form a **37**° angle with the head unit or table-top.
- Position the **midsagittal plane perpendicular** to the midline of the table, preventing rotation and/or tilting of head. (One way to check for rotation is to palpate the mastoid processes on each side and the lateral orbital margins with the thumb and fingertips and ensure that these lines are symmetrical and the same distance from the table-top.)
- Center cassette to CR and to acanthion.

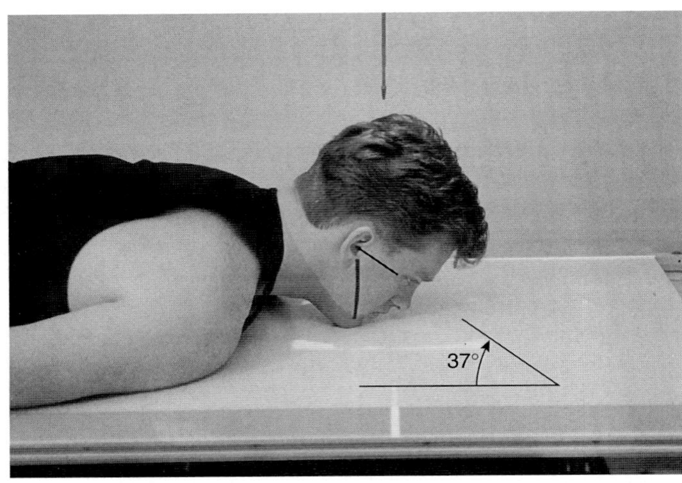

Fig. 12-12. Parietoacanthial (Waters)–**MML perpendicular** (OML 37°).

Central Ray

- Align CR **perpendicular** to film, to **exit at acanthion.**
- Center cassette to CR.
- SID: Head unit, 36 in. (91 cm); Table, minimum 40 in. (102 cm).

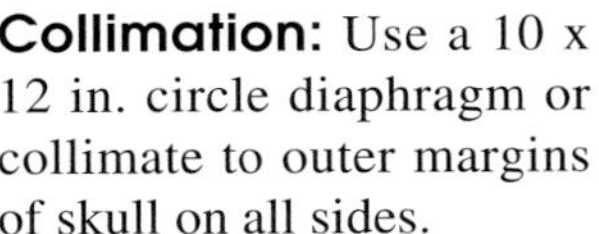

Collimation: Use a 10 x 12 in. circle diaphragm or collimate to outer margins of skull on all sides.

Respiration: Suspend respiration.

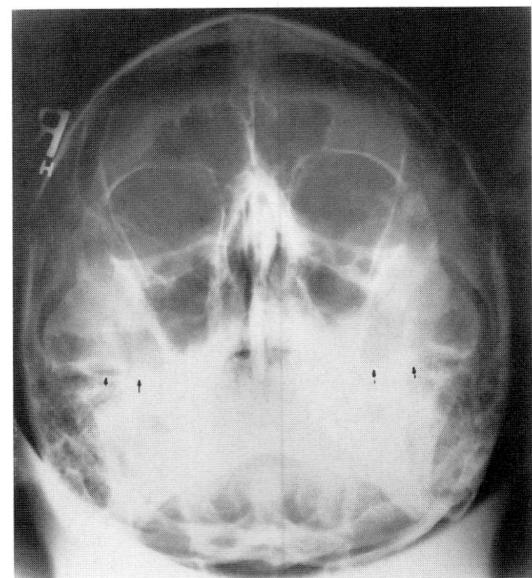

Fig. 12-13. Parietoacanthial (Waters).

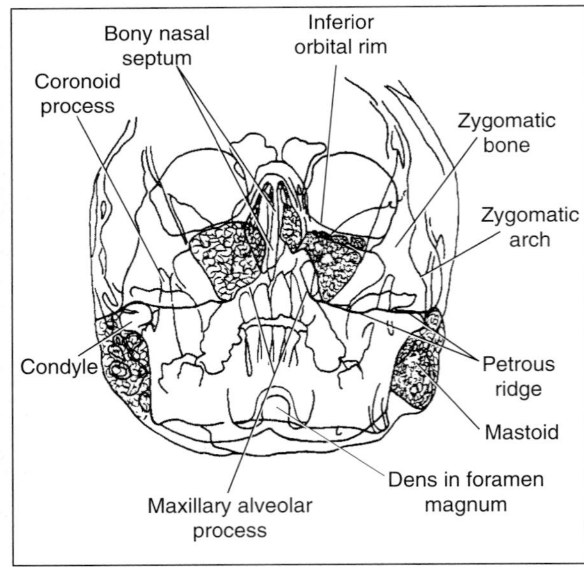

Fig. 12-14. Parietoacanthial (Waters).

Evaluation Criteria

- **Petrous ridges are just below the maxillary sinuses.**
- Inferior orbital rim is clearly identified.
- Sufficient penetration and exposure, without motion, to visualize maxillary region.
- Entire skull visualized on radiograph.
- Cranium seen without rotation:
  –Equal distance from midsagittal plane, identified by the bony nasal septum, to the outer skull margin on each side.
  –Equal distance from lateral orbital margins to the lateral margins of the skull.
- Inferior maxillary sinuses are free from superimposing maxillary alveolar processes.

PA Axial Projection

Caldwell Method

Facial bones
Basic
• Lateral
• Parietoacanthial (Waters method)
• **PA axial (Caldwell method)**

Structures Best Shown

Orbital rim, maxillae, nasal septum, zygomatic bones, and anterior nasal spine. (For floor of orbits, see Note below.)

Technical Factors

- Film size –10 x 12 in. (24 x 30 cm), lengthwise.
  or –8 x 10 in. (18 x 24 cm).
- Moving or stationary grid.
- 70-80 kVp range.
- Use small focal spot.
- Technique and dose:

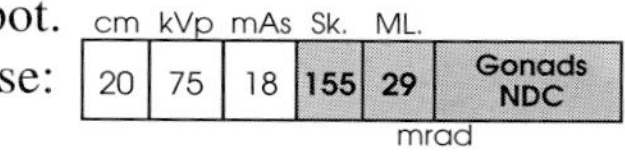

cm	kVp	mAs	Sk.	ML.	
20	75	18	155	29	Gonads NDC
			mrad		

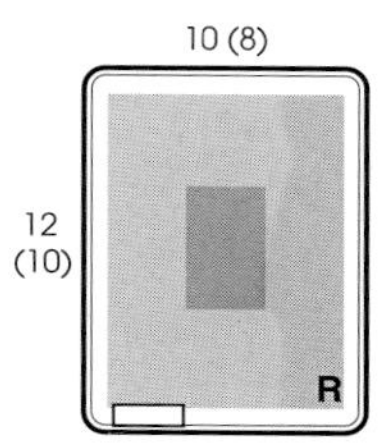

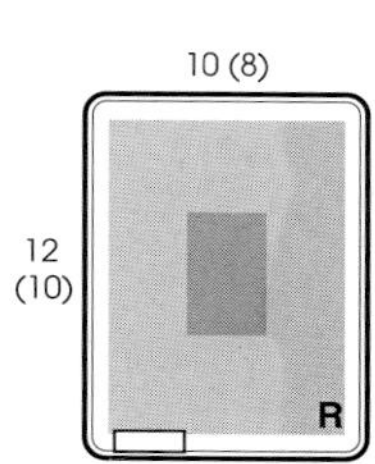

Patient Position

- Remove all metal, plastic or other removable objects from head.
- Patient erect or prone. (Erect preferred if patient's condition allows.)

Part Position 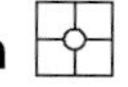

- Rest patient's nose and forehead against table-top.
- Tuck chin, bringing **OML perpendicular** to film.
- Align **midsagittal plane perpendicular** to midline of table-top. Ensure **no rotation** or tilt of head.
- Center cassette to CR and to nasion.

Central Ray

- Angle **CR 15° caudad**, to **exit at nasion**. (See Note).
- Center CR to cassette.
- SID: Head unit, 36 in. (91 cm).
  Table, minimum 40 in. (102 cm).

Fig. 12-15. PA axial Caldwell –**OML perpendicular, CR 15° caudad** –Erect.

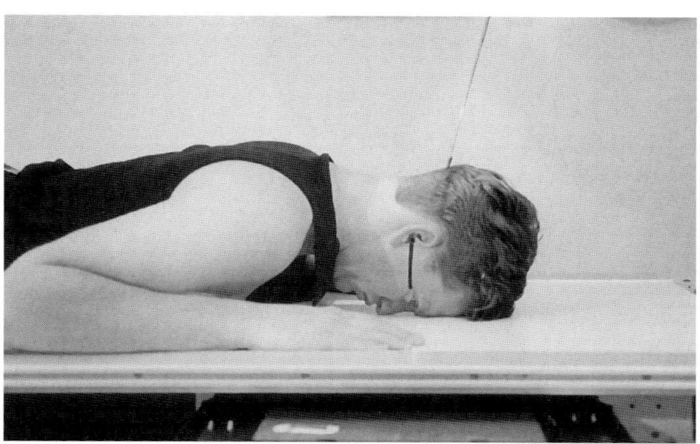

Fig. 12-16. PA axial Caldwell –**OML perpendicular, CR 15° caudad** –Recumbent.

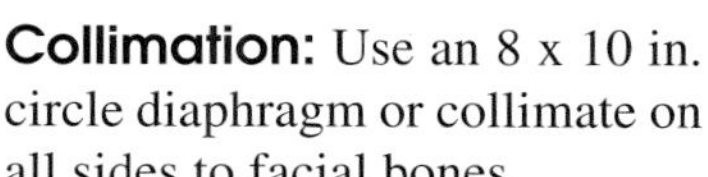

Collimation: Use an 8 x 10 in. circle diaphragm or collimate on all sides to facial bones.

Respiration: Suspend respiration.

Note: Optional method if interest is in orbital floors: Use a **30°** caudad angle to project the petrous ridges below the inferior orbital margin.

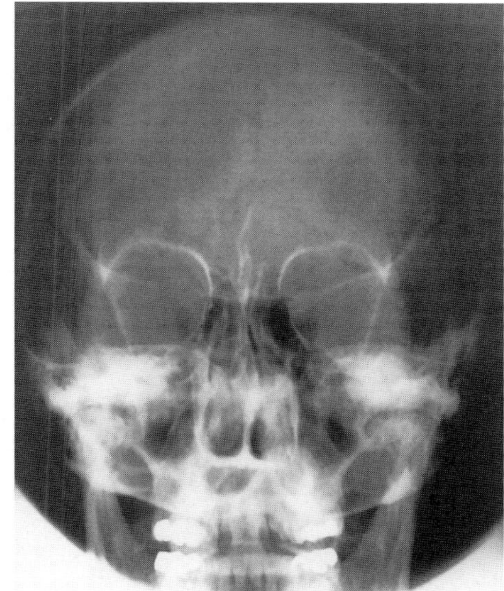

Fig. 12-17. PA axial Caldwell–CR 15°.

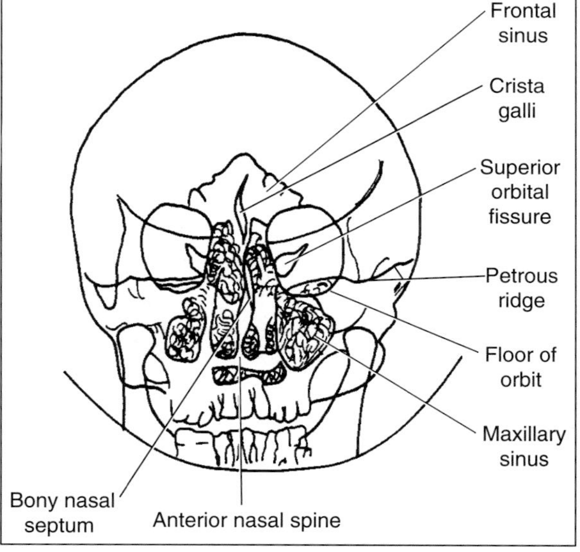

Fig. 12-18. PA axial Caldwell–CR 15°.

Evaluation Criteria

- **Petrous ridges** are projected into **lower one-third of orbits** with 15° caudad CR. (See Note above.)
- Frontal sinus is projected above frontonasal suture.
- Sufficient penetration and exposure, without motion, to visualize maxillary region and orbital floor.
- The inferior orbital rim is located in the center of the radiograph, with the entire orbital rim and maxillary bones within the collimated field.
- Cranium is not rotated:
  –Equal distance from midsagittal plane, identified by the crista galli, to the outer orbital margin on each side.
  –Superior orbital fissures are symmetrically visualized within the orbits.

12

Modified Parietoacanthial Projection

Modified Waters Method

Facial bones
Special
• **Modified parietoacanthial (modified Waters method)**

Structures Best Shown

Best demonstrates orbital floors, also provides a more direct view of entire orbital rims than with Waters projections.

Technical Factors

- Film size–8 x 10 in. (18 x 24 cm), lengthwise.
- Moving or stationary grid.
- 70-80 kVp range.
- Use small focal spot.
- Technique and dose:

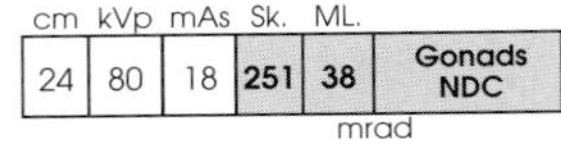

cm	kVp	mAs	Sk.	ML.	
24	80	18	251	38	Gonads NDC

mrad

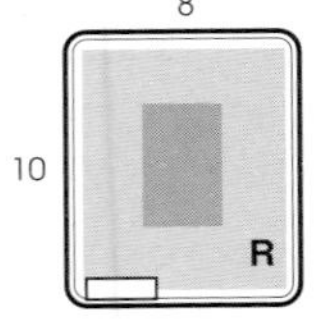

Patient Position

- Remove all metal, plastic or other removable objects from head.
- Patient erect or prone. (Erect preferred if patient's condition allows.)

Part Position 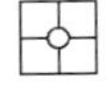

- Extend neck, resting chin and nose against head unit or table-top.
- Adjust head until **lips-meatal line (LML) is perpendicular;** OML will form a **55°** angle with the film.
- Position **midsagittal plane perpendicular** to the midline of the head unit or table. Ensure **no rotation** of head.
- Center cassette to CR and to acanthion.

Central Ray

- Align CR **perpendicular**, centered to **exit at acanthion**.
- Center cassette to CR.
- SID: Head unit, 36 in. (91 cm).
  Table, minimum 40 in. (102 cm).

Collimation: Use an 8 x 10 in. circle diaphragm or collimate to within 1 in. (2.5 cm) of facial bones.

Respiration: Suspend respiration during exposure.

Note: This projection is excellent for evaluating the possibility of a "blowout" fracture of the orbits.

Fig. 12-19. Modified parietoacanthial (Waters)–Erect. –**LML perpendicular (OML 55°)**.

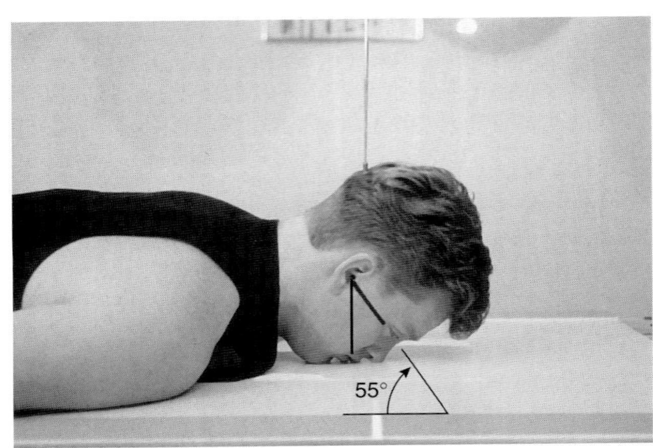

Fig. 12-20. Modified parietoacanthial (Waters)–Recumbent. –**LML perpendicular (OML 55°)**.

Evaluation Criteria

- **Petrous ridges** are projected into the **lower half of the maxillary sinuses, below the inferior orbital rim.**
- The inferior orbital rim is located in the center of the radiograph, with the entire orbital rim and maxillary bones within the collimated field.
- The cranium is not rotated:
  –Equal distance from the midsagittal plane, identified by the bony nasal septum, to the outer orbital margin on each side.
- Sufficient penetration and exposure, without motion, to visualize the orbital floors.

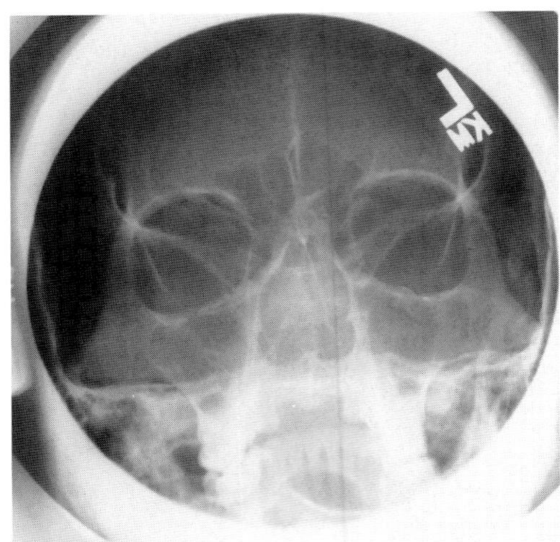

Fig. 12-21. Modified parietoacanthial (Waters).

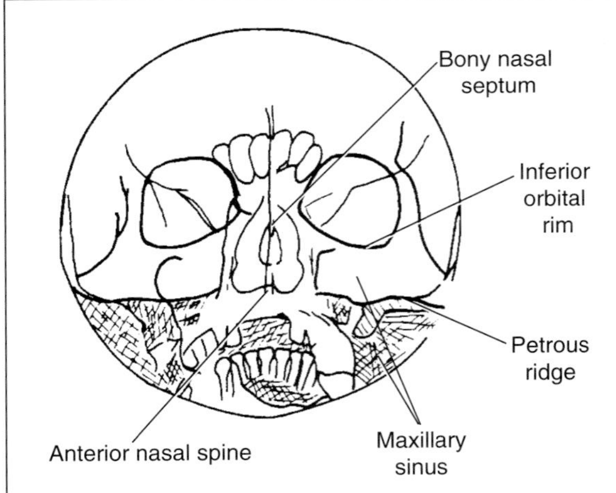

Fig. 12-22. Modified parietoacanthial (Waters).

Lateral Position

Nasal bones
Basic
• **Lateral**
• Parietoacanthial (Waters method) (see page 364: Facial bone–Waters method)

Structures Best Shown

Nasal bone and soft tissue nose structures.
Both sides are generally taken for comparison, with the side closest to film demonstrated best.

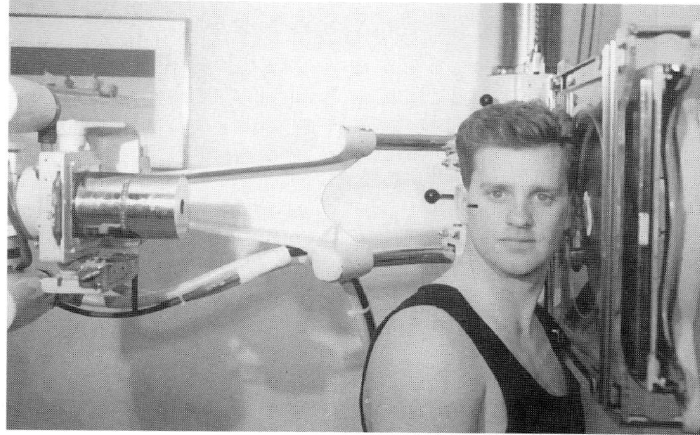

Fig. 12-23. Left lateral.

Technical Factors

- Film size–8 x 10 in. (18 x 24 cm).
- Place film crosswise and divide in half.
- **Detail screen,** table-top.
- 50-60 kVp range.
- Use small focal spot.
- Technique and dose:

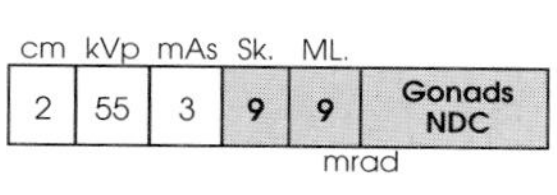

cm	kVp	mAs	Sk.	ML.	
2	55	3	9	9	Gonads NDC

mrad

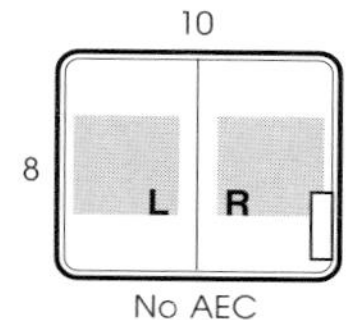

Patient Position

- Remove all metal, plastic or other removable objects from head.
- Patient in an erect or prone position.

Part Position 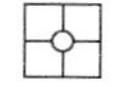

- Rest lateral side of head against head unit or table-top, with side of interest closest to cassette.
- Position nasal bone to center of unmasked half of cassette.
- Adjust head into a **true lateral position,** oblique body as needed for patient's comfort (place sponge block under chin if needed).
- Align **midsagittal plane parallel** with head unit or table-top.
- Align **interpupillary line perpendicular** to head unit or table-top.
- Position **infraorbitomeatal line perpendicular** to front edge of cassette.

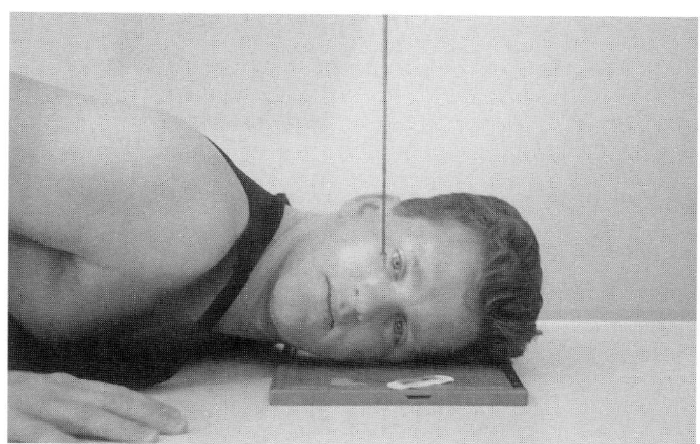

Fig. 12-24. Left lateral.

Central Ray

- Align CR **perpendicular** to film.
- Center CR to **½ in. (1.25 cm) inferior to nasion.**
- SID: Head unit, 36 in. (91 cm).
  Table, minimum 40 in. (102 cm).
- Center portion of film being exposed to CR.

Collimation: Use a circle diaphragm or collimate on all sides to within 2 in. (5 cm) of nasal bone.

Respiration: Suspend respiration during exposure.

Note: To obtain a sharply detailed image of the nasal bone, the utilization of a small focal spot, detail screens and close collimation is essential.

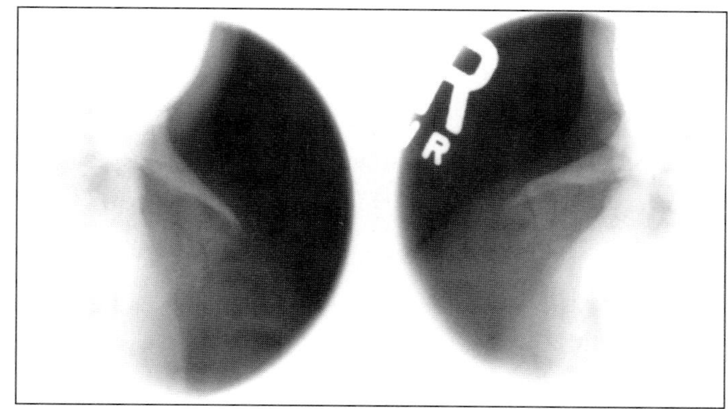

Fig. 12-25. Lateral (R and L).

Evaluation Criteria

- The nasal bone is located in the center of the unmasked half of film, with the nasal soft tissue, anterior nasal spine and frontonasal suture located within the collimated field.
- The nasal bone is demonstrated without rotation.
- Sufficient penetration and exposure, without motion, to visualize nasal bone and soft tissue structures without overexposure.

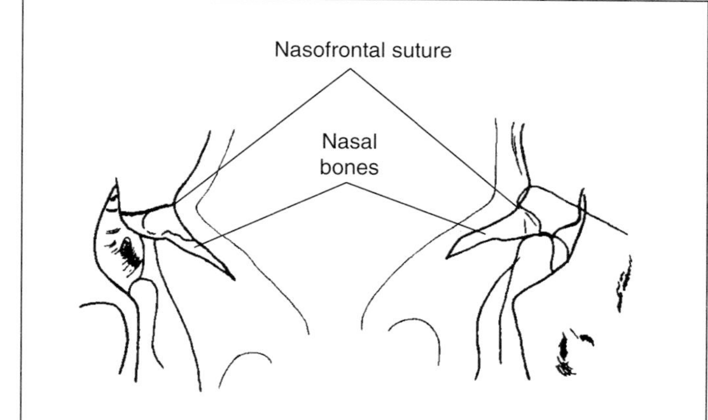

Fig. 12-26. Lateral.

Superoinferior Tangential (Axial) Projection

Nasal bones
Special
- PA Caldwell
  (See page 365)
- **Superoinferior (axial)**

Structures Best Shown

Demonstrates mid to distal nasal bones in a tangential perspective.

Technical Factors

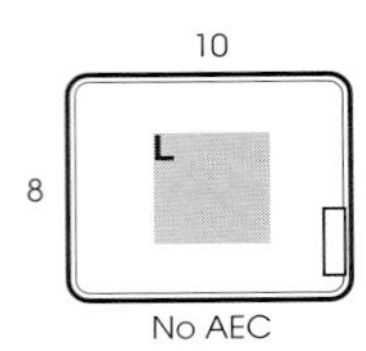

- Film size –8 x 10 in. (18 x 24 cm), crosswise.
  Optional –Occlusal film packet.
- Detail screen, table-top.
- 50-60 kVp range.
- Use small focal spot.
- Accessories: Sponge or sand bag and occlusal film if available.
- Technique and dose:

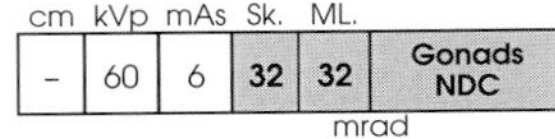

cm	kVp	mAs	Sk.	ML.	
-	60	6	32	32	Gonads NDC
			mrad		

Shielding

Place lead shield over lap or pelvic region to shield gonads.

Patient Position

- Seated in a chair at end of table, or prone on table.

Part Position

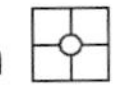

Upright Seated on Chair or Prone on Table-top:
- Extend chin and rest on cassette. Place angled support under cassette as demonstrated to **place film perpendicular to GAL,** (glabelloalveolar line).
- Align midsagittal plane perpendicular to CR and to cassette midline.

Optional with Occlusal Film:
- Elevate head on sponge.
- Place occlusal film between teeth, extend film beyond nasal soft tissue.
- Align film center to nasion (midsagittal plane) and to CR.
- Glabelloalveolar line is perpendicular to film and parallel to CR.

Central Ray

- Center CR to nasion and angle as needed to be **parallel to GAL** (glabelloalveolar line). (CR must just skim glabella and anterior upper front teeth.)
- Minimum 40 in. (102 cm) SID.

Collimation: Collimate on all sides to nasal bones.

Respiration: Suspend respiration during exposure.

Notes: The optional occlusal film packet may be used, if available, due to decreased OID with increased resolution. However, it does result in increased patient dose.

Any combination of prominent forehead, small nose or protruding front incisors may make visualization of the nasal bones impossible with this projection.

Fig. 12-27. Superoinferior projection-Erect.

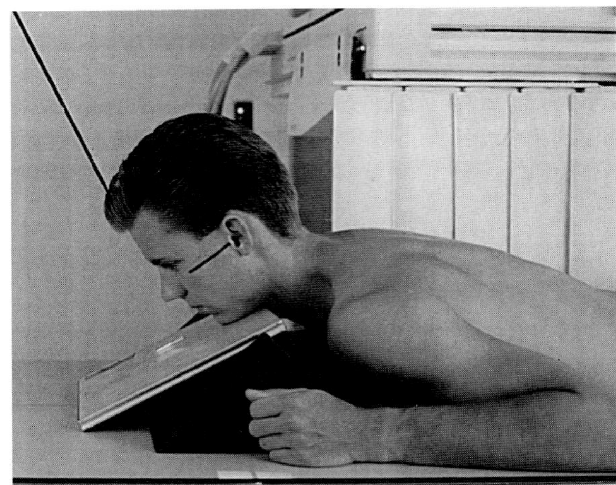

Fig. 12-28. Superoinferior projection-Prone.

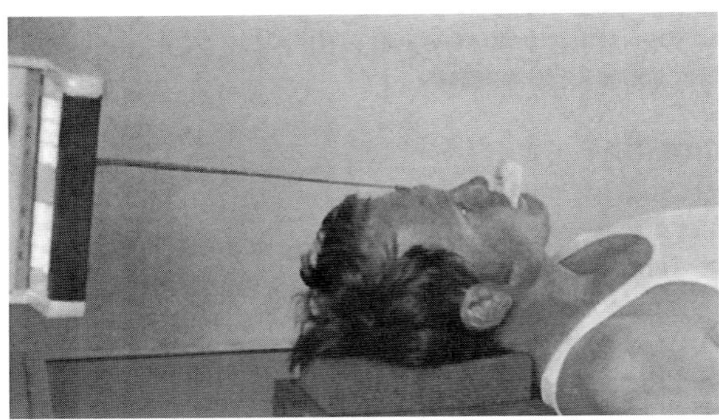

Fig. 12-29. Optional-With occlusal film.

Evaluation Criteria

- Included on radiograph are nasal soft tissue and nasal bones.
- Nasal bones are visualized with little superimposition of the glabella or alveolar ridge. (Excessive extension results in visualization of alveolar ridge and excessive flexion visualizes too much of the glabella.)
- No rotation: Equal distance from anterior nasal spine to outer soft tissue borders on each side.
- Sufficient penetration and exposure, without motion, to visualize nasal bones and nasal soft tissue.

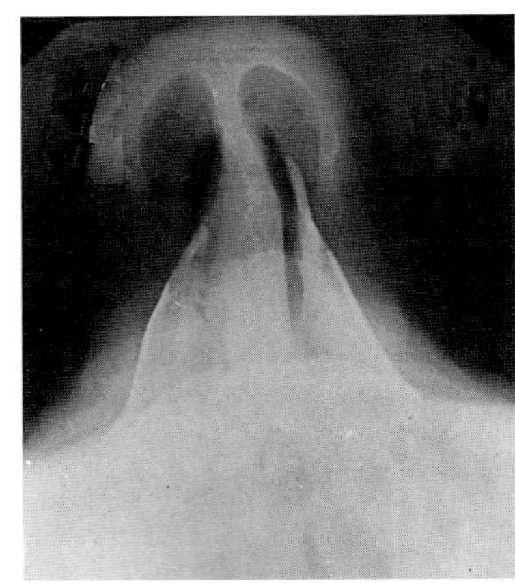

Fig. 12-30. Superoinferior projection.

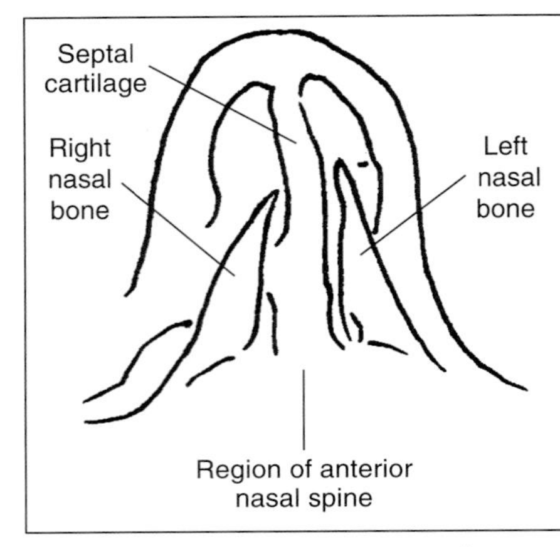

Fig. 12-31. Superoinferior projection.

Submentovertex (SMV) Projection

Zygomatic arches
Basic
- **Submentovertex**
- Oblique tangential
- AP axial (modified Towne)

Special (See Facial bones)
- Parietoacanthial (p. 364) (Waters method)
- Lateral (p. 363)

Structures Best Shown

Bilateral zygomatic arches.

Technical Factors

- Film size–8 x 10 in. (18 x 24 cm), crosswise.
- Detail screen, non grid cassette.
- 60-70 kVp range (soft-tissue technique, no AEC).
- Use small focal spot.
- Technique and dose:

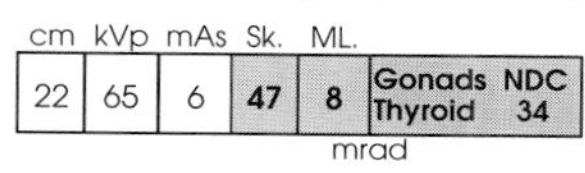

cm	kVp	mAs	Sk.	ML.	
22	65	6	47	8	Gonads NDC Thyroid 34

mrad

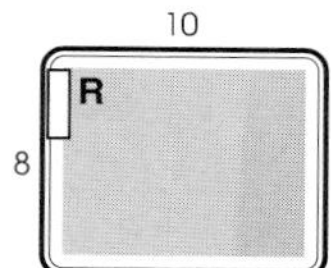

Patient Position

- Remove all metal, plastic or other removable objects from head.
- Patient in an erect or supine position.
- Erect, which is easier for patient, may be done with dedicated head unit if available or with erect table or other erect grid-film holder device.

Part Position

- Raise chin, hyperextending neck until **infraorbitomeatal line is parallel** to film. (See Notes.)
- Head rests on vertex of skull.
- Align **midsagittal plane perpendicular** to midline of head unit or vertical table, thus **avoiding all tilt and/or rotation**.

Central Ray

- Align CR **perpendicular** to film. (See Notes.)
- Center CR **midway between zygomatic arches**, at a level **1½ in.** (4 cm) **inferior to mandibular symphysis.**
- Center cassette to CR with plane of film parallel to IOML.
- SID: Head unit, 36 in. (91 cm). Table, minimum 40 in. (102 cm).

Collimation: Collimate to outer margins of skull on all sides.

Respiration: Suspend respiration during exposure.

Notes: If patient is unable to sufficiently extend neck, angle CR **perpendicular to IOML.** The cassette should also be angled if possible as needed to maintain the film perpendicular to CR.

Position is very uncomfortable for patient; move quickly.

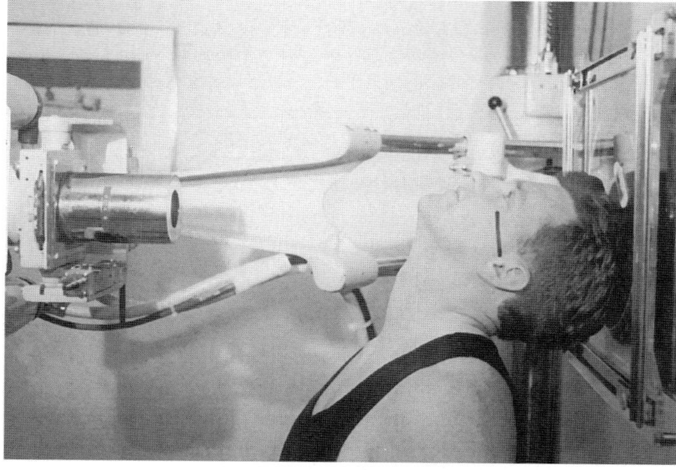

Fig. 12-32. SMV projection–**IOML parallel to film.** –**CR perpendicular to IOML.**

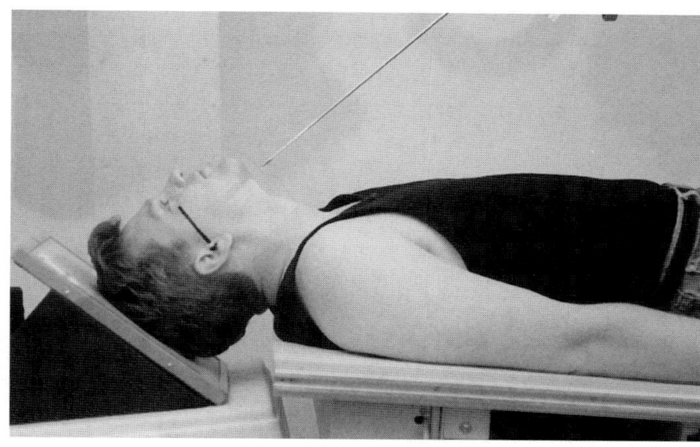

Fig. 12-33. SMV projection–**IOML parallel to film.** –**CR perpendicular to IOML.**

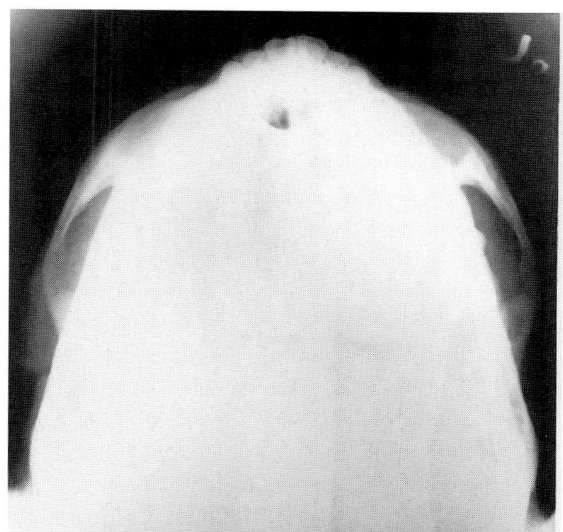

Fig. 12-34. SMV projection.

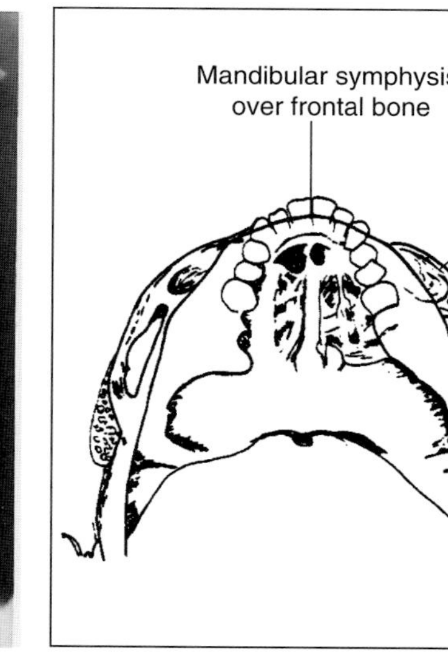

Fig. 12-35. SMV projection.

Evaluation Criteria

- Zygomatic arches are demonstrated, projecting laterally from each zygomatic and temporal bone, unless trauma prevents their visualization.
- Mandibular symphysis superimposes anterior frontal bone.
- Zygomatic arches are symmetrically visualized, without rotation.
- Sufficient penetration and exposure, without motion, to visualize zygomatic arches.

Oblique Inferosuperior (Tangential) Projection

Zygomatic arches
Basic
- Submentovertex
- **Oblique tangential**
- AP axial (modified Towne)

Special (See Facial bones)
- Parietoacanthial (p. 364) (Waters method)
- Lateral (p. 363)

Structures Best Shown

Single zygomatic arch free of superimposition. A good projection for "flat" or depressed zygomatic arches due to trauma or skull morphology.

Both sides are generally taken for comparison.

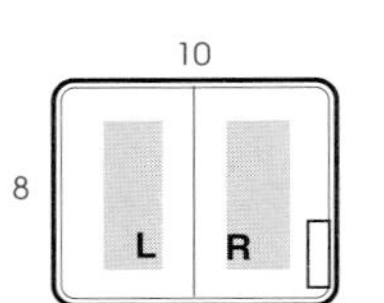

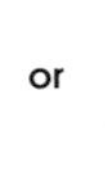

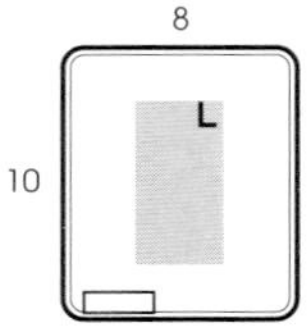

Technical Factors

- Film size–8 x 10 in. (18 x 24 cm), lengthwise. (May use one film crosswise divided in half or two single films lengthwise.)
- Detail screen, non grid cassette.
- 60-70 kVp range (soft-tissue technique no AEC).
- Use small focal spot.
- Technique and dose:

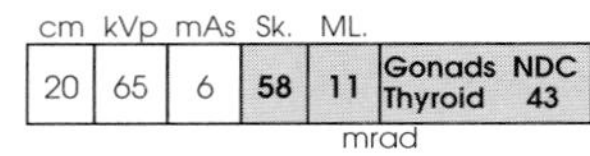

cm	kVp	mAs	Sk.	ML.	
20	65	6	58	11	Gonads NDC Thyroid 43

mrad

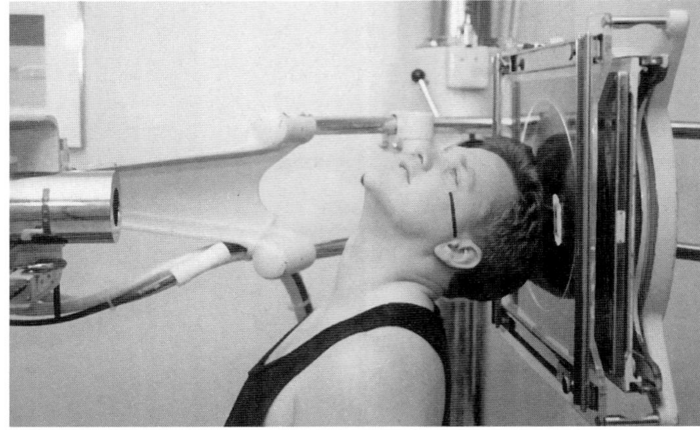

Fig. 12-36. Oblique tangential.

Patient Position

- Remove all metal, plastic or other removable objects from head.
- Patient in an erect or supine position.
- Erect, which is easier for patient, may be done with dedicated head unit if available or with erect table or other erect grid-film holder device.

Part Position 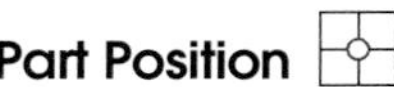

- Raise chin, hyperextending neck until **infraorbitomeatal line is parallel** to film. (See Notes.)
- Rest head on vertex of skull.
- **Rotate head 15° toward side to be examined; then also tilt chin 15° toward side of interest.**

Central Ray

- Align **CR perpendicular** to **film and IOML**. (See Notes).
- Center CR to **zygomatic arch of interest.** (CR will skim parietal eminence and body of mandible.)
- Adjust cassette to be parallel to IOML and perpendicular to CR.
- SID: Head unit, 36 in. (91 cm).
  Table, minimum 40 in. (102 cm).

Collimation: Collimate on all sides to within 1 in. (2.5 cm) of zygomatic bone and arch.

Respiration: Suspend respiration.

Notes: If patient is unable to sufficiently extend neck, angle CR **perpendicular to IOML**. If possible, angle cassette as needed to maintain the film perpendicular to CR.

Position is very uncomfortable for patient; move quickly.

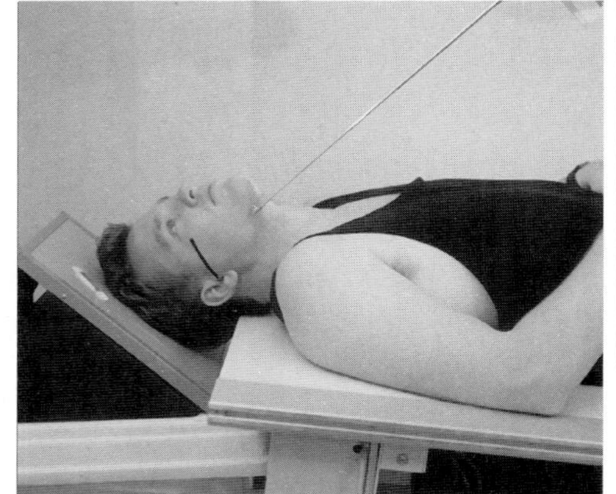

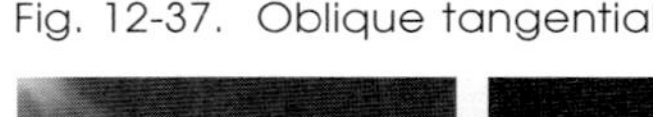

Fig. 12-37. Oblique tangential.

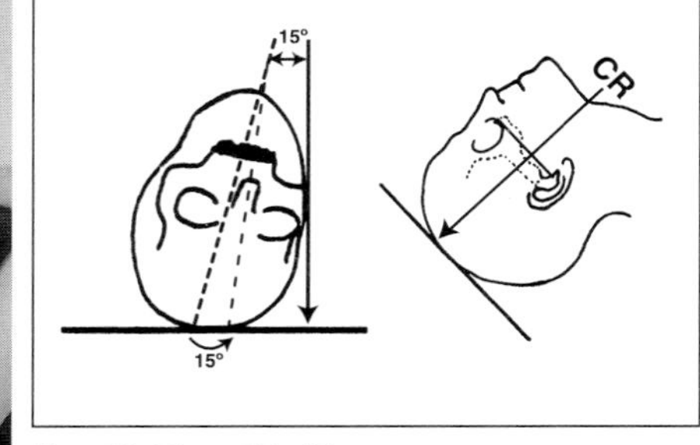

Fig. 12-38. –15° tilt.
–15° rotation.
–CR perpendicular to IOML.

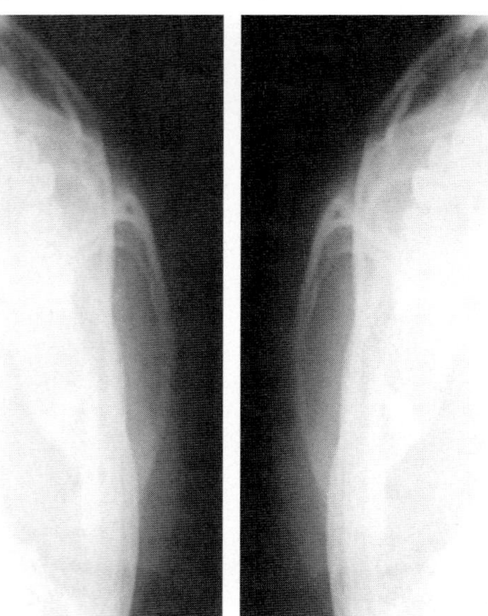

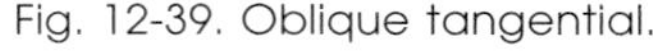

Fig. 12-39. Oblique tangential.

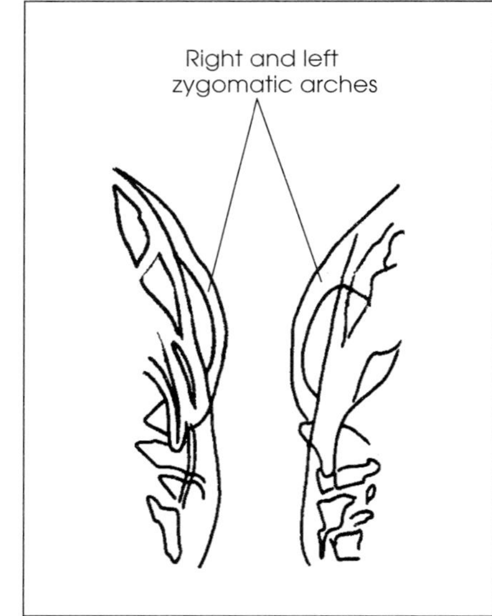

Fig. 12-40. Oblique tangential.

Evaluation Criteria

- Zygomatic arch visualized in the center of collimation field.
- Zygomatic arch is demonstrated **without superimposition of parietal or mandible.**
- Sufficient penetration and exposure, without motion, **to visualize zygomatic arch.**

AP Axial Projection

Modified Towne Method

Zygomatic arches
Basic
- Submentovertex
- Oblique axial (tangential)
- **AP axial (modified Towne)**

Special (See Facial bones)
- Parietoacanthial (p. 364) (Waters method)
- Lateral (p. 363)

Structures Best Shown

Bilateral zygomatic arches.

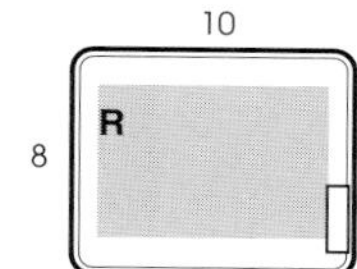

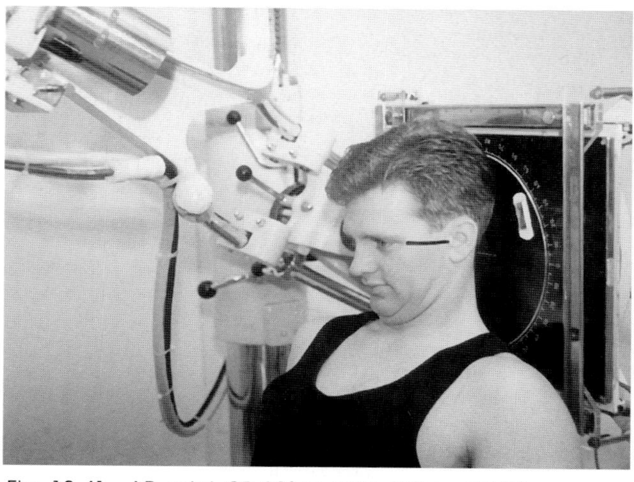

Fig. 12-41. AP axial–**CR 30° to OML** (37° to IOML).

Technical Factors

- Film size–8 x 10 in. (18 x 24 cm), crosswise.
- Moving or stationary grid (near soft-tissue technique, no AEC).
- 60-70 kVp range.
- Use small focal spot.
- Technique and dose:

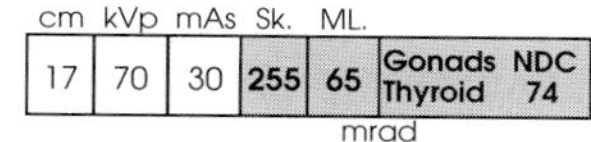

cm	kVp	mAs	Sk.	ML.	
17	70	30	255	65	Gonads NDC Thyroid 74
			mrad		

Patient Position

- Remove all metal, plastic or other removable objects from head.
- Patient in an erect or supine position.

Part Position

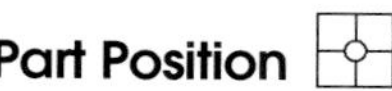

- Rest patient's posterior skull against head unit or table-top.
- Tuck chin, bringing **OML (or IOML) perpendicular** to film. (See Note below.)
- Align **midsagittal plane perpendicular** to midline of head unit or table-top to prevent head rotation or tilt.

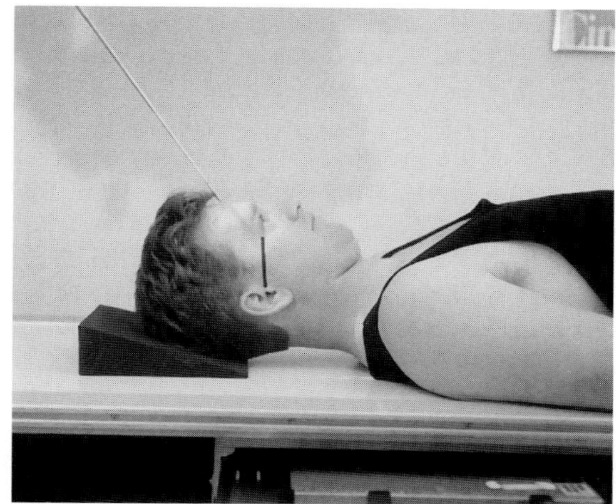

Fig. 12-42. AP axial–**CR 30° to OML** (37° to IOML).

Central Ray

- Angle CR **30° caudad to OML**, or **37° to IOML** (see Note).
- Center CR to 1 in. (2.5 cm) superior to glabella (to pass through mid arches).
- Center cassette to projected CR.
- SID: Head unit, 36 in. (91 cm). Table, minimum 40 in. (102 cm).

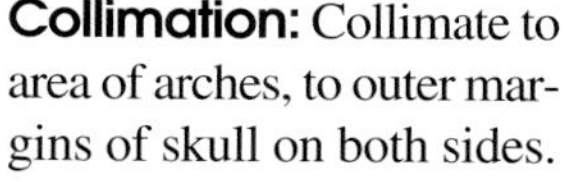

Collimation: Collimate to area of arches, to outer margins of skull on both sides.

Respiration: Suspend respiration during exposure.

Note: If patient is unable to depress the chin sufficiently to bring the OML perpendicular to the film, the infraorbitomeatal line (**IOML**) can be placed perpendicular instead and the CR angle increased to 37° caudad. This maintains the 30° angle between OML and CR and demonstrates the same anatomical relationships. (There is a 7° difference between the OML and IOML.)

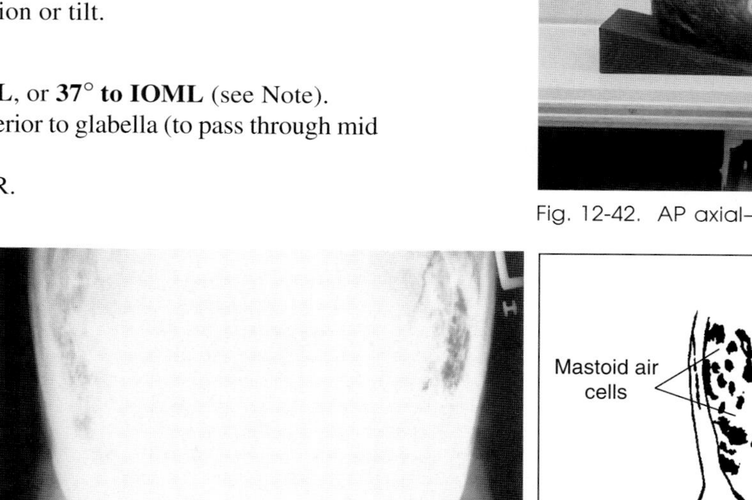

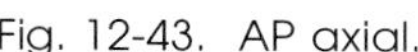

Fig. 12-43. AP axial.

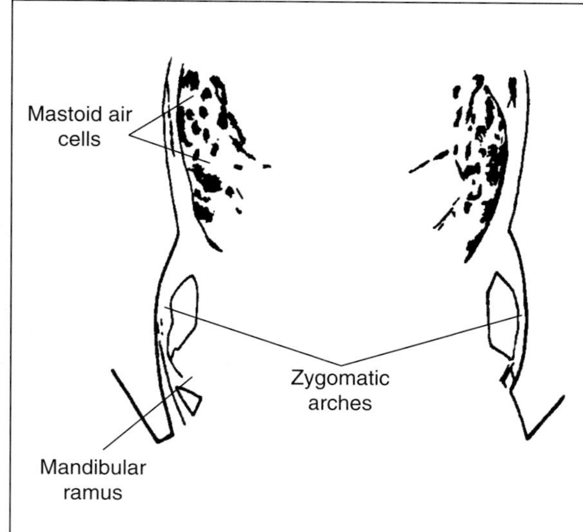

Fig. 12-44. AP axial.

Evaluation Criteria

- Zygomatic arches are in center of radiograph, visualized lateral to each mandibular ramus.
- Zygomatic arches are seen without rotation:
  - –Arches are not superimposing mandible.
  - –Arches are symmetrical.
- Sufficient penetration and exposure, without motion, to visualize zygomatic arches.

Parieto-Orbital Projection

Rhese Method

Optic foramina
Basic
• **Parieto-orbital (Rhese)**
• Parietoacanthial (Waters method), p. 364
• PA (Caldwell method)
Special
• Modified parietoacanthial (modified Waters method), p. 366

Structures Best Shown

Cross section of each optic canal, with a non-distorted view of optic foramen.

Both sides are generally taken for comparison.

Fig. 12-45. Parieto-orbital projection.

Technical Factors

- Film size–8 x 10 in. (18 x 24 cm)
- Crosswise, divided in half, or two separate films.
- Moving or stationary grid.
- 70-80 kVp range.
- No AEC due to small exposure field.
- Use small focal spot.
- Technique and dose:

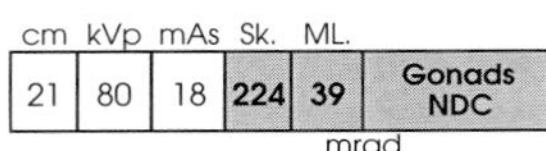

cm	kVp	mAs	Sk.	ML.	Gonads
21	80	18	224	39	NDC
			mrad		

Patient Position

- Remove all metal, plastic or other removable objects from head.
- Patient in an erect or supine position.

Part Position 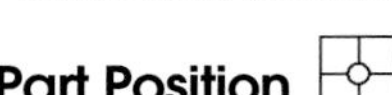

- As a starting reference, position patient's chin, cheek and nose against head unit or table-top. (See Note.)
- Adjust head as needed so that the midsagittal plane forms a **53° angle** with film. (An angle indicator should be used to obtain an accurate angle of 53° from a lateral position.)
- Position **acanthiomeatal line perpendicular** to plane of film.
- Center mid point of downside orbit to CR and to center of unmasked half of cassette. (Use spacer as needed in Bucky tray to center the half of cassette being exposed to center line and to CR, or use separate cassettes for each side.)

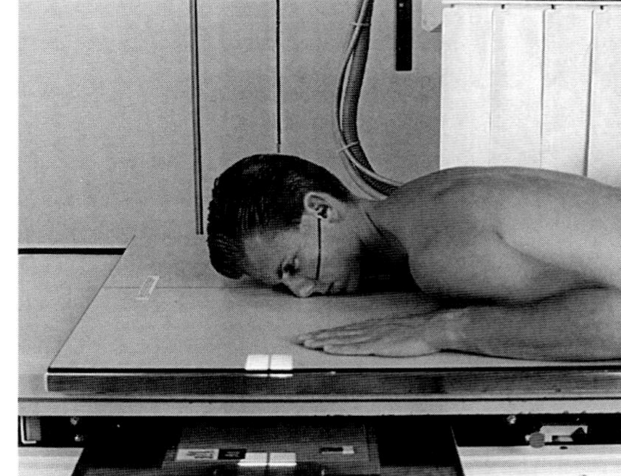

-53° rotation (from film).
-Acanthiomeatal line perpendicular.
-CR perpendicular.

Fig. 12-46. Parieto-orbital projection.

Central Ray

- Align CR **perpendicular** to film, centered to **downside orbit**.
- SID: Head unit, 36 in. (91 cm).
  Table, minimum 40 in. (102 cm).

Collimation: Use a circle diaphragm or collimate on all sides to yield a field size of approximately 4 in. (10 cm) square.

Respiration: Suspend respiration during exposure.

Notes: This is sometimes called a "three-point landing" position. This, however, is not an accurate final positioning reference.

A view of both orbits are taken for comparison. When positioning for the opposite orbit, oblique head in the opposite direction.

To obtain a sharply detailed image of the optic foramen, the utilization of a **small focal spot** and **close collimation** is essential.

Fig. 12-47. Bilateral parieto-orbital.

Evaluation Criteria

- **Optic foramen** is projected into the **lower outer quadrant of orbit.** (Results when acanthiomeatal line is perpendicular to plane of film. This slight extension of the neck moves the foramen from upper to lower aspect of orbit.)
- The optic foramen is located in the center of unmasked half of film, with the orbital margins also included within the collimated field.
- Sufficient penetration and exposure, without motion, to visualize the optic foramen.

Fig. 12-48. Bilateral parieto-orbital.

Axiolateral Projection

Mandible
Basic
• **Axiolateral**
• PA (or PA axial)
• AP axial (Towne)

Structures Best Shown

Mandibular rami, body and mentum of mandible positioned closest to film. Both sides taken for comparison.

10
8
R
No AEC

Technical Factors

- Film size–8 x 10 in. (18 x 24 cm), crosswise.
- Moving or stationary grid.
- 70-80 kVp range.
- Use small focal spot
- Technique and dose:

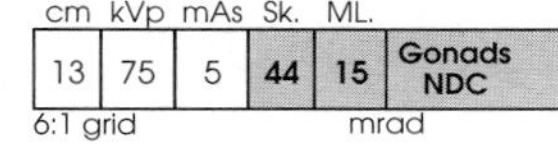

cm	kVp	mAs	Sk.	ML.	Gonads
13	75	5	44	15	NDC

6:1 grid   mrad

Patient Position

- Remove all metal, plastic or other removable objects from head.
- Patient erect, supine or prone. (If supine, place cassette on wedge sponge to minimize OID.)

Part Position

- Place head in a lateral position, with side of interest against film holder.
- If possible, have patient close mouth and bring teeth together.
- Extend chin, to prevent cervical spine superimposition.
- Oblique (rotate) head. The degree of obliquity will depend on which section of the mandible is of interest. (Area of interest if known should be positioned parallel to film).
  –Head in **true lateral** position best demonstrates **ramus.**
  –**30°** rotation toward film best demonstrates **body.**
  –**45°** rotation best demonstrates **mentum**.
  –**10 to 15°** rotation for **general survey** of mandible.

Central Ray

- Angle CR **25° cephalad**.
- Direct CR to pass through mandibular region of interest.
- Center cassette to projected CR.
- SID: Head unit, 36 in. (91 cm). Table, minimum 40 in. (102 cm).

Collimation: Use a circle diaphragm or collimate on all sides to region of mandible.

Respiration: Suspend respiration.

Note: For trauma patient who cannot assume this position, see Chapter 19 on trauma radiography.

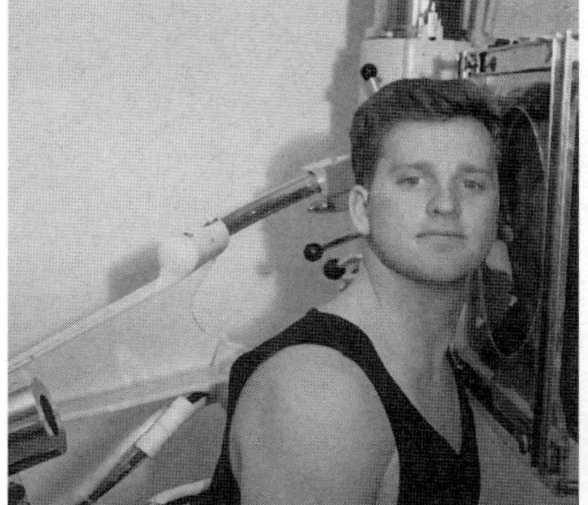

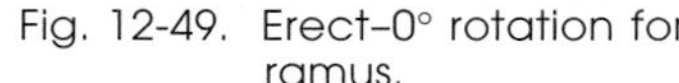

Fig. 12-49. Erect–0° rotation for ramus.

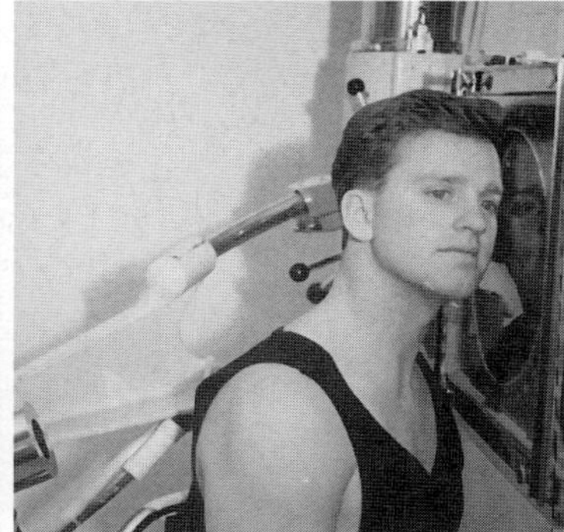

Fig. 12-50. Erect–30° rotation for body.

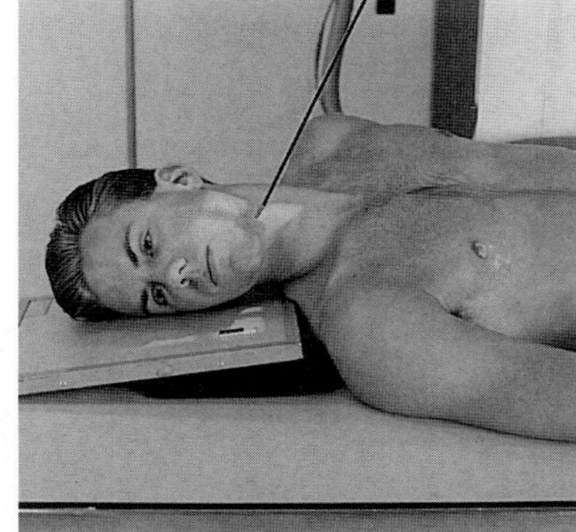

Fig. 12-51. Semisupine.

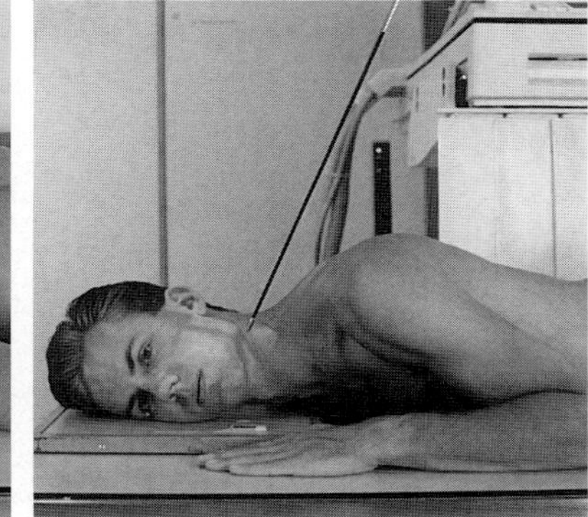

Fig. 12-52. Semiprone.

–General survey, 15° rotation.

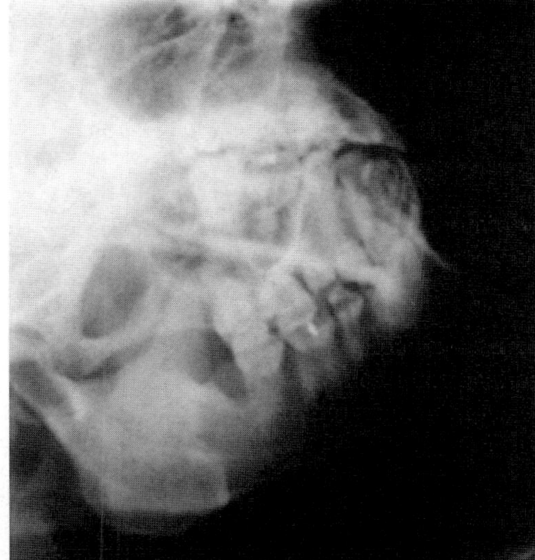

Fig. 12-53. Axiolateral (general survey).

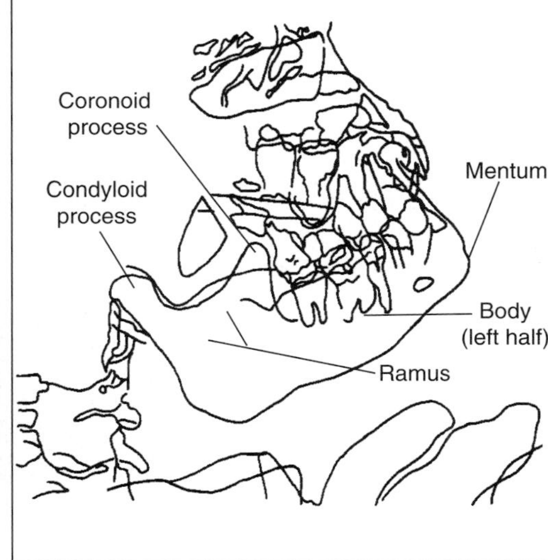

Fig. 12-54. Axiolateral (general survey).

Evaluation Criteria

- The entire mandible is located within the collimated field.
- If radiograph taken in a position for the **ramus** and **body**:
  –Opposite mandible does not superimpose ramus of interest, (from insufficient CR angle).
  –Ramus is visualized without superimposing the cervical spine, (from insufficient extension of chin).
  –Condylar and coronoid processes are well visualized.
  –Mandibular ramus and body are demonstrated without foreshortening (from improper rotation of head).
- If radiograph is taken at 45° head rotation for the mentum:
  –Mentum area of interest is seen with less superimposition.
  –Mandibular mentum is demonstrated with less foreshortening.
- Sufficient penetration and exposure, without motion, to visualize the mandibular area of interest.

PA or PA Axial Projection

Mandible
Basic
• Axiolateral
• **PA (or PA axial)**
• AP axial (Towne)

Structures Best Shown

PA:
Mandibular rami and lateral portion of body.
PA Axial:
Proximal rami and lateral aspects of body, elongated view of condyloid processes.

Technical Factors

- Film size–8 x 10 in. (18 x 24 cm), lengthwise.
- Moving or stationary grid.
- 70-80 kVp range.
- Use small focal spot.
- Technique and dose:

cm	kVp	mAs	Sk.	ML.	Gonads
17	75	12	120	32	NDC
			mrad		

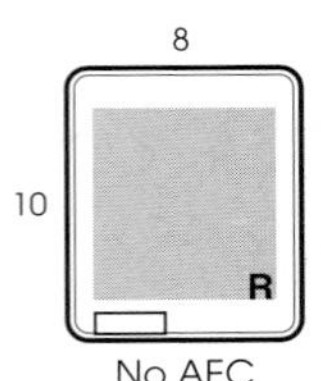

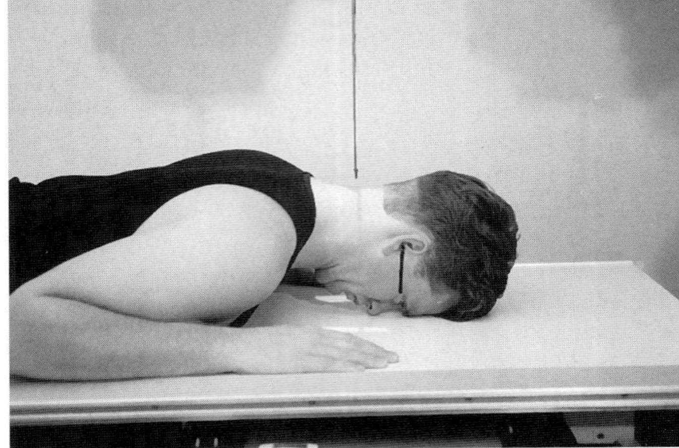

Fig. 12-55. PA–CR perpendicular.
–CR to exit at junction of lips.

Patient Position

- Remove all metal, plastic or other removable objects from head.
- Patient erect or prone.

Part Position

- Rest patient's forehead and nose against head unit or table-top.
- Tuck chin, bringing **OML perpendicular** to film. (See Note.)
- Align **midsagittal plane perpendicular** to midline of head unit or table-top. (Ensure no rotation or tilt of head.)
- Center cassette to projected CR (to junction of lips).

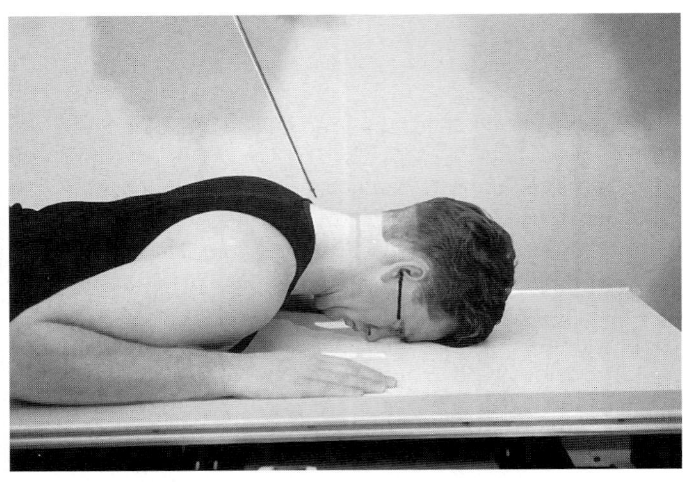

Fig 12-56. Optional: PA Axial–CR 20 to 25° cephalad.
–CR to exit at acanthion.

Central Ray

- *PA:* CR **perpendicular** to film, centered to **exit at junction of lips.**
- SID: Head unit, 36 in. (91 cm).
  Table, minimum 40 in. (102 cm).
- *PA Axial:* CR 20 to 25° cephalad, centered to **exit at acanthion**.

Collimation: Collimate to area of mandible.

Respiration: Suspend respiration during exposure.

Note: For a true frontal view of body (if this is area of interest), raise chin to bring acanthiomeatal line perpendicular to film.

Evaluation Criteria

- Radiograph includes TMJs, mandibular rami and mentum.
- Mandible is demonstrated without rotation when:
  –Mandibular rami are symmetrically visualized on each side of the cervical spine.
- Midbody and mentum are faintly visualized, superimposing the cervical spine.
- Sufficient penetration and exposure, without motion, to visualize mandibular body and rami.
- *PA Axial:* TMJ region and heads of condyles should be visible through mastoid process; condyloid processes are well visualized.

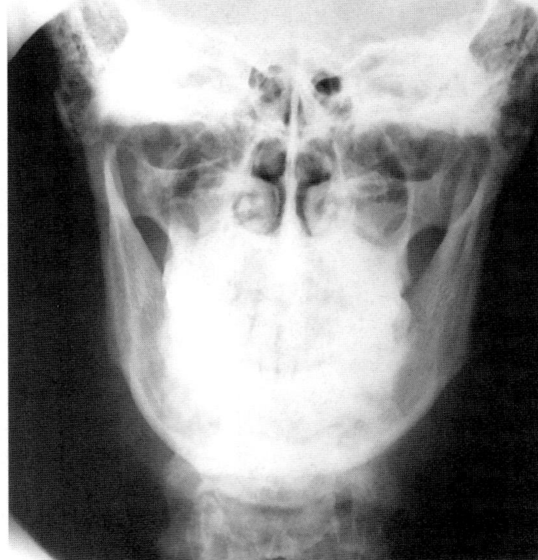

Fig. 12-57. PA.

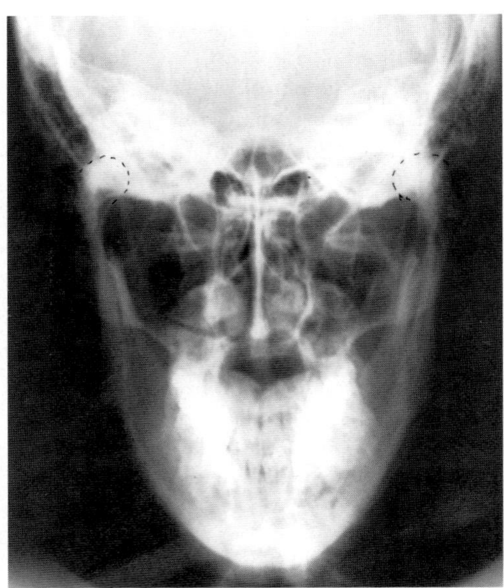

Fig. 12-58. PA axial, CR 20° cephalad.

AP Axial Projection

Towne Method

Mandible
Basic
• Axiolateral
• PA (or PA axial)
• **AP axial (Towne)**

Structures Best Shown

Condyloid processes of mandible and temporomandibular fossae.

Technical Factors

- Film size–8 x 10 in. (18 x 24 cm), lengthwise.
- Moving or stationary grid.
- 70-80 kVp range.
- Use small focal spot.
- Technique and dose:

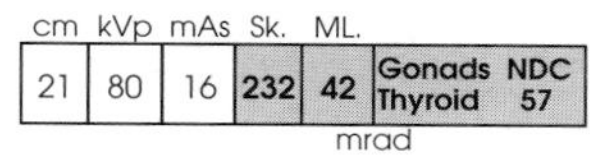

cm	kVp	mAs	Sk.	ML.	
21	80	16	232	42	Gonads NDC Thyroid 57
			mrad		

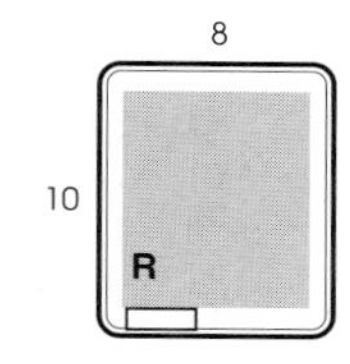

Patient Position

- Remove all metal, plastic or other removable objects from head.
- Patient in an erect or supine position.

Part Position

- Rest patient's posterior skull against head unit or table-top.
- Tuck chin, bringing **orbitomeatal line perpendicular** to film, or place IOML perpendicular and add 7° to CR angle. (See Note.)
- Align **midsagittal plane perpendicular** to midline of head unit or table-top to prevent head rotation or tilting.

Central Ray

- Angle CR **35 to 40° caudad**. (See Notes.)
- Center CR to **glabella**, to pass through **midway between EAMs and angles of mandible.**
- Center cassette to CR.
- SID: Head unit, 36 in. (91 cm).
  Table, minimum 40 in. (102 cm).

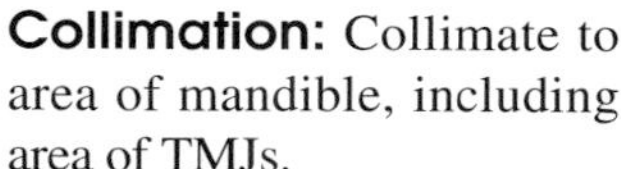

Collimation: Collimate to area of mandible, including area of TMJs.

Respiration: Suspend respiration during exposure.

Notes: If patient is unable to bring OML perpendicular to film, increase the CR angle 7° with the IOML perpendicular.

If the area of interest is the TM fossae, angle 40° to the OML to reduce superimposing the TM fossae and mastoid portions of the temporal bone.

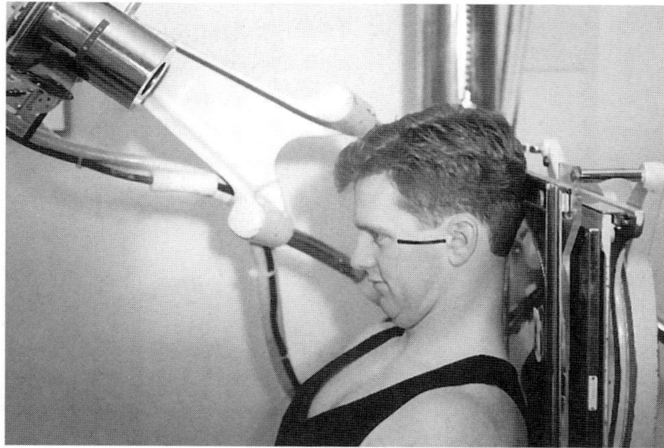

Fig. 12-59. AP axial–CR 35 to 40° to OML.

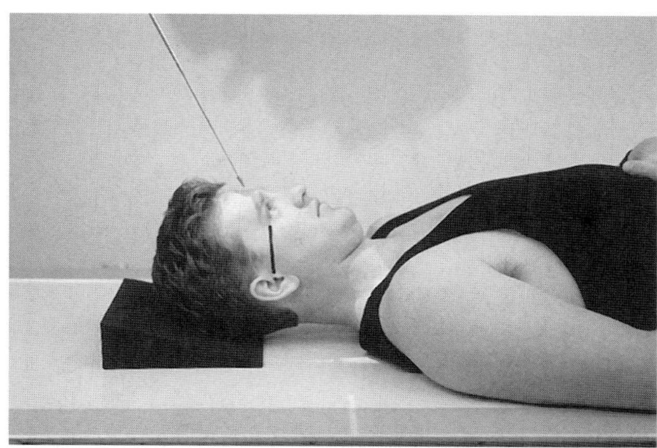

Fig. 12-60. AP axial–CR 35-40° to OML.

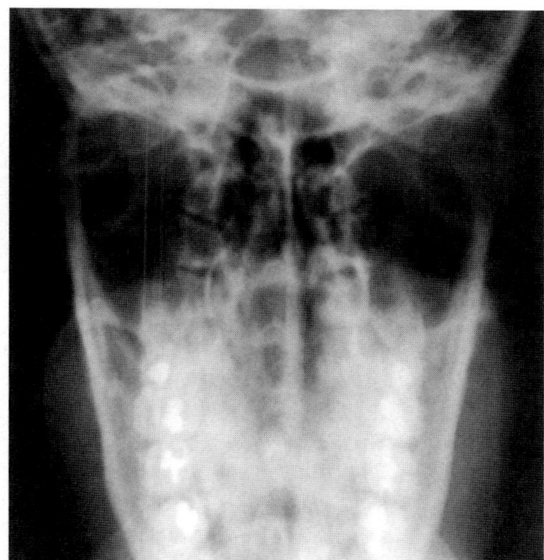

Fig. 12-61. AP axial.

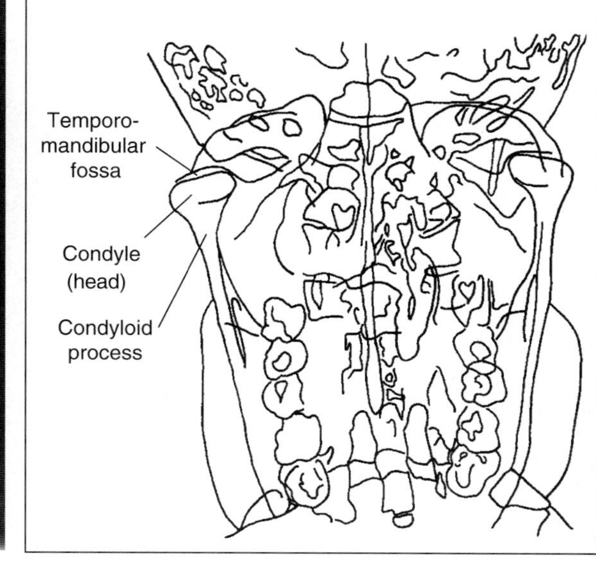

Fig. 12-62. AP axial.

Evaluation Criteria

- Included on the radiograph are the condyloid processes of the mandible and the temporomandibular fossae.
- Mandible is visualized without rotation when:
  –Condyloid processes are symmetrically visualized on each side of cervical spine.
- Clear visualization of condyle and temporomandibular fossae relationship with minimal superimposition of the TM fossae and mastoid portions.
- Sufficient penetration and exposure, without motion, to visualize condyloid process and temporomandibular fossa.

Submentovertex (SMV) Projection

Mandible
Special
- **Submentovertex (SMV)**
- Panorex
  (mandible and/or TMJs)

Structures Best Shown

Entire mandible, coronoid and condyloid processes.

Technical Factors

- Film size–8 x 10 in. (18 x 24 cm), lengthwise.
- Stationary or moving grid.
- 70-80 kVp range.
- Use small focal spot.
- Technique and dose:

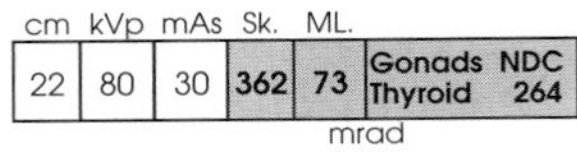

cm	kVp	mAs	Sk.	ML.	Gonads	NDC
22	80	30	362	73	Thyroid	264

mrad

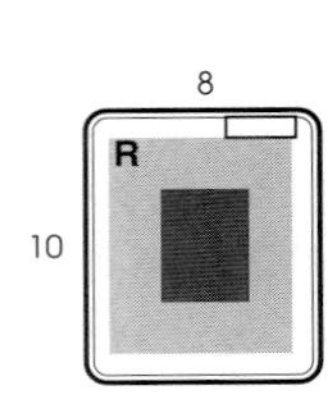
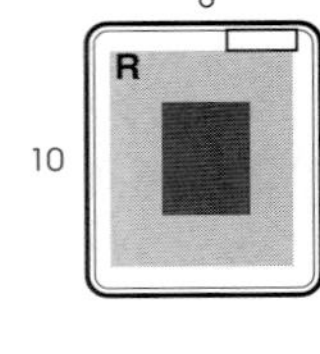

Patient Position

- Remove all metal, plastic or other removable objects from head and neck.
- Patient erect or supine (erect preferred, if patient's condition allows).
- Erect (which is easier for patient) may be done with dedicated head unit if available or with erect table or other erect grid-film holder device.

Part Position 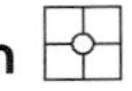

- Raise chin, hyperextending neck until **infraorbitomeatal line is parallel** to film.
- Rest head on vertex of skull.
- Align **midsagittal plane perpendicular** to midline of head unit or vertical table to prevent head rotation or tilt.

Central Ray

- Align CR **perpendicular to film or IOML**. (See Notes.)
- Center CR to a point **midway between angles of mandible**, at a level **1½ in.** (4 cm) **inferior to mandibular symphysis.**
- Center cassette to projected CR.
- SID: Head unit, 36 in. (91 cm).
  Table, minimum 40 in. (102 cm).

Collimation: Collimate to area of mandible.

Respiration: Suspend respiration.

Notes: If patient is unable to sufficiently extend neck, angle tube **perpendicular to IOML.** Angle film as needed to maintain the film perpendicular to CR.

This position is very uncomfortable for patient; move quickly.

Fig. 12-63. Submentovertex.

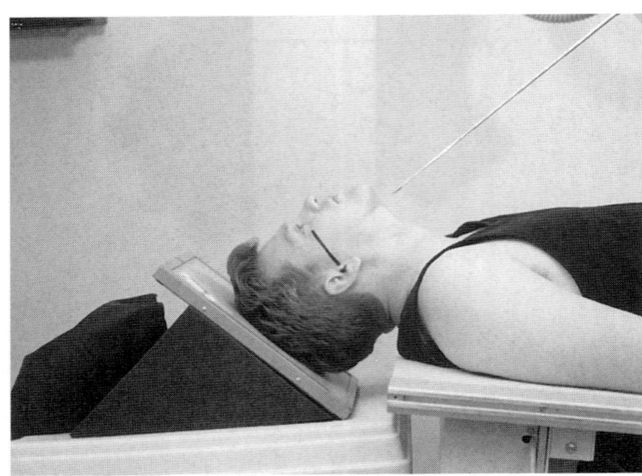

Fig. 12-64. Submentovertex.

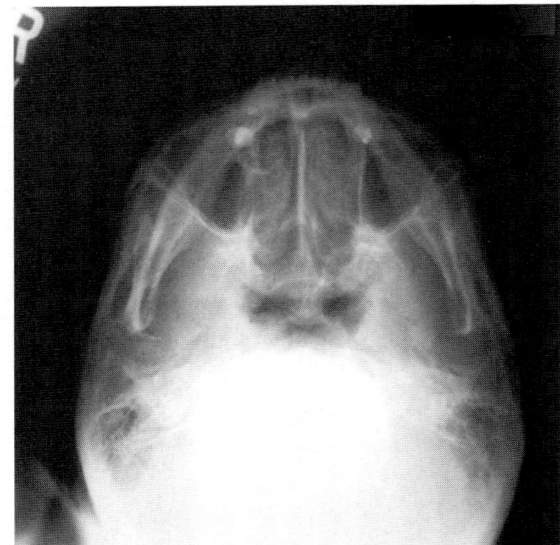

Fig. 12-65. Submentovertex.

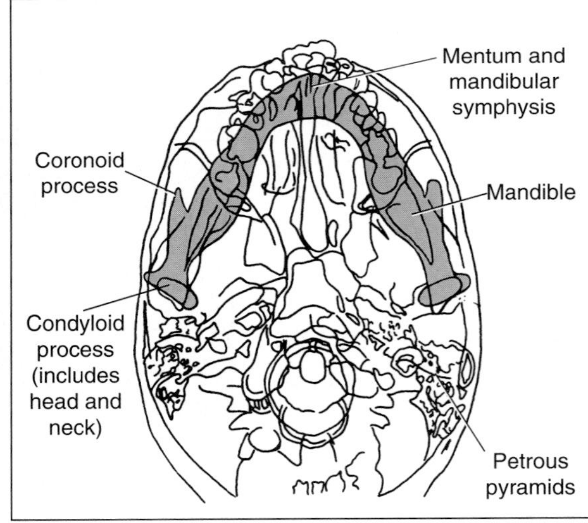

Fig. 12-66. Submentovertex.

Evaluation Criteria

- Entire mandible is visualized on radiograph.
- Mandibular symphysis superimposes anterior frontal bone.
- Cranium is not rotated: Distances along coinciding mandibular surfaces to lateral border of skull are equal.
- Mandibular condyles are projected anterior to petrous ridges.
- Mandibular coronoid processes are visualized, projecting laterally from the rami area, on each side of mandible.
- Sufficient penetration and exposure, without motion, to visualize entire mandible.

Panorex – Panoramic Tomography

Mandible
Special
• Submentovertex (SMV)
• **Panorex (mandible and/or TMJ's)**

Structures Best Shown

A single frontal projection of the teeth, mandible, nasal fossae, maxillary sinus, zygomatic arches and maxillae. (This may be performed for either the mandible and/or the TMJs; see Note.)

Technical Factors

- Film size–9 x 12 in. (23 x 30 cm), crosswise.
- Curved nongrid cassette.
- 70-80 kVp range.

Unit Preparation

- Attach cassette to panorex unit.
- Position tube and cassette at starting position.
- Raise chin rest to approximately same level as patient's chin.

Shielding: Wrap vest type lead apron around patient.

Patient Position

- Remove all metal, plastic or other removable objects from head and neck.
- Explain to patient how tube and film will rotate and the time span needed for exposure.
- Guide patient into unit resting patient's chin on bite block.
- Position patient's body, head and neck as demonstrated in Fig. 12-67. Do not allow head and neck to stretch forward but have patient stand in close with spine straight and hips forward (Fig. 12-70).

Part Position

- Adjust height of chin rest until **IOML is aligned parallel with floor**. The occlusal plane (plane of biting surface of teeth) will decline 10° from posterior to anterior.
- Align **midsagittal plane** with the vertical center line of the chin rest.
- Position bite block between patient's front teeth. (See Note.)
- Instruct patient to place lips together and position tongue on roof of mouth.

Central Ray

- X-ray beam direction is fixed and is directed slightly cephalic in order to project anatomical structures, positioned at the same height, on top of one another.
- Fixed SID as per panorex.

Collimation: A narrow vertical slit diaphragm is attached to tube, providing inherent collimation.

Note: When the temporomandibular joints are of interest, a second panorex is taken with the mouth open. This requires a larger bite block to be placed between the patient's teeth.

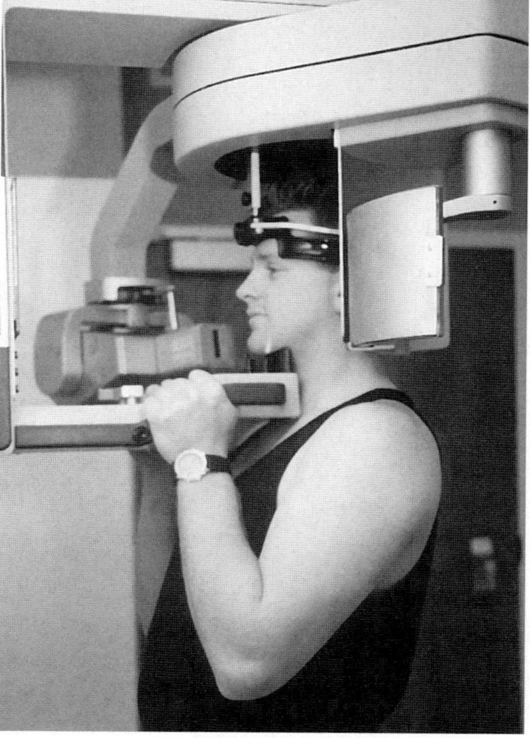

Fig. 12-67. Panorex–Head correctly positioned.

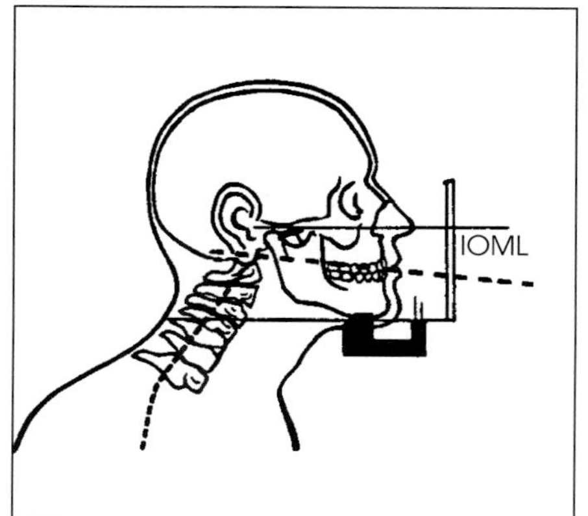

Fig. 12-68. **Incorrect** position.

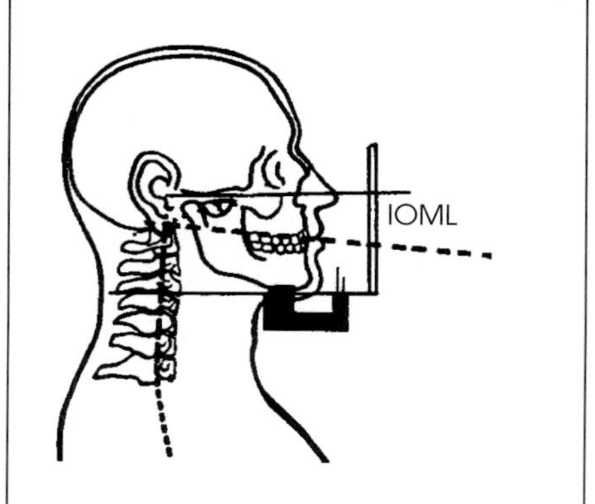

Fig. 12-69. **Correct** position.

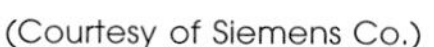
(Courtesy of Siemens Co.)

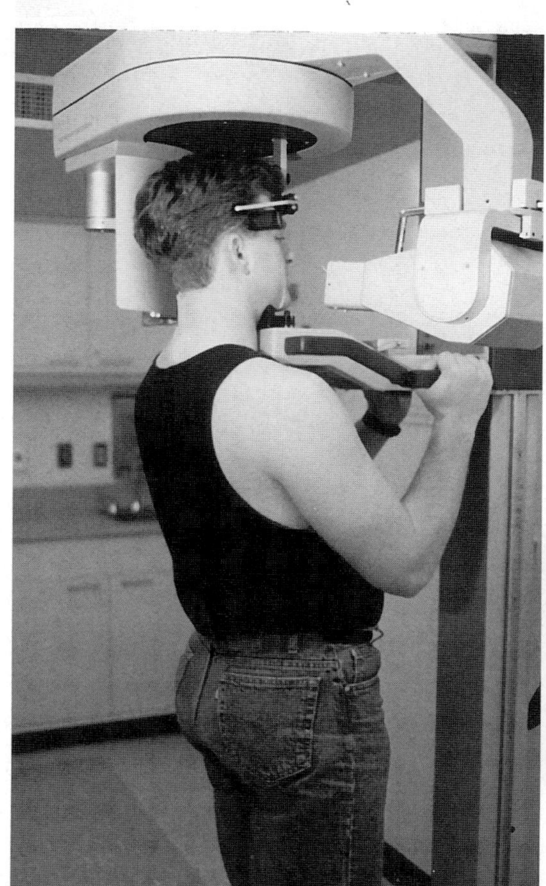

Fig. 12-70. Panorex–Correct body position.

Panorex continued

Evaluation Criteria

- Included on radiograph is entire mandible, nasal fossae and maxillary sinuses.
- The mandible is oval in shape, with the mandibular symphysis projected slightly below the mandibular angles.
- The occlusal plane is aligned parallel with the long axis of radiograph.
- The upper and lower teeth are positioned slightly apart with no superimposition.
- A portion of the cervical spine is visualized on each side of the radiograph.
- The cervical spine is demonstrated erect without superimposing the temporomandibular joints.
- Mandible is visualized without rotation or tilting:
  - –TMJs are at the same level on the radiograph.
  - –Rami and posterior teeth are equally magnified on each side.
  - –Image is located in the center of film.
- The anterior and posterior teeth are sharply visualized with uniform magnification.
- Density of mandible and teeth are uniform across entire radiograph, no density loss is seen in center of radiograph.
- No artifacts are seen blurring over image.
- Patient ID information with R or L marker is visible within collimated field without superimposing essential anatomy.

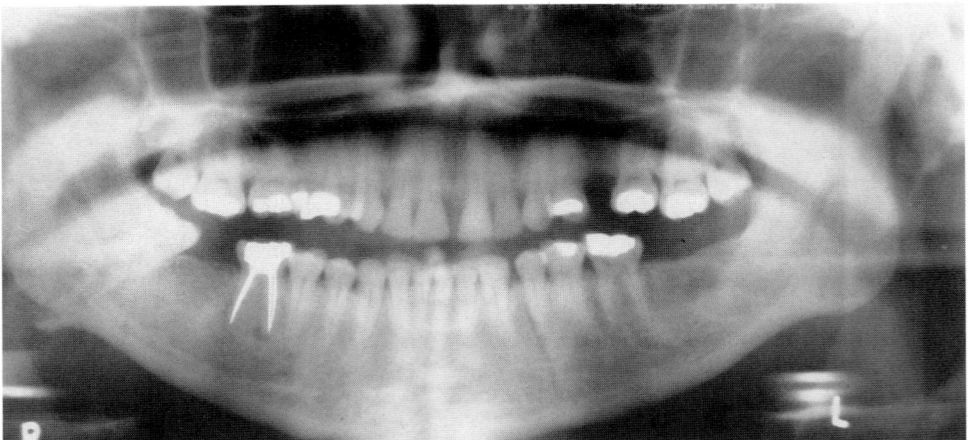

Fig. 12-71. Panorex.

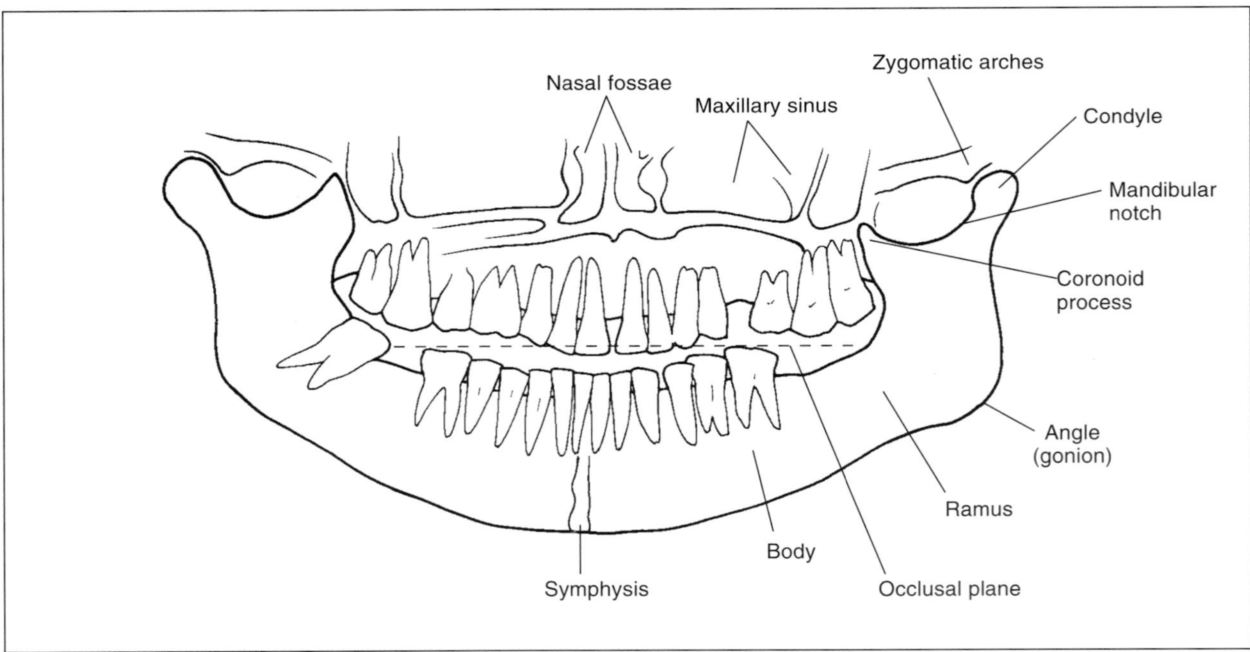

Fig. 12-72. Panorex.

12

AP Axial Projection - TMJs

Modified Towne Method

Warning: Open mouth should not be attempted with possible fracture.

> **TMJs**
> Special
> • **AP axial (modified Towne)**
> • Axiolateral oblique (modified Law)
> • Axiolateral (Schuller)
> • Tomography
> • Panorex (p. 377)

Structures Best Shown

Condyloid processes of mandible and temporomandibular fossae. See Note 1 concerning open and closed mouth comparisons.

Technical Factors

- Film size–8 x 10 in. (18 x 24 cm), lengthwise.
- Moving or stationary grid.
- 70-80 kVp range.
- Use small focal spot.
- Technique and dose:

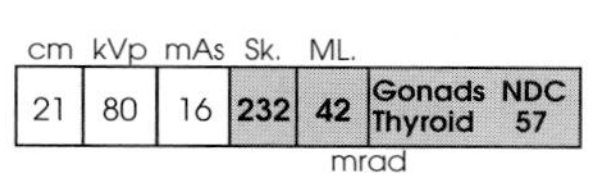

cm	kVp	mAs	Sk.	ML.	
21	80	16	232	42	Gonads NDC Thyroid 57

mrad

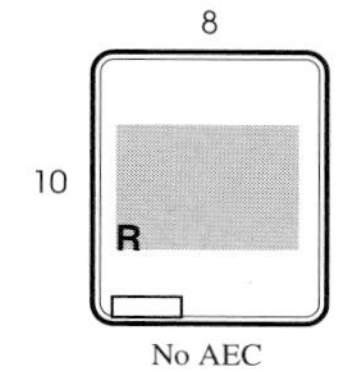

Patient Position

- Remove all metal, plastic or other removable objects from head.
- Patient in an erect or supine position.

Part Position

- Rest patient's posterior skull against head unit or table-top.
- Tuck chin, bringing **orbitomeatal line perpendicular** to head unit or table-top, or bring IOML perpendicular and increase CR angle 7°. (See Note 2.)
- Align **midsagittal plane perpendicular** to midline of head unit or table-top to prevent head rotation or tilt.

Central Ray

- Angle CR **35° caudad from the orbitomeatal line**, or **42° from IOML**.
- CR to pass through **level of TMJs** (1 in. [2.5 cm] anterior to EAMs).
- Center cassette to projected CR.
- SID: Head unit, 36 in. (91 cm). Table, minimum 40 in. (102 cm).

Collimation: Collimate on all sides to TMJ region.

Respiration: Suspend respiration during exposure.

Note 1: Some departmental protocols indicate, when patient's condition allows, these be taken in both closed and open mouth positions for comparison purposes.

Note 2: An additional 5° increase of CR may best demonstrate the TM fossae and joint area on some patients.

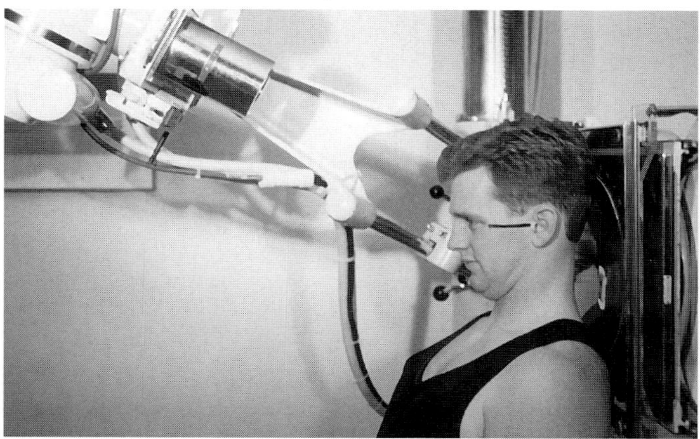

Fig. 12-73. AP axial–CR 35° to OML or 42° to IOML (Closed mouth position).

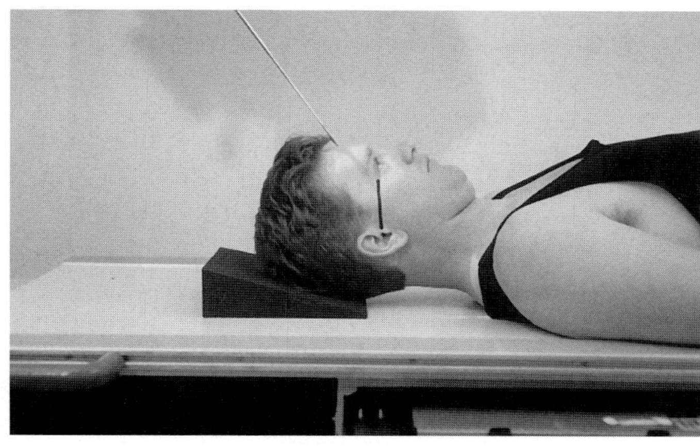

Fig. 12-74. AP axial–CR 35° to OML (closed mouth position).

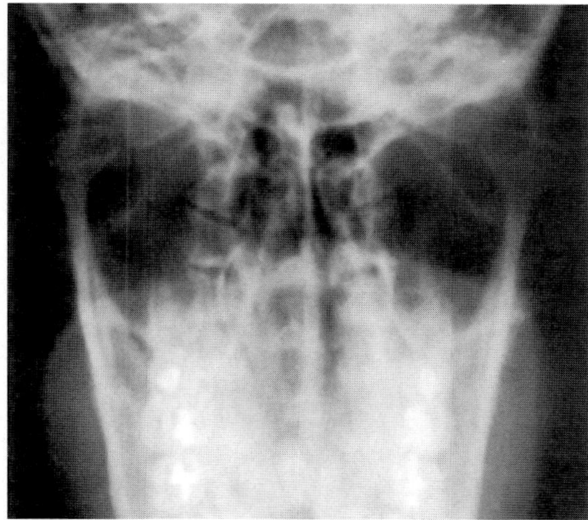

Fig. 12-75. AP axial (closed mouth position).

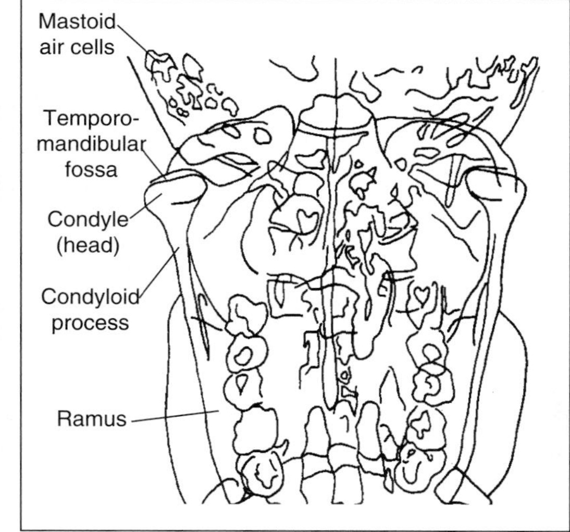

Fig. 12-76. AP axial.

Evaluation Criteria

- Included on the radiograph are the condyloid processes of the mandible and the temporomandibular fossae.
- Mandible is visualized without rotation when:
  - Condyloid processes are symmetrically visualized on each side of cervical spine.
- Clear visualization of condyle and temporomandibular fossae relationship.
- Sufficient penetration and exposure, without motion, to visualize condyloid process and temporomandibular fossa.

Axiolateral Oblique Projection - TMJs

Modified Law Method

TMJs
Special
- AP axial (modified Towne)
- **Axiolateral 15° oblique (modified Law)**
- Axiolateral (Schuller)
- Tomography
- Panorex (p. 377)

Structures Best Shown

Temporomandibular joint closest to film. Projects TMJ of interest posterior to upside TMJ. Generally taken **bilateral** with **open and closed mouth** positions to demonstrate relative positions of condyles with respect to TM fossae.

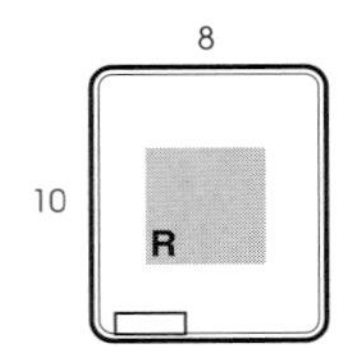

or

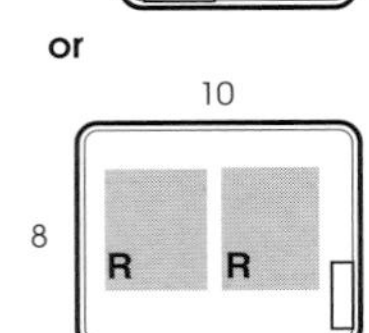

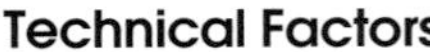

Technical Factors

- Film size –2 ea. 8 x 10 in. (18 x 24 cm), lengthwise.
  or –1 ea. 8 x 10 in. crosswise divided in half.
- Stationary or moving grid.
- 70-80 kVp range.
- Use small focal spot and detail screen.
- Technique and dose:

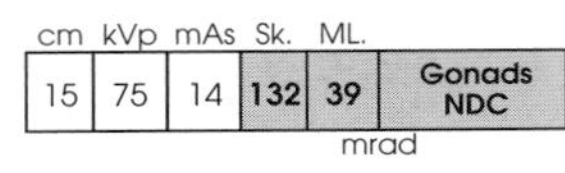

cm	kVp	mAs	Sk.	ML.	
15	75	14	132	39	Gonads NDC

mrad

Shielding: Secure lead shield around waist to protect gonads.

Patient Position

- Patient erect or prone. (Erect preferred if patient's condition allows.)
- Rest lateral side of head against head unit or table-top, with side of interest closest to cassette.

Part Position

- Oblique body as needed for patient's comfort.
- Prevent tilt by maintaining **interpupillary line perpendicular** to film with the anterior aspect of head rotated 15° toward film.
- Align **infraorbitomeatal line perpendicular** to front edge of cassette.
- From lateral position, **rotate face toward film 15°**. (Midsagittal plane of head is rotated 15° from plane of film.)

Fig. 12-77. Right TMJ-Closed mouth. **-15° oblique, CR 15° caudad.**

Fig. 12-78. Right TMJ-Open mouth. **-15° oblique, CR 15° caudad.**

Central Ray

- Angle CR **15° caudad**, centered to **1½ in. (4 cm) superior to upside EAM** (to pass through downside TMJ).
- Center cassette to projected CR.
- SID: Head unit, 36 in. (91 cm). Table-top, minimum 40 in. (102 cm).

Collimation: Use a circle diaphragm and cone or collimate on all sides to yield a field size of approximately 4 in. (10 cm) square.

Respiration: Suspend respiration during exposure.

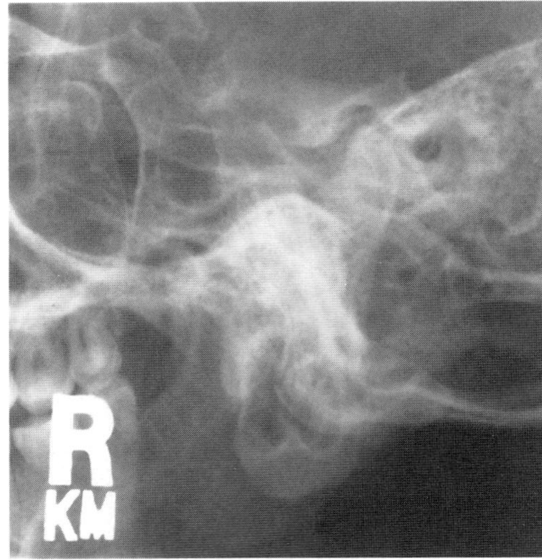

Fig. 12-79. TMJ-Closed mouth.

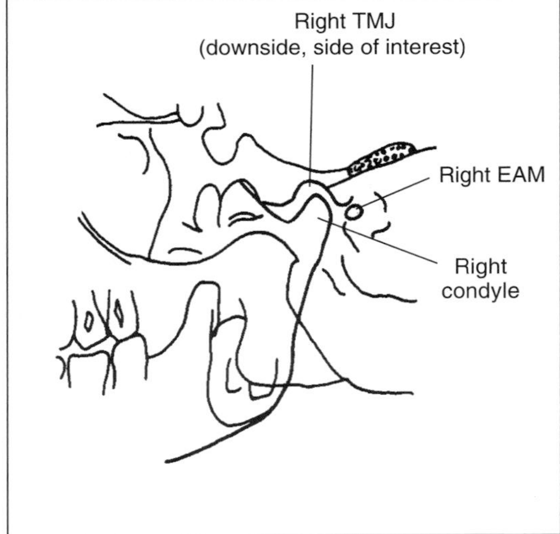

Fig. 12-80. TMJ-Closed mouth.

Evaluation Criteria

- TMJ closest to film is located in the center of collimation field.
- TMJ closest to film is clearly demonstrated without superimposition of opposite TMJ (15° rotation prevents superimposition).
- TMJ of interest does not superimpose cervical spine.
- On closed mouth radiograph, condyle will lie within mandibular fossa.
- On open mouth radiograph, condyle will move anterior within the mandibular fossa.
- Sufficient penetration and exposure, without motion, to visualize TMJ.

Axiolateral Projection - TMJs

Schuller Method

TMJs
Special
- AP axial (modified Towne)
- Axiolateral 15° oblique (modified Law)
- **Axiolateral (Schuller)**
- Tomography
- Panorex (p. 377)

Structures Best Shown

Temporomandibular joint closest to film. Generally taken **bilateral** with **open** and **closed mouth** positions to demonstrate relative positions of condyles with respect to TM fossae.

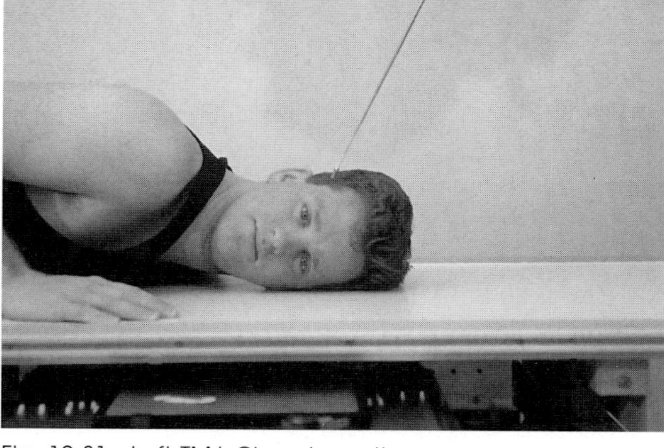

Fig. 12-81. Left TMJ–Closed mouth.
–**True lateral**.
–**25 to 30° caudad angle**.

Technical Factors

- Film size –2 ea. 8 x 10 in. (18 x 24 cm), lengthwise.
  or –1 ea. 8 x 10 in. crosswise divided in half.
- Stationary or moving grid.
- 70-80 kVp range.
- Use small focal spot and detail screen.
- Technique and dose:

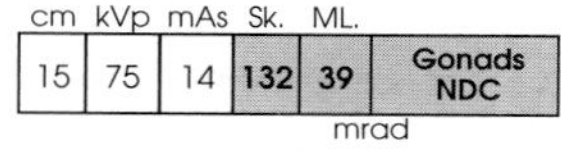

cm	kVp	mAs	Sk.	ML.	Gonads
15	75	14	132	39	NDC

mrad

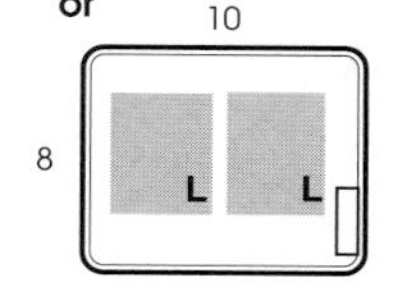

Patient Position

- Patient in an erect or prone position.
- Rest lateral side of head against head unit or table-top, with side of interest closest to cassette.

Part Position 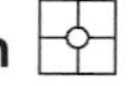

- Adjust head into a **true lateral position**, oblique body as needed for patient's comfort.
- Align **interpupillary line perpendicular** to film.
- Align **midsagittal plane parallel** with table-top.
- Position **infraorbitomeatal line perpendicular** to front edge of cassette.

Fig. 12-82. Open mouth.

Central Ray

- Angle CR **25° to 30° caudad**, centered to ½ in. (1.3 cm) anterior and 2 in. (5 cm) superior to upside EAM.
- Center cassette to projected TMJ.
- SID: Head unit, 36 in. (91 cm).
  Table, minimum 40 in. (102 cm).

Collimation: Use a circle diaphragm and cone or collimate on all sides to yield a field size of approximately 4 in. (10 cm) square.

Respiration: Suspend respiration during exposure.

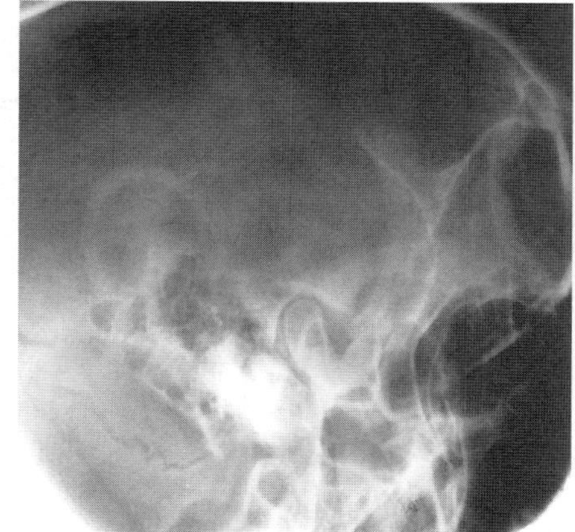

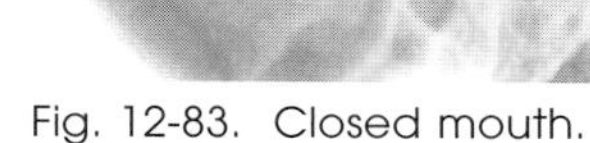

Fig. 12-83. Closed mouth.

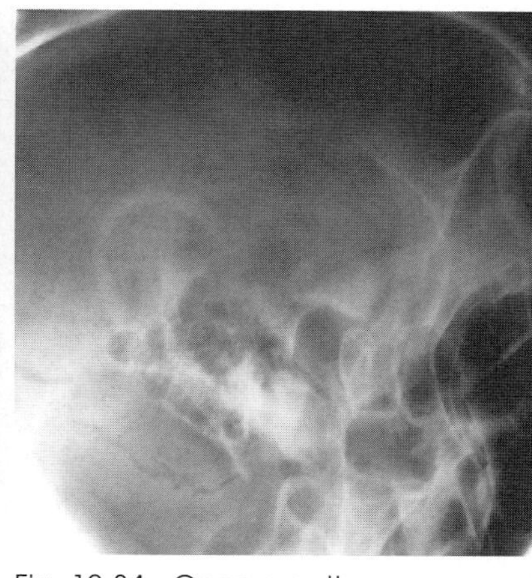

Fig. 12-84. Open mouth.

Evaluation Criteria

- TMJ closest to film is located in the center of collimation field.
- TMJ closest to film is visualized anterior to EAM.
- On closed mouth radiograph, condyle will lie within mandibular fossa.
- On open mouth radiograph, condyle will move to anterior margin of fossa.
- Sufficient penetration and exposure, without motion, to visualize TMJ.

Note: This projection results in more elongation of the condyle as compared to the modified Law method.

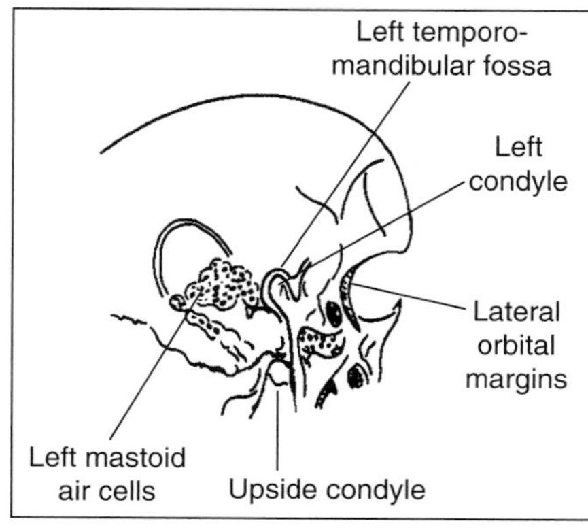

Fig. 12-85. Closed mouth.

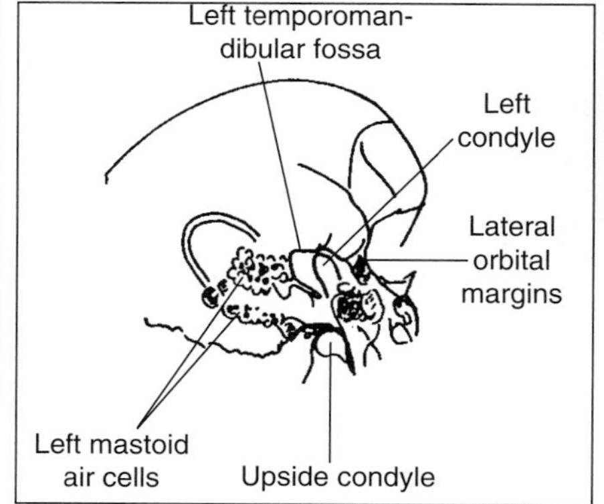

Fig. 12-86. Open mouth.

12

Tomography

TMJs
Special
• AP axial (modified Towne)
• Axiolateral 15° oblique (modified Law)
• Axiolateral (Schuller)
• **Tomography**
• Panorex (p. 377)

Structures Best Shown

Condyloid process of mandible and temporomandibular fossae. (Generally taken bilaterally with open and closed mouth positions.)

Side of interest should be placed **upside** for best blurring effect (see Chapter 21, Conventional Tomography).

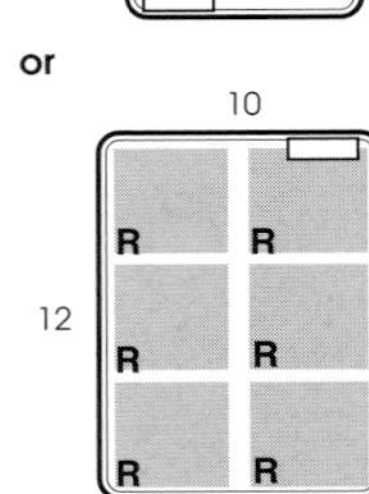

Technical Factors

- Film size –8 x 10 in. (18 x 24 cm),
  or –10 x 12 in. (24 x 30 cm), lengthwise.
- Moving grid.
- Low kVp range to produce high contrast.
- Long exposure time to provide time for machine movement.
- Small focal spot.

Unit Preparation

- With x-ray tube perpendicular to table, connect x-ray source to film holder.
- Set the most complex motion available in your facility.
- Use a wide tube angle in order to obtain thin cuts of the TMJs.
- Place a pad on table for patient's comfort.

Shielding: Place shield over thorax and pelvis.

Patient Preparation

- Remove all metal, plastic or other removable objects from head.
- Explain to patient how tube will move during the exposure and the importance of holding still while radiographs are being taken, as well as in between radiographs.
- Patient in a prone position.
- Rest lateral side of head against table-top, with **side of interest placed up**, away from the cassette, which should be the side to be in focus as set by the fulcrum height.

Part Position

- Adjust head into a **true lateral position**, oblique body as needed for patient's comfort.
- Align **interpupillary line perpendicular** to table-top.
- Align **midsagittal plane parallel** with table-top.
- Position **infraorbitomeatal line perpendicular** to front edge of cassette.
- Instruct patient to close mouth.
- Use radiolucent sponges, tape, etc. where needed to help patient maintain position.

Central Ray

- Center to a point **½ in.** (1.3 cm) **anterior to the EAM**.
- Mark centering point on patient, with a water-soluble marker, to ensure centering between radiographs.
- Position tube and cassette to starting position.
- Take 3 scout tomograms, vary fulcrum height between exposures:
  –**1st radiograph**: Take with the fulcrum set at the **level of the outer canthus** of affected TMJ (upside).
  –**2nd radiograph**: Take a cut **5 mm above** initial radiograph.
  –**3rd radiograph**: Take a cut **5 mm below** initial radiograph.
- Mark radiograph with a R or L marker and fulcrum height used.

Collimation: Tightly collimate to TMJ.

Respiration: Suspend respiration during exposure.

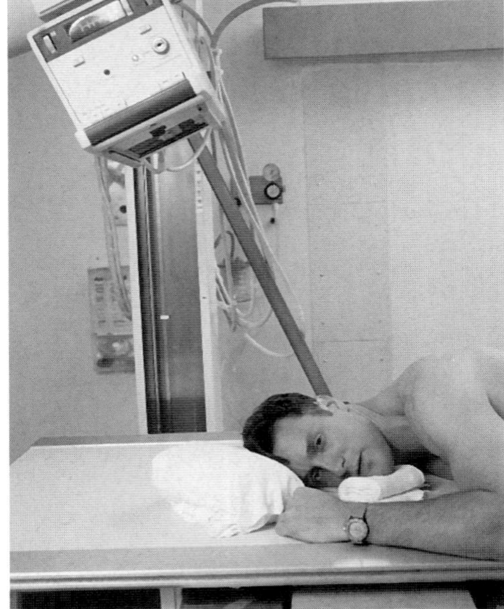

Fig. 12-87. TMJ tomogram – left side (upside). (Tube in left position, ready to begin arch movement.)

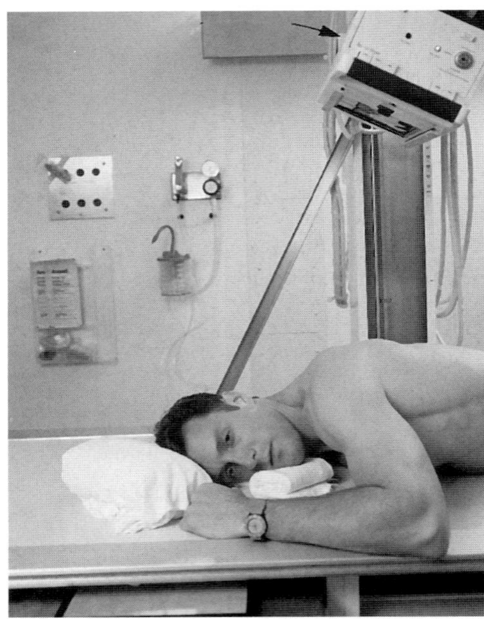

Fig. 12-88. TMJ tomogram. (Tube has moved across to right position.)

Tomography continued

Evaluation Criteria

- The TMJ is located in the center of the radiograph, with the condyloid process and EAM included within the collimated field.
- The cranium is visualized without rotation.
- The condyloid process and temporomandibular fossae are clearly visualized, in focus, on at least one radiographic cut.
- Sufficient penetration and exposure, without motion, to visualize temporomandibular joint.

Closed Mouth:

- Condyle lies within the mandibular fossa.

Open Mouth:

- Condyle is visualized anterior to the mandibular fossa.

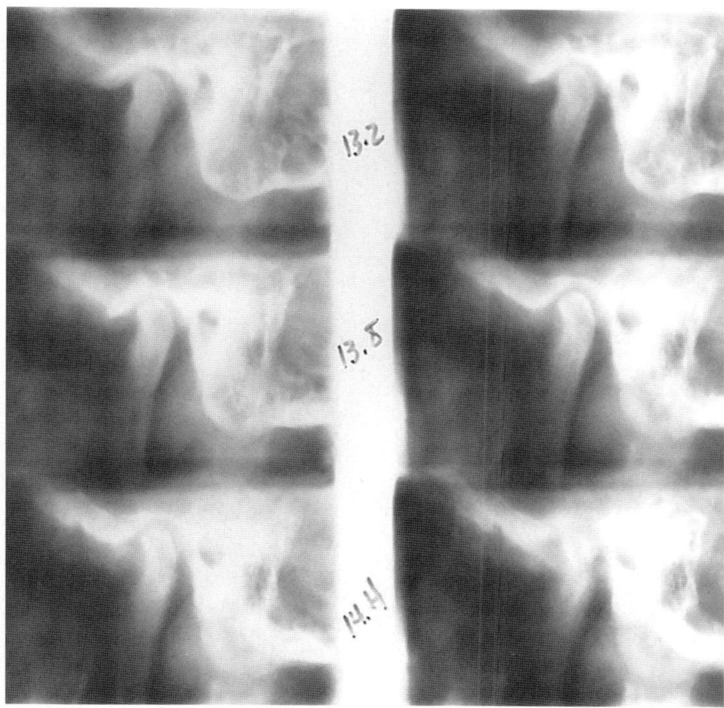

Fig. 12-89. Closed mouth (right TMJ, left side down).

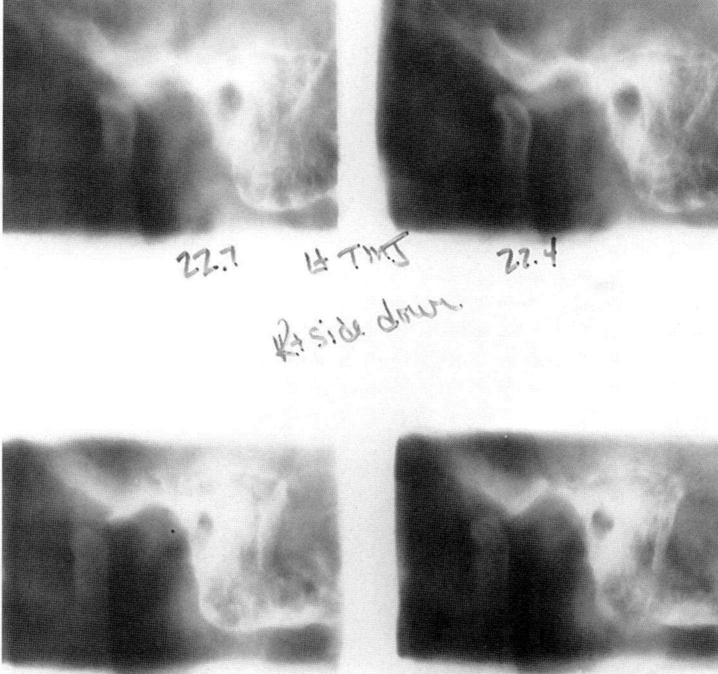

Fig. 12-90. Open mouth (left TMJ, right side down).

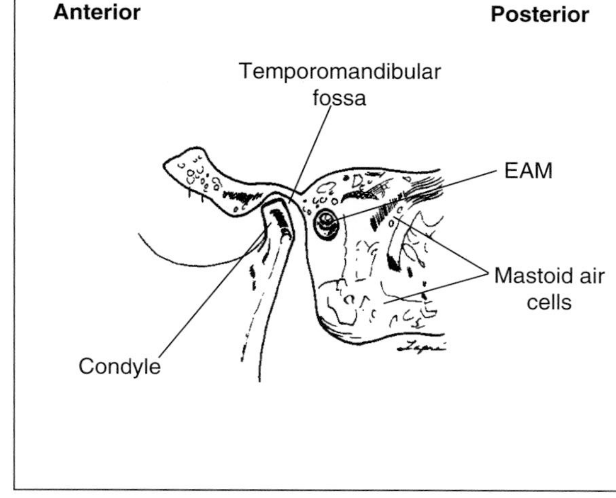

Fig. 12-91. Closed mouth.

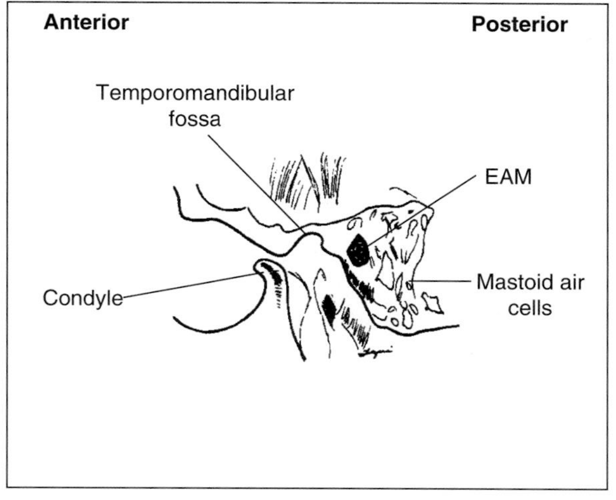

Fig. 12-92. Open mouth.

12

Radiographs for Critique

Each of these facial bone radiographs demonstrates some error in positioning which requires a repeat. These, along with accompanying lecture slides of these and other radiographs, will provide a basis for classroom and/or positioning lab discussion. Questions with answers based on these specific critique radiographs are provided in the accompanying student workbook/lab manuals to help prepare students for classroom and/or lab discussions on film critique.

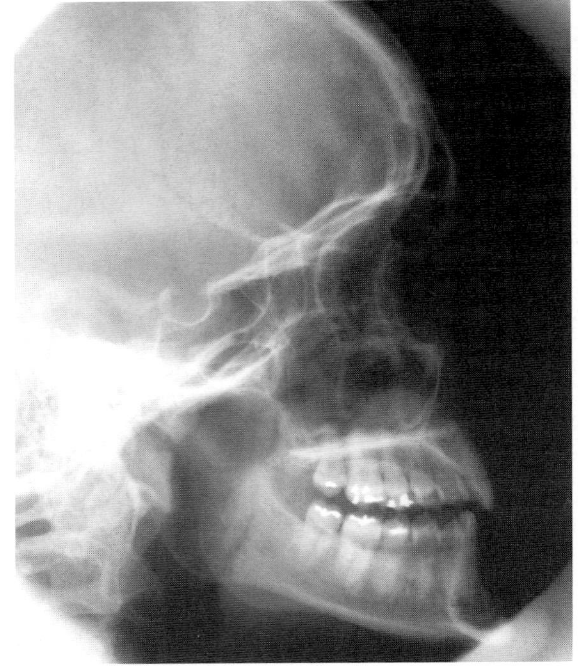

Fig. C12-93. Lateral facial bones.

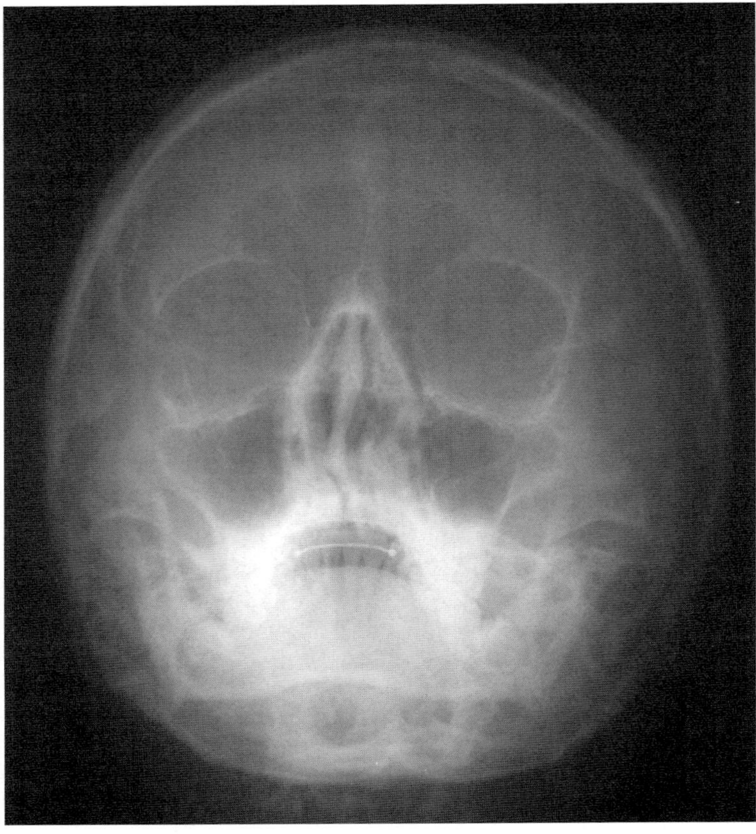

Fig. C12-94. PA Waters–facial bones.

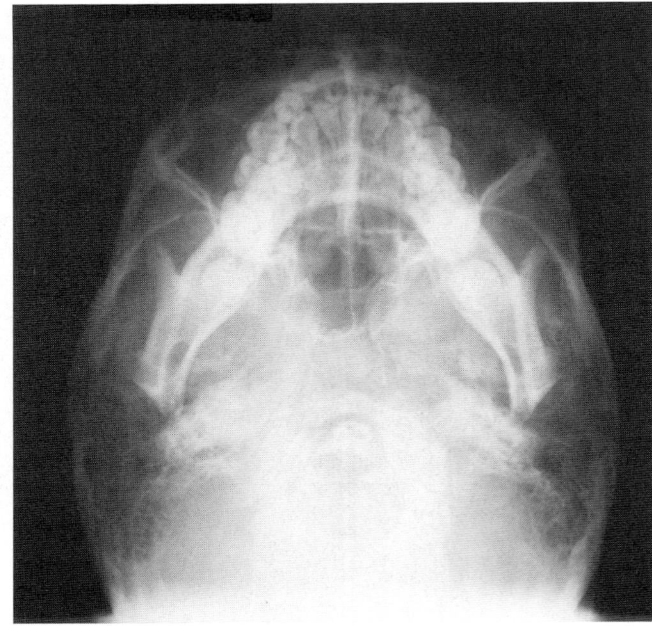

Fig. C12-95. SMV mandible.

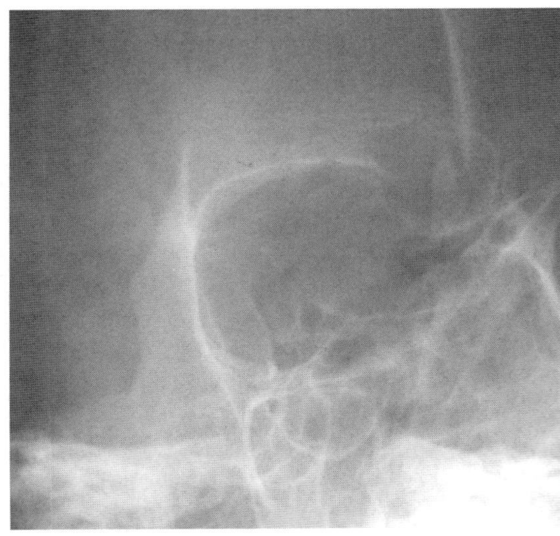

Fig. C12-96. Optic foramina–Rhese method.

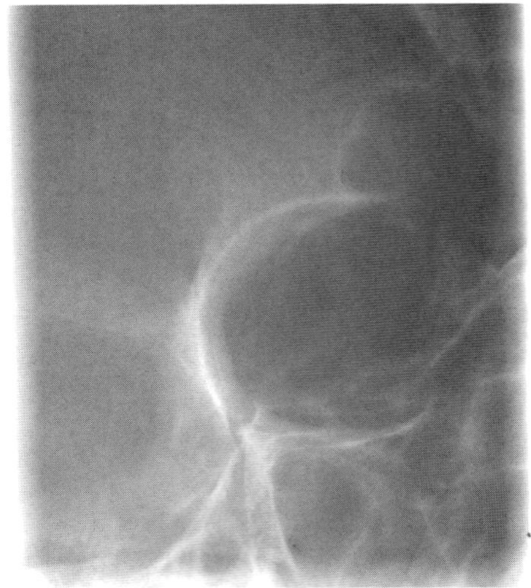

Fig. C12-97. Optic foramina–Rhese method.

CHAPTER 13

Paranasal Sinuses, Mastoids and Temporal Bone

CONTRIBUTIONS BY:
Kathy Martensen, BS, RT (R)
Barry T. Anthony, RT (R)

CONTENTS

Radiographic Anatomy

Paranasal sinuses:
- Maxillary **386**
- Frontal, ethmoid and sphenoid **387**

Anatomy review (radiographs) **388**

Temporal bones:
- Radiographs **389**
- External and middle ear **390**
- Internal ear **392**

Anatomy review (radiographs) **393**

Radiographic Positioning

Positioning considerations:
- Paranasal sinuses and temporal bone–Mastoids **394**
- Tomography and anatomical relationships **395**

Survey results and basic and special projections **396**

Paranasal sinuses:
- Lateral **397**
- PA 15° (Caldwell method) **398**
- Parietoacanthial (Waters method) **399**
- Submentovertex (SMV) **400**
- Parietoacanthial transoral (open-mouth Waters method) **401**

Mastoids:
- Axiolateral 15° oblique (modified Law method) **402**
- Axioanterior oblique–posterior profile (Stenvers method) **403**
- AP axial (Towne method) **404**
- Axiolateral (Schuller method) **405**
- Axioposterior oblique–anterior profile (Arcelin method–reverse Stenvers) **406**
- Axioposterior oblique (Mayer method and Owen modification) **407**

Petrous pyramids:
- AP axial (Towne method) **408**
- Submentovertex (SMV) **408**

Radiographs for critique **409**

Radiographic Anatomy

Skull

Chapter 11 included a study of the anatomy of the bony skeleton of the head, which includes the 8 cranial bones and the 14 facial bones. Two exceptions that were not described are the **paranasal sinuses**, and the **mastoid** and **petrous portions of the temporal bone**. The petrous portion contains the organs of hearing and equilibrium. The anatomy and related radiographic positioning for these parts will be described and illustrated in this chapter along with the paranasal sinuses.

PARANASAL SINUSES

The large, air-filled cavities of the **paranasal sinuses** are sometimes called the accessory nasal sinuses because they are lined with mucous membrane, which is continuous with and communicates with the nasal cavity. These sinuses are divided into four groups according to the bones that contain them:

1. **Maxillary** (2) –Maxillary (facial) bones
2. **Frontal** (usually 2)–Frontal (cranial) bones
3. **Ethmoid** (many) –Ethmoid (cranial) bones
4. **Sphenoid** (1 or 2) –Sphenoid (cranial) bone

Only the **maxillary sinuses** are part of the **facial bone** structure. The **frontal**, **ethmoid** and **sphenoid** are contained within the respective **cranial bones**.

The paranasal sinuses begin developing in the fetus, but only the maxillary sinuses exhibit a definite cavity at birth. The frontal and sphenoid sinuses begin to be visible on radiographs at age six or seven. The ethmoid sinuses develop last. All the paranasal sinuses are generally fully developed by the late teenage years.

Each of these groups of sinuses will be studied, beginning with the largest, the maxillary sinuses.

Maxillary Sinuses

The large **maxillary sinuses** are paired structures, one being located within the body of each maxillary bone. An older term for maxillary sinus is antrum, an abbreviation of "Antrum of Highmore."* Each maxillary sinus is shaped somewhat like a pyramid on a frontal view. Laterally, they appear more cubical in shape. The average total vertical dimension is between 3 and 4 cm, and the other dimensions are between 2.5 and 3 cm.

The bony walls of the maxillary sinuses are thin. The floor of each maxillary sinus is slightly below the level of the floor of each nasal fossa. The two maxillary sinuses are variable in size from one person to another and from one side to the other.

Projecting into the floor of each maxillary sinus are several conical elevations relating to roots of the first and second upper molar teeth (Fig. 13-2). Occasionally, the floor is perforated by one or more of these roots, and infections originating in the teeth, particularly the molars and premolars, may travel upward into the maxillary sinus.

All of the paranasal sinus cavities communicate with each other and with the **nasal cavity,** which is divided into two equal chambers or **fossae.** In the case of the maxillary sinuses, this site of communication is located at the upper or superior aspect of the sinus cavity itself, as demonstrated in Fig. 13-3. When a person is erect, any mucus or fluid trapped within the sinus will tend to stay there and layer out, forming an air-fluid level. Therefore, radiographic positioning of the paranasal sinuses should be accomplished with the patient in the **erect position** to demonstrate any possible air-fluid levels.

*Nathaniel Highmore, English physician, 1613-1685.

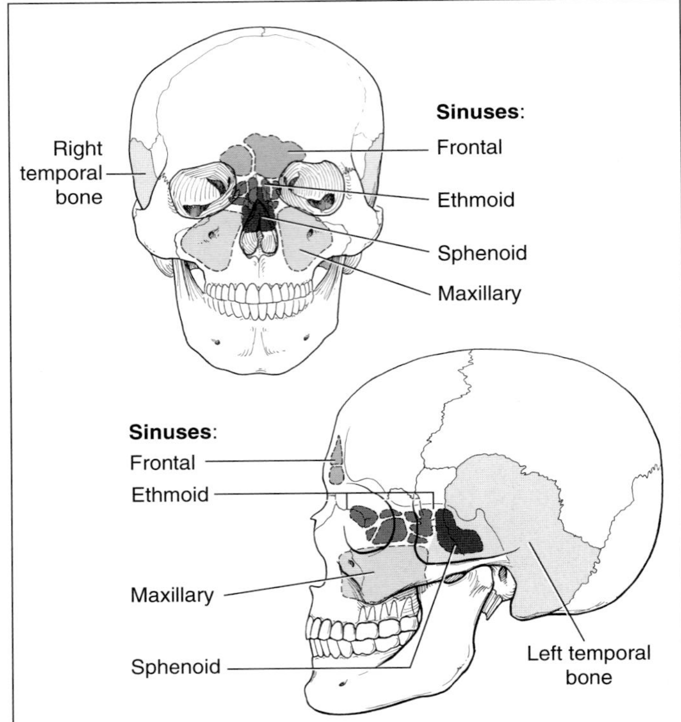

Fig. 13-1. Skull–Paranasal sinuses and temporal bone.

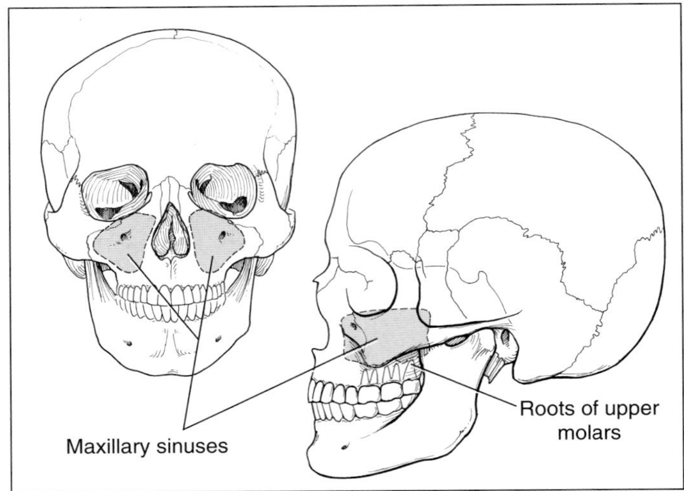

Fig. 13-2. Maxillary sinuses (2).

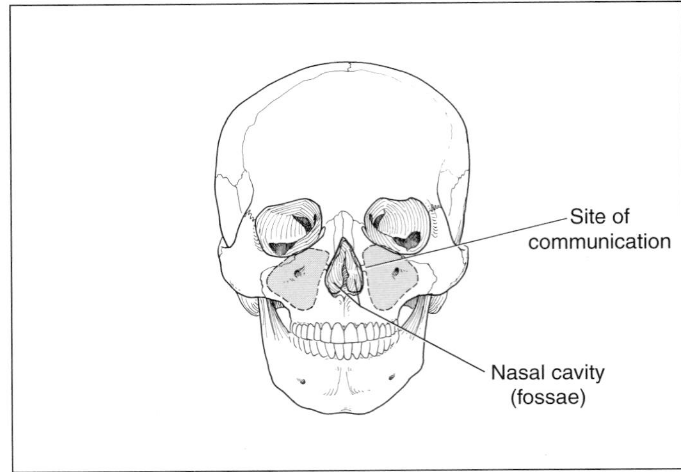

Fig. 13-3. Maxillary sinuses.

13

Frontal Sinuses

The **frontal sinuses** are located between the inner and outer tables of the skull, posterior to the glabella. Whereas the maxillary sinuses are always paired and are usually fairly symmetrical in size and shape, the frontal sinuses are rarely symmetrical. The frontal sinuses are usually separated by a septum, which deviates from one side to the other or may even be absent entirely, resulting in one single cavity. Generally, however, there are two cavities with a wide variation in their sizes and shapes. They are generally larger in men than in women.

The frontal sinuses, which **rarely become aerated before age 6,** communicate with the nasal cavity by way of a duct that empties into the anterior part of the mid nasal cavity or meatus. The size or even the presence of the frontal sinuses vary greatly among individuals. They may be only singular on either the right or left side only, or they may be paired as shown, or they may even be totally absent.

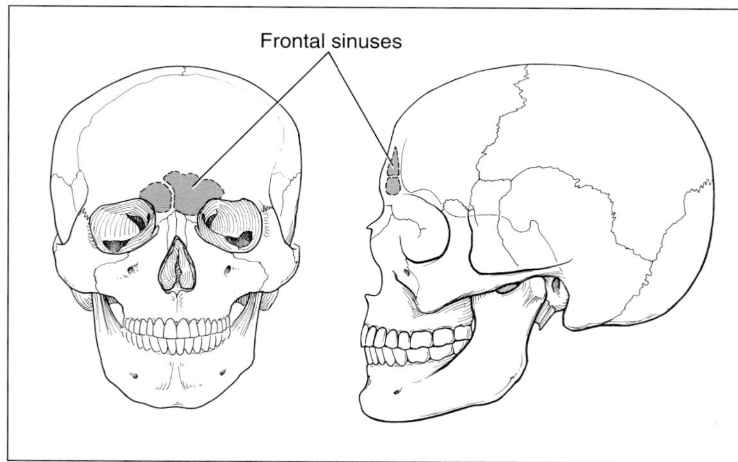

Fig. 13-4. Frontal sinuses.

Ethmoid Sinuses

The **ethmoid sinuses** are made up of many air cells contained within the lateral masses or labyrinths of the ethmoid bone. These air cells are grouped into **anterior**, **middle** and **posterior collections**, but they all intercommunicate. These cells also communicate with the nasal cavities via a single passageway from each side.

As seen from the side, it would appear that the anterior ethmoid sinuses fill the orbits. A portion of these sinuses are medial to the orbits, however, and are contained in the lateral masses of the ethmoid bone, which helps to form the medial wall of each orbit.

The ethmoid sinuses extend posteriorly within the labyrinths to communicate with the sphenoid sinuses contained in the sphenoid bone.

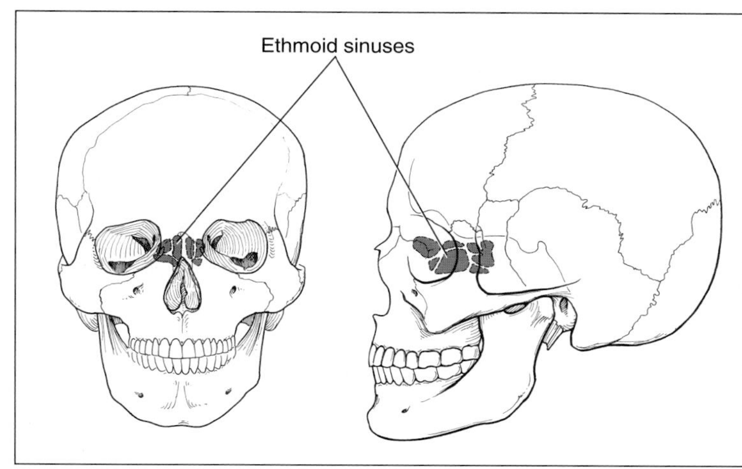

Fig. 13-5. Ethmoid sinuses.

Sphenoid Sinuses

The **sphenoid sinus** lies in the body of the sphenoid bone, directly below the sella turcica. The body of the sphenoid containing these sinuses is cubical in shape and is frequently divided by a thin septum to form two cavities. This septum may be incomplete or absent entirely, however, resulting in only one cavity. If there are two cavities or sinuses, they are generally asymmetrical in shape.

Anteriorly, the sphenoid sinuses communicate through rounded openings with the spheno-ethmoidal recess of the nasal cavity.

Since the sphenoid sinuses are so close to the base or floor of the cranium, sometimes a pathologic process makes its presence known by its effect on these sinuses. An example of this occurrence is the demonstration of an air-fluid level within the sphenoid sinuses following skull trauma. This demonstration could be the only radiographic proof obtainable that the patient has a basal skull fracture, and that either blood or cerebrospinal fluid is leaking through the fracture into the sphenoid sinuses, a condition referred to as **sphenoid effusion**.

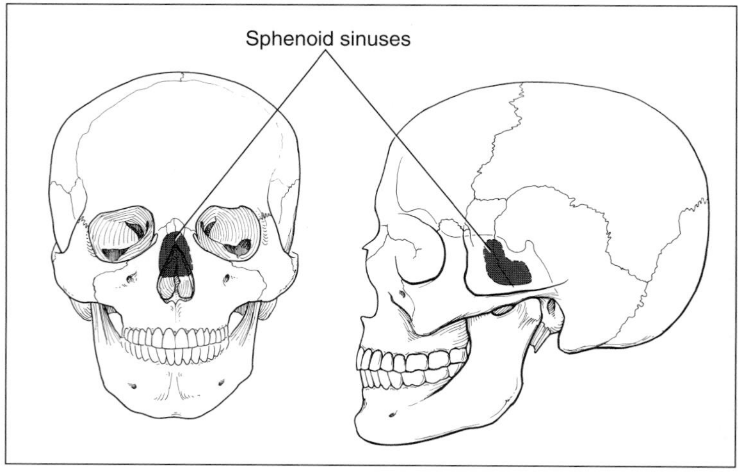

Fig. 13-6. Sphenoid sinuses.

RADIOGRAPHS–PARANASAL SINUSES

Drawings of the sinuses on preceding pages included definite sizes and shapes of the sinuses with clear-cut borders. In actual radiographs these borders are not nearly as definite since the various sinuses overlap and superimpose each other as seen on these radiographs of four common sinus projections. Relative locations and relationships of each of these sinuses are clearly demonstrated on these labeled radiographs: (**F**–Frontal sinuses, **E**–Ethmoid sinuses, **M**–Maxillary sinuses, **S**–Sphenoid sinuses).

Lateral Sinuses (Fig. 13-7)

The frontal sinuses are clearly visualized between the inner and outer tables of the skull.

The sphenoid sinuses appear to be continuous with the ethmoid sinuses anteriorly.

The large maxillary sinuses are clearly visualized. Note that the roots of the molars and premolars of the upper teeth appear to extend up through the floor of the maxillary sinuses.

PA (Caldwell) Projection (Fig. 13-8)

The frontal, ethmoid and maxillary sinuses are clearly illustrated in this frontal view radiograph. The sphenoid sinuses are not demonstrated specifically because they are located directly behind the ethmoid sinuses. This relationship is demonstrated on the lateral view (Fig. 13-7), and the SMV projection (Fig. 13-10).

PA Axial Transoral Projection (Open-mouth Waters) (Fig. 13-9)

All four groups of sinuses are clearly demonstrated on this projection taken with mouth open and the head tipped back to separate and project the sphenoid sinuses below the ethmoids. The open mouth also removes the upper teeth from direct superimposition of the sphenoids. The pyramid-shaped maxillary sinuses are clearly seen.

The mastoid air cells also appear on each side, posterolateral to the mandible (see arrows). They appear as small air-filled clusters within the mastoid portions of the temporal bone as described on following pages, but they are not part of the paranasal sinuses.

Submentovertex (SMV) Projection (Fig. 13-10)

This projection is taken with head tipped back so the top (vertex) of the head is touching the table-top and the CR is directed from below the chin (mentum).

The centrally located sphenoid sinuses are seen anterior to the large opening, the foramen magnum. The multiple clusters of ethmoid air cells are also clearly seen extending to each side of the nasal septum. Parts of the maxillary sinuses are seen on each side as superimposed by the mandible and teeth.

The mastoid portions containing air cells are visualized in Fig. 13-9 (labeled as **A**). Fig. 13-10 also demonstrates these air-filled mastoids, and the dense petrous portions of the temporal bones (labeled **B**), as described on the following page.

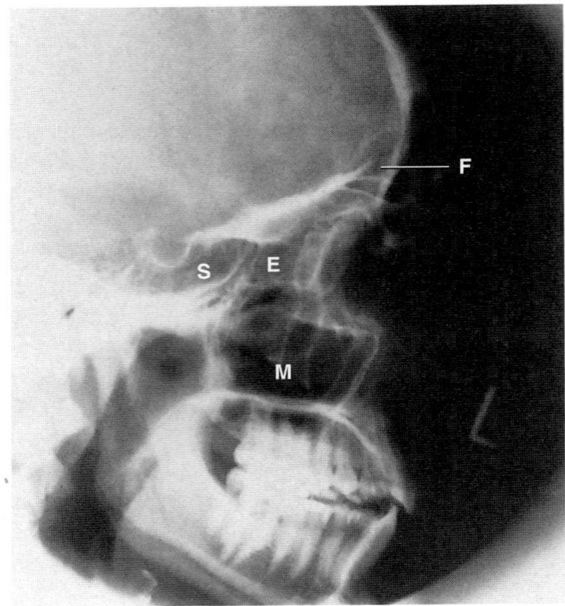

Fig. 13-7. Lateral sinuses.

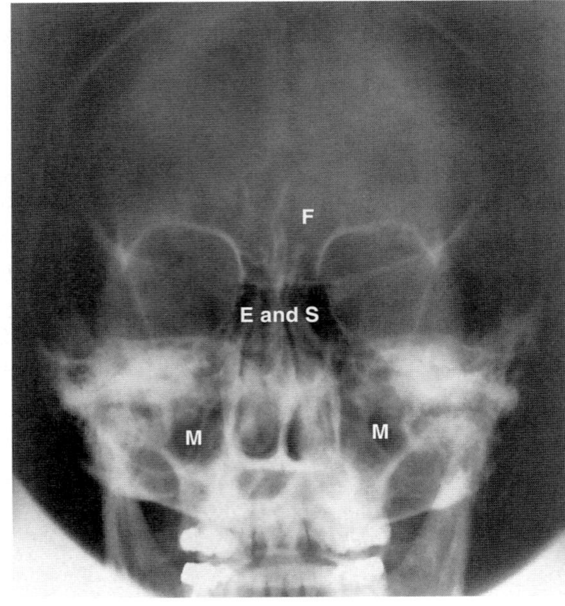

Fig. 13-8. PA Caldwell.

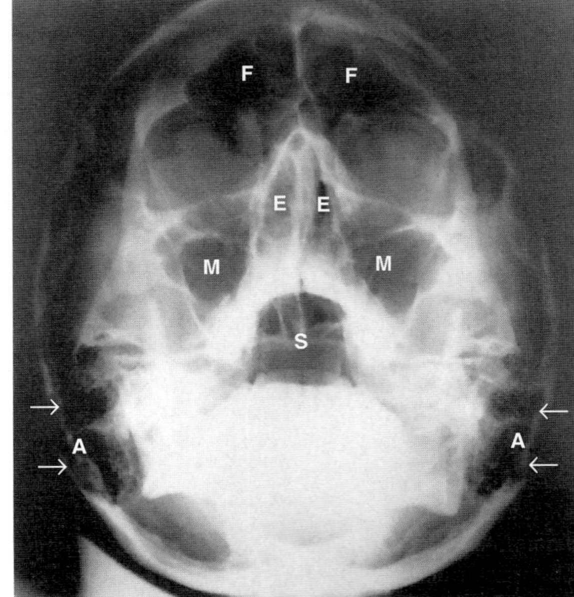

Fig. 13-9. PA axial transoral projection (open-mouth Waters).

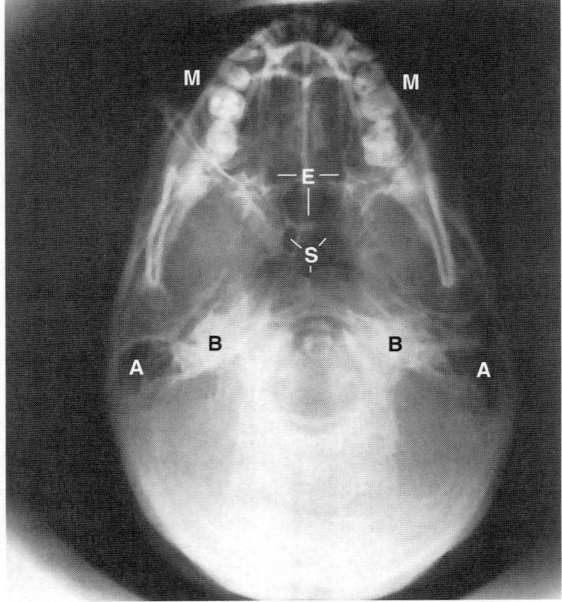

Fig. 13-10. SMV projection.

13

TEMPORAL BONES

Due to their dense inner structure and location, the mastoids and petrous portions of the temporal bones are very difficult to visualize with conventional radiography. Therefore, body section radiography, and CT or MRI have largely replaced conventional radiography of these parts. However, the air-filled mastoid sinuses can be demonstrated with specific projections as described in the positioning section of this chapter. CT and/or MRI sectional radiographs require a good understanding of specific anatomy and relationships of structures within the temporal bones.

As previously described in Chapter 11, each **temporal bone** is divided into three main portions. (1) The thin upper portion forming part of the wall of the skull is the **squamous portion,** which was well demonstrated in Chapter 11. (2) The area posterior to the external acoustic meatus (EAM) is the **mastoid portion**, with its prominent mastoid process or tip (Fig. 13-11). (3) The third main portion is the dense **petrous portion**, also called the **petrous pyramid** or **pars petrosa**.

The upper border or ridge of the petrous pyramids are clearly seen on certain conventional skull radiographs and are commonly called the **petrous ridges**.

These portions, which house the organs of hearing and equilibrium, are described in detail in the pages that follow.

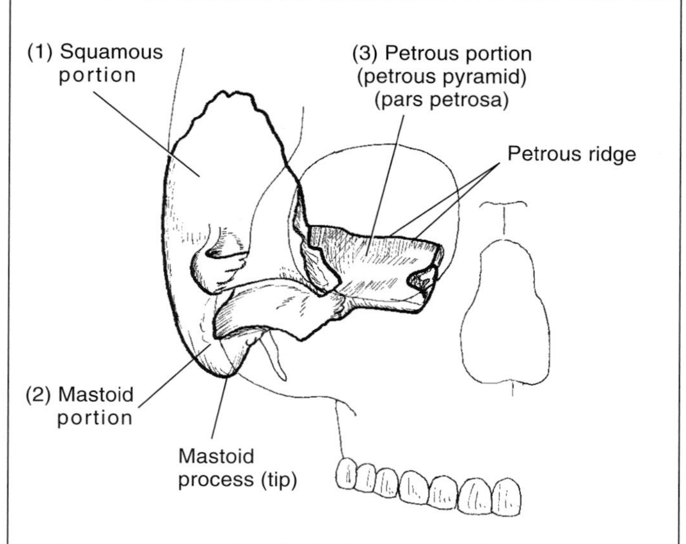

Fig. 13-11. Temporal bone–frontal view.

Radiographs–Mastoids & Petrous Pyramids

Various structures of the temporal bone are labeled on these radiographs of two projections most commonly taken to demonstrate the mastoids and petrous pyramids.

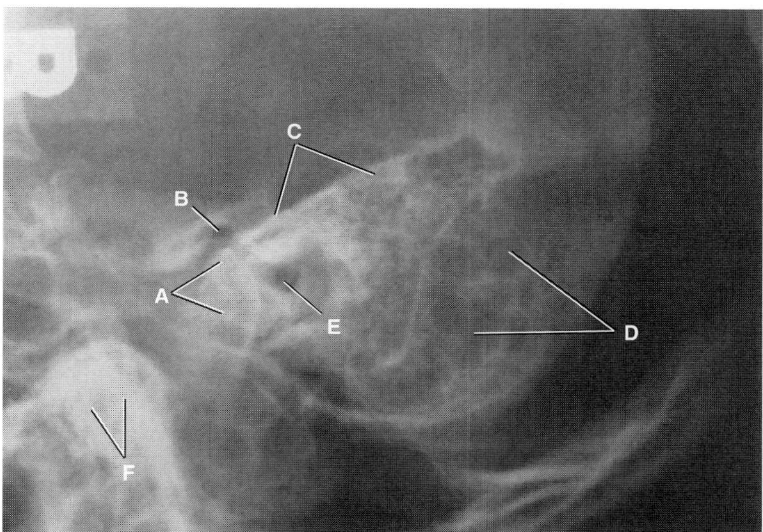

Fig. 13-12. Axiolateral 15° oblique (Law).

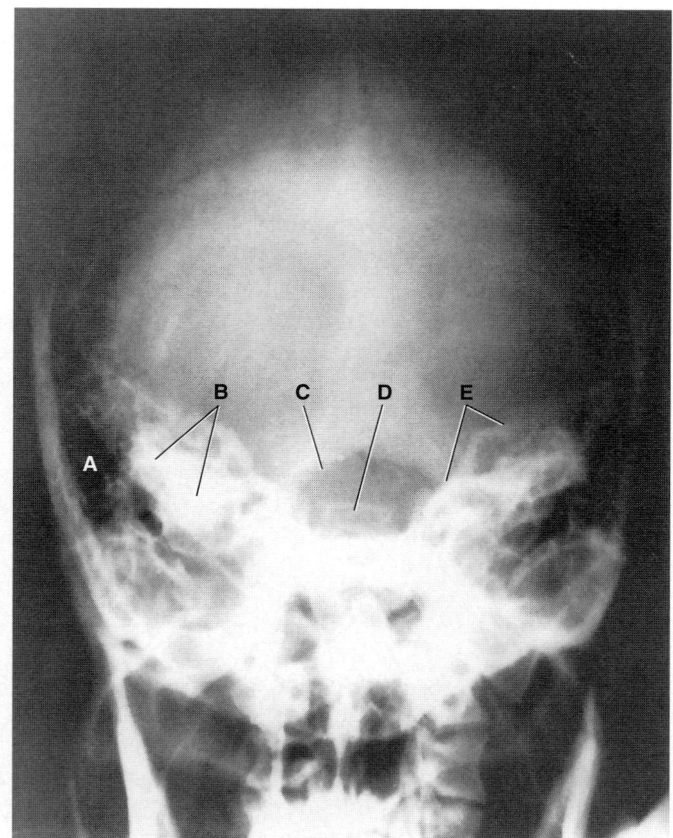

Fig. 13-13. AP axial (Towne).

Axiolateral 15° Oblique Position (Law Method):
A. Condyle of mandible (downside).
B. Temporomandibular fossa.
C. Petrous portion (petrous ridge), an end-on view.
D. Mastoid air cells.
E. External acoustic meatus (EAM).
F. Upside (magnified) condyle of mandible.

AP Axial (Towne Method):
A. Mastoid air cells.
B. Petrous portions (pars petrosa).
C. Foramen magnum.
D. Dorsum sellae.
E. Petrous ridge.

Anatomy of Organs of Hearing and Equilibrium

(Contained Within Petrous Portion of Temporal Bones)

EAR

The organs of hearing and equilibrium are the main structures found within the petrous portion of the temporal bones. As previously described, these small, delicate structures are difficult to visualize radiographically, due not only to their small size, but also to the increased density of the temporal bones surrounding them. The internal structures of the temporal bone, including the three important divisions of the ear (the external, middle and internal portions) are illustrated in Fig. 13-14.

The **external ear** begins outside the head with the **auricle** or **pinna**, which channels sound waves into a tubelike opening, the **external acoustic (auditory) meatus (EAM)**. This tubelike meatus ends at the eardrum, which is properly called the **tympanic membrane**.

The **middle ear**, located between the tympanic membrane and the inner ear, contains the **three** small bones called **auditory ossicles**. These small bones, which will be described individually later in this chapter, transmit sound vibrations from the tympanic membrane to the sensory apparatus of hearing in the **internal ear**. Certain nerves and blood vessels pass through an opening, the **internal acoustic meatus** or canal, to connect the inner ear with the brain.

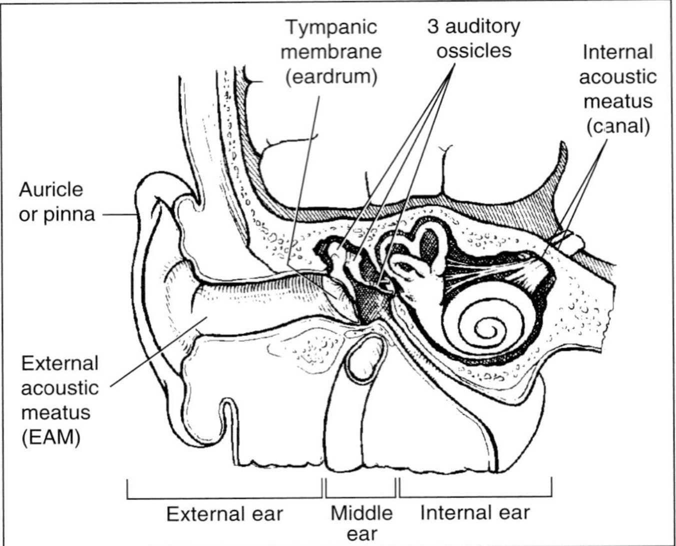

Fig. 13-14. Ear.

External Ear

The **external ear** begins with the **auricle** or **pinna** on each side of the head. The **tragus** is part of this external structure. It is the small liplike structure located anterior to the EAM. This acts as a partial shield to the ear opening.

The canal of the external ear is termed the **exterior acoustic meatus** (EAM). Some references refer only to the external opening as the **external acoustic meatus**, and the canal as the **external acoustic canal**. By definition meatus describes **an opening** or **passageway**,* and throughout this text the opening, as well as the entire canal, is referred to as the external acoustic meatus. The external acoustic canal or meatus is about 2.5 centimeters long, half of which is bony in structure and half of which is cartilaginous.

The **mastoid process** or **tip** of the temporal bone is posterior and inferior to the EAM, while the **styloid process** is inferior and slightly anterior. The meatus narrows somewhat as it meets the tympanic membrane. The eardrum is situated at an oblique angle, forming a depression or well at the lower medial end of the meatus.

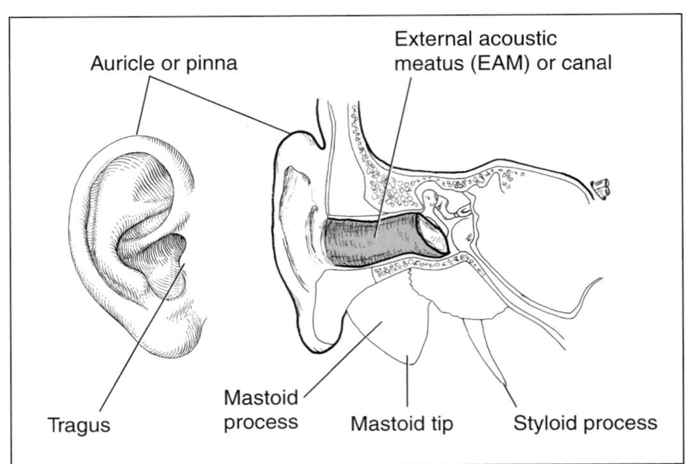

Fig. 13-15. External ear.

Middle Ear

The middle ear is an irregularly shaped, air-containing cavity located between the external and the internal ear portions. The three main parts of the middle ear are the **tympanic membrane,** the three small bones called **auditory ossicles**, and the **tympanic cavity.** The tympanic membrane is considered part of the middle ear even though it serves as a partition between the external and middle ears.

The tympanic cavity, is further divided into two parts. The larger cavity opposite the eardrum is called the **tympanic cavity proper**. The area above the level of the external auditory meatus and the eardrum is called the **attic** or the **epitympanic recess**. A structure important radiographically is the **drum crest** or **spur**. The tympanic membrane is attached to this sharp, bony projection. The drum crest or spur separates the external acoustic meatus from the epitympanic recess.

The tympanic cavity communicates anteriorly with the nasopharynx by way of the **Eustachian tube** or the **auditory tube**.

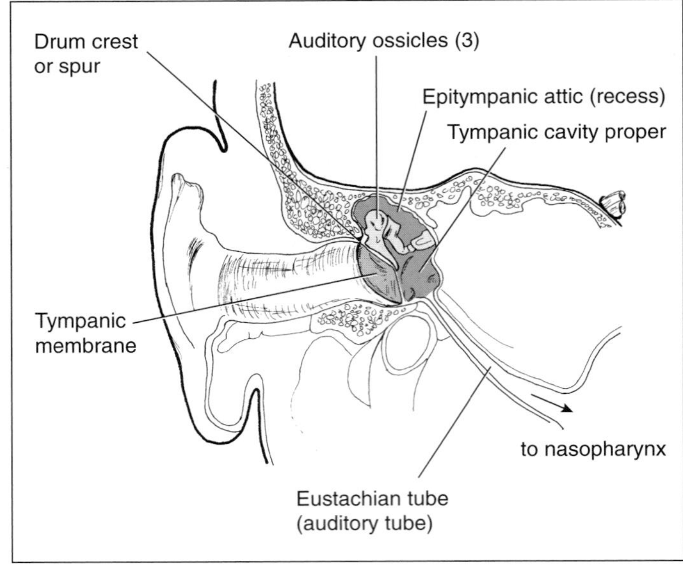

Fig. 13-16. Middle ear.

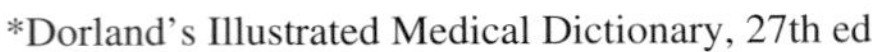

*Dorland's Illustrated Medical Dictionary, 27th ed.

Eustachian Tube: The frontal drawing in Fig. 13-17 illustrates the general relationships of the **external acoustic meatus** and **eustachian tube** to the external features. As seen, the **eustachian tube** is the passageway between the middle ear and the nasopharynx. This tube is about 4 centimeters long and serves to equalize the pressure within the middle ear to the outside atmospheric air pressure through the nasopharynx. The sensation of one's ears popping is caused by the pressure being adjusted internally in the middle ear to prevent damage to the eardrum.

A problem associated with this direct communication between the middle ear and the nasopharynx is that disease organisms have a direct passageway from the throat to the middle ear. Therefore, ear infections often accompany sore throats, especially in children whose immune system is still in development.

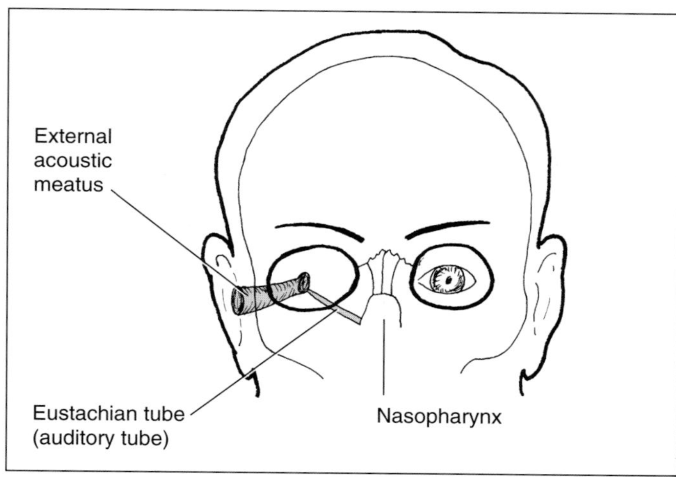

Fig. 13-17. Middle ear.

Internal Acoustic Meatus: The drawing in Fig. 13-18 demonstrates the ear structures as they would appear in a **modified PA (Caldwell) projection**. A 5 to 10° caudad angle to the orbitomeatal line will project the petrous ridges to the mid orbital level as shown in this drawing. This results a special transorbital view, which may be taken to demonstrate the **internal acoustic meatus**. The opening to the internal acoustic meatus is an oblique aperture, smaller in diameter than the opening to the external acoustic meatus, and is very hard to demonstrate clearly on any conventional radiographic projection. It is an important structure to demonstrate, however, for specific purposes because certain auditory and facial nerves, as well as blood vessels, pass through the internal acoustic meatus.

Note that in this PA projection the internal acoustic meatus is projected into the orbital shadow slightly below the petrous ridge, allowing it to be visualized on radiographs taken in this position. Remember that the lateral portions of the petrous ridges are at approximately the level of the **TEA** (top of ear attachment). These external relationships to the internal structures are important to remember.

The tubelike internal acoustic canal may be best demonstrated on an **anterior oblique projection**, also referred to as a posterior profile projection or Stenvers method taken for the mastoids as demonstrated on page 403. Therefore, both the modified PA Caldwell (with 5 to 10° CR angle) and the anterior oblique (Stenvers) may be taken to demonstrate the internal acoustic meatus or canal. However, as noted earlier in this chapter, CT and MRI have largely replaced conventional radiography in visualizing these hard-to-see temporal bone structures, and these two projections are rarely performed today for demonstrating these structures.

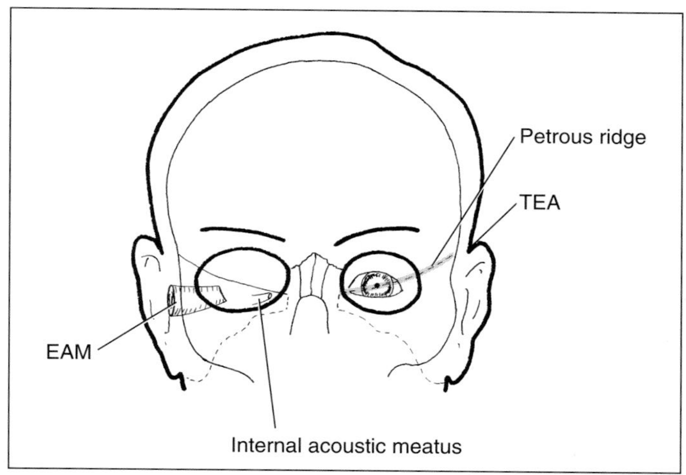

Fig. 13-18. Modified PA Caldwell (5 to 10° caudad).

Mastoids: A second direct communication into the middle ear occurs posteriorly from the **mastoid air cells**. The schematic drawing in Fig. 13-19 is a sagittal section showing the relationships of the mastoid air cells to the **attic** or **epitympanic recess** and the **tympanic cavity proper**. The **aditus** is the opening between the epitympanic recess and the mastoid portion of the temporal bone.

The aditus connects directly to a large chamber within the mastoid portion termed the **antrum**. The antrum then connects to the various mastoid air cells. This communication allows infection in the middle ear, which may have originated in the throat, to pass into the mastoid area. Once within the mastoid area, infection is separated from brain tissue by only thin bone. Before the common use of effective antibiotics, this was often a pathway for a serious infection of the brain, termed **encephalitis**. The thin plate of bone forming the roof of the antrum, aditus and attic area of the tympanic cavity is called the **tegmen tympani**.

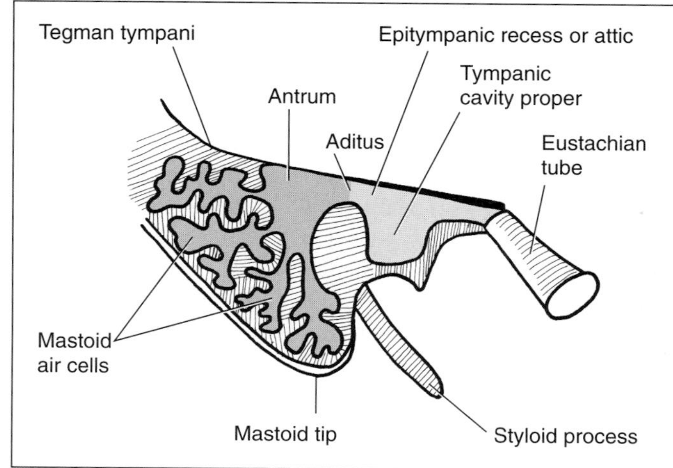

Fig. 13-19. Mastoid connection.

Middle Ear continued

Auditory Ossicles: The **auditory ossicles** are three small bones that are prominent structures within the middle ear. The drawing in Figs. 13-20 and 13-21 demonstrate that these three small bones are articulated to permit vibratory motion. The three auditory ossicles are located partly in the attic or epitympanic recess, and partly in the tympanic cavity proper. These delicate bones bridge the middle ear cavity to transmit sound vibrations from the tympanic membrane to the oval window of the internal ear.

Vibrations are first picked up by the **malleus**, meaning hammer, which is attached directly to the inside surface of the tympanic membrane. The head of the malleus articulates with the central ossicle, the **incus**. The incus receives its name from a supposed resemblance to an anvil, but it actually looks more like a premolar tooth with a body and two roots. The incus then connects to the stirrup-shaped **stapes**, which is the smallest of the three auditory ossicles. The foot plate of the stapes is then attached to another membrane called the **oval window** leading into the inner ear.

Auditory Ossicles–Frontal and Lateral View: The drawings in Fig. 13-21 illustrate the relationship of the **auditory ossicles** to one another in both a close-up frontal view and a lateral view. As seen from the front, the most lateral of the three bones is the **malleus**, while the most medial of the three bones is the **stapes**. The lateral-view drawing demonstrates how the ossicles would appear if one looked through the **external acoustic meatus** to see the bony ossicles of the middle ear. Note that the malleus, with its attachment to the eardrum, is located slightly anterior to the other two bones.

The resemblance of the **incus** to a premolar tooth with a body and two roots is well visualized in the lateral drawing. The longer root of the incus connects to the stapes, which in turn connects to the oval window of the cochlea, resulting in the sense of hearing as described in a lateral section.

Internal Ear

The very complex **internal ear** contains the essential sensory apparatus of both **hearing** and **equilibrium**. Lying within the densest portion of the petrous pyramid, it can be divided into two main parts, the **osseous** or **bony labyrinth**, important radiographically, and the **membranous labyrinth**. The osseous labyrinth is a bony chamber housing the membranous labyrinth, a series of intercommunicating ducts and sacs. One such duct is the **endolymphatic duct**, a blind pouch or closed duct contained in a small canal-like, bony structure. The canal of the endolymphatic duct arises from the medial wall of the vestibule and extends to the posterior wall of the petrous pyramid, located both posterior and lateral to the **internal acoustic meatus.**

Osseous (Bony) Labyrinth: The osseous or bony labyrinth is divided into **three** distinctly shaped parts, the **cochlea** (meaning snail shell), the **vestibule** and the **semicircular canals**. The osseous labyrinth completely surrounds and encloses the ducts and sacs of the membranous labyrinth. As illustrated on the frontal cutaway view in Fig. 13-22, the snail-shaped, bony cochlea houses a long coiled tubelike duct of the membranous labyrinth.

The **cochlea** is the most anterior of the three parts of the osseous labyrinth. This is best shown on the lateral view of the osseous labyrinth in Fig. 13-23. The **round window**, sometimes called the cochlear window, is shown to be at the base of the cochlea.

The **vestibule** is the central portion of the bony labyrinth and contains the **oval window**, sometimes called the vestibular window.

The three **semicircular canals** are located posterior to the other inner ear structures.

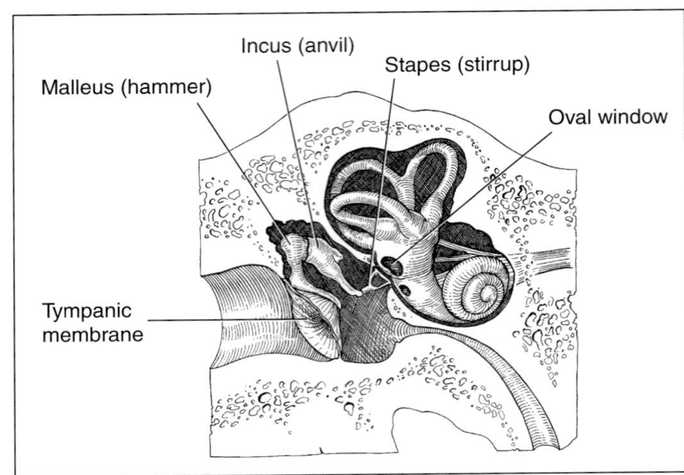

Fig. 13-20. Auditory ossicles–Malleus, incus and stapes.

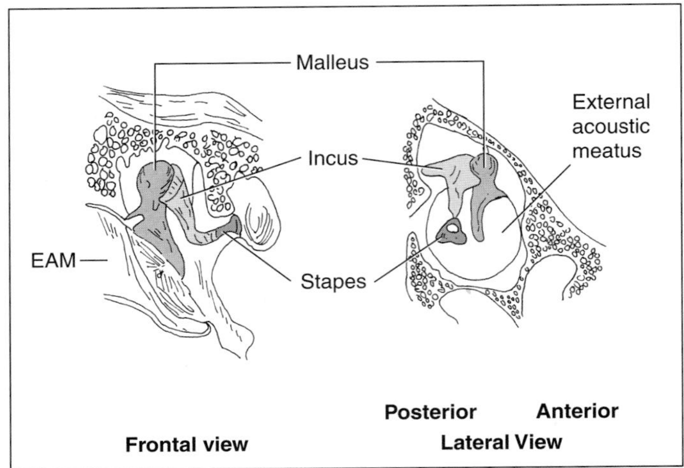

Fig. 13-21. Auditory ossicles.

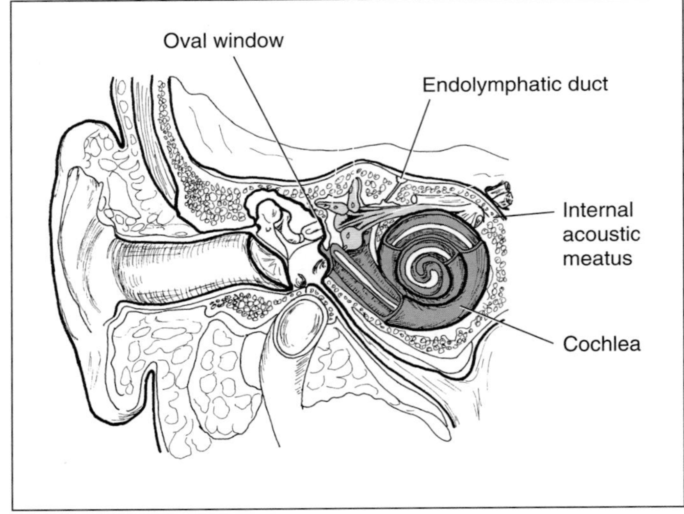

Fig. 13-22. Internal ear, osseous labyrinth–Frontal view.

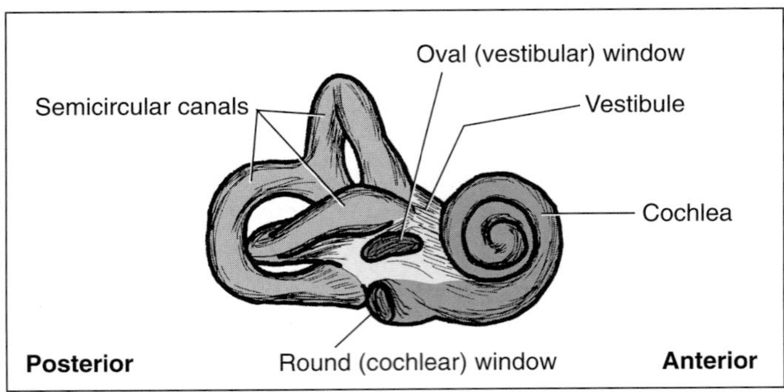

Fig. 13-23. Osseous (bony) labyrinth–Lateral view.

13

Osseous Labyrinth continued

A lateral view of the **osseous labyrinth** is again shown in Fig. 13-24. The three semicircular canals are named according to their position, thus they are called the **superior, posterior** and **lateral semicircular canals**. Observe that each is located at right angles to the other two, allowing a sense of equilibrium as well as a sense of direction. It is important to remember that the **semicircular canals relate to the sense of direction or equilibrium**, and the **cochlea relates to the sense of hearing** due to its connection to the stapes through the oval window.

"Windows" of Inner Ear: The two openings into the inner ear are covered by membranes. The **oval or vestibular window** receives vibrations from the external ear through the foot plate of the stapes of the middle ear and transmits these vibrations into the **vestibule** of the internal ear. The **round or cochlear window** is located at the base of the first coil of the cochlea. The round window is a membrane that allows movement of fluid within the closed duct system of the membranous labyrinth. As the oval window moves slightly inward with a vibration, the round window moves outward since this is a closed system and fluid does not compress. Vibrations and associated slight fluid movements within the cochlea produce impulses, which are transmitted to the auditory nerve within the internal acoustic meatus, creating the sense of hearing.

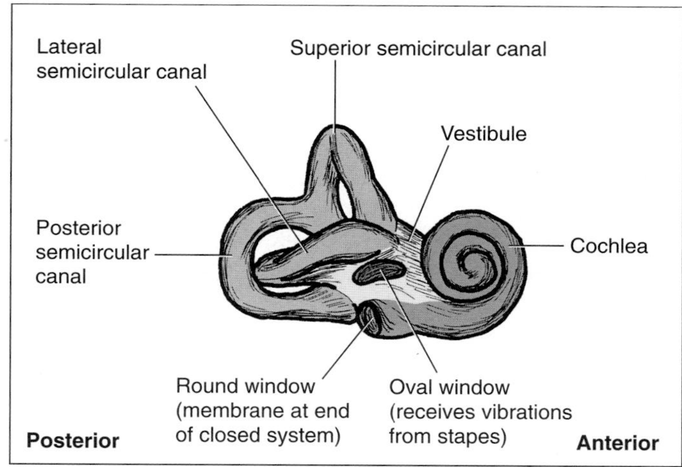

Fig. 13-24. Osseous labyrinth
–Cochlea, vestibule and semicircular canals.

ANATOMY REVIEW ON RADIOGRAPHS

Specific anatomy of the temporal bone is difficult to recognize on conventional radiograph. However, by knowing general shapes and relationships to recognizable structures, one can recognize certain structures as follows:

Axiolateral Projection (Fig. 13-25)

A. EAM (external auditory meatus).
B. Mastoid antrum.
C. Mastoid air cells.
D. Downside mandibular condyle (just anterior to EAM).
E. Upside (magnified) mandibular condyle.

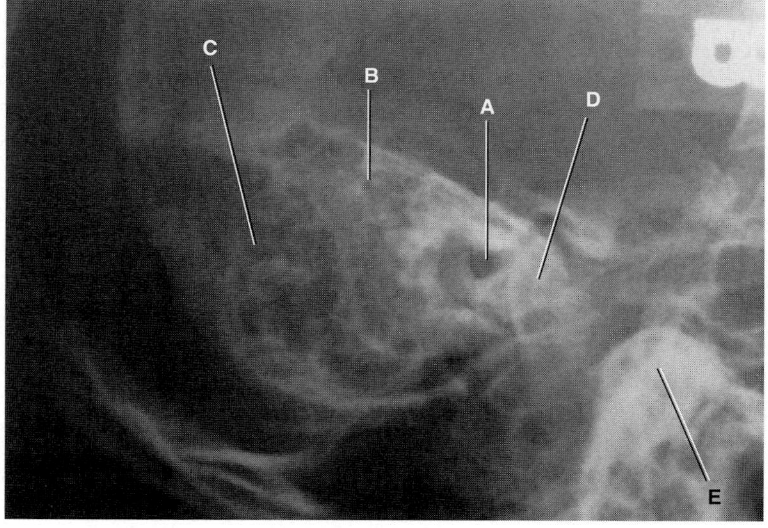

Fig. 13-25. Axiolateral projection for mastoids (modified Law method).

Posterior Profile Projection (Fig. 13-26)

A. Petrous ridge.
B. Bony (osseous) labyrinth (semicircular canals).
C. EAM.
D. Region of internal acoustic canal.

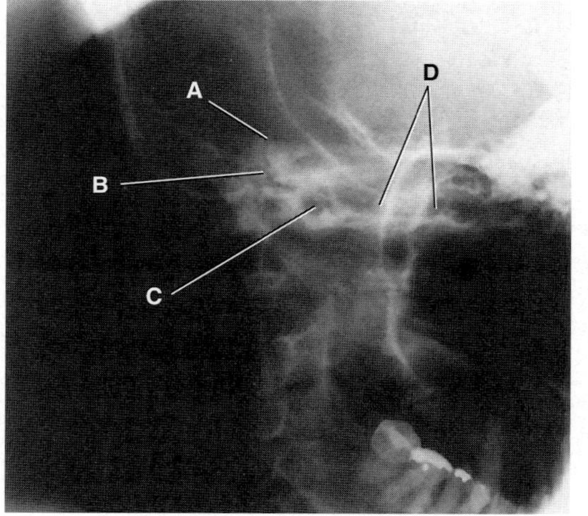

Fig. 13-26. Posterior profile projection for mastoids (Stenvers method).

Radiographic Positioning

POSITIONING CONSIDERATIONS

Paranasal Sinuses

Technical Factors: A medium kVp range of 70 to 80 is commonly used to provide sufficient contrast of the air-filled paranasal sinuses. Optimum density as controlled by the mAs is especially important for sinus radiography to be able to visualize possible pathology within the sinus cavities. Because of overlying structures in some of the sinus projections, it is sometimes more difficult to evaluate for optimum density. Comparing the more uniform density within the orbits to that of the various sinuses is one way to do this.

A small focal spot should be used, if possible, along with short exposure times for maximum detail.

As with cranial and facial bones, gonadal shielding is not useful in reducing gonadal exposure but shields over the pelvic area may be used for patient assurance and satisfaction. The gonadal doses in the dose icon boxes are listed as NDC, no detectable contribution. Good collimation and elimination of unnecessary repeats are the best protective measure for sinus and mastoid radiography.

Erect Position: Radiography of the paranasal sinuses should be **taken erect whenever possible** to demonstrate air-fluid levels if present within the sinuses. This also requires the use of a **horizontal x-ray beam**. If the x-ray beam is not completely horizontal, air-fluid levels will not be demonstrated as clearly defined straight lines but will be seen as a gradual density changes. Therefore, rather than angling the central ray (CR) for a specific projection (such as for a PA Caldwell, which generally requires a 15° CR caudad angle), the CR remains horizontal and the head is tilted back as needed (Fig. 13-27).

If the patient's condition does not allow an upright position, then a horizontal beam lateral of the sinuses can be taken with a horizontal x-ray beam to demonstrate air-fluid levels.

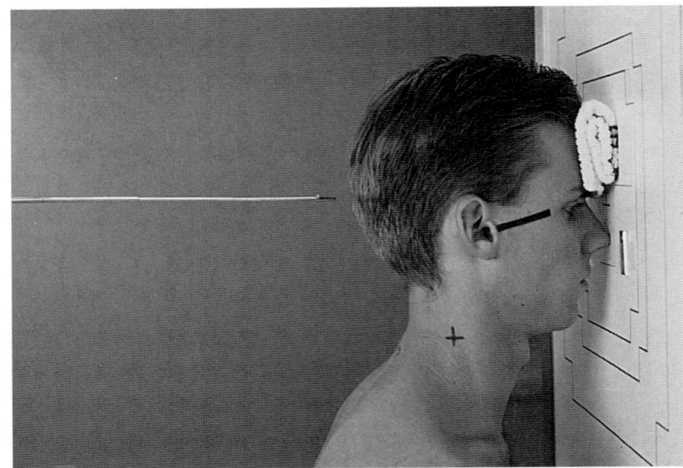

Fig. 13-27. Modified PA Caldwell–**Horizontal CR**, OML tilted 15° from perpendicular.

Temporal Bone–Mastoids

Basic conventional radiographic examinations for the temporal bone and/or mastoids are being performed less and less with the increased use of specialized imaging modalities such as body section radiography (tomography), CT or MRI, which demonstrate these delicate structures more clearly. However, requests for certain basic radiographic exams for the mastoids may be encountered in some institutions, and the more common basic projections for demonstrating these structures are included in this chapter.

Due to superimposition of the dense petrous pyramid structure, the mastoid process is best demonstrated on certain lateral oblique projections (Fig. 13-28).

Both right and left sides are examined for comparison purposes. Due to the small structures which need to be visualized, the use of a **small focal spot, detail screens, tight collimation** and **complete immobilization** is essential.

The auricles of the ear are taped forward on certain lateral projections to prevent shadows of the ear cartilage from superimposing temporal bone structures. Figure 13-28 demonstrates the axiolateral oblique projection (modified Law) for demonstrating the right (downside) mastoids. Note that auricles of the ear are taped forward.

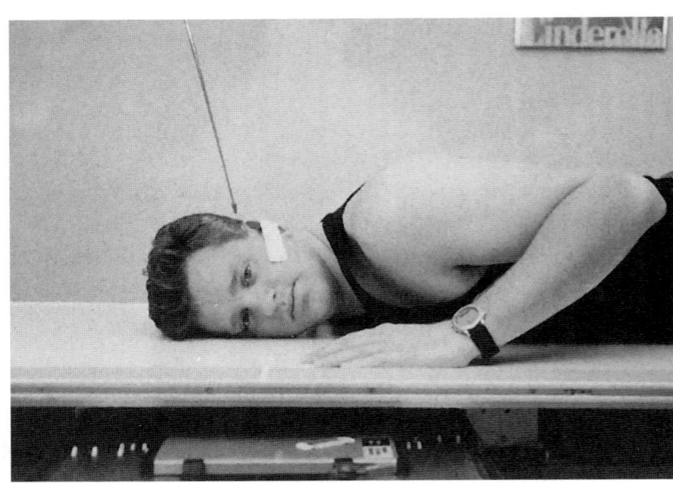

Fig. 13-28. Axiolateral 15° oblique (modified Law method).

TOMOGRAPHY–ANATOMICAL RELATIONSHIPS

Tomography or body section radiography is one way to visualize the delicate structures of the middle and internal ear. Tomography requires a good understanding of not only the specific anatomy, but also the distances between various structures in both frontal and lateral projections, as shown on these drawings.

Superior View–AP Projection

Certain structures labeled **A** through **I** are identified in Fig. 13-29. Distances and relationships between these structures should be noted as positioned for this AP projection. Part **A** is the cochlea; **B** is the eustachian or auditory tube; **C** is the bony ossicles in the tympanic cavity of the middle ear; **D** is the external acoustic meatus; **E** is the antrum; **F** is the semicircular canals; **G** is the endolymphatic duct; **H** is the vestibule; and **I** is the internal acoustic meatus.

It is important to note that almost all of the structures of the ear are located between the cochlea (toward the anterior) and the antrum (toward the posterior) in a distance of approximately 1 centimeter or 10 millimeters. The distance from the back of the head to the center of the external acoustic meatus is approximately 10 centimeters.

Average distances between structures are based on the average-shaped skull with the OML perpendicular to the table-top, and they will vary with the shape and size of the skull. If the OML were not kept perpendicular to the table-top, these distances would also vary.

Generally speaking, however, the most important structures of the middle and internal ear can be located in the **1 centimeter distance between 9.5 cm and 10.5 cm from the table-top**. Therefore starting focal plane distances for an AP projection on an average skull would be 9.5 to 10.5 cm.

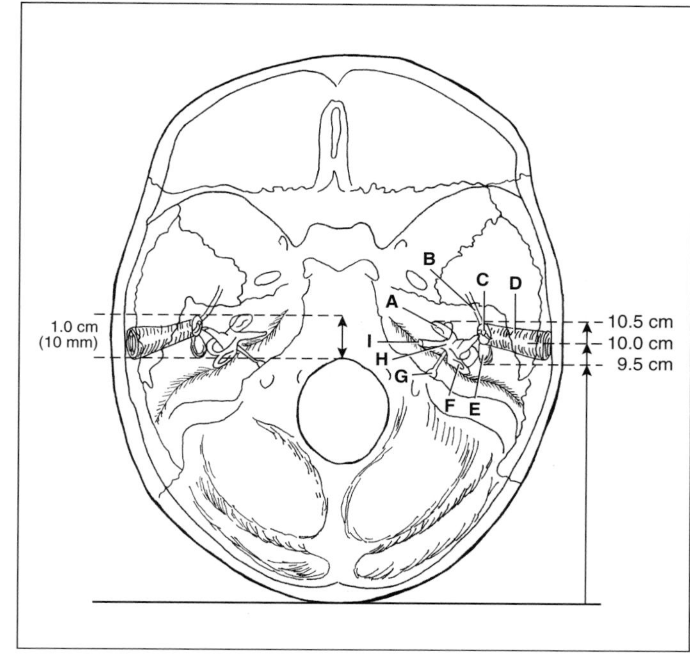

Fig. 13-29. Ear structures–As positioned for an AP tomogram.

Superior View–Lateral Projection

Fig. 13-30 gives a top view of the head with the patient in a lateral position. The various ear structures are again shown with important distances identified. From the table-top, the average distance to the midline is 7 centimeters, and to the internal acoustic meatus, 9 centimeters. The internal acoustic meatus extends 1 centimeter or 10 millimeters toward the inner ear. The inner ear extends another 1 centimeter and the middle ear extends approximately 5 millimeters farther. The distance from the tympanic membrane to the external acoustic opening is 2.5 centimeters or 25 millimeters.

These figures demonstrate that the **distance from the external opening of the external acoustic meatus to the internal acoustic meatus is approximately 5 centimeters** in the average-shaped skull. Starting focal plane distances on a lateral projection would be from 9 to 14 cm.

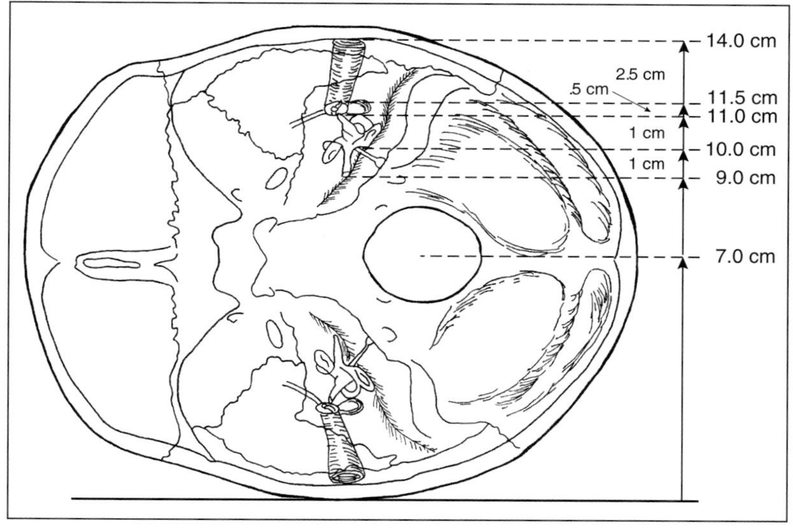

Fig. 13-30. Ear structures–As positioned for a lateral tomogram.

NATIONAL SURVEY

Departmental routines for exams of the paranasal sinuses, mastoids and temporal bone were quite consistent throughout the United States as follows:

Paranasal Sinuses Routine

Paranasal sinuses	U.S. Average	
	Basic 1995 (1989)	Special 1995 (1989)
• Lateral	95% (99%)	
• PA Caldwell	95% (97%)	
• PA Waters	95% (93%)	
• Submentovertex (SMV)	53% (57%)	15% (9%)
• Open mouth Waters	– (30%)	– (13%)

Petrous Pyramids Routine*

Petrous pyramids	U.S. Average	
	Basic 1995 (1989)	Special 1995 (1989)
• AP axial (Towne)	(83%)	
• Submentovertex (SMV)	(64%)	(7%)
• Anterior profile (reverse Stenvers)	(5%)	(9%)

*This was not included in the 1995 survey because of the infrequency of them being performed today.

Mastoids and Temporal Bones Routine

Mastoids	U.S. Average	
	Basic 1995 (1989)	Special 1995 (1989)
• Axiolateral 15° oblique (Law)	65% (81%)	
• Posterior profile (Stenvers)	69% (84%)	
• AP axial (Towne)	65% (30%)	
• Axiolateral (Schuller)	33% (7%)	15% (9%)
• Submentovertex (SMV)	31% –	18% –
• Axiolateral 45° oblique (Mayer)	27% (12%)	27% –
• Anterior profile (Arcelin)	20% –	23% –

STANDARD AND SPECIAL OPERATING PROCEDURES

Certain basic and special projections for the paranasal sinuses, mastoids and petrous pyramids are demonstrated and described on the following pages as suggested standard and special departmental procedures.

Basic Projections

Standard or basic projections, also sometimes referred to as routine projections or departmental routines, are those projections commonly taken on average patients who are helpful and can cooperate in performing the procedure.

Special Projections

Special projections are those more common projections taken as extra or additional projections to better demonstrate certain pathologic conditions or specific body parts.

Basic and Special Projections

Paranasal Sinuses
Basic
- Lateral **397**
- PA (Caldwell) **398**
- Parietoacanthial (Waters) **399**
- Submentovertex (SMV) **400**

Special
- Parietoacanthial transoral (open-mouth Waters) **401**

Mastoids
Basic
- Axiolateral oblique (modified Law) **402**
- Axioanterior oblique (posterior profile) (Stenvers) **403**
- AP axial (Towne) **404**

Special
- Axiolateral (Schuller) **405**
- Axioposterior oblique (anterior profile) (Arcelin–reverse Stenvers) **406**
- AP axial oblique (Mayer method and Owen modification) **407**

Temporal Bones and/or **Petrous Pyramids**
Basic
- AP axial (Towne) **408**
- Submentovertex (SMV) **408**

13

Lateral Position–Right or Left Lateral

Sinuses
Basic
- **Lateral**
- PA (Caldwell)
- Parietoacanthial (Waters)
- Submentovertex (SMV)

Structures Best Shown

Sphenoid sinuses, superimposed frontal, ethmoid and maxillary sinuses, sella turcica and orbital roofs.
Unilateral position.

Technical Factors

- Film size–8 x 10 in. (18 x 24 cm), lengthwise.
- Moving or stationary grid.
- 70-80 kVp range.
- Use small focal spot.
- Technique and dose:

cm	kVp	mAs	Sk.	ML.	Gon.
15	70	5	39	10	NDC

mrad

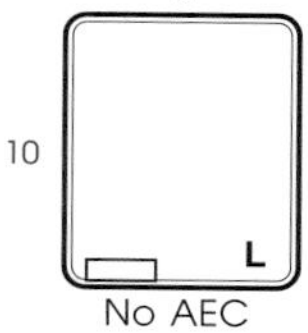

Patient Position

- Remove all metal, plastic or other removable objects from head.
- Patient in an **erect position**. (See Notes.)

Part Position

- Rest lateral side of head against head unit or table-top, with side of interest closest to cassette.
- Adjust head into a **true lateral** position, oblique body as needed for patient's comfort (midsagittal plane parallel to film).
- Align **interpupillary line perpendicular to film** (ensures no tilt).
- Adjust chin to bring IOML perpendicular to front edge of cassette.

Central Ray

- Align a **horizontal CR** perpendicular to the film.
- Center CR to a point **midway between outer canthus and EAM**.
- Center cassette to CR.
- SID: Head unit, 36 in. (91 cm).
  Upright table or grid unit, minimum 40 in. (102 cm).

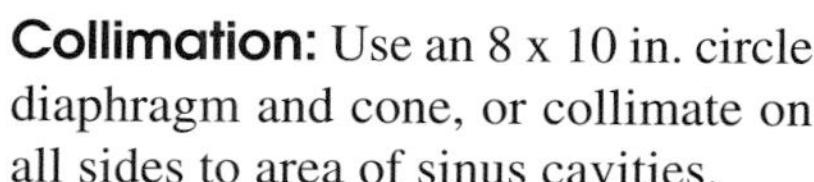

Collimation: Use an 8 x 10 in. circle diaphragm and cone, or collimate on all sides to area of sinus cavities.

Respiration: Suspend respiration during exposure.

Notes: To visualize air-fluid levels, an erect position is required. Fluid within the paranasal sinus cavities is thick and gelatin-like, causing it to cling to the cavity walls. In order to visualize this fluid, a short time (at least 5 minutes) must be allowed for the fluid to settle after a patient's position has been changed. If an upright head or grid unit is not available, the x-ray table can be placed in a vertical position and used in the same manner as the erect grid unit.

If patient cannot sit or stand, this can be taken with patient supine utilizing a horizontal beam x-ray, similar to trauma lateral facial bones, as described in Chapter 19 on mobile and trauma radiography.

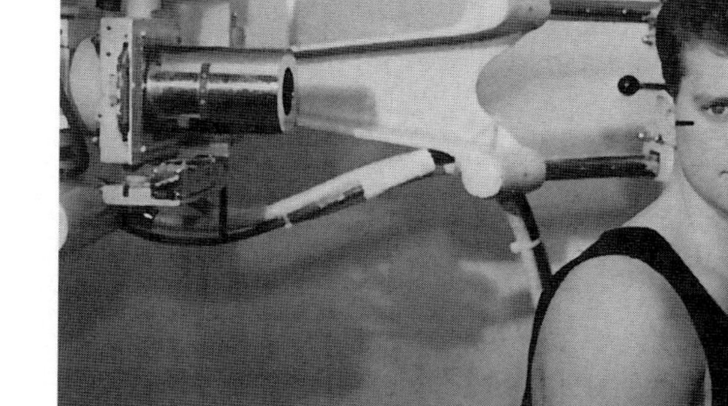

Fig. 13-31. Erect left lateral (head unit).

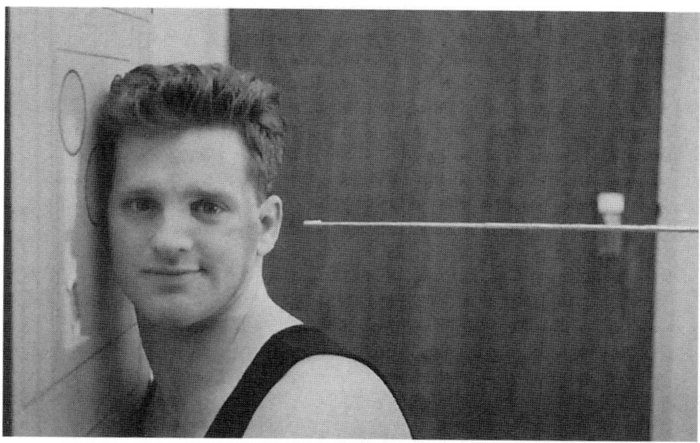

Fig. 13-32. Erect right lateral (upright grid).

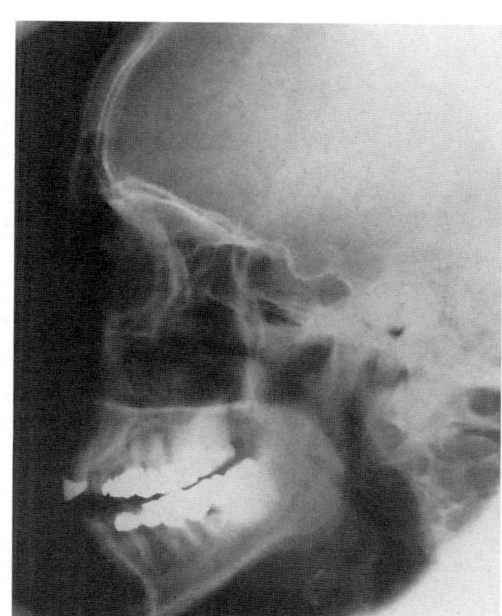

Fig. 13-33. Lateral.

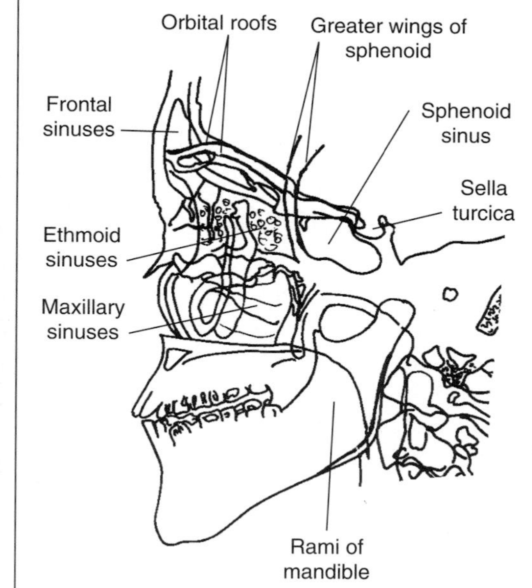

Fig. 13-34. Lateral.

Evaluation Criteria

- Included and centered to the collimation field and film are the frontal, sphenoid, ethmoid and maxillary sinuses. **Sphenoid sinuses** are of primary interest in the lateral position.
- The cranium is not rotated or tilted:
  - The mandibular rami, the orbital roofs and the greater wings of the sphenoid are superimposed.
  - The sella turcica is demonstrated without rotation.
- Sufficient penetration and exposure, without motion, to visualize the sphenoid sinuses without overexposing the maxillary and frontal sinus regions.

PA Projection

Caldwell Method

Sinuses
Basic
• Lateral
• **PA (Caldwell)**
• Parietoacanthial (Waters)
• Submentovertex (SMV)

Structures Best Shown

Frontal sinuses and anterior ethmoid sinuses.

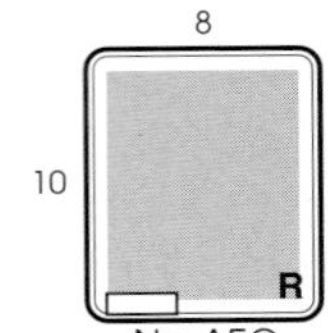

Technical Factors

• Film size–8 x 10 in. (18 x 24 cm), lengthwise.
• Moving or stationary grid.
• 70-80 kVp range.
• Use small focal spot.
• Upright head unit is angled 15°, CR is horizontal. (See Note.)
• Technique and dose:

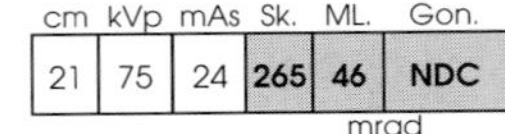

cm	kVp	mAs	Sk.	ML.	Gon.
21	75	24	265	46	NDC

mrad

Patient Position

• Remove all metal, plastic or other removable objects from head.
• Patient in an **erect position**. (See Note).

Part Position 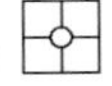

• Rest patient's nose and forehead against film holder with top of film tilted back toward patient 15° if possible.
• Extend head as needed, bringing **OML perpendicular** to film.
• Align **midsagittal plane perpendicular to midline** of film.
• Center cassette to CR and to nasion, ensure **no rotation**.

Central Ray

• Align **CR horizontal**, parallel with the floor. (See Note.)
• Center CR to **exit at nasion**.
• SID: Head unit, 36 in. (91 cm).
Upright table or grid unit, minimum 40 in. (102 cm).

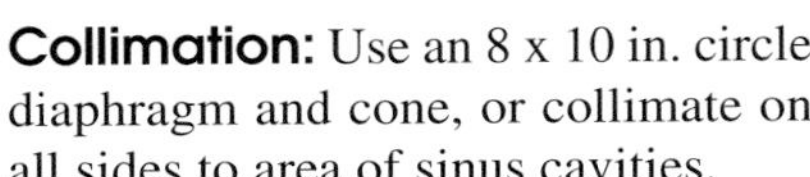

Collimation: Use an 8 x 10 in. circle diaphragm and cone, or collimate on all sides to area of sinus cavities.

Respiration: Suspend respiration.

Note: To measure air-fluid levels, the **CR must be horizontal** and the **patient must be erect.**

Modified PA (Fig. 13-36): If the vertical-grid film holder cannot be tilted and remains vertical, a radiolucent sponge or pad can be used to support the head tilted back to place the **OML 15°** from horizontal. **CR remains horizontal**.

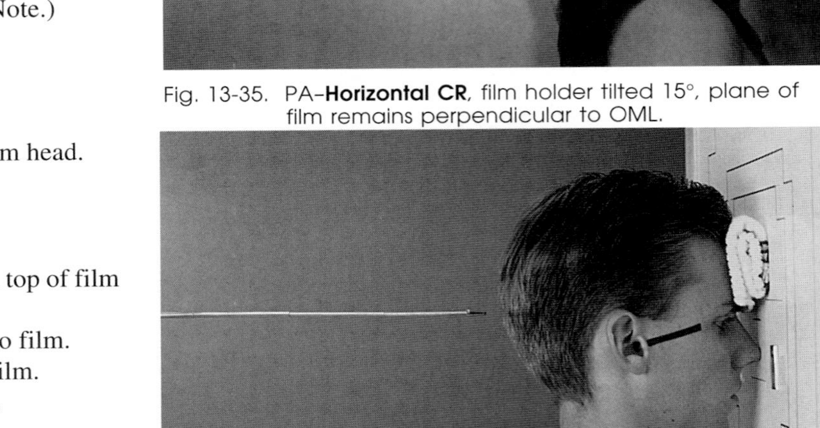

Fig. 13-35. PA–**Horizontal CR**, film holder tilted 15°, plane of film remains perpendicular to OML.

Fig. 13-36. Modified PA–**CR horizontal**, OML 15° to CR (if film holder cannot be tilted).

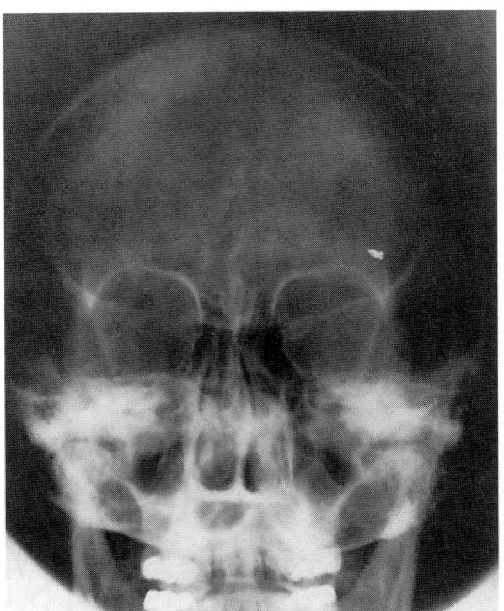

Fig. 13-37. PA.

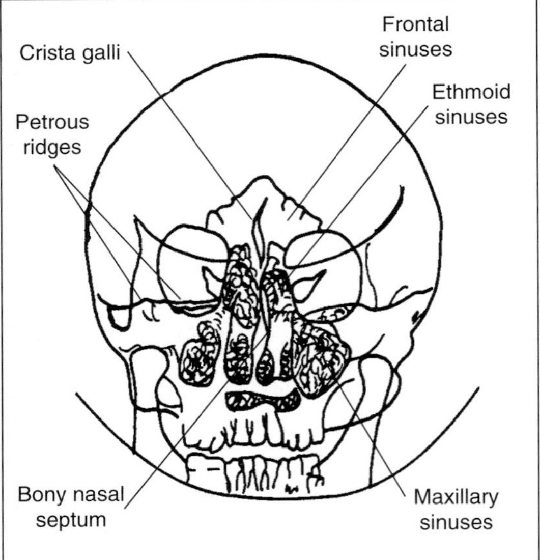

Fig. 13-38. PA.

Evaluation Criteria

• Petrous ridges are projected into lower one-third of orbits.
• Included and centered to the collimation field and film are the frontal and anterior ethmoid sinuses.
• The cranium is not rotated or tilted:
  –Equal distance from the midsagittal plane, identified by the crista galli, to the outer orbital margin.
  –Superior orbital fissures are symmetrically visualized within the orbits.
• Frontal sinuses are projected above the frontonasal suture.
• Anterior ethmoid air cells are visualized laterally adjacent to each nasal bone, directly below the frontal sinuses.
• Sufficient penetration and exposure, without motion, to visualize the frontal and ethmoid sinuses.

Parietoacanthial Projection

Waters Method

Sinuses
Basic
• Lateral
• PA (Caldwell)
• **Parietoacanthial (Waters)**
• Submentovertex (SMV)

Structures Best Shown

Maxillary sinuses and nasal fossae.

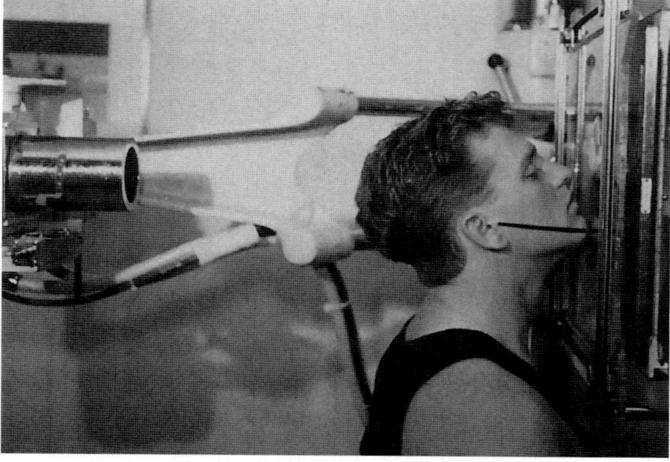

Fig. 13-39. Parietoacanthial projection (head unit) –CR and MML perpendicular to film.

Technical Factors

- Film size–8 x 10 in. (18 x 24 cm), lengthwise.
- Moving or stationary grid.
- 70-80 kVp range.
- Use small focal spot.
- Technique and dose:

cm	kVp	mAs	Sk.	ML.	Gon.
24	75	28	331	46	NDC

mrad

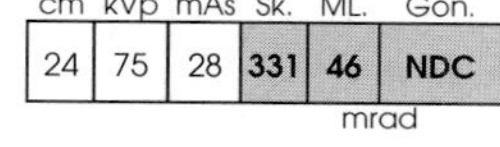

8 / 10 / R / No AEC

Patient Position

- Remove all metal, plastic or other removable objects from head.
- Patient in an **erect position**. (See Notes.)

Part Position

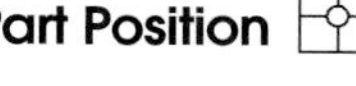

- Extend neck, resting chin and nose against head unit.
- Adjust head until **mentomeatal line (MML) is perpendicular** to film, OML will form a 37° angle with the plane of the film.
- Position the **midsagittal plane perpendicular** to the midline of film.
- Ensure **no rotation or tilt**.
- Center cassette to CR and to acanthion.

Central Ray

- Align a **horizontal CR perpendicular** to the film.
- Center CR to **exit at acanthion**.
- SID: Head unit, 36 in. (91 cm).
  Upright table or grid unit, minimum 40 in. (102 cm).

Collimation: Use an 8 x 10 in. circle diaphragm and cone, or collimate on all sides to area of sinus cavities.

Respiration: Suspend respiration during exposure.

Notes: CR must be horizontal and patient must be erect to demonstrate air-fluid levels within the paranasal sinus cavities.

In this position the average patient's nose tip will be approximately ¾ in. (2 cm) away from the head unit or table-top.

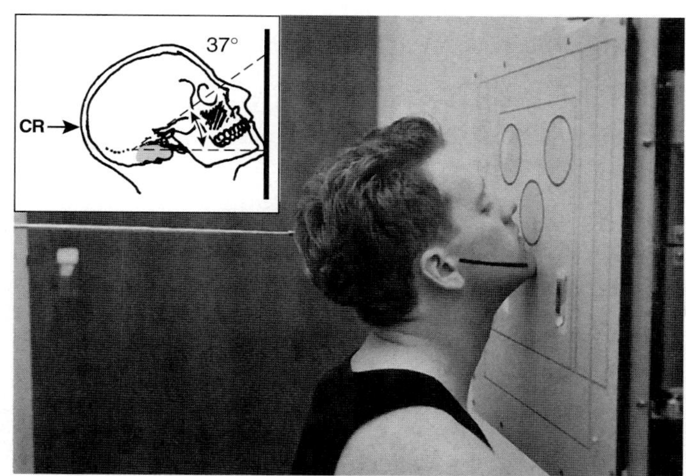

Fig. 13-40. Parietoacanthial projection (upright grid) –CR and MML perpendicular.

Evaluation Criteria

- Included on radiograph are the frontal and maxillary sinuses.
- Cranium seen without rotation:
  –Equal distance from midsagittal plane, identified by the bony nasal septum, to the outer orbital margin.
- Inferior maxillary sinuses are free from superimposing alveolar processes.
- Inferior orbital rim is clearly identified.
- Petrous ridges are below the maxillary sinuses. Each ridge is seen projecting laterally, from the posterior maxillary alveolar process.
- Sufficient penetration and exposure, without motion, to visualize maxillary sinuses.

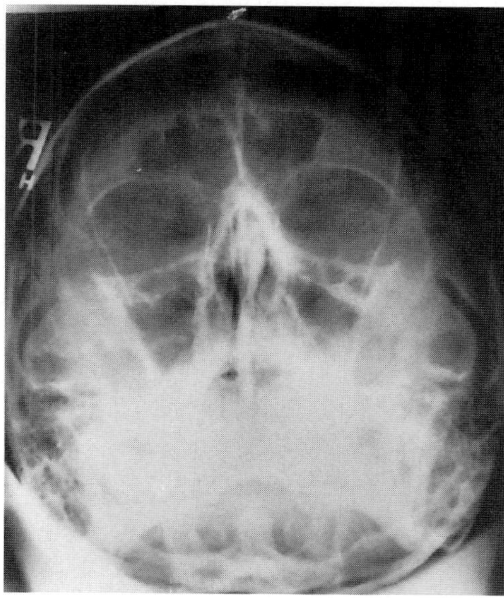

Fig. 13-41. Parietoacanthial projection.

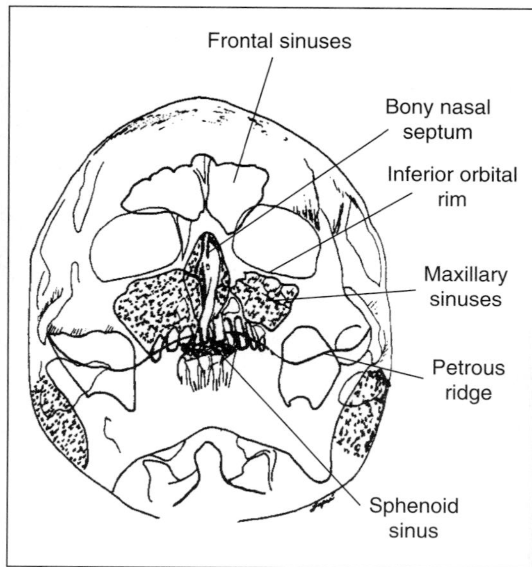

Fig. 13-42. Parietoacanthial projection.

13

Submentovertex (SMV) Projection

Sinuses
Basic
- Lateral
- PA (Caldwell)
- Parietoacanthial (Waters)
- **Submentovertex (SMV)**

Structures Best Shown

Sphenoid sinuses, ethmoid sinuses, nasal fossae and maxillary sinuses.

Technical Factors

- Film size–8 x 10 in. (18 x 24 cm), lengthwise.
- Moving or stationary grid.
- 70-80 kVp range.
- Use small focal spot.
- Technique and dose:

cm	kVp	mAs	Sk.	ML.	Gon.
22	75	34	363	69	NDC

mrad

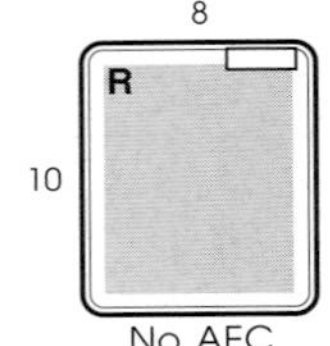

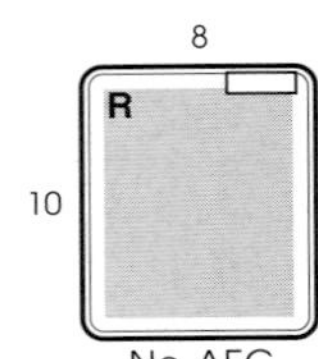

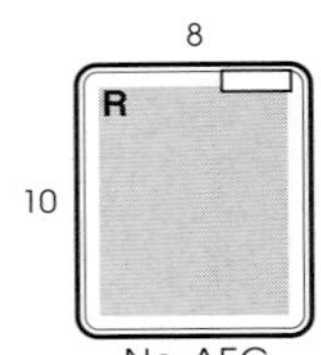

Fig. 13-43. SMV projection (head unit).

Patient Position

- Remove all metal, plastic or other removable objects from head and neck.
- Patient in an **erect position,** if possible, to show air-fluid levels.

Part Position

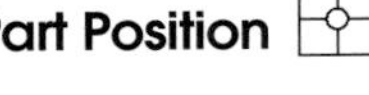

- Raise chin, hyperextending neck if possible until **IOML is parallel** to head unit or vertical table. (See Notes.)
- Head rests on vertex of skull.
- Align **midsagittal plane perpendicular** to midline of head unit or vertical table; ensure **no rotation or tilt**.

Central Ray

- CR directed **perpendicular to IOML**. (See Notes.)
- Center CR midway between angles of mandible, at a level 1½ in. (4 cm) inferior to mandibular symphysis.
- Center CR to cassette.
- SID: Head unit, 36 in. (91 cm). Upright table or grid unit, minimum 40 in. (102 cm).

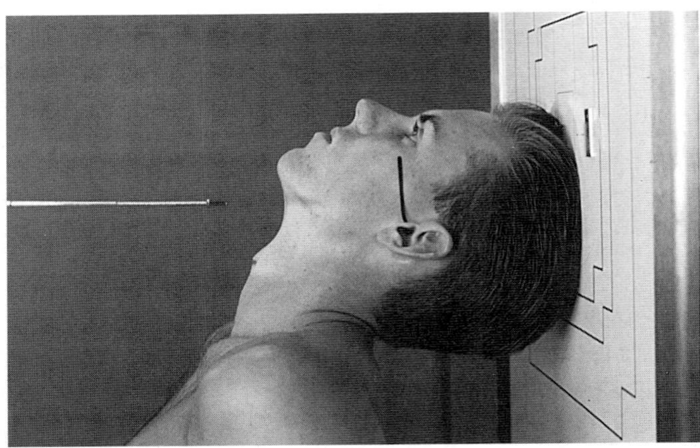

Fig. 13-44. SMV projection (upright grid).

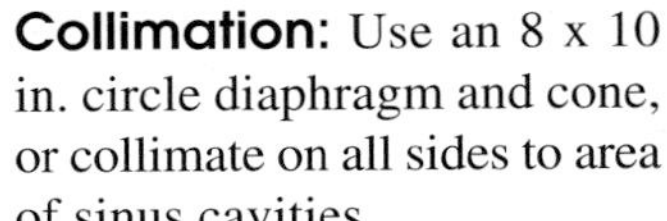

Collimation: Use an 8 x 10 in. circle diaphragm and cone, or collimate on all sides to area of sinus cavities.

Respiration: Suspend respiration during exposure.

Notes: If patient is unable to sufficiently extend neck, angle the tube from horizontal slightly as needed to be perpendicular to IOML. With head unit, the film can then also be angled as needed to maintain the film perpendicular to CR. This, however, should be avoided if possible, due to need of horizontal beam for fluid levels.

Position is very uncomfortable for patient; move quickly.

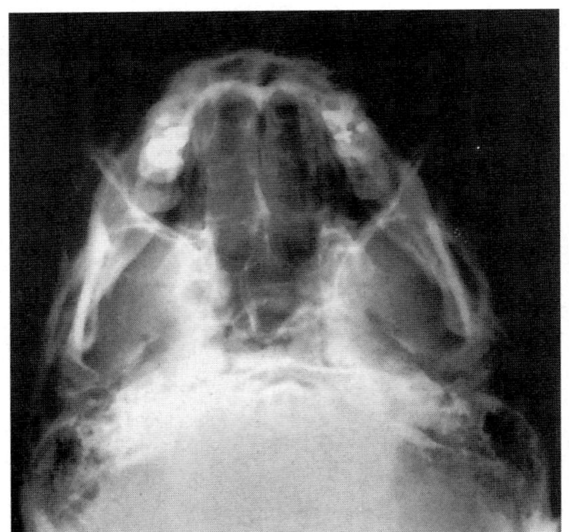

Fig. 13-45. SMV projection.

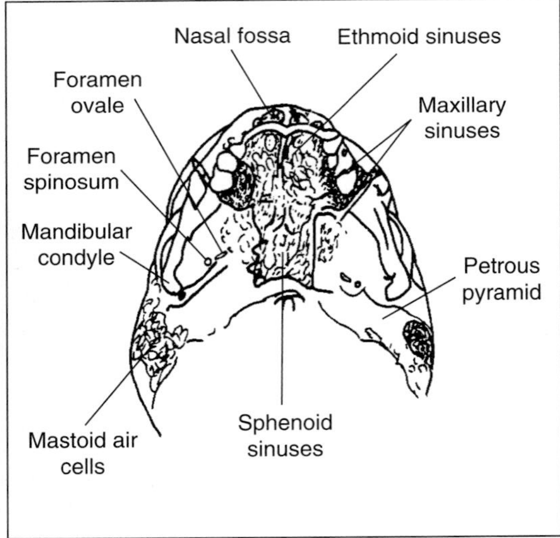

Fig. 13-46. SMV projection.

Evaluation Criteria

- **Mandibular condyles are projected anterior to petrous ridges**.
- Anatomy anterior to foramen magnum visualized and centered to collimation field and film.
- Mandibular symphysis superimposes anterior frontal bone.
- The cranium is not rotated or tilted:
  –Distance along coinciding mandibular surfaces to lateral border of skull are equal (tilt).
  –Petrous pyramids are visualized symmetrically (rotation).
- Sufficient penetration and exposure, without motion, to visualize sphenoid and ethmoid sinuses and foramen ovale and spinosum.

Parietoacanthial Transoral Projection

Open-mouth Waters Method

Sinuses
Special
• **Parietoacanthial transoral (open-mouth Waters)**

Structures Best Shown

Sphenoid and maxillary sinuses and nasal fossae. (Sphenoid sinuses are clearly seen through the "open mouth.")

Technical Factors

- Film size–8 x 10 in. (18 x 24 cm), lengthwise.
- Moving or stationary grid.
- 70-80 kVp range.
- Use small focal spot.
- Technique and dose:

cm	kVp	mAs	Sk.	ML.	Gon.
24	75	28	331	46	NDC

mrad

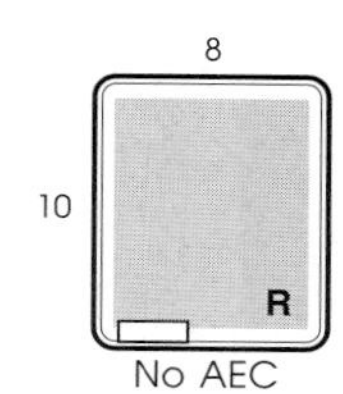

Fig. 13-47. Parietoacanthial transoral projection (head unit).

Patient Position

- Remove all metal, plastic or other removable objects from head.
- Patient in an **erect position**. (See Note.)

Part Position

- Extend neck, resting chin and nose against head unit.
- Adjust head until **OML forms a 37° angle** with film holder (**mentomeatal line will be perpendicular** with mouth closed).
- Position the **midsagittal plane perpendicular** to the midline of the head unit; ensure **no rotation or tilt**.
- Instruct patient to open mouth by telling him/her to "drop jaw without moving head." (Mentomeatal line is no longer perpendicular.)
- Center cassette to CR and to **acanthion.**

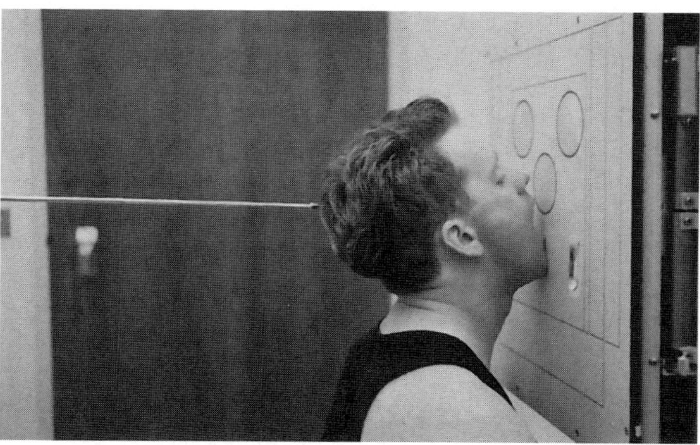

Fig. 13-48. Parietoacanthial transoral projection (upright grid).

Central Ray

- Align a **horizontal CR perpendicular** to the film.
- Center CR to **exit at acanthion**.
- SID: Head unit, 36 in. (91 cm). Upright table or grid unit, minimum 40 in. (102 cm).

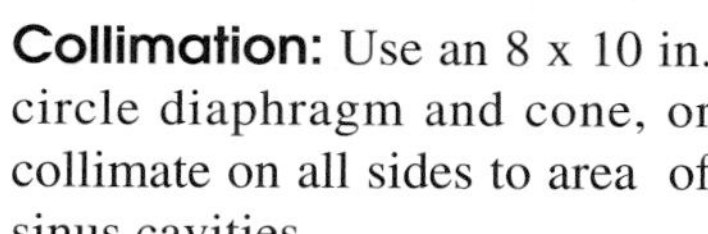

Collimation: Use an 8 x 10 in. circle diaphragm and cone, or collimate on all sides to area of sinus cavities.

Respiration: Suspend respiration during exposure.

Note: CR must be horizontal and patient erect to demonstrate air-fluid levels within the paranasal sinus cavities.

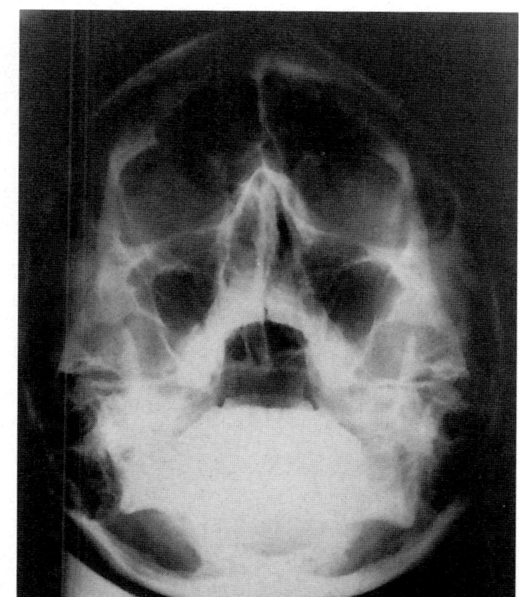

Fig. 13-49. Parietoacanthial transoral projection.

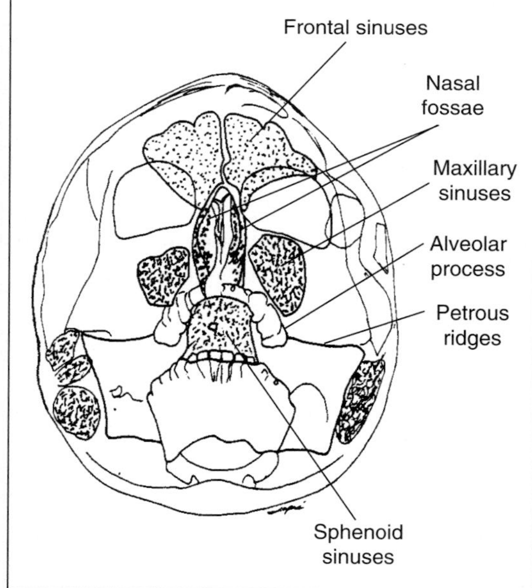

Fig. 13-50. Parietoacanthial transoral projection.

Evaluation Criteria

- Sphenoid sinus is visualized within shadow of open mouth.
- Included on radiograph are the frontal, maxillary and sphenoid sinuses.
- Cranium seen without rotation or tilt:
  - Equal distance from the midsagittal plane (identified by the bony nasal septum) to the outer orbital margin.
- Inferior maxillary sinuses are free from superimposing alveolar processes.
- Inferior orbital rim is clearly identified.
- Petrous ridges are below the maxillary sinuses. Each ridge is seen projecting laterally, from the posterior maxillary alveolar process.
- Sufficient penetration and exposure, without motion, to visualize the maxillary and sphenoid sinuses.

Axiolateral Oblique Projection

Modified Law Method

Mastoids
Basic
• **Axiolateral oblique (modified Law)**
• Axioanterior oblique (Stenvers)
• AP axial (Towne)

Structures Best Shown

Lateral prospective of mastoid air cells closest to film.

Both sides are generally taken for comparison.

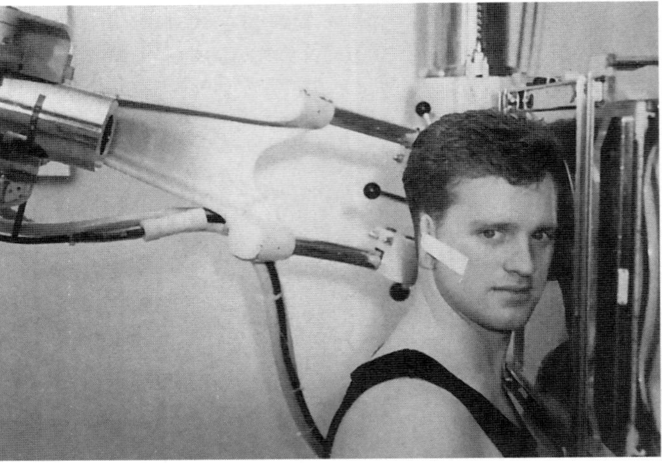

Fig. 13-51. Axiolateral oblique.
-15° oblique (head rotation).
-15° caudad angle.

Technical Factors

- Film size–2 each 8 x 10 in. (18 x 24 cm), lengthwise.
- Moving or stationary grid.
- 70-80 kVp range.
- Use small focal spot.
- Technique and dose:

cm	kVp	mAs	Sk.	ML.	Gon.
15	75	14	129	38	NDC

mrad

8 × 10, R, No AEC

Patient Position

- Remove all metal, plastic or other removable objects from head.
- Patient in an erect or prone position.
- **Tape each auricle forward** to prevent superimposing mastoid.

Part Position

- Rest lateral side of head against head unit or table-top, with side of interest closest to cassette; oblique body as needed for patient comfort.
- Align midsagittal plane parallel with head unit or table-top in a lateral position, then **rotate face 15° toward film.** Prevent tilt by maintaining the **interpupillary line perpendicular** to head unit or table-top.
- Adjust chin to bring **IOML perpendicular** to front edge of cassette.

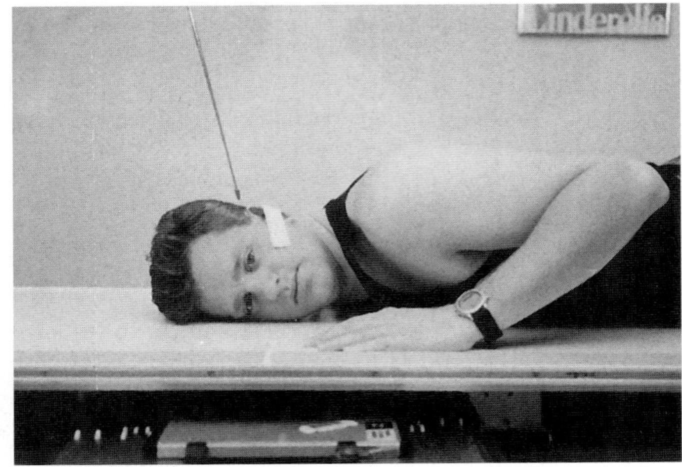

Fig. 13-52. Axiolateral oblique.
-15° oblique (head rotation).
-15° caudad angle.

Central Ray

- Angle CR **15° caudad.**
- Center CR to **exit at downside mastoid tip,** to **enter 1 in. (2.5 cm) posterior and superior to upside EAM.**
- Center cassette to projected CR.
- SID: Head unit, 36 in. (91 cm).
  Table, minimum 40 in. (102 cm).

Collimation: Use a circle diaphragm and cone, or collimate on all sides to yield a field size of approximately 4 in. (10 cm) square.

Respiration: Suspend respiration during exposure.

Note: To obtain a sharply detailed image of the mastoid cells, the utilization of a small focal spot and close collimation is essential.

Evaluation Criteria

- The mastoid air cells of interest are located in the center of collimation field and film, posterior to the EAM.
- Opposite mastoid does not superimpose mastoid of interest but is seen inferior to it.
- Ear auricle does not superimpose mastoid.
- Temporomandibular joint is visualized anterior to mastoid cell of interest.
- Sufficient penetration and exposure, without motion, to visualize mastoid air cells.

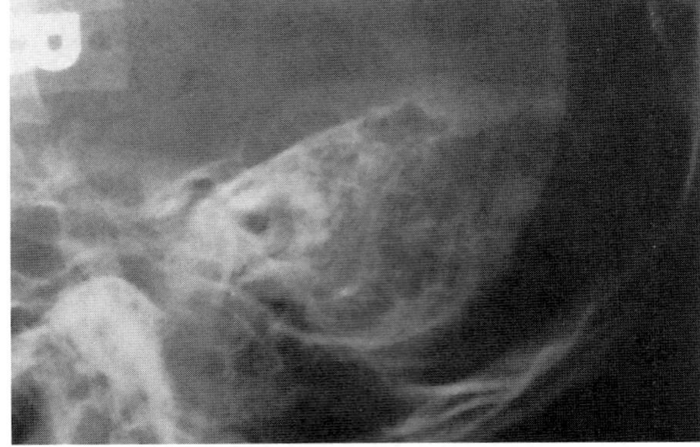

Fig. 13-53. Axiolateral oblique.

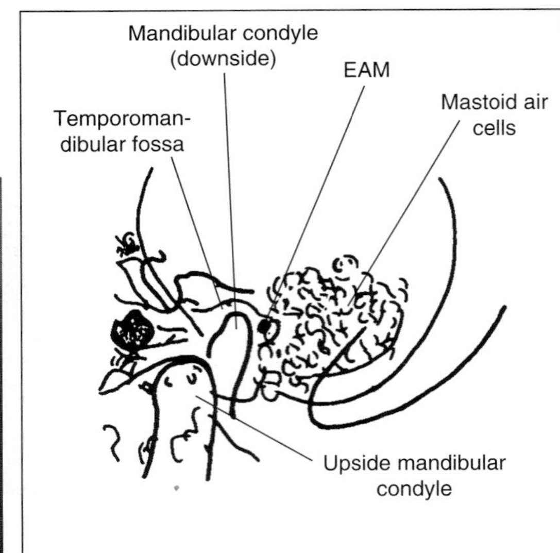

Fig. 13-54. Axiolateral oblique.

Axioanterior Oblique–Posterior Profile Position

Stenvers Method

Mastoids
Basic
• Axiolateral oblique (modified Law)
• **Axioanterior oblique (Stenvers)**
• AP axial (Towne)

Structures Best Shown

Downside petrous bone in profile (positioned parallel to film), the bony labyrinth, the tympanic cavity, the internal auditory canal and the mastoid air cells with mastoid tip projected clear of occipital bone.

Both sides are generally taken for comparison.

Technical Factors

- Film size–2 each 8 x 10 in. (18 x 24 cm), lengthwise.
- Moving or stationary grid.
- 70-80 kVp range.
- Use small focal spot.
- Technique and dose:

cm	kVp	mAs	Sk.	ML.	Gon.
16	75	20	184	55	NDC

mrad

8 / 10 / R / No AEC

Patient Position

- Determine skull morphology for degree of rotation.
- Remove all metal, plastic or other removable objects from head.
- Patient in an erect or prone position, facing the film as for a PA.

Part Position

- Adjust chin to bring **IOML perpendicular** to plane of film.
- Rotate head **45° (mesocephalic) with the side of interest downside.**
- Align downside mastoid region to CR and to center line of cassette.

Central Ray

- Angle CR **12° cephalad**, centered to enter at about **3 to 4 in. (7 to 10 cm) posterior, and ½ in. (1.25 cm) inferior to upside EAM**, to exit through downside mastoid process.
- Center cassette to projected CR.
- SID: Head unit, 36 in. (91 cm);
  Table, minimum 40 in. (102 cm).

Collimation: Use a circle diaphragm and cone, or collimate on all sides to yield a field size of approximately 4 in. (10 cm) square.

Respiration: Suspend respiration during exposure.

Note: To obtain a sharply detailed image of the mastoid air cells the utilization of a small focal spot and close collimation is essential.

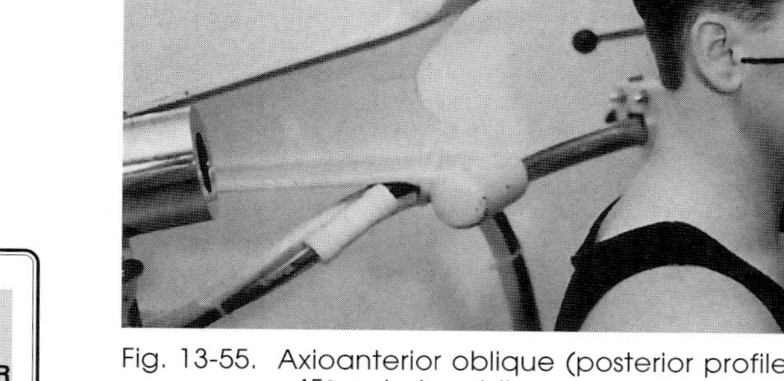

Fig. 13-55. Axioanterior oblique (posterior profile downside).
-45° anterior oblique.
-12° cephalad angle.

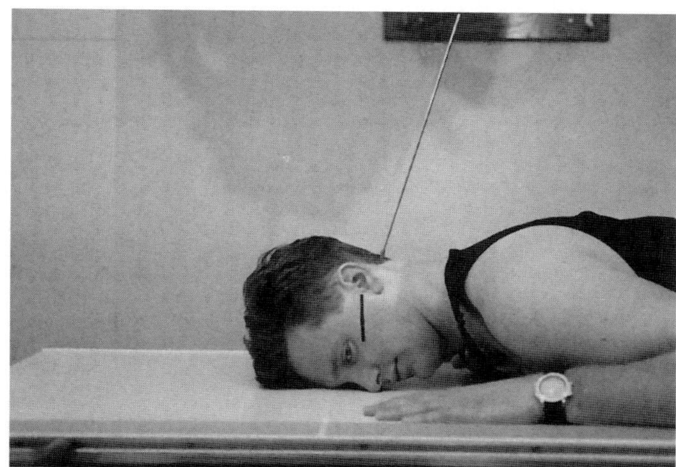

Fig. 13-56. Axioanterior oblique (posterior profile downside).
-45° anterior oblique.
-12° cephalad angle.

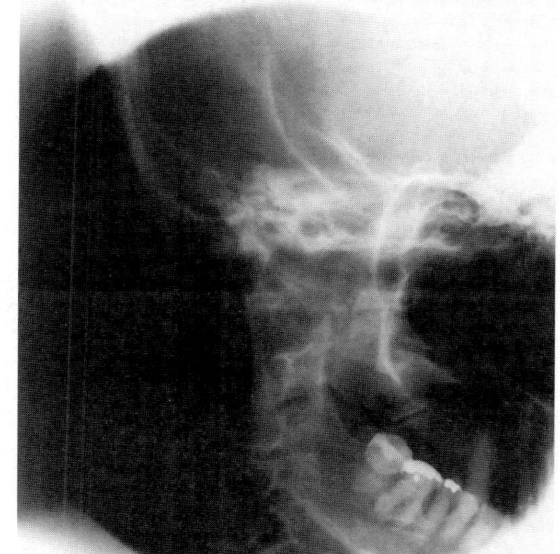

Fig. 13-57. Posterior profile position.

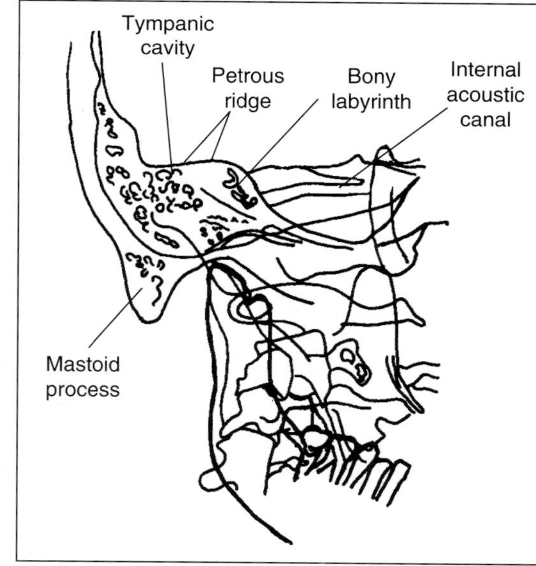

Fig. 13-58. Posterior profile position.

Evaluation Criteria

- Downside petrous bone is clearly visualized in profile.
- Included and centered to collimation field and film are the petrous ridge and mastoid process of side of interest.
- Mastoid process is seen in profile below the cranial margin.
- Posterior margin of mandibular ramus borders the posterior margin of the cervical spine.
- Mandibular condyle superimposes cervical spine.
- The internal acoustic canal, cochlea and semicircular canals (bony labyrinths) are visualized below petrous ridge.
- Sufficient penetration and exposure, without motion, to visualize the structures within bony labyrinth and petrous portions without overexposing mastoid process.

13

AP Axial Projection

Towne Method

Mastoids
Basic
• Axiolateral oblique (modified Law)
• Axioanterior oblique (Stenvers)
• **AP axial (Towne)**

Structures Best Shown

Bilateral appearances of petrous pyramids, mastoid air cells, and bony labyrinth.

Technical Factors

- Film size–8 x 10 in. (18 x 24 cm), lengthwise.
- Moving or stationary grid.
- 70-80 kVp range.
- Use small focal spot.
- Technique and dose:

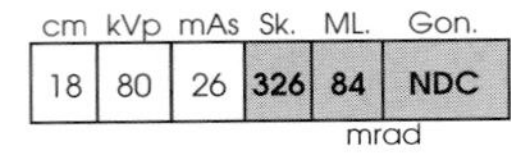

cm	kVp	mAs	Sk.	ML.	Gon.
18	80	26	326	84	NDC

mrad

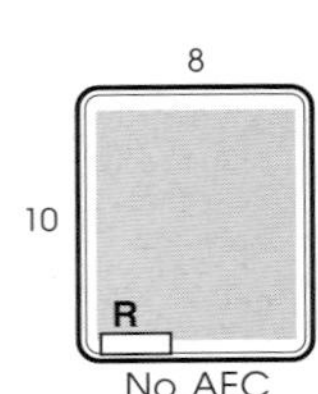
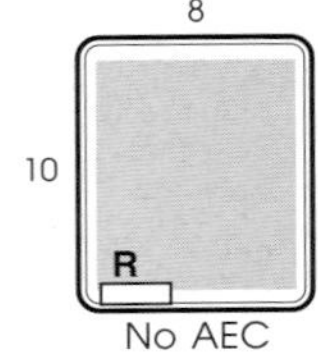

Fig. 13-59. AP axial–CR 30° to OML or 37° to IOML.

Patient Position

- Remove all metal, plastic or other removable objects from head.
- Patient in an erect or supine position with posterior skull against head unit or table-top.

Part Position 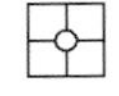

- Depress chin, bringing **OML or IOML perpendicular** to film. (See Note.)
- Align **midsagittal plane perpendicular** to midline of head unit or table to prevent head rotation and/or tilt.

Central Ray

- Angle **CR 30° caudad to OML, or 37° to IOML.**
- Center CR to the **midsagittal plane,** at a level **2 in.** (5 cm) **above glabella, to pass through level of EAMs**.
- Center cassette to projected CR.
- SID: Head unit, 36 in. (91 cm); Table, minimum 40 in. (102 cm).

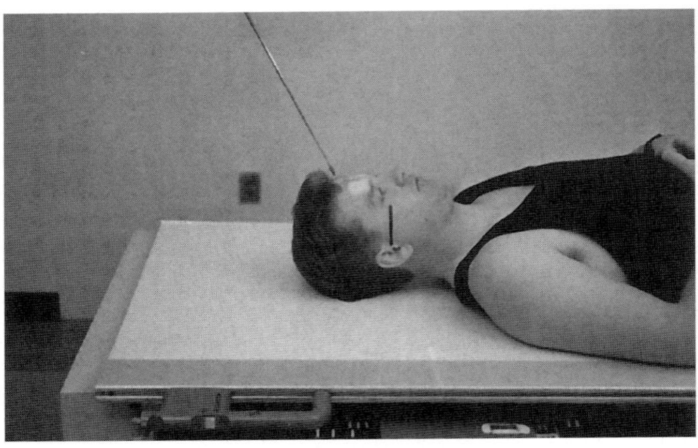

Fig. 13-60. AP axial–CR 30° to OML or CR 37° to IOML.

Collimation: Use an 8 x 10 in. circle diaphragm and cone, or collimate to outer margins of skull.

Respiration: Suspend respiration during exposure.

Note: If patient is unable to depress the chin sufficiently to bring the **OML** perpendicular to the film, the **IOML** can be placed perpendicular instead and the CR angle increased to 37° caudad. This maintains the **30° angle between OML and CR** and demonstrates the same anatomical relationships. (There is a 7° difference between the OML and the IOML.)

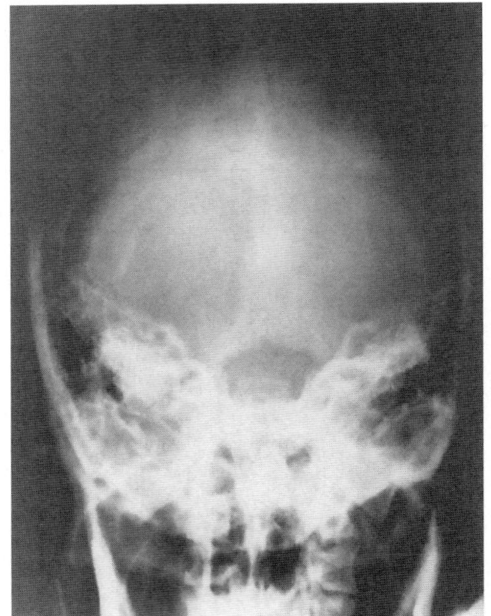

Fig. 13-61. AP axial.

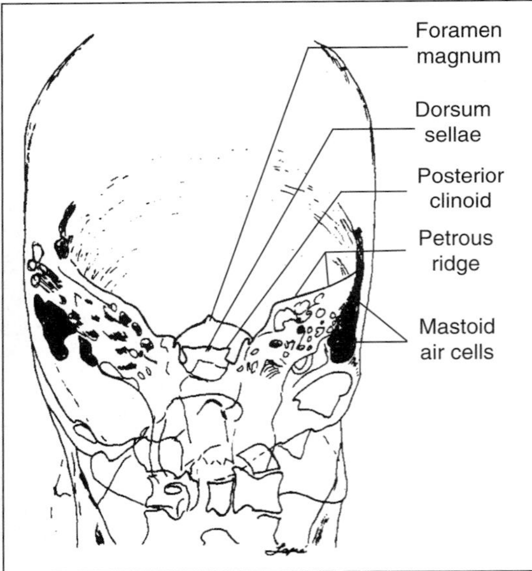

Fig. 13-62. AP axial.

Evaluation Criteria

- Dorsum sellae and posterior clinoids are projected into foramen magnum.
- Included on the radiograph are both petrous ridges and both mastoid air cells.
- The cranium is seen without rotation or tilt:
  - –Petrous ridges are symmetrical (rotation).
  - –Equal distance from foramen magnum to lateral margin of skull on each side (tilt).
- Sufficient penetration and exposure, without motion, to visualize bony labyrinth without overexposing mastoid air cells.

Axiolateral Projection

Schuller Method

Mastoids
Special
- **Axiolateral (Schuller)**
- Axioposterior oblique–anterior profile (Arcelin–reverse Stenvers)
- AP axial oblique (Mayer method and Owen modification)

Structures Best Shown

Mastoid air cells and bony labyrinth closest to film.

Both sides are generally taken for comparison.

Technical Factors

- Film size–2 each 8 x 10 in. (18 x 24 cm), lengthwise.
- Moving or stationary grid.
- 70-80 kVp range.
- Use small focal spot.
- Technique and dose:

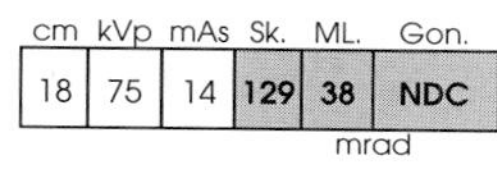

cm	kVp	mAs	Sk.	ML.	Gon.
18	75	14	129	38	NDC

mrad

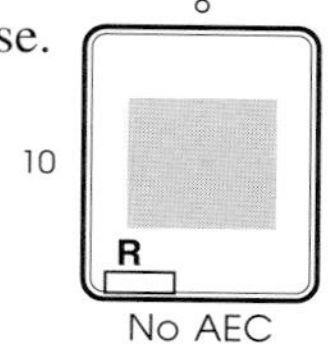

Fig. 13-63. Axiolateral, true lateral–CR 25 to 30° caudad.

Patient Position

- Remove all metal, plastic or other removable objects from head.
- Patient in an erect or semiprone position.
- Tape each auricle forward to prevent superimposing mastoid if this is the area of interest.

Part Position

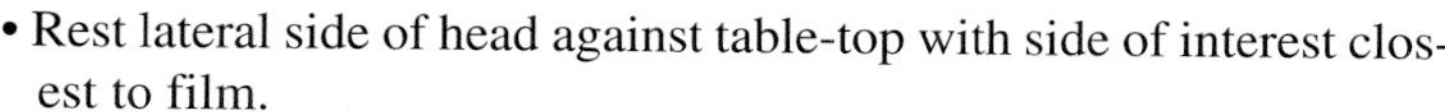

- Rest lateral side of head against table-top with side of interest closest to film.
- Adjust head into a **true lateral** position, oblique body as needed for patient comfort.
- Align **interpupillary line perpendicular** to film.
- Align **midsagittal plane parallel to film**.
- Position **infraorbitomeatal line perpendicular** to front edge of cassette.

Central Ray

- Angle **CR 25 to 30° caudad**, centered to **exit at downside mastoid tip**, enters at ≈**1½ in. (4 cm) superior and posterior to upside EAM**.
- Center cassette to projected CR.
- SID: Minimum 40 in. (102 cm).

Collimation: Collimate on all sides to yield a field size of approximately 4 in. (10 cm) square.

Respiration: Suspend respiration during exposure.

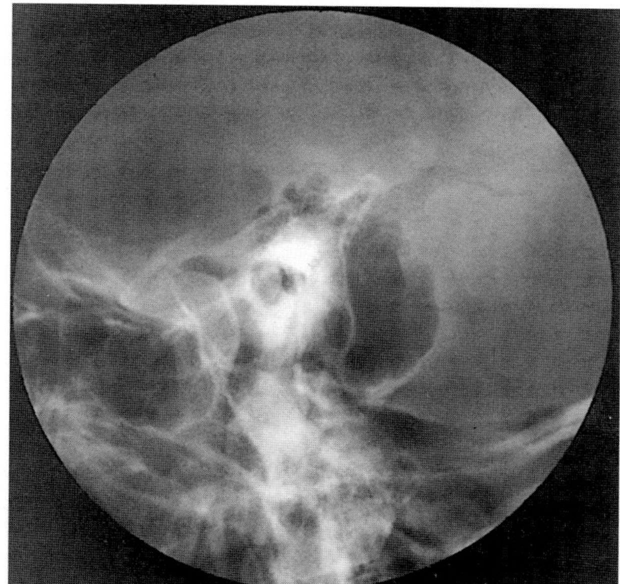

Fig. 13-64. Axiolateral.

Evaluation Criteria

- The mastoid air cells of interest are located in center of collimation field.
- Opposite mastoid is projected inferiorly to mastoid area of interest. (Underangulation will lead to some superimposition of mastoids.)
- Ear auricle does not superimpose mastoid of interest.
- Condyle of mandible and TMJ is visualized anterior to mastoid cells of interest.

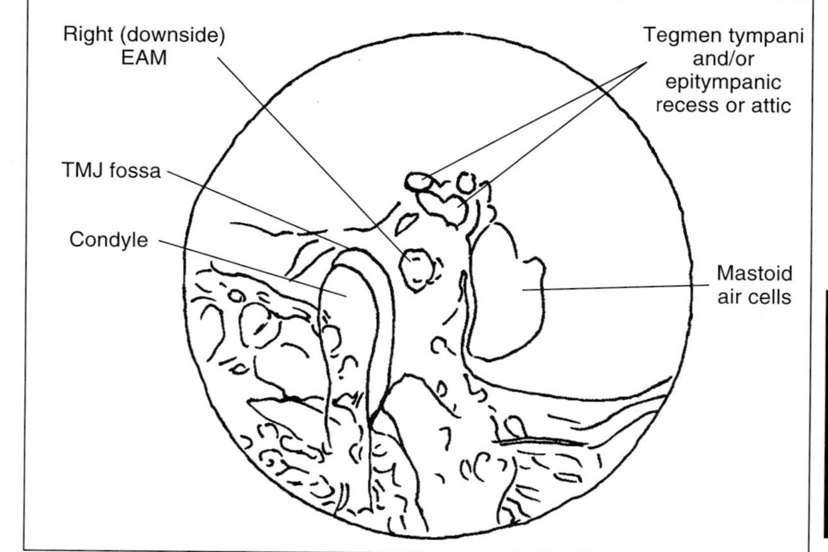

Fig. 13-65. Axiolateral.

Axioposterior Oblique–Anterior Profile Projection

Arcelin Method (reverse Stenvers Method)

> **Mastoids**
> Special
> • Axiolateral (Schuller)
> • **Axioposterior oblique (anterior profile) (Arcelin–reverse Stenvers)**
> • AP axial oblique (Mayer method and Owen modification)

Structures Best Shown

Provides a full view of upside petrous portion with petrous ridge aligned parallel to film.

Primarily for those patients in the supine position who cannot be placed in a prone position for posterior profile (Stenvers) projection.

Both sides are generally taken for comparison.

Fig. 13-66. Anterior profile–Right side up (upside). -45° oblique, CR 10° caudad.

Technical Factors

- Film size–2 each 8 x 10 in. (18 x 24 cm), lengthwise.
- Moving or stationary grid.
- 70-80 kVp range.
- Use small focal spot.
- Technique and dose:

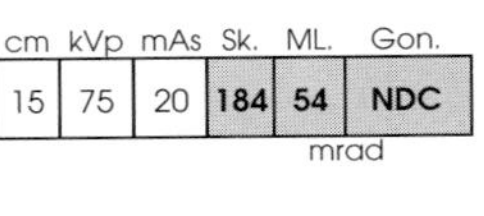

cm	kVp	mAs	Sk.	ML.	Gon.
15	75	20	184	54	NDC

mrad

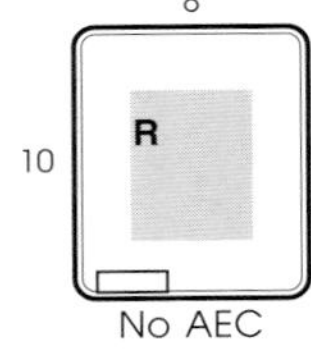

Patient Position

- Remove all metal, plastic or other removable objects from head.
- Patient in an erect or supine position.

Part Position 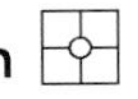

- Rotate head 45° away from side of interest (upside).
- Adjust chin, bringing IOML perpendicular to table-top.
- Align upside mastoid region to CR and to center line of table.

Central Ray

- Angle **CR 10° caudad**, centered to enter at **1 in. (2.5 cm) anterior and ¾ in. (2 cm) superior to upside EAM**.
- Center cassette to projected CR.
- SID: Minimum 40 in. (102 cm).

Collimation: Collimate on all sides to a rectangle area of upside petrous pyramid.

Respiration: Suspend respiration during exposure.

Fig. 13-67. Anterior profile.

Evaluation Criteria

- Upside petrous pyramid and petrous ridge are clearly visualized in profile.
- The petrous ridge and mastoid portion of side of interest are centered to collimation field.
- Mastoid process is seen in profile below the cranial margin.
- Posterior margin of mandibular ramus borders the posterior margin of the cervical spine.
- Temporomandibular joint is visualized anterior to mastoid cell of interest.
- Sufficient penetration and exposure, without motion, to visualize mastoid air cells.

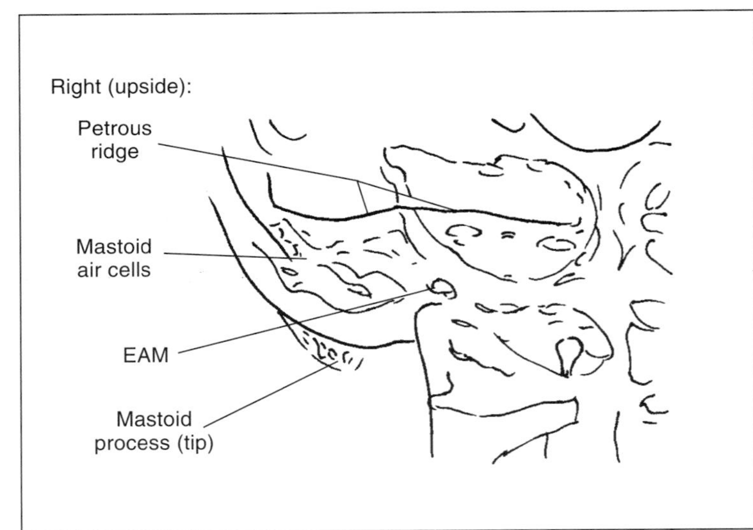

Fig. 13-68. Anterior profile.

AP Axial Oblique Projection

Mayer Method and Owen Modification

Mastoids
Special
- Axiolateral (Schuller)
- Anterior profile (posterior oblique) (Arcelin–reverse Stenvers)
- **AP axial oblique (Mayer method and Owen modification)**

Structures Best Shown

Provides an **end-on view of downside petrous portion**, visualizes the external acoustic meatus (canal), mastoid air cells, mastoid antrum and bony labyrinth.

Both sides are generally taken for comparison.

Technical Factors

- Film size–2 each 8 x 10 in. (18 x 24 cm), lengthwise.
- Moving or stationary grid.
- 70-80 kVp range.
- Use small focal spot.
- Technique and dose:

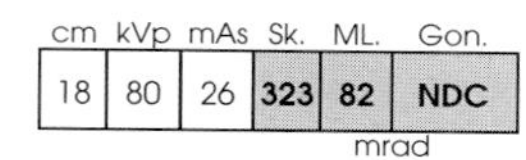

cm	kVp	mAs	Sk.	ML.	Gon.
18	80	26	323	82	NDC

mrad

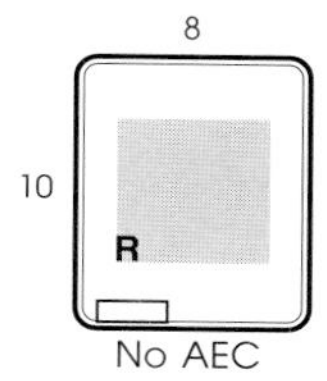

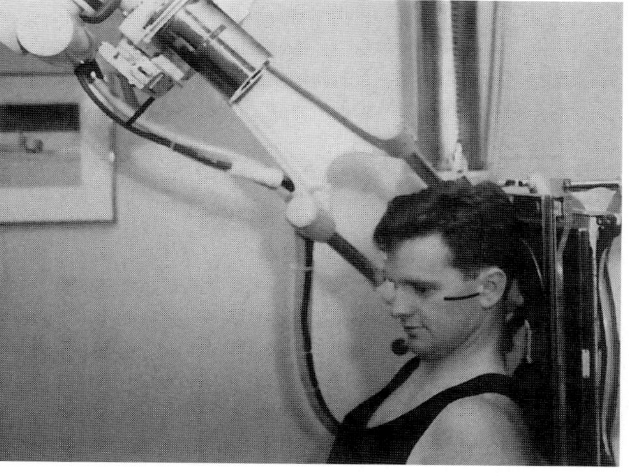

Fig. 13-69. Axioposterior oblique, erect (downside).
-45° posterior oblique.
-45° caudad CR.

Patient Position

- Remove all metal, plastic or other removable objects from head.
- Patient in an erect or supine position, start with back of head against table as for an AP projection.

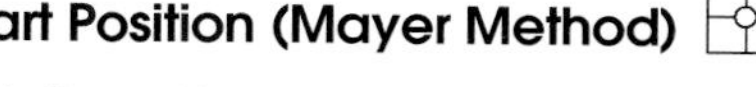

Part Position (Mayer Method)

- Adjust chin, bringing **IOML perpendicular** to front edge of cassette.
- Rotate head **45° toward side of interest.** (Side closest to film.)
- Align downside petrous portion to CR and to center line of table or cassette.

Central Ray

- Angle **CR 45° caudad**, centered to enter at approximately **3 in.** (7.5 cm) **above the superciliary arch**, to pass through about **1 in. (2.5 cm) anterior to level of downside EAM**.
- Center cassette to CR.
- SID: Head unit, 36 in. (91 cm). Table, minimum 40 in. (102 cm).

Alternate Owen Modification: A variation of the above Mayer method with less obliquity of head, and less CR angle. (Head rotation varies from 30 to 40° from lateral, and CR angle 30 to 40° caudad.)

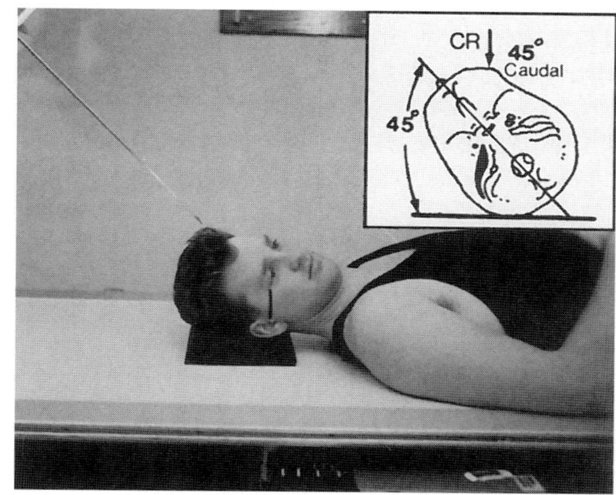

Fig. 13-70. Axioposterior oblique, supine.
-45° posterior oblique.
-45° caudad CR.
Owen modification: -30 to 40° oblique.
-30 to 40° caudad CR.

Collimation: Use a circle diaphragm or collimate on all sides to yield a field size of approximately 4 in. (10 cm).

Respiration: Suspend respiration during exposure.

Notes: To obtain a sharply detailed image of the mastoid air cells, the utilization of a small focal spot and close collimation is essential.

Evaluation Criteria

- The mastoid air cell of interest is located in the center of collimation field and film.
- The petrous portion is located inferior to the mastoid portion (as seen with end-on view).
- Sufficient penetration and exposure, without motion, to visualize the bony labyrinth without overexposing the mastoid air cells.

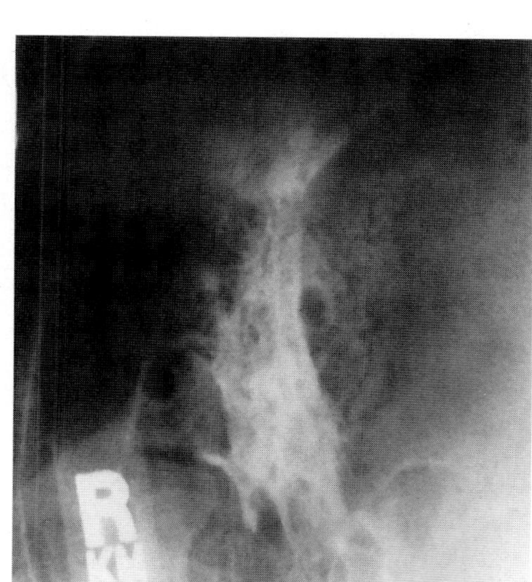

Fig. 13-71. Axioposterior oblique.

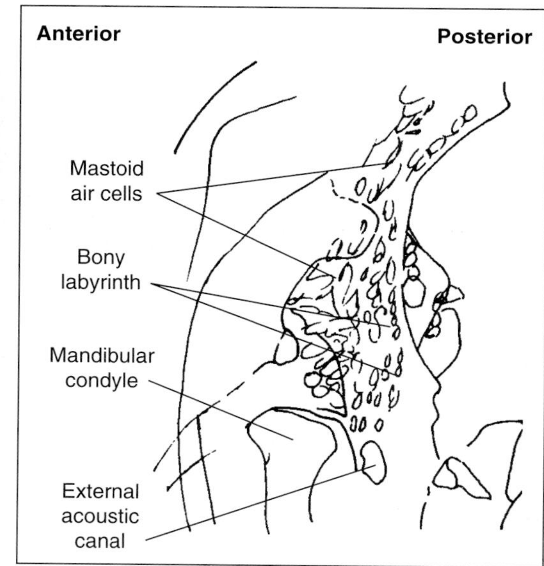

Fig. 13-72. Axioposterior oblique.

AP Axial (Towne) and Submentovertex (SMV) Projections

Temporal Bones and/or Petrous Pyramids
Basic
• **AP axial (Towne)**
• **Submentovertex (SMV)**

Structures Best Shown

Bilateral petrous pyramids, including internal acoustic canals, bony labyrinths and tympanic cavities.

Technical Factors

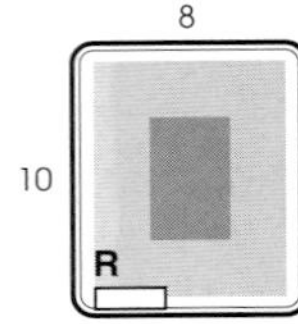

- Film size–8 x 10 in. (18 x 24 cm), lengthwise.
- Moving or stationary grid.
- 70-80 kVp range.
- Use small focal spot.

Patient Position

AP Axial Projection: Same positioning as for AP Towne mastoids, page 404.)

SMV Projection:

- Remove all metal, plastic or other removable objects from head and neck.
- Patient in erect position (or supine, only if erect is not possible).

Part Position 

- Raise chin, hyperextending neck if possible until **IOML is parallel** to head unit or vertical table. (See Notes.)
- Head rests on vertex of skull.
- Align **midsagittal plane perpendicular** to CR and to midline of head unit or vertical table.

Central Ray

- CR directed **perpendicular to IOML**. (See Notes.)
- Center CR **midway between angles of mandible**, at a level 2½ to 3 in. (6 to 8 cm) inferior to mandibular symphysis.
- Center cassette to projected CR.
- SID: Head unit, 36 in. (91 cm).
  Upright table or grid unit, minimum 40 in. (102 cm).

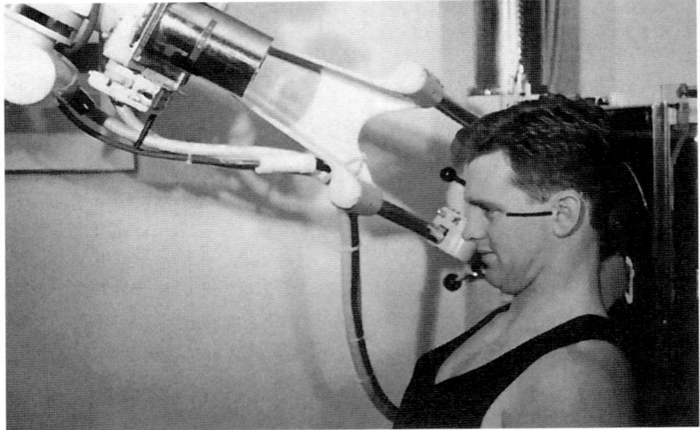

Fig. 13-73. AP axial projection.
-OML perpendicular.
-CR 30° caudad.

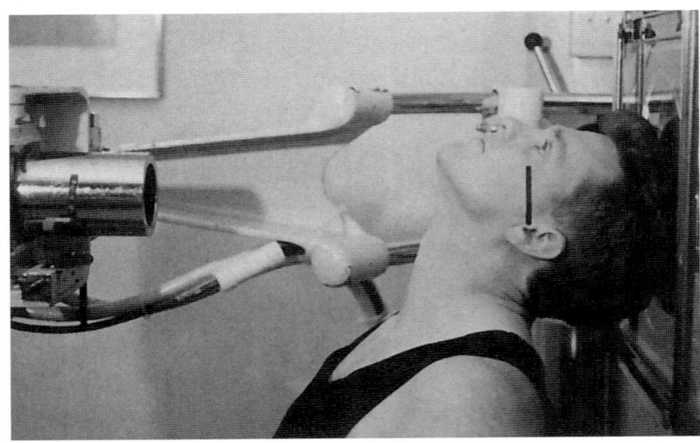

Fig. 13-74. SMV projection–CR perpendicular to IOML.

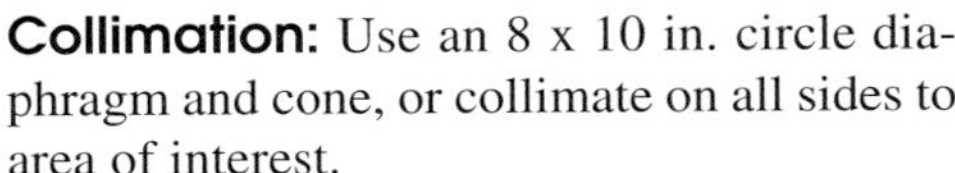

Collimation: Use an 8 x 10 in. circle diaphragm and cone, or collimate on all sides to area of interest.

Respiration: Suspend respiration during exposure.

Notes: If patient is unable to sufficiently extend neck, angle tube **perpendicular to IOML**. With head unit the film can then also be angled as needed to maintain the film perpendicular to CR.

Position is very uncomfortable for patient; move quickly.

Evaluation Criteria

- Entire skull visualized and centered to collimation field and film.
- Mandibular symphysis superimposes anterior frontal bone.
- The cranium is not rotated or tilted:
  - –Distance along coinciding mandibular surfaces to lateral border of skull are equal.
  - –Petrous pyramids are visualized symmetrically.
- Mandibular condyles are projected anterior to petrous pyramids.
- Internal acoustic canal, foramen ovale and spinosum are visualized.
- Sufficient penetration and exposure, without motion, to visualize petrous pyramids.

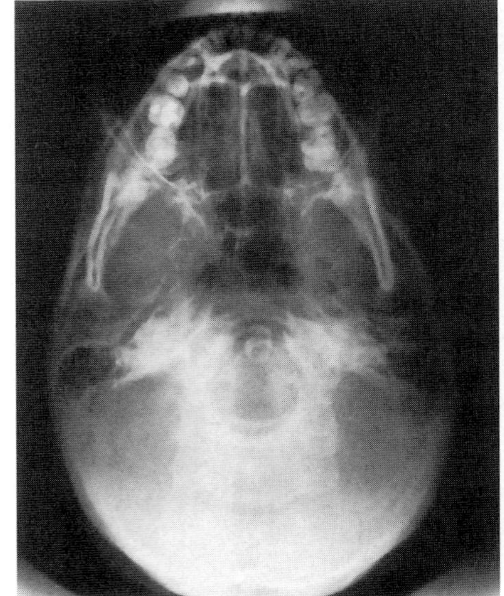

Fig. 13-75. SMV projection.

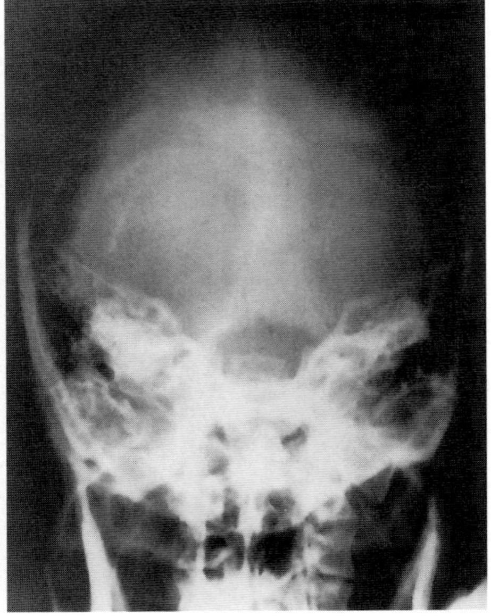

Fig. 13-76. AP axial projection.

Radiographs for Critique

Each of these sinus radiographs demonstrates some error in positioning which requires a repeat. These, along with accompanying lecture slides of these and other radiographs, will provide a basis for classroom and/or positioning lab discussion. Questions with answers based on these specific critique radiographs are provided in the accompanying student workbook/lab manuals to help prepare students for classroom and/or lab discussions on film critique.

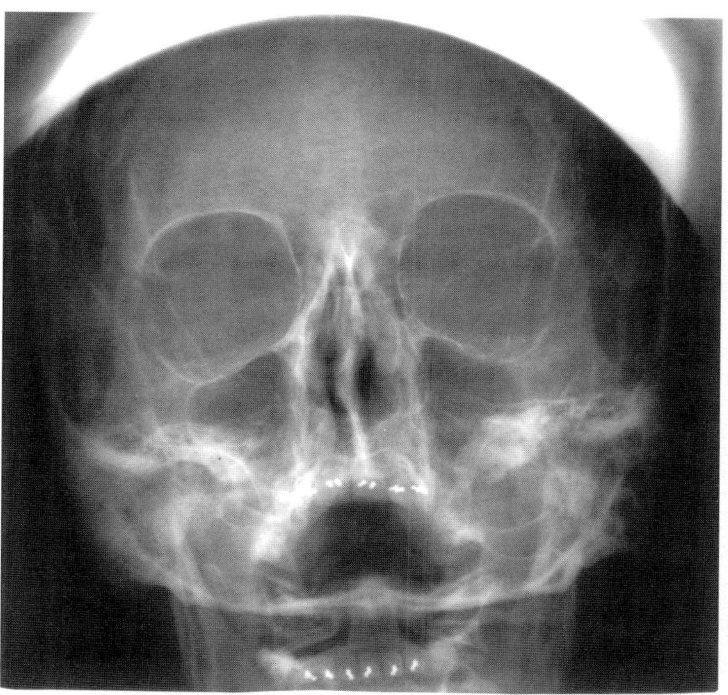

Fig. C13-77. Sinuses–Parietoacanthial transoral projection. (Open-mouth Waters)

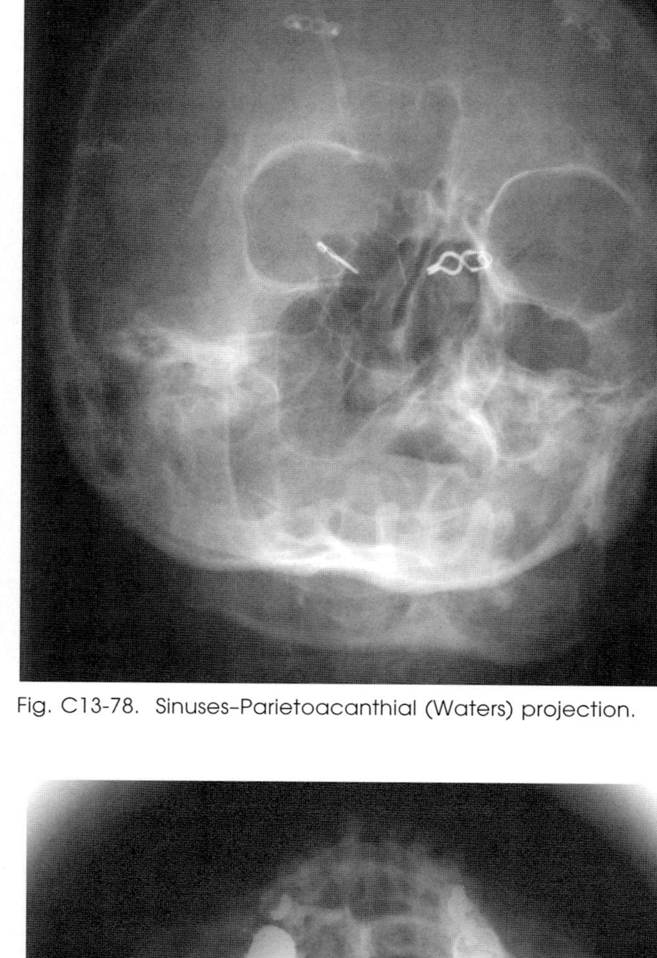

Fig. C13-78. Sinuses–Parietoacanthial (Waters) projection.

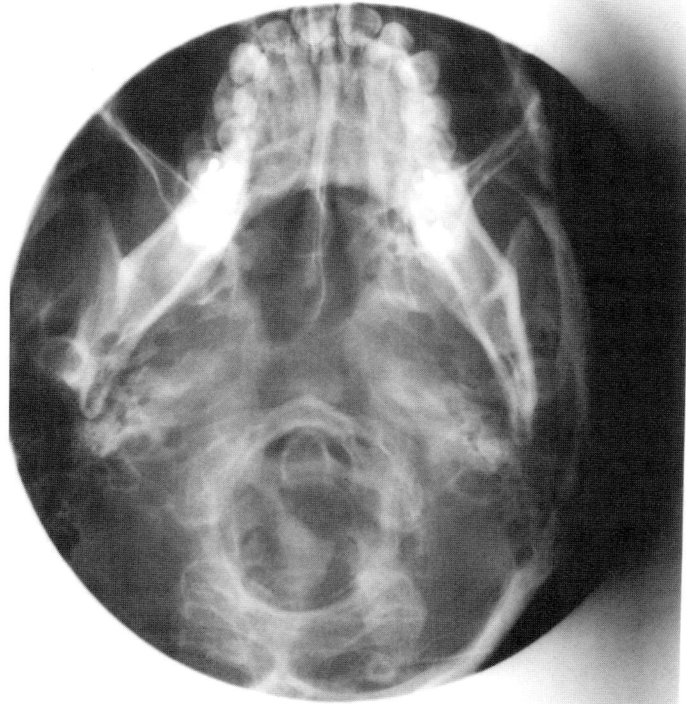

Fig. C13-79. Sinuses–SMV projection.

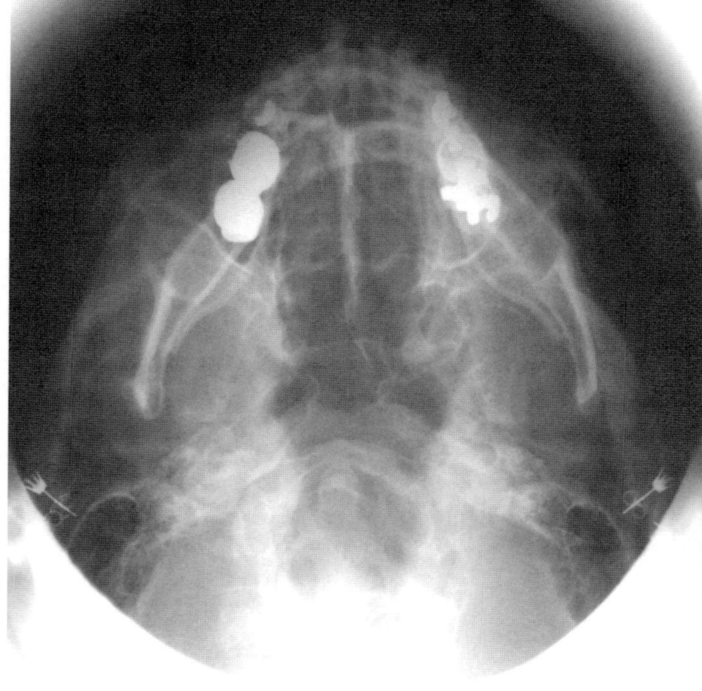

Fig. C13-80. Sinuses–SMV projection.

CHAPTER 14

Upper Gastrointestinal System

CONTRIBUTIONS BY:
John P. Lampignano, M Ed, RT (R)
Barry T. Anthony, RT (R)

CONTENTS

Radiographic Anatomy

Digestive system and common radiographic procedures **412**

Oral cavity and pharynx **413**

Esophagus **414**

Stomach **416**

Duodenum **418**

Anatomy review (radiographs) **418**

Digestion **419**

Body habitus **420**

Radiographs and models demonstrating body type **421**

Radiographic Procedures

Radiographic examinations of alimentary canal **422**

Contrast media **423**

Double contrast **424**

Radiography–Fluorography equipment **425**

Digital fluoroscopy (DF) **426**

Esophagram **427**

Upper GI series **431**

Radiographic Positioning

Survey results, basic and special projections **434**

Esophagram–Basic:
- RAO **435**
- Lateral **436**
- AP (PA) **437**

Esophagram–Special:
- LAO **438**
- Soft tissue lateral **439**

Upper GI series-Basic:
- RAO **440**
- PA **441**
- Right lateral **442**
- LPO **443**
- AP **444**

14

Radiographic Anatomy

DIGESTIVE SYSTEM

The digestive system includes the entire **alimentary canal** and several **accessory organs**. The alimentary canal begins at the (1) **oral cavity** (mouth), continues as the (2) **pharynx**, (3) **esophagus**, (4) **stomach**, (5) **small intestine** *(in-tes′ tin)*, and ends as the (6) **large intestine**, which terminates as the (7) **anus** *(a′ nus)*.

Accessory organs of digestion include the **salivary glands**, **pancreas**, **liver and gallbladder**.

Anatomy and positioning of parts (1) oral cavity, through (5) duodenum, will be covered in this chapter. The remainder of the small intestine, the large intestine and the anus will be covered in Chapter 15.

Functions: The digestive system performs three primary functions.

1. The first function is the intake of water, vitamins and minerals, plus the **intake and digestion** of food. Food is ingested in the form of carbohydrates, lipids and proteins. These complex food groups must be broken down or digested so that absorption can take place.
2. The second primary function of the digestive system is to **absorb** digested food particles, along with water, vitamins and essential elements from the alimentary canal into the blood or lymphatic capillaries.
3. The third function is to **eliminate** any unused material in the form of semisolid waste products.

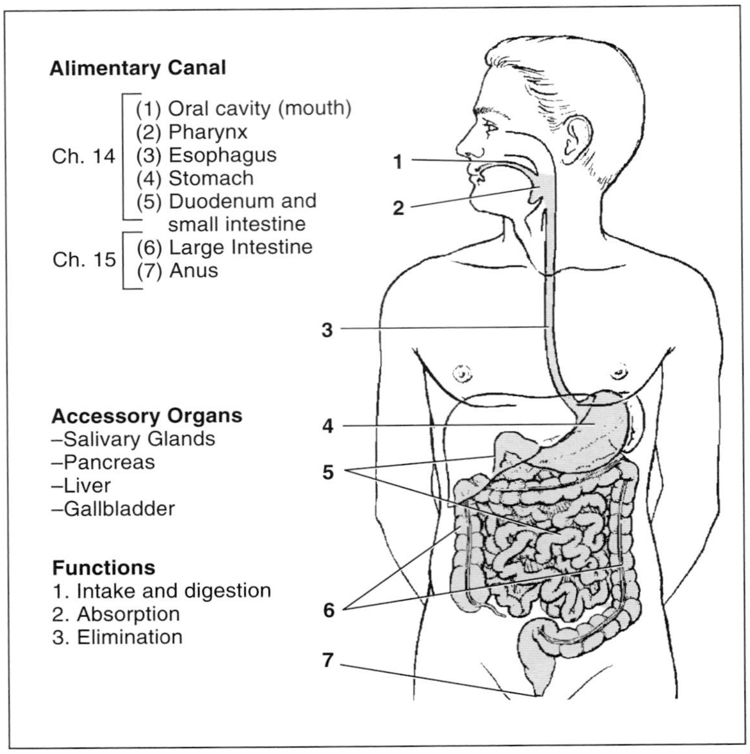

Alimentary Canal

Ch. 14
(1) Oral cavity (mouth)
(2) Pharynx
(3) Esophagus
(4) Stomach
(5) Duodenum and small intestine

Ch. 15
(6) Large Intestine
(7) Anus

Accessory Organs
–Salivary Glands
–Pancreas
–Liver
–Gallbladder

Functions
1. Intake and digestion
2. Absorption
3. Elimination

1 2 3 4 5 6 7

Fig. 14-1. Digestive system.

Common Radiographic Procedures

Two common radiographic procedures involving the upper gastrointestinal system are presented in this chapter. Common radiographic procedures are those examinations performed routinely in large and small radiology departments, as well as in certain clinics and physicians' offices. These common radiographic examinations involve the administration of a contrast medium.

1. Esophagram or Barium Swallow:
–Study of pharynx and esophagus.

A radiographic examination specifically of the pharynx and esophagus is termed an **esophagram** or **barium swallow**. This procedure studies the form and function of the swallowing aspect of the pharynx and esophagus.

2. Upper Gastrointestinal Series (UGI) (Upper GI):
–Study of distal esophagus, stomach and duodenum.

The procedure designed to study the distal esophagus, stomach and duodenum in one examination is termed an **upper gastrointestinal series**. Alternative designations for upper gastrointestinal series include UGI, upper, GI or, most commonly, **upper GI**. A PA radiograph from an upper GI series is shown in Fig. 14-2. Barium sulfate mixed with water is the preferred contrast medium for the entire alimentary canal. The negative density area (white appearing) on the radiograph indicates the stomach and duodenum area filled with the barium sulfate contrast media.

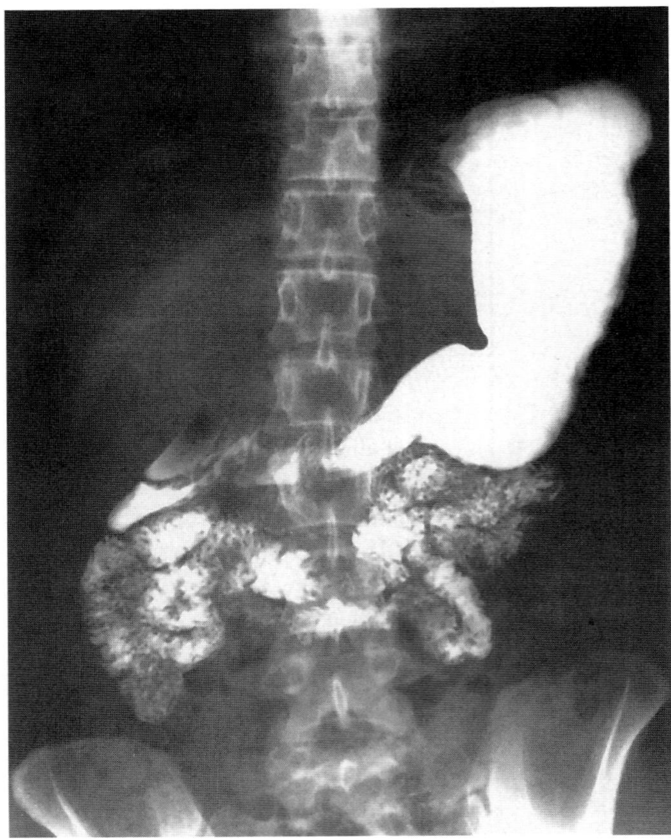

Fig. 14-2. PA–Upper GI series (barium in stomach and duodenum).

MOUTH (ORAL CAVITY)

The alimentary canal is a continuous hollow tube, beginning with the **oral cavity** (mouth). The oral cavity and surrounding structures are visualized in midsagittal section in Fig. 14-3.

The main cavity of the mouth is bounded in front and on the sides by the inner surfaces of the **upper** and **lower teeth**. The roof of the oral cavity is formed by the **hard** and **soft palates**. Hanging from the mid posterior aspect of the soft palate is a small conical process termed the **palatine uvula**, commonly referred to as just the **uvula** *(u′ vu-lah)*. The main part of the floor of the oral cavity is formed by the **tongue**. The oral cavity connects posteriorly with the **pharynx** *(far′ inks)*, as described below.

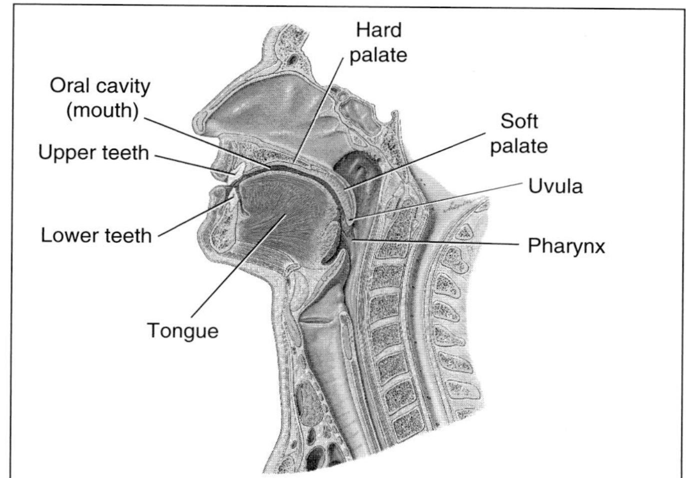

Fig. 14-3. Midsagittal section of mouth (oral or buccal cavity).

Accessory Organs in the Oral Cavity (Mouth)

The **salivary glands** are accessory organs of digestion associated with the mouth. The teeth and tongue cooperate in chewing movements to reduce the size of food particles and to mix food with saliva. These chewing movements, termed **mastication** *(mas″ ti-ka′ shun)*, initiate the mechanical part of digestion.

Three pairs of glands secrete most of the saliva in the oral cavity (Fig. 14-4). These are: (1) **parotid** *(pah-rot′ id)*, meaning near the ear, (2) **submandibular,** sometimes called submaxillary (below mandible or maxilla) and (3) **sublingual** *(sub-ling′ gwal)*, below the tongue.

Saliva is 99.5% water and 0.5% solutes or salts and certain digestive enzymes. Between 1000 and 1500 milliliters are secreted daily by the salivary glands. Saliva dissolves foods so that digestion can begin. It also contains an enzyme to begin digestion of starch.

Specific salivary glands secrete a thickened fluid which contains mucus. This lubricates food being chewed so that the food can form into a ball or bolus for swallowing. The act of swallowing is termed **deglutition** *(deg″ loo-tish′ un)*.

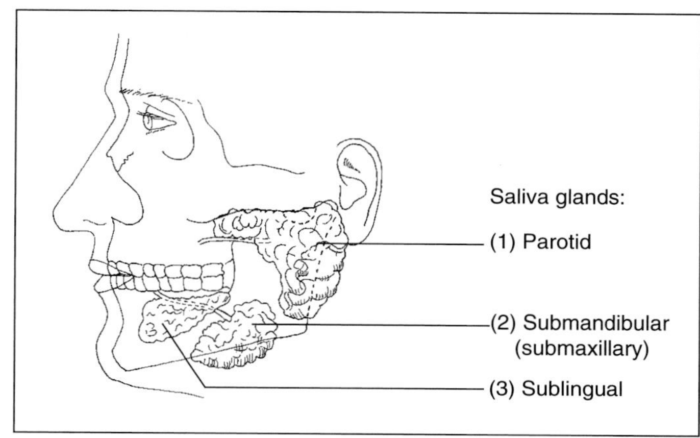

Fig. 14-4. Accessory organs in the mouth,

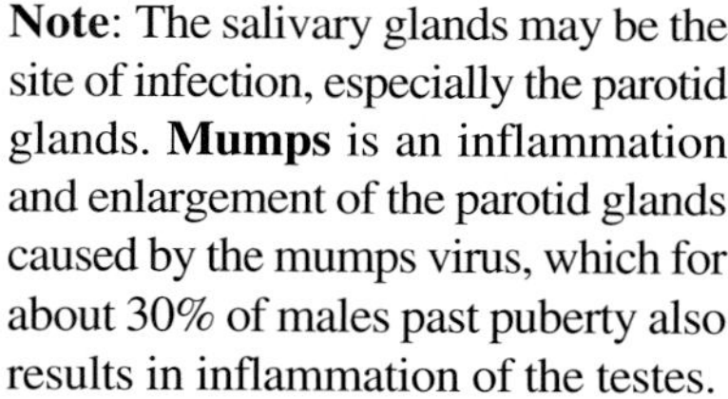

Note: The salivary glands may be the site of infection, especially the parotid glands. **Mumps** is an inflammation and enlargement of the parotid glands caused by the mumps virus, which for about 30% of males past puberty also results in inflammation of the testes.

PHARYNX

The alimentary canal continues as the pharynx posterior to the oral cavity. The **pharynx** is about 12.5 centimeters long, and is that part of the digestive tube found posterior to the nasal cavity, mouth and larynx. A midsagittal and a coronal section of the pharynx, as seen from the side and posterior, are shown in Fig. 14-5. The three parts of the pharynx are named according to their location.

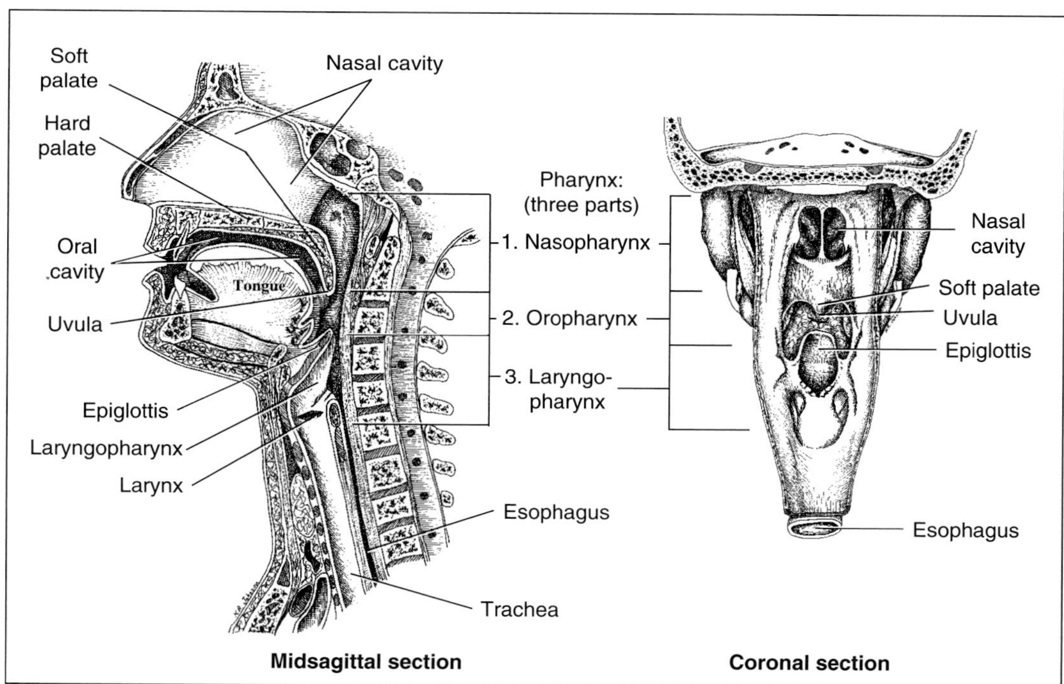

Fig. 14-5. Pharynx.

The **nasopharynx** is posterior to the bony nasal septum and nasal cavities, and soft palate.

The **oropharynx** is directly posterior to the oral cavity proper. The oropharynx extends from the **soft palate** to the **epiglottis** *(ep″ i-glot′ is)*. The epiglottis is a membrane-covered cartilage that moves down to cover the opening of the larynx during swallowing.

The third portion of the pharynx is termed the **laryngopharynx** or hypopharynx. The laryngopharynx extends from the level of the epiglottis to the level of the lower border of the cricoid cartilage (level of C6). From this point it continues as the **esophagus**. The **trachea** is seen anterior to the esophagus.

Pharynx continued

Cavities Communicating with the Pharynx

The drawing in Fig. 4-6 illustrates that there are **seven cavities or openings** communicating with the three portions of the pharynx. The two **nasal cavities** and the two **tympanic cavities** connect to the **nasopharynx**. The tympanic cavities of the middle ears connect to the nasopharynx via the **auditory** or **eustachian tubes** (not shown on this drawing).

The oral cavity (mouth) connects posteriorly to the oropharynx. Inferiorly, the **laryngopharynx** connects to the openings of both the **larynx** and the **esophagus**.

Deglutition (Swallowing)

It is most important that food and fluid travel from the oral cavity directly to the esophagus during the act of swallowing or deglutition. During swallowing, the **soft palate closes off the nasopharynx** to prevent swallowed substances from regurgitating into the nose. The tongue prevents the material from re-entering the mouth.

During swallowing, the **epiglottis is depressed to cover the laryngeal opening** like a lid. The vocal folds or cords also come together to close off the epiglottis. These actions combine to prevent food and fluid from being aspirated (entering the larynx, trachea and bronchi).

Also, respiration is inhibited during deglutition to help prevent swallowed substances from entering the trachea and lungs. Occasionally, bits of material pass into the larynx and trachea during deglutition. A forceful episode of reflex coughing is usually necessary to reject these offensive intruders.

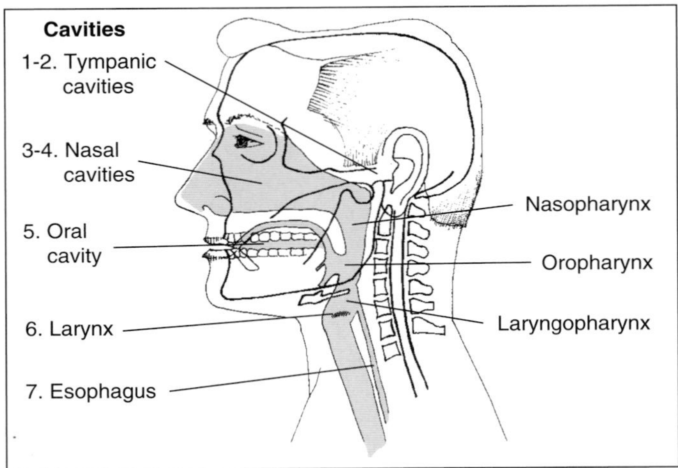

Fig. 14-6. Seven cavities or openings communicating with the pharynx.

ESOPHAGUS

The third part of the alimentary canal is the **esophagus**, or gullet as it is sometimes called. The esophagus is a muscular canal, about 9¾ inches (25 cm) long, extending from the laryngopharynx to the stomach. The esophagus begins posterior to the level of the lower border of the **cricoid cartilage of the larynx** (C5-6), which is at the level of the upper margin of the thyroid cartilage. The esophagus terminates at its connection to the stomach, at the level of the **eleventh thoracic vertebra** (T 11).

In Fig. 14-7, one can see that the esophagus is located posterior to the larynx and trachea. The spatial relationship of the esophagus to both the trachea and the thoracic vertebrae is an important relationship to remember. The esophagus is posterior to the trachea, and just anterior to the cervical and thoracic vertebral bodies.

The descending **thoracic aorta** is between the distal esophagus and the lower thoracic spine. The **heart**, within its pericardial sac, is immediately posterior to the sternum, anterior to the esophagus, and superior to the diaphragm.

The esophagus is essentially vertical as it descends to the stomach. This swallowing tube is the narrowest part of the entire alimentary canal. The esophagus is most constricted, first, at its proximal end where it enters the thorax, and second, where it passes through the diaphragm at the esophageal hiatus or opening. The esophagus pierces the diaphragm at the **level of T10**. Just before passing through the diaphragm, the esophagus presents a distinct dilatation as shown in Fig. 14-8.

As the esophagus descends within the posterior aspect of the mediastinum, **two indentations** are present. One indentation occurs at the **aortic arch**, and the second is found where the esophagus crosses the **left primary bronchus**.

The lower portion of the esophagus lies close to the posterior aspects of the heart.

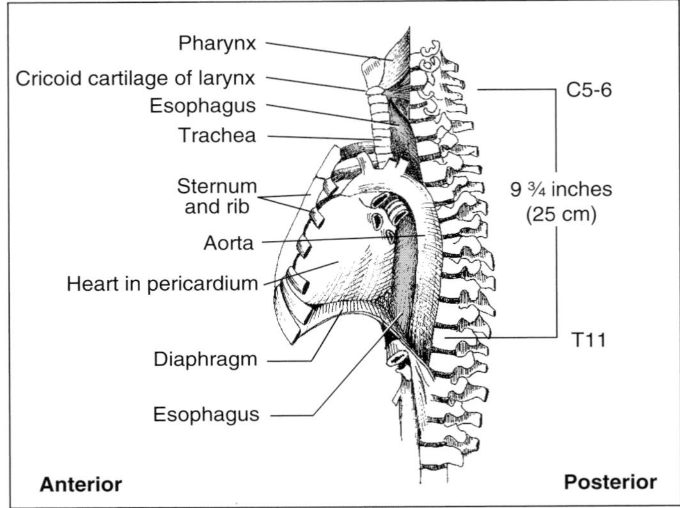

Fig. 14-7. Esophagus in mediastinum–Lateral view.

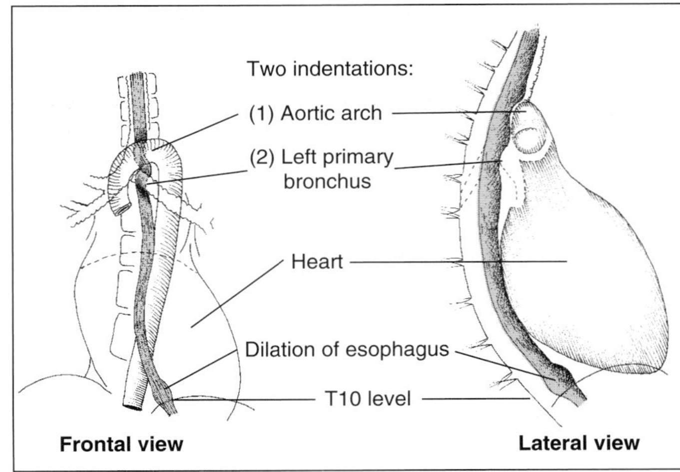

Fig. 14-8. Esophagus in mediastinum, demonstrating two indentations.

14

Diaphragm Openings

The **esophagus** passes through the **diaphragm** slightly to the left and somewhat posterior to the midpoint of the diaphragm. The drawing on the left in Fig. 14-9 represents the inferior surface of the diaphragm and indicates the relative positions of the **esophagus**, **inferior vena cava** and **aorta**.

The drawing on the right shows the short abdominal portion of the esophagus below the diaphragm. The **abdominal segment of the esophagus**, termed the **cardiac antrum**, measures between 1 and 2 centimeters. The cardiac antrum curves sharply to the left after passing through the diaphragm to attach to the stomach.

The opening between the esophagus and the stomach is termed the **esophagogastric junction** (cardiac orifice). This is best shown in the drawing on the following page, Fig. 14-13. Cardiac is an adjective denoting a relationship to the heart, therefore the cardiac antrum and the cardiac orifice are located near the heart.

The junction of the stomach and the esophagus is normally securely attached to the diaphragm, so the upper stomach tends to follow the respiratory movements of the diaphragm.

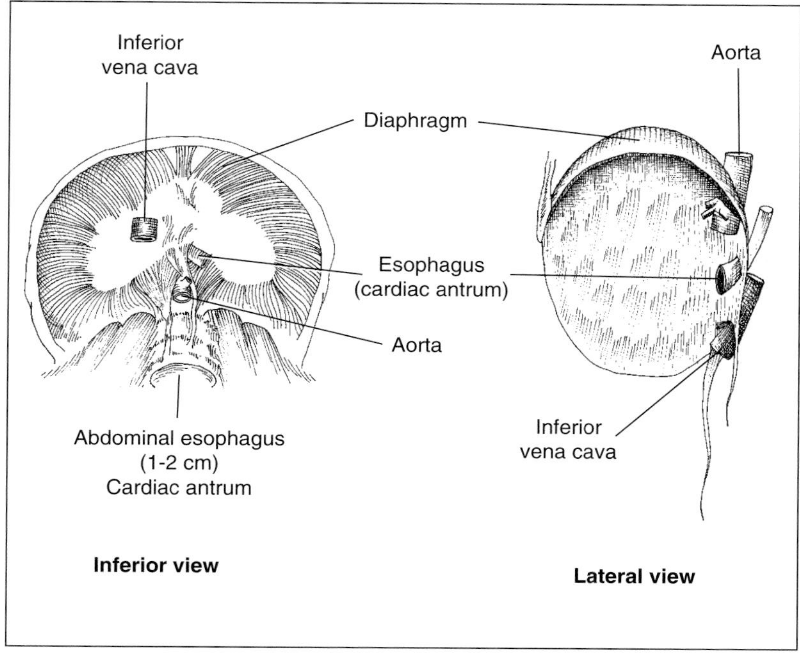

Fig. 14-9. Esophagus passing through diaphragm.

Swallowing and Peristalsis

The **esophagus** contains well-developed skeletal muscle layers (circular and longitudinal) in its upper third, skeletal and smooth muscle in its middle third, and smooth muscle in its lower third. Unlike the trachea, the esophagus is a collapsible tube that only opens when swallowing occurs. The process of deglutition continues in the esophagus after originating in the mouth and pharynx. Fluids tend to pass from the mouth and pharynx to the stomach primarily by gravity. A bolus of solid material tends to pass both by gravity and by peristalsis.

Peristalsis is a wavelike series of involuntary muscular contractions propelling solid and semisolid materials through the tubular alimentary canal. The bolus of barium sulfate, seen in the esophagus in Fig. 14-10 and 14-11, is descending to the stomach both by gravity and by peristalsis.

The esophagus in Fig. 14-11 is also seen filled with barium with a normal peristaltic constricture in the lower esophagus. This patient also has a pacemaker with attached wires evident in the upper mid-chest. Accumulation of barium in the stomach is seen on both of these radiographs.

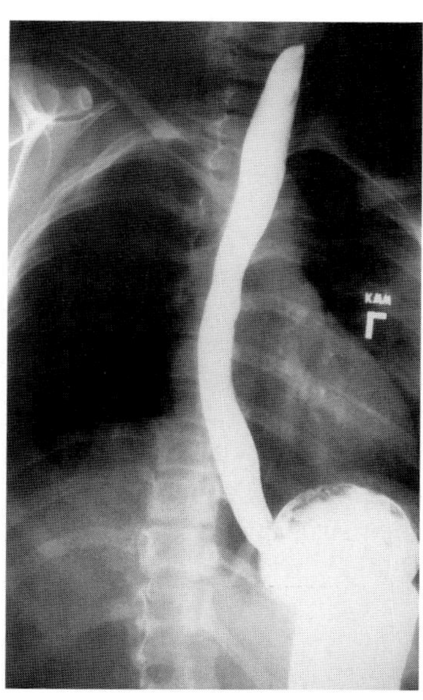

Fig. 14-10. PA esophagram. (slightly obliqued).

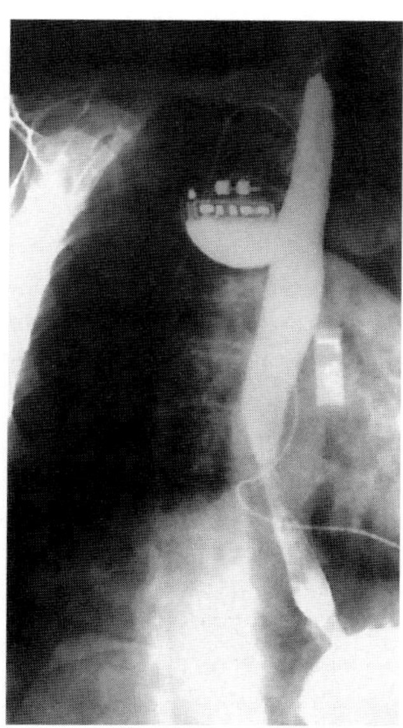

Fig. 14-11. RAO esophagram.

14

STOMACH

The **stomach**, located between the **esophagus** and the **small intestine**, is the most dilated portion of the alimentary canal. When empty, the stomach tends to collapse. When the stomach must serve as a reservoir for swallowed food and fluid, it is remarkably expandable. After a very full meal the stomach will stretch to what would appear to be almost the point of rupture.

Synonyms for stomach are the Latin word *ventriculus,* meaning "little belly," and the Greek word *gaster,* meaning "stomach." *Gastro* is a common term denoting stomach.

Since the shape and position of the stomach are highly variable, the average shape and location will be utilized in the following illustrations, with variations to follow later in this chapter.

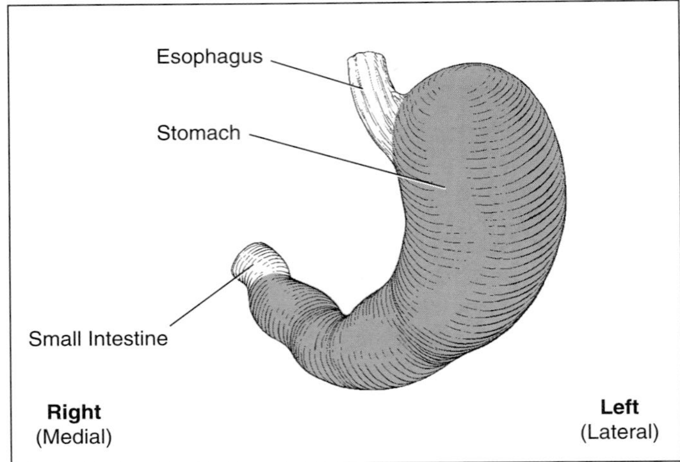

Fig. 14-12. Stomach–Frontal view.

Stomach Openings and Curvatures

The **esophagogastric junction** (cardiac orifice) is the aperture or opening between the esophagus and the stomach, which is guarded by circular muscles of the cardiac sphincter. This opening (the esophagogastric junction) in practice is commonly called the **cardiac orifice**, referring to the relationship of this orifice to that portion of the diaphragm near the heart upon which the heart rests. Directly superior to this orifice is a notch called the **cardiac notch** (incisura cardiaca). This distal abdominal portion of the esophagus curves sharply into a slightly expanded portion of the esophagus called the **cardiac antrum**.

The opening or orifice leaving the distal stomach is termed the **pyloric orifice**, sometimes just called pylorus. The pyloric sphincter at this orifice is a thickened muscular ring that relaxes periodically during digestion to allow stomach or gastric contents to move into the first part of the small intestine, the duodenum.

The **lesser curvature**, extending along the right or medial border of the stomach, forms a concave border as it extends between the cardiac and pyloric openings.

The **greater curvature** extends along the left or lateral border of the stomach. This greater curvature is four to five times longer than the lesser curvature.

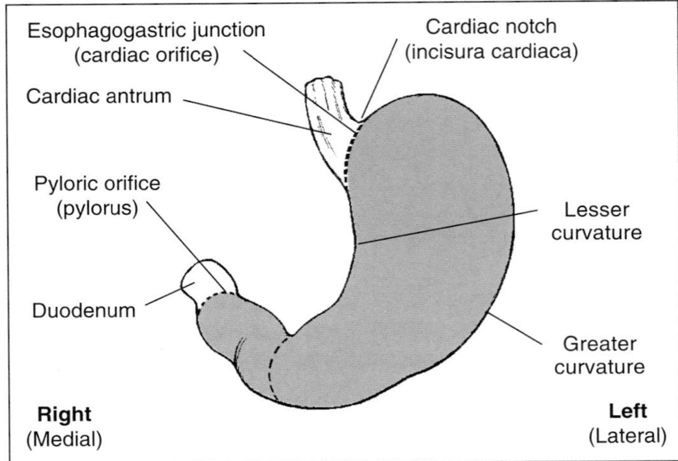

Fig. 14-13. Stomach–Openings and lesser curvature.

Stomach Subdivisions

The stomach is composed of three main subdivisions: (l) the **fundus**, (2) the **body** or **corpus**, and (3) the **pyloric portion**. The fundus is that ballooned portion lying lateral and superior to the cardiac orifice. The upper portion of the stomach, including the cardiac antrum of the esophagus, is relatively fixed to the diaphragm and tends to move with motion of the diaphragm. In the upright or erect position, the fundus is usually filled by a bubble of swallowed air.

The lower end of the large **body** or corpus portion of the stomach has a partially constricted area separating the body from the **pyloric portion** of the stomach. This "notch" or constricted ring-like area is called the **angular notch** (incisura angularis). The smaller terminal portion of the stomach to the right or medial of the angular notch is the pyloric portion of the stomach, which terminates at the **pyloric orifice** or sphincter.

The **pyloric portion** of the stomach is frequently divided into two parts, (1) the **pyloric antrum**, shown as a slight dilation immediately distal to the angular notch, and (2) the narrowed **pyloric canal**, ending at the pyloric sphincter.

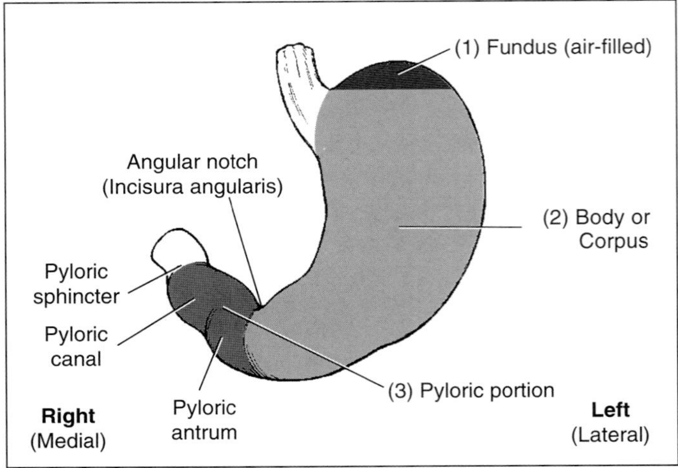

Fig. 14-14. Stomach–Subdivisions.

Gastric Folds Within Stomach–Rugae

When the stomach is empty, the internal lining is thrown into numerous longitudinal folds termed **gastric folds**, commonly called **rugae**, pronounced *roo′je,* (plural of ruga, *roo′gah*). A **gastric canal**, formed by rugae along the lesser curvature, is believed to funnel fluids directly to the pylorus.

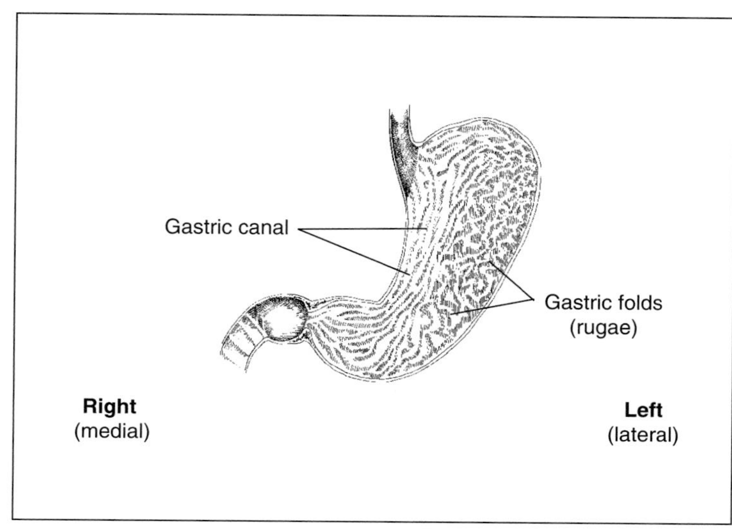

Fig. 14-15. Stomach–Coronal section.

Stomach Position

The illustration in Fig. 14-16 shows the typical orientation of an average, empty stomach in a frontal and lateral view. The **fundus**, in addition to being the most superior portion of the stomach in general, is located posterior to the **body** of the stomach. The body can be seen to curve inferior and anterior from the fundus.

The **pyloric portion** is directed posteriorly. The pyloric valve (sphincter) and the first part of the small bowel are very near the posterior abdominal wall. The relationship of these components of the stomach will be important in the distribution of air and barium in the stomach in specific body positions.

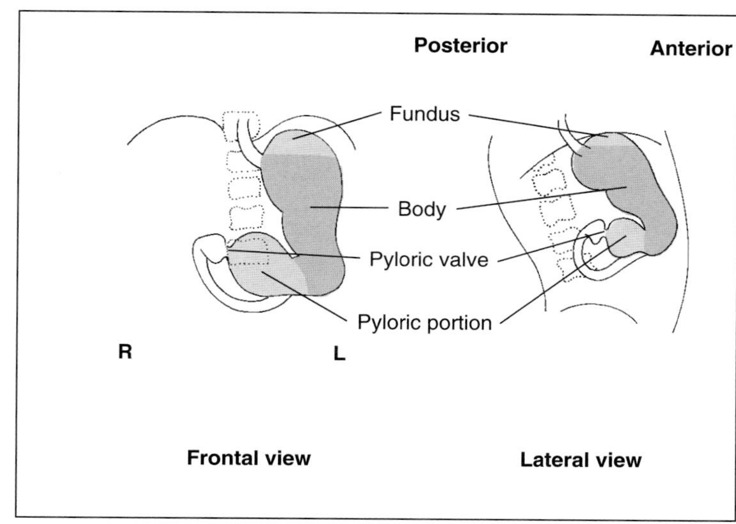

Fig. 14-16. Average empty stomach orientation.

Air-Barium Distribution in Stomach

If an individual were to swallow a barium sulfate and water mixture, along with some air, the position of the person's body would determine the distribution of the barium and air within the stomach. The illustrations in Fig. 14-17 show air as black, and the barium sulfate mixture as white.

The drawing on the left depicts the stomach of a person in a **supine** position. In a supine position, barium will travel to the fundus and upper portions of the stomach, while air will rise to the distal end of the stomach including the pyloric portion.

When studying recumbent radiographs of a stomach containing both air and barium sulfate, one can determine the patient's position by the relative locations of air versus barium within the stomach.

The middle drawing shows the stomach of a person in a **prone** position. Since the fundus is more posterior than the lower body of the stomach, air will be found primarily in the fundus, while barium will gravitate to the lower body and the pyloric portion of the stomach.

The drawing on the right depicts the stomach of a person who is in an **erect** position. In the erect position, air will rise to fill the fundus, while barium will descend by gravity to fill the pyloric portion of the stomach. The air-barium line will tend to be a straight line in the erect position compared to the prone and supine positions.

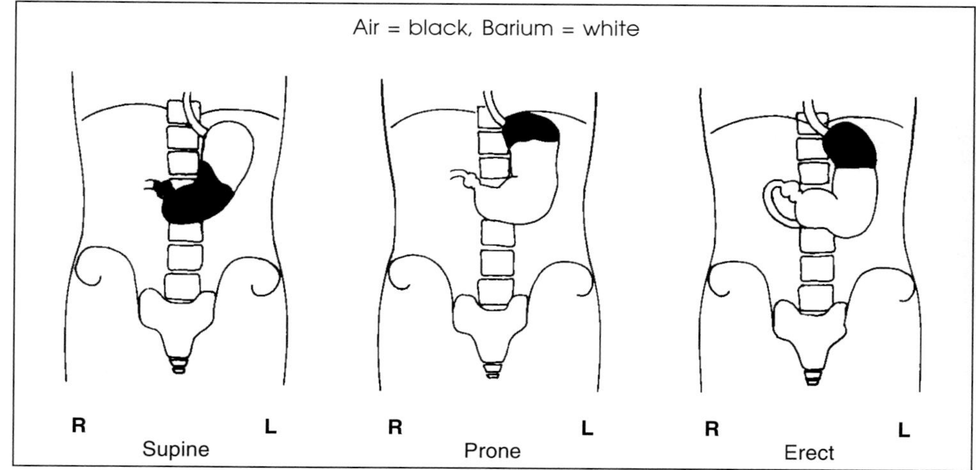

Fig. 14-17. Air-barium distribution in the stomach–Frontal views in various body positions.

DUODENUM

The fifth and final part of the upper GI system to be studied in this chapter is the **duodenum** *(du″ o-de′ num)*, which is the first portion of the small intestine commonly called the small bowel. Since the duodenum is examined radiographically during the routine upper GI series, the duodenum will be studied in this chapter, while the remainder of the small bowel will be studied in Chapter 15 with the lower GI system.

The duodenum is about 10 inches (25 cm) long, and is the shortest, widest and most fixed portion of the small bowel.

The drawing in Fig. 14-18 demonstrates that the C-shaped duodenum is closely related to the **head of the pancreas**. The head of the pancreas, nestled in the C-loop of the duodenum, has been affectionately labeled the "romance of the abdomen" by certain authors.

The duodenum and the pancreas are retroperitoneal structures, that is, they are located posterior to or behind the parietal peritoneum as described and illustrated in the following chapter on the lower GI system.

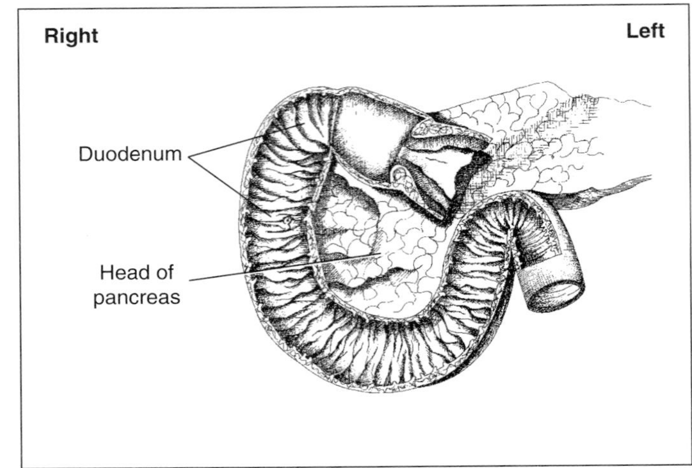

Fig. 14-18. Duodenum.

Four Parts of the Duodenum

The duodenum is shaped like a letter C and consists of four parts. The **first (superior) portion** begins at the pylorus. The first part of the superior portion is termed the **duodenal bulb** or **cap**. It is shaped somewhat like an arrowhead. The duodenal bulb is easily located during barium studies of the upper GI tract and must be carefully studied since this area is a common site of ulcer disease.

The next part of the duodenum is the **second (descending) portion**, the longest segment. The descending portion of the duodenum receives both the common bile duct and the main pancreatic duct.

The third part of the duodenum is called the **third (horizontal) portion**. This portion curves back to the left to join the final segment, termed the **fourth (ascending) portion**. The junction of the duodenum with the second portion of small bowel, the **jejunum** *(jĕ-joo′ num)*, is termed the **duodenojejunal flexure** (**angle of Treitz**). This portion is relatively fixed and held in place by a fibrous muscular band, the **ligament of Treitz**. This is a significant reference point in certain radiographic small bowel studies.

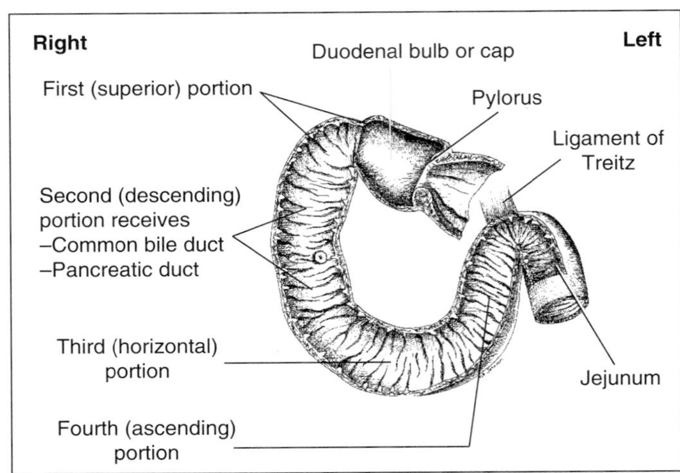

Fig. 14-19. Duodenum (cut away view to show internal surface).

ANATOMY REVIEW

Radiograph of Stomach and Duodenum

This PA radiograph of the stomach and duodenum provides a good review of important radiographic anatomy. Identify the structures labeled on the radiograph and then compare your answers with those listed below:

A. Distal esophagus.
B. Area of esophagogastric junction (cardiac orifice).
C. Lesser curvature of stomach.
D. Angular notch (incisura angularis) of stomach.
E. Pyloric portion of stomach.
F. Pyloric valve or sphincter.
G. Duodenal bulb of duodenum.
H. Second (descending) portion of duodenum.
I. Body of stomach.
J. Greater curvature of stomach.
K. Gastric folds or rugae of stomach.
L. Fundus of stomach.

Note: A pathologic constricture termed a "Schatzke's ring" is evident at the distal esophagus (see arrows). This is a type of hiatal hernia wherein the esophagogastric junction has herniated through the diaphragmatic opening.

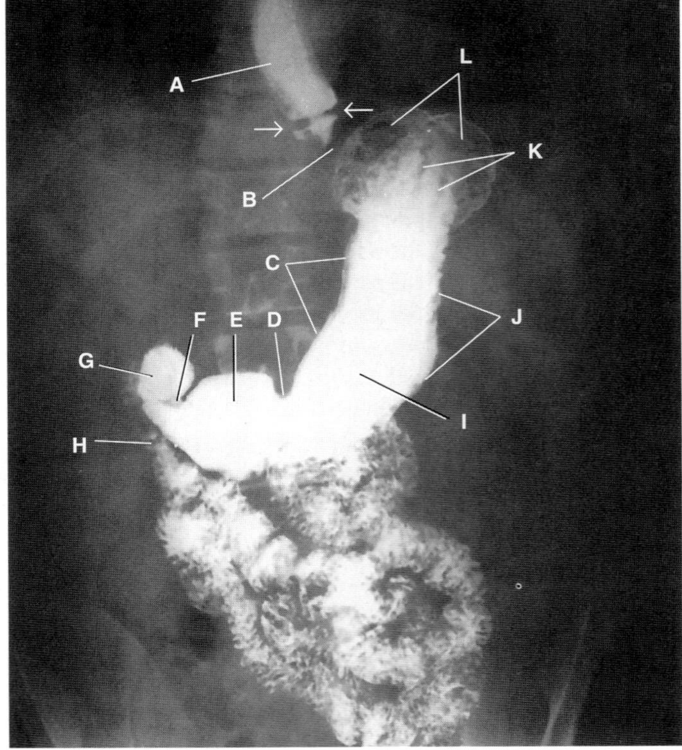

Fig. 14-20. PA projection.

DIGESTION

Mechanical Digestion

Digestion can be divided into a mechanical process and a chemical component. Mechanical digestion includes all movements of the GI tract, beginning in the oral cavity (mouth) with chewing or **mastication** *(mas″ ti-ka′ shun)*, and continuing in the pharynx and esophagus with swallowing or **deglutition**. **Peristaltic activity** can be detected in the lower esophagus as well as in the remainder of the alimentary canal. The passage of solid or semisolid food from the mouth to the stomach takes from 4 to 8 seconds, while liquids pass in about 1 second.

The stomach, acting as a reservoir for food and fluid, also acts as a large mixing bowl. Peristalsis tends to move the gastric contents toward the pyloric valve, but this valve opens selectively. If it is closed, the stomach contents are churned or mixed with stomach fluids into a semifluid mass termed **chyme** *(kim)*. When the valve opens, small amounts of chyme are passed into the duodenum by **stomach peristalsis**. Gastric emptying is a fairly slow process, taking 2 to 6 hours to totally empty after an average meal. Food with high carbohydrate content leaves the stomach in several hours, while food with high protein or fat content moves through much slower.

The small intestine (small bowel) continues mechanical digestion with a churning motion within segments of the small bowel. This churning or mixing activity is termed **rhythmic segmentation**. Rhythmic segmentation tends to thoroughly mix food and digestive juices, and to bring the digested food into contact with the intestinal lining or mucosa to facilitate absorption. **Peristalsis** is again present to propel intestinal contents along the alimentary canal. Peristaltic contractions in the small intestine, however, are much weaker and slower than in the esophagus and stomach and the chyme moves through the small intestine at about 1 cm/min. Therefore the chyme will normally take 3 to 5 hours to pass through the entire small intestine.

Summary of Mechanical Digestion	
Oral cavity (teeth and tongue)	• Mastication (chewing) • Deglutition (swallowing)
Pharynx	• Deglutition
Esophagus	• Deglutition • Peristalsis (waves of muscular contraction) (1 to 8 secs)
Stomach	• Mixing (chyme) • Peristalsis (2 to 6 hrs)
Small intestine (small bowel)	• Rhythmic segmentation (churning) • Peristalsis (3 to 5 hrs)

Chemical Digestion

Chemical digestion includes all of the chemical changes that food undergoes as it travels through the alimentary canal. Six different classes of substances are ingested: (1) **carbohydrates** or complex sugars, (2) **proteins**, (3) **lipids** *(lip′ id)* or **fats**, (4) **vitamins**, (5) **minerals** and (6) **water**. Only the carbohydrates, proteins and lipids need to be chemically digested in order to be absorbed. Vitamins, minerals and water are used in the form in which the body ingests them.

Chemical digestion is speeded up by various **enzymes**. Enzymes are **biological catalysts** found in the various digestive juices that are produced by salivary glands in the mouth and by the stomach, small bowel and pancreas. The various enzymes are organic compounds, which are proteins. They accelerate chemical changes in other substances without actually appearing in the final products of the reaction.

Summary of Chemical Digestion

Substances ingested, digested and absorbed:

1. Carbohydrates (complex sugars) → simple sugars (mouth and stomach)
2. Proteins → amino acids (stomach and small bowel)
3. Lipids (fats) → fatty acids and glycerol (small bowel only)

Substances ingested but NOT digested:

4. Vitamins
5. Minerals
6. Water

Enzymes (digestive juices)
• Biological catalysts
Bile (from GB)
• Emulsifies fats

Digested Substances and Resultant By-products:

(1) **Carbohydrate** digestion of starches begins in the mouth and stomach and is completed in the small intestine. The end products of digestion of these complex sugars are **simple sugars**.

(2) **Protein** digestion begins in the stomach and is completed in the small intestine. The end products of protein digestion are **amino acids**.

(3) **Lipid** or fat digestion essentially takes place only in the small bowel, although small amounts of the enzyme necessary for fat digestion are found in the stomach.

Bile, manufactured by the liver and stored in the gallbladder, is discharged into the duodenum to assist in the breakdown of lipids. Bile contains no enzymes, but it does serve to emulsify fats. During emulsification, large fat droplets are broken down to small fat droplets, which have greater surface area (to volume) and give enzymes greater access for the breakdown of lipids. The end products of fat or lipid digestion are **fatty acids** and **glycerol** *(glis′ er-ol)*.

Most absorption of digestive end products takes place in the small intestine. Simple sugars, amino acids, fatty acids, glycerol, H_2O and most salts and vitamins are absorbed into the bloodstream or the lymphatic system through the lining of the small intestine. Limited absorption takes place in the stomach and may include some water, alcohol and certain drugs but no nutrients. Any residues of digestion or unabsorbed digestive products are eliminated from the large bowel as a component of feces.

Digestion continued

Summary

In general, **three primary functions** of the digestive system are accomplished within the alimentary canal.

First, **ingestion** and/or **digestion** takes place in the oral cavity, pharynx, esophagus, stomach and small intestine.

Second, digestive end products along with water, vitamins and minerals are **absorbed** primarily by the small intestine and, to a very small degree by the stomach, and are transported into the circulatory system.

Third, unused or unnecessary solid material is **eliminated** by the large intestine. (Digestive functions of large intestine are described in Chapter 15.)

Summary: Primary Functions of Digestive System

1. **Ingestion** and/or **Digestion**
   - Oral cavity
   - Pharynx
   - Esophagus
   - Stomach
   - Small intestine
2. **Absorption**
   - Small intestine (and stomach)
3. **Elimination**
   - Large intestine

BODY HABITUS

The type of body habitus has a great effect on the location of the GI organs within the abdominal cavity. To be able to accurately and consistently position for these GI procedures, one must know and understand the characteristics of each of these classes of body habitus.

The four general classes of body habitus are shown in Fig. 14-21.

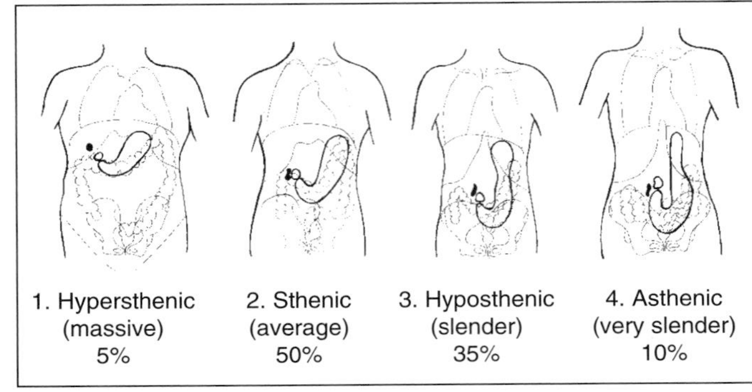

Fig. 14-21. Body habitus–Four body types.

Hypersthenic vs. Hyposthenic/Asthenic (Fig. 14-22)

Hypersthenic: The hypersthenic type designates 5% of the population which are those with the most **massive body build**, with the chest and abdomen being very broad and deep from front to back. The lungs are short and the diaphragm is high. The transverse colon is quite high, and the entire **large intestine** extends to the periphery of the abdominal cavity. This generally requires two films placed crosswise to include the entire large intestine.

The **gallbladder** (GB) tends to associate in location to the duodenal bulb and pylorus region of the stomach. For the hypersthenic the GB is high and almost transverse, and lies well to the right of the midline. The **stomach** is also very high and assumes a transverse position. The level of the stomach extends from approximately T9 to T13 with the center of the stomach about 1 inch (2.5 cm) distal to the xiphoid process. The duodenal bulb is at approximately the level of T11 or T12, to the right of midline.

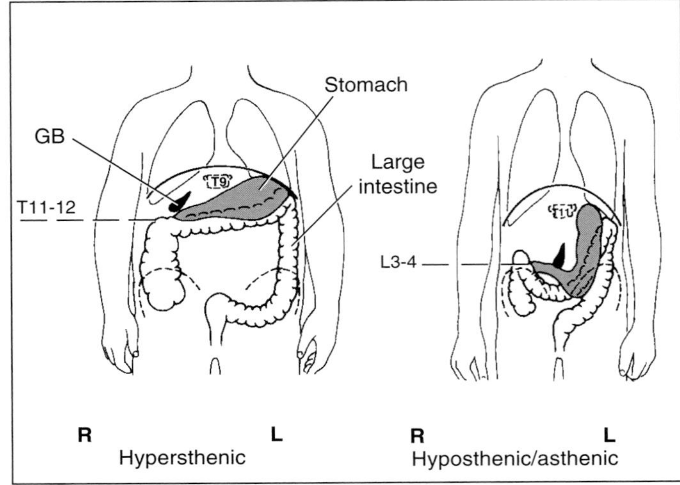

Fig. 14-22. Hypersthenic compared with hyposthenic/asthenic.

Hyposthenic/Asthenic: These represent the opposite body types, which are more slender and have narrow and longer lungs with a low diaphragm. This causes the **large intestine** to be very low in the abdomen, which has its greatest capacity in the pelvic region.

The **stomach** is J-shaped and low in the abdomen, extending from about T11 down below the level of the iliac crests to approximately L5 or even lower. The vertical portion of the stomach is to the left of midline, with the duodenal bulb near the midline at the level of L3 or L4.

The **gallbladder** is near midline or slightly to the right and just above, or at the level of the iliac crest, or approximately at L3-4.

Sthenic (Fig. 14-23): The **average body build** is the sthenic type, which is a more slender version of the hypersthenic classification. The **stomach** is also somewhat J-shaped and is located lower than in the massive body type and generally extends from the level of T10 or T11 down to about L2. The duodenal bulb is at the approximate level of L1-2, to the right of midline. The **gallbladder** is less transverse and lies midway between the lateral abdominal wall and the midline. The **left colic (splenic) flexure** of the **large intestine** is often quite high, resting under the left diaphragm.

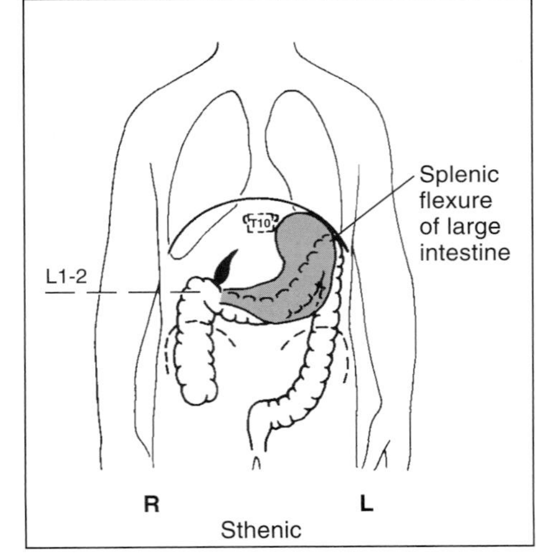

Fig. 14-23. Sthenic (average)

Additional Factors

In addition to body habitus, other factors affecting the position of the stomach include **stomach contents**, **respiration**, **body position** (erect vs. recumbent) and **age**. Since the upper stomach is attached to the diaphragm, whether one is in full inspiration or expiration affects the superior extent of the stomach. All abdominal organs tend to drop 1 to 2 inches in an erect position, or even more with age and loss of muscle tone. As a radiographer, correct localization of the stomach and other organs for different body types in various positions will come with positioning practice.

RADIOGRAPHS OF UPPER GI DEMONSTRATING BODY TYPES

Most persons do not fall clearly into one of the distinct four body types but are a combination of these types, and one needs to be able to evaluate each patient for probable stomach and/or gall bladder locations.

The three body type examples below with radiographs demonstrate the position and location of the stomach on these three most common body types. The location of the stomach and duodenal bulb to specific vertebra should be noted in relationship to the level of the iliac crest and lower costal margin positioning landmarks.

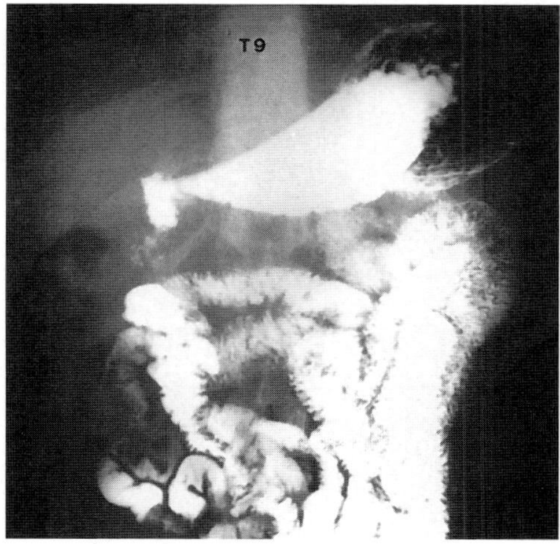

Fig. 14-24. Hypersthenic.

General stomach-High and transverse, level T9-T12.

Pyloric portion-Level of T11-12, at midline.

Duodenal bulb location-Level of T11-12, to right of midline.

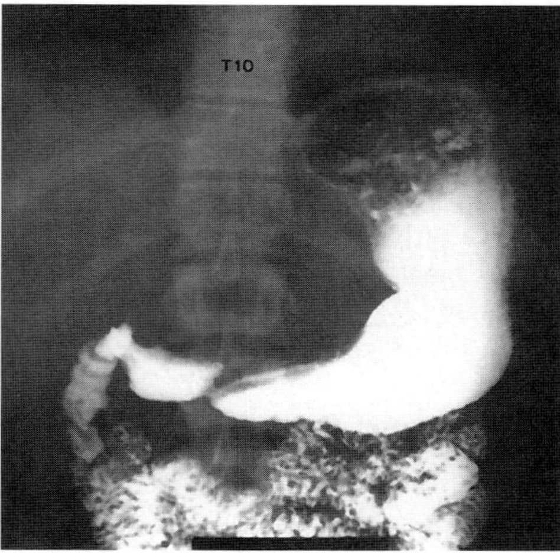

Fig. 14-25. Sthenic.

General stomach-Level T10 to L2.

Pyloric portion-Level of L2, near midline.

Duodenal bulb location-Level of L2, near midline.

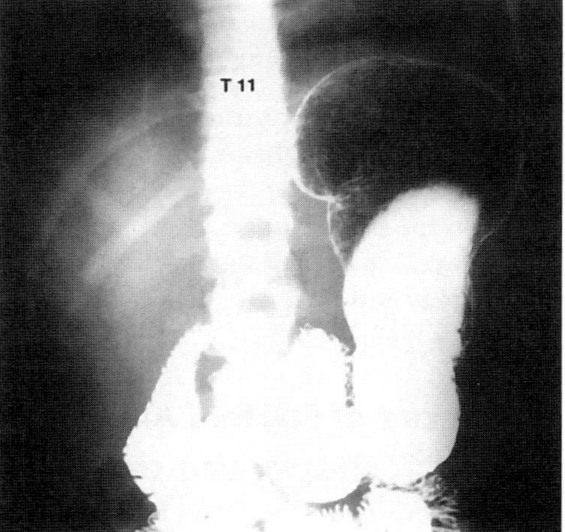

Fig. 14-26. Asthenic.

General stomach-Low and vertical, level T11 to L4.

Pyloric portion-Level of L3-4, to left of midline.

Duodenal bulb location-Level of L3, at midline.

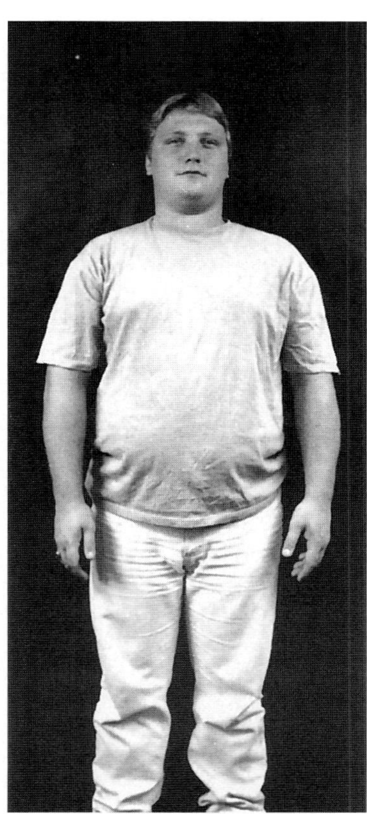

Fig. 14-27. Hypersthenic.

Generally shorter in height with broad shoulders and hips and short torso (less distance between lower rib cage and iliac crest). Abdominal cavity is widest at upper margin.

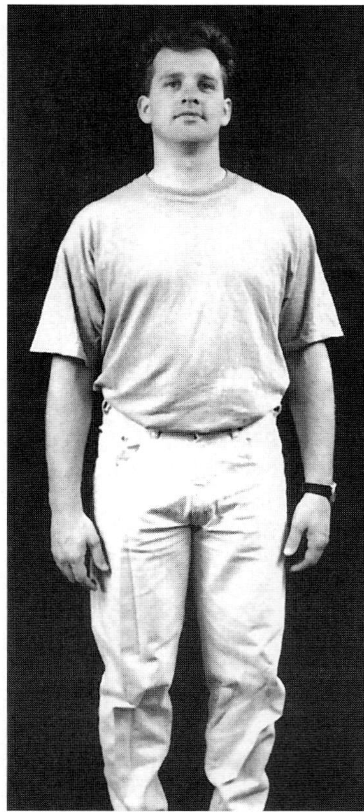

Fig. 14-28. Sthenic.

Near average in height, weight and length of torso. (May be somewhat heavier than average with some hypersthenic characteristics.)

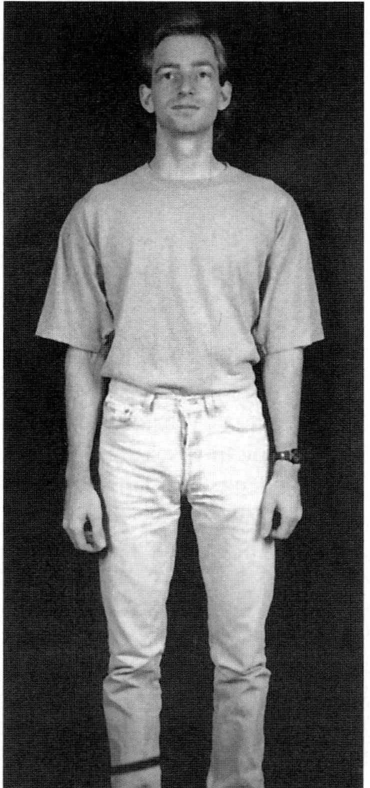

Fig. 14-29. Hyposthenic/asthenic.

Generally tall and thin with long torso. (This example is somewhere between a hyposthenic and asthenic.) Abdominal cavity is widest at lower margin for a true asthenic.

Radiographic Procedures

SIMILARITIES

Radiographic procedures or examinations of the entire alimentary canal are similar in three general aspects.

First, since most parts of the GI tract are comparable in density to those tissues surrounding them, some type of **contrast medium** must be added to visualize these structures. Ordinarily, the only parts of the alimentary canal that can be seen on plain radiographs are the fundus of the stomach (in the upright position) due to the gastric air bubble, and parts of the large intestine due to pockets of gas and collections of fecal matter.

Most of the alimentary canal simply blends in with the surrounding structures and cannot be visualized without the use of contrast media. This fact is illustrated by comparing a plain abdominal radiograph (Fig. 14-30) to an upper GI series radiograph using barium sulfate as a contrast medium (Fig. 14-31).

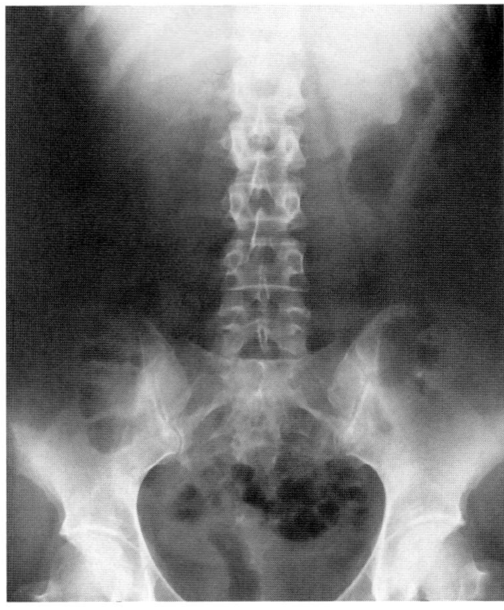

Fig. 14-30. Plain abdomen.

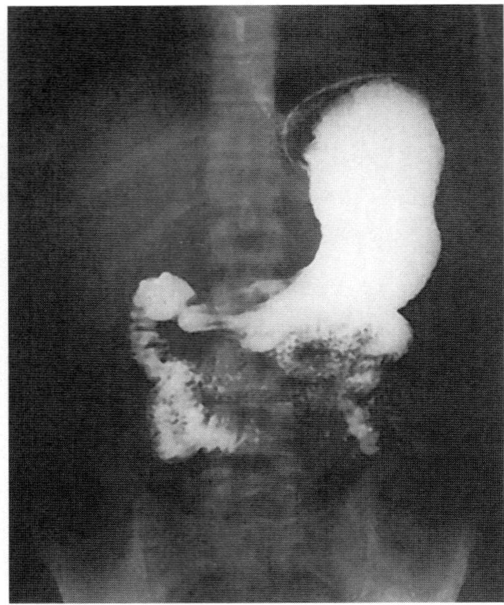

Fig. 14-31. Barium in stomach.

A **second** similarity is that the initial stage of each radiographic examination of the alimentary canal is carried out utilizing **fluoroscopy**. Fluoroscopy allows the interested physician to (1) observe the GI tract in motion, (2) produce radiographs during the course of the examination, and (3) determine the most appropriate course of action to take for the complete radiographic examination. To be able to view organs in motion and to isolate anatomical structures is absolutely essential for radiographic examination of the upper GI tract. The structures in this area assume a wide variety of shapes and sizes depending on the body habitus, age, and other individual differences.

In addition, the functional activity of the alimentary canal exhibits a wide range of differences that are considered within normal limits. In addition to these variations, a large number of abnormal conditions exist, making it important that these organs be viewed directly by fluoroscopy.

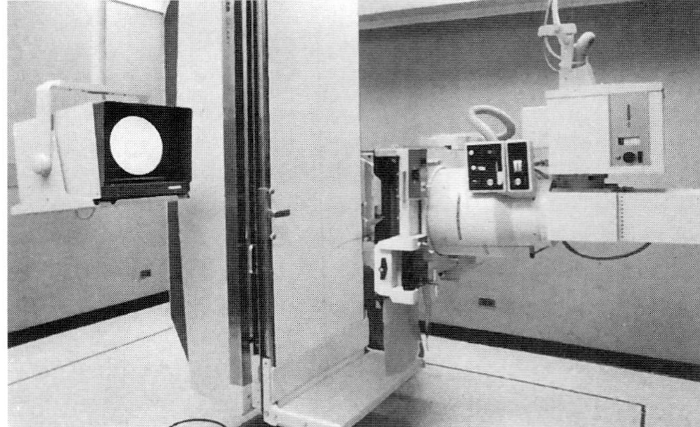

Fig. 14-32. Fluoroscopy room.

A **third** similarity is that **radiographs are produced during and after the fluoroscopic examination** of any specific parts of the alimentary canal to provide a permanent record of the normal or abnormal findings. A radiograph from an upper GI series is shown in Fig. 14-33, demonstrating a duodenal ulcer, a type of mucosal erosion or "out pouching."

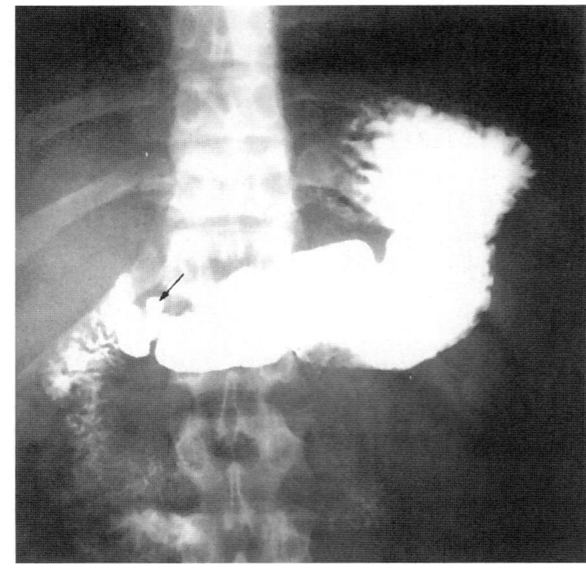

Fig. 14-33. Radiograph of stomach demonstrating duodenal ulcer (see arrow).

CONTRAST MEDIA

Radiolucent and radiopaque contrast media are utilized to render the GI tract visible radiographically. **Radiolucent** or **negative contrast media** include **swallowed air**, **CO_2 gas crystals**, and the normally present **gas bubble** in the stomach. Calcium and magnesium citrate carbonate crystals are most commonly used in producing CO_2 gas.

Note: Radiopaque contrast media absorb more x-rays, and **radiolucent media absorb less**, making structures filled with these contrast media more visible than surrounding tissue.

Barium Sulfate (Barium)

The most common **positive or radiopaque contrast medium** used to visualize the gastrointestinal system is **barium sulfate**, ($BaSO_4$), commonly referred to as just **barium**. As illustrated in Fig. 14-34, barium sulfate is a powdered, chalk-like substance. The powdered barium sulfate is mixed with water prior to ingestion by the patient. This particular compound, which is a salt of barium, is relatively inert because of its extreme insolubility in water and other aqueous solutions, such as acids. All other salts of barium tend to be toxic or poisonous to the human system. Therefore, the barium sulfate used in radiology departments must be chemically pure.

A mixture of barium sulfate and water forms a **colloidal suspension**, not a solution. In order to be a solution, the molecules of the substance added to water must actually dissolve in the water. **Barium sulfate never dissolves in the water**. In a colloidal suspension, however, (such as barium sulfate and water) the particles suspended in the water may tend to settle out when allowed to sit for a period of time.

The radiograph shown in Fig. 14-35 shows cups of four different brands of barium that were mixed with a ratio by volume of one part water to one part barium sulfate and then allowed to sit for 24 hours. Since different brands of barium sulfate were used, some cups exhibit more separation or settling out than others. This demonstrates that when the barium sulfate and water are mixed before they are actually needed, each cup must be well stirred before actual use.

Many special barium sulfate preparations are available commercially. Most of these preparations contain finely divided barium sulfate in a special suspending agent, so these preparations tend to resist settling out and, therefore, stay in suspension longer. Each of these suspensions must be well mixed before use, however. Various brands have different smells and different flavors, such as chocolate, chocolate malt, vanilla, lemon, lime or strawberry.

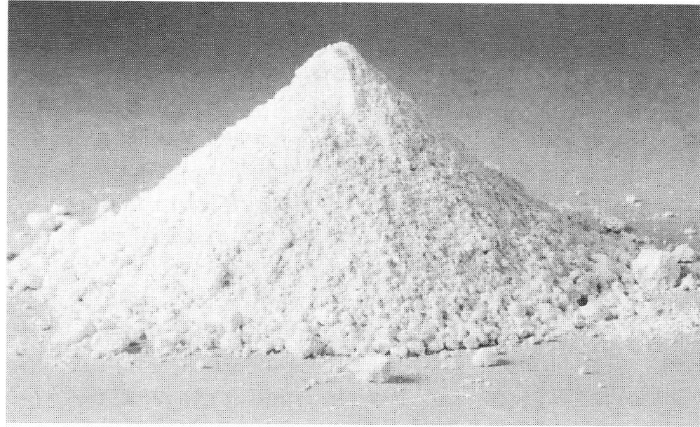

Fig. 14-34. Barium sulfate ($BaSO_4$).

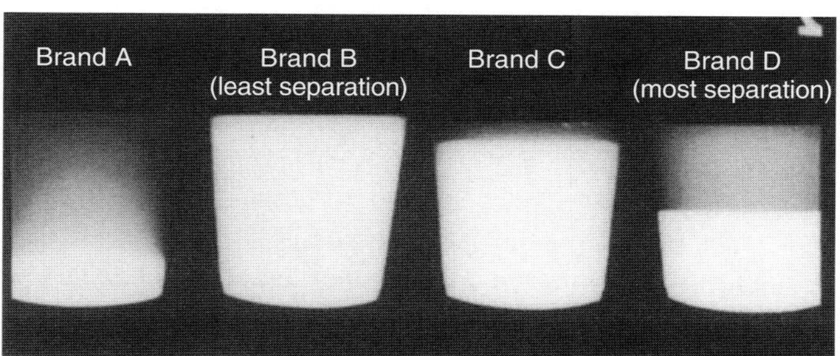

Fig. 14-35. Cups of barium.

Thin Barium

Barium sulfate may be prepared or purchased in a relatively thin or thick mixture. The thin barium sulfate and water mixture contained in a cup, as illustrated in Fig. 14-36, contains one part $BaSO_4$ to one part of water. Thin barium is the consistency of a thin milk shake and is used to study the entire GI tract.

The motility, or speed with which barium sulfate passes through the GI tract, depends on the suspending medium and additives, the temperature and the consistency of the preparation, as well as upon the general condition of the patient and the GI tract. It is most important to mix the preparation exactly according to radiologist preferences and departmental protocol. When the mixture is cold, the chalky taste is much less objectionable.

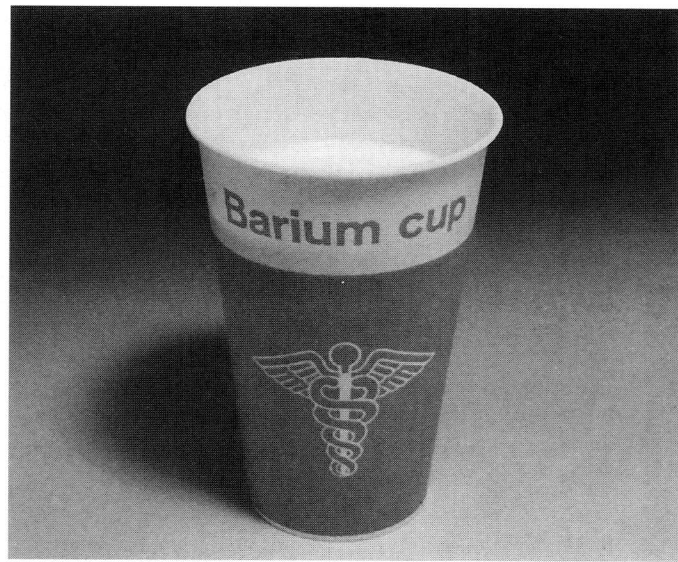

Fig. 14-36. Thin barium sulfate and water mixture.

Thick Barium

Thick barium contains three or four parts of $BaSO_4$ to one part of water and should be the consistency of cooked cereal. Thick barium is more difficult to swallow but is well suited for use in the esophagus since it descends slowly and tends to coat the mucosal lining.

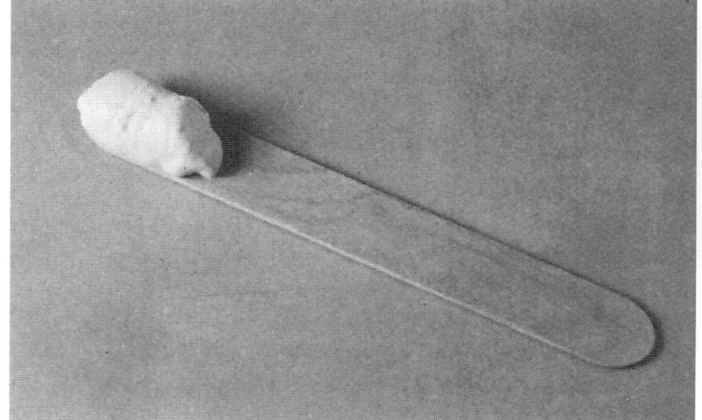

Fig. 14-37. Thick barium sulfate mixture.

Contrast Media continued

Contraindications to Barium Sulfate

Barium sulfate mixtures are contraindicated if there is any chance that the mixture might escape into the peritoneal cavity. This may occur through a perforated viscus, or it can occur during surgery if the surgery follows the radiographic procedure. In either of these two cases, **water-soluble, iodinated contrast media** should be used. An example of this type is MD-Gastroview®, shown in Fig. 14-38 in a 240 ml bottle. Other examples are Gastrografin® or Oral Hypaque®, all of which can be easily removed by aspiration before or during surgery. Should any of this water-soluble material escape into the peritoneal cavity, the body can readily absorb it. Barium sulfate, on the other hand, will not be absorbed and must be removed by the surgeon wherever it is found outside the alimentary canal.

One drawback to the water-soluble materials is their bitter taste. Although these iodinated contrast media are sometimes mixed with carbonated soft drinks to mask the taste, they are often used "as is" or diluted with water. The patient should be forewarned that the taste may be slightly bitter.

Warning: Water-soluble iodinated contrast media **should not be used** if the patient is sensitive to iodine.

It has also been reported that a small number of patients are hypersensitive to barium sulfate. Although this is a rare occurrence, the patient should be observed for any signs of allergic reaction.

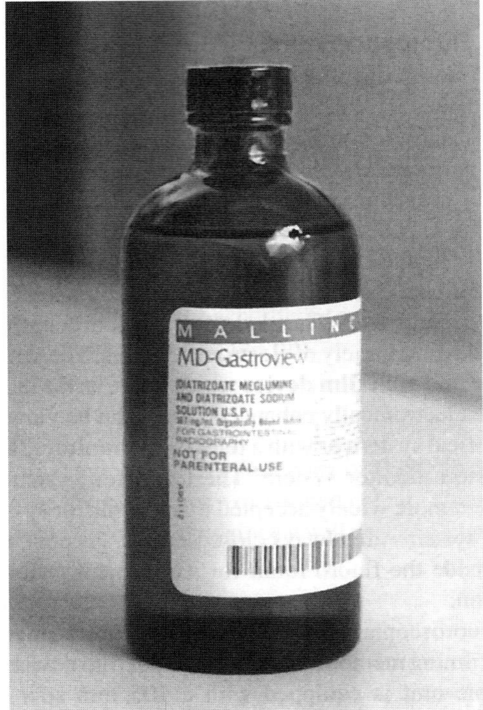

Fig. 14-38. Example of water-soluble iodinated contrast medium.

Double Contrast

The use of double-contrast techniques has been employed widely to enhance the diagnosis of certain diseases and conditions during upper GI's. Some departments are also performing double contrast esophagrams. The use of double contrast procedures employing both radiolucent and radiopaque contrast media was developed in Japan, where there is a high incidence of stomach carcinoma.

The **radiopaque** contrast medium is **barium sulfate**. A high-density barium is used to provide good coating of the stomach mucosa. A pre-measured, commercially produced cup of barium sulfate is most often provided by the department, where the technologist needs only to add water and mix thoroughly.

The **radiolucent** contrast medium is either **room air** or **carbon dioxide gas**. To introduce room air, small pin prick holes are placed in the patient's straw. As the patient drinks the barium mixture, air is drawn in.

Carbon dioxide gas is created when the patient ingests gas-producing crystals. Two common forms of these crystals are **calcium and magnesium citrate**. Upon reaching the stomach these crystals **form a large gas bubble**. The gas forces the barium sulfate against the stomach mucosa, providing better coating and visibility of the mucosa and its patterns (Fig. 14-39). Potential polyps, diverticulae, and ulcers will be demonstrated better with a double-contrast technique.

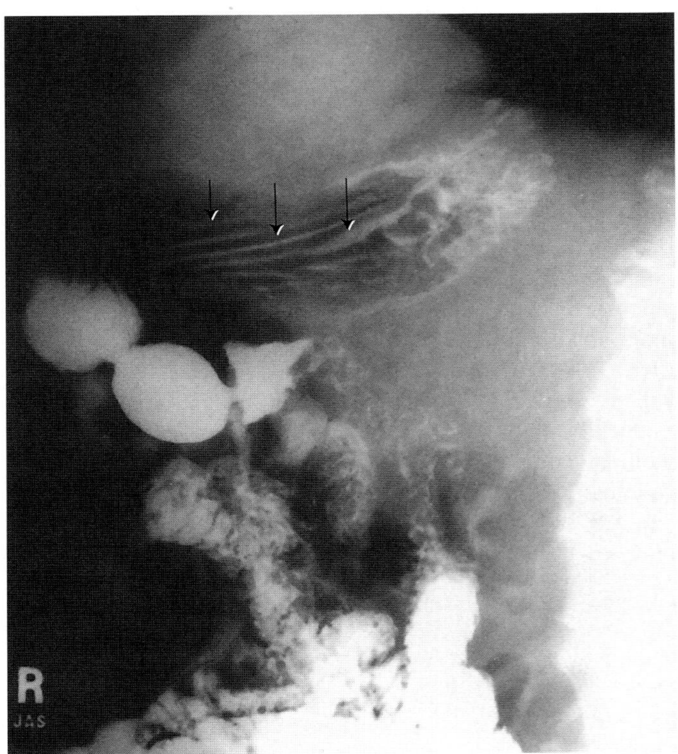

Fig. 14-39. UGI–Double contrast (R lateral position). Demonstrates air-filled stomach with mucosal folds lined with barium (see arrows).

Post-exam Elimination (Defecation)

One of the normal functions of the large intestine is the absorption of water. Any barium sulfate mixture remaining in the large intestine after either an upper GI series or a barium enema may become hardened and somewhat solidified in the large bowel, and consequently be difficult to evacuate. Certain patients may require a laxative after these examinations to help remove the barium sulfate. If laxatives are contraindicated, the patient should force fluids or use mineral oil until stools are free from all traces of white.

RADIOGRAPHY–FLUOROGRAPHY EQUIPMENT

General Fluoroscopy Unit

During fluoroscopy, the viewer is able to position a part so that the anatomy in question can be best seen by isolating it from objectionable overlying shadows. The fluoroscopic unit is equipped with a **spot cassette device** to permanently record optimum images. Cassettes of various sizes can be moved into position to permit a conventional, phototimed radiographic exposure. When fluoroscopy is being performed, these cassettes are in a lead-protected park position within the fluoroscopic unit.

A conventional combination radiography-fluorography (R/F) unit is illustrated in Fig. 14-40. The x-ray fluoro tube is located under the table. The modern general purpose fluoroscopy room is equipped with a variety of electronic devices. These include an **image intensifier** and **spot film devices,** which move as the table is tilted up or down. The electronically enhanced image can be viewed either with a **direct viewing mirror optical system** or with a **television monitor**.

Television Fluoroscopy: The equipment shown in Fig. 14-40 includes television monitor system. The video pickup tube (television camera) is generally located in the fluoro tower unit in combination with the image intensifier. The television system is much more versatile and more widely accepted than direct viewing with the mirror system. Since these television video systems are always closed-circuit, monitors can also be placed outside the fluoro room for simultaneous viewing during the examination.

Photospot Images or Cinefluorography: Some fluoroscopic systems also utilize a **spot film camera** for either photospot images (small stationary spot frame radiographs taken on 105 mm film) or cinefluorography (multiple frames exposed in succession viewed as movie film). These photospot or cine images are recorded by the spot film camera on the **output side** of the image intensifier, whereas conventional spot cassette films taken on 8 x 10 inch or similar sized cassettes are direct images taken on the **input side** of the image intensifier (Fig. 14-40). Therefore spot cassette images don't use the image intensifier and lack the brightness of spot film and cine images.

Spot film cameras are similar to movie cameras, but the framing frequency is slower and the film size is larger. These spot film cameras are generally 16 mm or 35 mm cameras, or cameras with 70, 90 or 105 mm film (film width).* Framing can be adjusted from a single exposure (photospots) to 6 or 12 frames per second (cine or movie film). Imaging with spot film cameras became possible with the brighter fluoroscopic images resulting from the use of image intensification.

Image Intensification

Conventional early fluoroscopy had two serious limitations: (1) the image was inferior and (2) the amount of light given off prevented the use of daylight or photopic vision. This required the use of colored eye goggles by the radiologist prior to beginning fluoroscopy to adapt the eyes to the low light level image. In the early 1950s, the invention of the **image intensifier** revolutionized fluoroscopy.

The image intensifier utilizes the radiation that passes through the patient and enhances the resultant image by electronically making this image 1,000 to 6,000 times brighter than the older fluoroscopy screen techniques. The image produced through image intensification is bright enough to be seen with photopic or day vision. The room lights are dimmed and the fluoroscopic examination is carried out in a comfortably illuminated room.

The image intensifier is located in the fluoro tower above the tabletop, while the x-ray tube is located beneath the tabletop (Fig. 14-40).

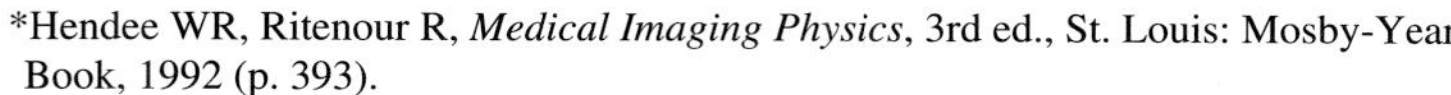

*Hendee WR, Ritenour R, *Medical Imaging Physics*, 3rd ed., St. Louis: Mosby-Year Book, 1992 (p. 393).

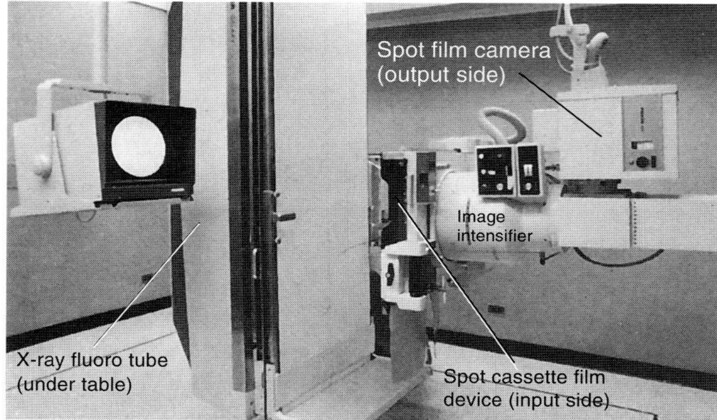

Fig. 14-40. General fluoroscopy room.

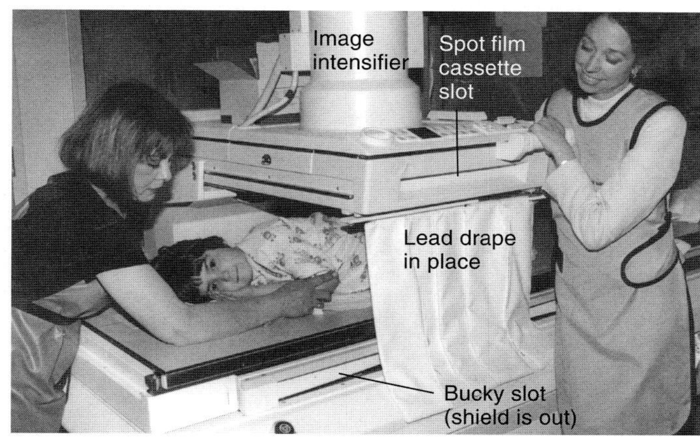

Fig. 14-41. Preparing pediatric patient for GI fluoroscopy.

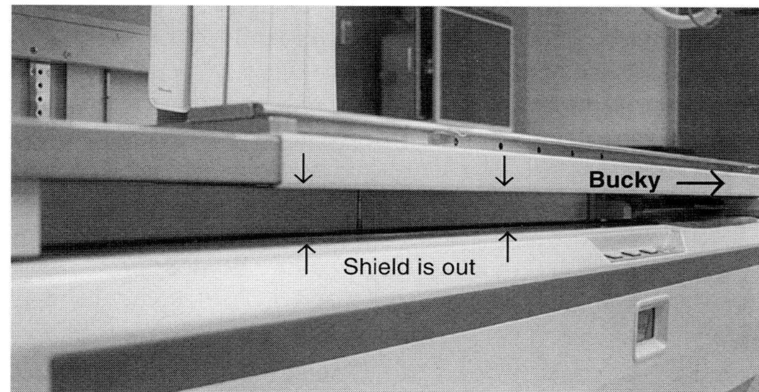

Fig. 14-42. Bucky slot shield completely out, Bucky tray at end of table.

Worker Protection During Fluoroscopy

Radiation protection practices during fluoroscopy were described in Chapter 1 (page 40). **Exposure patterns** and related doses within the fluoro room are given indicating where one should stand or not stand in the room during fluoroscopy (Fig. 1-127).

The flexible **lead drape shield** attached to the front of the fluoro and spot-film device is very important and should be inspected regularly. The technologist should ensure that the **Bucky is all the way to the end of the table**, which then brings out the metal **Bucky slot shield** to cover the ≈2 inch space directly under the table-top (Fig. 14-42). This significantly reduces the scatter radiation resulting from the fluoro x-ray tube located under the table. Leakage or scatter rays can escape through this waist-high Bucky space if the Bucky shield is not completely out.

This Bucky-at-end-of-table requirement during fluoroscopy is not only important for worker protection, but also is necessary to keep the Bucky mechanism out of the path of the fluoro x-ray tube under the table.

Digital Fluoroscopy (DF)

With the increased use of computers and digital imaging, the use of digitized fluoroscopy equipment is becoming more common. This system is similar to the television fluoroscopy system described on the preceding page with the addition of a computer for image manipulation and/or storage. A high-resolution video camera and a processor are incorporated into the fluoroscopy tower on the **output side** of the image intensifier. From here the image information is transmitted into a computer for manipulation and/or storage. A computer workstation, as illustrated in Fig. 14-43, provides a keyboard and usually a mouse or trackball for image manipulations. Images can then be displayed on a high-resolution monitor located in the fluoro room as well as on monitors located in other locations for remote viewing.

These digital fluoroscopy images can then also be printed to film by a laser-type printer for conventional viewing and/or storage as a "hard copy."

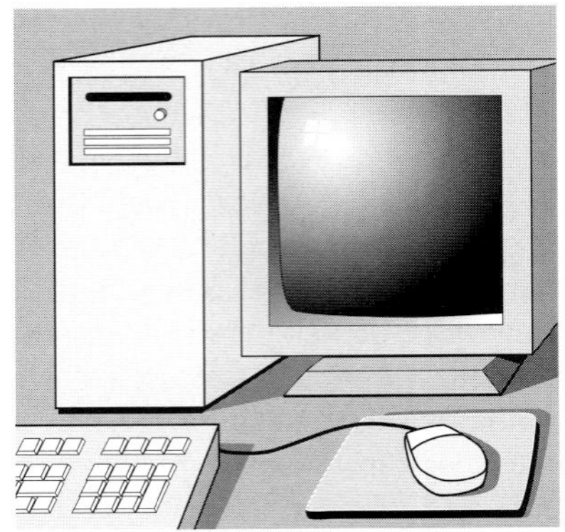

Fig. 14-43. Workstation for digital imaging.

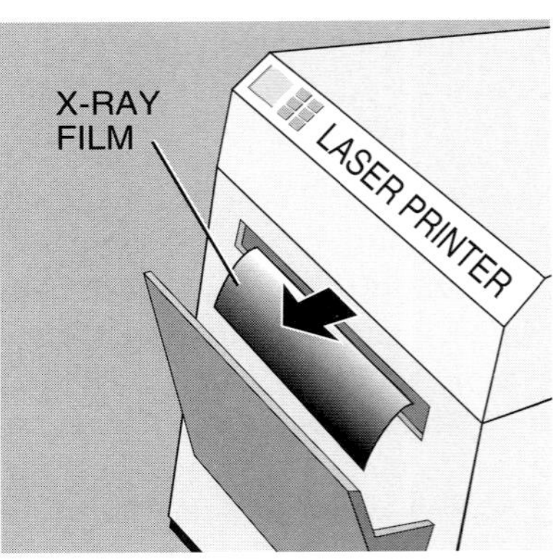

Fig. 14-44. Printer.

Unique Features and Capabilities of Digital Fluoroscopy

No Cassettes are Required: Radiographic images can be recorded during the fluoroscopy procedure similar to "spot films," except no cassettes are required. Specific images are captured instead in digital form for display on monitors and/or for storage and manipulation as needed, then printed on film if desired. Thus these digital still-frame images replace the conventional spot films taken on cassettes on the input side of the image intensifier. They also can replace photo spots or cine films from spot film cameras such as the 105 mm spot film cameras described on the preceding page.

Multiple Frame Formatting and Cine Loop Capability: Multiple images can be formatted and printed on one film. This can be four on one (Fig. 14-45), six on one, nine on one, or even twelve on one if the images are small enough.

Images can also be recorded in rapid succession (such as four images per second), which can then be displayed as moving or cine images. This is beneficial for certain studies such as an esophagram for possible esophageal reflux or impaired swallowing mechanisms. This replaces the need for spot film cameras for cinefluorography, which requires the use of "hard film" recording as well as developing and viewing on separate movie projectors.

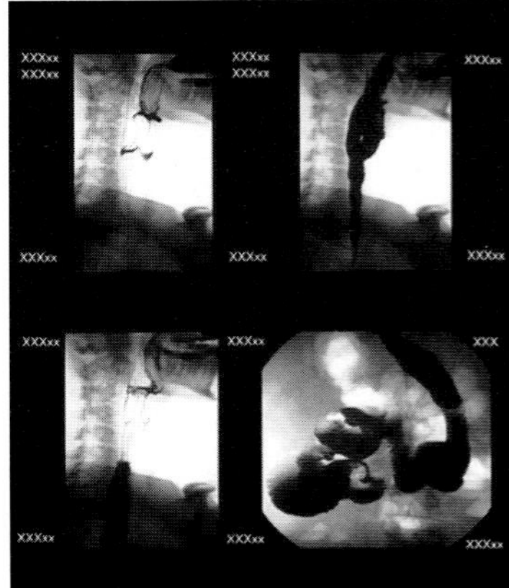

Fig. 14-45. Multiple-frame images (four images on one 14 x 17 film).

Image Enhancement and Manipulation: Digital fluoro images can be enhanced and/or manipulated by the use of equalization filters (Figs. 14-46 and 14-47). These image enhancement and manipulation features include edge enhancement, overall brightness and contrast controls, masking and digital subtraction study possibilities.

Multiple "Original" Films: "Hard-copy" films can be printed at any time and as often as desired. Therefore if radiographs are lost or misplaced or if duplicates are needed, additional "original" films can be printed at any time.

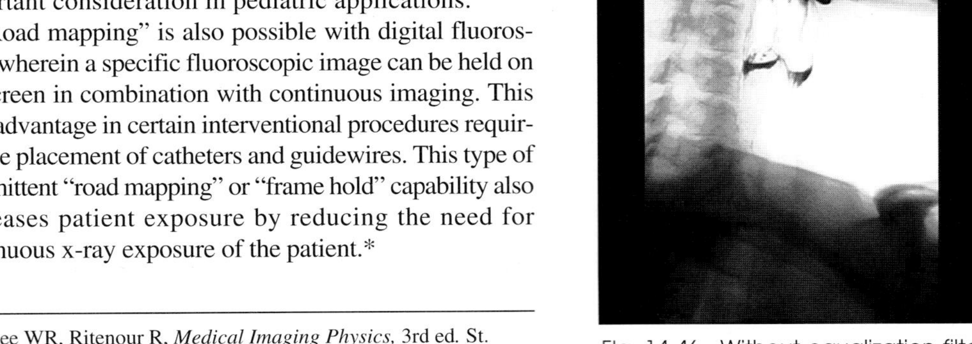

Reduced Patient Exposure: Digital fluorographic imaging **can reduce patient exposure 30 to 50%** compared to conventional fluoroscopy due to the increased sensitivity of image receptors resulting from a "pulsed progressive" scanning process.* This can be an important consideration in pediatric applications.

"Road mapping" is also possible with digital fluoroscopy wherein a specific fluoroscopic image can be held on the screen in combination with continuous imaging. This is an advantage in certain interventional procedures requiring the placement of catheters and guidewires. This type of intermittent "road mapping" or "frame hold" capability also decreases patient exposure by reducing the need for continuous x-ray exposure of the patient.*

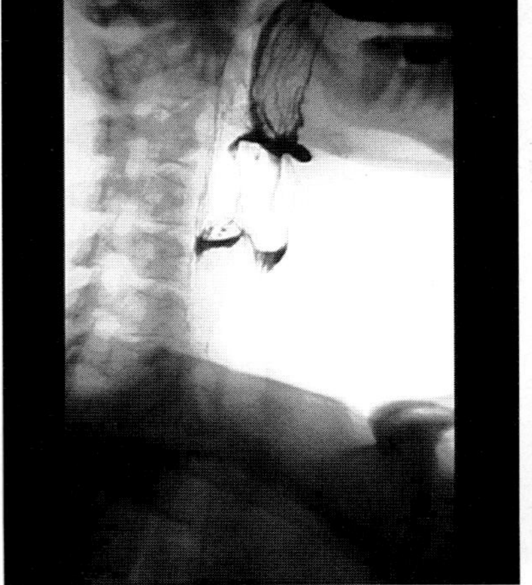

Fig. 14-46. Without equalization filter.

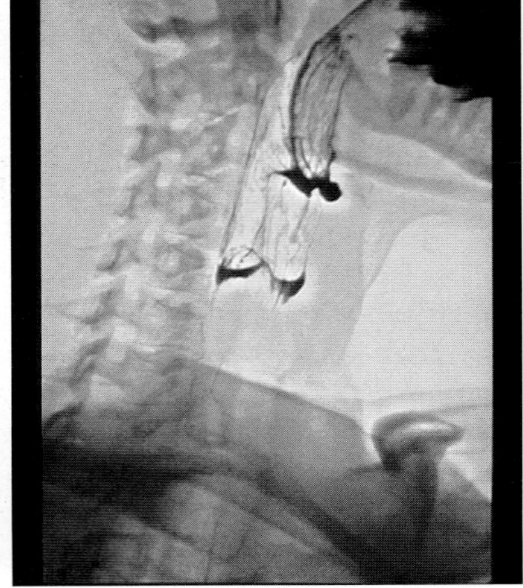

Fig. 14-47. With equalization filter.

*Hendee WR, Ritenour R, *Medical Imaging Physics,* 3rd ed. St. Louis: Mosby-Year Book, 1992.

ESOPHAGRAM

Two common radiographic procedures of the upper gastrointestinal system involving the administration of contrast media are the **esophagram**, or barium swallow as it is sometimes referred to, and the **upper GI series**. Each of these procedures will be described in detail beginning with the esophagram.

Definition

An esophagram or barium swallow is the common radiographic procedure or examination of the **pharynx** and **esophagus**, utilizing a radiopaque contrast medium. Occasionally a negative or radiolucent contrast medium may be used.

Purpose

The purpose of an esophagram is to study radiographically the form and function of the swallowing aspects of the pharynx and esophagus.

Indications

Some clinical indications for an esophagram include:

- Anatomical anomalies
- Impaired swallowing mechanics
- Foreign body obstruction
- Esophageal reflux
- Esophageal varices

Anatomical anomalies may be congenital or acquired due to lifestyle or disease, such as cancer involving the esophagus. Patients suffering from a stroke often develop **impaired swallowing mechanisms**.

Patients may ingest a variety of **foreign bodies** that may include a bolus of food, metallic objects, and other materials. Their location and dimensions may be determined during the esophagram. Radiolucent foreign bodies such as fish bones may require the use of additional materials and techniques to detect them.

Esophageal reflux is reported as heartburn by many patients. Gastric contents will return back through the gastric orifice and irritate the lining of the esophagus.

Esophageal varices are the dilation of the veins in the distal esophagus. This condition is often seen with acute liver disease such as cirrhosis. In advanced cases the veins may begin to bleed.

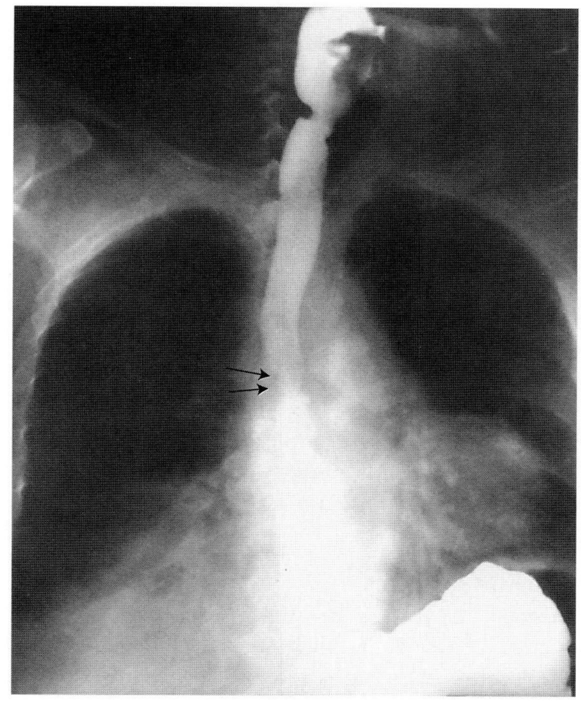

Fig. 14-48. Esophagram–Demonstrates a constricted area of the esophagus; probable carcinoma (see arrows).

Contraindications

No major contraindications exist for esophagrams except possible sensitivity to the contrast media used. The radiographer should determine if the patient has a history of sensitivity to barium sulfate, or water-soluble contrast media if it is utilized.

Patient Preparation

Radiographic examination of any part of the alimentary canal requires that the portion of the tract to be studied be empty. Since the esophagus is empty most of the time, there is **no patient preparation for an esophagram unless an upper GI series is to follow**. When combined with an upper GI, or if the primary interest is the lower esophagus, preparation for the UGI takes precedence.

For an esophagram only, all clothing and anything metallic between the mouth and the waist should be removed and the patient should wear a hospital gown. Prior to the fluoroscopic procedure, a pertinent history should be taken and the examination should be carefully explained to the patient.

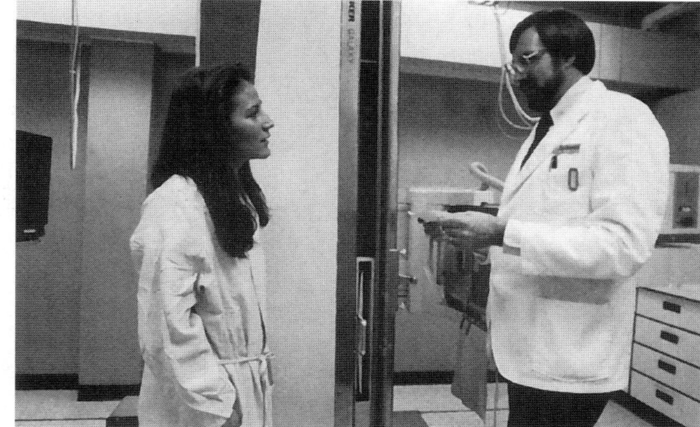

Fig. 14-49. Patient preparation.

Esophagram continued

Room Preparation

The first part of an esophagram involves fluoroscopy with a positive contrast medium. The examination room should be clean and tidy, and appropriately stocked before the patient is escorted to the room. The appropriate amount and type of contrast medium should be ready. Esophagrams utilize both thin and thick barium. Additional items useful in the detection of a radiolucent foreign body are (1) cotton balls soaked in thin barium, (2) barium pills or gelatin capsules filled with $BaSO_4$ and (3) marshmallows followed by thin barium.

The control panel should be set for fluoroscopy with the appropriate technical factors selected. The fluoroscopy timer should be set for its maximum, usually 5 minutes. The spot film mechanism should be in proper working order and a supply of spot film cassettes should be handy. The appropriate number and size of conventional cassettes should be provided. The spot film camera should be loaded and in working condition.

Since the esophagram begins with the table in the vertical position, the footboard should be in place and tested for security. Lead aprons and lead gloves should be provided for the radiologist, as well as lead aprons for all other personnel to be in the room. Proper radiation protection methods must be observed at all times during fluoroscopy.

In most fluoroscopy units, the Bucky tray must be positioned at the foot end of the table. Appropriately place the radiation foot switch and provide the radiologist a stool, except where the examination is controlled from a remote area. Tissues, towels, emesis basins, spoons, drinking straws and a waste receptacle should be readily accessible.

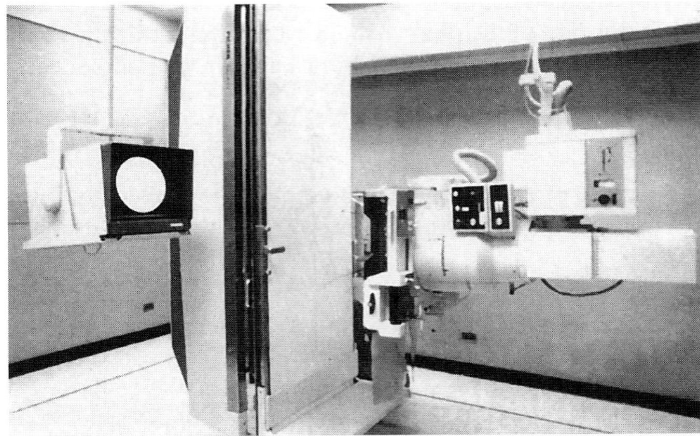

Fig. 14-50. Room preparation.

General Procedure

Fluoroscopy: With the room prepared and the patient ready, the patient and radiologist are introduced, and the patient's history and the reason for the exam are discussed. The fluoroscopic examination usually begins with a general survey of the patient's chest, including heart, lungs and diaphragm, and the abdomen (Fig. 14-51).

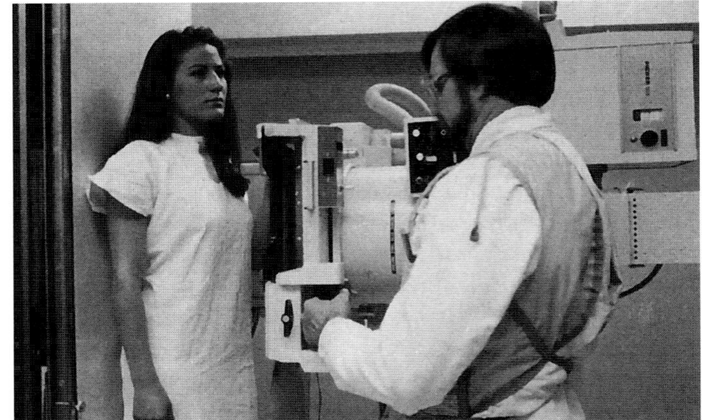

Fig. 14-51. Fluoroscopy.

During fluoroscopy, the radiographer's duties, in general, are to follow the radiologist's instructions, to assist the patient as needed and to expedite the procedure in any manner possible. Since the examination is begun in the upright or erect position, a cup of thin barium is placed in the patient's left hand close to the left shoulder. The patient is then instructed to follow the radiologist's instructions concerning how much to drink and when. The radiologist will observe the flow of barium with the fluoroscope.

Swallowing (deglutition) of thin barium is observed with the patient in various frontal and oblique positions. Similar positions may be utilized while the patient swallows thick barium. The use of thick barium allows better visualization of mucosal patterns and any lesion within the esophagus. The type of barium mixture to be used, however, will be determined by the radiologist.

After the upright studies, horizontal and Trendelenburg positions with thick and thin barium may follow. A patient is shown in position for an RAO projection with a cup of thin barium (Fig. 14-52). The pharynx and cervical esophagus are usually studied fluoroscopically with spot films, while the main portion of the esophagus down to the stomach is studied both with fluoroscopy and with overhead radiographs. Radiographs using a spot film device or the spot film camera are exposed to document any abnormalities or suspicious areas.

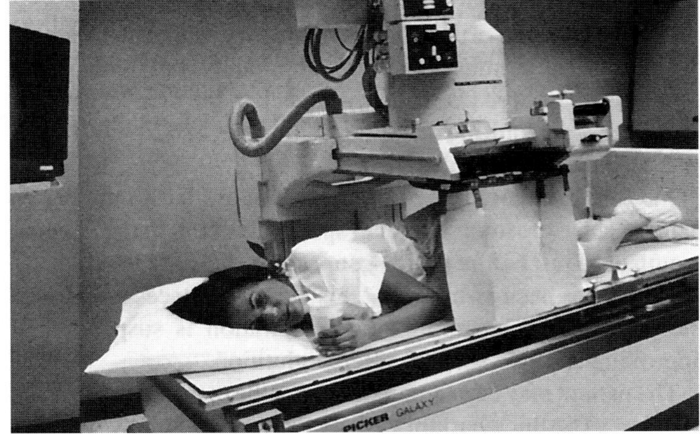

Fig. 14-52. RAO, with cup of thin barium.

Esophageal Reflux

The diagnosis of possible esophageal reflux or regurgitation of gastric contents may occur during fluoroscopy of an esophagram. One or more of the following procedures to detect esophageal reflux.

1. Breathing exercises
2. The water test
3. Compression paddle technique
4. The toe-touch test

1. Breathing Exercises

The various breathing exercises are all designed to increase both the intrathoracic and intra-abdominal pressures. The most common breathing exercise is the **Valsalva maneuver**. The patient is asked to take in a deep breath and, while holding the breath in, to bear down as though trying to move the bowels. This maneuver forces air against the closed glottis. A modified Valsalva maneuver is accomplished by having the patient pinch off the nose, close the mouth and try to blow his nose. The cheeks should expand outward as though the patient were blowing up a balloon.

A **Mueller maneuver** can also be performed by having the patient exhale and then try to inhale against a closed glottis.

2. Water Test (Fig. 14-53)

The water test is done with the patient supine and turned up slightly on his/her left side. This slight LPO position will fill the fundus with barium. The patient is asked to swallow a mouthful of water through a straw. Under fluoroscopy, the radiologist closely observes the esophagogastric junction. A positive water test occurs when significant amounts of barium regurgitate into the esophagus from the stomach.

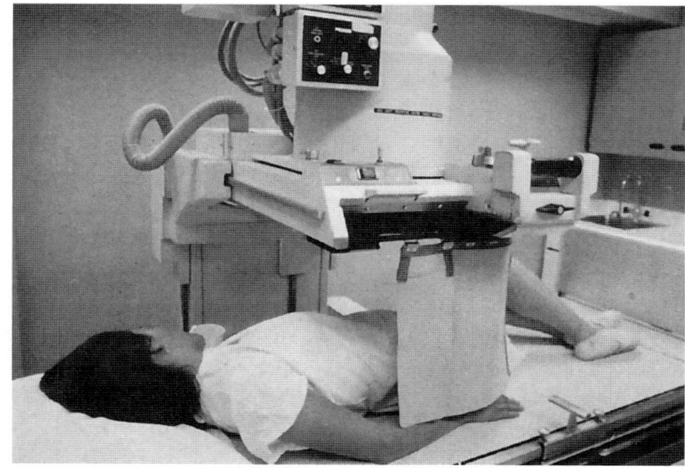

Fig. 14-53. Water test.

3. Compression Technique (Fig. 14-54)

A compression paddle can be placed under the patient in the prone position and inflated as needed to provide pressure to the stomach region. The radiologist can obscure the esophagogastric junction during this process to detect possible esophageal reflux.

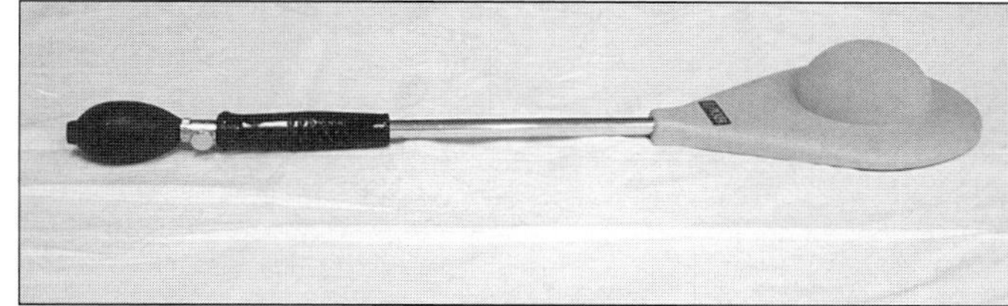

Fig. 14-54. Compression paddle.

4. Toe-touch Maneuver (Fig. 14-55)

The toe-touch maneuver is also performed to study possible regurgitation into the esophagus from the stomach. Under fluoroscopy, the cardiac orifice is observed as the patient bends over and touches his or her toes. Esophageal reflux and hiatal hernias are sometimes demonstrated using the toe-touch maneuver.

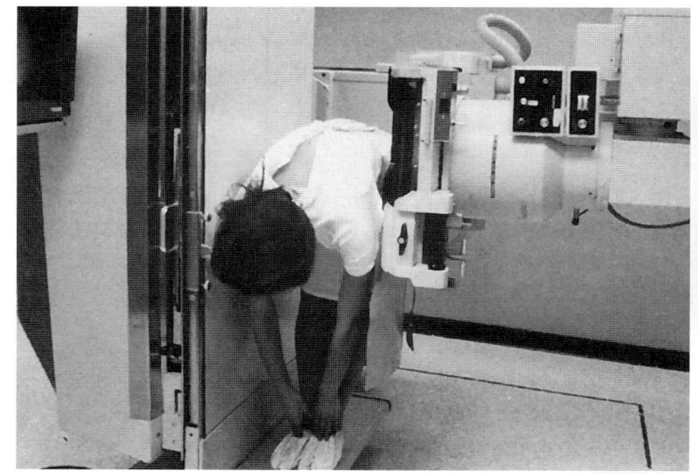

Fig. 14-55. Toe-touch maneuver.

Esophagram continued

Post Fluoroscopy Imaging

Following the fluoroscopy portion of the esophagram, radiographs are obtained of the entire barium-filled esophagus. General positioning is similar to chest radiography but with higher centering. The area from the lower neck to the diaphragm must be visualized, requiring centering at the level of T5 or T6 (1 inch or 2.5 cm below sternal angle).

One to three spoonfuls of thick barium are fed to the patient before each exposure. The final spoonful is held in the patient's mouth until just before the exposure. The exposure is made after the bolus has been swallowed. It is usually unnecessary to have the patient stop breathing since respiration is suspended for approximately 2 seconds after deglutition.

The patient may be examined in either the recumbent or upright position. The thick barium will not descend as rapidly when the patient is lying down, and more complete filling of the esophagus will be accomplished.

Three projections are considered routine for an esophagram or barium swallow. These include: (1) **RAO**, (2) **left lateral** and (3) **AP**.

Variations of the routine lateral are sometimes required. One variation is the soft tissue lateral position. When a foreign body is suspected high in the respiratory or digestive tracts, a soft tissue lateral is often the initial radiograph. Positioning is similar to an upright lateral of the cervical spine, although technical factors are adjusted so that approximately 10 kVp less is used. Radiopaque foreign bodies and some nonopaque foreign bodies can be demonstrated with this position. (A lower kVp is used to provide higher contrast and not overpenetrate small, less radiopaque foreign objects.)

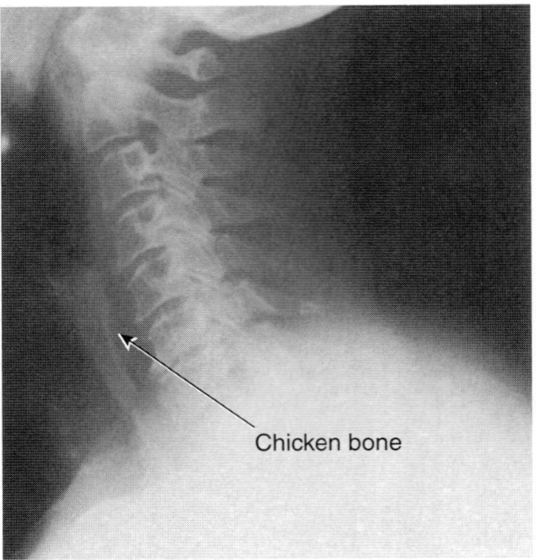

Fig. 14-56. Soft tissue lateral. (Demonstrates a chicken bone lodged in esophagus.)

CARDIAC SERIES

The cardiac series is a radiographic examination very similar to the esophagram. The cardiac series consists of four views of the esophagus, well filled with a thick barium mixture. These are (1) a PA, (2) a left lateral, (3) a 45° RAO and (4) a 60° LAO. The filled esophagus indicates the size and configuration of the heart as seen on these four radiographs. The left lateral (Fig. 14-57) illustrates a massively enlarged heart. This patient suffered from rheumatic fever as a young person. Rheumatic fever attacks and damages the valves of the heart so that the myocardium or heart muscle has to work very hard to pump adequate blood through the arteries. Whenever individual fibers of a muscle overwork, the result is an enlargement of the entire muscle, termed hypertrophy. This radiograph is an excellent demonstration of cardiac hypertrophy.

The **cardiac series, however, is rarely performed today** because of the greater accuracy with other imaging modalities. One example is echocardiography, the use of ultrasound wave energy to study the heart. This is considered an ideal method to study the size of the heart and its components. It will measure accurately the ventricles and intraventricular septum and demonstrate the heart valves.

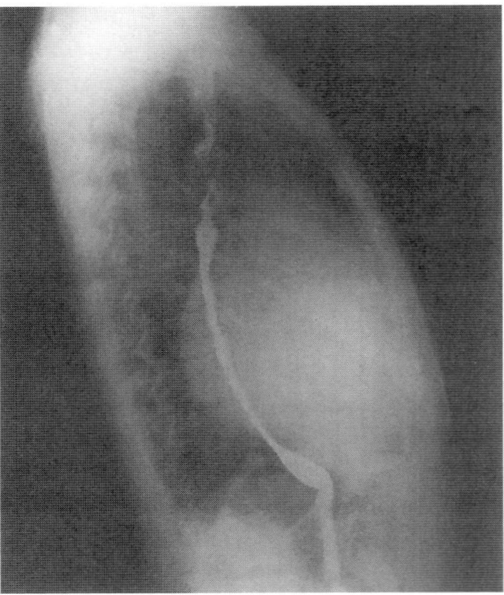

Fig. 14-57. Cardiac series, left lateral. (Demonstrates an enlarged heart.)

UPPER GI SERIES

In addition to the esophagram, the second and very common radiographic procedure or examination of the upper gastrointestinal system involving contrast media is the **upper gastrointestinal series** (UGI).

Definition

Radiographic examination of the **distal esophagus**, **stomach**, and **duodenum** is termed an upper GI series (UGI).

Purpose

The purpose of the upper GI is to study radiographically the form and function of the distal esophagus, stomach, and duodenum, as well as to detect abnormal anatomical and functional conditions.

Clinical Indications

Some clinical indications for an upper GI series include:

- Peptic ulcers
- Hiatal hernia *(hi-a′ tal her′ ne-ah)*
- Acute or chronic gastritis
- Tumor, carcinoma and benign
- Diverticula *(di′ ver-tik′ u-lah)*
- Bezoar *(be′ zor)*

Peptic ulcers, which include gastric and duodenal ulcers, are erosions of the stomach or duodenal mucosa due to various physiological or environmental conditions, such as excessive gastric secretions, stress, diet, and smoking. Some more recent studies suggest that ulcers may be caused by bacteria and thus can be treated with antibiotics. If untreated, the ulcer may lead to a perforation of the stomach or duodenum. The mucosal ulcer will usually fill with barium sulfate during the upper GI. A small peptic ulcer is demonstrated in Fig. 14-58.

A **hiatal hernia** is a condition where a portion of the stomach will herniate through the diaphragmatic opening. It may be a slight herniation or a severe form where a majority of the stomach is found within the thoracic cavity above the diaphragm. A moderate-size hiatal hernia is shown in Fig. 14-59.

Gastritis is inflammation of the lining or mucosa of the stomach. Gastritis may develop in response to various physiological and environmental conditions. **Acute gastritis** will present severe symptoms of pain and discomfort. **Chronic gastritis** is an intermittent condition that may be brought on by changes in diet, stress, or other factors.

Tumors in the stomach or duodenum may be either a carcinoma or benign. A **polyp** is a small mass growing from the mucosal wall. It could be either a cancerous or benign growth.

Diverticulae are a weakening and outpouching of a portion of the mucosal wall. Although benign, they can lead to perforation if untreated. A double-contrast upper GI is best to diagnose any tumors or diverticulae. An air-filled, barium-lined diverticulum of the duodenal bulb is shown in Fig. 14-60.

A **bezoar** is a mass of undigested material that gets trapped in the stomach. This mass is usually made up of hair, certain vegetable fibers, or wood products. The material builds up and may form an obstruction in time. Although a rare condition, it may be seen during an upper GI.

Contraindications

Contraindications for upper GI examinations apply primarily to the type of contrast media used. If the patient has a history of bowel perforation, laceration, or viscus rupture, the use of barium sulfate may be contraindicated. An oral water-soluble iodinated contrast media may be used in place of barium sulfate.

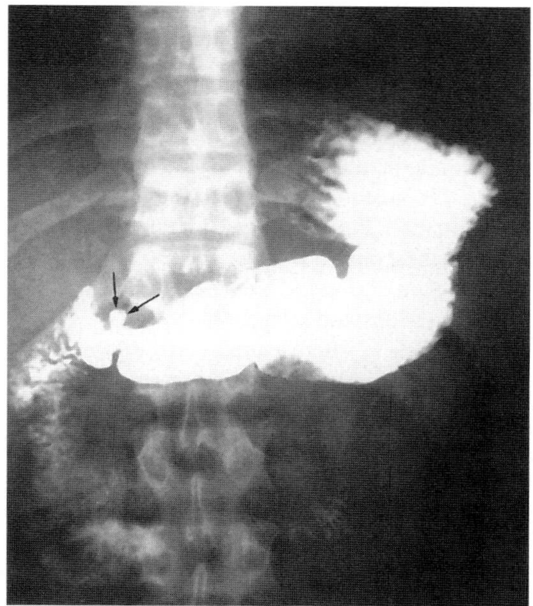

Fig. 14-58. PA projection–Peptic ulcer (see arrows).

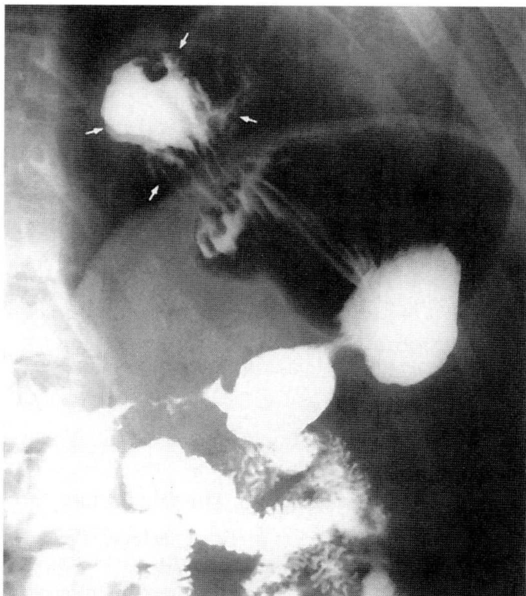

Fig. 14-59. Obli. projection–Hiatal hernia (see arrows).

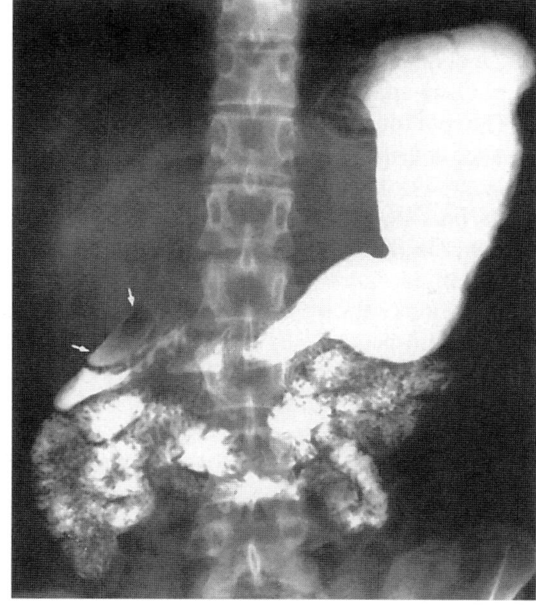

Fig. 14-60. PA projection–Diverticulum in duodenum (see arrows).

14

Upper GI Series continued

Patient Preparation

The goal of patient preparation for an upper GI series is for the patient to arrive in the radiology department with a completely empty stomach. For an examination scheduled in the morning hours, the patient should be **NPO** *(Non Per Os*, meaning nothing by mouth) from midnight until time for the examination. Food and fluids should be withheld for at least 8 hours prior to the exam. **The patient is also instructed not to smoke cigarettes or chew gum during the NPO period**. These activities tend to increase gastric secretions and salivation, which prevents proper coating of the barium to the gastric mucosa.

The upper GI series is often a time-consuming procedure so the patient should be forewarned of the time the examination may take when the appointment is made. This is especially true if the UGI is to be followed by a small bowel series. The importance of an empty stomach should also be stressed when the appointment is made so that the patient will arrive properly prepared both physically and psychologically.

Pregnancy Precautions

If the patient is a female, then a menstrual history must be obtained. Irradiation of an early pregnancy is one of the most hazardous situations in diagnostic radiography.

X-ray examinations such as the upper GI series that include the pelvis and uterus in the primary beam and which include fluoroscopy should only be done on pregnant females when absolutely necessary.

Any x-ray examination of the abdomen of a potentially pregnant female should be governed by the "**10-day rule**" as described in Chapter 1 (page 44) or by an elective booking policy wherein the benefits must outweigh the potential danger from radiation. In general, however, abdominal radiographs of a known pregnancy should be delayed at least until the third trimester, or if patient's condition allows as determined by the physician, until after the pregnancy. This is especially important if fluoroscopy, which greatly increases patient exposure, is involved.

Room Preparation

Responsibilities of the radiographer prior to the patient's arrival include setting up the room for fluoroscopy. Room setup for a UGI series is very similar to that for an esophagram. The thin barium sulfate mixture is the usual contrast medium necessary for an upper GI series. On occasion, thick barium may be used in addition to some type of gas-forming preparation. On rare occasions, water-soluble contrast media will be used in preference to the barium sulfate mixture.

The fluoroscopy table is raised to the vertical position, although with some very ill patients the exam must be started with the table horizontal. Therefore, the foot board should be placed at the end of the table. The room should be clean and tidy, and the control panel should be set for fluoroscopy. The spot film mechanism and the spot film camera should be properly loaded and in working condition. All cassettes for the entire exam should be provided. Lead aprons, lead gloves, and compression paddle should be provided for the radiologists, as well as lead aprons for all other personnel in the room. Any other equipment to be utilized during the examination should be readily accessible.

Prior to introduction of the patient and the radiologist, the examination procedure should be carefully explained to the patient and the patient's history should be obtained.

Patient Instructions

___ **I.V. CHOLANGIOGRAM AND/OR INTRAVENOUS PYELOGRAM**

1. Fleet's Prep Kit III - 24 hour prep. All instructions are contained in kit.

___ **BARIUM ENEMA**

1. Fleet's Prep Kit III - 24 hour prep. All instructions are contained in kit. May have a clear liquid breakfast.

___ **GALLBLADDER SERIES (ORAL CHOLECYSTOGRAM)**

1. Fat free supper evening before examination.
2. Take one Cholebrine tablet every 1/2 hour starting at 2:00 p.m. day before exam.
3. Nothing by mouth after midnight.

___ **UPPER G.I. SERIES AND/OR SMALL BOWEL SERIES**

1. Do not eat, drink, smoke or chew gum after midnight. Any antispasmodic medication should be preferably discontinued at least 24 hours before exam. Fleet's Prep Kit III may be purchased at most drug stores. Baptist Medical Center Pharmacy carries this kit along with Revco and Thrifty Drugs. Please call ahead to your pharmacy if you have any questions.

ULTRASOUND PREPS:

Ultrasound of the ABDOMEN: **Fat free clear** liquid diet from 6:00 p.m. the evening before examination.

Ultrasound of the PELVIS: **MUST** have a full bladder. Finish drinking 38 to 42 ounces of liquid one hour before exam. **DO NOT** empty bladder until after exam.

C.T. PREPS:

Abdomen - Clear liquids after midnight
Chest - Clear liquids only four hours prior to exam
Head - Clear liquids only four hours prior to exam
Pelvis - Clear liquids after midnight
Spine - no prep

Appointment date ______________ Appointment time ____________

Fig. 14-61. Sample patient instruction form.
(Courtesy of Phoenix Baptist Hospital and Medical Center, Phoenix, AZ.)

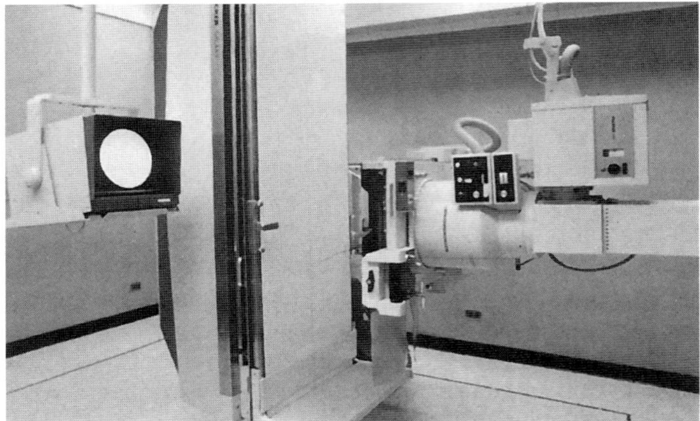

Fig. 14-62. Room preparation.

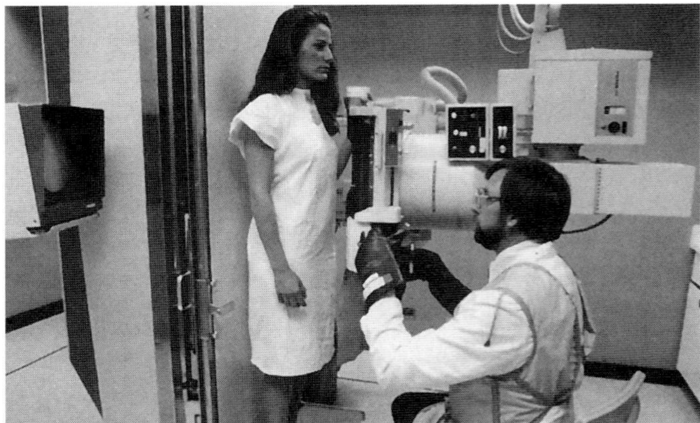

Fig. 14-63. Fluoroscopy.

General Routine Procedure

General duties during fluoroscopy for an upper GI series are similar to those for an esophagram. The radiographer should follow the radiologist's instructions, assist the patient as needed and expedite the procedure in any manner possible. The fluoroscopic routine followed by radiologists varies greatly. The general routine of each physician may also vary since each patient and each examination is different. The fluoroscopy routine is usually begun with the patient in the upright position. A wide variety of table moves, patient moves and special maneuvers follows until fluoroscopy is complete.

Table Moves

Since a large number of position changes are made during the fluoroscopic examination, the radiographer must help the patient with the barium cup, provide a pillow when the patient is lying down and keep the patient adequately covered at all times. The barium cup should be held by the patient in the left hand near the left shoulder whenever he (she) is upright. The cup must be taken from the patient when the table is tilted up or down.

Part of the technologist's responsibility is to watch the patient's hands and fingers during table movements. Sometimes holding onto the edge of the table can result in pinched fingers. The radiologist is occupied watching the fluoro screen or the monitor during these moves and doesn't see the patient's hands.

Patient Moves

Various patient moves combined with table moves are made during the fluoroscopic procedure. The right anterior oblique position, illustrated in Fig. 14-65, allows barium to migrate toward the pyloric portion or distal stomach, while any air in the stomach will shift toward the fundus.

Post Fluoroscopy Routines

Following fluoroscopy, certain routine positions or projections are obtained to further document any tentative diagnosis concluded fluoroscopically. These overhead radiographs, such as the RAO shown being positioned in Fig. 14-66, must be obtained immediately following fluoroscopy, before too much of the barium meal has passed into the jejunum (second part of small intestine).

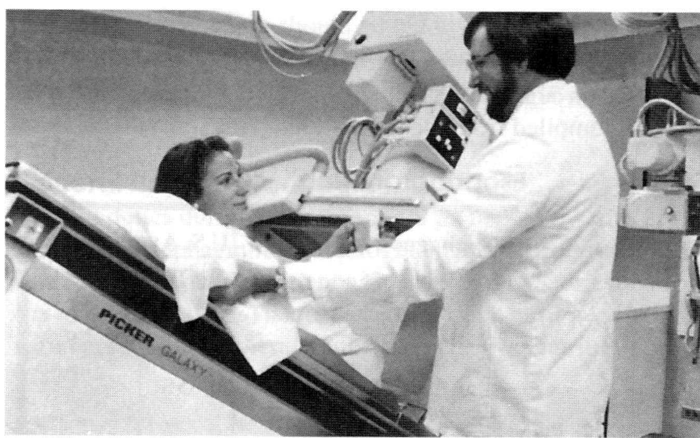

Fig. 14-64. Table moves.

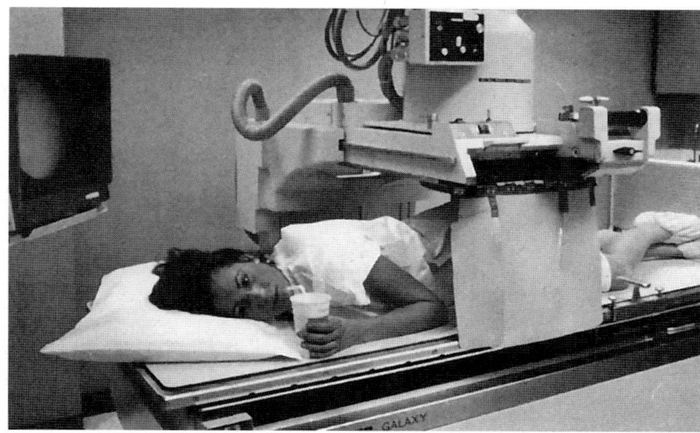

Fig. 14-65. Patient moves.

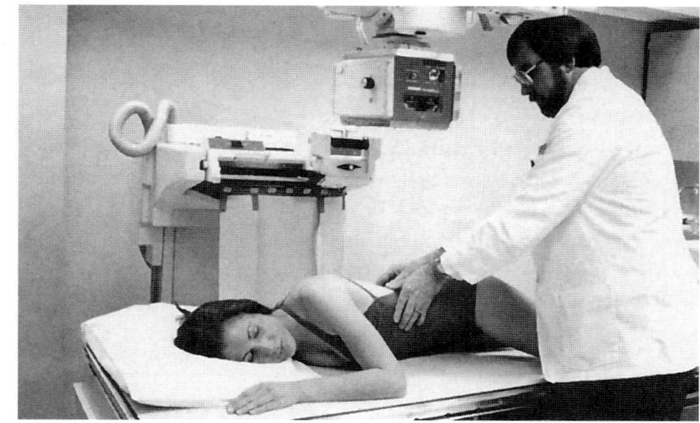
Fig. 14-66. RAO positioning.

SUMMARY OF POSITIONING TIPS FOR UPPER GI EXAMINATIONS

(1) Clinical History: Gain clinical history from the patient or his chart to determine clinical indications for the study and any past or recent abdominal surgery of the GI tract. Surgery or resection of the bowel or stomach will alter its normal position. Pay close attention to the fluoro monitor to detect such differences, which may affect positioning and centering on the post fluoroscopy filming.

Review the patient's chart to ensure that the correct procedure has been ordered. Also identify specific allergies and determine other pertinent information.

(2) Body Habitus: Consider the body habitus of the patient. Remember, the stomach will be high and transverse with the hypersthenic patient and low and vertical with the hyposthenic patient. The sthenic or average patient will have the duodenum bulb near the L2 region. Usually, L2 is located 1 to 2 in. (2.5 to 5 cm) above the lower lateral rib cage margin. Centering points in this text are designed for the average sthenic patient.

(3) Fluoroscopy: During fluoroscopy, identify the stomach on the fluoro monitor. Pinpoint surrounding structures to gain clues about location of the stomach and duodenum. For example , if the body of the stomach is adjacent to the iliac wing, then you need to center lower than the average or sthenic patient.

(4) High kVp and short exposure time: High kVp of 100 to 125 is required to penetrate adequately to provide high contrast of barium filled structures. Short exposure times are needed to control peristaltic motion.

Radiographic Positioning

NATIONAL SURVEY

A survey of the operating procedures (department routines) was conducted throughout the United States. The following information was compiled from the survey indicating the national norm for basic and special positions for esophagrams and upper GI exams. The survey results were very consistent throughout all regions of the United States.

Esophagram Routine

Esophagus	U.S. Average Basic 1995 (1989)	U.S. Average Special 1995 (1989)
• RAO	87% (88%)	
• Left lateral	65% (55%)	
• AP	59% (48%)	
• PA	32% (30%)	
• LAO	44% –	13% (14%)

Upper GI Routine

Stomach and Duodenum	U.S. Average Basic 1995 (1989)	U.S. Average Special 1995 (1989)
• AP scout (supine)	54% –	
• RAO (recumbent)	89% (93%)	
• PA (recumbent)	79% (85%)	
• Right lateral (recumbent)	82% (80%)	
• LPO (recumbent)	59% (55%)	19% (14%)
• AP (recumbent)	63% (50%)	19% (10%)
• AP (Trendelenburg)		20% –
• Dorsal decubitus		15% –
• Double-contrast techniques*	– (62%)	– (13%)

*Double-contrast techniques involve the use of both positive (barium sulfate) and negative (usually carbon dioxide gas) contrast media.

Summary

Upper GI Routine: The **AP scout** projection for an upper GI series is commonly taken throughout the U.S. by ≈54% of the responding institutions. Positioning would be similar to an AP abdomen as described in Chapter 3.

The **dorsal decubitus** is indicated to be used as a special projection by only 15% of institutions and therefore is not included as a separate projection in the positioning pages of this chapter. The **Trendelenburg** position is demonstrated as an alternate for the AP recumbent position (see page 444).

The **double-contrast technique** for the upper GI is a common procedure as indicated on the survey conducted in 1989. This question was not included in the 1995 survey but the results are presumed to be similar. This procedure is described on page 424 under radiographic procedures, but is not specifically described in the positioning pages which follow. Generally the double contrast positioning routines are similar to the regular single-contrast upper GI, with the only difference being the exposure techniques as described.

Basic and Special Projections

Certain basic and special positions or projections of the esophagus, stomach and duodenum are described and demonstrated on the following pages. The five projections for the upper GI series are listed in order of suggested clinical usefulness. While the routine of each radiologist or other clinical specialist may vary, the RAO and PA are considered a **minimum** series. The routine may also include other projections in addition to these five.

Esophagram
(barium swallow)
Basic
• RAO (35-40°) **435**
• Lateral **436**
• AP (PA) **437**
Special
• LAO **438**
• Soft tissue lateral **439**

Upper GI series
Basic
• RAO (recumbent) **440**
• PA (recumbent) **441**
• Right lateral (recumbent) **442**
• LPO (recumbent) **443**
• AP (recumbent) **444**

RAO Position

Esophagram
Basic
- **RAO** (35-40°)
- Lateral
- AP (PA)

Structures Best Shown

Esophagus between the vertebral column and heart. (RAO provides more visibility of pertinent anatomy between vertebrae and heart than does the LAO).

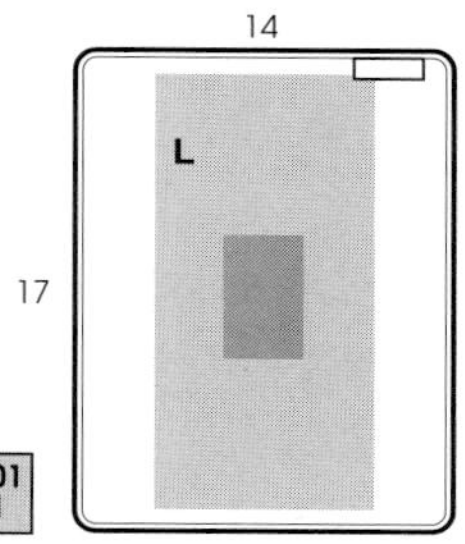

Technical Factors

- Film size–14 x 17 in. (35 x 43 cm), lengthwise.
- Moving or stationary grid.
- 100-125 kVp range.
- Technique and dose:

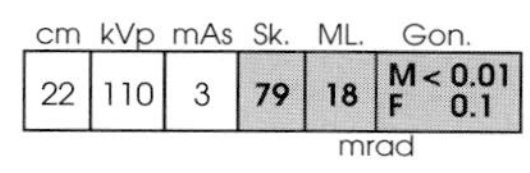

cm	kVp	mAs	Sk.	ML.	Gon.
22	110	3	79	18	M< 0.01 F 0.1

mrad

Shielding: Place lead shield over patient's pelvic region to protect gonads.

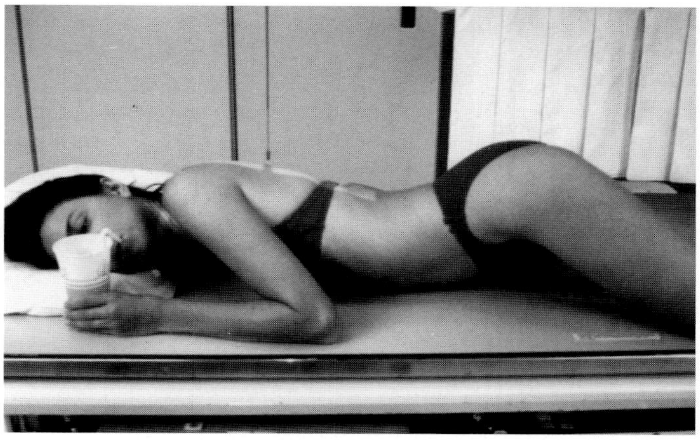

Fig. 14-67. 35 to 40° RAO–Recumbent.

Patient Position

- Recumbent or erect. Recumbent preferred because of more complete filling of esophagus (due to gravity factor with erect).

Part Position

- Rotate **35 to 40°** from a prone position with the right anterior body against film holder or table.
- Right arm down; left arm flexed at elbow and up by the patient's head, holding cup of barium, straw in patient's mouth.
- Flex left knee for support.
- Align midline of thorax in the oblique position to midline of film holder and/or table.
- Top of cassette about 2 in. (5 cm) above level of shoulders to place center of film at CR.

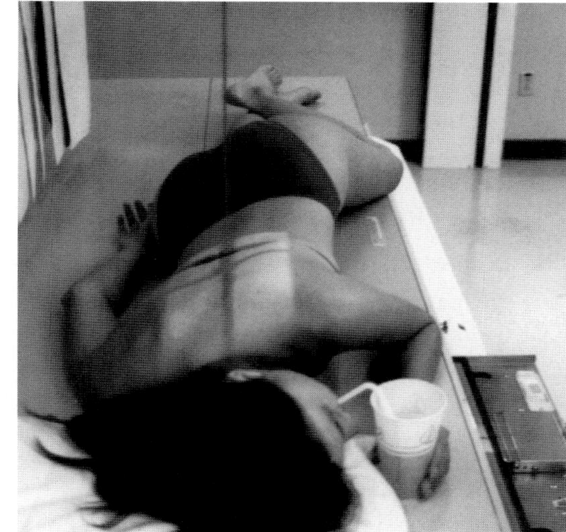

Fig. 14-68. RAO–Recumbent (demonstrates front-to-back centering).

Central Ray

- CR **perpendicular** to film holder.
- CR to center of cassette at **level of T5 or T6** (2 to 3 in. or 5 to 7.5 cm inferior to jugular notch).
- Minimum 40 in. (102 cm) SID; or 72 in. (183 cm) if erect.

Collimation: Collimate the lateral borders to create two-sided collimation about 5 or 6 in. (12 to 15 cm) wide. Collimate end borders to film margins with L or R placed within collimation field.

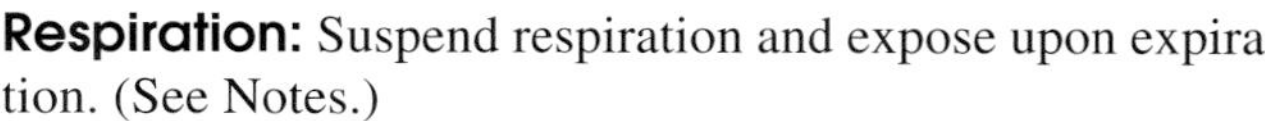

Respiration: Suspend respiration and expose upon expiration. (See Notes.)

Notes: **Thick barium**–Two or three spoonfuls of thick barium should be ingested and the exposure made immediately after last bolus is swallowed. (Patient will not be breathing immediately after a swallow.)

Thin barium–For complete filling of the esophagus using thin barium, it may be necessary for the patient to drink through a straw with continuous swallowing and exposure made after three or four swallows without suspending respiration (use as short exposure time as possible).

Evaluation Criteria

- Esophagus seen midway between heart and T spine.
- Upper limbs should not superimpose the esophagus.
- Entire esophagus is filled or lined with contrast media.
- Appropriate technique employed to clearly visualize borders of the contrast media filled esophagus.

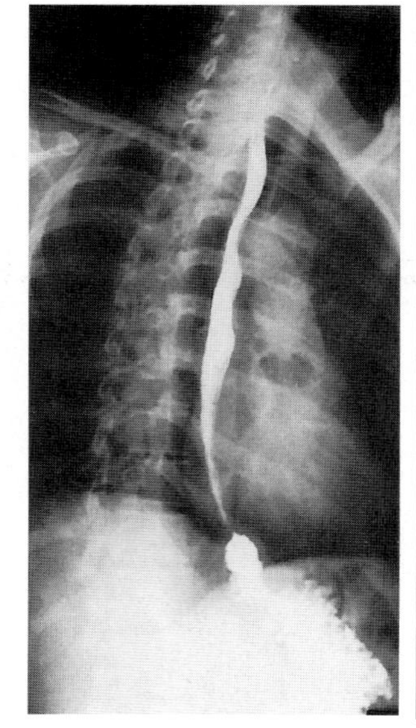

Fig. 14-69. RAO.

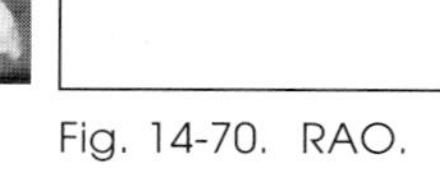

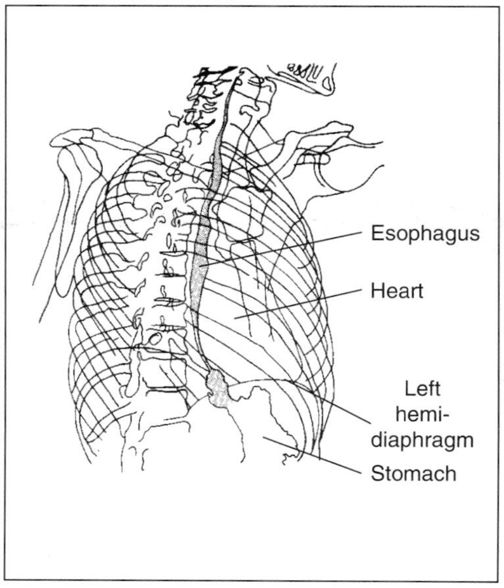

Fig. 14-70. RAO.

Lateral Position

Esophagram
Basic
• RAO (35-40°)
• **Lateral**
• AP (PA)

Structures Best Shown

Esophagus between the vertebral column and heart.

Technical Factors

- Film size–14 x 17 in. (35 x 43 cm), lengthwise.
- Moving or stationary grid.
- 100-125 kVp range.
- Technique and dose:

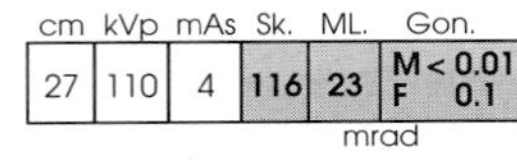

cm	kVp	mAs	Sk.	ML.	Gon.
27	110	4	116	23	M < 0.01 F 0.1

mrad

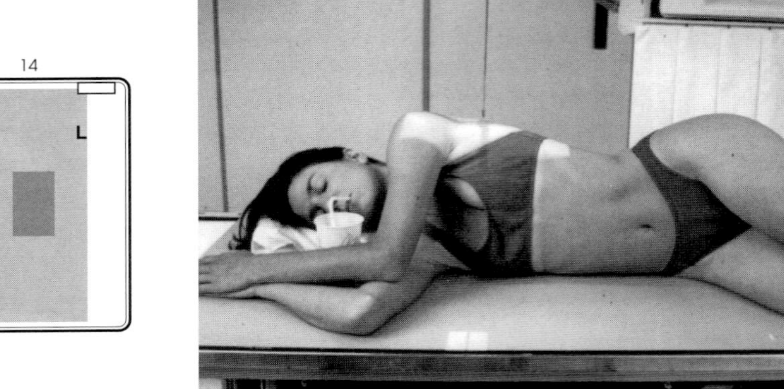

Fig. 14-71. Right lateral–Arms up.

Shielding: Lead shield over gonadal area.

Patient Position

- Recumbent or erect (recumbent preferred).

Part Position 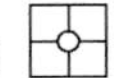

- Arms placed over the head with the elbows flexed and superimposed.
- Align **midcoronal plane to midline** of film holder and/or table.
- Shoulders and hips in a true lateral position.
- Top of cassette about 2 in. (5 cm) above level of shoulders, to place center of film at CR.

Central Ray

- CR **perpendicular** to film holder.
- CR to **level of T5 or T6** (2 to 3 in. or 5 to 7.5 cm inferior to jugular notch).
- Minimum 40 in. (102 cm) SID; or 72 in. (183 cm) if erect.

Collimation: Collimate along the lateral borders to create two-sided collimation about 5 or 6 in. (12 to 15 cm) wide.

Respiration: Suspend respiration and expose upon expiration (see Note).

Note: See preceding page for barium swallow instructions.

Optional swimmer's lateral (Fig. 14-72): Allows for better demonstration of the upper esophagus without superimposition of arms and shoulders.

Patient holds cup of barium while swallowing during or immediately before exposure.

Position hips and shoulders in true lateral position, then separate shoulders from esophagus region by placing top shoulder down with arm behind back. Downside shoulder and arm up and in front to hold cup of barium.

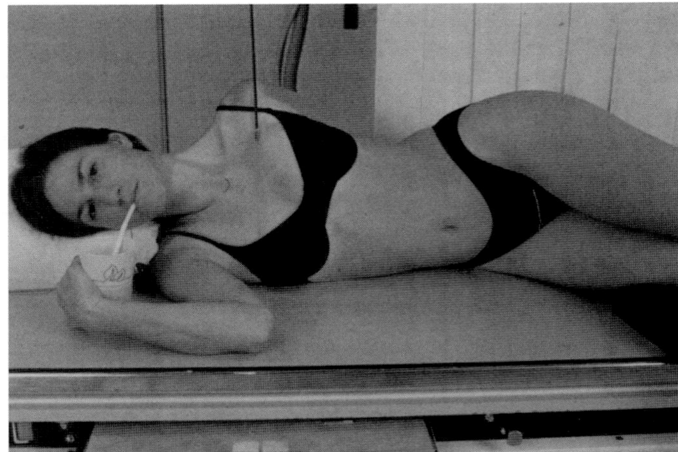

Fig. 14-72. Optional; swimmer's lateral for better visualization of upper esophagus.

Evaluation Criteria

- Esophagus seen between thoracic spine and heart.
- True lateral as indicated by direct superimposition of posterior ribs.
- The patient's arms should not superimpose the esophagus.
- Entire esophagus is filled or lined with contrast media.
- Appropriate technique employed to clearly visualize borders of the contrast media filled esophagus.

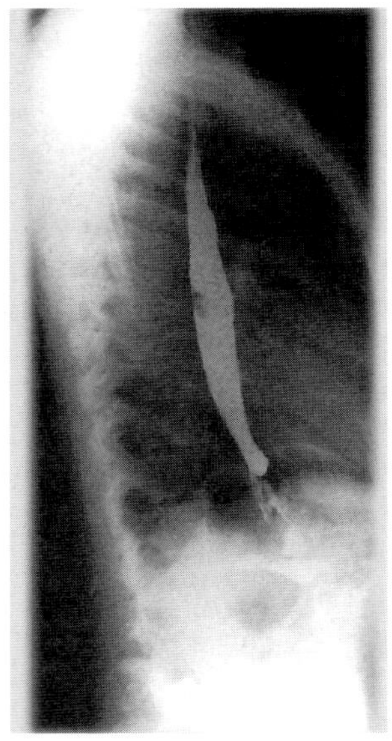

Fig. 14-73. Lateral –Arms up.

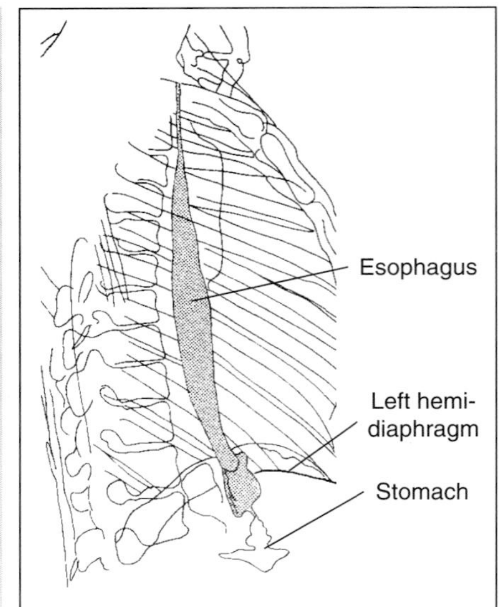

Fig. 14-74. Lateral.

14

AP (PA) Projection

Esophagram
Basic
- RAO (35-40°)
- Lateral
- **AP (PA)**

Structures Best Shown

A frontal image of the esophagus, the majority of which is superimposed over the thoracic vertebrae.

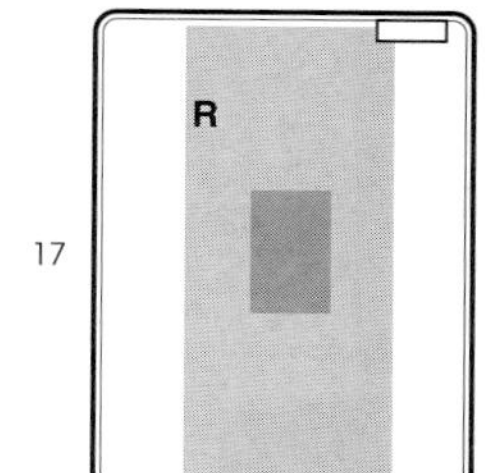

Technical Factors

- Film size–14 x 17 in. (35 x 43 cm), lengthwise.
- Moving or stationary grid.
- 100-125 kVp range.
- Technique and dose:

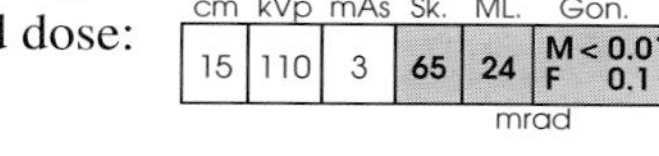

cm	kVp	mAs	Sk.	ML.	Gon.
15	110	3	65	24	M < 0.01 F 0.1
				mrad	

Shielding: Place lead shield over patient's pelvic region to shield gonads.

Patient Position

- Recumbent or erect (recumbent preferred).

Part Position

- Align **midsagittal plane to midline** of film holder and/or table.
- Ensure shoulders and hips are **not rotated**.
- Right arm up to hold cup of barium.
- Top of cassette about 2 in. (5 cm) above top of shoulder, to place CR at center of film.

Central Ray

- CR **perpendicular** to film holder.
- CR to midsagittal plane, **1 in**. (2.5 cm) **inferior** to **sternal angle** (T5-6) or approximately 3 in (7.5 cm) inferior to jugular notch.
- Minimum 40 in. (102 cm); or 72 in. (183 cm) SID if erect.

Collimation: Use tight side collimation to result in about 5 or 6 in. (12 to 15 cm) wide collimation field. Collimate end borders to film margins.

Respiration: Suspend respiration and expose upon expiration.

Alternate PA: This can also be taken as a PA projection with similar positioning, centering and CR locations.

Notes: Two or three spoonfuls of thick barium should be ingested and the exposure made immediately after last bolus is swallowed. (Patient will not be breathing immediately after a swallow.)

For complete filling of the esophagus using thin barium, it may be necessary for the patient to drink through a straw with continuous swallowing and exposure made after three or four swallows without suspending respiration.

Evaluation Criteria

- The entire esophagus is filled with barium.
- No rotation of the patient's body evidenced by the symmetry of the sternoclavicular (SC) joints.
- Appropriate technique utilized to visualize the esophagus through the superimposed thoracic vertebrae.

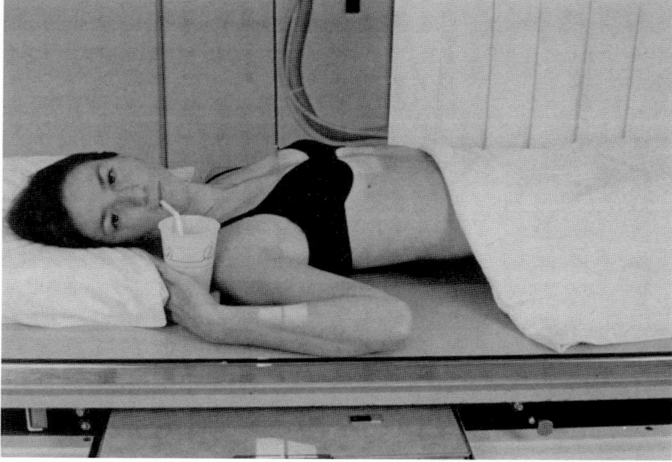

Fig. 14-75. Recumbent AP.

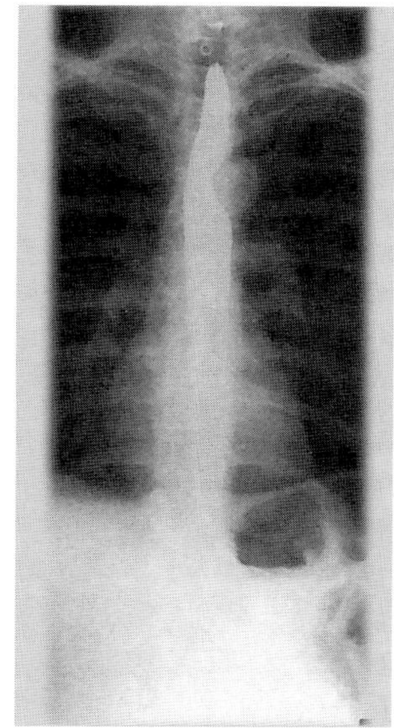

Fig. 14-76. AP.

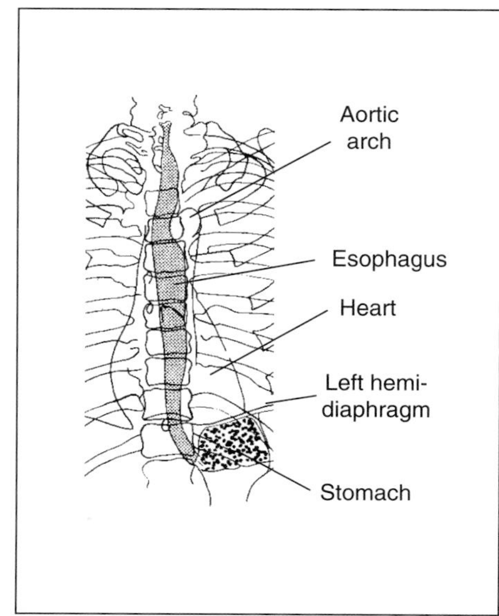

Fig. 14-77. AP.

LAO Position

Esophagram
Special
• **LAO**
• Soft tissue lateral

Structures Best Shown

Esophagus between the vertebral column and hilar region.

Technical Factors

- Film size–14 x 17 in. (35 x 43 cm), lengthwise.
- Moving or stationary grid.
- 100-125 kVp range.
- Technique and dose:

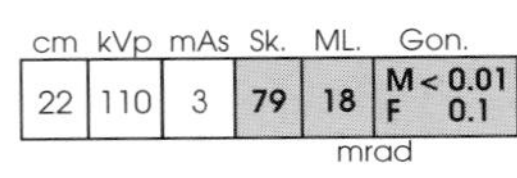

cm	kVp	mAs	Sk.	ML.	Gon.
22	110	3	79	18	M < 0.01 F 0.1

mrad

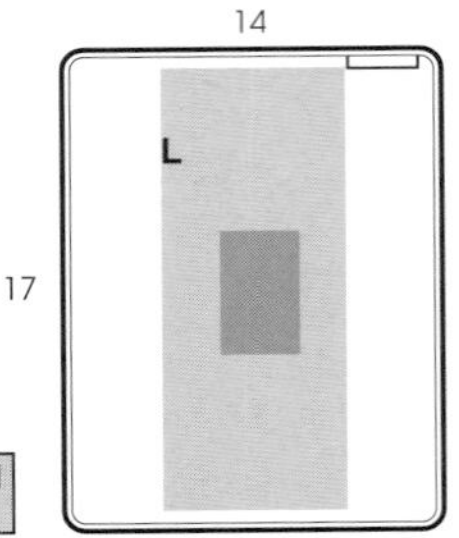

Shielding: Place lead shield over gonadal area.

Patient Position

- Recumbent or erect (recumbent preferred).

Part Position

- Rotate **35 to 40**° from a PA with the left anterior body against film holder or table.
- Left arm down by the patient's side, right arm flexed at elbow and up by the patient's head.
- Flex right knee for support.
- Top of cassette about 2 in. (5 cm) above level of shoulders, to place CR at center of film.

Central Ray

- CR **perpendicular** to film holder.
- CR to level of **T5** or **T6** (2 to 3 in. or 5 to 7.5 cm inferior to jugular notch).
- Minimum 40 in. (102 cm); or 72 in. (183 cm) SID if erect.

Collimation: Collimate lateral borders to create two-sided collimation about 5 or 6 in. (12 to 15 cm) wide. Collimate end borders to film margins.

Respiration: Suspend respiration and expose upon expiration.

Notes: Thick barium–Two or three spoonfuls of thick barium should be ingested and the exposure made immediately after last bolus is swallowed. (Patient will not be breathing immediately after a swallow.)

Thin barium–For complete filling of the esophagus using thin barium, it may be necessary for the patient to drink through a straw with continuous swallowing and exposure made after three or four swallows without suspending respiration (use as short an exposure time as possible).

Evaluation Criteria

- Esophagus seen between hilar region of lungs and thoracic spine.
- The patient's upper limbs should not superimpose the esophagus.
- The entire esophagus is filled with contrast medium.
- Appropriate technique employed to clearly visualize borders of the contrast media-filled esophagus.

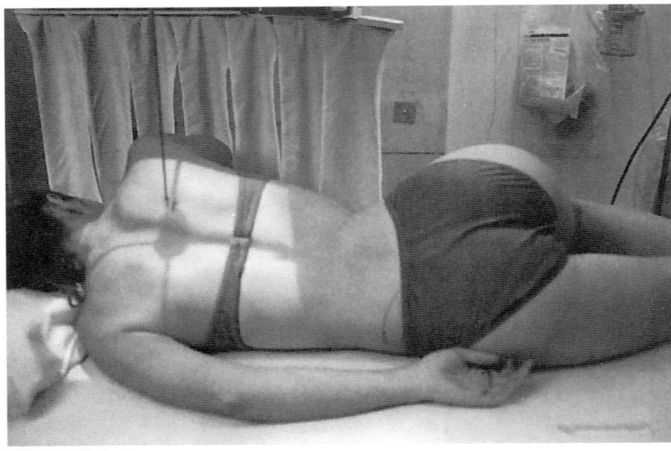

Fig. 14-78. Recumbent LAO.

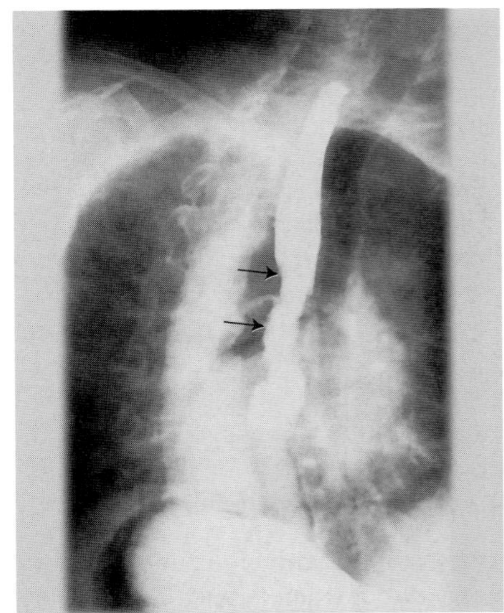

Fig. 14-79. LAO. (Demonstrates a constricted area of esophagus, probably carcinoma, see arrows.)

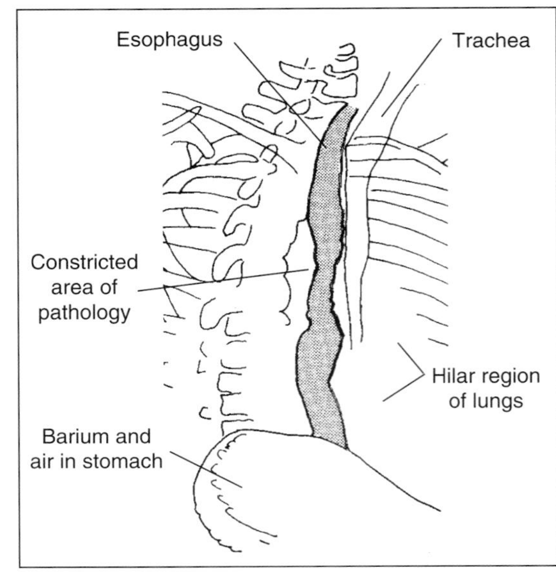

Fig. 14-80. LAO.

14

Soft Tissue Lateral Position

Esophagram
Special
• LAO
• Soft tissue lateral

Structures Best Shown

Laryngopharynx, larynx, upper esophagus and upper trachea, good for demonstrating small foreign bodies in the larynx or upper esophagus.

Technical Factors

• Film size–10 x 12 in. (24 x 30 cm), lengthwise.
• Moving or stationary grid.
• 60-70 kVp range.
• Short exposure time and small focal spot.
• Technique and dose:

cm	kVp	mAs	Sk.	ML.	Thyroid
15	80	6	**18**	**8**	**12**

mrad

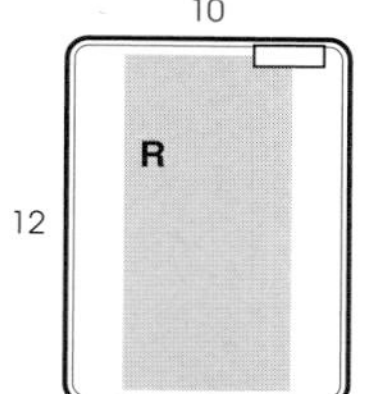

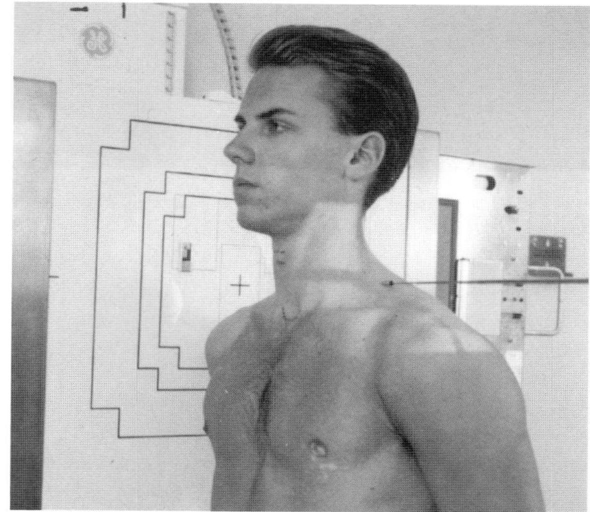
Fig. 14-81. Soft tissue lateral.

Patient Position

• Erect if possible, seated or standing with arms down by side, shoulders pulled back in a lateral position.

Part Position 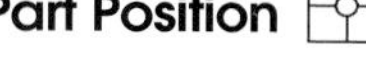

• Shoulders depressed and back as much as possible.
• Extend chin to remove ramus of mandible away from the laryngopharynx area.
• Adjust film height to place top of cassette at about the level of EAM (external auditory meatus), centered to CR.
• Position patient to center proximal airway and esophagus to CR and center of film. (Proximal airway and esophagus lie anterior to cervical vertebrae.)

Central Ray

• CR **perpendicular** to film holder.
• Center to **level of inferior margin of laryngeal prominence** (C6).
• Minimum 72 in. (183 cm) SID if possible to minimize magnification and increase definition.

Collimation: Closely collimate along the anteroposterior borders of the proximal airway and esophagus.

Respiration: See Notes.

Notes: Exposure should be made during a slow deep inspiration to ensure filling trachea and proximal airway with air to distinguish trachea from esophagus.

In case of radiolucent foreign bodies, additional material such as shredded cotton soaked in barium is swallowed. Expose after last bolus of contrast medium is swallowed.

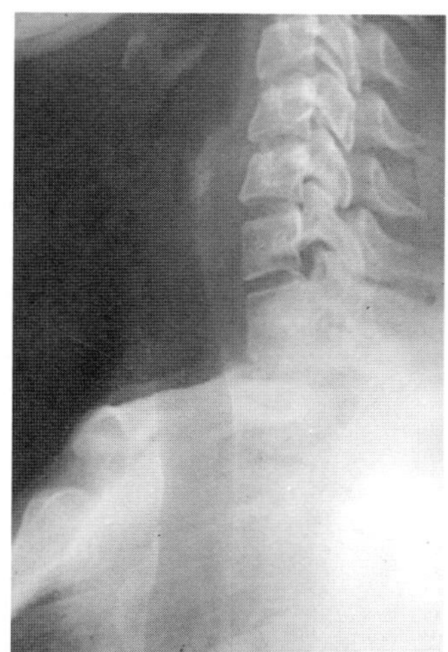
Fig. 14-82a. Soft tissue lateral. (Larynx and trachea visualized) (65 to 70 kVp range)

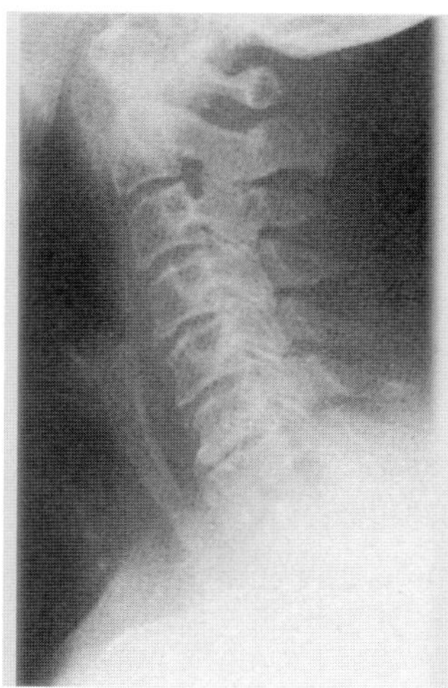
Fig. 14-82b. Soft tissue lateral. (Larynx and esophagus visualized) (70 t0 80 kVp range)

Evaluation Criteria

• The entire proximal airway and esophagus is filled with contrast media (with barium and/or air).
• No rotation of the cervical spine.
• Ramus of mandible not superimposed over proximal airway.
• Appropriate technique utilized to demonstrate the soft tissues of the pharynx and proximal esophagus. (Margins of the air-filled proximal airway should be visible.)

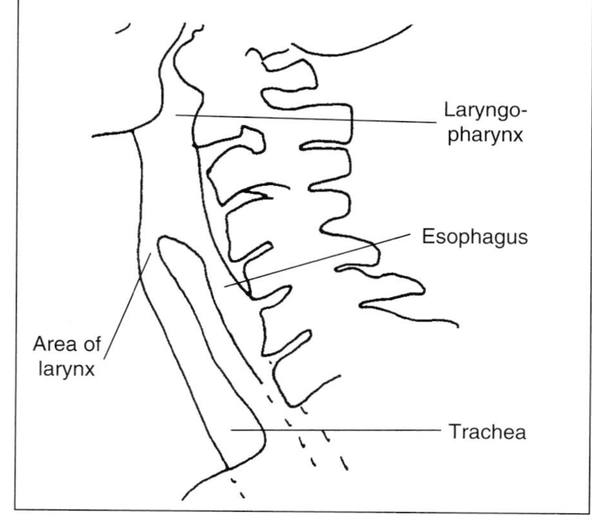

Fig. 14-83. Lateral.

RAO Position

Upper GI Series
Basic
• **RAO**
• PA
• Right lateral
• LPO
• AP

Structures Best Shown

Pylorus of stomach and C-loop of the duodenum. A profile image of the duodenal bulb.

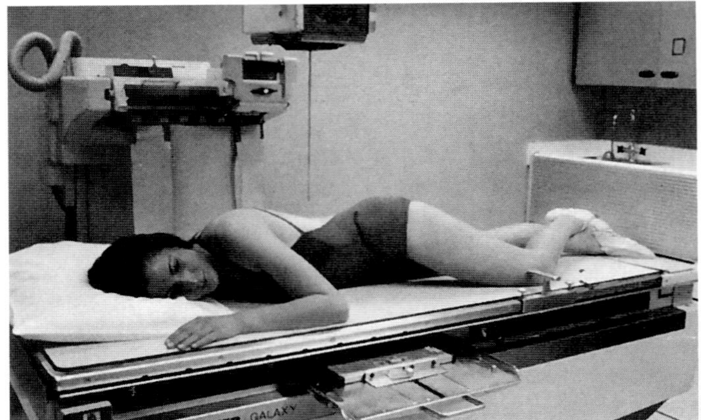

Fig. 14-84. RAO.

Technical Factors

10 (11)
12 (14)
R

- Film size–10 x 12 in. (24 x 30 cm), lengthwise.
  or –11 x 14 in. (30 x 35 cm).
- Moving or stationary grid.
- 100-125 kVp range.
  (80-100 kVp for double-contrast study.)
- Technique and dose:

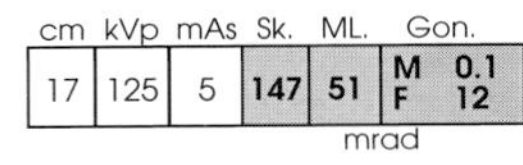

cm	kVp	mAs	Sk.	ML.	Gon.
17	125	5	147	51	M 0.1 F 12

mrad

Shielding: Place lead shield over patient's pelvic region to protect gonads **without covering pertinent anatomy**.

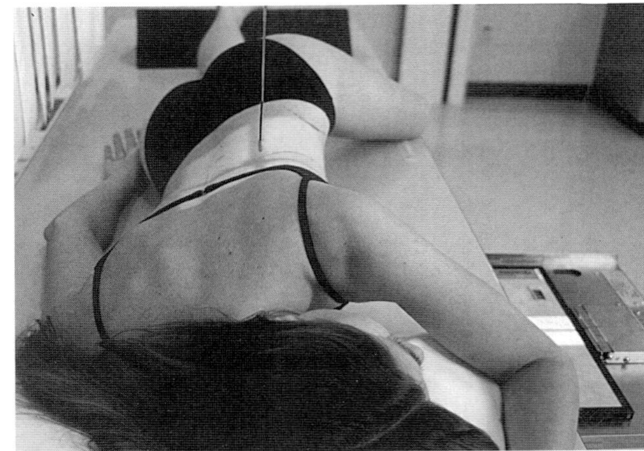

Fig. 14-85. RAO.

Patient Position

- Recumbent with the body partially rotated into a RAO position, provide pillow for head.

Part Position 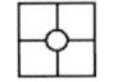

- From a prone position rotate **40 to 70°** with right anterior body against film holder or table (more rotation may be required for heavy hypersthenic-type patients and less for thin-asthenic type).
- Right arm down, left arm flexed at elbow and up by the patient's head.
- Flex left knee for support.

Central Ray

- CR **perpendicular** to film holder.
  Average Body Type:
- Center CR and film to duodenal bulb at **level of L2** (1 to 2 in. or 2.5 to 5 cm above lower lateral rib margin), **midway between spine and lateral border of abdomen**. (See Note for body variations.)
- Center cassette to CR.
- Minimum 40 in. (102 cm) SID.

Collimation: Collimate on four sides to outer margins of film, or to area of interest on larger film.

Respiration: Suspend respiration and expose upon expiration.

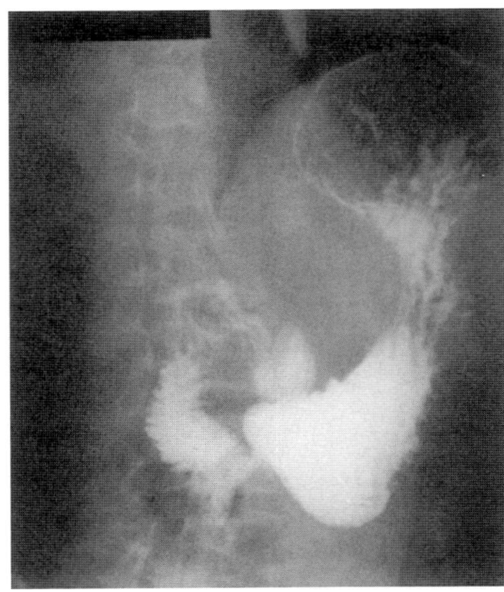

Fig. 14-86. RAO.

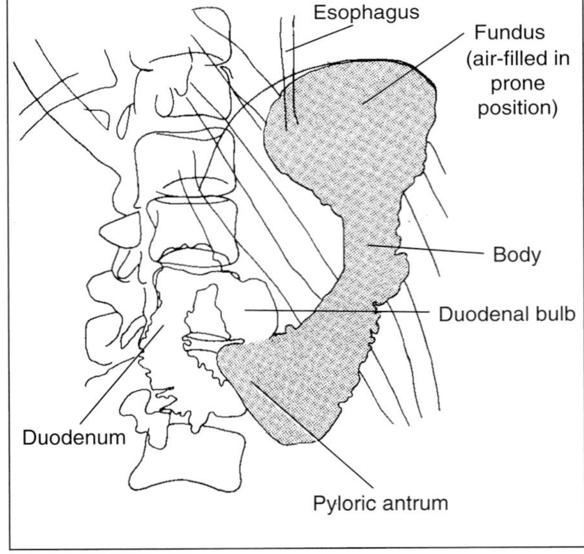

Fig. 14-87. RAO.

Evaluation Criteria

- Entire stomach and C-loop of duodenum is visualized.
- Body and pylorus of stomach is filled with contrast medium.
- Duodenal bulb is in profile.
- Appropriate technique employed to clearly visualize the gastric folds without overexposing other pertinent anatomy.

PA Projection

Upper GI Series
Basic
• RAO
• **PA**
• Right lateral
• LPO
• AP

Structures Best Shown

Stomach and duodenum with barium in the body and pylorus of the stomach.

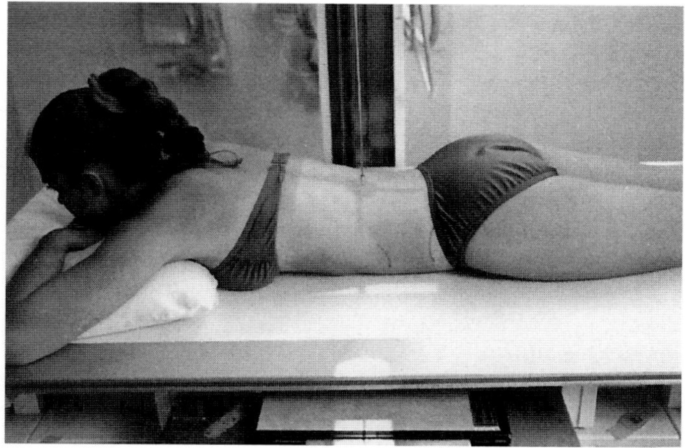

Fig. 14-88. PA.

Technical Factors

- Film size–10 x 12 in. (24 x 30 cm), lengthwise.
  or –11 x 14 in. (30 x 35 cm)
  or –14 x 17 in. (35 x 43 cm) if small bowel is to be included.
- Moving or stationary grid.
- 100 to 125 kVp range.
  (80-100 kVp range for double-contrast study)
- Technique and dose:

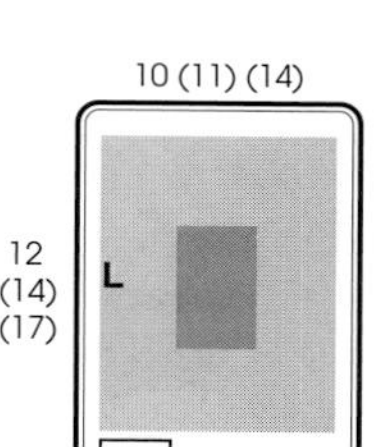

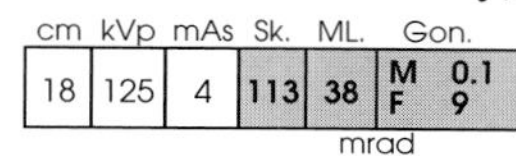

cm	kVp	mAs	Sk.	ML.	Gon.
18	125	4	113	38	M 0.1 F 9

mrad

Shielding: Place lead shield over patient's pelvic region to protect gonads **without covering pertinent anatomy**.

Patient Position

- Patient prone with arms up beside head, provide pillow.

Part Position

- Align midsagittal plane to CR and to table.
- Ensure there is **no body rotation**.

Central Ray

- CR **perpendicular** to film holder.
- ***Average Body Type:*** Center CR and film to level of pylorus and duodenal bulb at **level of L2** (which is 1 to 2 in. or 2.5 to 5 cm above lower lateral rib margin) and about **1 in. (2.5 cm) left of the vertebral column**.
  Asthenic: Center about 2 in. or 5 cm lower .
  Hypersthenic: Center about 2 in. or 5 cm higher and nearer midline.
- Center cassette to CR.
- Minimum 40 in. (102 cm) SID.

Collimation: Collimate on four sides to outer margins of film, or to area of interest on a larger film.

Respiration: Suspend respiration and expose upon expiration.

Alternate PA axial: The position of the high transverse stomach on a **hypersthenic** type patient causes almost an end on view with much overlapping of the pyloric region of the stomach and the duodenal bulb with a 90° PA projection. Therefore, a **35 to 45° cephalad angle** of the central ray separates these areas for better visualization. The greater and lesser curvatures of the stomach are also better visualized in profile.

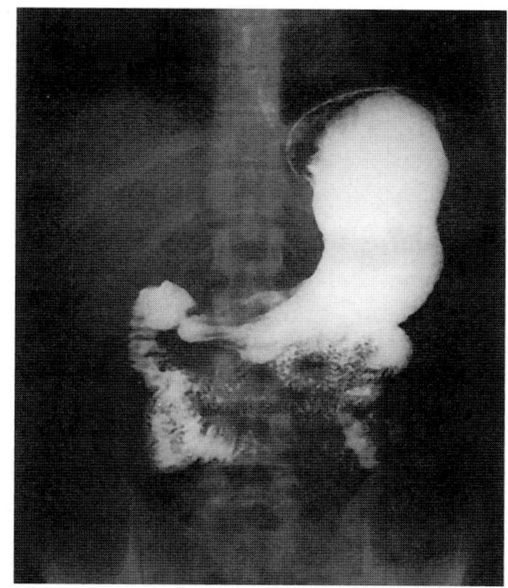

Fig. 14-89. PA.

Evaluation Criteria

- Entire stomach and duodenum are visualized.
- Pylorus region is near center of film.
- Body and pylorus of the stomach is filled with barium.
- Appropriate technique employed to visualize the gastric folds without overexposing other pertinent anatomy.

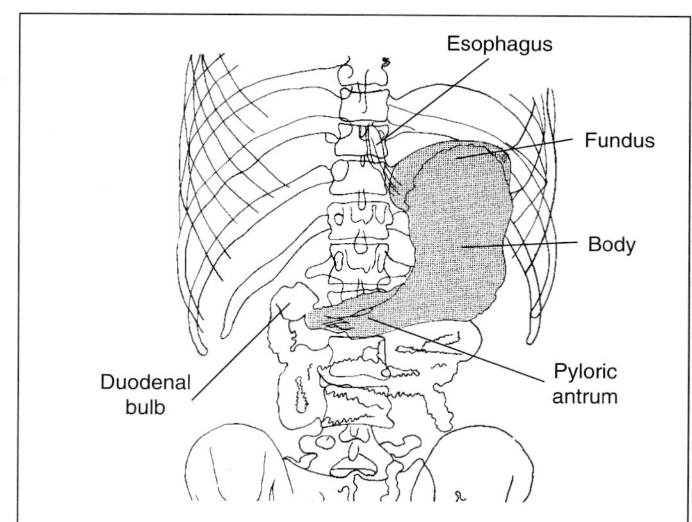

Fig. 14-90. PA.

Right Lateral Position

Upper GI Series
Basic
- RAO
- PA
- **Right lateral**
- LPO
- AP

Structures Best Shown

Stomach and duodenum with a view of the retrogastric space with barium primarily in mid and distal stomach and duodenum.

Technical Factors

- Film size–10 x 12 in. (24 x 30 cm), lengthwise.
  or –11 x 14 in. (30 x 35 cm)
- Moving or stationary grid.
- 100 to 125 kVp range.
  (80-100 kVp range for double-contrast study)
- Technique and dose:

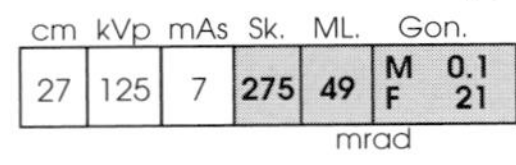

cm	kVp	mAs	Sk.	ML.	Gon.
27	125	7	275	49	M 0.1 F 21

mrad

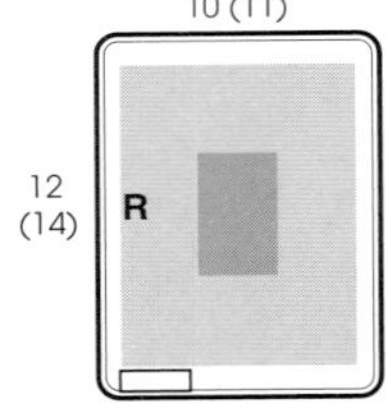

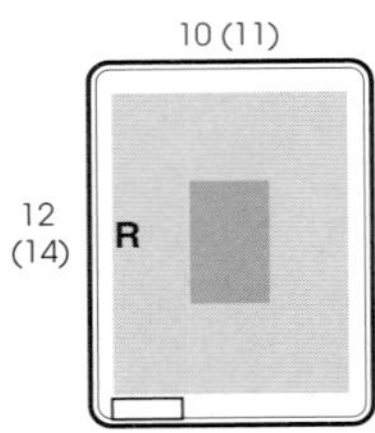

Fig. 14-91. Right lateral.

Shielding: Place lead shield over patient's pelvic region to protect gonads **without covering pertinent anatomy**.

Patient Position

- Recumbent in a right lateral position. Provide pillow for head. Arms up by the patient's head and knees flexed.

Part Position

- Ensure shoulders and hips are in a true lateral position.
- Center of cassette at CR.
  (Bottom of cassette should be about at level of iliac crest.)

Central Ray

- CR **perpendicular** to film holder.
- ***For Average Body Type:*** Center CR and film to duodenal bulb at level of **L1** (level of lower lateral margin of ribs) and **1 to 1½ in. or 2.5 to 4 cm anterior to midcoronal plane** (near midway between anterior border of vertebrae and the anterior abdomen).
  Hypersthenic: Center about 2 in. or 5 cm higher.
  Asthenic: Center about 2 in. or 5 cm lower.
- Minimum 40 in. (102 cm) SID.

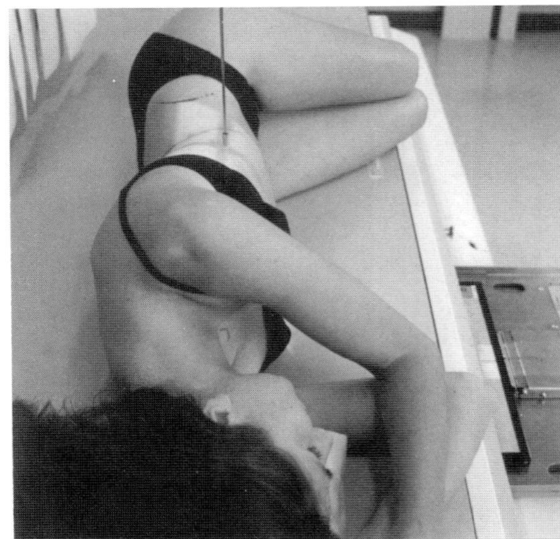

Fig. 14-92. Right lateral.

Collimation: Collimate on four sides to outer margins of film, or to area of interest on larger film.

Respiration: Suspend respiration and expose upon expiration.

Note: Stomach generally is located about one vertebra higher in this position than in PA or oblique positions.

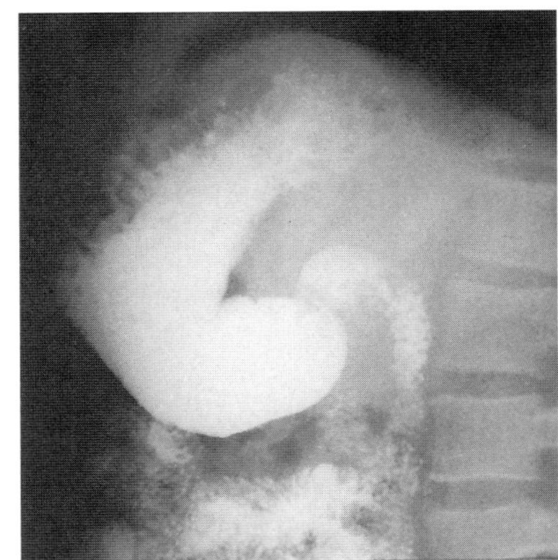

Fig. 14-93. Right lateral.

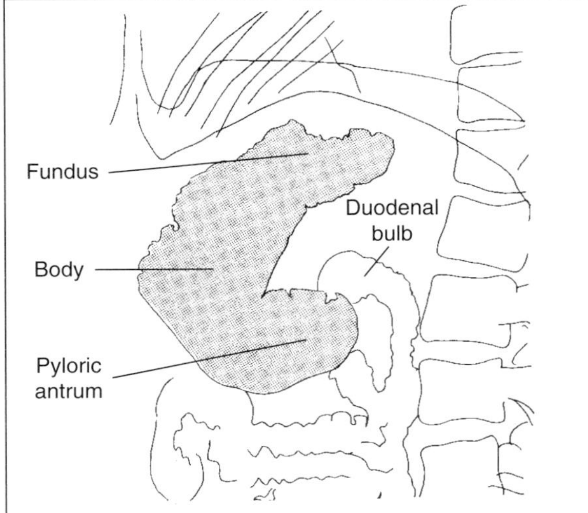

Fig. 14-94. Right lateral.

Evaluation Criteria

- Entire stomach and duodenum are visualized.
- Demonstration of the retrogastric space.
- Pylorus of stomach and C-loop of duodenum should be visualized well on hypersthenic type patients.
- Vertebral bodies should be seen for reference purposes. The intervertebral foramen should be open indicating a true lateral position.
- Appropriate technique employed to visualize the gastric folds without overexposing other pertinent anatomy.

LPO Position

Upper GI Series
Basic
• RAO
• PA
• Right lateral
• **LPO**
• AP

Structures Best Shown

Stomach with barium-filled body and fundus, with pylorus and duodenal bulb demonstrated with air-contrast in profile.

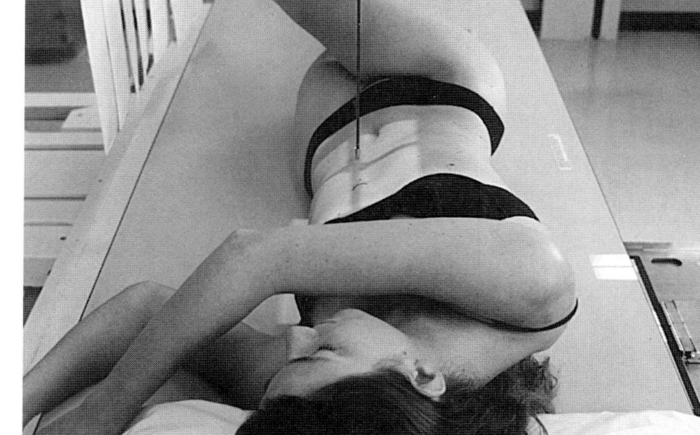

Fig. 14-95. LPO.

Technical Factors

- Film size–10 x 12 in. (24 x 30 cm), lengthwise.
  or –11 x 14 in. (30 x 35 cm)
- Moving or stationary grid.
- 100 to 125 kVp range.
  (80-100 kVp range for double-contrast study)
- Technique and dose:

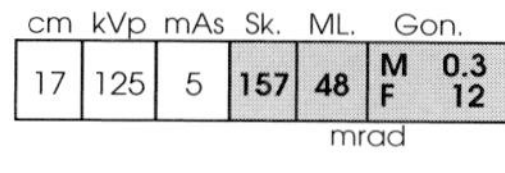

cm	kVp	mAs	Sk.	ML.	Gon.
17	125	5	157	48	M 0.3 F 12

mrad

10 (11)

12 (14)

L

Shielding: Place lead shield over patient's pelvic region to protect gonads without covering pertinent anatomy.

Patient Position

- Recumbent with the body partially rotated into a LPO position. Provide pillow for head.

Part Position

- Rotate **30 to 60°** from supine position with left posterior against film holder or table (more rotation may be required for heavy hypersthenic-type patients and less for thin-asthenic type).

- Flex right knee for support.
- Extend left arm away from body and raise right arm high across chest to grasp end of table for support (do not pinch fingers when moving Bucky).
- Center of cassette at CR.
  (Bottom of cassette should be about at level of iliac crest.)

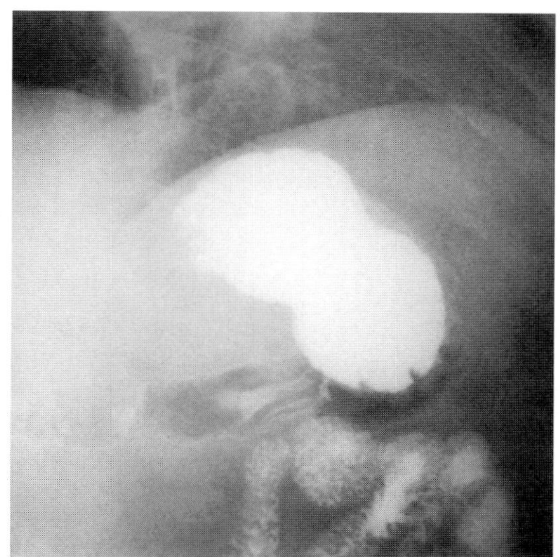

Fig. 14-96. LPO.

Central Ray

- CR **perpendicular** to film holder.
- ***Average Body Type:*** Center CR and film to **level of L1** (about midway between xiphoid tip and lower lateral margin of ribs), and **midway between midline of body** and **left lateral margin** of abdomen.
  Hypersthenic: Center about 2 in. or 5 cm higher
  Asthenic: About 2 in. or 5 cm lower and nearer to midline.
- Minimum 40 in. (102 cm) SID.

Collimation: Collimate on four sides to outer margins of film, or to area of interest on larger film.

Respiration: Suspend respiration and expose upon expiration.

Note: Stomach is generally located higher in this position than in the lateral; therefore, center one vertebra higher than on PA or RAO positions.

Evaluation Criteria

- Entire stomach and duodenum are visualized.
- An unobstructed view of the duodenal bulb without superimposition by the pylorus of the stomach.
- The fundus should be filled with barium.
- With a double-contrast procedure the body and pylorus and occasionally the duodenal bulb are air filled.
- Appropriate technique employed to visualize the gastric folds without overexposing other pertinent anatomy.

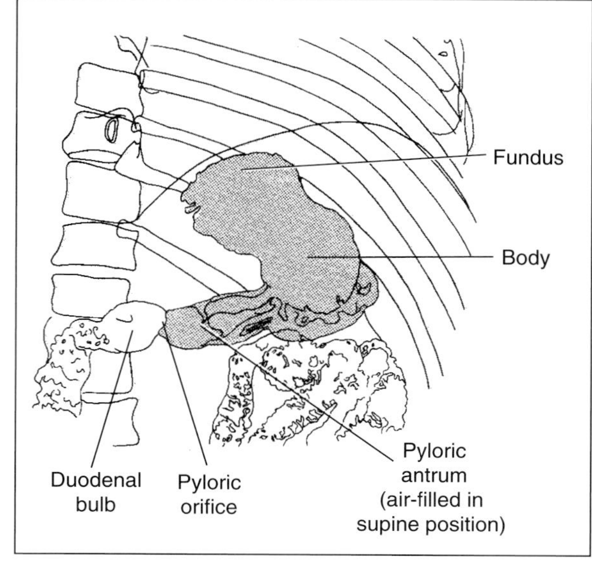

Fig. 14-97. LPO.

14

AP Projection

Upper GI Series
Basic
- RAO
- PA
- Right lateral
- LPO
- **AP**

Structures Best Shown

Fundus of stomach and duodenum with barium concentrated in the fundus of the stomach. Possible hiatal hernia may be demonstrated in Trendelenburg position.

Technical Factors

- Film size–11 x 14 in. (30 x 35 cm), lengthwise.
  or –14 x 17 in. (35 x 43 cm)
- Moving or stationary grid.
- 100-125 kVp range.
  (80-100 kVp range for double-contrast study.)
- Technique and dose:

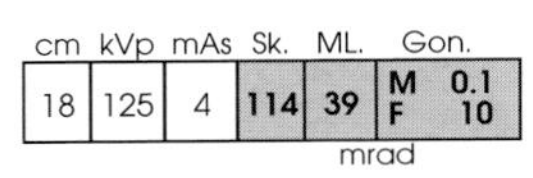

cm	kVp	mAs	Sk.	ML.	Gon. (mrad)
18	125	4	114	39	M 0.1 F 10

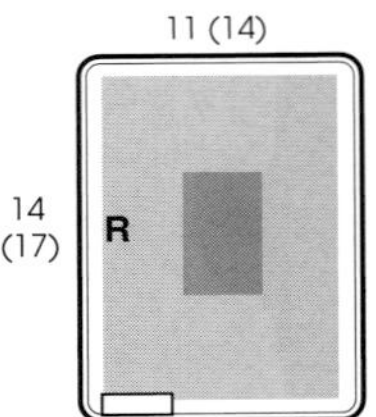
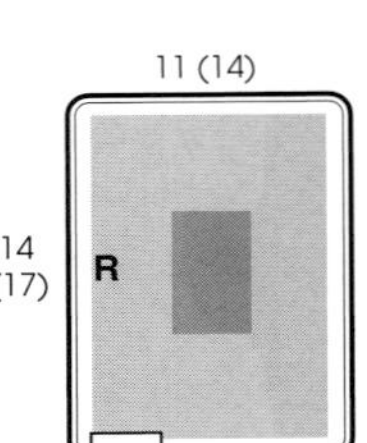

Shielding: Place lead shield over patient's pelvic region to protect gonads without covering pertinent anatomy.

Patient Position

- Patient supine, arms at sides; provide pillow for head.

Part Position

- Align **midsagittal plane to midline** of table.
- Ensure there is **no body rotation**.
- Center cassette to CR. (Bottom of 11 x 14 in. (30 x 35 cm) cassette should be about at level of iliac crest.)

Central Ray

- CR **perpendicular** to film holder.
- ***Average Body Type:*** Center CR and film to **level of L1** (about midway between xiphoid tip and lower margin of ribs), **midway between midline and left lateral margin** of abdomen.
  Hypersthenic: Center about 1 in. or 2.5 cm higher.
  Asthenic: About 2 in. or 5 cm lower and nearer to midline.
- Minimum 40 in. (102 cm) SID.

Collimation: Collimate on four sides to outer margins of film, or to area of interest on larger film.

Respiration: Suspend respiration and expose upon expiration.

Alternate AP Trendelenburg: A partial Trendelenburg (head down) position may be necessary to fill the fundus on a thin asthenic patient. A full Trendelenburg angulation facilitates the demonstration of hiatal hernia. (Install shoulder braces for patient safety.)

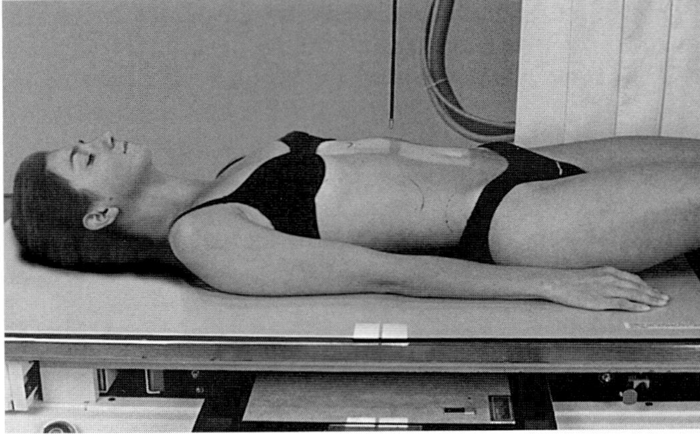

Fig. 14-98. AP recumbent.

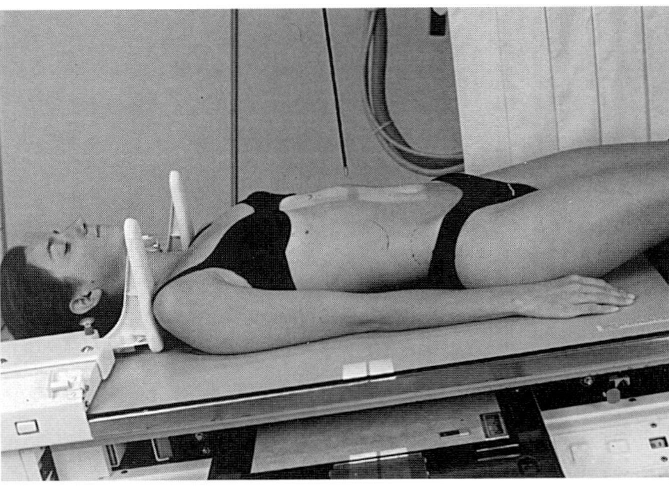

Fig. 14-99. AP Trendelenburg.

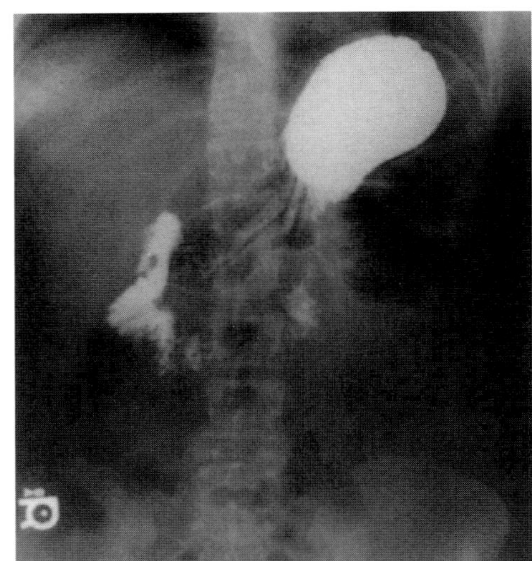

Fig. 14-100. AP.

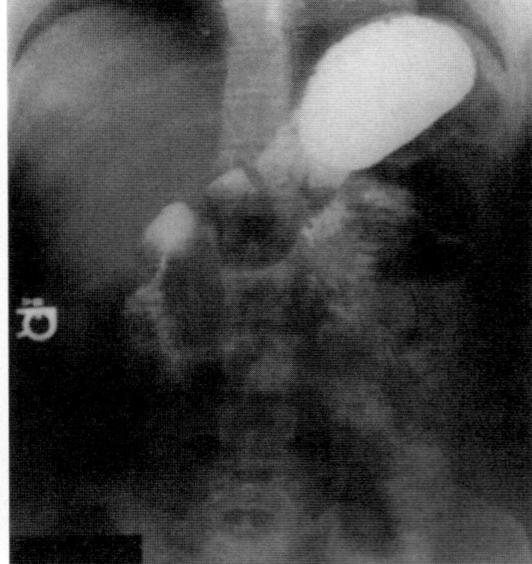

Fig. 14-101. AP Trendelenburg.

Evaluation Criteria

- Entire stomach and duodenum are visualized.
- Diaphragm and lower lung fields are included for demonstration of possible hiatal hernia.
- Fundus of the stomach is filled with barium and is near center of film.
- Appropriate technique employed to visualize the gastric folds without overexposing other pertinent anatomy.

CHAPTER 15

Lower Gastrointestinal System

CONTRIBUTIONS BY:
John P. Lampignano, M Ed, RT (R)
Barry T. Anthony, RT (R)

CONTENTS

Radiographic Anatomy

Digestive system and common radiographic procedures **446**

Small intestine **447**

Large intestine **448**

Colon **449**

Anatomy review (radiographs) **450**

Abdominal cavity (peritoneum, mesentery, and omentum) **451**

Anatomical relationships (retroperitoneal and infraperitoneal organs) **452**

Digestive functions **454**

Radiographic Procedures

Small bowel series **455**

Small bowel procedures:
- Upper GI/small bowel combination **456**
- Small bowel only series **456**
- Enteroclysis and intubation method **457**
- Patient and room preparation and method of imaging **458**

Barium enema **459**

Barium enema procedure:
- Patient and room preparation **460**
- Equipment and supplies **461**
- Enema tip insertion **462**

Types of lower GI procedures:
- Single and double-contrast **464**
- Post fluoroscopy radiography **465**
- Defecography **466**

Summary of safety concerns **467**

Radiographic Positioning

Survey results **468**

Basic and special projections **469**

Small bowel series:
- PA **470**

Barium enema–Basic:
- PA and/or AP projection **472**
- RAO **473**
- LAO **474**
- LPO and RPO **475**
- Lateral rectum **476**

Barium enema–Double-contrast:
- Right lateral decubitus **477**
- Left lateral decubitus **478**
- PA (AP) post-evac **479**

Barium enema–Special:
- AP or LPO axial **480**
- PA or RAO axial **481**

15

Radiographic Anatomy

DIGESTIVE SYSTEM

The first five parts of the alimentary canal (through the stomach and first part of the small intestine, the duodenum) were described in the preceding chapter.

This chapter continues with the alimentary canal of the digestive system beyond the stomach beginning with the **small intestine** (small bowel). If the entire small intestine were removed from the body at autopsy, separated from its mesenteric attachment, uncoiled and stretched out, it would average 7 meters or 23 feet in length. During life, with good muscle tone, the actual length of the small intestine is shorter, measuring between 4.5 and 5.5 meters or 15 to 18 feet. Tremendous individual variation does exist, however. In one series of 100 autopsies, the small bowel varied in length from 15 to 31 feet. It is about 1 inch in diameter.

The **large intestine** (large bowel) begins in the lower right quadrant near its connection with the small intestine. The large intestine extends around the periphery of the abdominal cavity to end at the **anus.** The large intestine is about 1.5 meters or 5 feet long and about 2.5 inches in diameter.

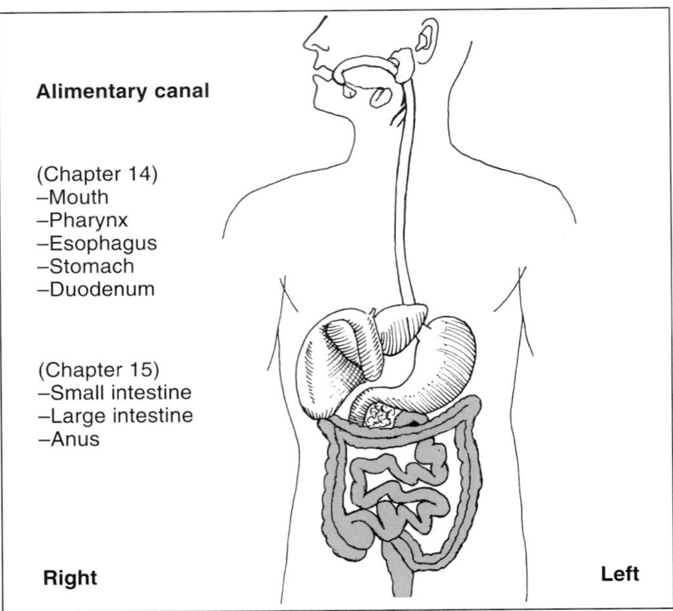

Fig. 15-1. Digestive system.

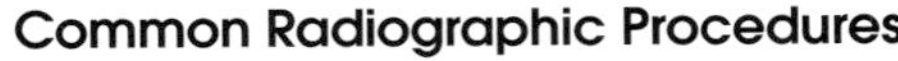

Common Radiographic Procedures

Two common radiographic procedures involving the lower gastrointestinal system are presented in this chapter. Both of these procedures involve administration of a contrast medium.

1. Small Bowel Series (SBS)–Study of Small Intestine: Radiographic examination specifically of the small intestine is termed a **small bowel series** or SBS. This examination is often combined with an upper GI series and, under these conditions, may be termed a small bowel follow-through. A radiograph of the barium-filled small bowel is shown in Fig. 15-2.

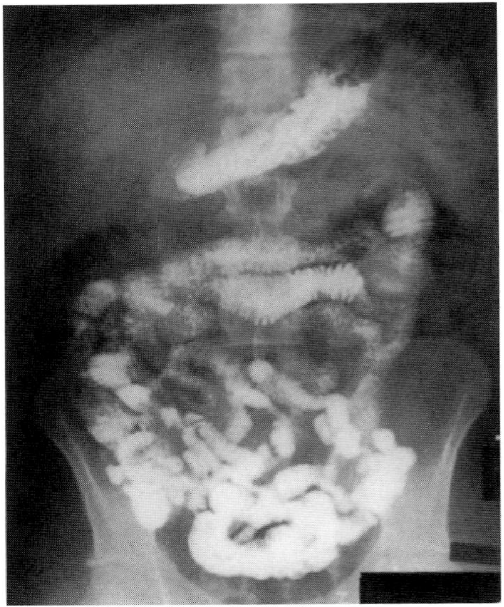

Fig. 15-2. Small bowel series–PA.

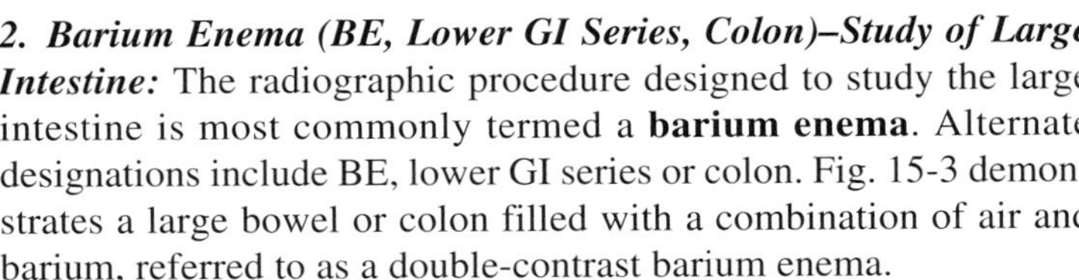

2. Barium Enema (BE, Lower GI Series, Colon)–Study of Large Intestine: The radiographic procedure designed to study the large intestine is most commonly termed a **barium enema**. Alternate designations include BE, lower GI series or colon. Fig. 15-3 demonstrates a large bowel or colon filled with a combination of air and barium, referred to as a double-contrast barium enema.

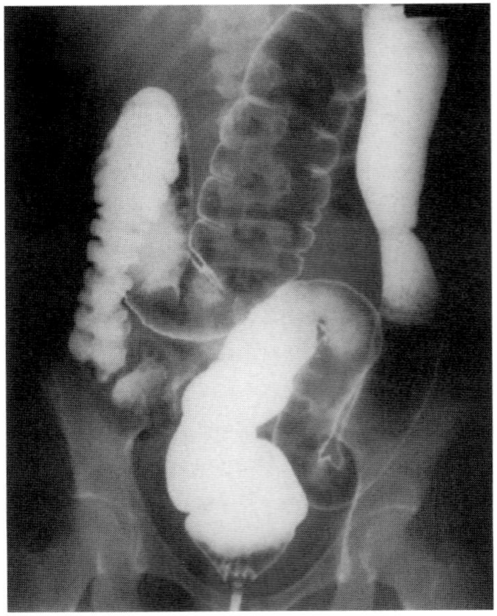

Fig. 15-3. Double-contrast barium enema–AP.

SMALL INTESTINE

The small intestine is located primarily in the central portion of the abdominal cavity. Beginning at the pyloric valve of the stomach, the three parts of the small intestine, in order, are **duodenum**, **jejunum** and **ileum**. The duodenum is the first part of the small intestine as studied in detail in Chapter 14, and is the shortest, widest and most fixed portion of the small bowel. Since the jejunum and ileum are much longer than the duodenum, and since the duodenum is posteriorly located, the many loops of small bowel looped over each other in the central abdomen, as shown in Fig. 15-4, are jejunum and ileum. The relative location of the three parts of the small intestine in relationship to the four abdominal quadrants is shown in Figs. 15-4 and 15-5.

Duodenum (RUQ and LUQ)

The **duodenum** measures a fairly constant 10 inches (25 centimeters) in length and is much shorter than the other two sections of the small intestine. The duodenum is primarily located in the RUQ but also extends into the LUQ where it joins the jejunum.

Jejunum (LUQ and LLQ)

The **jejunum** (light gray region in Figs. 15-4 and 15-5) is located primarily to the left of midline in the LUQ and LLQ of the abdomen, making up about **two-fifths** of the small bowel remaining after the duodenum.

The jejunum begins at the site of the **duodenojejunal junction** which is firmly held in position by a fibrous muscular band, the **ligament of Treitz**, slightly to the left of the midline in the left upper quadrant (under the transverse colon on this drawing). This relatively fixed site of the small bowel becomes a radiographic reference point for certain small bowel studies.

Ileum (RUQ, RLQ and LLQ)

The **ileum** is located primarily in the right upper and right lower quadrants, but also includes part of the left lower quadrant as shown by the darker gray region. Approximately **three-fifths** of the small bowel remaining after the duodenum is ileum. Therefore the ileum is the longest portion of the small intestine. The terminal ileum joins the large intestine at the ileocecal valve in the right lower quadrant.

***Sectional Differences** (Fig. 15-6):* The various sections of small intestine can be identified radiographically by their location and appearance. The C-shaped duodenum is fairly fixed in position. The proximal duodenum with its bulb or cap is unique and can be easily recognized on radiographs of the duodenum immediately distal to the stomach. The internal lining of the second portion (descending) of the duodenum is thrown into circular folds.

The circular folds continue throughout the remainder of the duodenum and are found in the jejunum as well. Radiographically, when the distal duodenum and the jejunum contain air, and especially when the bowel is distended, the internal lining of the duodenum and jejunum resemble a coiled spring or a stack of coins. When it contains barium, the appearance is described as feathery. While there is no abrupt end to the circular folds, the ileum tends not to have these indentations. Consequently, the internal lining of the ileum as it appears on a radiograph is smoother and does not have the feathery appearance.

A final observable difference in the three sections of small intestine is that the internal diameter gets progressively smaller from duodenum to ileum.

Radiographs demonstrating these sectional differences are shown in the anatomy review page which follows this section.

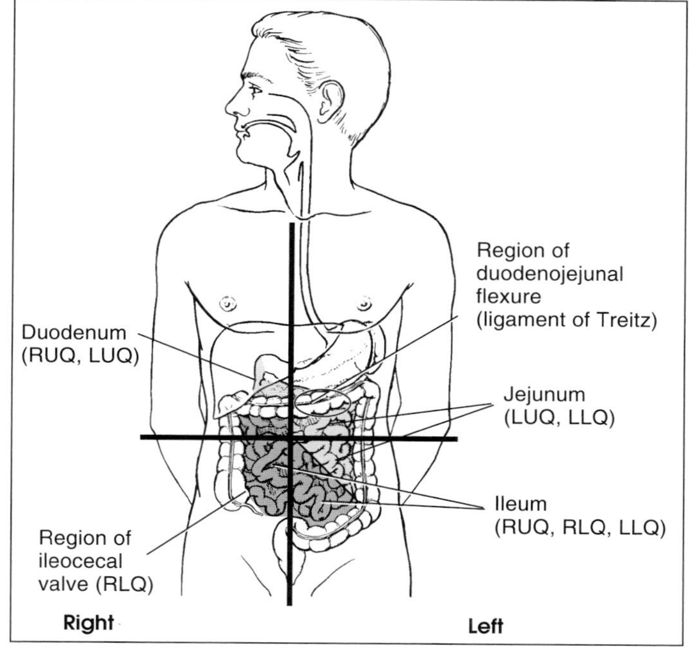

Fig. 15-4. Small intestines–Four quadrants.

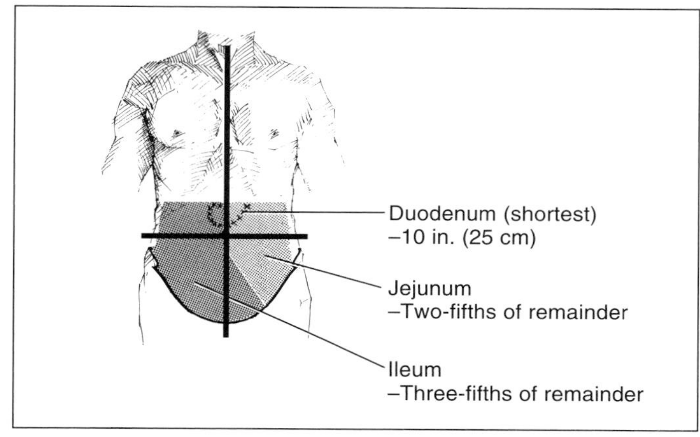

Fig. 15-5. Small intestine.

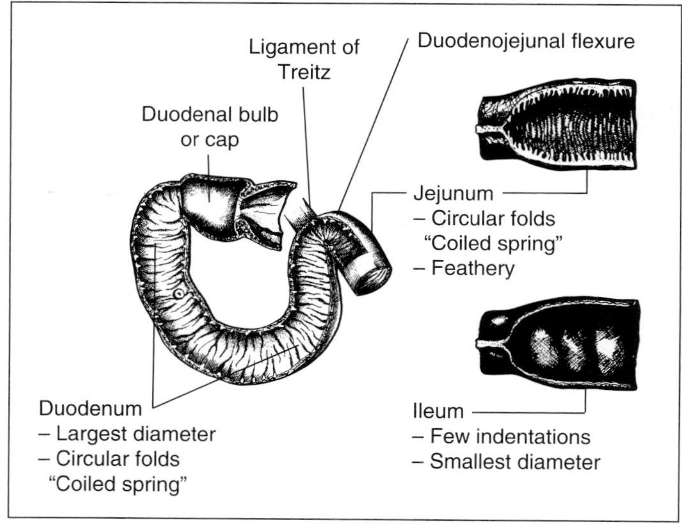

Fig. 15-6. Small intestine (cutaway drawing).

15

LARGE INTESTINE

The large intestine begins in the right lower quadrant just distal to the ileocecal valve. The vertical portion of the large intestine superior to the cecum is the **ascending colon,** which continues as the **transverse colon** after the **right colic** *(kol′ lik)* **(hepatic) flexure.** The **descending colon** continues from the transverse colon after another sharp bend termed the **left colic (splenic) flexure.** The descending colon continues as the S-shaped **sigmoid** *(sig′ moid)* **colon** in the left lower quadrant. The distal portion of the descending colon is sometimes called the iliac colon, while the sigmoid colon may also be called the pelvic colon.

The final segment of the large intestine is the **rectum.** The distal rectum contains the **anal canal** which ends at the **anus.**

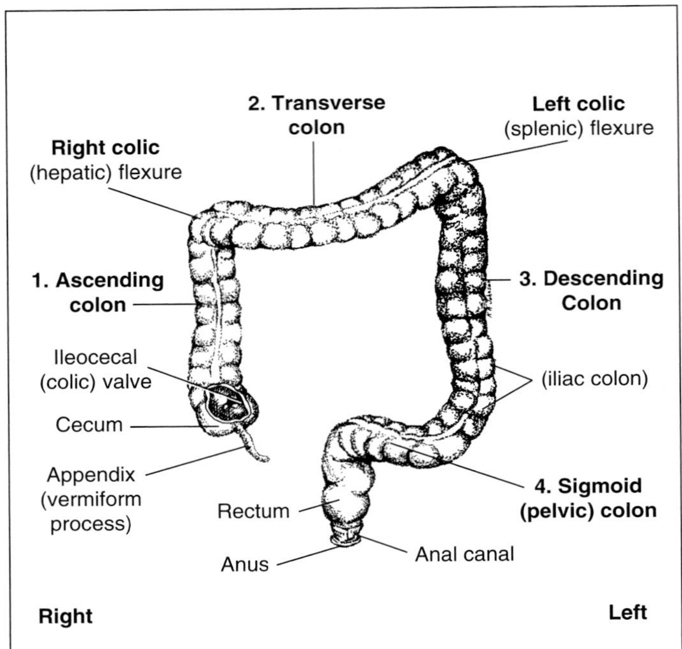

Fig. 15-7. Large intestine (includes colon).

Large Intestine vs. Colon

Large intestine and colon are NOT synonyms, although many persons use these terms interchangeably. The **colon** consists of **four sections** and **two flexures**, and does **not** include the cecum and rectum. The four sections of the colon are (1) the **ascending colon,** (2) the **transverse colon,** (3) the **descending colon,** and (4) the **sigmoid colon.** The **right** and **left colic flexures** thus are also included as part of the colon. The cecum and rectum (including the anal canal and anus), however, are part of the large intestine but are not part of the colon.

The total large intestine, which includes the colon, also consists of **four parts**, (1) **cecum**, (2) **colon**, (3) **rectum** and (4) **anal canal**. Each of these parts will be described beginning with the cecum.

1. Cecum

At the proximal end of the large intestine is the **cecum**, a large, blind pouch located inferior to the level of the ileocecal valve. The **appendix**, (vermiform process) is attached to cecum. The internal appearance of the cecum and **terminal ileum** is shown in Fig. 15-8. The most distal part of the small intestine, the ileum, joins the cecum at the **ileocecal valve.** The ileocecal valve consists of two lips that extend into the large bowel.

The ileocecal valve acts as a sphincter to prevent the contents of the ileum from passing too quickly into the cecum. A second function of the ileocecal valve is to prevent reflux, or a backward flow of large intestine contents, into the ileum. The ileocecal valve does only a fair job of preventing reflux since some barium can almost always be refluxed into the terminal ileum when a barium enema is performed. The cecum is the widest portion of the large intestine and is fairly free to move about in the lower right quadrant.

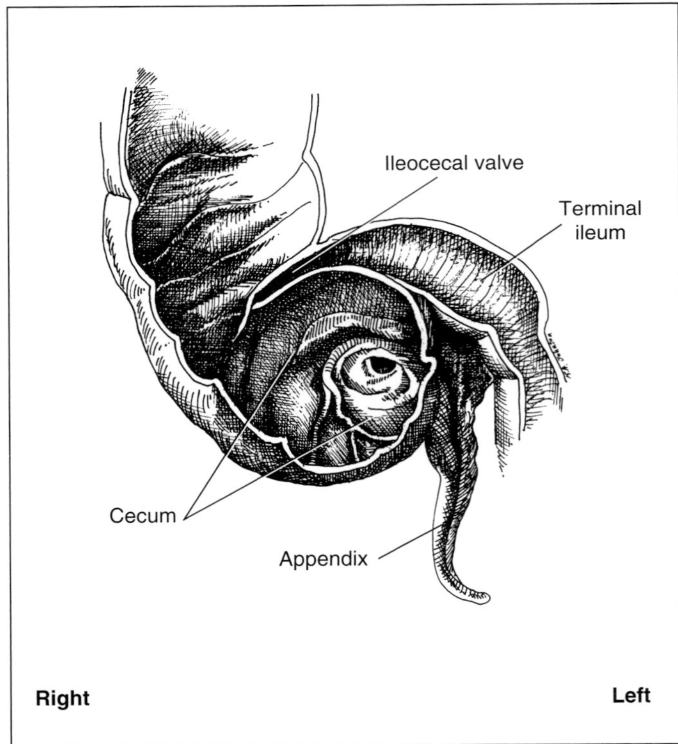

Fig. 15-8. Cecum, terminal ileum and appendix.

Appendix: The **appendix** or vermiform process is a long (2 to 20 cm), narrow, worm shaped tube extending from the cecum. The term, vermiform, in fact, means wormlike. The appendix is usually attached to the posteromedial aspect of the cecum and commonly extends toward the pelvis. It may, however, pass posterior to the cecum.

Since the appendix has a blind ending, infectious agents may enter an appendix, which cannot empty itself. The result is appendicitis. An inflamed appendix may require surgical removal, termed an appendectomy, before the diseased structure ruptures and causes peritonitis. Peritonitis is inflammation of the lining of the abdomen.

Occasionally, fecal matter or barium sulfate from a GI tract study may fill the appendix and remain there indefinitely.

2. Colon

After the cecum is the second part of the large intestine, the **colon.** As shown in Fig. 15-9, the colon is the major part of the large intestine surrounding the many loops of small intestine. Beginning with the **ascending colon**, the **four parts** of the colon are all slightly smaller in diameter than is the cecum.

The **transverse colon** is the second and the longest part of the colon and possesses considerable up and down movement. It normally loops more downward than shown on the drawing (see arrows), as it passes across the anterior surface of the abdominal cavity. Since the liver is such a large, solid organ, the right colic (hepatic) flexure usually lies lower in the abdomen than does the left colic (splenic) flexure, which lies beneath the inferior pole of the spleen.

The **descending colon** is the third part, which extends down from the left colic flexure to where it curves inward to become the sigmoid colon. The lower aspect of the descending colon is sometimes called the iliac colon.

The fourth and last part of the colon is the **sigmoid colon,** which normally lies in the pelvis, but does possess a wide freedom of motion. The sigmoid colon and the cecum are the two parts of the large intestine that possess the widest freedom of motion.

The sigmoid colon finally passes posteriorly and inferiorly along the curve of the sacrum to continue as the **rectum**, and **anal canal**. The location and position of these components of the colon will be important to remember during the barium enema procedure.

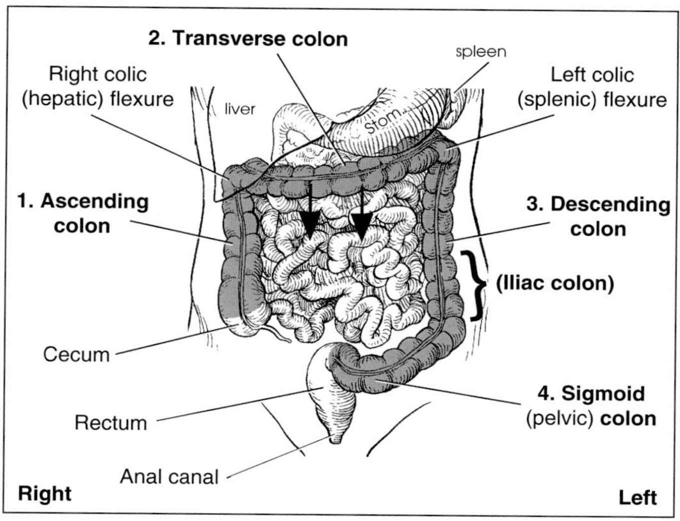

Fig. 15-9. Colon–Four parts.

3 & 4. Rectum and Anal Canal

The third and fourth parts of the large intestine are the **rectum** and the **anal canal.** The rectum extends from the sigmoid colon to the **anus.** The rectum begins at the level of S3 and is about 4½ inches (12 cm) long. The final 1 to 1½ in. (2.5 to 4 cm) of large intestine is constricted to form the anal canal. The anal canal terminates as an opening to the exterior, the anus. The rectum closely follows the sacrococcygeal curve as demonstrated in the lateral view in Fig. 5-10.

The **rectal ampulla** is a dilated portion of the rectum located anterior to the coccyx. The initial direction of the rectum along the **sacrum** is down and back; however, in the region of the rectal ampulla, the direction changes to down and forward. A second abrupt change in direction occurs in the region of the anal canal, which is directed downward and backward. Therefore, the rectum presents **two anteroposterior curves.** This fact must be remembered when a rectal tube or enema tip is inserted into the lower GI tract by the radiographer for a barium enema procedure. Serious injury can occur if the enema tip is forced into the anus and anal canal incorrectly at the wrong angle.

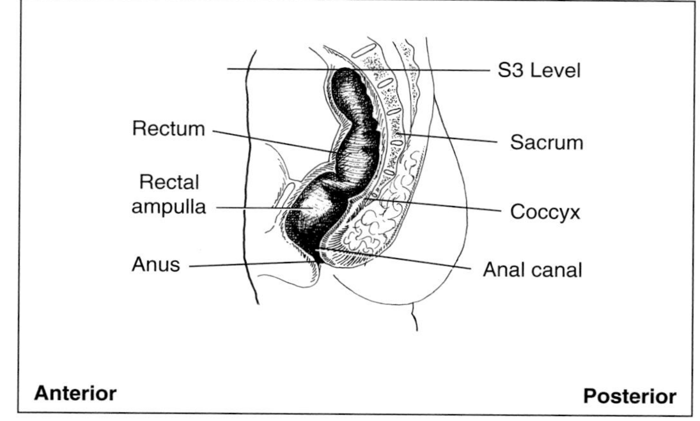

Fig. 15-10. Rectum–Lateral view.

Characteristics (Differences) of the Large Intestine

Three characteristics readily differentiate the large intestine from the small intestine. First, the **internal diameter** of the large intestine is usually greater than the diameter of the small bowel.

Second, the longitudinal muscle fibers of the large bowel form three bands of muscle called **taeniae coli,** which tend to pull the large intestine into pouches. Each of these pouches or sacculations is termed a **haustrum.** Therefore a second primary identifying characteristic of the large bowel is the presence of haustra.

The third differentiation is the **relative positions** of the two structures. The **large intestine** extends around the **periphery** of the abdominal cavity, while the **small intestine** is more **centrally** located.

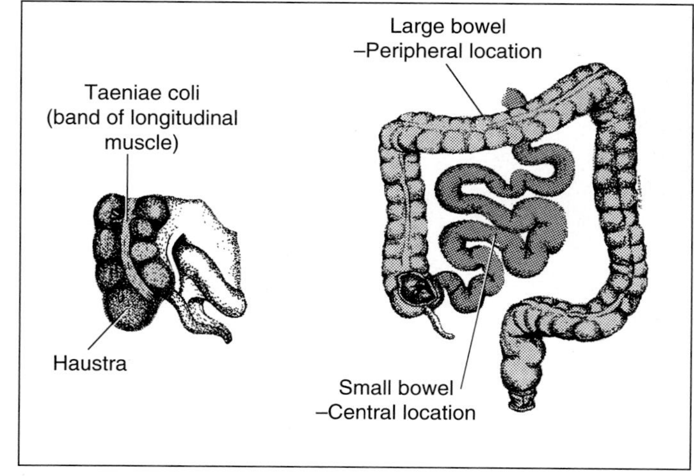

Fig. 15-11. Intestine differences–Large vs. small intestine.

ANATOMY REVIEW

Small Bowel Radiographs
(Figs. 15-12, 15-13a, and 15-13b)

Three parts of the small bowel are demonstrated in these 30 min. and 2 hour small bowel radiographs (taken 30 min. and 2 hours after ingestion of barium). Note the characteristic feathery-appearing sections of duodenum (A) and jejunum (C). The smoother appearance of the ileum is evident as section D.

The terminal portion of the ileum (D), the ileocecal valve (E) and the cecum of the large intestine are best shown on a spot film of this area (Fig. 15-13b). A spot film such as this using a compression cone is frequently taken of the ileocecal valve area at the end of a small bowel series to best visualize this region.

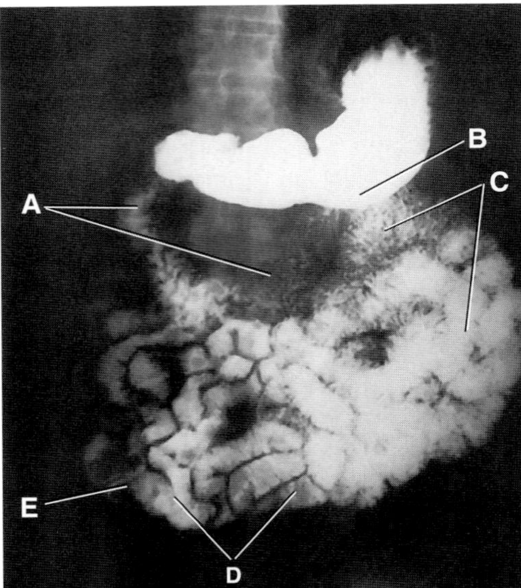

Fig. 15-12. PA, 30-min. small bowel.

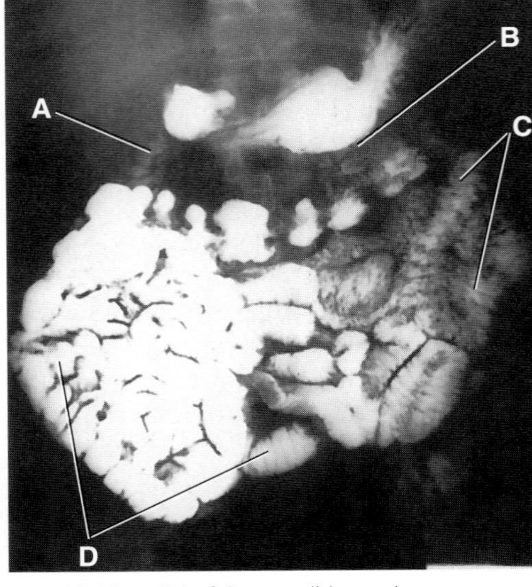

Fig. 15-13a. PA, 2-hr. small bowel.

Labeled Parts of Small Intestine:

A. Duodenum
B. Area of ligament of Treitz (site of duodenojejunal flexure, superimposed by stomach on these radiographs)
C. Jejunum
D. Ileum
E. Area of ileocecal valve

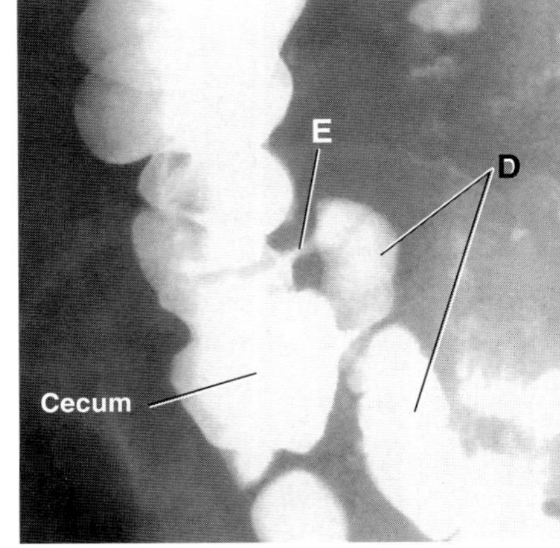

Fig. 15-13b. Spot film of ileocecal valve. (courtesy of Jim Sanderson, RT)

Barium Enema (Figs. 15-14, 15-15, and 15-16)

Anteroposterior (AP), lateral and right anterior oblique (RAO) radiographs of a barium enema exam illustrate the key anatomy of the large intestine labeled as follows:

a. Cecum
b. Ascending colon
c. Right colic (hepatic) flexure
d. Transverse colon
e. Left colic (splenic) flexure
f. Descending colon
g. Sigmoid colon
h. Rectum

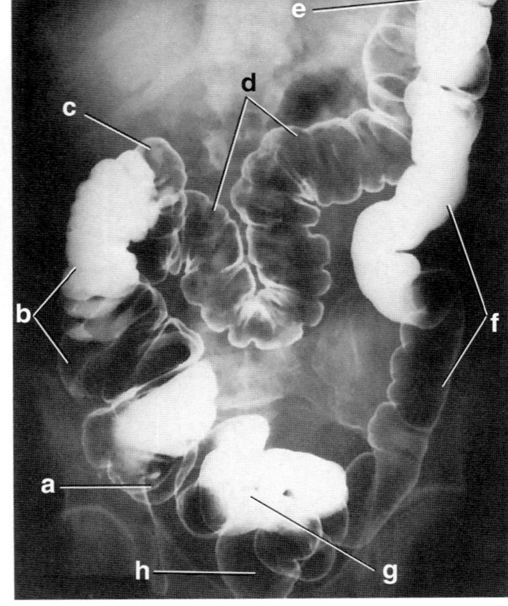

Fig. 15-14. AP, barium enema (double-contrast).

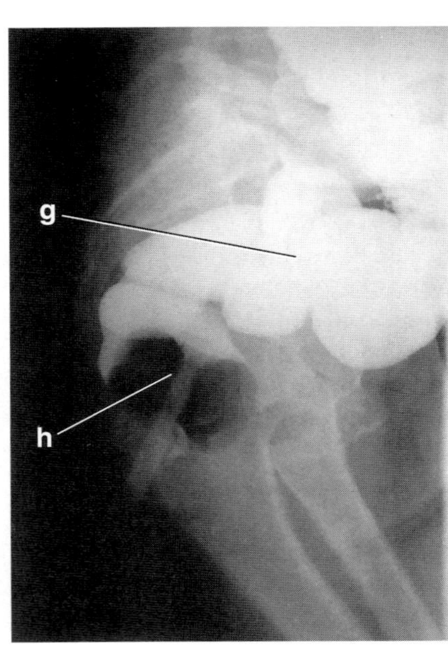

Fig. 15-15. Lateral rectum, barium enema.

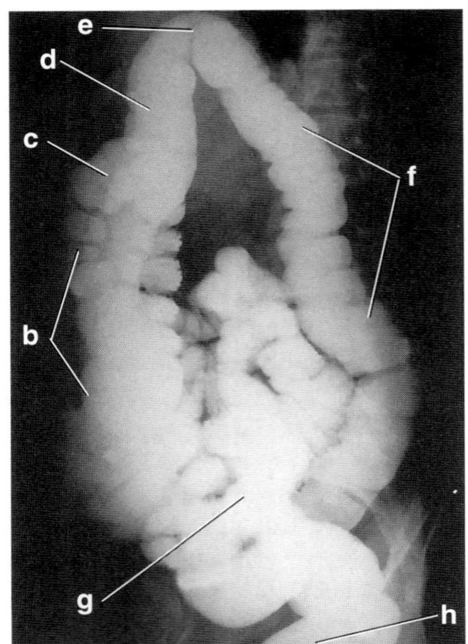

Fig. 15-16. RAO, barium enema (single contrast).

15

ABDOMINAL CAVITY

Peritoneum

The abdominal cavity contains many organs. Not only does this largest of all body cavities contain the major portion of the gastrointestinal system and its accessory organs, but it also contains certain organs of the endocrine, circulatory and urogenital systems. Most of these structures, as well as the wall of the abdominal cavity in which they are contained, are covered to varying degrees by an extensive serous membrane termed the **peritoneum** *(per″ i-to-ne′ um)*. In fact, the total surface area of peritoneum is about equal to the total surface area of the skin covering the entire body.

A simplified cross section of the abdominal cavity is shown in Fig. 15-17. There are two layers of the peritoneum; the parietal and the visceral. Peritoneum adhering to the cavity wall is termed **parietal peritoneum,** while that portion covering an organ is termed **visceral peritoneum.** The space or cavity between the parietal and visceral portions of the peritoneum is called the **peritoneal cavity,** which is really a potential cavity since normally this is filled with various organs. If all the loops of bowel and the other organs of the abdominal cavity were drawn in, there would be very little actual space left in the peritoneal cavity. This cavity contains some serous lubricating-type fluid, which allows organs to move against each other without friction.

The peritoneum forms large folds that bind the abdominal organs to each other and to the walls of the abdomen. Blood and lymph vessels and the nerves that supply these abdominal organs are contained within these folds of peritoneum. One of these double folds holding the small intestine in place is called the **mesentery** *(mes′ en-ter″ e)*.

Mesentery

The simplified cross section of the abdominal cavity, as again illustrated in Fig. 15-18, demonstrates three important facts. **First**, there is a **double fold of peritoneum** extending anteriorly from the region in front of the vertebral body at this level. This double fold of peritoneum completely envelops a loop of small bowel. The specific term for a double fold of peritoneum connecting the small intestine to the posterior abdominal wall is **mesentery.**

Second, a layer of parietal peritoneum **partially covers** certain organs. At this level, both the ascending colon and the descending colon are only partially covered as shown in this drawing, therefore they would **not** be considered mesentery.

Third, some structures, such as the aorta and inferior vena cava, are located **completely behind or posterior** to the parietal peritoneum. Organs or other structures located behind the peritoneum are termed **retroperitoneal structures.** These will be listed and described on the following page.

Greater Sac, Lesser Sac and Transverse Mesocolon

The midsagittal sectional drawing of an adult female, Fig. 15-19, shows peritoneum partially or completely covering various abdominal organs, as well as lining the abdominal cavity itself. The major portion of the peritoneal cavity, shown in dark gray, is termed the **greater sac**, commonly referred to as simply the **peritoneal cavity**.

A smaller portion of the upper posterior peritoneal cavity located posterior to the stomach is termed the **lesser sac**. This also has a special name, the **omentum bursa**.

In this drawing, **mesentery** is seen connecting a loop of small intestine (ileum) to the posterior abdominal wall.

Mesentery type folds from which other abdominal organs are suspended use the prefix **"meso"** such as the sigmoid mesocolon, or as shown on this drawing the **transverse mesocolon**, shown to be connecting the transverse colon to the posterior abdominal wall.

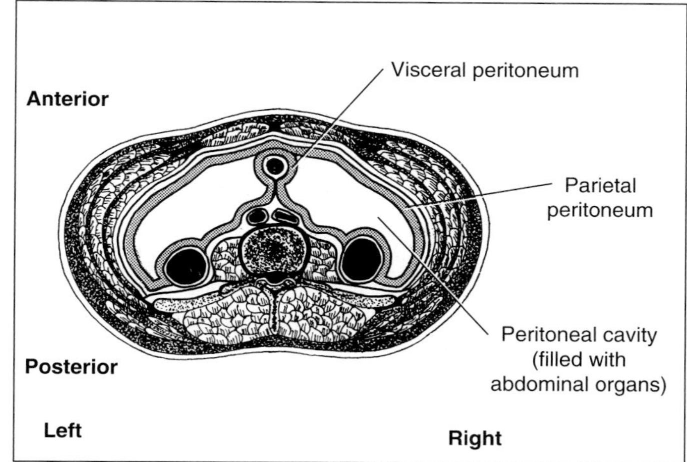

Fig. 15-17. Cross section–Abdominal cavity (demonstrates peritoneum).

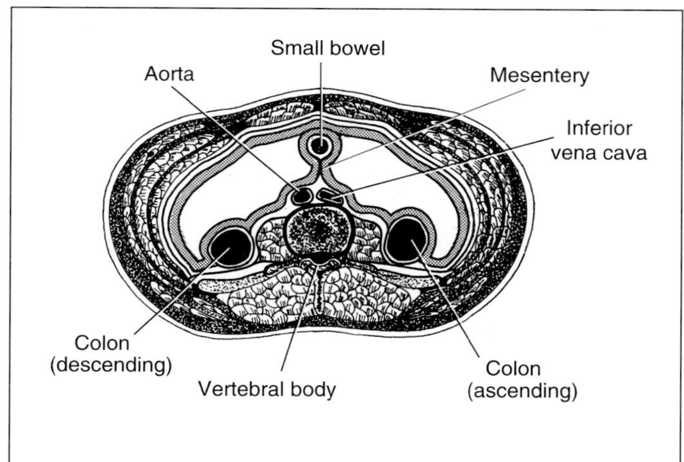

Fig. 15-18. Cross section–Abdominal cavity (demonstrates mesentery).

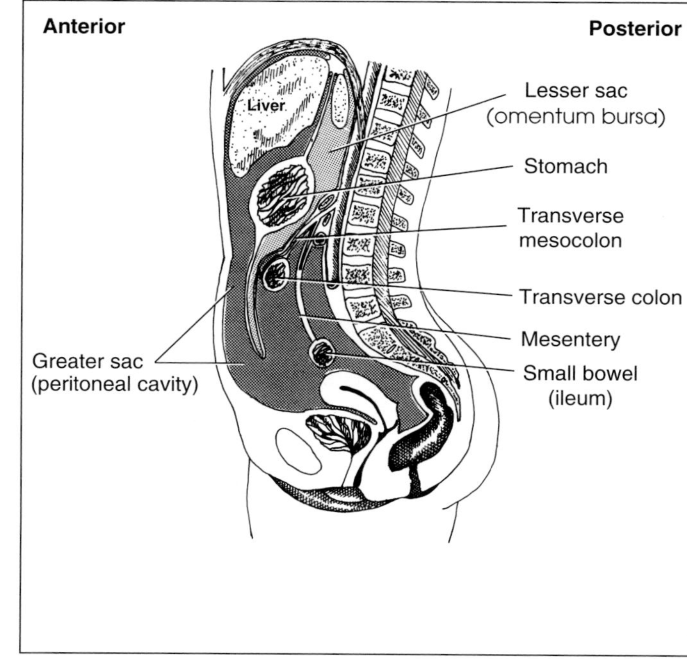

Fig. 15-19. Midsagittal section–Abdominal cavity (demonstrates greater and lesser sacs and transverse mesocolon).

Abdominal Cavity continued

Omentum

A different type of double fold of peritoneum, termed **omentum** *(o-men′tum)*, is shown in Fig. 15-20. Omentum is a **double fold of peritoneum extending from the stomach to another organ**.

The **lesser omentum** extends superiorly from the lesser curvature of the stomach to portions of the liver. The **greater omentum** connects the transverse colon to the greater curvature of the stomach inferiorly. The greater omentum drapes down over the small bowel to form an apron along the anterior abdominal wall. It then folds back on itself and connects to the transverse colon.

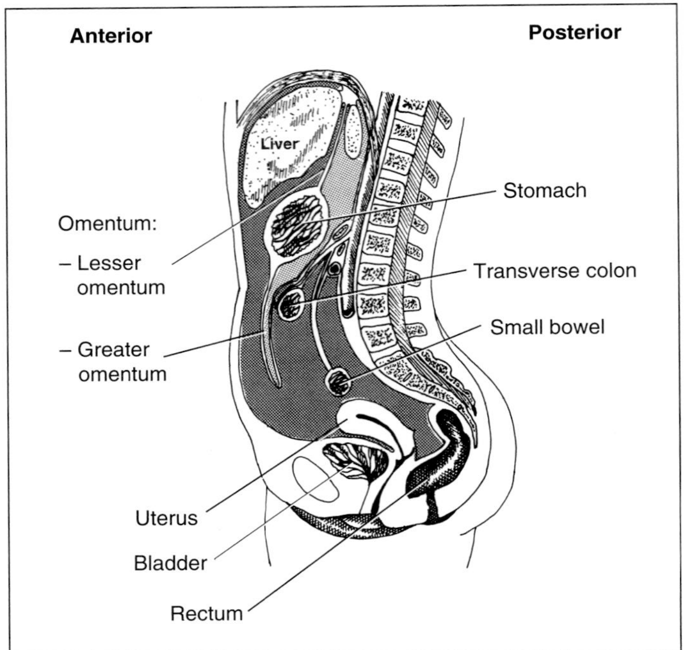

Fig. 15-20. Sagittal section–Abdominal cavity (demonstrates omentum).

Greater Omentum

The drawing on the left in Fig. 15-21 demonstrates the abdominal cavity with the anterior abdominal wall, muscles and parietal peritoneum removed. The first structure encountered beneath the parietal peritoneum is the **greater omentum.** Varying amounts of fat are deposited in the greater omentum, which serves as a layer of insulation between the abdominal cavity and the exterior. This is sometimes called the "fatty apron" due to its location and the amount of fat contained therein. A portion of the greater omentum has been omitted from this drawing to reveal the underlying organs.

The drawing on the right of Fig. 15-21 also illustrates the apron-like appearance of the greater omentum, the bottom edge of which is shown to be lifted up over the chest. This exposes the small bowel and shows the connection between the greater omentum and the transverse colon.

The **transverse mesocolon** is again seen on this drawing on the right as connecting the transverse colon to the posterior abdominal wall.

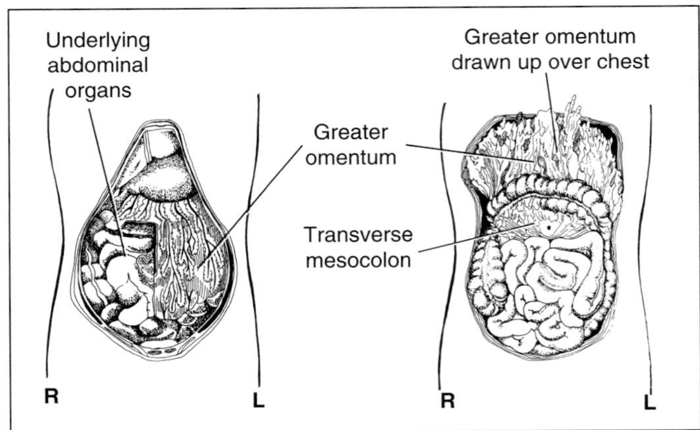

Fig. 15-21. Greater omentum.

ANATOMICAL RELATIONSHIPS

Retroperitoneal and Infraperitoneal Pelvic Organs (Fig. 15-22)

Organs within the abdominal cavity that are either partially or completely covered by visceral peritoneum are called **intraperitoneal** structures and include the liver, gallbladder, spleen, stomach, jejunum, ileum, cecum and parts of the colon. (These have been removed from the drawing in Fig. 15-22.) The remaining organs shown in this drawing are considered either **retroperitoneal** ("retro" meaning backward or behind), or **infraperitoneal** ("infra" meaning under or beneath). Therefore those structures lying entirely behind or posterior to the peritoneum are retroperitoneal, and those in the pelvic region under the parietal peritoneum are infraperitoneal pelvic organs.

Retroperitoneal Organs: Structures that are retroperitoneal are the **kidneys** and **ureters**, **adrenal glands**, **pancreas**, **duodenum**, **ascending** and **descending colon**, **upper rectum**, **abdominal aorta** and **inferior vena cava**. Two structures very often confused and erroneously thought to be located within the abdominal or peritoneal cavity are the **pancreas** and **duodenum**. These two structures are retroperitoneal, thus they are more fixed in their location since they are not suspended by folds of peritoneum.

Infraperitoneal Pelvic Organs: Located under or beneath the peritoneum in the true pelvis are the **lower rectum**, **urinary bladder** and **reproductive organs**.

Male vs. Female Peritoneal Enclosures

There are some differences between the male and female peritoneal enclosures. The lower aspect of the peritoneum is a **closed sac** in the **male** and **not in the female**, in that the uterine tubes in the female open directly into the peritoneal cavity. Further details of the orientation of these structures are beyond the scope of this textbook.

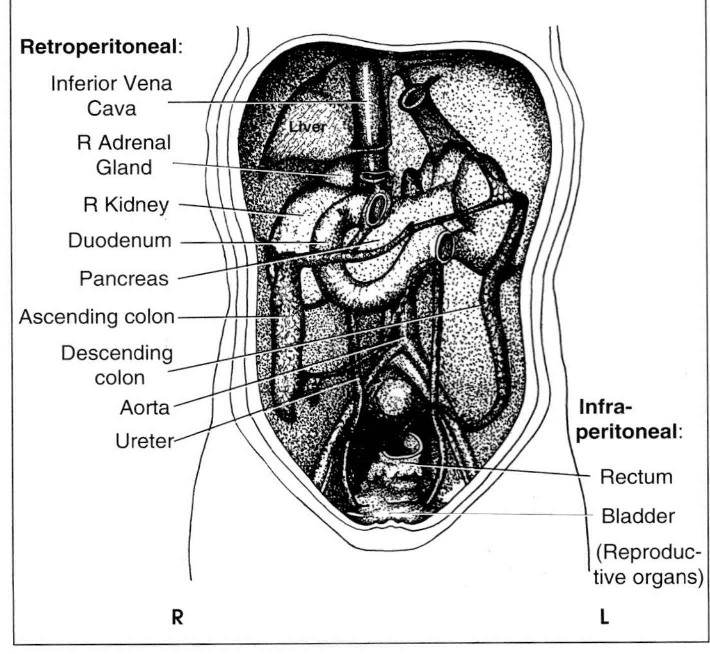

Fig. 15-22. Retroperitoneal and infraperitoneal pelvic organs.

Abdominopelvic Cavity (from left side)

The relative locations of various abdominal organs, as seen from the **left side,** are shown in Fig. 15-23. The **stomach** lies just inferior to the diaphragm, with its **fundus** much more posterior than the **body.**

The **spleen** of the circulatory system nestles between the stomach and the posterior abdominal wall. The spleen is ordinarily protected by the lower posterior rib cage.

The **transverse colon** lies underneath the greater omentum. The transverse colon is far anterior in the abdominal cavity, while its continuation, the **descending colon,** lies against the posterior abdominal wall. The S-shaped **sigmoid colon** first extends toward the anterior, then loops back posteriorly to continue as the rectum.

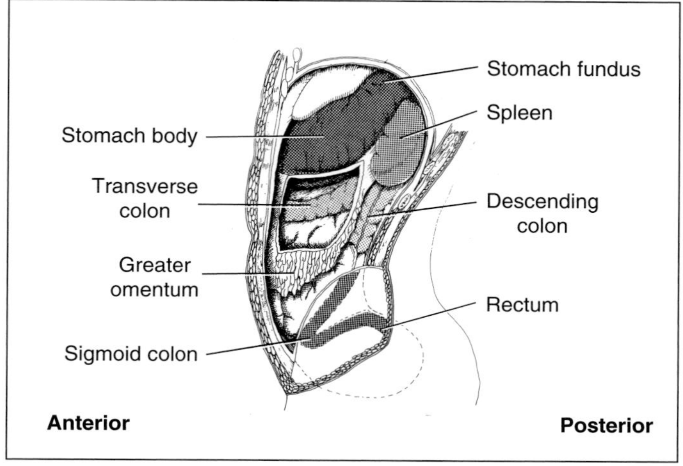

Fig. 15-23. Abdominopelvic cavity (left side).

Abdominopelvic Cavity (from right side)

The **abdominopelvic cavity** as seen from the **right side** is shown in Fig. 15-24. The large **liver** occupies most of the upper abdominal cavity on this right side. Lying beneath the liver, but **anterior** to the midaxillary line, is the **gallbladder.** The right **kidney,** right **adrenal gland, duodenum** and **head of the pancreas** are retroperitoneal structures, thus located more **posteriorly**.

The **transverse colon** is far anterior compared to the **ascending colon** and **cecum,** which lie more posteriorly. The **appendix** extends inferiorly from the cecum. The cecum and appendix lie below the level of the iliac crest. The relative positions of various abdominal organs, both side to side and front to back, are important for the radiographer to know.

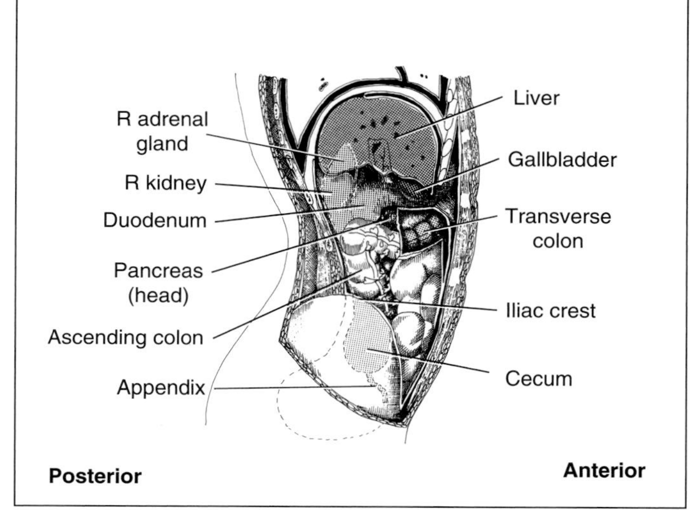

Fig. 15-24. Abdominopelvic cavity (right side).

Relative Locations of Air and Barium in Large Intestine

The simplified drawings in Fig. 15-25 represent the large intestine in **supine**, **prone** and **erect** positions. If the large intestine contained both air and barium sulfate, the air would tend to rise and the barium would tend to sink due to gravity. The displacement and ultimate location of air is shown as black, and the barium as white.

When a person is **supine**, air rises to fill those structures that are most anterior, which are the transverse and sigmoid colons. The barium sinks to fill primarily the ascending and descending portions of the colon and the rectum.

When a patient is **prone**, barium and air reverse positions. The drawing in the center illustrates the prone position, hence, air has risen to fill the rectum, ascending colon, and descending colon.

The **erect** position on the far right shows straight air/barium fluid lines with air naturally rising to the highest part of each portion of the large intestine.

Recognizing these spatial relationships is important both during fluoroscopy and during radiography when performing barium enema examinations.

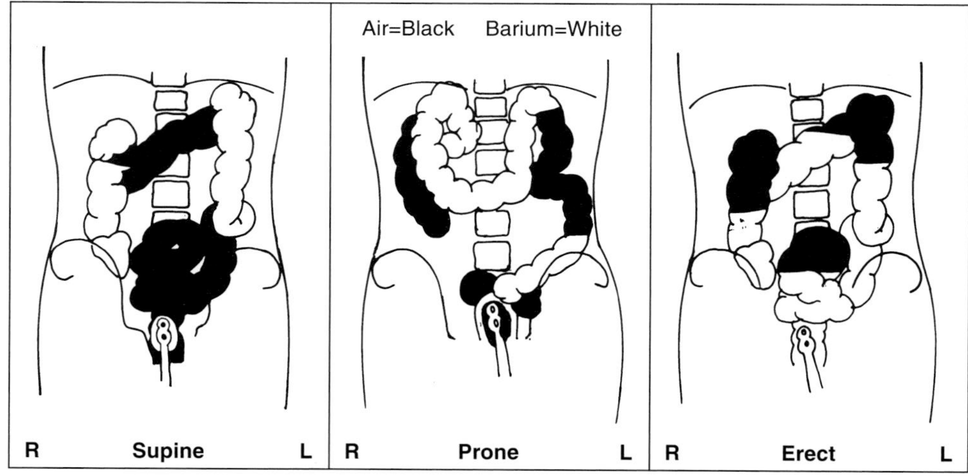

Fig. 15-25. Barium vs. air in large intestine.

DIGESTIVE FUNCTIONS

Digestive Functions of the Intestines

Four primary digestive functions that are accomplished largely by the small and large intestines are:

1. **Digestion** (chemical and mechanical)
2. **Absorption**
3. **Reabsorption** of water, inorganic salts, vitamin K and amino acids
4. **Elimination** (defecation)

Most **digestion** and **absorption** take place within the **small intestine**. Also the majority of the **salts** and approximately **95% of H_2O is reabsorbed** in the small intestine. Some minimal reabsorption of H_2O and inorganic salts also occurs in the large intestine along with the elimination of unused or unnecessary materials.

The primary function of the **large intestine**, however, is the **elimination of feces** (defecation). Feces consist normally of 40% water and 60% solid matter, such as food residues, digestive secretions and bacteria. Other specific functions of the large intestine are some absorption of water, absorption of inorganic salt, and absorption of vitamin K in addition to certain amino acids. These vitamins and amino acids are produced by a large collection of naturally occurring microorganisms (bacteria) found in the large intestine.

Therefore the last stage of digestion occurs in the large intestine through **bacteria action**, which converts the remaining proteins into amino acids. Some vitamins such as B and K are also synthesized by bacteria and absorbed by the large intestine. A by-product of this bacterial action is the release of hydrogen, carbon dioxide and methane gas. These gases are called **flatus** *(fla′ tus)* and aid in breaking down the remaining proteins to amino acids.

Summary: Lower Digestive System Functions

Responsible component of intestine:	***Function:***
Small intestine: –Duodenum and –Jejunum (primarily)	**1. Digestion**: Chemical and mechanical **2. Absorption**: Nutrients, H_2O, salts, proteins **3. Reabsorption**: H_2O and salts
Large intestine:	(Some reabsorption of H_2O and inorganic salts) –Vitamins B & K –Amino acids } Produced by bacterial action, releases gases (flatus) **4. Elimination** (defecation)

Movements of Digestive Tract

Of the various digestive functions of the intestine, digestive movements sometimes referred to as mechanical digestion, is best demonstrated and evident on radiographic studies.

Small Intestine: Digestive movements throughout the length of the small bowel consist of (1) **peristalsis** *(per″ i-stal′ sis)* to propel intestinal contents along the digestive tract, and (2) **rhythmic segmentation** to thoroughly mix digested food and facilitate absorption.

Large Intestine: In the large intestine, digestive movements continue with (1) **peristalsis**, (2) **haustral** *(haws′ tral)* **churning**, (3) **mass peristalsis** and (4) **defecation** *(def″ e-ka′ shun)*. Mass peristalsis tends to move the entire large bowel contents into the sigmoid colon and rectum, usually happening once every 24 hours. Defecation is a so-called bowel movement or emptying of the rectum.

Summary: Digestive Movements and Elimination

Responsible component of intestine:	***Function:***
Small intestine	**1. Peristalsis** **2. Rhythmic segmentation**
Large intestine	**1. Peristalsis** **2. Haustral churning** **3. Mass peristalsis** **4. Defecation**

Radiographic Procedures

LOWER GASTROINTESTINAL SYSTEM

The plain abdominal radiograph shown in Fig. 15-26 is of a healthy, ambulatory adult. The many meters of small intestine are not visible in the central portion of the abdomen. In the average ambulatory adult, any collection of gas in the small intestine is considered abnormal. Without any gas present, the small bowel simply blends in with other soft tissue structures.

Due to variable amounts of gas and fecal matter normally present in the large intestine, this structure is grossly, but inadequately, visualized on the plain radiograph. Therefore, radiographic examination of the alimentary canal distal to the stomach and duodenum requires the introduction of contrast media for diagnostic visualization.

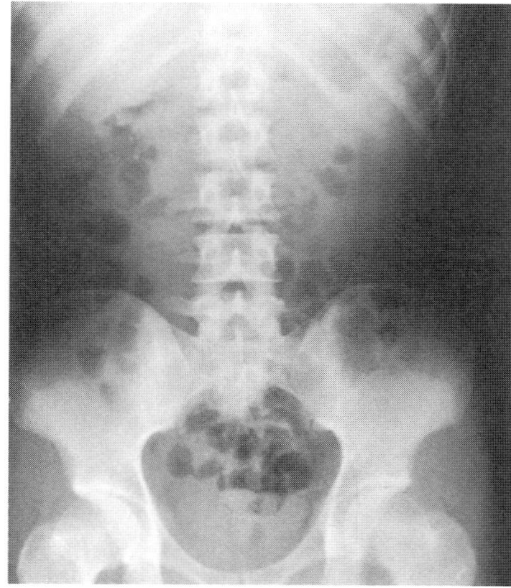

Fig. 15-26. Plain abdominal radiograph –Normal (some gas seen in large intestine).

SMALL BOWEL SERIES

Definition

A radiographic study specifically of the small intestine is termed a **small bowel series** or **SBS**. The upper GI and the small bowel series are most often combined. Under these circumstances, the small bowel portion of the exam may be called a small bowel follow-through. A radiopaque contrast media is required for this study.

Purpose

The purpose of the small bowel series is **to study the form and function of the three components of the small bowel**, as well as **detect any abnormal conditions**.

Since this study also examines **function** of the small bowel, the procedure **must be timed**. The time should be noted when the patient has ingested a substantial amount (at least ¾ cup) of the contrast media.

Clinical Indications

Some clinical indications for a small bowel series include:
- Enteritis or gastroenteritis
- Neoplasms
- Malabsorption syndromes
- Ileus

Enteritis *(en″ter-i′tis)* is a term describing the **inflammation and/or infection of the small bowel**. When the stomach is also involved, the condition is described as **gastroenteritis**.

Neoplasm *(ne′o-plazm)* is a term describing "new growth." This growth may be benign or malignant (cancerous). The small bowel series may demonstrate a stricture or blockage due to the neoplasm.

Malabsorption syndromes are conditions where the patient's GI tract is unable to process and absorb certain nutrients. During the small bowel series, the mucosa may appear to be thickened due to the constant irritation.

Ileus *(il′e-us)* is an **obstruction of the small intestine** as seen in Fig. 15-27 wherein the proximal jejunum is markedly expanded with air. There are **two types** of ileus: (1) **adynamic or paralytic**, and (2) **mechanical**. Adynamic or paralytic ileus is due to the cessation of peristalsis. Without these involuntary, wavelike contractions, the bowel is flaccid and unable to propel its contents forward. Causes for adynamic or paralytic ileus include infection such as peritonitis or appendicitis, presence of certain drugs, or a postsurgical complication.

A mechanical obstruction is a physical blockage of the bowel. It may be due to tumor, adhesions, or hernias.

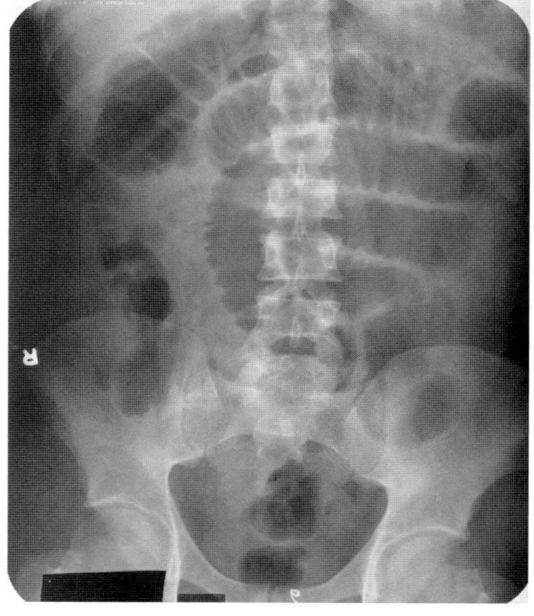

Fig. 15-27. Ileus (obstruction) of small bowel demonstrated by greatly extended air-filled loops of small bowel.

Contraindications

There are **two** strict contraindications to contrast media studies of the intestinal tract. **First,** presurgical patients and patients suspected of having a **perforated, hollow viscus** should **not** receive barium sulfate. The water-soluble, iodinated media should be used instead. With young or dehydrated patients, care must be taken when using a water-soluble contrast media. Because of their hypertonic nature, they tend to draw water into the bowel, leading to increased dehydration.

Second, barium sulfate by mouth is contraindicated in patients with a possible **large bowel obstruction**. An obstructed large bowel should first be ruled out with an acute abdominal series and a barium enema.

SMALL BOWEL PROCEDURES

Four methods are used to study the small intestine radiographically. Methods 1 and 2 are the more common methods. Methods 3 and 4 are special small bowel studies done if methods 1 and 2 are unsatisfactory, or if they are contraindicated.

1. UGI–small bowel combination
2. Small bowel only series
3. Enteroclysis
4. Intubation method

1. Upper GI-Small Bowel Combination

For an upper GI–small bowel combination procedure, a routine upper GI series is done first. After the routine stomach study, progress of the barium is followed through the entire small bowel. During a routine upper GI series, the patient generally should have ingested one full cup or 8 ounces of barium sulfate mixture. For any small bowel examination, the time that the patient ingested this barium should be noted because timing for sequential radiographs is based on the ingestion of this first cup during the UGI procedure.

After completion of fluoroscopy and routine radiography of the stomach, the patient is given one additional cup of barium to ingest. The time that this is done should also be noted. A full second cup of barium may be difficult for the patient to down since this is a large amount of barium to swallow. Thirty minutes after the initial barium ingestion, a PA radiograph of the proximal small bowel is obtained. This first radiograph of the small bowel series (marked "30 minutes") is usually obtained about 15 minutes after completion of the UGI series.

Radiographs are obtained at specific intervals throughout the small bowel series until the barium sulfate column passes through the ileocecal valve and progresses into the ascending colon. For the first 2 hours in the small bowel series, radiographs are usually obtained at 15 to 30 minute intervals. If it becomes necessary to continue the examination beyond the 2-hour time frame, then radiographs are usually obtained every hour until barium passes through the ileocecal valve.

Inspection of Radiographs: As soon as each radiograph in the small bowel series is processed, it should be inspected by the radiologist. The physician may wish to examine any suspicious area under the fluoroscope or request additional radiographs.

Fluoroscopic Study: The region of the terminal ileum and ileocecal valve is generally studied fluoroscopically. Spot filming of the terminal ileum usually indicates completion of the examination.

The patient shown in Fig. 15-28 is in position under the compression cone, which when lowered against the abdomen will spread out loops of ileum to better visualize the ileocecal valve.

Delayed Radiographs: The radiologist may request delayed radiographs in order to follow the barium through the entire large bowel. A barium meal given by mouth usually reaches the rectum in 24 hours.

2. Small Bowel Only Series

The second possibility for study of the small intestine is the small bowel only series as summarized on the right. For every contrast medium examination, including the small bowel series, a plain radiograph should be obtained before introduction of the contrast medium.

For the small bowel only series, 2 cups (16 ounces) of barium are generally ingested by the patient, and the time is noted. Depending on departmental protocol, the first radiograph is taken either 15 or 30 minutes after completion of barium ingestion. This first radiograph includes high centering to include the diaphragm. From this point on, the exam is exactly like the follow-up series of the UGI. Half-hour radiographs are taken for 2 hours, with 1-hour radiographs thereafter, until barium reaches the cecum and/or ascending colon.

Procedure Summary

1. Upper GI–Small bowel combination:

Basic:

- Routine UGI first.
- Note time patient ingested first cup (8 oz.) of barium.
- Ingest second cup of barium.
- 30-minute PA radiograph (center high for proximal SB).
- Half-hour interval radiographs, centered to iliac crest, until barium reaches large bowel (usually 2 hrs).
- One-hour interval radiographs, if more time is needed after two hours.

Special:

- Fluoroscopy and spot filming of ileocecal valve and terminal ileum (compression cone may be used).

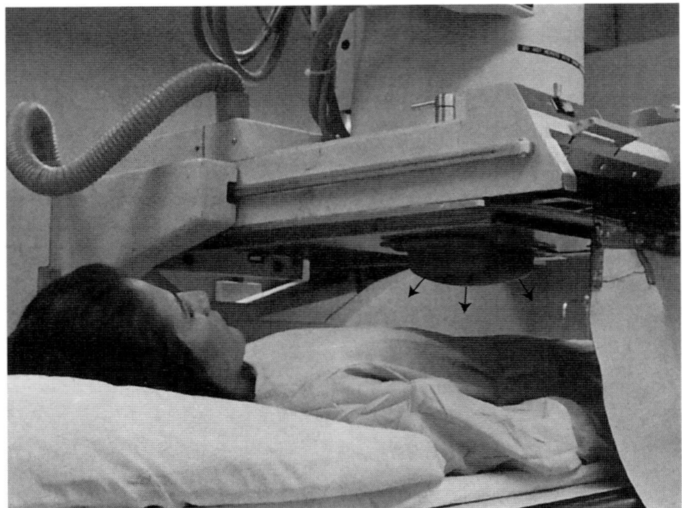

Fig. 15-28. Fluoroscopy of ileocecal region with compression cone.

Procedure Summary

2. Small bowel only series:

Basic:

- Plain abdomen radiograph (scout).
- 2 cups (16 oz.) of barium ingested (note time).
- 15- to 30-minute radiograph (centered high for proximal SB).
- Half-hour interval radiographs until barium reaches large bowel (usually 2 hrs).
- One-hour interval radiographs, if more time is needed.

Special:

- Fluoroscopy with compression may be required.

In the routine small bowel series, regular barium sulfate ordinarily reaches the large intestine within 2 or 3 hours, but this varies greatly among different patients.

Fluoroscopy with spot filming using a compression cone may again be an option to better visualize the ileocecal valve.

SPECIAL SMALL BOWEL PROCEDURES

In certain situations, a more comprehensive evaluation of the small bowel is required. The **enteroclysis** procedure is a **double-contrast method** of evaluating the small bowel. The **intubation method** provides for the direct introduction of contrast media into the small bowel.

3. Enteroclysis (Double-contrast Small Bowel Procedure)

Enteroclysis *(en″ ter-ok′ li-sis)* describes the injection of a nutrient or medicinal liquid into the bowel. In the context of a radiographic small bowel procedure, it refers to a study wherein the patient is intubated under fluoroscopic control with a special **enteroclysis catheter,** which passes through the stomach into the duodenum to the region of the duodenojejunal junction (ligament of Treitz). First a high-density suspension of **barium** is injected through this catheter. Then either **air** or **methylcellulose** is injected into the bowel to distend it and provide a double-contrast effect. Methylcellulose is preferred since it adheres to the bowel while distending it. This double-contrast effect dilates the loops of small bowel while increasing visibility of the mucosa. This leads to increased accuracy of the study.

The disadvantages of enteroclysis are increased patient discomfort, longer examination time compared to a standard small bowel series, and the possibility of bowel perforation during catheter placement.

Enteroclysis is ideal for patients with a clinical history of **small bowel obstruction**, **Crohn's disease**, or **malabsorption syndrome**.

Upon proper filling of the small bowel with the contrast media, the radiologist will take the appropriate fluoro spot films. The radiographer may be asked to produce various projections of the small bowel to include AP, PA, obliques, and possibly erect projections.

After the procedure is completed, the catheter is removed and the patient is encouraged to increase water intake and possibly laxatives.

The radiograph seen in Fig. 15-29 is an example of an enteroclysis. The end of the catheter (small arrows) is seen in the distal duodenum, not yet reaching the duodenojejunal junction (ligament of Treitz, see large upper arrow). The introduction of the methylcellulose dilates the lumen of the bowel, while the barium coats the mucosa.

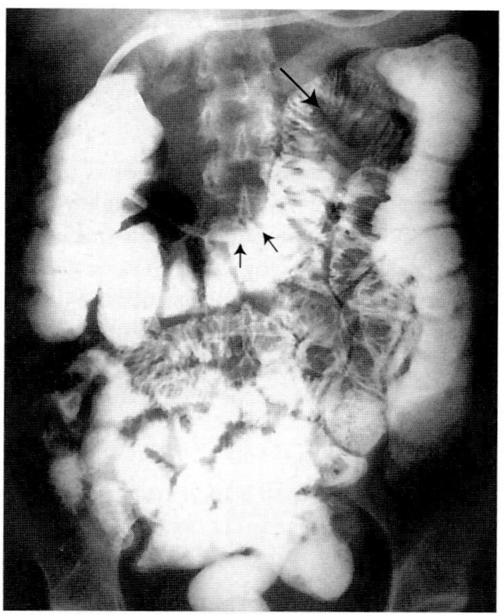

Fig. 15-29. PA radiograph–Enteroclysis.

Procedure Summary

3. Enteroclysis (Double-contrast small bowel series)

Procedure:

- Special catheter advanced to duodenojejunal junction.
- Thin mixture of barium sulfate is instilled.
- Air or methylcellulose is instilled.
- Fluoroscopic spot films and conventional radiographs are taken.
- Upon successful completion of exam, intubation tube is removed.

4. Intubation Method (Single-contrast Media Study)

Gastrointestinal **intubation** *(in″ tu-ba′ shun),* sometimes referred to as a small bowel enema, is a technique whereby a **nasogastric tube** is passed through the patient's nose and through the esophagus, stomach, duodenum and into the jejunum (Fig. 15-30). This radiograph demonstrates the end of the tube (small arrows) still looped in the lower part of the stomach, having not yet passed into the duodenum. The extended air-filled loops of small bowel demonstrating air-fluid levels indicate some type of small bowel obstruction.

This procedure is performed for both diagnostic and therapeutic purposes. The **diagnostic intubation** procedure may be referred to as a **small bowel enema**. A **single-lumen tube** is passed into the proximal jejunum. Placing the patient into a RAO position may aid in passing the tube from the stomach into the duodenum by gastric peristaltic action. Either a water-soluble iodinated agent or a thin barium sulfate suspension is then injected through the tube. Radiographs are taken at timed intervals similar to a standard small bowel series.

The **therapeutic intubation** procedure is often performed to relieve postoperative distention or decompress a small bowel obstruction. A **double lumen** catheter is advanced into the stomach. Mercury may be instilled on the outer lumen to aid in the advancement of the catheter. Through peristalsis, the catheter is advanced into the jejunum. The radiographer may be asked to take radiographs at timed intervals to determine if the catheter is advancing. Gas and excessive fluids can be withdrawn through the catheter.

An optional part of this study may include fluoroscopy wherein the tube can be guided into the duodenum by the use of compression and manual manipulation.

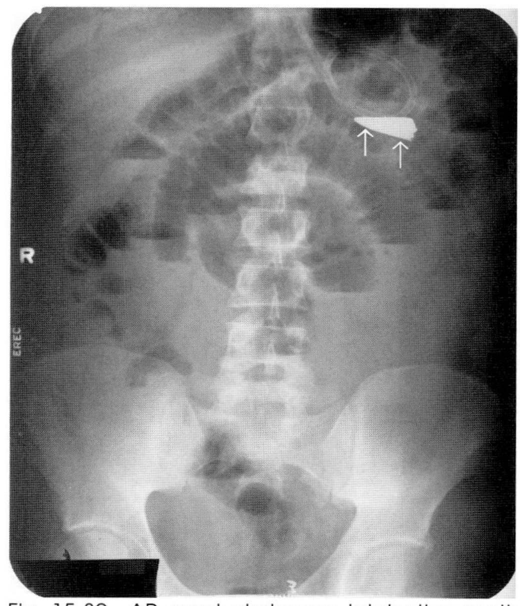

Fig. 15-30. AP erect abdomen–Intubation method.

Procedure Summary

4. Intubation method (Single-contrast small bowel series)

Procedure:

- Single lumen catheter advanced to proximal jejunum (double lumen catheter for therapeutic intubation).
- Water soluble iodinated agent or thin mixture of barium sulfate is instilled.
- Note time that contrast media is instilled.
- Conventional radiographs or optional fluoroscopic spot films taken at specific time intervals.

Small Bowel Series Procedure continued

Patient Preparation

Patient preparation for a small bowel series is identical to that for an upper GI series. In fact, the most common method of small bowel study is a combination of the two examinations into one long examination with the small bowel series following the UGI series.

The goal of patient preparation for either the upper GI series or the small bowel series is an **empty stomach**. Food and fluid must be withheld for at least **8 hours** prior to these exams. In addition, the patient should not smoke cigarettes or chew gum during the NPO period.

Pregnancy Precautions

If the patient is a female, then a menstrual history must be obtained. Irradiation of an early pregnancy is one of the most hazardous situations in diagnostic radiography. X-ray examinations such as the small bowel series or the barium enema that include the pelvis and uterus in the primary beam, and that include fluoroscopy, should **only be done on pregnant females if absolutely necessary**.

Any x-ray examination of the abdomen of a potentially pregnant female should be governed by the "10-day rule." This is the only time when pregnancy can be ruled out with any certainty. Abdominal radiographs and fluoroscopy of a known pregnancy should be delayed at least until the third trimester, if done at all. Generally the only time these GI exams are performed with known pregnancies is when the benefits outweigh the risks as determined by a radiologist in consultation with the referring physician.

Patient Instructions

___ **I.V. CHOLANGIOGRAM AND/OR INTRAVENOUS PYELOGRAM**

1. Fleet's Prep Kit III - 24 hour prep. All instructions are contained in kit.

___ **BARIUM ENEMA**

1. Fleet's Prep Kit III - 24 hour prep. All instructions are contained in kit. May have a clear liquid breakfast.

___ **GALLBLADDER SERIES (ORAL CHOLECYSTOGRAM)**

1. Fat free supper evening before examination.
2. Take one Cholebrine tablet every 1/2 hour starting at 2:00 p.m. day before exam.
3. Nothing by mouth after midnight.

___ **UPPER G.I. SERIES AND/OR SMALL BOWEL SERIES**

1. Do not eat, drink, smoke or chew gum after midnight. Any antispasmodic medication should be preferably discontinued at least 24 hours before exam. Fleet's Prep Kit III may be purchased at most drug stores. Baptist Medical Center Pharmacy carries this kit along with Revco and Thrifty Drugs. Please call ahead to your pharmacy if you have any questions.

ULTRASOUND PREPS:

Ultrasound of the ABDOMEN: **Fat free clear** liquid diet from 6:00 p.m. the evening before examination.
Ultrasound of the PELVIS: **MUST** have a full bladder. Finish drinking 38 to 42 ounces of liquid one hour before exam. **DO NOT** empty bladder until after exam.

C.T. PREPS:

Abdomen - Clear liquids after midnight
Chest - Clear liquids only four hours prior to exam
Head - Clear liquids only four hours prior to exam
Pelvis - Clear liquids after midnight
Spine - no prep

Appointment date ______________ Appointment time ______________

Fig. 15-31. Patient preparation.

Radiographic Room Preparation

Radiographic room preparation depends on the type of small bowel series to be performed. For the upper GI-small bowel combination, room preparation is exactly the same as for an upper GI series. One additional full cup (8 ounces) of barium sulfate mixture is needed. Initial radiographs for both the small bowel series can be made in any general radiographic room, unless the radiologist wishes to fluoroscope the patient's abdomen prior to ingestion of the barium sulfate mixture. Most of the sequentially timed radiographs in any small bowel series are performed in a general radiographic room.

For the enteroclysis and intubation methods, a general fluoroscopic room is necessary since a nasogastric tube must be advanced to the proximal small bowel.

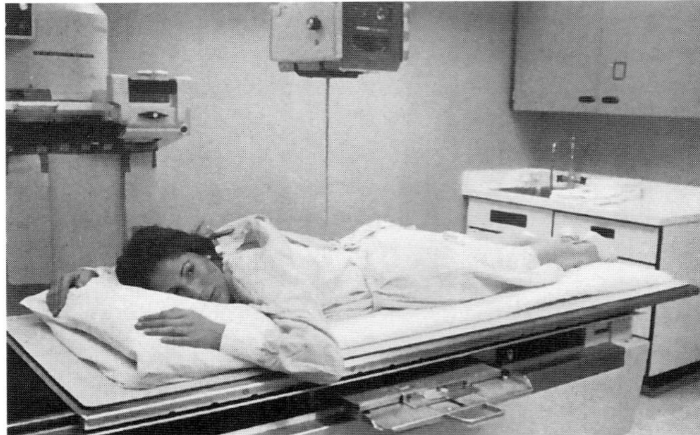

Fig. 15-32. Room preparation.

Method of Imaging

Imaging for any overhead radiograph during a small bowel series is done on 14 x 17 in. (35 x 43 cm) film in order to visualize as much of the small intestine as possible. Spot filming of selected portions of the small bowel is done on smaller-sized film.

The prone position is usually used during a small bowel series, unless the patient is unable to assume that position. The **prone position** allows abdominal compression **to separate the various loops of bowel and create a higher degree of visibility**.

For the 30-minute radiograph, the film is placed high enough to include the stomach on the finished radiograph. This requires longitudinal centering to the duodenal bulb and side-to-side centering to the midsagittal plane. Approximately three-fourths of the film should extend above the iliac crest. Since most of the barium will be in the stomach and proximal small bowel, a high kVp technique should be utilized on this initial radiograph.

All radiographs after the initial 30-minute exposure should be centered to the iliac crest. For the 1-hour and later radiographs, medium kilovoltage techniques may be used since barium is spread through more of the alimentary canal and not concentrated in the stomach. Spot filming of the terminal ileum usually completes the examination.

BARIUM ENEMA (BE OR LOWER GI SERIES)

Definition

The radiographic study of the large intestine is commonly termed a **barium enema**. It requires the use of a contrast media to demonstrate the large intestine and its components. Alternate designations include **BE** or **lower GI series**.

Types of Lower GI Examinations (Procedures)

There are three types of radiographic examinations of the large intestine that will be described and demonstrated in this chapter.
(1) Single-contrast barium enema.
(2) Double-contrast barium enema.
(3) Defecogram.

Purpose

The purpose of the barium enema is to **radiographically study the form and function of the large intestine**, as well as to **detect any abnormal conditions**. Both the single contrast and the double-contrast barium enema include a study of the entire large intestine, while the defecogram is a functional study of the distal portion, namely the anus and rectum.

Clinical indications

Clinical indications for the barium enema include:

- Colitis
- Diverticulosis/diverticulitis
- Neoplasms
- Volvulus
- Intussusception
- Appendicitis

Colitis *(ko-li′ is)*, is an inflammatory condition of the large intestine that may be caused by many factors including bacterial infection, diet, stress, and other environmental conditions. A severe form of colitis is **ulcerative colitis**. It is a chronic condition often leading to coin-like ulcers developing within the mucosal wall. These ulcers may be seen during the barium enema.

A **diverticulum** *(di″ ver-tik′ u-lum)* is an outpouching of the mucosal wall resulting from a herniation of the inner wall of the colon. Although a relatively benign condition, it may become widespread throughout the colon. The condition of having numerous diverticula is termed **diverticulosis**. If these diverticula become infected, the condition is now referred to as **diverticulitis**. A patient may develop peritonitis if a diverticulum perforates through the mucosal wall.

Diverticula will appear as small circular defects on the colon wall.

Neoplasms or tumors are common in the large intestine. While benign tumors do occur, carcinoma of the large intestine is a leading cause of death in both males and females. These cancerous tumors often encircle the lumen of the colon. The radiographic appearance leads to descriptive terms such as "apple core" or "napkin ring" lesions. Both benign and malignant tumors may begin as **polyps** *(pol′ ips)*. A polyp is a small growth extending from the mucosal wall. (These are not the same as diverticulum described above.) The double-contrast barium enema is valuable in detecting polyps.

Volvulus *(vol′ vu-lus)* is a twisting of a portion of the intestine on its own mesentery. Blood supply to the twisted portion is compromised leading to obstruction and necrosis or localized death of tissue. While a volvulus may be found in portions of the jejunum or ileum, the most common sites are the cecum and sigmoid colon.

Intussusception *(in″ tus-sus-sep′ shun)* is the telescoping of one part of the bowel into another. It is often seen with infants. A barium enema or an air enema may play a therapeutic role in re-expanding the involved bowel. Intussusception must be resolved quickly or it may lead to obstruction and necrosis of the bowel (see Chapter 20, pediatric radiography).

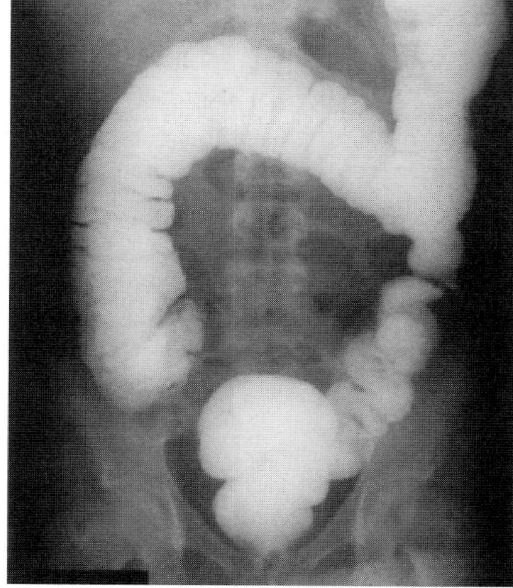

Fig. 15-33. BE, single contrast.

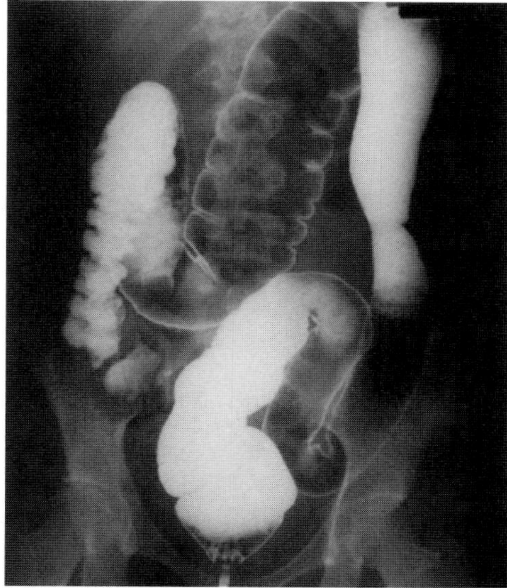

Fig. 15-34. BE, double contrast.

Appendicitis: A barium enema may be performed to rule out appendicitis. Appendicitis may be caused by infection or a blockage of the blood vessels that feed the appendix. Sometimes a fecal mass may develop near the proximal aspect of the appendix cutting off the blood supply to it. This mass is termed an appendolith. The barium enema may be helpful in identifying a possible appendolith or an inflamed appendix.

Contraindication

The contraindications for the barium enema are similar to those described for the small bowel series. A careful review of the patient's chart and clinical history may help prevent problems during the procedure.

It is important to review the patient's chart to determine if the patient had a sigmoidoscopy or colonoscopy prior to the barium enema. If a biopsy of the colon was performed during these procedures, the involved section of the colon wall may be weakened, which may lead to perforation during the barium enema. The radiologist must be informed of this situation prior to beginning the procedure.

BARIUM ENEMA PROCEDURE

Patient Preparation

Preparation of the patient for a barium enema is more involved than is preparation for the stomach and small bowel. The final objective, however, is the same. The **section of alimentary canal to be examined must be empty**. Thorough cleansing of the entire large bowel is of paramount importance to the satisfactory contrast medium study of the large intestine.

Contraindications to Cathartics *(kah-thar′ tiks)*

Certain conditions contraindicate the use of very effective cathartics or purgatives needed to thoroughly cleanse the large bowel. These exceptions are: (1) gross bleeding, (2) severe diarrhea, (3) obstruction and (4) inflammatory lesions such as appendicitis.

A cathartic or purgative is a substance that produces frequent, soft or liquid bowel movements. These substances increase peristalsis in the large bowel, and occasionally in the small bowel as well, by irritating the sensory nerve endings in the intestinal mucosa. This increased peristalsis dramatically accelerates intestinal contents through the digestive system.

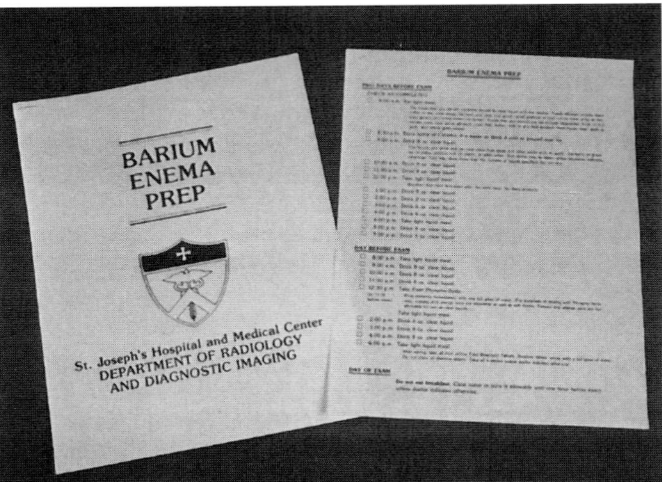

Fig. 15-35. Patient preparation instructions.
Courtesy of St. Joseph's Hospital and Medical Center, Phoenix, AZ

Two Classes of Cathartics

Two different classes of cathartics may be prescribed. First are the irritant cathartics such as castor oil; and second are the saline cathartics such as magnesium citrate or magnesium sulfate. For best results, bowel-cleansing procedures should be specified on patient instruction sheets for both inpatients and outpatients. A radiographer should be completely familiar with the type of preparation used in each radiology department. The importance of a clean bowel for a barium enema, and especially for a double-contrast barium enema, cannot be overstated. Any retained fecal matter may obscure the normal anatomy or give false diagnostic information and may lead to a rescheduling of the procedure after the colon has been properly cleaned.

Radiographic Room Preparation

The radiographic room should be prepared in advance of the patient's arrival. The fluoroscopic room and examination table should be clean and tidy for each patient. The control panel should be set for fluoroscopy with the appropriate technical factors selected. The fluoroscopy timer should be set at its maximum, usually 5 minutes. The spot film mechanism should be in proper working order and a supply of spot film cassettes should be handy. The appropriate number and size of conventional cassettes should be provided. Protective lead aprons and lead gloves should be provided for the radiologist, as well as lead aprons for all other personnel to be in the room. The fluoroscopic table should be placed in the horizontal position, with waterproof backing or disposable pads placed on the table-top. Waterproof protection is essential in case of premature evacuation of the enema.

The footboard is generally not necessary for the BE and may be removed. The Bucky tray must be positioned at the foot end of the table if the fluoroscopy tube is located beneath the table-top. Place the radiation foot control switch appropriately for the radiologist or prepare the remote control area. Tissues, towels, replacement linen, bedpan, extra gowns, a room air freshener and a waste receptacle should be readily available. Prepare the appropriate contrast medium or media, container, tubing and enema tip. A proper lubricant should be provided for the enema tip. The type of barium sulfate used and the concentration of the mixture varies considerably depending on radiologist preferences and the type of examination to be performed.

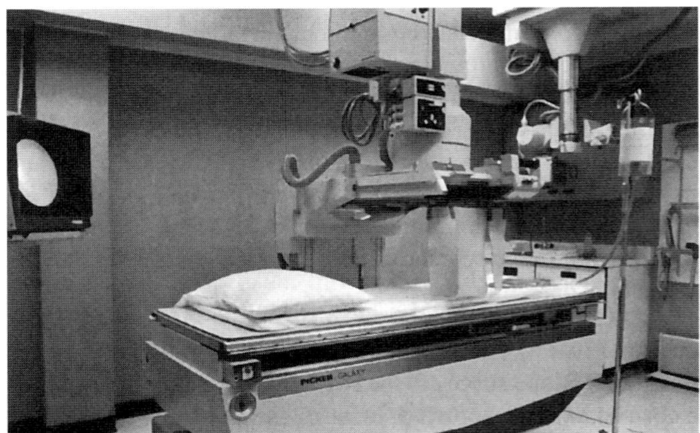

Fig. 15-36. Room preparation.

Equipment and Supplies

Barium Enema Containers: A closed system-type enema container is used to administer the barium sulfate or barium sulfate and air combination during the barium enema (Fig. 15-37). This closed type disposable barium enema bag system has replaced the older open type system for convenience and to reduce the risk of cross infection.

This system seen in the photograph demonstrates the disposable enema bag with a pre-measured amount of barium sulfate. Once mixed, the suspension travels down its own connective tubing and flow is controlled by a plastic stopcock. An enema tip is placed on the end of the tubing which is inserted in the patient's rectum.

After the examination, much of the barium can be drained back into the bag by lowering the system below table-top level. The entire bag and tubing are disposed of after a single use.

Enema Tips: Various types and sizes of enema tips are available (Fig. 15-38). The three most common enema tips are (A) the plastic disposable, (B) the rectal retention, and (C) air contrast retention enema tips. All of these are considered single use, disposable enema tips.

Rectal disposable retention tips (B) and (C) (sometimes called retention catheters) are used on those patients who have a relaxed anal sphincter, or those who cannot for any reason, retain the enema. These rectal retention catheters consist of a double lumen tube with a thin rubber balloon at the distal end (2). This balloon can be carefully inflated with air through a small tube (3) to assist the patient in retaining the barium enema. These retention catheters should be **fully inflated only with fluoroscopic guidance by the radiologist** because of the potential dangers of intestinal rupture. Due to the discomfort to the patient, the balloon should not be fully inflated until the fluoroscopy procedure begins.

A special type of rectal tip (C) is needed to inject air through a separate tube (5), which mixes with the barium tube (4) as it passes into the colon for a double-contrast BE exam.

Contrast Media Preparation

The preparation of the contrast media for a closed system barium enema kit is specified by the manufacturer. The mixing instructions as supplied by the manufacturer should be followed precisely.

A debate has evolved over the temperature of the water that is used to prepare the barium sulfate suspension. Some experts recommend the use of cold water (40 to 45° F) in the preparation of the contrast media. The cold water is reported to have an anesthetic effect on the colon and increase retention of the contrast media. Critics have stated that the cold water may lead to colonic spasm.

Room-temperature water is recommended by most experts to produce a more successful examination with maximum patient comfort. The radiographer should NEVER use hot water to prepare the contrast media. The hot water may scald the mucosal lining of the colon.

Since the barium sulfate produces a colloidal suspension, it is important to shake the enema bag prior to tip insertion to prevent separation of the barium sulfate and water.

Glucagon is a drug given intravenously to control colonic spasm. It should be kept in the department for these situations.

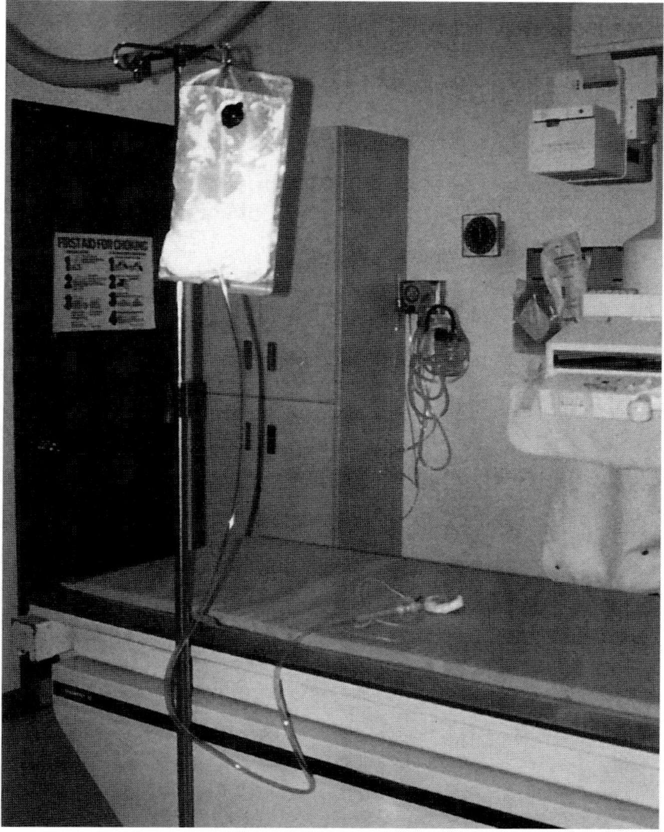

Fig. 15-37. Closed system enema container.

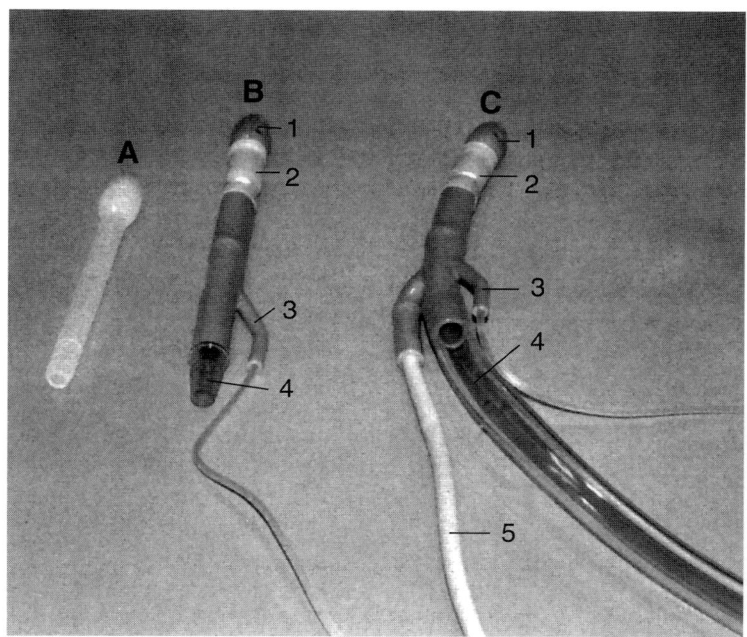

Fig. 15-38. Enema tips.

Description of above:

A. Plastic enema tip.

B. Rectal retention tip:
1. Enema tip with side and end holes.
2. Inflatable retention balloon.
3. Air tube for inflating balloon.
4. End attaching to enema bag tubing to introduce barium.

C. Air contrast retention tip:
1 - 4. Same as above.
5. Tube to introduce air into colon.

15

BE Procedure continued

Procedure Preparation

A barium enema patient is examined in an appropriate hospital gown. A cotton gown with the opening and ties in the back is preferable. Never use the type of gown that must be pulled over the patient's head to remove. Sometimes the gown will become soiled during the examination. The outpatient is instructed to remove all clothing, including shoes and socks or hose. Disposable slippers should be provided in case some barium is lost on the way to the rest room.

After the fluoroscopic room is completely prepared and the contrast medium is ready, the patient is escorted to the examination room. Prior to insertion of the enema tip, a pertinent history should be taken and the examination should be carefully explained. Since complete cooperation is essential, and since this examination can be somewhat embarrassing, every effort should be made to reassure the patient at every stage of the exam.

Any previous radiographs should be available for the radiologist. The patient is placed in the Sims position prior to insertion of the enema tip.

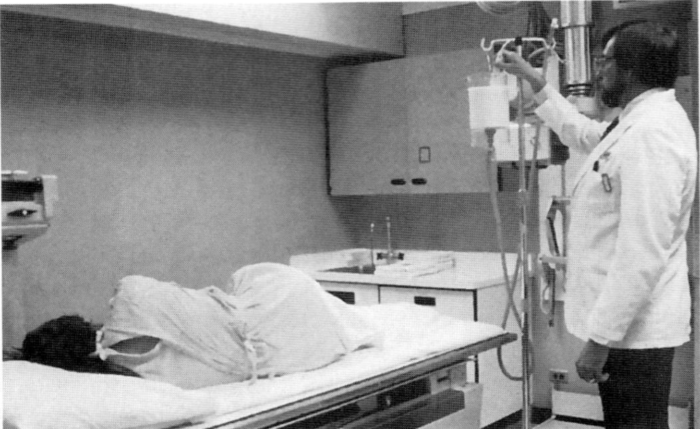

Fig. 15-39. Procedure preparation.

Sims Position

The Sims position is shown in Fig. 15-40. The patient is asked to roll onto the left side and to lean well forward. The right leg is flexed at the knee and hip and is placed in front of the left leg. The left knee is comfortably flexed. The Sims position relaxes the abdominal muscles and decreases pressure within the abdomen.

During the procedure, each phase of the rectal tube insertion must be explained to the patient. Prior to rectal tube insertion, the barium sulfate solution should be well mixed. Before insertion, a little of the barium mixture should be run into a waste receptacle to ensure that no air remains in the tubing or enema tip.

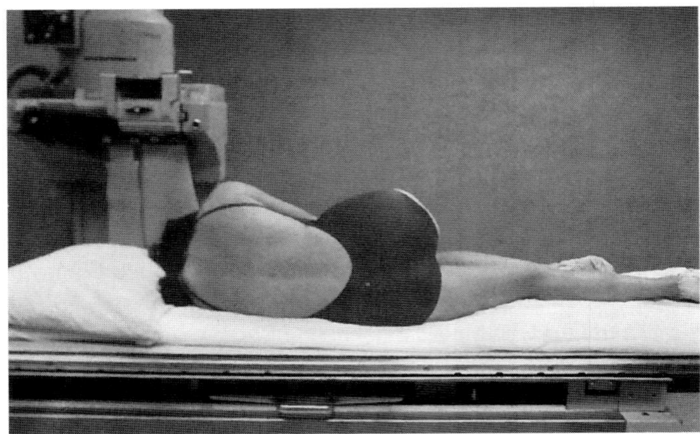

Fig. 15-40. Sims position.

Rectal Tube

The radiographer wears a rectal glove and enfolds the enema tip in several sheets of paper toweling. The rectal tip is well lubricated with a water-soluble lubricant. Before the examination, the patient should be instructed to (1) keep the anal sphincter tightly contracted against the rectal tube to hold it in position and prevent leakage, (2) relax the abdominal muscles to prevent increased intra-abdominal pressure and (3) concentrate on breathing by mouth to reduce spasms and cramping. The patient must be assured that barium flow will be stopped during cramping.

Enema Tip Insertion

To insert the enema tip, adjust the opening in the back of the patient's gown to expose only the anal region. The rest of the patient should be well covered when inserting the rectal tube. Protect the patient's modesty in any way you can during the barium enema examination. The right buttock should be raised to open the gluteal fold and expose the anus. The patient should take in a few deep breaths prior to actual insertion of the enema tip. If the tip will not enter with gentle pressure, the patient should be asked to relax and assist if possible. The tip should **NEVER** be forced in such a manner that could cause injury to the patient. Since the abdominal muscles relax on expiration, the tip should be inserted during the exhalation phase of respiration.

The rectum and anal canal present a double curvature, therefore the tube is first inserted in a forward direction approximately 1 to 1½ inches (2.5 to 4 cm). This initial insertion should be **aimed toward the umbilicus**. After the initial insertion, the rectal tube is directed **superiorly and slightly anteriorly** to follow the normal curvature of the rectum. The total insertion of the tip should **not exceed 3 to 4 centimeters** to avoid possible injury to the wall of the rectum. The rectal tube may be taped in place or held to prevent it from slipping out while the patient turns back into a supine position ready for the start of fluoroscopy. This position is usually supine, but may be prone depending on the preference of the radiologist.

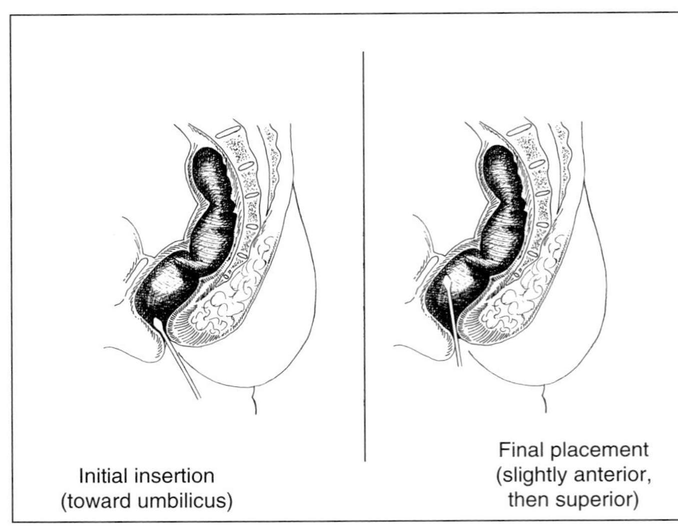

Fig. 15-41. Enema tip insertion.

If the retention type tip is necessary, most departments allow the radiographer to instill one or two puffs of air into the balloon end to help hold it in place. However, the bulb should be filled to its maximum only under fluoroscopic control as the fluoroscopy procedure begins.

Fluoroscopy Routine

The radiologist is summoned to the radiographic room when all room and patient preparations are completed. Following introduction of the physician and patient, the patient's history and the reason for the examination are discussed.

During barium enema fluoroscopy, the general duties of the radiographer are to follow the radiologist's instructions, to assist the patient as needed and to expedite the procedure in any way possible. The radiographer must also control the flow of barium and/or air, and change fluoro spot cassettes. The flow of barium will be started and stopped several times during the BE. Each time the radiologist asks that the flow be started, the radiographer should say "barium on" after the clamp or hemostat is released. Each time the radiologist requests that the flow be stopped, the radiographer should say "barium off" after the tubing is clamped.

Many changes in patient position are made during fluoroscopy. These positional changes are made to better visualize superimposed sections of bowel, as well as to aid in advancement of the barium column. Areas of the large intestine best studied by positional changes include the rectosigmoid area, the two flexures and the cecal area. The radiographer may need to assist the patient with positional moves and make sure that the tubing is not kinked or accidentally pulled out during the examination.

The fluoroscopic procedure begins with a general survey of the patient's abdomen and chest. If the retention-type enema tip is required, the air balloon is inflated under fluoroscopic control at this point. Various spot radiographs are obtained of selected portions of the large intestine as the barium column proceeds in retrograde fashion from rectum to cecum. At the end of the fluoroscopic procedure, a little barium is refluxed through the ileocecal valve and fluoro spots are obtained of that area. Moderate discomfort is usually experienced when the large bowel is totally filled, so the examination must be concluded as rapidly as possible. Routine overhead radiographs are obtained with the bowel filled.

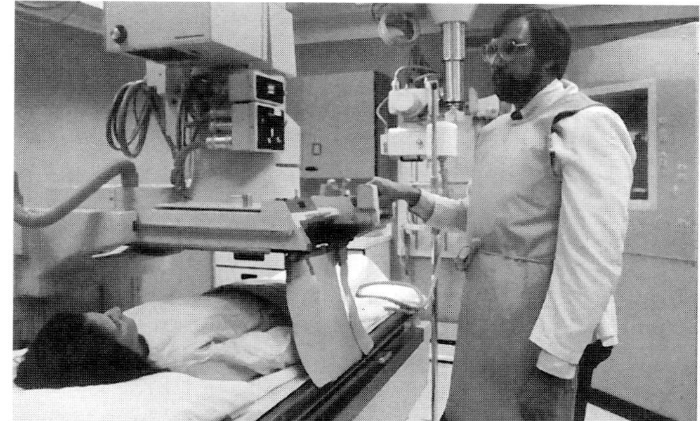

Fig. 15-42. Fluoroscopy.

TYPES OF LOWER GI EXAMINATIONS (PROCEDURES)

Three specific types of radiographic examinations or procedures of the lower GI are as follows:
(1) Single-contrast barium enema.
(2) Double-contrast barium enema.
(3) Defecogram.

(1) Single-contrast Barium Enema Procedure

The single-contrast barium enema utilizes only a positive contrast medium. In most cases the contrast material is barium sulfate in a thin mixture. Occasionally, the contrast medium will have to be a water-soluble contrast material. If the patient is to be taken to surgery following the BE, then a water-soluble contrast medium must be used. An example of a single-contrast barium enema utilizing barium sulfate as the contrast medium is shown in Fig. 15-43.

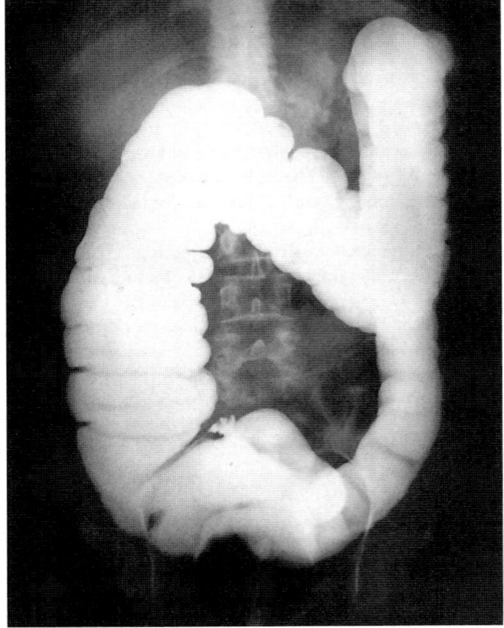

Fig. 15-43. Single-contrast barium enema.

(2) Double-contrast Barium Enema Procedure

Radiographic and fluoroscopic procedures for a double-contrast barium enema are somewhat different in that both air and barium must be introduced into the large bowel. Fig. 15-44 is a double-contrast BE radiograph taken in the right lateral decubitus position. An absolutely **clean large bowel is essential** to the double-contrast study, and a **much thicker barium mixture is required**. Although exact ratios depend on the commercial preparations utilized, the ratio approaches a one-to-one mix so that the final product is like heavy cream.

Two-Stage Procedure: One preferred method of coating the bowel is to utilize a two-stage, double-contrast procedure. Initially, the thick barium is allowed to fill the left side of the bowel. (The purpose of the thick barium mixture is to facilitate adherence to the mucosal lining.) Air is then instilled into the bowel, pushing the barium column through to the right side. The patient is then allowed to evacuate as much of the barium as possible.

The second stage consists of inflating the bowel with a large amount of air which moves the main column of barium forward leaving only the barium adhering to the mucosal wall. These steps are carried out under fluoroscopic control since the air column cannot be allowed to get in front of the barium column.

This procedure demonstrates neoplasms that may be forming on the inner wall of the bowel projecting into the lumen or opening of the bowel. These generally would not be visible during a single-contrast, full-column barium enema study.

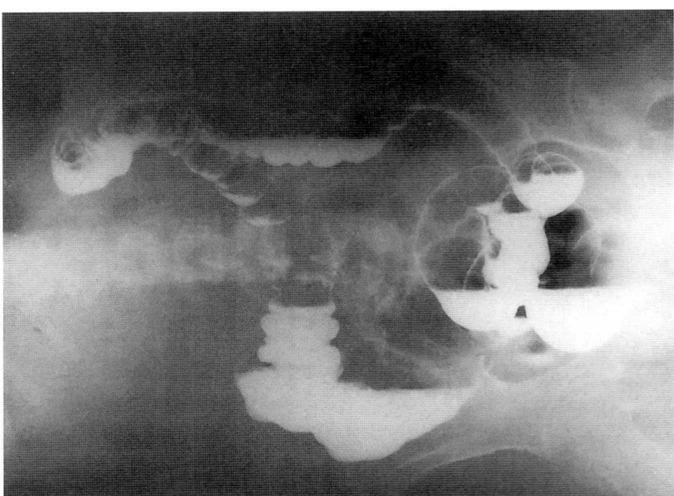

Fig. 15-44. Double-contrast barium enema (right lateral decubitus).

Single-Stage Procedure: A single-stage, double-contrast procedure may also be used wherein the barium and air are instilled in a single procedure, which reduces time and radiation exposure to the patient. With this method some high-density barium is first instilled into the rectum with the patient in a slightly Trendelenburg position. The barium tube is then clamped, and with the table in a horizontal position the patient is placed into the various oblique and lateral positions following the addition of various amounts of air with the double-contrast procedure.

Spot Films (During Fluoroscopy): With both the single-contrast and the double-contrast studies, spot radiographs are obtained to document any suspicious area. The patient may be asked to rotate several times to distribute the barium and air better with the double-contrast procedure.

Post Fluoroscopy Radiographs: After fluoroscopy and before the patient is allowed to empty the large bowel, one or more radiographs of the filled bowel should be obtained for either single-contrast or double-contrast procedures. The standard enema tip can be removed prior to these radiographs since this may make it easier to hold in the enema. However, some departmental routines keep the enema tip in during the overhead filming procedure. The retention-type tip, however, is generally not removed until the large bowel is ready to be emptied when the patient is placed on a bed pan or on the commode.

Figure 15-45 demonstrates the most common position for a routine barium enema. This is the PA projection with a full-sized 14 x 17 in. cassette centered to the iliac crest. The PA projection with the patient in a prone position is preferred over an AP in a supine position because compression of the abdomen in the prone position results in a more uniform radiographic density of the entire abdomen.

The film and cassette should be centered to include the rectal ampulla on the bottom of the finished radiograph. This positioning will usually include the entire large intestine with the exception of the left colic flexure. It may be acceptable to cut off the left colic flexure on the radiographs if this area is well demonstrated on a previously obtained spot film. However, some departmental routines may include a second film centered higher to include this area on larger patients.

Other projections are also obtained prior to evacuation of the barium. Double-contrast procedures generally require right and left lateral decubitus projections with a horizontal x-ray beam to better demonstrate the upside or air-filled portions of the large intestine. All post-fluoro radiographs must be obtained as rapidly as possible since the patient may have difficulty retaining the barium.

Once the routine pre-evacuation radiographs and any supplemental radiographs have been obtained, the patient is allowed to expel the barium. For the patient who has had the enema tip removed, a quick trip to a nearby rest room is necessary. For the patient who cannot make such a trip, a bedpan should be provided. For the patient who is still connected to a closed system, simply lowering the plastic bag to floor level and allowing most of the barium to drain back into the bag is helpful. Department protocol determines how a retention tip should be removed. One way is to first clamp off the retention tip, then disconnect it from the enema tubing and container. Once the patient is safely on a bedpan or commode, air is released from the bulb and the tip is removed.

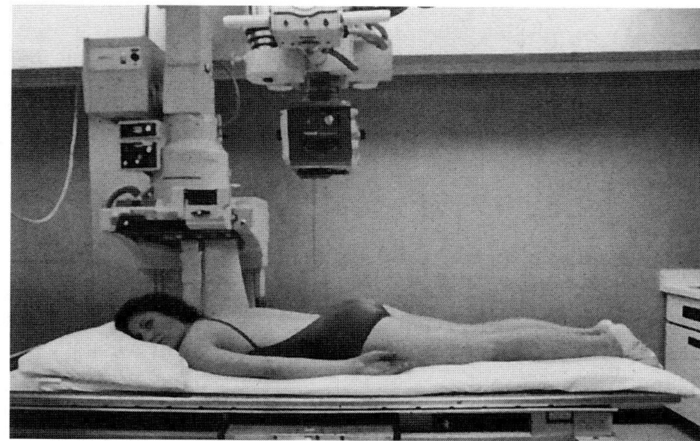

Fig. 15-45. Post fluoroscopy radiography–PA projection.

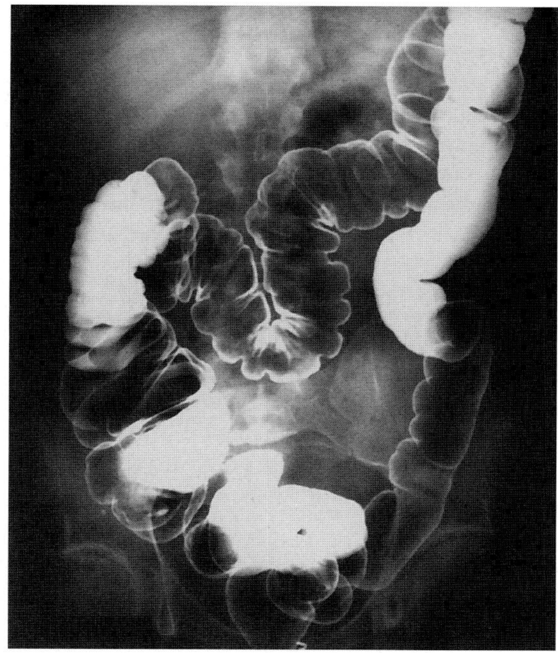

Fig. 15-46. AP, double-contrast barium enema.

Post-evac Radiograph: After most of the barium has been expelled, a post-evacuation radiograph is obtained. The post-evac radiograph is usually taken prone, but may be taken supine if needed. Most of the barium should have been evacuated. If too much barium is retained, the patient is given more time for evacuation and a second post-evac film is taken.

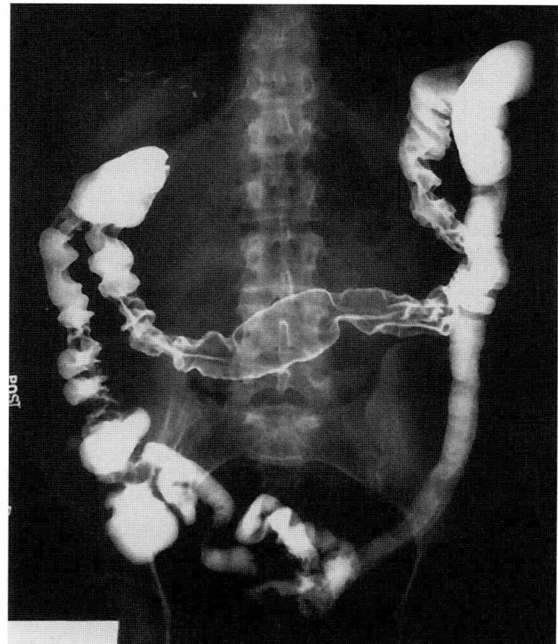

Fig. 15-47. AP, post-evac.

(3) Defecography

A third type of radiographic study involving the lower GI tract is **defecography**, sometimes called **evacuative proctography**. This is a newer type of procedure being performed in many departments, especially on children or younger patients.

Definition and Purpose: The defecogram is **a functional study of the anus and rectum during the evacuation and rest phases of defecation** (bowel movement).

Clinical Indications: Clinical indications for defecography include **rectoceles**, **rectal intussusception**, and **prolapse of the rectum**. The rectocele, a common form of pathology, is a blind pouch of the rectum due to weakening of the anterior or posterior wall. These rectoceles may retain fecal material even after evacuation.

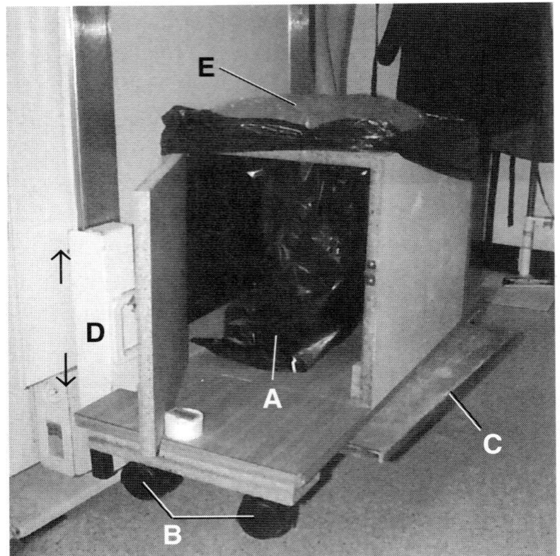

Fig. 15-48. Commode for defecogram.

Special Equipment: A special commode is required for this study (Fig. 15-48). It consists of a toilet seat built onto a frame that contains a waste receptacle or a disposable plastic bag (A). The commode demonstrated has wheels or casters (B) so it can be rolled into position over the extended foot board and platform (C) attached to the table-top (D). The entire commode with patient can then be raised or lowered by raising the table-top with the attached footboard and commode during the procedure (see arrows). Clamps should be used (not shown in these visuals) to secure the commode to the foot board platform for stability during the procedure. The clamps allow the commode to be attached to the footboard to be raised as needed to utilize the table Bucky and fluoroscopy unit. The seat is often cushioned (E) for patient comfort. The filters found beneath the seat (not shown) compensate for tissue differences and help maintain acceptable levels of density and contrast.

E

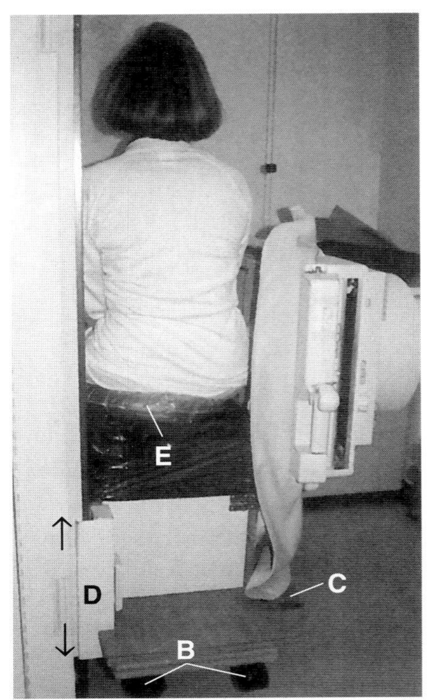

Fig. 15-49. Patient in position.

Contrast Media: To study the process of evacuation, a very high-density barium sulfate mixture is required. Some departments will produce their own contrast media by mixing barium sulfate with either potato starch or commercially produced additives. The potato starch thickens the barium sulfate to produce a mashed potato consistency. The normal barium sulfate suspension evacuates too quickly to detect any pathology.

A ready-to-use contrast media, **Anatrast®**, is available (Fig. 15-50). This contrast media is premixed and packaged in a single use tube. Some departments will also introduce a thick liquid barium, such as **Polibar Plus®**, prior to the Anatrast to determine the appearance and alignment of the rectum.

Applicator: The mechanical applicator (Fig. 15-50) resembles a caulking gun similar to that used in the building industry. The premixed and prepackaged tube of Anatrast is inserted in the applicator and a flexible tube with an enema tip is attached to the opened tip of the tube (B-1).

The thick liquid Polibar is drawn into a syringe and inserted through a rectal tube and tip. In this example an inner plastic tube (C) is being used, inserted in an outer rectal tube (D) to which the enema tip is attached. The syringe is then used to instill the thick liquid Polibar Plus® contrast media. The inner plastic tube is attached to the syringe filled with the Polibar and inserted within the rectal tube to which is attached a standard enema tip for insertion into the rectum.

Labeled parts (Fig. 15-50):
A. Mechanical applicator.
B. Tube of Anatrast (B-1 tip to be opened).
C. Inner plastic tube (for insertion of syringe or tube of Anatrast).
D. Rectal tube (to which enema tip is attached, D-1).
E. Syringe.

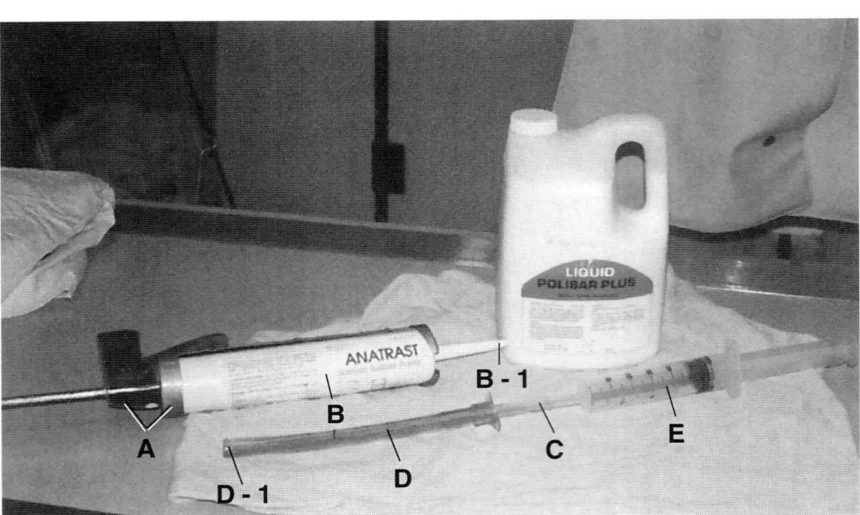

Fig. 15-50. Applicator.

Defecogram Procedure: With the patient in a lateral recumbent position on a cart, the contrast media is instilled into the rectum with the applicator. The patient is quickly placed on the commode for filming during defecation. Fluoroscopy spot films and standard radiographic projections are taken during the study. The lateral rectum projection is usually preferred by most radiologists (Fig. 15-51).

It is vital that the anorectal angle is demonstrated during the procedure. This angle is the alignment between the anus and rectum that shifts between the rest and evacuation phases. The radiologist will measure this angle during these phases to determine if any abnormalities exist.

A lateral post-evac radiograph is taken as the final part of this procedure (Fig. 15-52).

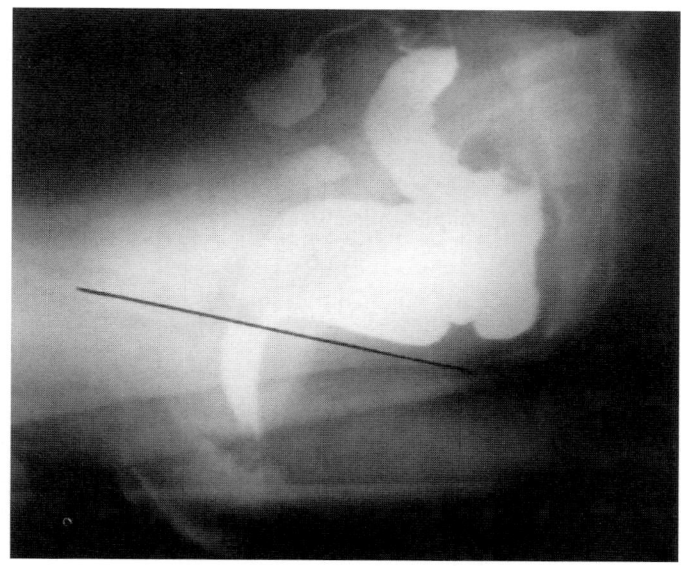

Fig. 15-51. Lateral defecogram (during strain or evacuation).

Summary of Defecogram Procedure

1. Place radiographic table vertical and attach commode with clamps.
2. Prepare contrast medium according to department specifications.
3. Set up imaging equipment (fluoroscopy, 105 mm spot film camera, spot cassette, or video recorder).
4. Have patient remove all clothing and change into a hospital gown.
5. Take a scout film using conventional x-ray tube (scout film must include the region of the anorectal angle).
6. Place patient in a lateral recumbent position on a cart and instill contrast medium.
7. Position patient on the commode and film patient in the rest and strain phases. Patient is in a lateral position and filmed using conventional x-ray tube.
8. Using fluoroscopy imaging devices or video recorder, patient is filmed while defecating.
9. Post-evacuation film is taken.

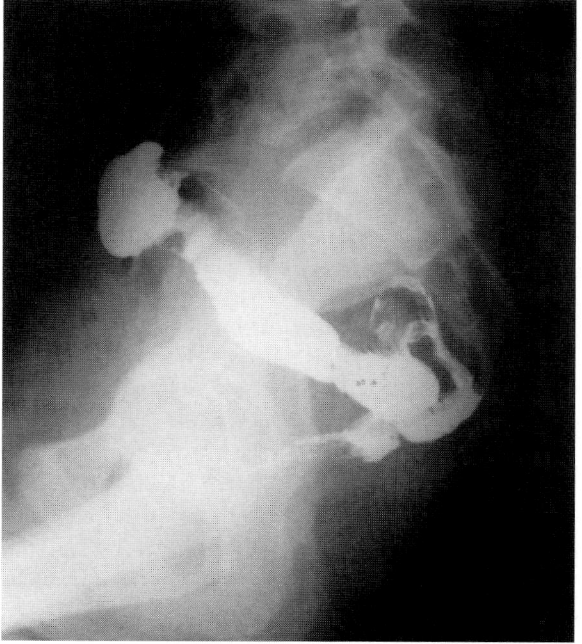

Fig. 15-52. Lateral defecogram (same patient as above-post-evac).

Summary of Safety Concerns During the Barium Enema Procedure

Safety during the barium enema procedure is of utmost importance. Five of these important safety concerns are as follows:

(1) **Review the patient's chart**. Note any pertinent clinical history on the exam requisition and inform the radiologist if the patient had a sigmoidoscopy or colonoscopy prior to the barium enema, especially if a biopsy was performed.

(2) **Never force an enema tip into the rectum**. This may lead to a perforated rectum. The radiologist will insert the enema tip under fluoroscopy guidance if needed.

(3) **The height of the enema bag should not exceed 24 inches above the table**. This distance should be maintained prior to the beginning of the procedure. The radiologist may wish to raise bag height during the procedure based upon the rate of flow of the contrast media.

(4) **Verify the water temperature of the contrast media**. Too hot or cold water may injure your patient or compromise the procedure.

(5) **Escort the patient to the rest room after completion**. A barium enema can be very stressful for certain patients. Patients have been known to faint during or after evacuation.

Radiographic Positioning

NATIONAL SURVEY

A survey of the operating procedures (department routines) was conducted throughout the United States. The following information was compiled from the survey indicating the national norm for basic and special projections for small bowel and barium enema series. The results were very consistent throughout all regions of the US. (637 institutions responded to this part of the survey in 1995, and 533 in 1989.)

Small Bowel Series

Small bowel series	U.S. Average			
	Basic		Special	
	1995	(1989)	1995	(1989)
• PA scout	71%	–		
• PA (½ hr. to 2 hrs., hourly after 2 hrs.)	93%	(85%)		
• Ileocecal spots	69%	(79%)		
• Enteroclysis procedure	13%	(12%)	38%	(25%)
• Intubation method	4%	(4%)	21%	(17%)

Barium Enema Routine

Barium enema	U.S. Average			
	Basic		Special	
	1995	(1989)	1995	(1989)
• Double-contrast	87%	(76%)	14%	–
• Single-contrast	81%	(72%)	16%	–
• PA	93%	(86%)		
• L lateral rectum	89%	(77%)		
• R lateral decubitus	76%	(73%)		
• L lateral decubitus	85%	(73%)		
• LPO & RPO	78%	(18%)	8%	(10%)
• RAO & LAO	58%	(58%)		
• PA post-evac	85%	(71%)		
• AP axial (butterfly)	45%	(18%)	14%	(7%)
• PA axial (butterfly)	40%	(15%)	11%	(4%)
• Chassard-Lapine axial	–	(13%)	–	(11%)
• Ventral decubitus	16%	–	15%	–

Summary

Small Bowel Series: The survey indicated that **ileocecal spots** are generally included as part of a routine small bowel series. This has not changed significantly in 1995 as compared to 1989. However, this does not indicate whether this includes fluoroscopy along with spot films or just localized overhead radiographs of this area.

Enteroclysis procedures are shown to be increasingly performed as special small bowel procedures (38% in 1995 and 25% in 1989). The **intubation method** also shows a slight increase in usage (21% in 1995 and 17% in 1989).

Barium Enema Routine: The survey indicated that both the **double-contrast** and the **single-contrast** barium enema are considered basic or routine in most departments in the US, with the double-contrast continuing to receive a slightly higher indication of usage.

The **Chassard-Lapine axial** (Fig. 15-53 and 15-54) is no longer included in this chapter as a separate projection in the positioning pages because of the very low percentage of survey respondents who indicated it as a basic or special projection. Also, because of the high gonadal dose, this is not a preferred projection for younger patients; older patients have difficulty with sphincter control in this position.

For information purposes, this projection and the resultant radiograph, which primarily demonstrates the rectosigmoid portion of the large intestine, are shown on the right.

As a preferred alternate to this axial Chassard-Lapine projection, the **AP axial** or **PA axial** (butterfly) also demonstrates the rectosigmoid region as shown and described in this chapter with more comfort to the patient and a much lower gonadal dose.

Another BE projection with a low percentage of usage is the **ventral decubitus** projection, which indicated less than 20% usage. Therefore it is not described as a separate projection but is included as an alternate projection for the lateral rectum with a double-contrast exam (page 476).

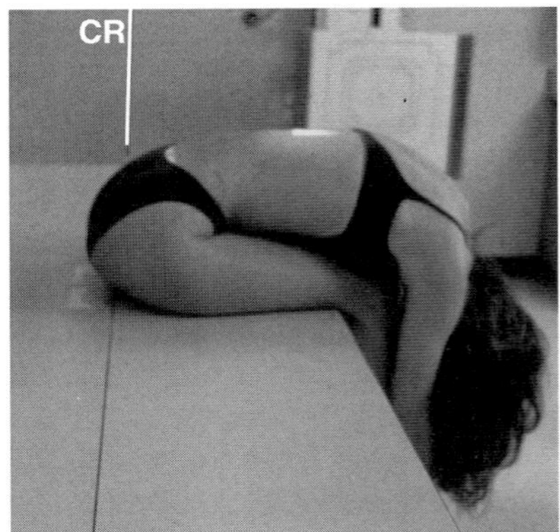

Fig. 15-53.Chassard-Lapine axial projection.

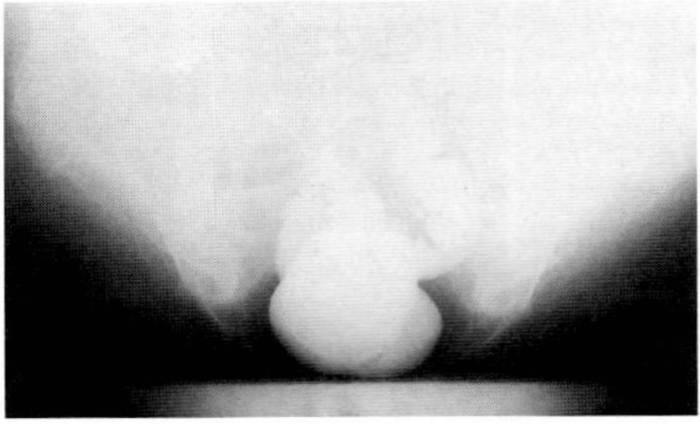

Fig. 15-54. Chassard-Lapine axial projection.

Not recommended due to gonadal dose and discomfort for patient. (AP axial or PA axial "butterfly" projections demonstrate same region.)

Basic and Special Projections

Certain basic and special projections of the small and large intestine are demonstrated and described on the following pages. The radiologist and radiographer must closely coordinate their efforts during both the small bowel series and the barium enema. A great deal of individual variation exists among radiologists. The routine or basic projections listed may vary from hospital to hospital. The radiographic routine for the barium enema, in particular, must be thoroughly understood by the radiographer in advance of the examination since any radiographs needed must be obtained as rapidly as possible.

Small bowel series
Basic
- PA (every 15 to 30 min) **470**

Special
- Enteroclysis and intubation **457**

Barium enema
Basic
- PA and/or AP **472**
- RAO **473**
- LAO **474**
- LPO and RPO **475**
- Lateral rectum and ventral decubitus (double-contrast) **476**
- R lateral decubitus (double-contrast) **477**
- L lateral decubitus (double-contrast) **478**
- PA (AP) post-evac **479**

Barium enema
Special
- AP or LPO axial (butterfly) **480**
- PA or RAO axial (butterfly) **481**

PA Projection–Small Bowel Series

Small bowel series
Basic
- **PA** (every 15 to 30 min)

Special
- Enteroclysis
- Intubation

Structures Best Shown

Contrast-filled small intestine.

- ***Upper GI-Small Bowel Combination:***
  The small bowel series is commonly done in combination with the upper GI wherein additional barium is ingested following completion of the upper GI. (See page 456.)
- ***Small Bowel Only Series:***
  Includes a scout abdomen radiograph followed by ingestion of barium and timed interval radiographs. (See page 456.)
- ***Enteroclysis and Intubation Procedures:***
  (See descriptions on page 457.)

14
17
30 min.
L

Technical Factors

- Film size–14 x 17 in. (35 x 43 cm), lengthwise.
- Moving or stationary grid.
- 100 -125 kVp range.
- Time markers to be used.
- Technique and dose:
  –PA, 30 min. SB

	cm	kVp	mAs	Sk.	ML.	Gon.
–PA, 30 min. SB	16	125	4	**116**	**33**	**M 27 F 33**

mrad

Shielding: Shield gonads only if such shielding does not cover pertinent anatomy.

Patient Position

- Prone (or supine if patient can't lie in prone position), pillow for head.

Part Position

- Align midsagittal plane to midline of table and/or film.
- Arms up beside head, legs extended with support under ankles.
- Ensure there is **no rotation**.

Central Ray

- CR **perpendicular** to film holder.
  (1) **15 or 30 min**: Center to about **2 in.** (5 cm) **above iliac crest** (see Notes).
  (2) **Hourly**: Center CR and mid point of film to **iliac crest**.
- Center cassette to CR.
- Minimum 40 in. (102 cm) SID.

Collimation: Collimate on four sides to outer margins of film.

Respiration: Suspend respiration and expose on expiration.

Notes: Timing begins with ingestion of barium.

Timed intervals of radiographs are dependent on transit time of specific barium preparation used and upon departmental protocol.

First 30-minute radiograph: Center high to include entire stomach. (Some departmental routines include the first radiograph at 15 minutes, then every 30 minutes thereafter.)

Thirty-minute interval radiographs taken until barium reaches large bowel (usually 2 hours). If this goes beyond 2 hours, then radiographs are generally taken at 1-hour intervals.

The study is generally completed once the contrast media reaches the cecum and/or the ascending colon.

Fluoroscopy and spot filming of the ileocecal valve and terminal ileum after barium reaches this area is a common part of SBS routine. This however is determined by radiologist preference and departmental routines.

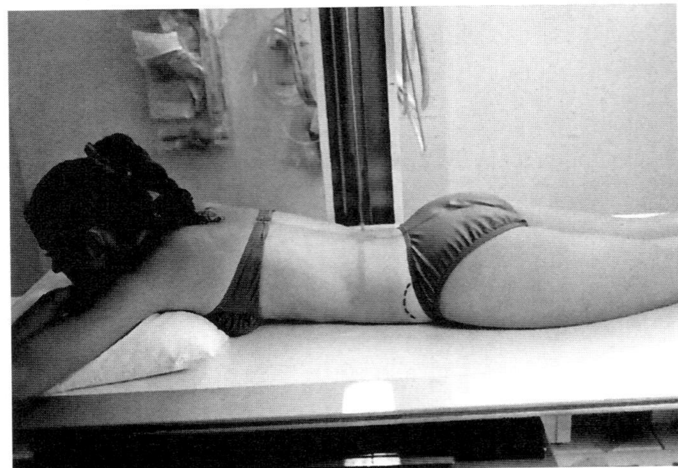

Fig. 15-55. PA, 15 or 30 min.
–Centered ≈2 inches above iliac crest.

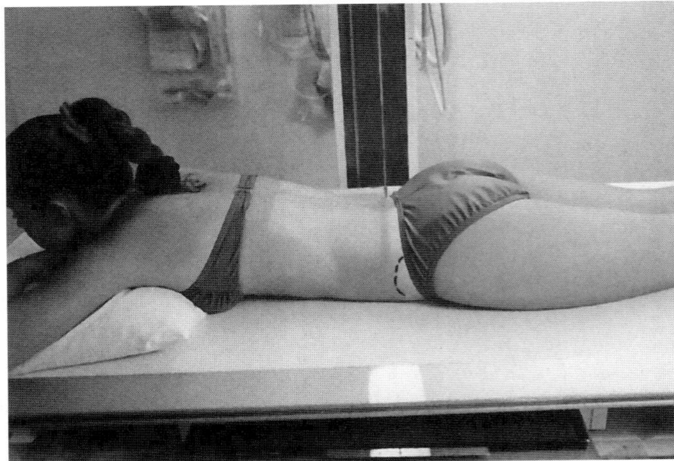

Fig. 15-56. PA, hourly–Centered to iliac crest.

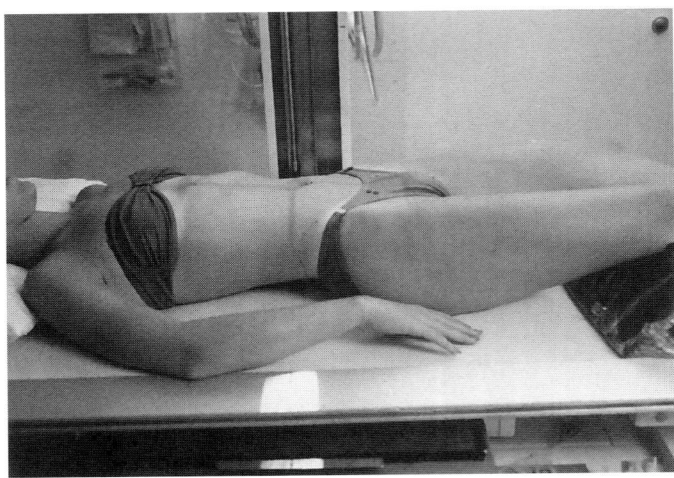

Fig. 15-57. AP, supine (if necessary).

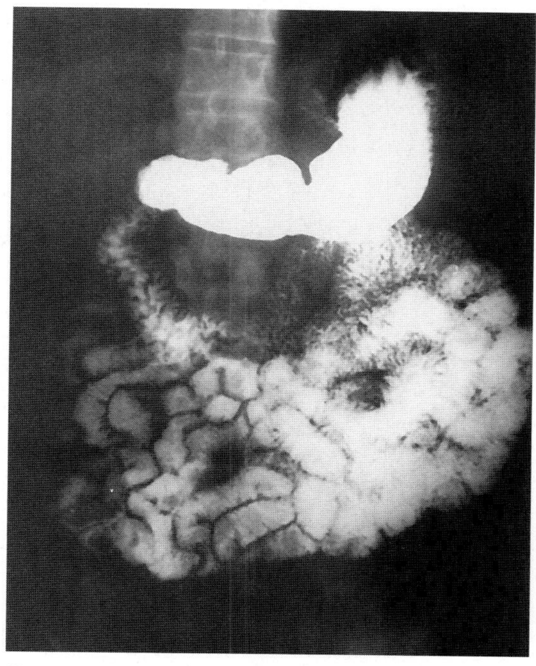

Fig. 15-58. PA SBS–30 min. (Most of barium in stomach, duodenum and jejunum.)

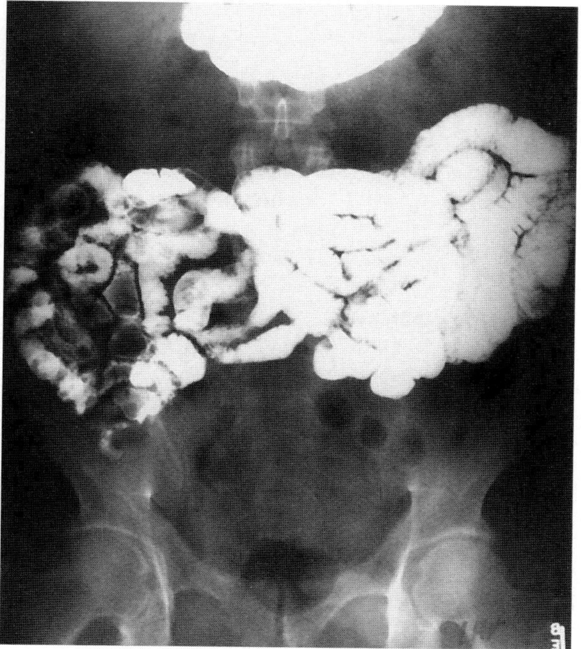

Fig. 15-59. PA SBS–1hr. (Most of barium in jejunum.)

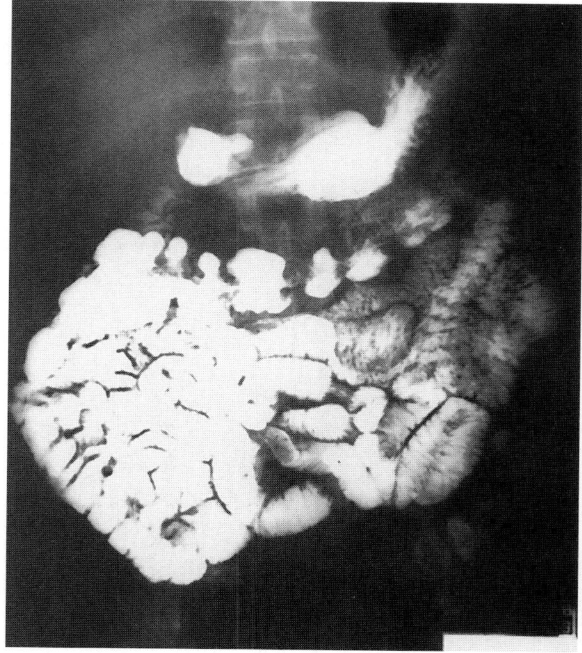

Fig. 15-60. PA 2 hr. (Most of barium in ileum.)

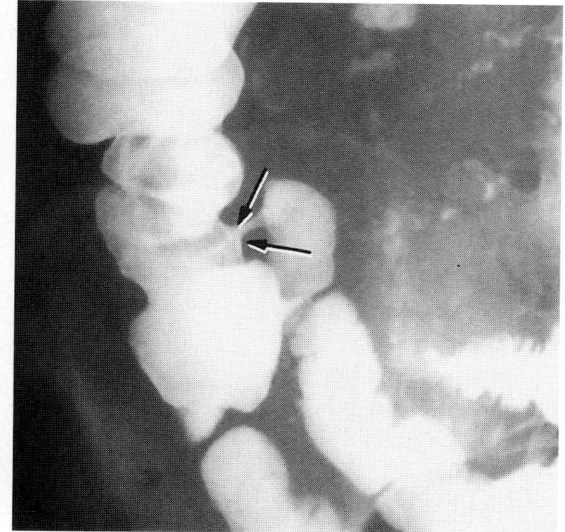

Fig. 15-61. PA (ileocecal spot). (Barium in ileum and in cecum of large intestine and ascending colon. Ileocecal valve demonstrated by arrows.) (Courtesy of James Sanderson, RT)

Evaluation Criteria

- Entire small intestine is demonstrated on each radiograph with the stomach included on the first 15- and/or 30-minute radiograph.
- No rotation evident by symmetry of iliac wings and lumbar vertebra.
- Appropriate technique employed to visualize the contrast-filled small intestine without overexposing those parts that are only partially filled with barium.
- Patient ID info, **time interval markers** and R or L marker are visible without superimposing essential anatomy.

PA and/or AP Projection

Barium enema
Basic
- **PA and/or AP**
- RAO
- LAO
- LPO and/or RPO
- Lateral rectum
- R and L lat. decub. (double-contrast)
- PA post-evac

Structures Best Shown

Entire contrast-filled large intestine. (Exception may be colic left flexure; see Notes below.)

Both PA and **AP** are generally taken with **double-contrast study.**

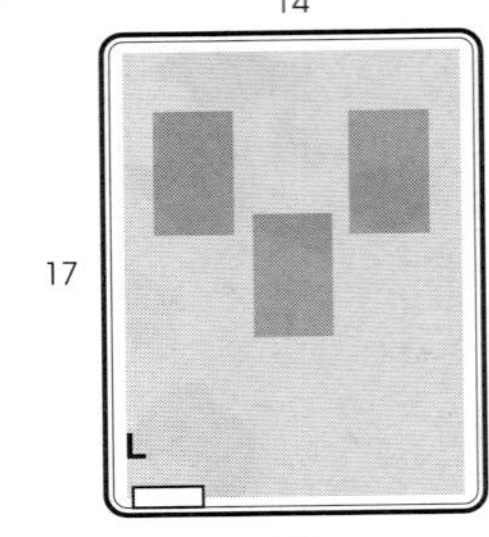

PA

Technical Factors

- Film size–14 x 17 in. (35 x 43 cm), lengthwise.
- Moving or stationary grid.
- 100-125 kVp range (single-contrast)
  80-90 kVp range (double-contrast)
- Technique and dose:

cm	kVp	mAs	Sk.	ML.	Gon.
16	125	4	116	33	M 27 F 33

mrad

Shielding: Place lead shields over gonads **only** if such shielding does not cover pertinent anatomy. (Generally female ovarian shielding is not possible for full-size BE radiographs.)

Patient Position

- Prone or supine, pillow for head.

Part Position

- Midsagittal plane aligned to midline of table.
- **No** body **rotation**.

Central Ray

- CR **perpendicular** to film holder.
- Center CR to level of **iliac crest**.
- Center cassette to CR.
- Minimum 40 in. (102 cm) SID.

Collimation: Collimate on four sides to margins of film.

Respiration: Suspend respiration and expose on expiration.

Notes: Proceed as rapidly as possible.

For most patients the enema tip can be removed before overhead filming, unless a retention-type tip is being used, which should generally not be removed until the patient is ready to evacuate.

Include rectal ampulla at lower margin of radiograph. Determine departmental policy regarding inclusion of the left colic flexure on all patients if this area is adequately included in spot films during fluoroscopy (most adult patients require 2 films if this area is to be included).

For hypersthenic patient use 2 ea. 14 x 17 films placed crosswise to include entire large intestine.

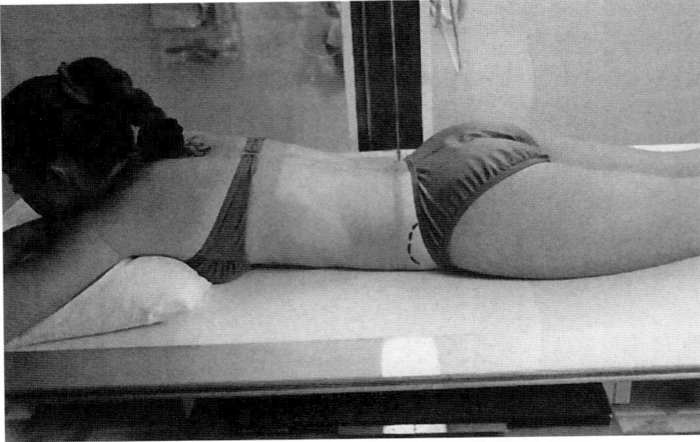
Fig. 15-62. PA.

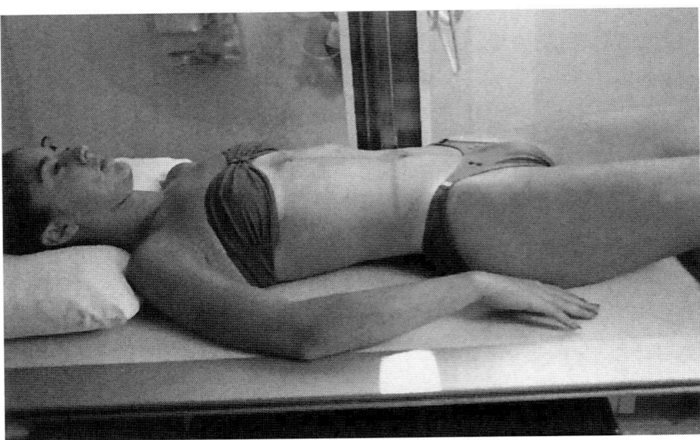
Fig. 15-63. AP.

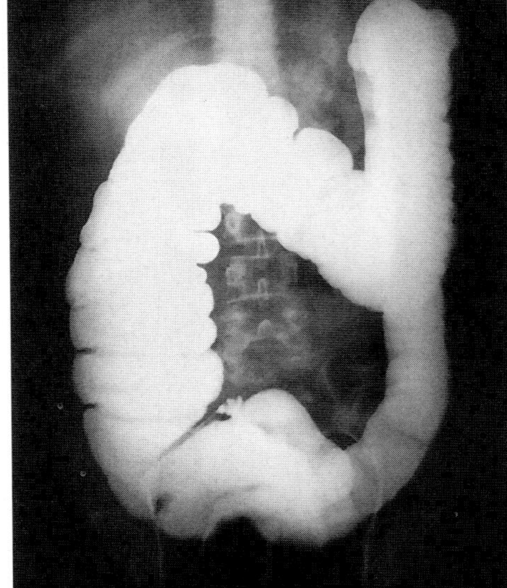
Fig. 15-64. PA.

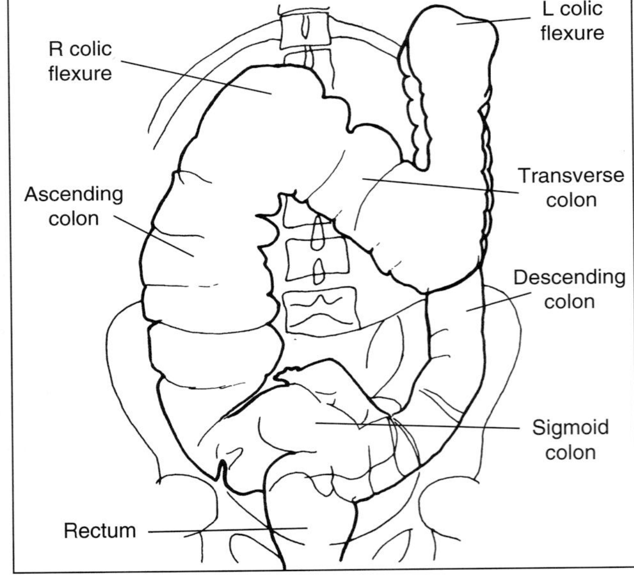

Fig. 15-65. PA.

Evaluation Criteria

- The transverse colon should be primarily barium-filled on the PA, and air-filled on the AP with a double-contrast study.
- Entire large intestine should be demonstrated with the possible exception of the left colic flexure. (See Notes above.)
- No rotation as evidenced by symmetry of hips and iliac wings.
- Appropriate technique should visualize the entire air and barium filled large intestine without overexposing the mucosal outlines of those sections of primarily air-filled bowel on a double-contrast study.

RAO Position

Barium enema
Basic
• PA and/or AP
• **RAO**
• LAO
• LPO and/or RPO
• Lateral rectum
• R and L lat. decub. (double-contrast)
• PA post-evac

Structures Best Shown

Best demonstrates the **right colic** (hepatic) **flexure**, the cecum and the ascending and sigmoid colon.

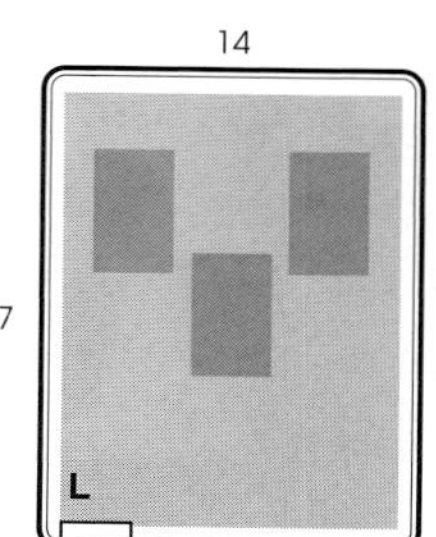

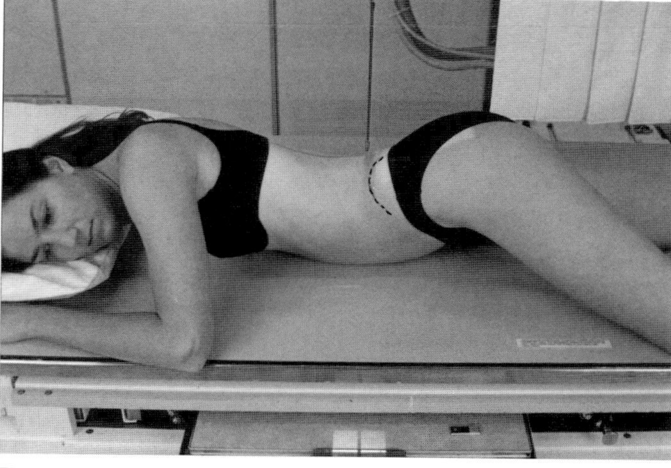

Fig. 15-66. 35 to 45° RAO.

Technical Factors

• Film size–14 x 17 in. (35 x 43 cm), lengthwise.
• Moving or stationary grid.
• 80-90 kVp range (double-contrast study) (100-125 kVp range if single-contrast study).
• Technique and dose:

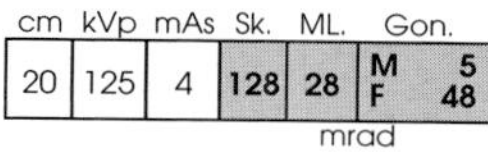

cm	kVp	mAs	Sk.	ML.	Gon.
20	125	4	128	28	M 5 F 48
					mrad

Shielding: Shield gonads only if this is possible without covering pertinent anatomy.

Patient Position

• Semiprone, rotated into a 35 to 45° right anterior oblique.
• Provide pillow for head.

Part Position 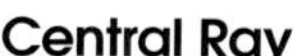

• Align midsagittal plane along long axis of table, with right and left abdominal margins equal distance from center line of table.
• Left arm up on pillow, right arm down behind patient, left knee partially flexed.
• Check posterior pelvis and trunk for **35 to 45° rotation**.

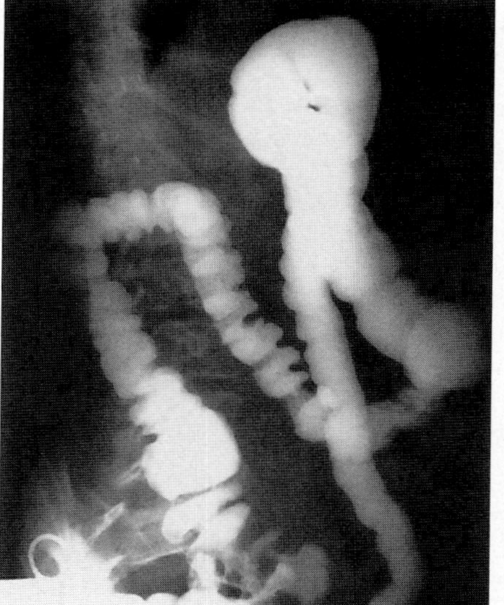

Fig. 15-67. RAO (centered high to include R and L colic flexures).

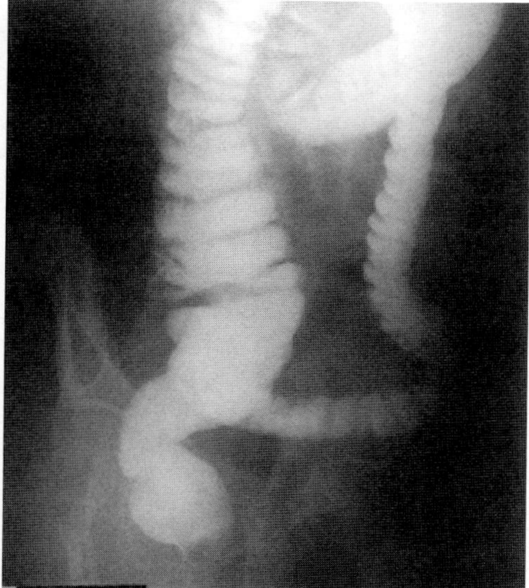

Fig. 15-68. RAO (centered low to include rectal ampulla).

Central Ray

• CR **perpendicular** to film holder to a point about **1 in.** (2.5 cm) **to the left** of midsagittal plane.
• CR and center of film to **level of iliac crest.** (See Notes.)
• Minimum 40 in. (102 cm) SID.

Collimation: Collimate on four sides to outer margins of film.

Respiration: Suspend respiration and expose on expiration.

Notes: Proceed as rapidly as possible.

Ensure that rectal ampulla is included on lower margin of film. This may require centering 1 or 2 in. (5 to 10 cm) below the iliac crest on larger patients and taking a second film centered 1 to 2 in. (5 to 10 cm) above the crest to include the right colic flexure (Figs. 15-67 and 15-68).

A hypersthenic patient may require two films crosswise to include all the large intestine.

If patient cannot lie prone, may also be taken as LPO to visualize the right colic flexure.

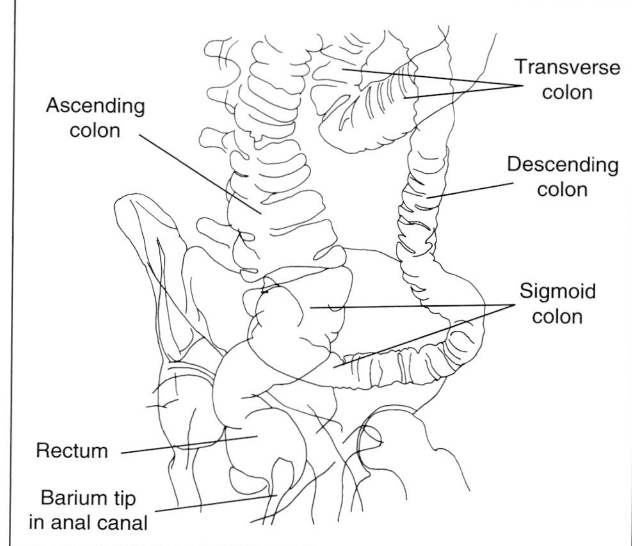

Fig. 15-69. RAO (to include rectal ampulla).

Evaluation Criteria

• The **right colic flexure** and the **ascending** and **sigmoid colon** are seen "open" without significant superimposition.
• Entire large intestine is included with the possible exception of the left colic flexure which is best demonstrated in LAO position.
• The rectal ampulla should be included on lower margin of radiograph.
• Appropriate technique should visualize the contrast-filled large intestine without significant overexposure of any portion.

LAO Position

Barium enema
Basic
- PA and/or AP
- RAO
- **LAO**
- LPO and/or RPO
- Lateral rectum
- R and L lat. decub. (double-contrast)
- PA post-evac

Structures Best Shown

Best demonstrates the **left colic** (splenic) **flexure** and the descending colon.

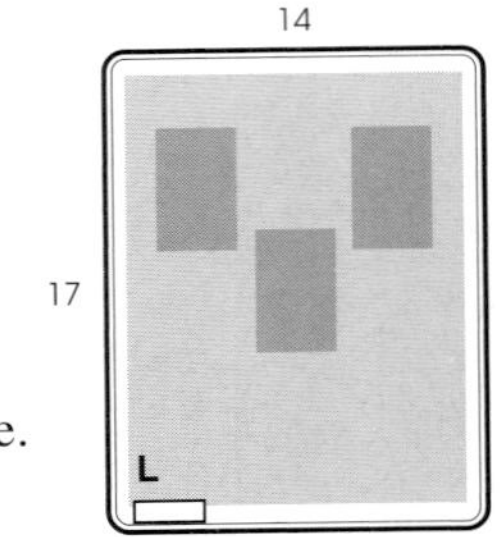

Technical Factors

- Film size–14 x 17 in. (35 x 43 cm), lengthwise.
- Moving or stationary grid.
- 100-125 kVp range (single-contrast).
  80-90 kVp range (double-contrast).
- Technique and dose:

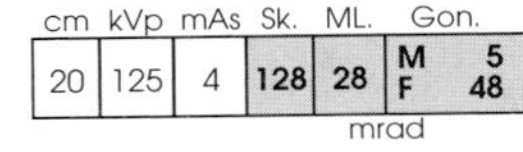

cm	kVp	mAs	Sk.	ML.	Gon.
20	125	4	128	28	M 5 F 48

mrad

Shielding: Place lead shield over gonads only if possible without covering pertinent anatomy.

Patient Position

- Semiprone, rotated into a 35 to 45° left anterior oblique.
- Provide pillow for head.

Part Position

- Align midsagittal plane along long axis of table, with right and left abdominal margins equal distance from center line of table.
- Right arm up on pillow, left arm down behind patient, left knee partially flexed.
- Check posterior pelvis and trunk for **35 to 45° rotation**.

Central Ray

- CR **perpendicular** to film holder to a point about **1 in.** (2.5 cm) **to the right** of midsagittal plane.
- CR and film centered to **1 to 2 in**. (2.5 to 5 cm) **above iliac crest** (see Notes).
- Center cassette to CR.
- Minimum 40 in. (102 cm) SID.

Collimation: Collimate on four sides to outer margins of film.

Respiration: Suspend respiration and expose on expiration.

Notes: Proceed as rapidly as possible.

Most adult patients require about 2 inches (5 cm) higher centering to include the **left colic flexure**, which will generally cut off lower large bowel; then a second film centered 2 or 3 inches (5 to 7.5 cm) lower is required to include the rectal area.

If patient cannot lie prone, may also be taken as an **RPO** to visualize left colic flexure.

Evaluation Criteria

- The **left colic flexure** should be seen as open without significant superimposition.
- Descending colon should be well demonstrated.
- Entire large intestine should be included (see Notes).
- Appropriate technique should visualize the contrast-filled large intestine without significant overexposure of any portion.

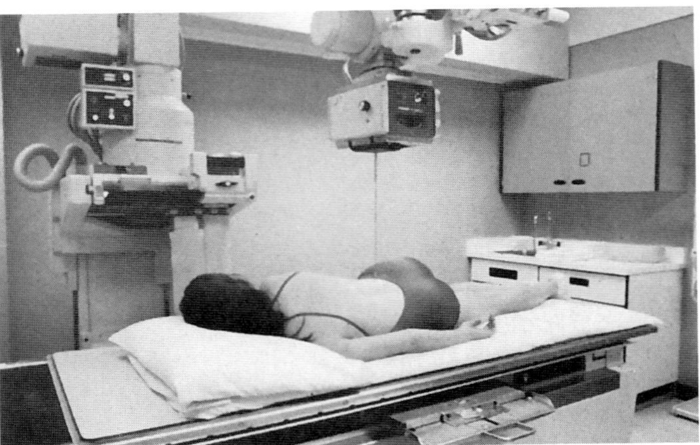

Fig. 15-70. LAO.

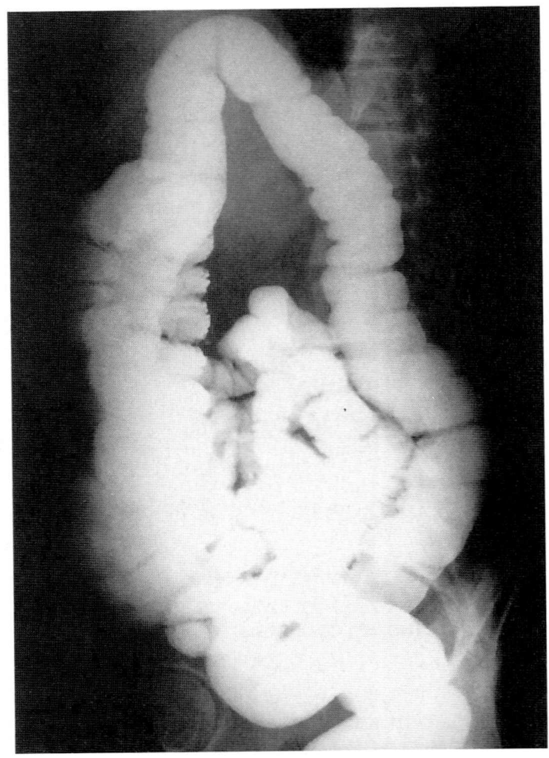

Fig. 15-71. LAO (centered high to include L colic flexure).

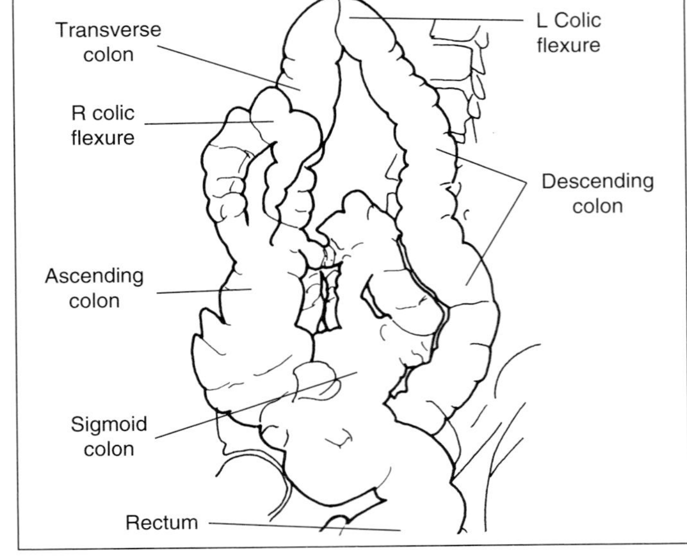

Fig. 15-72. LAO.

15

LPO and RPO Positions

Barium enema
Basic
- PA and/or AP
- RAO
- LAO
- **LPO and/or RPO**
- Lateral rectum
- R and L lat. decub. (double-contrast)
- PA post-evac

Structures Best Shown

Contrast-filled large intestine.
LPO: Best demonstrates **right colic** (hepatic) **flexure**, ascending, cecum and sigmoid portions (similar to RAO position).
RPO: Best demonstrates **left colic** (splenic) **flexure** and descending portion (similar to LAO position).

Technical Factors

- Film size–14 x 17 in. (35 x 43 cm), lengthwise.
- Moving or stationary grid.
- 100-125 kVp range (single-contrast)
  80-90 kVp range (double-contrast)
- Technique and dose:

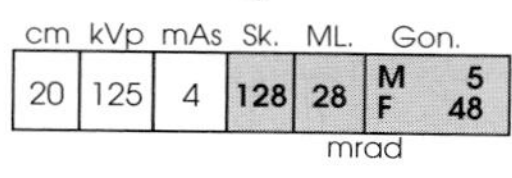

cm	kVp	mAs	Sk.	ML.	Gon.
20	125	4	128	28	M 5 F 48

mrad

14
17
R

Shielding: Place lead shield over gonads only if possible without covering pertinent anatomy.

Patient Position

- Semisupine, rotated 35 to 45° into right and left posterior obliques.
- Provide pillow for head.

Part Position

- Flex elevated side elbow and place in front of head, place opposite arm down by patient's side.
- Partially flex elevated side knee for support to maintain this position.
- Align **midsagittal plane along long axis of table** with right and left abdominal margins equal distance from center line of table.

Central Ray

- CR **perpendicular** to film holder.
- CR and center of film to level of **iliac crests** and about **1 in.** (2.5 cm) **lateral to elevated side** of midsagittal plane (see Notes).
- Minimum 40 in. (102 cm) SID.

Collimation: Collimate on four sides to outer margins of film.

Respiration: Expose on expiration.

Notes: Proceed as rapidly as possible.
Ensure that rectal ampulla is included.
Most adult patients require a second film centered 2 or 3 in. (5 to 7.5 cm) higher on the **RPO** if the left colic (splenic) flexure is to be included (Fig. 15-76).
A hypersthenic patient may require two films crosswise to include all of large intestine.

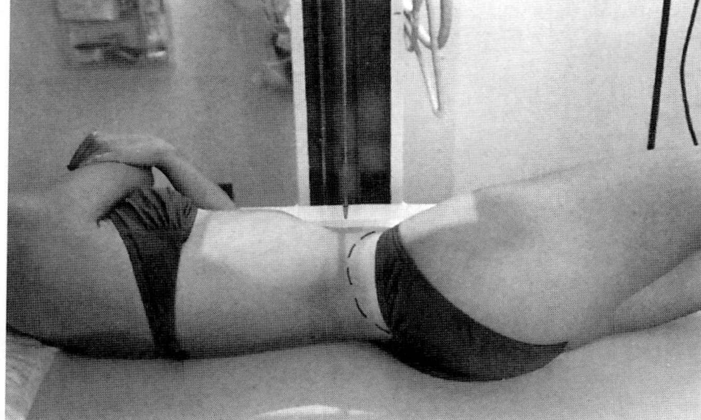

Fig. 15-73. LPO.

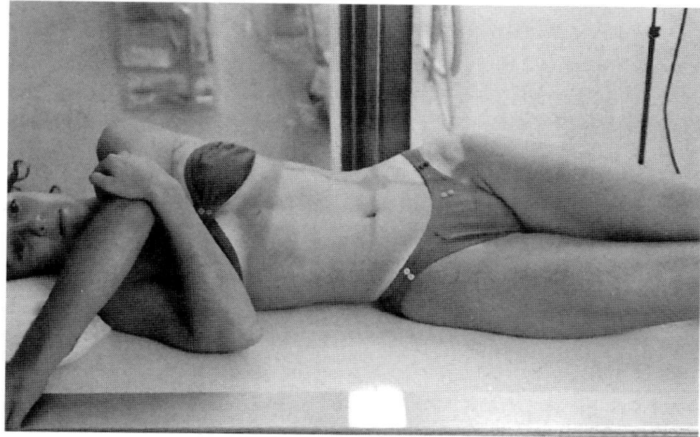

Fig. 15-74. RPO.

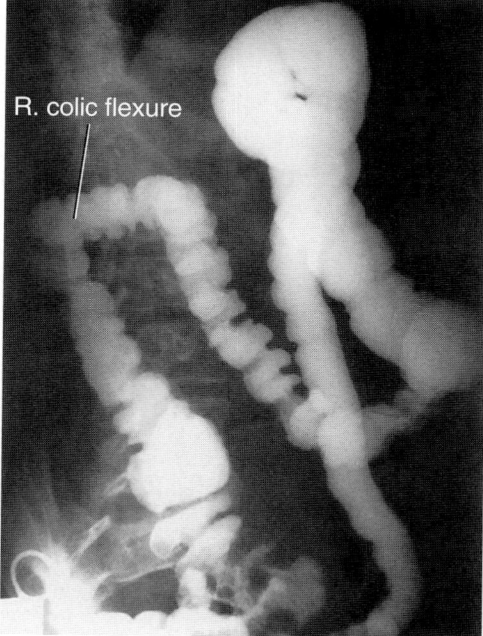

Fig. 15-75. LPO–For right colic flexure.

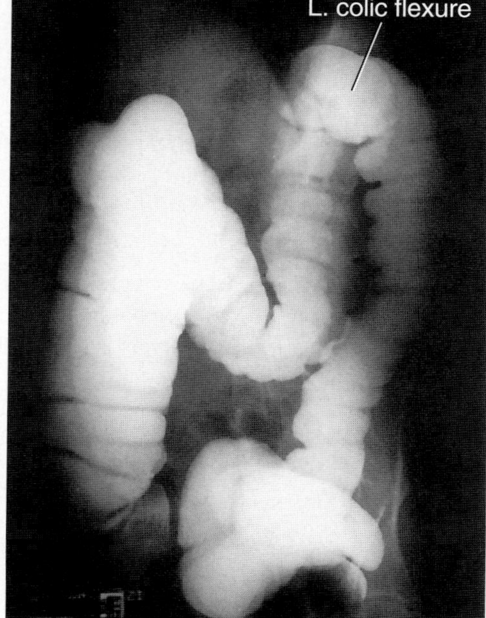

Fig. 15-76. RPO–For left colic flexure.
(Centered high to include both right and left colic flexures.)

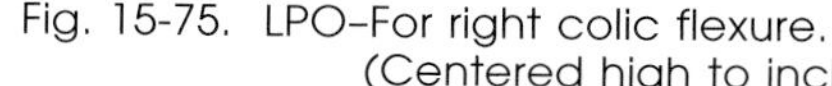

Evaluation Criteria

LPO: The **right colic** (hepatic) **flexure, ascending** and **rectosigmoid portions** should appear "open" without significant superimposition.
- Entire contrast-filled large intestine including the rectal ampulla should be included (see Notes).
- Appropriate technique should visualize the contrast-filled large intestine without significant overexposure of any portion.

RPO: The **left colic** (splenic) **flexure** and the **descending portions** should appear "open" without significant superimposition. (A second film centered lower to include the rectal area is required on most adult patients if this area is to be included on these post-fluoroscopy overhead radiographs, see Notes.)

15

Lateral Rectum Position – Lateral or Ventral Decubitus

Barium enema
Basic
- PA and/or AP
- RAO
- LAO
- LPO and/or RPO
- **Lateral rectum**
- R and L lat. decub. (double-contrast)
- PA post-evac

Structures Best Shown

Lateral view of the rectosigmoid region. Either a left or right lateral of rectum may be taken to demonstrate this area. Ventral decubitus laterals may also demonstrate this region, especially with double contrast study.

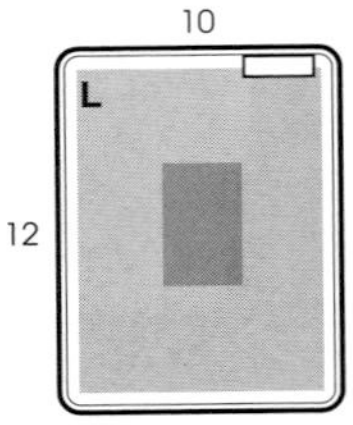

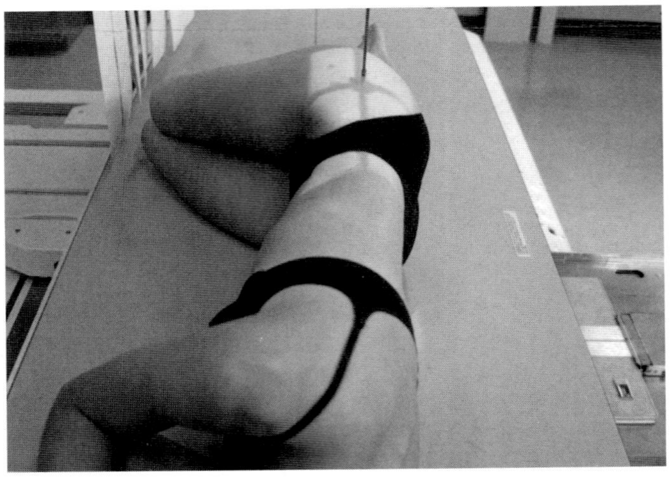

Fig. 15-77. Left lateral rectum.

Technical Factors

- Film size–10 x 12 in. (24 x 30 cm), lengthwise.
- Moving or stationary grid.
- 100-125 kVp range (for both single and double-contrast studies).
- A compensating or wedge filter may be used for more uniform density.
- Technique and dose:

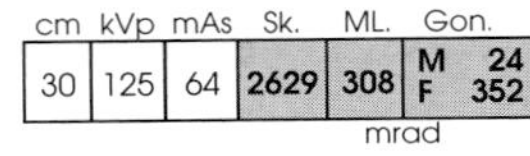

cm	kVp	mAs	Sk.	ML.	Gon.
30	125	64	2629	308	M 24 F 352

mrad

Shielding: Lead shielding of gonads without covering pertinent anatomy may not be possible, especially for females. This makes close and accurate collimation especially important.

Patient Position

- Lateral recumbent position, pillow for head.

Part Position

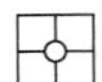

- Align midaxillary plane to midline of table and/or film.
- Flex and superimpose knees; arms up in front of head.
- Ensure **no rotation**, superimpose shoulders and hips.

Central Ray

- CR **perpendicular** to film holder. (CR **horizontal** for ventral decubitus.)
- Center CR to level of **ASIS** and **midaxillary plane** (midway between ASIS and posterior sacrum).
- Center cassette to CR.
- Minimum 40 in. (102 cm) SID.

Alternate Ventral Decubitus: Lateral horizontal beam projections are beneficial for double-contrast studies. Centering for the ventral decubitus is similar to the lateral rectum projection.

Collimation: Collimate on four sides to area of interest, generally near outer margins of film.

Respiration: Suspend respiration and expose on expiration.

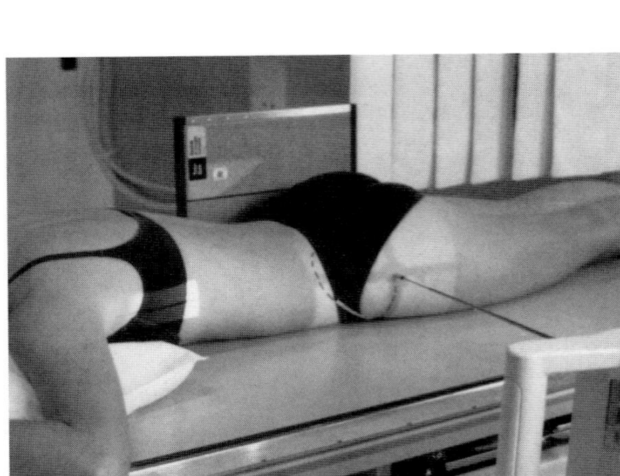

Fig. 15-78. Ventral decub. lateral rectum (alternate projection for double-contrast study).

Evaluation Criteria

- Contrast-filled rectosigmoid region is demonstrated centered to film.
- No rotation as evidenced by superimposed hips.
- Appropriate technique employed to visualize both the contrast-filled rectum and sigmoid regions, with adequate penetration to demonstrate these areas through the superimposed pelvis and hips.

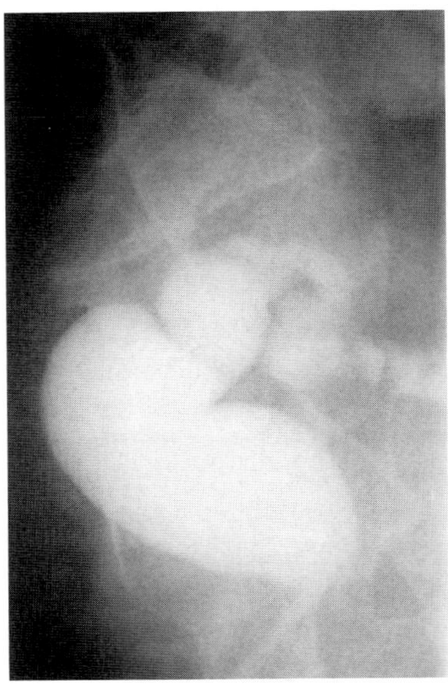

Fig. 15-79. Left lateral rectum.

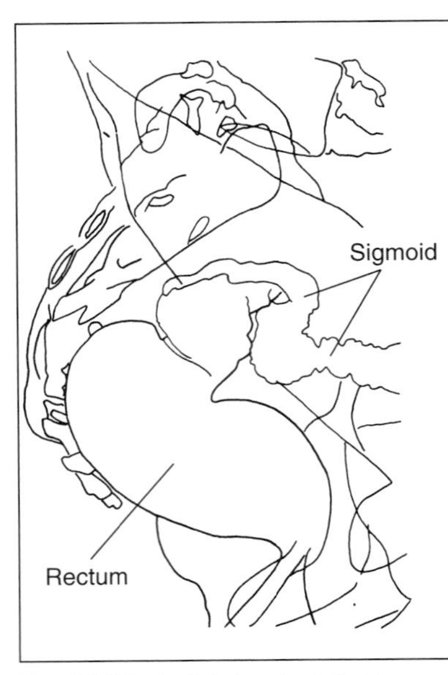

Fig. 15-80. Left lateral rectum.

Right Lateral Decubitus Position (AP)

Barium enema
Basic
- PA and/or AP
- RAO
- LAO
- LPO and/or RPO
- Lateral rectum
- **R and L lat. decub. (double-contrast)**
- PA post-evac

Structures Best Shown

Entire contrast-filled large intestine, especially helpful in demonstrating polyps. Best demonstrates the up side or air-filled portions of the large bowel.

Both right and left decubitus position are generally taken with double-contrast study (see following page).

Technical Factors

- Film size–14 x 17 in. (35 x 43 cm), lengthwise with patient.
- Bucky or grid cassette.
- 80-90 kVp (double-contrast study) (100-125 kVp if single-contrast study).
- Place compensating filter on upside of abdomen (attach to collimator face with magnets.
- Technique and dose:

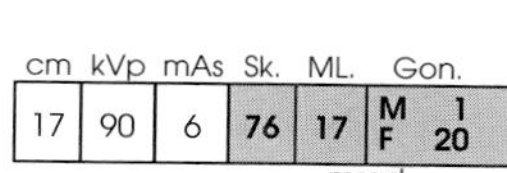

cm	kVp	mAs	Sk.	ML.	Gon. (mrad)
17	90	6	76	17	M 1 / F 20

Shielding: Place lead shield over gonadal region only if possible without covering pertinent anatomy.

Patient Position

- Lateral recumbent position, pillow for head, lying on **right** side on a radiolucent pad with portable grid placed behind patient's back. May also be taken with patient on cart with back against vertical table. (If on a cart, **lock wheels** or secure cart to prevent patient from falling.)
- Arms up, knees flexed.

Part Position

- Position patient and/or film so that iliac crest is to center of film and to CR.
- Ensure **no rotation**, superimpose shoulders and hips from above.

Central Ray

- CR **horizontal,** perpendicular to film holder.
- CR centered to **level of iliac crest** and **midsagittal plane.**
- Minimum 40 in. (102 cm) SID.

Collimation: Collimate on four sides to outer margins of film.

Respiration: Suspend respiration and expose on expiration.

Notes: Proceed as rapidly as possible.

For hypersthenic patient use 2 ea. 14 x 17 in. (35 x 43 cm) films placed crosswise to include all of large intestine.

Evaluation Criteria

- Entire large intestine is demonstrated with **air-filled left colic flexure** and **descending colon.**
- No rotation as evidenced by symmetrical appearance of pelvis and rib cage.
- Appropriate technique used to visualize borders of entire large intestine including barium-filled portions but to not over penetrate the air-filled portion of the large intestine. Mucosal patterns of air-filled colon should be clearly visible.

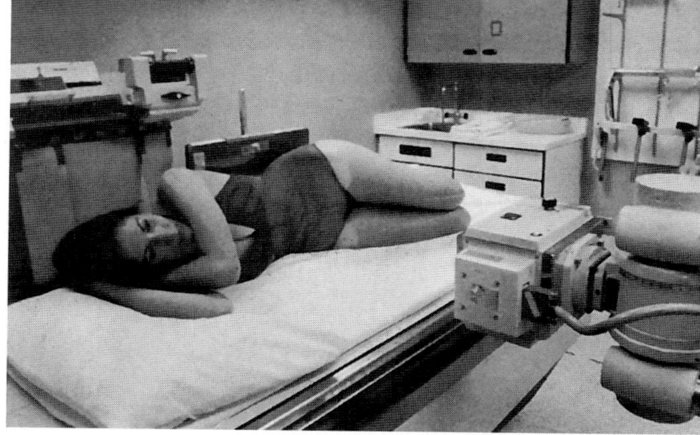

Fig. 15-81. Right lateral decubitus–AP (with portable grid).

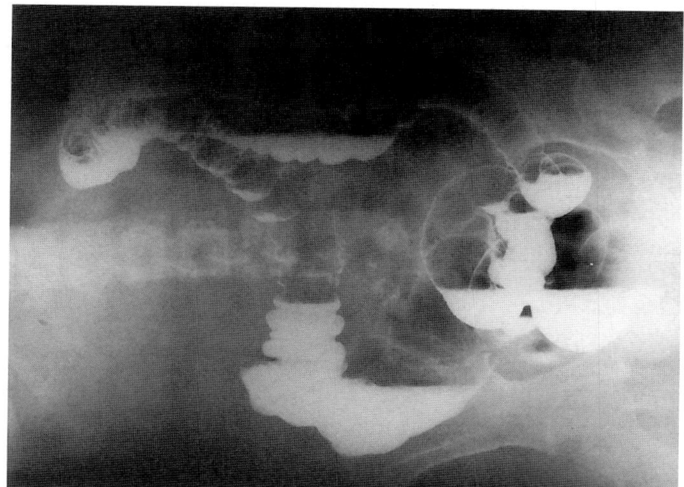

Fig. 15-82. Right lateral decubitus.

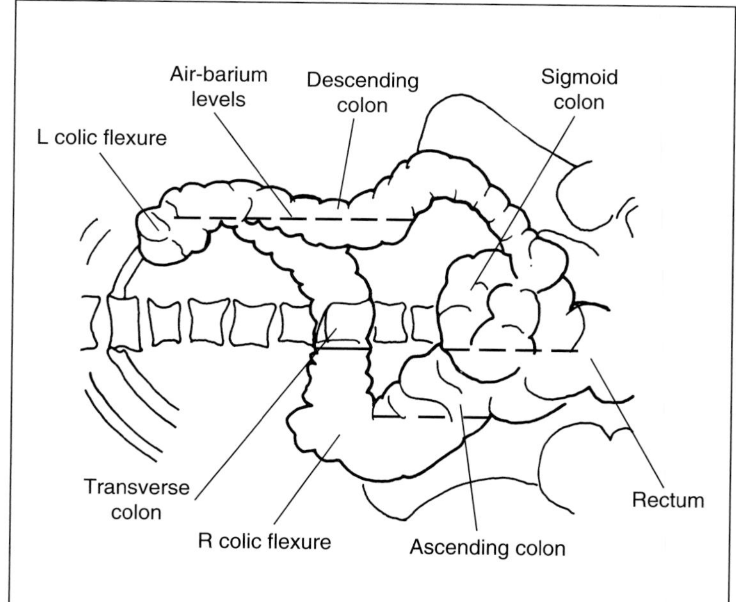

Fig. 15-83. Right lateral decubitus.

Left Lateral Decubitus Position (AP)

Barium enema
Basic
- PA and/or AP
- RAO
- LAO
- LPO and/or RPO
- Lateral rectum
- **R and L lat. decub. (double-contrast)**
- PA post-evac

Structures Best Shown

Entire contrast-filled large intestine, especially helpful in demonstrating polyps. Best demonstrates the up side or air-filled portions of the large bowel.

Both right and left decubitus position are generally taken with double-contrast study.

Technical Factors

- Film size–14 x 17 in. (35 x 43 cm), lengthwise with patient.
- Bucky or grid cassette.
- 80-90 kVp range (double-contrast study). (100-125 kVp range if single-contrast).
- Technique and dose:

cm	kVp	mAs	Sk.	ML.	Gon. (mrad)
17	90	6	76	17	M 1, F 20

Shielding: Place lead shield over gonadal region only if possible without covering pertinent anatomy.

Patient Position

- Lateral recumbent position, pillow for head, lying on **left** side on a radiolucent pad. (If on a cart, **lock wheels** or secure cart to prevent patient from falling.)
- Arms up, knees flexed.

Part Position

- Position patient and/or film so that iliac crest is to center of film and to CR.
- Ensure **no rotation**, superimpose shoulders and hips from above.
- Arms up, knees flexed.

Central Ray

- CR **horizontal,** perpendicular to film holder.
- CR centered to **level of iliac crest** and **midsagittal plane.**
- Minimum 40 in. (102 cm) SID.

Collimation: Collimate on four sides to outer margins of film.

Respiration: Suspend respiration and expose on expiration.

Notes: Since most double-contrast BE studies include both R and L lateral decubitus positions, it is generally easier to take one projection with the back against the table or film holder; then have the patient roll over on the other side and move the cart around with patient's head at other end of table. This may be easier than sitting the patient up and turning them end to end on the cart or table.

For hypersthenic patient use 2 ea. 14 x 17 in. films placed crosswise to include all of large intestine.

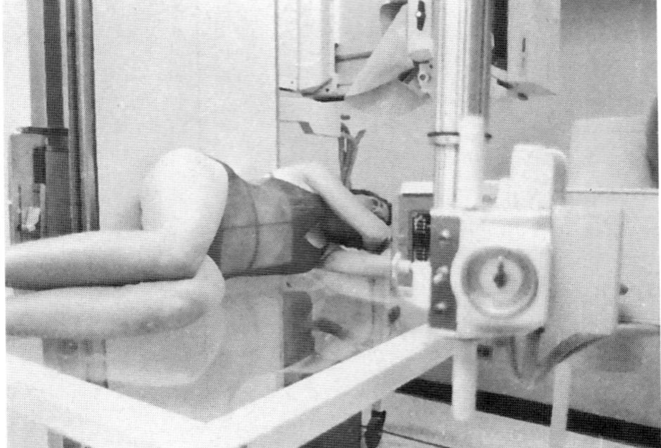

Fig. 15-84. Left lateral decubitus –AP (with vertical Bucky).

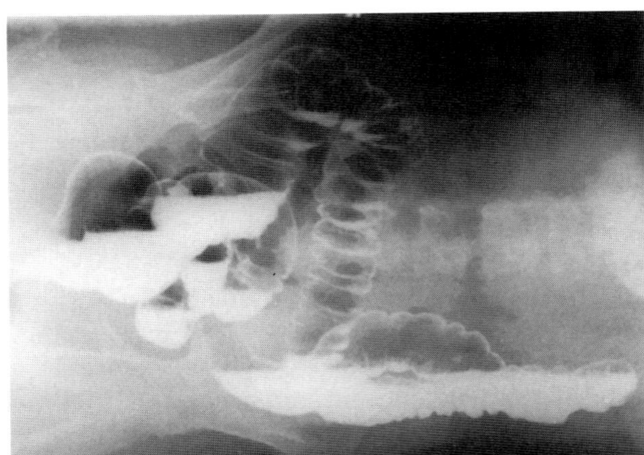

Fig. 15-85. Left lateral decubitus.

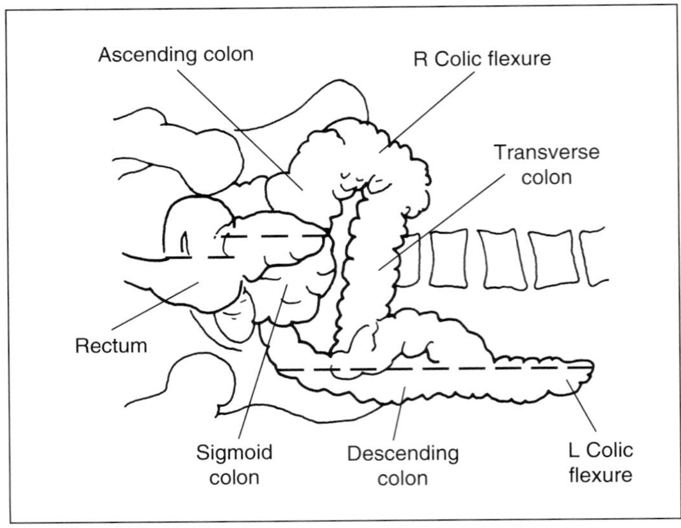

Fig. 15-86. Left lateral decubitus.

Evaluation Criteria

- Entire large intestine is demonstrated with air-filled right colic flexure, ascending colon and cecum.
- No rotation as evidenced by symmetrical appearance of pelvis and rib cage.
- Appropriate technique used to visualize borders of entire large intestine including barium-filled portions but to not over-penetrate the air-filled portion of the large intestine. Mucosal patterns of air-filled colon should be clearly visible.

PA (AP) Projection–Post-Evacuation

> **Barium enema**
> Basic
> • PA and/or AP
> • RAO
> • LAO
> • LPO and/or RPO
> • Lateral rectum
> • R and L lat. decub. (double-contrast)
> • **PA post-evac**

Structures Best Shown

Mucosal pattern of large intestine with residual contrast media.

Most commonly taken prone as a PA, but may be taken with patient supine as an AP if necessary.

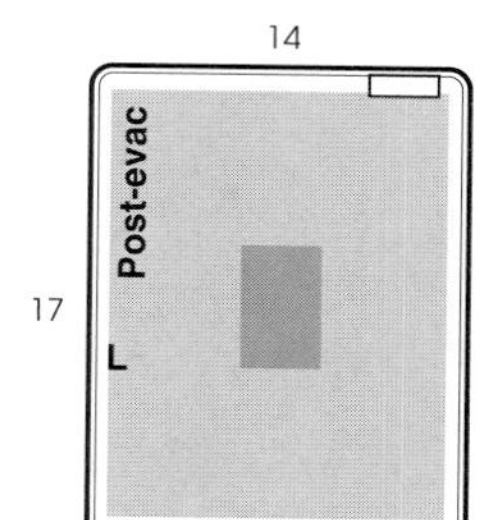

Technical Factors

- Film size–14 x 17 in. (35 x 43 cm), lengthwise.
- Moving or stationary grid.
- 80-90 kVp range.
- Use post-evac marker.
- Technique and dose:

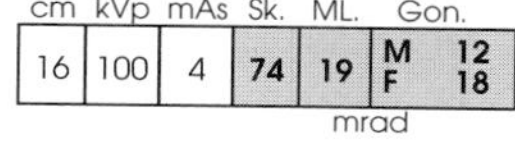

cm	kVp	mAs	Sk.	ML.	Gon.
16	100	4	74	19	M 12 F 18

mrad

Shielding: Place lead shield over gonads only if possible without covering pertinent anatomy.

Patient Position

- Prone or supine, pillow for head.

Part Position

- Midsagittal plane aligned to midline of table.
- **No** body **rotation.**

Central Ray

- CR **perpendicular** to film holder.
- Center CR and center of film to **iliac crest.**
- Minimum 40 in. (102 cm) SID.

Collimation: Collimate on four sides to outer margins of film.

Respiration: Suspend respiration and expose on expiration.

Notes: Taken after patient has had sufficient time for adequate evacuation.

If radiograph shows insufficient evacuation to clearly visualize mucosal pattern, the patient can be given hot tea or coffee to stimulate further evacuation, after which this radiograph should be repeated.

Include rectal ampulla on lower margin of radiograph.

Lower kVp is used to prevent over-penetration with only the residual contrast media remaining in large bowel.

Evaluation Criteria

- Entire large intestine should be visualized with only a residual amount of contrast media.
- No rotation as evidenced by symmetry of ilia wings and parts of the lumbar vertebrae.
- Appropriate technique employed to visualize outline of entire mucosal pattern of the large intestine without overexposure of any parts.

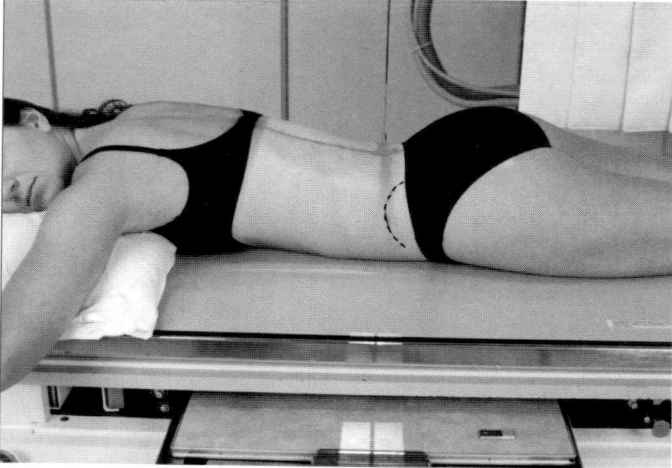

Fig. 15-87. PA post-evac.

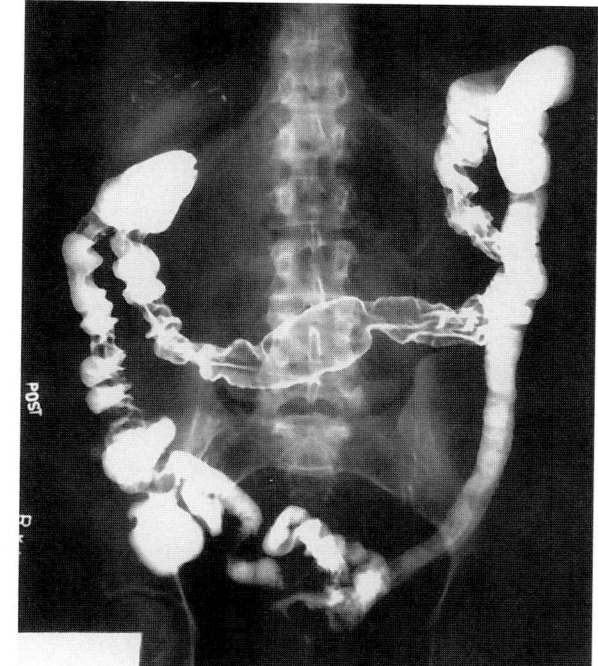

Fig. 15-88. PA post-evac.

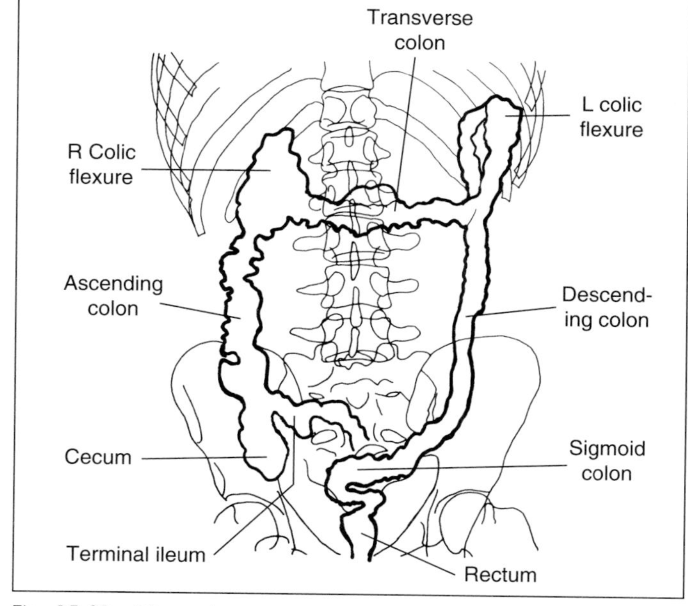

Fig. 15-89. PA post-evac.

15

AP Axial or AP Axial Oblique (LPO) Projections

"Butterfly" Positions

Barium enema
Special
- **AP or LPO axial**
- PA or RAO axial

Structures Best Shown

Elongated views of the rectosigmoid segments of large intestine.

Technical Factors

- Film size –14 x 17 in. (35 x 43 cm), lengthwise
- or –11 x 14 in. (28 x 35 cm), lengthwise.
- Moving or stationary grid.
- 100-125 kVp range for single-contrast, (or 90-100 kVp range, double-contrast).
- Technique and dose:

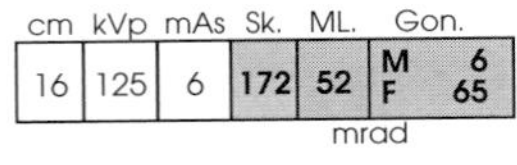

cm	kVp	mAs	Sk.	ML.	Gon.
16	125	6	172	52	M 6 F 65

mrad

14 (11)

17 (14)

L

Shielding: Place lead shield over gonads without covering pertinent anatomy (this may not be possible).

Patient Position

- Supine or partially rotated into a LPO position.
- Provide pillow for head.

Part Position

AP Axial:
- Patient supine, align midsagittal plane to midline of table.
- Extend legs, arms down by patient's side; ensure **no rotation**.

LPO:
- Rotate patient **30 to 40°** into LPO (left posterior side down).
- Raise right arm, left arm extended, right knee partially flexed.

Central Ray

- CR angled **30 to 40° cephalad**.

AP:
- CR **2 in.** (5 cm) **inferior** to **level of ASIS**, and to **midsagittal plane**.

LPO:
- CR **2 in.** (5 cm) **inferior** and **2 in.** (5 cm) **medial to right ASIS.**
- Center film holder to CR.
- Minimum 40 in. (102 cm) SID.

Collimation: Collimate on four sides to outer margins of film.

Respiration: Suspend respiration and expose on expiration.

Notes: Proceed as rapidly as possible.

Similar views can also be obtained with a **PA axial** and **RAO** with **30 to 40° caudad** CR angle (see following page).

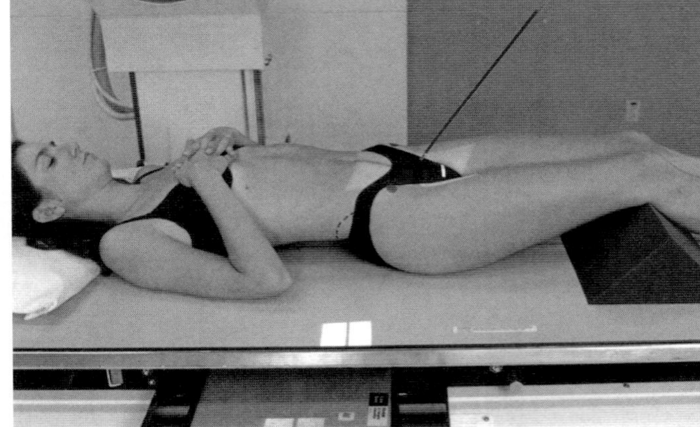

Fig. 15-90. AP axial–CR 30 to 40° cephalad.

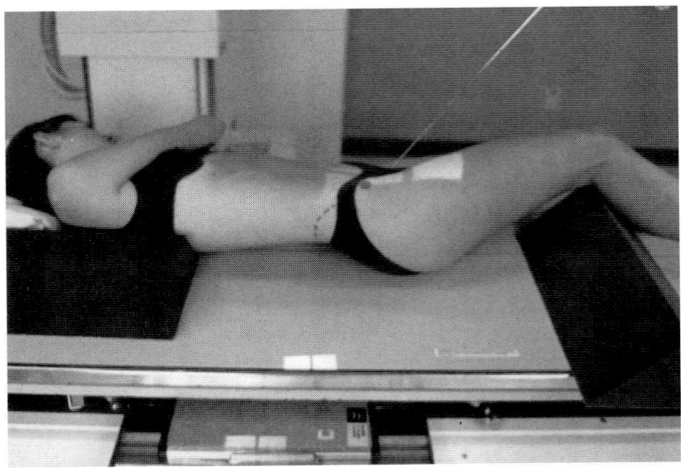

Fig. 15-91. 30 to 40° LPO –CR 30 to 40° cephalad.

Evaluation Criteria

AP Axial:
- Adequate CR angulation evidenced by elongation of rectosigmoid segments of large intestine.
- No rotation as evidenced by symmetrical appearance of pelvis.

LPO Axial:
- Adequate CR angulation and patient obliquity evidenced by elongation and less superimposition of rectosigmoid segments of large intestine.
- Appropriate technique used to visualize outlines of all rectosigmoid segments of large intestine. With air-contrast study, the kVp should be decreased so as not to over-penetrate the air-filled outlines of these segments of large bowel.

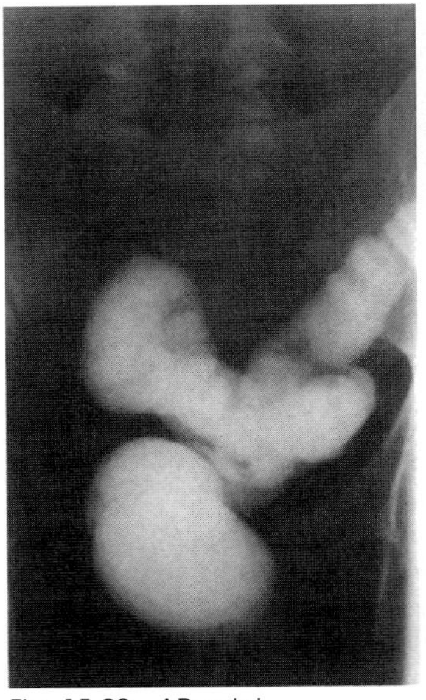

Fig. 15-92. AP axial.

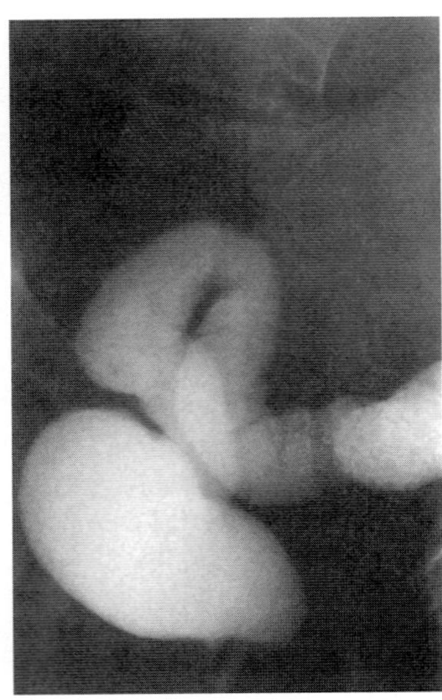

Fig. 15-93. AP axial oblique (LPO).

PA Axial or PA Axial Oblique (RAO) Projections

"Butterfly" Positions

Barium enema
Special
• AP or LPO axial
• **PA or RAO axial**

Structures Best Shown

Elongated views of the rectosigmoid segments of large intestine.

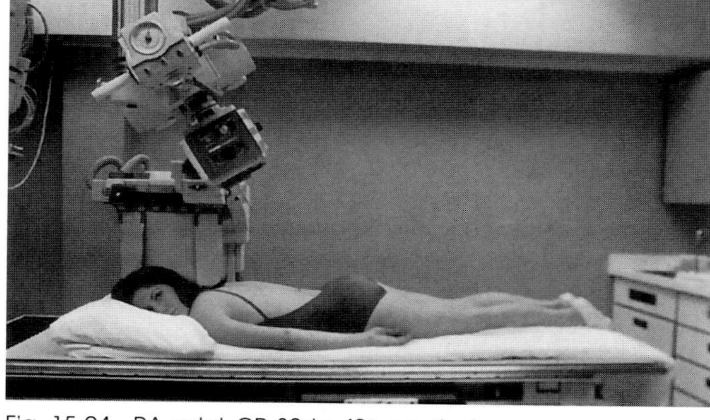

Fig. 15-94. PA axial–CR 30 to 40° caudad.

Technical Factors

- Film size –14 x 17 in. (35 x 43 cm), lengthwise
- or –11 x 14 in. (28 x 35 cm), lengthwise.
- Moving or stationary grid.
- 100-125 kVp range for single-contrast, (or 90-100 kVp range, double-contrast).
- Technique and dose:

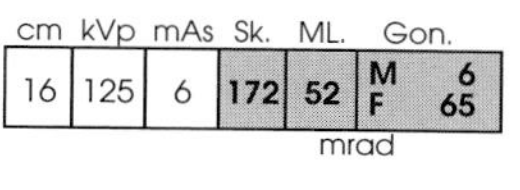

cm	kVp	mAs	Sk.	ML.	Gon.
16	125	6	172	52	M 6 F 65

mrad

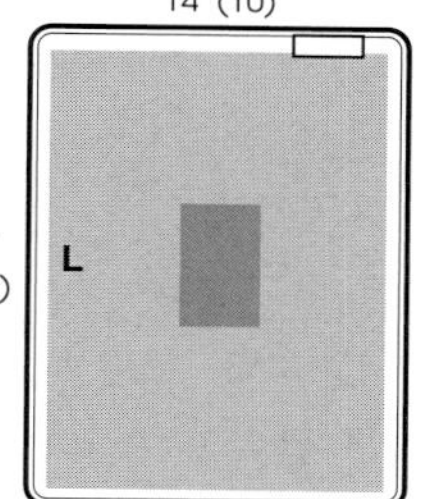

Shielding: Place lead shield over gonads without covering pertinent anatomy (this may not be possible).

Patient Position

- Prone or partially rotated into a RAO position.
- Provide pillow for head.

Part Position

PA:
- Patient prone, align midsagittal plane to midline of table.
- Arms up beside head or down by sides away from body.
- **No rotation** of pelvis or trunk.

RAO:
- Rotate patient **35 to 45°** into **RAO** (right anterior side down).
- Left arm up, right arm down by side, left knee partially flexed.

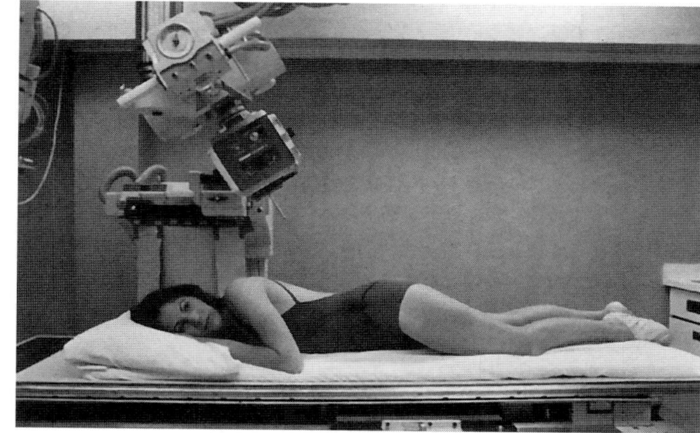

Fig. 15-95. 35 to 45° RAO –CR 30 to 40° caudad.

Central Ray

- CR angled **30 to 40° caudad.**

PA:
- CR to exit at **level of ASIS** and to **midsagittal plane**.

RAO:
- CR to exit at **level of ASIS** and **2 in.** (5 cm) to **left of lumbar spinous processes.**

- Center film holder to CR.
- Minimum 40 in. (102 cm) SID.

Collimation: Collimate on four sides to outer margins of film.

Respiration: Suspend respiration and expose on expiration.

Notes: Proceed as rapidly as possible.

Similar views of rectosigmoid region as AP and LPO with 30 to 40° cephalad angle as described on preceding page.

Evaluation Criteria

PA Axial:
- Adequate CR angulation evidenced by elongation of rectosigmoid segments of large intestine.
- No rotation as evidenced by symmetrical appearance of pelvis.

RAO Axial:
- Adequate CR angulation and patient obliquity evidenced by elongation and less superimposition of rectosigmoid segments of large intestine.
- Appropriate technique used to visualize outlines of all rectosigmoid segments of large intestine. With air-contrast study, the kVp should be decreased so as not to over-penetrate the air-filled outlines of these segments of large bowel.

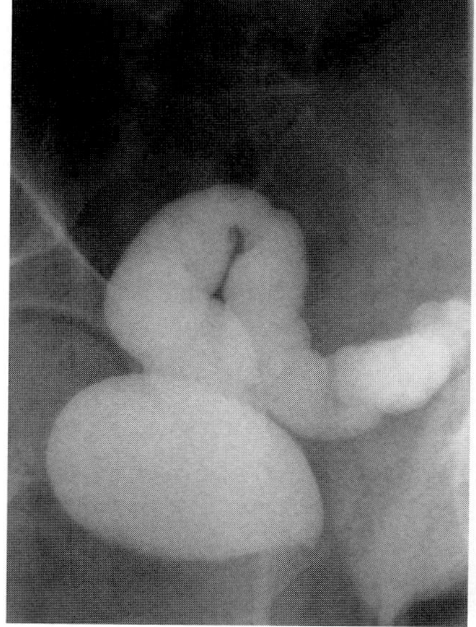

Fig. 15-96. PA axial.

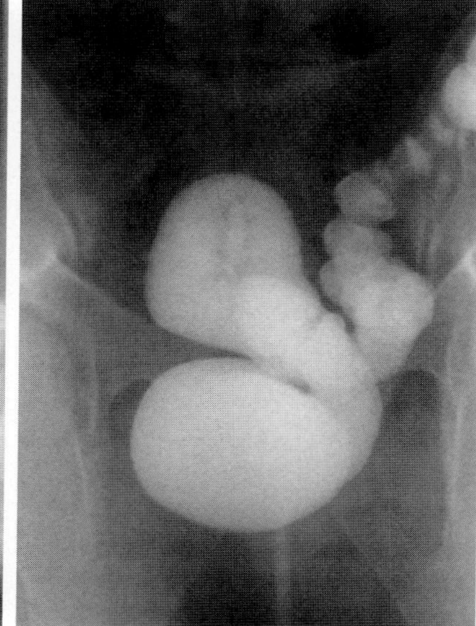

Fig. 15-97. RAO axial.

15

CHAPTER 16

Gallbladder and Biliary Ducts

CONTRIBUTIONS BY:
John P. Lampignano, M Ed, RT (R)
Barry T. Anthony, RT (R)

CONTENTS

Radiographic Anatomy

Liver **484**

Gallbladder and biliary ducts **485**

Anatomy review (radiographs) **486**

Radiographic Procedures

Cholecystography (oral cholecystogram) **487**

Oral cholecystogram procedure **488**

Sonography (Ultrasound) **489**

Operative cholangiogram **490**

Laparoscopic cholangiogram **491**

T-tube cholangiogram **491**

Percutaneous transhepatic cholangiogram (PTC) **492**

Endoscopic retrograde cholangiopancreatogram (ERCP) **493**

Summary–Table of gallbladder and biliary system procedures **494**

Radiographic Positioning

Survey results **495**

Special biliary duct procedures **496**

Basic and special projections **496**

Gallbladder–Oral cholecystogram:
- PA scout **497**
- LAO **498**
- R lateral decubitus (PA) **499**
- PA erect **500**

Biliary ducts–Operative cholangiogram:
- AP and/or RPO **501**

Radiographic Anatomy

LIVER

Radiographic examination of the biliary system involves studying the manufacture, transport and storage of bile. Bile is manufactured by the liver, transported by the various ducts and stored in the gallbladder. In order to understand radiographic examination of the biliary system, one should understand the basic anatomy and physiology of the liver, gallbladder and connecting ducts.

The liver is the largest solid organ in the human body and weighs 3 or 4 pounds (1.5 kg), or one thirty-sixth of the total body weight in an average adult. It occupies most of the **right upper quadrant**. Of the nine abdominal regions, it occupies almost all of the right hypochondrium, a major part of the epigastrium and a significant part of the left hypochondrium.

As viewed from the front in Fig. 16-1, the liver is triangular in shape. The upper border is the widest part of the liver (approximately 8 to 9 inches or 20 to 23 cm) and is convex to conform to the inferior surface of the right hemidiaphragm.

The right border of the liver is its greatest vertical dimension, approximately 6 to 7 inches or 15 to 17.5 cm. In the average person it extends to slightly below the lateral portion of the tenth rib just above the right kidney. The liver is fairly well protected by the lower right rib cage. Since the liver is highly vascular and easily lacerated, protection by the ribs is very necessary.

The distal end of the gallbladder extends slightly below the anterior, inferior margin of the liver. The rest of the gallbladder lies along the inferior and posterior surface of the liver (Fig. 16-3).

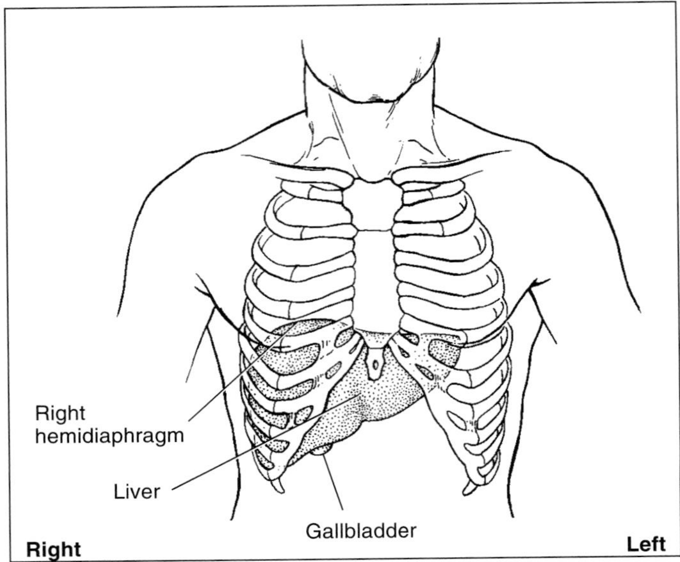

Fig. 16-1. Liver and gallbladder–Anterior view.

Lobes of the Liver

The liver is partially divided into two major lobes and two minor lobes. As viewed from the front in Fig. 16-2, only the two major lobes can be seen. A much larger **right lobe** is separated from the smaller **left lobe** by the **falciform** *(fal′ si-form)* **ligament.**

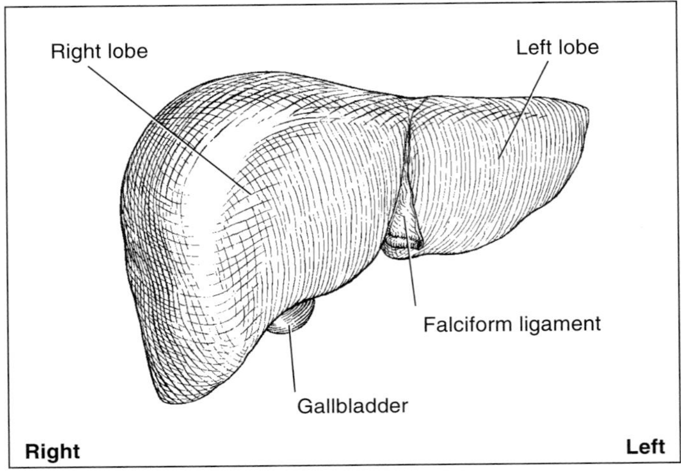

Fig. 16-2. Liver–Anterior view.

Associated with the large right lobe posteriorly are the two minor lobes, which can only be seen when viewing the visceral or inferior and posterior surface of the liver (Fig. 16-3). The first of these is the small **quadrate lobe** located on the inferior surface of the right lobe between the gallbladder and the falciform ligament. Just posterior to the quadrate lobe is the second minor lobe, the **caudate lobe,** which extends **superiorly** to the diaphragmatic surface. The large **inferior vena cava** vein is seen to contour over the surface of this caudate lobe. The other arteries and veins carrying blood to and from the liver are seen on the mid inferior surface, as well as the hepatic bile ducts which are described and illustrated on the following page.

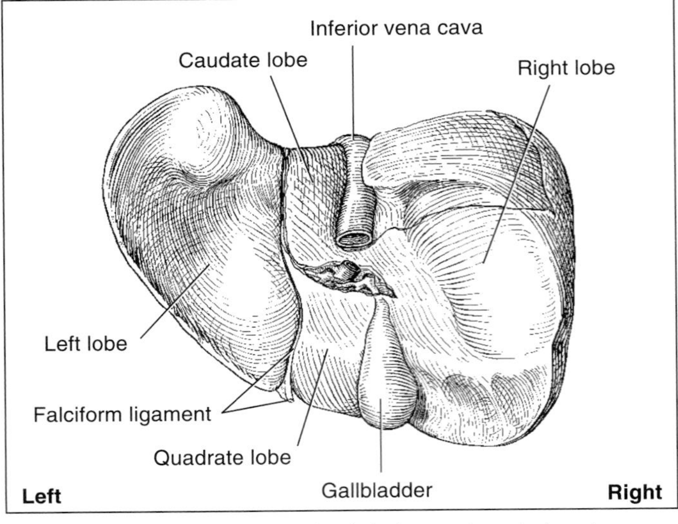

Fig. 16-3. Liver and gallbladder–Inferior and posterior view.

Function: The liver is an extremely complex organ and is absolutely essential to life. The liver performs over 100 different functions, but the one function most applicable to radiographic study is the production of large amounts of bile. It secretes from 800 to 1,000 ml, or about 1 quart of bile per day.

The major function of bile is to aid in the digestion of fats by emulsifying or breaking down fat globules, and the absorption of fat following its digestion. Bile also contains cholesterol which is made soluble in the bile by the bile salts.

GALLBLADDER AND BILIARY DUCTS

The gallbladder and the biliary ducts located outside of the gallbladder are shown in Fig. 16-4. Bile is formed in small lobules of the liver and travels by small ducts to either the **right** or **left hepatic duct.** The right and left hepatic ducts join to continue as the **common hepatic duct.** Bile is either carried to the **gallbladder** via the **cystic duct** for temporary storage, or poured directly into the **duodenum** by way of the **common bile duct**, which is joined by the main **pancreatic duct**.

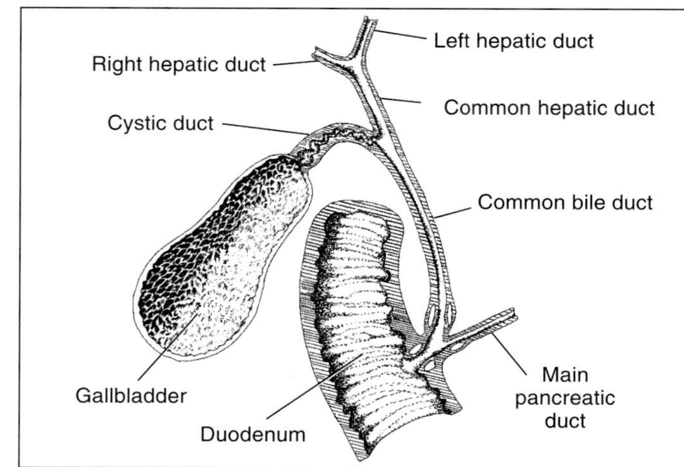

Fig. 16-4. Gallbladder and extrahepatic biliary ducts.

Gallbladder and Cystic Duct

The gallbladder and cystic duct are shown in Fig. 16-5. The gallbladder (GB) is a pear-shaped sac composed of three parts: **fundus, body** and **neck**. The fundus is the distal end and the broadest part of the gallbladder. The main section of the gallbladder is termed the body. The narrow proximal end is termed the neck, which continues as the **cystic duct.** The cystic duct is 3 to 4 centimeters long, containing several membranous folds along its length. These folds are termed the **spiral valve**, which functions to prevent distension or collapse of the cystic duct.

The normal gallbladder is from 7 to 10 centimeters long, about three centimeters wide and normally holds 30 to 40 ccs of bile.

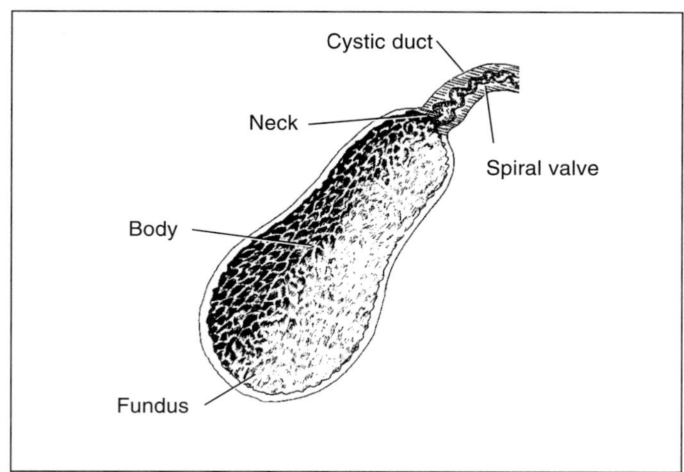

Fig. 16-5. Gallbladder and cystic duct.

Functions of the Gallbladder

The **three** primary functions of the gallbladder are to **store** and **concentrate** bile, and to **contract when stimulated**.

First: If bile is not needed for digestive purposes, it is stored for future use in the gallbladder.

Second: Bile is concentrated within the gallbladder due to hydrolysis (removal of water). In the abnormal situation, if too much water is absorbed or if the cholesterol becomes too concentrated, gallstones (choleliths) may form in the gallbladder. (Cholesterol coming out of solution forms gallstones.)

Third: The gallbladder normally contracts when foods such as fats or fatty acids are in the duodenum. These foods stimulate the duodenal mucosa to secrete the hormone cholecystokinin (CCK). Increased levels of CCK in the blood cause the gallbladder to contract and the terminal opening of the common bile duct to relax. In addition, CCK causes increased exocrine activity by the pancreas.

Common Bile Duct

The common hepatic duct draining the liver joins with the cystic duct of the gallbladder to form the **common bile duct.** The common bile duct averages about 7.5 centimeters in length and has an internal diameter about the size of a drinking straw. The common bile duct descends behind the superior portion of the duodenum and the head of the pancreas to enter the second or **descending portion of the duodenum**.

The end of the common bile duct is closely associated with the end of the **main duct** of the **pancreas (duct of Wirsung)**, *(Ver′soongz)** as shown in Fig. 16-6.

In about 40% of individuals these two ducts remain separated by a thin membrane as they pass into the duodenum. In the remaining 60%, the common bile duct joins the pancreatic duct to form an enlarged chamber just proximal to the terminal opening termed the **hepatopancreatic ampulla (ampulla of Vater)** *(fah′terz)*.† Near this terminal opening, the duct walls contain circular muscle fiber, termed the **hepatopancreatic sphincter (sphincter of Oddi)** *(Od′ez)*.‡ This sphincter relaxes when there are increased levels of CCK in the bloodstream. The presence of this ring of muscle causes a protrusion into the lumen of the duodenum. This protrusion is termed the **duodenal papilla**, which is the narrowest part of this passageway and therefore a common site for impaction of gallstones.

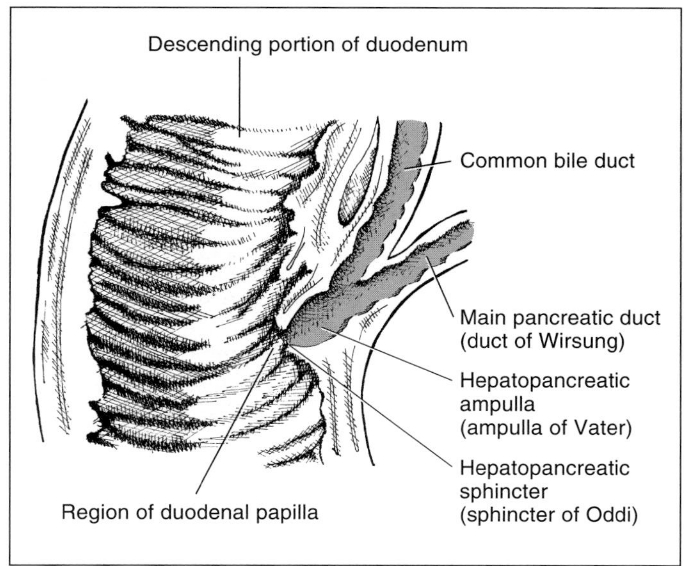

Fig. 16-6. Common bile duct.

*Wirsung, German physician, 17th century.
†Abraham Vater, German anatomist, 1684-1751.
‡Ruggero Oddi, 19th century Italian physician.

Gallbladder and Biliary Ducts

The simplified lateral drawing in Fig. 16-7 illustrates the arrangement of the **liver, gallbladder** and **biliary ducts** as seen from the right side. The gallbladder is **anterior** to the midcoronal plane, while the duct system is about midway between the front and the back. This spatial relationship influences optimal positioning of either the gallbladder or the biliary ducts. If it were necessary to place the gallbladder as close to the film surface as possible, the prone position would be much better than the supine position. If the primary purpose is to **drain the gallbladder** into the duct system, the patient would be placed **supine** to assist this drainage.

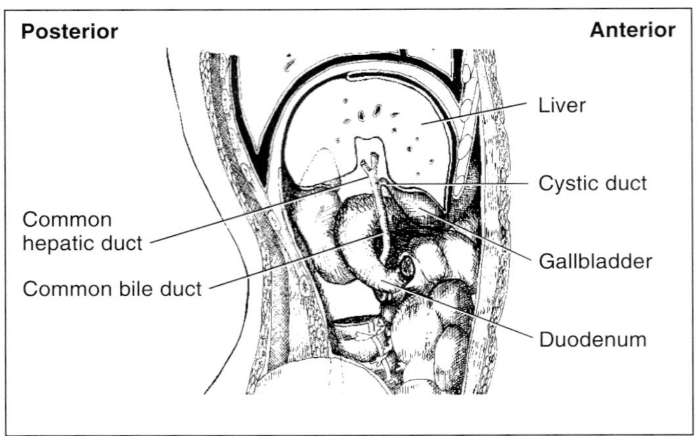

Fig. 16-7. Side view of gallbladder and biliary ducts.

Gallbladder Location Variation

The usual position of the gallbladder varies according to the body build of the patient. In the **hypersthenic** body habitus, the gallbladder is usually located higher and more lateral than average.

In the nearer average body build, which includes the **sthenic** and **hyposthenic** types, the gallbladder is usually located halfway between the xiphoid tip and the lower lateral rib margin.

In the **asthenic** body habitus, the gallbladder is much lower and near the midline.

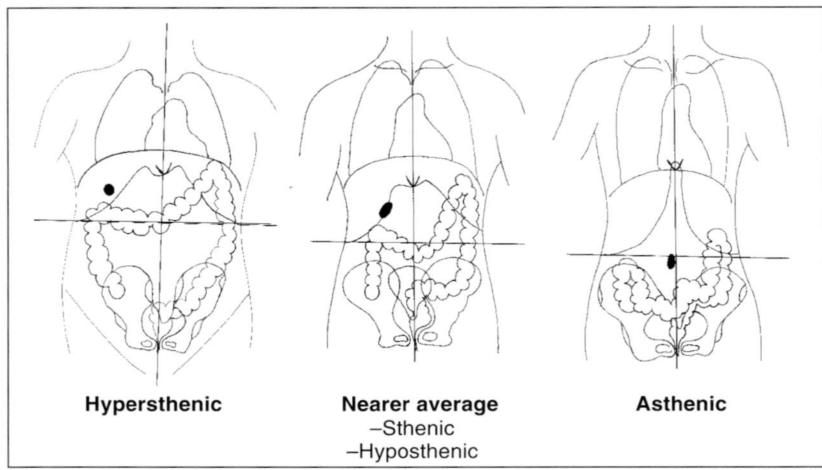

Fig. 16-8. Body habitus and gallbladder variation.

ANATOMY REVIEW

Radiograph of the Gallbladder

This PA projection of the gallbladder in Fig. 16-9 demonstrates the cystic duct and the three major divisions of the gallbladder as labeled:

A. Cystic duct
B. Neck
C. Body
D. Fundus

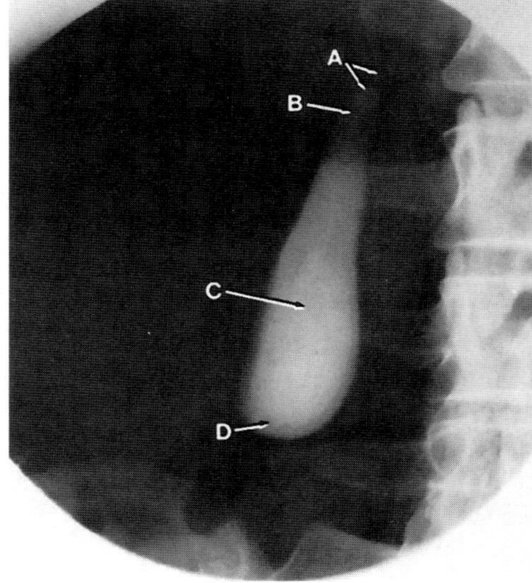

Fig. 16-9. Cholecystogram (gallbladder).
(Courtesy of Bill Collins, RT)

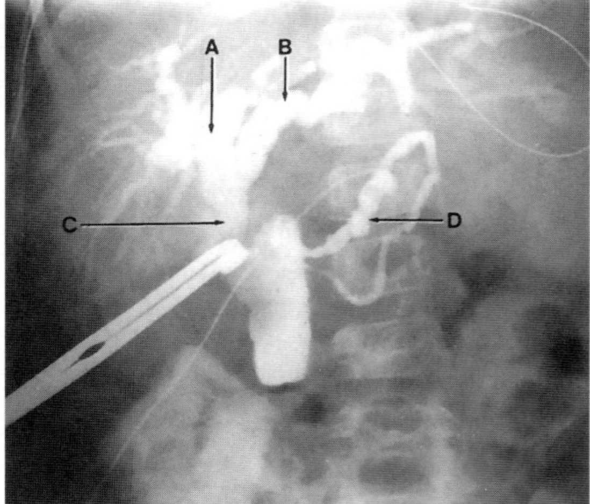

Fig. 16-10. Biliary ducts.

Radiograph of the Biliary Ducts

Radiograph 16-10 demonstrates the various divisions and components of the biliary tract. This was taken during a surgical procedure wherein contrast media was injected via a catheter directly into the biliary ducts. This does not represent normal duct positions but visualizes certain identifiable duct components and demonstrates the complexity of the biliary system as it may be seen on radiographs taken during an operative cholangiogram.

A. Right hepatic duct
B. Left hepatic duct
C. Common hepatic duct
D. Pancreatic duct (duct of Wirsung). This demonstrates an unusual and extra long loop of this duct.

Note: The common bile duct and the hepatopancreatic ampulla (ampulla of Vater) cannot be definitely determined from this radiograph alone.

Radiographic Procedures

GALLBLADDER AND BILIARY DUCT RADIOGRAPHY

Since the liver is such a large, solid organ, it can be easily located in the upper right quadrant on abdominal radiographs. The gallbladder and biliary ducts, however, blend in with other abdominal soft tissues and in most cases cannot be visualized without the addition of contrast media. Only about 15% of all gallstones contain enough calcium to be visualized on a plain abdominal radiograph.

Terminology

Radiographic examination of the gallbladder and biliary ducts is referred to by different terms. It is important to identify a specific examination by the correct term.

Radiographic examination specifically of the gallbladder is termed **cholecystography** *(ko″ le-sis-tog′ rah-fe)*. **Chole-** *(ko′ le)* is a prefix denoting a relationship to bile. **Cysto-** means sac or bladder. Therefore, chole combined with cysto literally translates as **bile sac** or **gallbladder**.

Cholangiogram is a radiographic examination of the **biliary ducts**. There are a number of techniques to study the bile ducts and these techniques will be discussed in a later section.

A study of both the **gallbladder** and **biliary ducts** is termed a cholecystocholangiogram *(ko″ le-sis″ to-ko-lan′ je-o-gram)*. Through the use of contrast media, both components are demonstrated.

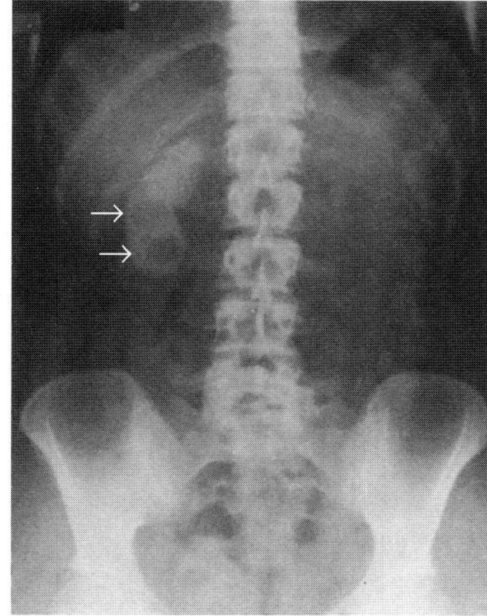

Fig. 16-11. Oral cholecystogram (OCG) (with gallstones–cholelithiasis, see arrows).

ORAL CHOLECYSTOGRAM

Contrast media is ingested orally for a **cholecystogram** *(ko′le-sis-to-gram)*, thus this procedure is termed an <u>O</u>ral <u>C</u>holecysto<u>G</u>ram, abbreviated, **OCG** (Fig. 16-11).

A common way to get contrast media into the biliary system has been orally (by mouth). Cholecystography of this type is accomplished following ingestion of four to six tablets or capsules during the evening preceding the examination. These oral contrast media for visualization of the gallbladder are termed **cholecystopaques**.

Note: The number of oral cholecystograms being ordered has declined greatly due to the increased use of sonography (see page 489). However they are still being performed in sufficient number that radiographers should be familiar with this procedure.

Purpose

The purpose of the oral cholecystogram is to study radiographically the anatomy and function of the biliary system. The oral cholecystogram measures: (1) the functional ability of the liver to remove the orally administered contrast medium from the bloodstream and to excrete it along with the bile, (2) the patency and condition of the biliary ducts and (3) the concentrating and contracting ability of the gallbladder.

Contraindications

Contraindications to cholecystography are few, but do include (1) advanced hepatorenal disease, especially those with renal impairment; (2) active gastrointestinal disease such as vomiting or diarrhea, which would prevent absorption of the oral contrast medium and (3) hypersensitivity to iodine-containing compounds.

Clinical Indications and Possible Radiographic Findings

Clinical indications for oral cholecystogram include **nausea**, **heartburn** and **vomiting**. A variety of abnormal conditions may be demonstrated during oral cholecystography. They include:

Cholelithiasis *(ko″ le-li-thi′ ah-sis) or* ***Biliary Calculi*** *(gallstones):* Cholelithiasis is the condition of having gallstones. Cholelithiasis is the most common abnormality diagnosed during an OCG. Increased levels of bilirubin, calcium, or cholesterol may lead to the formation of gallstones. Female and obese patients are at a higher risk of developing gallstones. Ninety percent of all gallbladder and duct disorders are due to cholelithiasis. Symptoms of cholelithiasis include right upper quadrant pain usually after a meal, nausea, and possibly vomiting.

Although drugs have been developed that will dissolve these stones, most patients will have their gallbladder removed. A new laparoscopic technique for removing the gallbladder (cholecystectomy) has greatly reduced the convalescence of the patient.

Cholecystitis *(ko″ le-sis-ti′ tis):* Cholecystitis, acute or chronic, is inflammation of the gallbladder. In acute cholecystitis, a blockage of the cystic duct restricts the flow of bile into the common bile duct. After a period of time, the bile begins to irritate the inner lining of the gallbladder and it becomes inflamed. Gas-producing bacteria may lead to a gangrenous gallbladder. The gallbladder with acute cholecystitis rarely becomes radiopaque during an OCG . Stenosis of the cystic duct prevents the contrast media from entering the gallbladder.

Chronic cholecystitis is almost always associated with gallstones, but may be an outcome of pancreatitis or carcinoma of the gallbladder. Symptoms of right upper quadrant pain, heartburn, and nausea may occur following a meal.

Neoplasms *(ne′ o-plazmz):* Neoplasms are new growths, which may be benign or malignant. Malignant or cancerous tumors of the gallbladder can be aggressive and spread to the liver, pancreas, or GI tract.

Biliary Stenosis *(ste-no′ sis):* Biliary stenosis is a narrowing of one of the biliary ducts. The flow of bile may be restricted by this condition. In the case of gallstones, the stenosis may prevent the passage of the small gallstones into the duodenum leading to obstruction of the ducts. Cholecystitis may result from biliary stenosis.

Congenital Anomalies *(ah-nom′ ah-les):* Congenital anomalies of the gallbladder are conditions that the patient possesses at birth. While most are benign, some may affect the production, storage, or release of bile.

ORAL CHOLECYSTOGRAM PROCEDURE

Patient Preparation

Patient preparation for the oral cholecystogram correlate well with preparations for an upper GI series, so these exams are commonly scheduled on the same morning. If the patient has been on a fat-free diet, he/she should eat some fats for one or two days before the gallbladder examination. Ingestion of fats causes the gallbladder to contract. By making sure that the gallbladder has emptied prior to the administration of contrast medium, chances are increased that the newly formed bile, with contrast medium added, will be stored in the gallbladder.

Laxatives are to be avoided during the 24-hour period before the exam. The evening meal before the examination should be a light one and should not contain any fats or fried foods. When combined with an upper GI, **the patient must be NPO** *(Non Per Os*, meaning nothing by mouth) for at least eight hours, and **must refrain from chewing gum or smoking** until after the exams.

Depending on the contrast medium used, either four or six tablets or capsules are taken after the evening meal, but before 9 P.M. The usual cholecystopaques are most effective **taken 10 to 12 hours before the exam**. No breakfast is permitted and the patient reports to radiology in the early A.M. The exact patient prep and amount of contrast medium utilized will vary from hospital to hospital.

When the patient arrives in the radiology department for oral cholecystography, they should be instructed to remove all clothing from the chest and abdomen areas and put on a hospital gown.

Patient Instructions

___ **I.V. CHOLANGIOGRAM AND/OR INTRAVENOUS PYELOGRAM**

1. Fleet's Prep Kit III - 24 hour prep. All instructions are contained in kit.

___ **BARIUM ENEMA**

1. Fleet's Prep Kit III - 24 hour prep. All instructions are contained in kit. May have a clear liquid breakfast.

___ **GALLBLADDER SERIES (ORAL CHOLECYSTOGRAM)**

1. Fat free supper evening before examination.
2. Take one Cholebrine tablet every 1/2 hour starting at 2:00 p.m. day before exam.
3. Nothing by mouth after midnight.

___ **UPPER G.I. SERIES AND/OR SMALL BOWEL SERIES**

1. Do not eat, drink, smoke or chew gum after midnight. Any antispasmodic medication should be preferably discontinued at least 24 hours before exam. Fleet's Prep Kit III may be purchased at most drug stores. Baptist Medical Center Pharmacy carries this kit along with Revco and Thrifty Drugs. Please call ahead to your pharmacy if you have any questions.

ULTRASOUND PREPS:

Ultrasound of the ABDOMEN: **Fat free clear** liquid diet from 6:00 p.m. the evening before examination.

Ultrasound of the PELVIS: **MUST** have a full bladder. Finish drinking 38 to 42 ounces of liquid one hour before exam. **DO NOT** empty bladder until after exam.

C.T. PREPS:

Abdomen - Clear liquids after midnight
Chest - Clear liquids only four hours prior to exam
Head - Clear liquids only four hours prior to exam
Pelvis - Clear liquids after midnight
Spine - no prep

Appointment date _______________ Appointment time _______________

Fig. 16-12a. Sample patient instruction form.
(Courtesy of Phoenix Baptist Hospital and Medical Center, Phoenix, AZ.)

Patient Interview

Before the scout radiograph, the patient must be questioned about taking the contrast medium. The patient should **first** be asked how many pills were taken and at what time. It may be necessary to have the patient describe the capsules or tablets to confirm that they were the correct ones.

Second, the patient should be questioned regarding any reaction from the pills. Nausea followed by vomiting would prevent adequate absorption, as would active diarrhea. Any anaphylactoid or hypersensitivity reactions should be noted.

Third, it should be determined that the patient has not had breakfast.

Fourth, make sure that the patient still has a gallbladder. There is no need to do a cholecystogram on those rare occasions when the patient has already had the gallbladder surgically removed.

Fifth, the female patient of childbearing age should be questioned regarding a possible pregnancy with precautions taken as for other abdominal radiographic exams.

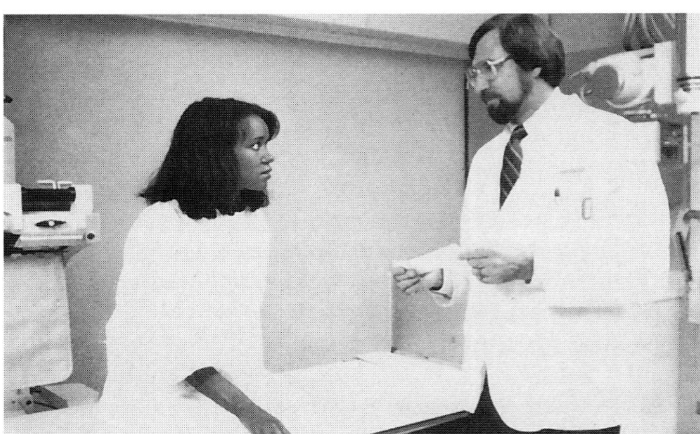

Fig. 16-12b. Patient interview.

Cholecystogram Scout

After appropriate questioning, a scout radiograph is taken on a 10 x 12 or 14 x 17 inch film depending, on departmental routines. The scout radiograph is made with the patient prone, as shown in Fig. 16-13. Since iodine is the major radiation-absorbing component of the contrast medium, a **kilovoltage of 70 to 76 should be used**. The scout radiograph must be checked to determine the presence or absence of an opacified gallbladder.

If the gallbladder shadow is present, the radiographer should determine (l) its exact location, (2) whether there is overlap by intestine or bone, (3) whether there is sufficient concentration of contrast medium for additional imaging, and (4) whether the exposure factors were optimal. If the gallbladder did not opacify adequately for imaging, the patient needs to be questioned again in detail about his preparation and, especially, about his diet for the past 24 hours.

Nonvisualization on the first day may result in a two-day study with a second dose of contrast medium or, perhaps, a trip to the sonography department for cholecystosonography.

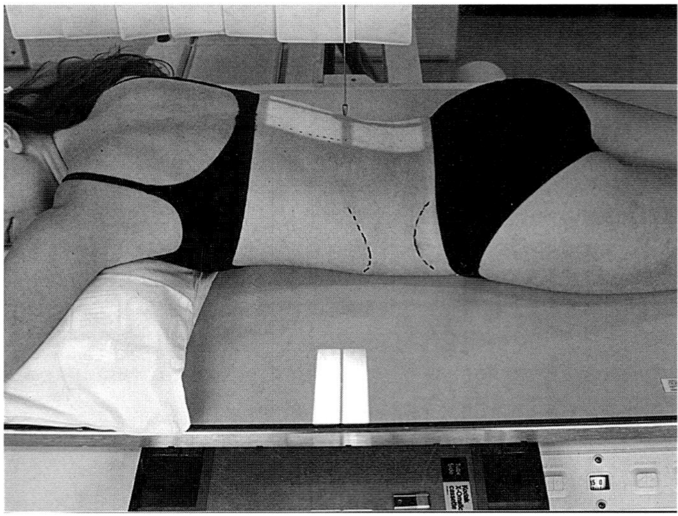

Fig. 16-13. Positioning for a cholecystogram scout.

General Routine Procedures

One or more positions may be utilized if the gallbladder visualizes adequately on the scout radiograph. At least one erect or decubitus projection utilizing a horizontal beam is essential. A wide range in both the location and the pathology of the gallbladder make cholecystography an individual examination.

The right lateral decubitus projection, as shown in Fig. 16-14, or the upright position is utilized to stratify or layer out gallstones. Depending on the density of the stones in relation to the specific gravity of bile, stones may sink, rise or layer out in these two positions. Additionally, these positions allow the gallbladder to assume a different position in the abdomen and, perhaps, allow better visualization.

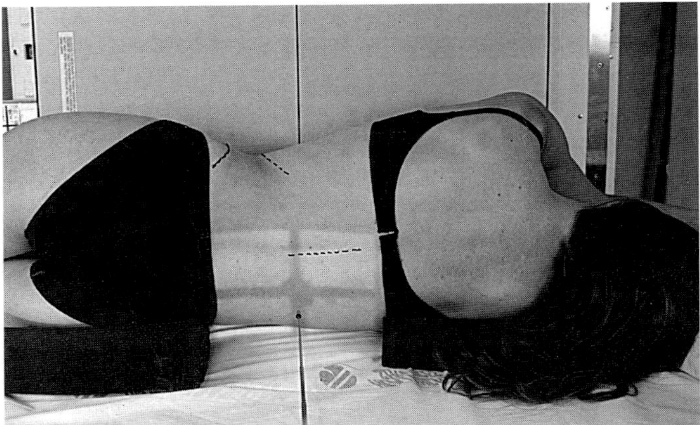

Fig. 16-14. Radiography–Right lateral decubitus projection.

Method of Imaging

Many radiologists request fluoroscopy and spot films of the gallbladder in the upright position in addition to a variety of conventional radiographs. Spot filming allows use of compression and small positional changes to optimally visualize the gallbladder. A model is shown in position for upright fluoroscopy of the gallbladder in Fig. 16-15. If an upper GI series is scheduled in addition to the oral cholecystogram, the patient would then be in position for ingestion of barium.

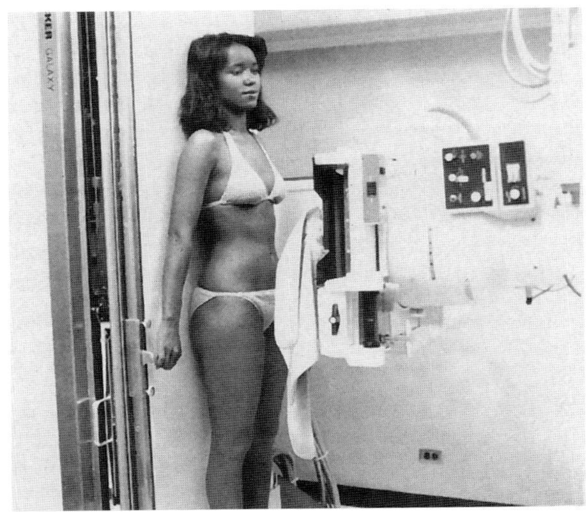

Fig. 16-15. Fluoroscopy.

With Fatty Meal or CCK

Occasionally, after adequate imaging of the filled gallbladder, the radiologist may wish to test the function of the gallbladder (ability to contract) and to study the extrahepatic biliary ducts.

The administration of a "fatty meal" will stimulate the duodenal mucosa to produce CCK (cholecystokinin) which, in turn, will cause the gallbladder to contract. Commercially available fatty meal substitutes are administered for this purpose. The patient is placed in an RPO position after the fatty meal so that the gallbladder can best drain (Fig. 16-16). Radiographs are obtained in the same RPO position every 15 minutes until satisfactory visualization of the duct system is obtained.

A second method for gallbladder stimulation and contraction is much faster and more direct. Either cholecystokinin (CCK) or a synthetic substitute is injected into the patient's venous system. This usually causes contraction of the gallbladder in 5 to 10 minutes. This method for visualizing the gallbladder, however, is seldom performed anymore due to advances in sonography imaging.

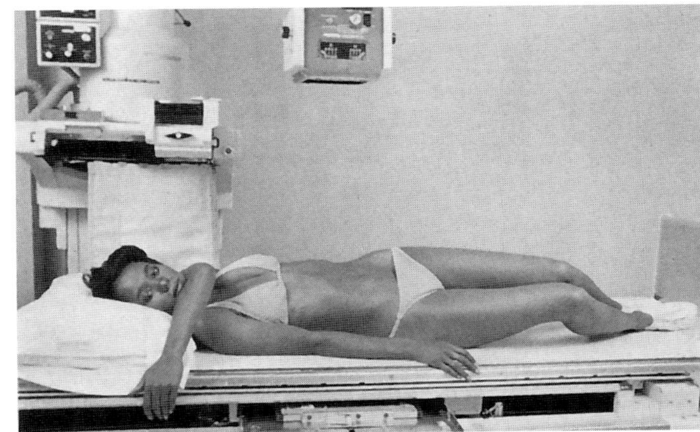

Fig. 16-16. Gallbladder drainage position–RPO.

SONOGRAPHY (ULTRASOUND)

The number of oral cholecystograms (OCGs) in general being ordered has declined greatly due to the increased use of diagnostic sonography. Sonography of the gallbladder provides a noninvasive means to study the gallbladder and the biliary ducts.

Four advantages of sonography over the conventional OCG are:

1. No Ionizing Radiation. Sonography is a nonionizing radiation imaging modality which eliminates radiation exposure to the patient, and also to the radiologist and technologist (if fluoroscopy is performed with conventional OCG).

2. Detection of Small Calculi. Sonography can detect small calculi in the gallbladder and biliary ducts that generally are not visualized during an OCG.

3. No Contrast Medium. No contrast medium is required with sonography. Therefore this is an ideal alternative for the patients who are sensitive to iodinated contrast agents.

4. Less Time-consuming Procedure. Patient preparation with sonography is greatly reduced as compared to the OCG. For sonography, the patient should be NPO 4 hours prior to the exam whereas the patient preparation and contrast media administration for an OCG can require two or more days to complete. Therefore sonography provides a quick diagnosis for gallbladder disease and the physician can make a surgical decision in hours rather than days.

OPERATIVE (OR IMMEDIATE) CHOLANGIOGRAM

The operative or immediate cholangiogram is performed during surgery, usually during a cholecystectomy. The surgeon may suspect that residual stones are located in one of the biliary ducts. After the gallbladder is removed, a small catheter is inserted into the remaining portion of the cystic duct. Iodinated contrast media is injected and conventional radiographs are taken. Most operative cholangiograms require the use of a high mA portable x-ray unit and grid cassettes.

Some surgeons prefer to use mobile fluoroscopy (C-arm) to provide a real-time image of the ducts during injection. Hard copy images (radiographs) can also be produced if requested by the surgeon. See Chapter 19 on trauma and mobile radiography for more information on the C-arm mobile digital fluoroscopy unit and its use in the operating room.

Purpose

Operative cholangiograms are performed to:

(1) Reveal any choleliths not previously detected (primary purpose).
(2) Investigate the patency of the biliary tract.
(3) Determine the functional status of the hepatopancreatic ampulla.
(4) Demonstrate small lesions, strictures or dilatations within the biliary ducts.

Procedure

Proper planning and preparation is essential for a successful cholangiogram. But many operative cholangiograms may be scheduled at the last moment and the technologist doesn't have the opportunity to even take a scout film. In these situations, the technologist must be resourceful to produce quality radiographs.

In the ideal situation, the following steps should occur:

(1) The radiographer changes into surgical attire and ensures that the portable unit or C-arm is functional and clean.
(2) Before the patient is surgically prepared, take a scout film. Note the distance the film is advanced from the head of the table. A special ruler-and-tray setup may be used in the positioning of the cassette.
(3) Process the scout film and adjust technique and film location accordingly.
(4) Once the catheter is in place, the surgeon will inject 6 to 8 ccs of contrast media.
(5) Images are obtained with the cooperation and synchronization of the surgeon, anesthesiologist, and radiographer. The anesthesiologist controls the breathing of the patient.
(6) Films are processed and may need to be reviewed by a radiologist. The radiographer may convey a written or oral report from the radiologist to the surgeon.

At least two and preferably three radiographs are obtained in slightly different positions. Each exposure is preceded by a fractional injection of contrast medium. Positions may include an AP, a slight RPO, and a slight LPO. The RPO is helpful in projecting the biliary ducts away from the spine, especially with a hyposthenic patient.

Notes:

(a) Protective aprons must be provided to those persons remaining in the room.
(b) Some surgeons will dilute the contrast media with saline to reduce the risk of spasm of the biliary ducts. Biliary duct spasm may mimic biliary stenosis or obstruction. Also, a contrast media that is too dense may obscure small stones.
(c) If the OR table is tilted for the oblique positions, place the grid cassette **crosswise** to avoid objectionable grid cutoff.

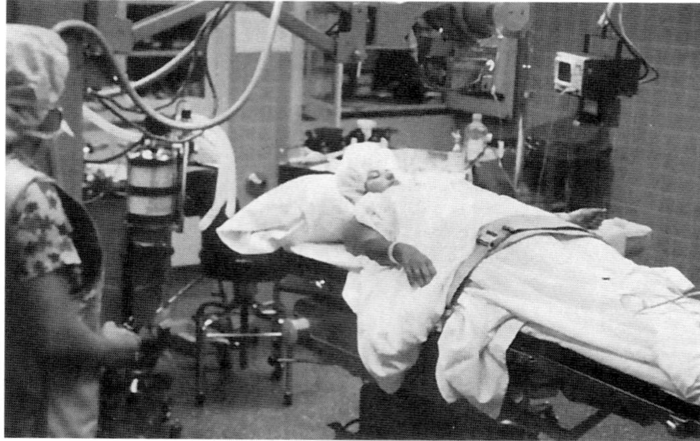

Fig. 16-17. Scout operative cholangiogram.

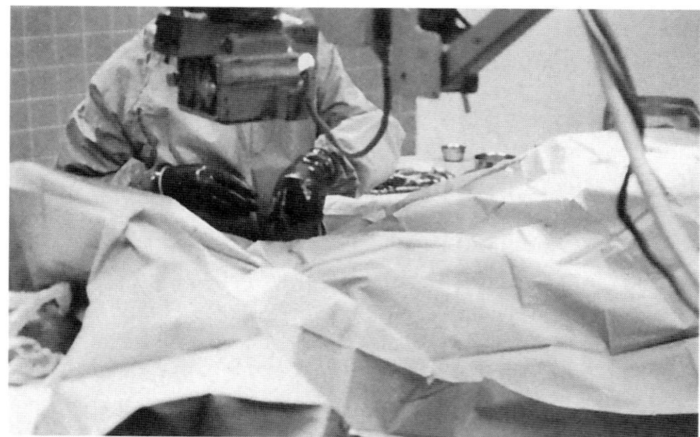

Fig. 16-18. Surgeon indicating CR centering.

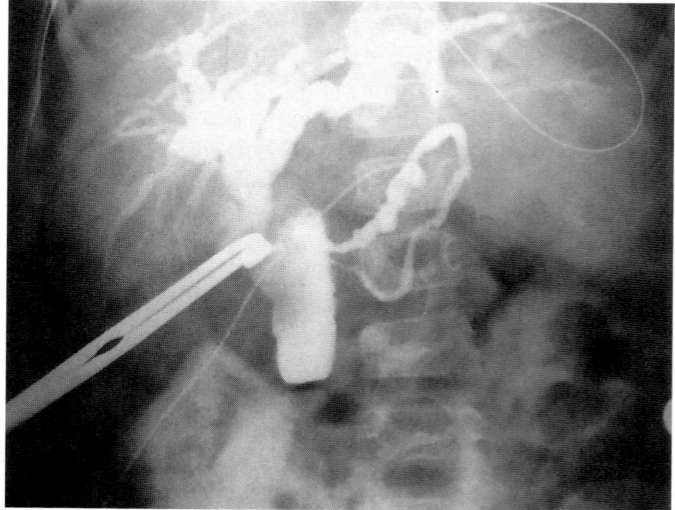

Fig. 16-19. Operative cholangiogram.

Centering Point

The surgeon should indicate the proper centering point on the sterile sheet covering the incision or, at least, indicate appropriate landmarks such as the xiphoid tip. In Fig. 16-18 the surgeon has twisted the sterile drape to identify the centering point.

Each fractional injection consists of 6 to 8 ccs of contrast medium. The exposure is made after the injection, after the surgeon steps back and after the anesthesiologist has stopped patient respiration.

LAPAROSCOPIC CHOLANGIOGRAPHY

New Surgical Procedure

A new technique has evolved over the past years that has simplified the removal of diseased gallbladders. The surgeon will make a small opening in the umbilicus and pass an endoscope into the abdominal cavity. This type of procedure has been used for years in the visual assessment of the abdomen to detect signs of pathology or trauma. It is referred to as a **laparoscopic** *(lap″ ah-ro-skop′ ik)* procedure. This technique has been modified to perform cholecystectomy and cholangiography with a minimal amount of surgical trauma to the patient.

Cholecystectomy

The endoscope (described on page 493) is inserted at the umbilicus and the surgeon advances it to the region of the gallbladder. Once the gallbladder is visualized, the surgeon can use special endoscopic tools to sever the diseased gallbladder, suction it out and cauterize (removal of tissue with a hot instrument) the remnant cystic duct. Additional openings may also be required to allow suction and to provide for other instruments to pass into the abdominal cavity.

Cholangiogram

If stones in the biliary ducts are suspected, the surgeon can then insert a catheter and inject contrast media into one of the ducts. The technologist would then perform the same imaging duties as outlined under the operative or immediate cholangiogram.

Advantages of Laparoscopy: Three advantages of laparoscopy are: (1) It can be performed as an outpatient procedure. (2) It is a less invasive procedure. Previous surgical techniques required a large opening be created to remove the gallbladder. This degree of invasive surgery required that the patient remain in the hospital for at least 2 days. (3) A third advantage then can be stated as **reduced hospital time** (reduced cost). Many patients having the laparoscopic technique can return home the same day, and in certain cases, return to work in 2 to 3 days.

The laparoscopic cholecystectomy however is not suited for every patient. More complex disease processes or involved procedures may require the more traditional surgical approach.

T-TUBE (POSTOPERATIVE OR DELAYED) CHOLANGIOGRAPHY

T-tube cholangiography, also termed postoperative or delayed cholangiography, is usually performed in the radiology department following a cholecystectomy. The surgeon may be concerned about residual stones in the biliary ducts that went undetected during the surgery. If these concerns exist, the surgeon will place a special T-tube catheter into the common bile duct. The catheter extends to the outside of the body and is clamped off.

Purpose

T-tube cholangiograms are performed to:

(1) Visualize any residual or previously undetected choleliths.
(2) Evaluate the status of the biliary duct system.
(3) Demonstrate small lesions, strictures or dilatations within the biliary ducts.

Procedure

On the average, the T-tube cholangiogram is performed 1 to 3 days following surgery. In certain cases, the patient may be discharged from the hospital and brought back for the study as an outpatient. The procedure requires the use of fluoroscopy. Spot films are generally also taken. Conventional radiographs may be taken during the course of the study.

The following steps are taken in the performance of a T-tube cholangiogram:

(1) Prepare the fluoroscopic suite.
(2) Set up examination tray.
(3) Select and prepare the contrast media. Determine if the patient is hypersensitive to iodinated contrast media.
(4) Take the appropriate scout films to verify position and technique.
(5) Provide lead aprons for those persons remaining in the room during the procedure.
(6) Monitor the patient during the procedure.
(7) Change fluoro spot films as needed.
(8) Produce conventional radiographs as requested.

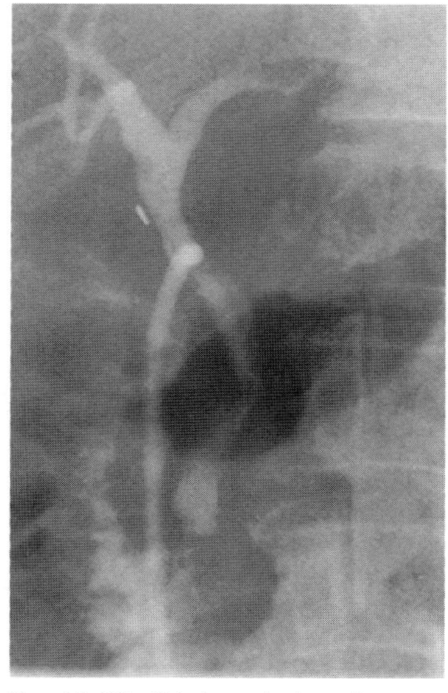

Fig. 16-20. T-tube cholangiogram.

Since the T-tube catheter has been clamped off, drainage of excess bile is performed at the beginning of the procedure. An emesis basin should be provided for this task. Follow universal precautions when handling bile.

After duct drainage and under fluoroscopic control, the iodinated contrast media is injected fractionally and fluoro spot films are taken.

If residual stones are detected, the radiologist may elect to remove them. Similar to the PTC, a basket catheter may be passed over a guide wire and the stones removed.

PERCUTANEOUS TRANSHEPATIC CHOLANGIOGRAPHY

Percutaneous Transhepatic Cholangiography (**PTC**) is another type of cholangiography that demonstrates the biliary ducts. It is also generally performed in the radiology department and is more invasive than other forms of cholangiography. However, it gives the radiologist more options in the diagnosis and treatment of biliary conditions.

The PTC involves **a direct puncture of biliary ducts** with a needle passing through the liver. Once within a duct, iodinated contrast media is injected under fluoroscopic control. Fluoroscopic spot films and conventional radiographs are taken during the procedure.

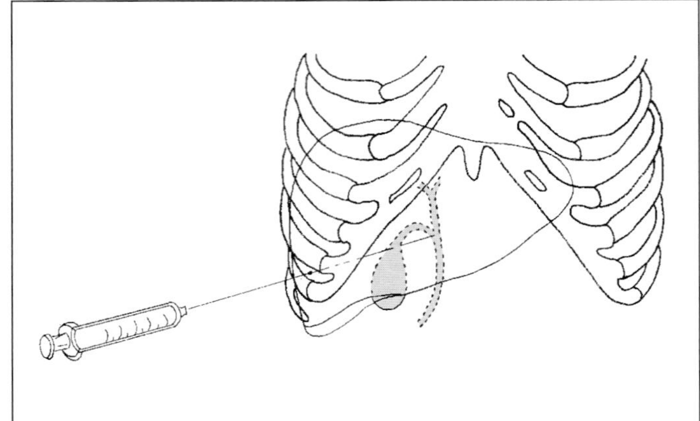

Fig. 16-21. PTC puncture through liver into biliary ducts.

Purpose

The PTC is performed for various clinical indications. The two most common indications are:

(1) Obstructive Jaundice: If the patient is jaundiced and the ducts are suspected to be dilated, an obstruction of the biliary ducts may be the cause. The obstruction may be due to calculi or biliary stenosis.

(2) Stone Extraction and Biliary Drainage: PTC allows the radiologist to diagnose the condition and, using specialized equipment, remove the stone or dilate the restricted portion of the biliary tract. Excess bile may be drained during a PTC to decompress the biliary ducts.

Procedure

There is a certain amount of risk associated with the PTC due to the needle puncture into the liver tissue. The liver may hemorrhage internally or bile may escape into the peritoneal cavity. Therefore, following the procedure, a chest radiograph may be ordered. Since the liver is near the right hemidiaphragm, the needle puncture may result in a pneumothorax. Both during and after the procedure, the patient's vital signs are closely monitored to detect deterioration.

While the percutaneous transhepatic puncture is performed by the radiologist, the radiographer has specific responsibilities. These responsibilities include:

(1) Prepare the fluoroscopic suite.
(2) Set up the sterile tray and include the long, thin-walled needle used for the puncture. (The needle is a Chiba or "Skinny" type. It has a flexible shaft that allows for easy manipulation of the needle during the puncture.)
(3) Select and prepare the contrast media. Determine if the patient is hypersensitive to iodinated contrast media.
(4) Provide lead aprons for those persons remaining in the room during the exposure.
(5) Take the appropriate scout films to verify position and technique.
(6) Monitor the patient during the procedure.
(7) Change fluoro spot films as needed.

The site of the puncture is surgically prepared. After the local anesthetic is given, the radiologist inserts the needle into the liver in the approximate location of the biliary ducts. More than one puncture may be necessary to locate the appropriate duct. Under fluoroscopic view, the radiologist adjusts the needle while slowly injecting the contrast media. Once the ducts are filled, fluoroscopic spot films and conventional radiographs are taken.

In addition to studying the biliary ducts, the PTC may serve as a therapeutic procedure to extract stones or decompress dilated ducts.

A larger needle may be inserted into a duct containing a stone. A special basket catheter is passed over a guide wire and is positioned near the stone. Under fluoroscopic control, the stone can be extracted from the duct.

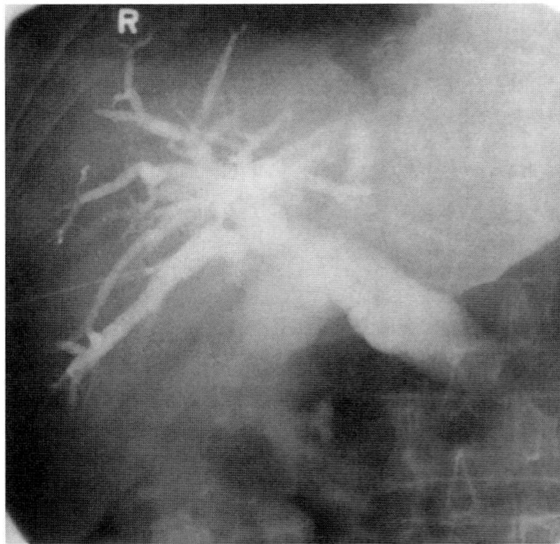

Fig. 16-22. Percutaneous transhepatic cholangiogram (PTC).

Summary of risks associated with PTC.

1. Possible liver hemorrhage.
2. Possible development of pneumothorax.
3. Bile may escape into peritoneal cavity leading to inflammation of surrounding tissue.

ENDOSCOPIC RETROGRADE CHOLANGIOPANCREATOGRAPHY (ERCP)

Another procedure for examination of the biliary and main pancreatic ducts, which is being performed more frequently, is Endoscopic Retrograde Cholangiopancreatography, or simply **ERCP**.

Endoscopy

Endoscopy *(en-dos′ko-pe)* is inspection of any cavity of the body by means of an endoscope, an instrument that allows illumination of the internal lining of an organ. Various fiber-optic endoscopes are available to examine the interior lining of the stomach, duodenum, and colon. Older type endoscopes allow for individual viewing only (Fig. 16-23), but newer **video endoscopes** project the image onto video monitors for multiple viewing. Also a special type of fiber-optic endoscope, called a **duodenoscope** is commonly used for an ERCP exam. This instrument when inserted into the duodenum through the mouth, esophagus and stomach, provides a wide-angle side view which is useful for locating and inserting a catheter or cannula into the small opening of the hepatopancreatic sphincter (sphincter of Oddi) leading from the duodenum into the common bile duct and the main pancreatic ducts.*

Diagnostic or Therapeutic

The ERCP can be either a diagnostic or therapeutic procedure. Therapeutically, ERCP can be performed to relieve certain pathologic conditions. This can be either the removal of choleliths or small lesions, or for other purposes such as to repair a stenosis (narrowing or blockage of a duct or canal) of the hepatopancreatic sphincter or associated ducts.*

For diagnostic purposes in general the ERCP procedure includes the insertion endoscopically, of the catheter or injection cannula into the common bile duct or main pancreatic duct under fluoroscopic control, followed by retrograde injection (backward or reverse direction) of contrast media into the biliary ducts. The procedure is usually performed by a gastroenterologist assisted by a team of the radiographer, one or more nurses and perhaps a radiologist.

Purpose of Diagnostic ERCP

The diagnostic ERCP is performed to:

(1) Investigate the patency of the biliary/pancreatic ducts.
(2) Reveal any choleliths not previously detected.
(3) Demonstrate small lesions, strictures or dilatations within the biliary/pancreatic ducts.

Procedure

The ERCP is primarily a fluoroscopic procedure that generally follows an oral cholecystogram or a sonogram exam of the gallbladder wherein the results have been inconclusive. Fluoroscopy, as operated by either the radiologist or the radiographer, is needed to aide with the cannulation of the hepatopancreatic ampulla and to provide spot films of the relevant anatomy.

The ERCP may involve the following steps:

(1) Prepare the fluoroscopic suite.
(2) Set up the examination tray.
(3) Select and prepare the contrast media. Determine if the patient is hypersensitive to iodinated contrast media.
(4) Take the appropriate scout films to verify position and technique.
(5) Assist the gastroenterologist with fluoroscopy for the placement of the catheter or injection cannula.
(6) Monitor the patient during the procedure.
(7) Change fluoro spot films as needed.
(8) Produce conventional radiographs as requested.

The gastroenterologist will spray an oral anesthetic in the patient's throat to suppress the gag reflex while the fiber-optic endoscope is advanced into the duodenum. Once the hepatopancreatic ampulla is isolated, a small catheter is passed through it and the contrast media is fractionally injected.

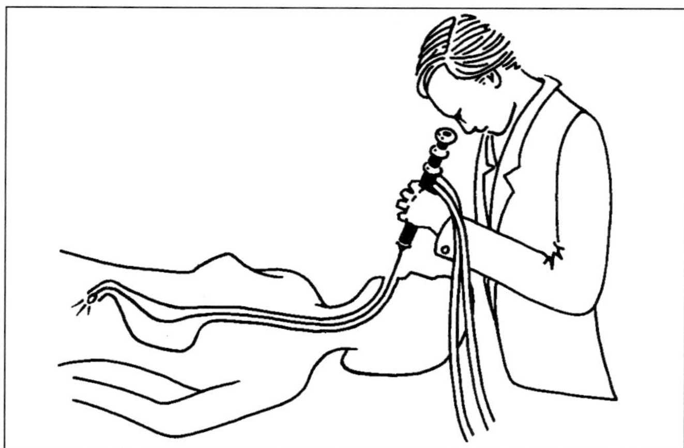

Fig. 16-23. Endoscopy.

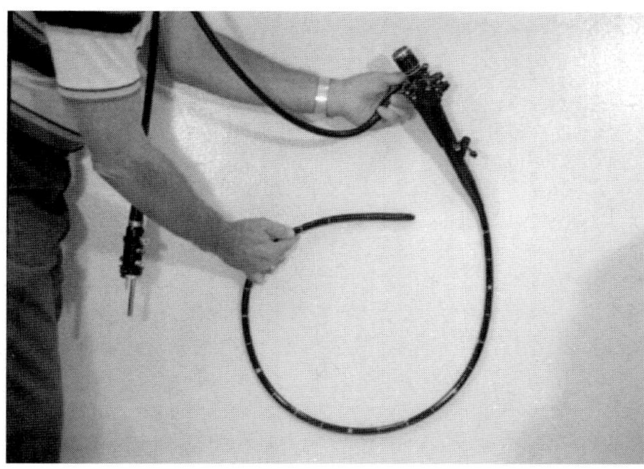

Fig. 16-24. Duodenoscope* (can be connected to video monitor). (Used with permission, F. A. Davis Company)

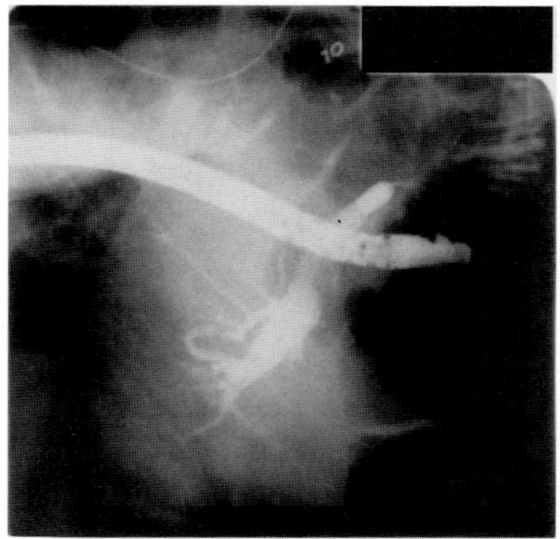

Fig. 16-25. ERCP radiograph demonstrating biliary tree.* (Used with permission, F. A. Davis Company))

The radiographer may be asked to perform fluoroscopy during the procedure to identify the location of the tip of the endoscope in relationship to the ampulla. A radiologist may be present to take the spot films during the injection of contrast media.

Precautions: (a) Since the patient's throat is anesthetized during the procedure, they should remain NPO for at least one hour (or more) following the procedure. This will prevent aspiration of food or liquid into the lungs.

(b) Review the clinical history of the patient to determine if the patient has pancreatitis or, specifically, a pseudocyst of the pancreas. Injecting contrast media into a pseudocyst may lead to a rupture.

(c) Ensure that all persons in the fluoroscopy room wear protective aprons.

*Tortorici, MR, Apfel, PJ: *Advanced Radiographic and Angiographic Procedures with an introduction to specialized imaging.* Philadelphia: F.A. Davis; 1995.

SUMMARY OF RADIOGRAPHIC PROCEDURES

Gallbladder and Biliary System Radiography

In summary, **cholecystography and cholangiography** may be categorized by the method of contrast medium administration. Contrast medium is usually administered orally for cholecystography (gallbladder exam). For cholangiography, the biliary ducts are usually studied following intravenous infusion or various methods of direct injection of contrast medium.

Summary Table of Gallbladder and Biliary System Procedures

Procedure	*Anatomy visualized*	*Administration of contrast media*
Cholecystography–Gallbladder:		
1. Oral cholecystogram (OCG)	Gallbladder	Oral ingestion
Cholangiography–Biliary ducts:		
1. Sonography procedure	Gallbladder and biliary ducts	None needed
2. Operative (immediate) cholangiogram or Laparoscopic cholangiogram	Biliary ducts	Direct injection through catheter during surgery
3. T-tube cholangiogram	Biliary ducts	Direct injection through indwelling drainage tube
4. Percutaneous transhepatic cholangiogram (PTC)	Biliary ducts	Direct injection by a needle puncture through the liver into the biliary ducts
5. Endoscopic retrograde cholangiopancreatogram (ERCP)	Biliary/pancreatic ducts	Direct injection through catheter placed during endoscopic procedure

Radiographic Positioning

NATIONAL SURVEY

A survey of the operating procedures (department routines) was conducted throughout the United States. The following information was compiled from the survey indicating the national norm for basic and special routines for oral cholecystography and operative cholangiography. The results were very consistent throughout all regions of the U.S.

Oral Cholecystogram (OCG or Gallbladder) Routine

Gallbladder (OCG)	U.S. Average	
	Basic 1995 (1989)	Special 1995 (1989)
• PA scout	70% (78%)	
• LAO	74% (63%)	
• R lat. decub.	34% (31%)	25% (30%)
• PA erect	30% (19%)	13% (13%)
• RAO	24% –	11% –
• Fatty meal or CCK-PZ injection	23% (20%)	28% (24%)
• Sonography in combination with oral cholecystogram	19% –	30% –

T-tube Postoperative Cholangiogram

T-tube	U.S. Average	
	Basic 1995 (1989)	Special 1995 (1989)
• Fluoro and spot films	86% –	
• AP	67% –	
• RPO	49% –	10% –
• LPO	15% –	12% –

Operative Cholangiogram Routine

OR cholangiogram	U.S. Average	
	Basic 1995 (1989)	Special 1995 (1989)
• AP	81% (87%)	
• RPO	27% (28%)	12% (16%)
• LPO	5% (5%)	11% (7%)

Percutaneous Transhepatic Cholangiogram (PTC)

PTC	U.S. Average	
	Basic 1995 (1989)	Special 1995 (1989)
• Post-injection AP fluoro and spots	65% –	8% –

Endoscopic Retrograde Cholangiopancreatogram (ERCP)

ERCP	U.S. Average	
	Basic 1995 (1989)	Special 1995 (1989)
• Post-injection AP fluoro and spots	75% –	3% –
• AP	42% –	7% –
• RPO	19% –	13% –
• LPO	10% –	13% –

Summary

Gallbladder: The gallbladder routines were generally consistent throughout the U.S. with no significant changes in 1995 as compared to 1989. The question concerning the use of sonography was not included in the 1989 survey but it appears its use has increased greatly in recent years. In 1995 19% indicated they used sonography routinely and 30% used it as optional or special.

With **sonography** there were some regional differences with a greater use of sonography for the gallbladder in the Mid U.S. (35%), as compared to the East (26%) and West (28%). (See Appendix in back pages of this text.)

T-tube, OR Cholangiogram and ERCP: Routine projections for these procedures were primarily the AP, with the RPO indicated as a second or special projection. The percentage using the LPO as routine or special was very low.

SPECIAL BILIARY DUCT PROCEDURES

Percutaneous transhepatic cholangiography (PTC), endoscopic retrograde cholangiopancreatogram (ERCP) and T-tube cholangiography are described in the preceding pages of this chapter. These exams are primarily performed by the radiologist, with the radiographer assisting, therefore they are not described in the positioning pages of this chapter. Certain of these procedures that may be performed in the operating room with the use of mobile fluoroscopy (C-arm) are described in Chapter 19 on mobile radiography.

T-tube cholangiogram
(fluoro spots, radiography optional)
Basic
• AP and RPO
Special
• LPO

Percutaneous transhepatic cholangiogram (PTC)
(fluoro spots, radiography optional)

Endoscopic retrograde cholangiopancreatogram (ERCP)
(fluoro spots, radiography optional)
Basic
• AP
Special
• RPO and LPO

BASIC AND SPECIAL PROJECTIONS

Certain basic and special projections or positions of the gallbladder and biliary ducts are demonstrated and described on the following pages. The radiologist and radiographer must closely coordinate their efforts during examinations of this part of the body. Individual variations exist among radiologists, and the routine or basic positions or projections listed may vary from hospital to hospital.

Gallbladder
(oral cholecystogram–OCG)
Basic
• PA scout **497**
• LAO **498**
Special
• Right lat. decub. (PA) **499**
• PA erect **500**

Biliary ducts
(OR cholangiogram)
Basic
• AP and/or RPO **501**

PA Projection

Scout

Gallbladder (oral cholecystogram)
Basic
• **PA scout**
• LAO
Special
• Right lat. decub. (PA)
• PA erect

Structures Best Shown

General survey of opacified gallbladder. The PA scout is taken to determine presence and location of gallbladder, adequate concentration of contrast media and adequacy of exposure factors.

Technical Factors

- Film size –10 x 12 in. (24 x 30 cm), lengthwise.
  or –11 x 14 in. (30 x 35 cm), lengthwise.
  or –14 x 17 in. (35 x 43 cm), lengthwise
- Moving or stationary grid.
- 70-76 kVp range.
- Technique and dose:

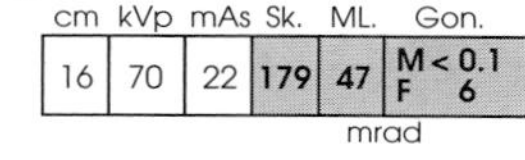

cm	kVp	mAs	Sk.	ML.	Gon.
16	70	22	179	47	M<0.1 F 6

mrad

10 (11) (14)
12 (14) (17)
L

Exception: Some departmental routines include a full abdomen scout on a 14 x 17 in. (35 x 43 cm), with positioning as for a PA abdomen centered to level of iliac crest or slightly above.

Shielding: Place lead shield over gonadal area, not obscuring area of interest.

Patient Position

- Patient prone, pillow for head, arms up beside head, legs extended with support under ankles.

Part Position

- Align midsagittal plane to long axis of table with right half of abdomen centered to CR and to midline of table for sthenic type patient (see Notes).
- No rotation of pelvis or trunk.

Central Ray

- CR **perpendicular** to film holder.
- For average sthenic patient, CR to **level of L2** (which is about ½ to 1 in. or 1.25 to 2.5 cm above lowest margin of rib cage) **about 2 in.** or 5 cm **to right of midsagittal plane**. (See Notes on body habitus).
- Center film holder to CR.
- Minimum 40 in. (102 cm) SID.

Collimation: Collimate on four sides to film margins.

Respiration: Suspend respiration upon expiration.

Notes: Body habitus variation: Hypersthenic (broad)–Gallbladder more horizontal, 2 inches (5 cm) higher and more lateral.

Asthenic (thin)–Gallbladder vertical, 2 inches (5 cm) lower, near the midline.

Evaluation Criteria

- Entire opacified gallbladder and area of cystic duct is demonstrated.
- No motion of gallbladder or abdominal contents is evident.
- Appropriate technique used with short scale contrast to clearly visualize gallbladder, even through overlying rib if present. Choleliths (gallstones) may be visible as indicated in Fig. 16-28.

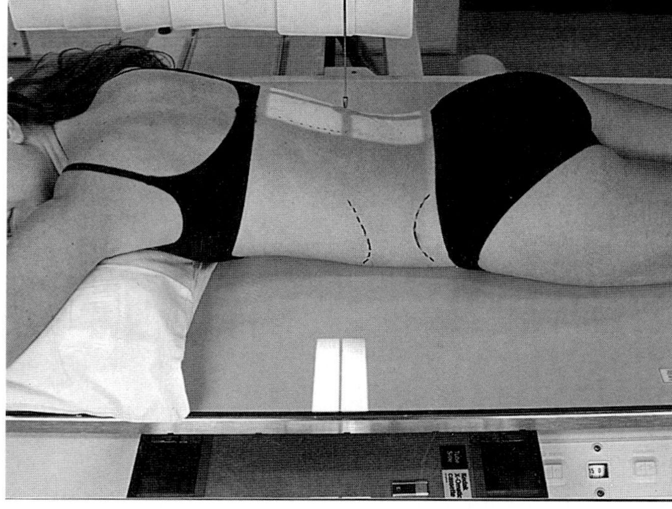

Fig. 16-26. PA scout (sthenic type)–Centered to GB.

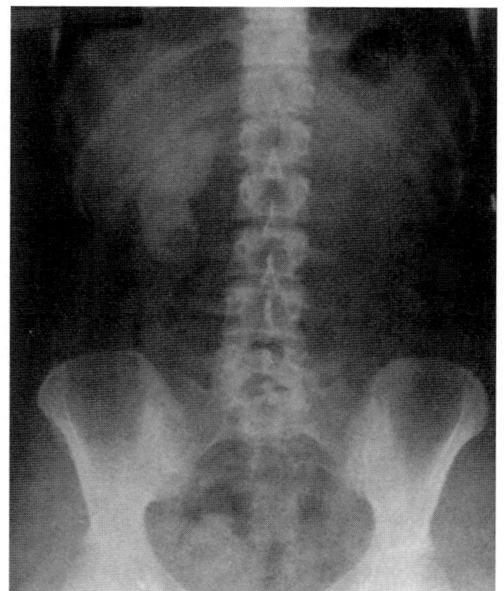

Fig. 16-27. PA scout.

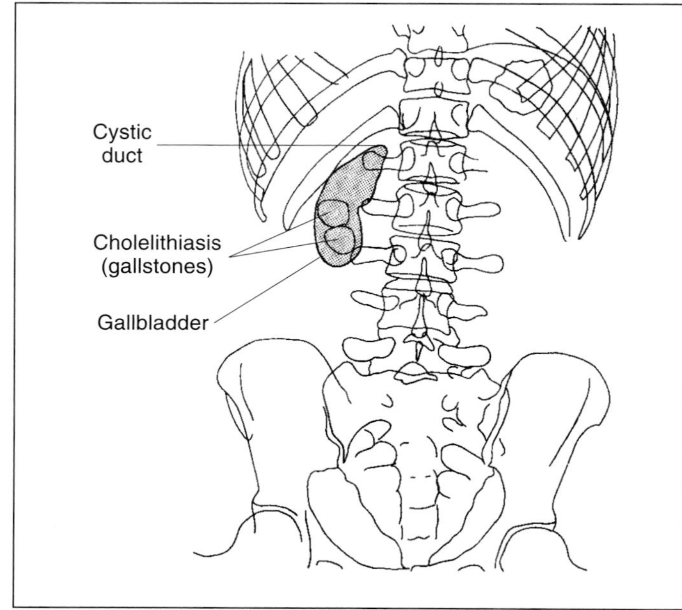

Fig. 16-28. PA scout.

LAO Position

Gallbladder (oral cholecystogram)
Basic
- PA scout
- **LAO**

Special
- Right lat. decub. (PA)
- PA erect

Structures Best Shown:

Opacified gallbladder projected away from vertebral column.

Technical Factors:

- Film size–10 x 12 in. (24 x 30 cm, lengthwise.
  or – 8 x 10 in. (18 x 24 cm), lengthwise.
- Moving or stationary grid.
- 70-76 kVp range.
- Technique and dose:

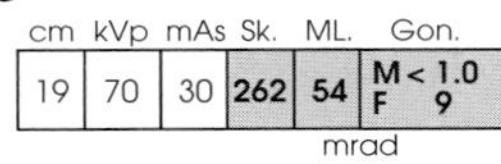

cm	kVp	mAs	Sk.	ML.	Gon.
19	70	30	262	54	M < 1.0 F 9

mrad

10 (8)
12 (10)
L

Shielding: Place lead shield over gonadal area, not obscuring area of interest.

Patient Position

- Patient semiprone, left anterior side down.
- Pillow for head, right arm up, left arm down, right knee partially flexed to maintain this position.

Part Position 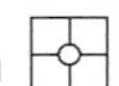

- Rotate patient **15 to 40°** into LAO (less rotation on broad hypersthenic, more rotation on thin asthenic type).
- Align midsagittal plane to long axis of table, approximate right half of abdomen to CR and to midline of table (determine from scout and resultant marking on skin).

Central Ray

- CR **perpendicular** to film holder.
- CR to gallbladder as determined from scout.
- Center film holder to CR.
- Minimum 40 in. (102 cm) SID.

Collimation: Four sided collimation to area of interest. (More collimation borders should be visible on larger film.)

Respiration: Suspend respiration upon expiration.

Note: Accurate centering and collimation should be possible with skin marking from preceding scout film.

An RPO may be performed if patient is not able to lie in a prone or semiprone position.

Evaluation Criteria

- Entire opacified gallbladder and area of cystic duct is included centered to film.
- Gallbladder is seen in profile without self superimposition and is not superimposed upon vertebral column which would indicate insufficient obliquity.
- No evidence of motion.
- Appropriate technique used with short scale contrast to clearly visualize gallbladder.

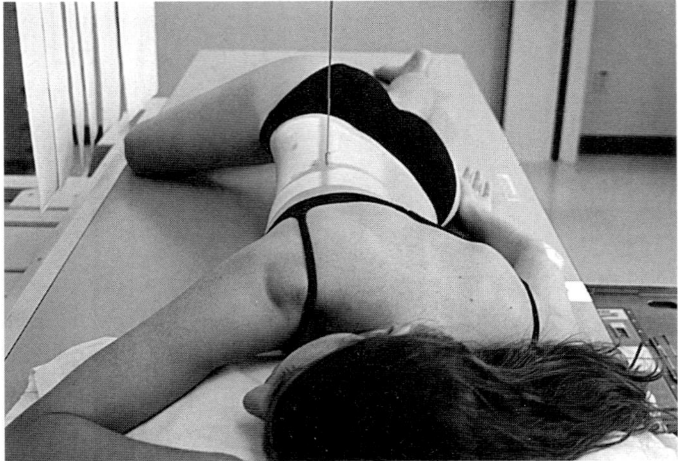

Fig. 16-29. LAO.

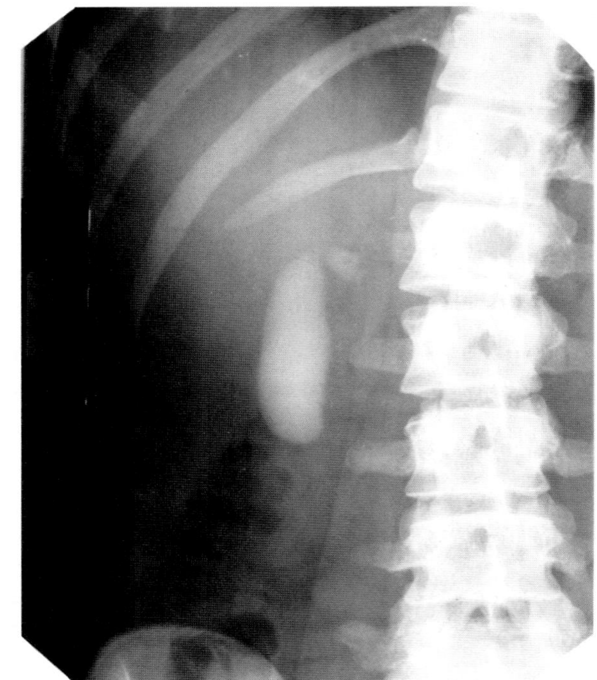

Fig. 16-30. LAO.

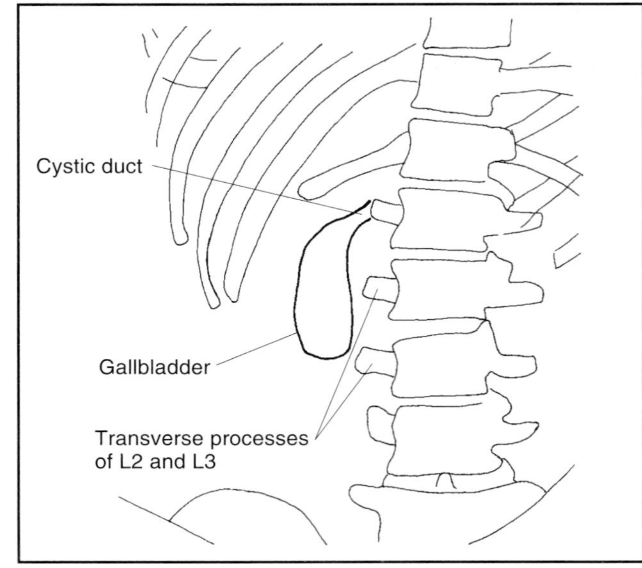

Fig. 16-31. LAO.

Right Lateral Decubitus Position (PA Projection)

Gallbladder (oral cholecystogram)
Basic
- PA scout
- LAO

Special
- **Right lat. decub. (PA)**
- PA erect

Structures Best Shown

Opacified gallbladder projected away from the vertebral column with stratification of possible choleliths (gallstones).
May be performed when the patient cannot stand erect.

Technical Factors

- Film size –10 x 12 in. (24 x 30 cm), lengthwise.
  or – 8 x 10 in. (18 x 24 cm), lengthwise.
- Moving or stationary grid.
- 70-76 kVp range.
- Use decubitus marker.
- Technique and dose:

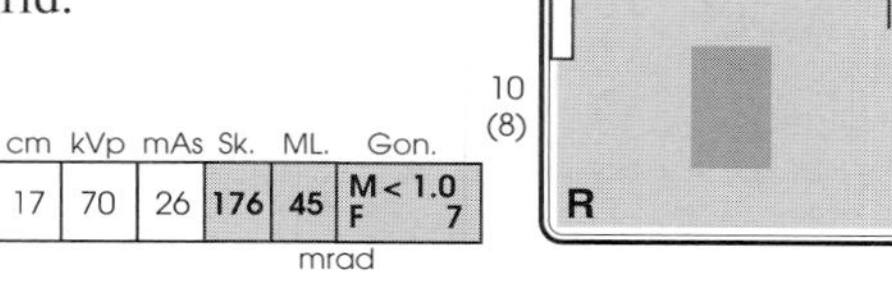

cm	kVp	mAs	Sk.	ML.	Gon.
17	70	26	176	45	M < 1.0 F 7

mrad

Fig. 16-32. Right lateral decubitus (PA).

Shielding: Place lead shield over gonadal area, not obscuring area of interest.

Patient Position

- Patient on radiolucent pads, lying on right side facing the table and/or film holder. (Separate pads for hips and shoulders allows gallbladder to drop more freely away from vertebrae.)
- Pillow for head, arms up above head, knees flexed one on the other.
- Secure cart wheels so patient will not fall.

Part Position

- Adjust cart and/or film holder to center gallbladder (GB) to film and to CR. (GB location determined from scout radiograph.)
- No rotation–Ensure that hips and shoulders are in a true lateral position.

Central Ray

- CR **horizontal**, directed to right half of abdomen to GB, location determined from scout radiograph.
- Center film holder to CR.
- Minimum 40 in. (102 cm) SID.

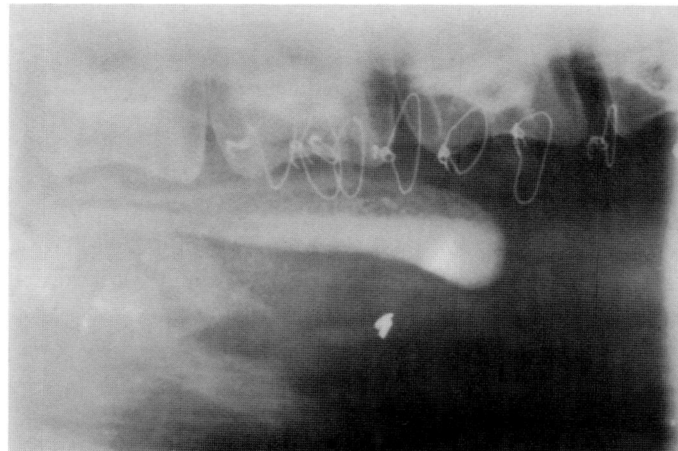

Fig. 16-33. Right lateral decubitus (PA).

Collimation: Four sided collimation to area of interest. (More collimation borders should be visible on larger film.)

Respiration: Suspend respiration upon expiration.

Notes: May be taken as an AP if necessary but a PA projection is preferred due to the more anterior location of GB.

Decubitus position provides for "dropping" of GB away from spine, and for stratification of gallstones wherein the stones heavier than bile layer out or separate from those lighter than bile (Fig. 16-33). These stones may not be visible on other projections.

Evaluation Criteria

- Entire opacified gallbladder and area of cystic duct is included centered to film.
- Gallbladder is seen without motion, located below vertebral column.
- Stratification lines of choleliths should be visible if present.
- Appropriate technique used with short scale contrast to clearly visualize gallbladder without over penetrating and burning out possible choleliths.

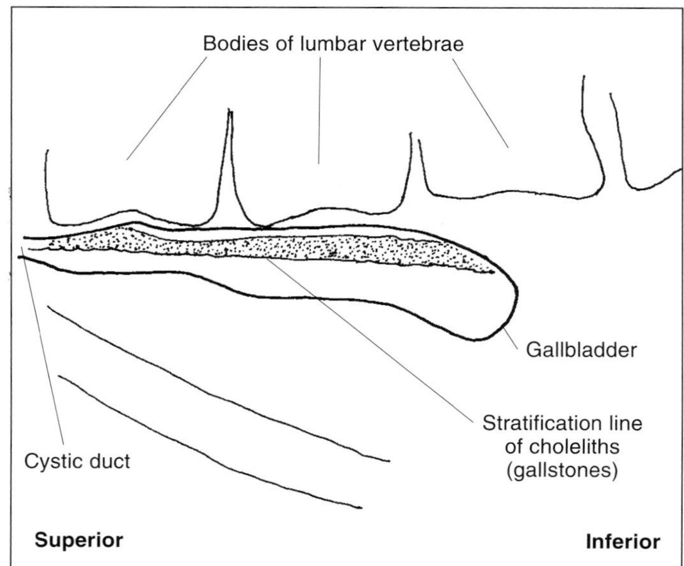

Fig. 16-34. Right lateral decubitus (PA).

PA Projection – Erect Position

Gallbladder (oral cholecystogram)
Basic
- PA scout
- LAO

Special
- Right lat. decub. (PA)
- **PA erect**

Structures Best Shown

Opacified gallbladder with stratification of possible choleliths (gallstones).

Technical Factors

- Film size –10 x 12 in. (24 x 30 cm), lengthwise.
  or – 8 x 10 in. (18 x 24 cm), lengthwise.
- Moving or stationary grid.
- 70-76 kVp range.
- Technique and dose:

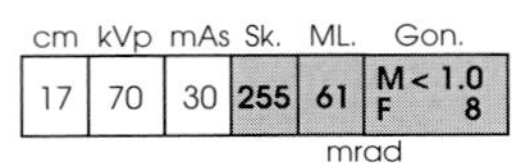

cm	kVp	mAs	Sk.	ML.	Gon.
17	70	30	255	61	M < 1.0 F 8

mrad

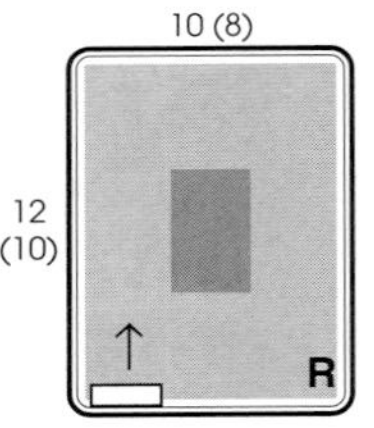

Fig. 16-35. PA erect.

Shielding: Place lead shield over gonadal area, not obscuring area of interest (may use freestanding shield as shown in Fig. 16-35).

Patient Position

- Patient erect, facing the table and/or film holder.
- Arms at side.

Part Position 

- Align a point on abdomen about **2 in.** (5 cm) **to right of midsagittal plane to CR and to midline of erect table**.
- Spread feet and distribute body weight evenly on both legs for stabilization.

Central Ray

- CR **horizontal**, directed to GB, which will be 1 to 2 in. (2.5 to 5 cm) more inferior than on scout radiograph taken recumbent.
- Center film holder to CR.
- Minimum 40 in. (102 cm) SID.

Collimation: Four sided collimation to area of interest. (More collimation borders should be visible on larger film.)

Respiration: Suspend respiration upon expiration.

Note: May be taken as an AP if necessary but the PA projection is preferred because of the more anterior location of GB.

Change centering as needed for extremes of body habitus.

Erect position with horizontal beam provides for stratification of possible gall stones similar to that of decubitus position. (Decubitus may be taken instead of erect if patient cannot stand.)

May be taken as a spot film with fluoroscopy (Fig. 16-37).

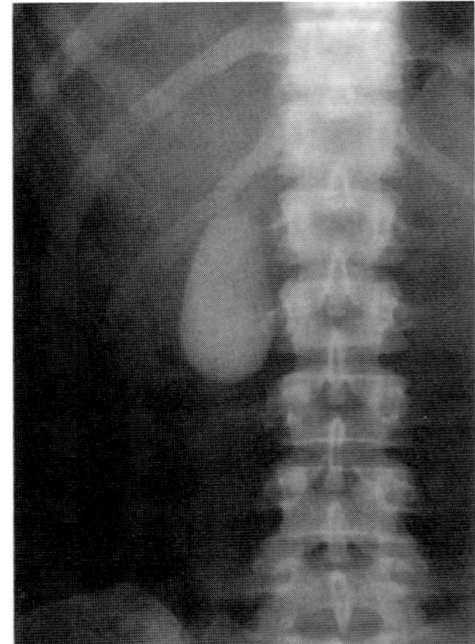

Fig. 16-36. PA erect.

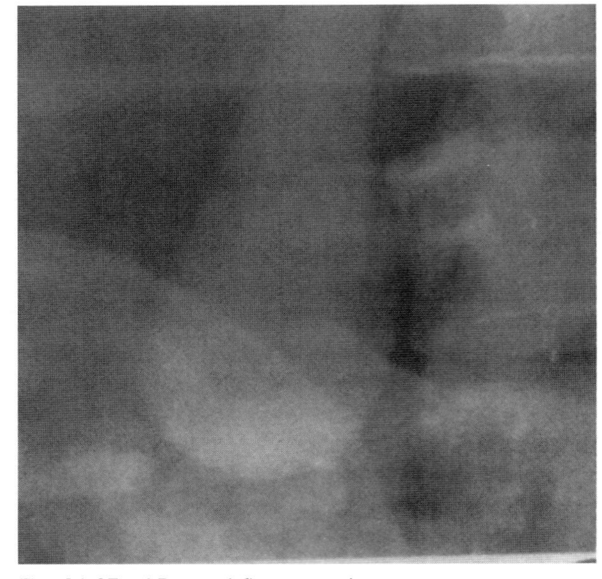

Fig. 16-37. AP erect fluoro spot.

Evaluation Criteria

- Entire opacified gallbladder and area of cystic duct is included centered to film.
- Gallbladder is seen without motion, located 1 to 2 in. (2.5 to 5 cm) more inferior than in recumbent position.
- Stratification lines of choleliths should be visible if present.
- Appropriate technique used with short scale contrast to clearly visualize gallbladder without over penetrating and burning out possible choleliths.

16

AP and/or RPO Projection

Biliary Ducts
(OR cholangiogram)
Basic
• AP and/or RPO

Structures Best Shown

Biliary duct system, drainage into duodenum and any residual gallstones.

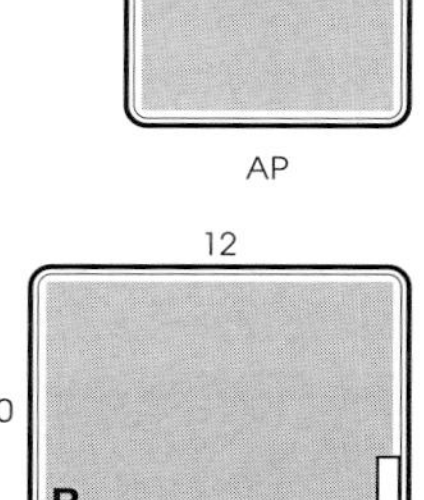

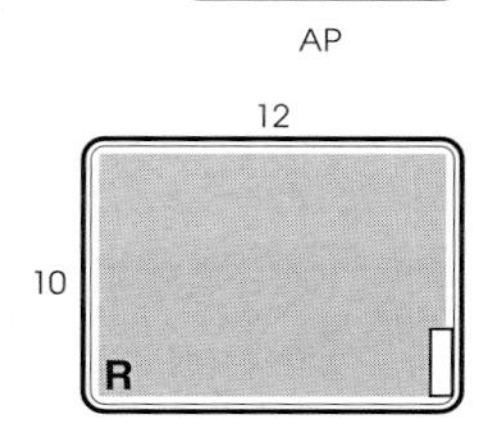

Technical Factors

- Film size–10 x 12 in. (24 x 30 cm), lengthwise (AP).
- Place grid **crosswise for oblique position** to prevent grid cutoff if table is tilted.
- Stationary grid.
- 70-80 kVp range.

Shielding: Due to sterile surgical field, gonadal shielding generally is not used.

Patient and Part Position

- Patient supine on surgery table.
- Table is tilted slightly for each oblique position.
- Communicate with surgical team regarding patient position, film placement and CR location.

Central Ray

- Center midway between right lower rib cage margin and xiphoid tip, or **to where surgeon indicates**.
- Minimum 40 in. (102 cm) SID.

Collimation: Collimate to approximate film borders.

Respiration: Expose after surgeon injects contrast media and anesthesiologist stops patient motion.

Optional RPO: This is not specifically demonstrated but centering is similar to AP projection. Patient is obliqued into a 15 to 25° RPO position by tilting the table to shift the biliary ducts away from the spine. The grid must be placed **crosswise** to prevent grid cutoff. The surgeon will instruct when this oblique should be taken and will have the table and patient tilted as needed for this oblique position.

Note: When possible, take a scout film prior to the beginning of surgery.

Evaluation Criteria

- Entire biliary duct system filled with contrast media is demonstrated.
- No motion evident on radiograph.
- Appropriate technique employed to visualize the biliary duct system.

Fig. 16-38. Scout AP.

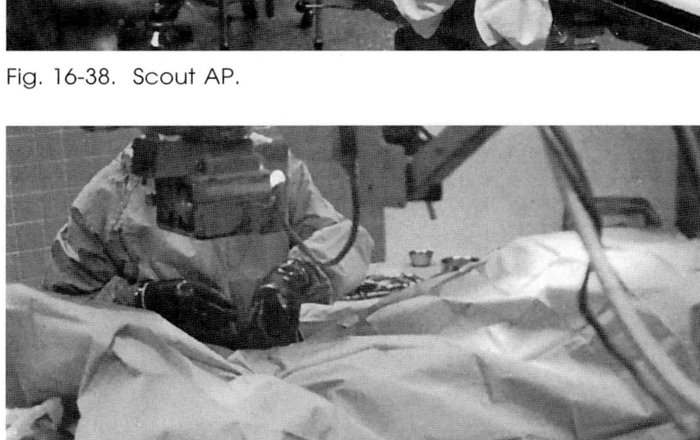

Fig. 16-39. AP (centering point indicated by surgeon).

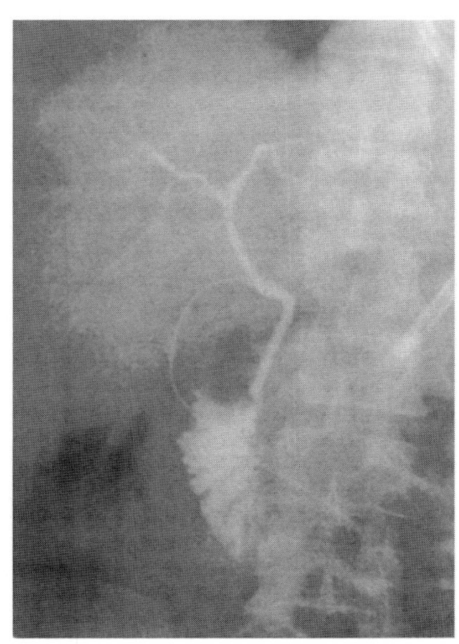

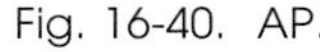

Fig. 16-40. AP.

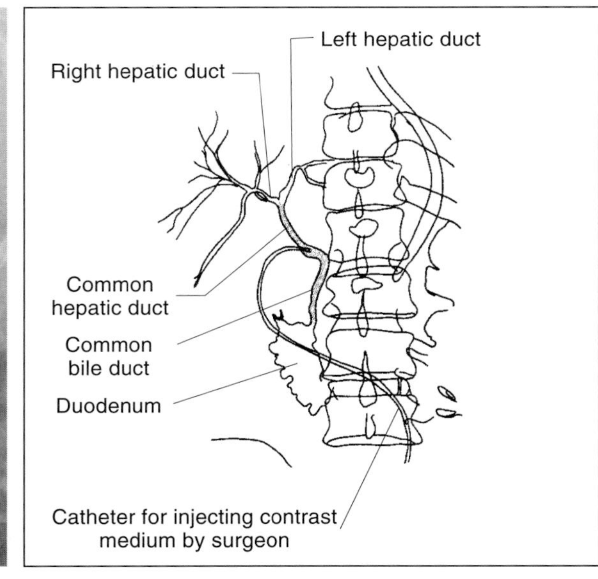

Fig. 16-41. AP.

CHAPTER 17

Urinary System

CONTRIBUTIONS BY:
John P. Lampignano, M Ed, RT (R)
Barry T. Anthony, RT (R)

CONTENTS

Radiographic Anatomy

Urinary system **504**
Kidneys **505**
Urine production **506**
Ureters and urinary bladder **508**
Male and female pelvic organs **509**
Anatomy review with radiographs **510**

Radiographic Procedures

- Urography **511**
- Contrast media **511**
- Reactions to contrast media **512**

Excretory Urography–
Intravenous urogram (IVU):
- Clinical indications and contraindications **514**
- Patient and room preparation **515**
- Ureteric compression **515**

General IVU procedures
- Basic filming routine **516**
- Alternates to routine **517**

Hypertensive IVU **517**
Retrograde urography **518**
Retrograde cystography **518**
Voiding cystourethrography **519**
Retrograde urethrography **519**
Summary of urinary system procedures **519**

Radiographic Positioning

Survey results **520**
Basic and special projections **520**

Intravenous urography:
- AP (scout and series) **521**
- Nephrotomogram **522**
- RPO and LPO **523**
- AP–Post-void **524**
- AP ureteric compression **525**

Retrograde urography:
- AP (scout, pyelogram and ureterogram) **526**

Cystography:
- AP (10 to 15° caudad) **527**
- Obliques **527**
- Lateral **527**

Voiding cystourethrography:
- Male–RPO (30°) **528**
- Female–AP **528**

17

Radiographic Anatomy

URINARY SYSTEM

Radiographic examinations of the urinary system are among the most common contrast medium procedures performed in radiology departments. The urinary system consists of **two kidneys, two ureters** *(u-re′ter* or yoo-ret′er†)*, **one urinary bladder** and **one urethra** *(u-re′thrah* or yoo-re′thra†)*.

Note: Determine which of these two possible pronunciations of these terms are most common in your region.

The two kidneys and the ureters are organs lying in the retroperitoneal space. These two bean-shaped organs lie on either side of the vertebral column in the most posterior part of the abdominal cavity. The right kidney is generally slightly lower or more inferior than the left due to the presence of the liver. Near the upper medial part of each kidney is a **suprarenal** (adrenal) **gland**. These important glands of the endocrine system are located in the fatty capsule surrounding each kidney.

Each kidney connects to the single urinary bladder by its own ureter. Waste material, in the form of urine, travels from the kidneys to the bladder via these two narrow tubes, termed ureters. The saclike urinary bladder serves as a reservoir to store urine until it can be eliminated from the body via the urethra.

The Latin designation for kidney is *ren*, and *renal* is a common adjective referring to kidney.

Kidneys

The various organs of the urinary system and their relationship to the bony skeleton are shown from the back in Fig. 17-2, and from the left side in Fig. 17-3. The posteriorly placed **kidneys** lie on either side of the vertebral column in the upper abdomen. The lower rib cage thus forms a protective enclosure for the kidneys.

Ureters

Most of each **ureter** lies anterior to its respective kidney. The ureters follow the natural curve of the vertebral column. Each ureter initially curves forward following the lumbar lordotic curvature and then curves backward upon entering the pelvis. After passing into the pelvis, each ureter follows the sacrococcygeal curve before entering the posterolateral aspect of the bladder.

Urethra

The **urethra** connects the bladder to the exterior. The urethra exits from the body inferior to the symphysis pubis.

The entire urinary system is either posterior to or below the peritoneum. The **kidneys and ureters are retroperitoneal structures,** while the **bladder and urethra are infraperitoneal structures**.

* Dorland's *Illustrated Medical Dictionary,* 27th Edition.
† *Webster's New World Dictionary,* Third College Edition, 1994.

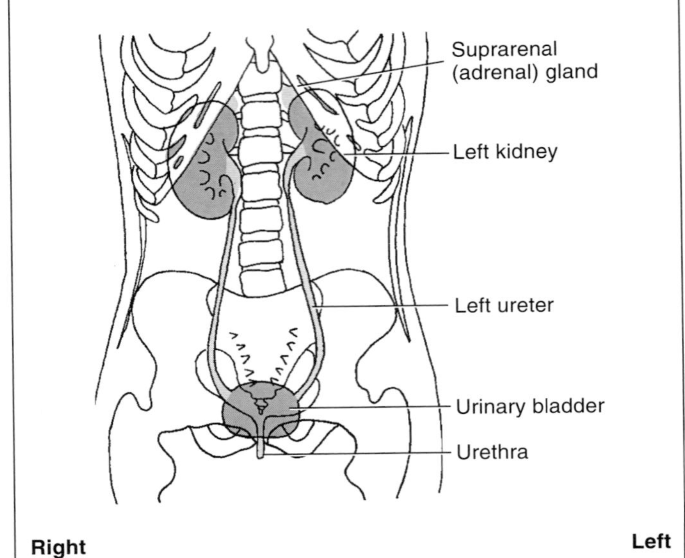

Fig. 17-1. Urinary system–Anterior view.

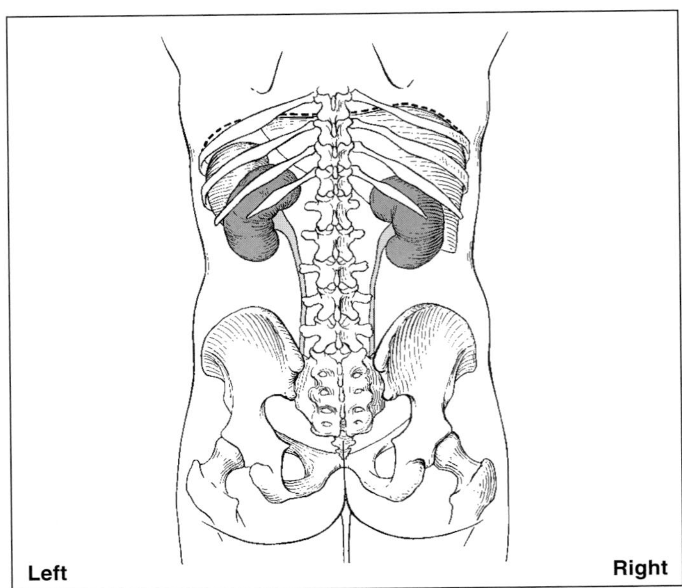

Fig. 17-2. Urinary system–Posterior view.

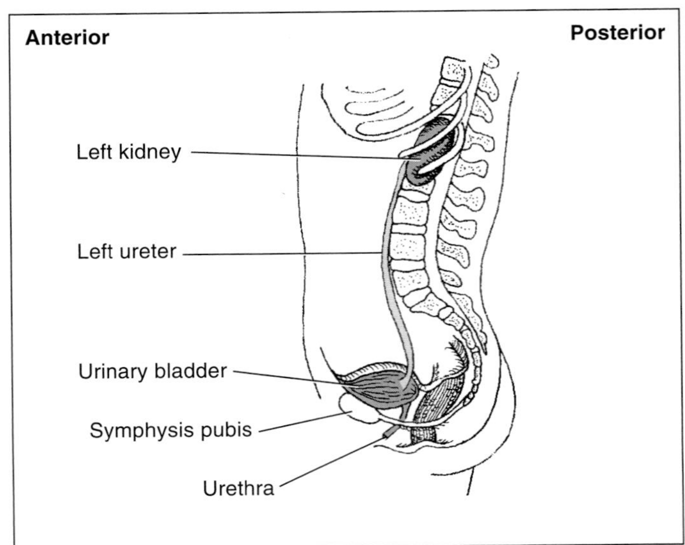

Fig. 17-3. Urinary system–Lateral view.

17

KIDNEYS

The average adult kidney is fairly small, weighing about 150 grams. The measurements are 4 to 5 inches (10 to 12 cm) long, 2 to 3 inches (5 to 7.5 cm) wide and 1 inch (2.5 cm) thick. The left kidney is a little longer but narrower than the right. Despite their small size, at least one functional kidney is absolutely essential for normal well-being. Failure of both kidneys, unless corrected, means inevitable death.

Kidney Orientation

The usual orientation of the kidneys in the supine individual is shown in Fig. 17-4. The large muscles on either side of the vertebral column cause the longitudinal plane of the kidneys to form a vertical angle of about 20° with the midsagittal plane. These large muscles include the two **psoas** *(so′es)* **major muscles**. These muscle masses get larger as they progress inferiorly from the upper lumbar vertebrae. This gradual enlargement causes the 20° angle wherein the upper pole of each kidney is closer to the midline than its lower pole (Fig. 17-4).

These large posterior abdominal muscles also cause the kidneys to rotate backward within the retroperitoneal space. As a result, the medial border of each kidney is more anterior than is the lateral border of each kidney (Fig. 17-5).

The aorta and inferior vena cava are also indicated to show their relationship to the kidneys.

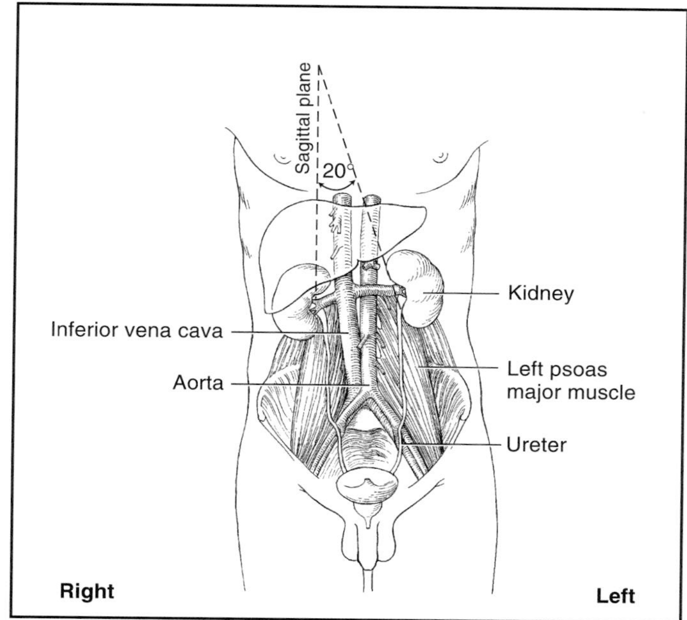

Fig. 17-4. Kidney orientation.

Cross Sectional View

Transverse cross-sectional views through the level of L2 illustrate the usual amount of backward rotation of the kidneys (Figs. 17-5 and 17-6). The normal kidney rotation of about 30° is due to the midline location of the vertebral column and the large muscles on either side.

When posterior oblique projections are utilized during radiographic studies of the urinary system, each kidney, in turn, is placed parallel to the film plane. The body is rotated about **30°** in each direction to place one kidney, and then the other, parallel to the film plane. A 30° LPO will position the right kidney parallel to the film, and a 30° RPO will position the left kidney parallel.

Each kidney is surrounded by a mass of fatty tissue termed the **adipose capsule** or **perirenal fat**. It is the presence of these fatty capsules around the kidneys that permits radiographic visualization of the kidneys on plain abdominal radiographs. There is sufficient density difference between fat and muscle to visualize the outline of each kidney on a technically satisfactory, abdominal radiograph.

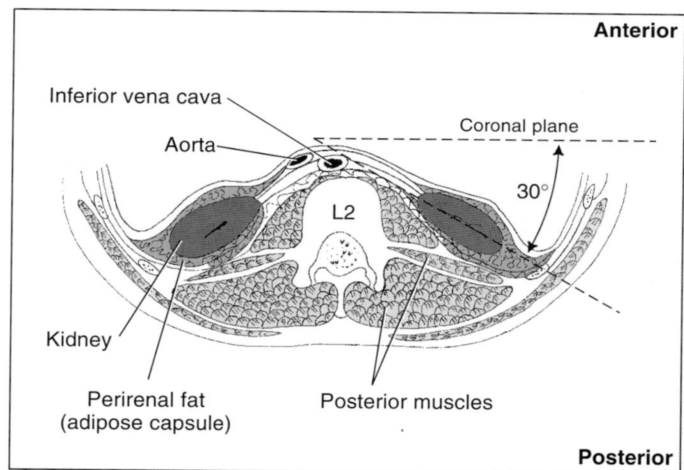

Fig. 17-5. Kidney orientation–Cross-sectional view.

CT Axial Section: Figure 17-6 represents a CT (Computed Tomogram) axial section through the level of the mid kidneys at L2. This demonstrates anatomical relationships of the kidneys to adjoining organs and structures. The anatomy that should be recognizable is as follows:

A. Pancreas
B. Gallbladder
C. Inferior portion of right lobe of the liver
D. Right kidney
E. Posterior abdominal muscles
F. L2 vertebra
G. Renal pelvis of left kidney
H. Abdominal aorta

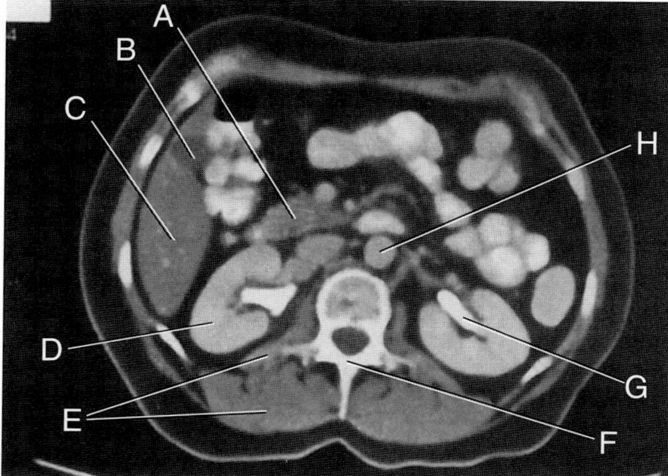

Fig. 17-6. CT axial section, level of L2.

17

Normal Kidney Location

Most abdominal radiographs, including urograms, are performed on expiration with the patient supine. The combined effect of expiration and a supine position allow the kidneys to lie fairly high in the abdominal cavity. Under these conditions, the kidneys normally lie about **halfway between the xiphoid process and the iliac crest**. The left kidney normally lies about 1 cm more superior than does the right one. The top of the left kidney is usually at the level of the **T11-12 interspace**. The bottom of the right kidney is most often level with the upper part of **L3**.

Kidney Movement: Since the kidneys are only loosely attached within their fatty capsule, they tend to move up and down with movements of the diaphragm and with position changes. When one inhales deeply or stands upright, the kidneys normally drop about one lumbar vertebra or 2 inches (5 cm). If the kidneys tend to drop more than this, a condition termed **nephroptosis** *(nef″ rop-to′ sis)* is said to exist. With some very thin and older patients, in particular, the kidneys may drop dramatically and end up within the pelvis, which may create problems from a "kinking" or twisting of the ureters.

Functions of Urinary System

The primary function of the urinary system is the **production of urine and its elimination** from the body. During production of urine, the kidneys:
(1) Remove nitrogenous wastes.
(2) Regulate water levels in the body.
(3) Regulate acid-base balance and electrolyte levels of the blood.
Nitrogenous waste products such as urea and creatinine are formed during the normal metabolism of proteins. Buildup of these nitrogenous wastes in the blood results in the clinical condition termed **uremia**.

Renal Blood Vessels

Large blood vessels are needed to handle the vast quantities of blood flowing through the kidneys daily. At rest about 25% of the blood pumped out of the heart with each beat passes through the kidneys. Arterial blood is received by the kidneys directly from the **abdominal aorta** via the left and right renal arteries. Each **renal artery** branches and rebranches until a vast capillary network is formed in each kidney.

Since most of the blood volume entering the kidneys is returned to the circulatory system, the **renal veins** must also be large vessels. The renal veins connect directly to the large **inferior vena cava** to return the blood to the right side of the heart.

Along the medial border of each kidney is a centrally located, longitudinal fissure termed the **hilum** *(hi′ lum)*. The hilum serves to transmit the renal artery and renal vein, lymphatics, nerves and the ureter.

Each kidney is arbitrarily divided into an upper part and a lower part, called the **upper pole** and the **lower pole**.

URINE PRODUCTION

The average water intake for humans during each 24-hour period is about 2.5 liters. This water comes from ingested liquids and foods, and from the end products of metabolism. These 2.5 liters of water eventually end up in the bloodstream. Vast quantities of blood are filtered every 24 hours. At rest, more than 1 liter of blood flows through the kidneys every minute of the day, which results in about 180 liters of filtrate being removed from the blood every 24 hours. Over 99% of this filtrate volume is reabsorbed by the kidneys and returned to the bloodstream. During the reabsorption process, the blood pH and amounts of various electrolytes such as sodium, potassium and chloride are regulated.

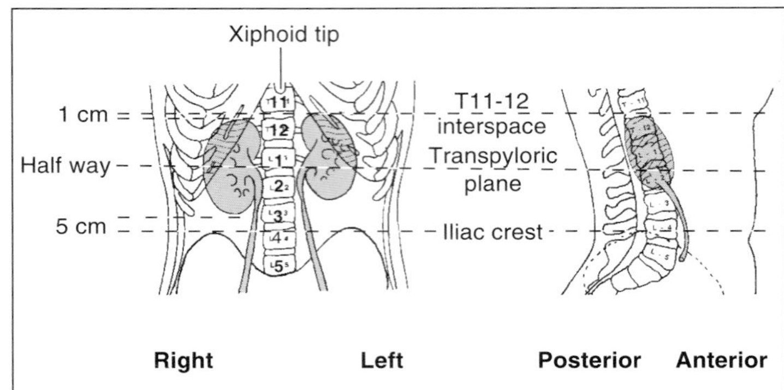

Fig. 17-7. Normal kidney location.

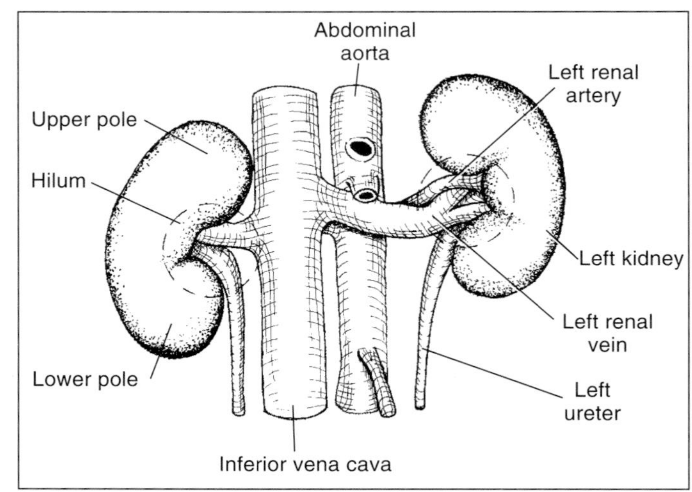

Fig. 17-8. Renal blood vessels.

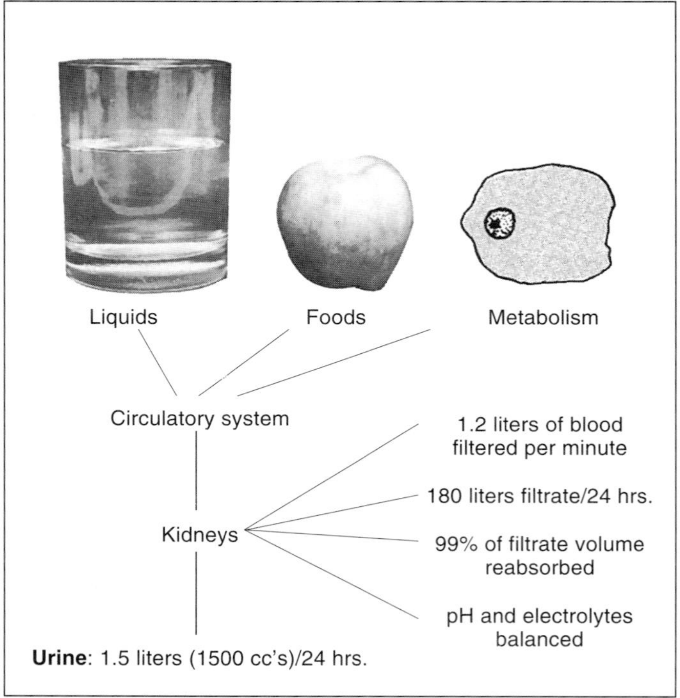

Fig. 17-9. Urine production.

From the large amount of blood flowing through the kidneys daily, about **1.5 liters or 1,500 cc's** of urine are formed. This is an average amount that varies greatly depending on fluid intake, amount of perspiration and other factors.

Macroscopic Structure

The macroscopic internal structure of the kidney is shown in Fig. 17-10. Directly under the **fibrous capsule** surrounding each kidney is the **cortex,** forming the peripheral or outer portion of the kidney substance. Under the cortex is the internal structure termed the **medulla,** which is composed of from 8 to 18 conical masses termed **renal pyramids.** The cortex periodically dips between the pyramids to form the **renal columns**, which extend to the **renal sinus**.

The renal pyramids are primarily a collection of tubules that converge at an opening at the **renal papilla** (apex), and drain into the **minor calyx** *(kal′ lis)*. Calyces appear as hollowed flattened tubes. There are from 4 to 13 minor calyces that unite to form 2 to 3 **major calyces.** The major calyces unite to form the **renal pelvis**, which appears in the shape of a larger flattened funnel. Each expanded renal pelvis narrows to continue as the **ureter.** Thus, urine formed in the microscopic or nephron portion of the kidney finally reaches the ureter by passing through the various collecting tubules, to a minor calyx, to a major calyx and then to the renal pelvis.

The term **renal parenchyma** *(par-eng′ ki-mah)* is a general term used to describe the total functional portions of the kidneys such as those which are visualized during an early phase of an intravenous urogram procedure.

Microscopic Structure

The structural and functional unit of the kidney is the microscopic **nephron.** There are over one million nephrons in each kidney. One such nephron is shown in Fig. 17-11, a greatly magnified but very small cut-away section of the kidney. A more detailed view of a single nephron and its collecting ducts is shown in Fig. 17-12. Small arteries in the kidney **cortex** form tiny capillary tufts, termed **glomeruli** *(glo-mer′ u-li)*. Blood is initially filtered through the many glomeruli.

Afferent arterioles supply blood **to** the glomeruli and **efferent** arterioles take blood away to a secondary capillary network in close relationship to the straight and convoluted tubules. Each glomerulus is surrounded by a **glomerular capsule** (Bowman's capsule), which is the proximal portion of each nephron collecting filtrate. (The glomerulus is also part of the **nephron** which is made up of the glomerulus **and** the long tubules.) The glomerular filtrate travels from the **glomerular capsule** to a **proximal convoluted tubule,** to the **descending** and **ascending limbs** of the **loop of Henle*** *(Hen′ lez)*, to a **distal convoluted tubule,** to a **collecting tubule** and, finally, into a **minor calyx.** The filtrate is termed urine by the time it reaches the minor calyx. Between Bowman's capsule and minor calyces, over 99% of the filtrate is reabsorbed into the kidney's venous system.

Microscopically, the glomeruli, glomerular capsules and the proximal and distal convoluted tubules of the many nephrons are located within the **cortex** of the kidney. The loop of Henle and the collecting tubules are located primarily within the **medulla**. The renal pyramids within the medulla are primarily a collection of tubules.

*Henle, Fredrich Gustav Jakob, a German anatomist 1809-1885.

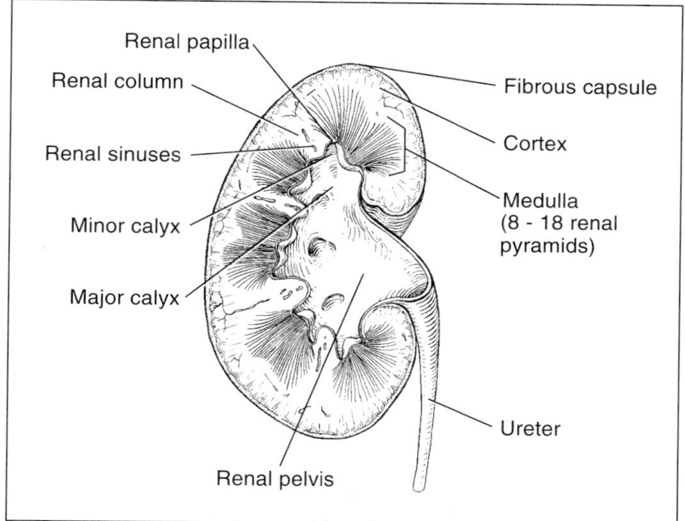

Fig. 17-10. Renal structure.

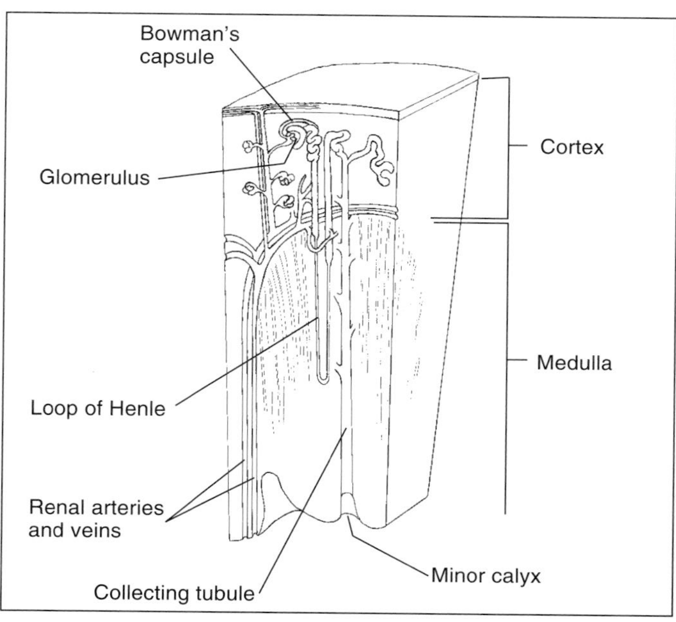

Fig. 17-11. Microscopic structure (nephron).

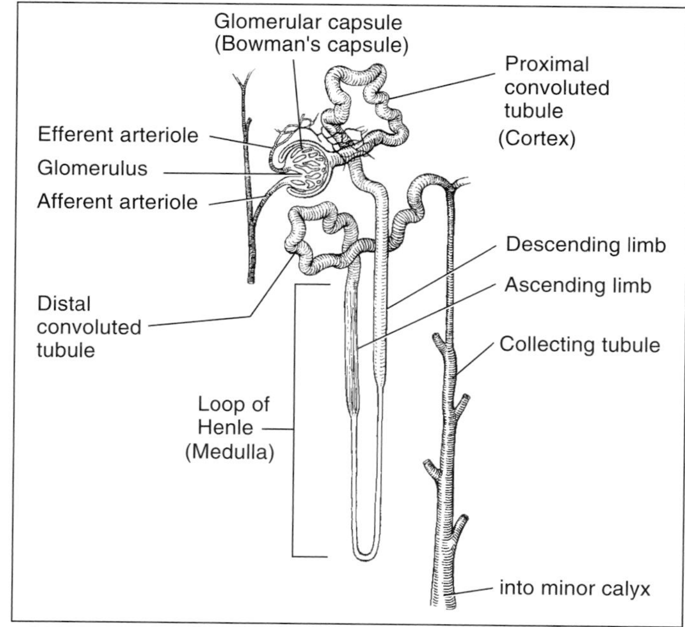

Fig. 17-12. Nephron and collecting duct.

17

URETERS

The **ureters** convey urine from the kidneys to the urinary bladder. Slow peristaltic waves along with gravity force urine down the ureters. The renal pelvis leaves each kidney at the hilum to become the ureter. The ureters vary in length from 28 to 34 centimeters, with the right one being slightly shorter than is the left. As the ureters pass inferiorly, they **lie on the anterior surface of each psoas major muscle**. Continuing to follow the curvature of the vertebral column, the ureters eventually enter the posterolateral portion of each side of the **urinary bladder.**

Prior to any pelvic surgery, the exact course of the ureters can be determined radiographically. The ureters are very narrow tubes and closely resemble surrounding tissue, therefore care must be exercised during surgery to leave the ureters intact. This is especially true during hysterectomies since the ureters are located close to the uterus.

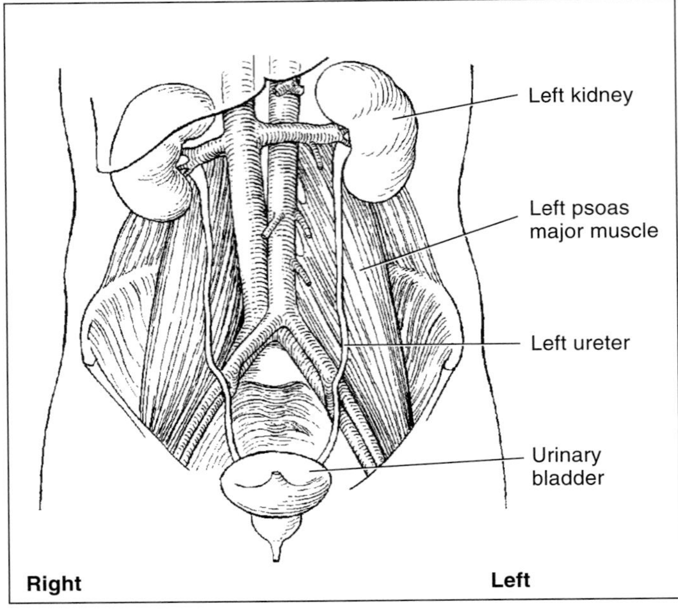

Fig. 17-13. Ureters.

Ureter Size and Points of Constriction

The ureters vary in diameter from one millimeter to almost one centimeter. Normally, there are **three constricted points** along the course of each ureter. Should a kidney stone attempt to pass from kidney to bladder, it would have trouble passing these three spots.

The first point is the **ureteropelvic** *(u-re′ ter-o-pel-vic)* **junction,** the second is near the **brim of the pelvis** where the iliac blood vessels cross over the ureters, and third where the ureter joins the bladder termed the **ureterovesical** *(u-re″ ter-o-ves′ i-kal)* **junction,** or UV junction. Most kidney stones passing down the ureter tend to hang up at the UV junction, and once the stone passes this point it will have little trouble passing through the bladder and urethra to the exterior.

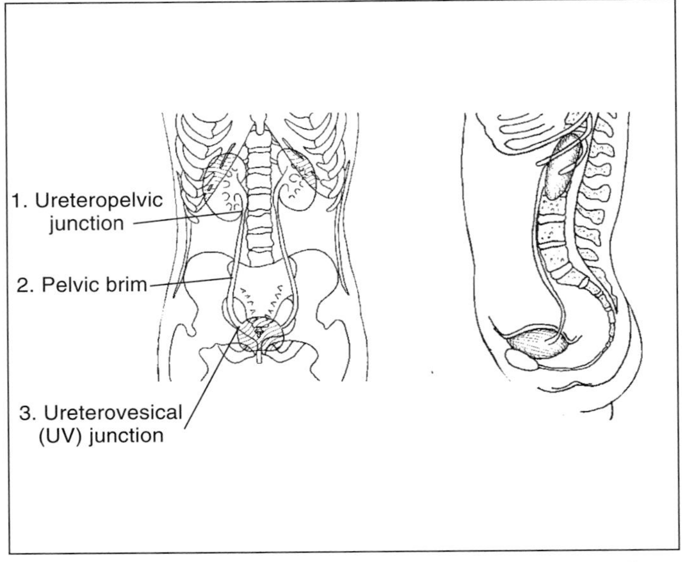

Fig. 17-14. Three possible points of constriction (possible sites for kidney stone lodging).

URINARY BLADDER

The urinary bladder is a musculomembranous sac that serves as a reservoir for urine. The empty bladder is somewhat flattened and only assumes the more oval shape as in this drawing when partially or fully distended.

The triangular portion of the bladder along the inner, posterior surface is termed the **trigone** *(tri′ gon)*. The trigone is the muscular area formed by the entrance of the two **ureters** from behind and the exit site of the **urethra** (Fig. 17-15). The trigone is firmly attached to the floor of the pelvis. As the bladder fills, the top of the bladder expands upward and forward toward the abdominal cavity.

The gland surrounding the proximal urethra is the **prostate gland.** Only males possess a prostate gland, so this drawing represents a male bladder, although the internal structure of the bladder in both sexes is similar.

Ureter
Ureteral opening
Trigone
Urethra
Prostate gland
R
L

Fig. 17-15. Urinary bladder–Anterior cutaway view.

Bladder Functions

The **bladder** functions as a reservoir for urine and, aided by the urethra, it expels urine from the body. There is normally some urine in the bladder at all times, but as the amount reaches 250 milliliters there is a desire to void. The act of voiding is termed **urination** or **micturition**. Normally, urination is under voluntary control and the desire to void may pass if the bladder cannot be emptied right away. The total capacity of the bladder varies from **350 milliliters** to **500 milliliters**. As the bladder becomes fuller and fuller, the desire to void becomes more and more urgent. If the internal bladder pressure rises too high, involuntary urination will occur. Involuntary urination, whether due to excessive pressure or to organic problems, is termed **incontinence**.

Retention is the inability to void, which may be due to an obstruction in the urethra or the lack of the sensation to urinate.

Size and Position of the Bladder: The size, position and functional status of the bladder depends somewhat on surrounding organs and on how full the bladder is. When the rectum contains fecal matter, the bladder is pushed up and forward. A term pregnancy, as shown in Fig. 17-16, exerts tremendous pressure on the bladder.

Note: This drawing is only to show anatomy and the location of the urinary bladder in relationship to the fetus. Remember there are **no** radiographic urinary system exams or procedures done during pregnancy unless in special cases wherein the benefits outweigh the risks as determined by a physician.

Male Pelvic Organs

The male pelvic organs are shown in midsagittal section in Fig. 17-17. When the **urinary bladder** is empty, most of the bladder lies directly posterior to the upper margin of the **symphysis pubis**. As the bladder distends, as it would during a cystogram or radiographic study of the bladder, more and more of the bladder will lie above the level of the symphysis pubis.

The male **urethra** extends from the internal urethral orifice to the external urethral orifice at the end of the penis. The urethra extends through the **prostate gland** and through the length of the penis. The male urethra averages 17.5 to 20 centimeters in length and serves two functions. Not only does the male urethra serve as the distal portion of the urinary tract, helping to eliminate urine stored in the bladder, but it also is the terminal portion of the reproductive system, serving as a passageway for semen.

Female Pelvic Organs

The female pelvic organs are shown in midsagittal section in Fig. 17-18. The **urinary bladder** lies behind or above the upper margin of the **symphysis pubis**, depending on the amount of bladder distension. The female **urethra** is a narrow canal, about 4 centimeters long, extending from the internal urethral orifice to the external urethral orifice. The single function of the female urethra is the passage of urine to the exterior.

There is a close relationship between the **urethra and bladder**, and the **uterus and vagina.** The urethra is imbedded in the anterior wall of the vagina. The spatial relationship of the three external openings becomes important during certain radiographic procedures. The anal opening is most posterior, the urethral opening is most anterior, and the vaginal opening is in between.

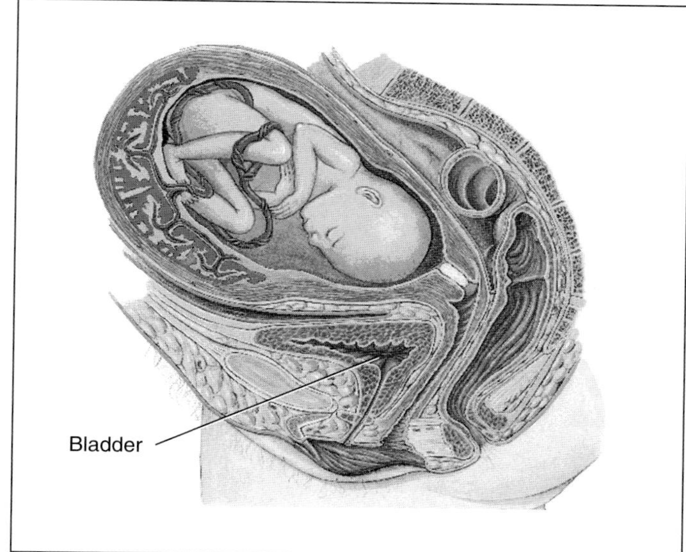

Fig. 17-16. Term pregnancy and relationship to bladder.

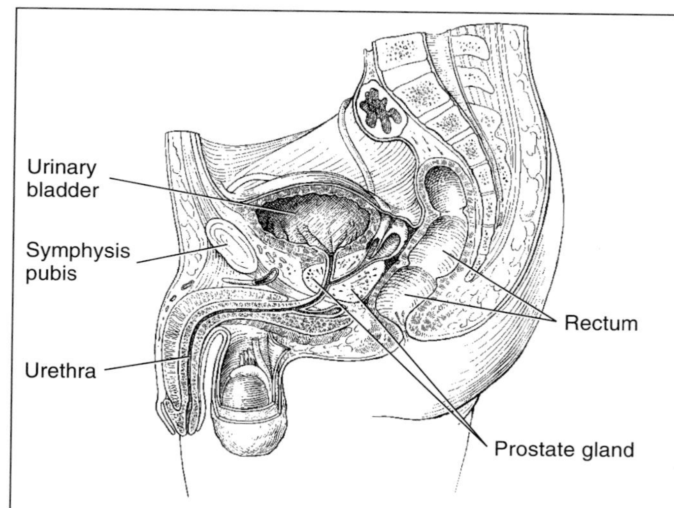

Fig. 17-17. Male pelvic organs.

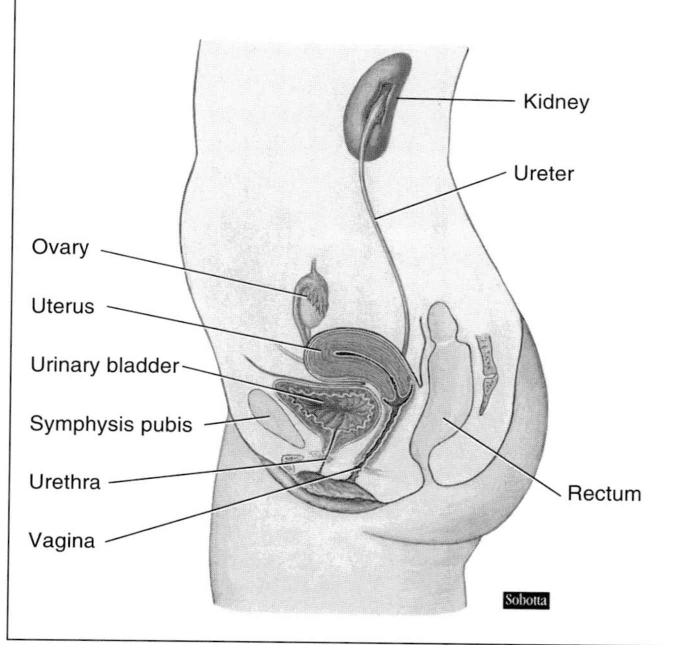

Fig. 17-18. Female pelvic organs

17

ANATOMY REVIEW (RADIOGRAPHS)

Excretory Urogram (Fig. 17-19)

An AP radiograph of an excretory or intravenous urogram (IVU) is demonstrated below with certain anatomy of the urinary system labeled A to H. Contrast media injected intravenously allows these parts of the urinary system to be visualized on a radiograph.

A. Minor calyces
B. Major calyces
C. Renal pelvis
D. Ureteropelvic junction (UPJ)
E. Proximal ureter
F. Distal ureter
G. Ureterovesical junction (UVJ) (Shown only in Fig. 17-19)
H. Urinary bladder (Shown only in Fig. 17-20)

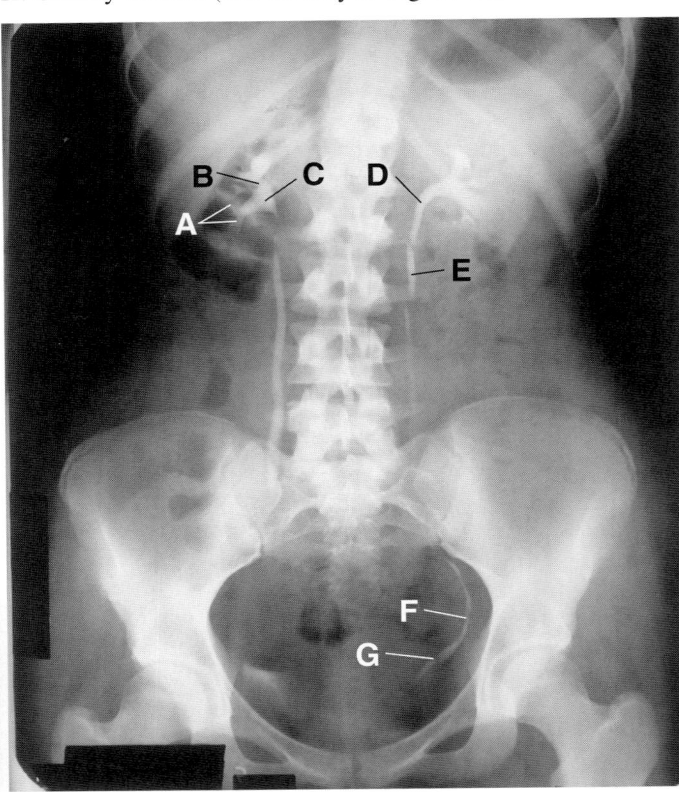

Fig. 17-19. Excretory (intravenous) urogram.

Retrograde Pyelogram (Fig. 17-20)

Anatomy is also labeled on this retrograde pyelogram wherein contrast media is being injected through a catheter inserted up (retrograde) through the urethra, bladder and the ureter to the level of the renal pelvis.

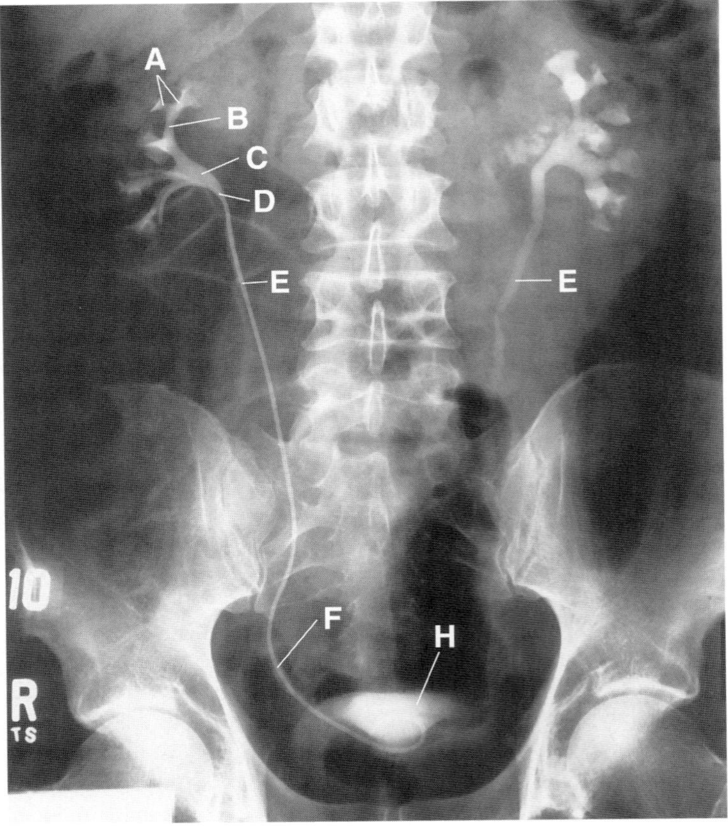

Fig. 17-20. Retrograde pyelogram (catheter in right ureter).

Voiding Cystourethrogram (Fig. 17-21)

Anatomy is labeled on this radiograph of the urinary bladder and urethra taken as the young male patient is voiding the contrast media.

A. Distal ureters
B. Urinary bladder
C. The trigone area of bladder
D. Area of prostate gland
E. Urethra

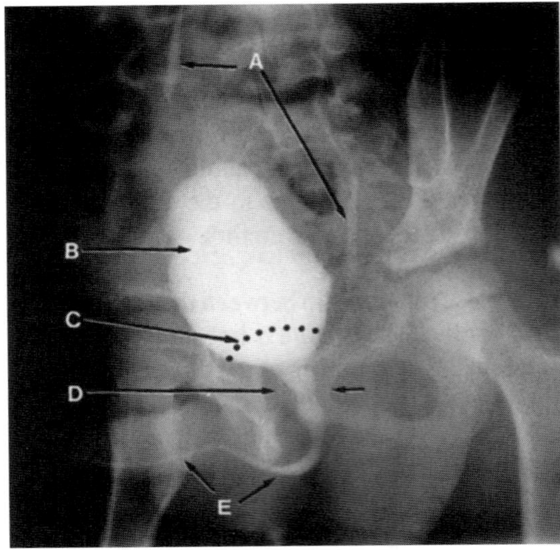

Fig. 17-21. Voiding cystourethrogram–RPO (male).

17

Radiographic Procedures

KIDNEY, URETER AND BLADDER (KUB)

The plain abdominal radiograph or KUB shown in Fig. 17-22 demonstrates very little of the urinary system. The gross outlines of the kidneys are generally faintly demonstrated due to the fatty capsule surrounding the kidneys. In general the urinary system blends in with the other soft tissue structures of the abdominal cavity, thus requiring contrast media to visualize the internal, fluid-filled portion of the urinary system radiographically.

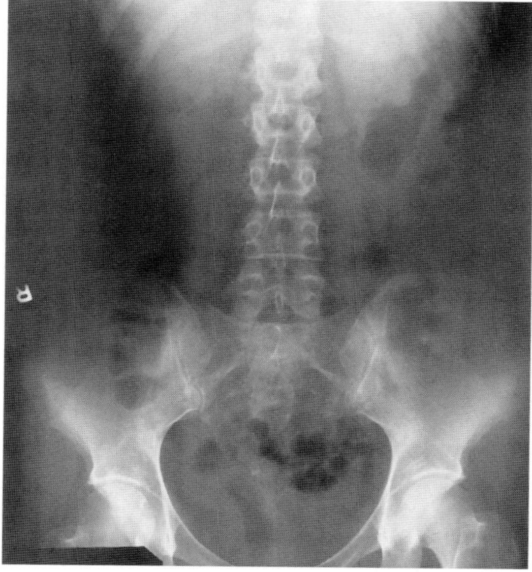

Fig. 17-22. Abdominal radiograph (KUB).

UROGRAPHY

Radiographic examination of the urinary system, in general, is termed **urography** *(u-rog′ rah-fe)*. Uro is a prefix denoting a relationship to urine or to the urinary tract. The contrast media utilized to visualize the urinary tract are introduced into the human system in one of two ways. First, the contrast medium may be introduced into the bloodstream by intravenous injection (Fig.17-19).

The second method requires some form of catheterization so that the contrast medium can be delivered directly into the structure to be studied radiographically (see Fig. 17-20). Radiographic examinations of the urinary system utilizing these two methods of contrast delivery are discussed in the remainder of this chapter.

CONTRAST MEDIA

The two major types of iodinated contrast media used in urology are **ionic** and **nonionic**. The chemical structure of the two types are somewhat different and behave differently in the body as follows:

Ionic Organic Iodides

For many years, patients received a type of organic, iodinated contrast media referred to as **ionic**. This contrast agent contains **iodine** as the **opacifying element**, and other chemical components to create a complex molecule. The parent compound of the molecule is a carboxyl group, in the form of benzoic acid to which other chemical components (side chains) are attached. Ionic, iodinated contrast media contain a positively charged side chain element called the **cation**. The cation is a salt, usually sodium or meglumine, or a combination of both. These salts increase the solubility of the contrast media.

The cation is combined with a negatively charged component called the **anion**. Diatrizoate and iothalamate are common anions, which help stabilize the contrast media compound. The cation and anion are side chains that attach to the parent, benzoic acid ring, along with **three iodine atoms**. These contrast media agents are referred to as tri-iodinated contrast media (Fig. 17-23).

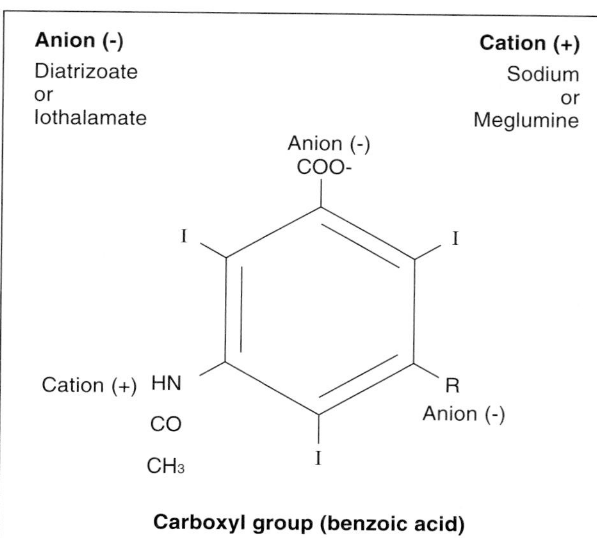

Fig. 17-23. Tri-iodinated contrast media.

Higher Osmolality and Greater Change of Reaction: Once injected, the cation will dissociate from the parent compound or anion, thus creating two separate ions in the blood. This creates a hypertonic condition, or an increase in the blood plasma **osmolality**. This increase in osmolality can cause vein spasm, pain at the injection site, and fluid retention. More importantly, ionic contrast agents may increase the probability that a patient will experience a contrast media reaction. Any disruption to the delicate balance of the bodies' physiological functions may result in a reaction. This is the basis of the Chemotoxic Theory, which states that any disruption to that physiological balance, called **homeostasis**, may lead to reaction. By increasing the number of ions in the plasma, it becomes hypertonic. Hypertonic agents in the blood can disrupt normal body fluid level, which can disrupt homeostasis and create a reaction.

Nonionic Organic Iodide

In the late 1960s, a new generation of contrast media was developed that also contains iodine as needed for opacity, but which contain **no positive charged cations**. The ionizing carboxyl group is replaced with a nondissociated group such as amide or glucose. When dissolved in water, a nonionic compound forms with each molecule containing three iodine atoms. Therefore, when injected into the blood or other body cavities, the contrast media **does not dissociate into two separate ions**, but remains intact. The term, **nonionic**, was coined to describe this type of contrast media based upon its nonionizing characteristic.

Low Osmolality and Less Change of Reaction: Due to their nonionizing nature, these contrast agents are of **low osmolality,** and therefore do not increase the osmolality of the blood plasma. Nonionic contrast media are thus near isotonic and are better tolerated by the body. Research indicates that patients are less likely to have contrast media reactions, or have less severe reactions or side effects when nonionic contrast agents are used. The cost for nonionic contrast media, however, is far greater than ionic. Therefore, while many radiology departments use nonionic contrast media exclusively, others will base their decisions to use nonionic contrast media on patient history and the potential for reactions.

Contrast Media continued

Common Side Effects

Side effects occur in many patients as an expected outcome to the injected iodinated contrast media. They are brief and self-limiting.

Two common side effects following an intravenous injection of iodinated contrast media are a **temporary hot flash** and a **metallic taste in the mouth**. Both the hot flash, particularly in the face, and the metallic taste in the mouth usually pass quickly. Discussion of these possible effects and careful explanation of the examination will help to reduce patient anxiety and help to prepare the patient psychologically.

Patient History: A careful patient history may serve to alert the medical team to a possible reaction. Patients with a history of allergy are more likely to experience adverse reactions to contrast media than those who have no allergies. Questions to ask the patient should include:

1. Are you allergic to anything?
2. Have you ever had hay fever, asthma or hives?
3. Are you allergic to any drugs or medications?
4. Are you allergic to iodine?
5. Are you allergic to seafood or shellfish?
6. Are you allergic to other foods?
7. Have you ever had an x-ray examination that required an injection into an artery or vein?

A positive response to any of these questions will alert the injection team to an increased probability of reaction.

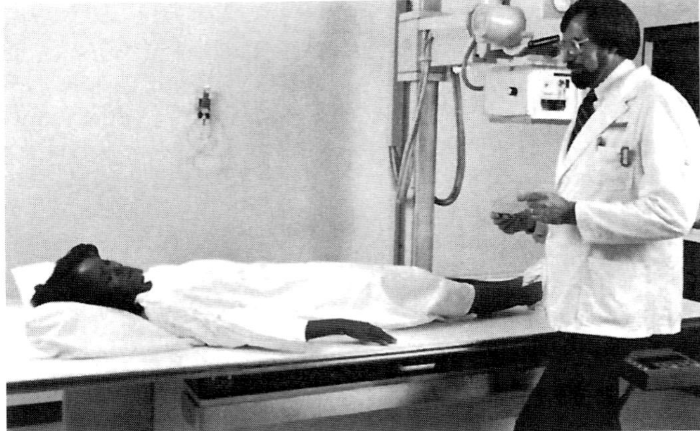

Fig. 17-24. Discussion of history.

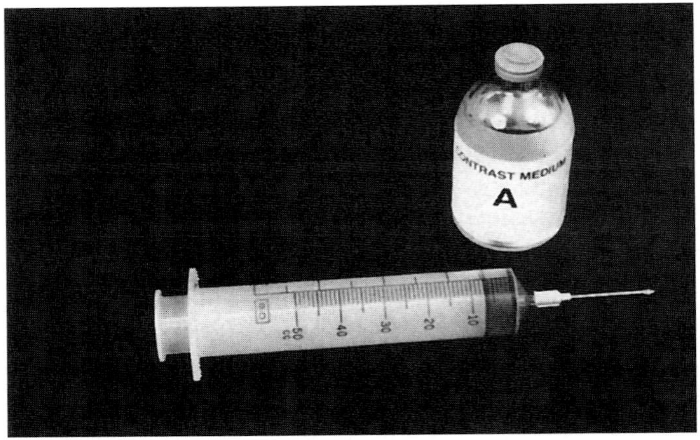

Fig. 17-25. Possible adverse reactions.

Selection and Preparation of Contrast Media

Selection and preparation of the correct contrast medium are important steps prior to injection. Since labels on various media containers are similar, one should **always read the label** three times. In addition, the **empty container should be shown to the radiologist or other person making the actual injection**. Whenever contrast medium is withdrawn into a syringe, be certain to maintain sterility of the medium, the syringe and the needle.

Preparation for Possible Reaction

Since contrast medium reaction is possible and unpredictable, a fully stocked emergency cart must be readily available whenever an intravenous injection is made. In addition to emergency drugs, the cart should contain cardiopulmonary resuscitation equipment, portable oxygen, suction and blood pressure apparatus, and possibly a defibrillator and monitor.

REACTIONS TO CONTRAST MEDIA

Research and past experiences indicate that patients have a greater risk of contrast media reactions if they have a history of one of the following conditions:

1. Hypersensitivity toward iodinated contrast media
2. Diabetes mellitus
3. Asthma or other respiratory conditions
4. Multiple myeloma
5. Severe dehydration
6. Chronic or acute renal or hepatic disease

One theory suggests that patients with fair complexion and red-hair may be more prone to contrast media reaction than other members of our population. While none of the above mentioned conditions indicate that these patients will have a contrast media reaction, they are at greater risk. Nonionic contrast media, as described on the preceding page, may minimize this risk for these patients.

Most reactions to contrast media occur rapidly if they are going to happen, but, on occasion, a delayed reaction may occur. Reactions to contrast media can be classed as **mild, moderate** or **severe.** Mild reactions are usually self-limiting and require no medication for relief of symptoms. A moderate reaction is one that requires treatment for both the symptoms and the comfort of the patient. Any reaction that produces life-threatening symptoms requiring vigorous, active treatment is classed as a severe reaction. Any reaction, however, regardless of how minor it may seem, deserves careful observation. Mild reactions sometimes signal a more serious reaction to follow.

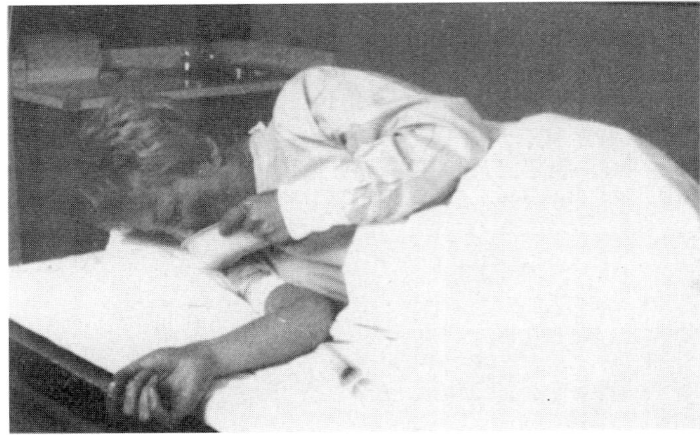

Fig. 17-26. Mild reaction.

The patient should **never be left alone** following an intravenous injection. As the necessary radiographs are produced, observe the patient and question the patient regarding any changes. The radiologist or other responsible physician should remain within immediate reach for 5 minutes following an injection, and within easy reach for one hour thereafter. **The physician must be summoned immediately for any moderate or severe reaction.**

Mild Reactions

The majority of reactions to contrast media are mild, usually requiring no treatment other than support and verbal reassurance. Mild reactions such as **nausea and vomiting** are fairly common. One should not forewarn the patient of their possible occurrence, however. Sometimes the power of suggestion is enough to bring on this type of reaction. Have an emesis basin handy in case of vomiting and a cold towel for the forehead in case of nausea. Take care that the patient does not vomit while supine. Either sit the patient up or turn the patient onto her side, as shown in Fig. 17-26 on preceding page.

Other mild reactions include **hives** or **urticaria** *(ur″ ti-ka′ re-ah)*, **itching** and **sneezing**. These reactions cause some concern because they may signal a more severe response.

Mild reactions may also occur at the injection site, particularly if some of the contrast medium leaks out of the vein into the surrounding tissue. Such leakage is termed **extravasation** *(eks-trav″ ah-sa′ shun)*. Pain, burning or numbness may result when extravasation occurs. A warm towel over the injection site may speed absorption of the contrast material.

Another mild reaction is a response to fear termed the **vasovagal** *(vas″ o-va′ gal)* **response**. Sometimes the sight of a needle or the sensation of a needle stick may trigger a vasovagal reaction. Symptoms include a sensation of weakness or dizziness, sweating and the feeling that precedes fainting. Explanation of the procedure and a confident injection team often deter this type of reaction. The patient's blood pressure should be taken during a vasovagal reaction since a marked drop in pressure indicates a more serious reaction.

Technologist Responsibilities:

1. Monitor and comfort patient
2. Provide warm towel for extravasation
3. Document patient reaction

Moderate Reactions

Moderate reactions require administration of some type of **medication** while the patient is still in radiology. Moderate reactions include **excessive urticaria** (hives), **tachycardia** *(tak″ e-kar′ de-ah)* or rapid heartbeat, **giant hives** and **excessive vomiting.** These symptoms usually respond rapidly and completely to the appropriate medication.

Technologist Responsibilities:

1. Call for medical assistance (nurse, radiologist, etc.)
2. Monitor and comfort patient
3. Document patient reaction

Severe Reactions

Severe reactions are **life-threatening** and require **immediate, intensive treatment**. Very **low blood pressure, cardiac or respiratory arrest**, **loss of consciousness, convulsions, laryngeal edema, cyanosis, difficulty in breathing** and **profound shock** are examples of severe reactions. Delayed or inappropriate treatment for any of these symptoms or conditions could result in the patient's death. If a moderate or severe reaction is suspected, get help and summon the physician immediately.

Technologist Responsibilities:

1. Call for immediate medical assistance.
2. Remove any physical obstacles (tube, monitors, etc.) that may impede the medical staff.
3. Assist medical staff in treating patient.

Mild Reactions

Reaction examples

- –Nausea and vomiting
- –Hives (urticaria)
- –Itching
- –Sneezing
- –Extravasation: burning or numbness at injection site
- –Vasovagal response (fear): weakness, dizziness, sweating, feeling of passing out

Moderate Reactions

Require medication

Reaction examples

- –Excessive urticaria (hives)
- –Tachycardia (rapid heartbeat)
- –Giant hives
- –Excessive vomiting

Severe Reactions

Life threatening–Require IMMEDIATE treatment!

Reaction examples

- –Very low blood pressure
- –Cardiac or respiratory arrest
- –Loss of consciousness
- –Convulsions
- –Laryngeal edema
- –Cyanosis
- –Difficulty in breathing
- –Profound shock

EXCRETORY UROGRAPHY–INTRAVENOUS UROGRAM (IVU)

The excretory or intravenous urogram (IVU) is the most common radiographic examination of the urinary system. This examination has often been referred to as an IVP or intravenous pyelogram. *Pyelo*, however, refers only to the renal pelves. Since the excretory urogram normally visualizes more anatomy than just the renal pelvis, the term IVP should not be used. The excretory (intravenous) urogram or the IVU exam as it will be commonly referred to in this text, visualizes the **minor** and **major calyces**, **renal pelves**, **ureters** and **urinary bladder** following an intravenous injection of contrast medium.

The IVU is a true functional test since the contrast medium molecules are rapidly removed from the bloodstream and are excreted completely by the normal kidney.

Purpose

The twofold purpose of an excretory urogram (IVU) is:

1. To visualize the collecting portion of the urinary system.
2. To assess the functional ability of the kidneys.

Clinical Indications

The IVU is one of the most common contrast media examinations performed in the radiology department. The major clinical indications for the IVU include:

1. Abdominal or pelvic mass.
2. Renal or ureteral calculi (kidney stones).
3. Kidney trauma.
4. Flank pain.
5. Hematuria or blood in the urine.
6. Hypertension.
7. Renal failure.
8. Urinary tract infections (UTIs).

The above includes certain conditions such as (2) **renal** or **ureteral calculi,** which is a very common indication for the IVU. Renal calculi (kidney stones) are insoluble stones formed from crystals of salts found in the urine. These result from conditions such as an excessive intake of mineral salts combined with an insufficient intake of water, an abnormal alkaline or acid urine and over activity of the parathyroid glands. They generally form in the pelvis of the kidney where they cause severe pain as they attempt to pass into or through the ureter where they may become lodged. This is a very painful condition that may require surgery or other invasive procedures to remove the obstruction.

(6) **Hypertension** or, more specifically, renal hypertension will often require an alteration of the normal IVU routine. The filming sequence for the study will allow for shorter spans of time between films. This procedure will be explained more completely in a later section.

(8) **Urinary tract infection** or **UTI** may be a chronic or acute condition. Bacteria entering the normally sterile urinary system may be difficult to control and eliminate. The most common bacteria is **Escherichia coli** or **E. coli**. The bacteria enters in a retrograde fashion through the bladder and may involve the ureters and kidneys. **Pyelonephritis** is inflammation of the collecting system due to bacterial invasion. During the intravenous urogram, the calyces become enlarged and asymmetrical with chronic pyelonephritis.

An IVU prior to pelvic surgery will confirm the location of the urinary system structures and their function.

Contraindications

Even though present-day contrast media are considered to be relatively safe, the technologist must take extra care in obtaining the patient history. Through the patient history, the technologist may become aware of certain conditions that will prevent the patient from having an IVU. The major contraindications include:

1. Hypersensitivity to iodinated contrast media.
2. Anuria *(ah-nu′ re-ah)* or absence of urine excretion.
3. Multiple myeloma.
4. Diabetes, especially mellitus.
5. Severe hepatic or renal disease.
6. Congestive heart failure.
7. Pheochromocytoma *(fe-o-kro″ mo-si-to′ mah)*.
8. Sickle cell anemia.

This list includes certain conditions such as (3) **multiple myeloma** and (7) **pheochromocytoma**. Multiple myeloma is a malignant condition of the plasma cells of the bone marrow; and a pheochromocytoma is a rare tumor of the kidney. Research indicates that these patients are at greater risk during the IVU. Since (8) **sickle cell anemia** can compromise the function of the kidney, these patients are also at a higher risk.

It is important to interview the patient completely prior to the procedure. Some departments require the technologist to review the inpatient chart and note BUN and creatinine levels. Both are indications of renal function.

A patient with one of the above contraindications may need to be examined using some other imaging modality. Certain high-risk patients may still have the IVU after a series of premedication or therapy have been given.

Patients with a suspected sensitivity toward the contrast medium may receive steroids, benadryl, or diuretics prior to the procedure. While many departments stress dehydration prior to the procedure, it is reported that a hydration therapy of a saline IV drip and diuretic prior to the procedure may reduce the risk for patients with multiple myeloma, diabetes mellitus, and other conditions.

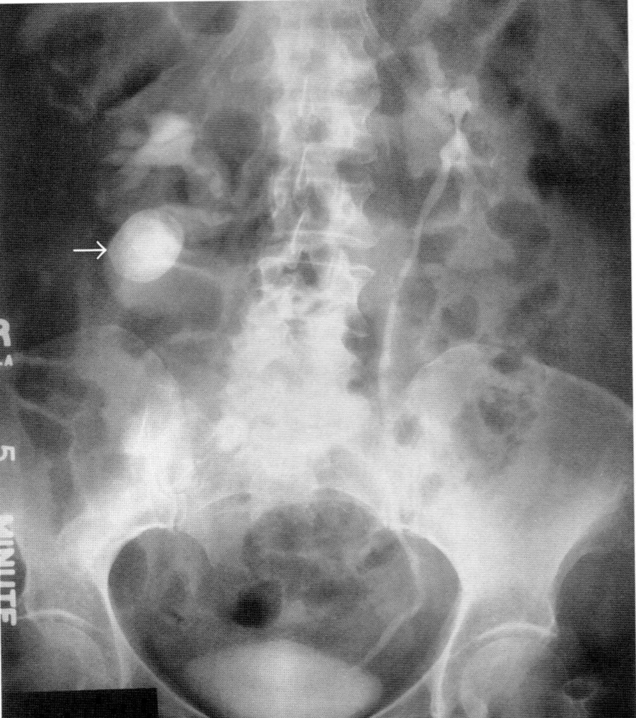

Fig. 17-27. AP IVU–Demonstrates unusually large calculus (stone) in right ureter.
(Courtesy of Gateway Community College)

Patient Preparation

Patient preparation for both the IVU and barium enema is similar. The intestinal tract should be free of gas and fecal material for both examinations. If both examinations are to be performed on the same patient, they can be done on the same day. The IVU is done first with the BE to follow.

The general patient preparation for the IVU includes:
1. Light evening meal prior to the procedure.
2. Bowel-cleansing cathartic.
3. NPO after midnight (a minimum of 8 hours).
4. Enema morning of the examination.

Many patient preparation routines exist among departments. Certain pediatric and emergency-situation adult patients may receive no bowel preparation. Become familiar with your department's protocol.

Prior to the excretory urogram, all clothing except shoes and socks should be removed and replaced with a short-sleeved hospital gown. The opening and ties should be in the back. Always make certain that the patient scheduled for this examination or any other radiographic procedure is the correct patient. Double check the inpatient identification band and verify the outpatient with appropriate questions. The patient should void just prior to the examination for two reasons:
1. A bladder that is too full could rupture, especially if compression is applied early in the exam.
2. Urine already present in the bladder dilutes the contrast medium accumulating there.

Pregnancy Precautions

If the patient is a female, then a menstrual history must be obtained. Irradiation of an early pregnancy is one of the most hazardous situations in diagnostic radiography.

X-ray examinations such as the IVU, which include the pelvis and uterus in the primary beam, should be done on pregnant females **only** when absolutely necessary and where the benefits exceed the risk.

Any x-ray examination of the abdomen of a potentially pregnant female should be governed by the "10-day rule." Any female of childbearing age should have such radiographic procedures **only** during the 10-day period after the start of menstruation. This is the only time when pregnancy can be ruled out with any certainty. Abdominal radiographs of a known pregnancy should be delayed at least until the third trimester, if done at all.

Radiographic Room Preparation

Equipment needed for urography, in addition to a suitable radiographic room, are:
1. Correct type and amount of contrast medium drawn up in an appropriate syringe.
2. The empty container of contrast medium to show the physician or assistant doing the injection.
3. A selection of sterile needles to include a 19-gauge butterfly needle and tubing.
4. Alcohol sponges or wipes.
5. Tourniquet.
6. Towel or sponge to support the elbow.
7. Male gonadal shield.
8. Emesis basin.
9. Lead numbers, minute marker, and R and L markers.
10. Emergency cart handy.
11. Epinephrine or benadryl ready for emergency injection.

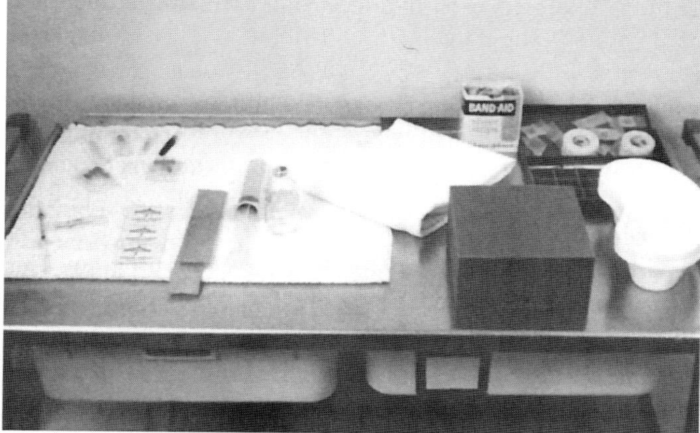

Fig. 17-28. Excretory urography equipment.

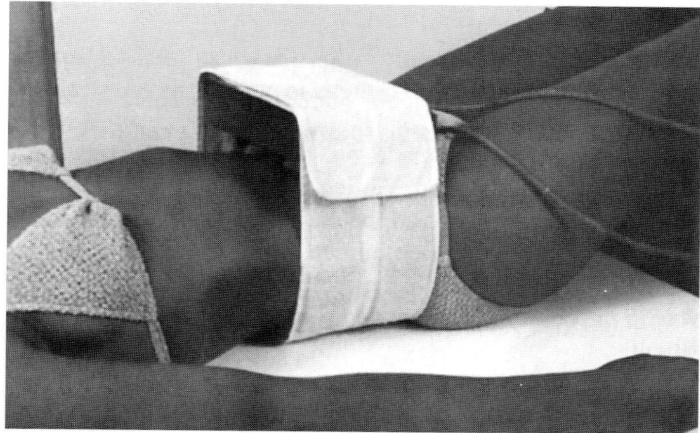
Fig. 17-29. Ureteric compression.

12. Ureteric compression device (if used by department).
13. A cold towel for the forehead or a warm towel for the injection site, if necessary.

These items should be assembled and ready before the patient is escorted to the radiographic room. Be certain that the room is clean and tidy for each patient, and make sure that the patient has voided prior to placing the patient on the radiographic table.

Ureteric Compression

A method utilized to enhance filling of the pelvicalyceal system and proximal ureters is ureteric compression. Furthermore, ureteric compression allows the renal collecting system to retain the contrast medium longer for a more complete study. One such compression device is shown on the model in Fig. 17-29. It is a Velcro band that wraps around two inflatable pneumatic paddles. These paddles are held in place by a piece of plexiglass and sponge.

Prior to injection of the contrast medium, the device is placed on the patient with the paddles deflated. It is vital that the paddles are placed at the pelvic brim to allow for compression of the ureters. Without proper placement of the paddles, the contrast medium will be excreted at its normal rate.

Once the contrast media is introduced, the paddles are inflated and will remain in place until the radiologist orders the release of compression.

Contraindications to Ureteric Compression

Certain conditions exist that will contraindicate the use of ureteric compression. These include:

1. **Possible ureteric stones.** It may be difficult to distinguish between the effects of compression versus the appearance due to a stone.
2. **Abdominal mass.** A mass may also present the same radiographic appearance as ureteric compression.
3. **Abdominal aortic aneurysm.** The compression device may lead to leakage or rupture of the aneurysm.
4. **Recent abdominal surgery.**
5. **Severe abdominal pain.**
6. **Acute abdominal trauma.**

Alternate Trendelenburg: The Trendelenburg position (wherein the head end of the table is lowered about 15°) will provide some of the same results as the compression procedure without as much risk to the patient with those symptoms that contraindicate ureteric compression.

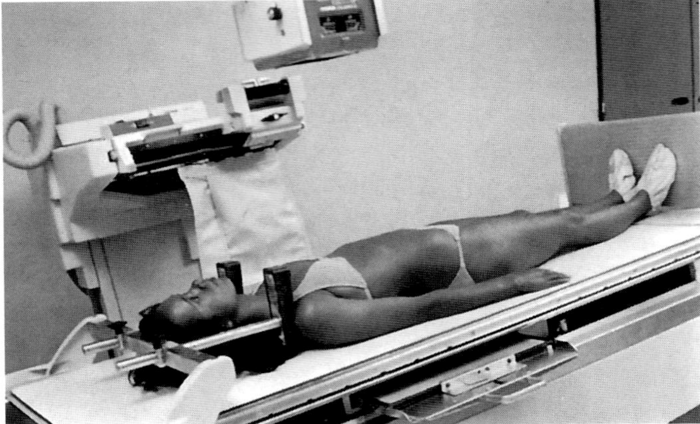

Fig. 17-30. IVU–Trendelenburg position.

GENERAL IVU PROCEDURE

Department routine will vary for the intravenous urogram. This section will introduce a generic procedure for the IVU. The department supervisor should be consulted for specific differences from the following description.

Scout Film and Injection

The patient's clinical history and other pertinent information is discussed with the radiologist prior to injection. The radiographs should be checked for technique, location of the kidneys and signs of motion. These scout radiographs should be shown to the radiologist prior to injection. If the patient has a catheter in place, it should be clamped prior to injection.

When the injection is made, one should note the exact starting time and the length of injection. Timing for the entire series is based on the start of the injection, not on the end of it. The injection usually takes between 30 seconds to one minute to complete. As the examination proceeds, carefully observe the patient regarding any physical changes. Note in the chart the amount and type of contrast medium given to the patient.

After the full injection of contrast medium, radiographs are taken at specific time intervals. Each film must be marked with a lead number indicating the time interval when the radiograph was taken.

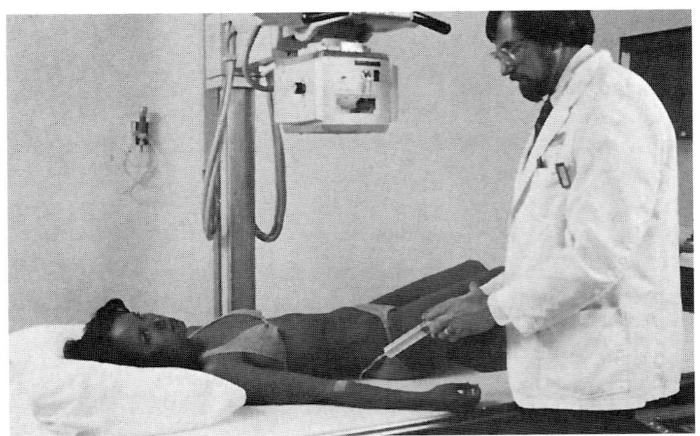

Fig. 17-31. IVU injection.

Basic Filming Routine

A common basic routine for an IVU is as follows:

1. **Nephrogram** or **nephrotomogram**: Taken immediately after completion of injection (or 1 minute after start of injection) to capture the early stages of the contrast medium entering the collecting system. (Additional description on following page.)
2. **Five-minute**: A full KUB to include the entire urinary system. The supine position (AP) is the preferred position.
3. **Fifteen-minute:** A full KUB to include the entire urinary system. Once again, the supine position (AP) is most commonly requested.
4. **Twenty-minute obliques**: The LPO and RPO positioning will provide a different perspective of the kidneys and remove the ureters from the spine.
5. **Post-void**: The post-void radiograph is taken after the patient has voided. The positions of choice may be a prone (PA), or an erect AP. Ensure that the bladder is included on this final radiograph.

IVU Basic Routine
1. **Clinical history taken**
2. **Scout radiograph taken**
3. **Injection of contrast media** (Note starting time of injection and type and amount of contrast media injected.)
4. **Basic filming routine** –1-minute Nephrogram or Nephrotomogram –5-minute AP supine –15-minute AP supine –20-minute posterior obliques –Post-void (prone or erect)

17

Alternates to Routine

Many variations or alternates to the basic routine exist and the radiologist may order specific positions at any time during the study. Some common variations include:

1. Post-release or "Spill" Procedure with Ureteric Compression: A full-size radiograph is taken after the release of compression. Explain to the patient what will be done, then release the air pressure as illustrated in Fig. 17-32. The spill radiograph or any other delayed imaging is usually done in the supine position.

To assess for asymmetric renal function, compression may be applied immediately after the 5-minute film is exposed (unless contraindicated), then removed immediately prior to the 15-minute film.

2. Erect Bladder Projection: If the patient has history of prolapse of the bladder or enlarged prostate gland, the erect bladder position taken before voiding may confirm these conditions.

3. Delayed Radiographs: Often with urinary calculi, the filling of the involved ureter is slow. The patient may be brought back to the department on a one or two hour basis. Ensure that the radiology staff is aware of when the next radiograph is due before leaving the department for the day.

After the completion of the usual IVU series, a post-void radiograph is often obtained in either the prone or upright position. By emptying the bladder, small abnormalities of the bladder may be detected. The upright position, will demonstrate any unusual movement of the kidneys.

Present all radiographs to the radiologist before releasing the patient from the department.

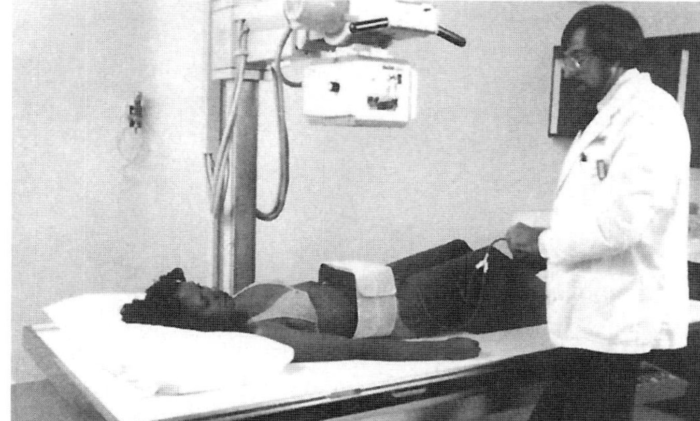

Fig. 17-32. Post-release or "spill" procedure.

Nephrogram or Nephrotomogram

Radiographs taken very early in the series are termed **nephrograms** *(nef′ ro-grams)*. The renal parenchyma or functional portion of the kidney consists of many thousands of nephrons. Since individual nephrons are microscopic, the nephron phase is a blush of the entire kidney substance. This blush results from contrast medium throughout the many nephrons, but not into the collecting tubules as yet. The usual nephrogram is obtained with a radiograph at 1 minute after the start of injection. Ureteric compression, if used, tends to prolong the nephron phase to as long as five minutes in the normal kidney.

With a **nephrotomogram**, (Fig. 17-33), three separate focal levels are commonly taken during this phase of the study.

Since the primary interest in nephrography is the two kidneys, centering and film size should be confined to the kidneys. Center halfway between the iliac crest and the xiphoid process unless a better centering point is determined after viewing the scout radiograph.

Timing is critical on this radiograph so be certain that the exposure is made exactly 60 seconds after the start of the injection. The table, film and control panel must be in readiness even before the injection is begun since the injection will sometimes take nearly 60 seconds to complete.

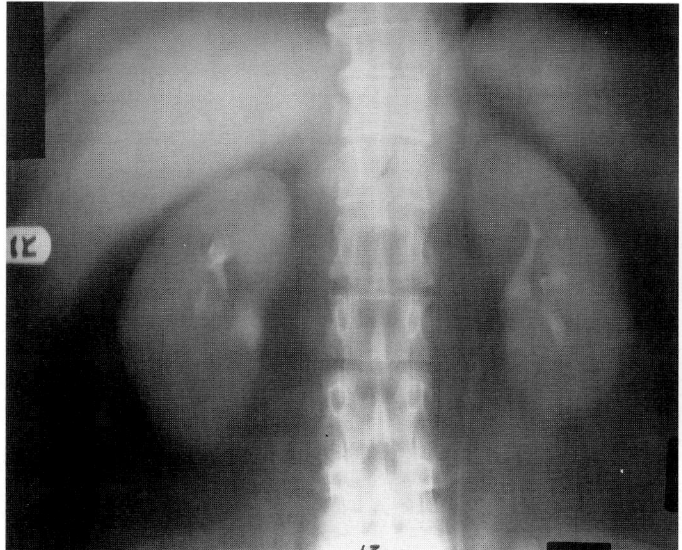

Fig. 17-33. Nephrotomogram–1 min.

HYPERTENSIVE IVU

Purpose

One special type of intravenous urogram is the **hypertensive urogram**. This examination is done on patients with high blood pressure (hypertension) to determine if the kidneys are the cause of the hypertension. There is a much shorter time between projections for a hypertensive IVU as compared to a standard IVU procedure.

Procedure

During the hypertensive urogram, several early radiographs must be obtained. It is important that all cassettes are available and marked with lead numbers to reflect the time sequence of each film. Once the procedure begins, radiographs must be taken at a set interval.

The hypertensive study will include, at least, **1-**, **2-**, and **3-minute radiographs** with the possibility of additional radiographs every 30 seconds. In most cases, timing begins at the start of injection.

After the very early radiographs, the film sequence may be similar to a standard IVU with imaging of the ureters and bladder.

17

RETROGRADE UROGRAPHY

Purpose

Retrograde urography is a **nonfunctional examination of the urinary system** during which contrast medium is introduced directly retrograde (backwards, against the flow) into the pelvicalyceal system **via catheterization** by a urologist during a minor surgical procedure. Retrograde urography is nonfunctional since the patient's normal physiologic processes are not involved in the procedure.

Procedure

Surgery personnel place the patient on the combination cystoscopic-radiographic table, usually located in the surgery department. The patient is placed in the modified lithotomy position, which requires that the legs be placed in stirrups as illustrated in Fig. 17-34. The patient is usually either sedated or anesthetized for this examination. The urologist inserts a cystoscope through the urethra into the bladder. After examining the inside of the bladder, the urologist inserts ureteral catheters into one or both ureters. Ideally, the tip of each ureteral catheter is placed at the level of the renal pelvis.

After catheterization, a **scout radiograph** is exposed. The scout radiograph allows the radiographer to check technique and positioning, and allows the urologist to check catheter placement. The **second radiograph** in the usual retrograde urographic series is a **pyelogram**. The urologist injects 3 to 5 ccs of any of the urographic contrast media directly into the renal pelvis of one or both kidneys. Respiration is suspended immediately after injection, and the exposure is made.

The **third and final radiograph** in the usual series is a **ureterogram**. The head end of the table may be elevated for this final radiograph. The urologist withdraws the catheters and simultaneously injects contrast material into one or both ureters. The urologist indicates when to make the exposure. This examination is used to directly visualize the internal structures of one or both kidneys and ureters.

The catheter is shown in place in Fig. 17-35 with contrast media being injected into the right kidney. The left kidney and proximal ureter also show residual contrast media present.

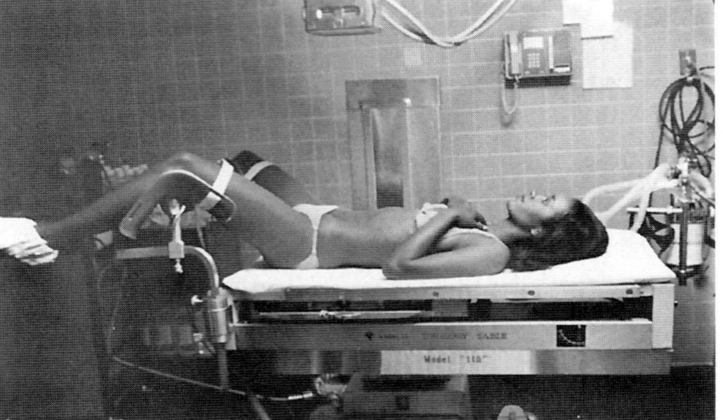

Fig. 17-34. Retrograde urogram (scout position).

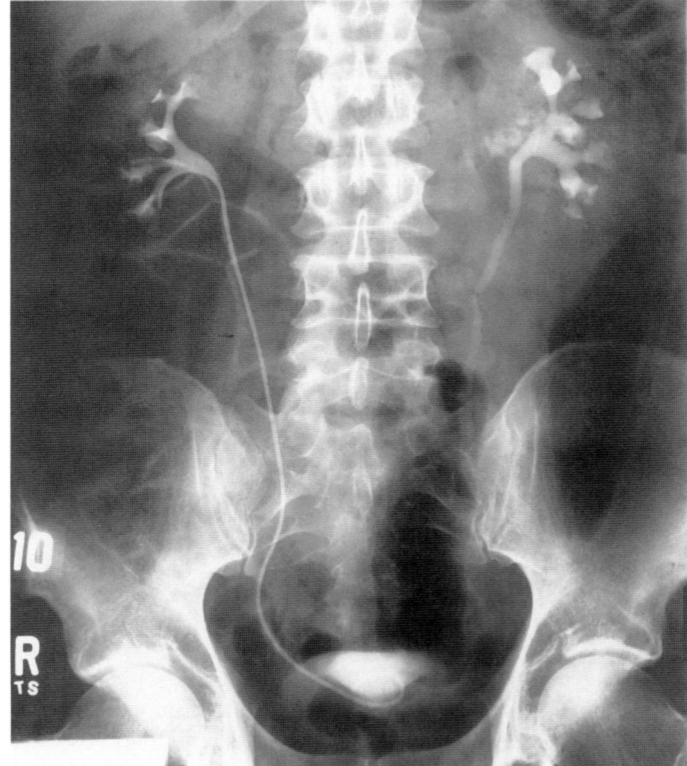

Fig. 17-35. Retrograde urogram.

RETROGRADE CYSTOGRAPHY (CYSTOGRAM)

Purpose

Retrograde cystography is another **nonfunctional** urinary system examination. A cystogram *(sis′ to-gram)* is a radiographic examination of the **urinary bladder** following instillation of an iodinated contrast medium via a urethral catheter.

Procedure

There is no patient preparation for this examination, although the patient should empty the bladder prior to catheterization. After routine bladder catheterization under aseptic conditions, the bladder is drained of any residual urine. The bladder is then filled with dilute contrast medium as illustrated in Fig. 17-36. The contrast material is allowed to flow in **by gravity only**. One should never get in a hurry and attempt to introduce the contrast medium under pressure. Bladders have been ruptured through the use of unnecessary pressure.

After the bladder is filled, which may require 150 to 500 ccs, either fluorographic spot radiographs are taken by the radiologist or various overhead positions are exposed by the radiographer.

Routine positioning for a cystogram includes an **AP with a 15° caudad angle** and **both posterior obliques**.

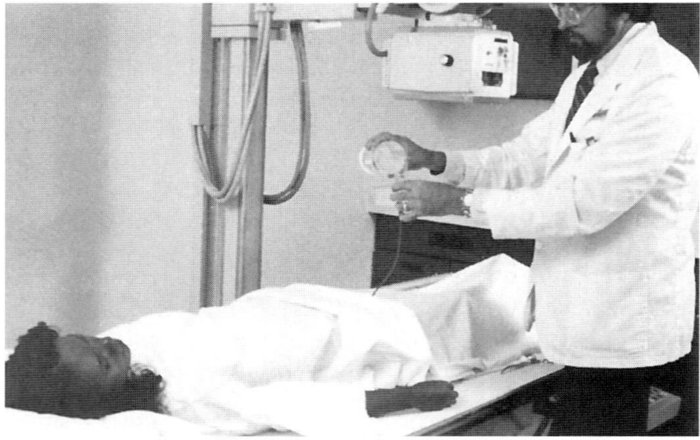

Fig. 17-36. Cystogram–Instilling contrast medium.

VOIDING CYSTOURETHROGRAPHY

Purpose

Voiding radiographs may be taken after the routine cystogram. When combined in this manner, the examination would be termed a cystourethrogram *(sist″ o-u-re′ thro-gram)* or voiding cystourethrogram (VCU). It will provide a study of the urethra and evaluate the patient's ability to urinate, therefore it is a **functional study** of the bladder and urethra.

Trauma or **involuntary loss of urine** are common **clinical indications**. The voiding phase of the examination is best done utilizing fluoroscopic control and a spot film camera.

Procedure

The procedure is sometimes done with the patient supine, although the upright position makes it easier to void. The key to a good voiding study is to gently remove the catheter from the bladder and urethra. First remove any liquid from the balloon portion of the catheter, if this type of catheter was used, and ever so gently remove the catheter. The urethra can be traumatized if care is not exercised.

The female is usually examined in the AP or slight oblique position, as shown on the radiograph in Fig. 17-37. The male is best examined in a 30° right posterior oblique position. An adequate receptacle or absorbent padding must be provided for the patient.

After voiding is complete and adequate imaging is obtained, a post-voiding AP may be requested.

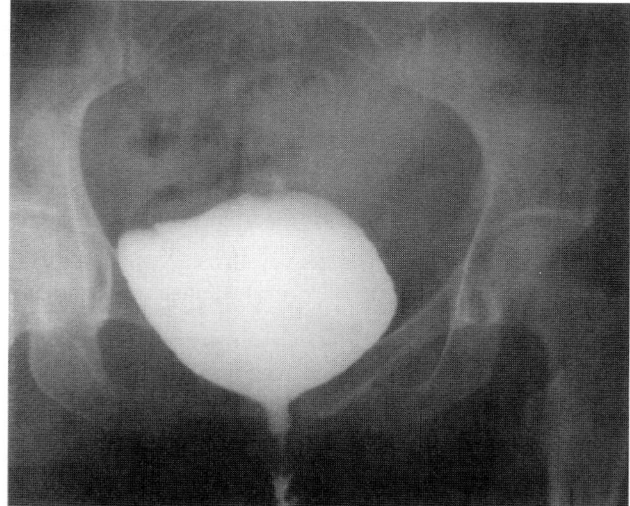

Fig. 17-37. Female voiding cystourethrogram.

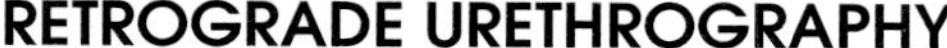

RETROGRADE URETHROGRAPHY

Purpose

A retrograde urethrogram is sometimes performed on the male patient to demonstrate the full length of the urethra. Contrast medium is injected into the distal urethra until the entire urethra is filled in retrograde fashion. This is **not** a commonly performed procedure today but radiographers should at least be aware of it in case it is requested.

Procedure

Injection of contrast material is sometimes facilitated by a special device termed a **Brodney clamp**, which is attached to the distal penis. A **30° right posterior oblique** is the position of choice; and centering is to the symphysis pubis. The tip of the syringe is inserted into the distal urethra and the injection is made. Ample contrast medium is used to fill the entire urethra and exposures are made. An RPO retrograde urethrogram on a male patient is shown in Fig. 17-38. Ideally, the urethra is superimposed over the soft tissues of the right thigh. This prevents superimposition of any bony structures except for the lower pelvis.

Because this procedure is rarely done today, it is not included in the positioning section of this chapter. However, the voiding cystourethrogram, as described above, provides much of the same diagnostic information and is described and demonstrated in the positioning section which follows.

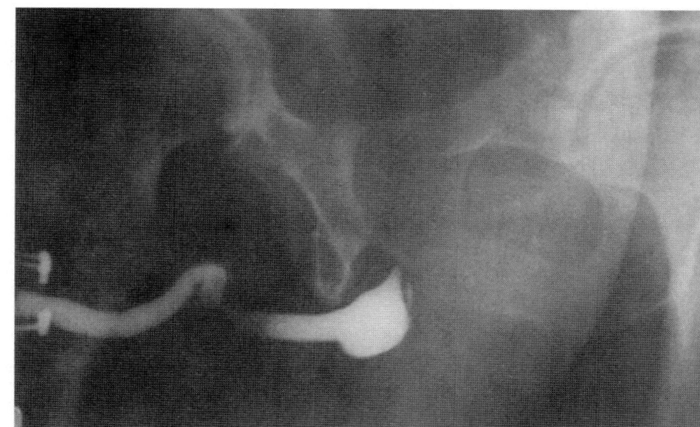

Fig. 17-38. Male retrograde urethrogram.

SUMMARY OF URINARY SYSTEM PROCEDURES

Urographic procedures may be categorized by the method of contrast medium administration. Contrast medium is introduced either (1) into the circulatory system, or (2) directly into the structure to be studied.

1. **Into the bloodstream** (usually intravenous injection):
   –Intravenous (excretory) urography (IVU)

2. **Directly into the structure to be studied** (requires catheterization):
   –Retrograde urography
   –Retrograde cystography (cystogram)
   –Voiding cystourethrography
   –Retrograde urethrography (rarely performed today)

Radiographic Positioning

NATIONAL SURVEY

A survey of the operating procedures (department routines) was conducted throughout the United States. The following information was compiled from the survey indicating the national norm for basic and special routines for intravenous urography and cystography.

Intravenous Urogram Routine

IVU	U.S. Average	
	Basic 1995 (1989)	Special 1995 (1989)
• AP (scout and series)	94% (99%)	
• Nephrotomography	– (77%)	(13%)
• RPO and LPO (30°)	71% (70%)	
• Tomograms	77% –	
• AP post-void (erect)	49% (51%)	(21%)
• PA post-void (prone)	– (38%)	(15%)
• AP ureteric compression	31% (33%)	(19%)

Retrograde Urogram Routine

Retrograde Urogram	U.S. Average	
	Basic 1995 (1989)	Special 1995 (1989)
• AP Scout	87% –	
• AP Pyelogram	71% –	
• AP Ureterogram	57% –	

Cystogram Routine

Cystogram	U.S. Average	
	Basic 1995 (1989)	Special 1995 (1989)
• AP (no angle)	– (85%)	
• AP 10-15° caudad	64% –	
• LPO and RPO (60°)	69% (70%)	
• Lateral	45% (51%)	12% (13%)

Voiding Cystourethrogram Routine

Voiding cystourethrogram	U.S. Average	
	Basic 1995 (1989)	Special 1995 (1989)
• Male–RPO 30°	75% –	
• Female–AP	79% –	

Summary

The survey responses for these two procedures were very consistent throughout the U.S.

BASIC AND SPECIAL PROJECTIONS

Certain basic or special projections of the urinary system are demonstrated and described on the following pages. The radiologist and radiographer must closely coordinate their efforts during examinations of this anatomy.

Intravenous (excretory) urography–IVU
Basic
- AP (scout and series) **521**
- Nephrotomogram **522**
- RPO and LPO (30°) **523**
- AP–Post-void **524**

Special
- AP ureteric compression **525**

Retrograde urography
Basic
- AP (scout) **526**
- AP (pyelogram) **526**
- AP (ureterogram) **526**

Cystography
Basic
- AP (10-15° caudad) **527**
- Both obliques (45-60°) **527**

Special
- Lateral **527**

Voiding cystourethrography
Basic
- Male–RPO (30°) **528**
- Female–AP **528**

AP Projection (Scout and Series)

> **Intravenous (excretory) urography–IVU**
> Basic
> • **AP (scout and series)**
> • Nephrotomogram
> • RPO and LPO (30°)
> • AP–Post-void
> Special
> • AP ureteric compression

Structures Best Shown

Collecting system of the kidneys, ureters, and urinary bladder filled with contrast medium.

Scout verifies patient preparation and correct exposure factors and detects any abnormal calcifications prior to injection of contrast medium.

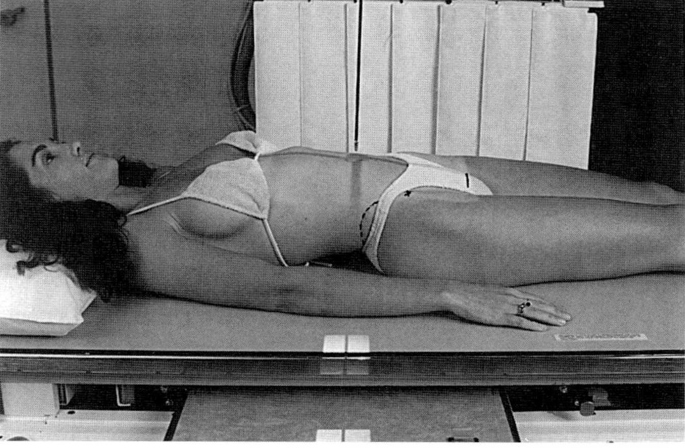

Fig. 17-39. IVU scout and series.

See pages 516 and 517 for basic IVU procedure routines.

14

17

R

Technical Factors

- Film size–14 x 17 in. (35 x 43 cm), lengthwise. For nephrogram: 10 x 12 in. (24 x 30 cm), or 11 x 14 in (28 x 35 cm), crosswise.
- Moving or stationary grid.
- 65-75 kVp range.
- Include minute markers where applicable.
- Technique and dose:

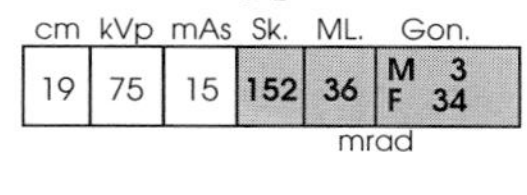

cm	kVp	mAs	Sk.	ML.	Gon.
19	75	15	152	36	M 3 F 34

mrad

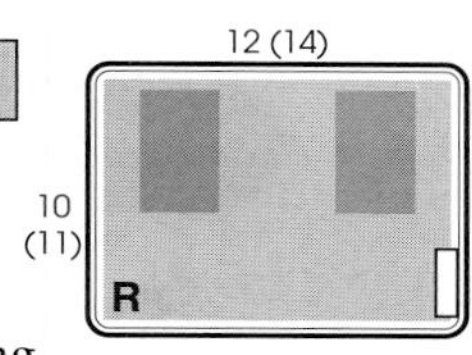

Nephrogram

Shielding: Shield gonads on males (females generally cannot be shielded without obscuring area of interest).
Shield both male and female for nephrogram.

Patient Position

- Patient supine, pillow for head, arms at sides away from body.

Part Position

- Align midsagittal plane to center line of table and to CR.
- Flex and support knees to reduce lordotic curvature.
- Ensure **no rotation** of trunk or pelvis.
- Include symphysis pubis on bottom of cassette without cutting off upper kidneys. (A second smaller film of bladder area may be necessary on large patients.)

Central Ray

- CR **perpendicular** to film holder.

For Entire Urinary System:

- Center CR and film to **level of iliac crest**, or 1 in. (2.5 cm) above crest, and to midsagittal plane.

For Nephrogram:

- See following page for centering.
- Minimum 40 in. (102 cm) SID.

Collimation: Collimate to film size or smaller if possible.

Respiration: Suspend respiration and expose upon expiration.

Notes: Have patient empty bladder immediately before beginning exam.

Explain procedure and obtain clinical history prior to injection of contrast medium.

Be prepared for possible reaction to contrast medium. (See page 513.)

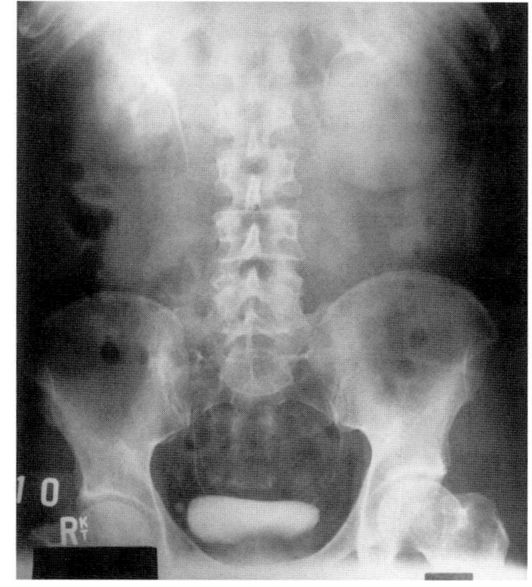

Fig. 17-40. IVU (10 min.).

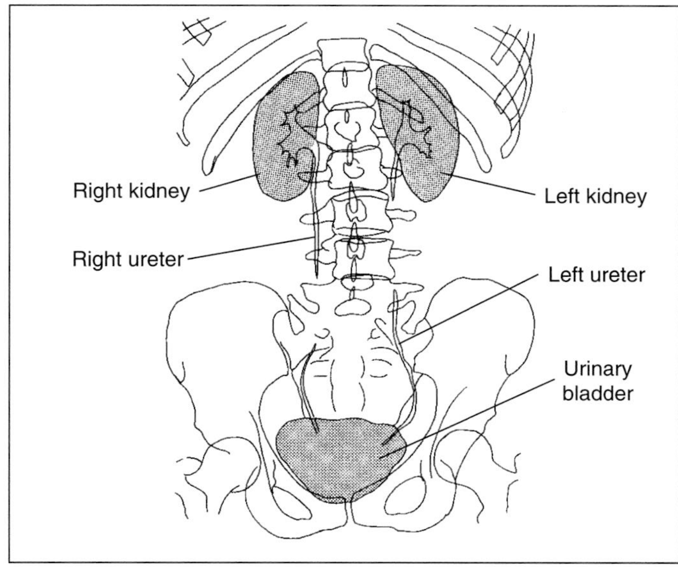

Fig. 17-41. IVU.

Evaluation Criteria

- Entire urinary system is visualized from upper renal shadows to distal urinary bladder. The symphysis pubis should be included on lower margin of the film.
- Only a portion of the urinary system may be opacified on a specific radiograph in the series.
- No rotation evidenced by symmetry of iliac wings and rib cage.
- No motion due to respiration or movement.
- Appropriate technique with short scale contrast should visualize the urinary system.
- Minute markers along with R or L markers should be visible on all series radiographs.

Nephrotomogram (Tomogram) and Nephrogram

Intravenous (excretory) urography–IVU
Basic
- AP (scout and series)
- **Nephrotomogram**
- RPO and LPO (30°)
- AP–Post-void

Special
- AP ureteric compression

Structures Best Shown

Renal parenchyma during early stages of IVU.

A **nephrogram** involves one single AP radiograph taken of the kidney region within 60 seconds following injection (taken as conventional AP radiograph centered to kidneys, not as a tomogram).

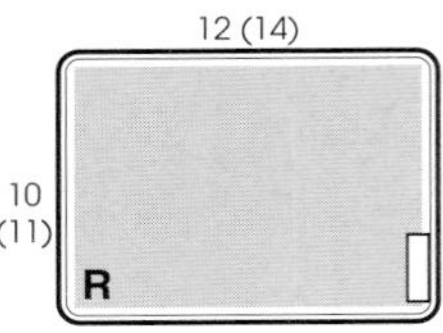

Technical Factors

- Linear or multidirectional tomography
- Film size–10 x 12 in. (24 x 30 cm), or 11 x 14 in. (28 x 35 cm) crosswise.
- Moving or stationary grid.
- 70-75 kVp range.
- Select the correct exposure angle:
  - –10° or less angle produces larger section of tissue in relative focus.
  - –40° exposure angle produces thinner sections of tissue in relative focus.
  - –If only three tomograms are to be taken, use a 10° or less exposure angle (actually known as **zonography).**

Shielding: Shield gonadal area for both males and females.

Patient Position

- Patient supine, pillow for head, arms at side away from body.

Part Position

- Align midsagittal plane to center line of table.
- Flex and support knees to reduce lordotic curvature.
- Ensure **no rotation** of trunk or pelvis.

Central Ray

- Center **midway between xiphoid tip and iliac crest.**
- 40 in. (102 cm) SID (or distance as required by specific equipment).

Collimation: Collimate to film size or smaller if possible.

Respiration: Suspend respiration and expose upon expiration.

Notes: Explain tomographic procedure to reduce anxiety for patient. Obtain clinical history prior to injection of contrast medium.

Remind patient to remain immobile between exposures.

Check scout film to verify focus level, optimum technique and position of kidneys.

Tomography procedures including equipment setup and procedure are described in Chapter 21.

Evaluation Criteria

- Entire renal parenchyma is visualized with some filling of collecting system with contrast medium.
- No motion due to respiration or movement.
- Appropriate technique employed to visualize renal parenchyma.
- The specific focus level markers should be visible on each radiograph along with R or L markers.

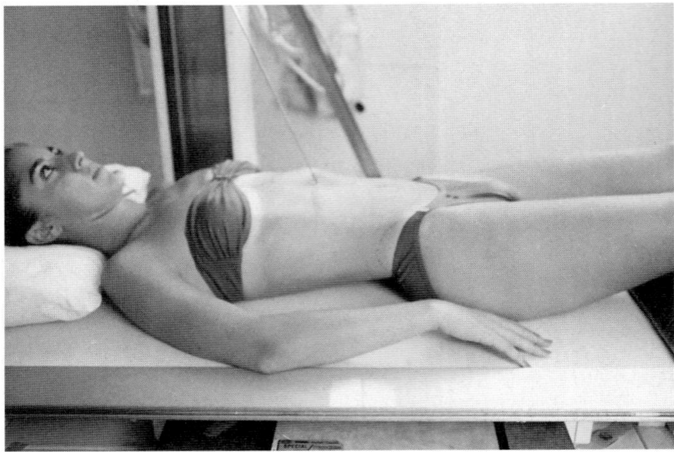

Fig. 17-42. Nephrotomogram.

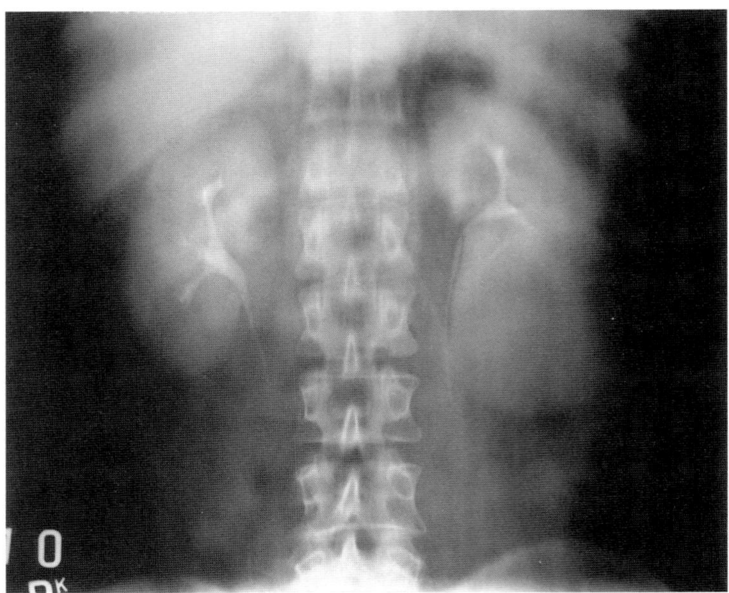

Fig. 17-43. Nephrotomogram.

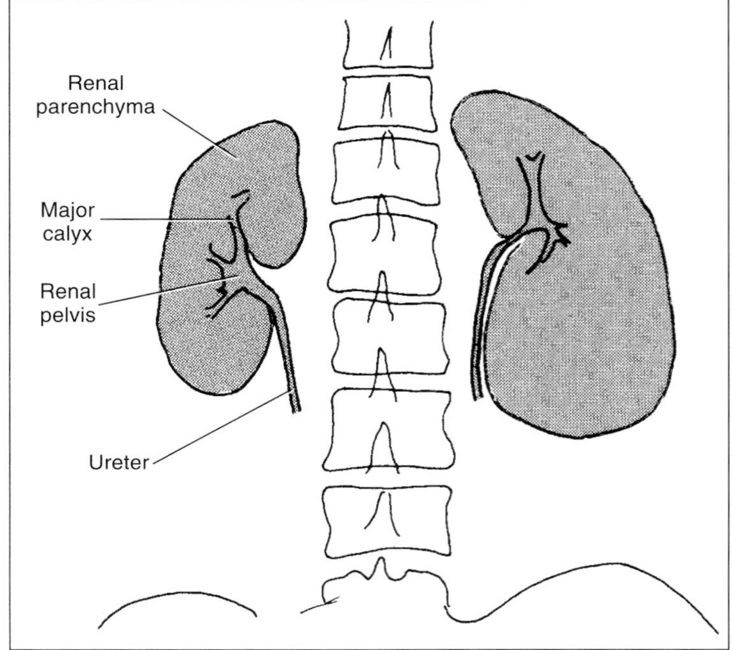

Fig. 17-44. Nephrotomogram.

17

RPO and LPO Positions

Intravenous (excretory) urography–IVU
Basic
- AP (scout and series)
- Nephrotomogram
- **RPO and LPO (30°)**
- AP–Post-void

Special
- AP ureteric compression

Structures Best Shown

The kidney on **elevated side** is placed in profile or parallel to the film and is best demonstrated with each oblique. (See anatomy Fig. 17-5.)

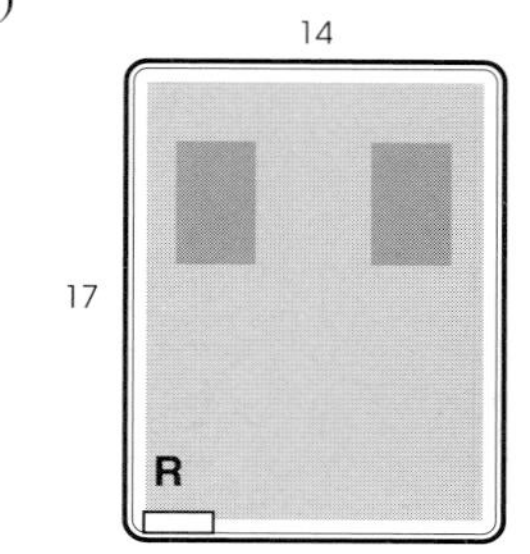

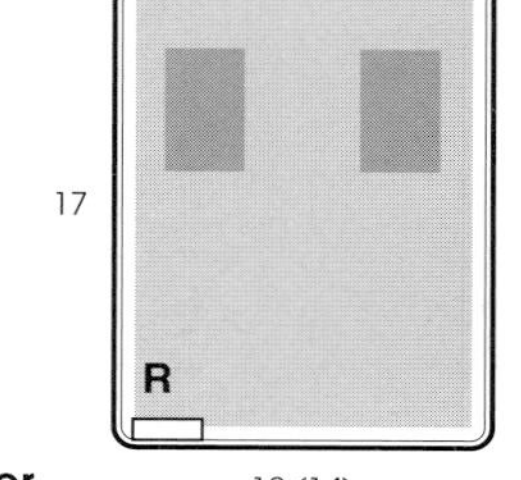

or

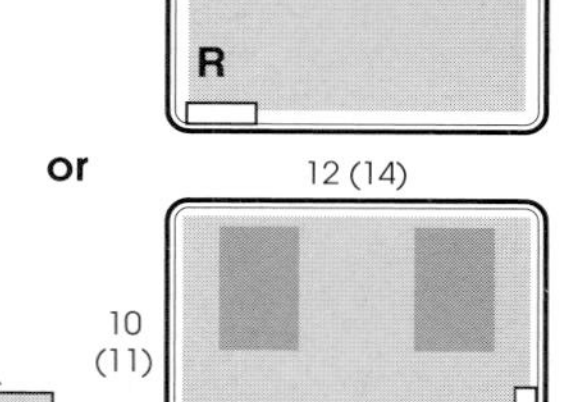

Technical Factors

- Film size–14 x 17 in. (35 x 43 cm), lengthwise or 11 x 14 in. (28 x 35 cm), crosswise (see Note).
- Moving or stationary grid.
- 70-75 kVp range.
- Include minute marker.
- Technique and dose with 14 x 17 in. (35 x 43 cm) film:

cm	kVp	mAs	Sk.	ML.	Gon.
19	75	25	**266**	**53**	M 5 F 60

mrad

Shielding: Shield gonads on males. (Females generally cannot be shielded without obscuring area of interest, see Note).

Patient Position

- Patient supine and partially rotated toward the right or left posterior side.

Part Position

- Rotate body into a 30° posterior oblique for both R and L oblique projections.
- Flex elevated side knee for support of lower body.
- Raise arm on elevated side and place across upper chest.
- Center vertebral column to midline of table and to CR.

Central Ray

- CR **perpendicular** to film holder.
- Center CR and film holder to **level of iliac crest**, and vertebral column.
- Minimum 40 in. (102 cm) SID.

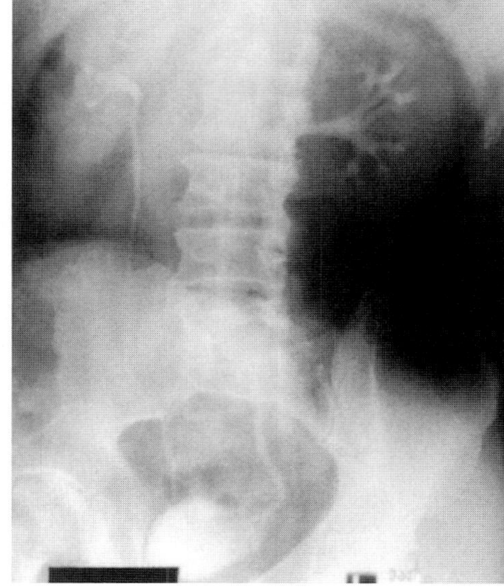

Fig. 17-47. RPO.

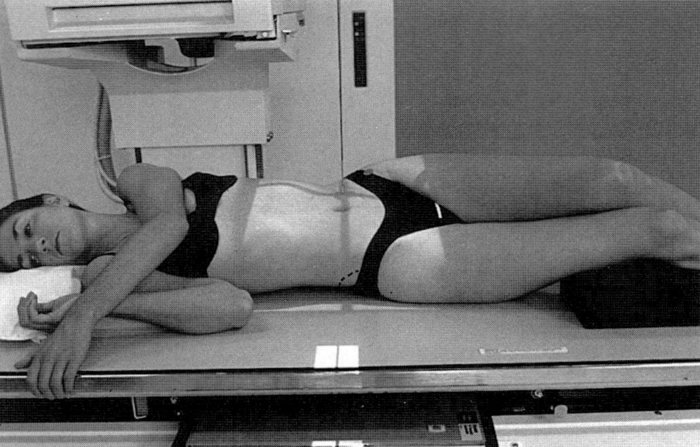

Fig. 17-45. RPO–30°.

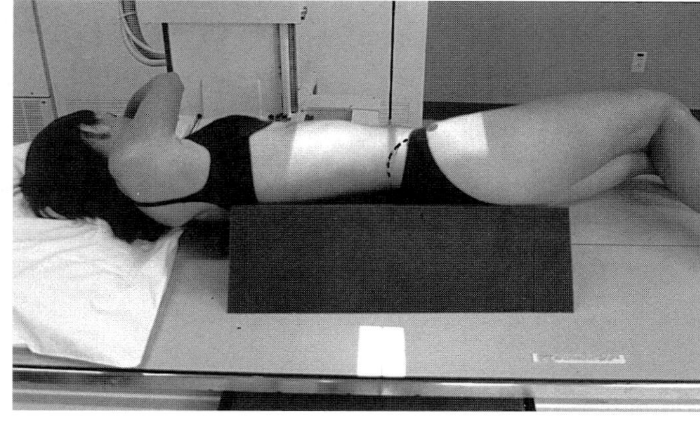

Fig. 17-46. LPO–30°.

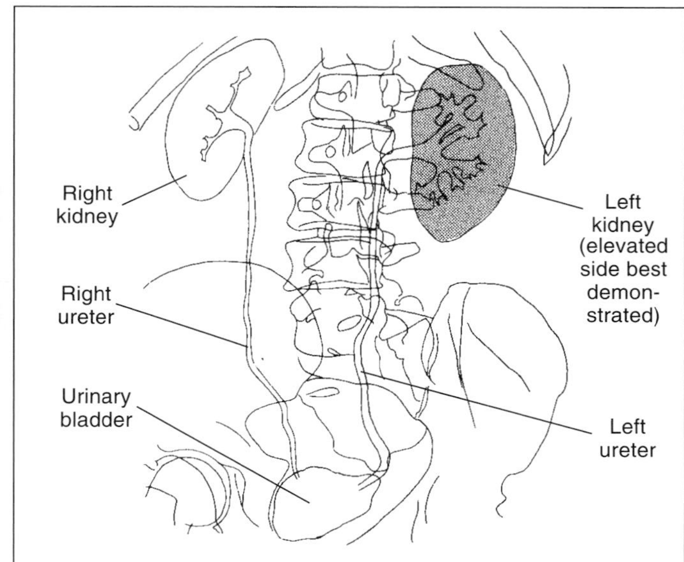

Fig. 17-48. RPO.

Collimation: Collimate to film size or smaller if possible.

Respiration: Suspend respiration and expose upon expiration.

Note: Some departmental routines include a smaller film placed crosswise to include the kidneys and proximal ureters thus allowing gonadal shielding for both males and females. Centering would be midway between xiphoid and iliac crests.

Evaluation Criteria

- The elevated side kidney is parallel to plane of film, not superimposed by vertebral column.
- The down side ureter is free of superimposition of the spine.
- Entire urinary system is visualized.
- Upper margin of kidneys should be included, as well as bladder and lower ureters if size permits. (See Note for exception.)
- No motion due to respiration or movement.
- Appropriate technique with short scale contrast employed to visualize the urinary system.
- Minute markers along with R or L markers should be visible.

AP Projection

Post-void

Intravenous (excretory) urography–IVU
Basic
- AP (scout and series)
- Nephrotomogram
- RPO and LPO (30°)
- **AP–Post-void**

Special
- AP ureteric compression

Structures Best Shown

Kidneys (positional change) and nearly empty bladder.

The erect position will demonstrate nephroptosis (positional change of kidneys).

The erect post-void position may also help demonstrate an enlarged prostate gland pushing up on the floor of the bladder.

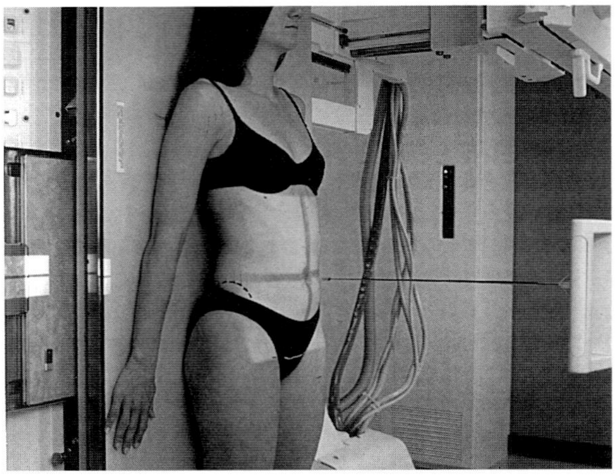

Fig. 17-49. AP erect (post-void)–Center at iliac crest to include symphysis pubis.

Technical Factors

- Film size–14 x 17 in. (35 x 43 cm), lengthwise.
- Moving or stationary grid.
- 70-75 kVp range.
- Use erect and/or post-void markers.
- Technique and dose:

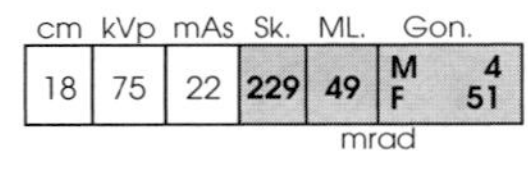
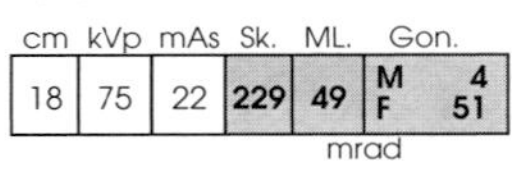

cm	kVp	mAs	Sk.	ML.	Gon.
18	75	22	229	49	M 4 F 51
			mrad		

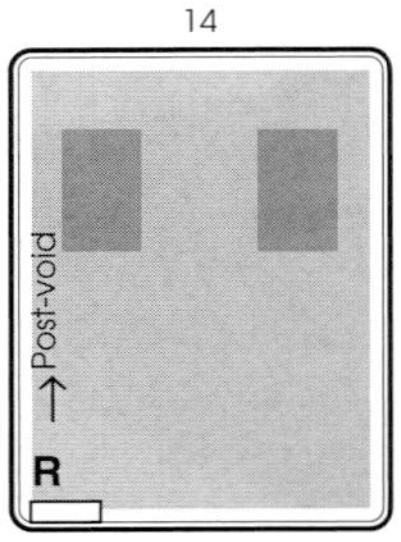

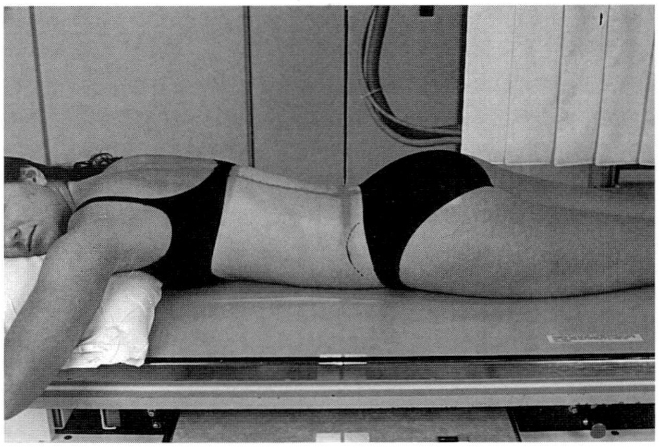

Fig. 17-50. Alternate: PA (post-void).

Shielding: Shield gonads on males (female gonads generally cannot be shielded without obscuring area of interest).

Patient Position

- Patient in erect position, back against table or prone position.

Part Position:

- Midsagittal plane to center of table or film holder, no rotation.
- Position arms away from body.
- Ensure symphysis pubis is included on bottom of cassette.
- Center low enough to include prostate area, especially on older males

Central Ray

- CR **perpendicular** to film holder.
- Center to level of **iliac crest** and midsagittal plane.
- Minimum 40 in. (102 cm) SID.

Collimation: Collimate to film size or smaller if possible.

Respiration: Suspend respiration and expose upon expiration.

Alternate PA prone or AP recumbent: This may also be taken as a PA or AP projection in the recumbent position with centering similar to that described above.

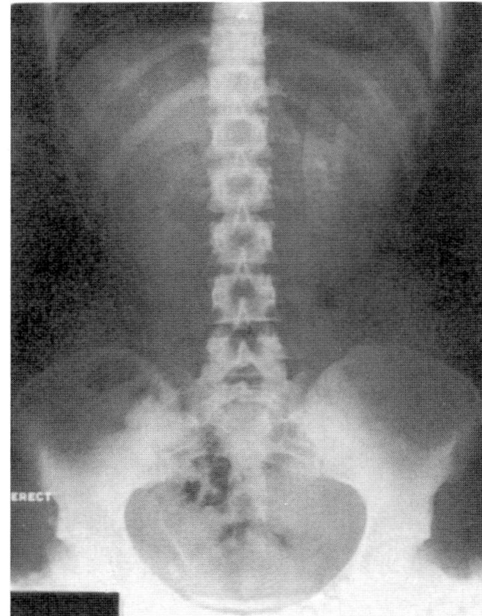

Fig. 17-51. AP erect (post-void).

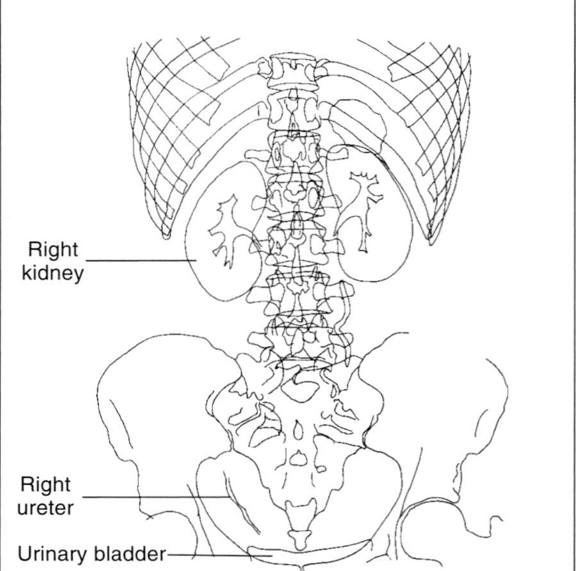

Fig. 17-52. AP erect (post-void).

Evaluation Criteria

- Entire urinary system is included with only residual contrast media visible.
- All of symphysis pubis (to include prostate area on males) is included on radiograph.
- No rotation evident by symmetry of iliac wings.
- No motion due to respiration or motion.
- Appropriate technique employed to visualize residual contrast media in the urinary system.
- Erect and/or post-void markers along with R or L markers are visible.

AP Projection
Ureteric Compression

Intravenous (excretory) urography–IVU
Basic
- AP (scout and series)
- Nephrotomogram
- RPO and LPO (30°)
- AP–Post-void

Special
- **AP ureteric compression**

Structures Best Shown

Renal pelvis and calyces with enhanced pelvic calyceal and proximal ureter filling.

Warning: Compression should **NOT** be used with acute problems, abdominal masses or recent surgery. See contraindications to ureteric compression, page 515. (A Trendelenburg position with 15° tilt, which approximates the same effect, can be used for such patients.)

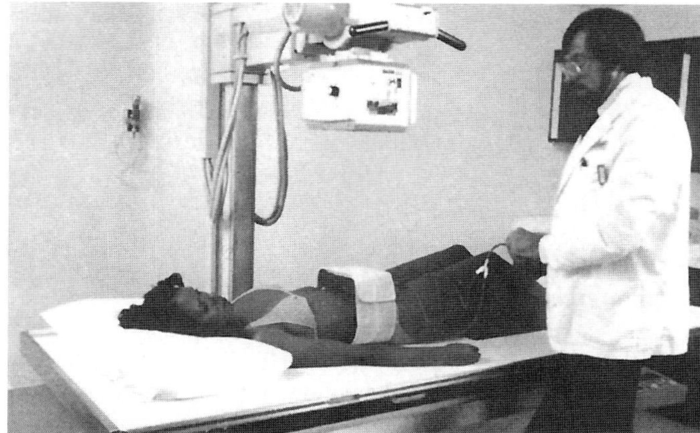

Fig. 17-53. AP–Ureteric compression.

Technical Factors

- Film size–14 x 17 in. (35 x 43 cm), lengthwise or 11 x 14 in. (30 x 35 cm), crosswise (see Notes).
- Moving or stationary grid.
- 70-75 kVp range.
- Technique and dose with 14 x 17 in. (35 x 43 cm) film:

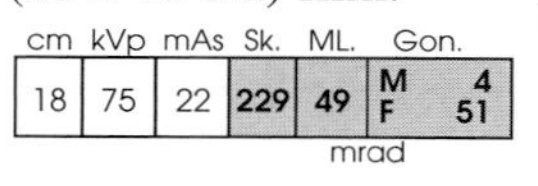

cm	kVp	mAs	Sk.	ML.	Gon.
18	75	22	229	49	M 4 F 51

mrad

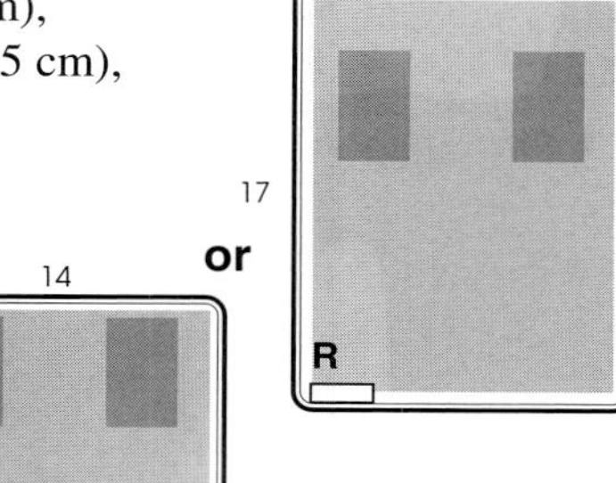

Shielding:
Place lead shield over gonadal area unless it obscures area of interest.

Patient Position

- Patient supine with compression device over lower abdomen.

Part Position

- Align midsagittal plane to center line of table.
- Flex and support knees.
- Position arms away from body.
- Ensure symphysis pubis is included on lower margin of film holder.

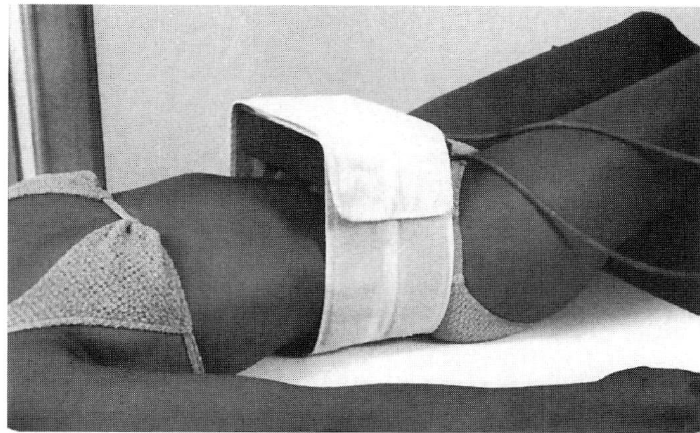

Fig. 17-54. AP–Ureteric compression.

Central Ray

- CR **perpendicular** to film holder.
- Center to **level of iliac crest** and midsagittal plane.
- Minimal 40 in. (102 cm) SID.

Collimation: Collimate to film size or smaller if possible.

Respiration: Suspend respiration and expose upon expiration.

Notes: Alternate centering with a smaller film placed crosswise is midway between xiphoid and iliac crests to center to kidneys and proximal ureters. (This allows gonadal shielding and tighter collimation for both males and females, which also results in better image quality.)

Place compression paddles just medial to ASISs.

Evaluation Criteria

- Entire urinary system visualized with enhanced pelvic calyceal filling.
- No rotation evident by symmetry of iliac wings.
- No motion due to respiration or movement.
- Appropriate technique employed with short scale contrast to visualize the urinary system.

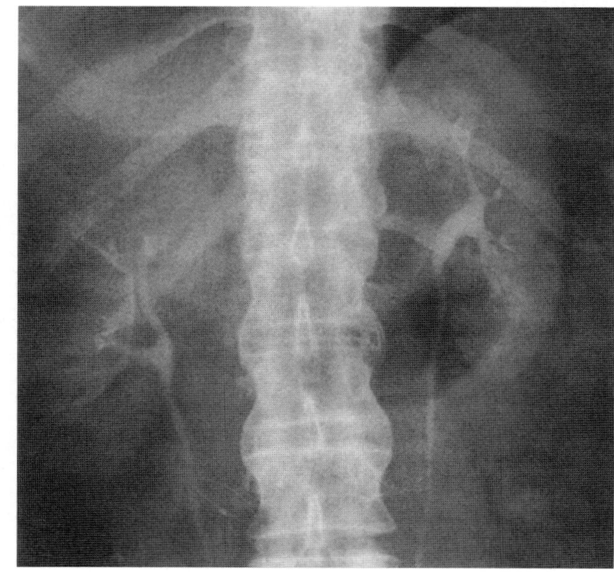

Fig. 17-55. AP–Ureteric compression.

AP Projection
(Scout, Pyelogram, Ureterogram)

Retrograde urography
Basic
- **AP (scout)**
- **AP (pyelogram)**
- **AP (ureterogram)**

Structures Best Shown

Contrast-filled renal pelvis, major and minor calyces, and ureter(s).

This is considered an operative procedure carried out by a urologist under aseptic conditions (see page 518 for procedure details).

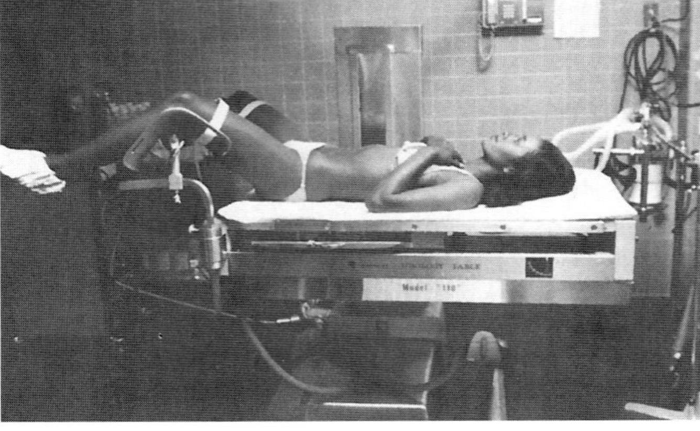

Fig. 17-56. Retrograde urography position.

Technical Factors

- Film size–14 x 17 in. (35 x 43 cm), lengthwise.
- Moving or stationary grid.
- 70-75 kVp range.
- Taken with special cystoscopic radiographic equipment.
- Technique and dose:

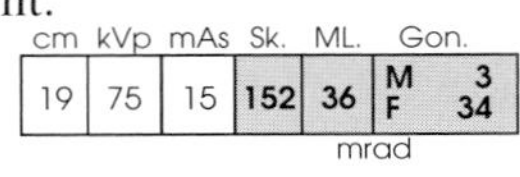

cm	kVp	mAs	Sk.	ML.	Gon.
19	75	15	152	36	M 3 F 34
					mrad

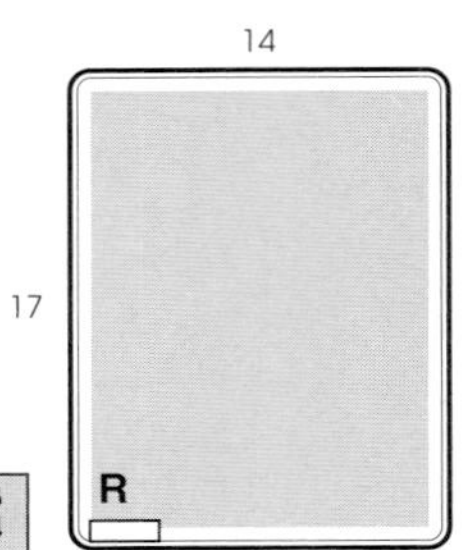
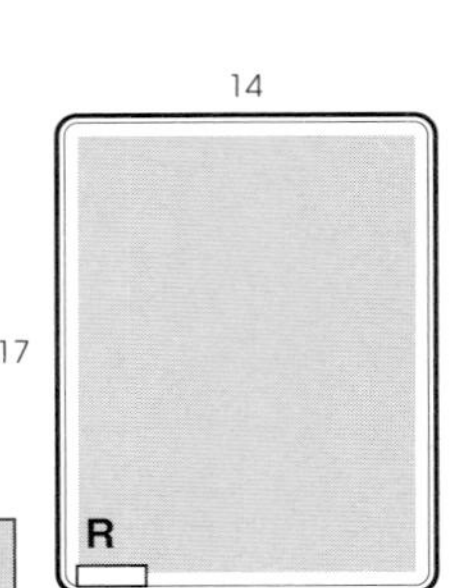

Shielding: Because of anatomy studied and sterile surgical field, gonadal shielding generally isn't practical.

Patient Position

- Modified lithotomy position with knees flexed over adjustable leg supports.

Part Position

- Ensure symphysis pubis is included on bottom of cassette.
- **No rotation** of pelvis or trunk.

Central Ray

- CR **perpendicular** to film holder.
- Center CR and film holder to **level of iliac crest** and midsagittal plane.
- Minimum 40 in. (102 cm) SID.

Collimation: Collimate to film size or smaller if possible.

Respiration: Expose after anesthetist suspends respiration if patient is under general anesthesia. The urologist generally indicates when to make exposure.

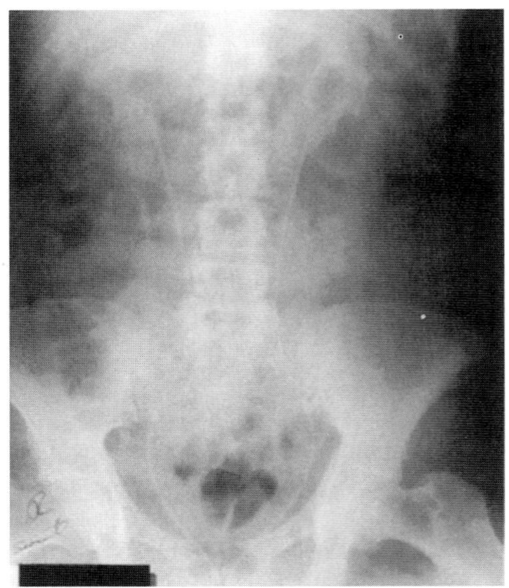

Fig. 17-57. Retrograde urogram scout (scout with catheters in place).

Notes: Take scout film after insertion of catheters but prior to injection of contrast media.

Pyelogram demonstrates the renal pelvis, major and minor calyces.

Ureterogram demonstrates the ureter.

Ureterogram exposed as catheters are withdrawn.

Evaluation Criteria

- Contrast-filled renal pelvis, major and minor calyces, and ureters visualized.
- No rotation evident by symmetry of iliac wings and rib cage.
- No motion due to respiration or movement.
- Appropriate technique with short scale contrast to visualize urinary system.

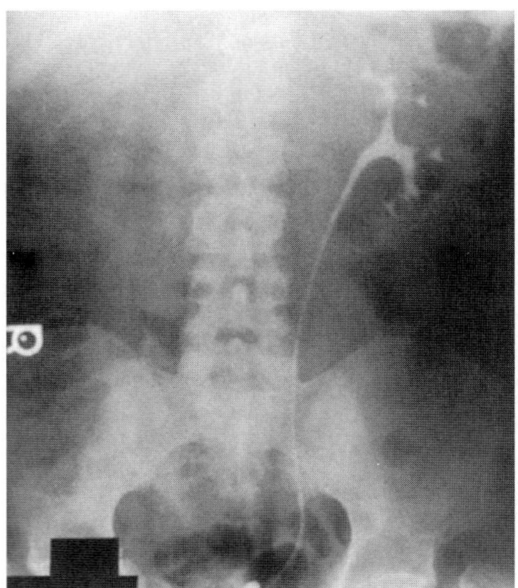

Fig. 17-58. Pyelogram–Left only (catheter in place).

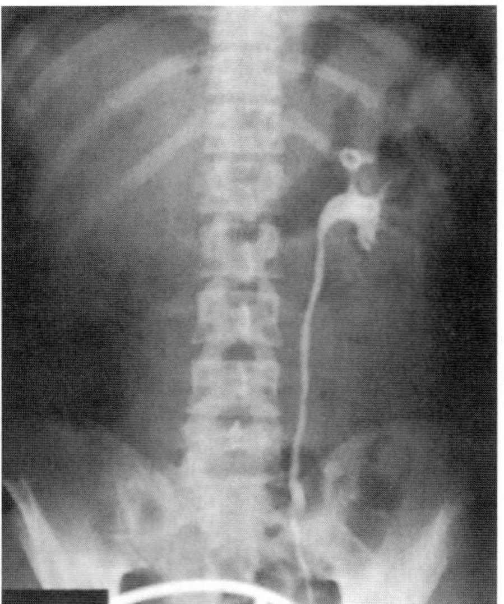

Fig. 17-59. Ureterogram–Left only (catheter withdrawn).

AP Projection • LPO and RPO Positions • Lateral Position (Optional)

Cystography
Basic
- **AP (10-15° caudad)**
- **Both obliques (45-60°)**

Special
- **Lateral**

Structures Best Shown:

Contrast-filled urinary bladder and distal ureters for possible reflux, prostate and proximal male urethra.

See page 518 for detailed procedure descriptions.

Technical Factors:

- Film size–11 x 14 in. (30 x 35 cm) or 14 x 17 in. (35 x 43 cm), lengthwise (to demonstate reflux).
- Moving or stationary grid.
- 70-75 kVp range. (80-90 kVp for lateral)

11 (14)
14 (17)
R

• Technique and dose	cm	kVp	mAs	Sk.	ML.	Gon.
AP:	16	75	15	143	41	M 56 F 27
Obliques:	20	75	20	215	42	M 83 F 41
Lateral:	31	90	48	1084	101	M 101 F 101

mrad

Patient and Part Position

AP:
- Supine, with legs extended, midsagittal plane to center of table.

Posterior Obliques:
- 45 to 60° body rotation. (Steep obliques are used to visualize posterolateral aspect of bladder, especially UV junction.)
- Partially flex downside leg for stabilization.

Note: Do not flex elevated side leg more than necessary to prevent superimposition of leg over bladder.

***Lateral** (Optional due to large gonadal radiation dose):*
- True lateral (no rotation). May be performed to demonstrate possible fistulae between bladder, rectum or uterus.

Central Ray

AP:
- Center **2 in.** (5 cm) **superior to symphysis pubis** with **10 to 15° caudad** tube angle (to project symphysis pubis inferior to bladder.)

Posterior Obliques:
- Center **2 in.** (5 cm) **superior to symphysis pubis** and **2 in.** (5 cm) **medial to ASIS**.

Lateral
- Center **2 in.** (5 cm) **superior to and posterior to symphysis pubis**.

Collimation: Collimate to film size or smaller if possible.

Respiration: Suspend respiration and expose upon expiration.

Notes: Unclamp and drain bladder prior to filling with contrast medium.

Contrast medium should **never** be injected under pressure but allowed to fill slowly by gravity in presence of an attendant.

Include prostate area just distal to pubis on older males.

Evaluation Criteria

- Distal ureters, urinary bladder and proximal urethra on males should be included.
- Appropriate technique employed to visualize the urinary bladder.

AP:
- Urinary bladder is **not** superimposed by pubic bones.

Posterior Obliques:
- Urinary bladder is **not** superimposed by partially flexed elevated side leg.

Lateral:
- Hips and femurs are superimposed.

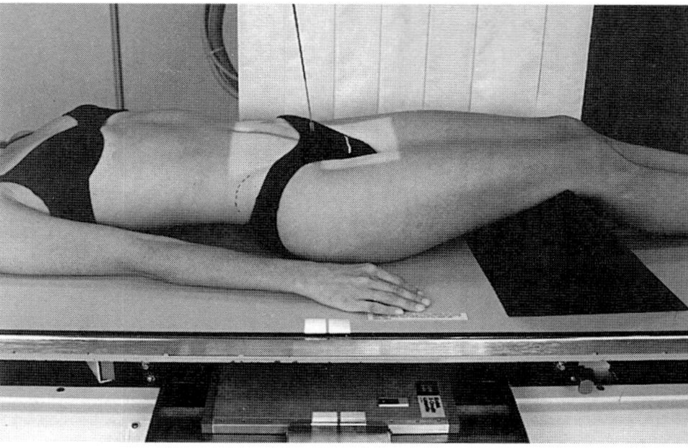

Fig. 17-60. AP (10 to 15° caudad).

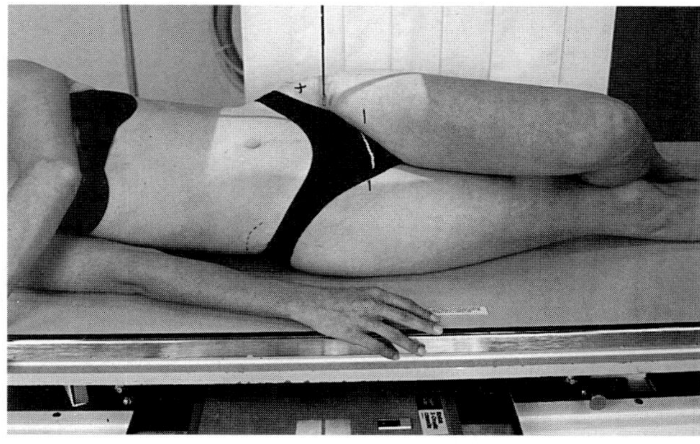

Fig. 17-61. RPO (45 to 60°).

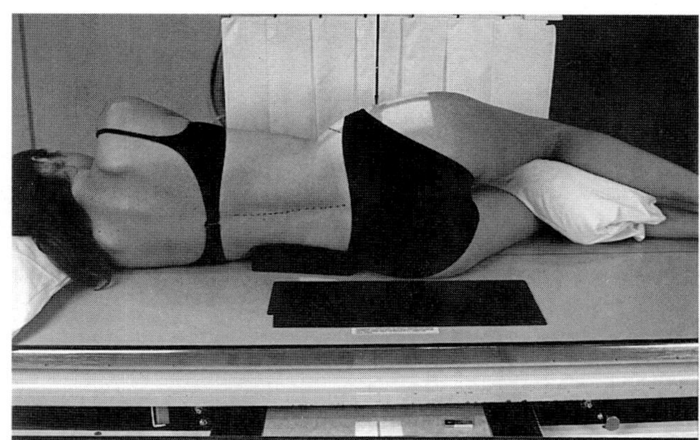

Fig. 17-62. Left lateral (optional).

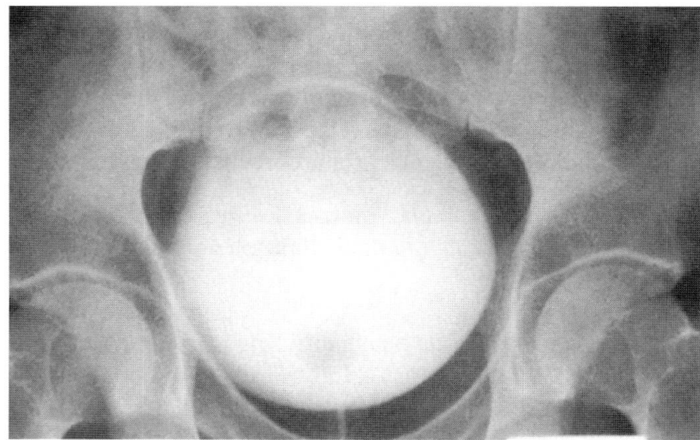

Fig. 17-63. AP (10 to 15° caudad).

RPO (30°) Position–Male • AP Projection–Female

Voiding cystourethrography
Basic
• **Male–RPO (30°)**
• **Female–AP**

See page 519 for additional procedure descriptions.

Structures Best Shown

Functional study of the urinary bladder and urethra with possible ureteral reflux.

Technical Factors

- Film size–10 x 12 in. (25 x 35 cm), lengthwise.
- Moving or stationary grid.
- 70-75 kVp range.
- Technique and dose:

(Oblique)

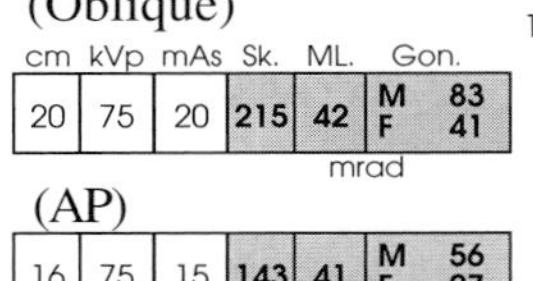

cm	kVp	mAs	Sk.	ML.	Gon.
20	75	20	215	42	M 83 F 41
				mrad	

(AP)

cm	kVp	mAs	Sk.	ML.	Gon.
16	75	15	143	41	M 56 F 27
				mrad	

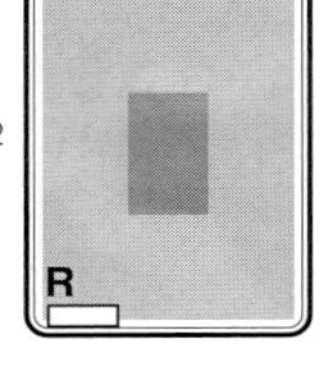

Shielding: Since bladder and urethra are primary area of interest, gonadal shielding isn't possible.

Patient Position

- May be taken **recumbent or erect.**

Part Position

Male:

- Oblique body **30° to the right** (RPO).
- Superimpose urethra over soft tissues of right thigh.

Female:

- Supine or erect.
- Center midsagittal plane to table or film holder.
- Extend and slightly separate legs.

Central Ray

- CR **perpendicular** to film holder.
- Center CR and film holder to **symphysis pubis.**
- Minimum 40 in. (102 cm) SID.

Collimation: Collimate to film size or smaller if possible.

Respiration: Suspend respiration and expose upon expiration.

Notes: Fluoroscopy and spot filming is best for this procedure. Catheter must be gently removed prior to voiding procedure. Provide radiolucent receptacle or absorbent padding for patient. After voiding is complete, a post-voiding AP may be requested.

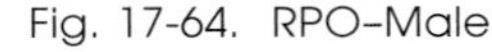

Fig. 17-64. RPO–Male.

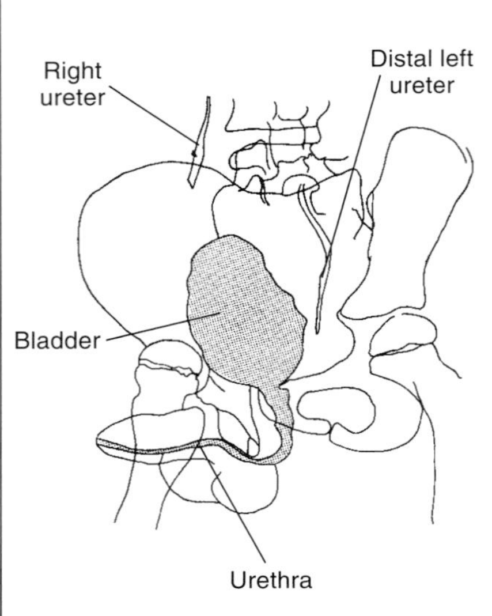

Fig. 17-65. RPO–Male.

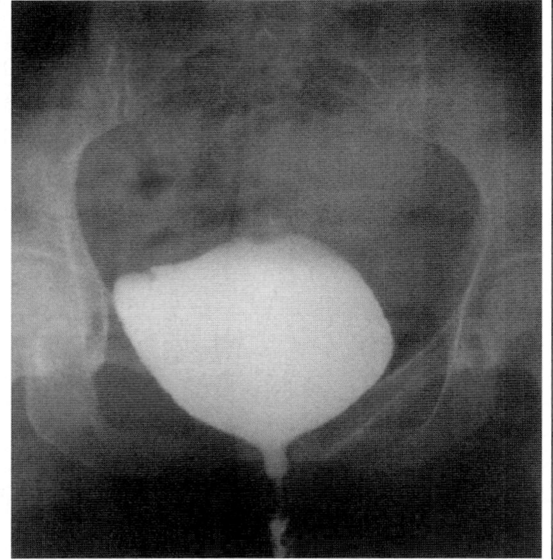

Fig. 17-66. AP–Female.

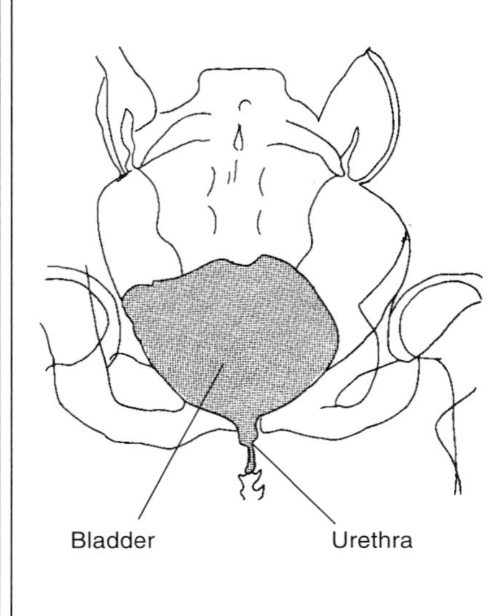

Fig. 17-67. AP–Female.

Evaluation Criteria

- Contrast-filled urinary bladder and urethra is visualized.
- Appropriate technique employed to visualize the urinary bladder without overexposing the male prostate area and the contrast-filled urethra of either male or female.

RPO: Male urethra containing contrast medium is superimposed over soft tissues of right thigh.

AP: Female urethra containing contrast medium is demonstrated inferior to the symphysis pubis.

CHAPTER 18

Mammography

CONTRIBUTIONS BY:
Eugene D. Frank, MA, RT (R), FASRT
Nancy L. Dickerson, RT (R) (M)

CONTENTS

Radiographic Anatomy

Introduction and Mammography Quality Standards Act (MQSA) **530**

Anatomy of the breast:
- Surface anatomy **530**
- Methods of localization **531**
- Sagittal section anatomy **531**
- Frontal view anatomy **532**
- Breast tissue types **532**

Breast classifications **533**

Radiographic Positioning

Breast positioning:
- X-ray tube **534**
- Compression **534**
- Magnification **535**

Imaging modalities:
- Film-screen mammography **535**
- Sonography **535**

New imaging modalities:
- Magnetic resonance imaging (MRI) **536**
- Breast implants **536**
- Digital mammography **536**

Terminology and abbreviations (ACR nomenclature) **537**

Basic and special projections **537**
- Craniocaudal (CC) projection **538**
- Mediolateral oblique (MLO) **539**
- Laterally exaggerated craniocaudal (XCCL) **540**
- Mediolateral (ML) projection **541**
- Implant procedure (Eklund technique) **542**

Radiographs for critique **543**

Radiographic Anatomy

Introduction

Until recently, breast cancer was the leading cause of death from cancer among women. Lung cancer has now become the leader. Breast cancer accounts for 32% of all cancers detected in women and 18% of all cancer deaths. Currently 1 in 9 American women will develop breast cancer sometime in her life. The best defense against the disease is to have regular mammograms so that early detection is possible.

Mammography in the 1990s has evolved into one of the most critical and demanding x-ray examinations performed. Accurate and careful positioning of the breast during mammography is imperative in diagnosing breast cancer. The maximum amount of breast tissue must be demonstrated on each view. Mammography images must contain maximum contrast, superb resolution, and have no artifacts. Mammographers must be certified through professional training, experience, and continuing education in mammography.

Mammography Quality Standards Act

In 1992, as a result of the American Cancer Society's high visibility public relations campaign that all women over 40 undergo screening mammography, and also because of federal legislation that provided reimbursement for screening mammography in women eligible for Medicare, the federal government enacted the Mammography Quality Standards Act (MQSA). The act was written because of lobbying from the American College of Radiography (ACR) due to the great concern about the poor quality mammography being performed. The act went into effect on October 1, 1994, and requires all sites (except VA facilities) that provide mammography service to meet quality standards and become certified for operation by the secretary of the Department of Health and Human Services (DHHS). Enactment of the MQSA marks the first time the use of an x-ray machine and a specific examination are regulated by the federal government.

The technical aspects of mammography are tightly controlled and mammography must be performed on a dedicated mammography unit. The x-ray machine, processor, screens, and cassettes must be state-of-the-art and monitored regularly through an intensive quality control program.

ANATOMY OF THE BREAST

In the adult female, each of the mammary glands or breasts is a conical or hemispherical eminence located on the anterior and lateral chest walls. There is a great deal of variation in breast size from one individual to another and even in the same woman, depending on her age and the influence of various hormones. However, the usual breast extends from the anterior portion of the **second rib** down to the **sixth** or **seventh rib,** and from the lateral border of the sternum well into the axilla.

Surface Anatomy

The surface anatomy includes the **nipple**, a small projection containing a collection of duct openings from the secretory glands within the breast tissue. The pigmented area surrounding the nipple is termed the **areola,** defined as a circular area of different color surrounding a central point. The junction of the inferior part of the breast with the anterior chest wall is called the **inframammary crease**. The **axillary tail** is a band of tissue that wraps around the pectoral muscle laterally, (Fig. 18-1).

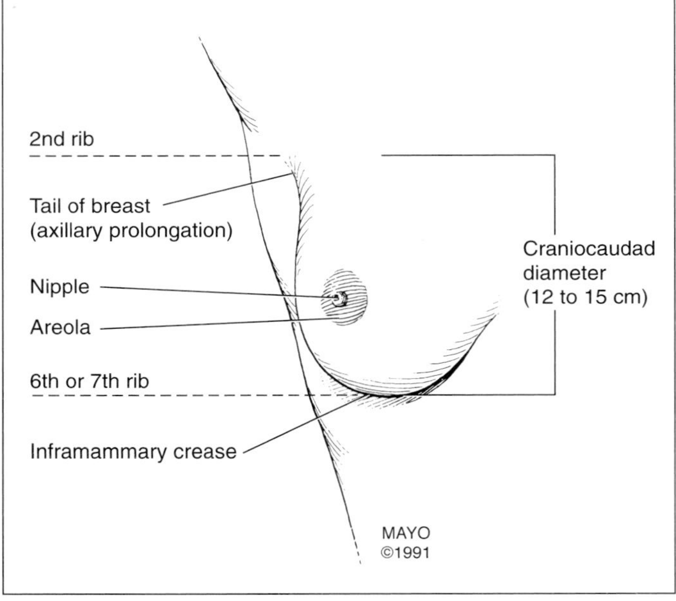

Fig. 18-1. Surface anatomy.

The width of the breast on most patients is greater than the vertical measurement, from top to bottom. The vertical measurement, which may be described as the **craniocaudad diameter**, averages from 12 to 15 centimeters at the chest wall. The radiographer must realize that there is more breast tissue than the tissue that extends obviously from the chest. There is mammary tissue overlying the costocartilages near the sternum and breast tissue extending well up into the axilla. The breast tissue extending into the axilla is called the **tail of the breast** or the **axillary prolongation** of the breast.

Methods of Localization

Two methods are commonly used to subdivide the breast into smaller areas for localization purposes. The **quadrant system**, shown in Fig. 18-2, is easiest to use. Four quadrants can be described by using the nipple as the center. These quadrants are the **UOQ** (upper outer quadrant), the **UIQ** (upper inner quadrant), the **LOQ** (lower outer quadrant), and the **LIQ** (lower inner quadrant).

A second **clock system** method, shown on the right in Fig. 18-2, compares the surface of the breast to the face of a clock. A problem with the clock method arises when a medial or lateral portion of either breast is described. What is described at 3 o'clock in the right breast has to be described at 9 o'clock in the left breast.

If either the referring physician or the patient has felt a mass of any suspicious area in either breast, one of these methods is used to describe the area of special interest to radiology personnel.

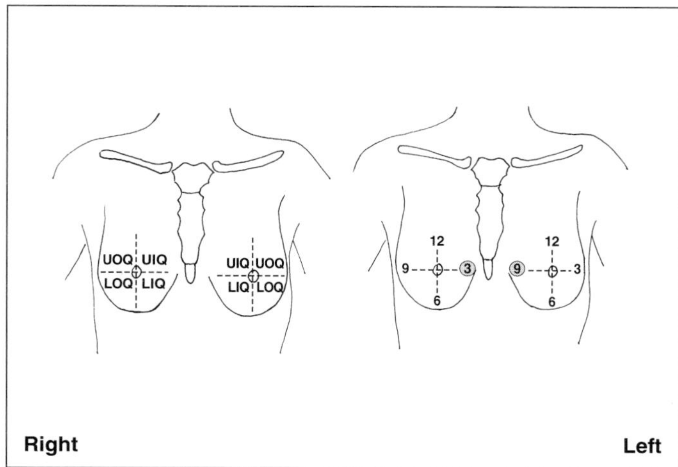

Fig. 18-2. Breast localization
-Quadrant and clock system methods.

Sagittal Section Anatomy

A sagittal section through a mature breast is illustrated in Fig. 18-3, showing the relationship of the mammary gland to the underlying structures of the chest wall. On this drawing the **inframammary crease** is at the level of the sixth rib, but a great deal of variation does exist among individuals.

The large **pectoralis major muscle** is seen overlying the bony thorax. A sheet of fibrous tissue surrounds the breast below the skin surface. A similar sheet of tissue covers the pectoralis major muscle. These two fibrous sheets connect in an area termed the **retromammary space.** This retromammary space must be demonstrated on at least one projection during the radiographic study of the mammary gland. Since the connections within the retromammary space are fairly loose, the normal breast exhibits considerable mobility on the chest wall.

The relative position of glandular tissue versus adipose (fatty) tissue is illustrated in Fig. 18-4. The central portion of the breast is primarily **glandular tissue.** Varying amounts of **adipose** or **fatty tissue** surround the glandular tissue. Size variation from individual to individual is due primarily to the amount of adipose or fatty tissue in the breast. The amount of glandular tissue is fairly constant from one female to another.

Since lactation or the secretion of milk is the primary function of the mammary gland, the amount of glandular and fatty tissue, or the size of the female breast, has no bearing on the functional ability of the gland.

The skin covering the breast is seen to be uniform in thickness, except in the area of the areola and nipple where the skin is somewhat thicker.

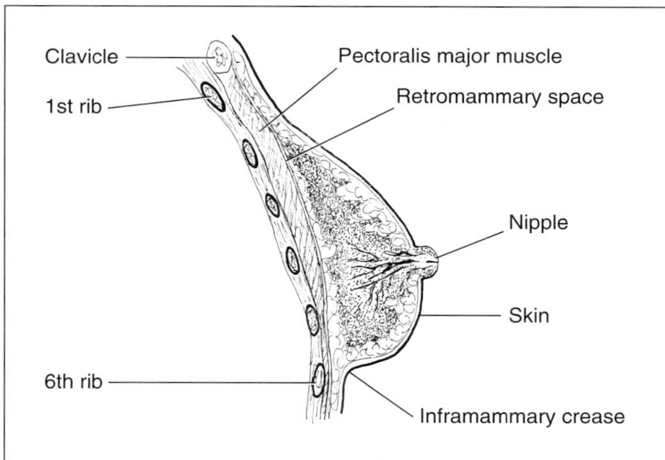

Fig. 18-3. Breast sagittal section.

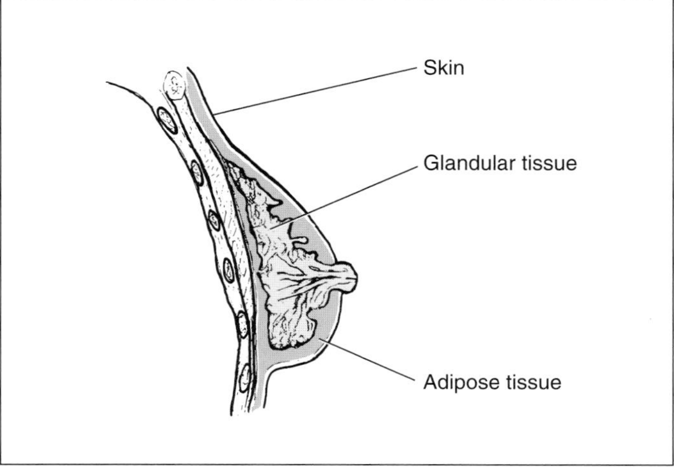

Fig. 18-4. Breast sagittal section.

18

Frontal View Anatomy

The glandular tissue of the breast is divided into **15** or **20 lobes** arranged like the spokes of a wheel surrounding the nipple (Fig. 18-5).

The glandular **lobes**, made up of a number of individual **lobules,** are not clearly separated, but are grouped in a radial arrangement as shown on this drawing. Distally, the smallest lobules consist of clusters of rounded **alveoli**. Upon glandular stimulation, peripheral cells of the alveoli form oil globules in their interior, which when ejected into the lumen of the alveoli constitute milk globules. The clusters of alveoli that make up the lobules are interconnected and drain by individual **ducts**. Each duct enlarges into a small **ampulla** that serves as a reservoir for milk just prior to terminating in a tiny opening on the surface of the **nipple.**

The various subdivisions of these ducts and associated ampullae are activated during pregnancy to prepare for lactation and following birth, to produce milk for the newborn.

A layer of adipose tissue just under the skin surrounds and covers the glandular tissue. Lobular mammary fatty tissue, **subcutaneous fat,** is interspersed between the glandular elements. **Interlobular connective** or fibrous tissues surround and support the lobes and other glandular structures. Band-like extensions of this fibrous tissue are known as **Cooper's** (suspensory) **ligaments** of the breast, and function to provide support for the mammary glands.

Each breast is abundantly supplied by blood vessels, nerves, and lymphatic vessels. The veins of the mammary gland are usually larger than the arteries, and are located more peripherally. Some of the larger veins can usually be seen distinctly on a mammogram. The term **trabeculae** is used by radiologists to describe various small structures seen on the finished radiograph, such as small blood vessels, fibrous connective tissues, ducts, and other small structures that cannot be differentiated.

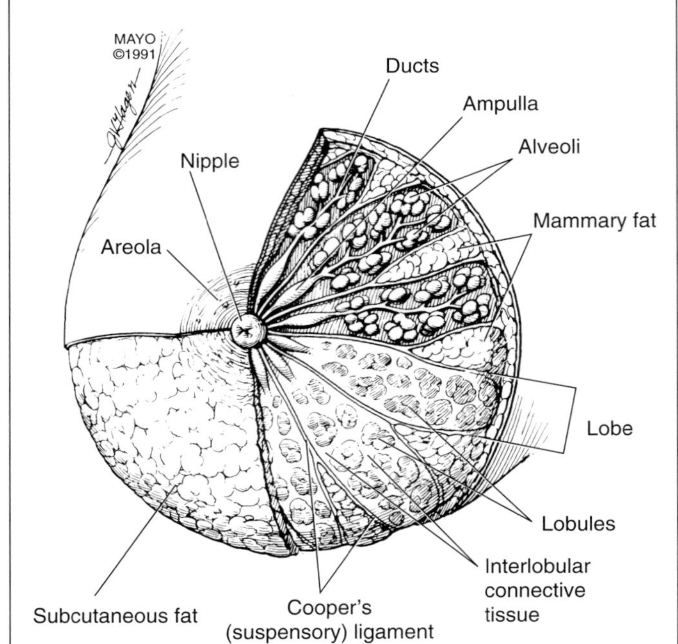

Fig. 18-5. Breast–Anterior view (glandular tissue).

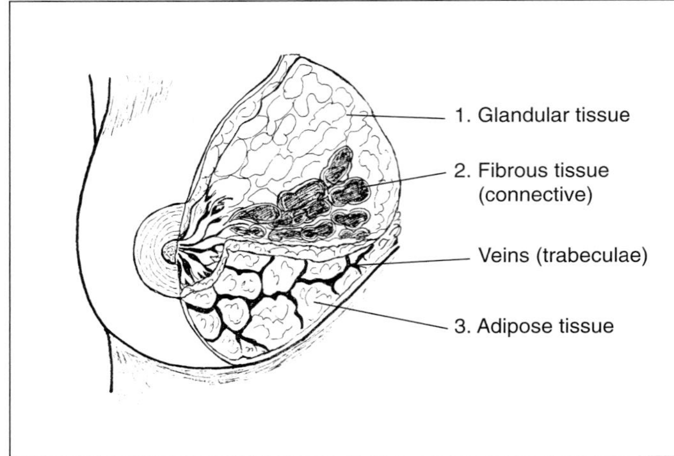

Fig. 18-6. Breast–Anterior view (three tissue types).

Breast Tissue Types

One of the major problems in radiography of the breast is that the various tissues have very low inherent subject contrast. Breast tissue can be divided into three main types of tissues: (1) **glandular,** (2) **fibrous** or **connective,** and (3) **adipose** (Fig. 18-6). Since these tissues are all "soft tissues," there is no bone or air-filled tissue to provide contrast. The fibrous and glandular tissues are of similar density—that is, radiation is absorbed by these two tissues in a similar fashion.

The major difference in the breast tissues is the fact that adipose or fatty tissue is less dense than either the fibrous or glandular tissue. This difference in density between the fatty tissue and the remaining tissues provides for the photographic density differences apparent on the finished radiograph.

Summary

Three types of breast tissue:

1. Glandular } Similar density
2. Fibrous or connective } Similar density
3. Adipose -------------------- Less density

The final mammogram (Fig. 18-7) demonstrates differences in tissue densities. These differences provide the basis for the radiographic image of the breast. Note that the more dense glandular and fibrous or connective tissues appear as "light" structures or regions. The less dense adipose or fatty tissues appear light to dark gray, depending on the thickness of these tissues.

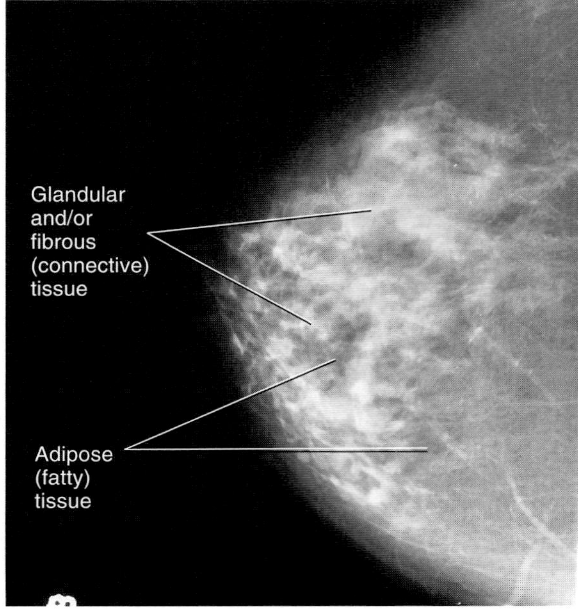

Fig. 18-7. Film-screen mammogram.

BREAST CLASSIFICATIONS

Technical radiographic factors for any one part of the body are determined mainly by the thickness of that particular part. A large elbow, for example, will require greater exposure factors than a small elbow. In mammography, however, **both** the **compressed breast thickness** and the **tissue density** contribute to technique selection. The breast size or thickness is easy to determine, but breast density is less obvious and requires additional information.

The relative density of the breast is primarily affected by the patient's inherent breast characteristics, hormone status, age, and pregnancies. The mammary gland undergoes cyclic changes associated with the rise and fall of hormonal secretions during the menstrual cycle, changes during pregnancy and lactation, and gradual changes that occur throughout a woman's lifetime.

Generally speaking, however, breasts can be classified into **three broad categories**, depending on the relative amounts of fibro-glandular tissue versus fatty tissue.

(1) Fibro-Glandular Breast

The first category is the fibro-glandular breast. The younger breast is usually quite dense, since it contains relatively little fatty tissue. The common age grouping for the fibro-glandular category is post-puberty to about age thirty. However, those females over the age of 30 who have never given birth to a live infant will probably also be in this general grouping. Pregnant or lactating females of any age are also placed in this grouping because they possess a very dense type of breast.

(2) Fibro-Fatty Breast

A second general category is the fibro-fatty breast. As the female ages and more changes occur in the breast tissues, there is a gradual shift from a low amount of fatty tissue to a more equal distribution of fat and fibro-glandular tissue. Therefore, in a 30- to 50-year-old group, the breast is not quite as dense as in the younger group.

Radiographically, this breast is of average density and requires less exposure than the fibro-glandular type of breast.

Several pregnancies early in a woman's reproductive life will accelerate her breast development toward this fibro-fatty category.

(3) Fatty Breast

A third and final grouping is the fatty breast that occurs following menopause, commonly age 50 and above. Following a female's reproductive life, most of the glandular breast tissue atrophies and is converted to fatty tissue in a process called involution. Even less exposure is required on this type of breast than is required on the first two types of breasts.

The breasts of children and most males contain mostly fat in small proportions and therefore fall into this category also. While most mammograms are performed on the female patient, it is well to realize that between 1 and 2 percent of all breast cancer is found in the male; therefore, mammograms will occasionally be performed on a male.

Summary: In summary, in addition to breast size or thickness upon compression, the average density of the tissues of the breast will determine exposure factors. The most dense breast is the fibro-glandular type. The least dense is the fatty type, and the breast with equal amounts of fatty and fibro-glandular tissue is termed fibro-fatty.

Breast Classifications
(1) Fibro-glandular breast
Common age group–15 to 30 years (and childless females over age 30)
Pregnant or lactating females
Radiographically dense
Very little fat
(2) Fibro-fatty breast
Common age group–30 to 50 years
Young women with 3 or more pregnancies
Average density, radiographically
50% fat and 50% fibro-glandular
(3) Fatty breast
Common age group–50 years and over
Postmenopausal
Minimal density, radiographically
Atrophic
Breasts of children and males

Fig. 18-8. Summary–Breast classifications.

Radiographic Positioning

BREAST POSITIONING

In mammography, the great variability of the breast, with respect to the proportion of fatty tissue to fibroglandular tissue, presents certain technical difficulties. In producing a superior quality mammogram, the shape and contour of the normal breast poses additional problems to the radiographer.

The **base** of the breast is that portion near the chest wall, while the area near the nipple is termed the **apex**. In either the craniocaudad or the mediolateral projection, the base of the breast is much thicker and contains much denser tissues than the apex.

To overcome this anatomical difference, compression is used in combination with a specially designed tube so the more intense central portion of the x-ray beam (CR) penetrates the thicker base of the breast.

X-ray Tube

The most distinctive aspect of the mammography machine is the unique design of the x-ray tube, which has a molybdenum target with small focal spots of 0.3 and 0.1 mm. The anode configuration produces a **prominent heel effect** due to the short source-to-image receptor distance (SID), and the use of a narrow reference target angle. Because the x-ray tube is aligned with the cathode placed over the base of the breast (at chest wall) and the anode outward toward the apex (nipple area), the heel effect fortunately can be used to maximum advantage (Fig. 18-9). Since the cathode side of the x-ray beam has significantly greater intensity of x-rays compared to the anode side, a more uniform-density breast image can be produced because the more intense x-rays are at the base, where there is greater tissue thickness. The primary reason the cathode end of the mammography x-ray tube is placed directly over the base or chest wall edge of the image is to take advantage of the prominent heel effect of the anode.

Grids are commonly used for most mammograms, along with **automatic exposure control** (AEC) and the important breast **compression device**.

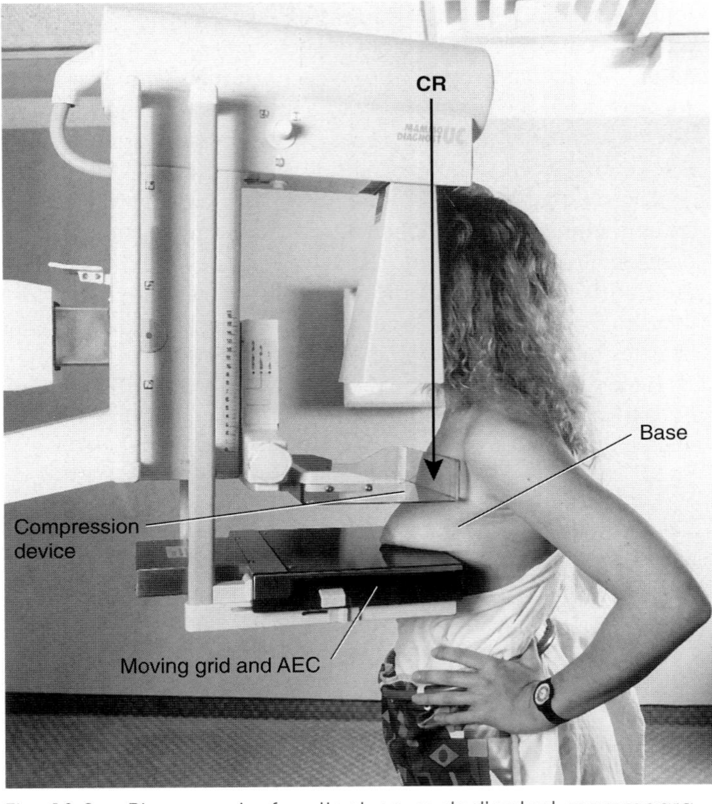

Fig. 18-9. Placement of patient on a dedicated mammography unit for a craniocaudal (CC) projection. (Compression is not firmly applied for this photo.)

Note: Vertical CR is placed directly over the chest wall structures, which allows the posterosuperior breast structures to be imaged.

18

Compression*

All mammography machines contain a compression device that is used to compress the breast. Improvements in breast compression technology in recent years have greatly improved the visibility of detail in breast images. The compression device is made of a plastic that allows transmission of the low energy x-rays. The device should have a straight chest wall edge to allow the compression to grasp the breast tissues close to the chest wall. Compression is controlled by the radiographer and is typically applied at **25 to 40 pounds** of force.

In addition to the standard compression device, a smaller "spot" device may be used to compress localized areas. The compression device should be checked regularly to ensure that it is working properly and applying the correct amount of pressure.

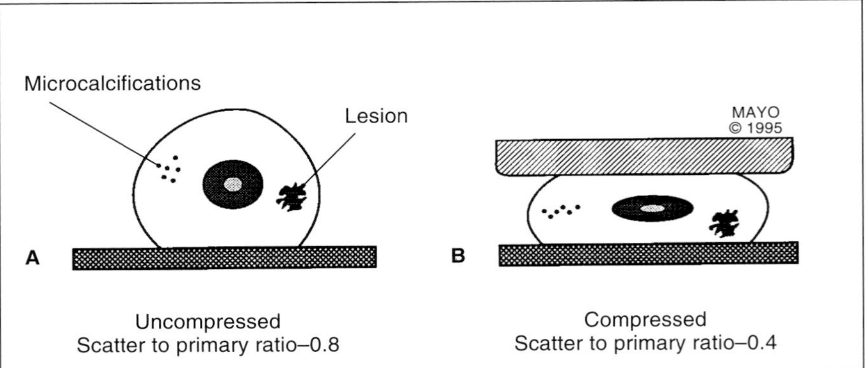

Fig. 18-10. The effect of breast compression.
(1) Decreased tissue thickness (less scatter, better resolution).
(2) Breast structures closer to film.

Appropriately applied compression is one of the critical components in the production of a high quality mammogram. The **two-part function of compression** is to (1) decrease the thickness of the breast and (2) bring the breast structures as close to the film as possible. These two factors improve image quality or resolution by reducing scatter and also by reducing magnification of breast structures. This is illustrated by comparing the uncompressed and compressed drawings above. Note the location of the microcalcifications and lesion which are surrounded by dense breast tissue in drawing A, and how compression has brought them closer to the film (drawing B). Therefore, the overall breast thickness has also been greatly reduced, which reduces the scatter to primary radiation ratio by one-half.

* Frank, ED, "Technical Aspects of Mammography," Ch. 40 in *Principles of Radiographic Exposure, 2nd ed.* by Carlton, R.L. and Adler, A.M.; Delmar Publishers, 1996.

Magnification (Fig. 18-11)

The magnification method is used to enlarge specific areas of interest such as small lesions or microcalcifications. This requires an x-ray tube with a **0.1 mm focal spot** to maintain image resolution. Enlargements of 1½ to 2 times can be used by inserting a magnification platform between the film and the breast, thereby magnifying the part. This magnification technique can be used with most mammogram projections.

Patient Dose

Patient dose is significant in mammography, as seen by the dose icon boxes included on each positioning page. A skin dose of 800-900 mrad is common for mammograms, which is much higher than for most other body parts. For example, a lateral lumbar spine at 90 kVp, 50 mAs, has a skin dose of 700-800 and a midline dose of ≈100 mrad (page 291). This is one of the highest dose projections of any body part. The reason for the relatively high dose for mammograms is the very low kVp (25 to 28) and the high mAs (75 to 85) required.

The principal way patient dose is controlled in mammography is by careful and accurate positioning, which minimizes the need for repeats. The ACR (American College of Radiology) recommends a repeat rate of **less than 5%** for mammography.

Shielding: The only shielding possible is a waist apron for shielding the gonadal region.

Note: The patient dose icon boxes in this chapter include an **MGD** (**Mean Glandular Dose**), which is the average breast tissue dose, rather than a specific midline dose as for other body parts.

IMAGING MODALITIES

Various modalities for studying the tissues of the breast have been developed. Xeromammography, which was used in the 70s and 80s is no longer used for mammography due to major technical advances in screen-film mammography and machine design. **Film-screen mammography** and **sonography** (ultrasound) are currently the primary imaging modalities used. Film-screen mammography, however, remains the most important and the most widely used. In a modern mammography department, film-screen mammography and sonography are used together to diagnose breast disease.

Mammography

Mammography is the **x-ray examination of the breast**. Many factors contribute to the overall quality of a mammogram. Some of these are the x-ray machine characteristics such as focal spot size, target material, beam filtration, kVp and mAs selection, film or other material selection, intensifying screens, breast position and compression, image processing, and the training and qualifications of the operator.

Film-screen Mammography: Film-screen mammography is the standard in current breast radiography. The greatest benefit of the film-screen system is an **excellent image with the lowest radiation dose possible,** allowing women to have this examination regularly. The ability to see **fine detail**, **edge sharpness**, and **soft tissue** is a hallmark of a good film mammogram.

Sonography

Sonography has been used to image the breast since the mid 1970s. It provides valuable adjunct information for the radiologist along with the screen-film mammogram and physical examination. Today sonography is an integral part of the mammography department and the mammogram examination. Its major value is its ability to **distinguish a cyst from a solid lesion**. It is also used extensively to determine fluid, abscess, hematoma, and silicone gel. Mammographers may also be trained to perform sonography of the breast in addition to screen-film mammography.

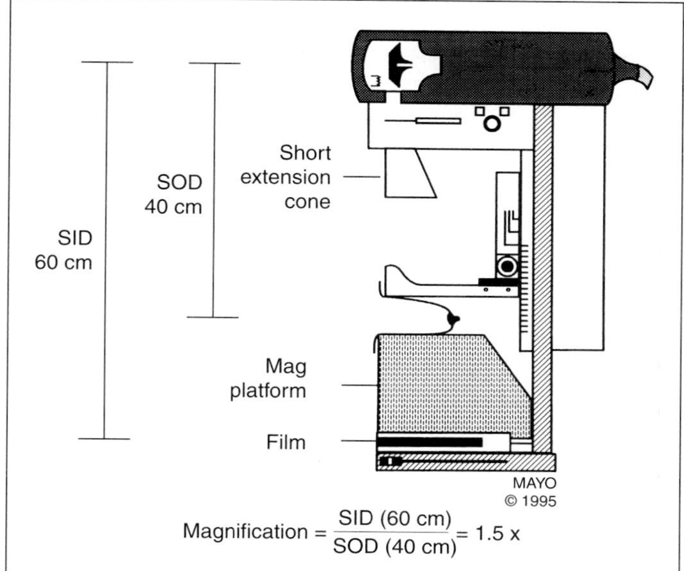

Fig. 18-11. Breast magnification–Breast in position on a raised platform to produce a 1.5x magnification image.

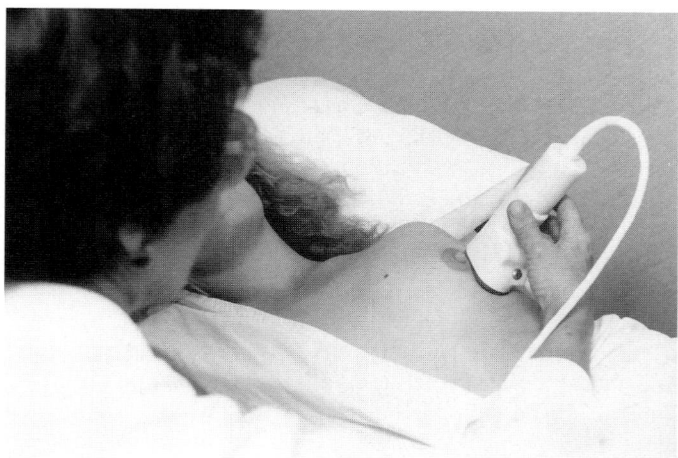

Fig. 18-12. Conventional scanner with hand-held transducer.

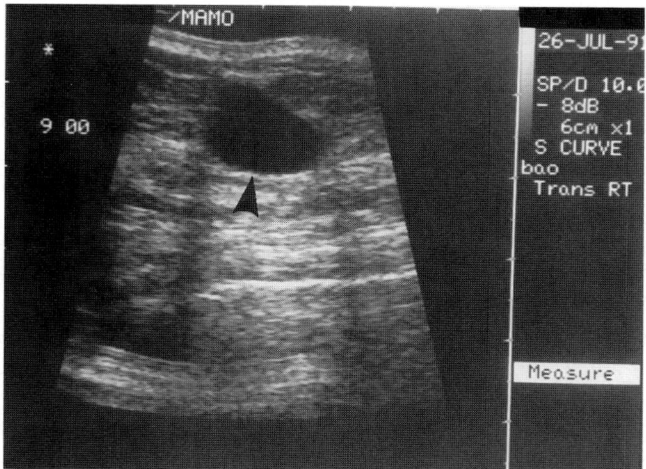

Fig. 18-13. Breast sonogram obtained with conventional scanner showing a cyst (arrow).

Conventional Scanner and Hand-Held Transducer: With a high-resolution conventional scanner (Fig. 18-12), the patient is supine or rolled up slightly on a side. The hand-held transducer is placed on a palpable mass or an area noted on a mammogram. Fig. 18-13 shows an image from such a scanner. Sonographic imaging is not recommended for routine screening.

18

NEW BREAST IMAGING MODALITIES

Magnetic Resonance Imaging (MRI)

MRI is generally not yet an acceptable method of diagnosing breast cancer. Breast MRI techniques have not yet been standardized and at the time of this writing the lack of commercially available techniques and equipment makes this a speculative breast imaging modality. In addition its cost makes it prohibitive for general clinical use. However, for certain applications, MRI has been clinically proven to be very effective.

Dense Breast Tissue: As an adjunct to mammographic studies, MRI has shown to be useful for classifying suspicious lesions and micro-calcifications that have been identified on mammograms. MRI is especially helpful in evaluating small and very dense breast tissue (see Figs. 18-14 to 18-17).

Breast Implants: Over 1 million women in the U.S. have breast augmentation (implants). Silicone and saline implants are radiopaque, requiring implant-displaced views (Eklund technique). Compression is more difficult with implants, and extra care must be taken by the radiographer not to rupture the implant. Automatic exposure control (AEC) also cannot be used with augmented breasts, all of which makes imaging of breast tissue with implants a challenge using conventional screening mammograms or ultrasound techniques.

MRI has been clinically proven to be most effective in diagnosing problems related to breast implant imaging. For example, with MRI it is possible to exclude the possibility of intracapsular and extracapsular rupture, including the area posterior to the implant, which is very problematic with either mammography or sonography studies. The MRI image in Fig. 18-18 clearly demonstrates an extracapsular rupture of a silicone implant.

In addition to diagnosing implant rupture, it is also important to demonstrate the breast tissue surrounding and posterior to the implants for possible malignant growth. Physical examination is more difficult with implants, which also increases the risk of cancer growth without detection. MRI, unlike mammography or sonography, is not hindered by the presence of an implant.

Clinical testing is being done with a new kind of radiolucent implant that will allow more effective use of film-screen mammography, including the use of automatic exposure controls. However, the over 1 million women with radiopaque implants, many of whom are nearing the life expectancy limits of the implants, will require more and more evaluations of breast implants for possible rupture or other related problems. This in turn increases the potential role of MRI with breast implant imaging.

Digital Mammography

Digital mammography is very promising at this time. Many believe this technique will eventually replace screen-film mammography. As with other forms of digital radiography, the advantages include the ability to enhance and modify the digital images without additional radiation exposure to the patient. Overall dose to the patient can also be decreased without compromising image quality. However, at the time of this writing, additional development of equipment, along with clinical testing, needs to occur before this becomes a viable breast imaging technique.

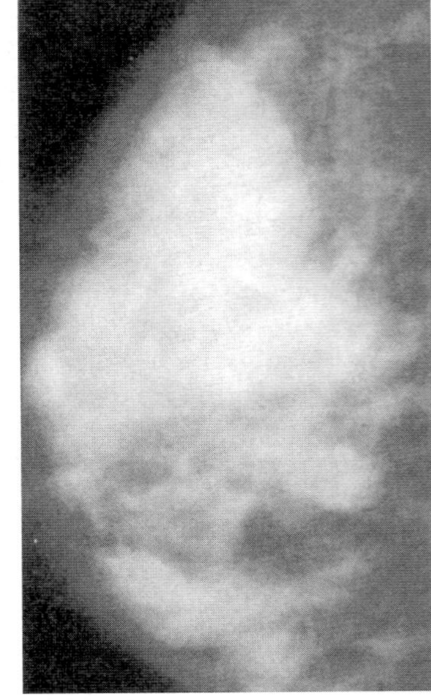

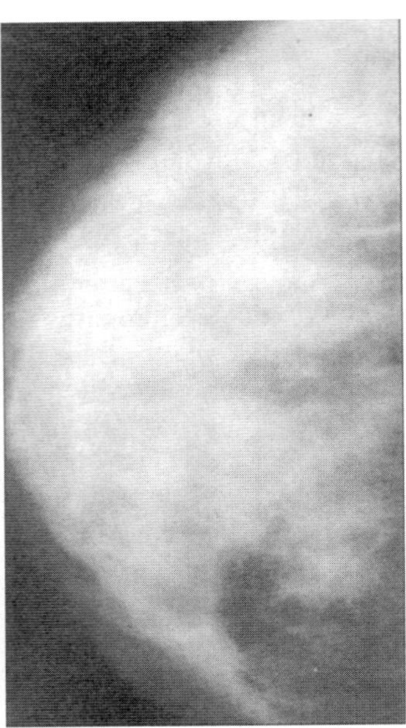

Fig. 18-14. CC mammogram. Fig. 18-15. MLO mammogram. Palpable mass not demonstrated–Very dense breast tissue.

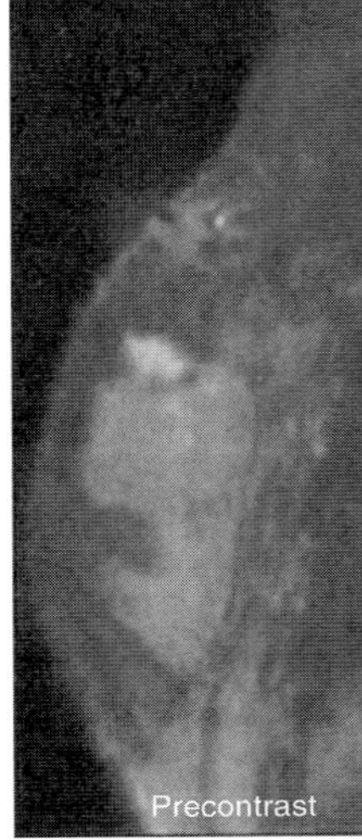

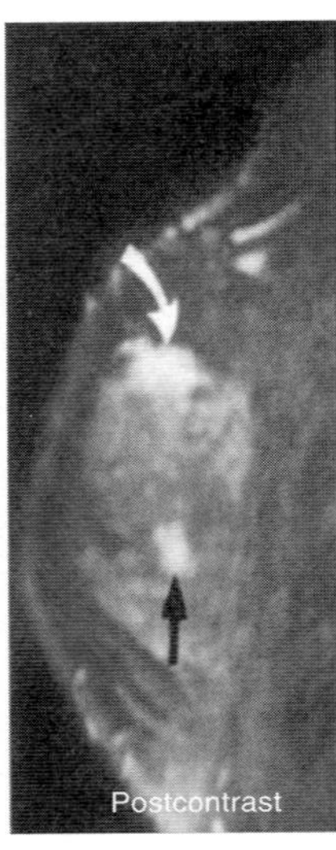

Fig. 18-16. MRI sagittal images. Fig. 18-17. Patient with dense breast tissue with palpable mass in upper outer quadrant. Not identified in mammogram films above but demonstrated on MRI sagittal image as carcinoma (arrows).

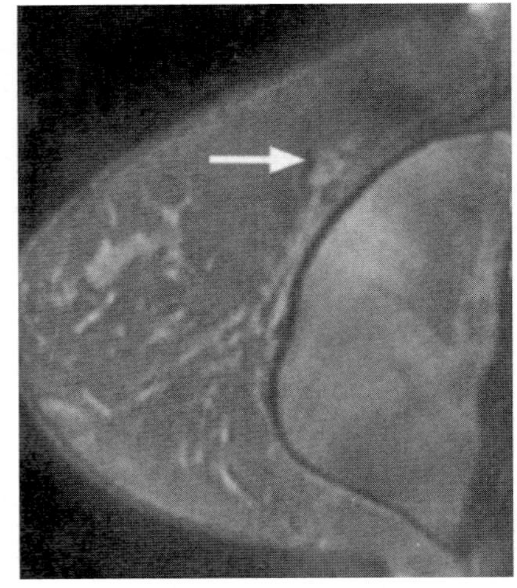

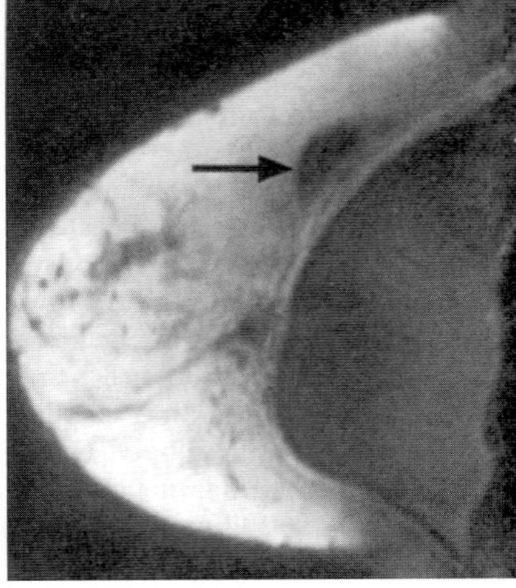

Fig. 18-18. MRI image demonstrating extracapsular rupture of silicone implant. Arrow indicates a collection of free silicone anterior to the subpectoral implant.

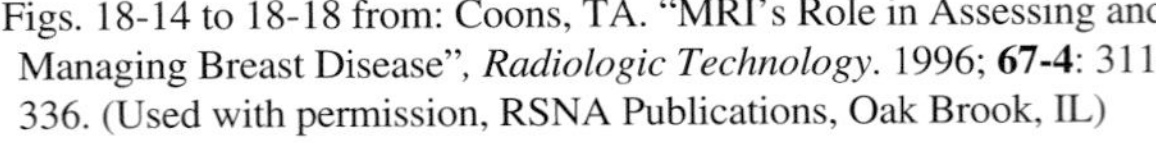

Figs. 18-14 to 18-18 from: Coons, TA. "MRI's Role in Assessing and Managing Breast Disease", *Radiologic Technology.* 1996; **67-4**: 311-336. (Used with permission, RSNA Publications, Oak Brook, IL)

Terminology and Abbreviations

Certain positioning terminology, some of which is unique to mammography, needs to be understood and used correctly. These terms with their abbreviations are used to identify films and are standard nomenclature as approved by the ACR in October 1995. These **terms** and **abbreviations** should be used correctly when applying for ACR accreditation.

Mammography Teminology Chart

ACR nomenclature	*Description*
CC	**Craniocaudal**: A basic superior to inferior projection.
MLO	Superomedial-inferolateral oblique, **mediolateral oblique,** the basic oblique.
XCCL*	**Laterally exaggerated craniocaudal**: A special CC projection with emphasis on the axillary tissue.
ML	**Mediolateral** projection.
LM	**Lateromedial** projection.
ID	**Implant displaced** (for Eklund technique views).
AX	**Axillary view** (for lymph nodes and other axillary content).
CV	**Cleavage view**, a double breast compression view. (Demonstrates breast tissue anterior to the sternum and the medial aspects of both breasts.)
AT	**Axillary tail view**, Cleopatra view, 20-30° oblique.
LMO	**Inferolateral-superomedial**, with pacemaker.
SIO	**Superolateral-inferomedial oblique**, reverse oblique.
TAN	**Tangential** (also mark film with view and degree of angulation).
RL†	**Rolled lateral.**
RM†	**Rolled medial.**
FB	Caudocranial, **from below** (sometimes in practice also abbreviated as CCFB). Film should be marked with any deviation from 0° with LMO or SIO.

*XCCL is the correct official ACR abbreviation for this projection. In practice, however, and in some literature it has been abbreviated as XLCC (exaggerated lateral craniocaudal).
†Used as a suffix after the projection.

18

Basic and Special Projections

The most **basic** or primary screening projections currently performed in mammography are the **craniocaudal** (CC) and **mediolateral oblique** (MLO).

In addition, the **laterally exaggerated craniocaudal (XCCL)** and the **mediolateral (ML)** are described because of their frequent use as additional or special projections. Also, because of the increasing number of patients who have breast implant procedures, the **Eklund technique** procedure is included.

Mammogram
Basic
- Craniocaudal (CC) **538**
- Mediolateral oblique (MLO) **539**

Special
- Laterally exaggerated craniocaudal (XCCL) **540**
- Mediolateral (ML) **541**
- Implant procedure (Eklund technique) **542**

Craniocaudal (CC) Projection

Mammogram
Basic
• **Craniocaudal (CC)**
• Mediolateral oblique (MLO)

Structures Best Shown

Entire breast tissue.

Both breasts are imaged on separate films for comparison.

Technical Factors

- Film size –8 x 10 in. (18 x 24 cm), crosswise
  or –10 x 12 in. (24 x 30 cm), crosswise.
- Moving grid.
- 25 to 28 kVp.
- Technique and dose:

kVp	mAs	Sk.	MGD
25	75	867	133
		mrad	

8 (10)
10 (12)
L

Shielding: Waist apron.

Patient Position

- Standing; if not possible, seated.

Part Position

- Film tray height is determined by **lifting the breast** to achieve a 90° angle to the chest wall. The tray will be at the level of **the inframammary crease at its upper limits**.
- The breast is pulled forward onto the film holder centrally with the **nipple in profile**.
- The arm on the side being imaged is relaxed and the shoulder is back out of the way.
- The head is turned away from the side being imaged.
- Wrinkles and folds on the breast should be smoothed out and compression applied until taut.
- The marker and patient ID information is always placed on the **axillary side**.

Central Ray

- Perpendicular centered to the base of the breast, the chest wall edge of the cassette. The CR is not moveable.
- **SID**: Fixed, varies with manufacturer, about 60 cm (23.6 in).

Collimation: Use appropriate cone.

Respiration: Suspend breathing.

Evaluation Criteria

- No motion is evident.
- The central, subareolar, and medial breast should be visualized (sometimes pectoral muscle is included).
- Nipple is seen in profile.
- Tissue thickness is distributed evenly on the film.
- Optimum compression is noted.
- Dense areas are adequately penetrated.
- High tissue contrast and optimal resolution noted.
- Absence of artifacts.
- Marker is in proper position and patient identification is accurate with date included.

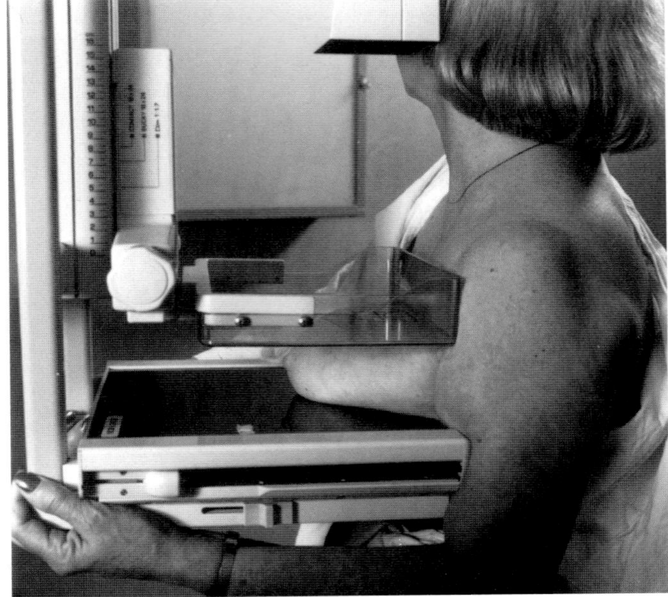

Fig. 18-19. CC projection.

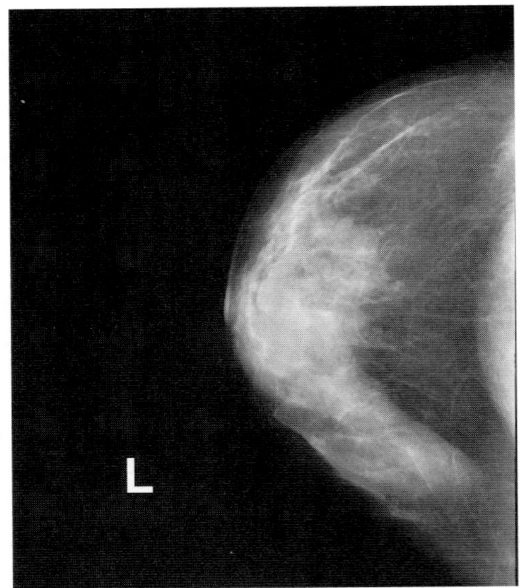

Fig. 18-20. CC projection.

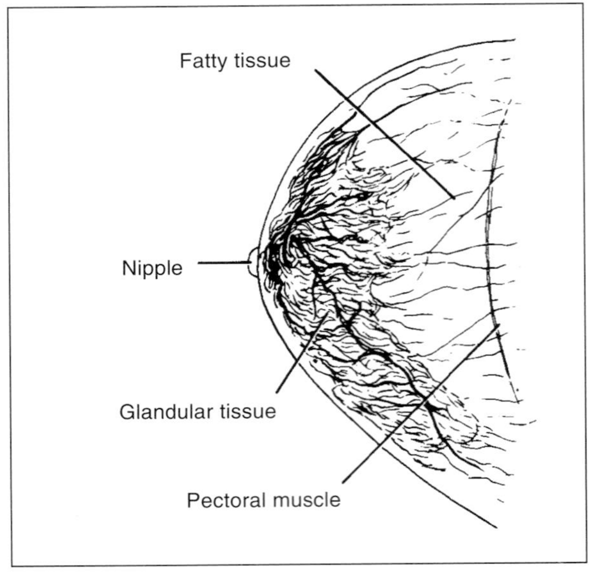

Fig. 18-21. CC projection.

Mediolateral Oblique (MLO) Projection

(Superomedial-Inferolateral Oblique)

Mammogram
Basic
• Craniocaudal (CC)
• **Mediolateral oblique (MLO)**

Structures Best Shown

Entire breast tissue.

Both breasts are imaged on separate films for comparison.

Technical Factors

• Film size –8 x 10 in. (18 x 24 cm), crosswise
  or –10 x 12 in. (24 x 30 cm), crosswise.
• Moving grid.
• 25 to 28 kVp.

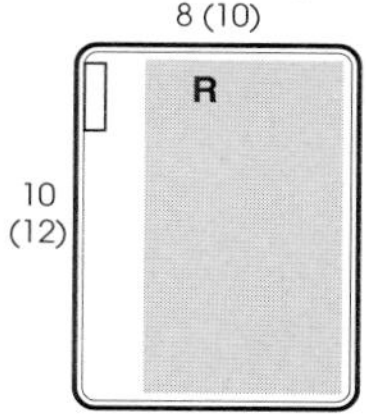

• Technique and dose:

kVp	mAs	Sk.	MGD
25	85	983	151
		mrad	

Shielding: Waist apron.

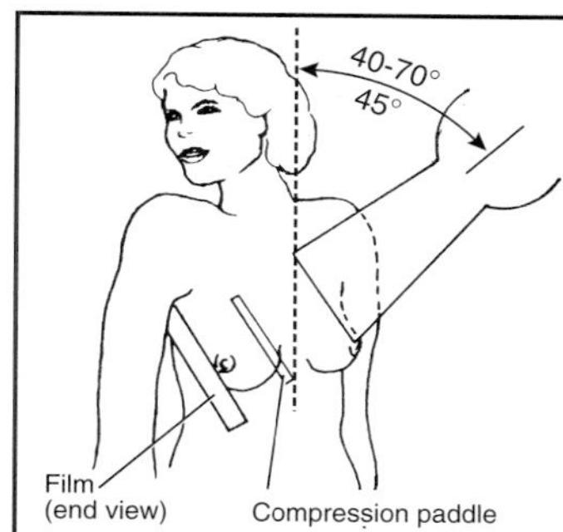

Fig. 18-22. MLO projection.

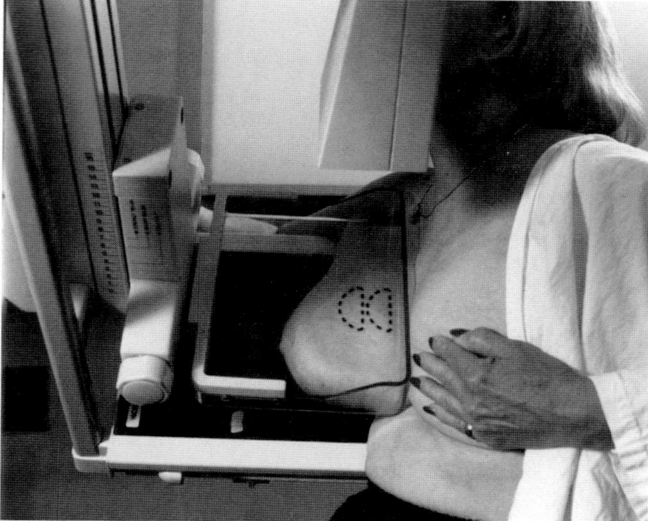

Fig. 18-23. MLO projection. (Note x-ray tube/film unit angled about 45°, see Fig. 18-22.)

Patient Position

• Standing; if not possible, seated.

Part Position

• Tube and film holder remain at right angles to each other as **CR is angled about 45°**. CR enters the breast **medially,** perpendicular to the patient's pectoral muscle.
  –Heavy and large-breasted women, angle 40 to 60° from vertical.
  –Thin and small-breasted women, angle 60 to 70° from vertical.
• Adjust film height so top of film will be at the level of the axilla.
• With the patient facing the unit and feet forward exactly like CC view, place the arm of the side being imaged forward and the hand on the bar toward the front.
• Pull breast tissue and pectoral muscle **anteriorly** and **medially away from chest wall.** Push the patient slightly toward the angled film holder until the inferolateral aspect of the breast is touching the film holder. The nipple should be in profile.
• Apply compression slowly with the **breast held away from the chest wall and up**, to prevent sagging.
• The upper edge of the compression device will rest under the clavicle and the lower edge will include the inframammary fold.
• Wrinkles and folds on the breast should be smoothed out and compression applied until taut.
• If necessary, have patient gently retract opposite breast with other hand to prevent superimposition.
• The marker should be placed high and at the axilla.

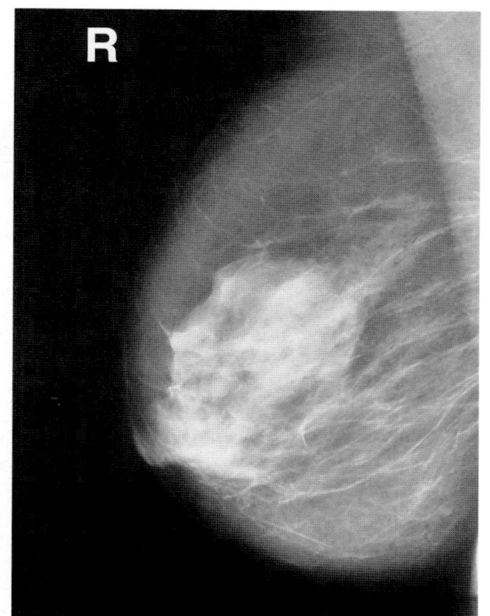

Fig. 18-24. MLO projection.

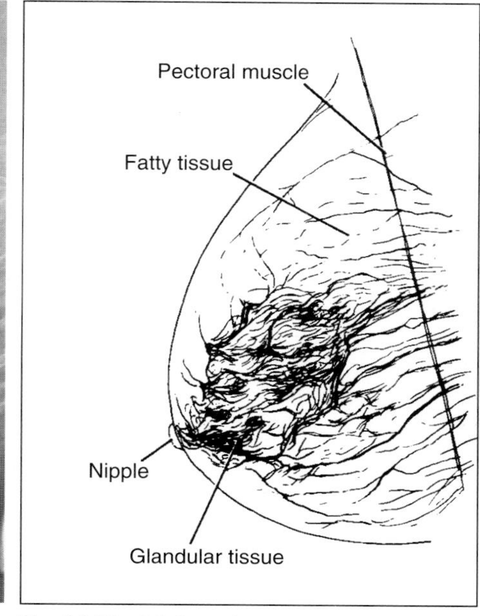

Fig. 18-25. MLO projection.

Note: To show **all** of the breast tissue on this projection with a large breast, two films may be needed, one positioned higher to get all of the axillary region and a second film positioned lower to include the main part of the breast.

Central Ray

• Perpendicular centered to the base of the breast, the chest wall edge of the cassette. The CR is not movable.
• **SID**: Fixed, varies with manufacturer, about 60 cm (23.6 in).

Collimation: Use appropriate cone.

Respiration: Suspend breathing.

Evaluation Criteria:

• No motion is evident.
• A correctly positioned MLO will visualize the pectoral muscle down to the level of the nipple.
• Breast must be shown to be pulled out and away from the chest so as not to droop, with nipple in profile.
• Optimum compression is noted.
• Dense areas are adequately penetrated.
• High tissue contrast and optimal resolution noted.
• Absence of artifacts.
• Marker is in proper position and patient identification is accurate with date included.

Laterally Exaggerated Craniocaudal (XCCL) Projection

Mammogram
Special
- **Laterally exaggerated craniocaudal (XCCL)**
- Mediolateral (ML)
- Implant procedure (Eklund technique)

Structures Best Shown

Breast tissue with emphasis on the **axillary tissue**.

This is the most frequently requested optional projection. It is done if the CC projection does not show all the axillary tissue. In addition it is usually requested when a lesion is seen on the MLO but not on the CC.

Technical Factors

- Film size –8 x 10 in. (18 x 24 cm), crosswise or –10 x 12 in. (24 x 30 cm), crosswise.
- Moving grid.
- 25 to 28 kVp.
- Technique and dose:

kVp	mAs	Sk.	MGD
25	75	867	133

mrad

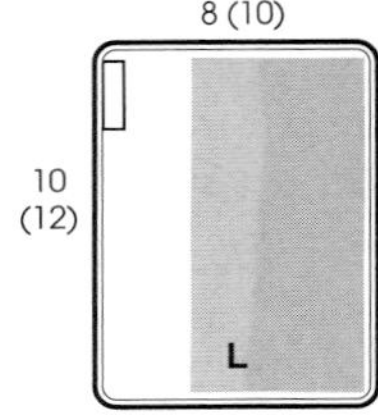

Shielding: Waist apron.

Patient Position

- Standing. If not possible, seated.

Part Position

- Begin as if to do a CC projection but **rotate the body** slightly as needed to include more of the **axillary** aspect of breast (Fig. 18-26).
- Put the patient's hand on the bar toward the front and relax the shoulder. (Some recommend angling the tube 5° mediolaterally.)
- The head is turned away from the side being imaged.
- The breast is pulled forward onto the film holder, wrinkles and folds should be smoothed out, and compression applied until taut. The nipple should be in profile.
- The marker is always placed on the axillary side.

Central Ray

- Perpendicular, centered to the base of the breast, the chest wall edge of the cassette. The CR is not movable.
- SID: Fixed, varies with manufacturer, about 60 cm (23.6 in).

Collimation: Use appropriate cone.

Respiration: Suspend breathing.

Notes: If a lesion is deeper, do an **AT** (**axillary tail** or **Cleopatra**) view.

If a lesion is not found on lateral aspect of breast, do **medially exaggerated craniocaudad** view.

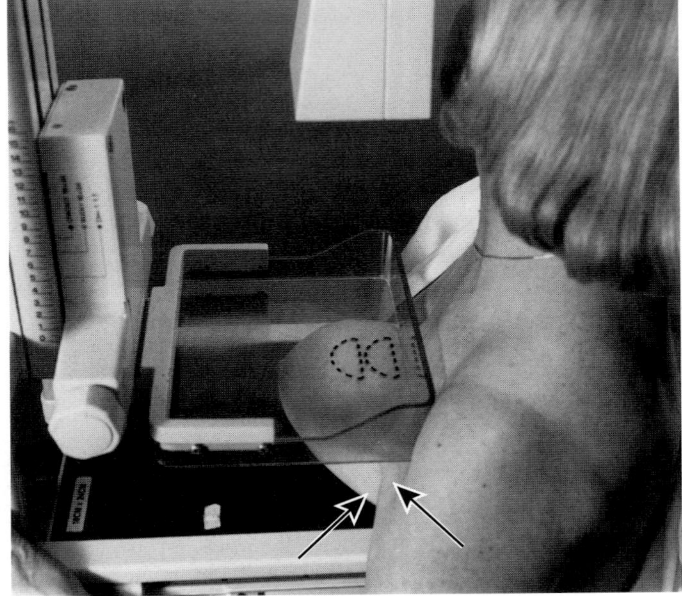

Fig. 18-26. XCCL projection.
Note: Patient is turned so axillary tissue (arrows) is included on the image. Note arm and hand is forward for ease in turning body.

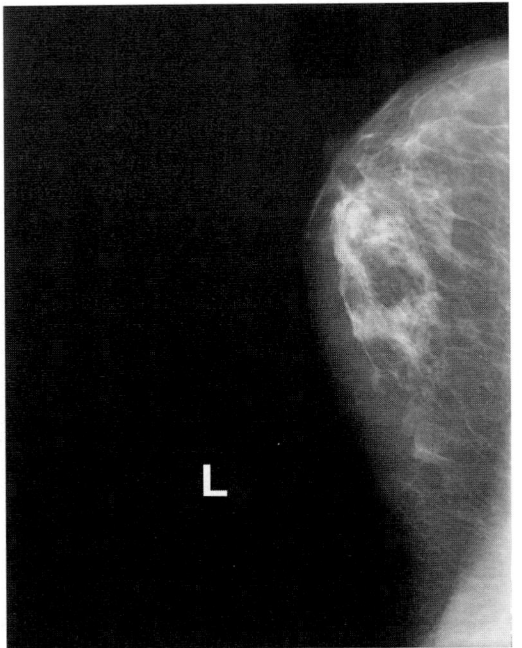

Fig. 18-27. XCCL projection.

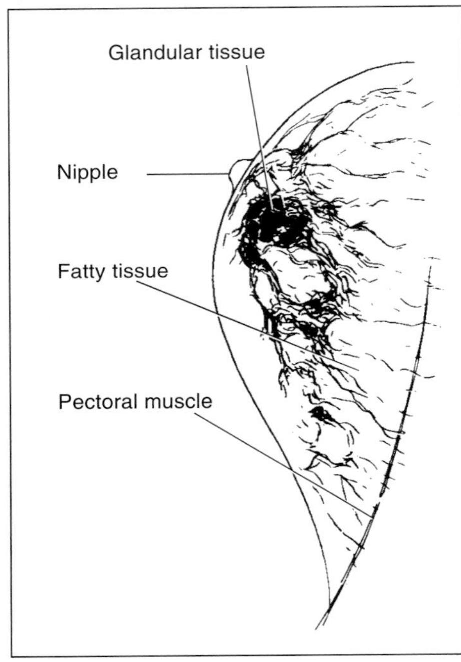

Fig. 18-28. XCCL projection.

Evaluation Criteria

- No evidence of motion.
- Evaluation criteria from CC projection also applies to this projection.
- Nipple should be seen in profile.
- The axillary aspect of the breast should be well visualized.
- May see pectoral muscle.
- Marker is in proper position and patient identification is accurate with date included.

Mediolateral (ML)–True Lateral Projection

Mammogram
Special
- Laterally exaggerated craniocaudal (XCCL)
- **Mediolateral (ML)**
- Implant procedure (Eklund technique)

Structures Best Shown

Milk of calcium (an inflammation process of the breast).

This projection may be requested by the radiologist as an optional projection to check whether an abnormality is real when seen only on the MLO.

Technical Factors

- Film size –8 x 10 in. (18 x 24 cm), crosswise or –10 x 12 in. (24 x 30 cm), crosswise.
- Moving grid.
- 25 to 28 kVp.
- Technique and dose:

kVp	mAs	Sk.	MGD
25	85	983	151

mrad

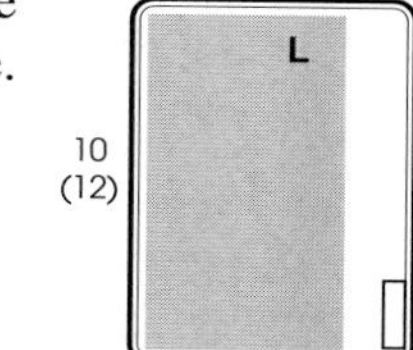

Shielding: Waist apron.

Patient Position

- Standing. If not possible, seated.

Part Position

- Tube and film holder remain at right angles to each other as **CR is angled 90°** from vertical.
- Adjust film height to be centered to mid breast.
- With patient facing the unit feet forward, place arm of the side being imaged forward and the hand on the bar toward the front.
- Pull breast tissue and pectoral muscle anteriorly and medially away from the chest wall. Push the patient slightly toward film holder until the inferolateral aspect of the breast is touching the film holder. The nipple should be in profile.
- Apply compression slowly with the breast held away from the chest wall and up to prevent sagging. After paddle has passed the sternum, rotate patient until breast is in a true lateral position.
- Wrinkles and folds on the breast should be smoothed out and compression applied until taut.
- Open inframammary fold by pulling abdominal tissue down.
- If necessary, have patient gently retract opposite breast with other hand to prevent superimposition.
- The marker should be placed high and at the axilla.

Central Ray

- Perpendicular, centered to the base of the breast, the chest wall edge of the cassette. The CR is not movable.
- SID: Fixed, varies with manufacturer, about 60 cm (23.6 in).

Collimation: Use appropriate cone.

Respiration: Suspend breathing.

Evaluation Criteria

- No evidence of motion.
- Tissue thickness is distributed evenly on the film.
- Nipple is seen in profile.
- Optimum compression is noted.
- Dense areas are adequately penetrated.
- High tissue contrast and optimal resolution noted.
- Absence of artifacts.
- Marker is in proper position and patient identification is accurate with date included.

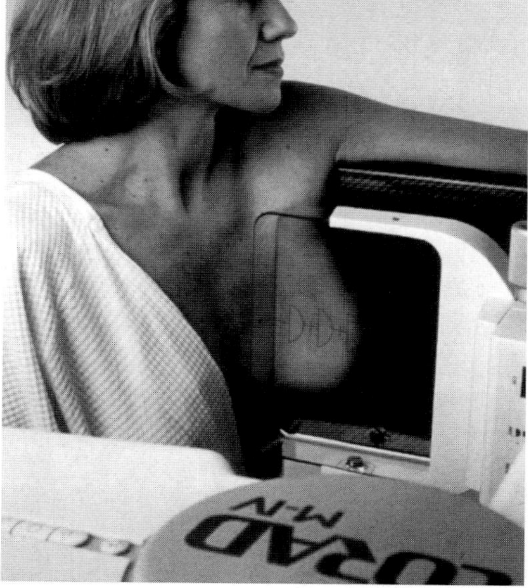

Fig. 18-29. ML projection.

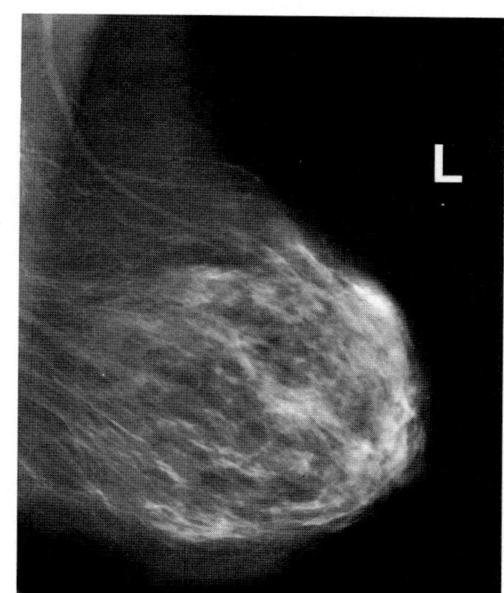

Fig. 18-30. ML projection.

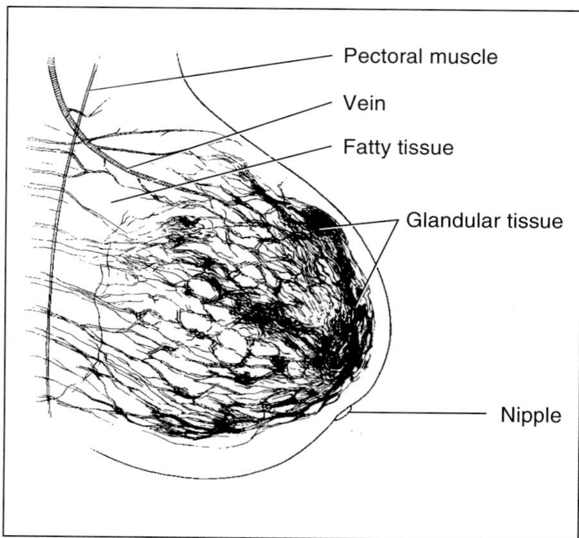

Fig. 18-31. ML projection.

Implant Procedure with the Ecklund Technique*

Mammogram
Special
- Laterally exaggerated craniocaudal (XCCL)
- Mediolateral (ML)
- **Implant procedure (Eklund technique)**

Patients who have breast implant procedures done for size and shape enhancement also require routine mammography. However, a slightly different technique is used as follows:

Standard CC and MLO Projections:

Standard CC and MLO projections, as previously described, are done first with the implant device in place (Fig. 18-32). Caution must be used with the compression device—firm compression cannot be accomplished.

Ecklund Technique:

The Eklund technique of "pinching" the breast (Figs. 18-34 and 18-35) is performed after the basic CC and MLO projections. During this procedure, the implant is pushed posteriorly to the chest wall so that the anterior breast tissue can be compressed and visualized in the usual manner (Fig. 18-33).

Exception: The Eklund technique can be performed on most patients with implants; however, some implants become encapsulated and only the routine views with the implant in place can be done. An additional projection such as the mediolateral or lateromedial may be helpful to demonstrate all the tissue.

Manual exposure techniques: For those projections done with the implant in place, only **manual exposure techniques can be set** on the generator because the implant device will prevent the x-ray photons from reaching the phototimer sensor. **This will cause overexposure of the breast** and the AEC system may possibly go to maximum backup time, overexposing the radiograph.

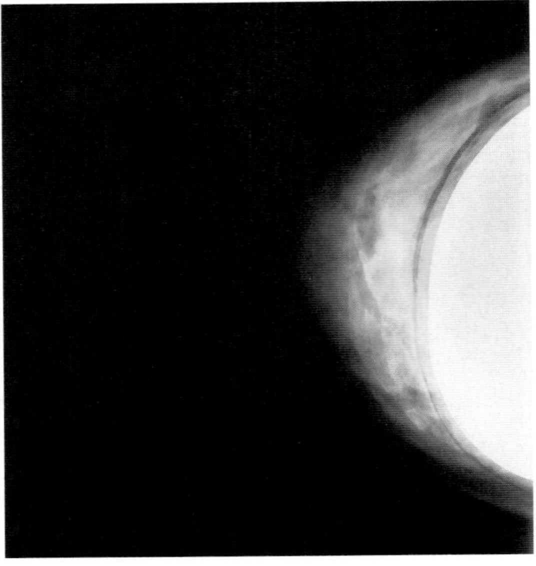

Fig. 18-32. Standard CC projection with implant in place.

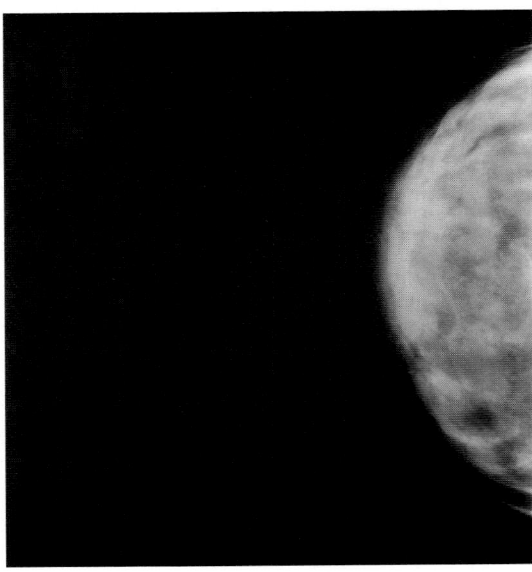

Fig. 18-33. Standard CC projection with implant pushed back. (Same patient as in Fig. 18-32).

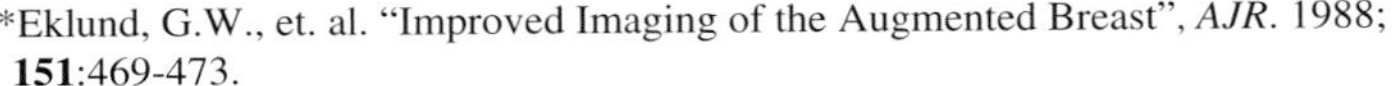

*Eklund, G.W., et. al. "Improved Imaging of the Augmented Breast", *AJR*. 1988; **151**:469-473.

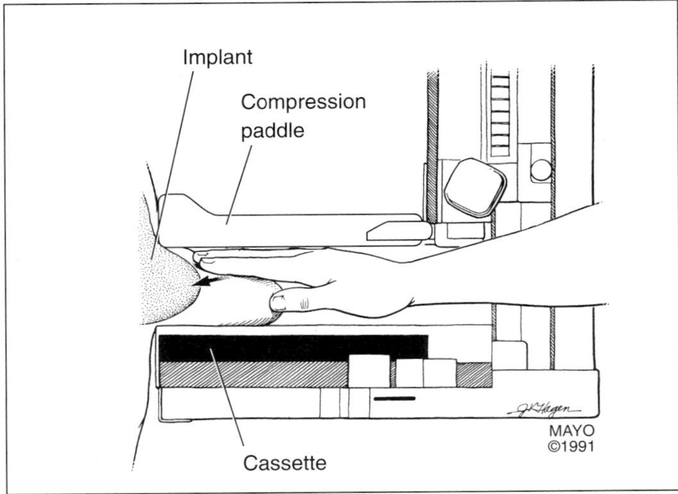

Fig. 18-34. Positioning with Eklund "pinch" technique.

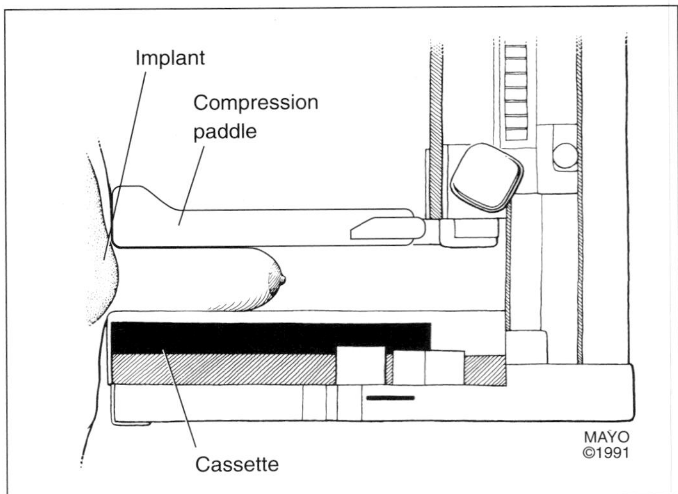

Fig. 18-35. Breast in place for CC projection with implant pushed back.

Radiographs for Critique

Each of these radiographs demonstrates some errors that required a repeat. These radiographs (which are also available as part of the lecture slide set) can provide a basis for classroom or lab discussions. Questions concerning the reasons for these to be repeated, along with answers, are included in the student workbook/lab manuals that accompany this textbook.

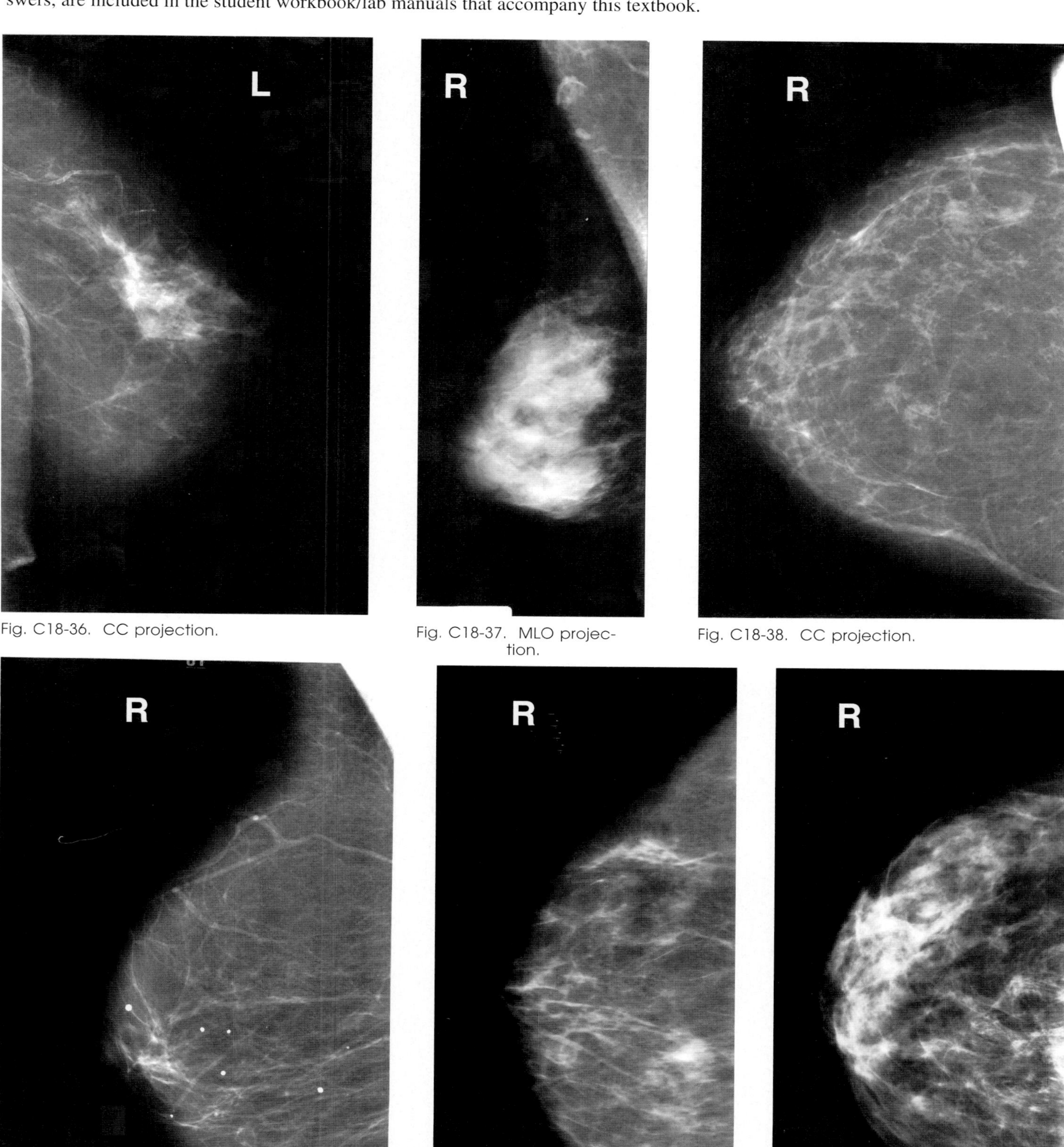

Fig. C18-36. CC projection.

Fig. C18-37. MLO projection.

Fig. C18-38. CC projection.

Fig. C18-39. MLO projection.

Fig. C18-40. CC projection.

Fig. C18-41. CC projection.

CHAPTER 19

Trauma and Mobile Radiography

CONTRIBUTIONS BY:
James A. Sanderson, BS, RT (R)

CONTENTS

Terminology, Principles and Equipment

Trauma and Fracture Terminology
- Dislocation, sprain and fracture **546**
- Fracture alignment terminology **547**
- Types of fractures **548**
- Specific "named" fractures **549**
- Additional fracture types **550**
- Post reduction radiographs **551**

Positioning Principles and Grid Use

Two positioning principles:
(1) Two projections at 90°, with true CR-part-film alignment **551**
(2) Include entire structure or trauma area on film **552**

Use of grids:
- Grid use rules **553**
- Special nonlinear wafer type portable grid **553**

Mobile X-ray Equipment

Types of mobile x-ray systems:
- Battery-driven, battery-operated mobile x-ray units **554**
- 110 V, capacitor-discharge mobile x-ray units **554**
- Mobile C-arm digital fluoroscopy systems:
  –Equipment types and uses **555**
  –Image orientation and sterile fields **556**

Radiation protection:
- Three cardinal rules–distance, time and shielding **557**
- Exposure patterns surrounding C-arm **557**

Trauma and Mobile Positioning

Chest:
- AP (supine, semierect and decub.) **558**

Bony thorax:
- Sternum–AP oblique and lateral **559**
- Ribs–AP and oblique **560**

Abdomen:
- AP supine and lateral decubitus **561**

Upper limb and shoulder:
- Fingers, thumb, hand and wrist **562**
- Forearm, wrist, and post reduction in cast **563**
- Elbow–PA and lateral **564**
- Humerus–AP and lateral **565**
- Shoulder, scapula and clavicle –AP and lateral **566**

Lower limb and pelvis:
- Toes and foot–AP and lateral **567**
- Ankle and leg (tibia/fibula)–AP and lateral **568**
- Knee–AP and lateral (oblique) **569**
- AP and lateral mid and distal femur, and AP pelvis **570**
- Lateral proximal femur and hip (Danelius-Miller and Sanderson methods) **571**

Cervical spine:
- AP and horizontal beam lateral **572**
- Double-angle oblique (biplane angulation method) **573**

Thoracic and lumbar spine:
- AP and horizontal beam lateral **574**

Skull:
- Lateral (horizontal beam) **575**
- AP 0°, AP 15° and AP 30° axial (Towne) **576**

Facial bones:
- Lateral, AP acanthioparietal (reverse Waters) and modified acanthioparietal **578**
- Mandible–AP axial, AP and horizontal beam axiolateral obliques **579**

Terminology, Principles and Equipment

INTRODUCTION

Situations arise in which the radiographer encounters patients who are very ill and in a weakened condition, or have experienced severe trauma, all of which require major adaptations in positioning and handling. It may mean that they cannot be brought to the radiology department for radiographic procedures as described in other sections of this text. Even if the patient is brought to the radiology department, they may be strapped to a backboard with a cervical collar in place, or may have one or more splints, indicating possible limb fractures or dislocations. In these cases the patients cannot be moved into the usual routine positions, therefore requiring **major adaptation of CR angles and film placement**. This may be done with a mobile (portable) x-ray unit taken to the emergency room or to the patient's room. Even if these patients can be brought into a conventional radiographic room, they frequently cannot be turned into lateral or prone positions. Therefore, all projections must be taken in the supine position, requiring the use of grids and cross-table laterals, and/or other special projections.

This chapter introduces the radiographer to trauma and mobile radiography. Also described and illustrated are commonly used terminology and positioning principles and methods of radiographing various body parts when routine projections cannot be achieved. Common types of mobile (portable) x-ray equipment are described as well as certain grid use principles and rules essential in trauma and mobile radiography.

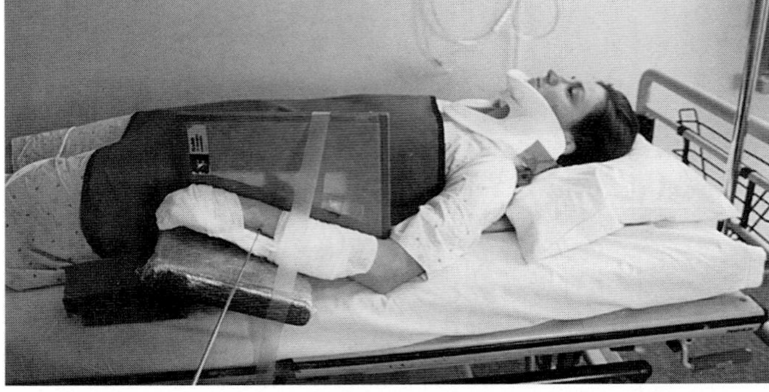

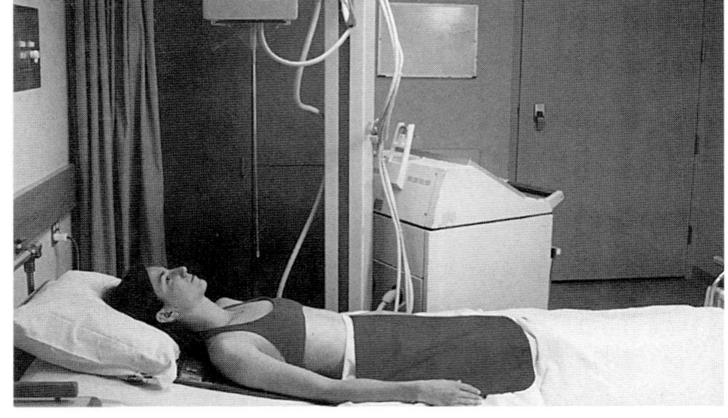

Fig. 19-1. Trauma and bedside mobile radiography.

Trauma and Fracture Terminology

Trauma radiography requires an understanding of certain terms that are unique to these situations, such as injury descriptions and fracture or dislocation terminology. Knowing and recognizing this terminology on patient histories or exam requisitions will allow the radiographer to know which type of injury or fracture is suspected and which projections are most important for that injury. It will also help in knowing how to avoid certain positioning methods or body positions which may result in additional injury.

***1. Dislocation or Luxation** (luk-sa′ shun):*

- The **displacement of a bone from a joint**, or the complete loss of articular contact of bones comprising a joint.*

  The most common dislocations encountered in trauma radiography are of the shoulder, fingers or thumb, patella and hip.

  Dislocations can frequently be recognized by the abnormal shape or alignment of the body parts, and **any movement of these parts can be very painful and must be avoided**. As with fractures, dislocations should also be radiographed in two directions, 90° or right angles from each other to demonstrate the direction and amount of dislocation.

  Also, even if a bone has relocated itself, damage has frequently occurred, and a minimum of two projections of the affected joint are generally required to assess for damage and/or possible associated avulsion fractures.

- ***Subluxation:*** **Partial dislocation**, such as with the spine, in which a vertebrae is displaced posteriorly (Fig. 19-4).

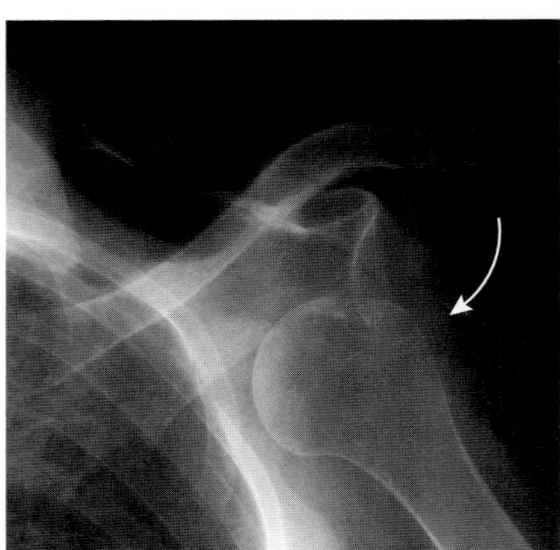

Fig. 19-2. Shoulder dislocation (AP projection).

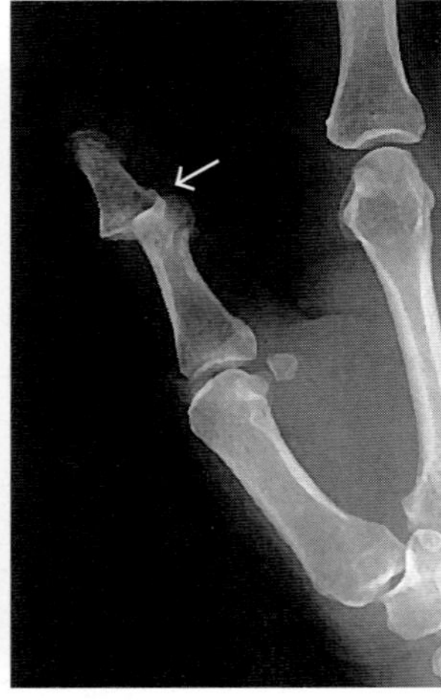

Fig. 19-3. Thumb dislocation (distal phalanx).

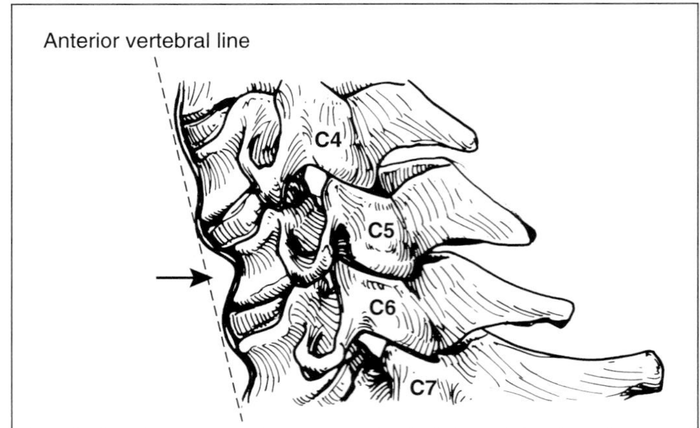

Fig. 19-4. Subluxation of cervical vertebra (C5 vertebra displaced posteriorly).

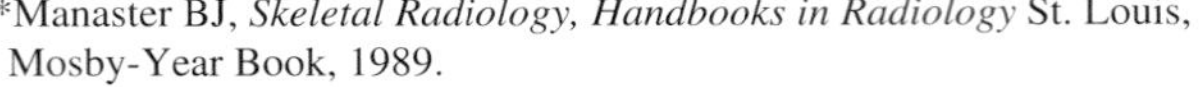

*Manaster BJ, *Skeletal Radiology, Handbooks in Radiology* St. Louis, Mosby-Year Book, 1989.

2. Sprain:

- **A forced wrenching or twisting of a joint resulting in a partial rupture or tearing of supporting ligaments without dislocation** (luxation).

  Even if there is no fracture, there can be severe damage to associated blood vessels, tendons, ligaments or nerves. A severe sprain can be very painful and must be handled with great care during the radiographic examination. Severe swelling and discoloration, due to hemorrhage from ruptured blood vessels, frequently accompany a severe sprain. Symptoms are very similar to fractures and radiographs aid in differentiating a sprain from a fracture.

3. Fracture:

- A fracture indicates a **break in a bone**.

  With any possible fracture the radiographer must take extra caution in moving and positioning the patient so as not to cause further injury or dislocation of fracture fragments. The radiographer should **never** force a limb or body part into position. If the fracture is obvious, or if severe pain accompanies any movement even if done gently, one should adapt positioning as needed to **not rotate the body part** and only lift the part gently as needed for film placement.

4. Contusion (kon-tu′zhun):

- This is also a type of injury **without a fracture** of a bone, or **without a break in the skin**. This is a "bruise" type of injury. An example is a **hip pointer**, a football type injury involving a contusion of bone at the iliac crest of the pelvis.

Fracture Alignment Terminology

5. Apposition (ap″o-zish′un):

- An alignment or disalignment describing the **relationship of the long axes of fracture fragments**.

  Three types of apposition are:

  (1) **Anatomic apposition**: Refers to anatomical alignment of ends of fractured bone fragments, wherein the ends of the fragments make end-to-end contact.

  (2) **Lack of apposition (distraction)**: The ends of fragments have been pulled apart and do not make contact (such as may occur from excessive traction (*Fig 19-5*).

  (3) **Bayonet apposition**: A fracture wherein the fragments overlap and the shafts make contact but not the fracture ends (*Fig 19-6*).

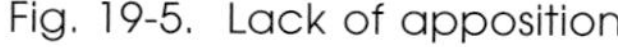

Fig. 19-5. Lack of apposition.

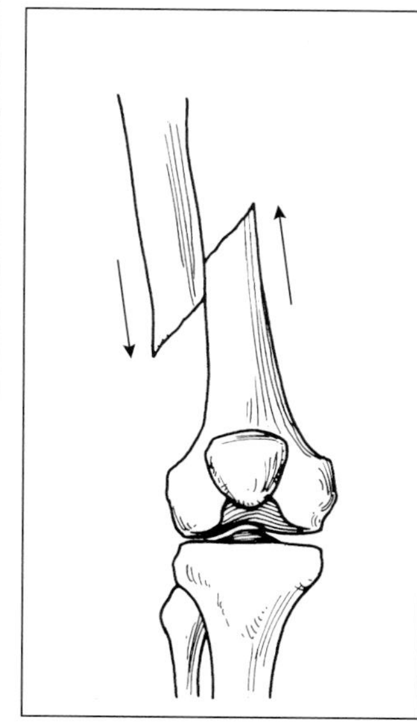

Fig. 19-6. Bayonet apposition.

6. Angulation:

- Refers to the **loss of alignment**. Three terms describing the type or direction of angulation are as follows:

  (1) **Apex angulation**: Describes the direction or angle of the apex of the fracture, such as a medial or lateral apex wherein the point or apex of the fracture points medially or laterally.

  (2) **Varus deformity**: The distal part of the distal fragments angled **toward the midline** of the body, a lateral apex which points away from the midline.

  (3) **Valgus deformity**: The opposite of varus, the apex is directed toward the midline (medial apex), and the distal fragment **away from** midline.

  Note: Varus and valgus are also used as inversion and eversion stress movement terms (see Terminology, Chapter 1, page 25).

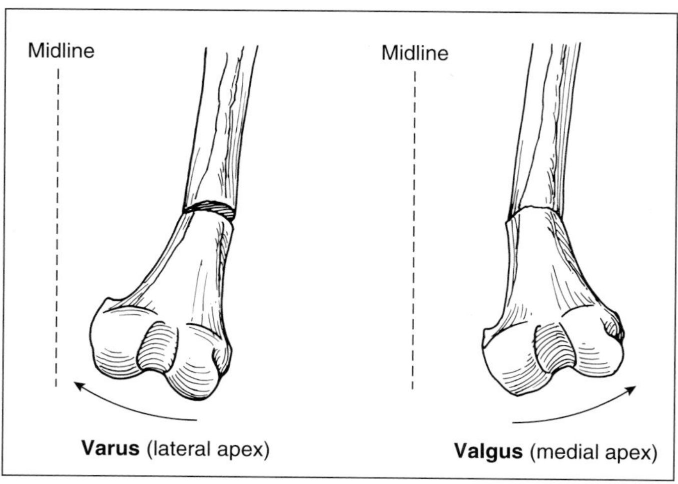

Fig. 19-7. Varus vs. valgus deformity.

Types of Fractures

There are many different terms used in describing fractures. Those terms that radiographers are most likely to encounter are described as follows:

7. Simple (Closed) Fx:

- A fracture wherein the bone **does not break through the skin.**

8. Compound (Open) Fx: (Fig. 19-8)

- A fracture wherein the **bone protrudes through the skin.**

9. Incomplete (Partial) Fx:

- Fracture **does not traverse through entire bone**. (The bone is not broken into two pieces.)

  Three major types of incomplete fractures (child type fractures) are:

  (1) **Torus Fx**: A buckle of the cortex in which there is localized expansion or torus of the cortex. There may be little or no displacement and there is **no complete break in the cortex**.

  (2) **Greenstick Fx (hickory or willow stick)**: **Incomplete fracture on one side only**. The cortex on one side of bone is broken and the other side is bent. When the bone straightens, a very faint fracture line in the cortex may be seen on one side of bone, and a slight bulging or wrinkle-like defect on the opposite side (Fig. 19-9).

  (3) **Plastic Fx**: A **bending type fracture** without specific angular deformity and without a need for straightening by splinting or casting.

10. Complete Fx:

- A fracture in which the **break is complete** and includes the entire cross-section of bone. The bone is **broken into two pieces**.

  Three major types of complete fractures:

  (1) **Transverse Fx**: Fracture line is transverse at a **near right angle** to the long axis of the bone.

  (2) **Oblique Fx:** Fracture line passes through bone at an **oblique angle**.

  (3) **Spiral Fx**: A fracture in which the bone has been twisted apart and the fracture line is **spiral in shape** (Fig. 19-10).

11. Comminuted (kom′i-nut-ed) Fx:

- A fracture in which the bone is **splintered or crushed** at the site of impact, resulting in **two or more fragments** (Fig. 19-11).

  Following are three types of comminuted fractures that have specific implications for treatment and prognosis due to the possible substantial disruption of blood.

  (1) **Segmental Fx**. A type of double fracture with **two fracture lines isolating a distinct segment of bone**.

  (2) **Butterfly Fx.** A type of comminuted fracture in which there are **two fragments on each side of a main, wedge-shaped separate fragment**. Has some resemblance to the wings of a butterfly.

  (3) **Splintered Fx.** A comminuted fracture in which the bone is **splintered into thin sharp fragments**.

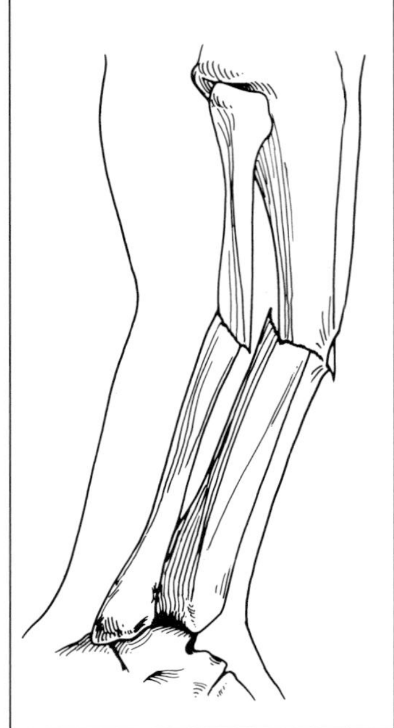

Fig. 19-8. Compound fx (tibia-fibula).

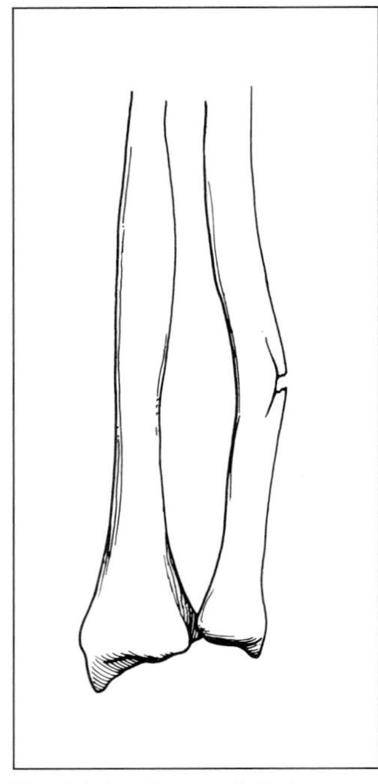

Fig. 19-9. Greenstick fx (ulna).

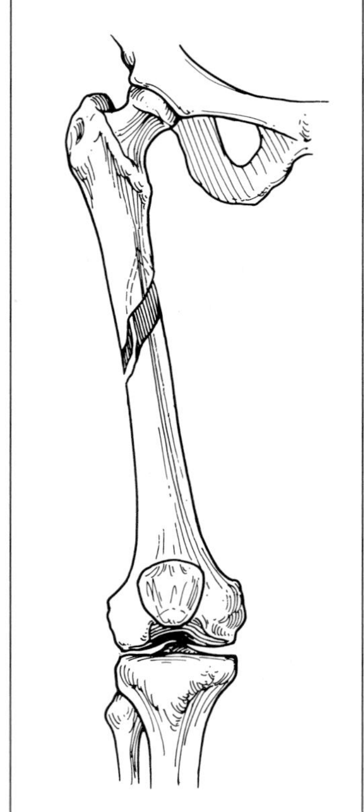

Fig. 19-10. Spiral fx (femur).

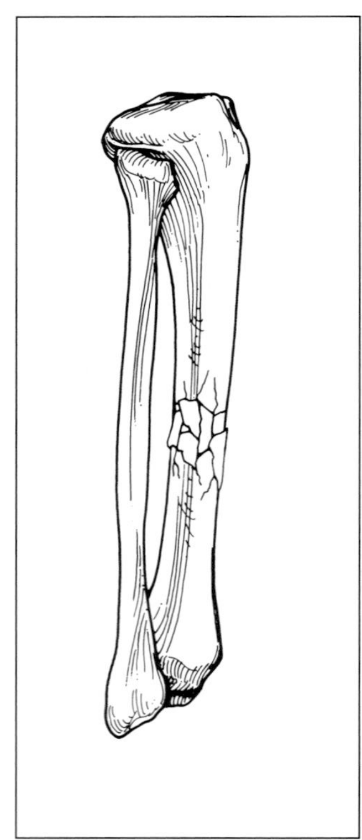

Fig. 19-11. Comminuted fx (tibia).

12. Impacted Fx:

- A fracture in which **one fragment is firmly driven into the other**, such as the shaft of the bone being driven into the head or end segment. Most commonly occur at distal or proximal ends of femur, humerus or radius.

Specific "Named" Fractures

Following are some examples of "named" fractures, usually named by the type of injury or after the person identifying them.

13. Baseball (Mallet) Fx:

- A fracture of the **distal phalanx** from a ball striking end of extended finger. The DIP joint is partially flexed and an avulsion fracture frequently is present at the posterior base of the distal phalanx.

14. Barton's Fx:

- An intra-articular fracture of the **posterior lip of the distal radius**.

15. Bennett Fx:

- A longitudinal fracture at the **base of the first metacarpal** with the fracture line entering the **carpometacarpal joint**. Generally includes posterior dislocation or subluxation.

16. Boxer's Fx:

- A fracture most commonly involving the **distal 5th metacarpal** with an apex posterior angulation best demonstrated on the lateral view.

17. Colles (kol′ ez) Fx:

- A fracture of an adult wrist in which the **distal radius is fractured** with the distal fragment **displaced posteriorly** (apex anterior angulation). Results from a fall on outstretched arm.

18. Hangman's Fx:

- A fracture through the pedicles of the axis (C2), with or without displacement of C2 on C3.

19. Hutchinson's (Chauffeur's) Fx:

- An **intra-articular fracture of the radial styloid process**. (Name originates from the time hand-cranked cars would backfire with the crank striking the lateral side of the distal forearm.)

20. Monteggia's (mon-tej′ ahz) Fx:

- A fracture of the **proximal half of the ulna** along with **dislocation of the radial head**. (May result from defending against blows with the raised forearm.)

21. Nursemaid's Elbow ("Jerked Elbow"):

- Not a fracture but a traumatic **subluxation or partial dislocation of the radial head of a child**, caused by a hard pull on the hand and wrist of a child by an adult. This frequently is cured spontaneously by reducing itself when the forearm is supinated for the AP elbow.

22. Pott's Fx:

- A complete fracture of the **distal fibula** with major injury to ankle joint including ligament damage and **frequent fracture of distal tibia or medial malleolus**.

23. Smith's (Reverse Colle's) Fx:

- A fracture of the **distal radius with anterior displacement** (apex posterior angulation).

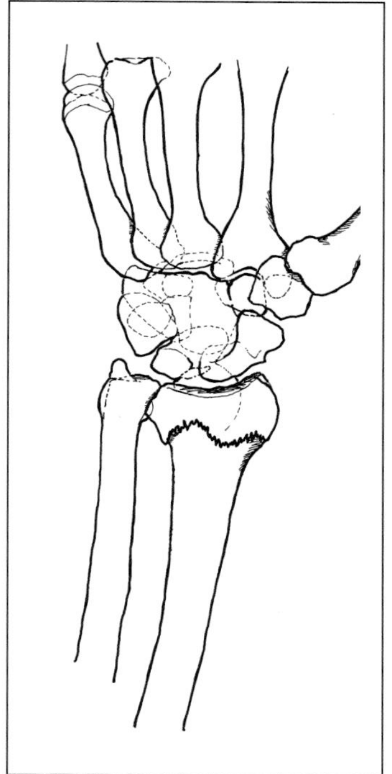

Fig. 19-12. Impacted fx (radius).

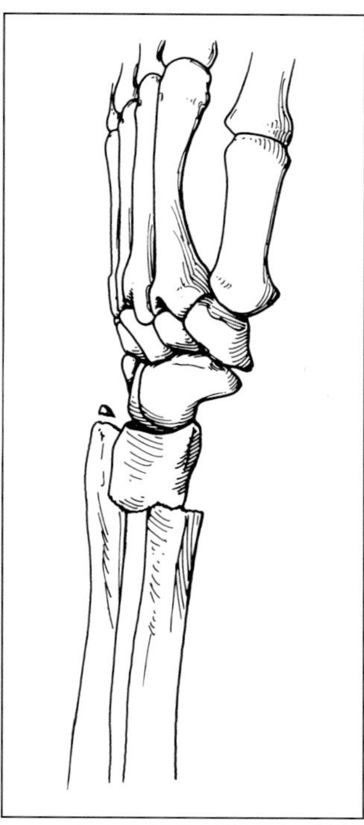

Fig. 19-13. Colles fx (radius).

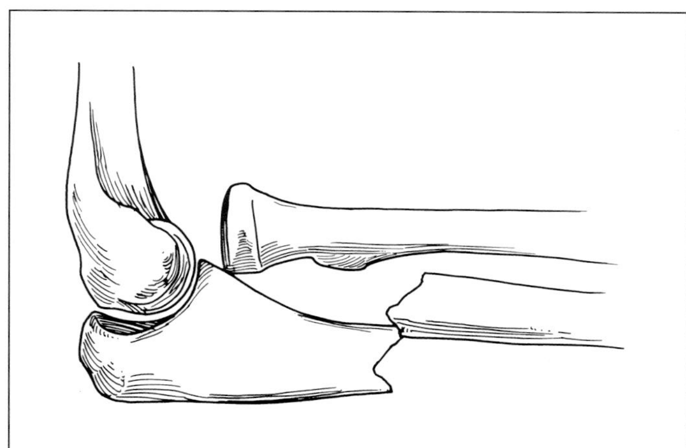

Fig. 19-14. Monteggia's fx (ulna).

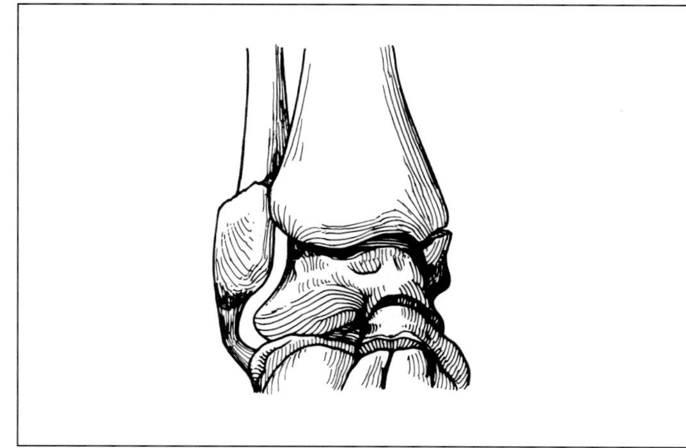

Fig. 19-15. Pott's fx (distal tibia-fibula).

19

Additional Fracture Types

24. Avulsion Fx:

- A fracture resulting from severe stress to a tendon or ligament in a joint region. A **fragment of bone is separated or pulled away** by the attached tendon or ligament rather than tearing the tendon or ligament.

25. Blowout and/or Tripod Fx:

- Fractures from a **direct blow to the orbit** and/or facial region as described and illustrated in Chapter 11 (p. 339).

26. Chip Fx:

- A fracture involving an **isolated bone fragment**. (This is **not** the same as an avulsion fracture.)

27. Compression Fx:

- A **spinal fracture produced by compression** in which the vertebral body collapses or is compressed.
  Generally, it is most evident radiographically by a decreased vertical dimension of the **anterior vertebral body**.

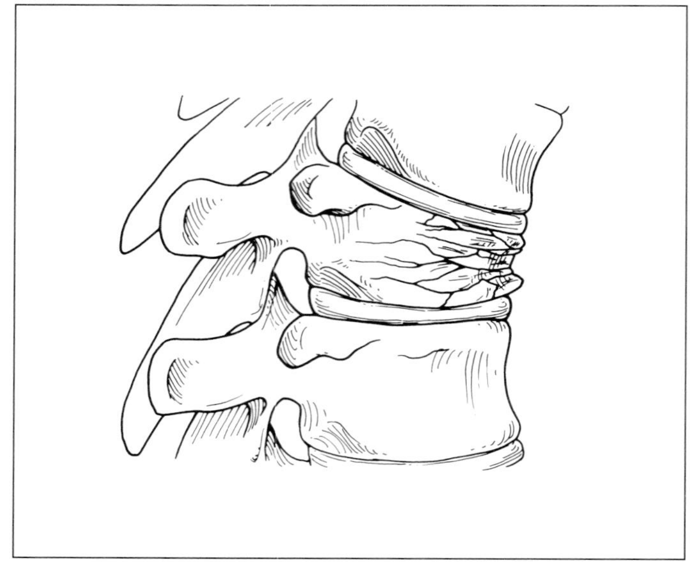

Fig. 19-16. Compression fx (body of vertebra).

28. Depressed Fx (Sometimes Called a Ping-pong Fx):

- An **indented fracture of the skull** in which a fragment is depressed inward. Appearance is similar to a ping-pong ball that has been pressed in by the finger, but if the indentation can be elevated again it can assume its near-original position.

29. Epiphyseal Fx:

- A fracture **through the epiphyseal plate**, the point of union of the epiphysis and shaft of a bone.
  This is one of the most easily fractured sites in long bones of children. Radiologists commonly use the Salter-Harris classification (Salter 1-5) for describing these fractures as to their severity and reasonable indication of prognosis.*

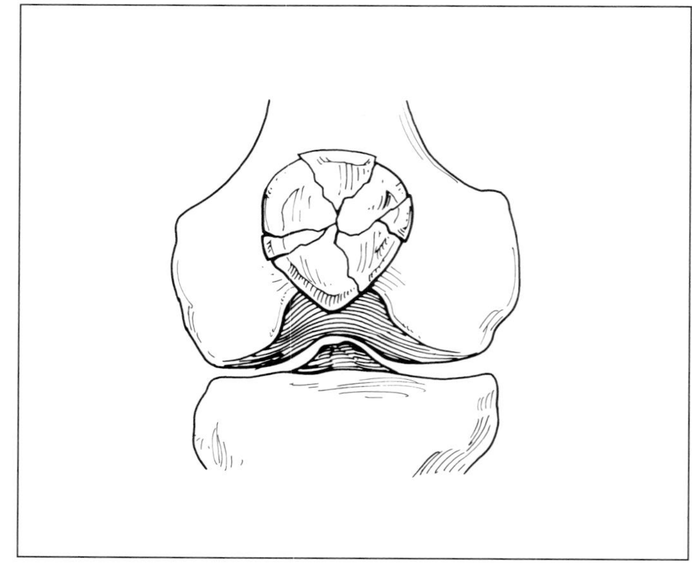

Fig. 19-17. Stellate fx (patella).

30. Pathologic Fx's:

- Fractures due to **disease process within the bone**, such as from tumors, cancers or other bone diseases.

31. Stress or Fatigue Fx (Sometimes Called a "March" Fx.):

- A type of pathologic fracture that is **nontraumatic in origin**.
  Results from repeated stress such as from marching or running. Such fractures, if from marching, usually are in the midshafts of metatarsals; and if from running are in the distal shaft of tibia. These types of fractures are frequently very difficult to demonstrate radiographically and may be visible only by subsequent callus formation at the fracture site, or by a nuclear medicine bone scan.

32. Stellate Fx:

- A fracture in which the **fracture lines radiate from a central point** of injury with a starlike pattern. The most common example of this type of fracture is the patella of the knee hitting the dashboard in an auto accident.

33. Trimalleolar Fx:

- A fracture of the ankle involving both the **medial and lateral malleoli**, and the **posterior tip of the distal tibia**.

34. Tuft or Burst Fx:

- A **comminuted fracture of the distal phalanx** such as from a crushing blow to the distal finger or thumb.

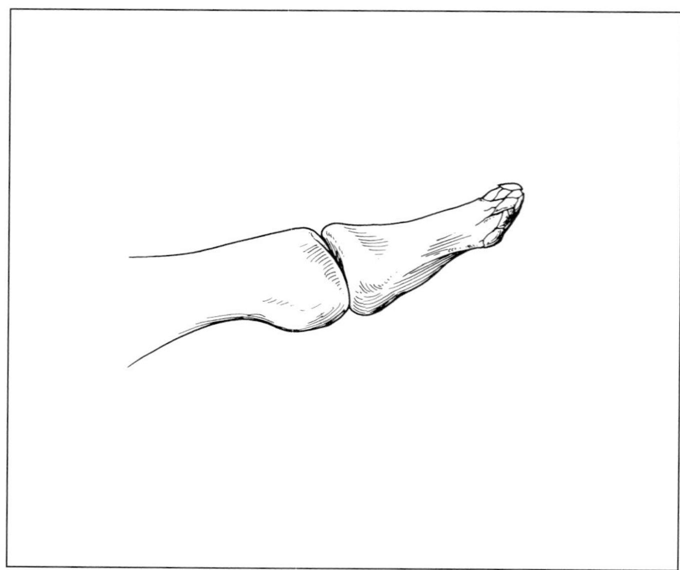

Fig. 19-18. Tuft fx (distal phalanx).

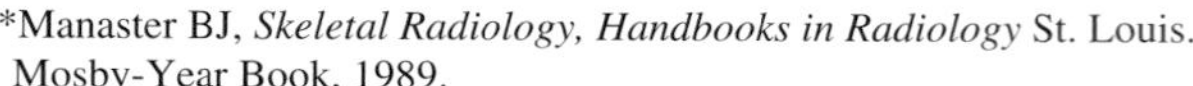

*Manaster BJ, *Skeletal Radiology, Handbooks in Radiology* St. Louis. Mosby-Year Book, 1989.

Post Reduction Radiographs

Closed Reduction: Those fractures in which there is misalignment requiring restoration to a normal position by manipulation. These are generally performed by an orthopedic surgeon. If this can be done without surgery, the procedure is called a **closed reduction**.

Open Reduction: For severe fractures with significant displacement or fragmentation, a surgical procedure is required. The fracture site is exposed and screws, plates, or rods are installed as needed to align and retain the placement of the bony fragments and pieces until new bone growth can take place. This is called an **open reduction**. Radiographs are frequently taken during such surgical procedures to aid the surgeon.

Follow-up post reduction radiographs are generally required for both closed and open reductions with the body part in a cast or splint to retain correct alignment. These radiographs should also include an AP (or PA) and a lateral taken 90° or right angles from each other (Fig. 19-19 and 19-20).

C-arm fluoroscopy is being increasingly used for both open and closed reductions (page 555).

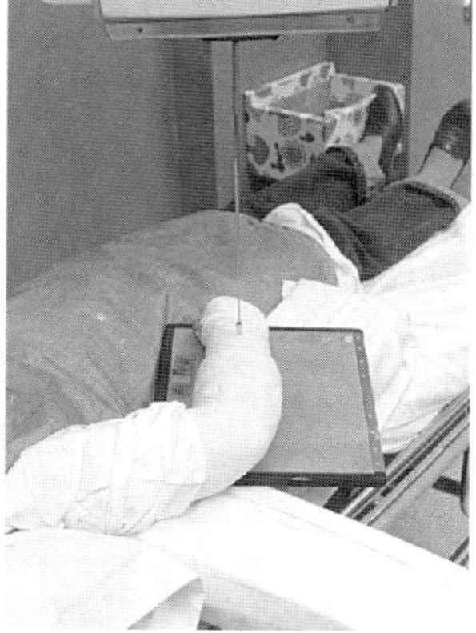

Fig. 19-19. Post reduction PA forearm and wrist.

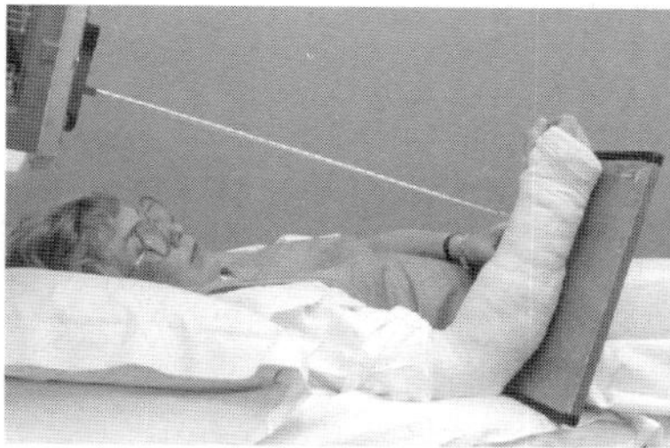

Fig. 19-20. Post reduction lateral forearm and wrist.

Positioning Principles and Grid Use

Positioning principles for trauma radiography are in many ways similar to that for general radiography as described in Chapter one of this text. The primary difference can be summed up with the word **"adaptation."** Each trauma patient is different and the radiographer must first evaluate the patient, then **adapt CR angles and film placement as needed** to demonstrate radiographically, with minimal patient movement, those injured body parts as requested by the referring physician.

Principle One -Two Projections 90° to Each Other with True CR-Part-Film Alignment

Principle One states that trauma radiography generally requires **two projections at 90° or right angles to each other** while maintaining a true CR-part-film alignment.

The preferred choices for the two projections are a **true AP or PA** and a **true lateral** achieved by either turning the body part (standard positioning) **or angling the CR and film as needed** (trauma adaptation positioning). In this way the **CR-part-film alignment can be maintained even if the patient cannot be turned or rotated**. An example is shown in Fig. 19-21 and 19-22 wherein true AP and lateral foot projections are achieved without flexing or moving the lower limb. This is done by angling the CR and film in relationship to the foot, thus maintaining a true CR-part-film alignment.

This same adaptation principle can be applied to **any body part** as will be demonstrated in this chapter. This appears to be a simple principle but inexperienced radiographers have a tendency to want to use the conventional vertical CR, AP and lateral or horizontal beam (cross-table) CR method, rather than adapting the CR and film angles as needed without moving the body part.

Exception to Two-projection True AP (PA) and Lateral Principle: Occasionally it may not be possible to maintain this standard CR-part-film relationship for both a true AP (PA) and lateral projection. If this is not possible due to unavoidable obstructions such as large bulky splints, back supports, traction bars or other paraphernalia, the radiographer should still attempt two projections as near 90° to each other as possible even if both projections are partially obliqued. **Only as a last resort should only one projection be taken.** When these exceptions are made, a note should be made on the patient's history sheet or exam requisition explaining the reason for this single projection. (An exception is the routine AP abdomen or KUB wherein one projection is standard policy.)

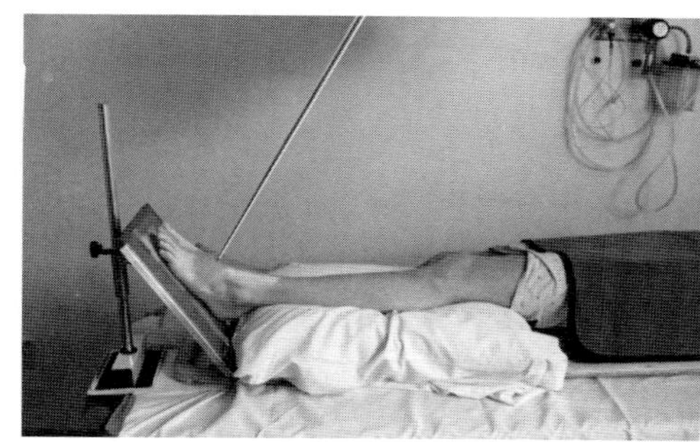

Fig. 19-21. AP foot (trauma adaptation positioning).

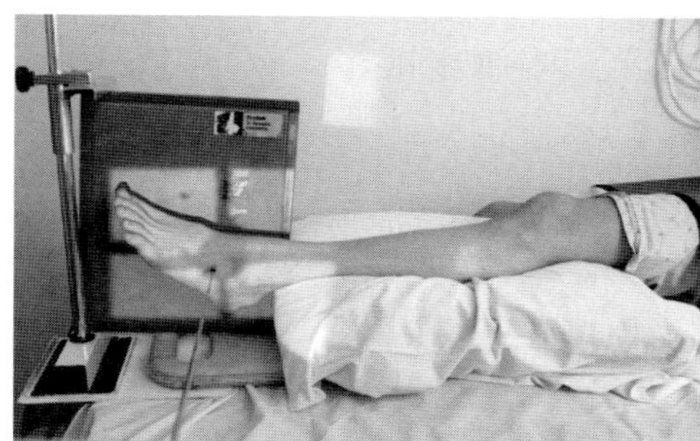

Fig. 19-22. Lateral foot.

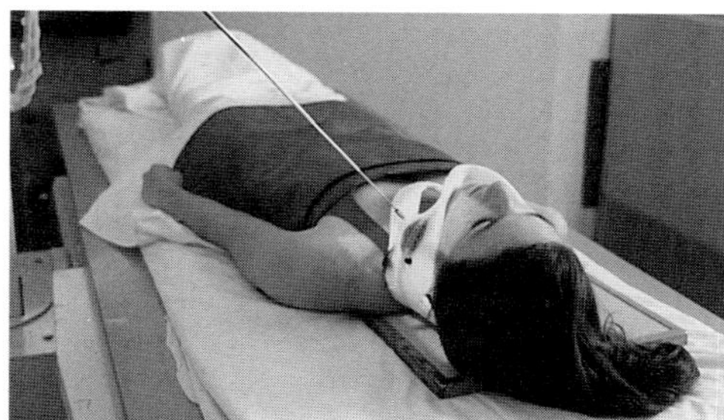

Fig. 19-23. Trauma oblique C-spine exception, film is not perpendicular to CR.

Exception to CR-Part-Film Alignment: Generally this principle includes placing the film at right angles or perpendicular to the CR for minimum part distortion. However, there may be situations as shown above (Fig. 19-23) wherein the CR-part relationship can be maintained but not the part-film relationship. In this example the above oblique cervical spine is taken supine table-top with the film remaining flat on the table under the patient rather than being tilted so as to be perpendicular to the CR. This will result in part distortion, but in trauma radiography it may be an acceptable option, even though attempts should be made whenever possible to place the film parallel with the part. A way to do this in certain situations for the trauma oblique cervical spine will also be demonstrated later in this chapter.

Principle Two–Include Entire Structure or Trauma Area on Film

Principle Two of trauma radiography states that it is important that the **entire structure being examined be included on the radiograph** to ensure that no pathology is missed. This requires selection of sufficiently large films, or the use of more than one film if needed.

Upper and Lower Limbs: If an initial exam request on a trauma patient includes long bones of the upper or lower limbs, then **both joints should be included** for possible secondary fractures away from the primary injury region. An example is an initial post-trauma exam request for a leg (tibia-fibula). This may require a second smaller film of the knee to include the proximal tibia-fibula region if the film is not long enough to include both the ankle and knee joints. Fractures of the distal tibia may also have a secondary fracture of the proximal fibula. This principle of including joints is true for both AP and lateral projections.

If, however, the exam request names a joint region (ankle, knee, wrist, elbow) and the injury obviously is near that joint, such as in Figs. 19-24 and 19-25, then generally only this one joint nearest the injury site is included.

Always Include a Joint Rule: For **all** upper and lower limb exams, **always include a minimum of one joint nearest the site of injury**. There are few if any exceptions to this rule, even if the obvious fracture site as shown on previous films is to the mid shaft region. The joint nearest the fracture site should **always** be included.

Bony Thorax, Chest and Abdomen: Principle Two of including the entire structure or trauma region includes these larger body areas also. For example the abdomen on a large patient may require two films placed crosswise to include the entire abdomen. This may also be true for the chest or bony thorax, such as for ribs.

Horizontal Beam Lateral: Trauma patients most often arrive in a supine position and horizontal beam or cross-table projections are commonly required for the lateral projections. Care must be taken so **the divergent x-ray beam doesn't project the body part off the film**, especially when the film cassette is placed on edge directly beside the patient. This is true for the spine, skull or other parts that rest directly on the tabletop. An example of this is demonstrated in Figs. 19-26 and 19-27 of a horizontal beam lateral skull with and without a possible spine injury. With a questionable spinal injury, the **head and neck cannot be moved or elevated** and therefore no support or pad can be placed between the head and tabletop. Therefore, if the film cassette is placed on edge next to the patient's head, the divergent x-ray beam will project the posterior part of the skull off the film. The film inside the cassette also does not extend all the way to the edge of the cassette due to the frame structure of the cassette, which also adds to the cutoff of the posterior part of the skull.

To avoid this cutoff, the patient can be moved to the back edge of the table, and the cassette placed below the table-top off the back edge of the table (Fig. 19-27). This results in some increase in part-film distance and the x-ray tube can be moved back to increase the SID to reduce part magnification. Exposure factors will need to be increased accordingly.

If cervical spine radiographs have ruled out cervical fracture or subluxation, then for a lateral skull the head may be raised and supported by a sponge block so as to prevent posterior skull cut-off (Fig. 19-26).

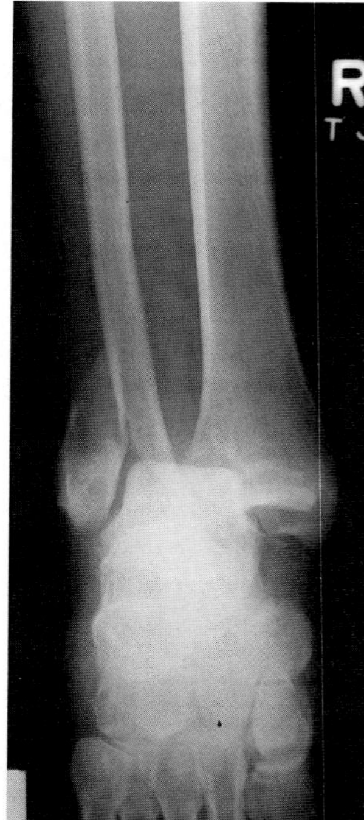

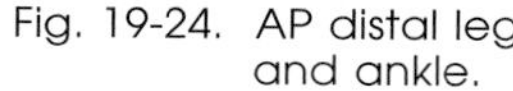
Fig. 19-24. AP distal leg and ankle.

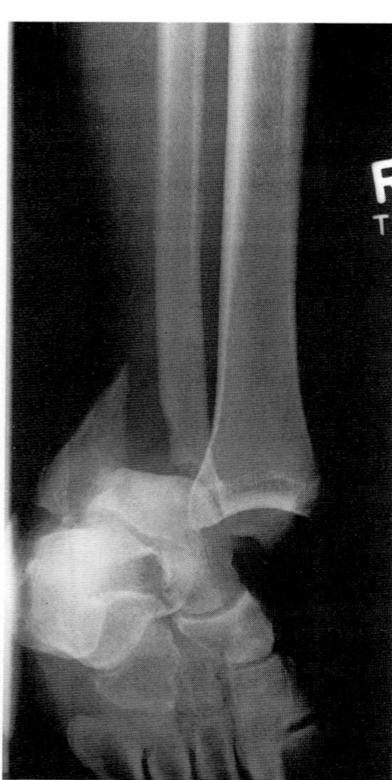

Fig. 19-25. Lateral distal leg and ankle.

(Example of severe Pott's fracture.)

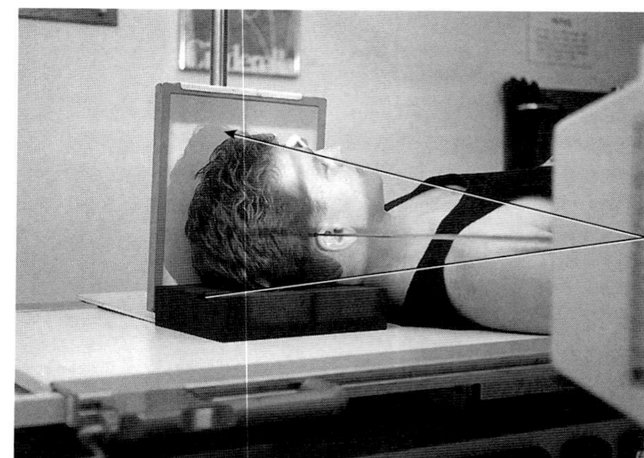
Fig. 19-26. Horizontal beam lateral skull **without** possible spine injury (head raised from table-top).

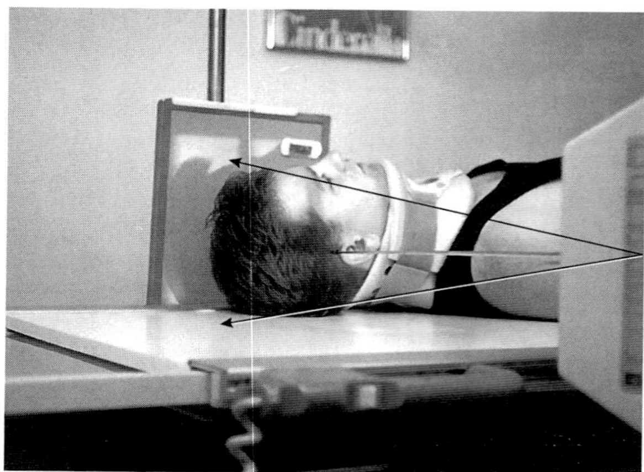
Fig. 19-27. **With** possible spine injury, head **cannot** be raised or moved (cassette is placed below table-top level to prevent posterior skull cutoff).

USE OF GRIDS

Grids should generally be used for all body parts measuring more than 10 cm, the same as for conventional radiography. This means that except for distal upper and lower limbs and for smaller children, grids are used for most trauma or mobile radiographs. Additional part swelling, splints, backboards and atypical projections also result in additional scatter due to the increase in part thickness and the higher kVp required, making the use of grids even more essential.

Preventing grid cutoff is a challenge in trauma and mobile radiography due to required adaptations in CR-part-film alignments.

Grid Use Rules

Successful use of grids requires an understanding of the principles and rules to prevent grid cutoff, which can occur when these principles and rules are violated. Slight grid cutoff caused by the lead strips is evident by the light, underpenetrated areas causing some loss of visible detail (Fig. 19-28). More severe grid cutoff will completely obliterate or eliminate all or part of the radiographic image (Fig. 19-29).

Grid cutoff can be avoided by understanding that when using a focused linear grid, there are certain limitations to CR-grid centering and alignment, and to the CR-grid distance, which must be adhered to. Three limitations or rules concerning grid cutoff relate to (1) **CR centering**; (2) **CR angling** and (3) **grid focal range** (SID range).

(1) CR Centering: **The CR must always be centered near the centerline** (within 1-1½ inches or 2.5-4 cm at 40 in. SID) **somewhere along the length of the grid**. When the CR cannot be centered to the central point of the grid, the grid must be turned in such a way (lengthwise or crosswise) so the CR will still be **centered somewhere near the length of the centerline**. Linear focused grids contain lead strips that are tilted or focused and run parallel to the centerline and long dimension of the grid (Fig. 19-30).

(2) CR Angle: **Any CR angling of more than 3 or 4° must be along the direction of the lead strips**. Therefore any time the CR is not perpendicular to the plane of the film, the grid must again be turned in such a way so the CR angle is along the length of the grid and not across the width, which would result in grid cutoff.

(3) Grid Focal Range: **Each linear focused grid has a certain range of focus which must be adhered to** (wherein the CR can pass through without excessive absorption). This is described as the **focal range** or **grid radius**. The focal range is determined by the **grid frequency** (number of grid strips per inch) and the **grid ratio** (height of lead strips compared to the space between them). Portable grids generally have a lower grid frequency and lower grid ratio than fixed grids or Bucky type grids. A common grid ratio for portable grids is **6:1** or **8:1** compared to 12:1 for Bucky grids. This results in a greater grid focal range for portable grids but there are still SID limitations to prevent grid cutoff. This varies depending on the grid manufacturer but typical ranges are from 12 to 15% on each side of the focal SID. For example, a **medium range portable grid** may have a focal range of **34 to 46 in.** (86 to 117 cm), or 6 in. (15 cm) on each side of 40 in. (102 cm). A typical **long focal range portable grid** has a focal range of from **48 to 72 in** (122 to 183 cm). Each radiographer should know the types of portable grids they have available and the focal range of each.

Special Nonlinear, Wafer-Type Portable Grid

A newer type of portable cassette-mounted grid consisting of very small circular openings is available as shown in Fig. 19-32, which has certain advantages in trauma and mobile use. This special purpose wafer-type grid is unique in its construction of a series of stacked sheets of lead foil with many very small circular openings (14,400 holes per square inch). The scatter absorption is equivalent to a 4:1 or 5:1 linear grid.*

Three advantages of this type of portable grid are its (1) **lightweight construction**, (2) **wide focal range** (20 inches to infinity) and (3) **wider tolerance** (10° in any direction) **of off-center and/or off-angle CR** without grid cutoff.

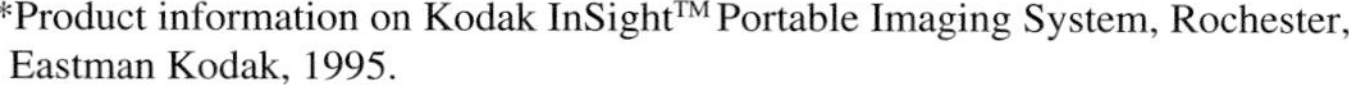

*Product information on Kodak InSight™ Portable Imaging System, Rochester, Eastman Kodak, 1995.

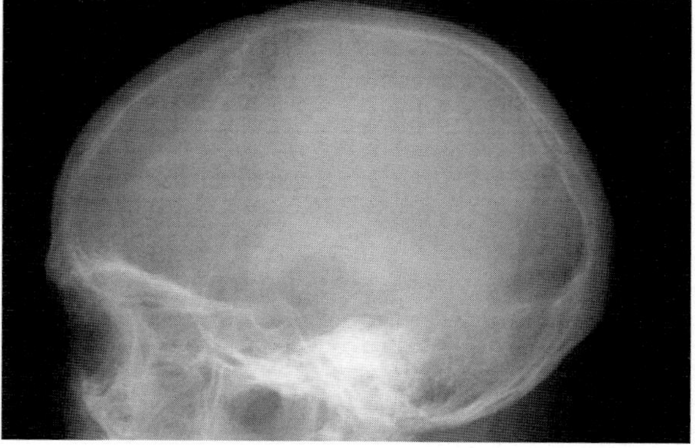

Fig. 19-28. Slight grid cutoff-CR 3 inches off center (appears underexposed).

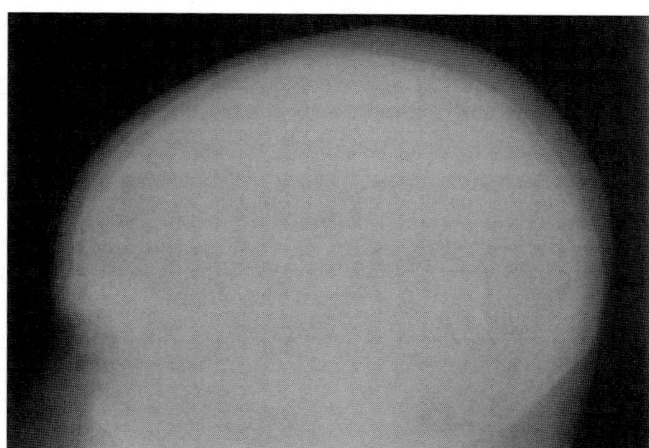

Fig. 19-29. Severe grid cutoff-CR 5 inches off center (appears severely underexposed).

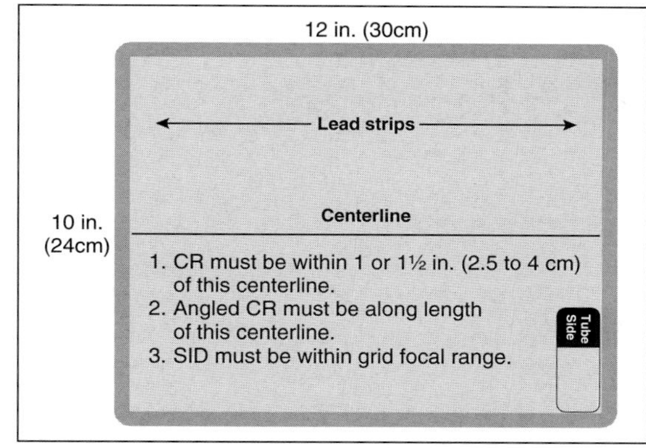

Fig. 19-30. Portable linear focused grid cassette.

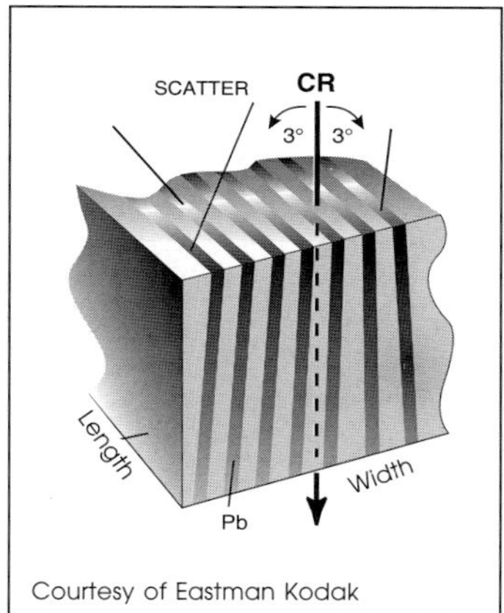

Fig. 19-31. Conventional linear focused grid.
-Limited cross-angle of **3 to 4°**.
-Unlimited CR angle along **length** of lead strips.
-Limited focal range of **±4 in.**

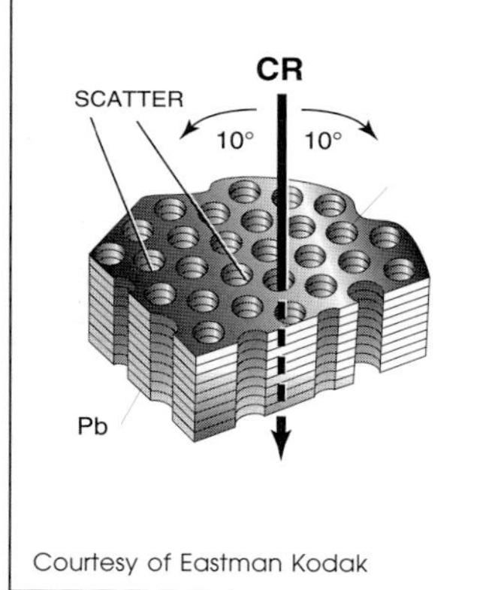

Fig. 19-32. InSight™ wafer grid.
-Limited ≈**10°** CR angle in **any direction**.
-Focal range of **20 in.** (50 cm) **to infinity**.

Mobile X-Ray Equipment

Introduction

A study of trauma and mobile radiography requires an understanding of the functions and operations of the equipment being used. Trauma radiography may be performed either with conventional overhead tube and x-ray table equipment, or with **mobile (portable) units** that are brought to the emergency room, or to the patient's bedside, or to the operating room for surgical procedures.

This type of mobile x-ray machine has commonly been called a "portable." However, this is not an accurate term because portable by definition means to be carried or easily movable, and the usual type of mobile units being used today may weigh up to 1,000 lbs. or more.

TYPES OF MOBILE X-RAY SYSTEMS

There have been major advances in mobile radiographic and fluoroscopic equipment in recent years, and examples of three general types which are now in common use will be described and illustrated.

Contemporary mobile radiographic x-ray equipment consist primarily of either (1) **a battery powered, battery driven type** (Fig. 19-33), or (2) **a 110 V capacitor-discharge**, plug-in, lighter weight, push type (Fig. 19-34). Each of these types have advantages and disadvantages and this is not intended to be an endorsement or recommendation of specific equipment. These two examples of mobile x-ray machines available today include a partial listing of specifications as provided by the manufacturer.

(1) Battery-Driven, Battery-Operated Mobile X-ray Units

These systems are powered by nine or ten 12-volt rechargeable sealed lead acid type batteries connected in series. The self-propelled system of these units are also battery powered with separate 12-volt rechargeable batteries and have variable travel speeds up to an average walking speed of 2½ to 3 mph. They have a driving range of up to ten miles on the level after a full charge.

They are driven and maneuvered by dual drive motors operating the two drive wheels. They also have a lower speed forward and reverse for maneuvering in close quarters. Parking brakes are automatically engaged when the control levers are not in use and when they are set in the charging mode.

They can be plugged in for recharging when not being used and can be recharged at either 110 or 220 volts. With 110 volt, 5 amp outlets, the charging time is about **8 hours** if fully discharged.

(2) 110 V, Capacitor-Discharge Mobile Radiographic X-ray Units

This type of mobile x-ray unit incorporates a capacitor-discharge system that generates sufficiently high voltage (kVp) and amperage (mAs) from a standard 110 volt household type outlet without the use of battery power. They are **not self powered** but can be manually moved due to their lighter weight because they don't have the weight of the batteries. Some larger units of this type may also have 220V capabilities for greater output.

The controls on both of these types of units generally include some type of optional **programmed memory system** based on anatomical parts, or they have **operator selected kV and mAs** technique controls.

Note: These are only two examples of types of mobile systems available at the time of this writing. Other manufacturers offer various modifications, features and options.

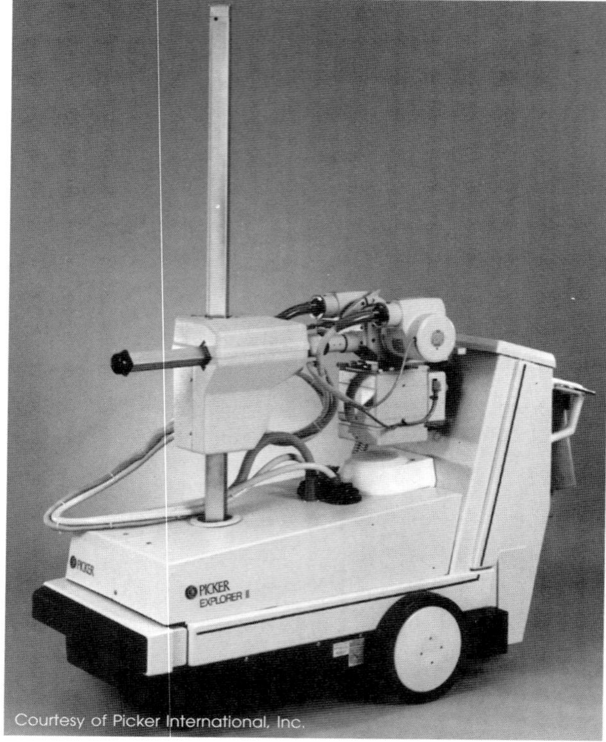

Courtesy of Picker International, Inc.

Fig. 19-33. Picker Explorer® II mobile x-ray system.
- Battery powered, battery driven.
- Weight: 950 lbs. (427 kgs).
- Output: -15.2 kw @ 100 kV, .01 sec.
  -40-125 kVp range.
  -.04-320 mAs (30 steps).

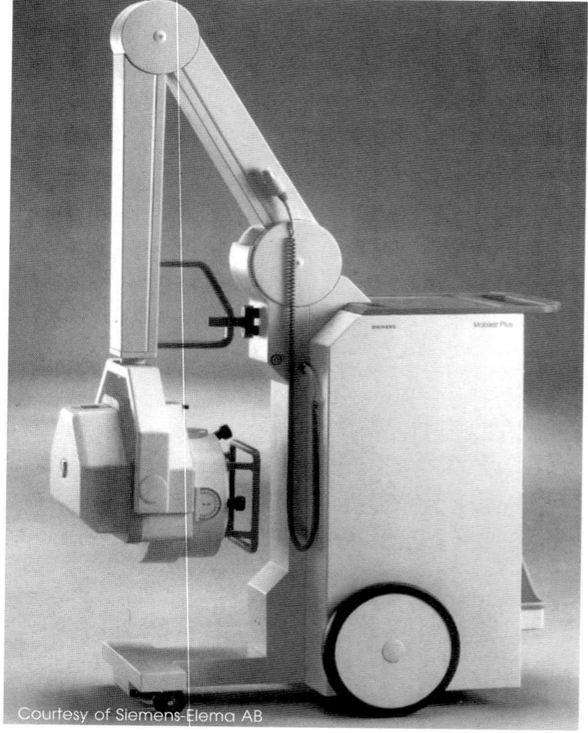

Courtesy of Siemens-Elema AB

Fig. 19-34. Siemens Mobilett Plus.
- 110 V capacitor-discharge.
- Weight: 463 lbs. (210 kgs).
- Output: -25 kw @ 102 kV, .01 sec.
  -40-133 kVp range.
  -.05-200 mAs (53 steps).

(3) Mobile C-arm Digital Fluoroscopy Systems

The term "C-arm" is very descriptive of this basic design of a mobile fluoroscopy unit, with the x-ray tube at one end of the C-arm and the image intensifier tower at the other end.

A familiarity with the C-arm and the monitor and image controls is essential for the radiographer. One must also become familiar with the various types of surgical beds or carts that are used in surgery with the C-arm. For example a surgical bed used for cholangiograms may not accommodate the C-arm x-ray tube under the table in the abdominal area due to the base supports unless the patient's head is placed at the correct end of the bed or cart as shown in Fig. 19-35.

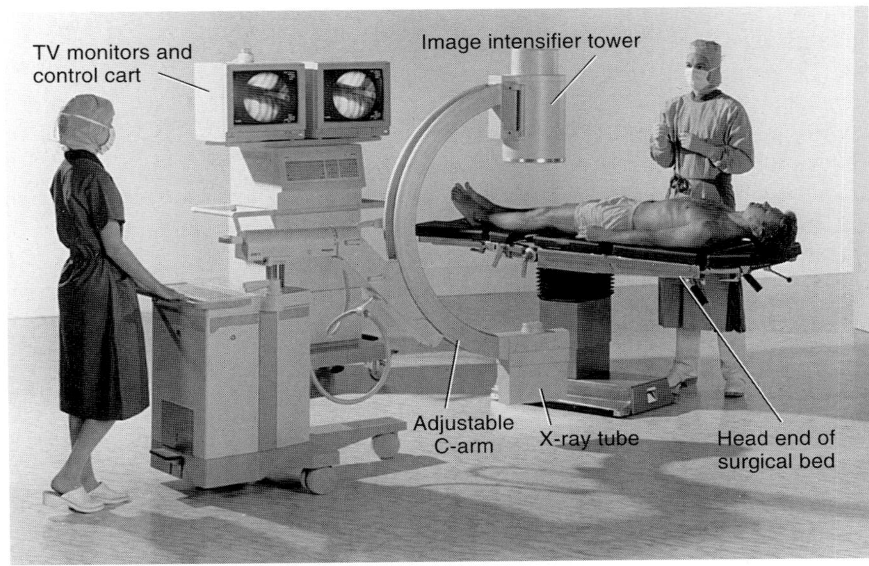

Fig. 19-35. Phillips BV29 C-arm with image processor and display stand demonstrating setup for PA projections for surgical and interventional cases.
-Output: 40-105 kVp range, 0.1-7.4 mA.
-6-, 9- or 12-inch image intensifier (9-inch shown above).
Courtesy of Phillips Medical Systems, Shelton, CT.

Maneuverability: The equipment is designed to be very maneuverable with the C-arm itself attached to an L shaped arm that can be raised and lowered or extended as needed. The counter balanced C-arm can also be rotated or tilted for cephalic or caudal angles, or rotated into a horizontal beam "cross-table" position for lateral hips or other lateral projections as needed (Fig. 19-36). It can also be rotated 180° to place the tube on top and the intensifier on the bottom for an AP projection even though **this is not recommended** because it increases the OID, which decreases image resolution and increases scatter radiation. The "tube on top" position also will result in **a significant increase in exposure to the head and neck area** of the surgeon or radiologist due to the exposure pattern of the C-arm in this AP orientation (see Fig. 19-44, page 557).

Overall, the unit is very flexible in use and the technologist must be familiar with the variety of built in joints, extensions and adjustments. With its three-wheel base with steerable rear wheels and a swiveling nose wheel, the operator can easily maneuver the unit into almost any possible configuration with reasonable space.

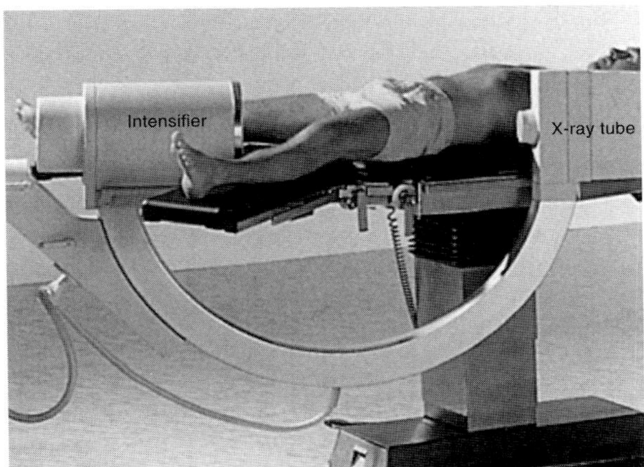

Fig. 19-36. Horizontal setup for lateral hip.
Courtesy of Picker International, Inc.

TV Monitors and Control Cart: Two monitors are needed so the active image can be displayed on one monitor while the second monitor can be used as an "image hold" for reference purposes. Generally the active monitor is on the left and the hold monitor on the right. Images can also be rotated or flipped as needed for preferred viewing by the surgeon and/or radiologist.

Uses of C-Arm: The technologist will use the C-arm unit with various types of procedures where portable fluoroscopy and/or still frame imaging is needed. Examples are surgical procedures such as cholangiograms and open reductions of fractures or hip pinnings. Other uses include various types of special procedures and interventional studies. Images can be stored temporarily with video memory, or on optional hard disks. Optional hard copy film printers are also available for print outs onto film. Cine loop capability is also possible wherein images are recorded in rapid succession then displayed as moving or cine image, such as for barium swallow examinations for swallowing disorders.

As with other types of digital imaging, image enhancement and manipulation is possible including overall brightness and contrast controls, magnification, edge enhancement, masking and digital subtraction studies.

Mini C-Arm Systems: Newer C-arm systems now available also include smaller **single component units** used for orthopedic and other uses in hospital OR and ER centers, clinics and doctor's offices. They include most of the features and operation modes of the larger C-arm systems but they combine the workstation and monitors with the small C-arm into a compact, single component unit. These mini C-arm units operate at lower x-ray energy levels for imaging smaller body parts, which also results in a much lower scatter radiation rate than the larger, high energy C-arm systems.

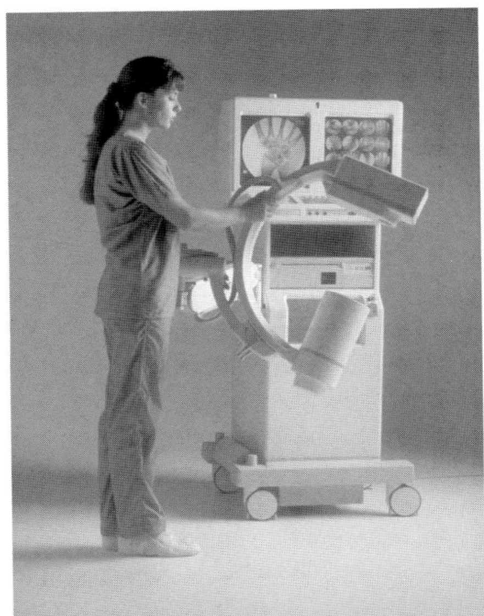

Fig. 19-37. OEC mini 6600™ digital mobile C-arm.
-Output: 40-75 kVp, 0.02-0.1 mA.
-4-inch or 6-inch image intensifier.
Courtesy of OEC Medical Systems, Salt Lake City, UT

Controls and Operation Modes: The digital C-arm fluoroscopy systems include a variety of operating mode option controls that the radiographer must be familiar with. These control panels may be on the TV monitor control cart, or with certain equipment the control panel may be on the C-arm unit itself (Fig. 19-38).

The **mag mode**, refers to the ability to magnify the image when requested by the surgeon to better visualize structures that they frequently have to view at a distance from the monitor.

The **pulse mode** is used to create a pulsating x-ray beam at timed increments to reduce exposure.

The **snapshot** or **digital spot mode** activates a "digital spot," which results in a higher quality **computer-enhanced image** as compared to a held fluoro image.

The **film mode** is for exposing standard cassettes placed in the optional holder placed on the image intensifier. This **cassette holder** can be attached to the image intensifier tower in which to place regular cassettes for conventional radiographs (Fig. 19-39). In this way the C-arm can also function as a conventional mobile radiography unit without using the digital imaging functions.

Auto/manual exposure control allows for manual exposure control by the operator if desired, or the use of AEC type controls.

Additional optional modes available on some equipment that allow more complicated procedures are **subtraction** (digital subtraction) and **roadmapping**. Roadmapping is a method of image display wherein a specific fluoro image is held on the screen in combination with continuous fluoro. This is especially useful in interventional procedures requiring placement of catheters and guidewires.

Foot Pedal: The foot pedal allows the physician or other operator hands free operation of the C-arm. A fully equipped foot pedal has multiple pedals for controlling various functions such as shown in the upper right of Fig. 19-38. This specific model has four controls. The **scout fluoro** pedal operates unprocessed or raw fluoro functions. The **digital process fluoro** activates selected computer enhanced processing functions such as averaging (fluoro image noise reduction). A third pedal is the **image save** control for saving the last image displayed. The pedal marked **snapshot** or **boost digital spot** when activated results in a higher quality computer enhanced image.

Image Orientation

The flexibility of the C-arm to image a variety of anatomical structures at virtually any conceivable angle from any side or direction **requires correct image orientation each time it is set up for use**. This needs to be done during setup time before the patient is brought into the room to avoid needless exposure to the patient and personnel after the procedure begins. For example, attempting to orient a smaller size image in the abdominal region which has few landmarks to indicate top or bottom, or right or left, can be very confusing and difficult.

Each radiographer should develop their own method of doing this. One method is to bring the C-arm into the room in the same position and orientation that will be used for the procedure. Place a lead marker R on the flat surface of the x-ray tube collimator oriented in the same way the patient will be oriented. The top of the R to the head end, to be displayed on the patient's right side to appear anatomically correct on the monitor to the viewer's left. (The same orientation as for viewing radiographs, the patient's right to the viewer's left.) A light exposure can be made during this setup with an apron or other shielding covering the C-arm to shield other personnel in the room. By viewing and orienting the test image of the R on the monitor correctly, one can be prepared when the procedure begins.

Sterile Fields

C-arm use in surgical settings requires special attention in maintaining sterile fields. The top location of the image intensifier often causes it to be placed over open incisions.

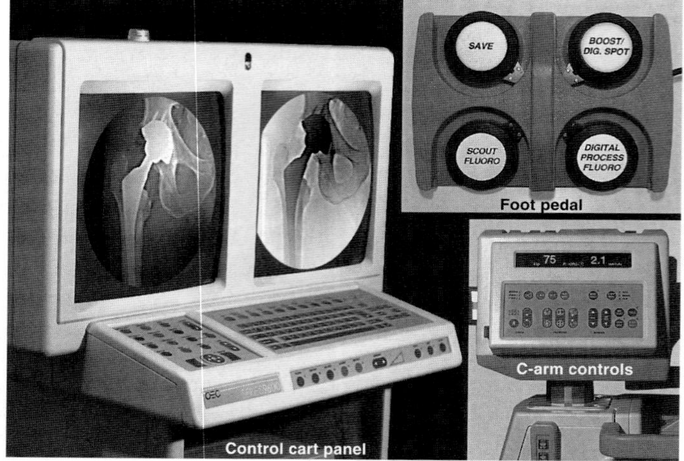

Fig. 19-38. Control panels and foot pedal of OEC 9600 series C-arm.

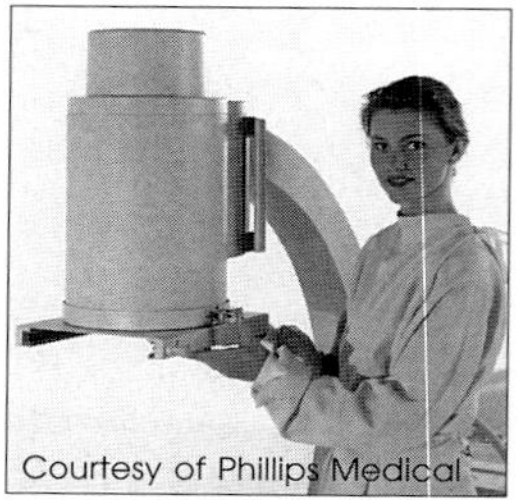

Courtesy of Phillips Medical

Fig. 19-39. Cassette holder attachment.

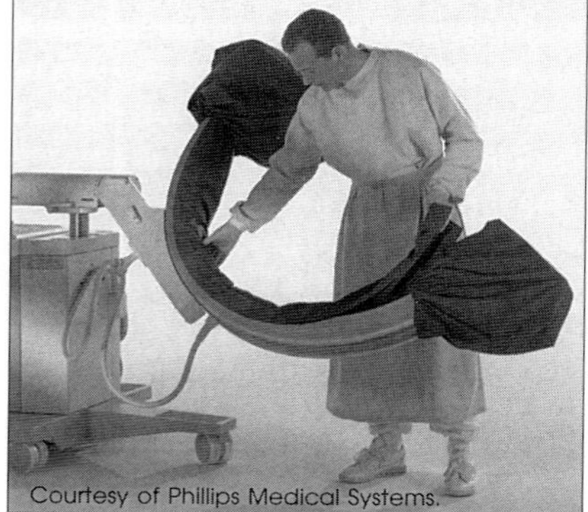

Courtesy of Phillips Medical Systems.

Fig. 19-40. Sterile field–Draping image intensifier and C-arm (snap cover).

There are **three** basic approaches to maintaining a sterile field: The most common method is **draping the image intensifier, x-ray tube and C-arm** using a sterile cloth and/or bags with a tension band holding the cloth and bags in place (Fig. 19-40). The cover is called a **snap cover** (the band makes a snapping sound when it is released into position). Snap covers make it possible for the surgeon to operate with the image intensifier over an open incision. It also provides the physician a way to move the C-arm for precise movement or centering.

A second, less commonly used approach is to **temporarily drape the patient** (or surgery site) with an additional sterile cloth before the undraped C-arm is positioned over the anatomy. Once positioned and a satisfactory image has been obtained and the C-arm is removed, the sterile cloth (or drape) is then removed from the patient and discarded. This process is repeated with a new (unused) sterile cloth if there is need to use the C-arm again. This approach is employed in cases where the physician does not need to interact with the surgical site during fluoro, or when snap covers are not available.

The third method of maintaining a sterile area uses what is called **a "shower curtain."** Hip pinnings or femur roddings require a lateral approach to the surgical incision making these procedures ideal for the shower curtain. A long horizontal metal bar attached to two vertical suspending rods is placed along the lateral longitudinal axis of the affected side. A large sterile, clear plastic sheet (a "shower curtain") is suspended from the horizontal bar which is about two feet above the patient. A special opening in the middle of the plastic is attached with a second adhesive strip to the lateral aspect of the hip/proximal femur and is used for access to the incision. The curtain forms a sterile barrier between the doctor and the patient as the C-arm is positioned for a standard PA and horizontal beam lateral hip from the non-affected side of the patient.

RADIATION PROTECTION

Radiation safety is a special concern with fluoroscopy of any type, especially with the C-arm when used in unshielded environments such as the operating room. Safety precautions for the C-arm follow the **three cardinal rules** of radiation protection; **distance, time** and **shielding**.

Distance (most effective means of reducing occupational exposure)

As demonstrated by the exposure fields in these drawings, the secondary fields from scatter radiation drop off dramatically as one moves away from the source (applying the inverse square law).

Before exposures are made the technologist should remind all personnel to stand back as far as possible even if wearing lead aprons. **Distance is key for reducing personnel exposure** as seen on these drawings. For example, someone standing 2 or 3 feet from the source (Zone C) will receive a dose equivalent of about 60 mR/hr. (1 mR/min.). If a total of 5 minutes of fluoro time was used on one procedure, the total dose received would be about **5 mR at 3 feet**, but only about **0.2 mR at 6 to 10 feet** (the exposure rate at 6 to 10 ft. in Zone F would be about 5 R/hr.).

Time

Limiting exposure time is also an effective means of radiation protection. This is especially true in fluoroscopy where fluoro exposure times and resultant scatter radiation can be excessive as compared to conventional still frame radiographs. Non-radiologists may not have the experience and training in the use of intermittent or "foot-tapping" fluoroscopy. This makes the use of the **pulse mode** more important with the C-arm in surgical procedures, which allows pulsed fluoroscopy at a rate of only one or two frames per second with the digital recorder holding this image on the monitor between pulses.

Shielding (least effective means)

In addition to time and distance, correct use of shielding is also important in trauma and mobile radiography. For example, before a surgical procedure begins, the radiographer should provide **lead aprons** for all persons remaining in the room during exposures, or should provide a mobile lead shield behind which they can stand. The surgeon or radiologist, the anesthesiologist and other personnel remaining in the room who cannot move behind a shield should be given lead aprons to wear under their sterile gowns.

C-Arm Orientation and Exposure Patterns

Vertical PA CR: Keeping the C-arm PA and directly vertical and perpendicular to the floor minimizes exposure to the neck and facial region (Fig. 19-41). If the C-arm is tilted as much as 30° as shown in Fig. 19-42, the configuration of the exposure fields change to significantly increase exposure to the upper body and facial region not shielded by the lead apron. Studies have shown that even a **30° C-arm tilt will increase the dose** to the face and neck region of the average height operator standing next to the C-arm **by a factor of four.**[†]

Horizontal CR: The configuration of the exposure fields with a horizontal beam is demonstrated in Fig. 19-43. Note that the **exposure region on the x-ray tube side of the patient is significantly greater than the region near the intensifier tower**. This should be an important consideration for the surgeon or other operator who may need to stay near the patient.

Vertical AP CR: Occasionally the radiographer may be asked to reverse the C-arm with the tube on top and the intensifier on the bottom. This provides the surgeon more room for manipulation but it is **not recommended** due to the **significant increase in exposure** to the operator as shown in Fig. 19-44.

Summary: Good radiation protection practices are especially important in trauma and mobile radiography where fixed lead barriers are not present behind which to stand during exposures. This is true with bedside portables, but even more so with C-arm mobile fluoroscopy which potentially results in considerably more scatter radiation to the immediate area. The radiographer must continually be aware of the three cardinal rules of radiation protection, **distance, time** and **shielding**.

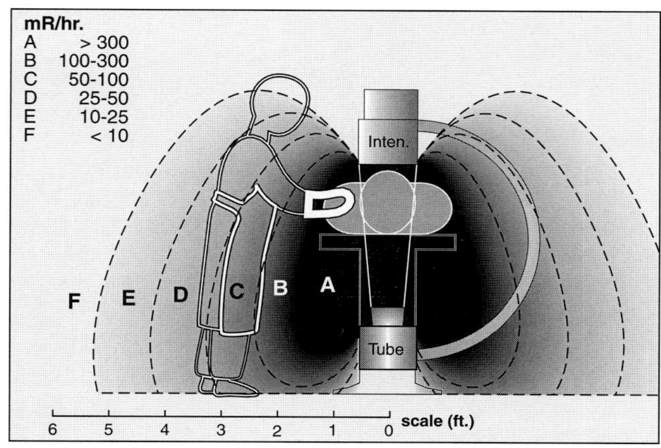

Fig. 19-41. Exposure levels–CR vertical, **PA projection**.*†

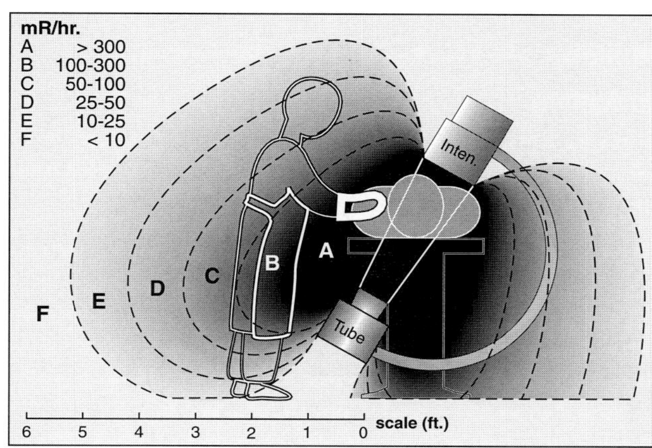

Fig. 19-42. Exposure levels–CR 30° from vertical.*†

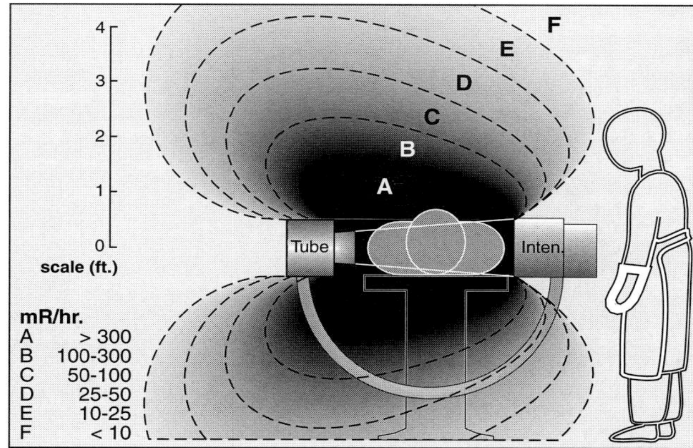

Fig. 19-43. Exposure patterns and levels–CR horizontal.*†

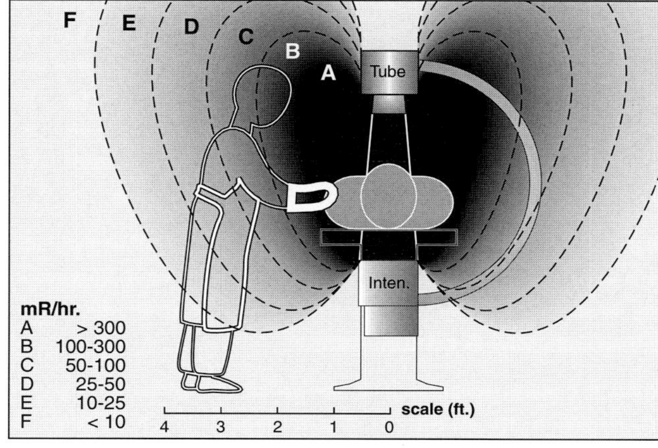

Fig. 19-44. Exposure levels, **AP projection** (tube on top).*† –**NOT** recommended.

*Technical reference, OEC Medical Systems, Salt Lake City, Utah, 1996.

†Geise, R.A., Hunter, D.W., Personnel Exposure During Fluoroscopy, *Postgraduate Radiology*, Vol. 8, 1988.

Radiographic Positioning

AP Chest

Warning: With possible spinal injury or severe trauma do not attempt to elevate patient for semierect or decubitus. Lift patient only with assistance of other medical personnel to place cassette under patient for AP supine. Some ER carts or tables have a tray under the patient into which to place the cassette.

Technical Factors

- Film size–14 x 17 in. (35 x 43 cm) **crosswise** for average to large patients (see Note 1).
- 70-80 kVp, screen–small to medium
  80-90 kVp, grid–large (see Note 2)

Shielding: Shield pelvic region if childbearing age.

Positioning

- Enclose cassette in a pillow slip or some other type of cover so it does not make contact with patient's bare skin (for hygiene purposes and for easier cassette placement).

  Bedside chest: Elevate head end of bed if possible into a semierect position (Fig. 19-46).
- Place top of cassette about 2 in. (5 cm) above the shoulders, which should center cassette to CR.
- Rotate arms internally if patient's condition allows to roll shoulders forward to move scapulae out of lung fields.
- Ensure **no** rotation (coronal plane parallel to film). (Place supports under parts of cassette as needed to keep film level in bed.)

Central Ray

- Direct CR to 3 to 4 in. (7 to 10 cm) below jugular notch.
- Angle CR 3 to 5° caudad, or raise head end of bed slightly to place the CR perpendicular to long axis of sternum (unless grid prevents this). This simulates the PA projection and prevents the clavicles from obscuring the apices of the lungs (Fig. 19-45).
- 48 to 72 in. (122 to 182 cm) SID. Use 72 in. (180 cm) if possible.

Respiration: Exposure at end of 2nd full inspiration.

Optional lateral chest (not demonstrated here): A lateral horizontal beam CR can be taken if patient can raise arms at least 90° from body. Place cassette parallel to MSP, top of film ≈2 in. (5 cm) above level of shoulders. Raise patient on radiolucent pad to center chest to film, center horizontal CR to level of T7.

Lateral decubitus AP projection: To determine air-fluid levels when patient cannot be elevated sufficiently for erect position, a lateral decubitus can be taken in bed with cassette placed behind patient, or on a cart in front of a film holder as shown in Fig. 19-47. Place radiolucent pads under thorax and shoulders, and raise arms above head. CR-part-film alignment and centering is similar to supine AP with necessary adaptations for decubitus position.

Note 1: Side cutoff is more of a problem with AP mobile chests taken at a shorter SID due to the increased angle of divergence of the x-ray beam. Therefore, unless the patient is quite small, a **crosswise film placement is recommended**.

Note 2: Linear focused grids are generally difficult to use for mobile chests due to the problems of grid cutoff. The nonlinear, wafer type grid is well suited for portable AP chests due to its tolerance for non-centering and for up to 10° CR angles without grid cutoff. (See page 553, Fig. 19-32).

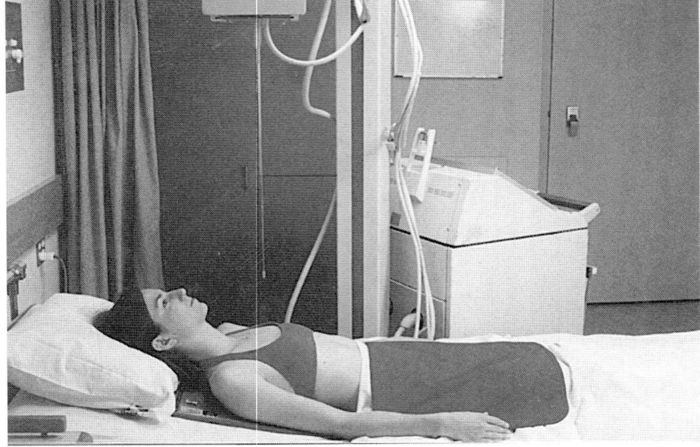

Fig. 19-45. AP supine–Bedside (film crosswise).
–CR 3-5° caudad, perpendicular to sternum.

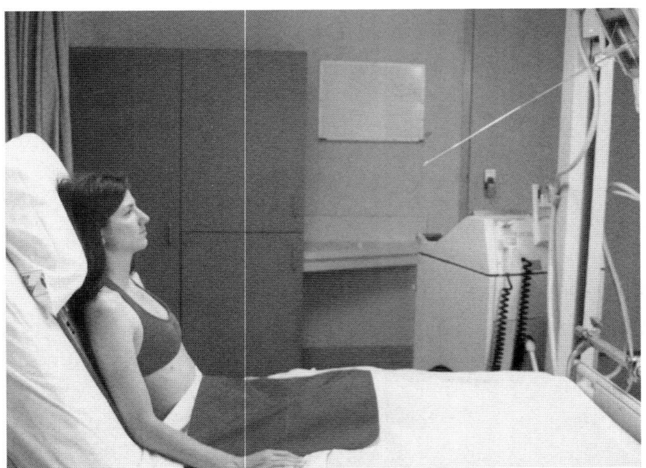

Fig. 19-46. AP semierect–Bedside.

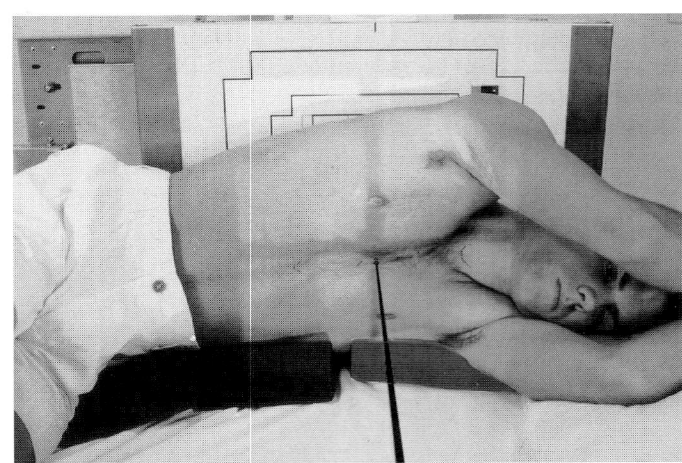

Fig. 19-47. Lateral decubitus (AP), horizontal beam for detecting possible air-fluid levels.

AP Oblique and Lateral Sternum

The sternum is nearly impossible to visualize radiographically on a straight frontal view due to the thin flat bone being superimposed by the thoracic vertebrae. It is possible to visualize, however, by superimposing the sternum over the homogenous heart shadow just to the left of the vertebrae, which requires an **LPO or an equivalent mediolateral angle** CR for a supine trauma patient.

Technical Factors

- Film size–10 x 12 in. (24 x 30 cm) or 11 x 14 in. (30 x 30 cm) (crosswise for AP supine with a mediolateral angle CR).
- 60-70 kVp range with grid.
- 2 to 3 second exposure breathing technique is commonly used to blur out lung structures and posterior ribs. If patient can cooperate, have them breathe gentle short breaths for movement of lungs and ribs with little movement of the sternum.
- 40 in (102) SID (Note 1).

Shielding: Shield pelvic region if childbearing age.

Positioning and Central Ray

***AP Oblique–LPO** (Fig. 19-48):*

- If patient cannot be rotated, maintain the CR-part-film alignment of a LPO position by angling the CR 15 to 20° mediolaterally, from right to left (see Note 2); or if patient's condition allows, rotate in a 15 to 20° LPO position with CR perpendicular to film.
- CR perpendicular to center of sternum with film centered to CR.
- Angle CR 15 to 20° from right to left to project sternum over heart shadow. Center CR to mid sternum.
- Place top of crosswise placed cassette about 1½ in. (4 cm) above jugular notch, with cassette centered to projected CR.

Respiration: See breathing instructions above.

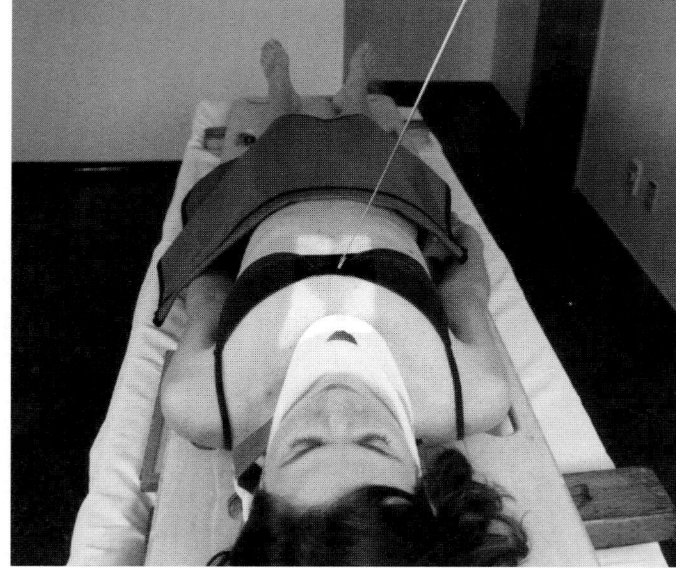

Fig. 19-48. AP supine (oblique) sternum.
-Patient remains supine.
-15 to 20° CR mediolateral angle.
-Grid crosswise to prevent cutoff.

***Lateral, Horizontal Beam** (Fig. 19-49):*

- With patient supine place arms at side, shoulders drawn back.
- Grid cassette at patient's side parallel to MSP centered to midpoint of sternum (midway between manubrial notch and xiphoid).
- Horizontal CR to mid sternum.
- Expose upon full inspiration.

Note 1: It is a common practice to use a shorter SID of ≈30 in. (77 cm) for the routine anterior oblique (RAO) which magnifies posterior ribs to better visualize the sternum. However, for this supine AP projection, a routine 40 in. (102 cm) SID should be used due to the distance of the sternum from the film, which with a shorter SID would result in increased magnification and resultant loss of visible detail.

Note 2: For the oblique sternum less body rotation or less mediolateral angle CR (≈15°) is required on large deep-chested thorax, and more rotation or CR angle (≈20°) for smaller thorax.

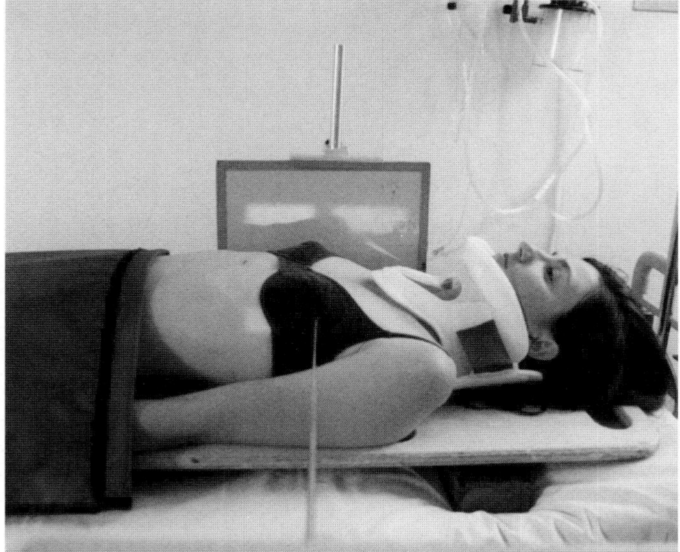

Fig. 19-49. Lateral sternum.
-Horizontal beam CR to mid sternum.

19

AP and Oblique Ribs–Above or Below Diaphragm

If the patient is able, it is less painful to radiograph ribs erect rather than recumbent, which places the weight of their body on possible fractured ribs. (See Chapter 10.) Anterior or posterior obliques would be determined by the site of injury. The oblique view that places the injury closest to the film should be taken if the patient's condition allows. Severe trauma requires adaptation for oblique position with cross-angle CR with patient supine as shown.

Above or below diaphragm is determined by region of injury.

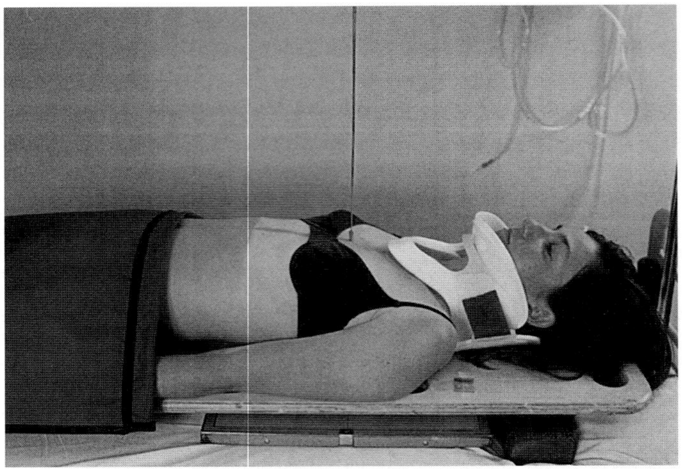

Fig. 19-50. AP ribs, above diaphragm.

Technical Factors

- Film size–14 x 17 in. (35 x 43 cm) crosswise for bilateral ribs (see Note).
- 65-70 kVp range, grid, above diaphragm.
  75-80 kVp range, grid, below diaphragm.
- 40-44 in. (102-112 cm) SID.

Shielding: Shield pelvic region.

Positioning and Central Ray

AP Above or Below Diaphragm:

- For above diaphragm, place grid cassette under patient, centered to thorax bilaterally and to CR.
- CR perpendicular to MSP, centered 3 to 4 in. (7 to 10 cm) below jugular notch as for an AP chest.
- For below diaphragm, place bottom of cassette at level of iliac crest.
- CR perpendicular to center of film.

Oblique above or below diaphragm:

- If patient is able, oblique patient 30 to 45°, injured side down.
- Center cassette to thorax bilaterally.
- Center cassette for above or below diaphragm centering.
- CR perpendicular to center of film.

Respiration: Above diaphragm – expose on inspiration.
Below diaphragm – expose on expiration.

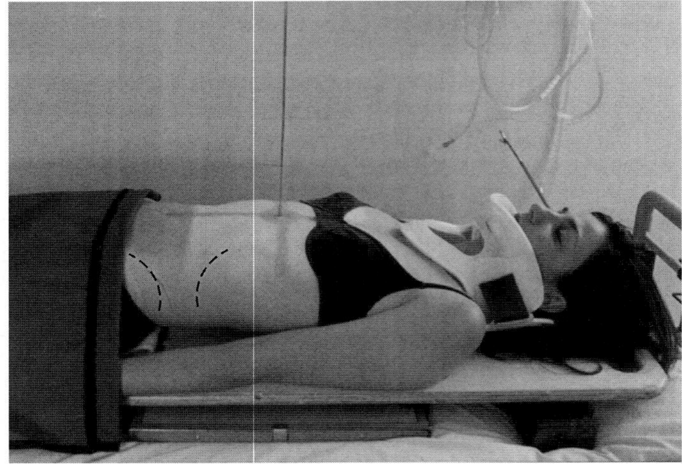

Fig. 19-51. AP ribs below diaphragm.

Alternate Mediolateral of CR (Supine Immobile Patient):

- If patient cannot be rotated, the CR can be cross-angled mediolaterally 30 to 40° with grid cassette crosswise, centered to include region of injury.
- To maintain CR-part-film relationship and decrease distortion, it is best to also angle the plane of the film to be near perpendicular to the CR. This can be done by placing supports under the patient so the smaller size cassette (10 x 12 or 11 x 14 in.) can also be propped up at an angle to be nearer perpendicular to CR. A full 45° oblique projection may not be possible, but even a 30° CR angle will provide a second oblique projection of ribs, which may demonstrate pathology not seen on the straight AP supine projection.
  (Provides a second perspective as an alternate to the routine 45° oblique when patient cannot be rotated.)

Note: Some departmental routines include unilateral obliques on a smaller film centered to the point of injury, in addition to the AP and oblique bilateral ribs on large films.

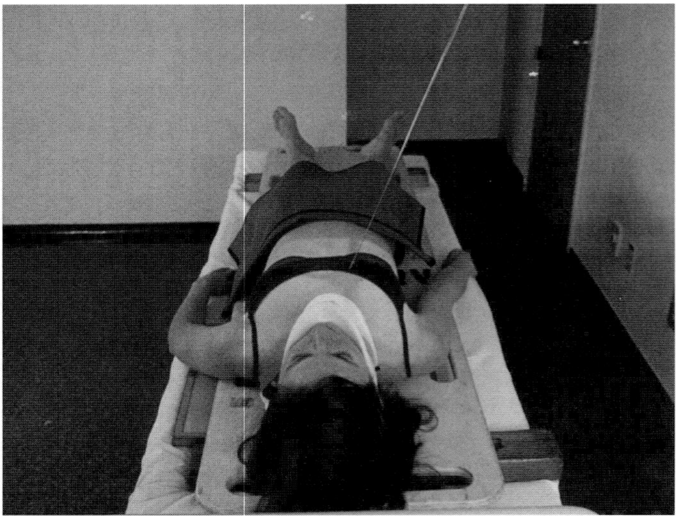

Fig. 19-52. Alternate 30 to 40° mediolateral CR–Grid crosswise.

AP Abdomen-Supine and Decubitus

Technical Factors

- Film size–14 x 17 in. (35 x 43 cm) lengthwise.
- 70-80 kVp range, with grid.
- Include decub and upside markers if applicable.
- 40-44 in. (102-112 cm) SID.

Shielding: Shield male gonads.

Positioning and Central Ray

AP Supine:

- Place cassette into pillow case or cover for easier placement under patient, if taken bedside.
- Align cassette lengthwise to MSP.
- Center cassette to CR at **level of iliac crest**. Ensure that both sides of upper and lower abdomen are equal distances from lateral cassette margins.
- Place pads under parts of cassette if needed to ensure that cassette is level and perpendicular to CR (to prevent rotation on soft bed surface which can cause rotation and grid cutoff).
- CR perpendicular, to level of iliac crest and to center of film.

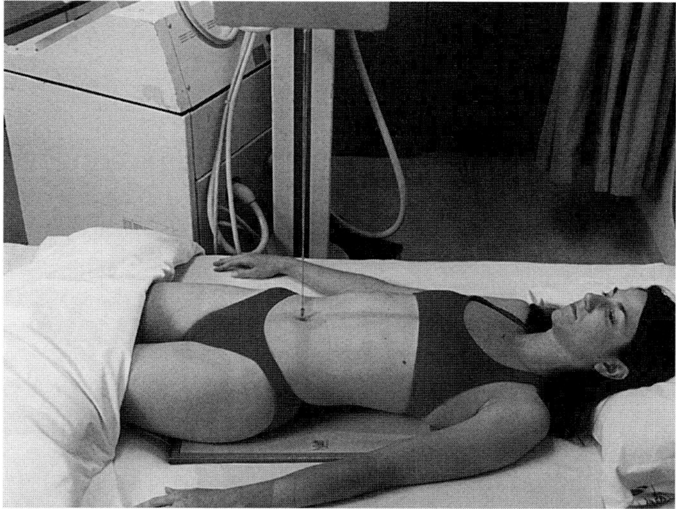

Fig. 19-53. Supine AP-Bedside.

Left Lateral Decubitus AP (or PA) Projection:

- To determine air-fluid levels and possible free intra-abdominal air when an upright is not possible. The lateral decubitus (AP) can be taken in bed, on a cart in ER, or on cart in radiographic room in front of erect grid device.
- Ensure that **diaphragm and upside of abdomen is included on film.** Place center of cassette 1 to 2 in. (3 to 5 cm) above level of iliac crests.
- Place pads or a positioning board under hips and thorax as needed to center abdomen to film for both lateral and dorsal decubitus, if done bedside.
- Ensure no rotation and that plane of film is perpendicular to CR.
- **Horizontal CR** to center of film.

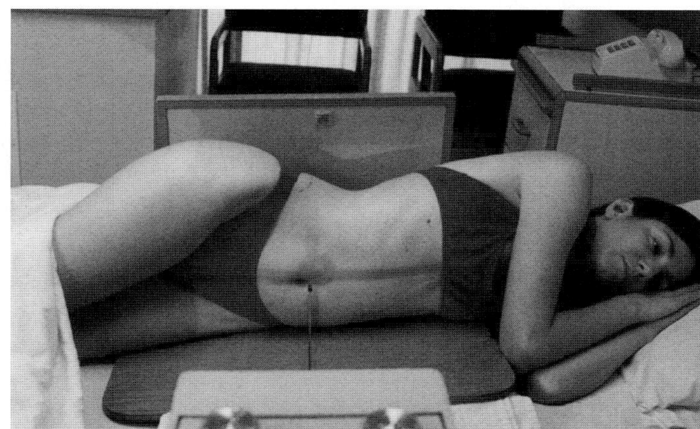

Fig. 19-54. Lateral decubitus (AP)-Bedside.

Respiration: Expose on expiration, ensure that breathing has ceased before making exposure.

Note: For lateral decubitus, have patient lie on side for **5 minutes** prior to making exposure to allow for air to rise to highest placement within abdomen.

Dorsal Decubitus, Lateral Position:

This is not a common bedside projection and when requested usually involves bringing the patient to radiology where it can be performed in front of an erect x-ray table as also shown and as described in Chapter 3 on the abdomen.

Note: This dorsal decubitus is a good projection to demonstrate a possible abdominal aortic aneurysm.

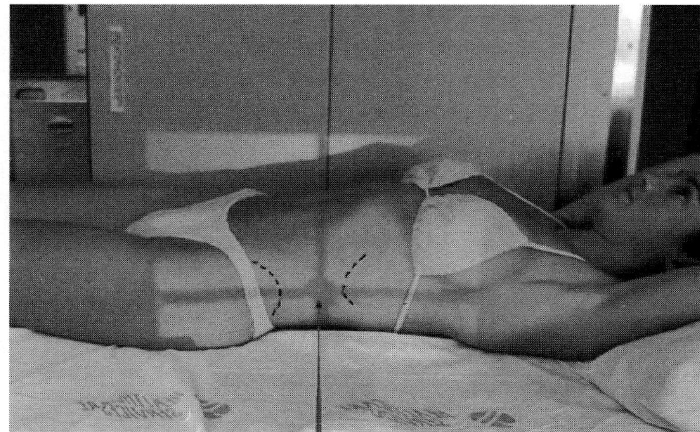

Fig. 19-55. Dorsal decubitus (lateral), on cart in front of erect x-ray table.

AP (PA) Oblique and Lateral–Fingers, Thumb, Hand and Wrist

Technical Factors

- Film size–8 x 10 in. (20 x 24 cm) or–10 x 12 in. (24 x 30 cm).
- 50-60 kVp range, detail (100 speed) screens.
- 40-44 in. (102 cm) SID.

Shielding: Shield pelvic region.

Positioning and Central Ray–Patient Supine

AP–Fingers, Hand and/or Wrist *(Fig. 19-56):*

- Generally the hand and/or fingers or wrist can be positioned as needed on the cassette placed on the cart or table beside the patient. Move patient to one side of cart or table as needed to provide room for film placement. If the fingers and hand can be fully extended, AP or PA projections can be readily achieved. Positioning, CR centering and collimation to parts of interest is similar to routine upper limb projections as described in Chapter 4.
- CR perpendicular to part and film, centered to:
  –Hand, CR to 3rd MP joint.
  –Finger, CR to PIP joint.

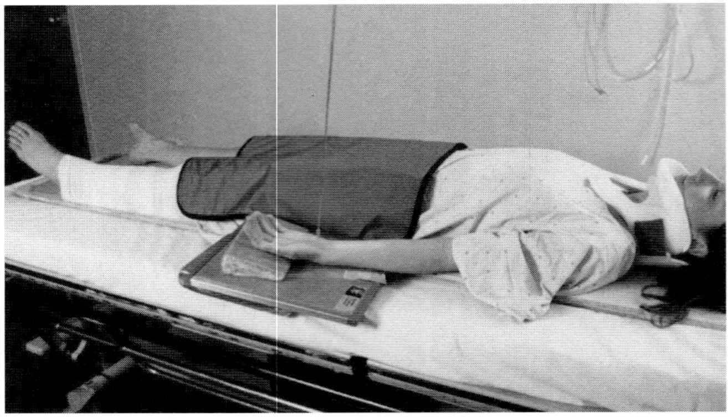
Fig. 19-56. AP hand and/or wrist.

Alternate AP of Fingers (With Fingers and Hand Partially Flexed) *(Figs. 19-57 and 19-58):*

- If patient cannot fully extend fingers, then specific AP projections can be done as shown with the **parts of interest placed parallel to the film**.
- CR perpendicular to part of interest and to film. Angle film and CR as needed.

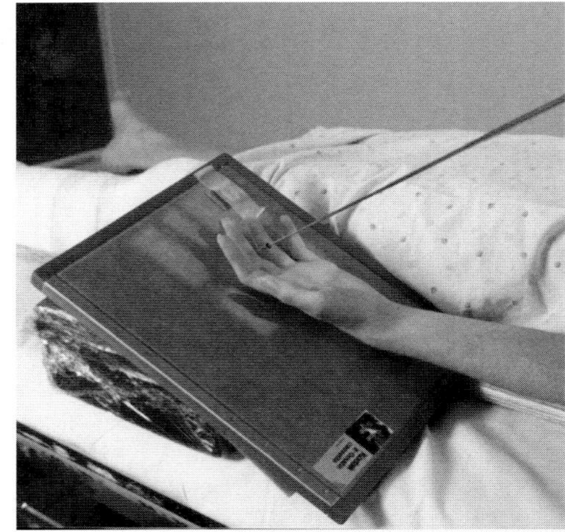
Fig. 19-57. AP hand and fingers for **distal phalanges**.

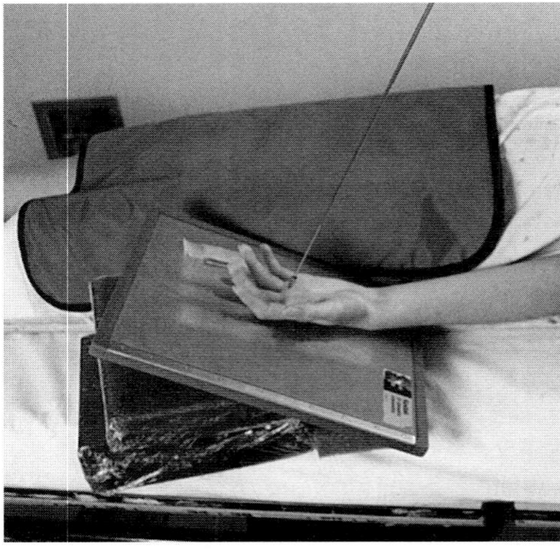
Fig. 19-58. AP hand and fingers for **proximal phalanges** and **metacarpals**.

PA and Lateral Thumb:

- If specific injury is to the thumb, a PA projection can be achieved using a radiolucent sponge as demonstrated (Fig. 19-59).
- Lateral positioning of the thumb can also be readily achieved by angling the CR as needed for a lateral projection (Fig. 19-60).
- Ensure that entire thumb including all of 1st metacarpal is included.
- CR to 1st MP joint.

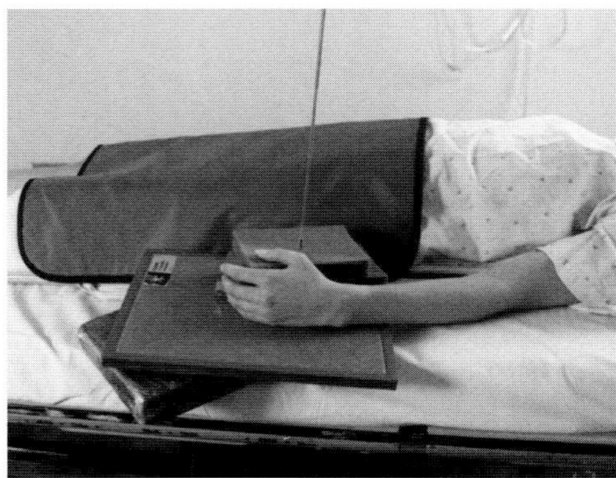
Fig. 19-59. PA thumb.

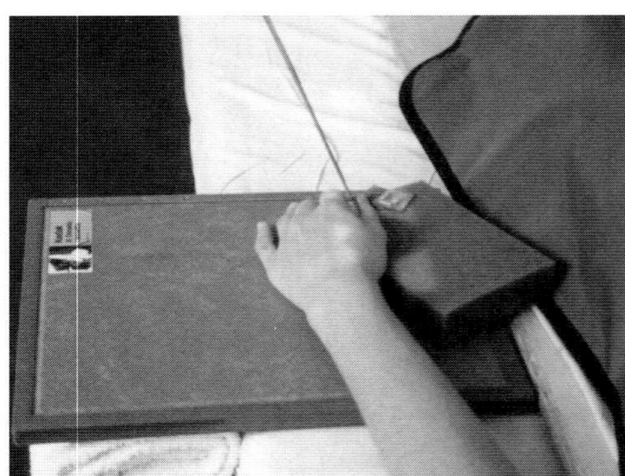
Fig. 19-60. Lateral thumb.

Oblique and Lateral –Fingers, Hand and/or Wrist:

- Obliques and laterals of the fingers, hand and/or wrist can be achieved by lateral rotation as with routine positioning of these parts as shown in Chapter 4, or by adjusting CR and film angles as needed (see lateral wrist, Fig. 19-62).
- CR centering and collimation to specific region of interest.

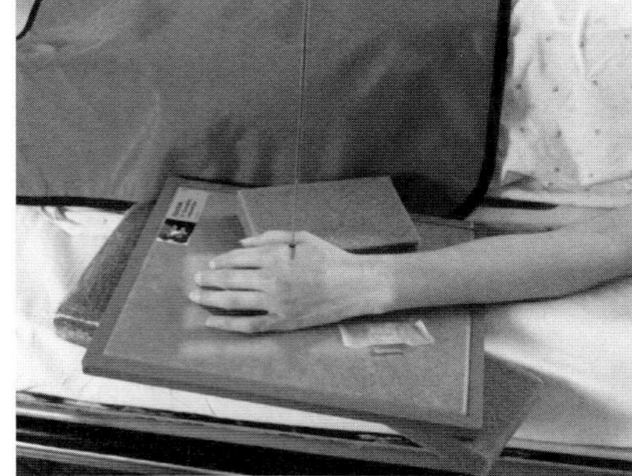
Fig. 19-61. Oblique –Fingers, hand and/or wrist.

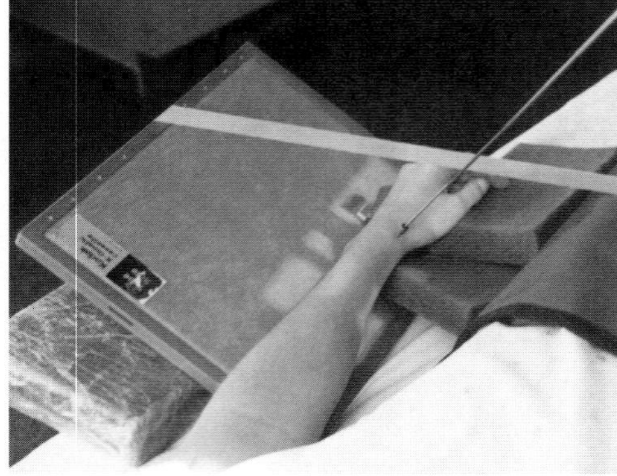
Fig. 19-62. Lateral wrist and hand.

19

AP and Lateral Forearm
Post Reduction Forearm and Wrist

Include both joints with original trauma films of forearm.
Post reduction film can include only the joint nearest fracture site.

Technical Factors

- Film size–11 x 14 in. (30 x 35 cm)
  or–14 x 17 in (35 x 43 cm) to include both joints.
- 65-70 kVp range, detail (100 speed) screens.
- 40-44 in (100-112 cm) SID.

Cast conversion: Dry cast, +5-7 kVp.
Wet cast, 2x mAs or +8-10 kVp.
Fiberglass, +5-7 kVp.

Shielding: Shield pelvis and chest region.

Positioning and Central Ray–Patient Supine

***PA** (Fig. 19-63):*

- Adjust plane of film and CR as needed for a true PA; center to wrist or mid forearm to include the area of interest.

***Lateral** (Fig. 19-64):*

- With hand pronated as much as possible, use supports to prop up hand and arm as needed for lateral projection with film-part-CR 90° from PA.

Note: If possible trauma region includes the elbow, use larger films to include both wrist and elbow joints on these projections.

***Post Reduction Forearm and Wrist** (Figs. 19-65 and 19-66):*

- Move patient to one side of cart for more room for film placement for PA and lateral projections.
- PA may be taken as demonstrated. (Cast generally holds wrist and forearm in place without radius-ulna crossover.) Include either the wrist or elbow, whichever is closest to known fracture site.
- For lateral, adjust arm, cassette and CR as needed for 90° projection from PA.

Alternate erect position (Figs. 19-69 to 19-71): If patient is already erect in a wheelchair, or can stand, these projections can be taken seated at the end of the x-ray table with arm, cassette and CR adjusted as needed for these two projections.

Postreduction radiographs: PA and lateral of distal forearm and wrist are shown below.

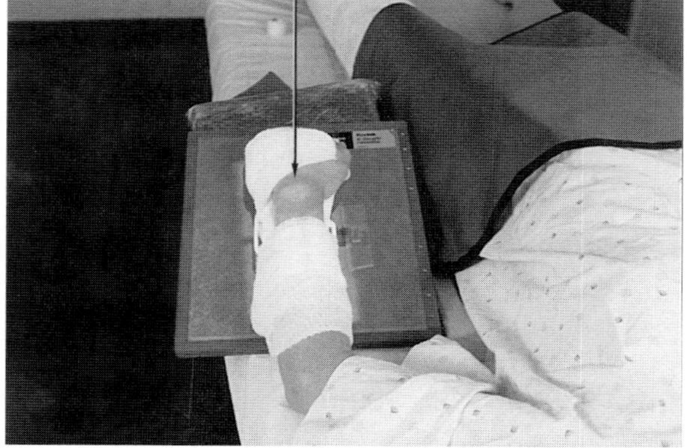

Fig. 19-63. PA wrist and forearm in splint.

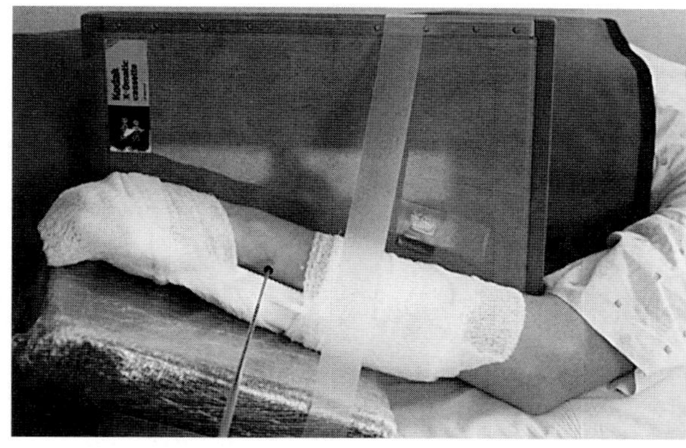

Fig. 19-64. Lateral wrist and forearm in splint.

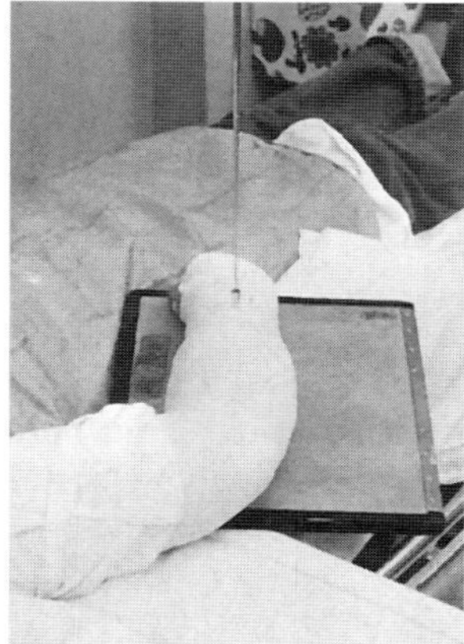

Fig. 19-65. With cast, PA forearm and wrist.

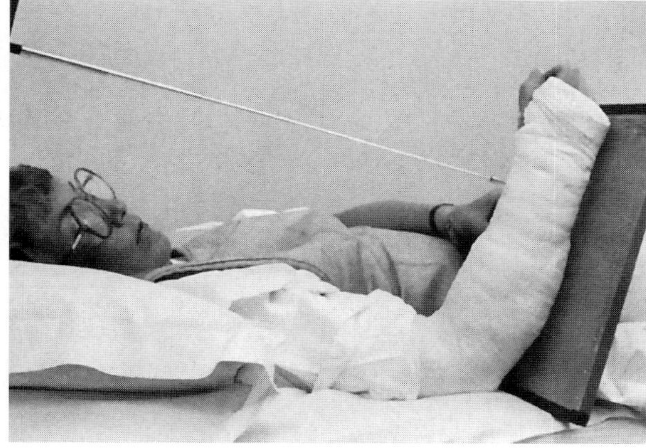

Fig. 19-66. With cast, lateral forearm and wrist (lateromedial).

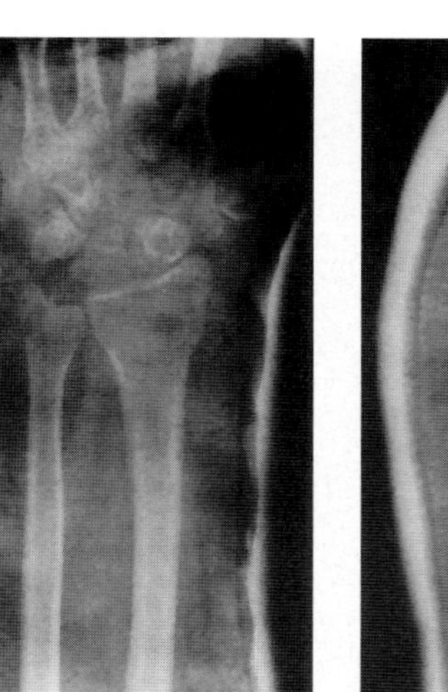

Fig. 19-67. PA wrist.

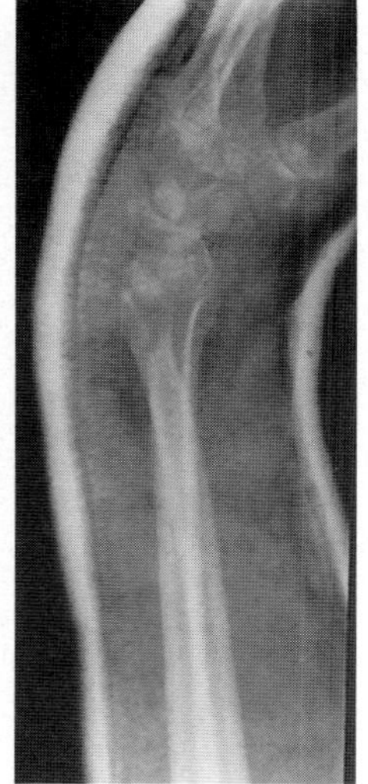

Fig. 19-68. Lateral wrist.

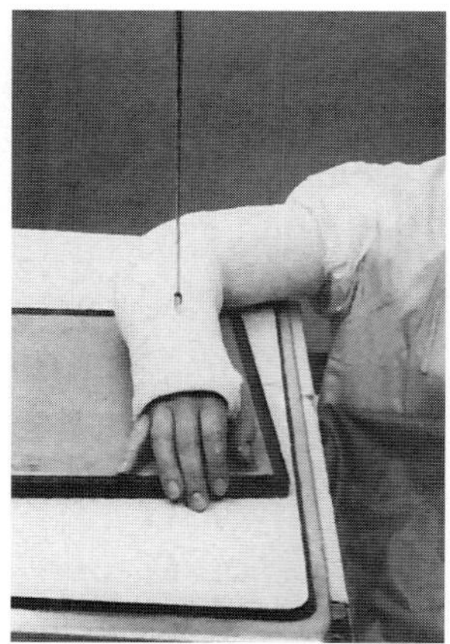

Fig. 19-69. PA erect.

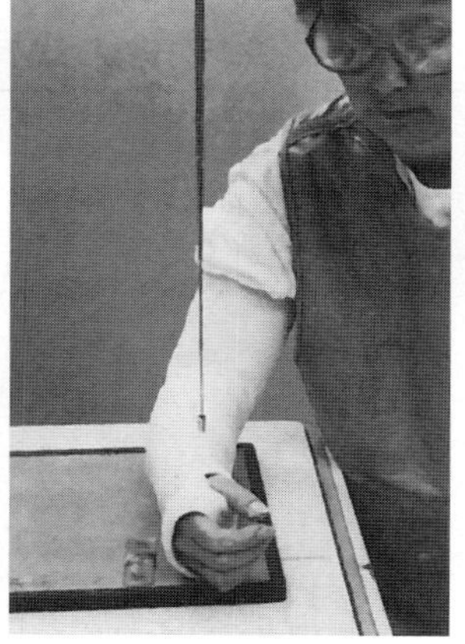

Fig. 19-70. Lateral erect.

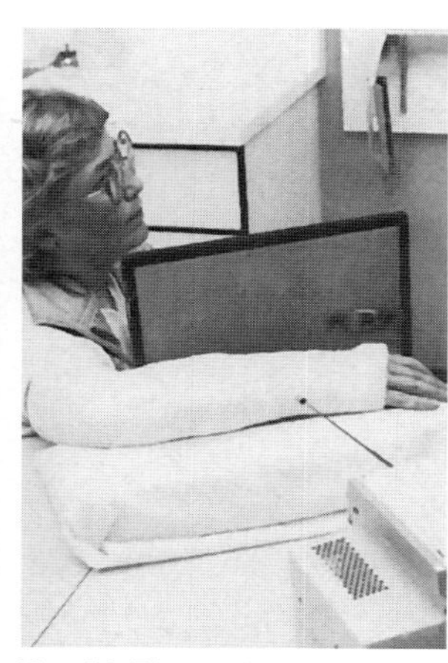

Fig. 19-71. Horizontal beam (lateral).

PA and Lateral Elbow

As with other trauma radiographic examinations a minimum of two projections should be completed if possible, an **AP or PA** and a **lateral**. For patients with multiple trauma injuries including possible trauma to thorax and/or spine and wherein the elbow remains partially flexed and the hand pronated, **horizontal beam PA** and **vertical beam lateral** projections may be performed as demonstrated for initial elbow examination.

Technical Factors

- Film size–8 x 10 in. (20 x 24 cm)
  or–10 x 12 in. (24 x 30 cm).
- 60-70 kVp range, detail (100 speed) screens.
- 40-44 in. (102-112 cm) SID.

Shielding: Shield pelvis and chest region.

Positioning and Central Ray With Hand Pronated and Elbow Partially Flexed).

PA (Fig. 19-72):

- Place vertical cassette between arm and patient. (Place shield between cassette and thorax.) Place support under arm and hand.
- Direct horizontal beam CR to be **perpendicular to interepicondylar plane** for true PA.

***Lateral** (Fig. 19-73 and 19-74):*

- With arm in similar position as for PA, with elbow partially flexed place cassette under elbow and forearm and angle the CR as needed to be **parallel to interepicondylar plane** (90° from PA). (Two possible lateral arm and cassette positions are shown in Figs. 19-73 and 19-74).

Note: If possible trauma region includes the proximal humerus or shoulder, take an AP of the entire humerus to include both elbow and shoulder joints as shown on following page along with a transthoracic lateral.

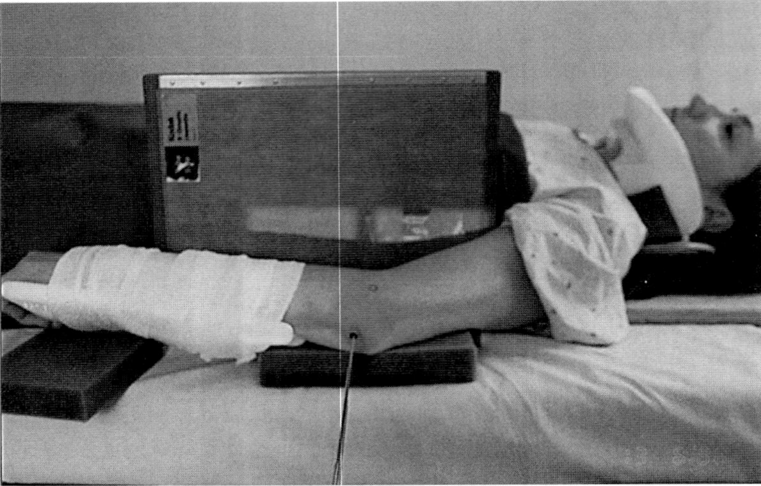

Fig. 19-72. **PA** horizontal beam elbow.
–CR **perpendicular** to interepicondylar plane.

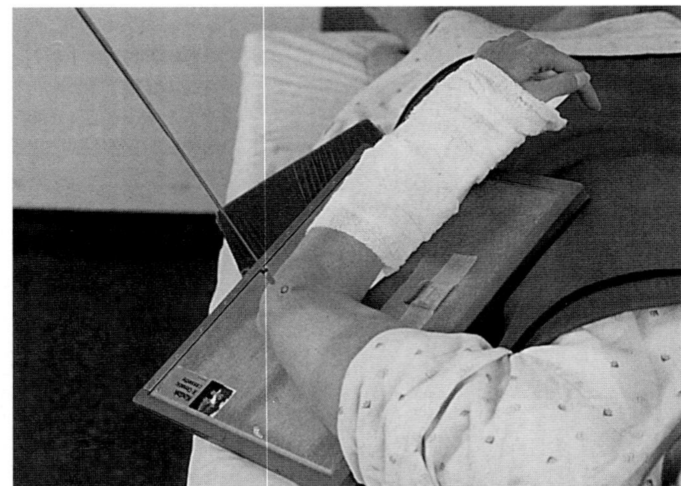

Fig. 19-73. Lateral elbow partially flexed.
–CR angled as needed to **be parallel** to interepicondylar plane.

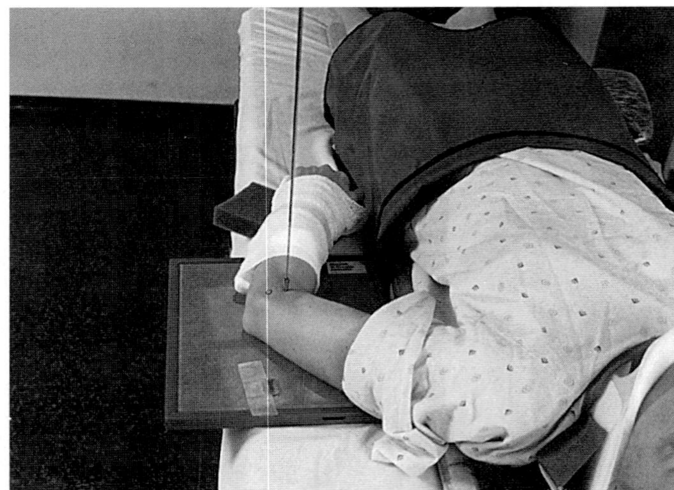

Fig. 19-74. Lateral elbow, hand remains pronated.
– CR perpendicular, **parallel** to interepicondylar plane.

AP and Lateral Humerus

Do not attempt to rotate arm for initial AP and lateral projections if evidence of fracture or dislocation is present. The AP should include both elbow and shoulder joints, but the lateral will include either the elbow or shoulder as demonstrated.

Technical Factors

- Film size–14 x 17 in. (35 x 43 cm)
  or–11 x 14 (30 x 35 cm).
- 65-70 kVp range with detail (100 speed) screens for AP, except for extra large patient over 10 cm, use grid and increase kVp accordingly.
- Grid required for transthoracic lateral, at 75-80 kVp.
- Transthoracic lateral generally taken with 2 to 3 sec. exposure and breathing technique if possible.
- 40-44 in (102-112 cm) SID.

Shielding: Shield pelvis and chest region.

Positioning and Central Ray –Patient Supine

AP *(Fig. 19-75):*

- With patient supine, carefully place cassette under shoulder and arm (large enough film to include both shoulder and elbow).
- Abduct arm slightly and supinate hand if patient's condition allows or take as is.
- Cross-angle CR as needed to be perpendicular to epicondyles if hand cannot be supinated. Center CR to mid humerus.

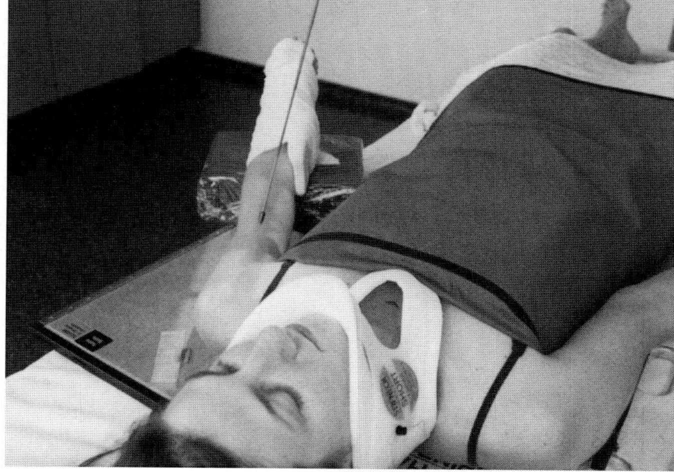

Fig. 19-75. AP humerus–To include both joints.

Lateral–Mid and Distal Humerus *(Fig. 19-76):*

- Place vertical cassette between arm and thorax with top of cassette as far into axilla as possible. Place shield between cassette and thorax.
- Flex elbow 90° if possible, or take as is.
- CR horizontal, and perpendicular to distal third of humerus and cassette.

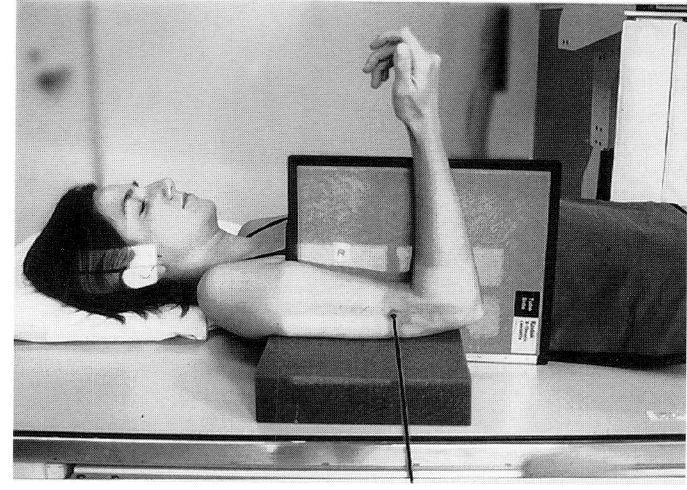

Fig. 19-76. Lateral–Mid and distal humerus to include elbow.

Lateral–Proximal Humerus (Horizontal Beam Transthoracic Lateral)
(Fig. 19-77):

- Place vertical grid next to injured shoulder and arm. Place grid lines vertically to prevent grid cutoff, if grid cassette is not low enough to center midline of grid to CR.
- Raise opposite arm above head, which also elevates this shoulder.
- Center horizontal CR through thorax to surgical neck and to centerline of grid. (A 10 to 15° cephalad angle may be required if shoulder of interest can't be lowered.)
- Have patient relax and lower shoulder of interest.

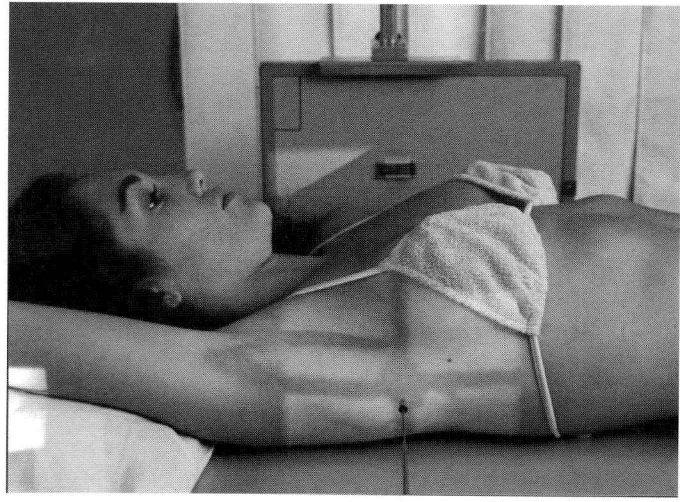

Fig. 19-77. Lateral–Transthoracic proximal humerus.

AP and Lateral–Shoulder, Scapula and Clavicle

Technical Factors

- Film size–10 x 12 in. (24 x 30 cm).
- 75-80 kVp range with grid.
- 40-44 in. (102-112 cm) SID.

Shielding: Shield pelvis and chest region.

Positioning and Central Ray –Patient Supine

***AP Shoulder** (Fig. 19-78):*

- With patient supine and arm in neutral rotation position at side, center cassette (grid cassette under patient if on cart) centered to shoulder joint and to CR.
- CR perpendicular to shoulder joint.

***AP Scapula** (Fig. 19-79):*

- With patient supine, gently abduct arm 90° from body if possible and center film and perpendicular CR to scapula.

Lateral Shoulder:

- See transthoracic lateral on preceding page; or take lateral scapular Y projection as shown in Fig. 19-81, but with CR centered to head of humerus.

***Lateral Scapular Y –AP Oblique (Lateromedial Scapula)** (Figs. 19-80 and 19-81):*

- Patient in posterior oblique position, side of interest elevated with arm raised and crossed to opposite shoulder. Palpate borders of scapula and turn patient until scapula is in profile in lateral position. (Generally requires about a 25 to 30° posterior oblique body position).
- Project CR perpendicular to film, or cross-angle CR as needed to be parallel to scapular blade (wing) as determined by palpation. (With CR cross-angled, turn grid crosswise to prevent grid cutoff.)
- CR centered to mid lateral (axillary) border of scapula.

***AP and AP Axial Clavicle** (Figs. 19-82 and 19-83):*

(In most trauma situations only one of these projections is required.)

- With patient supine and arm at side, center cassette placed crosswise to the clavicle.
- Direct CR perpendicular to mid clavicle and mid film for the AP; and 15 to 20° cephalad for the AP axial projection. A greater CR angle (20°) is required on a thin patient, and less angle (15°) for a thick patient.

Note: For the AP and/or axial clavicle a non-grid cassette can be used for a small to average patient, and a grid placed lengthwise to prevent grid cutoff from the CR angle on a large patient.

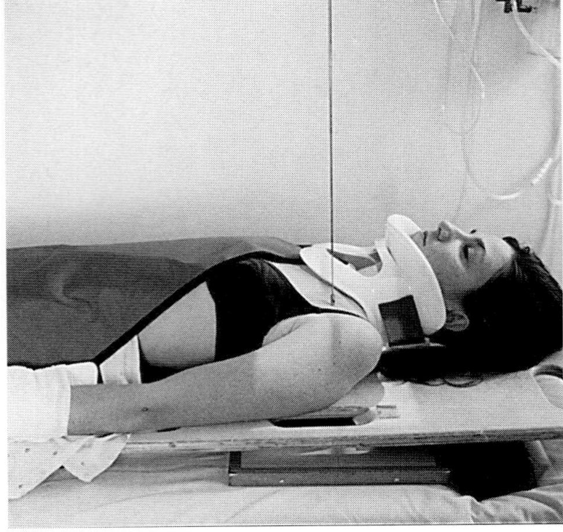

Fig. 19-78. AP shoulder.

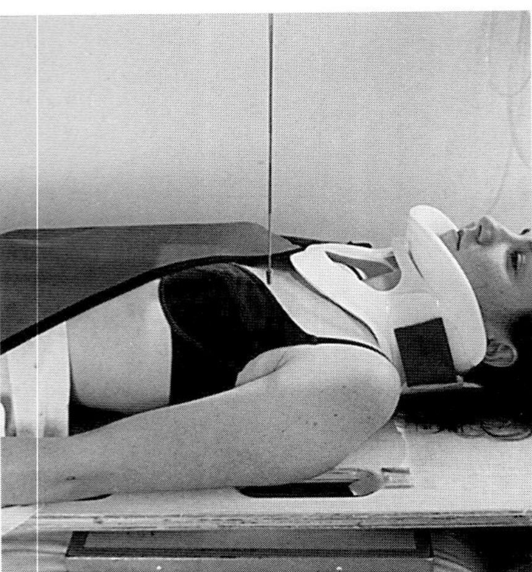

Fig. 19-79. AP scapula.

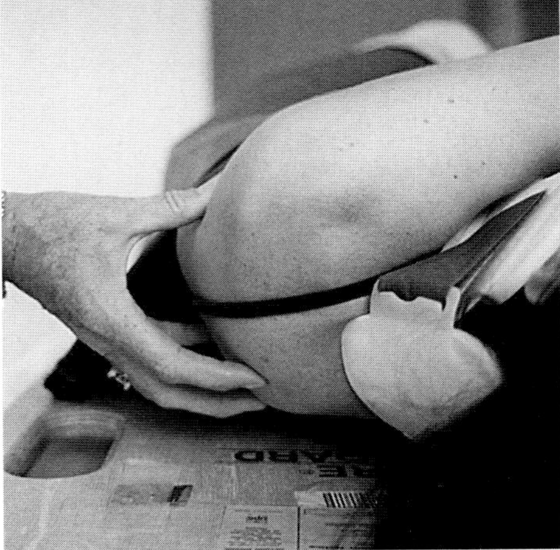

Fig. 19-80. Palpate borders of scapula to determine true lateral position.

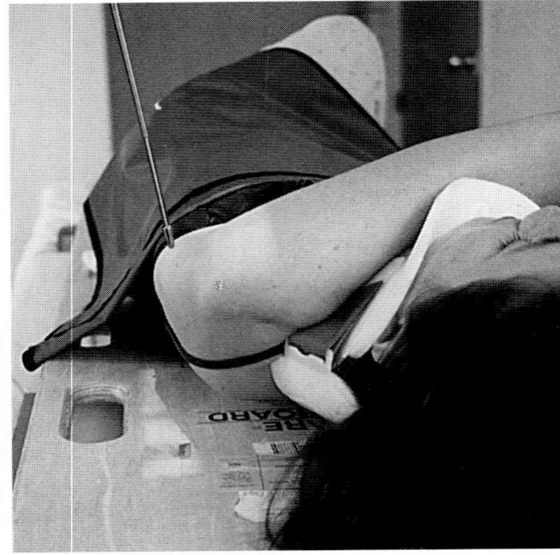

Fig. 19-81. AP oblique, scapular Y. –Lateromedial projection of scapula. –Cross-angle CR if needed.

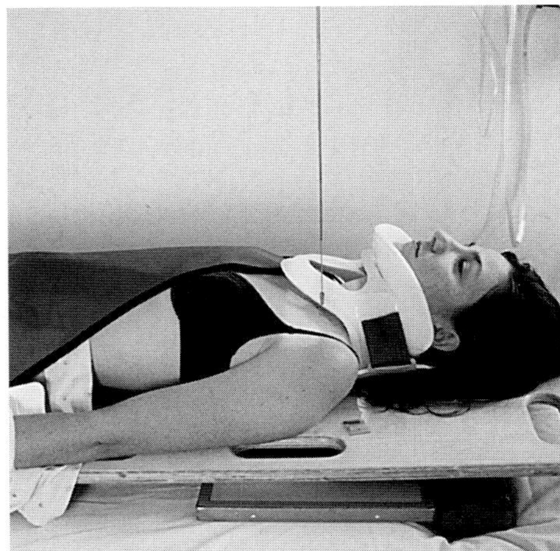

Fig. 19-82. AP clavicle–CR perpendicular.

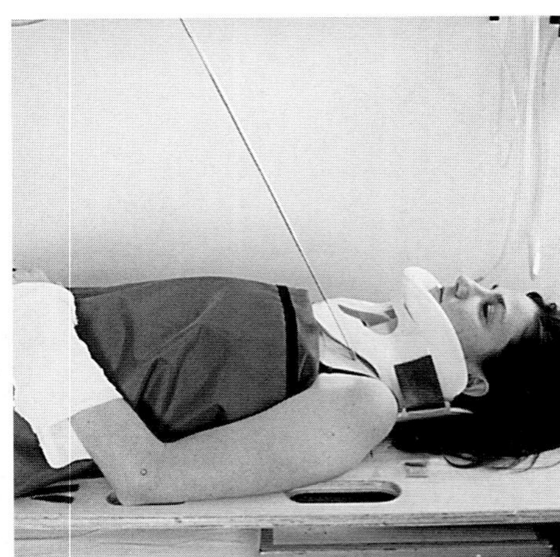

Fig. 19-83. AP axial clavicle. –CR 15 to 20° cephalad (grid lines lengthwise).

AP and Lateral–Toes and Foot

The general trauma rule applies for the lower limb radiographic procedures also, namely that a **minimum of two projections taken 90° to each other** are required. Therefore the oblique projection is generally not included with these initial trauma examinations.

Technical Factors

- Film size–10 x 12 in. (24 x 30 cm).
- 60-65 kVp range, detail (100 speed) screens.
- 40-44 in. (102-112 cm) SID.

Shielding: Shield gonadal region.

Positioning and Central Ray –Patient Supine, Leg Extended.

AP Foot and/or Toes (see Note):

- With leg extended toes up, place cassette vertically against plantar surface of foot. Use cassette holder device as shown, or use other means such as a pillow and/or sand bags, to hold cassette in place.
- Angle CR as needed to be ≈10° from perpendicular to plantar surface of foot and plane of film (Fig. 19-84). (Equivalent to a 10° posterior CR angle for routine AP foot with plantar surface flat on table-top.)
- Center CR to 3rd MT joint. For specific toes, center to PIP joint and collimate to area of interest; however, for general trauma cases the entire foot is generally included for injuries to specific toes.

Note: If patient can flex knee and place foot flat on table-top, routine AP (and oblique) toes and foot projections can be completed as described in Chapter 6.

Lateral Foot (Lateromedial Projection):

- Place support under foot and ankle with vertical cassette against medial surface.
- Direct horizontal CR to base of metatarsals for lateral foot.

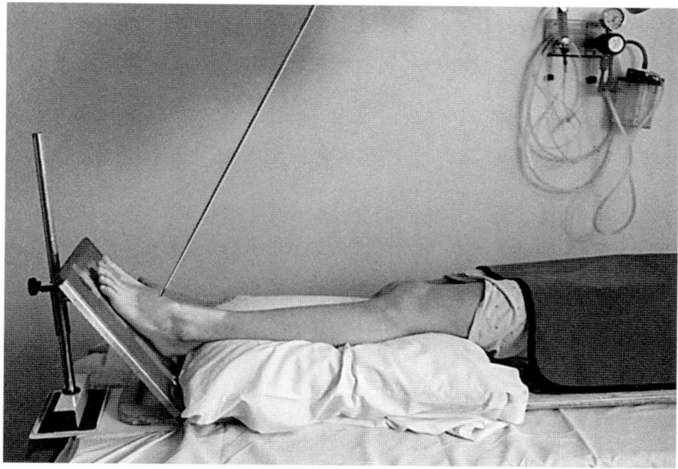

Fig. 19-84. AP foot and/or toes.

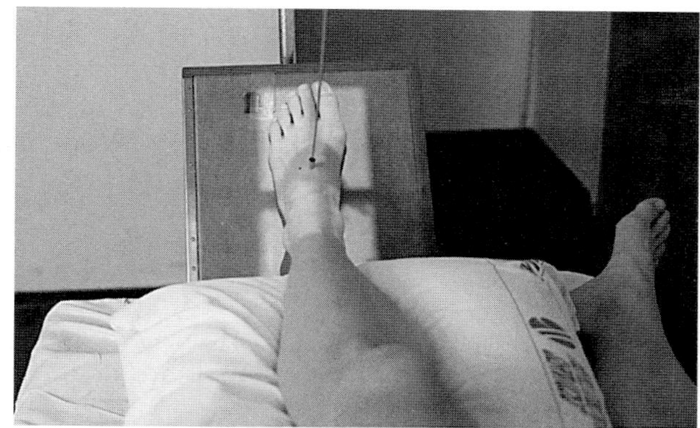

Fig. 19-85. AP foot and/or toes, end-on view.

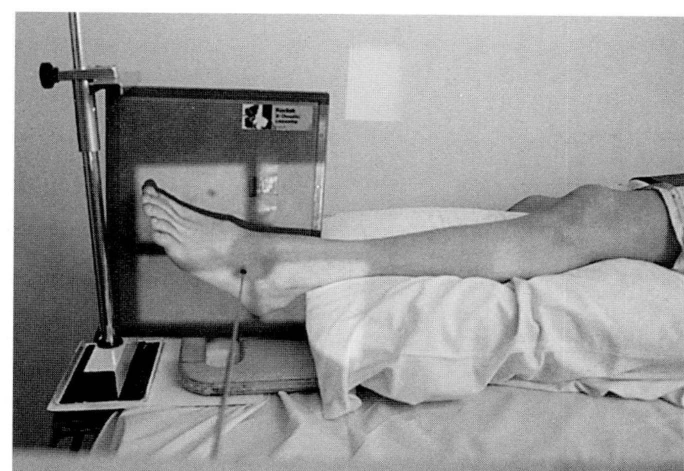

Fig. 19-86. Lateral foot or calcaneus.

AP Mortise (or AP) and Lateral–Ankle and Leg (Tibia-Fibula)

The AP mortise projection of the ankle is a common routine projection when potential trauma or sprains of the ankle joint are involved. (This is either in place of, or in addition to, a straight AP ankle.) Departmental policy concerning this should be determined. The basic lateral projection should always be included.

Technical Factors

- Film size–10 x 12 in. (24 x 30 cm) for ankle,
  or–14 x 17 in. (35 x 43 cm) for adult leg.
- 60-70 kVp range, detail (100 speed) screens.
- 40-44 in. (102-112 cm) SID.

Shielding: Shield gonadal region.

Positioning and Central Ray -Patient Supine, Leg Extended.

AP Ankle Mortise:

- Place cassette under ankle, centered to malleoli and CR.
- Do not dorsiflex the foot but allow to remain in a natural extended position, which aids in demonstrating the base of the 5th metatarsal on the AP ankle projection. (This is a common fracture site with trauma to foot and/or ankle, see Chapter 6, page 200.)
- Angle CR lateromedially as needed to be **perpendicular to the interepicondylar plane**. This requires a 15 to 20° lateromedial angle to the long axis of foot.
- CR is centered to midway between malleoli.

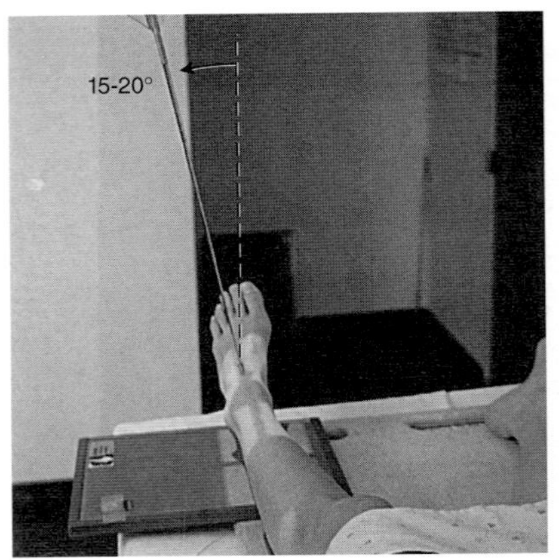

Fig. 19-87. AP mortise projection. -CR 15 to 20° lateromedial angle, perpendicular to interepicondylar line.

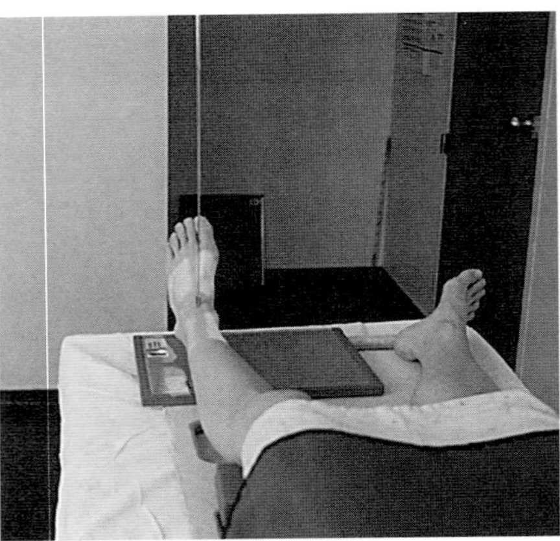

Fig. 19-88. Optional AP ankle. -CR perpendicular (parallel to long axis of foot).

Optional AP Ankle:

- Place cassette under ankle, centered to malleoli and CR.
- Do not dorsiflex the foot but allow to remain in a natural extended position, which aids in demonstrating the base of the 5th metatarsal on the AP ankle projection.
- CR parallel to long axis of foot. (Cross-angle CR if foot and ankle remain partially obliqued.) CR centered to midway between malleoli.

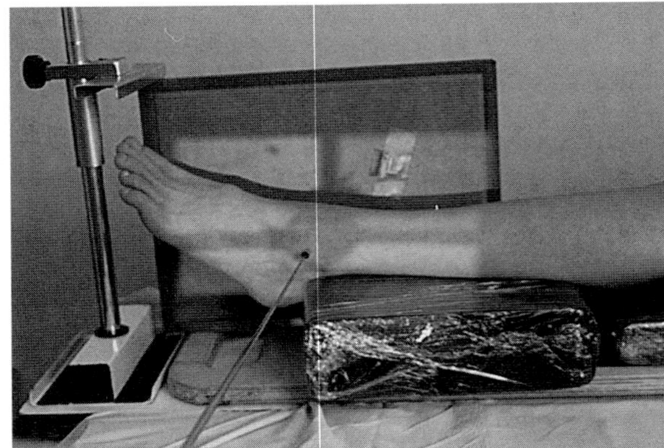

Fig. 19-89. Lateral ankle–CR horizontal.

Lateral Ankle (Lateromedial Projection):

- Place vertical cassette against medial aspect of ankle, centered to malleoli and CR.
- Place support under foot and ankle as needed.
- Direct horizontal CR to lateral malleolus, perpendicular to film. (Remember the lateral malleolus will be 15 to 20° more posterior than the medial malleolus on a true lateral ankle.)

AP Leg (Tibia and Fibula):

- Place large cassette under leg to include ample knee and ankle joints (place diagonally if necessary).
- CR **parallel to long axis of foot.** Cross-angle lateromedially if leg is partially rotated. CR centered to mid shaft of leg.

Note: SID may need to be increased to 44 in. (112 cm) to be able to cover the 14 x 17 in. diagonally placed cassette.

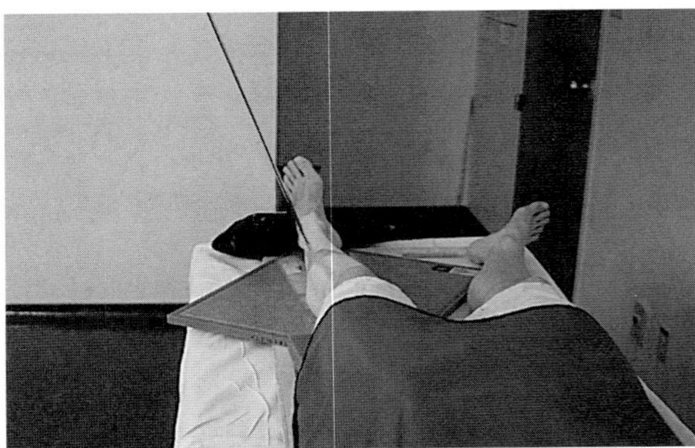

Fig. 19-90. AP leg–CR cross-angled lateromedially (parallel to long axis of foot).

Lateral Leg (Lateromedial Projection):

- Place support under knee, leg and ankle and support vertical cassette against medial surface of leg. Use tape or cassette holder to hold cassette.
- Direct horizontal CR (or 90° from AP), centered to midshaft of leg.

Note: A large adult patient will require a second smaller film of the proximal tibia-fibula to include the knee. This is especially true on this lateral because the cassette cannot easily be placed diagonally.

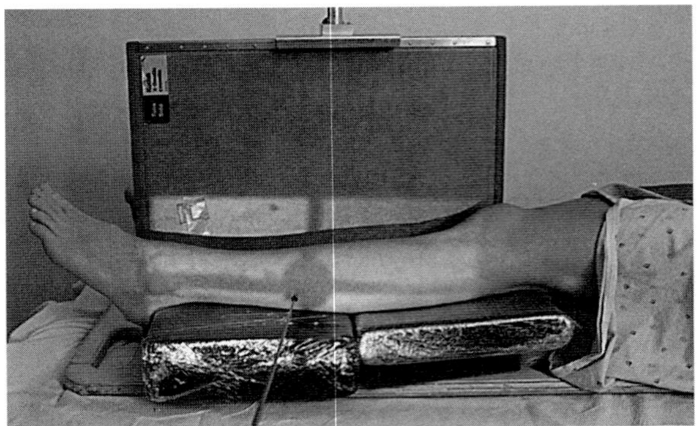

Fig. 19-91. Lateral leg.

AP and Lateral–Knee

Technical Factors

- Film size–10 x 12 in. (24 x 30 cm) lengthwise.
- 65-70 kVp range, grid (small knee, <10 cm, grid not required).
- 40-44 in. (102-112 cm) SID.

Shielding: Shield gonadal region.

Positioning and Central Ray–Patient Supine, Leg Extended

AP Knee:

- Place cassette under knee centered to knee joint (¾ in. or 2 cm distal to apex of patella).
- Direct CR to knee joint with some lateromedial cross-angle if needed to be parallel to long axis of foot (if leg is partially rotated externally).
- No cephalad CR angle is required for average patient. (Thick thigh and buttocks requires 3 to 5° cephalad angle and thin thigh and buttocks a 3 to 5° caudal angle, see Chapter 6, page 206.)
- Angle cassette as needed to be near perpendicular to CR.

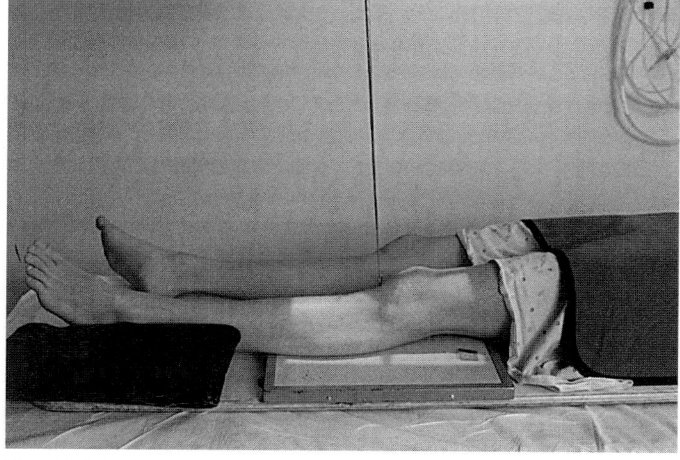

Fig. 19-92. AP knee.
–CR parallel to long axis of foot, lateromedially.
(No cephalic angle required on average patients.)

Lateral Knee:

- Place vertical cassette against medial aspect of knee centered to level of knee joint (¾ in. or 2 cm distal to apex of patella).
- Place support under knee to center leg and knee to cassette.
- Direct CR horizontally, angled up slightly as needed for true lateral to be parallel to epicondyles and perpendicular to long axis of foot if leg is partially externally rotated.

Note: A horizontal beam true lateral of the knee without knee flexion best demonstrates subpatellar bursa and associated fat pads for possible displacement or presence of fluid level. Effusion (fluid accumulation) within the articular cavity of the knee is a strong indicator of knee-joint pathology.

This also is a good projection for possible fracture or dislocation of patella.

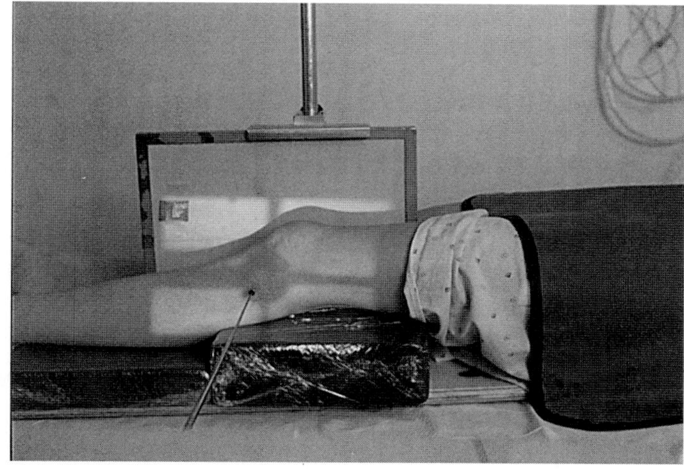

Fig. 19-93. Lateromedial knee–Horizontal CR.

Optional Medial Oblique Knee–Lateromedial CR Angle:

This may be requested to better demonstrate the **fibular head and neck** unobscured.

- Angle CR 45° lateromedially, with grid cassette angled as needed to be near perpendicular to CR. (Place grid crosswise to prevent grid cutoff).
- Direct CR to knee joint (¾ in. or 2 cm distal to apex of patella).
- Place props under leg and knee and support cassette as shown to place film as near perpendicular to CR as possible to minimize distortion.

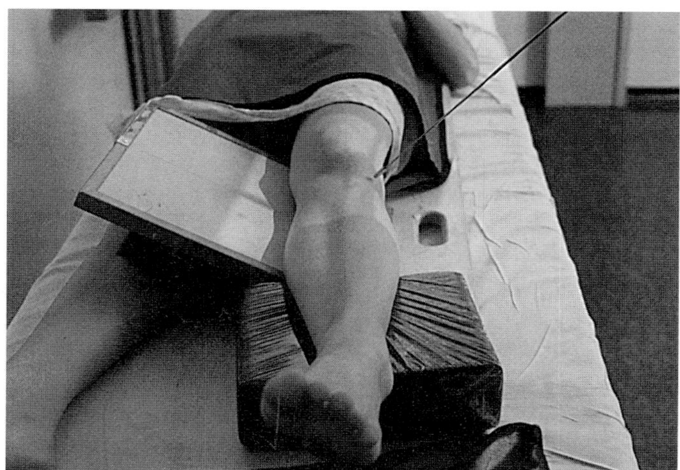

Fig. 19-94. Optional medial oblique knee.
–CR 45° lateromedial cross-angle.
–Grid crosswise.

AP and Lateral–Mid and Distal Femur
AP Pelvis and Proximal Femora

Warning: Do not attempt to internally rotate leg if hip fracture is suspected.

Technical Factors

- Film size–14 x 17 in. (35 x 43 cm).
- 70-75 kVp range, grid–Femur.
- 75-80 kVp range, grid–Pelvis.
- 40-44 in. (102-112 cm) SID.

Shielding: Shield gonadal region on both male and female without obscuring essential anatomy. (Ovarian shielding on females may not be possible for pelvis without obscuring essential pelvic anatomy unless interest is in area of hips and proximal femora only.)

Positioning and Central Ray–Patient Supine, Leg Extended

AP Mid and Distal Femur:

- Place cassette under knee and femur centered to ensure that all of knee joint is included on the film considering the divergence of the x-ray beam.
- Direct CR to mid cassette with some lateromedial cross-angle if needed to be parallel to long axis of foot (if leg is partially rotated externally).
- Collimate closely to femur and film margins.

Lateral Mid and Distal Femur:

- Place vertical grid cassette against medial aspect of leg, placed as high proximally as is comfortable for patient. Place support under leg and knee.
- Direct CR horizontally to distal one-third of femur to near centerline of grid to prevent grid cut-off, may require crosswise placement of grid with vertical centerline.
- Collimate closely to femur with proximal collimation border at upper edge of film.

AP Pelvis:

- Place pillow case or cover over grid cassette and slide under pelvis, film crosswise, centered to patient.
- Top of cassette about 1 in. (2.5 cm) above iliac crest. Ensure **no rotation**, equal distances from ASISs to film. Rotate feet 15° internally if possible. (See warning above.)
- CR perpendicular, to center of film and pelvis.

AP Hip:

- Shield gonads for both male and female without obscuring hip region.
- Place cassette under hip centered to hip and CR.
- CR perpendicular to film, centered to hip (2 in. or 5 cm medial to ASIS, at level of greater trochanter).
- Rotate leg 15° internally if possible (see warning above).

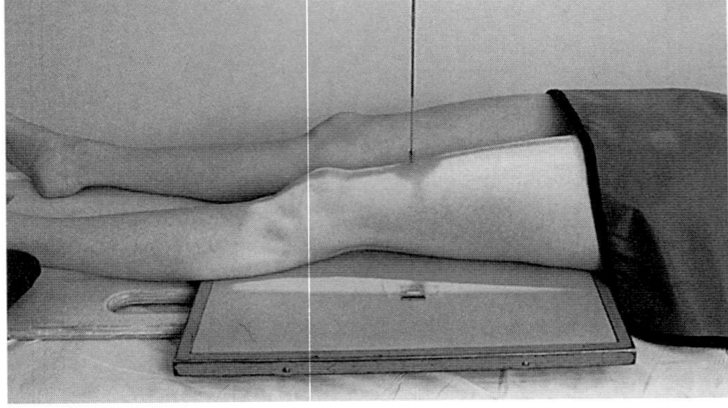

Fig. 19-95. AP mid and distal femur.

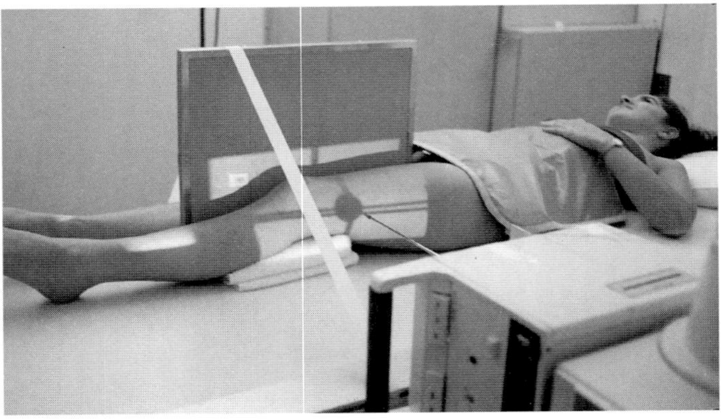

Fig. 19-96. Lateral mid and distal femur.
Note: More support should have been placed under leg to prevent grid cut-off with grid lengthwise.

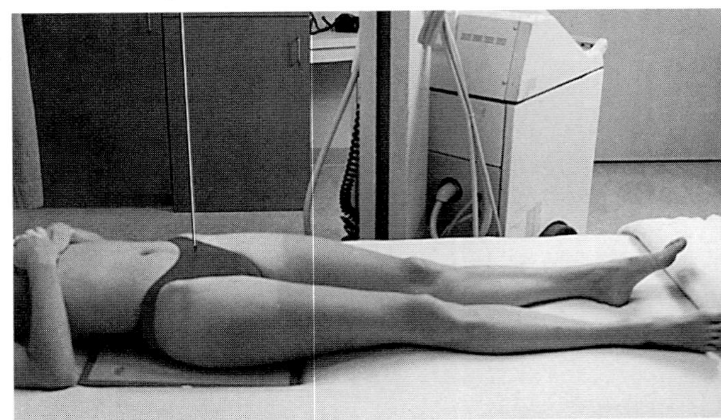

Fig. 19-97. AP pelvis–Bedside mobile. (Right leg is not internally rotated in this example.)

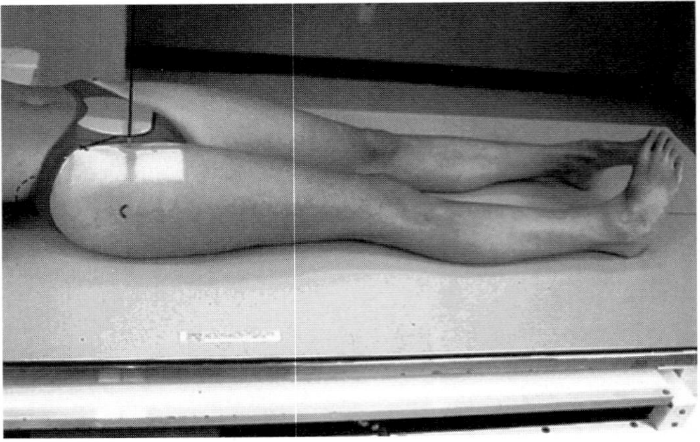

Fig. 19-98. AP hip.

Lateral-Proximal Femur and Hip

Inferosuperior Hip–Danelius-Miller Method
Mediolateral Hip–Sanderson Method*

Warning: Do not attempt to rotate or move leg if evidence of fracture is present.

Technical Factors

- Film size–10 x 12 in. (24 x 30 cm) hip,
  or–14 x 17 in. (35 x 43 cm) proximal femur and hip.
- 70-80 kVp range, grid
- 40-44 in. (102-112 cm) SID.

Shielding: Gonadal shielding generally not possible for male or female without covering area of interest.

Positioning and Central Ray–Patient Supine

***Inferosuperior Lateral Hip with Unilateral Hip Injury Only –Danelius-Miller Method** (Fig. 19-99):*

- Place vertical cassette on table top against patient's side just above iliac crest (grid lines vertical, unless patient is elevated with hip to near level of center of cassette). Internally rotate leg if possible. Elevate opposite leg.
- Direct horizontal CR perpendicular to femoral neck and to plane of film. With vertical grid lines, ensure that CR is to centerline of grid cassette.

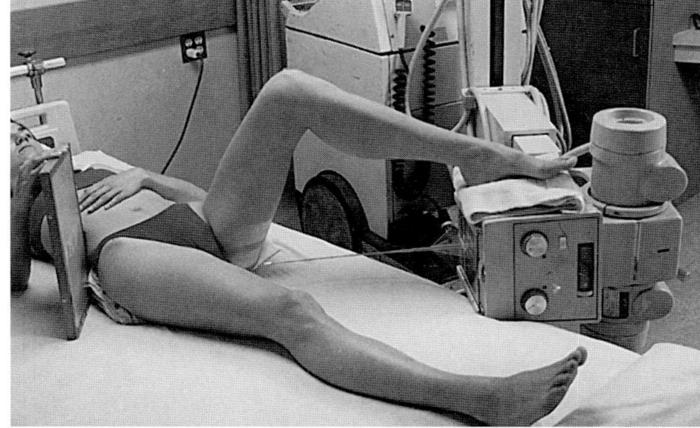

Fig. 19-99. Inferosuperior lateral. –Bedside mobile, Danelius-Miller method.

***Mediolateral Projection For Trauma or Bedside Mobile Lateral of Hip and Proximal Femur–Sanderson Method** (Fig. 19-100):*
This is a good method for postsurgical lateral hip and proximal femur for alignment of hip prosthesis or pin. Can be readily taken in bed or on stretcher with affected leg relaxed and partially externally rotated. Traction bars or other obstacles do not hinder this projection.

Generally, an AP pelvis or hip is taken first and as this cassette is being removed from under the patient, the cassette can be used to lift the patient **gently.** With the cassette still about halfway under the patient, it can be used as a lifting lever. A folded blanket or towels can then be placed under affected hip and femur. (Patient should be obliqued 20 to 30° from supine.)

- With grid lines vertical, place the grid cassette against and partially under the thigh as shown, at an angle as needed to be near perpendicular to CR. Support and hold cassette in place with 45° support blocks or other supports and/or tape as needed.
- Angle CR mediolaterally as needed to be **near perpendicular to long axis of foot** (90° from AP, see Note). A 10 to 20° cephalad CR angle is possible to better visualize the neck and head if the grid cassette can also be angled sufficiently to prevent grid cutoff.

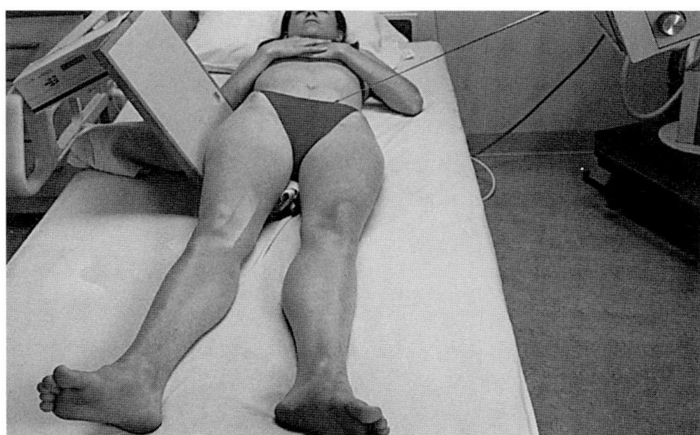

Fig. 19-100. Mediolateral proximal femur and hip.
–Bedside mobile, Sanderson method.*
–CR cross angled mediolaterally, perpendicular to long axis of foot.

Note: The amount of CR cross-angle will vary depending on the external rotation of affected leg.

Summary of Sanderson Method

- Support placed under affected hip as patient is lifted gently when removing cassette from AP projection.
- With cassette partially under hip, cassette is angled to be parallel to long axis of foot.
- CR angled mediolaterally to be perpendicular to long axis of foot.

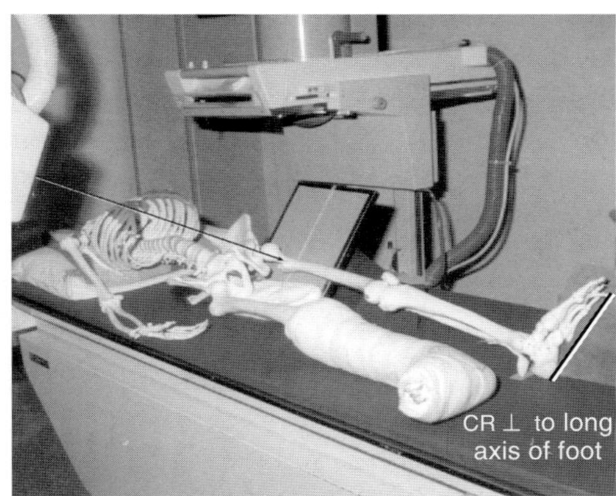

Fig. 19-101. Demonstration of Sanderson method.
Courtesy of Jim Sanderson BS, RT(R)

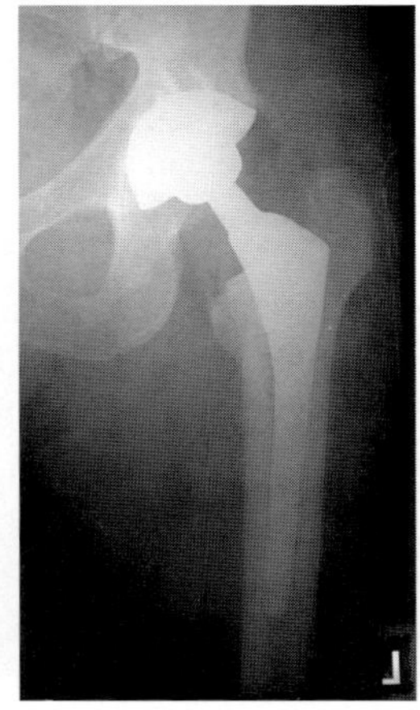

Fig. 19-102. AP hip.

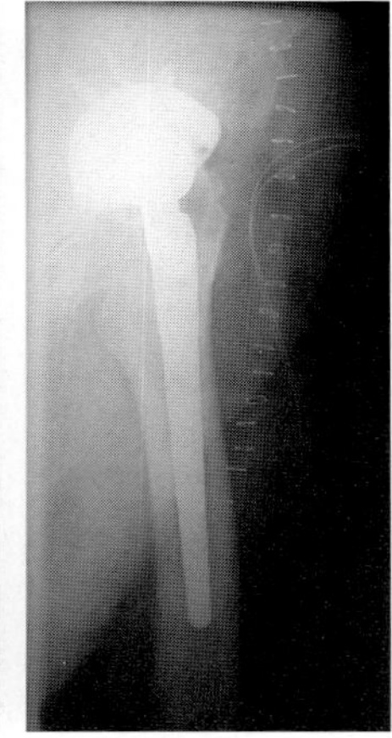

Fig. 19-103. Lat. hip. –Sanderson method.
Courtesy of Jim Sanderson BS, RT(R)

*Sanderson, James A., Phoenix, AZ. This method was first demonstrated and described by Sanderson to the author in April 1992.

AP and Lateral–Cervical Spine

Warning: Do not remove cervical collar or move patient's head or neck until cervical fractures have been ruled out. Generally this requires an AP and a lateral shown to a physician **before** the cervical collar is removed or before the patient is moved off a backboard.

Technical Factors

- Film size–10 x 12 in. (24 x 30 cm).
- 75-80 kVp range, grid (screens may be used on small patients).

  AP:
- 40-44 in. (102-112 cm) SID.

  Lateral:
- 60-72 in. (152-183 cm) SID.

Shielding: Shield pelvic region and chest region.

Positioning and Central Ray (Patient supine with potential spinal injury)

***AP Projection** (Fig. 19-104):*

- Place cassette in Bucky or grid cassette lengthwise under patient with top of cassette 1 to 2 in. (3 to 5 cm) above level of EAM.
- Angle CR 15 to 20° cephalad to enter at level of lower margin of thyroid cartilage (C5).

***AP Open Mouth–C1 and C2** (Fig. 19-105):*

- If patient's condition allows, have patient open mouth as far as possible without moving head or neck.
- CR angled if needed to be parallel to a line from the lower margin of upper teeth to base of skull (mastoid tips).

Optional AP Axial C1-2 Region –To demonstrate **dens within foramen magnum** when open mouth projection is not possible and interest is to upper cervical region *(Fig. 19-106):*

- Place cassette lengthwise as for AP projection, centered to projected CR.
- Angle CR cephalad 35 to 40°, or as needed to align CR parallel to a line from tip of mandible to base of skull. Center CR to enter just inferior to mandible.

Horizontal Beam Lateral:

- Vertical cassette against shoulder, parallel to MSP, with top of cassette 1 to 2 in. (3 to 5 cm) above level of EAM. Ensure that C7 region is included.
- Have patient relax and depress shoulders as much as possible. If needed, have non-radiology personnel pull down on both arms to further depress shoulders to visualize C7 region. (Supply with lead apron.)
- CR horizontal, to C4 (upper thyroid cartilage) and to centerline of grid to prevent grid cutoff, or grid turned with centerline vertical to prevent grid cutoff.
- Increase SID to 60 or 72 in. (152-183 cm) if equipment and room space allows to decrease beam divergence, to better visualize C7.

Note: For a small to average patient, a screen can be used rather than a grid if desired due to the air-gap absorption of scatter.

Swimmer's Lateral (If C7 is not visualized on C-spine lateral):

- Similar vertical film placement positioning as for horizontal beam lateral but elevate arm and shoulder closest to film, and depress opposite shoulder as much as possible.
- CR horizontal, centered to C7-T1 (about 1.5 in. or 4 cm above level of jugular notch). Center centerline of grid cassette to CR to prevent grid cut off (grid lines vertical).

Note: A 5° CR caudal angle may be required if patient cannot depress shoulder opposite cassette.

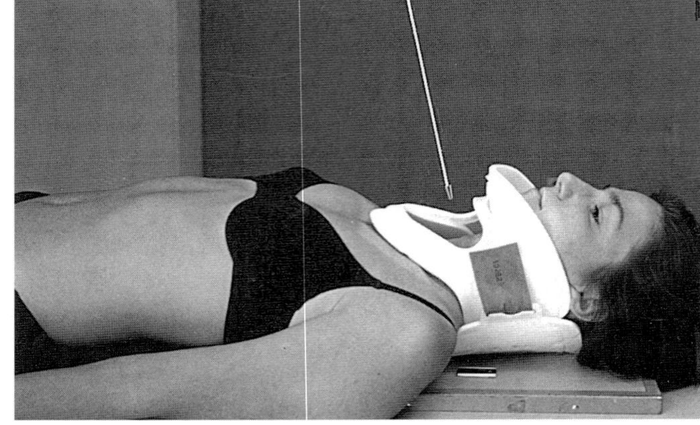

Fig. 19-104. AP cervical–CR 15 to 20° cephalad.

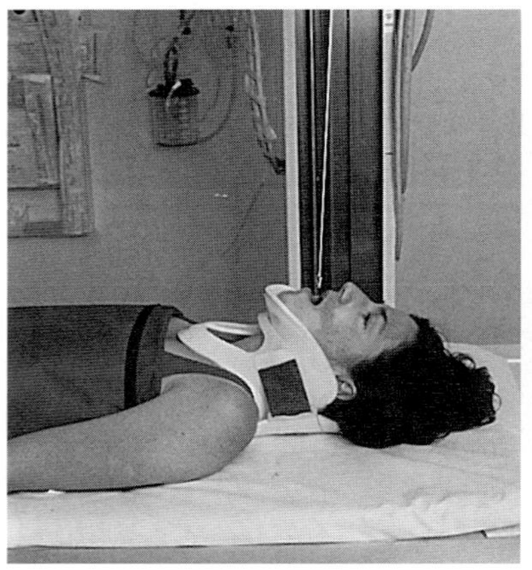

Fig. 19-105. AP open mouth of C1-2 region if patient can cooperate.

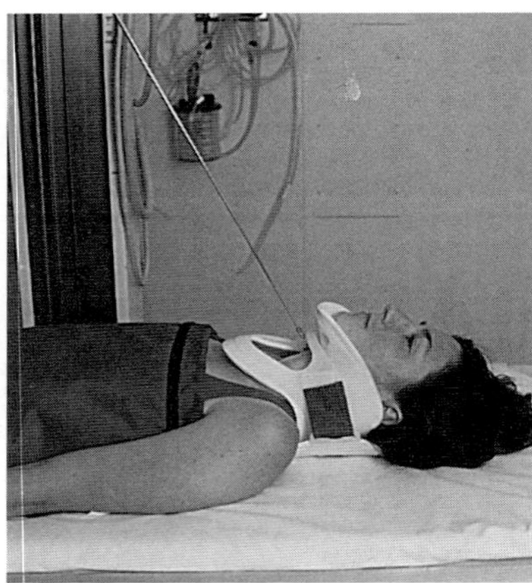

Fig. 19-106. Optional AP C1-2 region if open mouth AP is not possible. –CR 35 to 40° cephalad.

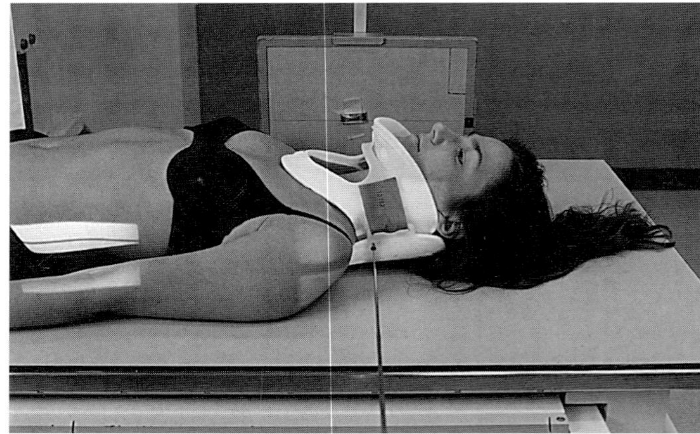

Fig. 19-107. Horizontal beam lateral.

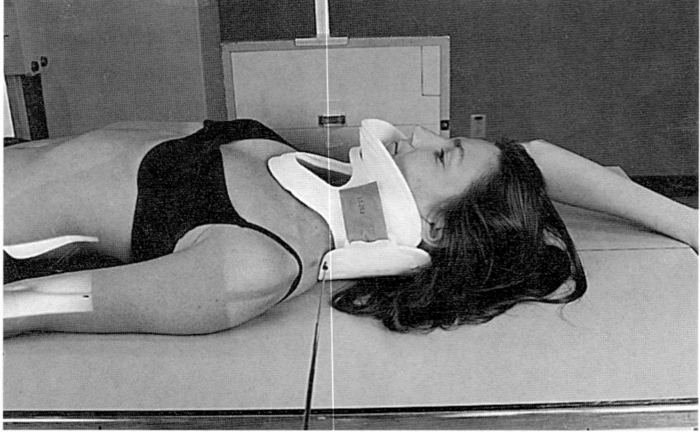

Fig. 19-108. Swimmer's lateral, C7-T1.

Overhead Trauma Obliques, Cervical Spine–RPO and LPO Biplanar Angulation Method*

Two Methods

Supine cervical oblique projections, to visualize pedicles and intervertebral foramina, can be achieved two ways:

Method one, wherein the screen cassette remains flat on the x-ray table, is easier and quicker but results in **more distortion** of the pedicles and the intervertebral foramina.

Method two results in **less distortion,** and the increase in OID (which acts as an air gap) improves image quality when the 45° angled cassette is placed under the table-top.

Biplanar Angulation: Where angulation is required along two planes and the overhead tube does not have transverse tube-swivel capacity, the cephalad or caudad angle must be achieved by rotating the tube yoke at the base of the vertical column. Compensation is then required to achieve the desired net angles; in this case, 45° medial and 15° cephalad for the trauma oblique cervical spine. Using the formula below, these actual angles have been calculated to be **52°** and **22°**, respectively.

Technical Factors

- Film size–10 x 12 in. (24 x 30 cm) lengthwise.
- 400-speed screens, small focal spot. Nongrid due to double angle.
- 66 in. (168 cm) or 72 in. (183 cm) SID.
- 70-75 kVp range

Compensation Formula for Biplanar Angulation

$\angle C$ = **Compensatory angle**, derived by simply dividing the product of the desired net angle (15° × 45°) by 90°, then adding this to both medial and cephalic angles.

$\angle C = (15° \times 45°) \div 90°$, $\angle C = \frac{(15° \times 45°)}{90°} = \mathbf{7.5°}$

7.5° + 15° cephalic angle = ***22.5° (22°)***

7.5° + 45° medial angle = ***52.5° (52°)***

Positioning–Patient Supine with Head and Neck Immobilized

Method one: Place cassette lengthwise flat on table-top under patient and to one side so as to be centered to projected CR. Align top of cassette to level of EAM.

Method two: Place cassette at a 45° angle just below table height on an adjustable stand or stool. With patient and table-top completely out of the way, and with longitudinal and transverse locks released, angle the CR as described below and center to cassette. Collimate to film borders, then drive the table-top and patient into place so the projected CR is centered to C4 (level of lower thyroid cartilage). (RPO visualizes left side foramina.) Make sure the area of interest does not overlie the metal reinforcement at the end of the table-top.

Central Ray (Methods One and Two)

- Set vertical tube height to **45 in.** (114 cm) from tabletop, or **47 in.** (119 cm) from Bucky. This will achieve a net 66 in. (168 cm) angled SID with method one, or a net 72 in. (183 cm) angled SID for method two.
- With tube at this height, bring tube yoke out to the side of, and parallel to, the long axis of the table. Angle the tube head **medially 52°** from vertical.
- Rotate the tube yoke back **22°**, away from the table and the side of the foramina to be demonstrated; that is, clockwise for the RPO (Fig. 19-111) and counterclockwise with tube on other side for the LPO. (45° and 15° net angles have now been achieved.)

Collimation: Rotate collimator as needed and collimate on four sides to area of interest.

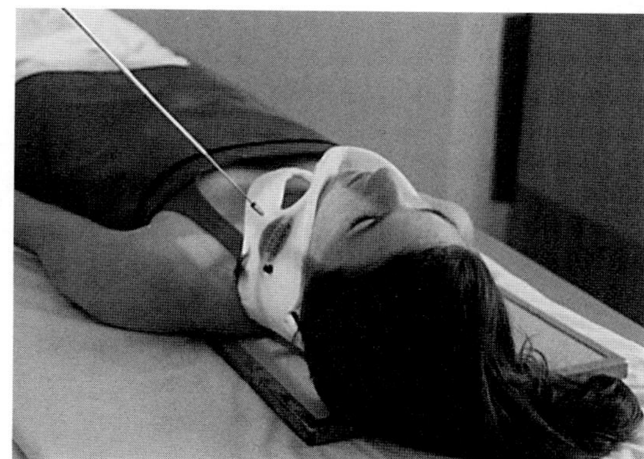

Fig. 19-109. **Method one:** Oblique cervical–Cassette flat on tabletop. –CR 52° medial and 22° cephalad, 66 in. (168 cm) SID.

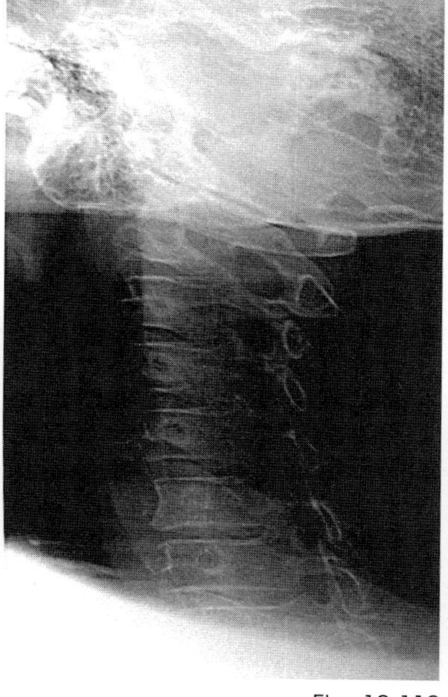

Fig. 19-110 (Courtesy of Susan C. Poulin, RT (R))

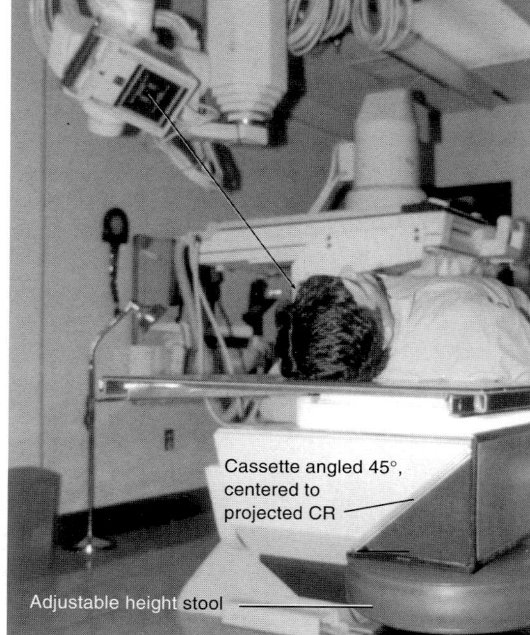

Fig. 19-111. **Method two:** Oblique cervical–Cassette angled 45°. –CR 52° medial and 22° cephalad, 72 in. (183 cm) SID. (Courtesy of N.J. Martin, M.Ed., RT (R) (CT))

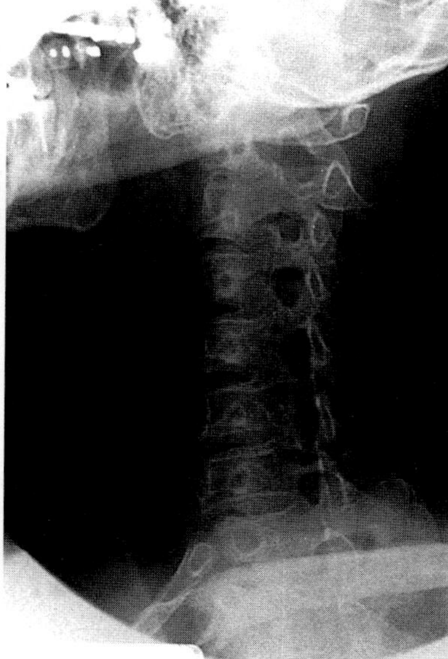

Fig. 19-112

*Martin, Napoleon J. Excerpt from "Composition 501," first presented June 1992 at 10th Annual Renew-Review-Revive Seminar. SUNY Health Science Center, Syracuse, New York.

AP and Horizontal Beam Lateral–Thoracic and Lumbar Spine

If patient can be turned on his/her side, conventional thoracic and lumbar spine projections can be achieved as described in Chapters 8 and 9.

Technical Factors

- Film Size—14 x 17 in. (35 x 43 cm) lengthwise.
- 75-85 kVp range, grid.
- 40-44 in. (102-112 cm) SID.
- Collimate long and narrow field to region of spine.

Shielding: Shield gonads.

Positioning and Central Ray–Patient Supine

AP Thoracic Spine:

- Place cassette in Bucky, or slide grid cassette under patient with top of cassette ≈1½ in. (3 cm) above shoulders.
- CR perpendicular, to center of cassette, at level of T7, 3 to 4 in. (8 to 10 cm) inferior to jugular notch.

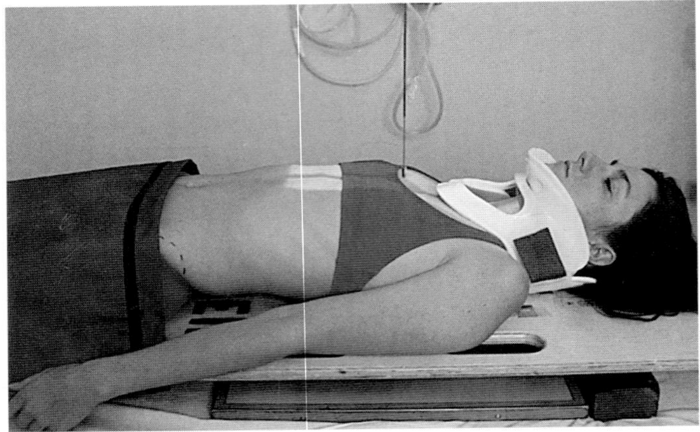

Fig. 19-113. AP thoracic spine.

AP Lumbar Spine:

- Same as for AP thoracic spine except move cassette down to center cassette to level of ≈1 in. (2.5 cm) above iliac crest. Knees up if patient's condition allows.
- CR perpendicular to center of cassette (level of L3).

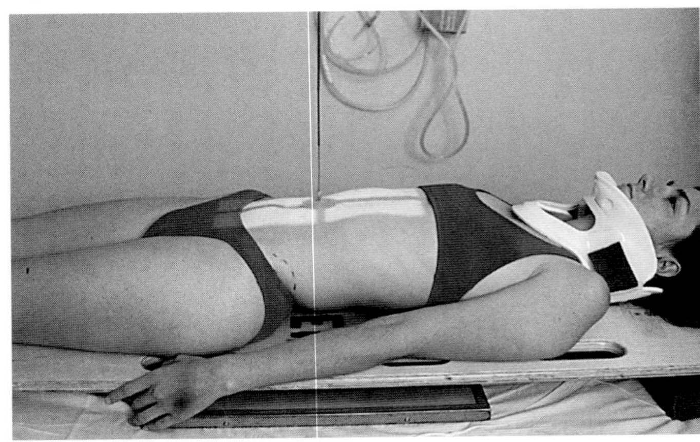

Fig. 19-114. AP lumbar spine.

Lateral Thoracic Spine:

- Move patient to edge of table so vertical cassette next to patient can be placed below level of table-top (Fig. 19-115). Use cassette holder device or tape and/or sandbags to hold cassette in position. Top of cassette about 1 in. (3 cm) above shoulders, which centers film to CR at level of T7. Have patient raise arms above head, or raise and cross over above chest so as not to obscure thoracic vertebra. Align cassette parallel to MSP.
- Horizontal CR centered to vertebral column, and to near centerline of grid at level of T7, 3 to 4 in. (8 to 10 cm) inferior to jugular notch.

Note: In these photographs the patient is on a raised backboard to allow the centerline of the grid to be near the CR to prevent grid cutoff. Grid may be placed crosswise to patient for better centering of CR to mid grid line if patient and backboard are not raised high enough to allow CR to be within 1 or 1 ½ in. (3-4 cm) of centerline of grid.

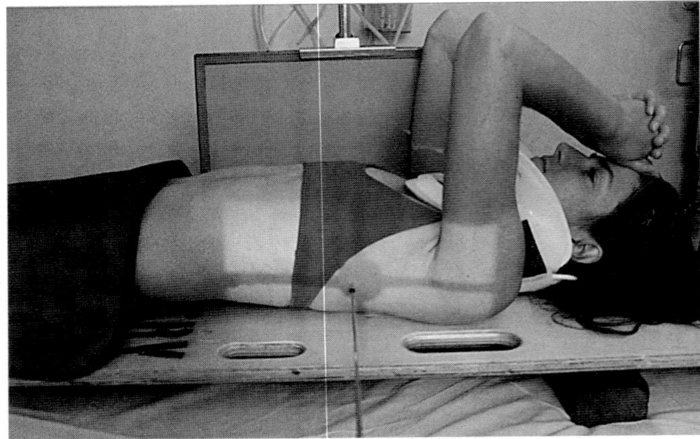

Fig. 19-115. Horizontal beam lateral thoracic spine.

Lateral Lumbar Spine:

- Same as lateral thoracic spine except move cassette down to be centered to level of ≈1 in. (2.5 cm) above iliac crest (L3). Align cassette parallel to MSP.
- Horizontal CR centered to vertebral column and to near centerline of grid at level of L3, or 1 in. (2.5 cm) above level of iliac crest.

Optional Lateral L5-S1 (not shown):

- 8 × 10 in. (20 to 24 cm) lengthwise.
- Vertical cassette on edge centered to ≈1 in. (2.5 cm) distal to level of iliac crest.
- Horizontal CR perpendicular to MSP, centered to cassette.

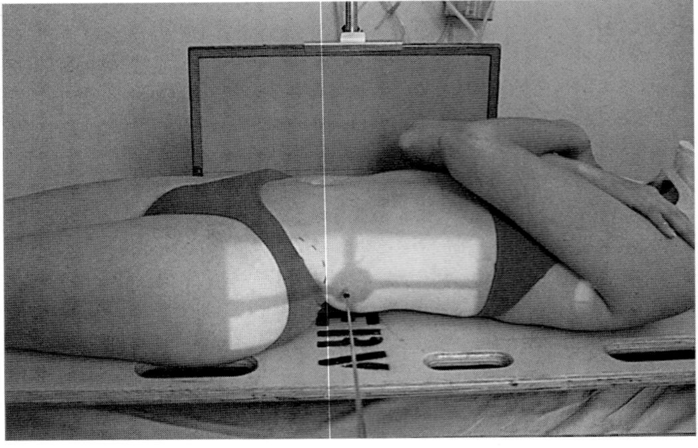

Fig. 19-116. Horizontal beam lateral lumbar spine.

Lateral Trauma Skull–Horizontal Beam Projection

Warning: It is essential that cervical spine fractures and dislocations be ruled out **before** attempting to move or manipulate the patient's head or neck. A good projection for demonstrating sphenoidal effusion (fluid within sphenoid bone may be an indication of intracranial trauma).

Technical Factors

- Film size–10 x 12 in. (24 x 30 cm)
- Place grid cassette vertically against affected lateral cranium, crosswise to patient.
- 70-80 kVp range.
- 40-44 in. (102-112 cm) SID.
- Use small focal spot.

Positioning–Patient Supine

- Remove all metal, plastic or other removable objects from head.
- If patient's head can be manipulated (see warning above), carefully elevate skull on a radiolucent sponge (Fig. 19-118).

  If one cannot manipulate head, move patient to back edge of table, then by moving the floating table forward the cassette can be placed on edge at least 1 in. (2.5 cm) below tabletop and occipital bone as shown in Fig. 19-117. The divergent beam then will not project posterior skull off the film.
- Place head in **true lateral position**, relative to cassette, with side of interest closest to cassette.
- Align MSP parallel with cassette, and interpupillary line perpendicular to cassette.
- Adjust cassette to assure that entire circumference of skull will be visualized on radiograph and centerline of grid is centered to CR.

Central Ray

- A **horizontal beam** (which is essential for visualization of inner cranial air/fluid levels), is directed **perpendicular** to cassette.
- Center to a point 2 in. (5 cm) superior to EAM.

Collimation: Collimate to outer margins of skull on all sides.

Note: On patient with cervical spine injury **do not** attempt to raise and place support under head, as shown in Fig. 19-118, until cervical trauma has been ruled out with a horizontal beam lateral.

Evaluation Criteria

- Entire skull visualized on radiograph.
- The cranium is seen without rotation or tilt:
  - –Mandibular rami, orbital roofs, greater and lesser wings of sphenoid and external auditory canals are superimposed.
  - –Sella turcica and clivus are demonstrated in profile without rotation.
- Sufficient penetration and exposure, without motion, to visualize parietal and temporal regions.

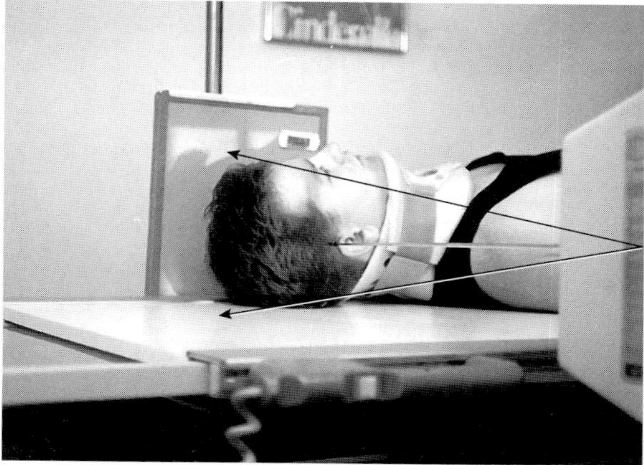

Fig. 19-117. Trauma lateral **without head manipulation**.

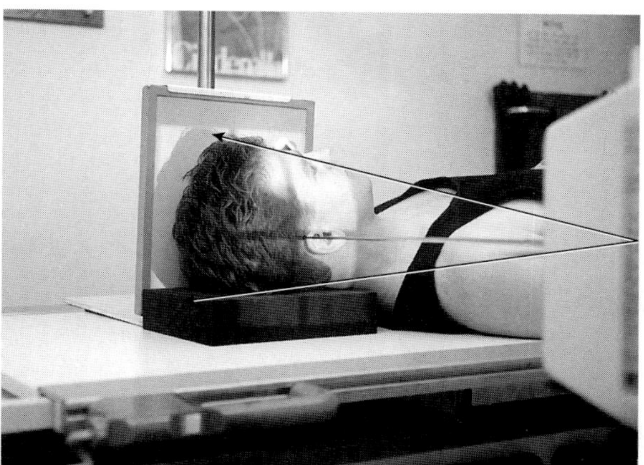

Fig. 19-118. Trauma lateral–**after cervical injury has been ruled out**. Place support under elevated head.

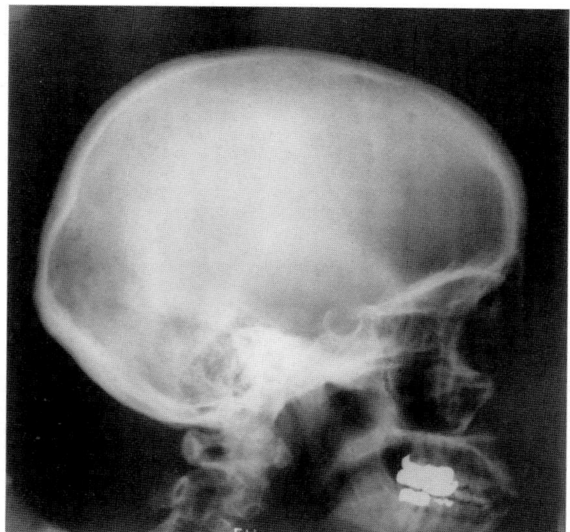

Fig. 19-119 Trauma lateral.

AP 0°, AP 15° (Reverse Caldwell) and AP 30° Axial (Towne)–Skull

Warning: It is essential that cervical spine fractures and dislocations be ruled out before attempting to move or manipulate the patient's head or neck.

For all three of the projections demonstrated on this page, the patient's head and neck are not moved. The degree of CR angulation is the only variation.

Exception: If a cervical spine injury has been ruled out, the chin may be depressed to bring the orbitomeatal line perpendicular to the film and the CR can then be adjusted accordingly.

Technical Factors

- Film size–10 x 12 in. (24 x 30 cm) lengthwise.
- Moving or stationary grid.
- 70-80 kVp range.
- 40-44 in. (102-112 cm) SID.
- Use small focal spot.

Positioning–Patient Supine

- If possible, slide patient onto x-ray table in one movement, do **NOT** move head or neck. May also be taken using a portable grid placed under patient's head or under the backboard. It is not necessary to remove collar or backboard in order to obtain these projections.
- Remove all metal, plastic or other removable objects from head.
- Slide patient's entire body to align MSP to midline of table.

Central Ray

AP 0° Projection *(Figs. 19-120 and 19-123):*

- Angle CR **parallel with OML**. With patient in a cervical collar this is approximately 10 to 15° caudad.
- Center CR to **glabella**; then center cassette to projected CR.

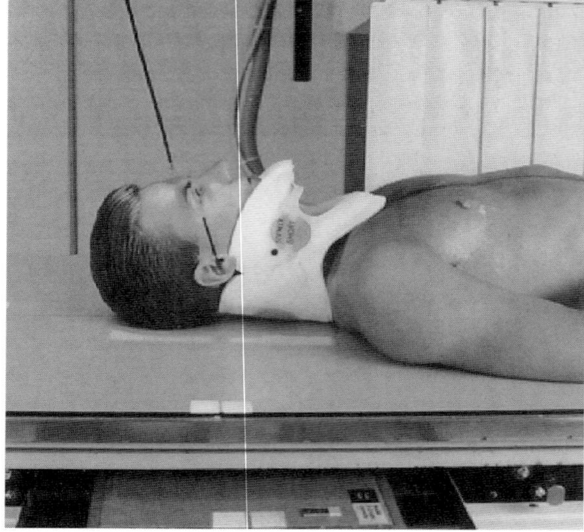

Fig. 19-120. AP 0° to OML.
-CR parallel to OML, centered to glabella.

19

AP "Reverse Caldwell" Projection *(Figs. 19-121 and 19-124):*

- Angle CR **15° cephalad to OML**, which is 15° more than angle used for AP. This requires determining the angle of the OML with chin extended as shown, then angle 15° cephalad to the OML. (If OML is 15° as shown, then the net CR is 0° or perpendicular to film. If the OML were 20°, then the CR would be 5° caudal.)
- Center CR to **nasion**; then center cassette to projected CR.

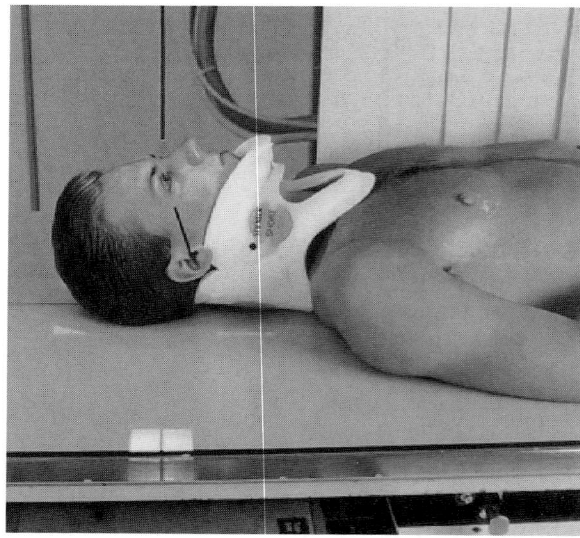

Fig. 19-121. AP 15° "reverse Caldwell".
-CR 15° cephalad to OML, centered to nasion.

AP Axial (Towne) Projection *(Figs. 19-122 and 19-126):*

- Angle CR **30° caudad to OML**, which is 30° more than angle used for AP. (See Note.)
- Center CR to pass **midway between EAMs**, which centers CR to midsagittal plane 2½ in. (6 cm) above superciliary arch; then center cassette to projected CR.

Collimation: Collimate to outer margins of skull on all sides.

Note: The CR for the AP axial, should not exceed 45° or excessive distortion will hinder the visualization of essential anatomy.

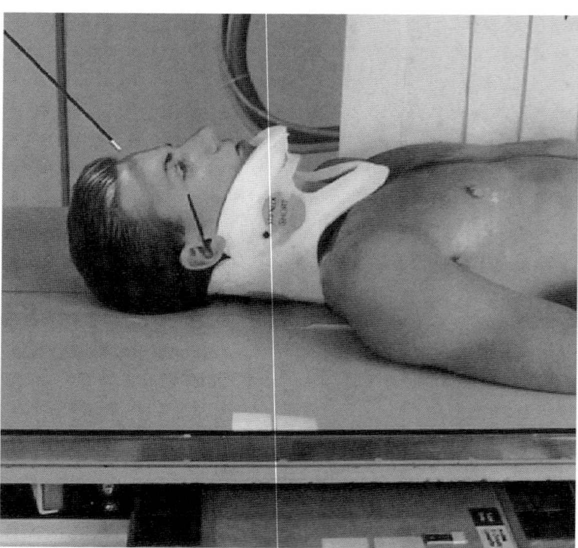

Fig. 19-122. AP axial Towne–CR 30° caudad to OML, centered to midpoint between EAMs.

AP 0°, AP 15° "Reverse Caldwell" and AP 30° Axial (Towne)–Skull continued

AP Versus PA

Trauma skull projections are performed AP while most of the nontrauma projections are taken PA. This variation will demonstrate reverse anatomical magnification. For example on a PA projection the orbits, being closest to the cassette, will be less magnified than the sagittal and lambdoidal sutures which are situated farther from the cassette. On the AP projection the opposite is true, the orbits are more magnified than the sutures. The PA projection will also demonstrate more distance from the oblique orbital line to the lateral margin of the skull than the AP projection. This is illustrated in Figs. 19-124 and 19-125, which compares an **AP reverse Caldwell** with a standard **PA Caldwell.**

Even though magnification differences exist between the PA and AP projections, causing them to look quite different from one another, the basic evaluation criteria remains the same.

Exposure to Neck and Thyroid: AP projections of the skull and facial bones obviously increase the exposure to more radiosensitive organs such as neck and the thyroid regions compared to PA projections. However, benefits outweigh these disadvantages for trauma patients who cannot be turned into a prone position due to possible spinal or other injuries.

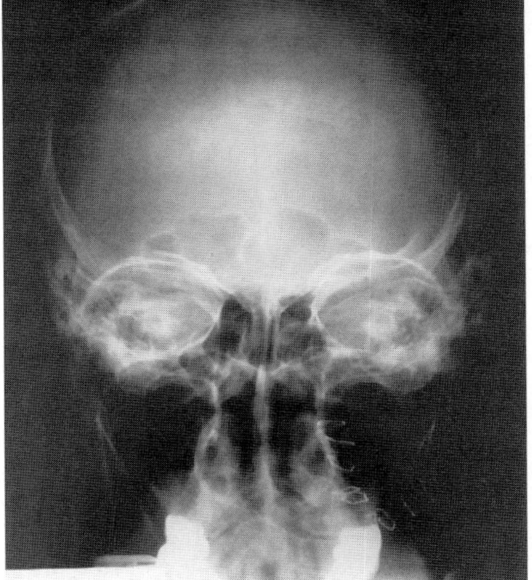

Fig. 19-123. AP 0° to OML.

Evaluation Criteria

Trauma AP 0° Projection:

- Entire skull visualized on radiograph.
- Petrous ridges superimpose superior orbital region.
- Petrous pyramids fill orbits with internal auditory canals seen horizontally through center of orbits.
- Distance from oblique orbital line to lateral margin of skull on each side is equal.
- Dorsum sellae and anterior clinoids are visualized superior to ethmoid sinuses.
- Sufficient penetration and exposure, without motion, to clearly visualize frontal bone.

Trauma AP "Reverse Caldwell" Position:

- Entire skull visualized on radiograph.
- Distance from oblique orbital line to lateral margin of skull on each side is equal.
- Superior orbital fissures are symmetrically visualized within orbits.
- Petrous pyramids and internal auditory canals are projected into the lower one-third of orbits.
- Superior orbital margin is visualized without superimposition.
- Sufficient penetration and exposure, without motion, to clearly visualize frontal bone.

Trauma AP Axial (Towne) Projection:

- Entire skull visualized on radiograph.
- Equal distance from foramen magnum to lateral margin of skull on each side.
- Dorsum sella and posterior clinoids are projected into foramen magnum. (See Note.)
- Petrous ridges are symmetrical and visualized superior to the mastoids.
- Sufficient penetration and exposure, without motion, to clearly visualize occipital bone.

Note: If one could not bring the CR 30° more caudal than the AP projection before the maximum angle of 45° was reached, the dorsum sella and posterior clinoids would be projected inferior to the foramen magnum instead of within it as seen in Fig. 19-127.

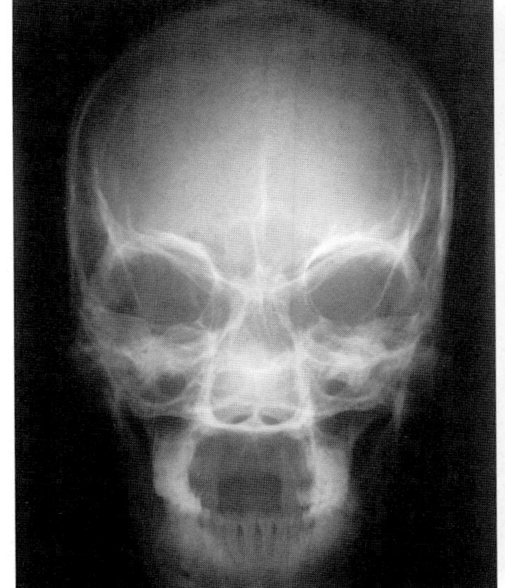

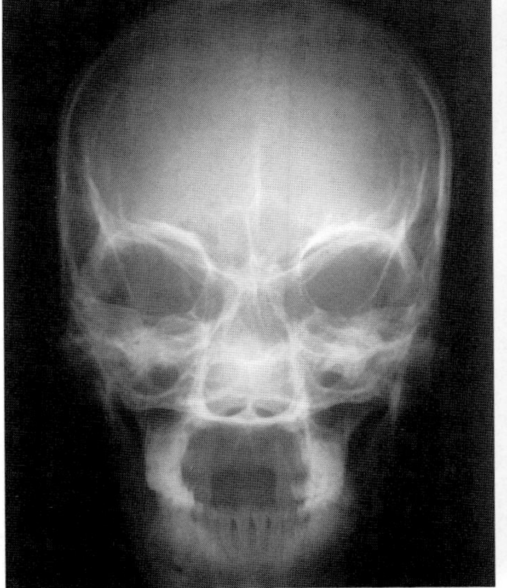

Fig. 19-124. AP "reverse Caldwell." –15° cephalad to OML.

Fig. 19-125. PA Caldwell (15° caudad) –Comparison radiograph.

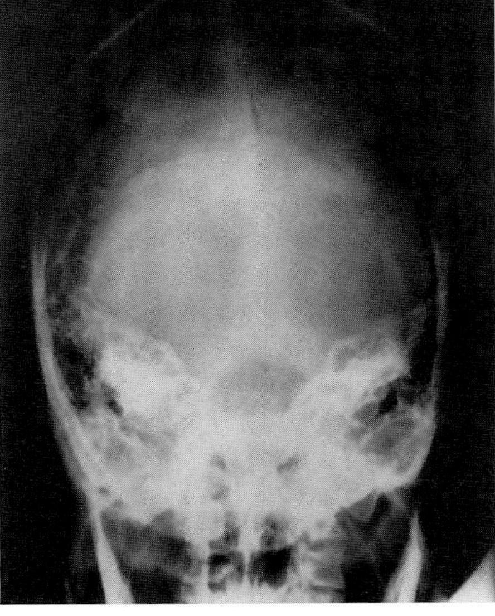

Fig. 19-126. Trauma AP axial "Towne." –30° caudad to OML (max. 45° angle).

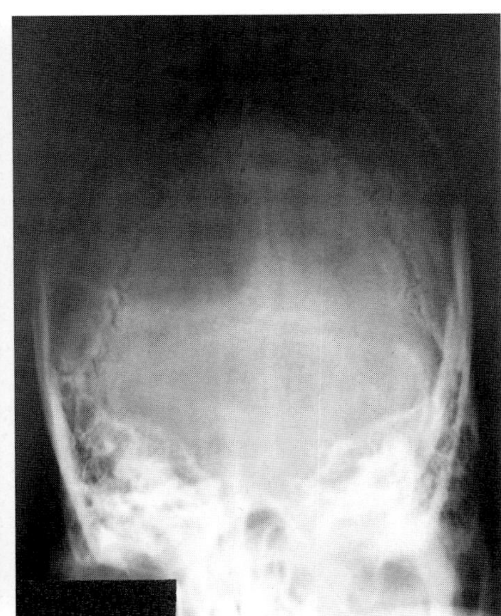

Fig. 19-127. Trauma AP axial –Less than 30° caudad to OML.

Lateral and AP Acanthioparietal–Facial Bones

Lateral, Reverse Waters Method and Modified Reverse Waters Method

Warning: It is essential that cervical spine fractures and dislocations are ruled out **before** attempting any manipulation of the patient's head or neck. All three of these projections can be achieved without any movement or adjustment of patient's head and neck.

Technical Factors

- Film size–10 x 12 in. (24 x 30 cm) lengthwise.
- Grid cassette on edge for lateral.
- 70-80 kVp range.
- Use small focal spot.
- 40-44 in. (102-112 cm) SID.

Positioning–Patient Supine

- If possible, slide patient onto x-ray table in one movement. The head should not be raised to position a grid cassette under patient. It is not necessary to remove cervical collar or backboard to obtain these projections.
- Remove all metal, plastic or other removable objects from head.
- Slide patient's entire body to bring MSP to midline of table.
- Assure no rotation or tilt, for lateral align MSP parallel with grid cassette.

Central Ray

Lateral:

- Horizontal beam is essential for visualization of intracranial air-fluid levels.
- Center CR to level of **midway between outer canthus and EAM**, which should be to about the centerline of grid cassette.

AP Acanthioparietal–Reverse Waters:

This projection best visualizes facial bone structure and the maxilla region by projecting the petrous ridge below the maxilla and maxillary sinuses (see small arrows, Fig. 19-131).

- Angle CR cephalad as needed to align **CR parallel to mentomeatal line (MML)**. (A 37° angle will be formed between CR and OML.)
- Center CR to **acanthion**, then center cassette to projected CR.

Optional AP Modified Acanthioparietal –Modified Reverse Waters:

This projection best visualizes the floor of orbits and provides a direct view of entire orbital rims. Petrous ridges are projected into mid maxillary sinus region (Fig. 19-133).

- Angle CR cephalad as needed to align **CR parallel to lips-meatal line (LML)**.
- Center CR to **acanthion**, then center cassette to projected CR.

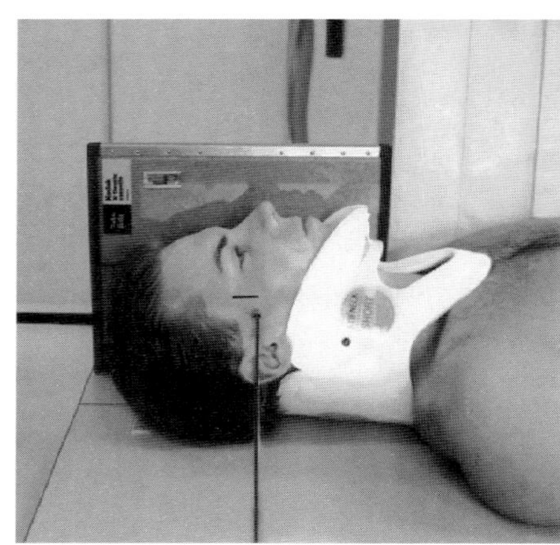

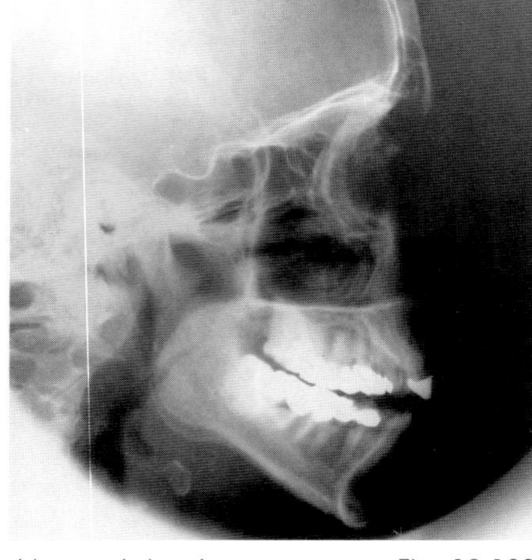

Fig. 19-128. Trauma horizontal beam lateral. Fig. 19-129.

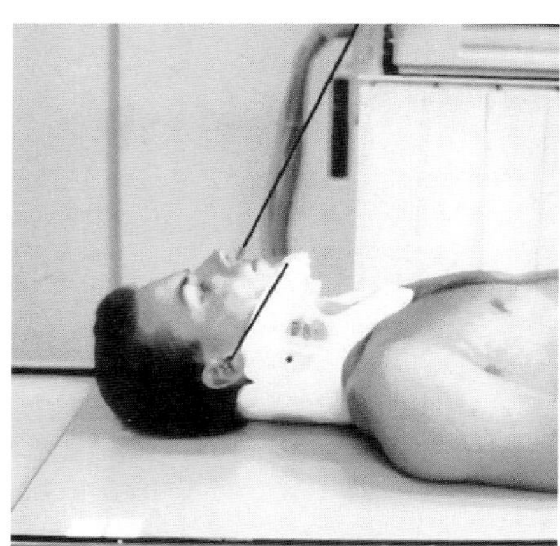

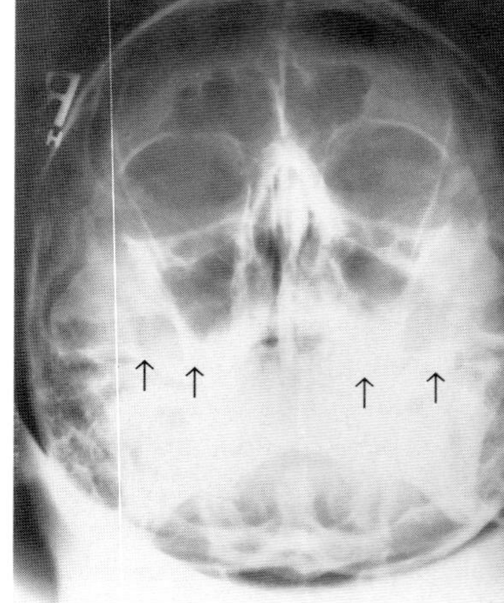

Fig. 19-130. Acanthioparietal (reverse Waters) –CR parallel to MML, centered to acanthion Fig. 19-131.

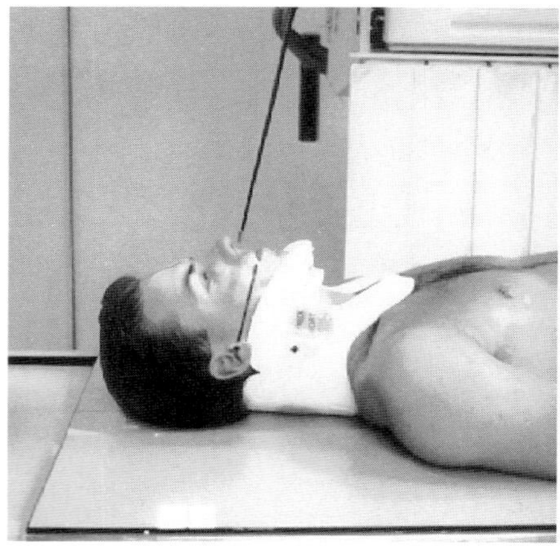

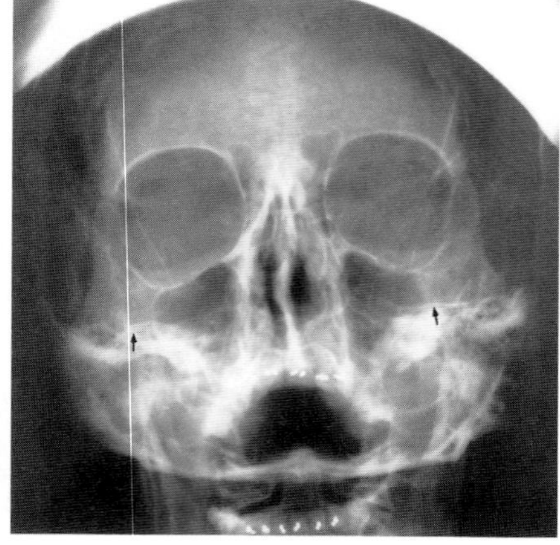

Fig. 19-132. Modified acanthioparietal (modified reverse Waters) –CR parallel to LML, centered to acanthion Fig. 19-133.

AP Axial, AP and Axiolateral Oblique–Mandible

Warning: With possible spinal injury do not attempt to move patient's head or neck. All projections for the mandible can be achieved as is with the patient supine.

Technical Factors

- Film size–8 x 10 in. (18 x 24 cm) lengthwise for APs, and crosswise for axiolateral obliques.
- Grid cassette on edge for axiolateral oblique.
- 40-44 in. (102-112 cm) SID.

Positioning–Patient Supine

- Place grid cassette under patient's head and shoulders, or under backboard. May be taken with cervical collar in place with possible neck injury
- Remove all metal, plastic or other removable objects from head and mandible area, if possible

Central Ray

AP Axial *(Best visualizes condyloid processes, condyles and TMJs):*

- Without manipulating patient's head, angle **CR 35 to 40° caudad to OML**.
- Center CR to pass through region of condyloid processes and condyles, **about 2 in. (5 cm) anterior to EAMs**.
- Center cassette to projected CR.

AP Projection *(Best visualizes rami and lateral body):*

- Angle CR caudad as needed to be **parallel to OML**.
- Center CR to mid mandible region, approximately at junction of lips.
- Center cassette to projected CR.

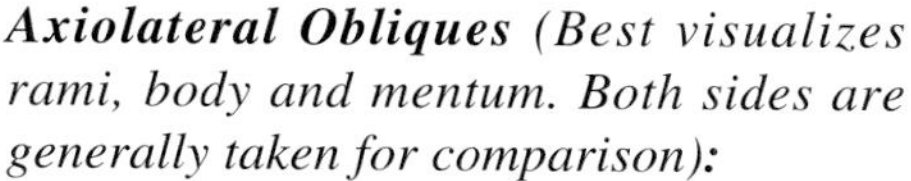

Axiolateral Obliques *(Best visualizes rami, body and mentum. Both sides are generally taken for comparison):*

- Place grid cassette on edge next to face, parallel to MSP with lower edge of cassette about 1 in. (2.5 cm) below mentum.
- Depress shoulders if possible and elevate chin. (Only if cervical fracture is **not** a consideration.)
- Angle horizontal beam CR 25 to 30° cephalad (from lateral), and angle CR posteriorly 5 to 10° if necessary to clear shoulder.
- CR centered to ≈2 in. (5 cm) inferior to angle of mandible on side away from film.

Note (axiolateral obliques): Head in true lateral position best demonstrates **ramus** and **proximal body**, and if head is rotated 10 to 20° toward film, the **mid and distal body** and **mentum** region are best visualized.

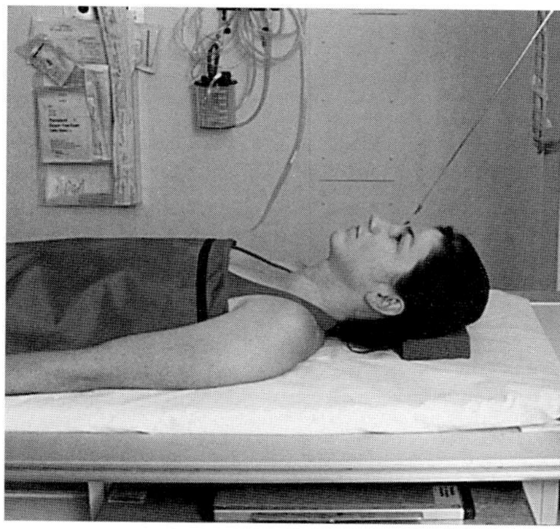

Fig. 19-134. AP axial –CR 35 to 40° caudad to OML.

Note: With cervical trauma, do **not** elevate head on sponge as shown (increase CR angle as needed instead).

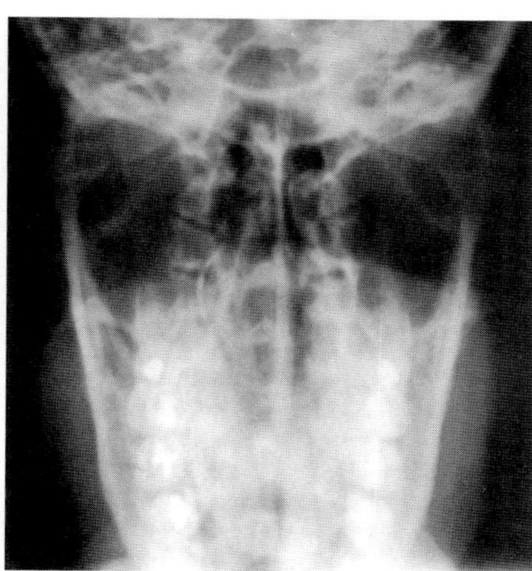

Fig. 19-135. AP axial.

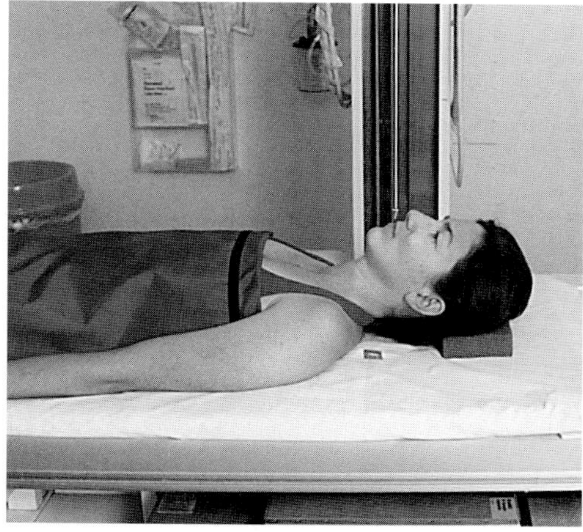

Fig. 19-136. AP projection–CR parallel to OML, to junction of lips.

Note: With cervical trauma, do **not** elevate head on sponge as shown (angle CR caudad as needed instead).

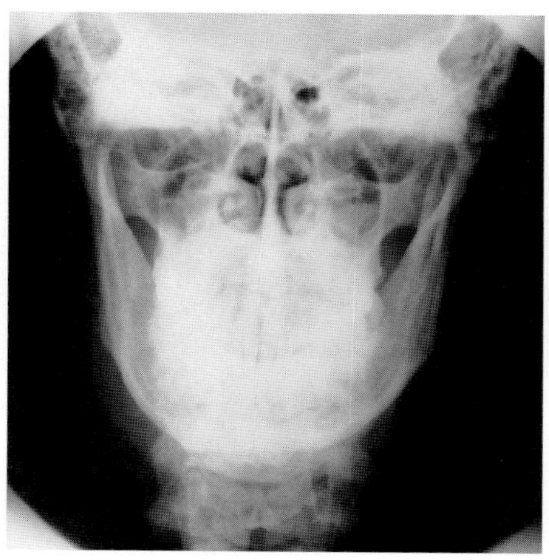

Fig. 19-137. AP projection.

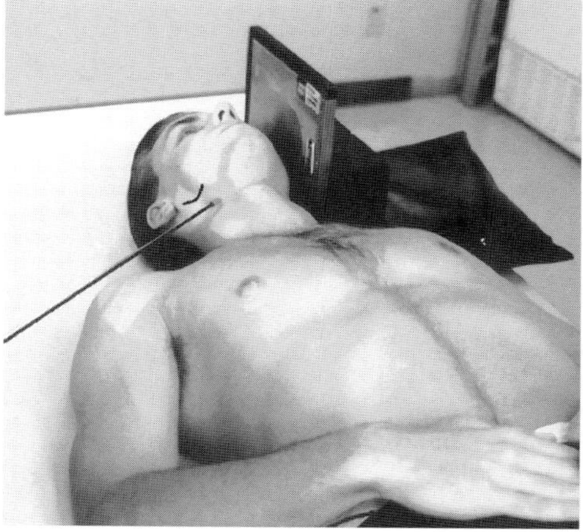

Fig. 19-138. Horizontal beam axiolateral oblique –CR horizontal (or 5 to 10° posteriorly) and 25 to 30° cephalad.

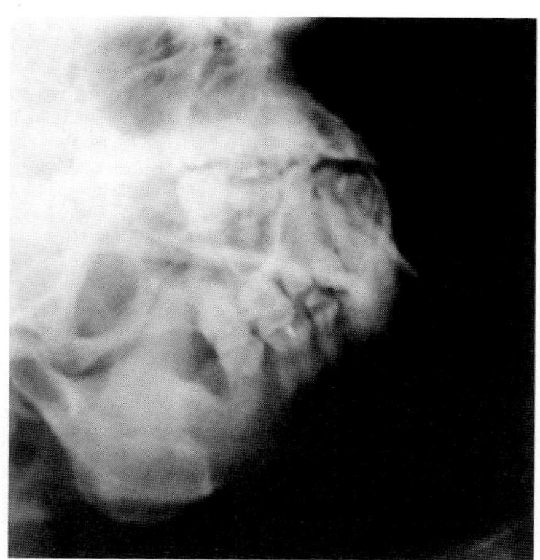

Fig. 19-139. Axiolateral oblique.

CHAPTER 20

Pediatric Radiography

CONTRIBUTIONS BY:
Claudia Calandrino, MPA, RT(R))
Jessie R. Harris, RT (R)
Cecilie Godderidge, BS, RT(R)

20

CONTENTS

Introduction and Principles

Introduction:
- Age of understanding **582**
- Pre-exam introduction **582**
- Reporting child abuse **582**

Immobilization:
- Tam-em board and plexiglass hold-down paddle **583**
- Pigg-O-Stat **583**
- Tape, sandbags, head clamps, etc. **584**
- Steps of "mummifying" **585**

Bone development **586**

Radiation protection and pre-exam preparation **587**

Radiographic Positioning –Chest and Skeletal System

Chest:
- AP supine **588**
- PA erect **589**
- Lateral recumbent **590**
- Lateral erect **591**

Upper limbs:
- AP and lateral **592**

Lower limbs:
- AP and lateral (infants and young children **594**
- AP and lateral leg **595**
- AP and lateral foot **595**

Pelvis and hips:
- AP and lateral **596**

Skull:
- AP **598**
- Lateral **599**

The Pediatric Abdomen

Difference between children and adults **600**
Patient preparation for contrast media procedures **600**

Abdomen:
- AP KUB supine **601**
- AP erect **602**
- Dorsal decubitus **603**

GI fluoroscopy:
- Barium swallow, upper GI and small bowel **604**
- Lower GI system **606** (single contrast, double contrast, air enema)

Genitourinary system:
- Voiding cystourethrogram (VCUG) **608**
- Intravenous urogram (IVU) **609**

Introduction and Principles

INTRODUCTION

The pediatric technologist sees children not just as adults in miniature but as very special human persons to be handled with care and special understanding. This requires patience and the necessary time to **talk to** and **make friends** with the child. Explaining instructions to the child in a way that they can understand is of great importance in developing trust and cooperation.

Age of Understanding and Cooperation

Children do not reach a sense of understanding at a specific predictable age. This varies greatly from child to child and the pediatric technologist must not assume that the small person lacks this capability. Generally, however, by the age of **two years**, most normal children can be talked through a diagnostic radiographic study without immobilization or parental aid. Most important is a sense of trust, which begins at the first meeting between the patient and the technologist; the first impression the child has of this stranger is everlasting and forges the bond of a successful relationship.

Successful radiographic studies are dependent on two things. First and most important is the **technologist's attitude and approach to a child.** Second and also important is the **technical preparation in the room**, which includes certain essential immobilization devices as will be described and illustrated in this chapter.

Pre-exam Introduction and Child/Parent Evaluation

Self Introduction: At the first meeting, most patients are accompanied by at least one parent. It is important to:

- Introduce yourself as the technologist who will be working with this child.
- Find out what information the attending physician has given the parent and patient.
- Explain what you are going to do and what your needs will be.

Tears, fear and combative resistance are perfectly normal reactions for a young child. The technologist must take the time to communicate to the parent and child, in a language they can understand, exactly what they are going to do. They must try to build an atmosphere of trust in the waiting room before the patient is taken into the radiographic room. The technologist should discuss the necessity of immobilization as a last resort if the child's cooperation is unattainable.

Evaluate Parent's Role: This is also the time to evaluate the parent's role. There are three possibilities:

(1) Parent in room as an observer who lends support and comfort by their presence.
(2) Parent as a participator who assists with immobilization.
(3) Parent asked to remain in the waiting area and not accompany child into radiography room.

Many times children who act fearful and combative in the waiting room with the parent present will be much more cooperative without the parent. This is the time when the technologist's skills in communication are necessary. At this time the technologist should also try to convince the parent that he or she is capable of radiographing the patient **without** parental assistance.

This assessment of the parent's role is very important and requires an objective evaluation by the technologist. If it is determined that the parent's anxiety will interfere with the child's cooperation, then option (3) would be chosen. Parents, however, generally do wish to assist in immobilizing the child, and if this option is chosen, the radiographer should carefully explain the procedures to both the parent and the patient. This includes instructions to the parent on correct immobilization techniques. Cooperation and the parent's effectiveness in assisting tends to increase when they understand how proper but firm immobilization will improve the diagnostic quality of the image, and also reduce radiation exposure to the patient.

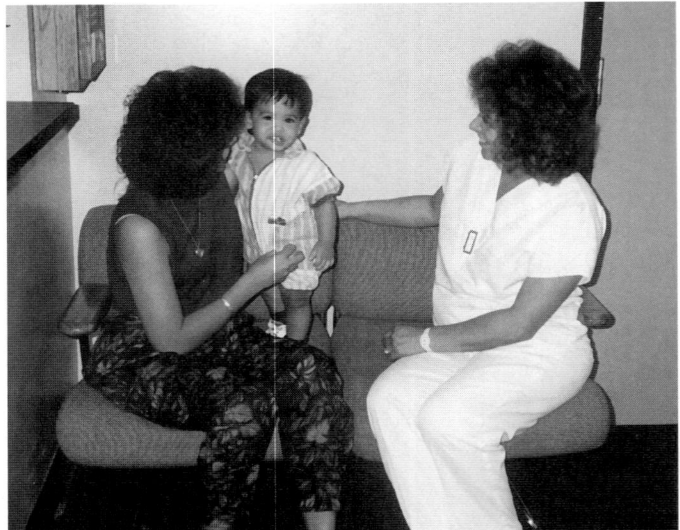

Fig. 20-1. Talking to patient and developing trust.

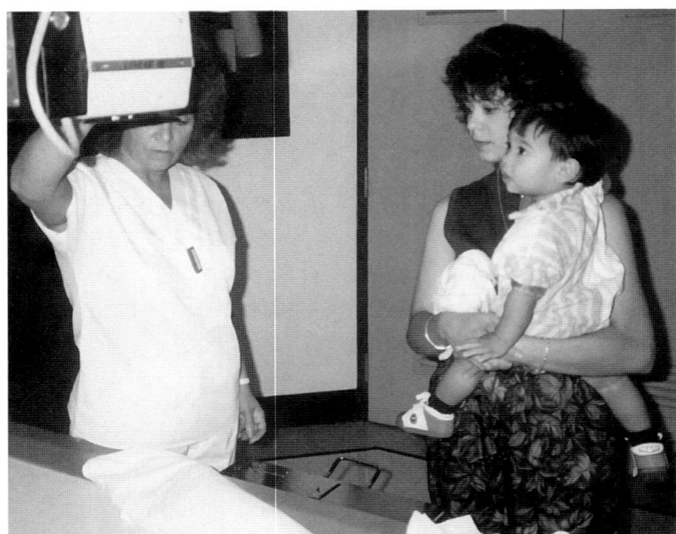

Fig. 20-2. Technologist introducing herself.

Reporting Child Abuse

Most medical facilities have a procedure in place to report suspected child abuse. In the past the term used for this was battered child syndrome (BCS). Today the acceptable term is **nonaccidental trauma (NAT).**

It is generally not the responsibility of the technologist to make a judgment as to whether or not child abuse has occurred, but rather to report the facts as they are seen or suspected. If NAT is suspected, the technologist should discuss this with the radiologist or such supervisor as determined by departmental protocol. State laws vary on technologists' responsibilities and it is most important that **every technologist know what their responsibilities are concerning this in the state in which they are working.**

IMMOBILIZATION

Pediatric patients in general can include infants through age 12 to 14. However, older children can be treated more like adults except for special care in gonadal shielding, and reduced exposure factors due to their smaller size. This chapter primarily describes and illustrates radiographing infants and toddlers who require special attention to prevent motion during the exposure. In general pediatric radiography should **always utilize exposure times as short as possible** to minimize image blurring resulting from patient motion. However, even with short exposure times, preventing motion during exposures is a constant challenge in pediatric radiography, and effective methods of immobilization are essential.

There are immobilization devices on the market today that can be purchased. These can generally be found in a radiology supply catalog. Examples of these are the **Tam-em Board** and **Pigg-O-Stat** as demonstrated. The **Posi-Tot** is another type of immobilization device also available commercially. The cost effectiveness of these devices is dependent on how often the devices are utilized.

Tam-em Board and Plexiglass Hold-down Paddle (Fig. 20-3)

The **Tam-em Board,** along with several short Velcro straps for immobilizing the upper and lower limbs, is shown. This is a commercially available immobilization device that is easy to use and will be demonstrated in this chapter.

A **plexiglass hold-down paddle** is also shown in front of the Tam-em Board. This can be cut from a clear sheet of plexiglass of sufficient thickness for necessary rigidity. It can be used in various applications such as to hold down upper or lower limbs without obscuring essential anatomy. This can be an aid for parents to utilize in assisting with immobilization.

Pigg-O-Stat (Fig. 20-4)

The **Pigg-O-Stat** is a commonly used immobilization apparatus for erect chest and abdomen procedures on infants and small children up to the approximate age of 2 years. The infant or child is seated on the small bicycle type seat (A) with their legs placed down through the opening. This seat is adjustable in height. The arms are then raised above the head and the two clear plastic body clamps (B) are adjusted firmly against each side of the body to prevent movement (see page 589). There are two sizes of these clamps, which are easily interchangeable depending on the size of the child, (B and G). The cassette is placed in the film holder mount (C).

The entire seat and body clamps are mounted on a swivel base (D), which can be rotated independent of the film holder. This places the patient into the desired position for erect AP, PA, lateral or oblique projections. The adjustable lead gonadal shield (E), is shown in position between the x-ray tube and patient. This shield also contains the necessary film markers. The entire Pigg-O-Stat device is mounted on a stand (F) with wheels and locks that allows it to be easily moved into position, and from room to room as needed.

Other Immobilization Forms (Fig. 20-5)

The simplest and least expensive form of immobilization is to utilize the paraphernalia that are commonly found in most departments. **Tape, sheets** or **towels, sandbags, covered radiolucent sponge blocks, compression bands, stockinette** and **ace bandages** if used correctly are very effective in immobilization.

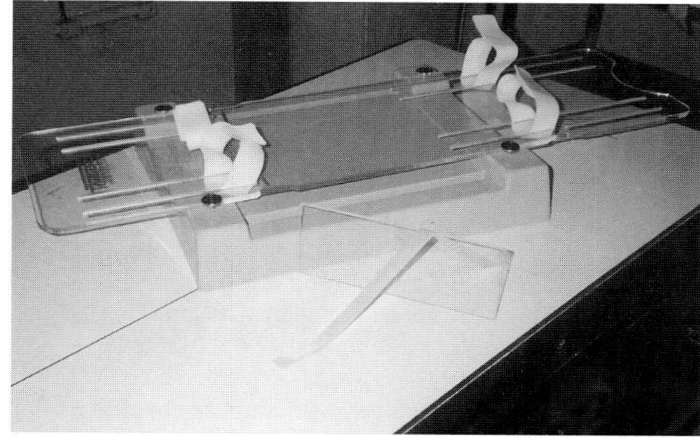

Fig. 20-3. Tam-em board (plexiglass hold-down paddle).

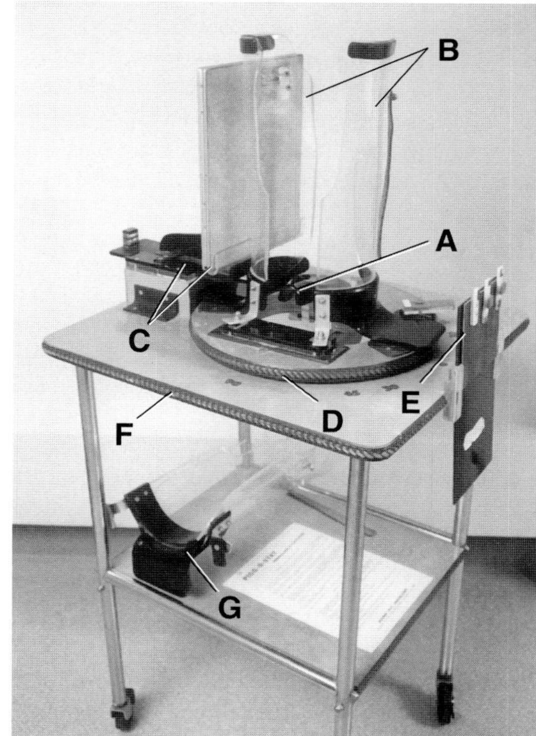

Fig. 20-4. Pigg-O-Stat (set for lateral chest).

A. Bicycle type seat.
B. Side body clamps.
C. Film holder mount.
D. Swivel base.
E. Adjustable lead shield with markers.
F. Mounting stand on wheels.
G. Extra set of smaller body clamps.

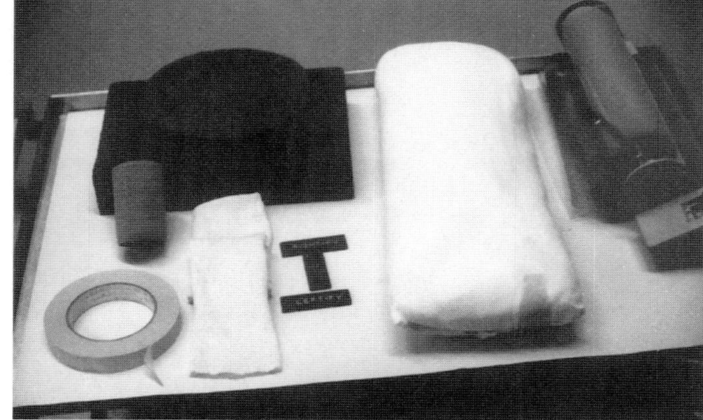

Fig. 20-5. Immobilization aids.

Immobilization continued

Sandbags

There are sandbags available for purchase. However most of these are used as weights or immobilization aids for adults. These bags are not as effective for immobilization of the pediatric patient as those bags that are made specifically for this purpose.

Strong canvas-type material and children's coarse sterilized playing sand should be utilized. Coarse sand is recommended because if the bag should break open the sand is easily cleaned up and the chance of causing artifacts on radiographs is minimized.

Two sandbag sizes are recommended, 8 x 18 in. (20 x 46 cm) and 13 x 20 in. (33 x 50 cm). The sandbags should not be overfilled with sand, which makes the bag stiff, rather **the bag should be pliable** so that when placed over a patient's limb it will mold to that part.

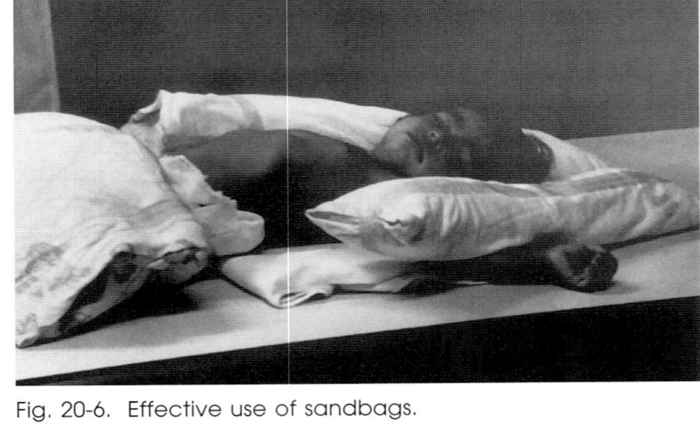

Fig. 20-6. Effective use of sandbags.

Tape

Masking or autoclave type tape is recommended. Adhesive tape may show on the radiograph and create an artifact that could obscure the anatomical part of interest. Also, there are accounts of patients who have had an allergic reaction to adhesive tape. The fragile skin of infants can also be injured by adhesive tape unless the tape is twisted so the adhesive surface is not against the skin. Gauze pads placed between skin and adhesive tape can also be used effectively.

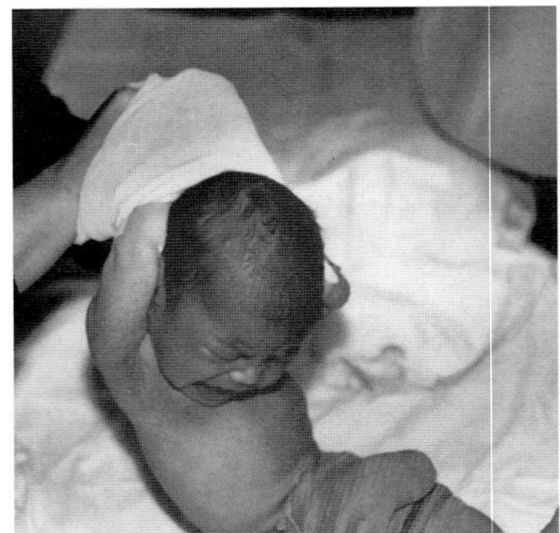

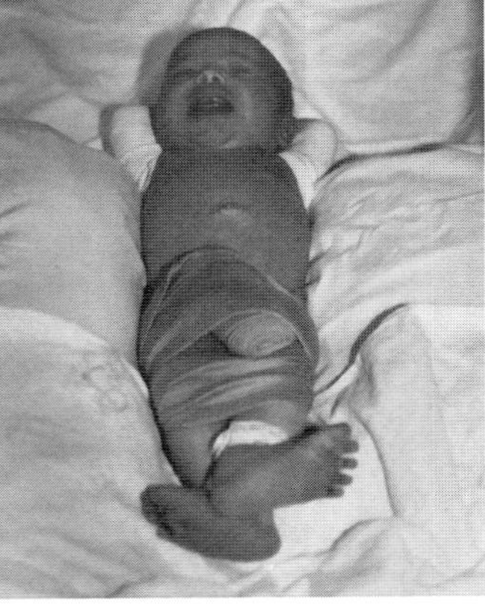

Fig. 20-7. Using stockinette and ace bandage. Fig. 20-8.

Stockinette

If stockinettes are utilized, they should be tubular. They come in various sizes; 3-inch is recommended for small infants and 4-inch for larger children.

When using the stockinette, double the stockinette and place over the patient's arms covering the arms up to the shoulders. Not only does this serve to immobilize the arms, but it also serves as a pillow (Fig. 20-8).

Ace Bandage

A 4-inch ace bandage is best for small infants and children while a six-inch bandage works well for older children. These are best used for immobilizing the legs. When starting the wrapping process, begin at the patient's hips and wrap down to the patient's mid calf (Fig. 20-8). Do not wrap too tightly to cut off circulation.

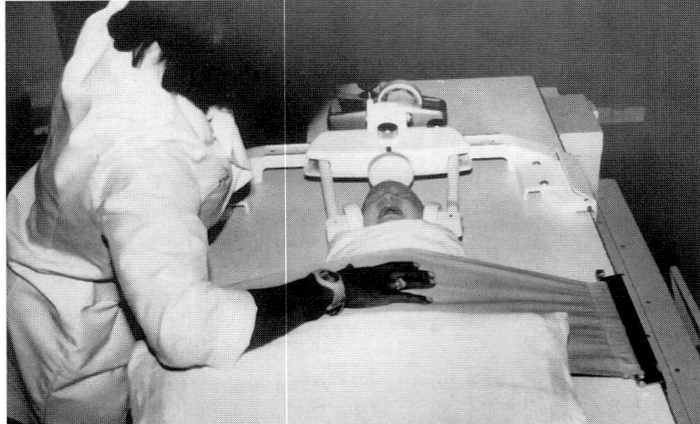

Fig. 20-9. Compression band and head clamps.

Compression Bands and Head Clamps

Compression or retention bands are also valuable aids for immobilization. Compression bands, however, are more effective with pediatrics when used in combination with sandbags as will be demonstrated later in this chapter.

Various types of adjustable head clamps are also available which attach to the table top as shown in Fig. 20-9.

Weighted Angle Blocks as Head Clamps

These are heavy steel angle blocks with thick radiolucent sponge pads attached (Fig. 20-10). They are relatively inexpensive to have made compared to the cost of commercially available head clamps but are very effective and versatile in immobilization, especially when used in combination with sandbags and/or tape, or if the patient is mummified as shown in Fig. 20-10.

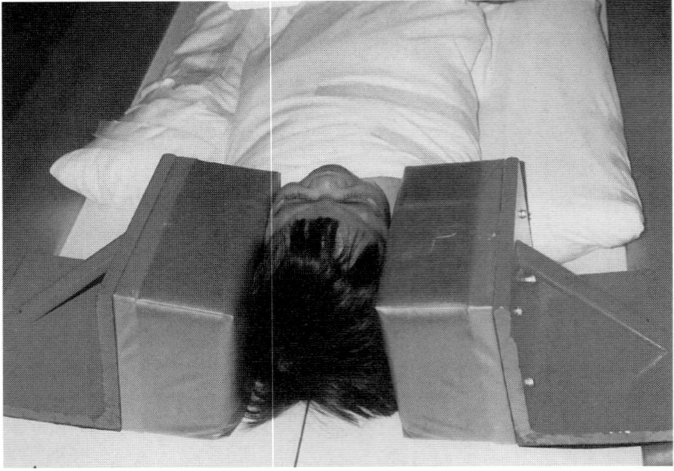

Fig. 20-10. Weighted angle blocks as head clamps (patient "mummified").

"Mummifying" or Wrapping with Sheets or Towels

In addition to some type of head clamps, "mummifying" or wrapping is often necessary to immobilize the child for certain radiographic procedures such as head exams. This is very effective for immobilization if done correctly. Following is a six-step method of how this is done. The room should be set up and prepared before bringing the patient into the room.

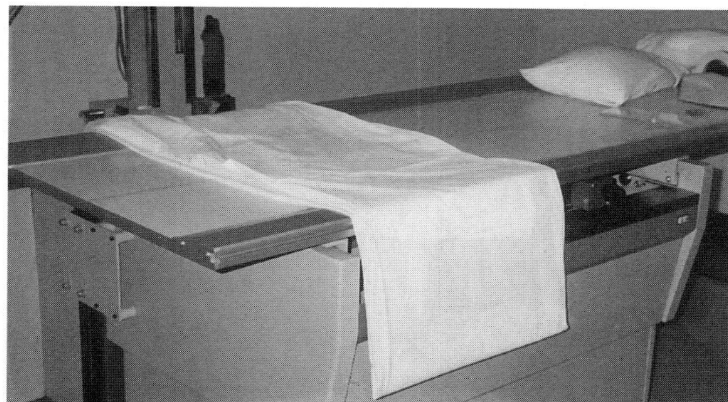

Fig. 20-11. **Step 1.** Place the sheet on the table folded in half or in thirds lengthwise, depending on the size of the patient.

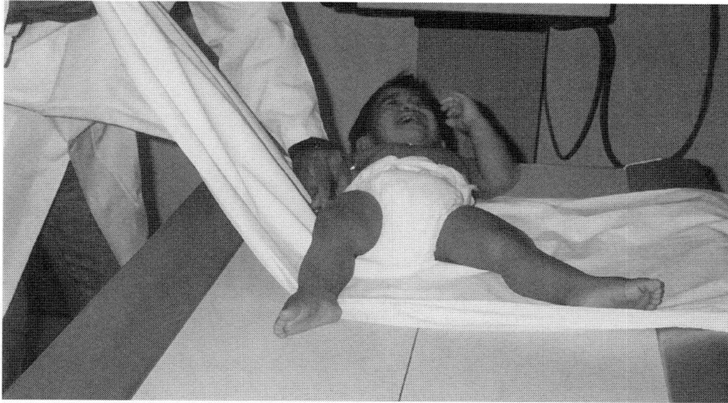

Fig. 20-12. **Step 2.** Place the patient in the middle of the sheet, then place the patient's right arm along side of his body. Take the end of the sheet closest to the technologist and pull the sheet across the patient's body tightly, keeping the arm next to the patient's body.

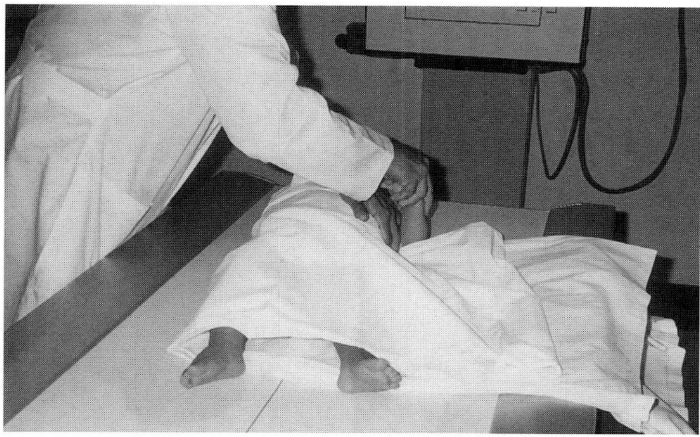

Fig. 20-13. **Step 3.** Place the patient's left arm along side of his body on top of the top sheet. Bring the free sheet over the left arm to the right side of the patient's body and around under the body as needed.

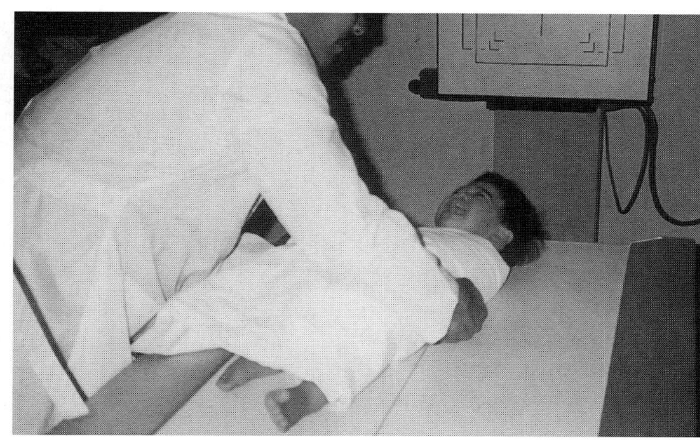

Fig. 20-14. **Step 4.** Complete the wrapping process by pulling the sheet tightly enough so that the patient cannot free his arms.

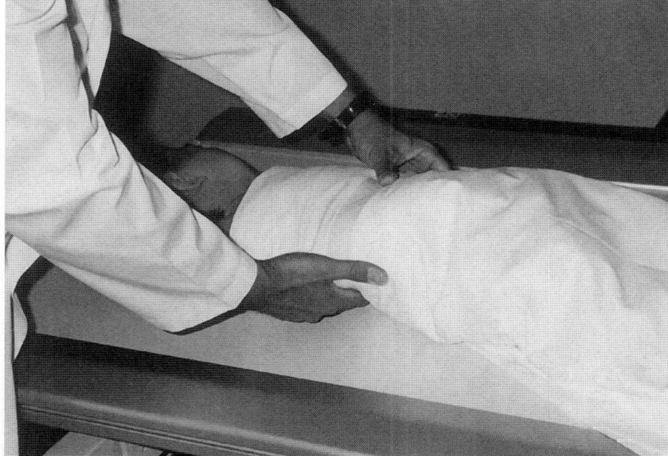

Fig. 20-15. **Step 5.** Pull the sheet and tape the end of the sheet. Place a long piece of tape from the back of the right wrapped arm to the left wrapped arm over the sheet. This will prevent the patient from breaking out of the sheet.

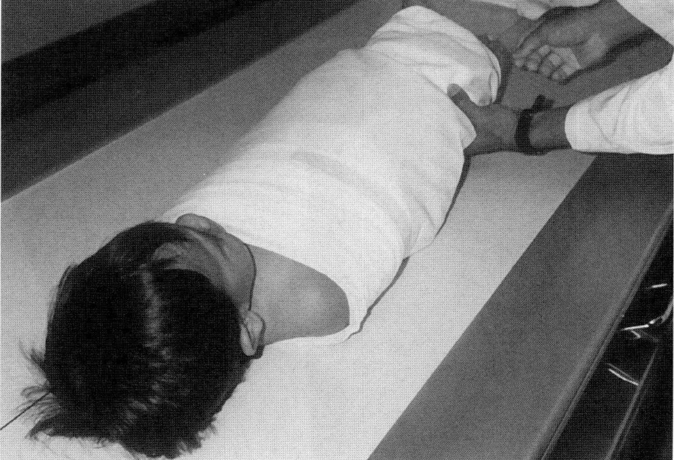

Fig. 20-16. **Step 6.** Place another piece of tape around the patient's knees. This will keep the patient's lower limbs from becoming free.

Bone Development (Ossification)

The bones of infants and small children go through various growth changes from birth through adolescence. The pelvis is an example where ossification changes are apparent in children. As shown in Fig. 20-17, the divisions of the hip bone between the ilium, ischium and pubis is evident. They appear as individual bones separated by a joint space, which is the cartilaginous growth region in the area of the acetabulum.

The heads of the femurs also appear to be separated by a joint space which should not be confused with fracture sites or other abnormalities. These are also normal cartilaginous growth regions.

Most primary centers of bone formation or ossification such as those involving the mid shaft area of long bones appear before birth. These primary centers become the **diaphysis** (shaft or body) (D) of long bones (Fig. 20-18 and 20-19). Each secondary center of ossification involves the ends of long bones and is termed an **epiphysis** (E). This is demonstrated on the PA hand radiograph of a 9-year old in Fig. 20-18, and the lower limb of a 1-year old in Fig. 20-19. Note the epiphyses at the ends of the radius and ulna as well as the metacarpals and phalanges (see small arrows).

The space between the diaphysis and epiphysis is made up of cartilage and is termed an **epiphyseal plate** (EP). These epiphyseal plates are found between each diaphysis and each epiphysis until skeleton growth is complete upon full maturity, which is normally at about 25 years.

The epiphyses are the parts of bones that increase in size and appearance as a child grows, as shown on the growth comparison radiographs below (Figs. 20-20 to 20-23). Note in these four knee radiographs the change in size and shape of the epiphyses of the distal femur and proximal tibia and fibula from age 3 to age 12. At age 3 the epiphysis of the fibula is not yet visible, but by 12 years old it becomes quite obvious (see arrows). The size and shape of the larger epiphysis of the proximal tibia also changes dramatically from age 3 to age 12 as evident on these knee radiographs.

Growth charts are available which list and demonstrate normal growth patterns. Radiographers need to be familiar with bone development in infants and children and recognize the appearance of these normal growth stages.

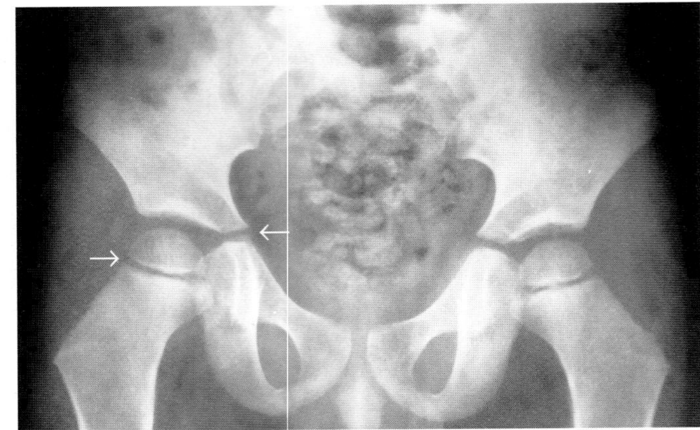

Fig. 20-17. Normal three-year-old pelvis.

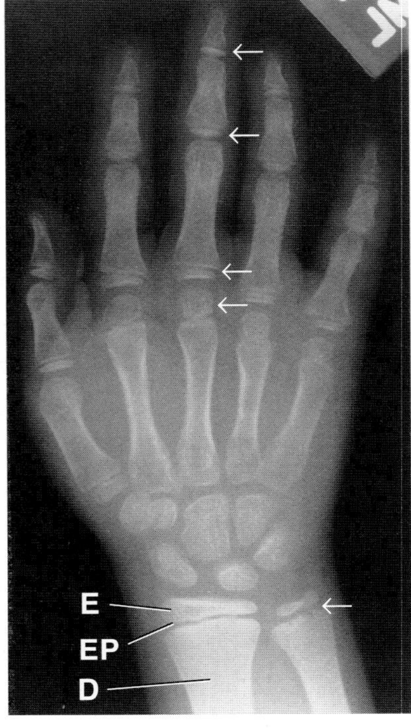

Fig. 20-18. Normal nine-year-old hand.

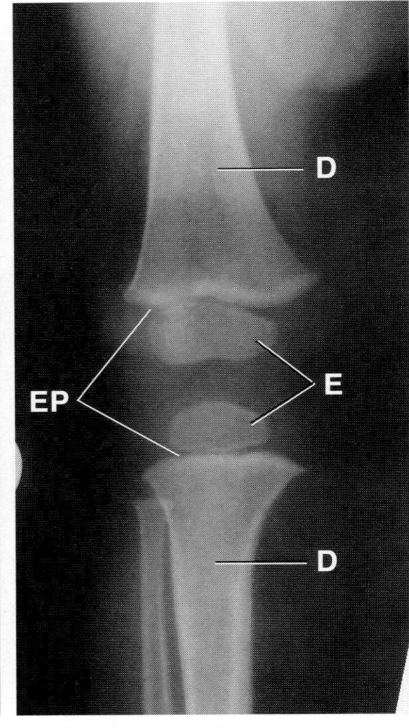

Fig. 20-19. Normal one-year-old lower limb.

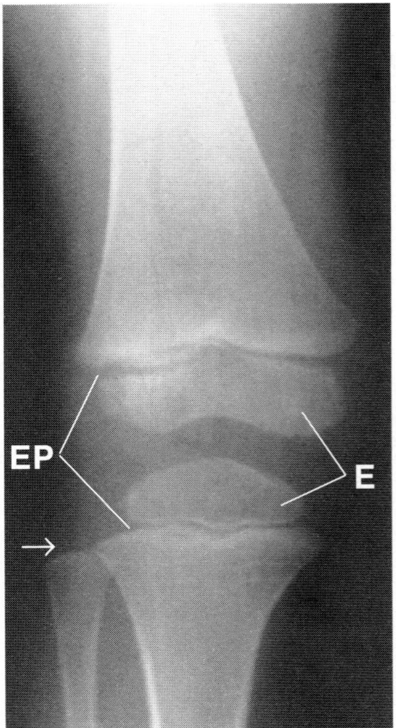

Fig. 20-20. Three-year-old.

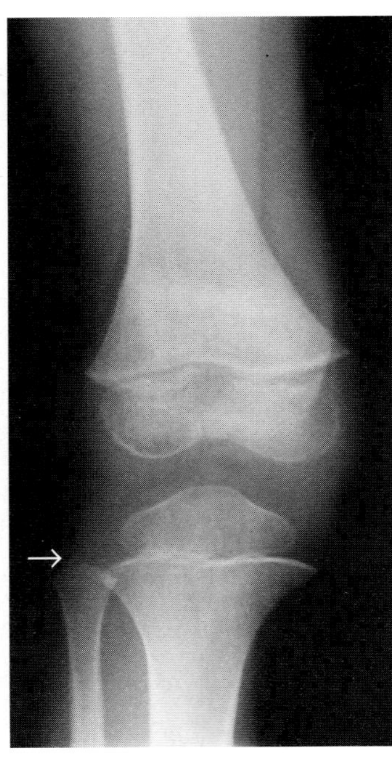

Fig. 20-21. Four-year-old.

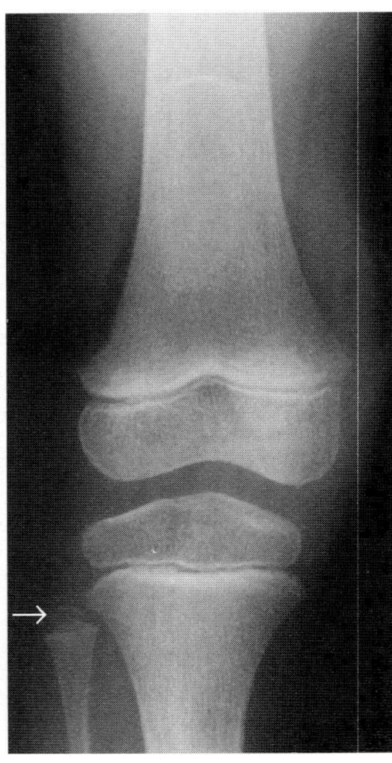

Fig. 20-22. Six-year-old.

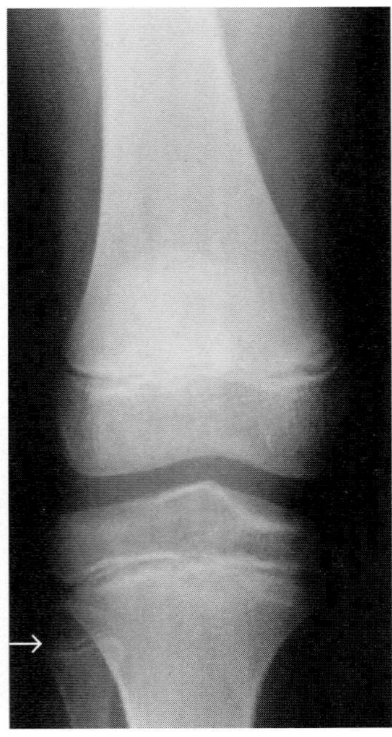

Fig. 20-23. Twelve-year-old.

RADIATION PROTECTION

Minimal Repeats

Reduction of repeat exposures is critical, especially in young children, whose developing cells are particularly sensitive to the effects of radiation. **Proper immobilization** and high mA, **short exposure time techniques** will reduce the incidence of motion blur. Accurate **technique charts with patient body weights** should be used. Radiographic grids should be used only when the body part examined is greater than 9 cm in thickness.

Each radiology department should also have a list of specific procedures for pediatric patients, including specialized views and limited examination series to ensure that appropriate projections and no unnecessary exposures are made.

Gonadal Protection

Gonads of the child should **always** be shielded with contact type shields in addition to close collimation unless such shields obscure essential anatomy of the lower abdomen or pelvic area. Various shapes and sizes of contact shields are shown in Fig. 20-24.

Since parents will often request shielding for their child's gonads, they should also be aware of other safeguards used for radiation protection such as **close collimation**, **low dosage techniques**, and a **minimum number of exposures**. To relieve the parents' fears, the technologist should explain in as simple language as possible, the protection practices being used and why.

Parent Protection

If parents are to be in the room, they must be supplied with **lead aprons**. If they are immobilizing the child and their hands are in/or near the primary beam, they should also be given **lead gloves**.

If the mother or other female guardian is in childbearing years and wishes to assist in the procedure, the radiographer must **ask if she is pregnant** before allowing her to remain in the room during the radiographic exposure. She should not be allowed in the room if she is pregnant.

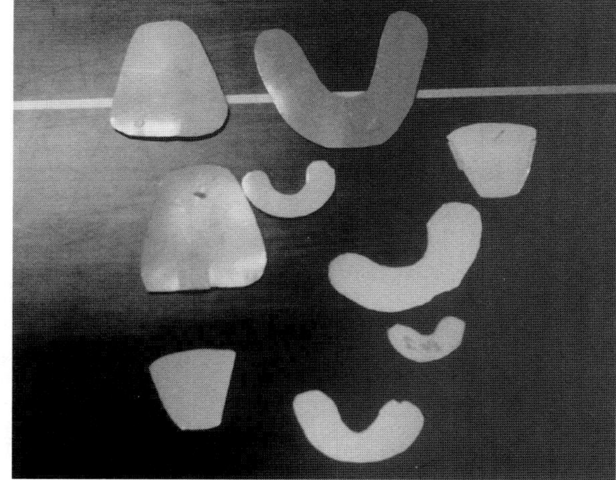

Fig. 20-24. Contact gonad shields.

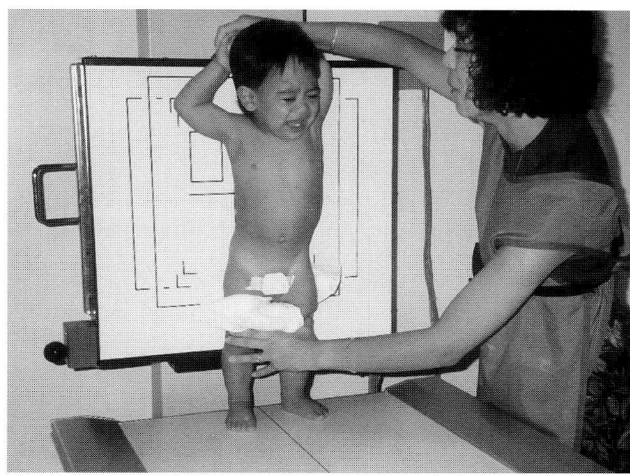

Fig. 20-25. Male gonadal shield in place for erect abdomen. **Note:** Lead gloves should have been provided for the parent holding this patient along with a lead apron.

PRE-EXAM PREPARATION

The following should be completed before the patient is brought into the room:

- The necessary immobilization and shielding paraphernalia should be in place (sandbags, tape, Tam-em Board if used, sheets or towels, stockinette, ace bandages and shielding devices for patient and for parents if assisting).
- Cassettes and film markers should be in place and techniques set (if a solo technologist is performing the exam).
- The specific projections should be determined, which may require consultation with the radiologist.
- If two technologists are working together, they should discuss the role each will perform during the procedure. A suggested division of responsibilities is:
  - –The assisting technologist sets techniques, makes exposures, changes the cassettes and processes the film.
  - –The primary technologist positions the patient and instructs parents (if assisting), positions tube, collimation and required shielding.

Child Preparation: After the child is brought into room and the procedure explained to both child and parent's satisfaction, then due to the low dosage technique used, the parent or technologist must remove from the body parts to be radiographed any clothing, bandages and/or diapers. This is necessary to prevent such from casting shadows and creating artifacts on the radiograph.

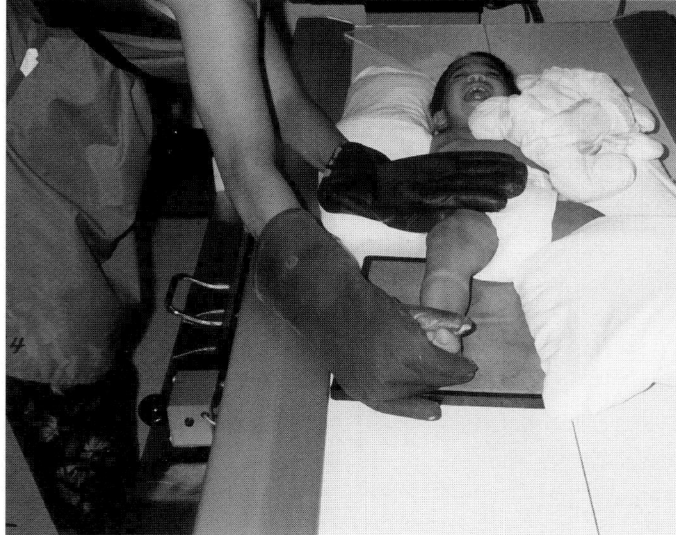

Fig. 20-26. Lead aprons and gloves for parents.

AP/PA Chest Projection

Erect if possible: Generally, pediatric chest patients, if old enough, should be examined in an erect position using a Pigg-O-Stat or similar erect immobilization device (see next page). Exceptions are infants in an isolette, or if too young to support head.

Chest
Basic
- **AP/PA**
- Lateral

Diagnostic Indications

Asthma
Adenopathy (enlarged glands)
Cystic fibrosis
CHF (congestive heart failure)
Emphysema
Foreign body
Hemoptysis (blood in sputum)
Meconium aspiration (dark green secretions)
Metastases
PFC (persistent fetal circulation)
Atelectasis (incomplete expansion of lung)
Bronchitis
Cough
Dyspnea (difficulty in breathing)
Embolus
Heart disease
Hyaline membrane disease
Neoplasm
Pleura effusion
Pneumothorax

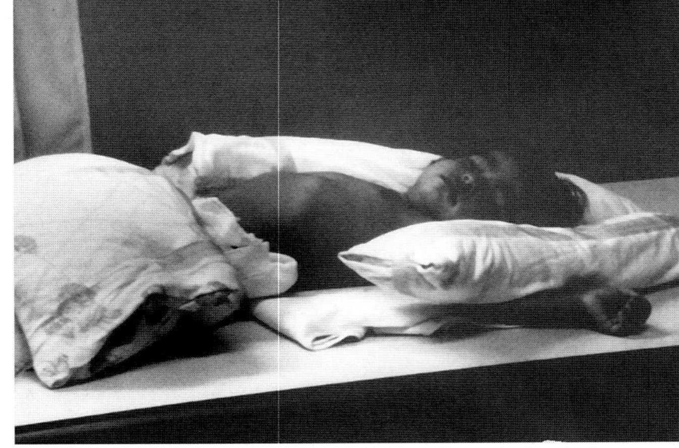

Fig. 20-27. Supine, immobilized with sandbags.

Technical Factors

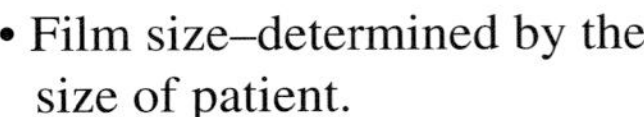

- Film size–determined by the size of patient.
- Film crosswise, if supine place cassette under patient.
- Grid not required.
- 65-70 kVp, shortest exposure time possible.

Shielding: Contact lead shielding should be placed over the pelvic area with upper margin to level of iliac crests.

Patient Position

- Generally taken **supine** unless a Pigg-O-Stat or similar erect immobilization device is available. (See next page.)
- Patient supine, arms extended to remove scapula from the lung fields.
- Arms are secured to the table with sandbags or velcro straps if using Tam-em Board.
- Legs extended to prevent rotation of pelvis. Hips and legs are secured by placing sandbags at the level of the hip to the top of the knee. If using Tame-em Board, hip and legs are velcro strapped to the board.
- If utilizing parental assistance:
  1. Have parent remove child's chest clothing.
  2. Provide parent with lead apron and gloves.
  3. Place child on cassette.
  4. Parent should extend child's arms over head with one hand while keeping head tilted back to prevent superimposing upper lungs. With other hand hold child's legs at level of the knees, applying pressure as necessary to prevent movement.
  5. Place parent in a position that will not obstruct technologist's view of patient while making exposure.
  6. Place lead gloves over the top of the parent's hands if parent is not wearing the gloves. (It may be easier to hold on to patient if not wearing the gloves.)

Part Position

- Place the patient in the middle of the cassette with the shoulders 2 in. (5 cm) below the top of the cassette.
- Insure that thorax is **not rotated**.

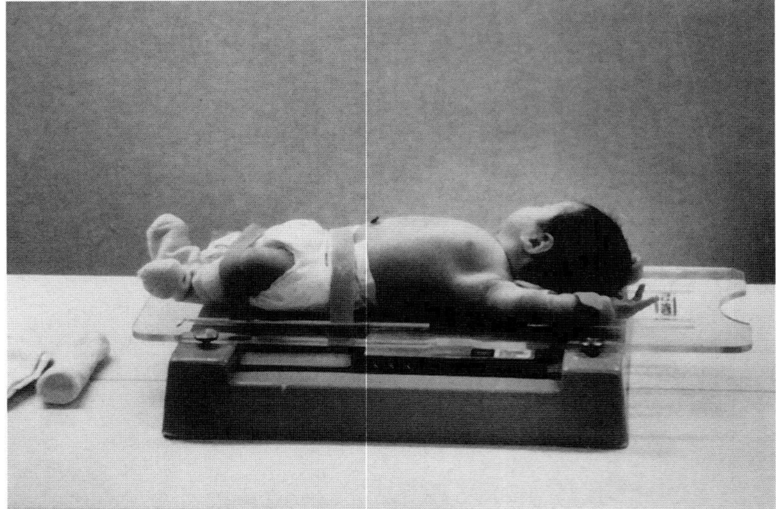

Fig. 20-28. Immobilized with Tam-em board.

Central Ray

- CR **perpendicular** to the film, centered to the midsagittal plane at the **level of mid-thorax** which is approximately at the **mammillary (nipple) line**.
- SID: 50 to 60 in. (127 to 212 cm). Tube raised as high as possible.

Collimation: Closely collimate on four sides to outer chest margins.

Respiration: Make exposure upon second full inspiration. If child is crying, watch respiration and make exposure immediately after the child fully inhales.

AP/PA Chest Projection continued

ERECT PA CHEST WITH PIGG-O-STAT

Patient Position

- Patient placed on seat with legs down through center opening. Adjust seat to correct height so top of cassette is about 1 in. (2.5 cm) above shoulders.
- Arms are raised and side body clamps placed firmly against patient and secured by base adjustment and by adjustable strap.
- Lead shield raised to a level about an inch above iliac crest.
- Correct R and L markers and insp (inspiration) marker are set to be exposed on film.
- Insure no rotation.

Central Ray

- CR **perpendicular** to film at **level of mid thorax** (at mammary line).
- SID: 72 in. (180 cm).

Collimation: Collimate closely on four sides to outer chest margins.

Respiration: If child is crying, watch respiration and make exposure as child fully inhales and holds his breath. (Can frequently hold their breath on inspiration after a practice session.)

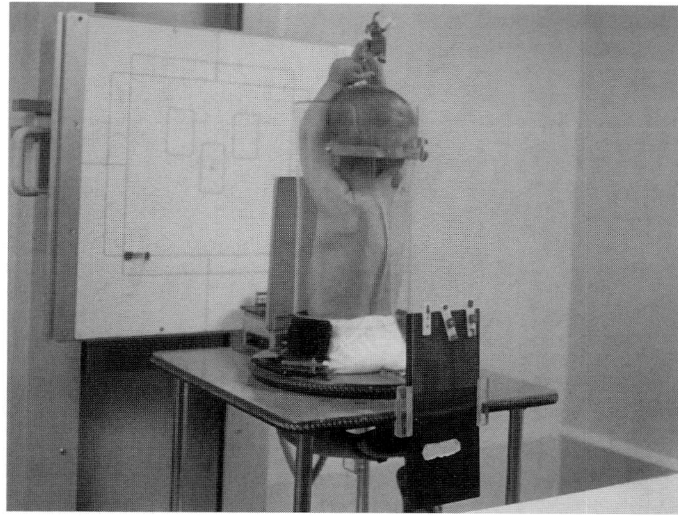

Fig. 20-29. Immobilized by Pigg-O-Stat.

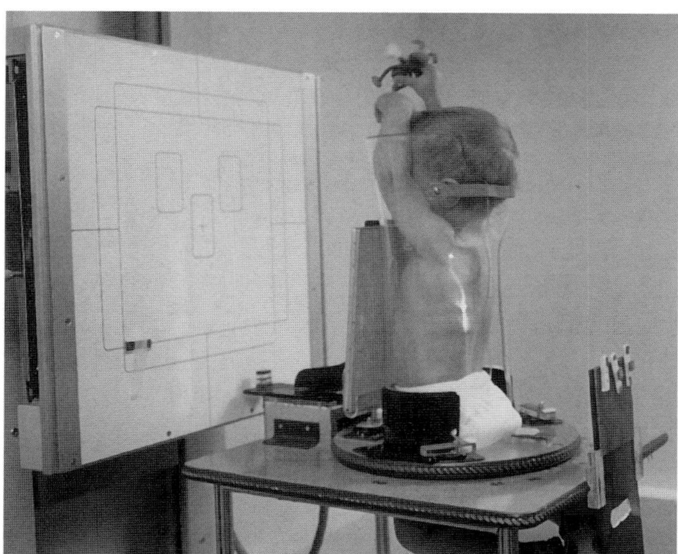

Fig. 20-30. Immobilized by Pigg-O-Stat.

Evaluation Criteria

- **No rotation**: Both sternoclavicular joints should be the same distance from the vertebral column. The distance from the lateral borders of the ribs to the spine should be the same on each side.
- The arms should be extended to remove the scapulae from the lung fields.
- Entire lungs, which must be fully expanded.
- Collimation margins should be apparent on four sides.
- **No motion** should result in clear lung markings and sharp outlines of diaphragm and heart and rib borders.
- Correct penetration and exposure should faintly visualize outlines of vertebra and ribs through the heart shadow without overexposing the fine vascular lung markings throughout lungs.
- Patient ID and right or left marker are placed correctly.

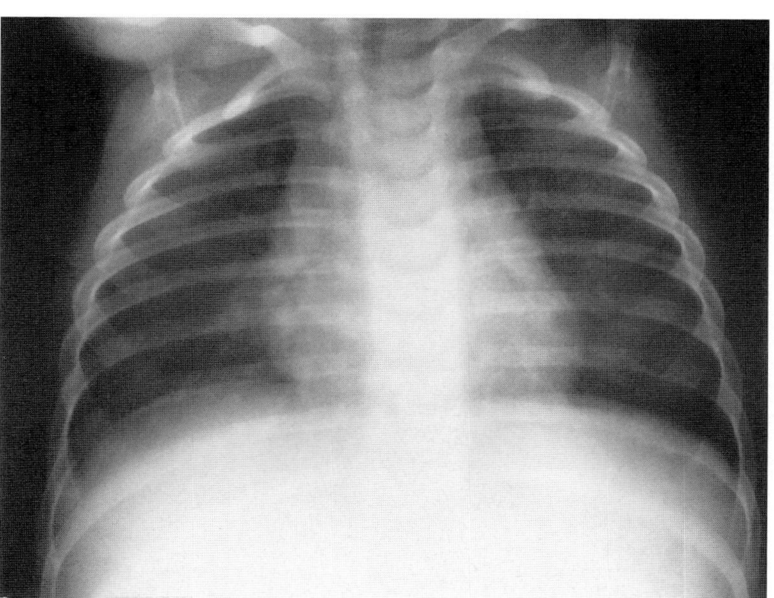

Fig. 20-31. AP (PA) chest.

Lateral Chest Position

Chest
Basic
• AP/PA
• **Lateral**

Diagnostic Indications

Same as for AP/PA chest.

Technical Factors

- Film size–determined by the size of patient.
- Film lengthwise under patient (unless horizontal beam is taken on Tam-em Board).
- Grid not required.
- 75-80 kVp, shortest exposure time possible.

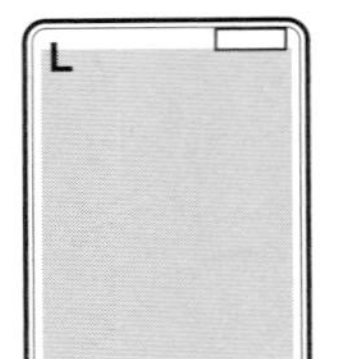

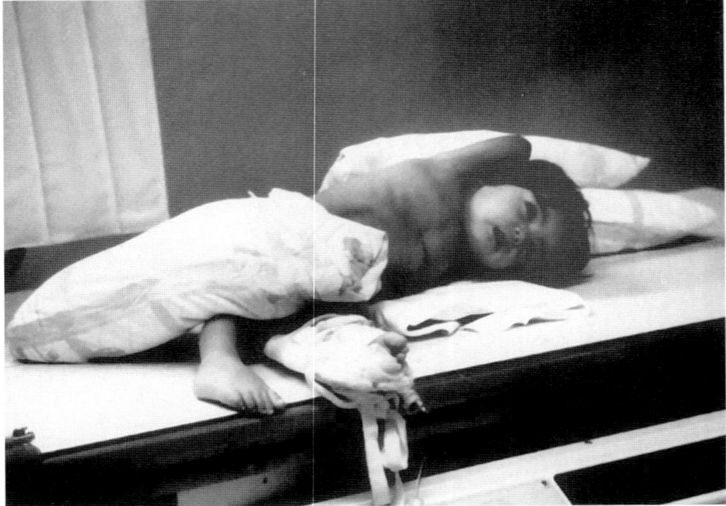

Fig. 20-32. Recumbent lateral chest (with immobilization aids).

Shielding: Contact lead shielding should be placed directly over pelvic area with upper margin at the top of the iliac crest.

Patient Position

- Patient lying on side in true lateral (generally left lateral) position with arms extended above head to remove arms from lung field. Bend arms at the elbows for patient comfort and stability with head placed between arms.
- Place one sandbag across arm that is closest to the film.
- Place a second sandbag over the top of the upside humerus .
- Place a third sandbag between the legs at the level of the knee while bending the legs forward.
- A fourth sandbag is placed across the top of the hips to further immobilize the patient.
- If using Tam-em Board, patient position does not change from the AP projection. Turn x-ray tube for horizontal beam projection and place vertical cassette against the lateral wall of the chest as shown (Fig. 20-33).
- If utilizing parent assistance:
  1. Place patient on cassette in left lateral position (unless right lateral is indicated).
  2. Bring arms above the head and hold with one hand. Place the other hand across patient's lateral hips to prevent child from rotating or twisting.
  3. Place parent in a position that will not obstruct technologist's view of patient while making exposure.
  4. Place lead gloves over the top of parent's hand if parent is not wearing the gloves.

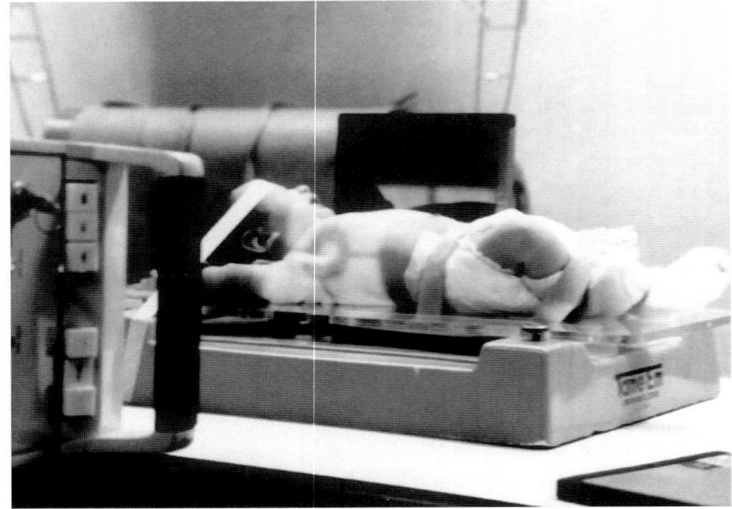

Fig. 20-33. Supine horizontal beam lateral chest (with Tam-em board).

Part Position

- Place the patient in the middle of the cassette with the shoulders about 2 in. (5 cm) below the top of cassette.
- No rotation, insure a true lateral position.

Central Ray

- CR **perpendicular** to the film **centered to the midcoronal plane** at the level of the mammillary (nipple) line.
- When using Tam-em Board, center the x-ray tube in horizontal beam lateral position to midcoronal plane of thorax at level of mammillary line.
- SID: 50 to 60 in. (127 to 212 cm).

Collimation: Closely collimate on four sides to outer chest margins.

Respiration: Make exposure upon 2nd full inspiration. If child is crying, watch respiration and make exposure when the child fully inhales.

Lateral Chest continued

ERECT LATERAL CHEST WITH PIGG-O-STAT

Can be used on infants and children up to approximately age 2 (age of this patient is 16 months). The larger size body clamps are being used on this patient and the seat is adjusted as low as it will go.

Patient Position

- Patient placed on seat and adjusted to correct height so top of film holder is about 1 inch (2.5 cm) above shoulders.
- Arms are raised and side body clamps placed firmly against patient and secured by base adjustment and by adjustable strap.
- Lead shield raised to a level about an inch above iliac crest.
- Correct R and L markers and inspiration marker are set to be exposed on film.
- Insure no rotation.

Procedure If Lateral Follows PA Projection:
If patient is already in position from the PA projection, then patient and swivel base are turned 90 degrees to lateral position. Lead shield remains in position and lead marker is changed to indicate correct lateral. Film cassette is placed in film holder mount.

Central Ray

- CR **perpendicular** to film at **level of mid thorax** (mammillary line).
- SID: 72 in. (180 cm).

Collimation: Collimate closely on four sides to outer chest margins.

Respiration: If child is crying, watch respiration and make exposure as child fully inhales and holds his breath.

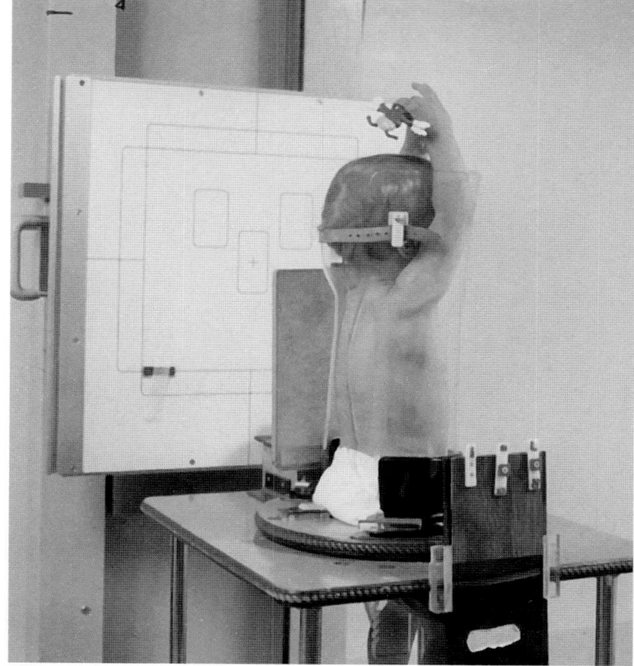

Fig. 20-34. Pigg-O-Stat–Left lateral.

Evaluation Criteria

- **No rotation**: ribs posterior to the vertebral column should be superimposed.
- Lungs must be fully expanded.
- Arms should be elevated and not superimpose apices of lungs.
- All of lung fields should be included with collimation margins appearing on all four sides of the film. The center of the field should be at the level of the lower margin of the scapula.
- **No motion**: Lung markings and other structural outlines should appear sharp and not blurred.
- Correct exposure and penetration should visualize rib margins and lung markings through the heart shadow without overexposing other regions of the lungs.
- Patient ID and right or left marker are placed correctly.

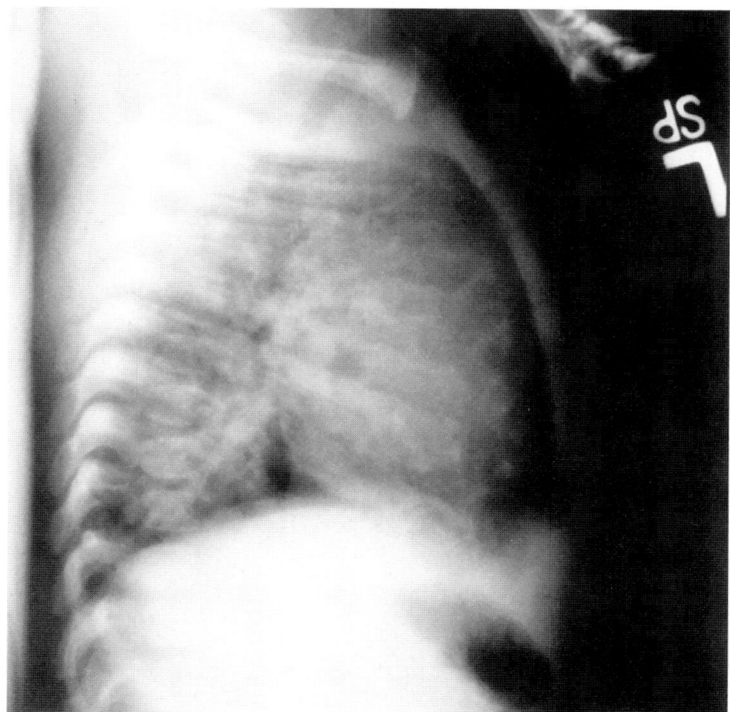

Fig. 20-35. Lateral chest (motion is evident on this radiograph, requires a repeat).

20

AP and Lateral Upper Limbs

Note: Department routines and protocols should be followed as to specific positioning routines for the upper limbs at various ages and for specific diagnostic indicators. The entire upper limb may be included on infants and very young children as shown in Fig. 20-36. For older children with more bone growth in the joint regions (except for general survey exams), individual joints such as the elbow or wrist are radiographed separately with the CR centered to the joint of interest. For older children, if the area of interest is the hand, generally a PA oblique and lateral hand should be taken, as for an adult.

Upper limbs
Basic
- **AP**
- **Lateral**

Diagnostic Indications

Arthritis
Avascular necrosis
Bone dysplasia
Bone age
Bowing
Congenital anomaly
Inflammation
Infection
JRA (juvenile rheumatoid arthritis)
Neoplasm
Non-accidental trauma
Osteodystrophy
Osteoporosis
Rickets
Short limbs
Trauma

Technical Factors

- Film size is determined by the size of patient.
- Grid is not used for any body part under 9 cm.
- Use extremity/detail screen if available.
- 55-65 kVp, shortest exposure time possible.

Shielding: Secure or place lead shield over entire pelvic area.

Patient Position

- Place patient in the supine position.
- Immobilize patient body part not to be radiographed either on the Tam-em Board or with sandbags before the part to be radiographed is positioned.
- When radiographing a long bone, place cassette under the limb to be radiographed including both proximal and distal joints.
- When radiographing a joint, place the cassette under the joint to be radiographed including a minimum of 1 to 2 in. (2.5-5 cm) of proximal and distal long bones.

Part To Be Positioned

- Align the part to be radiographed to the long axis of the film; or cross-cornered if necessary to include entire upper limb and both joints.

AP:
- Supinate the hand and forearm into the AP position (with hand and fingers extended).

Lateral:
- If patient is in the supine position, abduct the arm and turn the forearm and wrist into a lateral position.

Immobilization: Immobilize the hand, forearm, and humerus with either masking tape or compression band; or have parent immobilize wearing lead gloves.

Central Ray

- CR perpendicular to the film directed to the mid point of the part to be radiographed.
- Minimum 40 in. (102 cm) SID.

Collimation: Collimate closely on four sides to area of interest.

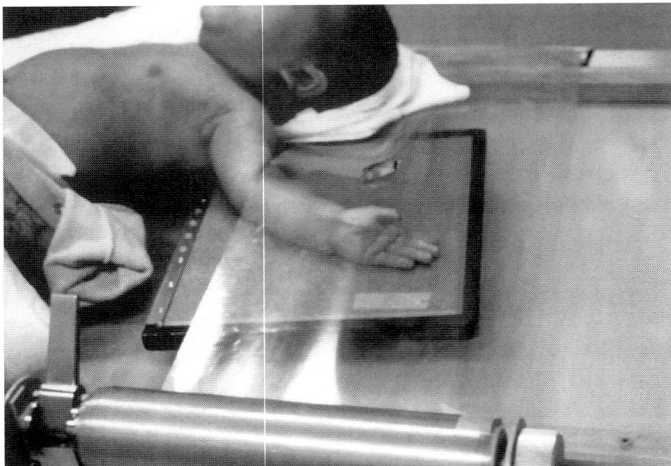

Fig. 20-36. AP upper limb (secured with retention board).

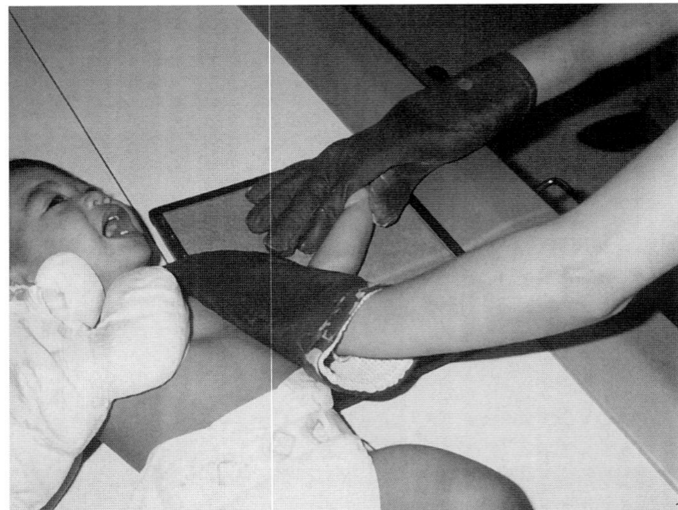

Fig. 20-37. Lateral forearm (parent immobilizing).

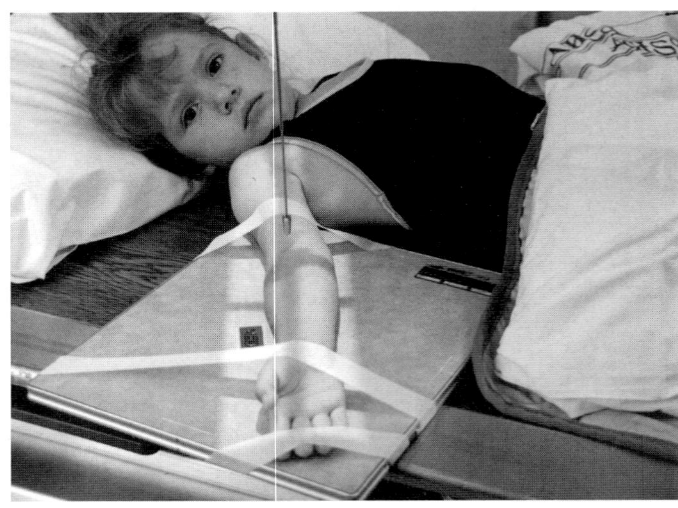

Fig. 20-38. AP forearm–four-year-old (secured with tape).

Upper Limbs continued

Evaluation Criteria

- **No motion**: Trabecular markings and bone margins should appear clear and sharp.
- Collimation borders should be evident on each side of upper limb without cutting off essential anatomy.
- Patient ID including date, should appear clear and legible, with correctly placed Right or Left markers without superimposing any body part pertinent to the diagnosis.

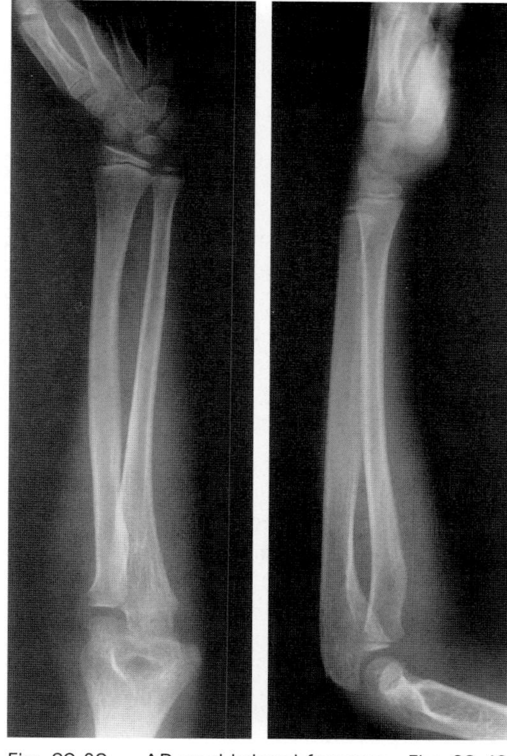

Fig. 20-39. AP and lateral forearm –Seven-year-old. Fig. 20-40.

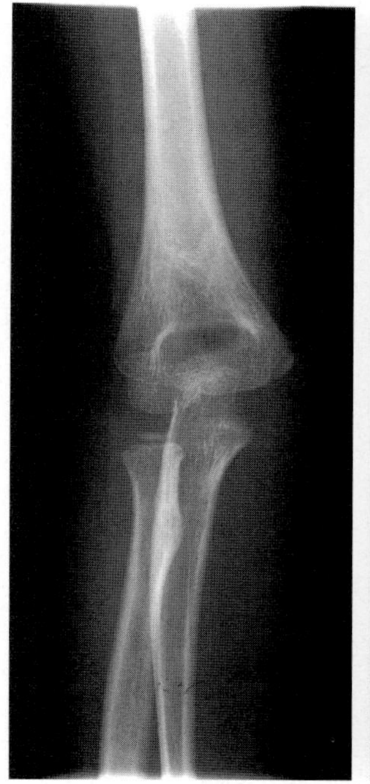

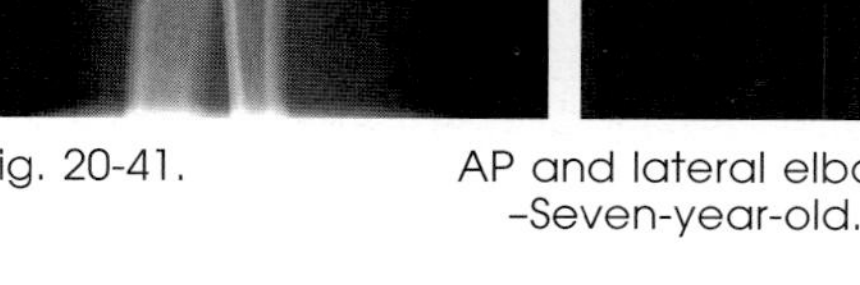

Fig. 20-41. AP and lateral elbow –Seven-year-old. Fig. 20-42.

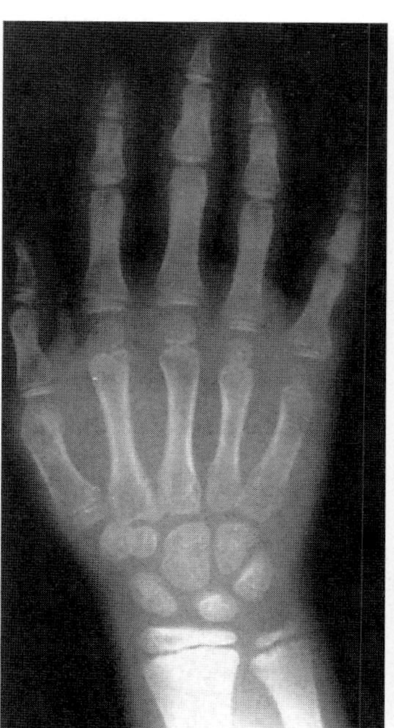

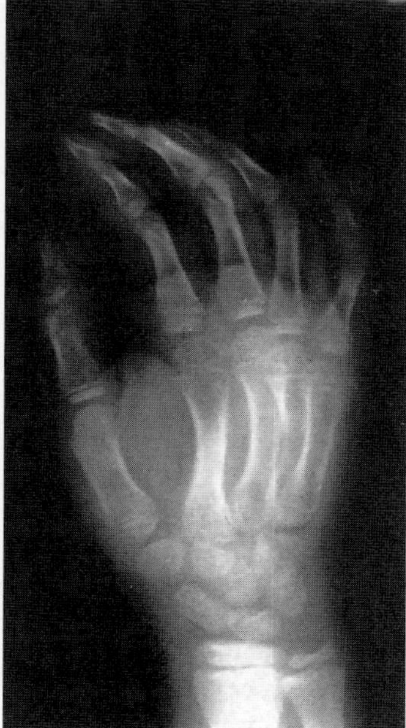

Fig. 20-43. PA and oblique hand –Nine-year-old. Fig. 20-44.

Note: A positioning angle sponge was not used with oblique hand on right; therefore, digits are not parallel to film, resulting in obscured interphalangeal joints.

AP and Lateral Lower Limbs

Note: For young infants, department routines may include entire lower limb as shown in Figs. 20-45 and 20-46. Also, for infants or young children, bilateral exams may be requested on one film for a bone survey or for comparison purposes (Figs. 20-47 and 20-48).

Lower limbs
Basic
- **AP**
- **Lateral**

Technical Factors:

- Film size is determined by the size of body part to be radiographed, film crosswise.
- Grid not necessary for infants and small children
- 60-65 kVp, shortest exposure time possible.

Shielding: Male or female gonadal shields correctly placed to not obscure hips and proximal femora.

Patient Position and Central Ray

AP and Lateral:

- Patient supine with cassette under patient centered to affected limb, or placed diagonally for bilateral limbs if needed to include entire limbs from hips to feet.
- Immobilize with tape and/or compression band, or have parent hold leg in position with one hand on the pelvis above the hip region and one hand holding the foot (wearing lead gloves and apron, Figs. 20-45 and 20-46).
- For lateral rotate leg externally and immobilize with tape or have parent hold as for AP projection.
- For bilateral limbs abduct both limbs into "frog-leg" position. Immobilize with tape or compression band across knees and/or ankles.
- CR perpendicular to mid area of limbs.

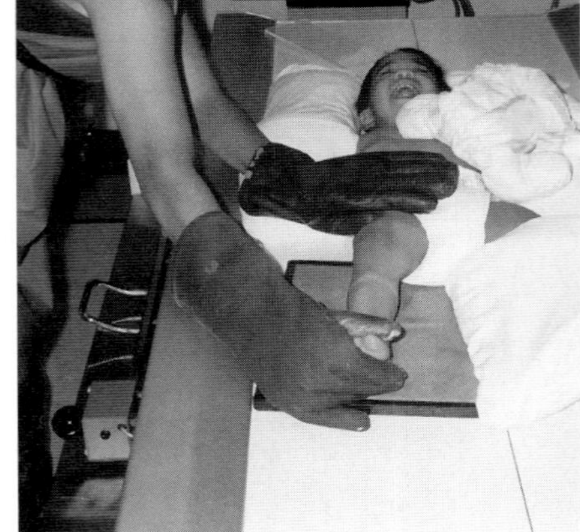
Fig. 20-45. AP leg.

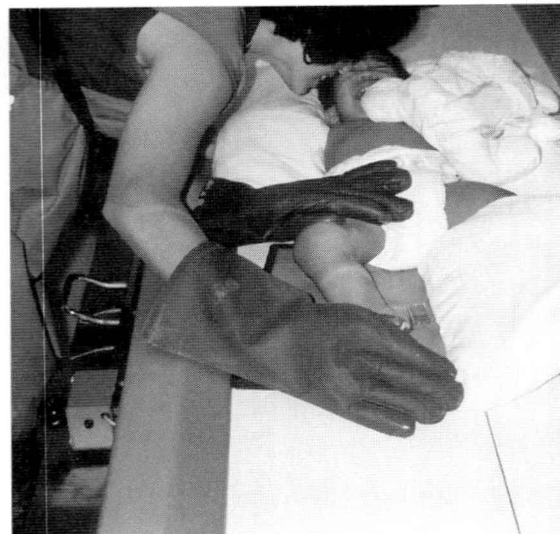
Fig. 20-46. Lateral leg.

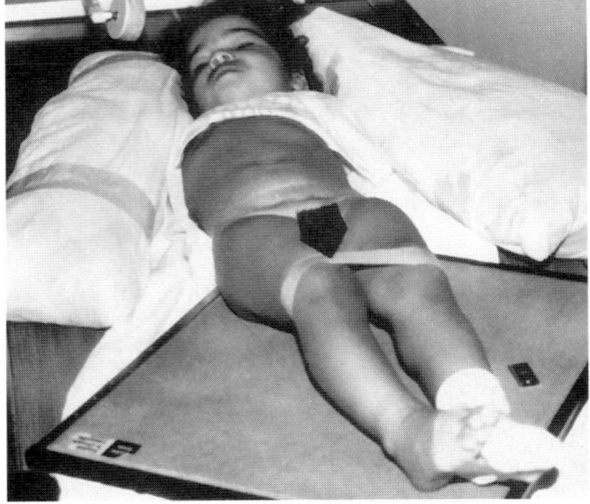
Fig. 20-47. AP (bilateral) lower limbs.

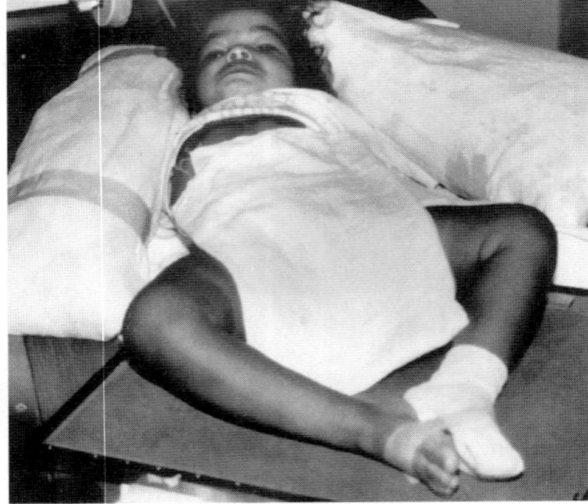
Fig. 20-48. Lateral (bilateral) lower limbs –"frog-leg."

Evaluation Criteria

- **No motion**: Trabecular markings and bone margins should appear clear and sharp.
- Patient ID information including date should be clear and legible with Right or Left markers not superimposing essential anatomy.

AP:

- Lateral and medial epicondyles of distal femur should appear symmetrical and in profile.
- Tibia and fibula should appear alongside each other with minimal overlap.

Lateral:

- Medial and lateral condyles and epicondyles of distal femur should be superimposed.
- Tibia and fibula should appear mostly superimposed.

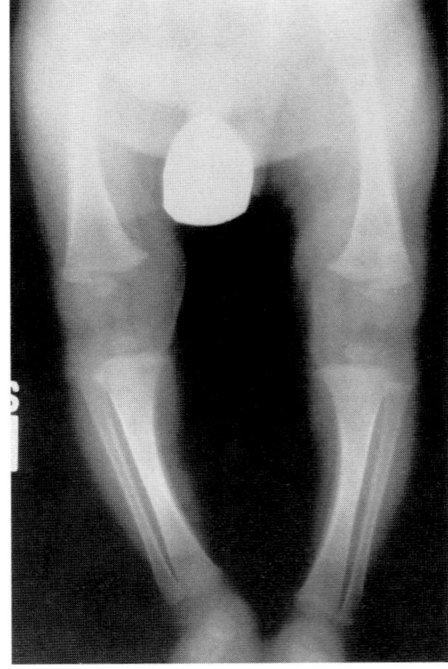
Fig. 20-49. AP (bilateral) lower limbs.

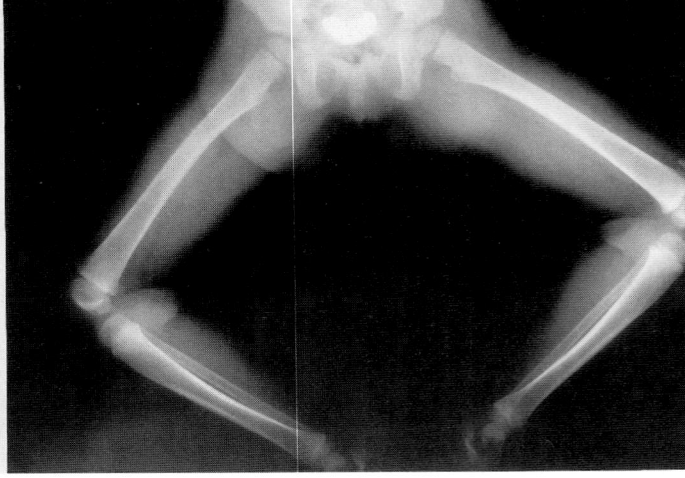
Fig. 20-50. Lateral (bilateral) "frog-leg" for lower limbs.

AP and Lateral Leg
AP and Lateral Foot–Kite Method

Leg
Basic
- **AP**
- **Lateral**

Foot
Basic
- **AP**
- **Lateral**

Note: Department routines and protocols should be followed as to specific positioning routines for the lower limbs at various ages and for specific diagnostic indicators. If the specific area of interest is to the **knee**, **ankle or foot region**, separate films should be obtained with the CR centered to the joint of interest (Figs. 20-53 and 20-54).

Diagnostic Indications

Arthritis
Avascular necrosis
Blount disease
CHD (congenital hip dislocation)
Club foot
Congenital anomaly
Foreign body
Fracture
Infection
Leg perthes
Neoplasm
Osteomyelitis
Pes cavas
Pes planus
Post reduction
Physiologic bowing
Septic arthritis
Slipped epiphysis
Swelling
Trauma

Technical Factors

- Film size is determined by the size of the body part to be radiographed.
- Grid not necessary for infants and small children.
- 55-65 kVp, shortest exposure time possible.

Shielding: Place lead gonad shield across pelvis, or specific gonadal shields for male and female, if proximal femurs are to be included.

Patient Position and Central Ray

AP Leg:

- With patient supine, immobilize arms and the leg not being radiographed if needed.
- Place cassette under limb being radiographed, include knee and ankle joints.
- Place leg as for a true AP projection rotating knee internally slightly until the interepicondylar line is parallel to plane of film. The feet and ankles should be in a true anatomical position.
- Immobilize the leg as needed in this position with sandbags, tape or compression band.
- If parent is being utilized for immobilization, have the parent hold the leg in this position with one hand firmly on the pelvis and the other holding the feet.
- CR perpendicular to mid leg.
- Minimum 40 in. (102 cm) SID.

Lateral Leg:

- Rotate patient toward affected side with leg in a frog lateral position, bending knee at an approximate 45 degree angle.
- Immobilize body parts not being radiographed.
- If parent is being utilized for immobilization, have parent hold the feet and hips in position.
- CR perpendicular to mid leg.
- Immobilize leg with sandbags, tape or compression band.

Collimation: Collimate closely on four sides to area of leg, including knee and ankle.

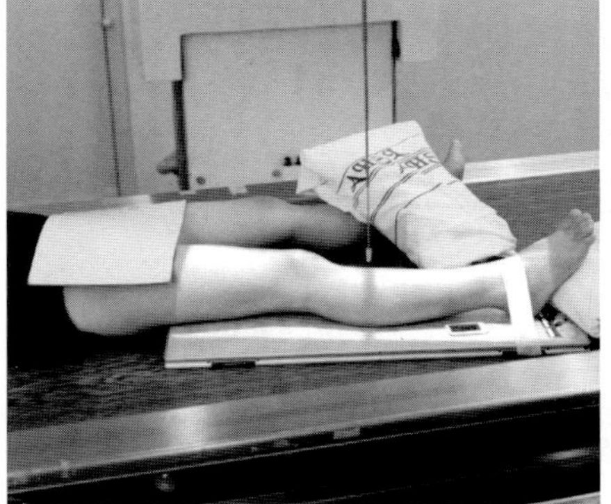

Fig. 20-51. AP leg.

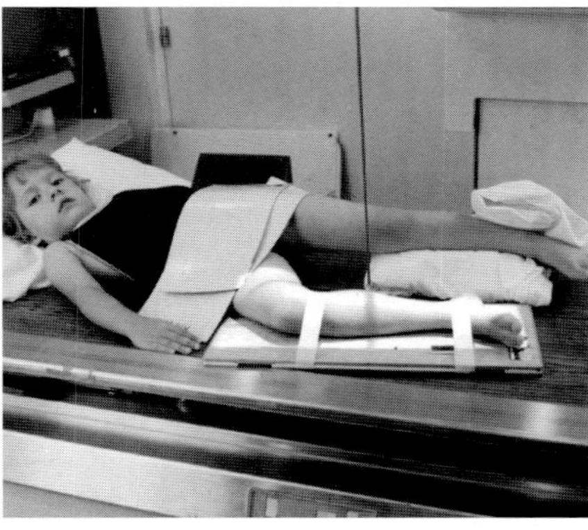

Fig. 20-52. Lateral leg.

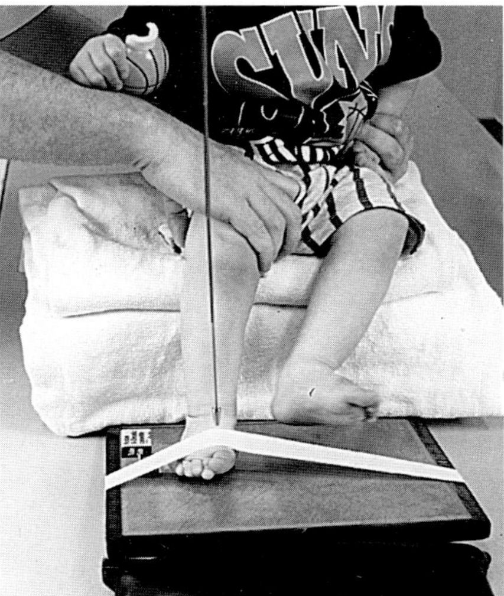

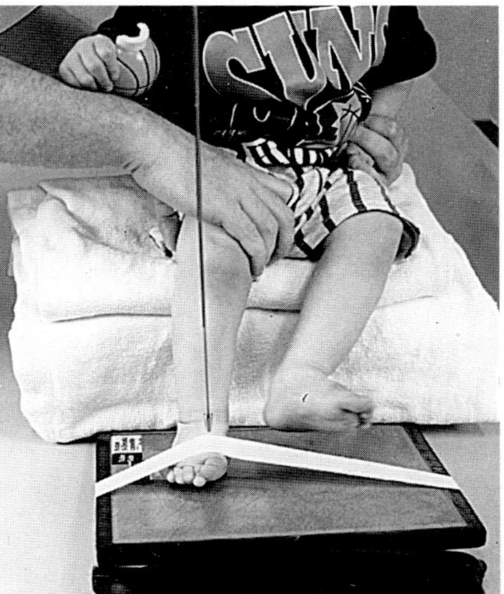

Fig. 20-53. AP foot.

Fig. 20-54. Lateral foot.

(Same patient as Fig. 20-55 below, but one year later after corrective treatment had been completed.)

AP and Lateral Foot

AP Foot:

- Seat child on elevated support with knee flexed and foot placed on cassette. Use tape to immobilize.
- Direct CR perpendicular to mid foot.

Lateral Foot:

- With patient lying or seated on table, rotate leg externally to place foot into lateral position. Use tape to immobilize.
- CR perpendicular to mid foot.

Collimation: Collimate closely on four sides to area of foot.

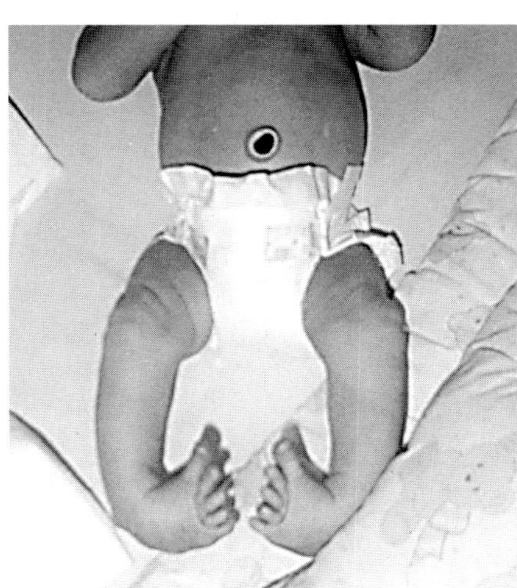

Fig. 20-55. Newborn–Clubfeet (before corrective treatment).

Congenital Clubfoot–Kite method:

The foot is positioned for AP and lateral positions as demonstrated above with **no attempt to straighten foot when placing on cassette**. Due to shape distortion (Fig. 20-55), it may be difficult to obtain a true AP and lateral but two projections 90° from each other should be obtained. Both feet are generally taken separately for comparison purposes.

AP and Lateral Pelvis and Hips

Warning: Do not attempt bilateral frog-leg hips on trauma patients until fractures have been ruled out from the AP pelvis projection.

Pelvis and hips
Basic
- **AP**
- **Lateral (bilateral frog-leg)**

Diagnostic Indications

Arthritis	Neoplasm
Avascular necrosis	Osteomyelitis
Blount disease	Pes cavas
CHD (congenital hip dislocation)	Pes planus
Congenital anomaly	Post reduction
Foreign body	Physiologic bowing
Fracture	Septic arthritis
Infection	Slipped epiphysis
Leg perthes	Swelling
	Trauma

Technical Factors

- Film size is determined by the size of body part to be radiographed, film crosswise.
- Use table Bucky or portable grid if more than 9 cm.
- 60-65 kVp, shortest exposure time possible.

Shielding

- Before radiographing the patient discuss the examination with the radiologist. Patient's history may require that a gonad shield not be used if it obscures an area of interest.
- **Female**: Carefully shield the gonadal area. Place the female pediatric shield under the umbilicus and above the pubis. This will avoid covering the hip joints.
- **Male**: Carefully place the upper border of the male pediatric shield at the level of the symphysis pubis.

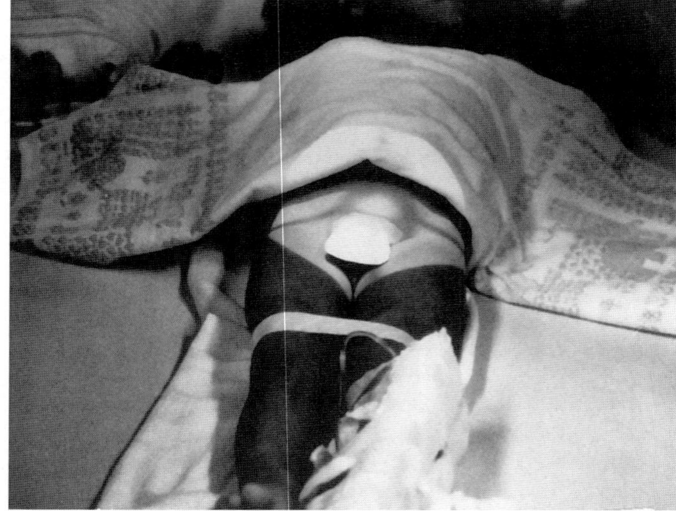

Fig. 20-56. AP pelvis (male gonadal shield taped in place).

Patient and Part Position

- Align patient to center of table and/or film holder.
- Immobilize patient so that pelvis is not rotated.
- Immobilize arms with sand bags or Tam-em Board.

AP:

With patient in supine position, position hips for the AP projection by rotating knees and feet internally so that the anterior feet cross each other.

- Immobilize lower limbs in this position with tape and sandbags.

Lateral:

- Abduct the legs by placing the soles of the feet together, knees bent and abducted. Tape soles of feet together, if needed.
- Keep the knees in the lateral position by securing tape to one side of the table crossing over both knees to the other side of the table. This can also be accomplished by using a compression band.

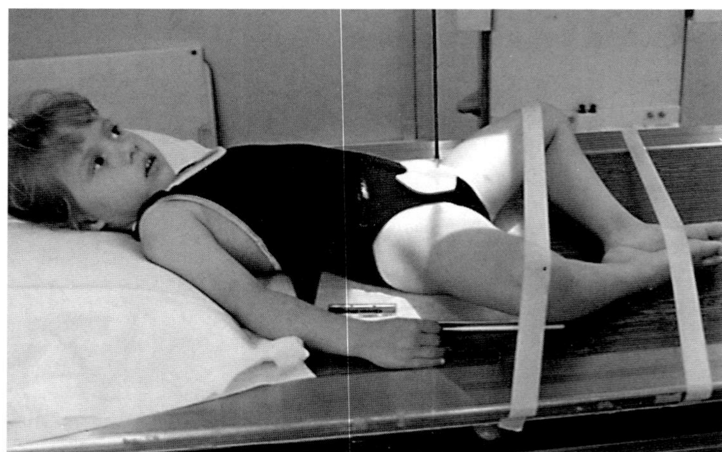

Fig. 20-57. Lateral hips and proximal femora-bilateral frog-leg. (female gonadal shield in place).

Central Ray

- CR perpendicular to film, centered at the level of the hips.
- Minimum 40 in. (102 cm) SID.

Collimation: Collimate closely on four sides to area of interest.

Respiration

- Infants and small children: Watch breathing pattern. When the abdomen is still, make the exposure.
- If the patient is crying, watch for the abdomen to be in full extension.

Pelvis and Hips continued

Evaluation Criteria

- **No rotation**: Both iliac crests should be equal in size and shape.
- Femoral heads should be perpendicular to the acetabula.
- **No motion**: Trabecular markings and margins of bones should appear clear and sharp.
- Correctly placed gonadal shielding should be evident on both male and female, without obscuring the hip joints (unless contraindicated by radiologist).
- Patient ID information including date should be clear and legible with correctly placed Right or Left marker not superimposing essential anatomy.

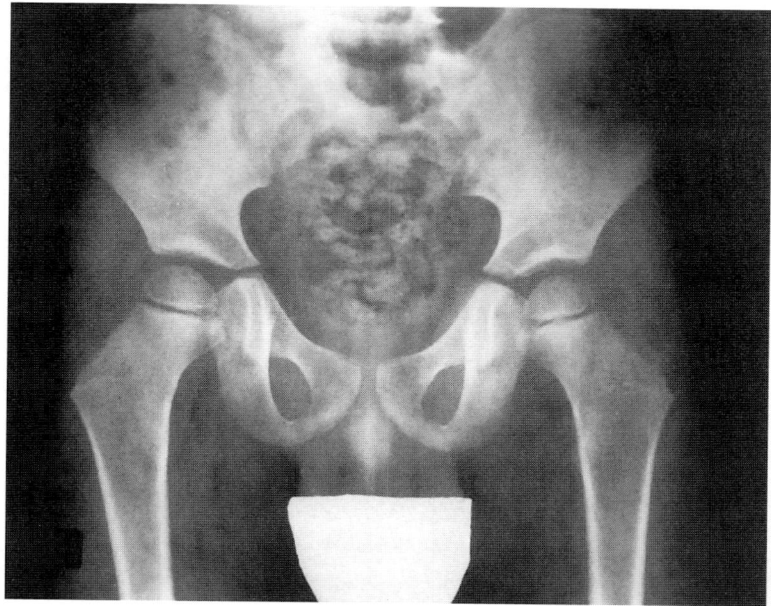

Fig. 20-58. AP hips and proximal femora (male). (Shielding error–Shield should have been placed higher, top of shield at lower margin of symphysis pubis unless pubic bones were in area of interest.)

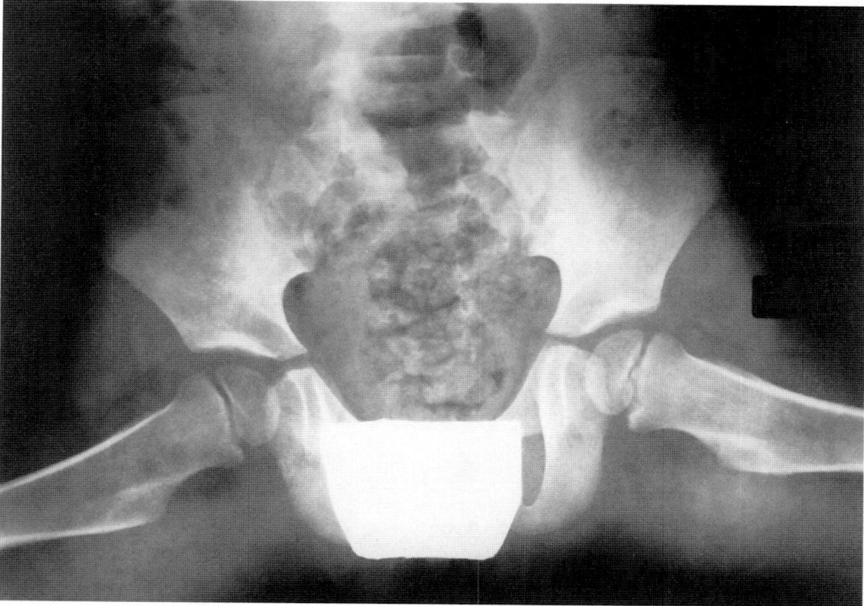

Fig. 20-59. Lateral hips and proximal femora (male). (Shield is placed too high on this radiograph, covers up symphysis area and doesn't extend low enough to cover all of genitals.)

AP, AP Reverse Caldwell and AP Towne Skull Projections

Skull (head)
Basic
• **AP**
AP Caldwell
AP Towne
• Lateral

Diagnostic Indications

Abnormal sella	Shunt check
Congenital anomalies	*Stridor
*Croup	Sinusitis
*Epiglottitis	Sidereal synosto
Headaches	Reconstruction
Hearing loss	*Retropharyngeal
Hydrocephalus	Abscess
Mastoiditis	Trauma
Post-Op	Tumor

*May require soft-tissue cervical spine procedure

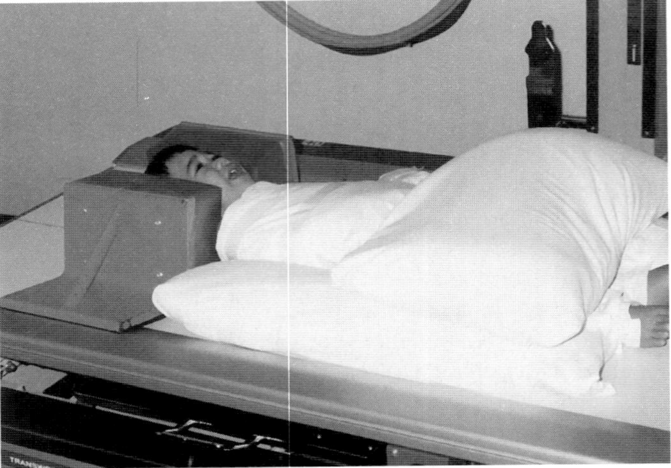

Fig. 20-60. Patient mummified, sandbags and head supports in use.

Technical Factors

- Film size–Infants and small children: 8 x 10 in. (18 x 24 cm), lengthwise. –Children and young adolescents: 10 x 12 in (24 x 30 cm), lengthwise.
- Use table Bucky, or portable grid if more than 9 cm.
- 65-70 kVp, shortest exposure time possible.

Shielding: Secure or place lead shield over entire pelvic area.

Patient Position

- Mummify patient's body and limbs if needed (may be necessary for infants and for some small children).
- Patient supine, aligned to midline of table.
- If needed, place sandbags over patient's legs and on each side of mummified body. Compression band can also be used if needed.

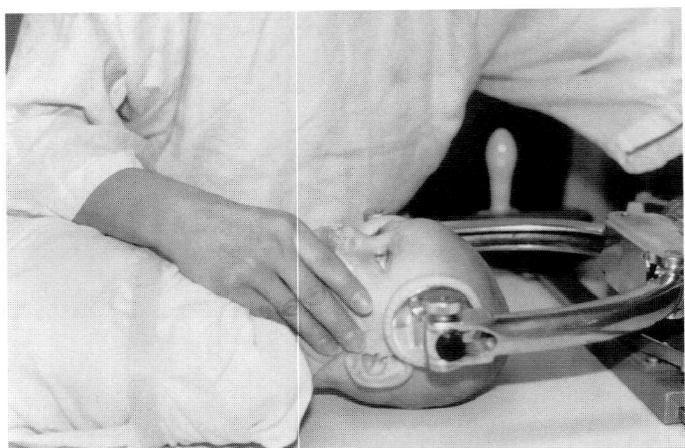

Fig. 20-61. Patient mummified, head clamps in use.

Part Position

- Position head with **no rotation.**
- Adjust chin so **orbitomeatal line (OML) is perpendicular to film.**
- Immobilize head with head clamps or head supports as demonstrated.
- Tape may also be used if necessary but turn adhesive side out over patient area so as not to adhere to skin.

Central Ray

- CR **centered to glabella.**
  - –AP skull: **CR parallel to OML.**
  - –AP reverse Caldwell: **CR 15° cephalad to OML.**
  - –AP Towne: **CR 30° caudad to OML.**
- Center cassette to CR.
- Minimum 40 in. (102 cm) SID.

Collimation: Collimate closely on four sides to outer margins of skull.

Note: Generally holding by parent is **not** needed for exams of the head if immobilization devices are used.

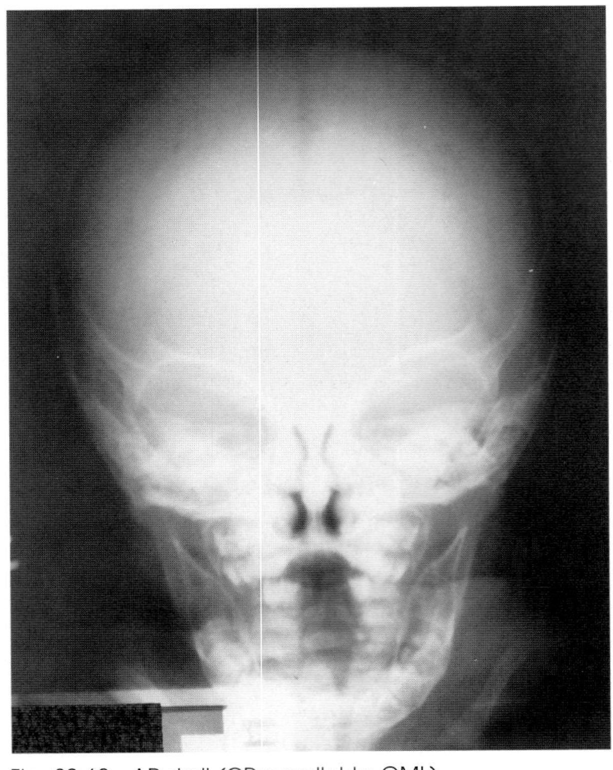

Fig. 20-62. AP skull (CR parallel to OML).

Evaluation Criteria

- **No motion**, as evidenced by sharp margins of bony structures.
- **No rotation**, as evidenced by symmetrical orbits at equal distances from outer skull margins.
- Sufficient penetration and exposure should be evident to visualize the frontal bone and the petrous pyramids and dorsum sellae on the 30° axial.
  AP 0°: Petrous ridges superimpose superior orbital margins.
  AP with 15° Cephalad Angle: Petrous pyramids and internal auditory canals are projected into lower one-half to one-third of orbits.
  AP with 30° Cephalad Angle: Petrous pyramids are projected below the inferior orbital rim, allowing visualization of the entire orbital margin.
- Dorsum sella and posterior clinoids are projected into foramen magnum.

Lateral Skull Position

Skull (head)
Basic
• AP
AP Caldwell
AP Towne
• **Lateral**

Diagnostic Indications

Same as AP projection on preceding page.

Technical Factors

10 (12)
8 (10)
R

- Film size–Infants and small children: 8 x 10 in. (18 x 24 cm) crosswise.
  –Children and young adolescents: 10 x 12 in. (24 x 30 cm) crosswise.
- Use table Bucky or portable grid if more than 9 cm.
- A screen can generally be used with a small infant.
- 65-70 kVp, shortest exposure time possible.

Shielding: Secure or place lead shield over pelvic area.

Patient Position

- Mummify patient's body and limbs (may be necessary for infants and for some small children).
- Patient in semiprone position, centered to midline of table. Place sandbags along patient's back and under elevated side of body.
- If necessary, place sandbag across buttocks and legs (Fig. 20-63). A compression band can be used across sandbags if needed.

Part Position

- Rotate head into true lateral position and maintain by placing a sponge or folded towel under mandible.
- Place weighted support or sponge and sandbag behind head to prevent from pushing their head backward.
- Use compression band across head, or use tape by securing tape to each side of table and crossing patient's head with adhesive side up to prevent adhering to skin. Sandbags can also be placed over tape to prevent patient from lifting head from tabletop.

Central Ray

- CR **perpendicular** to film, centered **midway between glabella and occipital protuberance or inion**.
- Center cassette to CR.
- Minimum 40 in. (102 cm) SID.

Collimation: Collimate closely on four sides to outer margins of skull.

Note: For infants, the Tam-em Board can be used for skull exams with the lateral taken with horizontal beam, as shown in Fig. 20-64. A small focal spot should be used due to the increased OID.

Evaluation Criteria

- **No motion**, as evidenced by sharp margins of bony structures.
- **No rotation**, as evidenced by superimposed rami of mandible, orbital roofs and greater and lesser wings of sphenoid.
- Sella turcica and clivus are demonstrated in profile without rotation.
- Sufficient penetration and exposure should visualize parietal region and the lateral view outline of the sella turcica without overexposing perimeter margins of skull.

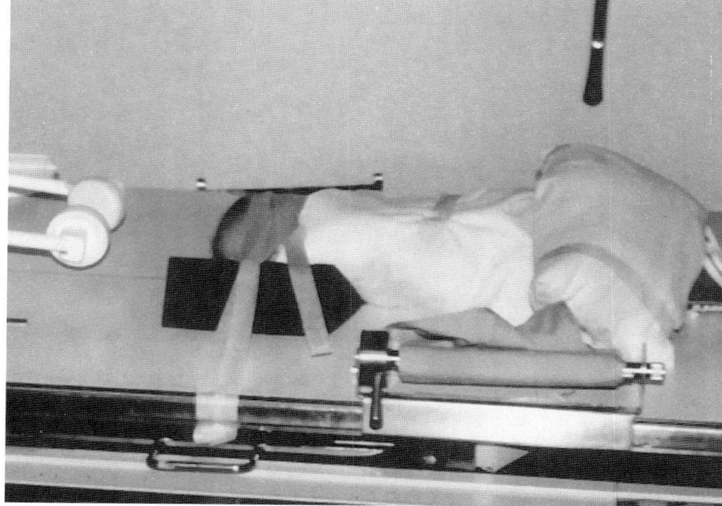

Fig. 20-63. Lateral skull.

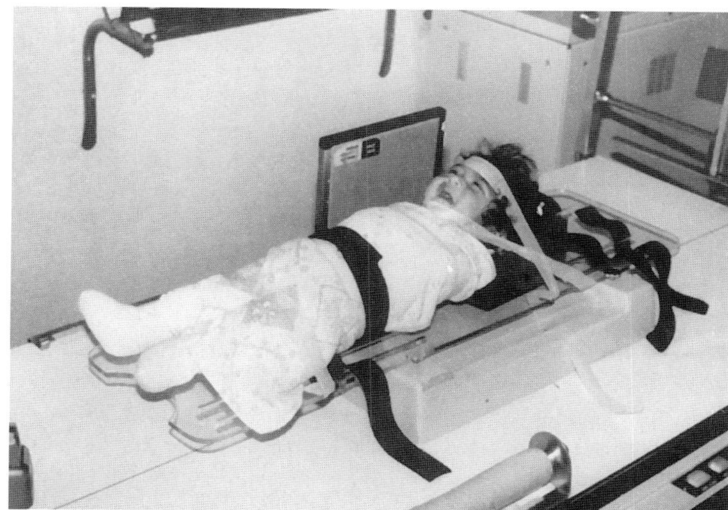

Fig. 20-64. Horizontal beam lateral with Tam-em board.

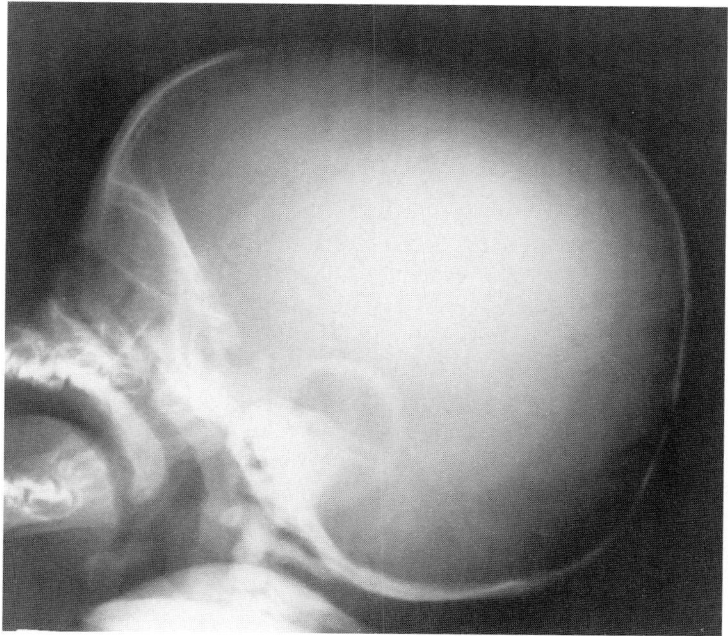

Fig. 20-65. Lateral skull.

20

The Pediatric Abdomen

with Cecilie Godderidge, BS, RT(R)

Differences Between Children and Adults

The difference between children and adults is not only in size but in the many developmental changes that take place from birth to puberty. The chest and abdomen are almost equal in circumference in the newborn. The pelvis is small and more cartilage than bone. The abdomen is more prominent and the abdominal organs are higher in infants than in older children. Accurate centering may be difficult for technologists more used to radiographing adults, utilizing the iliac crest and the anterior superior iliac spine as positioning landmarks, that for all practical purposes, are nonexistent in a young child. As a child grows, bone and musculature develop, the body outline and characteristics become distinctive and familiar landmarks are more easily located.

It is difficult to distinguish on a radiograph between small and large bowel in infants and toddlers, as the haustra of the large bowel are not as apparent as in older children and adults. There is also little intrinsic body fat so that an outline of the kidneys, for example, is not as well seen as in adults. Even so, visualization of the soft tissues is very important in children and a good plain radiograph of the abdomen provides valuable diagnostic information. Radiologists commonly say that the gas in the gastrointestinal tract may be the best contrast medium in evaluating the pediatric abdomen.

Precise collimation is important and in children the diaphragm, symphysis pubis and the outer edges of the abdomen should all be included in a plain supine radiograph. Radiographs of young children tend to look "flat" and there is less contrast than seen in those of adults. This is to be expected as bones are less dense, there is less fat, muscles are undeveloped and the range of soft tissues is softer and less defined. Exposure factors must be chosen that ensure subtle changes in soft tissues are not "burned out" at too high a kilovoltage.

Patient Preparation for Contrast Media Procedure

Patient history is important when evaluating the pediatric patient as this assists the radiologist in deciding the order and type of radiographic procedures to be performed. When it is necessary to withhold feeding for an upper gastrointestinal study, the examination should be scheduled early in the morning. Children become irritable when hungry and a crying baby whose feeding schedule has been disrupted is not easily consoled. Unable to feed the child, the harassed parent will have had to deal with this scenario long before arriving at the hospital. Technologists need to be understanding of the difficulties in having a young child fast for a long period of time and they must be supportive of both parent and child before and during fluoroscopic examinations of the GI tract. Not only is it important for an infant's stomach to be empty to ensure a good diagnostic barium swallow or upper GI, but babies and infants, when hungry, are more likely to drink the barium.

Upper Gastrointestinal Tract (Upper GI)

Infants and young children require minimal preparation for upper GI studies. Length of fasting is determined by age and the older the child, the slower the gastric emptying. **Infants under 1 year** should be **NPO for 4 hours before the exam**. Babies can have an early morning feed at 6:00 A.M. and be scheduled for a barium swallow and UGI at 10:00 A.M. Children **over 1 year**, nothing to eat or drink **(NPO) from 12:00 midnight** for an early morning exam, and **NPO for 6 hours** if the appointment is late morning or in the afternoon.

Written instruction should be given to the parent and the reason for "absolutely nothing by mouth" explained and emphasized.

Lower Gastrointestinal System (Lower GI)

Patient history determines the preparation for a lower GI examination. This is usually a single contrast barium enema in children. Double contrast enemas are performed less frequently than in adults and are mainly used to diagnose polyps in children.

Contraindications: Patients with the following clinical symptoms or diagnosis should **not** be given laxatives or enemas: **Hirschsprung's disease**, **extensive diarrhea**, **appendicitis**, **obstruction** and **patients who cannot withstand fluid loss**. Instructions for all other patients are as follows:

Newborn to 2 Years: No preparation necessary.

Children 2 to 10 Years: Low residue meal the evening before the exam. One (1) bisacodyl tablet or similar laxative whole, with water, before bedtime the evening prior to the examination. If no bowel movement in the morning, a Pedi-Fleet enema may be given on the advice of a physician.

Children 10 Years to Adult: Low residue meal the evening before. Two (2) bisacodyl tablets or similar laxative whole, with water, before bedtime the evening prior to the examination. If no bowel movement in the morning, a Pedi-Fleet enema may be given on the advice of a physician.

Intravenous Urogram (IVU)

The preparation of children for an IVU is simple. No solid foods 4 hours prior to the examination to diminish the risk of aspiration from vomiting. The patient should be encouraged to drink plenty of clear liquids until one hour prior to the examination.

Summary

Patient Preparation

- Good patient history is important.
- Early morning scheduling if feeding is withheld
  –Problem with irritable child with long fasting.
- Empty stomach required for GI study
  (also if hungry more likely to drink barium).

Upper GI Preparation

Minimum prep required:

Infants to 1-year-olds:
- NPO 4 hours before exam.

One year and older:
- NPO after midnight for early A.M. exam, or
- NPO 6 hours before for late A.M. or P.M exam.

Lower GI Preparation

Patient history determines required prep:

(Certain clinical symptoms or diagnoses preclude any prep.)

Infants to 2-year-olds:
- No prep required.

Two to ten years:
- Low residue meal evening before.
- One bisacodyl tablet or similar laxative before bedtime evening before.
- If no bowel movement in morning, upon advice of physician give a Pedi-Fleet enema.

Ten years to adult:
- Low residue meal evening before.
- Two bisacodyl tablets or similar laxative evening before.
- If no bowel movement in morning, upon advice of physician give a Pedi-Fleet enema.

IVU Preparation

- No solid food 4 hours before exam.
  (to lessen risk of aspiration from vomiting)
- Encourage drinking of clear liquids until 1 hour before exam.

Preparations for GI tract courtesy of Children's Hospital, Boston, MA.

AP Projection (KUB)

Abdomen
Basic
- **AP (KUB)**

Optional
- AP erect
- Dorsal decub.

Diagnostic Indications

Appendicitis
Bleeding
Constipation
Diarrhea
Distention
Foreign body
Intussusception (a telescoping of one part of intestine into another)
Hepatomegaly (enlargement of liver)
Abdominal mass
NEC (necrotizing enterocolitis, inflammation of small bowel or colon resulting in cell death)

Technical Factors:

- Film size–Determined by the size of patient, film lengthwise.
- 400 speed screen/film combination.
- Moving or stationary grid, if more than 9 cm.
- 65-85 kVp NB to 18 years, shortest exposure time possible.

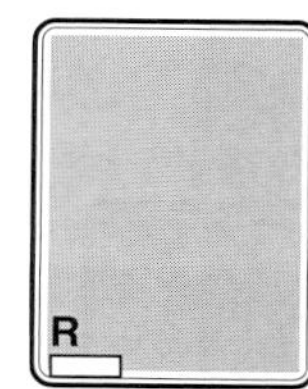

Shielding

- Gonadal shield on all males–Size appropriate for age (tape shield in place).
- No gonadal shielding on females.

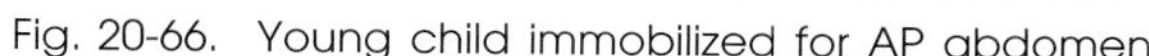

Fig. 20-66. Young child immobilized for AP abdomen.

Patient and Part Position

- Patient supine, aligned to midline of table and/or cassette.
- Immobilize with soft flexible sandbags and compression band.

Newborns and Young Infants:

- Position the arms away from the body and mold a large flexible sandbag over each arm. Since it is difficult to straighten the little, short legs of infants, place one sandbag under their knees and another over the top to immobilize their legs. Babies if they feel snug and warm are usually calm unless they are in pain. If a baby is crying a pacifier may help and will not interfere with the exam.

Infants and Toddlers:

- Restrain the arms the same as for younger infants. Place a sandbag under the knees and tighten a compression band over both femora and knees. Be sure to place padding under the band so it does not cut into the child's legs. Compression bands on most x-ray tables are designed for adults, so that this restraint works best if the spaces between the band and patient are padded with foam sponges or towels.
- If utilizing parental assistance:
  –Provide parent with lead apron and gloves.
  –Position tube and cassette and set exposure factors before positioning
  –Position parent so that technologist's view is not obstructed.
  –Usually it is only necessary to have a parent hold the child's arms. The legs can be satisfactorily immobilized as described above.

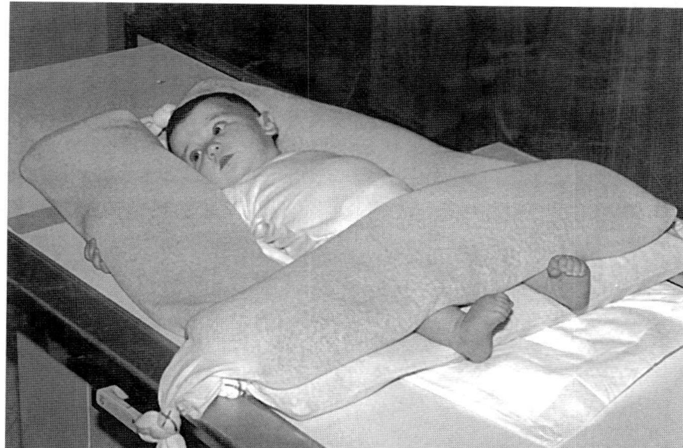

Fig. 20-67. Child immobilized with sandbags for AP abdomen. (Note sandbag under and over lower limbs.)

Central Ray

- Infants and small children: Center CR and cassette **1 inch (2.5 cm) above the umbilicus**.
- Older children and adolescents: Center CR at the **level of the iliac crest**.
- SID 40 in. (102 cm)

Respiration

- **Infants and children**: Watch the breathing pattern and when the abdomen is still, make the exposure. If the patient is crying make the exposure as the baby takes a breath in to let out a cry.
- Children over 5 years can usually hold their breath after a practice session.

Evaluation Criteria

- The vertebral column is aligned to the center of the radiograph.
- The diaphragm, symphysis pubis and lateral borders should be included.
- **No rotation**: Pelvis and hips should be symmetrical.
- **No motion**: Diaphragm and gas patterns should appear sharp.

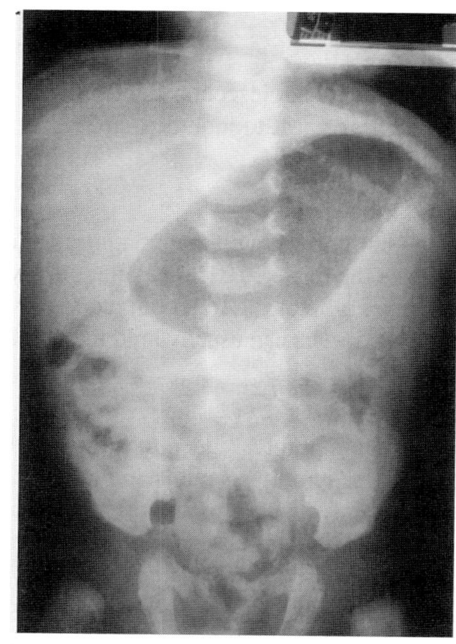

Fig. 20-68. AP abdomen, supine (demonstrates distended air-filled stomach).

Upper Gastrointestinal System (UGI) Study
Barium Swallow, UGI and Small Bowel Combination Study

Diagnostic Indications for GI Fluoroscopy

Congenital Anomalies:
Atresias (absence or closure of normal organ opening)
Pyloric stenosis
Malrotation
Intussusception
Hirschsprung's disease (congenital megacolon)
Imperforate anus

Diseases and Symptoms:
Abdominal pain
Bleeding
Constipation
Appendicitis
Inflammatory bowel disease
Meconium ileus
Tumor or mass

Patient Preparation

- **Infants under 1 year**: NPO for 4 hours.
- **Children over 1 year**: NPO for 6 hours, or nothing by mouth after midnight if exam is scheduled early A.M.

Room Preparation

The fluoroscopic procedure room should be prepared before the child is brought into the room. The table is placed in the horizontal position and the fluoroscopic controls set. A cotton or disposable sheet should be placed over the table. Depending on the exam, the appropriate barium or contrast medium, feeding bottle, nipple, straw, feeding catheter and syringe should be ready for use. Suction and oxygen should also be readily available in the event of an emergency.

Shielding: A piece of 1 mm lead vinyl is positioned to place under the child's buttocks to shield the gonads from scatter radiation from the "under table" fluoro tube.

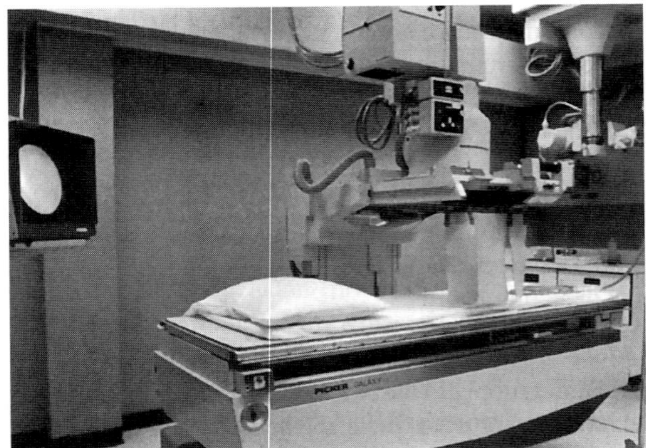

Fig. 20-74. Room setup for GI study.

Barium Preparation

Liquid barium may be used according to a particular manufacturer's instructions. The barium may be need to be diluted for younger children and infants. Dilution is usually necessary when using a feeding bottle and it is helpful to widen the hole in the nipple with a sterile needle or scalpel so that the baby can feed more easily.

The amount of barium given varies with the age of the child. The recommended amounts are as follows:*

- NB to 1 yr. – 2 to 4 oz.
- 1 to 3 yrs. – 4 to 6 oz.
- 3 to 10 yrs. – 6 to 12 oz.
- Over 10 yrs. – 12 to 16 oz.

Patient and Parent Preparation

Parents should accompany their child into the procedure room before the study is started. A few minutes spent explaining the exam and how the equipment works is of benefit to both parent and child. The large equipment and strange noises that a technologist is so used to, is terrifying to many young children. An explanation and demonstration of how the image intensifier is brought down over the chest and abdomen allays fears that the child might have of being crushed. Children can be shown how they can watch the "milk shake" going down into the stomach on the television monitor.

Barium procedures on children are usually performed with the patient lying down. Parents are given a lead apron and gloves so that they can sit at the head of the table with their child. Holding the child's hand and assisting the technologist in feeding the child reduces anxiety and helps in providing a supportive environment for both parent and child. Continual words of encouragement helps the barium go down.

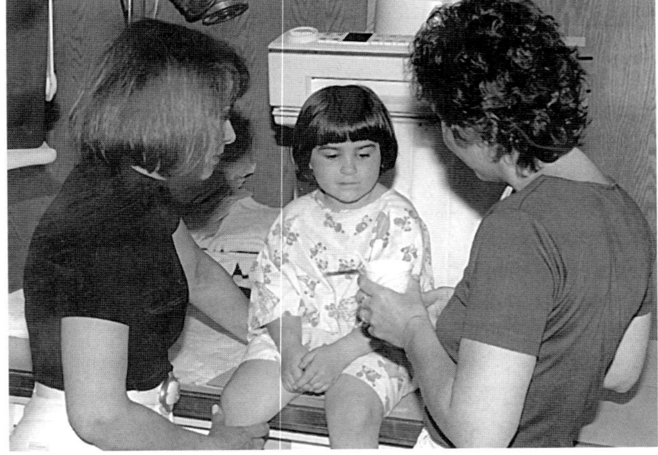

Fig. 20-75. Clear explanations to parent and child

*Courtesy of Department of Radiology, Children's Hospital, Boston, MA.

Upper GI Study continued

Procedure

Pre GI Exams:

- AP supine abdomen (KUB) before an UGI.
- PA and lateral chest before a barium swallow.

Drinking Barium: A baby or infant will drink from a feeding bottle. An older child will usually drink through a straw which prevents spillage.

In some cases a child may insist on drinking directly from a cup. This entails sitting the child up to drink and then lying down to be fluoroscoped. If the esophagus needs to be outlined, barium paste can be spooned onto the palate or tongue. Another tactic is to squirt barium into the child's mouth with a 10 ml syringe while gently holding the nose. If a child refuses to swallow the barium it may be necessary for the radiologist to pass a nasogastric tube into the stomach.

Fig. 20-76. "Drinking" barium.

Fluoro Positioning Sequence

Radiologists follow a particular sequence of positions for a UGI starting with the **patient supine**. This is generally followed by a **left lateral**, **LPO** and **RAO**, then a **right lateral** with the patient turned onto the right side; in this position the stomach empties quickly. It is important to check the location of the duodenojejunal junction to rule out malrotation before the jejunum fills. The final position is **prone**. This is a standard procedure even in patients whose symptoms are not necessarily of malrotation.

Permanent images are recorded during fluoroscopy on spot films of various types depending on the equipment. Young children generally do not require the usual overhead tube PA and RAO radiographs of the stomach following fluoroscopy that are standard for adults. If these projections are required, the radiologist should be asked to point out the level at which the film should be centered.

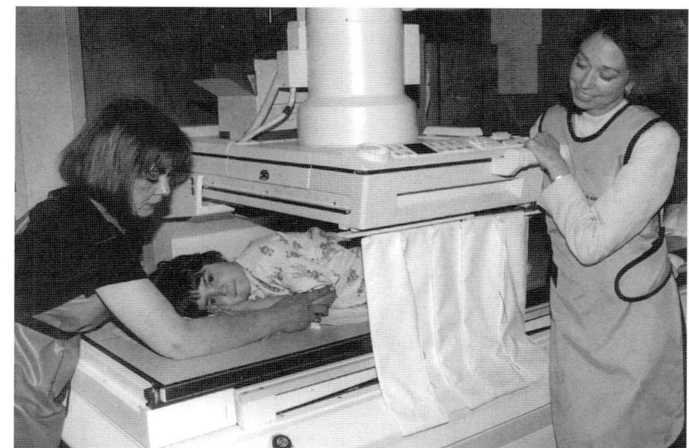

Fig. 20-77. Patient being positioned into RAO position in preparation for upper GI fluoro.

Small Bowel Follow-through

AP or PA abdomen are taken at **20 to 30-minute intervals**, either supine or prone, depending on the age and condition of the patient. Transit time is quite rapid in young children and the barium may reach the ileocecal region in **1 hour**.

Post Procedure Instructions

Once the examination is complete and the radiographs checked, the patient may eat and drink normally if diet permits. The child should be encouraged to drink plenty of water and fruit juices. The technologist should check that spot films and overheads are placed together in the patient's folder and appropriately labeled. Number of films and fluoroscopic time should be recorded on the requisition.

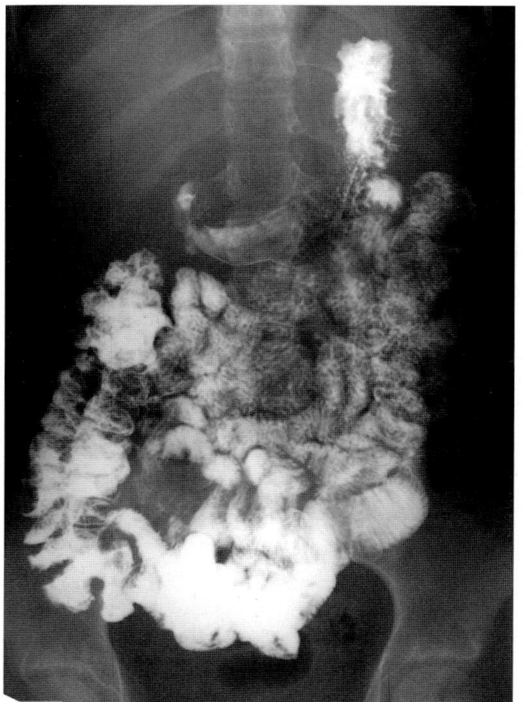

Fig. 20-78. Forty-five minute small bowel follow-through.

Lower Gastrointestinal System Study–Barium Enema

Single Contrast, Double Contrast and/or Air Enema

Patient Preparation

- **NB to 2 yrs**: No preparation necessary
- **2 yrs to 10 yrs**: Low-residue meal the evening before the exam. One bisacodyl tablet or similar laxative, whole with water before bedtime. If no bowel movement in the morning, a stimulant enema, such as a Pedi-Fleet enema, may be given on the advice of a physician.
- **10 yrs to adult**: Same as for 2 yrs to 10 yrs, except patient should take 2 bisacodyl tablets with water before bedtime.

Contrast and Materials–Barium Enema, Single Contrast

Children Over 1 Yr:

- Disposable enema bag with barium sulfate, tubing and clamp. Add tepid (not cold) water according to manufacturer's instructions.
- **Pediatric flexible enema tip**. Some of these catheters are designed so that they cannot be inserted beyond the rectum. Taping the tube in place will prevent leakage.
  Warning: Latex tips must **NOT** be used because of the potential of a life-threatening allergic response to latex. Inflatable balloon-type retention tips must also **NOT** be used as they may perforate the rectum.

Neonates and Infants:

- #10 French flexible silicone catheter and a 60 ml syringe. Barium should be injected manually and very slowly.

All Patients:

- Water-soluble lubricating jelly
- Hypoallergenic tape
- Gloves
- Washcloths and towels for clean-up

Contrast and Materials–Barium Enema, Double Contrast

- High density barium and air contrast enema kit or enema bag with double-line tip including tube through which air is introduced into the colon.
- Air insufflation device.
- Remainder of materials are the same as for a single contrast barium enema.

Air Enema

An air enema is performed under fluoroscopy for the pneumatic reduction of an intussusception. This condition occurs when one portion of the large bowel telescopes into an adjacent portion. The pneumatic reduction is most often performed as an emergency as the patient is in severe abdominal pain. It is a specialized procedure and must be done very carefully to avoid perforation of the bowel. When successful, the child's pain dissipates quickly and in many cases the reduction helps prevent an operative procedure. An intussusception may also be reduced by barium enema, depending on the preference of the radiologist.

Materials

- Air insufflation device.
- Aneroid air pressure gauge.
- Disposable tubing with three-way stopcock.
- Flexible enema tip.
- Hypoallergenic tape.
- Gloves.
- Washcloths and towels for clean-up.

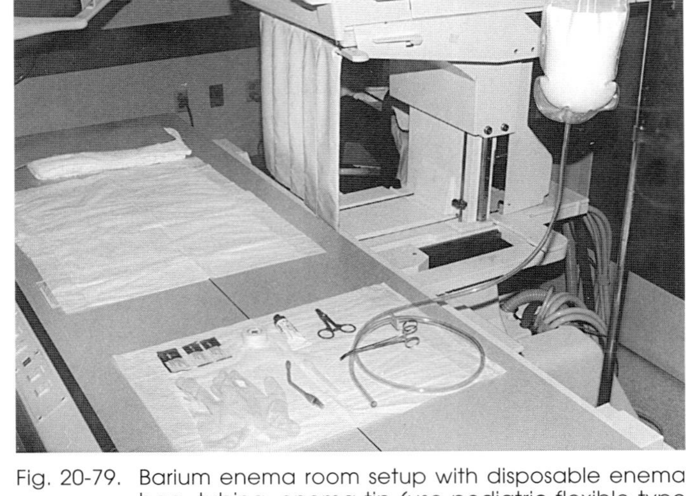

Fig. 20-79. Barium enema room setup with disposable enema bag, tubing, enema tip (use pediatric flexible type enema tip) and other supplies.

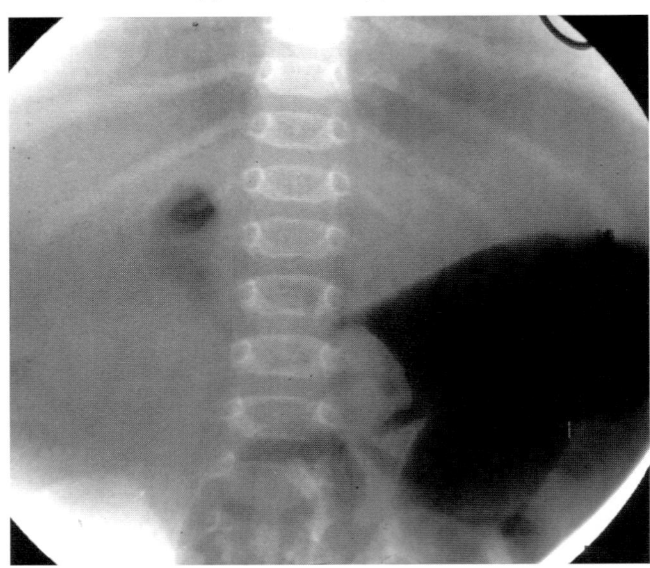

Fig. 20-80. Air enema demonstrating air in the transverse colon, the most common site of intussusception.*

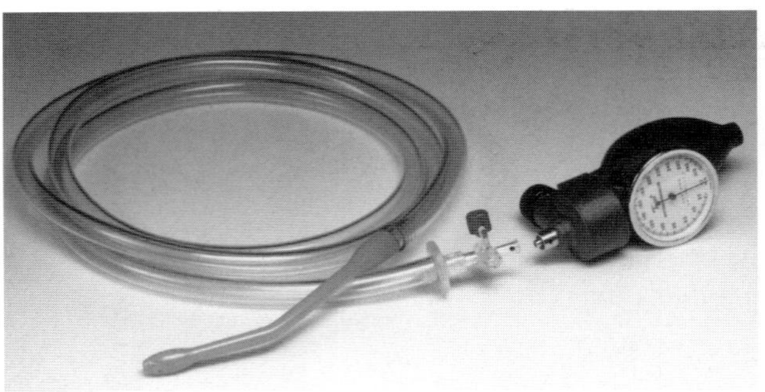

Fig. 20-81. Shiels™ Intussusception Air Reduction System.

Courtesy of Custom Medical Products, Maineville, Oh.

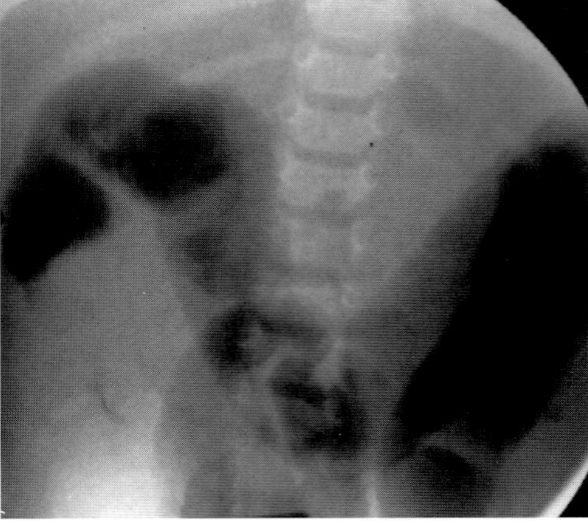

Fig. 20-82. Air enema spot film following the above showing the air having pushed out the telescoped bowel.*

*Reprinted with permission: Godderidge, C: *Pediatric Imaging*. Philadelphia, WB Saunders Company, 1995.

Room Preparation

The room should be prepared as for a UGI with the table horizontal, covered with a disposable or cotton sheet and the fluoroscopic controls set. The enema bag with barium, tubing, stand, clamp and tip should be assembled and ready for use. The barium is administered slowly, by gravity, from **3 feet** above the tabletop unless otherwise directed by the radiologist.

Shielding: The gonads cannot be shielded during a fluoroscopic examination of the large bowel.

Patient and Parent Preparation

The patient and the parent should be brought into the room and the procedure explained clearly and simply. It is particularly important to explain why the tube is being inserted into the rectum and how the barium enhances the bowel on the television screen. Appropriate technology and language should be used in the explanation depending on the age of the child. It is to be expected that a young child will be frightened by having someone touch their buttocks and genital area.

Technologists should be reassuring and supportive, and explain to parent and child that the exam does not hurt, though the child may feel as though he/she wants to go to the bathroom while the barium is passing into the bowel.

A parent should stay with their child throughout the exam. Talking and giving words of encouragement will help the exam go smoothly.

Procedure

Pre GI Exam:

- Preliminary supine AP (KUB) abdomen before beginning fluoroscopy procedure.

Fluoroscopy and Spot Filming:

- Spot films during fluoroscopy - film size depends on age of child and equipment.
- Supine or prone abdomen at completion of fluoroscopy.
- Right and left lateral decubitus films of the abdomen for double contrast.
- AP supine abdomen post-evacuation of barium.

Note: Unlike the follow-up films taken for adults, fewer radiographs, and sometimes none, are taken at the completion of fluoroscopy.

Post Reduction of Intussusception Following Air or Barium Enema:

- AP supine abdomen; to document that air or barium, depending on the contrast used, has passed through the ileocecal region into the ileum documenting that the intussusception has been reduced (Fig. 20-84).

Post-procedure Instructions

Once the examination is complete and the radiographs checked, the patient should be encouraged to drink plenty of water and fruit juices if diet permits. The technologist should ensure that the spot films and overheads are placed together on the patients folder and are appropriately labeled. The number of films taken and fluoroscopic time should be recorded.

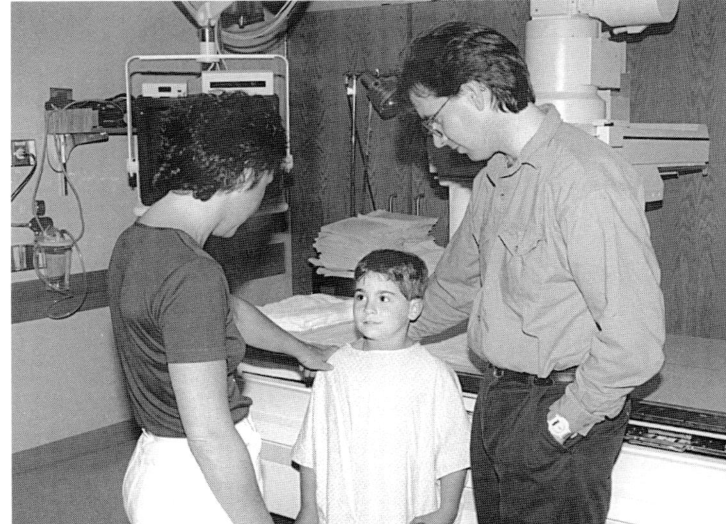

Fig. 20-83. Clear explanations to child and parent.

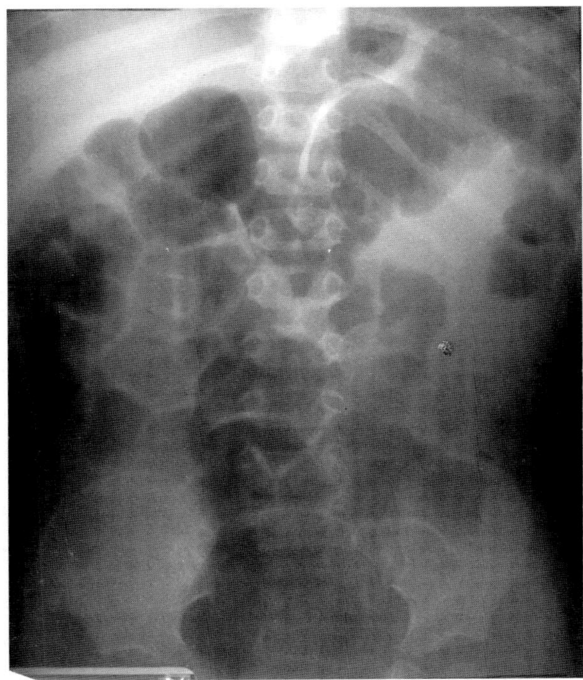

Fig. 20-84. Post reduction of intussusception demonstrating air in terminal ileum.*

*Reprinted with permission: Godderidge, C: *Pediatric Imaging*. Philadelphia, WB Saunders Company, 1995.

Genitourinary System Study
Voiding Cystourethrogram (VCUG) and Intravenous Urogram (IVU)

Diagnostic Indications

Congenital Anomalies:
Ureteral shortening
Vesicoureteral reflux (backward flow from bladder into ureters and kidneys)
Double ureter and/or kidney
Horseshoe kidney
Urethral valve
Hypospadia (developmental anomaly such as when urethra opens on underside of penis in male or into vagina in female)
Indeterminate sexual organs

Diseases and Symptoms:
Urinary tract infection (UTI)
Tumor
Kidney or Ureteral calculi
Abdominal pain
Hematuria

Technical Factors

- Film size–determined by size of patient
- 400 screen/film combination
- 8:1 grid (no grid if less than 9 cm)
- 65-85 kVp, NB to 18 yrs, shortest possible exposure time.

Shielding

- Gonadal shielding should always be used on males for plain films of the abdomen and for excretory urography except for voiding films. Shielding is not used during voiding cystourethrography.
- Gonadal shielding cannot be used on females except when radiographing the kidney area only since the ovaries of younger children are higher in the abdomen and their location is variable. The lower abdomen may be shielded for the 3-minute radiograph of the kidneys taken during an IVU unless shielding obscures the area of diagnostic interest.

20

VOIDING CYSTOURETHROGRAM (VCUG)

This examination may be performed prior to an IVU or an ultrasound of the kidneys. One of the most common conditions in young children is **urinary tract infection** (UTI), and this study is frequently performed to check or evaluate **vesicoureteral reflux**, a common cause of UTI.

Patient Preparation

There is no special preparation prior to a VCUG. If the procedure is to be followed by an IVU, then the child should follow the preparation for an IVU. It is important for this procedure to be described to the patient beforehand and, depending on the age of the child, the timing of this should be left to the parent. Written simple instructions given to the parent will assist them in their explanation.

Contrast Medium and Materials

- Contrast medium for cystography (such as iothalamate meglumine 17.2%).
- IV stand, tubing and clamp.
- Sterile tray with small bowls, sterile gauze and gloves.
- Urine specimen container.
- #8 French feeding tube (inflatable balloon retaining catheters should not be used for children).
- Lidocaine lubricating jelly.
- Skin cleanser - antiseptic, wash cloths and towels.
- 10 cc syringe and fistula tip for boys.
- Urine receptacle.

Room Preparation

The table should be in a horizontal position covered with a disposable or cotton sheet and the fluoroscopic controls set. The bottle of contrast should be warmed slightly and then hung from an IV stand with tubing and clamp attached. Warmed antiseptic skin cleanser is poured into a small sterile bowl ready for use and the tray covered until the patient is on the table.

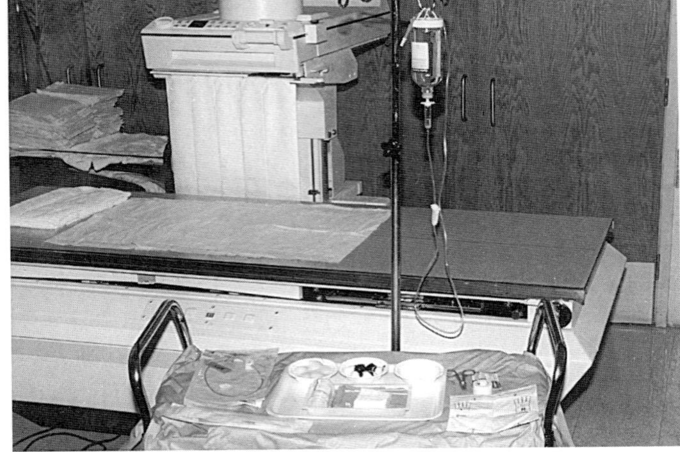

Fig. 20-85. Room setup and materials for VCUG.

Patient and Parent Preparation

The patient and parent should be brought into the room and the procedure again explained simply and clearly. The child should be shown the equipment and how it works, and reassured that the image intensifier will not squash or hurt them. The explanation of the procedure should be in language appropriate for the age of the child. Void or voiding is frequently used by technologists or radiologists, but a word such as "tinkle" or "pee" is more likely to be understood by a young child, enabling them to follow instructions. As there are so many terms used for urination, ask the parent for the word that is used at home.

A VCUG is just as embarrassing and difficult for a young child as it is for an adult. A child who has just been toilet-trained has difficulty in understanding why he/she may now urinate lying down on a table. There should be as much privacy as possible, and it is important to have only those staff in the room who are participating in the exam.

Procedure

An older child should be asked to empty their bladder before entering the room. An infant's bladder is drained at catheterization. After cleaning the perineum, the catheter is inserted into the bladder and a urine specimen taken. After running the contrast media to clear air from the tubing, the catheter is attached to the tubing and bottle of contrast and the bladder is slowly filled.

Spot films are taken when the patient's bladder is full and when voiding, as this is when reflux is most likely to occur. A post-void spot or overhead film is taken of the bladder and kidneys. If there is reflux, a late film of the abdomen may be taken to check if the kidneys have emptied. If a patient is being followed for reflux or postoperatively, a radionuclide voiding cystourethrogram, at a reduced radiation dose, may be performed instead of a fluoroscopic procedure.

Post-procedure Instructions

Parent and child should be told that there might be a slight burning sensation when the child first urinates after the procedure and that the urine might be pink. Drinking plenty of clear fluids quickly helps to alleviate this problem.

Radiographs should be appropriately labeled and placed in the patient's folder. The amount and type of contrast, number of films and fluoroscopic time should be recorded. A urine specimen should be sent for culture.

INTRAVENOUS UROGRAM (IVU)

Patient Preparation

Preparation for an IVU in children is simple. The patient needs to be hydrated, **NOT** dehydrated, and the child should be encouraged to drink plenty of water and clear fruit juices. No solid foods for 4 hours before the exam to diminish the risk of aspiration if the child vomits. Laxatives are not usually recommended for young children for this procedure as they can cause increased gas and discomfort.

Allergic Response to Contrast Media

Although studies of children have found that they have fewer and less severe allergic reactions to iodine-based contrast media than adults, an allergic response is still a possibility . The patient and/or parent must always be asked, prior to the exam, if the child has asthma, is allergic to iodine, pollens, dust or any foods, and if there is a family history of allergies. Even if the child does not have a history of allergies, it is important to be cautious if there is a close relative who does. If a patient has had other procedures using iodine-based contrast without incident, it is still possible for an allergic reaction to occur.

Resuscitation equipment and appropriate medications should be immediately available should there be a reaction and may consist of the following:

- Diphenhydramine hydrochloride for injection or by mouth.
- Epinephrine for injection.

Reactions may be slight to severe: warmth and reddening of the skin, nausea, hives, respiratory difficulties, and although rare, cardiac arrest. It is important that all personnel including students know how to call a "CODE" should a reaction occur.

Contrast Preparation

Low osmolality, nonionic contrast media such as ioversol, iopamidol or iohexal is preferred, for although allergic reactions tend to be less severe and occur less frequently in children, many radiology departments prefer not to take the risk. On the other hand, some departments may choose to use nonionic contrast for high risk patients and high-osmolality contrast for children with no prior history or family background of allergic response.

Dosage According to Weight*

Weight	Dose	*Metric system* Weight	Dose
0 to 12 lb.	2 cc/lb.	0 to 11 kg	3 ml/kg
13 to 25	25 cc	12 to 23 kg	2 ml/kg
26 to 50	1 cc/lb.	24 to 45 kg	50 ml
51 to 100	50 cc	> 45 kg	1 ml/kg
> 100	½ cc/lb.		

*Courtesy of Department of Radiology, Children's Hospital, Boston, MA.
(The metric system doses of ml/kg being used at Children's Hospital are slightly lower doses than the cc/lb doses.)

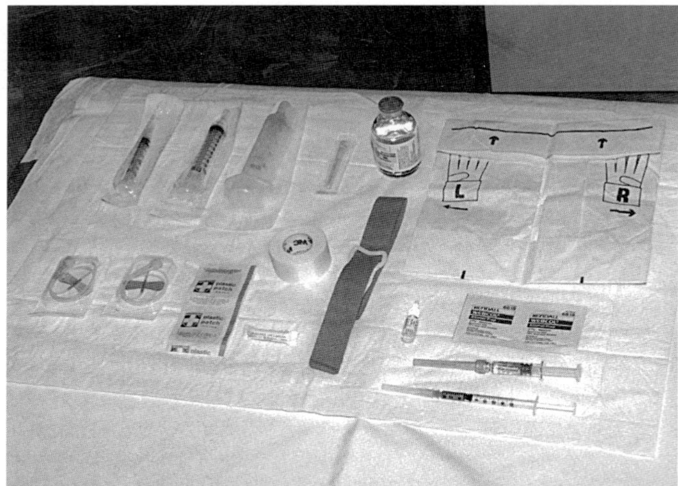

Fig. 20-86. Supplies and materials for injection, IVU.

Materials for Injection

- Syringes: 1, 5, 10, 20 and 50 cc
- Butterfly needles: 19, 23. 25, 27 G
- 16 G straight needle to draw contrast from vial
- Tourniquet
- Gloves
- Mask
- Alcohol swabs
- Band-Aids
- Emesis basin

The contrast should be drawn up and ready for use. Cover the tray and syringe before a child is brought into the injection or procedure room. Ensure that the appropriate medications and resuscitation equipment are readily available to respond to an allergic reaction.

20

Patient and Parent Preparation

Children at any age do not like having needle sticks. It is worth remembering that many adults do not like needles either and may have a problem staying with their child. If at all possible, a parent should stay with their child, to hold their hand and for emotional support. The procedure should be explained to the child beforehand and the timing of this should be left to the parent. Usually the best time for very young children is immediately prior to the procedure

When explaining a needle stick, it is important not to lie by saying it will not hurt. Suggesting that it is like a bee sting, or a pinch in the arm is realistic and less frightening. Babies and very young children may have to be swaddled or "mummified" to immobilize them.

As with any radiographic procedure, the child should be shown the x-ray equipment beforehand and the importance of not moving while the exposure is made explained. Holding a favorite toy or blanket is comforting for many children.

Procedure

Fewer radiographs are taken on children than on adults, and in some instances evaluation of kidneys may be made by ultrasound avoiding the use of ionizing radiation.

A filming sequence may be as follows:

- Preliminary AP supine abdomen (KUB).
- Post-injection (label times accurately):
  - –3 minute of kidneys (shield lower abdomen). Tomography may be used if there is gas or feces in the abdomen.
  - –15 minute supine or prone abdomen.
  - –A delayed film may be needed depending on etiology (factors causing the disease or disorder).
- Use gonadal shielding on male patients.

Giving a carbonated drink to depress the large bowel and create a radiolucent window to visualize the kidneys is not commonly recommended by pediatric radiologists. The gas passes quickly into the bowel, compounding the problem and causing discomfort to an infant or young child.

Post Procedure Instructions

The child should be told to continue drinking plenty of fluids to clear the contrast from their kidneys. Radiographs should be correctly labeled and placed in the patient's folder. The number of films taken, amount of contrast injection and type allergic response, if any, should be recorded on the requisition.

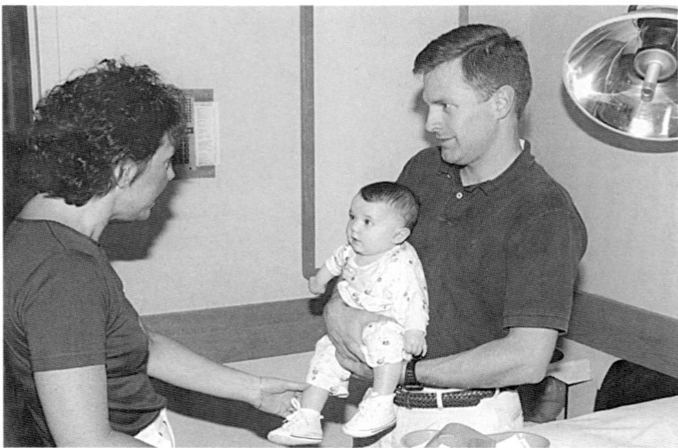

Fig. 20-87. Importance of talking to child and parent.

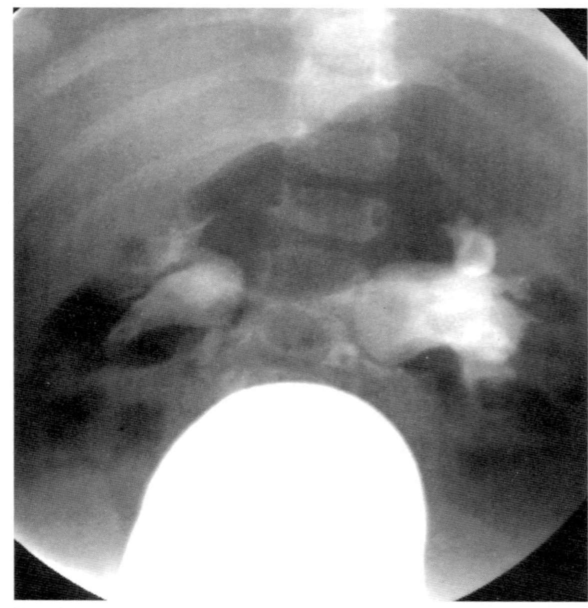

Fig. 20-88. AP demonstrates reflux of both kidneys, (18-month female).

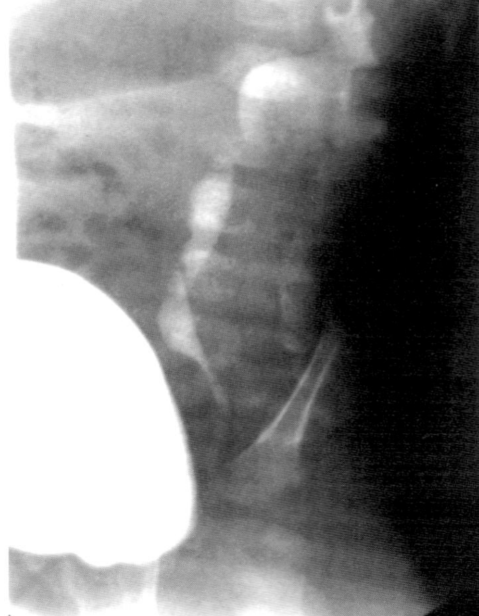

Fig. 20-89. Oblique, reflux of left kidney and ureter. 18-month female demonstrating vesicoureteral reflux (reflux is most likely to occur during voiding phase of voiding cystourethrogram).

CHAPTER 21

Additional Imaging Procedures

- ORTHOROENTGENOGRAPHY–Long Bone Measurement
- ARTHROGRAPHY
- MYELOGRAPHY
- CONVENTIONAL TOMOGRAPHY

Contributing Authors:
Marianne Tortorici, Ed.D., RT(R)
Patrick Apfel, M.Ed., RT(R)

CONTENTS

Orthoroentgenography –Long Bone Measurement

Computed tomography scanograms **612**

Orthoroentgenograms:
- Limb length discrepancies **612**
- Lower limb measurement **613**
- Upper limb measurement **614**

Arthrography

Introduction **615**

Knee arthrography:
- Anatomy, purpose, indications and contraindications **615**
- Patient preparation and equipment **615**
- Injection process and contrast media **616**
- Positioning routines **617**

Shoulder arthrography:
- Purpose **619**
- Equipment, injection process and contrast media **619**
- Positioning routines **619**

Myelography

Myelogram procedure:
- Anatomy, purpose, indications and contraindications **620**
- Patient preparation and equipment **620**
- Injection process **621**
- Contrast media **622**

Myelography cont.

Positioning routines:
- Fluoroscopy and spot filming **622**

Conventional radiographic myelography routines (following fluoroscopy):
- Cervical region **623**
- Thoracic region **623**
- Lumbar region **624**

Radiographs and evaluation criteria **624**

Additional myelographic special procedures **625**

Conventional Tomography

Purpose and terminology **626**

Tube trajectories:
- Introduction **626**
- Linear (unidirectional) **627**
- Control panel **627**
- Multidirectional **627**

Fulcrum:
- Variable vs. fixed fulcrum levels **628**
- Determination of focal level and centering **628**

Blur:
- Influencing and controlling factors **629**
- Sectional thickness **630**

Variations of conventional tomography:
- Autotomography (breathing technique) **631**
- Pantomography (panorex) **631**

Drawings in Figs. 21-50, 21-54, 21-55, 21-56, 21-59, 21-60, 21-61, 21-62, and 21-63 have been adapted with permission from: Tortorici, M.: *Concepts in Medical Radiographic Imaging*, Philadelphia; W.B. Saunders Co., 1992.

Orthoroentgenography

LONG BONE MEASUREMENT

Computed Tomography (CT) Scanograms

One-way limb length discrepancies can be determined is with CT (computed tomography) scanograms, in which CT cursors are placed over the respective joints of either the upper or lower limbs and measurements obtained. However, this requires the use of specialized and more costly equipment and is not as commonly performed as orthoroentgenograms, which utilize conventional radiography as described in this chapter.

Orthoroentgenograms

The term **orthoroentgenogram** *(or′ tho-rent-gen′ o-gram)* is a combination of the prefix "ortho" and the term "roentgenogram," (another term for radiograph). "Ortho" means **straight**, or at **right angles to**. Thus orthoroentgenogram literally means **a straight or right angle radiograph**. This is a very appropriate term, since this procedure is performed utilizing a straight or right angle CR to radiograph the long bones without magnification to determine accurate and comparative long bone measurements.

As described in Chapter 1 on principles of image formation, the usual long bone radiograph results in significant magnification and elongation due to the divergent ray principle. This is more pronounced with large films, especially with some distance between the body part and the film as occurs when the cassette is in the Bucky tray for an AP femur to include the hip or knee (Fig. 21-1). The distance "A" equals the magnification or elongation of the distal femur occurring with this AP projection.

A body part taken table-top has less object film distance but still results in some elongation as seen in Fig. 21-2. If the "straight" or "right angle" CR in Figs. 21-1 and 21-2 were centered directly over the joints, there would theoretically be no elongation on radiographs of these long bones. This is in essence what the orthoroentgenogram procedure of the lower or upper limb does by utilizing multiple exposures on one film with the CR centered directly over the limb joints. A long ruler with metallic markings is placed on the table-top directly beside or under each limb. The respective length of the bones of each limb can be measured by subtracting the numerical value as visualized on the ruler at one end of the bone, from the reading at the other end (Fig. 21-3).

Indications-Limb Length Discrepancies

This procedure is occasionally performed on **adults** for **leg length discrepancies** which may be a cause of back pain or other symptoms. However, this procedure is more common for **children** who sometimes **develop differences in length of their limbs** during periods of bone growth. This is most common for the lower limbs, but can also occur with the upper limbs.

Orthoroentgenography is a common and accurate way of diagnosing and monitoring limb length discrepancies. If the condition is too severe, it can be corrected by either shortening one limb, or lengthening the other. Limb shortening can be done with an operation called epiphysiodesis *(ep″ i-fiz″ e-od′ e-sis)*, a premature fusion of the epiphysis which retards the growth of that limb. Limb lengthening can also be done surgically by cutting and lengthening the shorter limb and stabilizing it until new bone growth occurs.

These conditions and remedies require multiple repeats of these radiographic exams, which on children especially requires careful collimation and shielding practices.

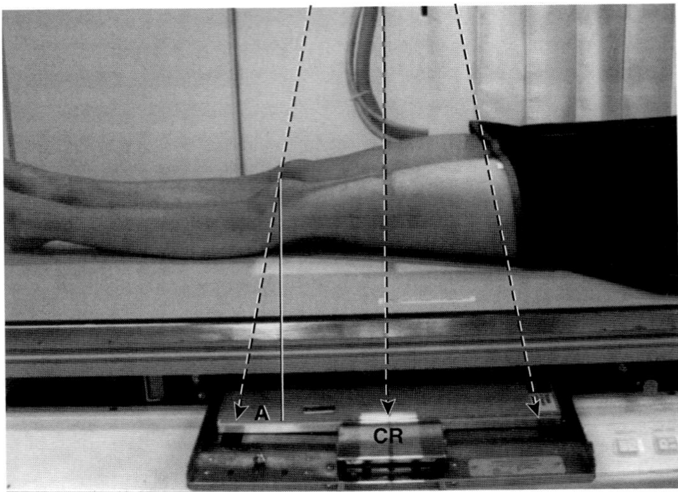

Fig. 21-1. Conventional AP distal femur.
-Demonstrates extensive image elongation of distal femur region.

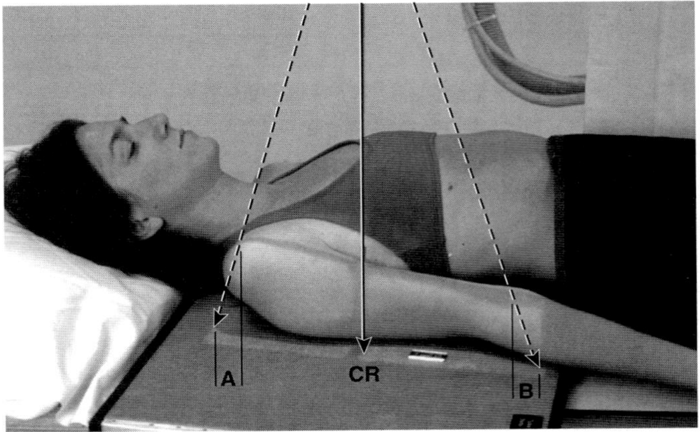

Fig, 21-2. Conventional AP humerus.
-Demonstrates some image elongation, regions A and B.

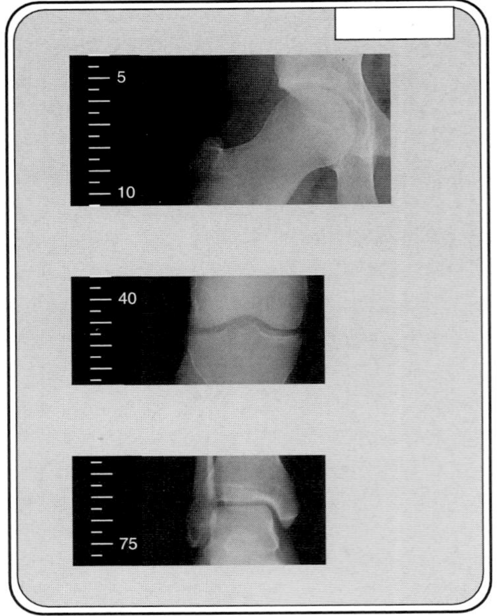

Fig. 21-3. Orthoroentgenogram of lower limb.
-Three exposures on one film.
-CR centered to joints.
-Metallic ruler placed beside limb.

Lower Limb – Long Bone Measurement

(Unilateral on Separate Films or Bilateral on Same Film)

This exam for the lower limbs is commonly performed on each limb separately and measurements are compared for limb length discrepancies. It can also be done bilaterally by placing a ruler under each limb (or one ruler midway between them) and radiographing both limbs simultaneously on a larger film placed crosswise. This requires centering the CR midway between the limbs at the level of the respective joints. More precise measurements are possible, however, if each limb is radiographed separately because of the more centrally located CR. This should be determined by departmental protocol but some references suggest that if the lower limb length discrepancy is more than 1 inch (2.5 cm), the limbs should be radiographed separately.*

Technical Factors

- Film size–10 x 12 in., 11 x 14 in., or 14 x 17 in. depending on age or size of patient and if taken unilaterally on one film or bilaterally on same film, placed crosswise.
- 70-80 kVp, Bucky grid with cassette in Bucky tray so it can be moved between exposures without moving patient or ruler.
- Requires a long "Bell-Thompson" type ruler with metallic markings.

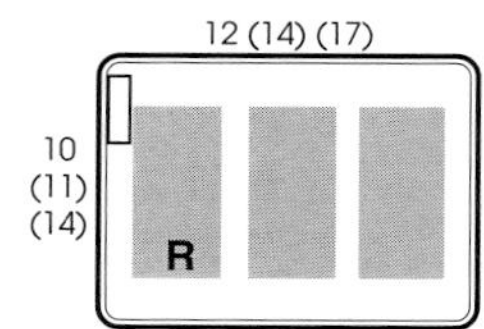

Shielding: Carefully place appropriate size ovarian or testes shield to **not obscure hips or ruler**.

Positioning and Central Ray–Unilateral Exposure

(See Note for bilateral exposure.)

- Patient supine, with leg extended and feet up. Center hip and entire leg to be examined to CR, ensure **no rotation** of pelvis.
- Place ruler directly beside or under the limb. Ensure that ruler is placed high enough lengthwise so the exposure at both ends includes calibrated reading portions of the ruler.
- Immobilize the foot and/or leg if needed to **ensure no movement of leg or ruler between exposures**. The ruler can be taped to the tabletop.

AP Hip

- Center **head and neck** (≈¾ in. or 2 cm above level of symphysis pubis or at upper level of greater trochanter) to perpendicular CR.
- Center upper portion of film to CR. (Ensure that three exposure areas of the hip, knee and ankle do not overlap.)
- Narrow collimation field to include head, neck and greater trochanter region. Ensure that upper margin of femoral head is included on film for total femur length measurement.

AP Knee

- Center **knee joint** (¾ in. or 2 cm distal to apex of patella) to perpendicular CR.
- Narrow collimation field, centered to mid film region.
- Reduce exposure factors from hip to knee technique.

AP Ankle

- Center **ankle joint** (midway between malleoli) to perpendicular CR.
- Narrow collimation field, centered to lower third of film.
- Reduce exposure factors to an ankle grid technique.

Note: If both the lower limbs are radiographed together on one film, two rulers are recommended, one placed under each limb rather than one ruler placed midway between them, which makes gonadal shielding difficult without obscuring the upper portion of the ruler.

For bilateral exposure, center entire patient and CR to midline of table. Ensure that hips and each leg is at an equal distance from center line. Use large enough film placed crosswise to ensure that both hips and both rulers are included.

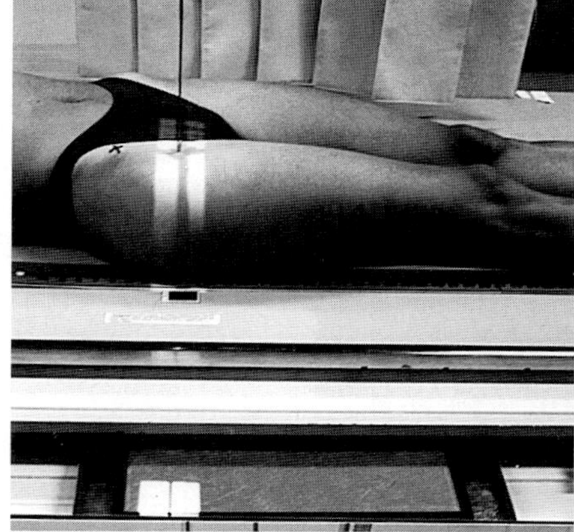

Fig. 21-4. Unilateral- AP hip.

Fig. 21-5.

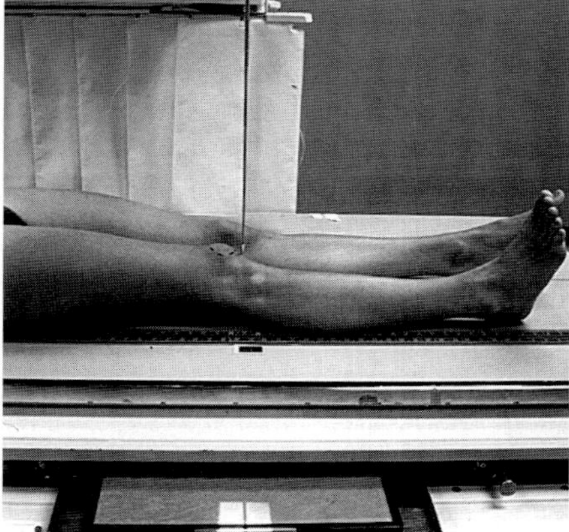

Fig. 21-6. Unilateral–AP knee.

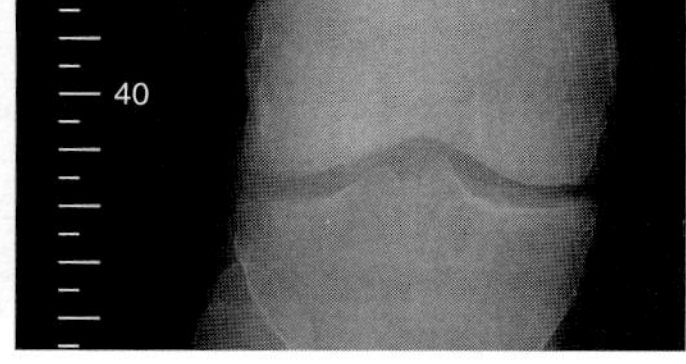

Fig. 21-7.

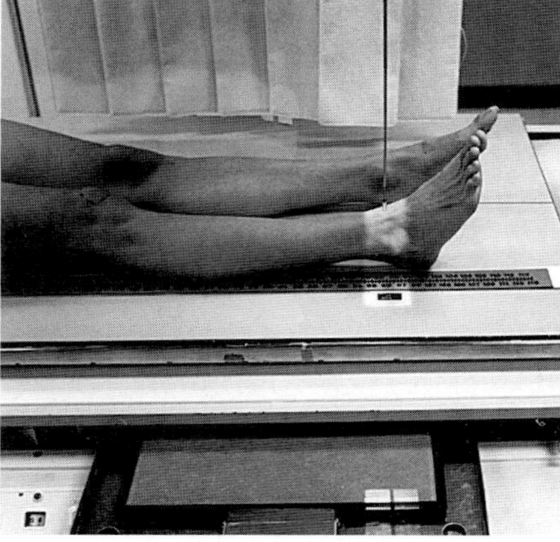

Fig. 21-8. Unilateral–AP ankle.

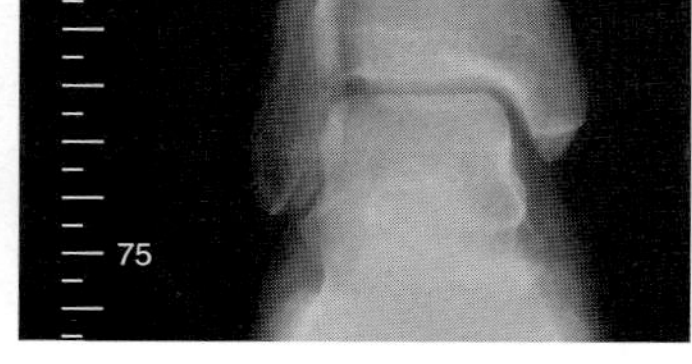

Fig. 21-9.

*Godderidge, C. *Pediatric Imaging*; Philadelphia, WB Saunders, 1995.

Upper Limb – Long Bone Measurement

Discrepancy of long bone lengths of the upper limbs is less common than that of the lower limbs, but the procedure is similar with three exposures made at the shoulder, elbow and wrist joints respectively. Each side is radiographed separately. The ruler is placed under each limb and it is important that neither the arm nor the ruler be moved between exposures.

Technical Factors

- Film size–10 x 12 in. (24 x 30 cm) lengthwise or 11 x 14 in. (30 x 35 cm) depending on age and size of patient.
- 60-70 kVp range, Bucky grid (cassette in Bucky tray).
- Ruler placed lengthwise under the outer edge of arm and shoulder.

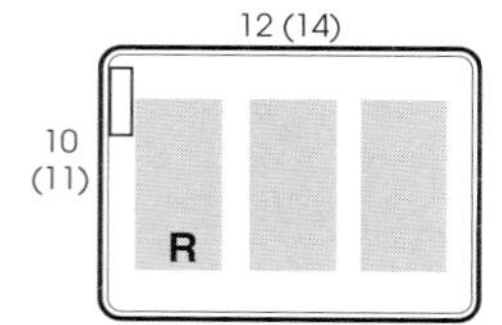

Shielding: Shield pelvis, and also breast region on females.

Positioning and Central Ray

- Patient supine, arm extended and hand supinated.
- Center shoulder, elbow and wrist respectively to CR.

AP Shoulder

- Center **mid shoulder joint** (≈2 in. or 5 cm inferior and medial to superolateral border of shoulder) to perpendicular CR.
- Ensure that ruler is placed high enough to include calibrated reading portion of ruler in exposure field.
- Narrow collimation field to include entire humeral head, centered to upper portion of film. (Ensure that collimator fields do not overlap.)

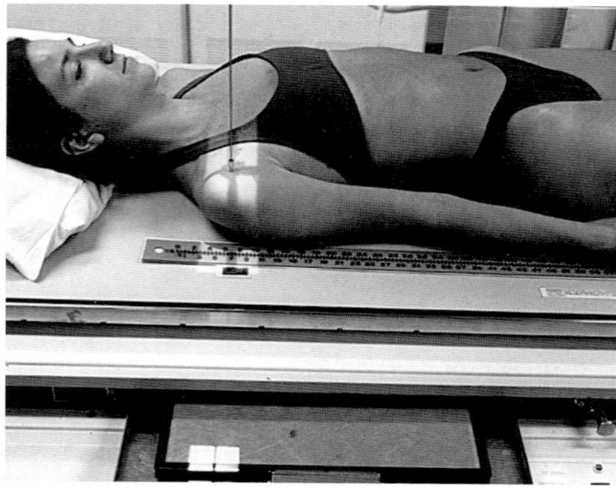

Fig. 21-10. AP shoulder.

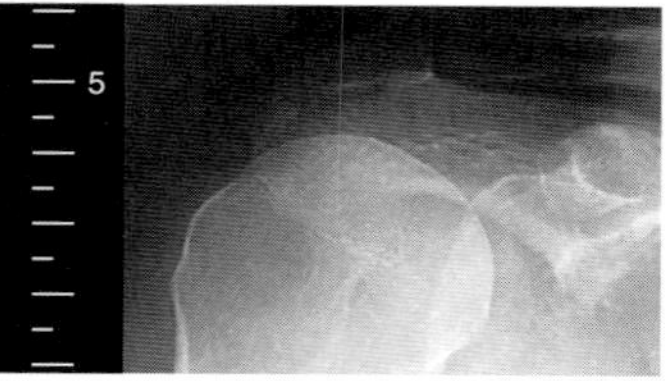

Fig. 21-11.

AP Elbow

- Center **mid elbow joint** to perpendicular CR.
- Narrow collimation field to elbow joint region, centered to midportion of film.

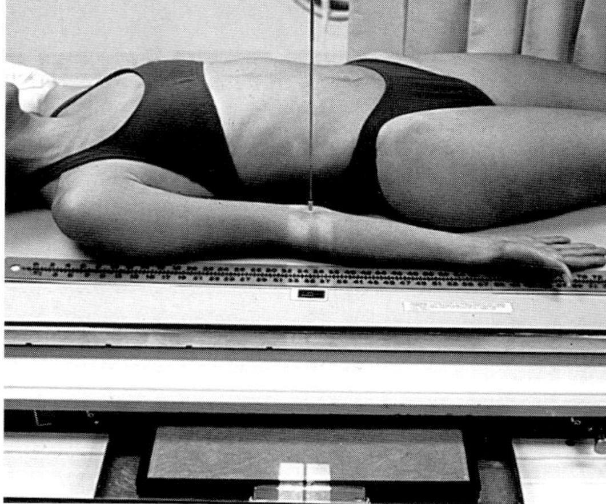

Fig. 21-12. AP elbow.

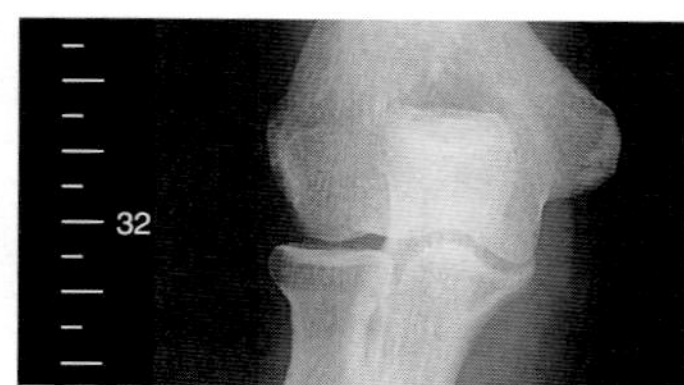

Fig. 21-13.

AP Wrist

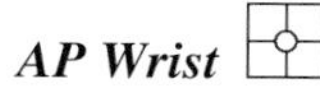

- Center **mid wrist joint** region to perpendicular CR.
- Narrow collimation field to wrist joint, centered to lower portion of film.

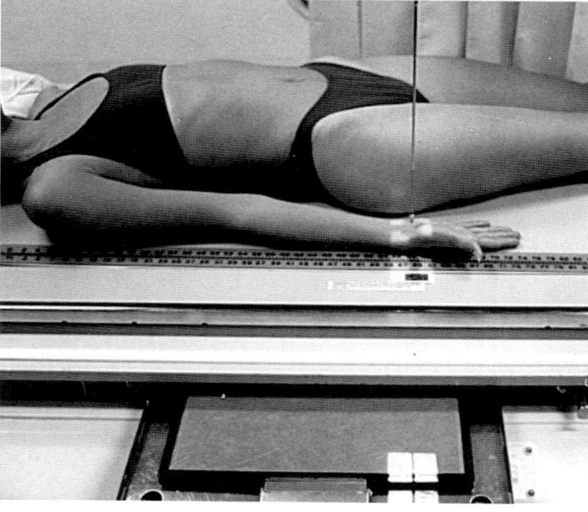

Fig. 21-14. AP wrist.

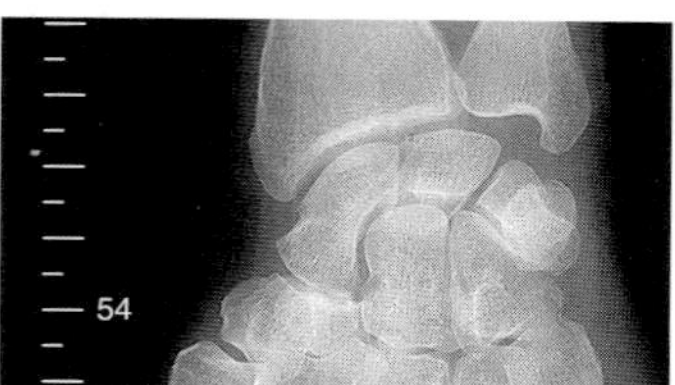

Fig. 21-15.

Arthrogram Procedures

INTRODUCTION

Arthrography *(ar-throg' rah-fe)* is a **contrast media study of synovial joints and related soft tissue structures.** The joints, which can be examined by this procedure, include the hip, knee, ankle, shoulder, elbow, wrist and temporomandibular joints.

It should be noted that although some physicians recommend arthrography as the method of choice for examination of the **knee** or **shoulder** joint, others prefer magnetic resonance imaging (MRI) to evaluate these joints.

In considering arthrography as a whole, the technique of examination is similar for all the joints with variations occurring primarily due to anatomical differences. Arthrogram studies of the temporomandibular joints (TMJs) are occasionally performed and examples are shown in Figures 21-16 and 21-17 wherein contrast media is seen in the temporomandibular joint space in lateral open and closed mouth positions. The mandibular condyle can be seen outlined by the contrast medium within the TMJ joint capsule (small arrows).

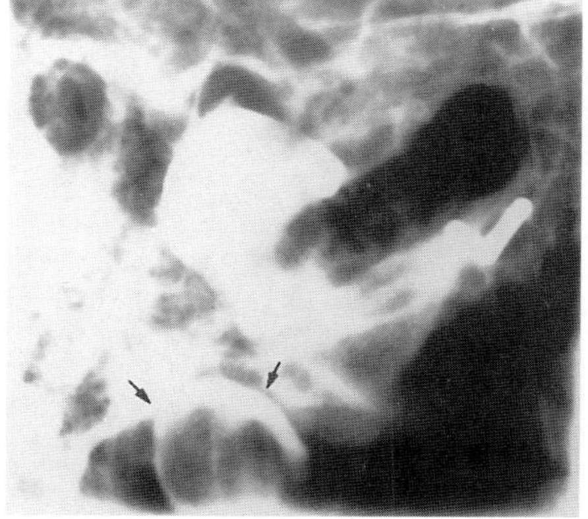

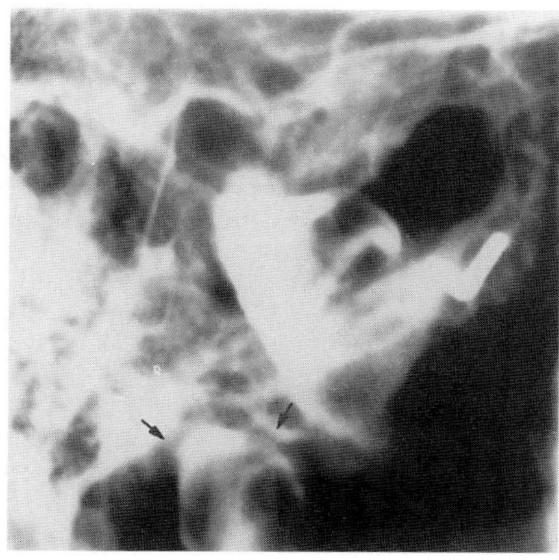

Fig. 21-16. Closed mouth. TMJ arthrograms. Open mouth. Fig. 21-17.

Arthrograms of the shoulder and the knee are the most common of arthrogram procedures being done today and will be described and illustrated in this chapter.

KNEE ARTHROGRAPHY

Anatomy

The anatomical structures demonstrated during arthrography of the knee are presented in Chapter 6.

Purpose

Knee arthrography is performed to **demonstrate and assess the knee joint and associated soft tissue structures for pathology**. The structures of major interest include the **joint capsule**, **menisci** and the **collateral**, **cruciate** and other **minor ligaments**. These structures are visualized through the introduction of a contrast medium into the joint capsule with fluoroscopic spot filming and/or routine radiographic filming utilized to record a permanent image.

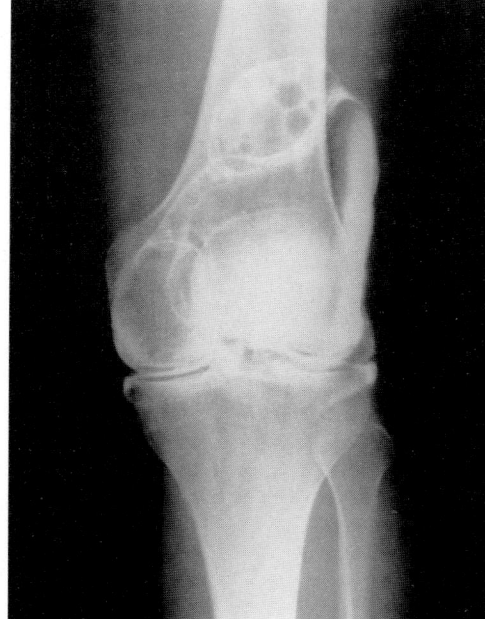

Fig. 21-18. AP knee arthrogram.

Indications

Knee arthrography is indicated when **tears of the joint capsule**, **menisci** or **ligaments are suspected**. The knee is a joint which is subject to considerable stress especially during sports activities. Therefore, much of the pathology seen in the knee is due to trauma. An example of nontraumatic pathology indicating arthrography is a Baker's cyst, which communicates with the joint capsule in the popliteal area.

Contraindications

In general, arthrography of any joint is contraindicated when the patient is known to be allergic to an iodine based contrast medium or to local anesthetics.

Patient Preparation

Any arthrographic procedure should be thoroughly explained before the examination proceeds to preclude unnecessary anxiety on the part of the patient. The patient should be advised of any complications, and must sign an informed consent form.

Major Equipment

The major equipment for knee arthrography varies with the method of filming. Filming may be accomplished by **fluoroscopic spot filming**, **conventional radiographic** (vertical or horizontal beam) **filming** or by a **combination of both**. If a conventional radiographic room is used, it must be equipped so that horizontal beam radiography can be accomplished. The patient should be advised of any complications and sign an informed consent.

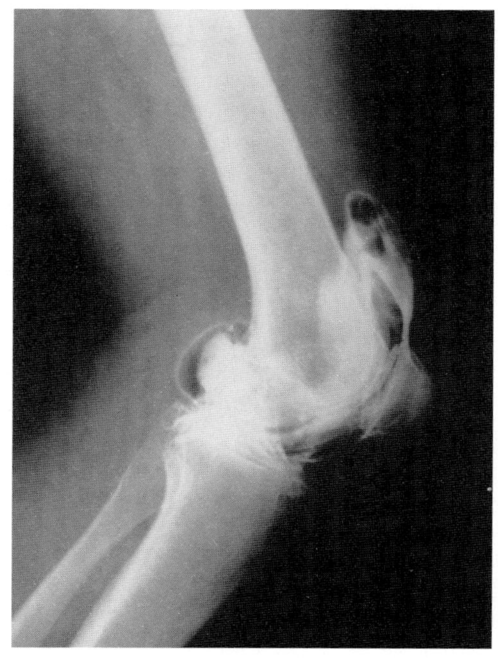

Fig. 21-19. Lateral knee arthrogram.

Accessory and Optional Equipment

Accessory and optional equipment for examination of the knee will vary according to the method of filming, except for those items needed for the contrast injection and preparation of the injection site. These are basically the same for any arthrogram tray (Fig. 21-20).

Arthrogram Tray: Generally, a **disposable tray** is used to prepare the site for injection, which is an aseptic procedure. Such a tray should contain **prep sponges**, **gauze sponges**, a **fenestrated drape**, **one 50 cc** and **two 10 cc syringes**, **a flexible connector**, **several hypodermic needles** (usually 18, 20, 21 and 25 gauge) and a **5 ml ampule of local anesthetic** such as xylocaine. Additionally, **sterile gloves** and **antiseptic solution** (such as betadine), **a razor** and the contrast media are needed. For knee arthrography, a **2 to 3 in. wide ace bandage** is also required.

The injection site is prepared by shaving the area with a razor, and cleansing the site by using the prep sponges and basin containing the antiseptic solution. The area is dried with the gauze sponges and draped with the fenestrated drape. The positive contrast medium is drawn up for injection later (approximately 5 cc) with a 10 cc syringe and 18 gauge needle. The physician injects the skin, underlying tissues and the joint capsule with the local anesthetic using a 10 cc syringe with a 21 or 25 gauge needle.

Needle Placement and Injection Process

A retropatellar, lateral or medial approach may be used during needle placement. The actual site of injection is the preference of the physician.

With the site prepared, draped and anesthetized the physician introduces the 20 gauge needle, mounted on a 10 cc syringe, through the skin and underlying tissues into the joint space. All joint fluid is aspirated. If it is normal in appearance (i.e., clear and tinged yellow), it may be discarded. If it appears abnormal (cloudy) it should be sent to the laboratory for assessment.

With all of the fluid aspirated, the positive contrast medium (drawn up earlier) is injected into the joint through the 20 gauge needle, which has been left in place for the injection. If the study is a dual contrast exam, the 50 cc syringe is used to inject the negative contrast medium.

Once the contrast medium is injected, the needle is removed and the ace bandage is wrapped around the distal femur to obliterate the area of the suprapatellar bursae.

Contrast Media

Knee arthrography can be accomplished by utilizing a radiolucent (negative) medium, a radiopaque (positive) medium or a combination of both media (dual contrast). The dual contrast study seems to be the method of choice. For this study, a very small amount (approximately 5 cc) of a relatively low density positive medium (ex. trade name: Renografin M 60®) is used along with 80 to 100 cc of a negative medium such as carbon dioxide, oxygen or room air.

With the media injected, the knee is gently flexed which produces a thin, even coating of the soft tissue structures with the positive medium.

Fluoroscopic or Overhead Filming: Either fluoroscopic or overhead radiography is used for filming. The accessory filming equipment is minimal and basically the same. Film holders include 8 x 10 in. cassettes or, for fluoroscopy, 9 x 9 in. cassettes. A table mounted patient restraining device arranged as a sling around the knee area should be available (Fig. 21-21). The sling is used to provide lateral or medial stress to "open up" the appropriate area of the joint to better visualize the meniscus during fluoroscopy. Overhead (vertical beam) radiography is the least used method for filming. Fluoroscopy is a more common method employed for filming and requires that the fluoroscopic tube have a small (fractional) focal spot to provide the detail necessary to adequately visualize the menisci.

Horizontal Beam Radiography: Horizontal beam radiography is another common form of filming as described and illustrated on a following page. This requires a 7 x 17 cassette, a lead diaphragm, a low small table or stand to support the knee, a firm pillow and a 5 lb. sandbag (Figs. 21-22 and 21-27).

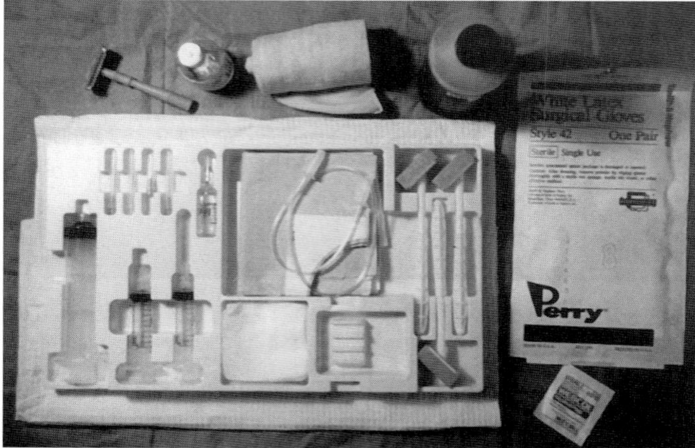

Fig. 21-20. Arthrogram tray.

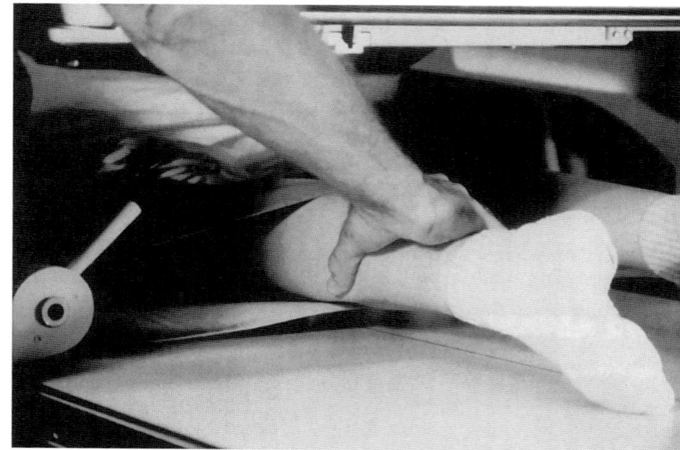

Fig. 21-21. Knee arthrogram (sling around knee in place).

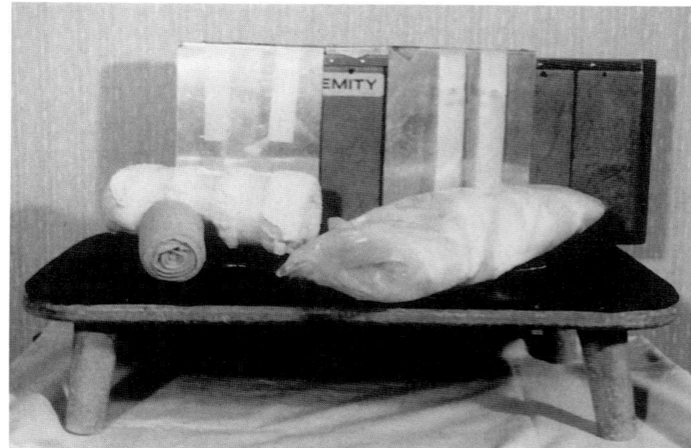

Fig. 21-22. Accessory equipment for horizontal beam radiograph of knee.

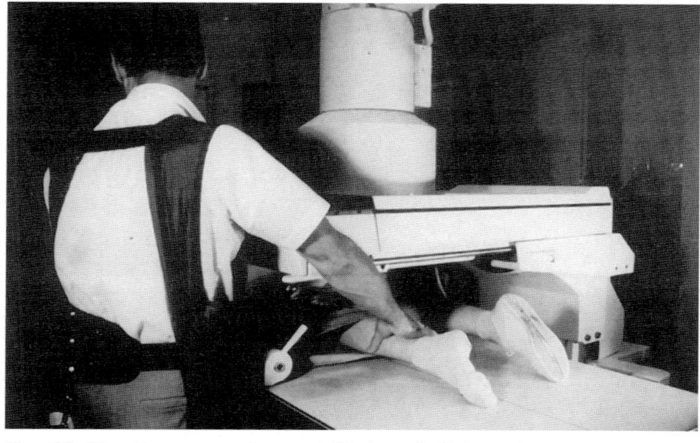

Fig. 21-23. Fluoroscopic spot filming (left knee).

POSITIONING ROUTINES

Radiographic Routines

The routine positioning and procedure for knee arthrography varies with the method of examination, i.e., fluoroscopy, conventional radiography or combination of both.

Fluoroscopy and Spot Filming

During fluoroscopy the radiologist usually takes a series of closely collimated views of **each meniscus**, rotating the leg approximately **20 degrees between each exposure**. The result is a spot film with nine exposures of each meniscus which demonstrates the meniscus in profile throughout its diameter (Fig. 21-24).

Evaluation Criteria

- Each meniscus should be clearly visualized in varying profiles on each of the nine exposed areas of the film. Additional exposures may be necessary to demonstrate pathology.
- The meniscus being visualized should be in the center of the collimated field.
- Correct exposure and adequate penetration should be evident to visualize the meniscus and contrast media.
- The meniscus under examination should be appropriately marked as M (medial) or L (lateral) using small lead markers (smaller than usual right and left markers to lessen chance of obscuring anatomy).
- Patient ID marker should be clear, and R or L marker should be visualized without superimposing anatomy.

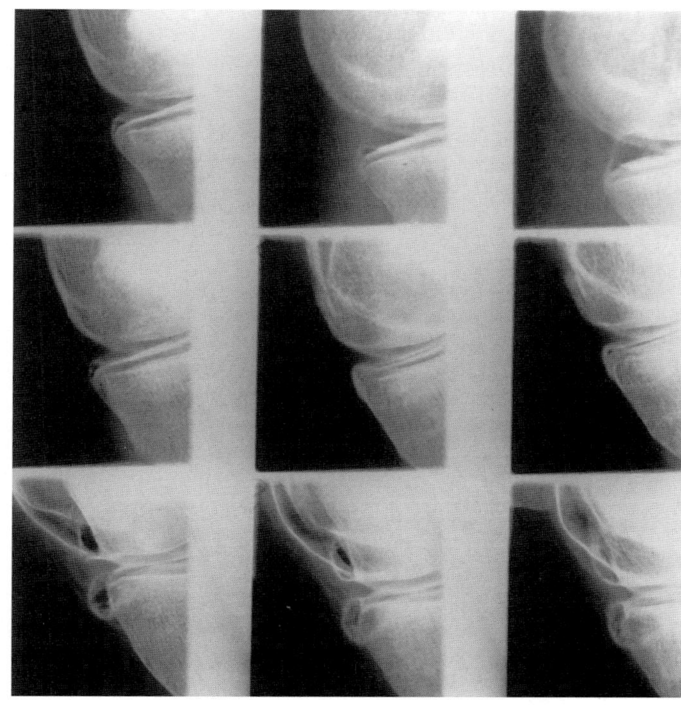

Fig. 21-24. Fluoroscopic spot film (approx. 20° rotation between exposures).

Conventional "Overhead" Projections

In addition to the spot films, routine AP and lateral films of the entire knee, utilizing the radiographic tube, are usually included (Figs. 21-25 and 21-26) These radiographs are taken after removing the ace bandage from the distal femur.

Evaluation Criteria

- The AP and lateral radiographs should demonstrate the entire articular capsule as outlined by the combination negative and positive contrast media.
- Positioning criteria should be similar to the conventional AP and lateral knee as described in Chapter 6.
- Patient ID marker should be clear, and R or L marker should be visualized without superimposing anatomy.

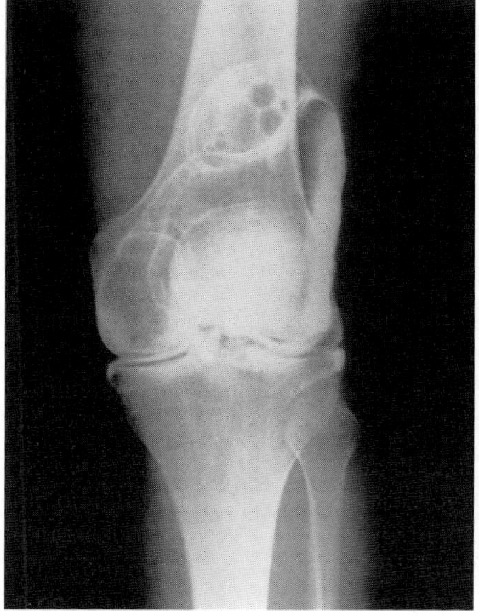

Fig. 21-25. AP knee.

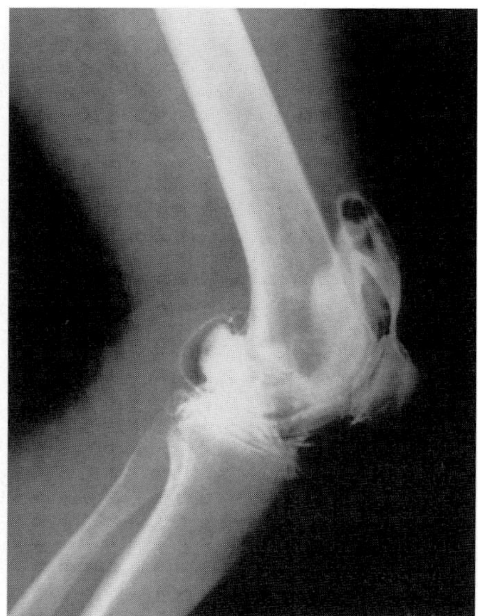

Fig. 21-26. Lateral knee.

Horizontal Beam Projections

Horizontal beam radiography is another common method of filming for knee arthrography and requires some special equipment (Fig. 21-27). This includes:

- A 7 x 17 in. cassette divided to accommodate six exposures.
- Lead diaphragm providing an opening limited to the size of the marked exposure sites on the cassette.
- Low, small table or stand used when radiographing the lateral meniscus; a firm pillow.
- 5 lb. sandbag.

These last two items are used to open up the appropriate area of the joint space to visualize the lateral and medial menisci.

Each meniscus is radiographed on one film with the patient's leg **rotated 30° between each exposure**. The resulting radiograph demonstrates **six views of each meniscus**, in profile, throughout its diameter (Fig. 21-28).

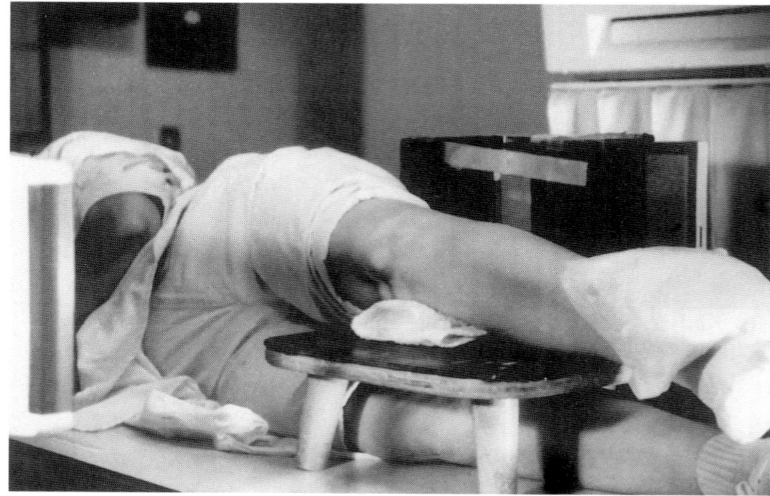

Fig. 21-27. Horizontal beam projection.

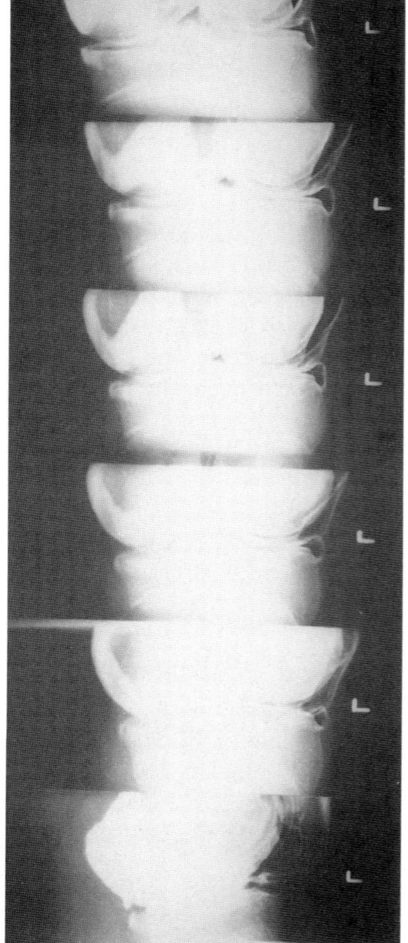

Fig. 21-28. Six views of lateral meniscus (AP on top to lateral on bottom).

Evaluation Criteria

- Each meniscus should be demonstrated in a different profile in six exposures on the 7 x 17 inch film.
- Collimated fields should not overlap.
- The joint/meniscus should be centered to the collimated field.
- Correct exposure and adequate penetration to visualize the meniscus and contrast media.
- The meniscus under examination should be appropriately marked as M (medial) or L (lateral).
- Patient ID marker should be clear, and R or L marker should be visualized without superimposing anatomy.

SHOULDER ARTHROGRAPHY

Purpose

Arthrography of the shoulder utilizes either a single or double contrast injection to **demonstrate the joint capsule, rotator cuff** (formed by conjoined tendons of four major shoulder muscles), the **long tendon of the biceps muscle** and the **articular cartilage**.

Equipment and Procedure

A radiographic/fluoroscopic room is needed for the procedure, similar to that of a knee arthrogram. Contrast injection is monitored under fluoroscopic control and conventional filming is done utilizing the overhead x-ray tube. Equipment and supplies needed include a standard disposable arthrogram tray and a 2½ to 3½ in. spinal needle.

Needle Placement and Injection Process (Fig. 21-29)

The injection site, directly over the joint, is prepared as in any arthrographic procedure. Once the area is anesthetized, the physician uses fluoroscopy to guide the needle into the joint space. Since the joint is quite deep, a spinal needle must be used. A small amount of contrast medium is injected to determine if the bursa has been penetrated. Once the contrast medium has been fully instilled, filming begins.

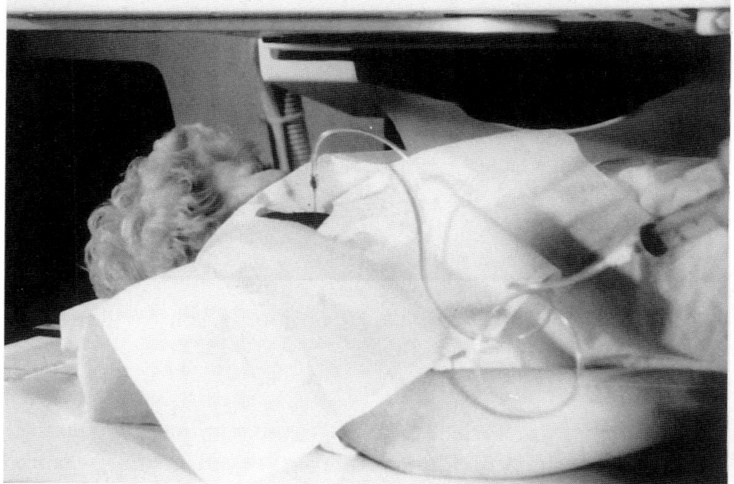

Fig. 21-29. Needle placement.

Contrast Media

Arthrography of the shoulder can be accomplished utilizing either a single, positive contrast medium or a combination of positive and negative (dual) contrast media. For a single contrast study, 10 to 12 cc of a positive medium such as Renographin M-60® is used. For a dual contrast study, 3 to 4 cc of the positive medium and 10 to 12 cc of a negative medium (e.g. room air) are used.

A dual contrast study is believed by some to better demonstrate specific areas, such as the inferior portion of the rotator cuff, when the views are done with the patient upright.

Routine Positioning and Filming Sequence

Routine radiography varies and filming can be done with the patient upright or supine. A suggested filming sequence can include **scout AP projections**, with **internal and external rotation** as standard, and a **glenoid fossa**, **transaxillary** or **bicipital groove projection** (per departmental routine or as indicated).

Once the contrast medium has been injected, the views are repeated (Fig. 21-30). If the radiographs appear normal, the patient is directed to exercise the shoulder and the radiographs are repeated a second time. Caudad angulations of 15 to 23° may be used on the AP projections per specific department routines.

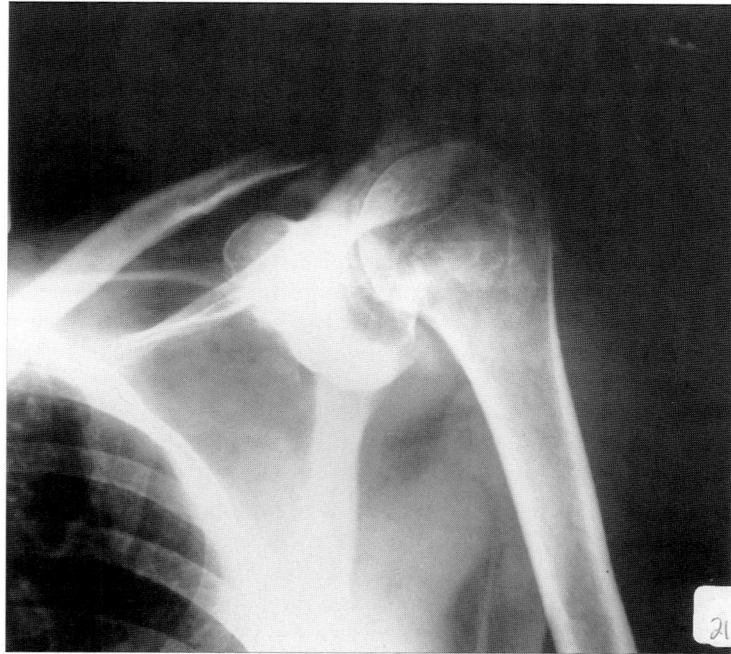

Fig. 21-30. AP shoulder with contrast media.

Myelogram Procedure

Anatomy

The bony anatomy related to **myelography** *(mi″e-log′rah-fe)* of the cervical, thoracic and lumbar level of the spine is presented in Chapters 8 and 9. Additional spinal cord and related brain anatomy is demonstrated in Chapter 22.

Purpose

A **myelogram** *(mi′e-lo-gram)* is a **radiographic study of the spinal cord and its nerve root branches utilizing a contrast medium**.

The spinal cord and nerve roots are outlined by injecting a contrast medium into the subarachnoid space of the vertebral canal. The shape and contour of the contrast medium is assessed to detect possible pathology. Since most pathology demonstrated by this procedure occurs in the lumbar and cervical areas, myelography of these areas of the spine are most common.

Indications

Myelography is performed when patient symptoms indicate the presence of **a lesion which may either be present within the spinal canal or protruding into the canal**. If the pathology impinges on the spinal cord, patient symptoms may include pain and numbness, often in the upper or lower limbs. The most common lesions demonstrated by myelography include **herniated nucleus pulposus (HNP)**, **cancerous or benign tumors**, **cysts** and (in the case of trauma) **possible bone fragments**. If a lesion is present, myelography serves to identify the extent, size and level of the pathology. Another important feature of myelography is in the identification of **multiple lesions**. The most common pathological finding of myelography is **HNP** (herniation of the inner portion of a spinal disk).

Contraindications

Myelography is contraindicated when there is **blood in the cerebrospinal fluid** (CSF), **arachnoiditis** (inflammation of the arachnoid membrane), **increased intracranial pressure**, or a **recent lumbar puncture** (performed within 2 weeks of the current procedure).

The presence of blood in the CSF indicates probable irritation within the spinal canal which can be aggravated by the contrast medium. Myelography is contraindicated in the case of arachnoiditis because the contrast medium may increase the severity of the arachnoiditis. In cases of elevated intracranial pressure, tapping the subarachnoid space during needle placement may cause severe complications to the patient as the pressure equalizes between the areas of brain and spinal cord. Performing myelography on a patient who had a recent lumbar puncture may result in the contrast medium extravasating outside the subarachnoid space through the hole left by the previous puncture.

Patient Preparation

Patients scheduled for myelography may be apprehensive about the procedure. To reduce anxiety and relax the patient, an injectable sedative/muscle relaxant is usually administered one hour prior to the examination. The type and amount of premedication used is determined by the radiologist performing the procedure.

Prior to the examination, the procedure and possible complications should be explained to the patient by the physician and an informed consent signed by the patient.

Major Equipment

The major equipment for myelography includes a radiographic/fluoroscopic room with a 90/15° tilting table, shoulder braces, and a footrest with myelography ankle restraints (Fig. 21-31). Shoulder braces and the ankle restraints are used to secure the patient during the procedure which may require tilting the table Trendelenburg (head lower than feet). It is advisable to use both the shoulder rests and ankle restraints together rather than one or the other separately. The footrest is utilized to support the patient when the table is moved to the upright position.

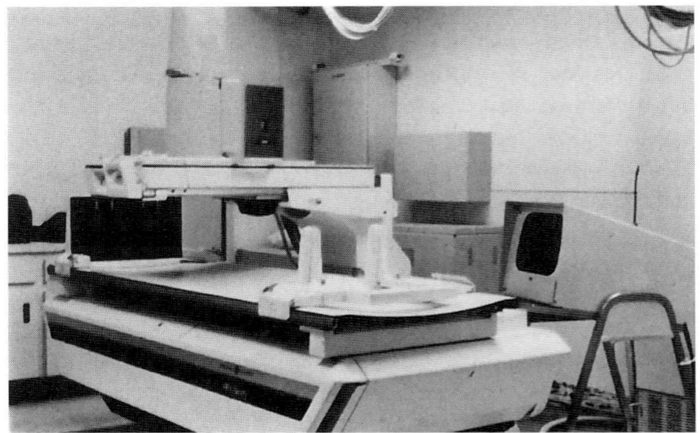

Fig. 21-31. Myelography equipped room.

Accessory and Optional Equipment

The accessory equipment for myelography includes appropriate **grid cassettes with holders** for horizontal beam radiography, a **myelography tray**, **sterile gloves**, an **antiseptic solution**, **appropriate laboratory requisitions** and a **large position sponge or pillow**. The number and sizes of grid cassettes used depends of the level of the spinal canal being examined.

The myelography tray is generally a commercial prepackaged, sterilized, disposable unit (Fig. 21-32). A typical tray should contain the following: a **razor**, **basin** and **prep sponges**; **sterile drapes**; **sterile gauze**; **5 cc** and **20 cc syringes**; **25 g** and **22 g needles**; **18 g spinal needle**; a **single dose vial of local anesthetic**; and **three test tubes**.

Needle Placement and Injection Process

Introduction of contrast medium for myelography is accomplished through a puncture of the subarachnoid space. There are generally two locations for the puncture site; the **lumbar** (L3-4) and **cervical** (C1-2) areas. Of the two locations, the lumbar area is safer, easier on the patient, and most commonly used for the procedure. A cervical puncture is indicated if the lumbar area is contraindicated, or if pathology indicates a complete blockage of the vertebral canal above the lumbar area obstructing the flow of contrast medium to the upper spinal region.

After the puncture site is selected, the radiologist may fluoroscope the patient to facilitate needle placement.

There are generally two possible body positions for a **lumbar puncture**. The patient may be in a **prone position** with a firm pillow or large positioning block placed under the abdomen to flex the spine (Fig. 21-33); or the patient may lie in a **left lateral position** with the spine flexed. Flexion of the spine widens the interspinous space which facilitates introduction of the spinal needle.

For a **cervical puncture**, the patient may be seated in an **erect position** (Fig. 21-34), or **prone** with the head flexed to open the interspinous space.

In both types of punctures the injection site is prepared for this sterile procedure by shaving any hair present with the razor and cleaning the skin using the basin, sponges and an antiseptic solution. The area is then dried with gauze pads and draped with a fenestrated drape (a drape with a central opening). The local anesthetic is administered using the 5 cc syringe with either the 22 g or 25 g needle. With the area anesthetized, the spinal needle is introduced through the skin and underlying tissues into the subarachnoid space.

The location of the needle in the subarachnoid space is verified by an unobstructed back flow of cerebral spinal fluid (CSF) which generally is allowed to flow through the needle. Allowing free flow of the CSF rather than drawing it out with a syringe reduces the risk of spinal cord trauma at the distal end of the needle within the canal. A sample of CSF is collected at this time and sent to the laboratory for analysis. The amount of CSF collected is dictated by the amount needed for the laboratory tests ordered. When the CSF is collected, the spinal needle is left in place for the contrast medium injection.

The contrast medium is injected through the spinal needle into the subarachnoid space, utilizing the 20 cc syringe. Once the injection is completed, the needle is removed. A band-aid is applied to the puncture site and fluoroscopic spot filming and conventional overhead filming begins.

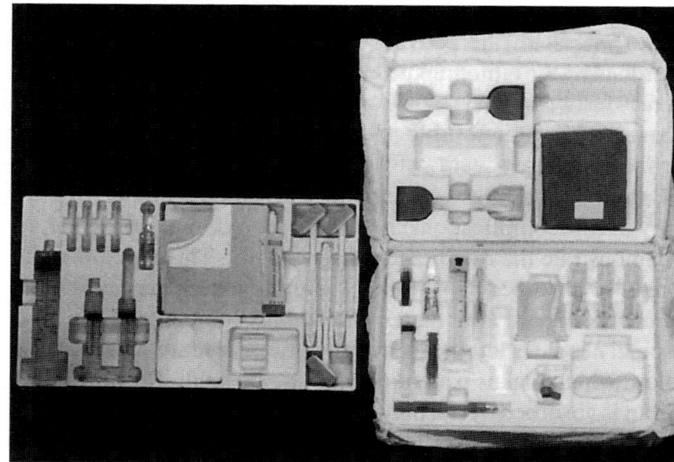

Fig. 21-32. Myelogram tray.

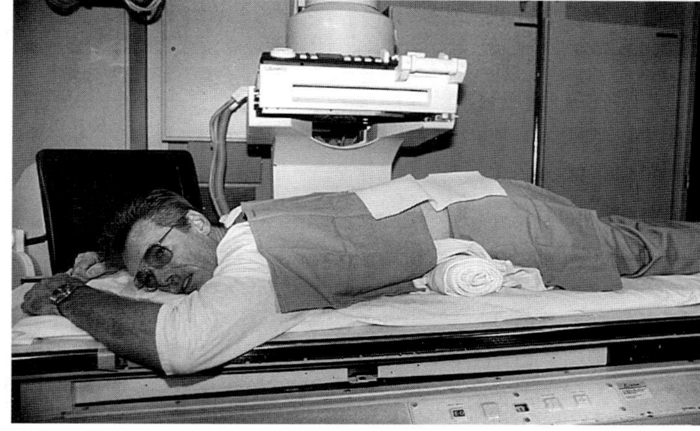

Fig. 21-33. Prone position for lumbar puncture.

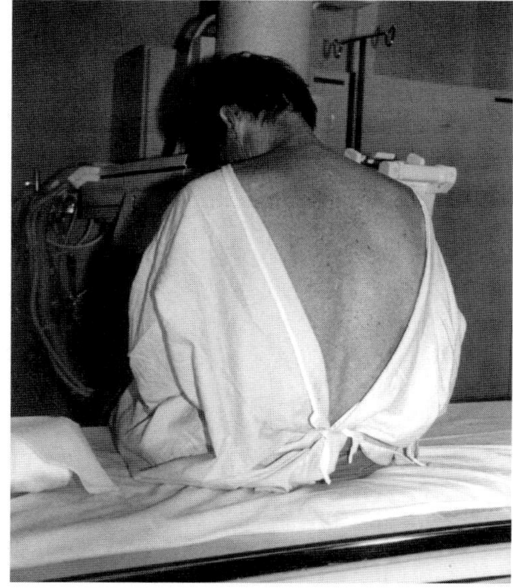

Fig. 21-34. Erect position for cervical (C1-2) puncture.

Contrast Media

The best type of contrast medium for myelography is one that is miscible (mixes well) with the cerebrospinal fluid, is easily absorbed, nontoxic, inert (non-reactive) and has good radiopacity. No one type of contrast medium meets all the above criteria. In the past, air or gas (radiolucent) and oil-based iodinated (radiopaque) media have been used for myelography. Currently, however, either **ionic** or **nonionic**, **water-soluble iodine based media** are used. Because of their relatively low osmolality (see Chapter 17) nonionic water soluble contrast media may be used to reduce the chances of patient reactions.

Water soluble contrast media provide excellent radiography visualization of the nerve roots; are easily absorbed into the vascular system; and are excreted by the kidneys. Absorption begins approximately 30 minutes after injection with good radiopacity up to about 1 hour post injection. After 4 to 5 hours, the contrast medium will have a hazy radiographic effect, and is radiographically undetectable after 24 hours.

Dosages: Dosage for myelographic contrast media is recommended by the manufacturer and will vary with the concentration of the medium used and the area of the spine under examination. In general, a range of approximately **6 to 17 cc** are used. Care should be taken to prevent the contrast medium from entering the area of the head. For example when examining the cervical area with the patient prone, or Trendelenburg, the chin is hyperextended to prohibit the medium from flowing into the cranial region of the subarachnoid space.

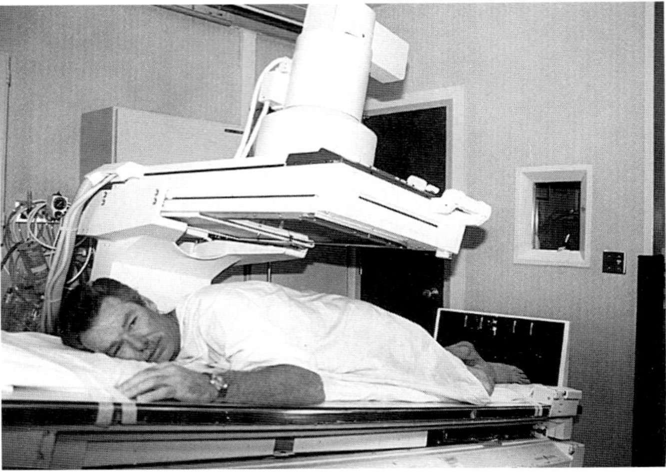

Fig. 21-35. Left posterior oblique for spot filming of lumbar myelogram (x-ray tube is under table making this a posterior oblique, AP projection).

POSITIONING ROUTINES

Fluoroscopy and Spot Filming

During fluoroscopy the table (and patient) are tilted from erect through Trendelenburg positions. This facilitates the flow of contrast medium to the area under examination.

Under fluoroscopic control, once the contrast medium has reached the desired area, the radiologist may film the patient with a spot film device or high-speed camera in a variety of positions from prone to supine, and in anterior or posterior oblique positions (Figs 21-35 and 21-36). Following fluoroscopy, the radiographer will take conventional radiographs appropriate for the area under examination.

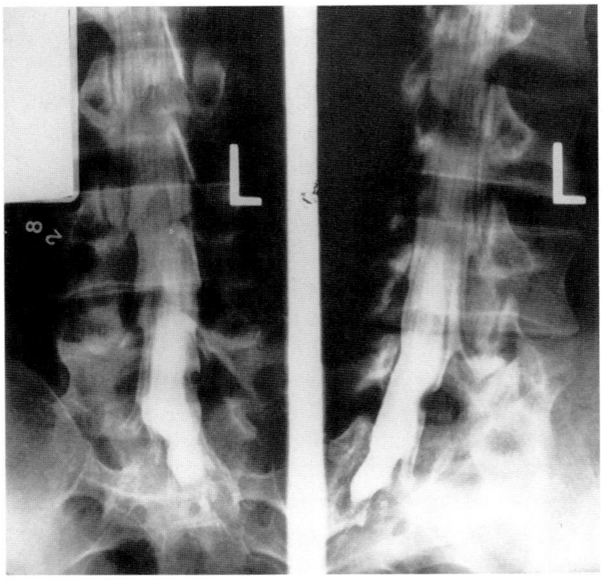

Fig. 21-36. Spot films of lumbar myelogram (AP and LPO).

Conventional Radiographic Myelography Routines (Following Fluoroscopy)

Although department radiographic routines for myelography may vary significantly, the following positions/projections as described represent suggested **basic** routines for the different levels of the spinal column. Additional positions/projections which may be considered routine or special are also listed.

Before routine radiography begins, the radiologist adjusts the table tilt as needed to concentrate the contrast medium to the level of the spinal cord being radiographed.

Cervical Region

Transcervical Lateral–Horizontal Beam *(Fig. 21-37):* The patient is prone with the arms extended along the sides of the body and the shoulders depressed. The chin is extended and resting on a small positioning sponge or folded linen for comfort and to maintain extension. The central ray is directed to the level of C5. The field should be collimated to reduce scatter radiation. Respiration is suspended during the exposure.

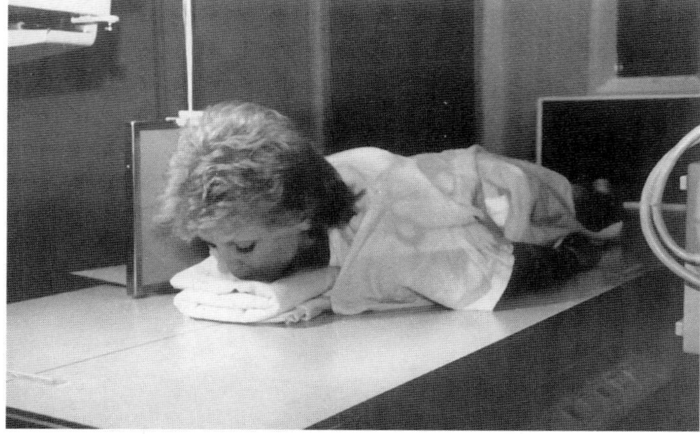

Fig. 21-37. Cervical region –Transcervical (horizontal beam) lateral.

Swimmers Lateral–Horizontal Beam *(Fig. 21-38):* The patient is prone with the chin extended. For a right lateral, the right arm is extended along the right side of the body with that shoulder depressed. The left arm is flexed (i.e., stretched superior to the head). The central ray is directed to the level of C7. The field is collimated to reduce scatter radiation. Respiration is suspended during the exposure.

Note: Additional positions may include prone anterior obliques with a horizontal beam.

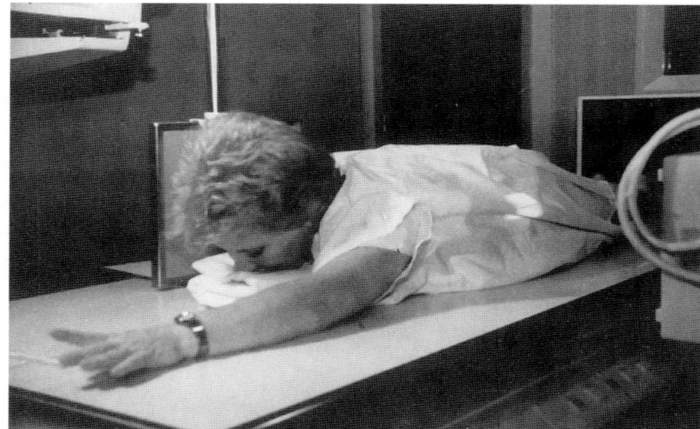

Fig. 21-38. Cervical region (C7 to T1 region) –Swimmer's (horizontal beam) lateral.

Thoracic Region

Right Lateral Decubitus–AP or PA Projection with Horizontal X-ray Beam *(Fig. 21-39):* The patient is positioned in a true right lateral with the right arm flexed, superior to the head. The left arm is extended and resting along the left side of the body. To maintain the alignment of the spine parallel to the table top, the patient may rest the head on the arm. If needed, a small positioning sponge or folded linen may be placed between the head and the arm to maintain alignment. The central ray is directed to the level of T7. Collimate the field to area of interest to reduce scatter radiation. Respiration is suspended during the exposure.

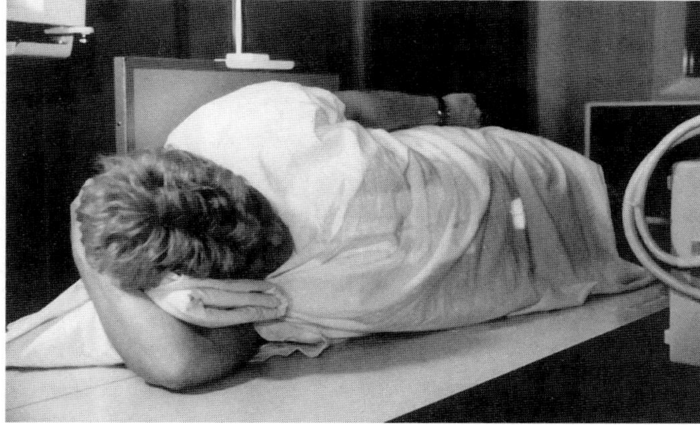

Fig. 21-39. Thoracic region–Right lateral decubitus (AP horizontal beam projection).

Left Lateral Decubitus–AP or PA Projection with Horizontal X-ray Beam: The patient is positioned in a true left lateral position with the left arm raised and flexed above head. The right arm is extended down resting on the right side of body as shown. The spine remains parallel to the table-top. The central ray is directed to T7 with close collimation to reduce scatter radiation. Respiration is suspended during the exposure.

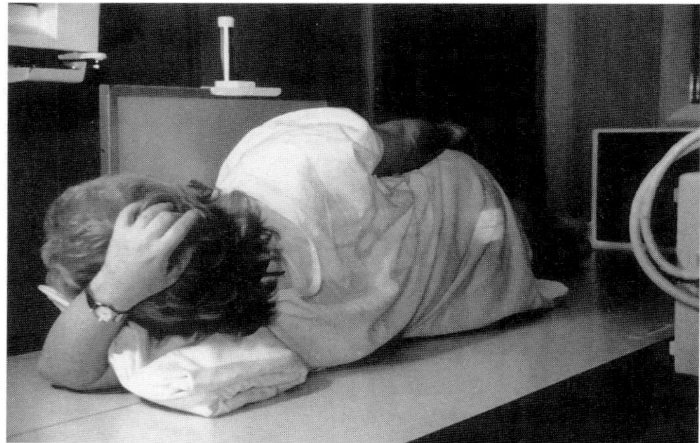

Fig. 21-40. Thoracic region–Left lateral decubitus (PA horizontal beam projection).

***Right or Left Lateral–Vertical Beam** (Fig. 21-41):* The patient is positioned in a true lateral with the knees flexed. Both arms are semi-flexed. The alignment of the spine should be maintained parallel to the table top. The patient may rest the head on the hands, or a small positioning sponge or folded linen may be placed between the hands and the head to maintain alignment of the spine. The central ray is directed to the level of T7. The field is collimated to reduce scatter radiation. Respiration is suspended during the exposure.

Additional positions may include a supine (AP projection) and a lateral with a horizontal beam.

Note: A supine AP and horizontal beam lateral are not generally recommended since, in the supine position, pooling of the contrast medium occurs in the mid thoracic region due to the usual thoracic curvature. This, of course, is more prominent in some patients. Therefore, to best demonstrate the entire spinal canal of the thoracic region, **AP and PA projections** should be taken in both the **right and left lateral decubitus positions**, in addition to the **vertical beam lateral position** as described and illustrated.

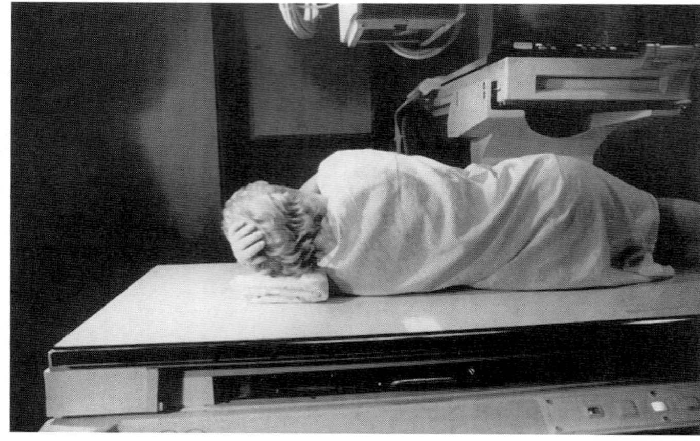

Fig. 21-41. Thoracic region–Left vertical beam lateral.

Lumbar Region

***Semierect Transabdominal Lateral–Horizontal Beam** (Fig. 21-42):* The patient is positioned prone with the arms flexed superior to the head. The table and patient are semierect. The radiologist, under fluoroscopic control, will adjust the angulation of the table to concentrate the contrast medium in the lumbar area.

The central ray is directed to L3. Collimation to the area of interest is important to reduce scatter radiation. Respiration is suspended during the exposure.

Additional positions may include obliques with either a vertical or horizontal beam and a supine AP projection.

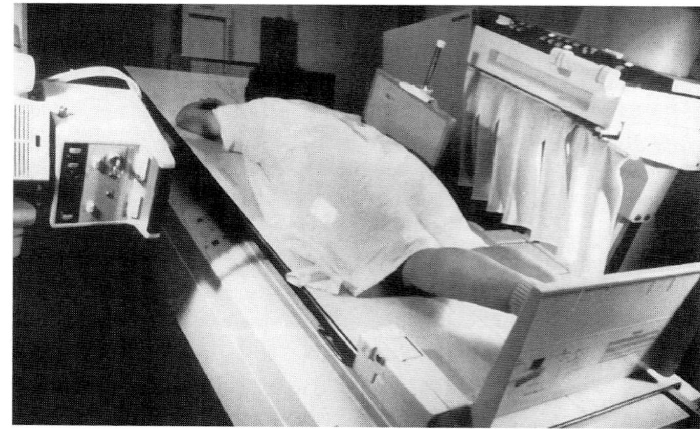

Fig. 21-42. Lumbar region–Semi-erect transabdominal (horizontal beam right lateral).

RADIOGRAPHS

Evaluation Criteria

(for all levels of the spinal column)

- The appropriate level of the spinal column, with contrast present, should be demonstrated.
- Correct exposure and adequate penetration to demonstrate anatomy and contrast medium.
- Patient ID markers and anatomic markers (right or left) should be clearly visualized without superimposing anatomy.
- Collimation should be evident.

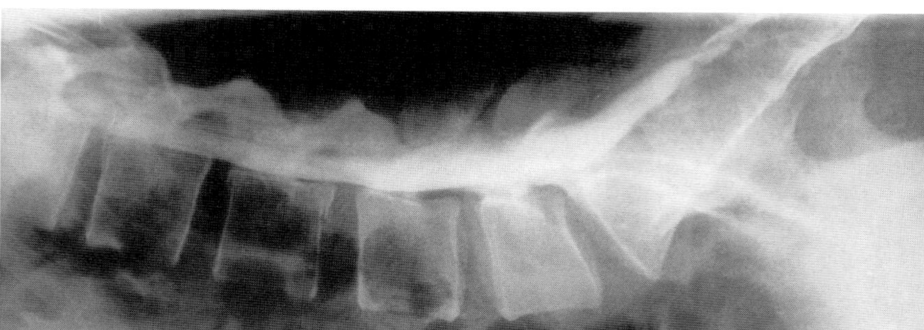

Fig. 21-43. Lumbar–Transabdominal.

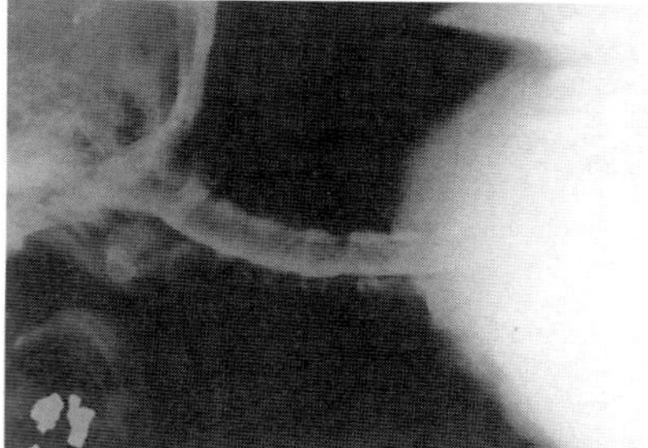

Fig. 21-44. Transcervical (horizontal beam) lateral.

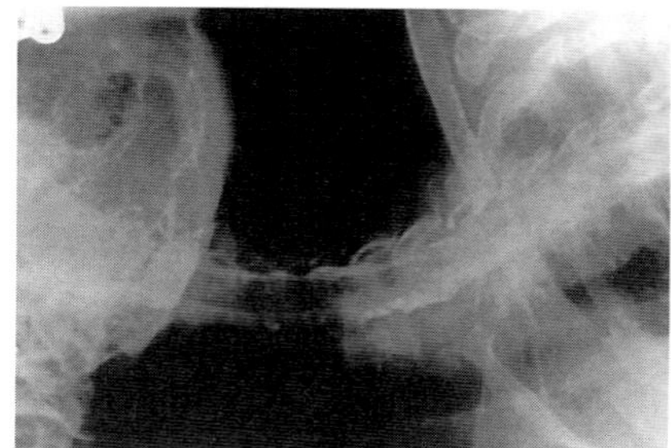

Fig. 21-45. Swimmer's (horizontal beam) lateral.

ADDITIONAL MYELOGRAPHIC SPECIAL PROCEDURES

The following are not commonly performed procedures in today's radiology departments due to the increased use of other imaging modalities such as MRI. Radiographers, however, should at least understand what these procedures are in case they are encountered.

Computed Tomography

Computed myelography is computer-enhanced radiographic examination of the vertebral column, spinal cord and spinal nerves following injection of a water-soluble contrast medium.

In addition, nonenhanced computed tomography of the vertebral column and its contents is often performed. An example of and axial section of part of a computed myelogram procedure is shown in Fig. 21-46.

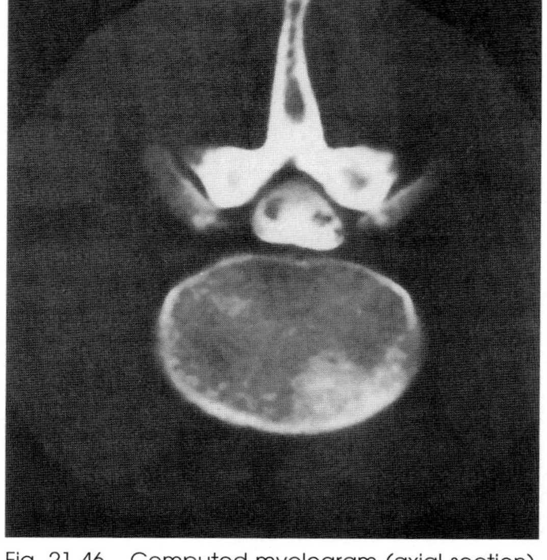

Fig. 21-46. Computed myelogram (axial section).

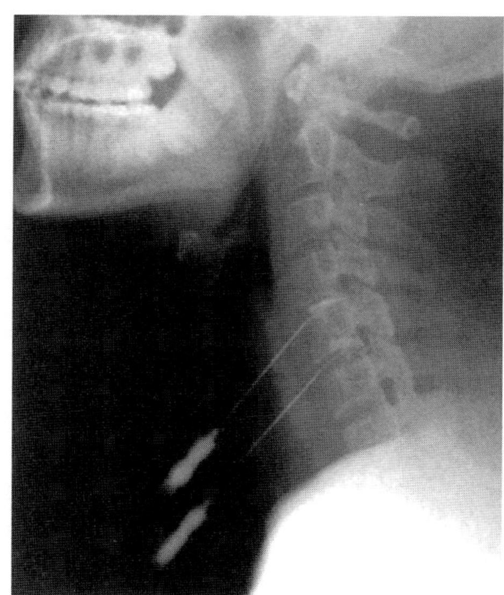

Fig. 21-47. Cervical diskogram.

Diskography

Diskography *(dis-kog′ rah-fe)* or nucleography is radiographic examination of individual intervertebral disks following injection of water-soluble, iodinated contrast medium into the center of the disk (nucleus pulposus). An example of a cervical diskogram is shown in Fig. 21-47.

Epidural Venography

Epidural venography *(ve-nog′ rah-fe)* is a radiographic examination of the collection of veins lining the spinal canal. This intricate plexus of veins is closely related to the intervertebral disks. This examination complements myelography in the diagnosis of intervertebral disk herniations. An example of an epidural venogram *(ve′ no-gram)* is shown in Fig. 21-48.

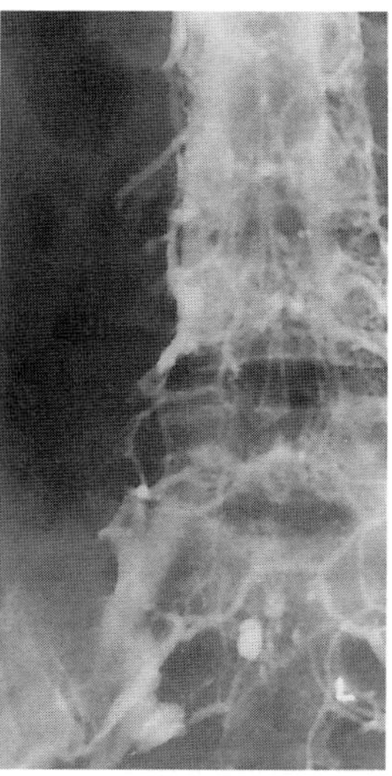

Fig. 21-48. Epidural venogram.

Conventional Tomography

Purpose

Tomography is a special type of imaging used to **obtain a diagnostic image of a specific layer of tissue or object, which is superimposed by other tissues or object(s)**. This is accomplished utilizing accessory equipment that allows the x-ray tube and film to move about a fulcrum point during film exposure. The resulting radiograph is called a **tomogram**, which demonstrates a clear image of an object lying in a specific plane while blurring the structures located above and below the specific plane. Figure 21-49 illustrates a patient in position on the x-ray table for a tomogram of the thoracic region. A basic linear tomographic equipment setup is shown in position behind the patient connecting the x-ray tube to the Bucky tray. The basic principles of conventional tomography will be described beginning with terminology.

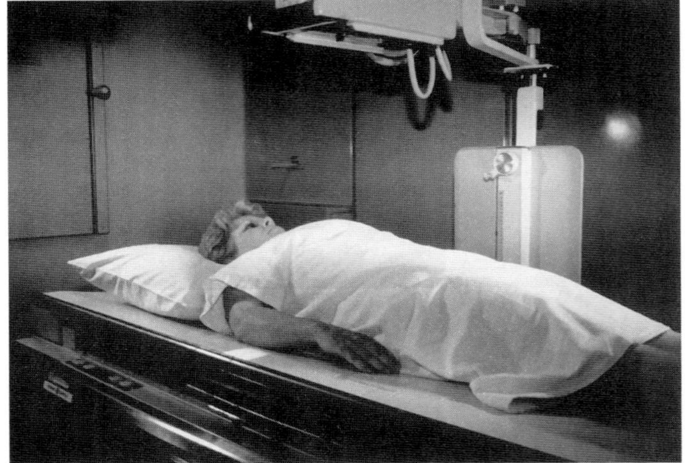

Fig. 21-49. Linear tomographic unit.

Terminology

Since the tomogram represents a section of the body, this type of filming is sometimes termed **body section radiography**. Other terms sometimes used to identify tomography are planigraphy, stratigraphy, and laminography. The International Commission on Radiological Units and Measures (ICRU) in 1962 established the term, **tomography**, to describe all forms of body section radiography.

Since terminology may differ, following is a list of terms and their definitions as used in this textbook:

Tomogram: The radiograph produced by a tomographic unit.
Fulcrum: The pivot point of the connecting rod between the x-ray tube and the film.
Fulcrum level: Distance, measured in centimeters or inches, from the table-top to the fulcrum.
Objective plane (focal plane): The plane in which the object is clear and in focus.
Sectional thickness: The thickness of the objective or focal plane. (This is variable, controlled by exposure angle and tube movement.)
Exposure angle: The angle resulting from the x-ray beam movement (Fig. 21-54 and 21-61).
Tube movement (or shift): The distance the tube travels.
Amplitude: The speed of tube movement measured in inches or centimeters per second.
Tube trajectory: The geometric configuration or blurring pattern of tube movement (Fig. 21-50).
Blur: The area of distortion of objects outside the objective plane.
Blur margin: The outer edge of the blurred object.

Each of these terms will be used and illustrated in this chapter beginning with tube trajectory.

Tube Trajectories

There are five basic types of trajectories for tube movement in tomography (Fig. 21-50). These are listed from simplest to most complex:

(1) **Linear** → (unidirectional)
(2) **Elliptical**
(3) **Circular**
(4) **Spiral**
(5) **Hypocycloidal**
} (multidirectional)

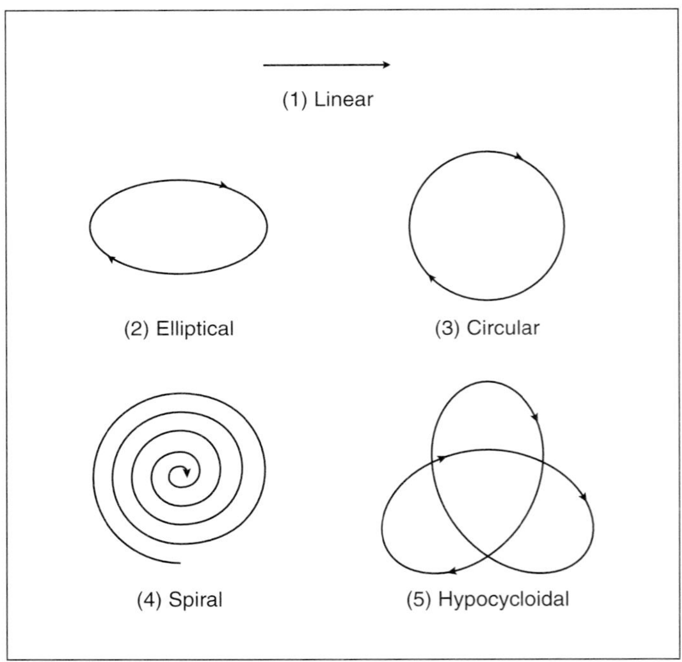

Fig. 21-50. Five basic trajectories (blurring patterns).

In **linear** trajectories (sometimes available as vertilinear and curvilinear) the tube moves in one direction. These trajectories are therefore identified as **"unidirectional."**

The tube trajectories for **elliptical**, **circular**, **spiral** and **hypocycloidal** all move in several directions and are therefore identified as **multidirectional** (pluridirectional).

Linear Unidirectional Tube Trajectories

Linear or unidirectional tomography involves the least complex type of equipment setup (Fig. 21-51). This utilizes a basic x-ray table with Bucky tray and overhead tube connected by a metal connecting arm or rod. This rod passes through an adjustable fulcrum level attachment (see Fig. 21-52). This attachment is used to manually or electrically adjust the height of the fulcrum level.

Tube movement is achieved by a motor attached to the unit. Since the tube moves along the longitudinal axis of the table, the longitudinal tube lock must be opened (unlocked). The Bucky tray and tube angle locks must also be opened to permit these items to move freely.

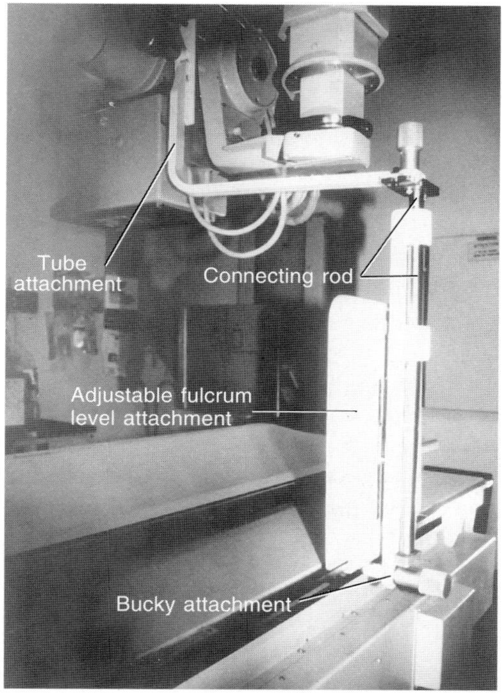

Fig. 21-51. Linear (unidirectional) tomographic equipment.

Control Panel

The tomographic unit is operated by its own control panel. The options on the control panel vary from unit to unit. Common features of the control apparatus regulate the:

- Tube travel speed (in inches or cm/sec) for those units with variable amplitude.
- Objective plane (focal plane thickness, or sectional thickness).
- Direction or type of tube trajectory or travel (on equipment with multidirectional capabilities).
- Tube center.
- Fulcrum level.

Some units are designed so that all features except the fulcrum level adjustment are on a control apparatus located in the x-ray room control area. In these units, it is common for the fulcrum level to be the adjustable type located directly on the fulcrum attachment connected to the x-ray table (Fig. 21-52). Other units may also have the exposure angle selector located in the x-ray table area rather than in the control booth area.

A large part of the object is parallel to the tube movement in unidirectional or linear tube trajectories. This limits the amount of blurring on the tomogram. It also creates an image having "streaks." The image clarity may be improved by maximizing the amount of perpendicular movement of the tube to the object. This is achieved by changing the type of tube trajectory to multidirectional. An example of multidirectional tomography is a specialized type of tomographic unit shown in Fig. 21-53 used primarily for tomographic exams involving the skull.

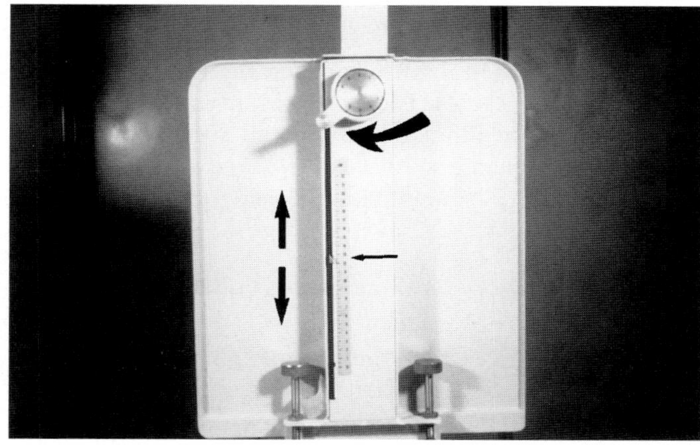

Fig. 21-52. Adjustable fulcrum level attachment.

Multidirectional Tube Trajectories

Of the four types of multidirectional movement, the least complex is the elliptical, which is a slight variation from the linear. The circular movement is "a step above" the elliptical pattern in complexity. The two most complex multidirectional movements are spiral and hypocycloidal. The more complex the multidirectional movement, the thinner the possible objective plane (see objective plane thickness section on a following page) and the clearer the image.

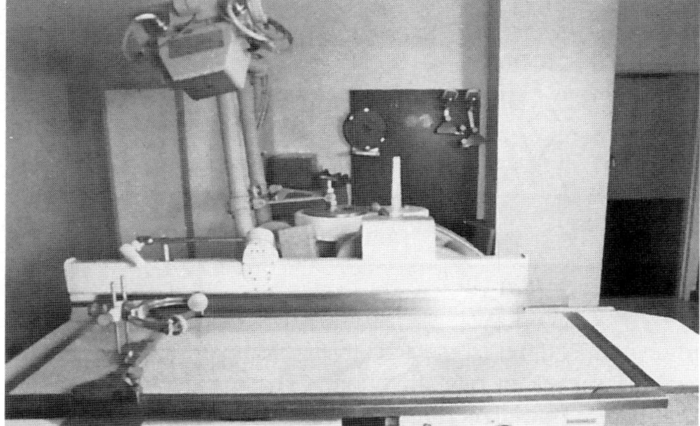

Fig. 21-53. Multidirectional tomographic unit.

21

FULCRUM

The fulcrum is the pivot point through which the x-ray tube and film move. This pivot point is important because all structures located in its plane (objective plane) and parallel to the tube trajectory or travel remain sharp and in focus because they are in the same position (structures do not move) on the film during the exposure (see B in Fig. 21-54). Conversely, all objects located outside the objective plane, either above or below, are projected from one point on the film to another. For example see point A in Fig. 21-54 as the tube and film move from position 1 to position 2. Point A starts out on the left edge of the film in position 1 but ends up on the right edge in position 2 resulting in movement or blurring of objects at point A.

Point C below the fulcrum level also in the same way is blurred as it is projected from one edge of the film to the other edge. (Point C is on the right edge of the film in position one, and finally ends up on the left edge of the film in position two.)

The amount of movement of these structures is determined by the distance the object is from the fulcrum. Consequently, the objects that remain stationary (do not move) appear well defined (sharp) on the tomogram while those objects above and below the fulcrum move and therefore are blurred. This is referred to as the **tomographic blurring principle**.

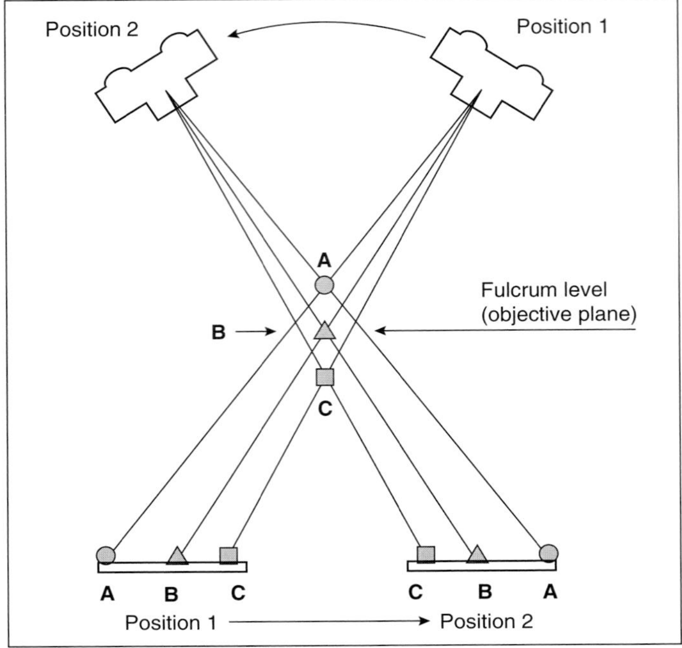

Fig. 21-54. Tomographic "blurring" principle.

Variable Vs. Fixed Fulcrum

The fulcrum level is used to determine the anatomical level of interest to be imaged. This may be achieved two ways. The most simple method utilizes a **variable fulcrum** (adjustable or movable) in which the **fulcrum level is moved** in relationship to the patient. This is shown in Fig. 21-55.

A second method involves a **fixed fulcrum** and an adjusting height table (Fig. 21-56). The fixed fulcrum adjusting height table is used most often with multidirectional or specialized tomographic units. In this system, the fulcrum level is changed by moving the patient and table up or down until the desired plane within the patient is at the level of the fixed fulcrum.

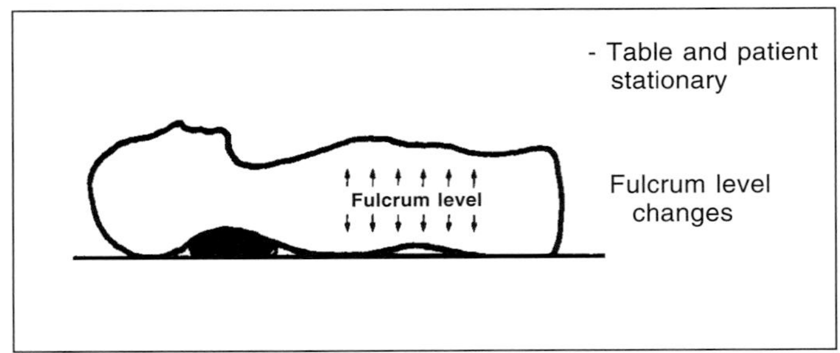

Fig. 21-55. Variable fulcrum.

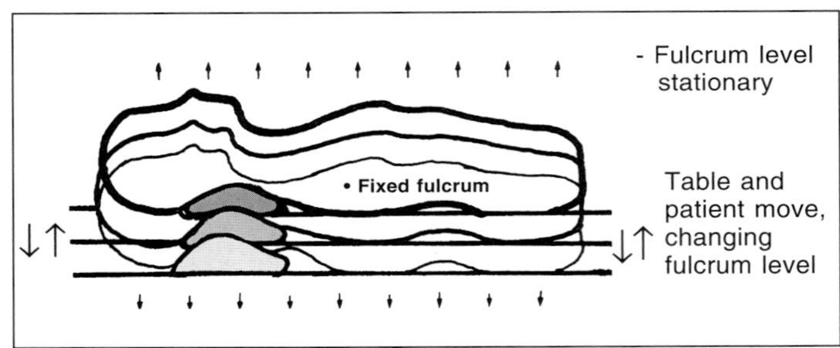

Fig. 21-56. Fixed fulcrum.

Determining Focal Level and Centering

To determine part centering, and where the starting fulcrum level should be set, two 90° conventional radiographs are taken, such as a PA or AP and a lateral chest for a tomogram of a suspect area in the lungs. One radiograph, the PA, locates the object of interest relative to its lateral (right or left) position, e.g., 5 cm to the right of the spine. The lateral radiograph is used to determine the anterior/posterior location, e.g., 10 cm posterior to the sternum. Both radiographs are useful in determining the superior/inferior location of the object. By using the PA and lateral radiographs as well as knowledge of the basic location of organs, the technologist can approximate the site of the object or area of specific interest. The initial scout tomogram would be taken with the fulcrum set at the estimated level of the specific area of interest. Centering would be done by determining specific distances as measured on the PA and/or lateral radiographs from known positioning landmarks.

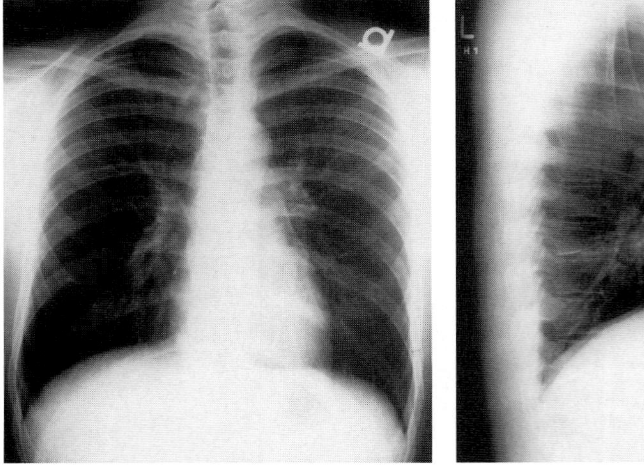

Fig. 21-57. AP. Localizing radiographs. Lateral. Fig. 21-58

BLUR

Blur was defined as the **area of distortion of objects outside the objective plane**. In tomography the structures which superimpose the object of interest are blurred. These blurred objects or structures within the patient are either above or below the level of interest at the fulcrum level.

Influencing and Controlling Factors

There are **four factors** which determine the amount of blurring. They are:

(1) **Distance the object is from the objective plane** (d).
(2) **Exposure angle** (Θ) (the degrees of angle of tube movement from position #1 to position #2).
(3) **Distance the object is from the film**.
(4) **Tube trajectory** (tube movement pattern).

The amount of blurring caused by the first two factors, (1) the distance the object is from the objective plane and (2) the exposure angle, is demonstrated in the following formula:

$$\text{Movement} = 2d \tan \Theta/2$$

Movement is a measurement of blurring wherein d is the distance of the object from the fulcrum, and Θ is the exposure angle. (Θ is the Greek symbol theta.)

(1) Distance of Object From Objective Plane (d): The above formula reveals that if all factors except d remain constant, then as d increases, movement or blurring increases. This is demonstrated by comparing Figs. 21-59 and 21-60 wherein the exposure angle remains constant at 30°, but "d" changes (distance from fulcrum plane to objects above and below). Fig. 21-59, with a greater "d" distance, has greater movement of objects "A" and "C" on the film from position one to position two, therefore it has increased blurring.

This demonstrates that those objects within the body that are farther from the focal plane have greater movement and therefore increased blurring.

(2) Exposure Angle (Θ): The formula also indicates that if only Θ (exposure angle) is increased and other factors remain constant, then the movement or blurring increases. This is demonstrated by comparing Fig. 21-61 at a 60° exposure angle, with the 30° angle of Fig. 21-60. The 60° exposure angle increases the movement of objects "A" and "C" even if "d" remains fixed, thereby increasing the blurring.

Formula summary: This formula demonstrates that as the **distance the object is from the objective plane increases** and/or as the **exposure angle is increased**, an increase in the amount of blurring occurs.

The net effect of this increased blurring is a **thinner focal plane** (objective plane) as described and demonstrated on the following page (Fig. 21-63).

(3) Object Film Distance: The third factor affecting blurring is the distance the object is from the film. **As the distance from the film increases, blurring increases**. This may not be an adjustable or controllable variable if it is determined by body part thickness, or by the general location or distance of the part being radiographed in relationship to the film. However, the body part may be placed on the table in such a way to increase the object film distance. For example, the head can be placed in a lateral position with the upside being examined rather than the downside.

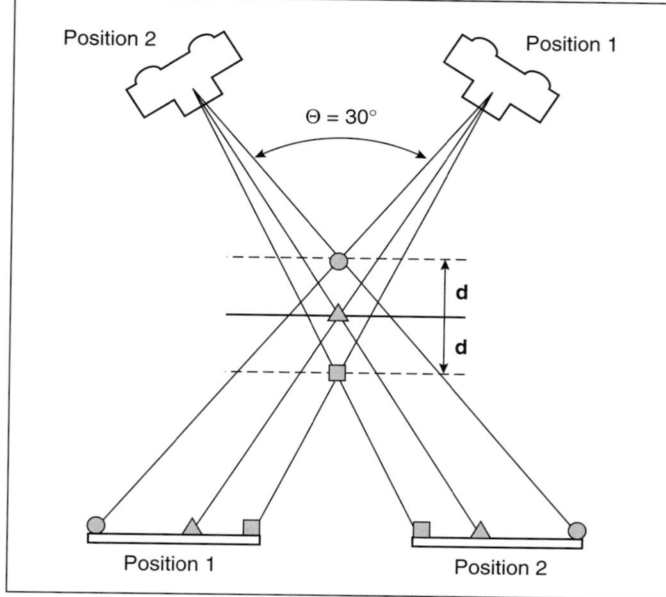

Fig. 21-59. Increase in "d" = Increase in movement or blurring.

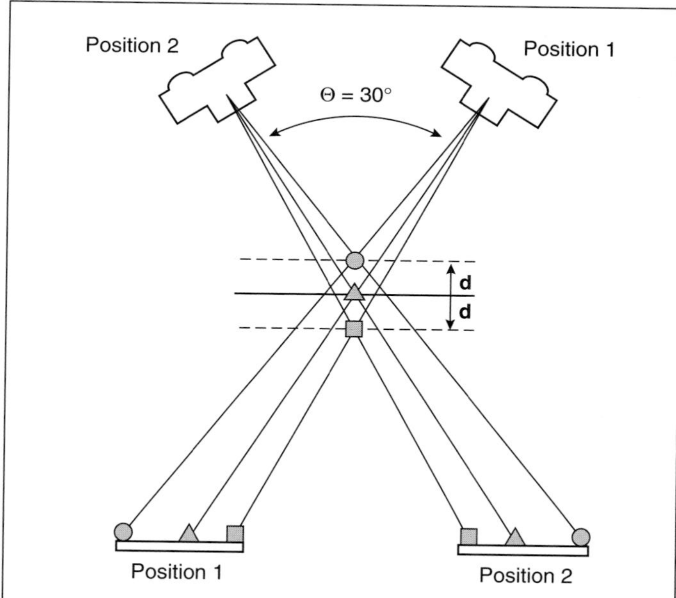

Fig. 21-60. Decrease in "d" = Decrease in movement or blurring.

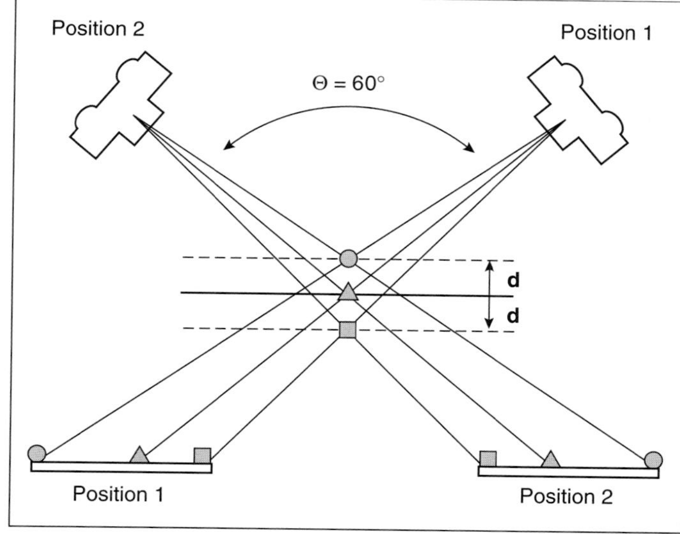

Fig. 21-61. Increase in exposure angle = Increase in movement and increase in blurring.

Blur continued

(4) Tube Trajectory or Tube Movement Pattern: The fourth and last influencing or controlling factor determining the amount of blurring is tube trajectory or movement pattern. Maximum blurring of an object occurs **when the structure is perpendicular to the direction of tube movement**. In unidirectional or linear tube trajectories, the tube moves in only one direction. This results in a large portion of the object being parallel to the tube movement. Therefore **less overall blurring** occurs with unidirectional tube trajectory.

Conversely, multidirectional tube trajectories result in few parts of the object being parallel to the total tube movement. Therefore elliptical or circular tube movements result in a **greater amount of blurring** than only linear movement.

Maximum Blurring Patterns: The spiral and hypocycloidal movement patterns result in **maximum blurring** in that these include a **vertical dimension** as part of their multitiered movement resulting in maximum blurring of those structures that are both close and farther away from the focal plane. These movements are most useful in tomographic procedures involving the skull, such as the small middle and inner ear structures, which require focal planes of 1 mm or less.

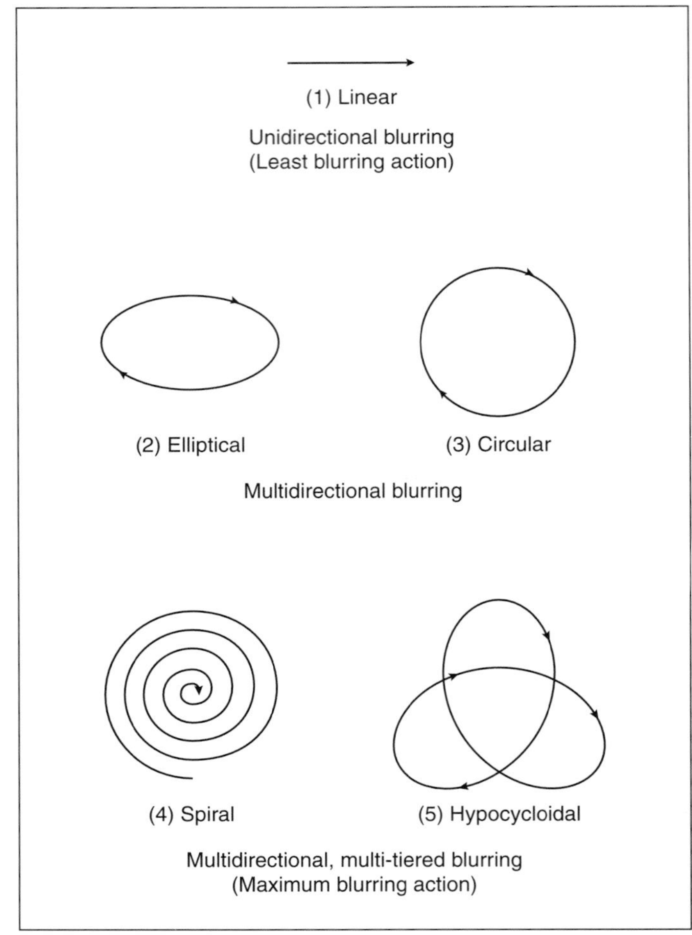

Fig. 21-62. Summary of tube trajectories.

Sectional Thickness (Objective Plane Thickness)

Blurring increases as the distance from the fulcrum level or objective plane increases as described above. Therefore, this results in a gradual process of blurring with those structures being the closest to the fulcrum level the least blurred, and those farthest away the most blurred. Also, the human eye is limited in its ability to distinguish blur from nonblur. Thus the human eye accepts a certain amount of blur as being well defined. The amount of blur the eye accepts as well defined is subjective and varies from one individual to another. These combined factors result in what is defined as **sectional thickness**, or **objective plane "thickness."**

The **more blurring** that occurs, **the thinner the objective plane**. The primary factor affecting sectional thickness, and which is under the control of the operator, is the **exposure angle** (Fig. 21-63). It is advantageous to adjust the thickness of the objective plane to correspond to the object being imaged. Small objects are best imaged using a thin objective plane with greater exposure angle, while large objects, such as the lung, should use a thick objective plane with less exposure angle.

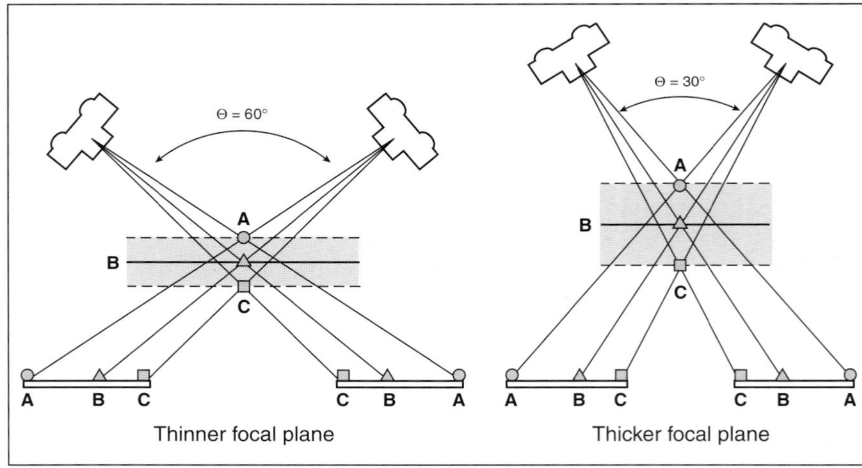

Fig. 21-63. Sectional thickness (objective plane thickness).

VARIATIONS OF CONVENTIONAL TOMOGRAPHY

There are various techniques and imaging modalities which evolved from the fundamental principles of conventional tomography. The following is a brief discussion on several tomographic applications.

Autotomography (Breathing Technique)

In **autotomography**, the **patient moves and the film and tube remain stationary**. This is commonly termed a "breathing technique," which is easily performed on a regular conventional radiographic unit and requires no special equipment. The objective is to blur out structures (by having the patient move them) which superimpose the object of interest. Examples of autotomography are the sternal oblique (Fig. 21-64) and the transthoracic lateral of the proximal humerus. For these examinations, the patient continues breathing during the exposure which blurs the ribs and pulmonary markings. Exposure times must be long enough (2 to 3 seconds) to allow sufficient movement of body parts during the exposure.

Autotomography may also be a nonbreathing method such as a moving mandible to show the upper C spine as demonstrated in Chapter 8, page 274.

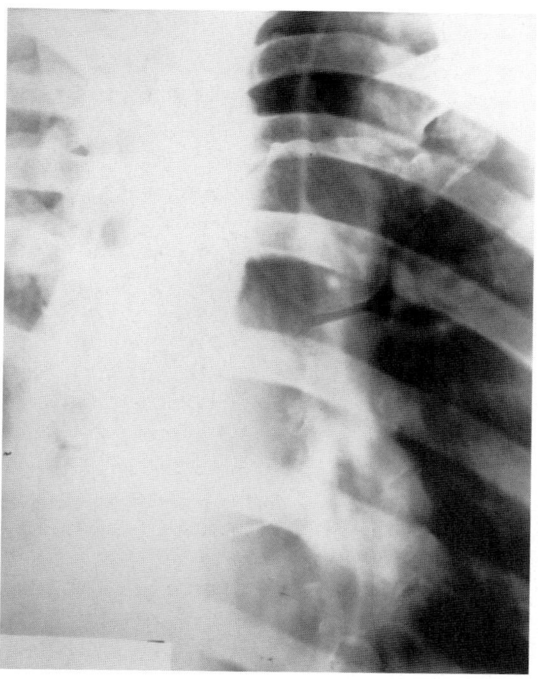

Fig. 21-64. Autotomogram–Sternum (breathing technique).

Pantomography (Panorex)

Pantomography is used for a curved body part, most commonly the mandible. An example of this is the **panorex unit** as illustrated in Figs. 21-65 and 21-66. In pantomography, the patient is stationary and the tube and film move. This is fully described and illustrated in Chapter 12 on the mandible.

The beam restrictor of a pantomographic unit has a thin narrow slit (see small white arrows Fig. 21-65), which is essential for eliminating the diverging x-rays that normally produce penumbra blurring. This results in a pantomogram, which has an image similar to a conventional radiograph (Fig. 21-67).

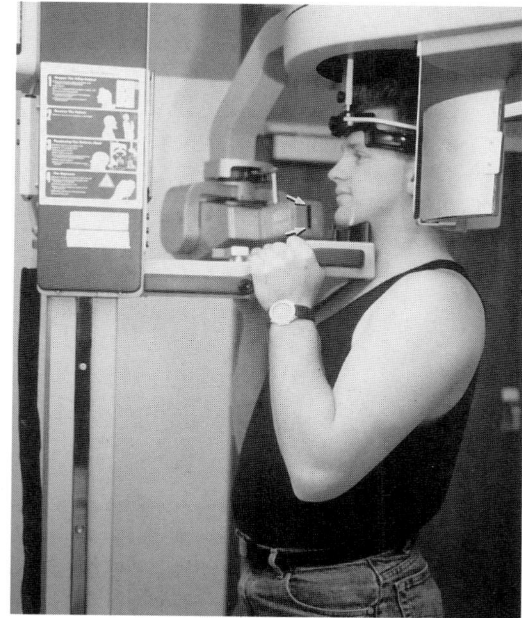

Fig. 21-65. Panorex unit.

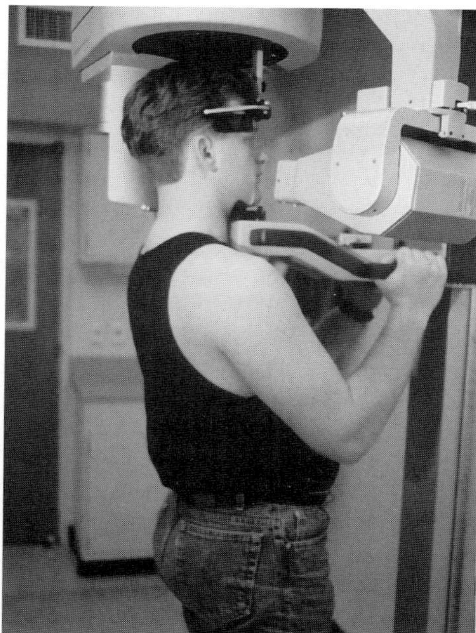

Fig. 21-66. Panorex unit.

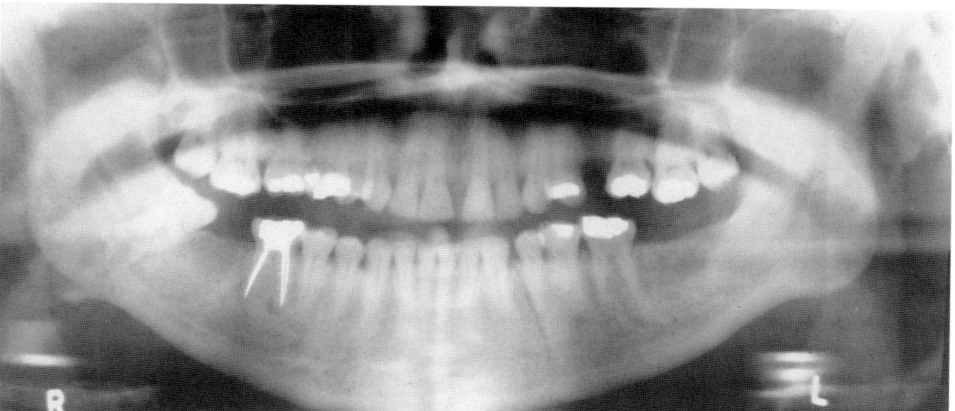

Fig. 21-67. Pantomogram (panorex) of mandible.

CHAPTER 22

Cranial Computed Tomography

CONTRIBUTIONS BY:
Barry T. Anthony, RT (R)

22

CONTENTS

Radiographic Anatomy

Anatomy of central nervous system (CNS) **634**

Brain divisions:
- Forebrain
  –Cerebrum, thalamus and hypothalamus **636**
- Midbrain and hindbrain
  –Pons, medulla and cerebellum **639**

Gray and white matter **640**

Cranial nerves **641**

Sectional anatomy of brain:
- Coronal sections **643**
- Axial sections **645**

Basic Principles and Procedures

Scanner principles **649**

Basic principle **651**

Principles of image reconstruction **651**

Computed tomographic image **653**

Computed tomographic system:
- Scan unit, processing unit, display unit, and storage system **654**

Cranial computed tomographic procedure **655**

CCT positioning **656**

Examples of positive CCT images **658**

Radiographic Anatomy

COMPUTED TOMOGRAPHY

The **general principles** of computed tomography (CT) are similar to conventional tomography as described in the preceding chapter in which the **x-ray tube and the image receptors move about a focal point during the exposure**. The primary difference, as described later in this chapter, relates to the use of computers to reconstruct the focused image or tomographic "slice" as received by the image receptors.

The development of computed tomography represents one of the most dramatic advances in radiology since Roentgen's discovery of x-rays in 1895. The person credited with the first successful clinical demonstration of CT was G. N. Hounsfield, a research scientist at EMI Research Laboratories in England, who in 1972 produced the first cranial scan, a computer reconstructed image displayed on a television monitor.

Prior to **cranial computed tomography** (CCT), direct imaging methods for the cranium could visualize very little except cranial bony anatomy. Occasionally a calcified structure, often the pineal gland, would visualize. Various brain tissues, cerebrospinal-fluid-filled spaces and blood vessels merged into a homogeneous gray shadow and could not be differentiated. Therefore, invasive special procedures utilizing some type of contrast medium were required to visualize the ventricles or blood vessels. A certain degree of risk was inherent in these special examinations.

The astounding success of CCT is based on the fact that direct information concerning the structure of normal and abnormal brain tissue can be obtained without subjecting the patient to painful and potentially fatal invasive procedures. Since individual anatomic structures can be visualized on computed tomograms, a good understanding of gross and sectional anatomy is essential. Since CTs are viewed in sectional form, various coronal and axial sections are described in this chapter.

ANATOMY OF THE CENTRAL NERVOUS SYSTEM

Central Nervous System (CNS)

The central nervous system can be divided into two main divisions: (1) the **brain or encephalon** *(en-sef′ ah-lon),* which occupies the cavity of the cranium, and (2) the **spinal cord or medulla spinalis,** *(me-dul′ lah spi-na′ lis),* which extends inferiorly from the brain and is protected by the bony vertebral column. The spinal cord terminates at the lower border of L1 with a tapered area called the **conus medullaris** *(ko′ nus med′ u-lar-is).*

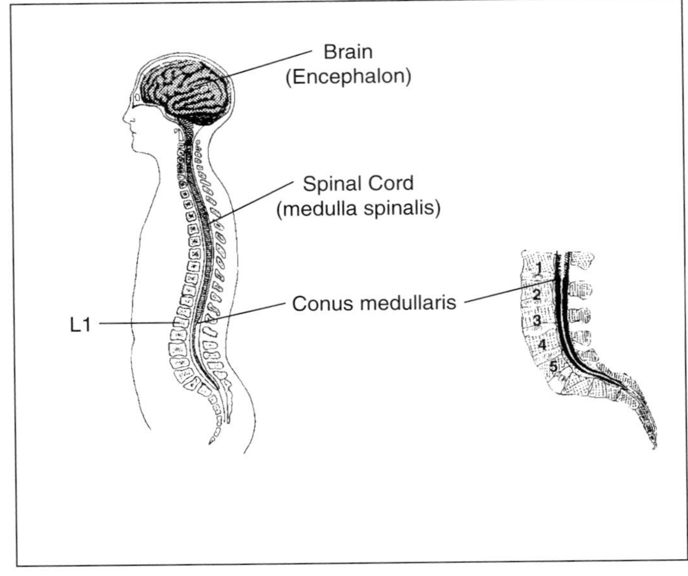

Fig. 22-1. Central nervous system (CNS).

Neurons

Neurons or nerve cells are the specialized cells of the nervous system that conduct electrical impulses. Each neuron is composed of an **axon, a cell body** and one or more **dendrites.** Dendrites are processes that conduct impulses toward the neuron cell body. The axon is a process leading away from the cell body.

A multipolar motoneuron is shown in Fig. 22-2. This type of neuron is typical of the neurons conducting impulses from the spinal cord to muscle tissue. A multipolar neuron is one with several dendrites and a single axon.

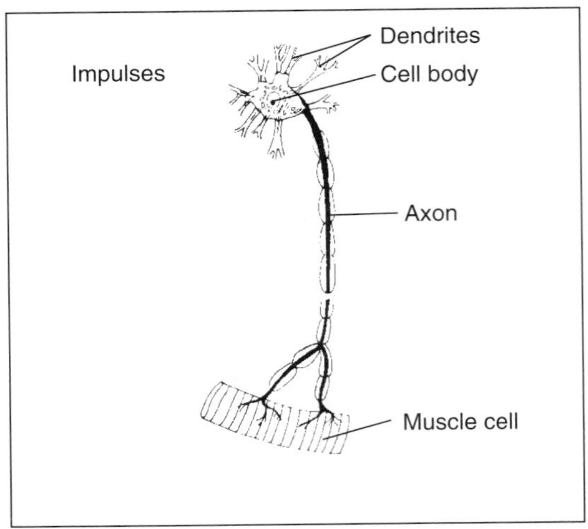

Fig. 22-2. Multipolar motoneuron (several dendrites, one axon).

Brain Coverings–Meninges

Both the brain and spinal cord are enclosed by **three** protective coverings or membranes termed **meninges**. Starting externally these three are the (1) **dura mater** *(du′ rah ma′ ter)*, (2) **arachnoid** *(ah-rak′ noid)*, and (3) **pia mater,** *(pi′ ah ma′ ter)*.

The outermost membrane is the **dura mater** which means "hard" or "tough mother." This strong fibrous brain covering has an **inner** and an **outer layer**. The outer layer of the dura mater is tightly fused to the inner layer, except for spaces that are provided for large venous blood channels called **venous sinuses.** The outer layer closely adheres to the inner table of the **cranium** or skull.

The innermost of these membranes is the pia mater**,** literally meaning "tender mother." This membrane is very thin and highly vascular and lies next to the brain and spinal cord. It encloses the entire surface of the brain, dipping into each of the fissures and sulci.

Between the pia mater and dura mater is a delicate avascular membrane called the **arachnoid** *(ah-rak′ noid)*. Delicate threadlike trabeculae attach the arachnoid membrane to the pia mater.

Meningeal Spaces: Immediately exterior to each meningeal layer is a space or potential space. Therefore there are three of these spaces or potential spaces, the (1) **epidural space**, (2) **subdural space**, and (3) **subarachnoid space**. Exterior to the dura mater, between the dura and the inner table of the skull, is a potential space termed the epidural space**.** Beneath the dura mater, between the dura and the arachnoid, is a narrow space called the subdural space, which contains a thin film of fluid. Both the epidural and the subdural spaces are potential sites for hemorrhage following trauma to the head.

Beneath the arachnoid membrane, between the arachnoid and the pia mater, is a comparatively wide space termed the subarachnoid space**.** The subarachnoid space of both the brain and spinal cord is normally filled with **cerebrospinal fluid (CSF)**.

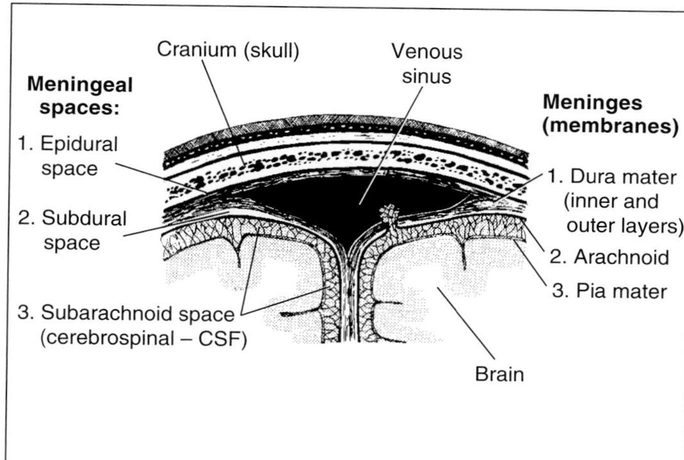

Fig. 22-3. Meninges and meningeal spaces.

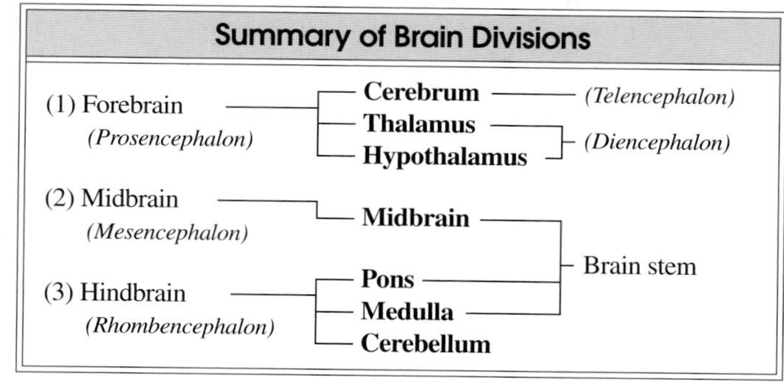

Summary of Brain Divisions

Division	Structures	Secondary terms
(1) Forebrain *(Prosencephalon)*	**Cerebrum**	*(Telencephalon)*
	Thalamus	*(Diencephalon)*
	Hypothalamus	*(Diencephalon)*
(2) Midbrain *(Mesencephalon)*	**Midbrain**	Brain stem
(3) Hindbrain *(Rhombencephalon)*	**Pons**	Brain stem
	Medulla	Brain stem
	Cerebellum	

THREE DIVISIONS OF THE BRAIN (ENCEPHALON)

The brain can be divided into three general areas: (1) the **forebrain,** (2) the **midbrain,** and (3) the **hindbrain.** These three divisions of the brain are further divided into specific areas and structures. Understanding relationships between the structures in each of these three divisions helps in understanding the anatomy of the brain. See summary chart of brain divisions on the right. Secondary terms found in earlier literature for these various divisions are included in this chart.

Each of these three brain divisions are shown on the midsagittal sectional drawing in Fig. 22-4. Note that the **forebrain** consists of three parts. First is the very large **cerebrum** *(ser′ e-brum),* then two small midsection portions called the **thalamus** *(thal′ ah-mus)* and the **hypothalamus** *(hi″po-thal′ ah-mus)*.

The **midbrain** is located centrally between the hypothalamus superiorly and the pons inferiorly. As the name implies, it connects the forebrain to the hindbrain.

The **hindbrain** consists of three parts also. First is the **cerebellum** *(se″ re-bel′ um)*, then the smaller **pons** *(ponz)* and **medulla** *(me-dul′ ah)*, meaning innermost part), which is also correctly called the **medulla oblongata** *(ob″ long-ga′ tah)*.

The combination of **midbrain**, **pons** and **medulla** make up the **brain stem**, which passes through the large opening at the base of the skull, the foramen magnum to become the **spinal cord**.

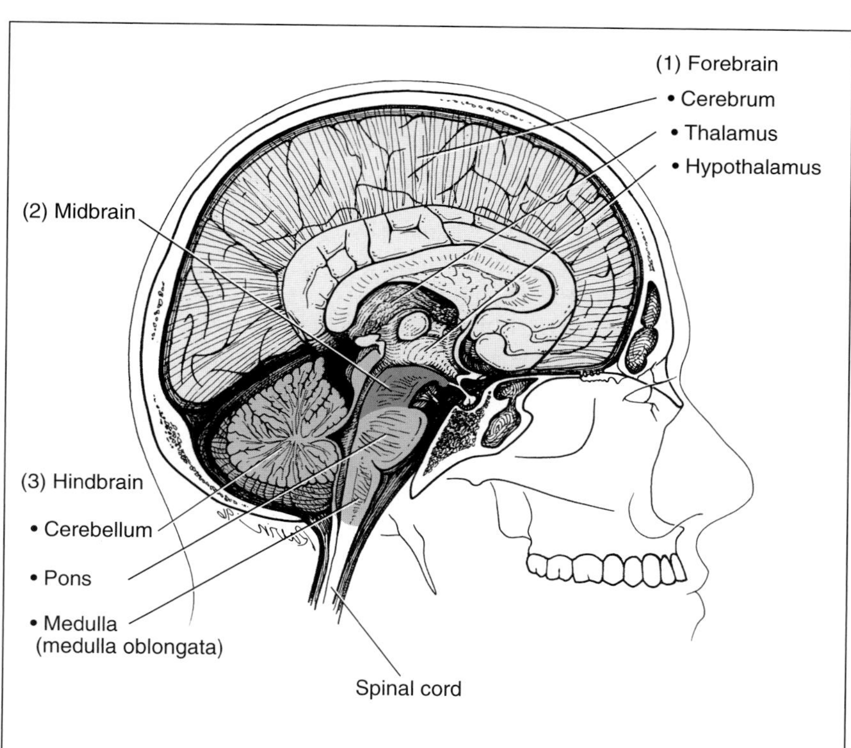

Fig. 22-4. Brain (midsagittal section).

FOREBRAIN

The first part of the forebrain to be studied is the large **cerebrum**, made up of right and left **cerebral hemispheres**.

Cerebrum

A sagittal section through the head and neck leaving the brain and upper spinal cord intact is demonstrated in Fig. 22-5, showing the relative size of the various structures including the **five lobes** of the cerebrum. The surface layer of the entire cerebrum, about 2 to 4 mm in thickness, is called the **cerebral cortex**. As can be seen, the total cerebrum occupies the majority of the cranial cavity.

Five Lobes of Each Cerebral Hemisphere: Each side of the cerebrum is termed a **cerebral** *(ser′ e-bral)* **hemisphere** and is divided into five lobes. The four lobes seen in Fig. 22-5 lie beneath the cranial bones of the same name. The **frontal lobe** lies under the frontal bone and the **parietal lobe** under the parietal bone. Similarly, the **occipital lobe** and the **temporal lobe** lie under their respective cranial bones. The fifth lobe, termed the **insula** or **central lobe**, is more centrally located and cannot be seen on a lateral view.

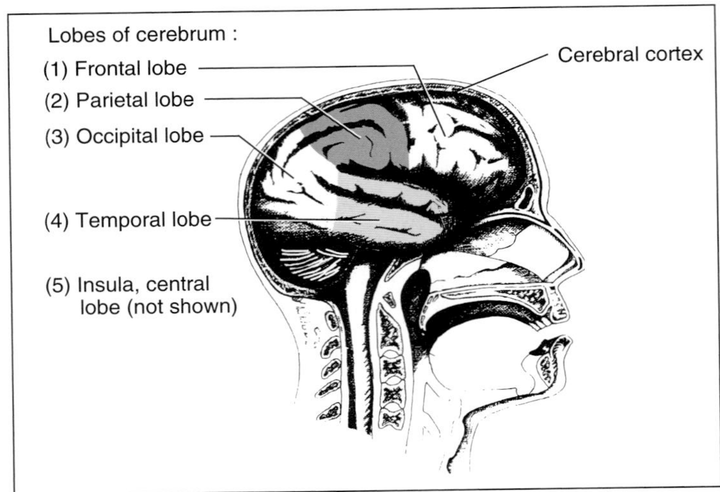

Fig. 22-5. Demonstrates four lobes of each cerebral hemisphere.

Cerebral Hemispheres

The top of the brain is shown in Fig. 22-6. The cerebrum is partially separated by a deep **longitudinal fissure** in the midsagittal plane. This fissure divides the cerebrum into a right and a left cerebral hemisphere. Parts of the **frontal, parietal** and **occipital lobes** are again visualized on this top-view drawing.

The surface of each cerebral hemisphere is marked by numerous grooves and convolutions, which are formed during the rapid embryonic growth of this portion of the brain. Each convolution or raised area is termed a **gyrus**. Two such gyri, an **anterior central (precentral) gyrus** and a **posterior central (post central) gyrus**, are shown on each side of the **central sulcus**. A sulcus is a shallow groove, and the central sulcus, which divides the frontal and parietal lobes of the cerebrum, is a landmark for identifying specific sensory areas of the cortex.

A deeper groove is called a **fissure**, such as the deep **longitudinal fissure** separating the two hemispheres.

The **corpus callosum**, located deep within the longitudinal fissure and not visible on this drawing, consists of an arched mass of transverse fibers (white matter) connecting the two cerebral hemispheres. (A midsagittal sectional view of the corpus callosum is shown on page 639 in Figs. 22-14 and 22-15.) A fold of dura matter, termed the **falx cerebri** (not visible on these drawings) extends downward into the longitudinal fissure separating the two cerebral hemispheres.

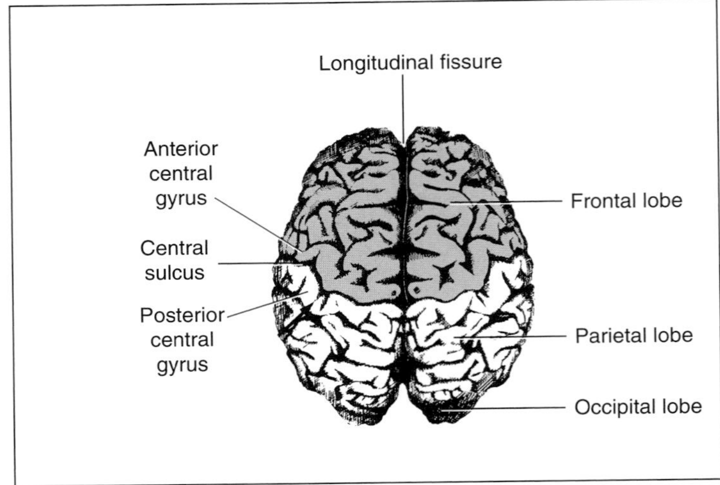

Fig. 22-6. Cerebral hemispheres (top view). Demonstrates the frontal, parietal and occipital lobes; and the relative differences between a gyrus, sulcus and fissure.

Cerebral Ventricles

A thorough understanding of the cerebral **ventricles** is important for cranial computed tomography. The ventricular system of the brain is connected to the subarachnoid space. There are **four cavities** in the ventricular system. These four cavities are filled with cerebrospinal fluid and interconnect through small tubes. The lateral drawing of the ventricular system in Fig. 22-7 demonstrates the **right and left lateral ventricles,** the **third ventricle** and the **fourth ventricle**. The two lateral ventricles are located within the right and left cerebral hemispheres, while the third and fourth ventricles are midline structures.

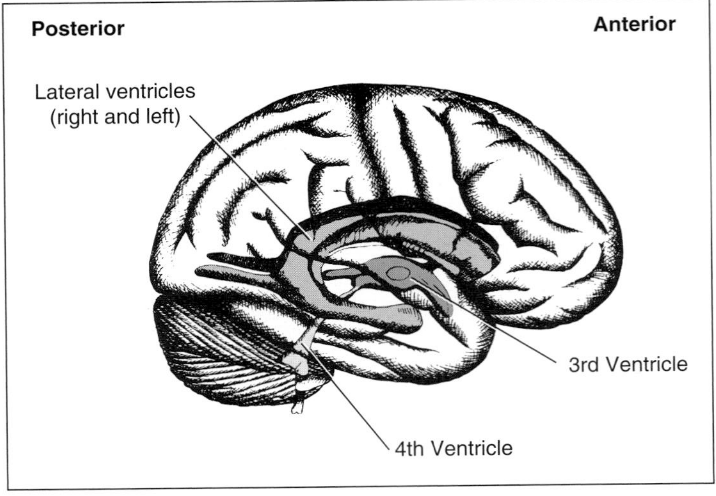

Fig. 22-7. Cerebral ventricles.

Lateral Ventricles

Each lateral ventricle is composed of four parts. The superior and lateral views in Fig. 22-8 demonstrate that each of the lateral ventricles has a centrally located **body** and three projections or horns extending from the body. The **anterior or frontal horn** is toward the front. The **posterior or occipital horn** is toward the back, and the **inferior or temporal horn** extends inferiorly.

The two lateral ventricles are located on each side of the midsagittal plane within the cerebral hemispheres and are mirror images of each other. Certain pathology, such as a space-occupying lesion or "mass lesion," would alter the symmetrical appearance of the ventricular system.

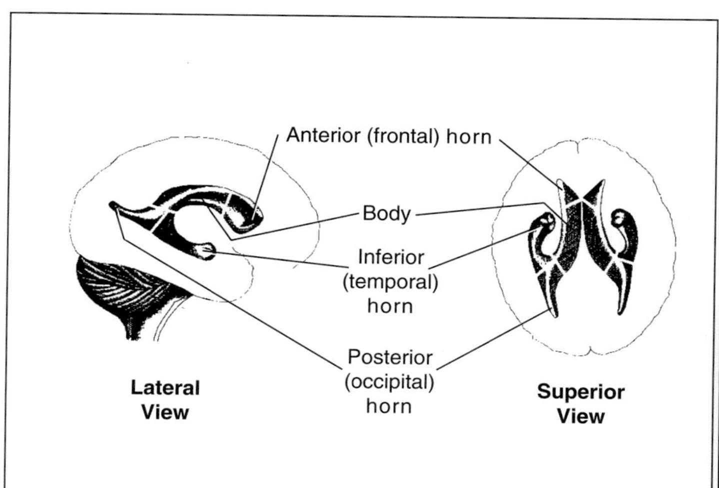

Fig. 22-8. Lateral ventricles.

Third Ventricle

Each of the lateral ventricles connects to the third ventricle through an **interventricular foramen (foramen of Monro). The third ventricle** is located in the midline and is roughly four-sided in shape. It lies just below the level of the bodies of the two lateral ventricles. The **pineal** *(pin′ e-al)* **gland** is attached to the roof of the posterior part of the third ventricle which causes a recess in the posterior part of this ventricle. (The pineal gland is also shown in Fig. 22-15 in relationship to the thalamus portion of the forebrain.)

Fourth Ventricle

The cavity of the third ventricle connects posteroinferiorly with the **fourth ventricle** through a passage known as the **cerebral aqueduct or aqueduct of Sylvius.** The diamond-shaped fourth ventricle connects with a wide portion of the subarachnoid space called the **cisterna magna.** On each side of the fourth ventricle is a lateral extension termed the **lateral recess (foramen of Luschka)**, which also connects with the subarachnoid space through an opening or foramen.

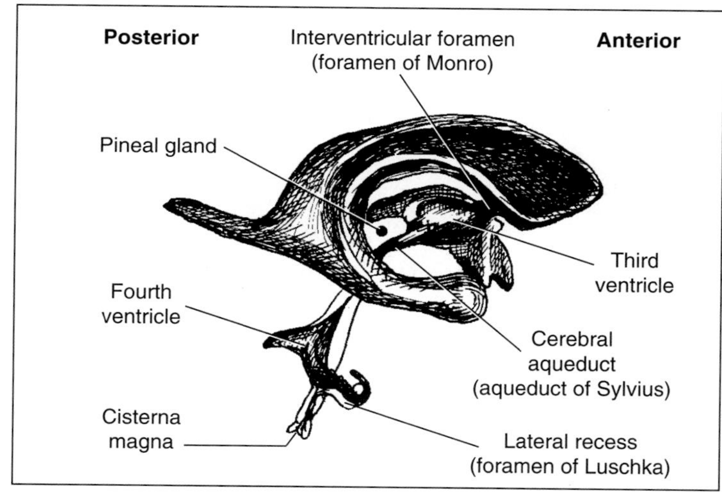

Fig. 22-9. Third and fourth ventricles (lateral view).

Superior View of Ventricles: A superior view of the ventricles is shown in Fig. 22-10. This view demonstrates the relationship of the **third and fourth ventricles** to the two **lateral ventricles.** The third ventricle is a narrow, slitlike structure lying in the midline between and below the bodies of the lateral ventricles. The **cerebral aqueduct** is clearly shown connecting the third ventricle to the fourth ventricle.

The **lateral recess** is shown on each side of the fourth ventricle providing a communication with the subarachnoid space. The **body**, **inferior horn** and the **anterior** and **posterior horns** of the lateral ventricles are again well demonstrated on this top view.

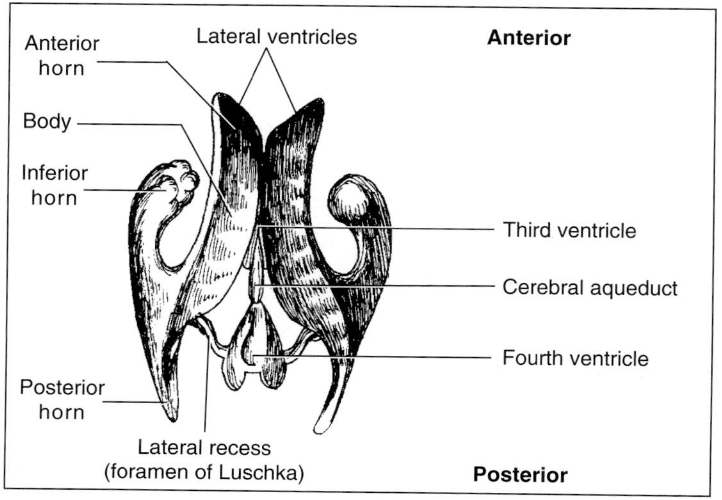

Fig. 22-10. Ventricles (superior view).

Anterior View of Ventricles: An anterior view of the ventricles with the outline of the brain in place is shown in Fig. 22-11. The **interventricular foramina** connect the body of each lateral ventricle to the third ventricle. This view emphasizes the fact that the **third** and the **fourth ventricles** are midline structures. The **anterior horn, body** and **inferior horn** of each lateral ventricle are shown on this drawing as they would appear on a frontal projection of a cerebral pneumogram. The region of the lateral recess connecting the fourth ventricle to the subarachnoid space is also shown.

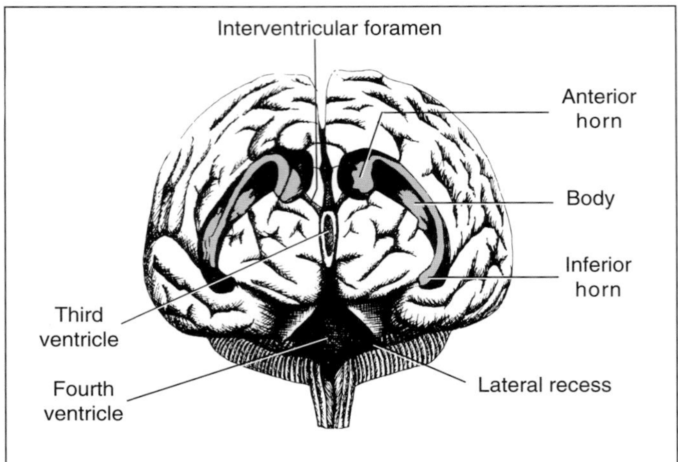

Fig. 22-11. Ventricles (anterior view).

Subarachnoid Cisterns

Cerebrospinal fluid is normally manufactured within each ventricle. After cerebrospinal fluid leaves the **fourth ventricle,** it completely surrounds the brain and spinal cord by filling the subarachnoid space, as shown by the dotted areas in Fig. 22-12. Any blockage along the pathway leading from the ventricles to the subarachnoid space may cause excessive accumulation of cerebrospinal fluid within the ventricles, a condition known as **hydrocephalus**.

There are various larger areas within the subarachnoid space or system called **cisterns**, the largest being the **cisterna magna**, located inferiorly to the fourth ventricle and the cerebellum. The **cisterna pontis** is located just inferior and anterior to the **pons.** Each of the larger black "dots" in these drawings indicate specific cisterns that are usually named according to their locations. The **chiasmatic cistern**, shown on the top view drawing of the brain (Fig. 22-13), is so called because of its relationship to the optic chiasma, the site of crossings of optic nerves as will be identified in later drawings.

Various other cisterns lie along the base of the brain and brain stem. Since the midbrain is totally surrounded by fluid-filled cisterns, this area can be well seen on a CT scan.

The cerebrospinal-fluid-filled subarachnoid space and ventricular system are very important in computed tomography, since these areas can be differentiated from tissue structures.

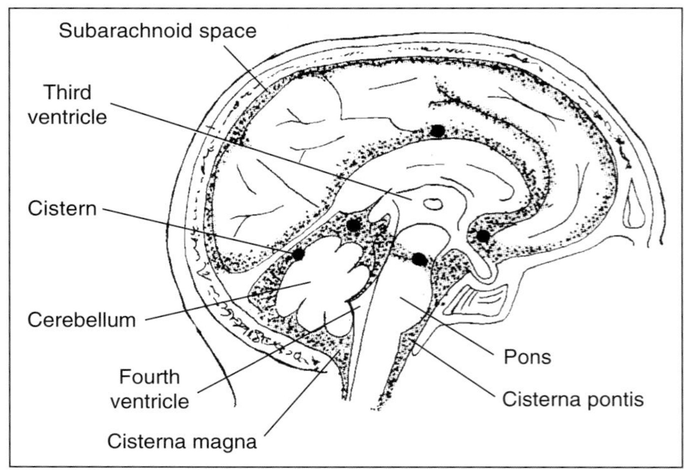

Fig. 22-12. Subarachnoid cisterns–side view.

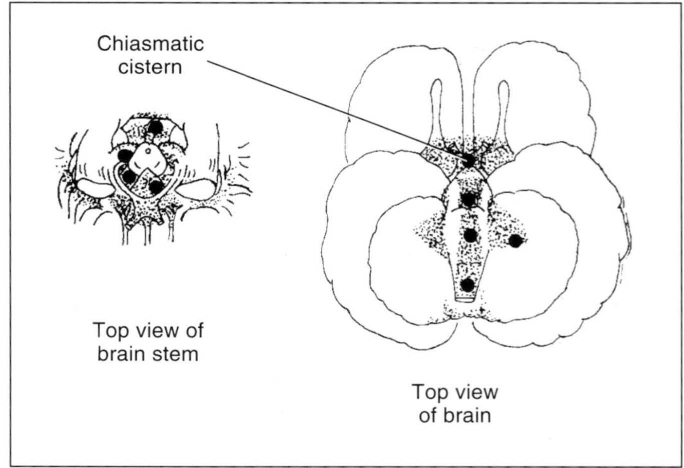

Fig. 22-13. Subarachnoid cisterns–top view.

Forebrain continued

Thalamus (Figs. 22-14 and 22-15)

Following the large cerebrum, the second part of the forebrain is the **thalamus**. The thalamus is a relatively small oval structure (about 1 inch in length) located just above the midbrain and under the corpus callosum. It consists of two oval masses of primarily gray matter or nuclei that **form part of the walls of the third ventricle**, just superior to the midbrain.

These groups of nuclei (gray matter) of the thalamus serve as relay stations for most of the sensory impulses as they pass from the spinal cord and midbrain structures into the cerebral cortex. Thus the thalamus serves as **an interpretation center** for certain sensory impulses such as **pain**, **temperature** and **touch**, as well as **certain emotions and memory**.

The thalamus and hypothalamus together make up the diencephalon portion of the forebrain as described previously.

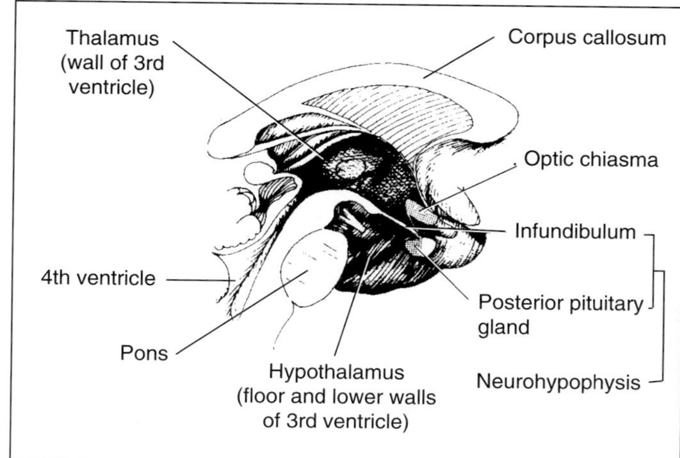

Fig. 22-14. Thalamus and hypothalamus (midsagittal section).

Hypothalamus (Figs. 22-14 and 22-15)

The third and final division of the forebrain is the **hypothalamus**, "hypo" meaning under, thus its location under the thalamus. The hypothalamus forms the floor and lower walls of the third ventricle. Three structures associated with the hypothalamus as labeled on the midsagittal section in Fig. 22-14 are the **infundibulum** *(in″ fun-dib′ u-lum)*, **posterior pituitary gland** and the **optic chiasma** *(kı-as′ mah)*.

The infundibulum is a conical process projecting downward and ending in the posterior lobe of the pituitary gland. The infundibulum plus the posterior pituitary are known as the **neurohypophysis** *(nu″ ro-hi-pof′ i-sis)*.

The optic chiasma, so named because it resembles the Greek letter X (chi), is located superior to the pituitary gland and anterior to the third ventricle.

The hypothalamus is small in size but it **controls important body activities** most of which are related to **homeostasis**, the tendency or ability of the body to stabilize its normal body states.

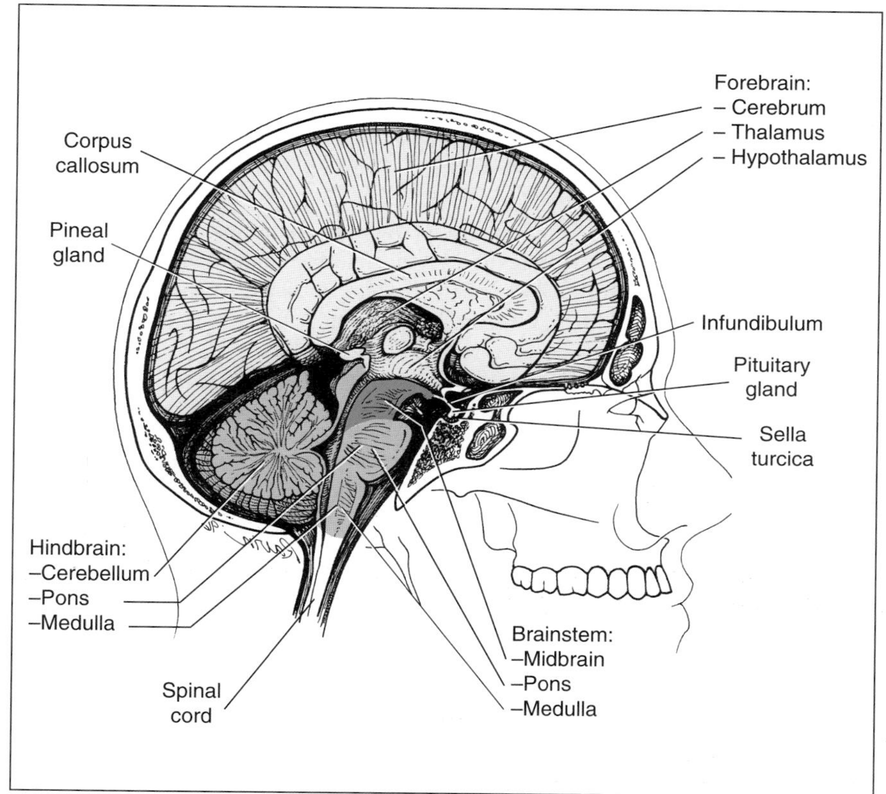

Fig. 22-15. Brain (midsagittal section).

MIDBRAIN AND HINDBRAIN

The **midbrain** is a short, constricted portion of the upper brain stem connecting the forebrain to the hindbrain.

The **hindbrain** consists of the **cerebellum**, **pons** and **medulla.** As seen in the drawing in Fig. 22-15, the cerebellum is the largest portion of the hindbrain and the second largest portion of the entire brain and will be described in detail on the following page.

Brain Stem

The brain stem includes the **midbrain** and the **pons** and **medulla.** The pons is a prominent oval structure inferior to the midbrain. The medulla is the final portion of the brain stem, located at the level of the foramen magnum, the opening at the base of the skull. Thus, the brain stem is composed of midbrain, pons and medulla, and serves to connect the forebrain to the spinal cord.

Pituitary and Pineal Glands

Two important midline structures are the pituitary and pineal glands. The **pineal gland** was demonstrated in its relationship to the third ventricle in Fig. 22-9. This small gland (≈5 mm or ¼ inch in length and width) is an **endocrine gland,** which secretes hormones that **aid in regulating certain secretory activities**.

The important **pituitary gland**, also called the **hypophysis** *(hi-pof′ i-sis)*, is referred to as the **"master" gland** because it regulates so many body activities. It is located in, and protected by, the **sella turcica** of the sphenoid bone, and is attached to the hypothalamus of the brain by the **infundibulum** (shown in Figs. 22-14 and 22-15). This gland which is also relatively small, about 1.3 cm or ½ inch in diameter, is divided into anterior and posterior lobes. The hormones secreted by this "master" gland **control a wide range of body functions, including growth and reproductive functions**.

Cerebellum

The last part of the brain to be described is the **cerebellum** which occupies the major portion of the inferior and posterior cranial fossa. In the adult, the size proportion between the cerebrum and cerebellum is about eight to one. The anterior and posterior surfaces of the cerebellum are shown in Fig. 22-16.

The cerebellum is shaped somewhat like a butterfly and consists of two **hemispheres** united by a narrow median strip, the **vermis**. Toward the superior end of the anterior surface is the wide, shallow **anterior cerebellar notch.** The fourth ventricle is located within the anterior cerebellar notch, separating the pons and medulla from the cerebellum (also shown in Fig. 22-14 on preceding page).

Inferiorly, along the posterior surface, the cerebellar hemispheres are separated by the **posterior cerebellar notch.** An extension of the dura mater, termed the **falx cerebelli**, is located within the posterior cerebellar notch.

The cerebellum primarily **coordinates the important motor functions** of the body such as **coordination**, **posture** and **balance**.

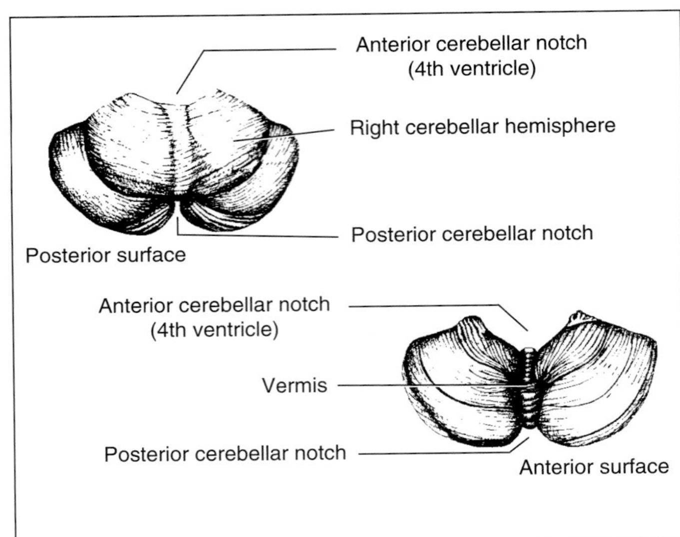

Fig. 22-16. Cerebellum.

GRAY MATTER AND WHITE MATTER

The central nervous system can be divided by appearance into white matter and gray matter. **White matter** in the brain and spinal cord is composed of **tracts**, which consist of bundles of **myelinated axons**. Myelinated axons are those wrapped in a myelin sheath, a fatty substance having a creamy-white color. Thus, axons comprise the majority of the white matter.

The **gray matter** is composed mainly of **neuron dendrites** and **cell bodies**. A section of brain tissue through the cerebral hemispheres is shown in Fig. 22-17. At this level of the brain, gray matter forms the **outer cerebral cortex,** while the brain tissue under the cortex is white matter. This underlying mass of white substance is termed the **centrum semiovale.** Deep within the cerebrum, inferior to this level, is more gray matter termed the **cerebral nuclei** or **basal ganglia**.

Since a cranial computed tomographic scan can differentiate between white and gray matter, a section through the cerebral nuclei provides a wealth of diagnostic information. The horizontal or axial section of the right cerebral hemisphere shown in Fig. 22-18 demonstrates those areas that can usually be visualized. Areas of white matter include the **corpus callosum** and the **centrum semiovale**. Gray matter areas include the **cerebral nuclei**, the **thalamus** and the **cerebral cortex**.

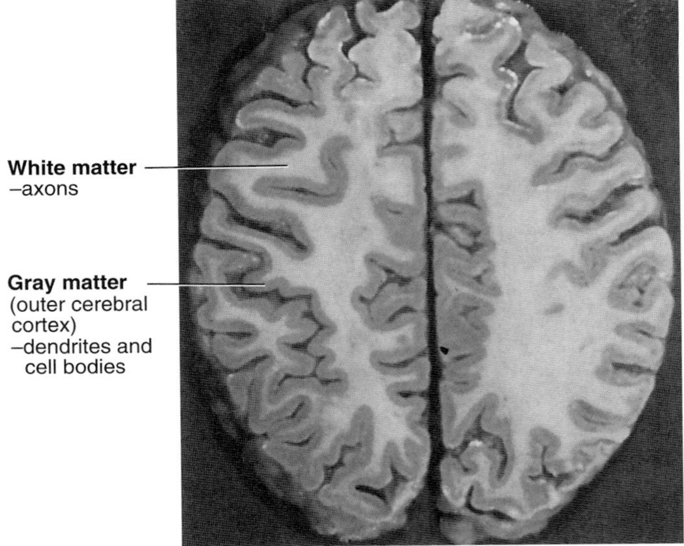

Fig. 22-17. Brain section demonstrating white and gray matter.

Summary–White Matter vs. Gray Matter

White Matter: White matter consists of **myelinated axons** commonly identified on CT brain sections as light or "white" appearing tissue. It is most commonly seen on sectional scans of the cerebral hemispheres as subcortical white masses of **centrum semiovale**, which are fibers connecting the gray matter of the cerebral cortex with the deep more caudal parts of the midbrain and spinal cord.

The second major white matter structure is the **corpus callosum**, a band of fibers connecting the right and left cerebral hemispheres deep within the longitudinal fissure.

Gray Matter: The thin outer layer of the folds of the **cerebral cortex** is gray matter, made up of dendrites and cell bodies.

Other gray matter of the brain includes more central brain structures such as the **cerebral nuclei** or **basal ganglia** located deep within the cerebral hemispheres, and the groups of **nuclei** making up the **thalamus**.

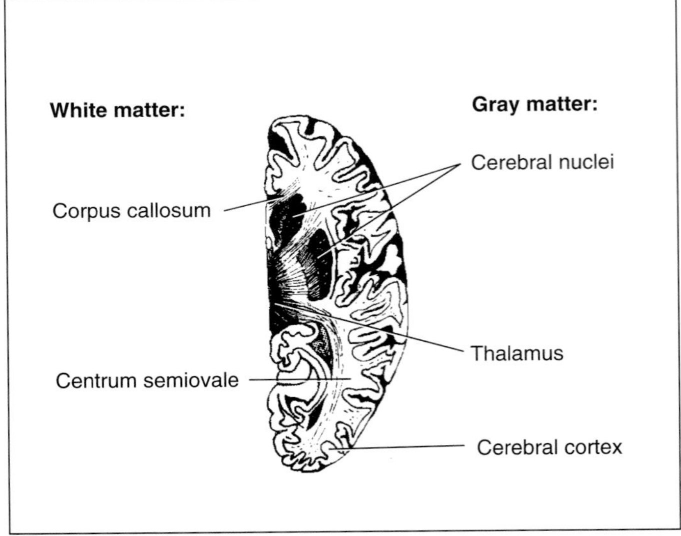

Fig. 22-18. White and gray matter.

Cerebral Nuclei (Basal Ganglia) (Gray Matter)

The cerebral nuclei or basal ganglia are paired collections of gray matter deep within each cerebral hemisphere. There are four specific areas or groupings of these cerebral nuclei as shown on this cutaway drawing. These are the (1) **caudate nucleus**, (2) the **lentiform nucleus**, composed of putamen and globus pallidus, (3) the **claustrum** (not visible on this drawing), and (4) the **amygdaloid nucleus** or body.

The relationship of the **brain stem** and **cerebellum** to three of the cerebral nuclei and to the **thalamus** is shown in Fig. 22-19. The cerebral nuclei are bilaterally symmetrical collections of gray matter located on **both sides of the third ventricle**.

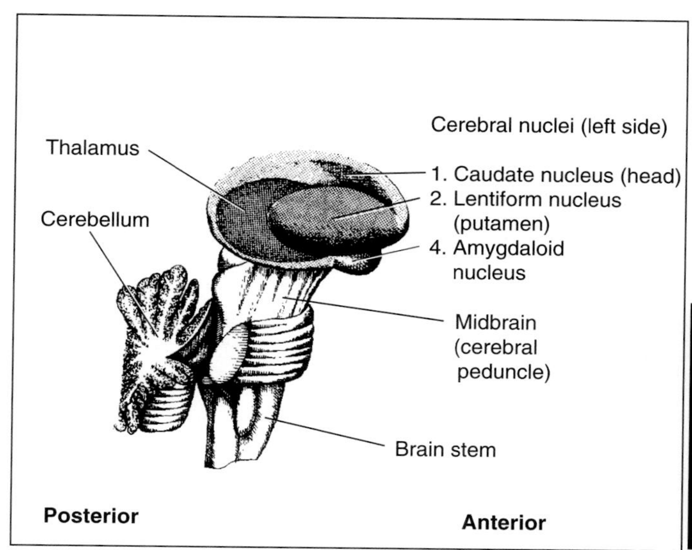

Fig. 22-19. Midsagittal view of cerebral nuclei (basal ganglia) deep within the cerebrum.

Brain–Inferior Surface

The inferior surface of the brain (Fig. 22-20) demonstrates the **infundibulum, pituitary gland** and **optic chiasma**, which are anterior to the **pons** and **midbrain**. Extending forward from the optic chiasma are the large **optic nerves,** and extending posterolaterally are the **optic tracts**. A portion of the **corpus callosum** is shown to be located deep within the longitudinal fissure.

Cranial Nerves

The 12 pairs of cranial nerves are shown on this drawing of the inferior surface of the brain. The pairs shown are:

1. **Olfactory nerve**	On
2. **Optic nerve**	Old
3. Oculomotor nerve	Olympus'
4. Trochlear nerve	Towering
5. **Trigeminal nerve**	Tops
6. Abducens nerve	A
7. Facial nerve	Finn
8. Acoustic nerve	And
9. Glossopharyngeal nerve	German
10. **Vagus nerve**	Viewed
11. Spinal accessory nerve	Some
12. Hypoglossal nerve	Hops

The more important of the cranial nerves are numbers 1, **2**, **5** and **10**.

The familiar mnemonic, "**On Old Olympus's Towering Tops**, **A Finn** and **German Viewed Some Hops**," gives the first letter of each of the 12 pairs of cranial nerves and can be used to help remember these names.

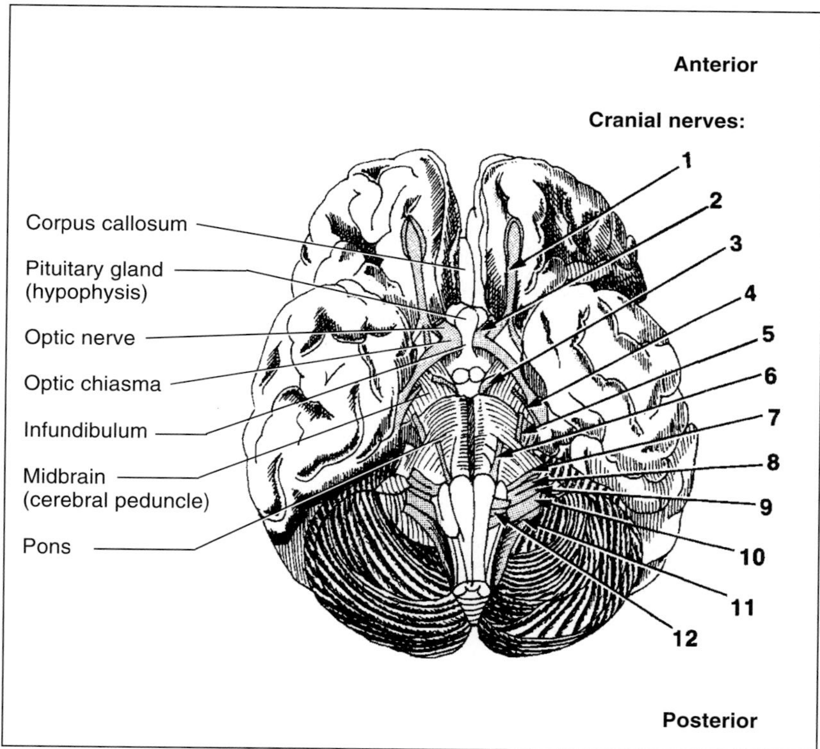

Fig. 22-20. Brain (inferior surface).

22

Orbital Cavity

The orbital cavities are often scanned as a routine part of cranial computed tomography. The orbital cavity as dissected from the front includes the **bulb** of the eye and numerous associated structures, as illustrated in Fig. 22-21. Orbital contents include the **ocular muscles**, **nerves** (including the large optic nerve), **blood vessels**, **orbital fat** and the **lacrimal gland**.

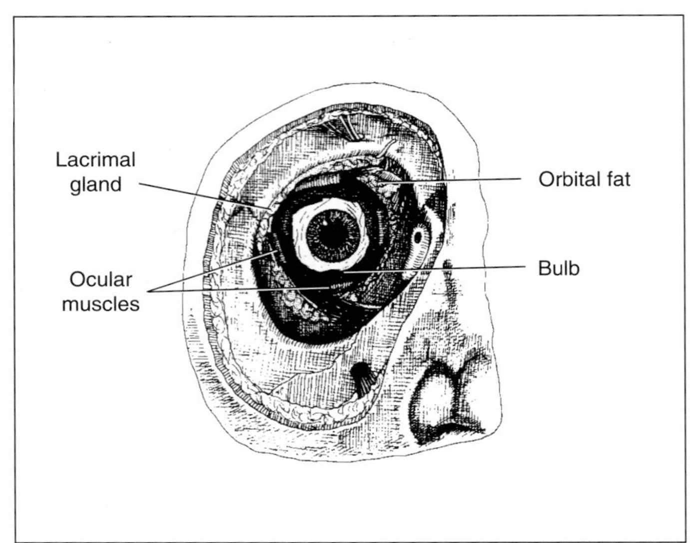

Fig. 22-21. Orbital cavity.

Orbital Cavities (Superior View)

The orbital cavities are exposed from above in Fig. 22-22 by removing the orbital plate of the frontal bone. The right orbit illustrates the normal fullness of the orbital cavity. The lacrimal gland in the upper outer quadrant, orbit fat, and ocular muscles help to fill the entire cavity. The internal carotid artery is seen entering the base of the skull. At this point, the internal carotid artery has already given off an artery that supplies the orbital contents.

The left orbital cavity, with fat and some muscles removed, illustrates the course of the larger **optic nerve** as it emerges from the bulb to course medially to the **optic chiasma.** Orbital tumors and foreign bodies can be readily detected through computed tomography of the orbits.

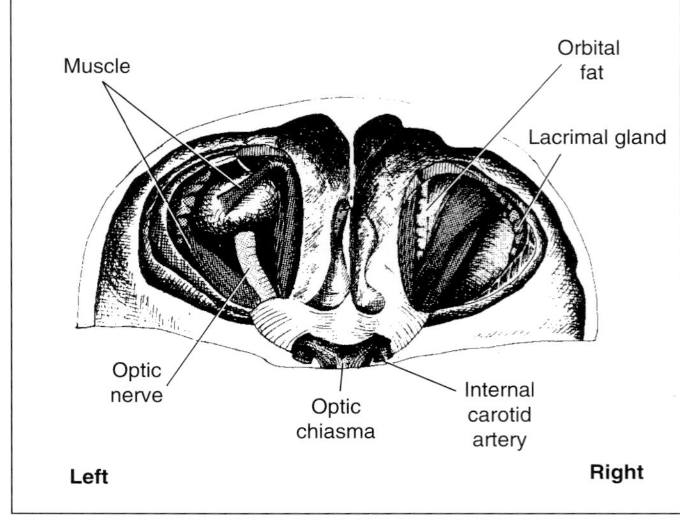

Fig. 22-22. Orbital cavities (superior view).

Visual Pathway

Axons leaving each eyeball travel via the **optic nerves** to the **optic chiasma.** Within the optic chiasma, some fibers cross to the opposite side and some remain on the same side, as shown in Fig. 22-23. After passing through the optic chiasma, the fibers form an **optic tract.** Each optic tract enters the brain and terminates in the thalamus.

In the thalamus, fibers synapse with other neurons, whose axons form the **optic radiations,** which then pass to the **visual centers** in the cortex of the occipital lobes of the cerebrum. Due to the partial crossing of fibers, sight can be affected in various ways depending on the location of a lesion in the visual pathway. An example is hemianopia, which causes blindness or defective vision in only half of the visual field of each eye.

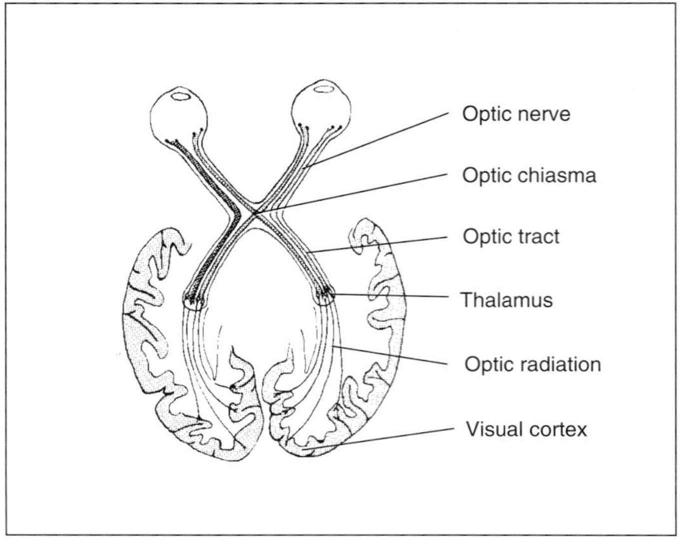

Fig. 22-23. Visual pathway.

Sectional Anatomy of the Brain

Familiarity with the gross structure of the central nervous system is important as well as the relative location of each because in CCT this anatomy is viewed primarily in cross-section. The rest of this part of the chapter on anatomy of the CNS now covers this anatomy viewed in various coronal and axial sections as seen on both drawings and CT scans. Those in parentheses are for information purposes of anatomy not yet covered in this textbook.

CORONAL SECTIONS

Coronal Section 1

Cranial computed tomography displays thin, cross-sectional, gray-scale images of cranial structures. Understanding this type of radiographic information requires a good understanding of cranial anatomy displayed in sectional form.

Beginning with Fig. 22-24, seven coronal or frontal sections of the cranium are shown. The first coronal section presented is the most anterior, passing through the eyeballs and frontal lobes of the cerebrum. Those structures labeled in Fig. 22-24 are:

A. Frontal bone
B. Falx cerebri
C. Gyrus or raised convoluted area of cerebral cortex
D. Centrum semiovale of the frontal lobe
E. Crista galli of the ethmoid bone
F. Ocular muscle
G. Bulb or eyeball
H. Periorbital fat

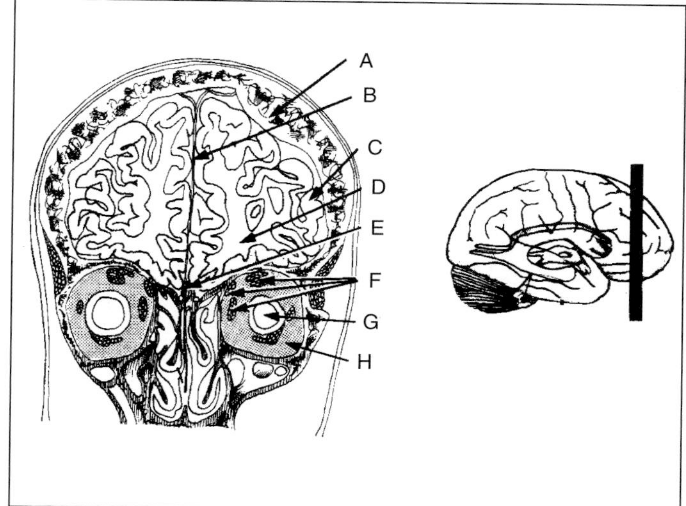

Fig. 22-24. Coronal section 1–Through eyes and frontal bone.

Coronal Section 2

Coronal section 2 is slightly posterior to the first coronal section. Those structures labeled are:

A. Superior sagittal sinus
B. Falx cerebri
C. Centrum semiovale of the frontal lobe
D. Corpus callosum
E. Anterior horn of the lateral ventricle
F. Temporal lobe
G. Optic nerve
H. Nasal septum
I. Maxillary sinus

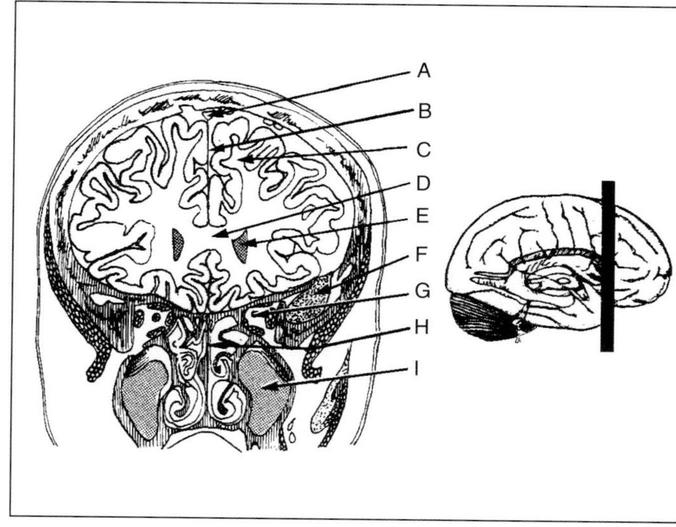

Fig. 22-25. Coronal section 2–Posterior to eyes.

Sectional Anatomy continued

Coronal Section 3

Coronal section 3, represents a section through the pituitary gland. Those parts labeled are:

A. Body of lateral ventricle
B. Cerebral nuclei
C. Pituitary gland
D. Sphenoid sinus
E. Greater wing of the sphenoid bone

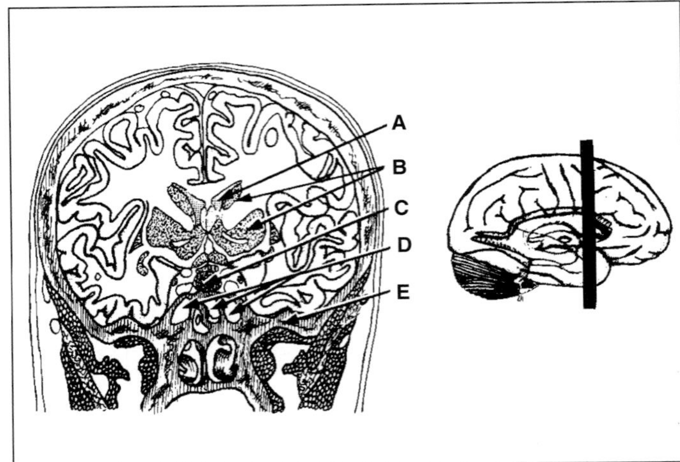

Fig. 22-26. Coronal section 3–Through pituitary gland.

Coronal Section 4

The drawing in Fig. 22-27 represents a coronal section through the main part of the thalamus. Those parts labeled are:

A. Parietal lobe of the cerebrum
B. Body of lateral ventricle
C. Thalamus
D. Inferior horn of lateral ventricle
E. Pons
F. (Internal carotid artery)
G. Condyle of the mandible

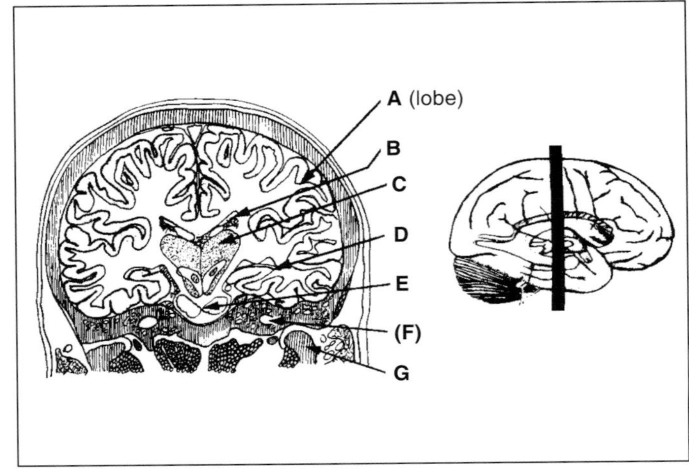

Fig. 22-27. Coronal section 4–Through thalamus.

Coronal Section 5

The drawing in Fig. 22-28 represents a coronal section through the posterior portion of the foramen magnum. Those labeled parts are:

A. Superior sagittal sinus
B. Inferior sagittal sinus
C. Cerebellar hemisphere
D. Midbrain
E. Sigmoid sinus
F. Mastoid process
G. Medulla

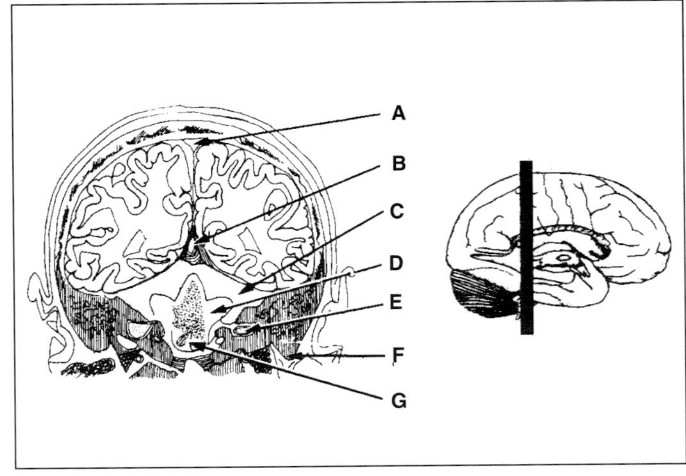

Fig. 22-28. Coronal section 5–Through posterior portion of foramen magnum.

Coronal Section 6

The sectional drawing shown in Fig. 22-29 depicts a section through the main substance of the cerebellum. Labeled parts are:

A. Superior sagittal sinus
B. Parietal bone
C. Falx cerebri
D. Parietal lobe of cerebrum
E. Inferior sagittal sinus
F. Sigmoid sinus
G. Cerebellar hemisphere
H. Cerebellar tonsi

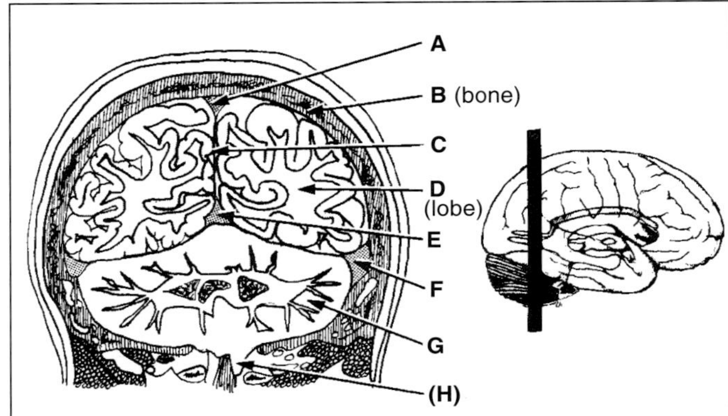

Fig. 22-29. Coronal section 6–Through cerebellum.

Coronal Section 7

The drawing in Fig. 22-30 represents a coronal section through the confluence of the sinuses and is the most posterior of the sectional coronal slices. Labeled parts are:

A. Occipital lobe of the cerebrum
B. Occipital bone
C. Confluence of sinuses
D. Transverse sinus
E. Cerebellar hemisphere

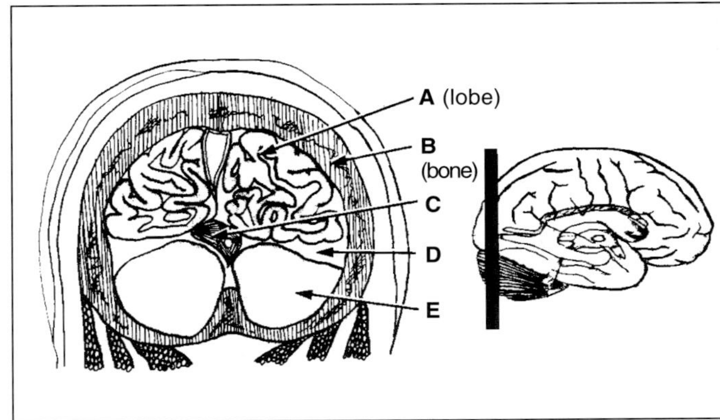

Fig. 22-30. Coronal section 7–Through posterior cerebellum.

AXIAL SECTIONS

Axial Section 1

Seven sectional drawings are now shown in axial orientation. Initial slices of the usual CCT scan are similar to the axial drawings. In computed tomography of the cranium, the patient's right is to the viewer's right, the same as in conventional radiography. Axial section number 1, shown in Fig. 22-31, is the most superior of the axial sections and is termed the extreme hemispheric level. Parts labeled are:

A. Anterior portion of the superior sagittal sinus
B. Centrum semiovale (white matter of the cerebrum)
C. Falx cerebri
D. Central sulcus
E. Cerebral cortex (gray matter of cerebrum)
F. Posterior portion of superior sagittal sinus
G. Cranium

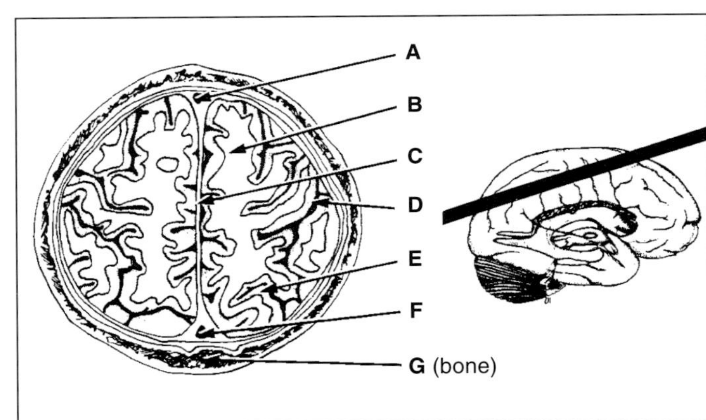

Fig. 22-31. Axial section 1–Extreme hemispheric level.

Brain Tissue and CT–Extreme Hemispheric Level

An actual slice of brain tissue and a computed tomogram corresponding to the extreme hemispheric level are shown in Figs. 22-32 and 22-33. Compare the brain tissue slice and the CT to the drawing in Fig. 22-31.

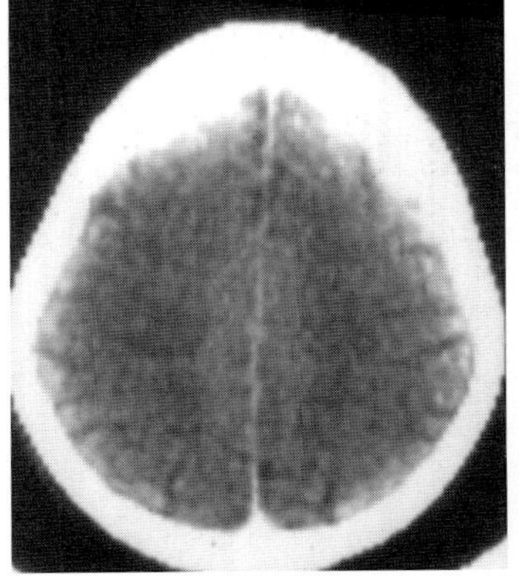
Fig. 22-32. CT section.

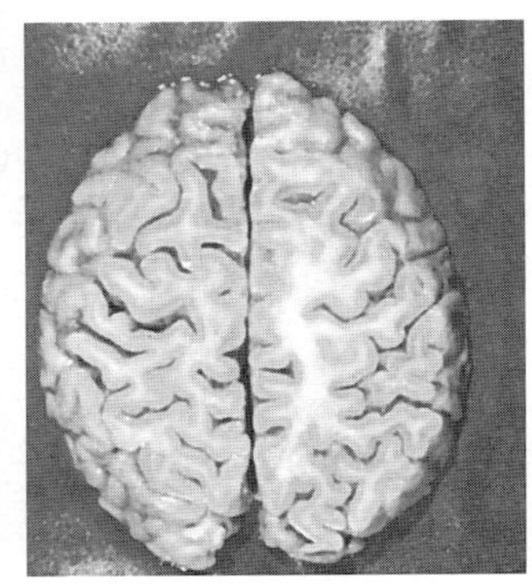
Fig. 22-33. Brain tissue.

Sectional Anatomy continued

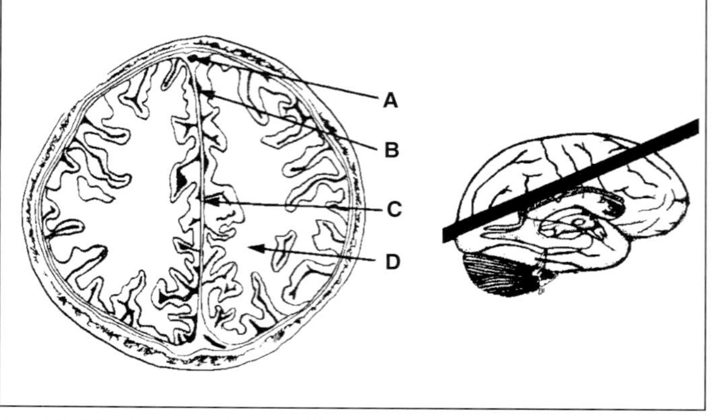

Fig. 22-34. Axial section 2–High hemispheric level.

Axial Section 2

Axial section number 2 (Fig. 22-34) is slightly caudad to axial section number 1. This level is just superior to the ventricles and is termed the high hemispheric level. The anatomy shown in axial sections 1 and 2 is similar.

A. Superior sagittal sinus
B. C. Longitudinal fissure with the Falx cerebri dipping down into the fissure
D. White matter of the cerebrum (centrum semiovale)

Brain Tissue and CT–High Hemispheric Level

A photograph of an actual slice of brain tissue and a computed tomogram corresponding to the high hemispheric level are shown in Figs. 22-35 and 22-36. This photograph and radiograph are at a similar level as the drawing in Fig. 22-34.

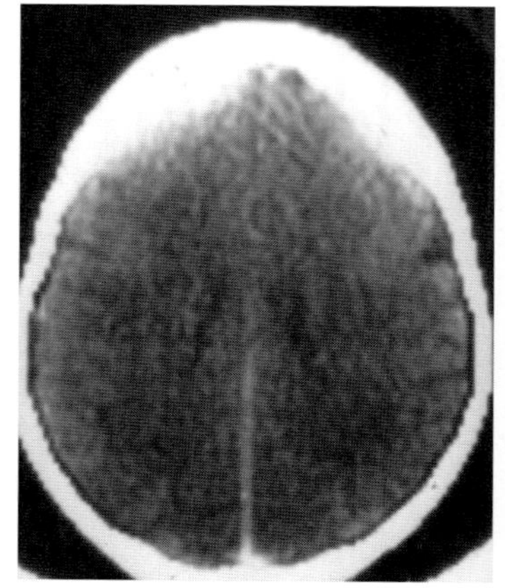

Fig. 22-35. CT section.

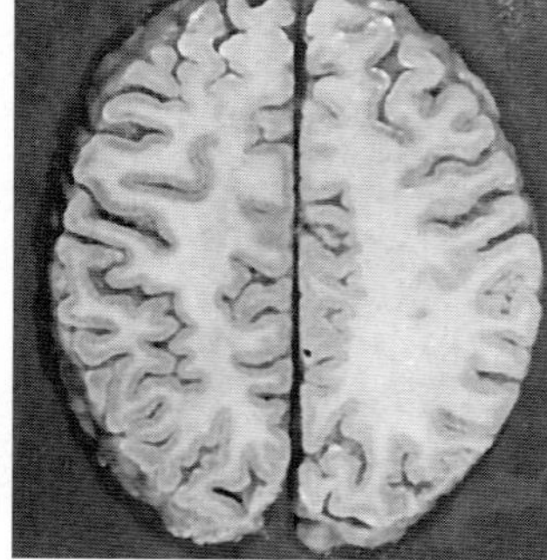

Fig. 22-36. Brain tissue.

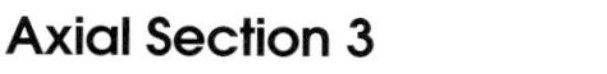

Axial Section 3

Progressing farther toward the base of the brain, the sectional drawing in Fig. 22-37 progresses into the lateral ventricles, termed the high ventricular level. Those structures labeled are:

A. Falx cerebri
B. Anterior central gyrus
C. Central sulcus
D. Posterior central gyrus
E. One lateral ventricle

The relationship of sulci and gyri are studied carefully by the neuroradiologist since the sulci are increased in size in cases of cerebral atrophy.

CT–High Ventricular Level

A computed tomogram through the high ventricular level is shown in Fig. 22-38. Each lateral ventricle assumes a characteristic banana shape on the CCT scan at this level. The prominent cerebral sulci on this CCT scan indicate some atrophy of cerebral tissue.

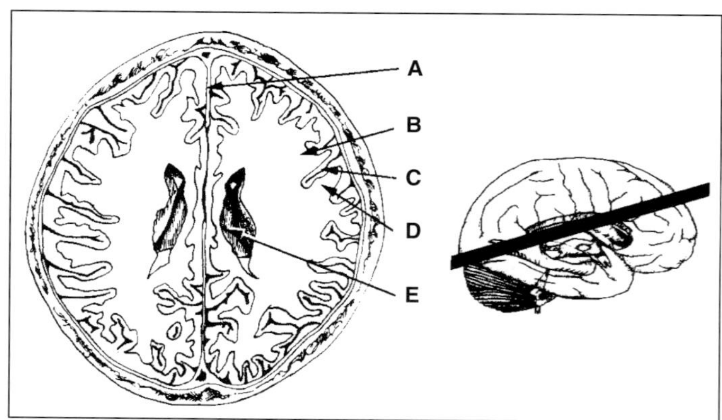

Fig. 22-37. Axial section 3–High ventricular level.

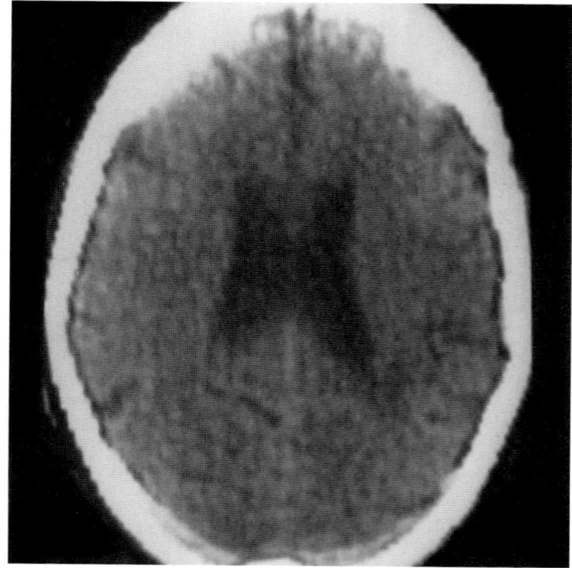

Fig. 22-38. CT section.

Axial Section 4

This drawing is of the mid ventricular level. The deep-lying cerebral nuclei are visible at this level.

A. Corpus callosum
B. Anterior horn of the right lateral ventricle
C. Cerebral nuclei
D. Thalamus
E. Third ventricle
F. Pineal gland or body
G. Corpus callosum
H. Inferior horn of the right lateral ventricle
I. Straight sinus

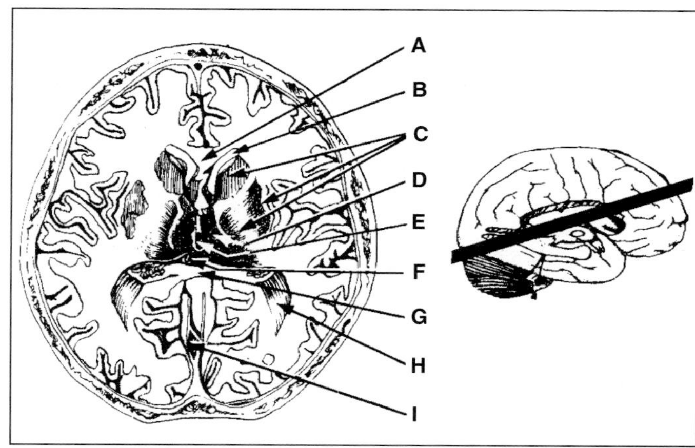

Fig. 22-39. Axial section 4–Mid ventricular level.

Brain Tissue and CT–Mid Ventricular Level

This photograph of brain tissue and the computed tomogram are at the level of the mid ventricles.

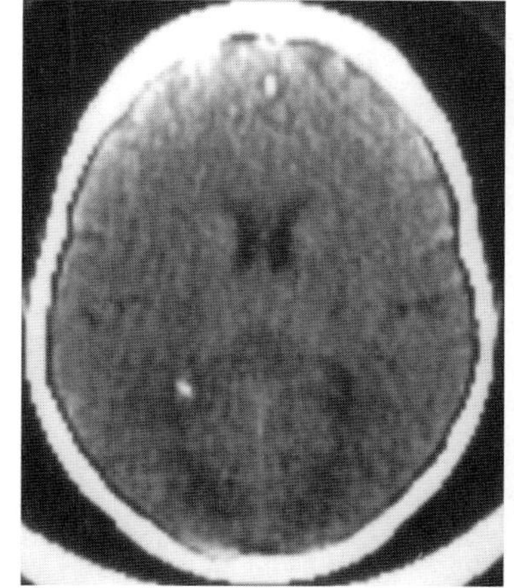
Fig. 22-40. CT section.

Fig. 22-41. Brain tissue.

Axial Section 5

The drawing in Fig. 22-42, titled Axial Section 5, represents a drawing of brain tissue through the mid third ventricle. Cerebral nuclei are visible in addition to structures of the midbrain. Those parts labeled are:

A. Corpus callosum
B. Anterior horn and body lateral ventricle
C. Cerebral nuclei
D. Third ventricle
E. (Right sigmoid sinus)
F. Cerebellar hemisphere
G. Internal occipital protuberance

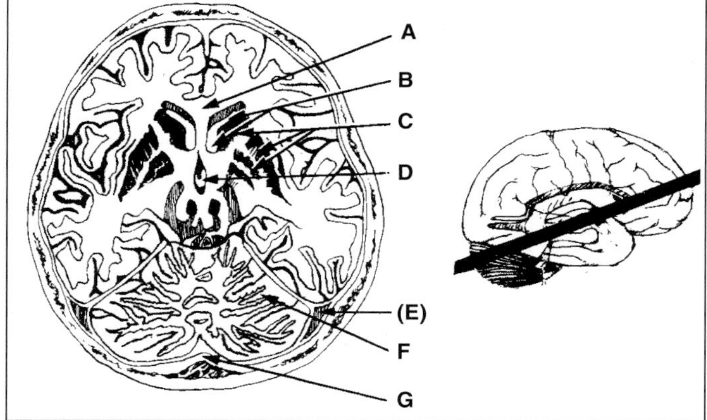
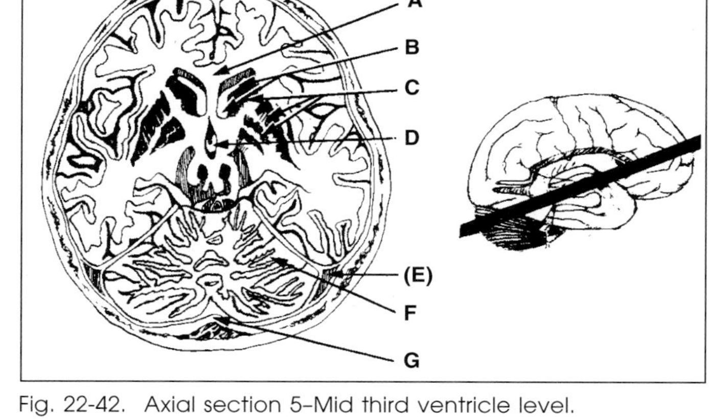

Fig. 22-42. Axial section 5–Mid third ventricle level.

Brain Tissue and CT–Mid Third Ventricle Level

A photograph of brain tissue and a computed tomogram through the mid-third ventricle level are shown in Figs. 22-43 and 22-44. This level corresponds to the drawing in Fig. 22-42.

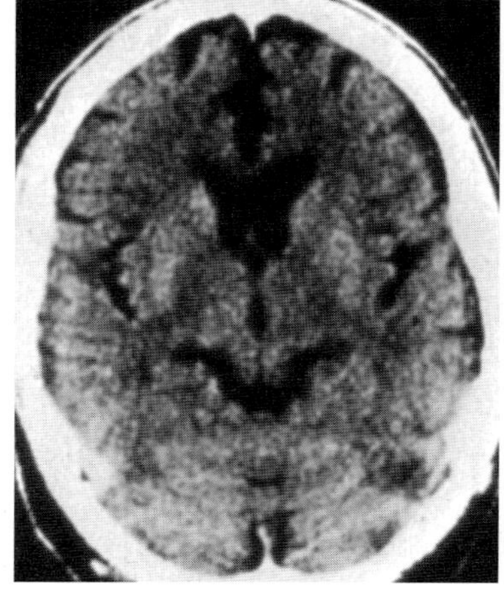
Fig. 22-43. CT section.

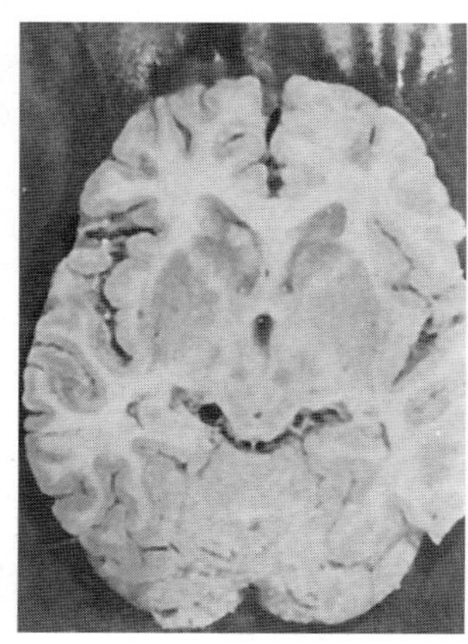
Fig. 22-44. Brain tissue.

Axial Section 6

The drawing in Fig. 22-45 represents the tissue plane through the sella turcica. Parts labeled are:

A. Right frontal lobe of the cerebrum
B. Pituitary gland
C. Right temporal lobe
D. Petrous pyramid
E. Pons
F. (Right sagittal sinus)

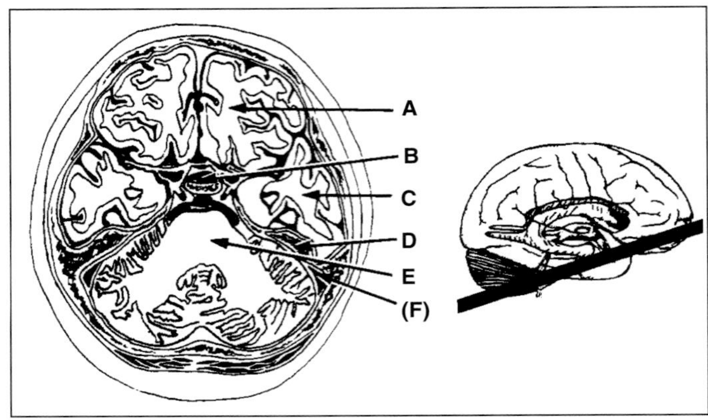

Fig. 22-45. Axial section 6–Through sella turcica.

Brain Tissue and CT–Sella Turcica Level

A photograph of actual brain tissue and a CCT scan through the level of the sella turcica are shown in Fig. 22-46 and 22-47.

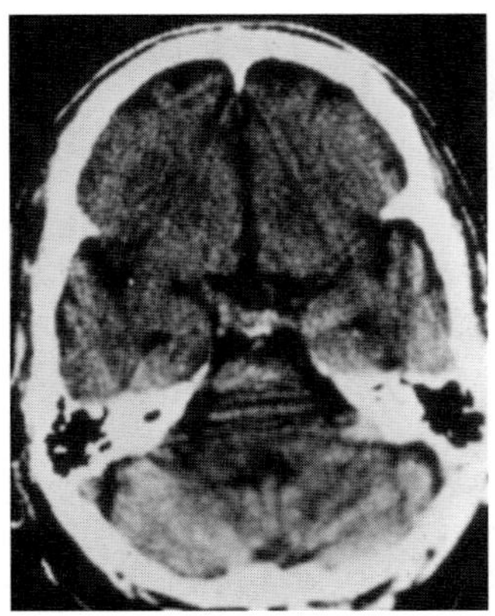

Fig. 22-46. CT section.

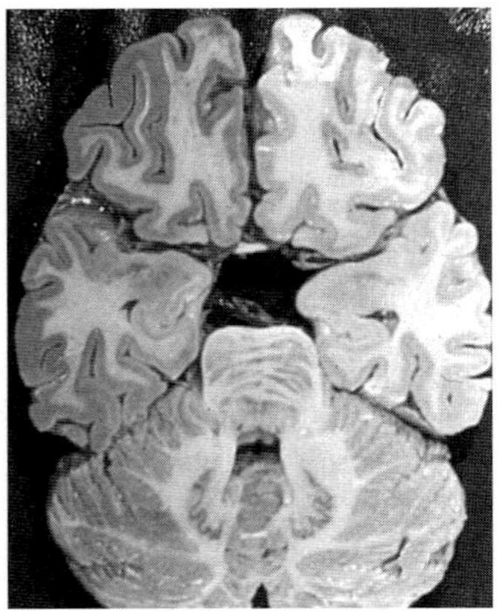

Fig. 22-47. Brain tissue.

Axial Section 7

Axial section number 7 represents a drawing of tissue in the orbital plane. Note in Fig. 22-48 that a different angle is used to better visualize the orbital cavities. Those structures labeled are:

A. Ocular bulb or eyeball
B. Optic nerve
C. Optic chiasma
D. Temporal lobe
E. Midbrain
F. Cerebellum
G. Occipital lobe
H. Falx cerebri
I. (Superior sagittal sinus)

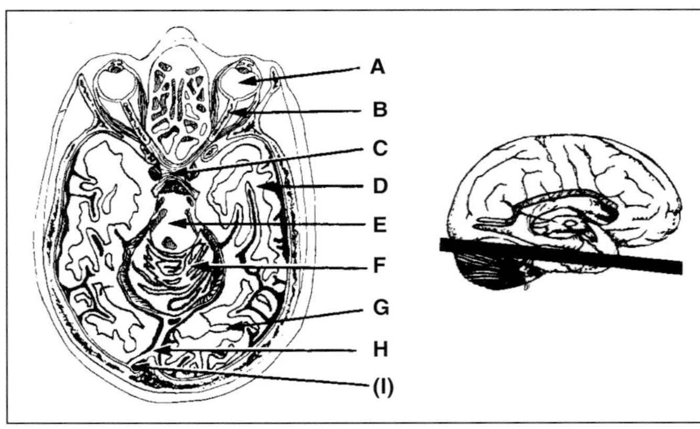

Fig. 22-48. Axial section 7–Through orbital plane.

CT–Orbital Level

A CCT scan through the orbital level is shown in Fig. 22-49. Compare the CT section through the orbital level with the drawing in Fig. 22-48. Note especially how clearly the ocular bulb and optic nerve are visualized.

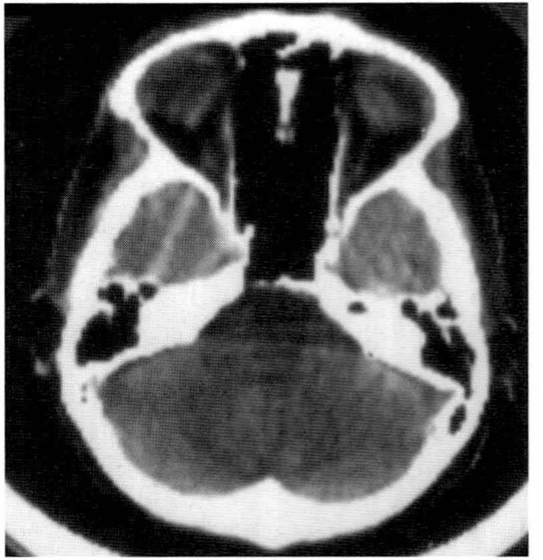

Fig. 22-49. CT section.

Basic Principles and Procedures

Definition

Cranial computed tomography (CCT) refers to **radiographic examination of the cranium displayed as a thin, cross-sectional, grayscale, tomographic image** representing a computer-assisted mathematical reconstruction of numerous x-ray absorption differences of the cranial contents.

Advantages over Conventional Radiography

Computed tomography has three distinct advantages over conventional radiography.

First, three-dimensional information is presented in the form of a series of thin slices of the internal structure of the part in question. Since the x-ray beam is closely collimated to that particular slice, the resultant information is not degraded by secondary and scatter radiation from tissue outside the slice being studied.

Second, the system is much more sensitive when compared to conventional radiography so that differences in soft tissue can be clearly delineated.

Third, CT measures x-ray absorption of individual tissues accurately, allowing the basic nature of tissue to be studied.

Changes and Advances in CT Systems

Since the introduction of clinical CT scanning in 1972, equipment systems have evolved through stages, commonly referred to as **generations**. Each generation of scanners decreased the scanning time, the time required to gather the information for each scan. The difference between the succeeding generations of scanning systems primarily involved the x-ray tube and detector arrangements. The addition of more detectors reduced the scanning times considerably.

First and Second-Generation Scanners: The **first generation scanners** with only **one or two detectors** required up to 4½ minutes to gather enough information for one slice from a 180° rotation of the tube and detector. **Second-generation scanners** included up to **30 or more detectors** with shorter scanning times of about 10 minutes for a 40 slice exam.

Third-Generation Scanner: The third generation scanner includes an arrangement of a bank of up to 852 detectors opposite the x-ray tube which together rotate around the patient in a complete **360° cycle** to create one slice of tissue data. The patient and table are then moved one increment superiorly or inferiorly and the tube and detectors rotate a full 360° cycle in the opposite direction to create a second slice of tissue data.

Fourth-Generation Scanner: Fourth generation scanners developed during the 1980s possess a ring of as many as 4800 detectors, completely surrounding the patient in a full circle within the gantry. A single x-ray tube rotates through a 360° arc during data collection. Throughout the continuous rotary motion, short bursts of radiation are provided by a pulsed, rotating-anode x-ray tube.

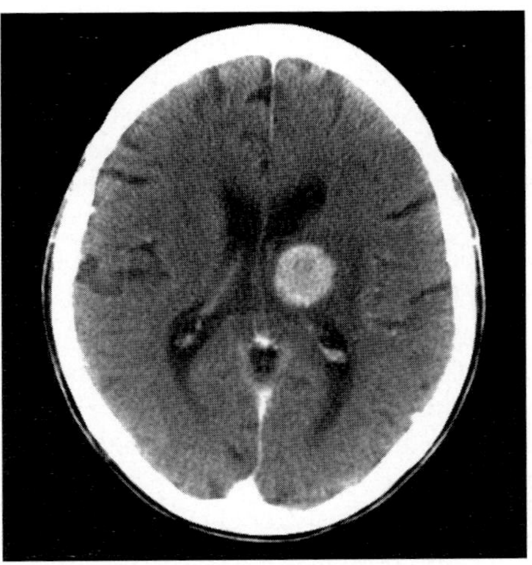

Fig. 22-50. Cranial computed tomogram (axial section).
(Courtesy of Imatron, Inc. San Francisco, CA.)

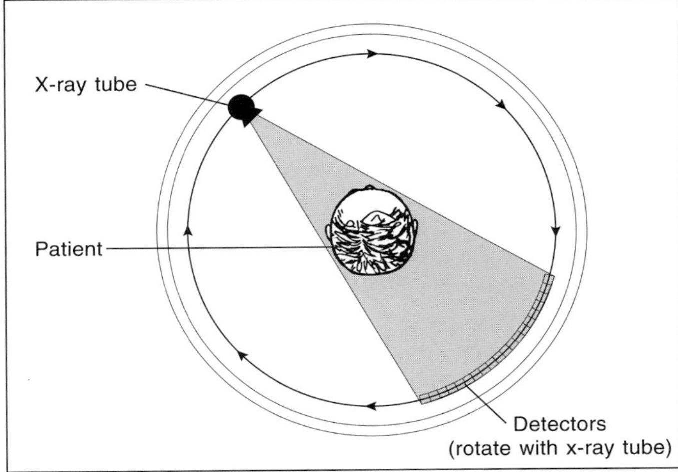

Fig. 22-51. Third generation scanner.
-Up to 852 detectors.
-360° simultaneous rotation of x-ray tube and detectors.

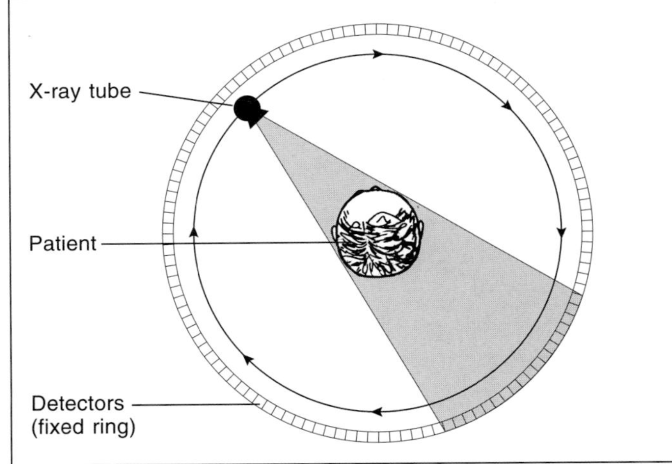

Fig. 22-52. Fourth generation scanner.
-Up to 4800 detectors on a fixed ring.
-X-ray tube rotating 360°.

Scanner Principles continued

Helical CT Scanners

During the early 1990s a new type of scanner was developed termed **helical CT scanners**. With this system the patient continuously moves slowly in or out during the 360° circling of the x-ray tube creating a helical or "coiled spring" type of data acquisition (Fig. 22-53). In this way a **volume of tissue** is examined and data collected rather than individual slices as with other systems.

Helical CT systems utilize either **third** or **fourth-generation** type detector arrangements with **most** helical systems utilizing the **third generation type**.

The development of **slip rings** to replace the high tension x-ray tube cables allows for continual tube rotation such as is necessary for helical type scanning. Formerly the x-ray tube with attached high tension cables was limited to one 360° rotation in one direction comprising one slice, followed by another 360° rotation in the opposite direction creating a second slice with the patient moved one increment between slices.

The development of slip ring engineering technology allows for continuing tube rotations, which when combined with patient movement creates a helical type scan data with total scan times that are one-half or less that of other third or fourth-generation type scanners.

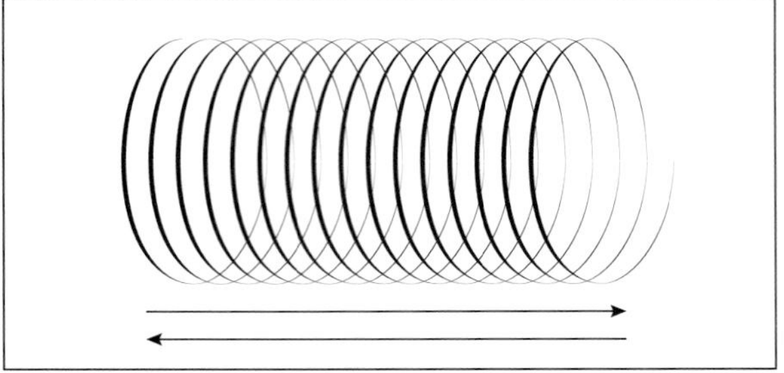

Fig. 22-53. Helical scan in either direction -With either third or fourth-generation scanners (depending on manufacturer).

Electron Beam Tomography–Ultrafast CT®

The 1980s have added another new CT scanner system termed **Electron Beam Tomography** or **Ultrafast CT®**, sometimes also described as **Cardiovascular Computed Tomography** (CVCT). A prototype of this system was first installed in 1983, and at the time of this writing in 1996, there are 75 of these systems in use world wide, with 33 installations in the United States. This system provides scan times as fast as **50 to 100 milliseconds,** and in the fast acquisition mode generates up to **34 scans per second**. These fast scan times freeze motion of organs, even that of the heart. The amount of contrast media required for invasive type studies is greatly reduced and the true arterial phase of organs such as the liver, spleen and pancreas can be visualized with this system. Noninvasive studies without the use of contrast media is possible including 3D visualization of the coronary arteries of the heart.

These systems are also well suited for pediatrics and/or trauma patients where immobility is a concern.

The principle of operation of electron beam tomography is radically different from other CT systems. X-rays are generated by an **electron beam gun** with the electron beam focused and deflected by **computer controlled electromagnets** to one of **four fixed tungsten rings.** This creates a **fan beam of x-rays** that pass through the patient into the two level stationary **detector rings** and the **data acquisition system**.

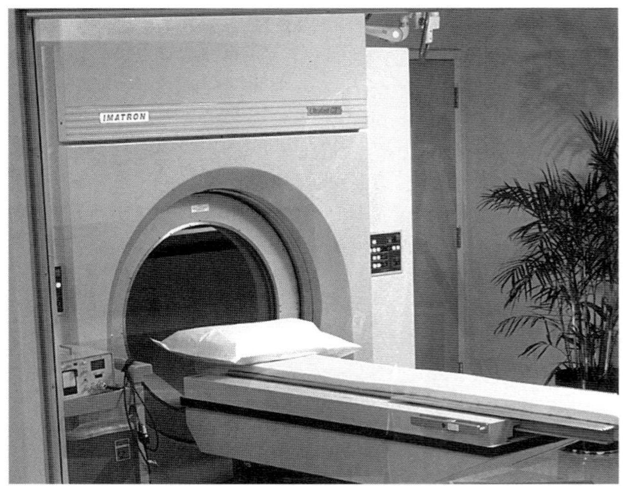

Fig. 22-54. Electron beam (Ultrafast®) tomographic system.
(Courtesy of Imatron, Inc. San Francisco, CA.)

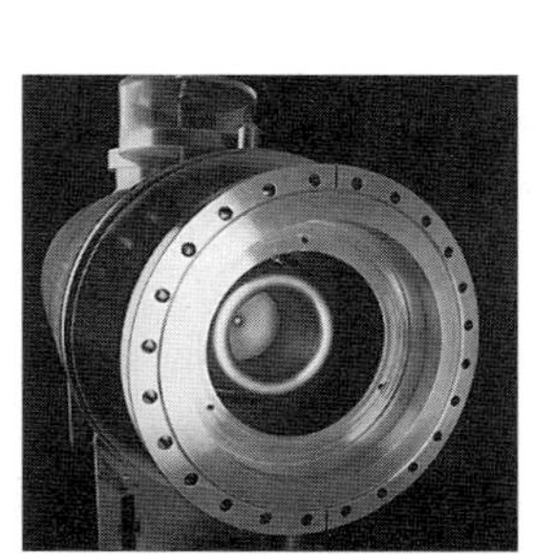

Fig. 22-55. Electron gun.

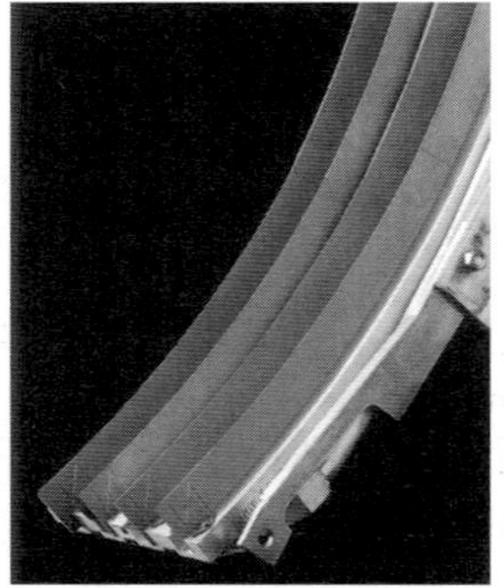

Fig. 22-56. Four track fixed tungsten (target) rings.

(Courtesy of Imatron, Inc. San Francisco, CA.)

Three types of scanning are possible with this system.

1. Single-slice scanning.
2. Multi-slice scanning. Through the combined use of the four tungsten target rings and the two detector rings, it is possible to scan up to 8 images simultaneously.
3. Continuous volume scanning (CVS). The patient and table can also be moved during the scanning process to create continuous volume scanning similar to that of helical CT systems.

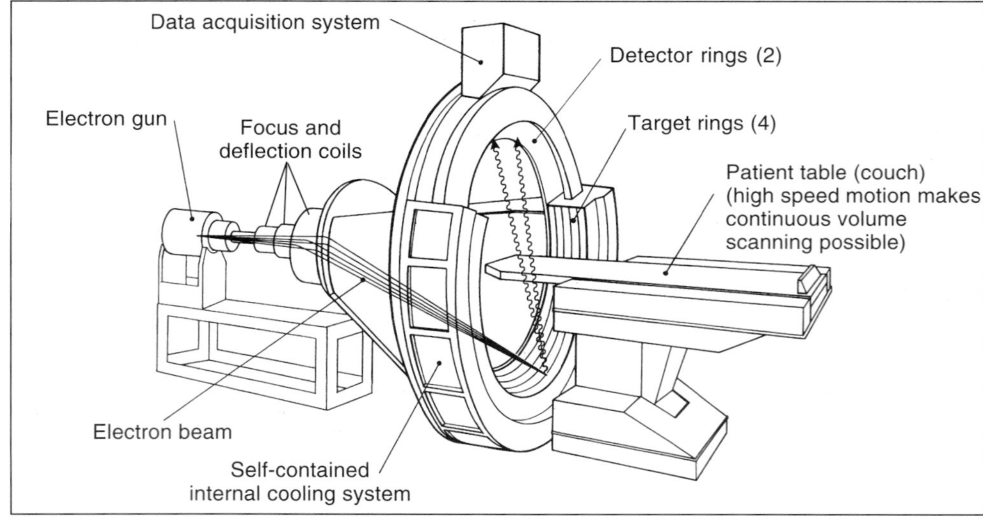

Fig. 22-57. Electron beam tomographic system.
(Adapted from drawing by Imatrom, Inc., San Francisco, CA.)

BASIC PRINCIPLE

The basic principle of computed tomography is that **the internal structure of any three-dimensional subject can be reconstructed from many different projections or views of that subject.** This necessitates the collection of large amounts of data in order to reconstruct an accurate picture of the original structure.

X-ray Transmission and Collection of Data

At least 180 different projections are required to obtain a diagnostically useful radiograph. This fact is demonstrated by assuming that the patient anatomy in question is a mass of homogeneous tissue with an air-filled cross in the center, as shown in Fig. 22-58. Narrow beams of x-rays are directed through the section of tissue and the photons that pass through are collected and processed.

Due to the shape and configuration of the air-filled cross in this illustration, more x-rays pass through the center of the slice than pass through either the top or the bottom. By plotting the intensity of radiation collected along the left side of the section, a profile of the emergent radiation is formed. If the x-ray beam were directed through the tissue at 1-degree intervals until 180 readings were made, 180 different profiles would be formed. Collecting this large amount of transmission data for processing by the computer is the function of the scan unit.

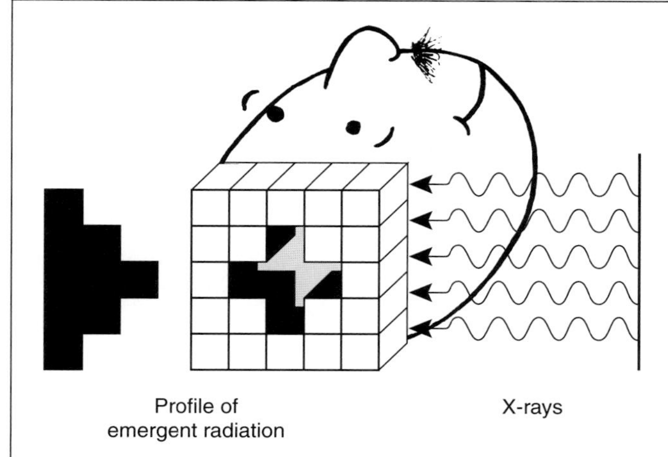

Fig. 22-58. One profile of emergent radiation.

Source and Detector Collimation

In CCT, very close collimation is necessary to limit the radiation beam to the area of interest. The x-ray beam is actually collimated on both sides of the patient's head. The **source collimator** is located very close to the x-ray tube, and a **detector collimator** is located close to each detector in the detector array. The actual **thickness of the tomographic slice is controlled by the source collimator** and ranges from 1 to several millimeters. The detector collimators limit the amount of scatter radiation picked up by the detectors. Since each section is very thin, little secondary and scatter radiation escapes to neighboring tissue.

The location of the two collimators is shown diagrammatically in Fig. 22-59. The width and length of each individual transmission of radiation is limited by the collimators.

Volume Element (Voxel): After many transmissions of x-ray data, the reconstructed anatomy appears to be composed of a large number of tiny, elongated blocks. Each of the tiny blocks shown in the drawing of the "blockhead" represents a volume of tissue as defined by the opening in the source collimator. In CT language, each block is termed a **volume element,** which is shortened to **voxel.** Any CT slice is composed of a large number of voxels.

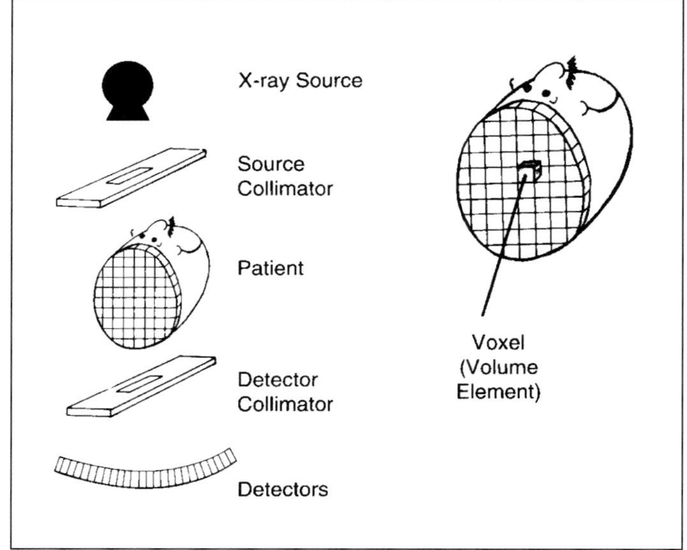

Fig. 22-59. Collimation and volume element (voxel).

PRINCIPLES OF IMAGE RECONSTRUCTION

The large amounts of data accumulated by the scan unit must be processed by the computer to provide a meaningful picture form. A simplified method of image reconstruction is shown in Figs. 22-60 through 22-63 to demonstrate the principle utilized by computed tomography. The actual methods of reconstruction are much more complex and extensive than shown, but the basic principle is the same.

Exposure and Information Profile

Our subject is the "blockhead" with an air-filled cross located within a mass of homogeneous tissue. The total tissue volume of the slice in question is divided into a 5 x 5 system of **25 voxels**, as shown in Step A of Fig. 22-60. Step B of this illustration shows two beams of **x-radiation** directed through the slice of tissue in question. One beam is directed from right to left, while the second beam is directed from top to bottom. The collected data produces two **profiles** of information, as shown in Step C.

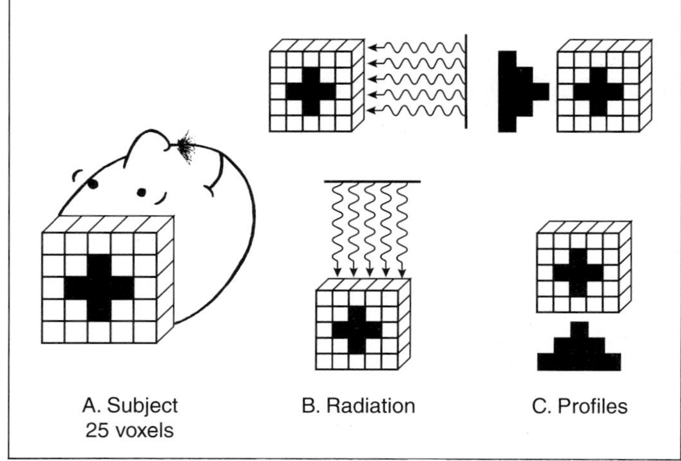

Fig. 22-60. Exposure and information profile.

Principles of Image Reconstruction continued

Attenuation

Radiation is attenuated or absorbed more readily by the tissue surrounding the cross than by the air in the cross. Assume that each voxel of tissue absorbs one unit of radiation, and each air-filled voxel absorbs no radiation. This is represented in Step D of Fig. 22-61 by assigning the **number 1 to each tissue voxel and O (zero) to each air-filled voxel.** Therefore, the two drawings in Step D represent relative attenuation values in very simplified form.

The next step, as shown by the two illustrations in Step E, is to **add the numbers in the direction of the two beams of radiation.** Each beam of radiation passes through a total of five voxels. The maximum number of 5 occurs along each border of the cross where the x-rays pass through five tissue voxels. Addition of numbers in the central portion of the cross results in the number 2 since only two voxels represent tissue in that direction. Addition of each row of numbers results in two profiles of radiation represented by the numbers, as shown in Step E of this illustration.

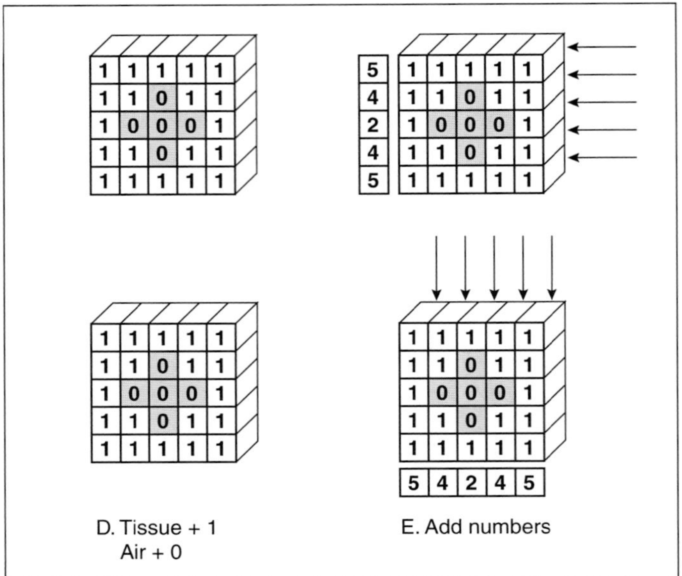

Fig. 22-61. Attenuation.

Summation

The next step involves **combining the two numerical profiles into one**, as shown in **Step F**. This is done by adding the numbers in each of the two directions. Therefore, the upper right voxel in Step F is represented by the number 10 since the transmission readings were 5 in each of the two directions. The sum for the lower voxel is 6, since 4 was obtained in one direction and 2 in the other direction.

The numerical composite, shown on the right in **Step G**, is the **sum of the numbers comprising each profile**. This addition process is essentially what the computer does with the large mass of transmission data accumulated by the scan unit.

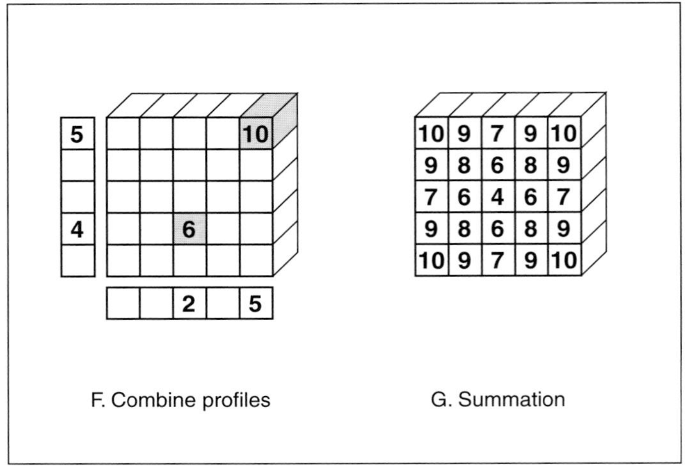

Fig. 22-62. Summation.

Picture Reconstruction

The large amount of numerical data obtained by summation must now be transformed into a picture. This is done by **assigning various shades of gray, black or white to various numbers**. As shown in **Step H** of this illustration, the number 4 is assigned white and the number 10 is black. Any numbers between 4 and 10 are assigned darker and darker shades of gray, as shown in the table to the right in Fig. 22-63. A projection of this reconstruction as an image looks like the gray-scale drawing in **Step H**.

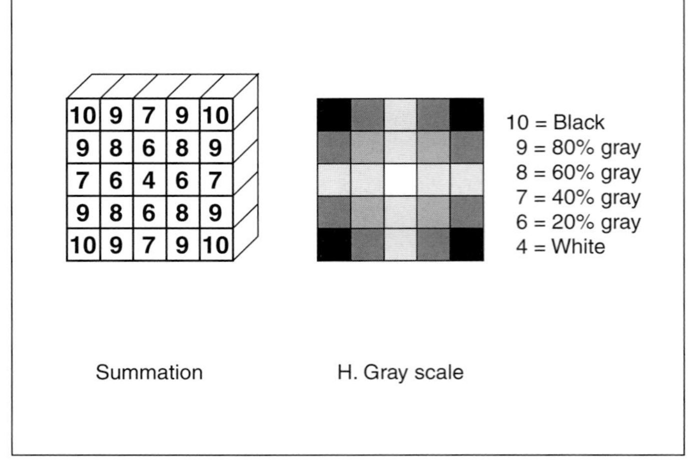

Fig. 22-63. Picture reconstruction.

Image Manipulation

Finally, the gray-scale image shown in Step H can be manipulated to give a more accurate reconstruction of the original image. Increasing the contrast or, in effect, removing the gray from the image results in a black and white image, shown in Step 1 of Fig. 22-64. This image results if any number equaling 6 or less is assigned white, and any number 7 or larger is assigned black. Basically, this describes cranial computed tomography. The internal structure of any three-dimensional structure can be reconstructed from many different projections of that subject.

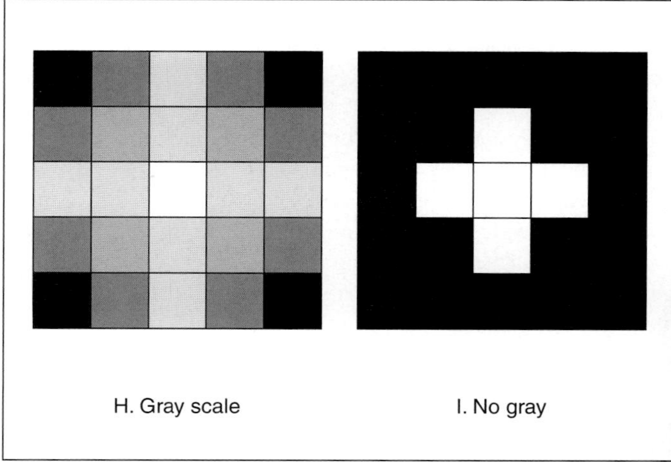

Fig. 22-64. Image manipulation.

COMPUTED TOMOGRAPHIC IMAGE

Degree of Attenuation of Each Voxel (Differential Absorption)

A computed tomographic image is shown in Fig. 22-65. Each voxel in the tissue slice is assigned a number proportional to the degree of x-ray attenuation of the entire chunk of tissue or voxel. Attenuation or differential absorption is defined as the reduction in the intensity of the x-ray beam as the beam passes through matter. X-ray photons are removed from the incident beam through absorption or scattering as a result of interaction with individual atoms or molecules comprising the matter. Many photons pass through the matter in question without any type of interaction.

Many variables affect the degree of attenuation. Variables include the energy of the x-ray beam, as well as the density, effective atomic number and number of electrons per gram of the subject matter. Generally, production of diagnostic images in radiology and in computed tomography depend entirely on the differential absorption or attenuation between adjacent tissues.

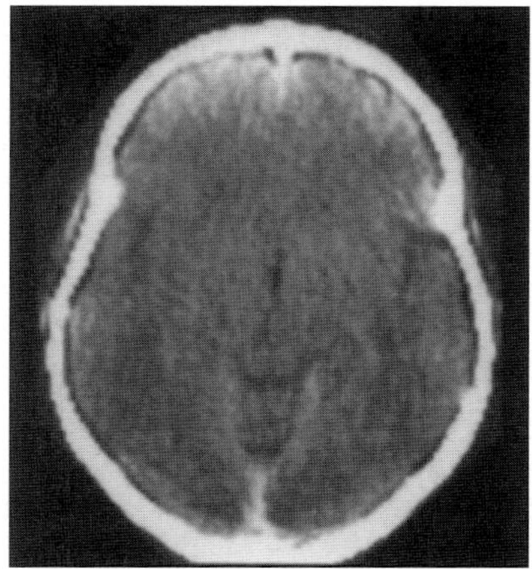

Fig. 22-65. Cranial computed tomogram (axial section).

Converting Three-dimensional Voxels to Two-dimensional Pixels

Once the degree of attenuation of each voxel is determined, each three-dimensional tissue slice is projected on the television screen as a **two-dimensional image**. This two-dimensional image is termed the **display matrix** and is composed of tiny picture elements termed **pixels**. Each voxel is represented on the television screen as a pixel. The number of individual elements or pixels comprising the display matrix is determined by the manufacturer and may range from a fairly coarse matrix of 80 x 80 pixels to a very fine matrix of 512 x 512 pixels.

Computed Gray Scale

After the CT computer (through thousands of separate mathematical equations) determines a relative linear attenuation coefficient for each pixel in the display matrix, the values are then converted to another numerical scale involving CT numbers. Shades of gray are then assigned to the CT numbers. The end result is a gray-scale, computed tomographic image, as shown in Fig. 22-65.

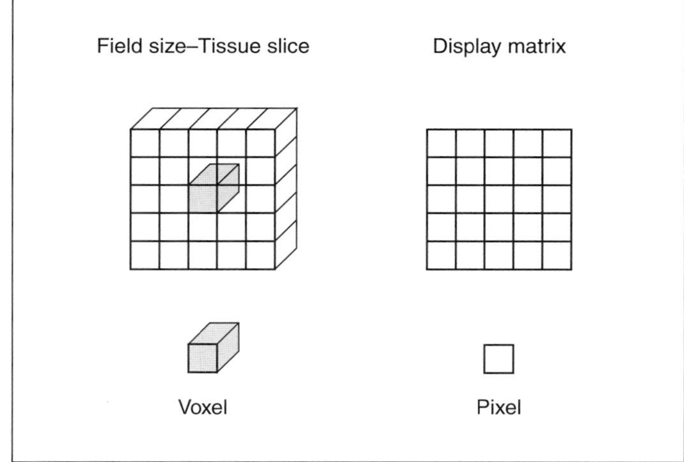

Fig. 22-66. Computed tomographic image.

COMPUTED TOMOGRAPHIC SYSTEM

1. Scan Unit

All computed tomographic systems consist of two major elements. One major element is the **scan unit.** The scan unit provides large amounts of information to the computer. The scan unit is usually housed in a room by itself and is the part of the computed tomographic system seen by the patient. This room is often termed the treatment room or scanner room.

The scan unit consists of two parts: (1) the **patient table** (couch), and (2) the **gantry.** The patient table or couch provides a fairly comfortable surface for the recumbent patient during the total scanning time. The gantry is a rigid support structure that encompasses the patient within a central opening termed the **gantry aperture.** The depth to which the patient is placed within the aperture determines the section to be studied. The gantry houses the x-ray tube or tubes and the radiation detector array.

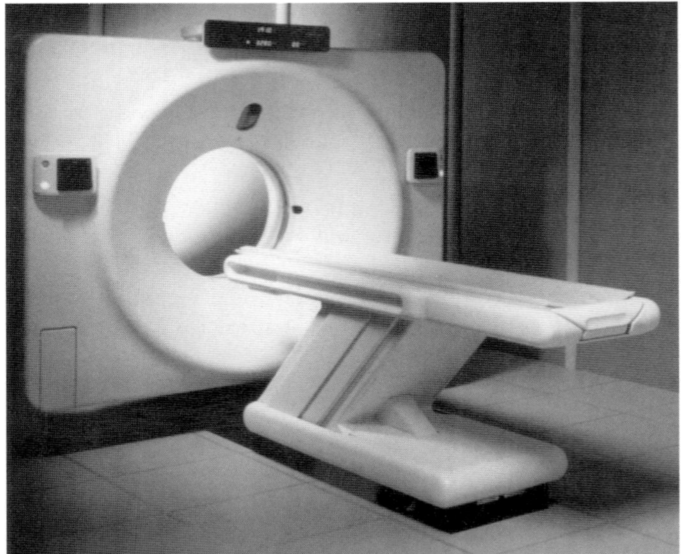

Fig. 22-67. Computed tomography scanning unit. -Patient table (couch) and gantry.
(Courtesy of GE Medical Systems, Milwaukee, WI.)

2. Operator Control Console

A second major element of any computed tomographic system is the operator control console, which includes the processing unit or **computer** that takes raw data and converts it into a meaningful picture form. It is the computer or processing unit that makes CT so different from conventional radiography and most other radiographic imaging modalities.

Huge amounts of raw data are received directly from the scan unit by the processor. This data consists of positional, reference and calibration information, in addition to all the individual absorption readings. The transmission readings alone can amount to more than 100 thousand bits of information. This mass of information is analyzed and converted to picture form for diagnosis. Modern ingenuity and computer technology allow the scanning and image reconstruction to be performed in a matter of seconds.

Modern control consoles include the processing unit or computer into the base of the console under the monitors and control shelf.

Operator Controls: All the necessary controls to proceed through each examination are located at the operator control console usually located just outside the scanning room. This includes controls for the exposure factors (kVp, mA, scan time) as well as slice thickness and pitch selections, scan directions and other variables that may be specific to the equipment being used. Image manipulation such as edge enhancement, zoom, brightness and contrast controls are also possible at the control console.

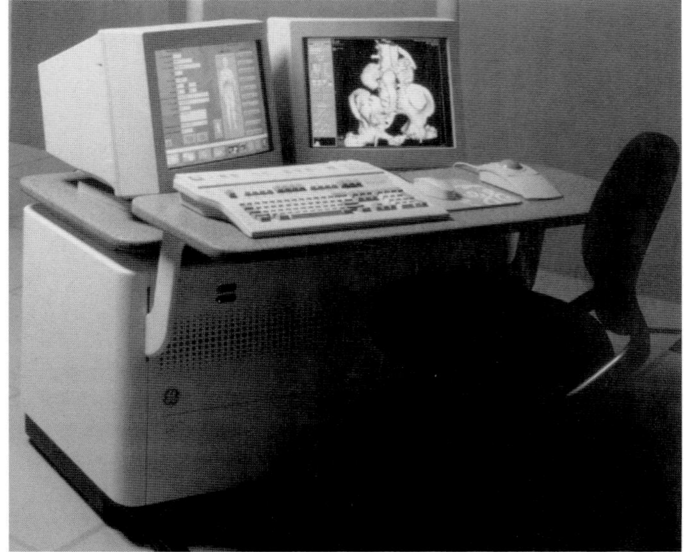

Fig. 22-68. Operator control console.
(Courtesy of GE Medical Systems, Milwaukee, WI.)

Monitors: Most modern control consoles include two color monitors, one for the icons and other control displays, and one for viewing the radiographic image. Networking is common where separate monitors may be situated in other locations for viewing by the radiologist. These may be in other offices or areas within the department, or in totally remote areas with transmission through telephone lines, fiberoptics or satellite transmission.

Image archiving or storage: Most modern systems utilize a combination of optical disks and hard disk drives as high capacity, immediate and permanent storage of data information in digital form. This information can be readily retrieved at any time. Laser printers are also available for print-out of hard copy onto film if desired.

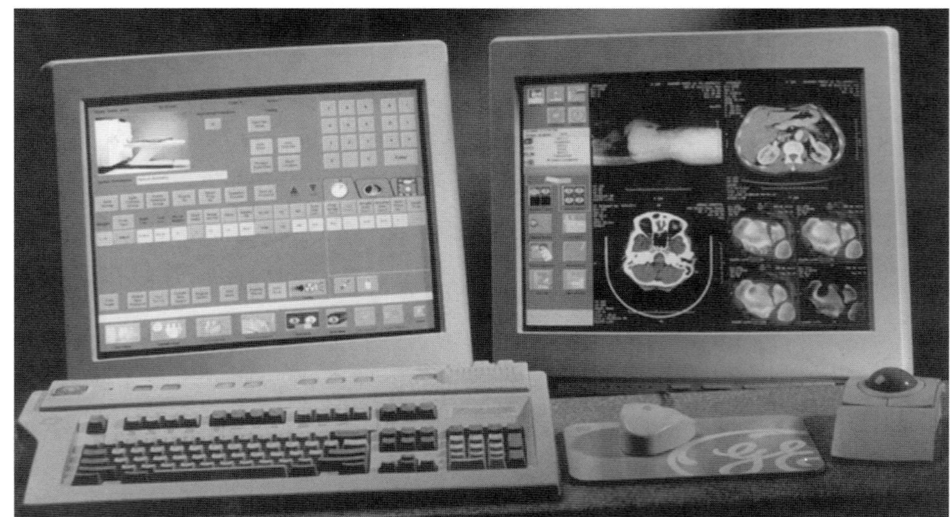

Fig. 22-69. Operator controls and monitors.
(Courtesy of GE Medical Systems, Milwaukee, WI.)

CRANIAL COMPUTED TOMOGRAPHY PROCEDURE

Purpose

The primary purpose of cranial computed tomography is to provide accurate diagnostic information, significantly improving the management of the patient. The ideal result is a definitive diagnosis that does not require collaborative tests for verification. CCT, in many instances, does provide this high degree of reliability. Acute trauma to the head, for example, may result in epidural or subdural hematoma formation. This type of lesion can be quickly, accurately and unequivocally diagnosed by CCT.

Indications

Virtually any suspected disease process involving the brain is an indication for cranial computed tomography. Since the first patient was scanned on a prototype CCT unit in 1972, neuroradiologic emphasis has greatly changed. CCT has virtually eliminated the need for cerebral pneumography and echoencephalography. Furthermore, a substantial decrease in the number of cerebral angiograms and radionuclide brain scans has resulted.

Some of the more common indications for cranial computed tomography include **suspected brain neoplasms or masses**, **brain metastases**, **intracranial hemorrhage**, **aneurysm**, **abscess**, **brain atrophy**, **post-traumatic abnormalities** such as epidural and subdural hematomas, and **acquired or congenital abnormalities**.

Contraindications

Contraindications to cranial computed tomography are few. **About 50% of all CCTs do not require contrast enhancement**; consequently, these examinations are noninvasive. If the patient can be transported to the CT treatment room, the examination can be performed. With some very ill or severely injured patients, the transfer from patient room to treatment room and the transfer from patient bed to CT patient table may be the most hazardous part of the examination.

For the other 50 percent of all CCTs that require contrast enhancement, injection of an iodinated contrast medium is necessary. A very small percentage of persons may react adversely to an injection of iodinated contrast medium. A careful history must be taken prior to such an injection. Should the patient's history indicate a possible severe reaction, the patient's physician may choose to medicate prior to the examination or cancel the contrast-enhanced portion of the study.

Except for the patient with an actual history of severe reaction to iodinated contrast medium, and the nontransportable patient, there are no real contraindications to cranial computed tomography.

Patient Preparation

There is usually no patient preparation for a CCT. Unpleasant side effects such as nausea and/or vomiting may occur whenever iodinated contrast medium is introduced into the human circulatory system. For the **contrast-enhanced examination**, it is prudent to examine the patient with an empty stomach to prevent complications associated with premature gastric emptying.

Patient preparation may be necessary for the uncooperative type of individual. **Patient motion** during the scan is a serious impairment to the diagnostic CCT, so some cooperation is essential. Many circumstances may render the patient less cooperative than usual. Brain lesions may affect the patient in bizarre ways, depending on the location and amount of brain tissue involved.

Events prior to an acute head injury may include ingestion or inhalation of a variety of substances that may also alter normal behavior. Therefore, should sedation or anesthesia be necessary to allow scan completion without unwanted patient motion, appropriate medication must be administered by medical personnel. Preparation for resuscitative measures, including endotracheal tube placement capabilities, are mandatory for the sedated patient.

Contrast Media

The contrast media utilized for cranial computed tomography are identical to those used for excretory urography. These iodinated contrast media are usually administered as a bolus injection, but may be introduced via an intravenous infusion.

Complications

True anaphylactoid reaction to currently used iodinated contrast media is rare, but possible minor or major reactions must be foremost in the minds of radiology staff members whenever such injections are necessary. Complications arising from such injections are treated according to a well-established departmental protocol.

Postprocedure care includes careful observation since delayed reactions to contrast media are possible, although most reactions will occur within the first 5 minutes following injection if they are going to happen.

Scanner Room Preparation

Room preparation for a CCT is fairly simple. Basically, three steps need to be taken. **First**, the scanner or treatment room should be clean and tidy. All patients, as they are brought into the scanner room, should be made to feel that they are the first patient to utilize the equipment. **Second**, assemble any patient support items necessary. If oxygen, suction or IV pole are necessary, these should be provided. If the patient must be ventilated during examination or anesthetized prior to the procedure, the appropriate personnel must be assembled.

Finally, the operator console, direct display console and computer must be activated. The computer must be instructed via the keyboard to prepare for the appropriate procedure. If the examination is to be a contrast-enhanced procedure, then it is necessary to prepare for injection or infusion in the standard, sterile manner.

CRANIAL COMPUTED TOMOGRAPHY POSITIONING

Basic Positioning

Routine positioning for cranial computed tomography is shown in Fig. 22-70. **The neck is flexed until a line 25° to the IOML is parallel to the x-ray beam.** This positioning requires that the chin be depressed and support be placed under the head. An exact 25° angle is not absolutely necessary since both sides are seen on the finished reconstruction. More important is placement of the head so that **no rotation** and **no tilt** are detected on the scan.

The basic principles of skull positioning used in conventional radiography apply equally to computed tomography, with one major exception. In CCT, the **section of interest is placed parallel to the x-ray beam** rather than perpendicular to it. With accurate positioning, interested physicians can examine bilateral symmetry in the normal scan and asymmetry in the abnormal reconstruction.

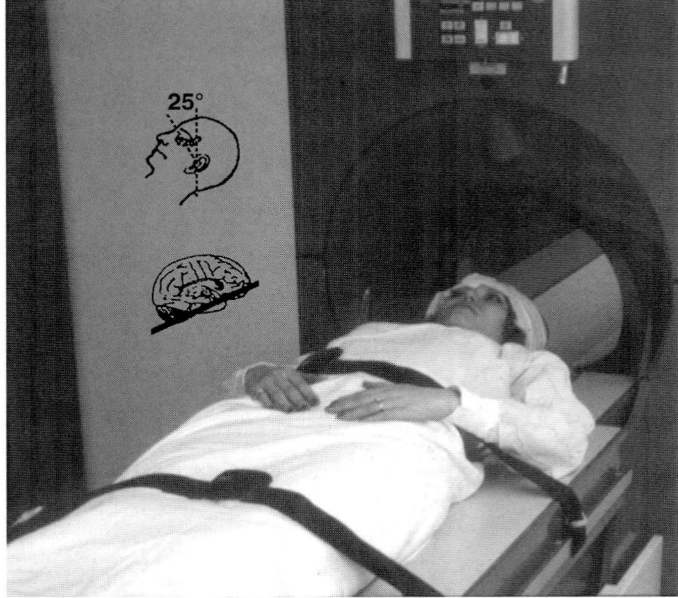

Fig. 22-70. Routine CCT positioning–IOML parallel to CR.

Alternate Positioning Method.

An alternate positioning method for routine cranial scanning is to use **a line connecting the** SOG (supraorbital groove) and the TEA (top of ear attachment). By placing this line parallel to the x-ray beam, similar results can be obtained when compared to the 25° to the IOML method. Placing the head in this position allows most of the cerebellum to be visualized on the same slice as the area of the sella turcica.

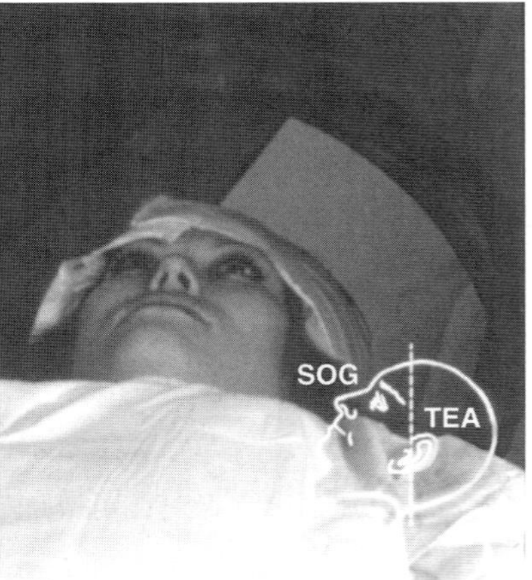

Fig. 22-71. Alternate positioning.

Procedure for Complete CCT

The procedure for a complete CCT scan may vary from facility to facility, but usually the initial sequence is six to ten scans. These **6 to 10 scans** cover the entire brain from base to vertex, in up to 13 millimeter sections. Depending on the scan unit in use, the sections may be thinner, such as 5, 8 or 10 millimeters.

The initial sequence is usually performed without contrast enhancement. Should enhancement be indicated, as determined by the provisional diagnosis and/or departmental routine, a second sequence is then performed. The same brain sections are again examined; but, for the second series, contrast medium is injected or infused.

CCT Scan

No Rotation: One of the axial sections in the cranial computed tomographic series is shown in Fig. 22-72. No rotation or tilt is detected on the section. The bilateral symmetry of the brain and cranial structures is demonstrated on this radiograph.

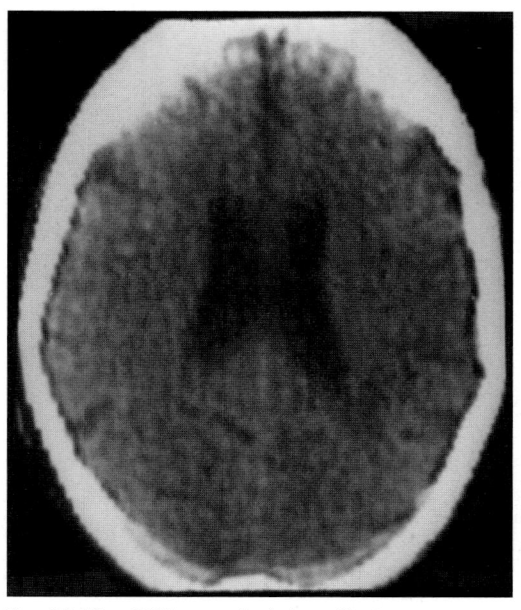

Fig. 22-72. CCT scan (axial section).

Orbital Scan Positioning

One variation to the basic CCT routine is **orbital scanning**. Some routines call for the automatic inclusion of approximately three sections through the orbits, utilizing a slightly different head position. The patient is shown in position for orbital scanning in Fig. 22-73. The head is in a neutral position so that the **radiation beam parallels the IOM line.** An alternative line used for the same result is one connecting the midlateral orbital margin and the TEA. This line is parallel to the IOML.

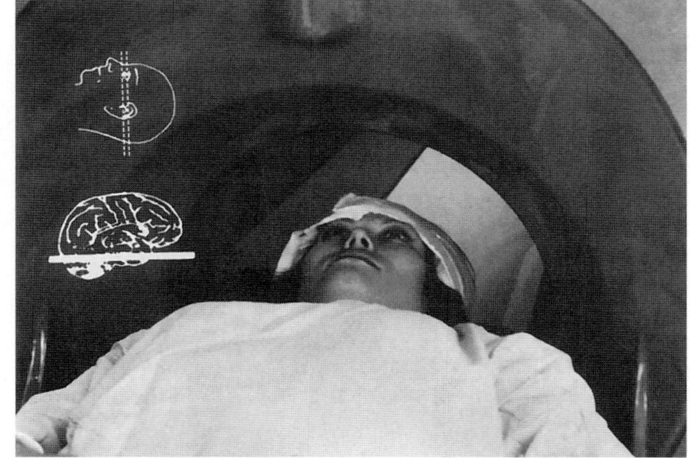

Fig. 22-73. Orbital scanning position–IOML parallel to CR.

Orbital Scan

The radiograph in Fig. 22-74 is an orbital scan utilizing the neutral head position. This radiograph clearly shows the orbital cavities, including the ocular bulbs and optic nerves.

Other positioning angles may be utilized to meet different needs. Certain scanners allow different positions to be assumed, including the submentovertex projection for coronal sections. Certain units allow reconstruction of coronal sections based on axial section data stored in the computer.

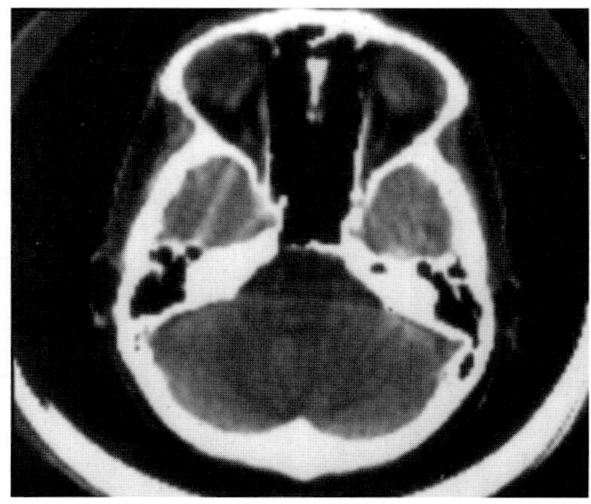

Fig. 22-74. Orbital scan.

Contrast Enhancement

The brain is well supplied with blood vessels that supply oxygen and nutrients. Oxygen must be in constant supply since total oxygen deprivation for the short time of 4 minutes can lead to permanent brain cell damage. Similarly, glucose must be continually available since carbohydrate storage in the brain is limited. Glucose, oxygen and certain ions pass readily from the circulatory blood into extracellular fluid, then into brain cells. Other substances found in the blood normally enter brain cells quite slowly. Still others, such as proteins, most antibiotics and contrast media, will not pass at all from the normal cranial capillary system into brain cells.

The brain is different from other tissues in that there is a natural barrier to the passage of certain substances. This natural phenomenon is termed the "blood-brain barrier." Contrast medium appearing outside the normal vascular system is an indication that something is wrong. A normal cranial computed tomograph is shown in Fig. 22-75, while the same level is shown in Fig. 22-76 with contrast enhancement. Both are normal, without any disruption of the blood-brain barrier.

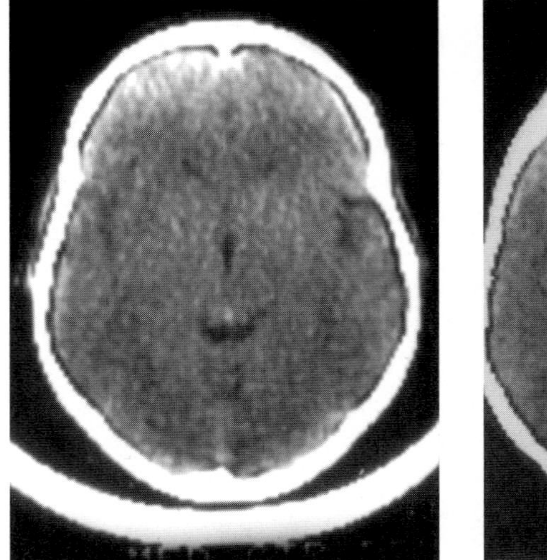

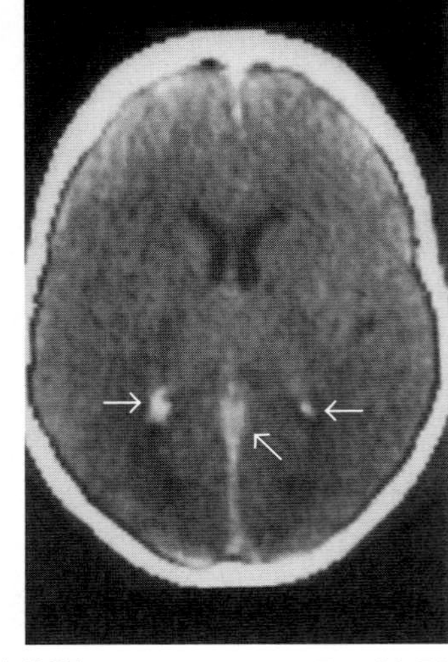

Fig. 22-75. Contrast-enhanced CCT. Fig. 22-76.

EXAMPLES OF POSITIVE CCT IMAGES

Glioma

An example of a positive CCT is shown in Figs. 22-77 and 22-78. This particular lesion is a glioma *(gli-o′mah)*, a type of brain tumor. A noncontrast tomogram is shown in Fig. 22-77, and a contrast-enhanced version of the same slice in Fig. 22-78. Contrast enhancement is necessary for all suspected neoplasia due to possible breakdown of the normal blood-brain barrier.

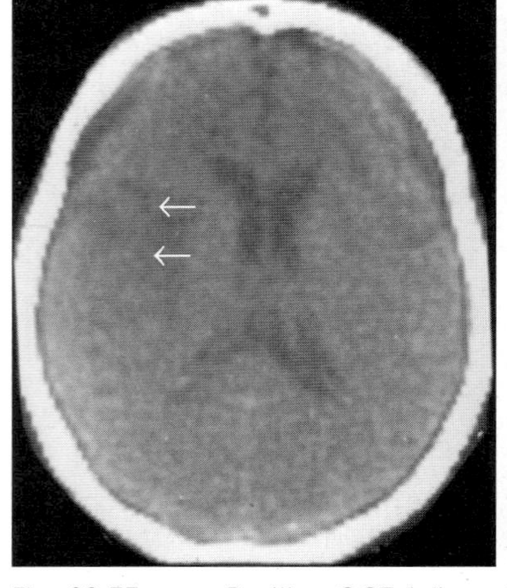

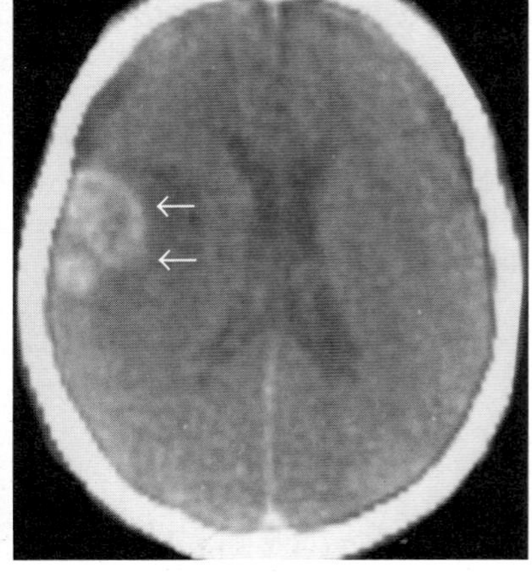

Fig. 22-77. Positive CCT (gliomatous tumor). Fig. 22-78.

Subdural Hematoma and Hydrocephaly

Two additional positive examples of cranial computed tomograms are illustrated in Figs. 22-79 and 22-80. A large bilateral, frontal, subdural hematoma of at least 3 weeks' duration is shown in Fig. 22-79. This type of lesion, whether acute or chronic, can be diagnosed without contrast enhancement.

Figure 22-80 demonstrates an example of hydrocephalus. Note the enlarged ventricles and how well they visualize on the CCT.

With well-maintained and properly functioning equipment, computed tomography of the head is not a difficult examination for the radiographer to perform, or for the neuroradiologist to interpret. CCT is an exciting diagnostic radiographic tool and is proving invaluable to the diagnosis of cranial disease.

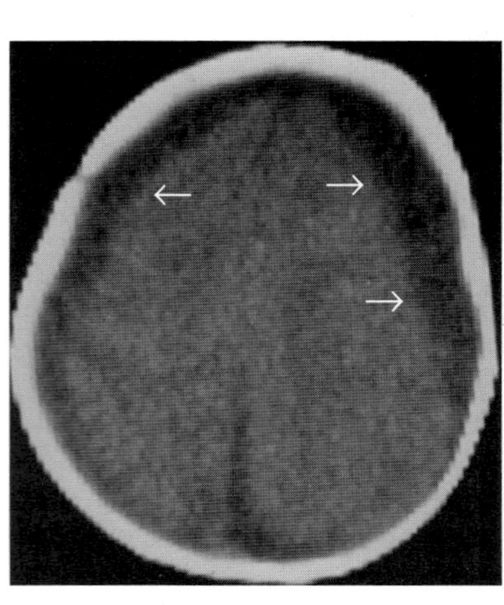

Fig. 22-79. Subdural hematoma.

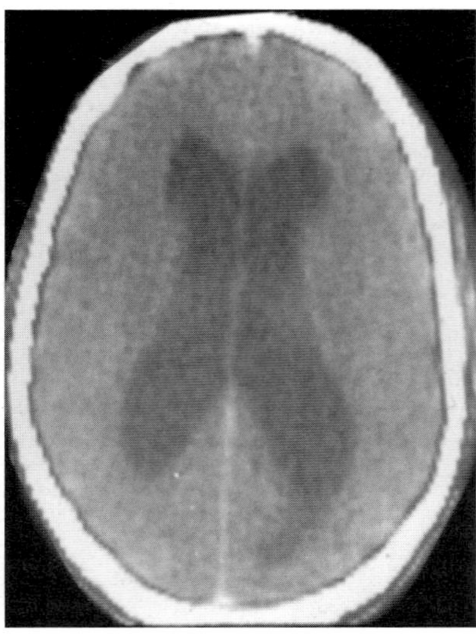

Fig. 22-80. Hydrocephalus.

CHAPTER 23

Thoracic, Abdominal & Pelvic Computed Tomography

CONTRIBUTIONS BY:
James D. Lipcamon, RT (R)

CONTENTS

Computed Tomography

Introduction **660**

Computed tomographic system **660**

Radiographic Anatomy–Thorax

Axial sections of chest **661**

Radiographic Positioning and Procedures–Thorax

Purpose and indications **664**

Contraindications and contrast media **665**

Positioning for CT of chest **665**

Procedure for CT of chest **666**

Radiographic Anatomy –Abdomen and Pelvis

Axial sections of the abdomen **667**

Axial sections of the pelvis **670**

Radiographic Positioning and Procedures–Abdomen and Pelvis

Purpose and indications **673**

Contraindications and patient preparation **674**

Types of contrast media **675**

Recommended oral and rectal contrast media volumes **676**

Procedure for complete CT of abdomen and pelvis **677**

Introduction

COMPUTED TOMOGRAPHY

Definition

Computed tomography refers to **a radiographic examination of a body cavity or body part in which x-rays and a computer are used to produce a sectional slice of anatomy free of superimposed structures.** The images are representations of different shades of gray that correspond to the amount of x-ray that was absorbed as described in the preceding chapter on cranial computed tomography, (CCT). **Axial** or **transverse sections** of the thorax and abdomen are shown on the following pages.

Advantages Over Conventional Radiography

Computed tomography (CT) has become a well-accepted imaging device in diagnostic medicine. Excellent visualization of the site, free of superimposed structures, is the foremost advantage over conventional radiographic procedures. Its ability to discriminate differences in tissue densities (from .5 % to 1% in most scanners) make it a superior method. Because the x-ray beam is closely collimated and the scatter radiation reduced, excellent image quality is obtained.

Additionally, collected data can be manipulated and measured. By measuring the attenuation value, it is often possible to determine if a lesion is fat, fluid or calcium in nature. The extent and relationship of abnormal pathology to surrounding structures can be determined because in addition to axial or transverse sections the area can also be visualized in two other dimensions as shown in Fig. 23-1. Due to the utilization of the computer, software programs provide the capability of manipulating the acquired data into **coronal** and **sagittal views**.

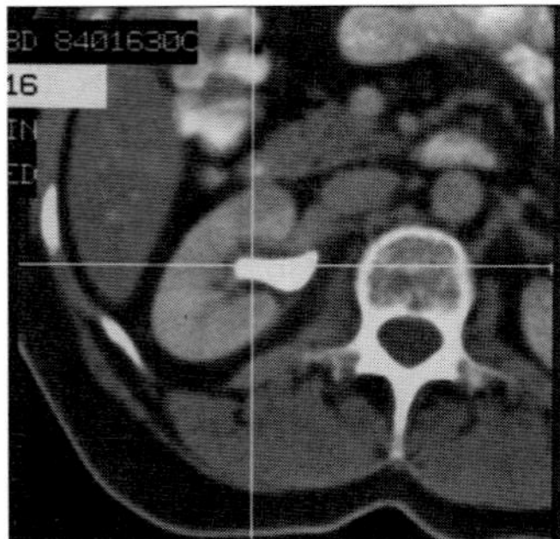

Axial (transverse)

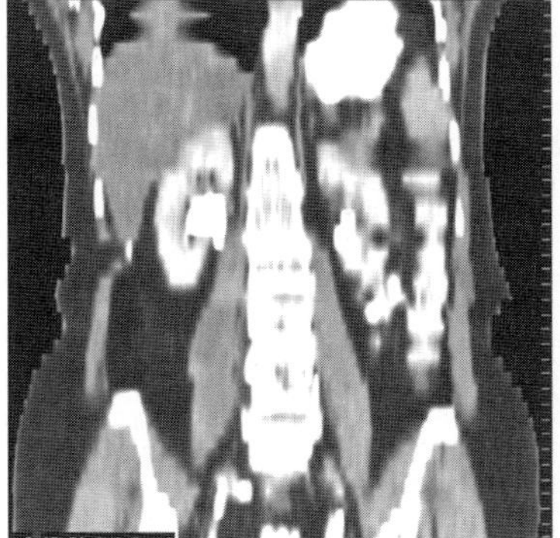

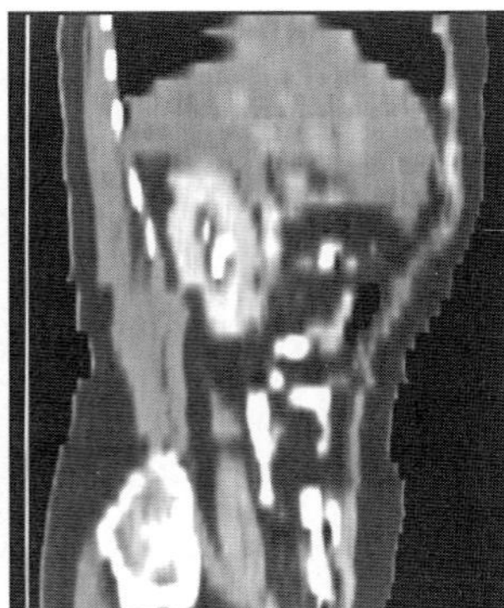

Fig. 23-1. Coronal Sagittal
Axial, coronal and sagittal reconstruction.

COMPUTED TOMOGRAPHIC SYSTEM

The preceding Chapter 22 on cranial computed tomography explains not only the basic principles of computed tomography but also the various **components** of a computed tomographic system. These components include the **scan unit** (made up of the patient table or couch and the gantry), and the **operator control console**, which includes the processing unit or computer, monitors, storage or archival systems in addition to operator controls.

The earlier models of CT systems included a scanning unit with smaller apertures so that only smaller parts such as patients' heads could be scanned. Later model whole body scanners (Fig. 23-2) have larger apertures so entire bodies including chest, abdomen and pelvic areas can be scanned, as described and illustrated in this chapter.

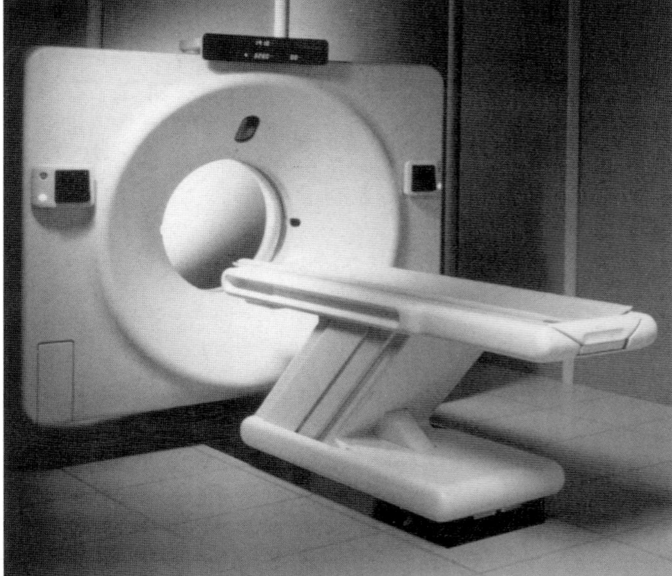

Fig. 23-2. Whole body scanner (gantry and table).
(Courtesy of GE Medical Systems, Milwaukee, WI.)

Radiographic Anatomy - Thorax

Thoracic Anatomy

The anatomy of the thorax is covered thoroughly in **Chapter 2** on general chest anatomy, **Chapter 10** on the bony thorax and **Chapter 24** on the heart and circulatory system of the thorax. The anatomy from these chapters should be mastered before continuing with this study of sectional anatomy of the thorax.

Thoracic computed tomography requires a thorough understanding of sectional anatomy of the thorax as viewed in **axial sections.**

AXIAL SECTIONS OF THE CHEST

Ten thorax CT scans of 10 mm thickness are shown in the axial orientation. The examination for these scans was obtained using bolus injections of intravenous contrast. The total volume used was 180 cc's. The patient's right is on the viewer's left as with conventional radiography.

Axial Section 1

Axial section number 1, shown in Fig. 23-3, represents a section at **the level of the sternal notch.** Parts labeled are:

A. Right internal jugular vein.
B. Right carotid artery.
C. Left internal jugular vein.
D. Left subclavian artery.
E. Left carotid artery.
F. Right subclavian artery.

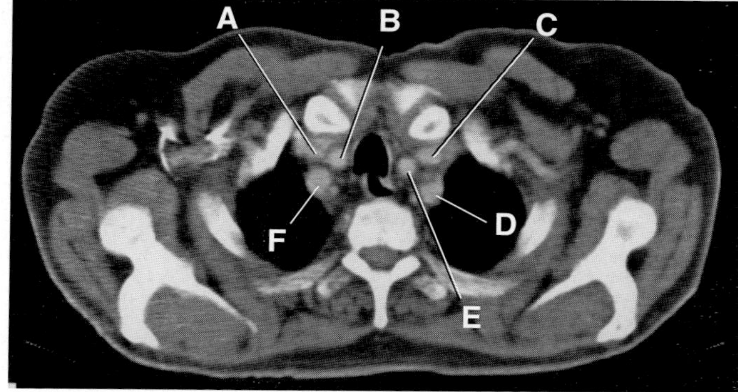

Fig. 23-3. Axial section 1.

Axial Section 2

Axial section 2 represents a section through the **superior portion of the manubrium.** Parts labeled are:

A. Right brachiocephalic vein.
B. Right carotid artery.
C. Left carotid artery.
D. Left subclavian artery.
E. Esophagus.
F. Trachea.
G. Right subclavian artery.

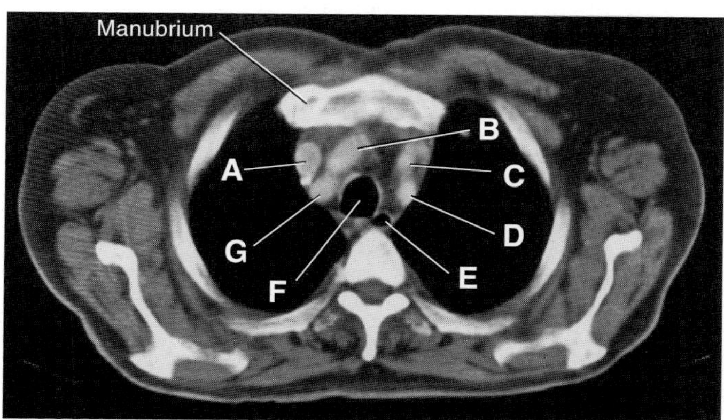

Fig. 23-4. Axial section 2.

Axial Section 3

Axial section 3 represents a section through the **inferior portion of the manubrium.** Parts labeled are:

A. Right brachiocephalic vein.
B. Brachiocephalic artery (innominate).
C. Left brachiocephalic vein.
D. Left carotid artery.
E. Left subclavian artery.
F. Esophagus.
G. Trachea.

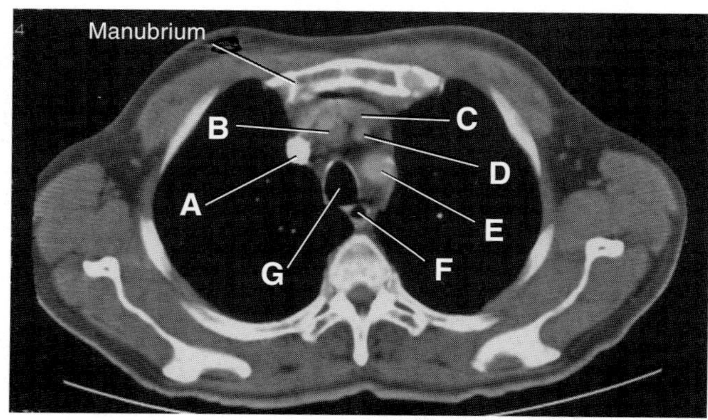

Fig. 23-5. Axial section 3.

Axial Section 4

Axial section 4 represents a section at the level of the **aortic arch.** The right and left brachiocephalic veins have united forming the superior vena cava. Parts labeled are:

A. Superior vena cava.
B. Aortic arch.
C. Esophagus.
D. Trachea.

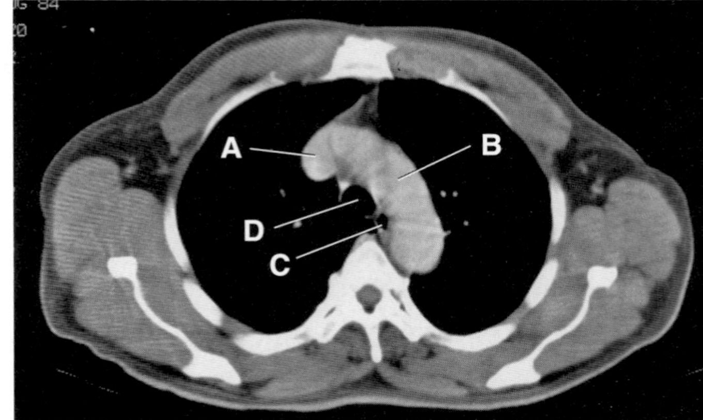

Fig. 23-6. Axial section 4.

Axial Section 5

Axial section 5 represents a section at the level of the **aortopulmonary window**. The aortopulmonary window is a space located between the ascending and descending aorta. Parts labeled are:

A. Superior vena cava.
B. Ascending aorta.
C. Aortopulmonary window.
D. Esophagus.
E. Descending aorta.
F. Trachea.

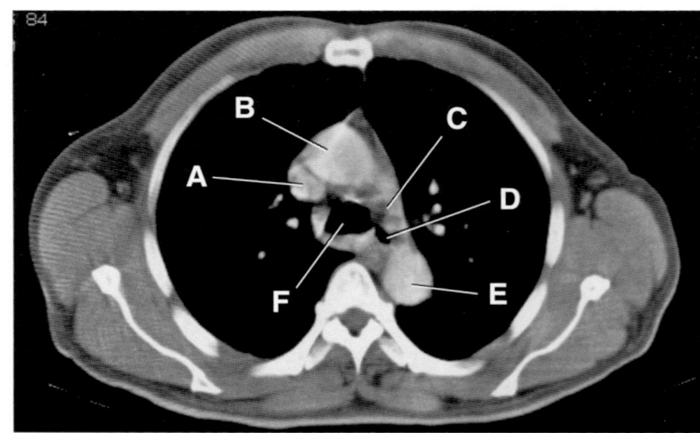

Fig. 23-7. Axial section 5.

Axial Section 6

Axial section 6 represents a section at the level of the **carina.** The carina is the lower level of where the trachea divides into the openings of the right and left bronchi (see Chapter 2). Parts labeled are:

A. Superior vena cava.
B. Ascending aorta.
C. Mediastinal fat.
D. Trunk of pulmonary artery.
E. Left pulmonary artery.
F. Left main stem bronchus.
G. Descending aorta.
H. Azygos vein.
I. Esophagus.
J. Right main stem bronchus.
K. Right pulmonary artery.

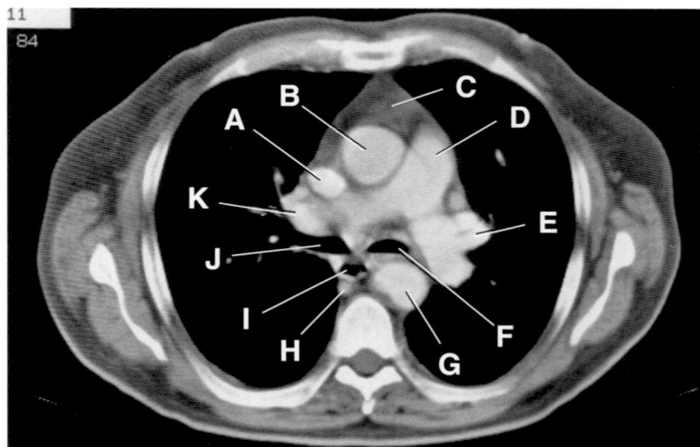

Fig. 23-8. Axial section 6.

Axial Section 7

Axial section 7 was taken at a level of **1 cm below the carina**. Parts labeled are:

A. Superior vena cava
B. Ascending aorta
C. Main pulmonary artery
D. Left pulmonary vein
E. Left pulmonary artery
F. Descending aorta
G. Azygos vein
H. Esophagus
I. Right pulmonary artery

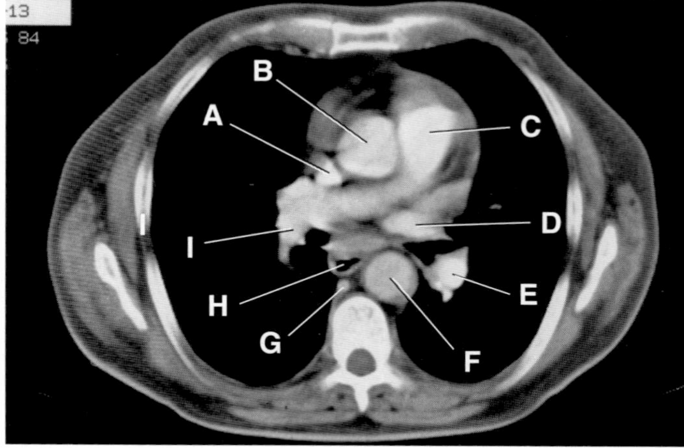

Fig. 23-9. Axial section 7.

Axial Section 8

Axial section 8 is through the level of the **left atrium**. Parts labeled are:

A. Right atrium.
B. Aortic root.
C. Pulmonary trunk.
D. Left ventricle.
E. Left pulmonary vein.
F. Descending aorta.
G. Azygos vein.
H. Esophagus.
I. Left atrium.

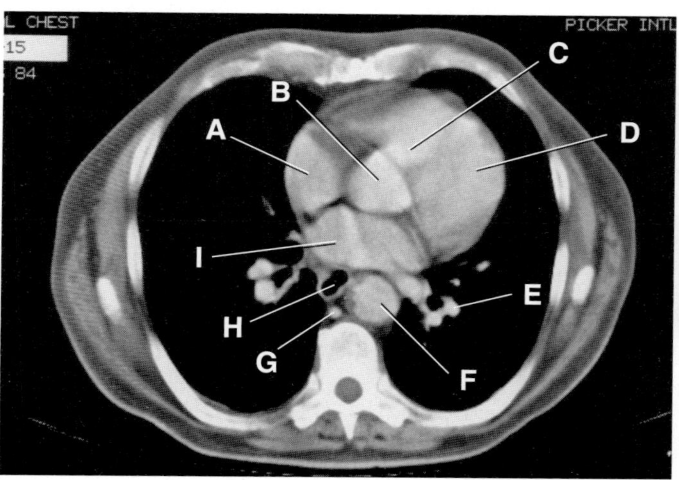

Fig. 23-10. Axial section 8.

Axial Section 9

In this section all **four cardiac chambers** are seen. The arrows pointing between the left atrium and left ventricle represent the approximate location of the mitral valve. Parts labeled are:

A. Inferior vena cava.
B. Right atrium.
C. Right ventricle.
D. Interventricular septum.
E. Left ventricle.
F. Left atrium.
G. Descending aorta.
H. Azygos vein.
I. Esophagus.

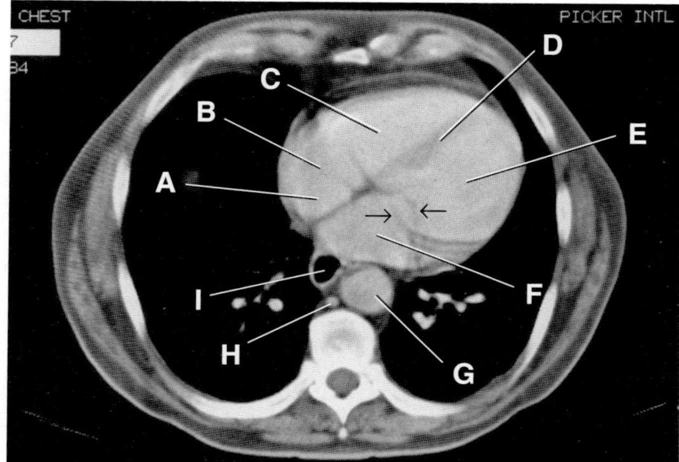

Fig. 23-11. Axial section 9.

Axial Section 10

At this level, **through the base of the heart,** the arrows between the right ventricle and right atrium are pointing to the area of the tricuspid valve. Parts labeled are:

A. Inferior vena cava.
B. Right atrium.
C. Pericardium.
D. Right ventricle.
E. Interventricular septum.
F. Left ventricle.
G. Left atrium.
H. Descending aorta.
I. Azygos vein.
J. Esophagus.
K. Right hemidiaphragm.

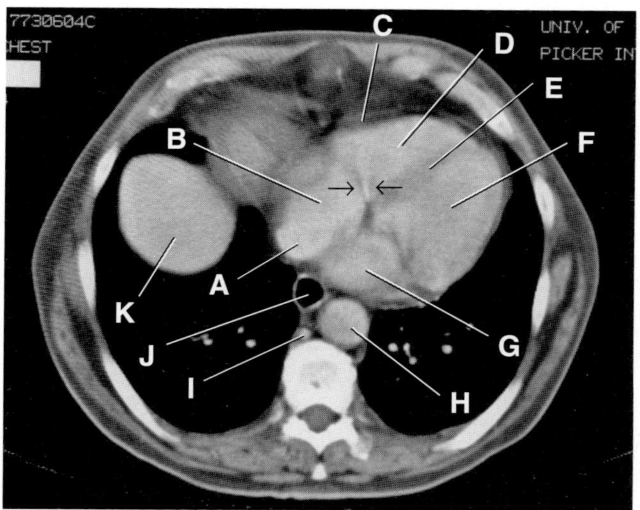

Fig. 23-12. Axial section 10.

Radiographic Positioning and Procedures - Thorax

Purpose

The primary purpose of thoracic computed tomography is to **serve as a diagnostic adjunct to conventional chest radiography.** However, because of its cost effectiveness, conventional chest radiography is still the primary screening tool in patients suspected of having chest disease. As a secondary purpose, CT serves as a valuable imaging modality in the staging and management of previously diagnosed conditions.

Indications

Most **mediastinal abnormalities** of the chest, as documented on plain radiographs, are an indication for computed tomography. This is demonstrated on the conventional chest radiograph in Fig. 23-13 showing a **mediastinal mass**, as marked by the arrows. Compare this with the CT image in Fig. 23-14 clearly defining the mediastinal mass; and the coronal and sagittal reconstruction in Fig. 23-15 showing the true location and relative size of this mass.

Some of the more common indications for CT of the chest are **mediastinal and hilar lesions**, **aneurysms**, **abscess**, **cardiac and pericardial disease**.

The innovation of computed tomography has made conventional tomography of the thorax a procedure of the past in most departments.

Clinically suspected disease does not always appear on plain radiographs, however. In fact, in many instances the radiograph will be negative. When the clinical history is suggestive of ongoing disease, CT can be a valuable diagnostic adjunct in such cases. Undetected or disguised abnormalities of mediastinal structures can be diagnosed before reaching advanced stages.

Another use of CT of the chest is in **the evaluation of pulmonary nodules where** CT can help to determine the benign or malignant nature of the node. Since benign nodes generally have evidence of calcium content, using thin collimation and measuring the attenuation value of the area can give an indication of the nature of the nodule.

Example of Thoracic Pathology

Figures 23-13 through 23-15 demonstrate how thoracic computed tomography can be used to provide diagnostic information on a mediastinal mass.

The AP radiograph (Fig. 23-13) of a 53-day-old male demonstrates mediastinal widening (arrows) of unknown cause. A CT axial scan (Fig. 23-14) shows a well circumscribed, homogeneous mass in the posterior mediastinum. Coronal and sagittal reconstructions (Fig. 23-15) give an additional 2 dimensions as to the mass's extent and relationship to adjacent structures. From the attenuation value of this mass, which is slightly above water, this mass was determined to be a bronchogenic cyst.

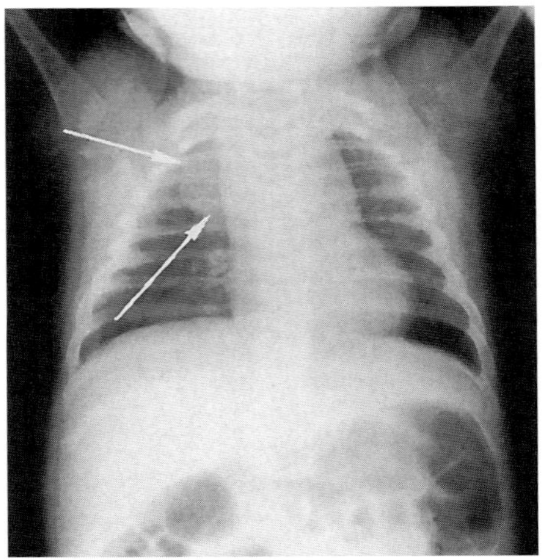

Fig. 23-13. AP radiograph.

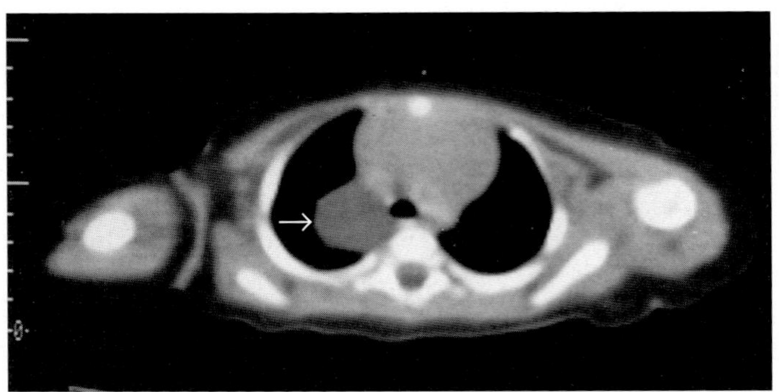

Fig. 23-14. CT image.

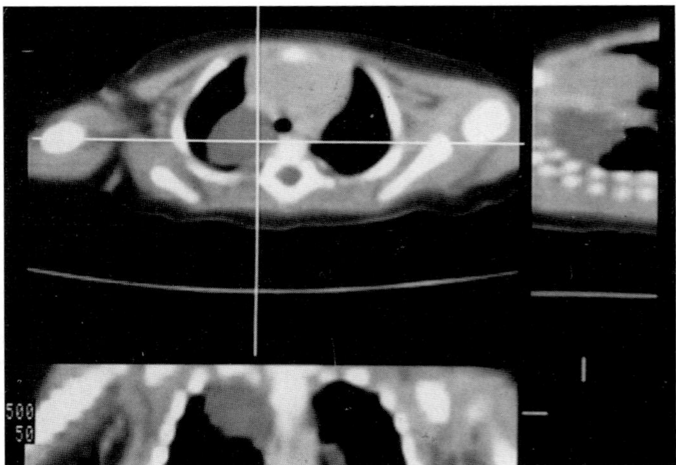

Fig. 23-15. Coronal and sagittal reconstructions.

Contraindications

There are no major contraindications to computed tomography of the chest. One relative contraindication to CT, however, as with any x-ray examination is **pregnancy**. In such cases, the benefits must be weighed against the risks.

With those patients who require a procedure with an injection of iodinated contrast media, a careful history must be taken in order to assess any possibility for **adverse reaction**.

Further, patients with a history of **renal failure**, **multiple myeloma**, **pheochromocytoma** or **diabetes** must be carefully evaluated. When the risk outweighs the benefit, the use of contrast media should be avoided.

Patient Preparation

There are no unusual patient preparation procedures to be followed for computed tomography examinations of the chest. To help reduce the incidence of nausea and/or vomiting following the introduction of intravenous contrast media, the patient should be examined with an empty stomach. To prevent the introduction of metal induced artifacts, patients are to change into clothing with cloth ties, and all opaque objects in the radiographic area of interest must be removed.

In order to obtain high quality examinations, patient cooperation is essential. Patient motion during the procedure seriously impairs the quality of the CT. Patients should be given brief instructions that are to the point and easy to understand. Factors such as breathing instructions and length of examination are important items to discuss.

Contrast Media

The identical contrast media used in excretory urography is utilized in computed tomography of the chest. Various methods are used for the administration of contrast media, including drip infusion, bolus injections, or combinations thereof. The method used is indicated by the clinical history or suspected site of the lesion.

Complications

The possibility of reaction to iodinated contrast material is ever present and although rare, has occurred after the administration of as little as 1 ml of contrast material.

Some common symptoms of minor anaphylactoid reaction are **urticaria** (hives), **nausea**, **vomiting**, and **flushing of the face**.

Moderate reactions include **urticaria**, **facial** and **laryngeal edema** and **hypotension**. Usually some treatment is required with moderate reactions.

Scanner Room Preparation

Proper preparation of the CT scanning room is essential. Particular emphasis should be placed on the readiness of equipment for emergency situations. Suction, blood pressure cuff, cardiac monitor, oxygen tanks and crash cart should be easily accessible. Emergency phone numbers should be placed near the phone and in easy to recognize colors.

The room should be clean. Contrast media, emesis, and blood should be cleaned immediately in order to reduce bacterial growth. All personnel working in the area should be trained in emergency procedures and be familiar with the workings of the unit.

POSITIONING FOR CT OF THE CHEST

For routine examinations of the chest the patient is placed in a supine position with arms elevated above the head. Keeping the arms above the head will help reduce scan artifacts, particularly beam hardening artifacts from the humeral heads. Patients need to be instructed to keep their arms extended and close to the head so their elbows do not hit the sides of the gantry.

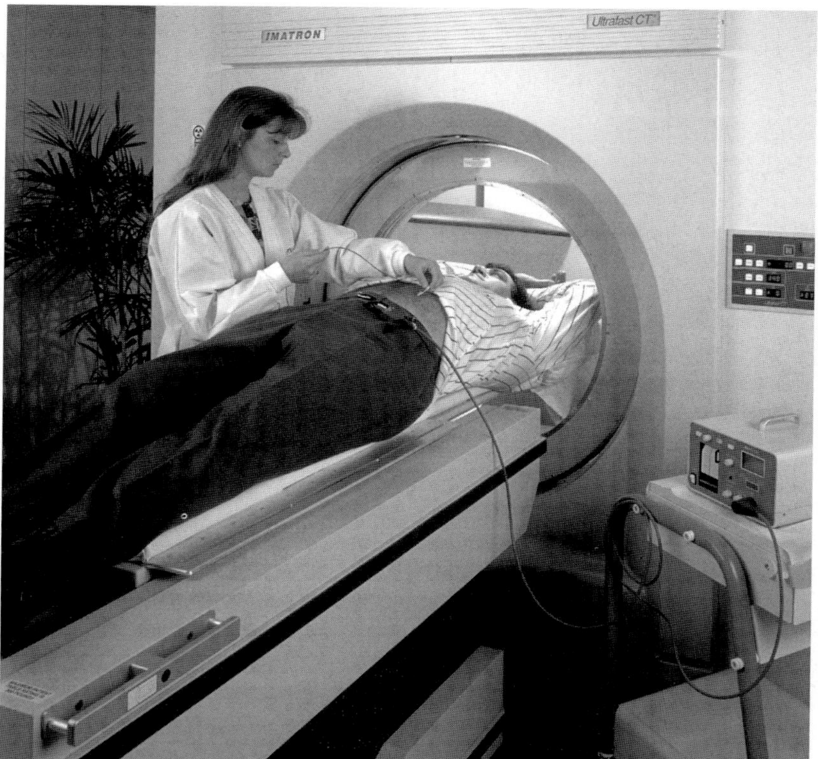

Fig. 23-16. Demonstration of preparation for CT of chest and/or abdomen.
(Courtesy of Imatron, Inc., San Francisco, CA.

PROCEDURE FOR COMPLETE CT OF THE CHEST

For positioning of where slices are to occur for an examination, a pilot or localizing scan is used. A pilot or localizing scan is taken in which the detectors and tube are stationary while the patient moves up through the gantry aperture on the patient couch (Fig. 23-17). As the patient moves through the gantry aperture, an exposure is made, the data is processed by the computer and an image is produced which looks similar to a conventional radiograph (Fig. 23-18).

Once this localizing radiograph (Fig. 23-18) is obtained, the location of the first slice is placed at the apices. Scanning continues to the level of the diaphragm in mediastinal pathology cases. If the primary concern is pulmonary malignancy, scanning continues to the level of the adrenal glands. This is done because a number of pulmonary malignancies will metastasize to the adrenal glands.

In routine CT examinations of the chest, a 10 mm slice thickness and couch incrementation is commonly used. Couch incrementation refers to how far the patient couch moves after each exposure is made. In instances of smaller lesions, smaller sections (3 to 5 mm) are used.

Soft tissue masses frequently constrict or compress the esophagus. To help distinguish the two, esophageal creams are used, which help opacify the esophagus by coating the mucosa.

With the advent of third and fourth generation scanners with exposure times as fast as 1 to 2 seconds, motion artifact produced by respiratory and cardiac motion has virtually been eliminated. However, the patient should be instructed in suspended respiration at inspiration, expiration or at resting volume. It is critical that the same method be used throughout the examination so anatomical fluctuation is avoided.

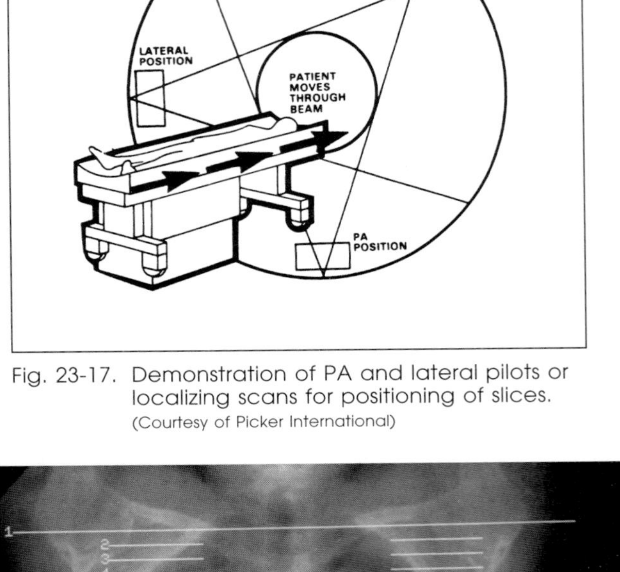

Fig. 23-17. Demonstration of PA and lateral pilots or localizing scans for positioning of slices. (Courtesy of Picker International)

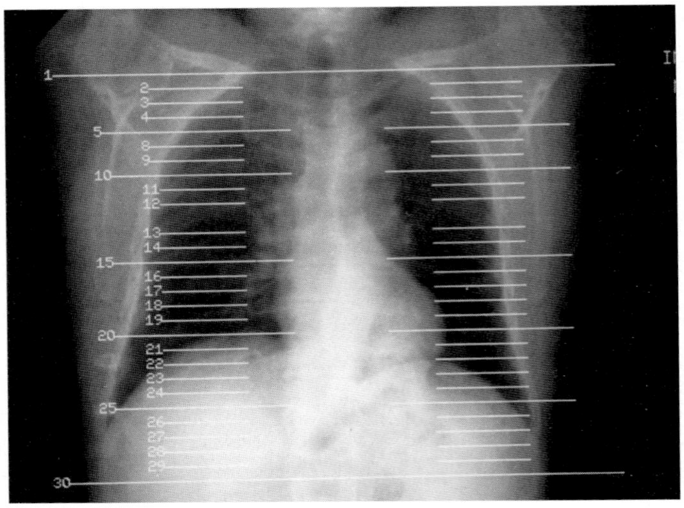

Fig. 23-18. Localizing radiograph (pilot scan).

Contrast Scales

When imaging and viewing chest scans from the display unit, two different contrast scales must be used. Mediastinal structures and lung parenchyma have differing attenuation values therefore necessitating two different mediastinal and lung contrast scales. **Mediastinal structures** are viewed and imaged using a **narrow contrast scale** as shown in Fig. 23-19.

When viewing and imaging lung structures such as **pulmonary parenchyma**, a **wide contrast scale** is used as demonstrated in Fig. 23-20.

Contrast Enhancement

The use of intravenous contrast media can provide valuable information to chest examinations, particularly when the area of concern is the mediastinum. Contrast media has proven to be diagnostically useful in the separation of soft tissue lesions from vascular structures and in the distinction of a vascular from nonvascular lesion.

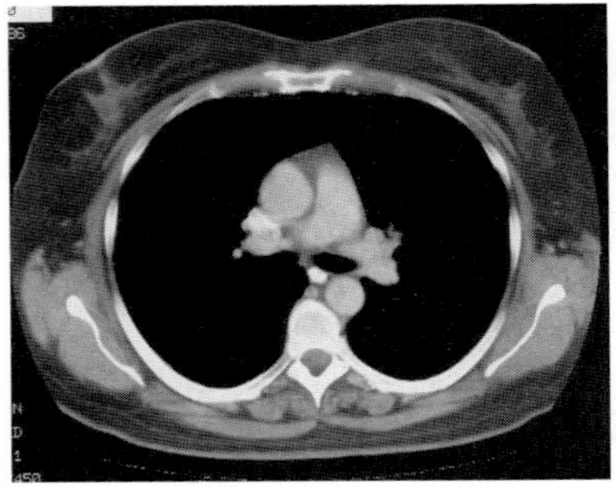

Fig. 23-19. Mediastinal (narrow) contrast scale.

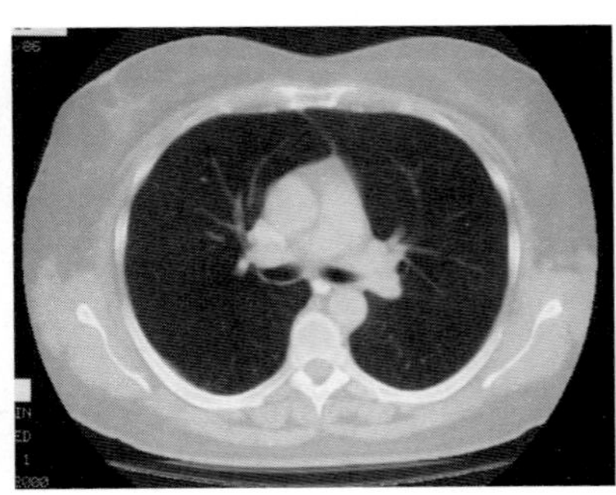

Fig. 23-20. Lung (wide) contrast scale.

Radiographic Anatomy - Abdomen and Pelvis

Abdominal and Pelvic Anatomy

The anatomy of the abdomen and pelvis is covered in **Chapters 3** and **7** respectively with additional anatomy of digestive, biliary and urinary systems in **Chapters 14, 15, 16** and **17**. The anatomy covered in these chapters should be mastered before beginning this chapter on sectional anatomy of the abdomen and pelvis.

AXIAL SECTIONS OF THE ABDOMEN

Eight CT axial scans of the abdomen are shown with 10 mm thick slices. The examination was obtained using a 50 cc bolus injection followed by a 100 cc drip infusion of intravenous contrast. An oral preparation of water-soluble contrast solution was used. Total volume was 900 ml. The patient's right is on the viewer's left.

Axial Section 1

Axial section number 1 is shown in Fig. 23-21. The scan is through the **upper portion of the liver.** The liver is divided into 2 lobes, the right (A) and left (B) lobes. The labeled parts are:

A. Right lobe of liver.
B. Left lobe of liver.
C. Stomach (fundus).
D. Spleen.
E. Aorta.
F. Inferior vena cava.

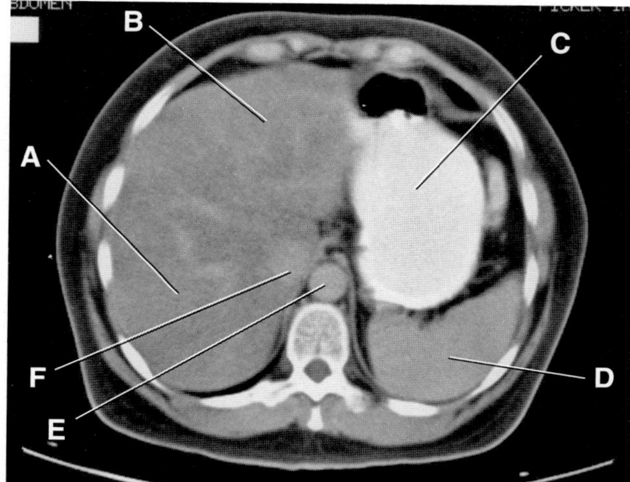

Fig. 23-21. Axial section 1.

Axial Section 2

This section represents the level of the **splenic hilus**. The splenic hilus is the area of the spleen where the splenic artery and vein enter and exit. Note that all four segments of the liver are easily seen. The right lobe is divided into anterior (B) and posterior (A) segments. The left lobe is divided into medial (C) and lateral (D) segments. Parts labeled are:

A. Right lobe, posterior segment of liver.
B. Right lobe, anterior segment of liver.
C. Left lobe, medial segment of liver.
D. Left lobe, lateral segment of liver.
E. Stomach (fundus).
F. Splenic artery.
G. Spleen.
H. Aorta.
I. Inferior vena cava.

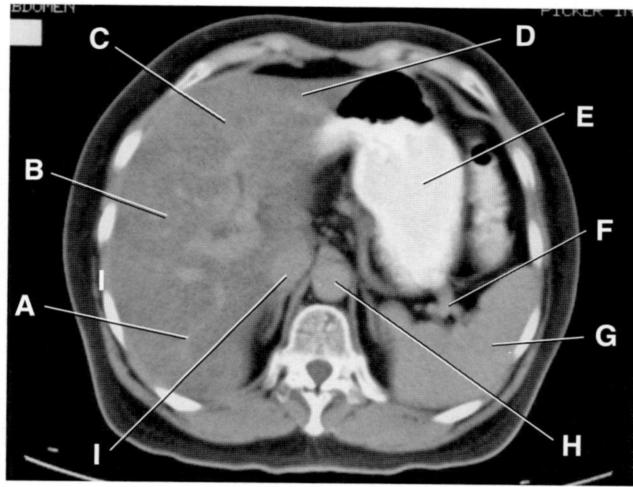

Fig. 23-22. Axial section 2.

Axial Sections of Abdomen continued

Axial Section 3

This scan is at the level of the **pancreatic tail** (G) . The pancreatic tail is in its general position, anterior to the left kidney. Note the excellent visualization of the adrenal gland (I). The adrenal glands are most often seen as an inverted V shape. The parts as labeled are:

A. Right lobe of liver (posterior segment).
B. Gallbladder.
C. Right lobe of liver (anterior segment).
D. Left lobe of liver (medial segment).
E. Left lobe of liver (lateral segment).
F. Stomach (body).
G. Pancreatic tail.
H. Spleen.
I. Left adrenal gland.
J. Inferior vena cava.
K. Upper lobe of right kidney.

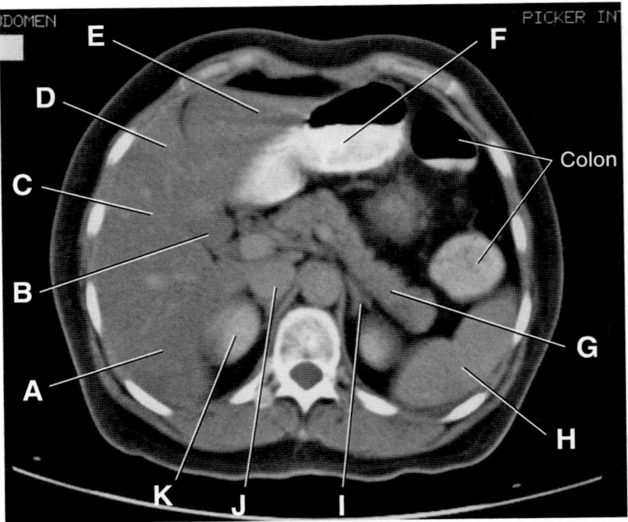

Fig. 23-23. Axial section 3.

Axial Section 4

This cross section is through **the body (F) and neck of the pancreas** (C). The splenic vein (G) runs posterior to the body and neck of the pancreas, joining the superior mesenteric vein to form the portal vein (B). The parts as labeled are:

A. Right lobe of liver (posterior segment).
B. Portal vein.
C. Neck of pancreas.
D. Left lobe of liver (lateral segment).
E. Stomach (pylorus).
F. Body of pancreas.
G. Splenic vein.
H. Spleen.
I. Aorta.
J. Inferior vena cava.
K. Right kidney.

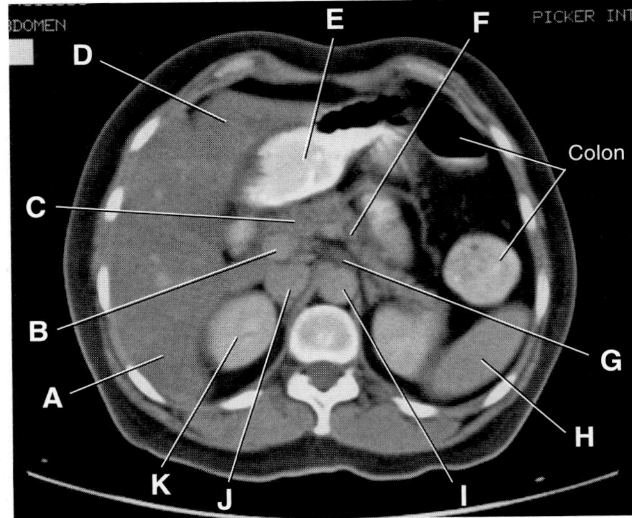

Fig. 23-24. Axial section 4.

Axial Section 5

This scan was taken at the level of the **second portion of the duodenum** (C). The head of the pancreas (I) is well outlined by the duodenum. If the second portion of the duodenum is inadequately opacified it can be confused for a pancreatic tumor. The parts as labeled are:

A. Right lobe of liver (posterior segment).
B. Gallbladder.
C. Second portion of duodenum.
D. Left lobe of liver (lateral segment).
E. Stomach.
F. Left kidney.
G. Aorta.
H. Inferior vena cava.
I. Head of pancreas.

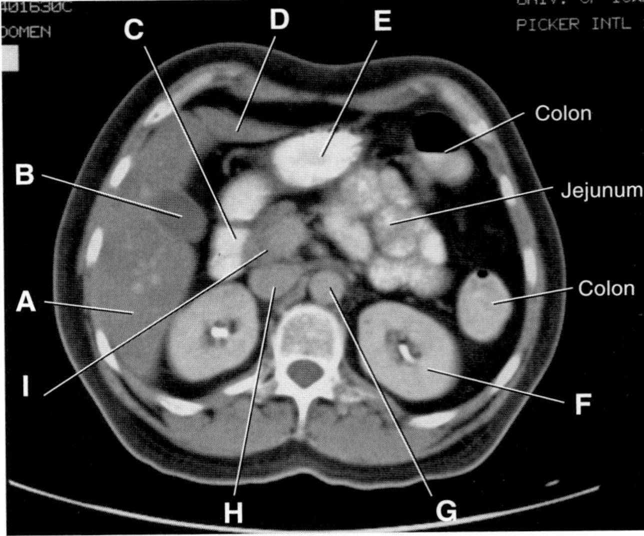

Fig. 23-25. Axial section 5.

Axial Section 6

This cross-section is through the **uncinate process of the pancreas** (B). The uncinate process is a hooklike extension of the head of the pancreas. Note the left renal vein (E) which is coursing anterior to the aorta (G) and entering into the inferior vena cava (H). The left renal vein usually is longer than the right. The labeled parts are:

A. Right lobe of liver.
B. Uncinate process of the pancreas.
C. Gallbladder.
D. Left lobe of liver.
E. Left renal vein.
F. Left kidney.
G. Abdominal aorta.
H. Inferior vena cava.

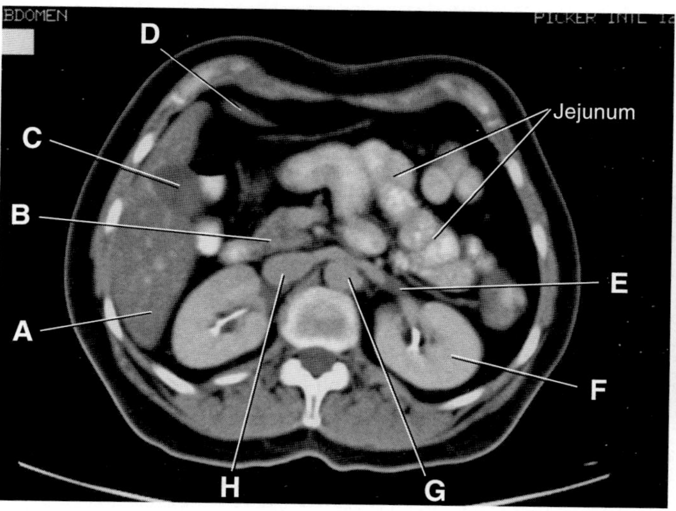

Fig. 23-26. Axial section 6.

Axial Section 7

This scan was taken through the **mid portion of the kidneys.** There is excellent visualization of the right and left renal pelvis (D). The parts as labeled are:

A. Right lobe of the liver.
B. Uncinate process of the pancreas.
C. Gallbladder.
D. Left renal pelvis.
E. Abdominal aorta.
F. Inferior vena cava.

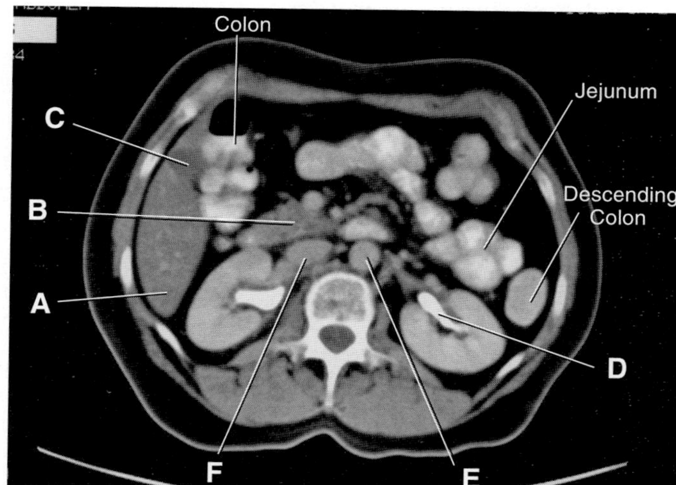

Fig. 23-27. Axial section 7.

Axial Section 8

This scan is 2 **cm caudal to the renal pelvis** and demonstrates the contrast filled ureters medial to the kidneys. The labeled parts are:

A. Right lobe of the liver.
B. Left kidney.
C. Left ureter.
D. Abdominal aorta.
E. Inferior vena cava.
F. Right ureter.

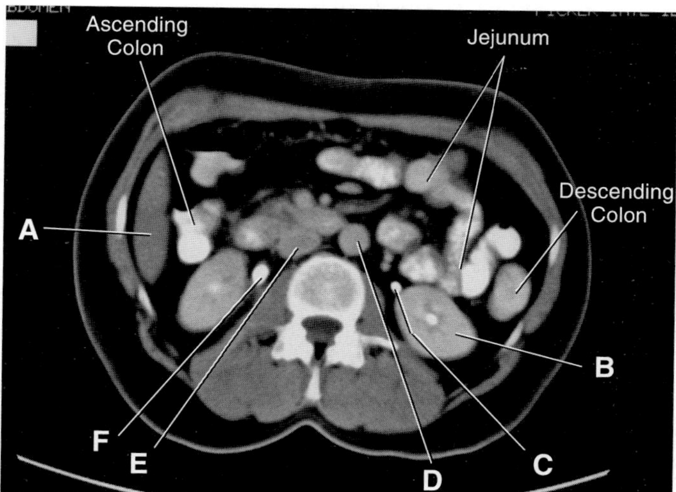

Fig. 23-28. Axial section 8.

Axial Sections of the Pelvis

MALE PELVIS

Ten sectional CT scans of 10 mm slice thickness are shown in the axial orientation. The male pelvis was obtained using a 150 cc drip infusion of intravenous contrast. Intravenous contrast was not used for the female examination due to the patient being in renal failure. Gastrointestinal opacification was obtained by administering barium sulfate orally and by enema for both patients. The patient's right is on the viewer's left.

Axial Section 1

Axial section number 1 is shown in Fig. 23-29. This cross-section is **2 cm caudal to the iliac crest.** This is a male pelvis. The labeled parts are:

A. Gluteus medius muscle.
B. Right iliac wing.
C. Ascending colon.
D. Rectus abdominus muscle.
E. Psoas muscle.
F. Iliacus muscle.

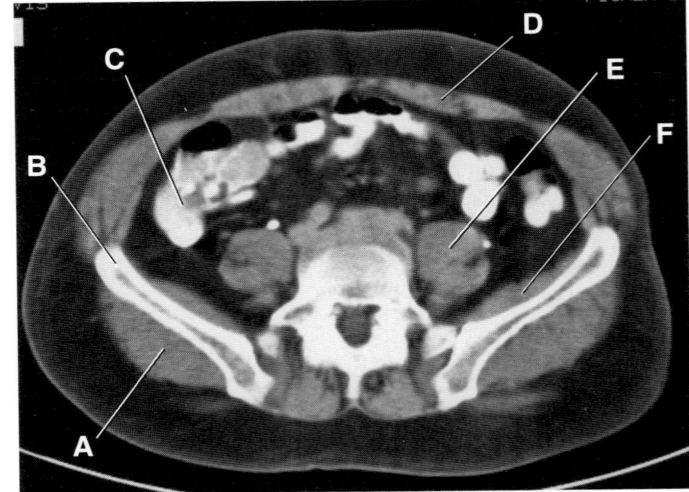

Fig. 23-29. Axial section 1.

Axial Section 2

This scan was taken at the level of the **sacroiliac joints** (H) . This is a male pelvis. Parts labeled are:

A. Gluteus maximus muscle.
B. Gluteus medius muscle.
C. Right iliac wing.
D. Cecum.
E. Rectus abdominus muscle.
F. Psoas muscle.
G. Iliacus muscle.
H. Sacroiliac joints.
I. Sacrum.

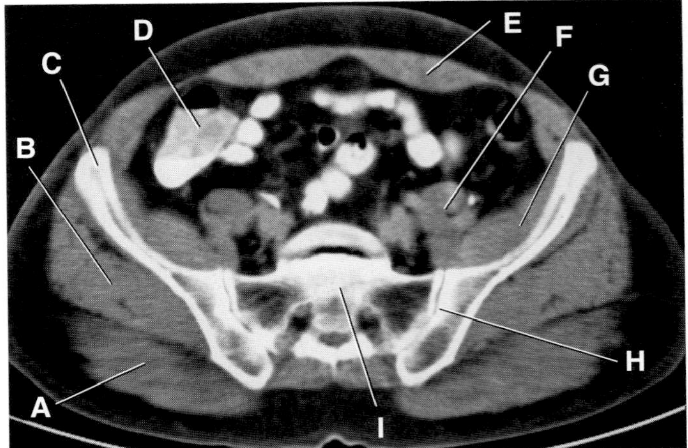

Fig. 23-30. Axial section 2.

Axial Section 3

At this level the **three gluteal muscles** are easily identified because of the excellent fat planes. The gluteal muscles assist in movement of the thigh. This is a male pelvis. Parts labeled are:

A. Gluteus maximus muscle.
B. Gluteus medius muscle.
C. Gluteus minimus muscle.
D. Rectus abdominus muscle.
E. Iliopsoas muscle.
F. Ilium.
G. Sigmoid colon.

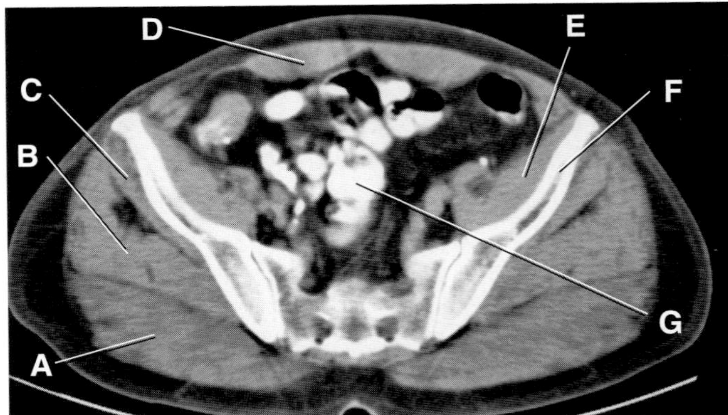

Fig. 23-31. Axial section 3.

Axial Section 4

This cross-section is at the level of the **ilium** (G). There is excellent visualization of the pyriformis muscles (I) which are located between the sacrum (J) and ilium (G). This is a male pelvis. The parts as labeled are:

A. Gluteus maximus muscle.
B. Gluteus medius muscle.
C. Gluteus minimus muscle.
D. Iliopsoas muscle.
E. Rectus abdominus muscle.
F. Bladder.
G. Ilium.
H. Rectum.
I. Pyriformis muscles.
J. Sacrum.
K. Right ureter.

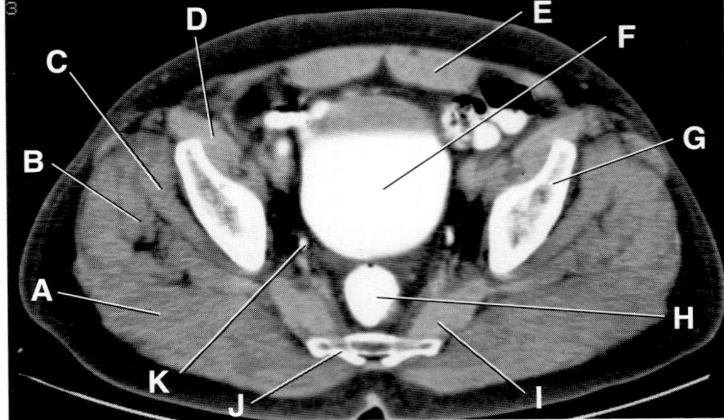

Fig. 23-32. Axial section 4.

Axial Section 5

This section is at the level of the **acetabular roof** (B). The paired, oval-shaped seminal vesicles (F) are seen posterior to the bladder (D). This obviously is a male pelvis. The labeled parts are:

A. Gluteus maximus.
B. Acetabular roof.
C. Rectus abdominus muscle.
D. Bladder.
E. Iliopsoas muscle.
F. Seminal vesicles.
G. Rectum.

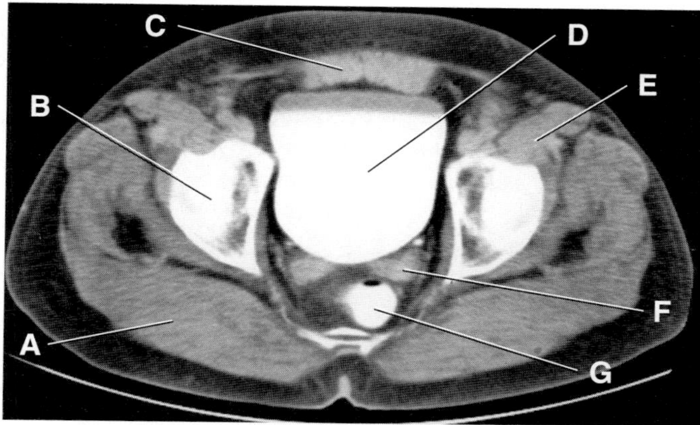

Fig. 23-33. Axial section 5.

Axial Section 6

At this level there is good demonstration of the **femoral heads** (C) **within the acetabulum** (D). Note also the greater trochanter (B). This is a male pelvis. The labeled parts are:

A. Gluteus maximus.
B. Greater trochanter.
C. Femoral head.
D. Acetabulum.
E. Bladder.
F. Pubic bone.
G. Rectum.

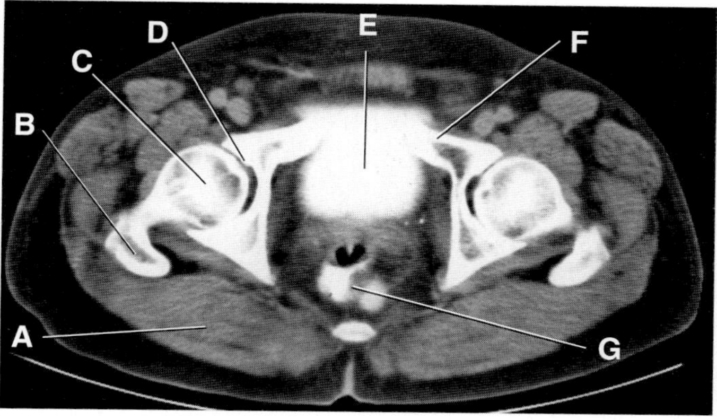

Fig. 23-34. Axial section 6.

Axial Section 7

This section, through the **symphysis pubis** (F) of this male pelvis, shows the prostate (L) between the symphysis (F) and the rectum (M). The size of the prostate varies with age. With progressive age the prostate increases in size. The labeled parts are:

A. Gluteus maximus.
B. Femur.
C. Femoral artery.
D. Femoral vein.
E. Pubic bone.
F. Symphysis pubis.
G. Pectineus muscle.
H. External obturator muscle.
I. Internal obturator muscle.
J. Tensor fascia lata muscle.
K. Ischial tuberosity.
L. Prostate.
M. Rectum.
N. Ischiorectal fat.

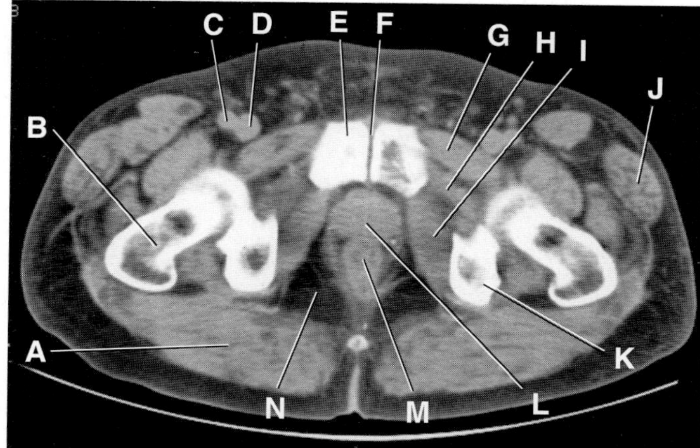

Fig. 23-35. Axial section 7.

Axial Section 8

This is a cross-section at the level of the **ischial ramus** (E). This is a male pelvis. The labeled parts are:

A. Gluteus maximus.
B. Femur.
C. Corpus cavernosum penis.
D. Adductor muscles.
E. Ischial ramus.

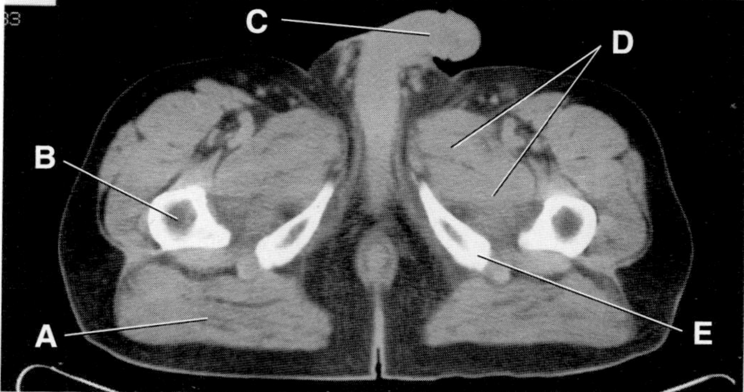

Fig. 23-36. Axial section 8.

FEMALE PELVIS

Axial Section 9

This scan is at the level of the **acetabulum** (C) of this female pelvis. There is good visualization of the uterus (H) which is bordered by the bladder (E) anteriorly and the rectum (I) posteriorly. The labeled parts are:

A. Gluteus maximus muscle.
B. Femoral head.
C. Acetabulum.
D. Rectus abdominus muscle.
E. Bladder.
F. Iliopsoas muscle.
G. Ischial spine.
H. Uterus.
I. Rectum.

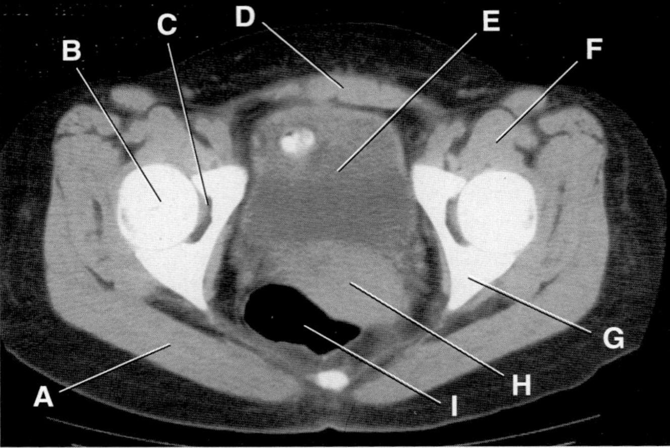

Fig. 23-37. Axial section 9.

Axial Section 10

This cross-section at the **symphysis pubis** (D) of this female pelvis gives excellent visualization of the vagina (I) due to insertion of a tampon. Other parts labeled are:

A. Gluteus maximus.
B. Femoral neck.
C. Pubic bone.
D. Symphysis pubis.
E. Pectineus muscle.
F. External obturator muscle.
G. Internal obturator muscle.
H. Ischial tuberosity.
I. Vagina (with tampon inserted).
J. Rectum.
K. Ischiorectal fat.

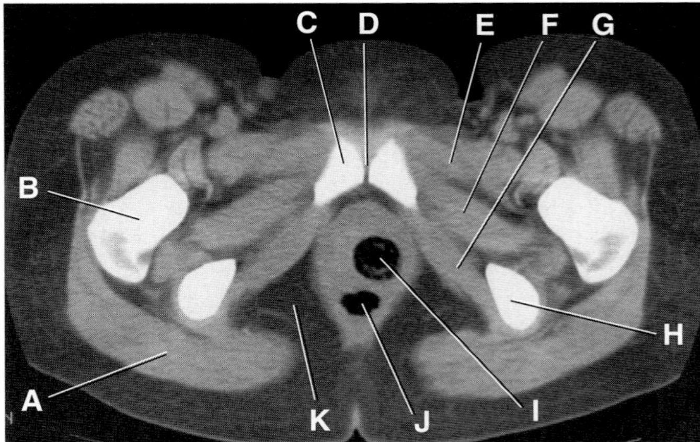

Fig. 23-38. Axial section 10.

Radiographic Positioning and Procedures - Abdomen and Pelvis

Purpose

With the advent of computed tomography, the ability to diagnose abdominal and pelvic morphology has been significantly enhanced. Due to its speed and accuracy, CT has become an effective management and treatment tool for **abdominal and pelvic disease** and has been especially useful in the **cases of malignancies**. The use of standard diagnostic tests such as endoscopic retrograde cholangiopancreatography (ERCP) have been greatly reduced due to the completeness and cost effectiveness of CT examination.

Indications

Any abnormality of the abdomen and/or pelvis is an indication for computed tomography.

Abdomen: Some of the more common indications for computed tomography of the abdomen include suspected primary or **metastatic lesions of the liver**, **pancreas**, **kidney** or **spleen**. Computed tomography is a preferred choice for examination of suspected **adrenal gland pathology** and has replaced lymphangiography in detecting lymph-node malignancies. Other common indications are suspected **pancreatitis**, **abscesses** and **hepatic** or **splenic hematomas**.

Pelvis: In the region of the pelvis, computed tomography is primarily used to provide information on the **state of advancement of pelvic disease**. Computed tomography has proven valuable in the evaluation of **prostatic**, **cervix**, **urinary bladder**, and **ovarian carcinomas**. Other indications are evaluation of **soft-tissue masses** and diseases of the **pelvic muscles**, **suspected abscesses** and **evaluation of the hip joint**, especially in trauma patients as shown in Fig. 23-40.

Additionally, CT has been found particularly valuable in the exclusion or detection of occult disease (hidden or concealed).

Examples of Abdominal Pathology Visualized by CT

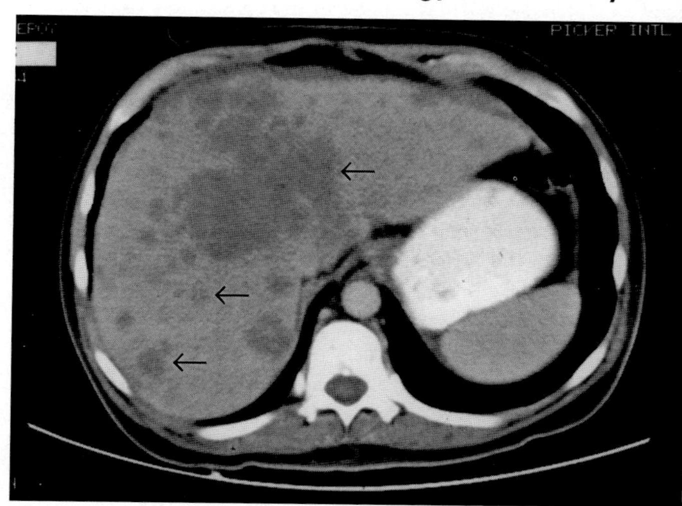

Fig. 23-39. **Liver metastasis**–There are multiple low-density lesions of variable size within the liver tissue representing metastatic disease. Note the opacification of the aorta due to a bolus injection of contrast media.

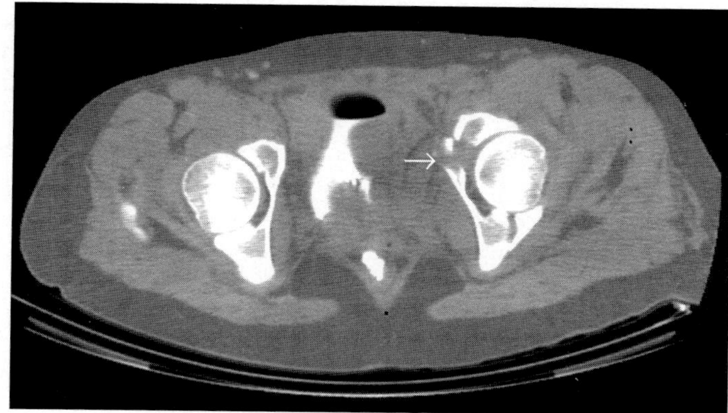

Fig. 23-40. **Left acetabular fracture**–Scan of an 18-year-old female show fractures of the anterior segment of the acetabulum.

Contraindications

There are almost no contraindications to computed tomography of the abdomen and pelvis. Any patient who can be transported to the scanning unit can have the examination performed. However, as with any x-ray examination, **pregnancy** is a contraindication to CT. In each case, **the benefits must be weighed against the risks.**

For those patients who require a procedure with an injection of iodinated contrast media, a careful history must be taken in order to assess any **possibility for adverse reaction to the contrast media**. Furthermore, patients with a history of **renal failure**, **multiple myeloma**, **pheochromocytoma** or **diabetes must be carefully evaluated**. When the risk outweighs the benefit, the use of contrast media should be avoided.

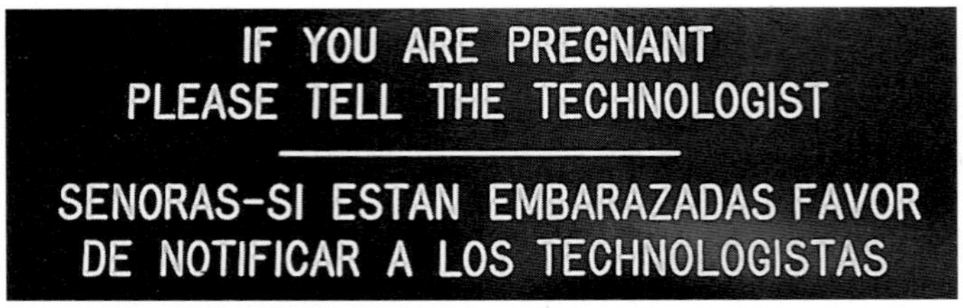

IF YOU ARE PREGNANT
PLEASE TELL THE TECHNOLOGIST

SENORAS-SI ESTAN EMBARAZADAS FAVOR
DE NOTIFICAR A LOS TECHNOLOGISTAS

Fig. 23-41. **Warning-Pregnancies:** Benefits must outweigh the risks.

Patient Preparation

Proper patient preparation for computed tomography of the abdomen and pelvis is crucial. Inadequate or incorrect preparation may produce an inaccurate diagnosis.

The use of oral and rectal contrast media to opacify the gastrointestinal tract is imperative for diagnostic examinations of the abdomen and pelvis. Unopacified portions of small and large bowel can be misdiagnosed as lymph nodes, abscesses or masses. This is demonstrated by comparing the scans in Figs. 23-42 and 23-43 of the lower abdomen, which show a questionable soft tissue mass on the left. After administering additional oral contrast media the mass is shown to be actually loops of small bowel. Questionable areas like this are seen frequently at the head or tail of the pancreas where unopacified loops of small bowel can be confused for pancreatic tumors.

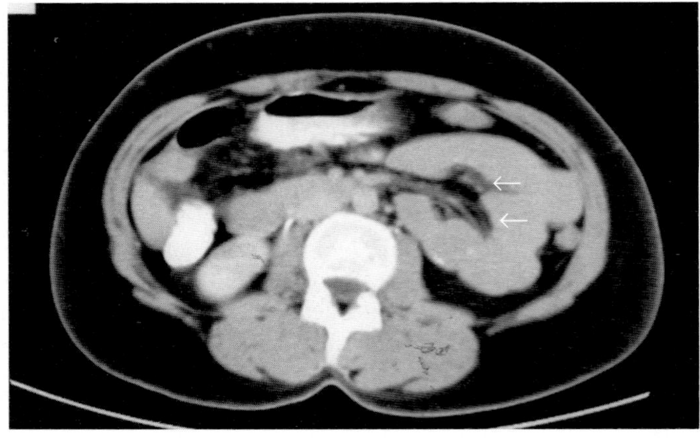

Fig. 23-42. Pseudotumors of the abdomen.

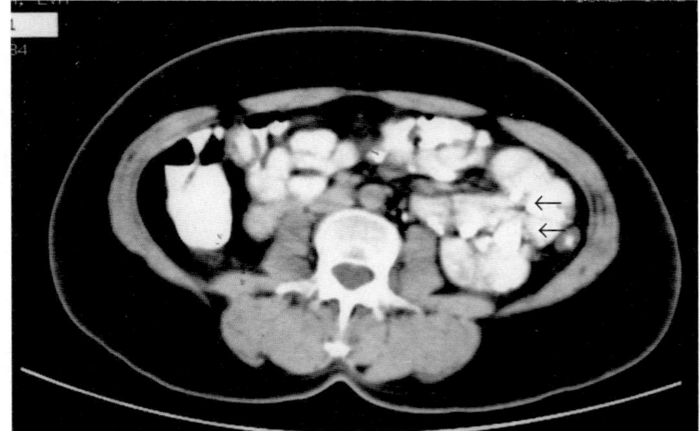

Fig. 23-43. After administration of contrast media.

Types of Contrast Media

There are **two types** of positive contrast agents used to opacify the gastrointestinal tract. They are **barium sulfate suspensions** and **water-soluble solutions** (diatrizoate meglumine and diatrizoate sodium). Each has been proven effective, but in certain clinical situations only barium sulfate or water-soluble solutions can be used.

Barium Sulfate Suspensions

There are numerous flavored barium sulfate suspensions made especially for abdominal CT. In order to be useful in abdominal CT, barium sulfate suspensions must be of low concentrations (1 to 3%) to avoid streaking artifacts due to beam hardening. Barium suspensions are effective, economical and, because they are premixed, are easy to administer.

The manufacturer's directions must be followed strictly when administering barium sulfate. Delays after ingestion allow water to be absorbed by the bowel which leaves residual barium and causes **beam hardening artifacts**, as shown by the scan in Fig. 23-44. Note the linear streaks arising from the stomach on this scan, which are examples of such beam hardening artifacts.

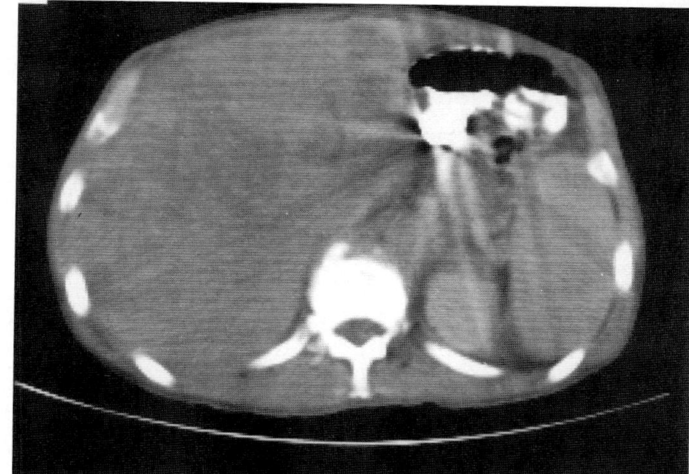

Fig. 23-44. Beam hardening artifacts.

Water-Soluble Solutions

An alternative to barium sulfate suspensions for opacification of the GI tract is the use of water-soluble contrast agents. These agents are a valuable alternative when barium sulfate suspensions are not feasible. They provide good coating of the gastrointestinal tract and, because they increase peristaltic motion, they have a fast transit time. They can prove to be a disadvantage, however, in examinations requiring long exposure times (5 seconds or more) due to increased motion artifact.

Extreme care must be used in the preparation of water-soluble solutions. Diatrizoate preparations containing 2 to 5% dilutions have been found to be generally safe and clinically useful. Preparations that contain 15 to 40% diatrizoate solution, however, are considered hypertonic. These may draw excessive amounts of fluid into the intestinal tract and may cause hypovolemia.

Other adverse reactions include diarrhea, nausea, and vomiting, occurring particularly when the solutions are used in large quantities and high concentrations. Urticaria (hives) may also occur.

Contraindications to Barium Sulfate

Barium sulfate is an insoluble material and therefore **should not be used in pre-operative patients** or patients suspected of having **gastrointestinal perforations.** Severe complications, such as barium peritonitis, can result from barium leakage into the abdominal and pelvic cavities.

Additional contraindications include patients with a **known hypersensitivity to barium sulfate** or patients with **diagnosed bowel obstruction.**

Contrast Media and Complications

The contrast media used and the possible complications due to reactions to iodinated contrast media is similar to that of intravenous urography as discussed in more detail in Chapter 17.

Recommended Oral and Rectal Contrast Media Volumes for Abdominal and Pelvic Scanning

(Water-Soluble and Barium Sulfate Solutions)

The following times when the oral contrast is initiated, and the volumes given, are dependent on the parts of the gastrointestinal tract to be included in the scanning area.

***Abdomen and Pelvis** (Oral and by Enema):*
- 700-900 ml orally 30-45 minutes prior to scan.
- 800-1000 ml enema immediately before scan.
- 300 ml orally immediately before scan.
- Patient in right decubitus position 3-5 minutes before scanning.

***Abdomen and Pelvis** (Oral only):*
- 1200-1500 ml 45-60 minutes prior to scan.
- 300 ml immediately before scan.
- Patient in right decubitus position 3-5 minutes before scanning.

Upper Abdomen Only:
- 400-600 ml orally 15-30 minutes prior to scan.
- 300 ml orally immediately before scan.
- Patient in right decubitus position 3-5 minutes before scanning.

Pelvis Only:
- 700-900 ml orally 30-45 minutes prior to scan.
- 800-1000 ml enema immediately before scan.

Oral or Enema Method: The choice to use the oral and enema method, or the oral only method for preparation of the patient for abdominal and pelvic scans is strictly personal preference. However, in cases where the oral only method was used and the colon is not completely opacified an enema may be necessary.

Use of Tampon: To aid in easier anatomical localization of the vagina a tampon should routinely be used. Insertion of a tampon produces an entrapment of air. This is demonstrated in Fig. 23-45.

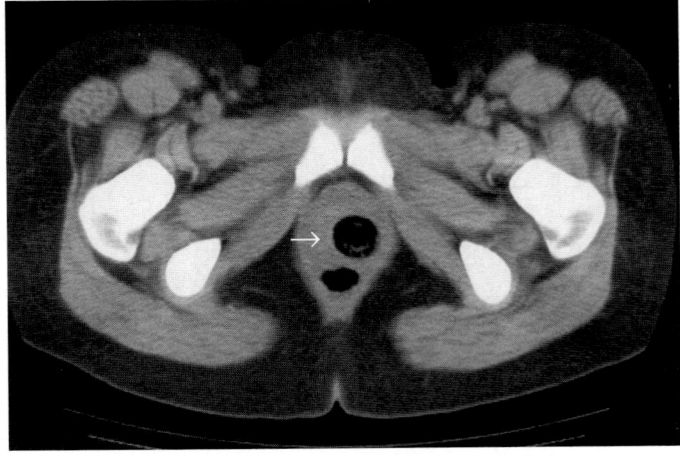

Fig. 23-45. Use of tampon with entrapment of air for localization purposes.

Patient Preparation

The abdominal tract should be as free from fecal matter as possible prior to examination. The patient should have taken a laxative and have had only clear liquids for supper the evening prior to exam. Fecal material restricts the flow of contrast and can also appear as a mass. Until the examination is performed the patient should continue to have clear liquids since solid food in the digestive tract can appear to be a gastric tumor.

Patients should change into clothing with cloth ties and all opaque objects in the radiographic area of interest must be removed.

In order to obtain high quality examinations, patient cooperation is essential. Patient motion during the procedure seriously impairs the quality of CT. Patients should be given brief instructions that are to the point and easy to understand. Items such as breathing instructions and length of examination are important to discuss.

Scanner Room Preparation

The room preparation, with equipment for possible emergency situations, room cleanliness, etc., is similar to that described earlier in this chapter on CT in the chest.

PROCEDURE FOR COMPLETE CT OF THE ABDOMEN AND PELVIS

Pilot or Localization

A localizing or pilot radiograph (Fig. 23-46) is obtained with the first slice starting at the xiphoid process. Scanning then continues to the symphysis pubis.

If only the upper abdomen is the area of interest, then scanning starts at the xiphoid process and continues to the iliac crest. If the pelvis is the only area of interest, then scanning starts at the iliac crest and continues to the symphysis pubis.

In certain examinations the decubitus position is valuable. This position frequently is used when the pancreas is the area of concern. Placing the patient in a right decubitus position immediately after drinking oral contrast causes the duodenum to fill because of gravitational flow. This technique helps eliminate false positives when pancreatic tumors are suspected.

Slice Thickness and Couch Incrementation

In routine examinations of the abdomen and pelvis a 10 mm thick slice is commonly used. The parameter used for couch incrementation will vary, depending on the clinical history. Couch incrementation refers to how far the couch or table moves after each slice. For most routine examinations a couch incrementation of 10 or 15 mm is used. A 20 mm incrementation occasionally will be used in detecting gross pathology and/or when a fast examination time is of importance. In certain instances small parameters (5 to 8 mm) may be used for detailed evaluation of organs such as the pancreas or kidney.

Exposure Times

Exposure times of **1 to 3 seconds** are needed for examination of the abdomen to reduce the effect of peristaltic and respiratory artifact on image quality.

Breathing Instructions

Suspended respiration is required in order to obtain high quality diagnostic images in abdominal examinations. It is essential that the same method of suspended respiration be used throughout the entire exam. Inconsistent suspended respirations can cause fluctuations in the exam by creating varying compressions of the diaphragm on abdominal organs.

Contrast Enhancement of Vascular Structures

Use of intravenous contrast is important in the evaluation of vascular structures of the abdomen and pelvis such as the abdominal aorta, inferior vena cava, portal vein and iliac arteries and veins.

Often lesions can be characterized and identified by their enhancement or by their attenuation when compared to normal enhanced adjacent tissue.

Occasionally, dual examinations will be performed with and without contrast. Some lesions may be isodense with normal tissue before or after contrast enhancement. This method is frequently used in evaluation of the liver and kidneys. Intravenous contrast is also important for visualizing the ureters and bladder.

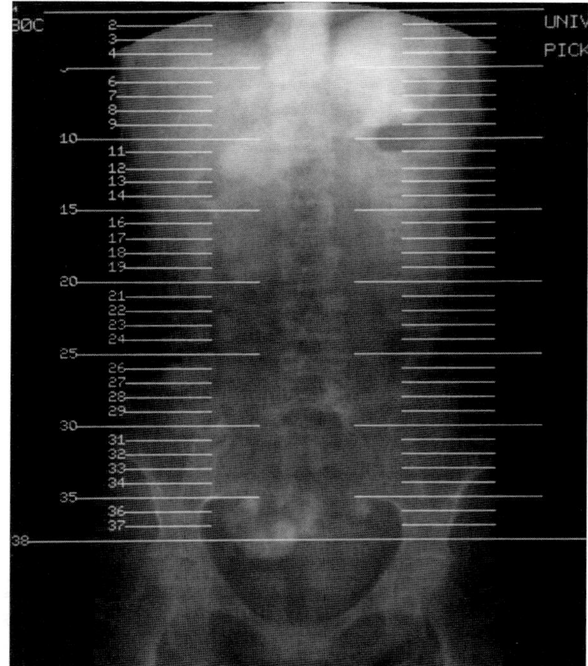

Fig. 23-46. Localizing (pilot) scan for abdomen and pelvis (solid white line represents the slice location).

Radiographic Anatomy

INTRODUCTION

Definition

Angiography refers to the **radiographic examination of the blood vessels following injection of a positive contrast medium**. Since the various soft tissues of the body possess similar radiographic densities, a positive contrast medium must be added in order to study normal and abnormal distribution of the circulatory system. For example, the routine lateral skull radiograph in Fig. 24-1 demonstrates none of the vessels of the cranial circulatory system, while the lateral carotid arteriogram in Fig. 24-2 clearly differentiates between brain and blood vessels. This is also true for the circulatory system of other body regions such as the thorax, abdomen and the upper and lower limbs (peripheral). Angiography of these body parts will be studied in this chapter also in which contrast media is injected into specific vessels of each of these regions.

A good understanding of the anatomy involved, as covered in Part I of this chapter, is essential for performing angiography of any body region.

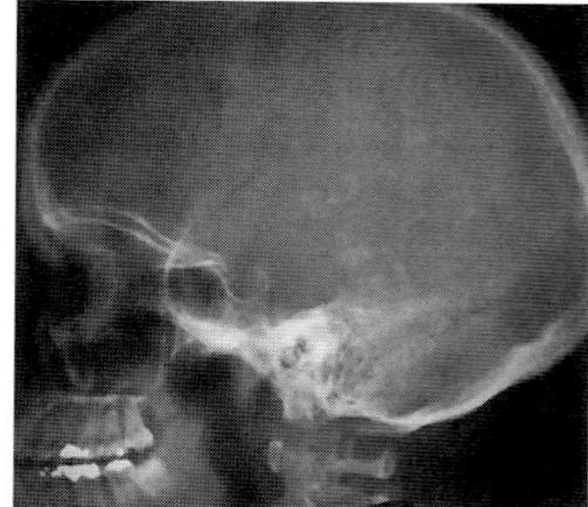

Fig. 24-1. Lateral skull radiograph.

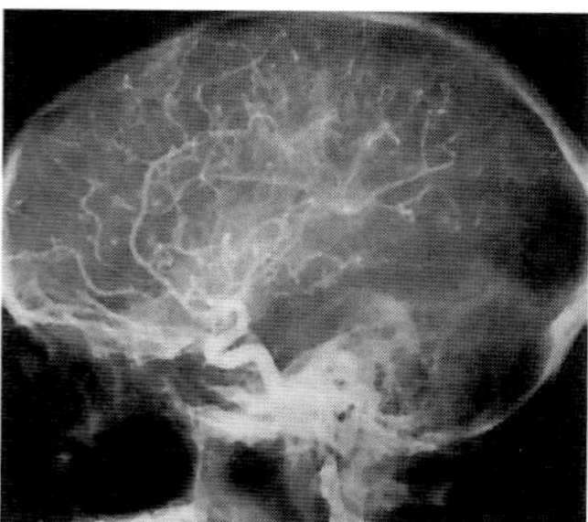

Fig. 24-2. Lateral carotid arteriogram.

Divisions or Components

The **circulatory system** consists of the **cardiovascular and lymphatic components.** The cardiovascular portion includes the heart, blood and vessels which transport the blood. The lymphatic element of the circulatory system is comprised of a clear watery fluid called lymph, lymphatic vessels, and lymphatic nodes. The cardiovascular and lymphatic components differ in the function and method of transporting the respective fluids within the vessels.

The **cardiovascular** or blood circulatory division may further be divided into the **cardio** (circulation within the heart) and **vascular** (blood vessel) components.

The vascular or vessel component is divided into the **pulmonary** (heart to lungs and back) and the general or **systemic** system (throughout the body).

Circulatory System Summary

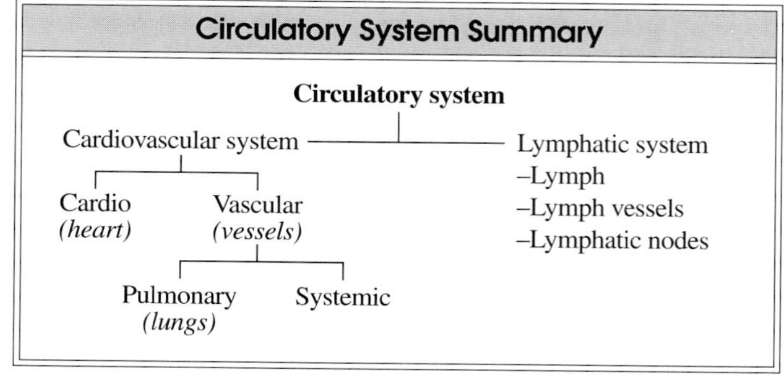

Cardiovascular System

The cardiovascular system (CVS) consists of the heart and vascular (blood and blood vessels) organs. The heart is the major organ of the cardiovascular system and functions as a pump to maintain circulation of blood throughout the body. The vascular component is a network of blood vessels that carry blood from the heart to body tissues and back to the heart again.

Functions: Functions of the cardiovascular system include:

1. Transportation of oxygen, nutrients, hormones and chemicals necessary for normal body activity.
2. Removal of waste products through the kidneys and lungs.
3. Maintenance of body temperature and water and electrolyte balance. These functions are performed by the following blood components; red blood cells, white blood cells, and platelets suspended in plasma.

Blood Components: **Red blood cells**, or **erythrocytes**, are produced in the red marrow of certain bones and transport oxygen via the protein hemoglobin to body tissues.

White blood cells, or **leukocytes**, formed in both bone marrow and lymph tissue, defend the body against infection and disease. **Platelets**, also originating from bone marrow, repair tears in blood vessel walls and promote blood clotting.

Plasma, the liquid portion of the blood, consists of 92% water and about 7% plasma protein and salts, nutrients, and oxygen.

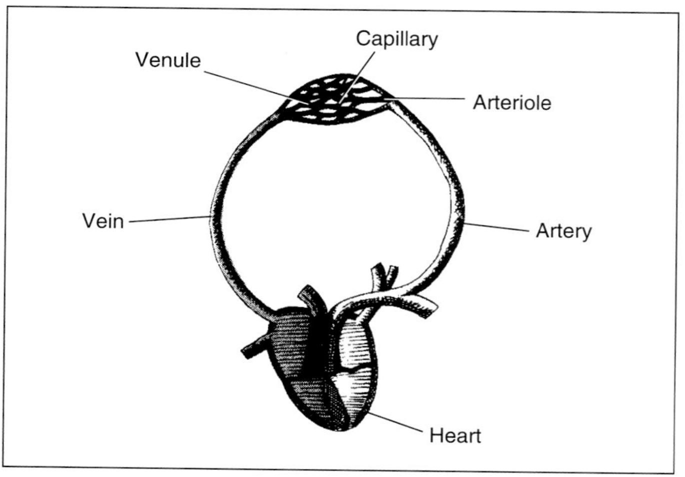

Fig. 24-3. General cardiovascular circulation.

Systemic Circulation

Arteries: Vessels transporting oxygenated blood from the heart to tissues are called **arteries.** Arteries that originate directly from the heart measure approximately 3 centimeters in diameter. These arteries then subdivide and decrease in size as they extend from the heart to the various parts of the body. The smaller arteries are termed **arterioles.** As the blood travels through the arterioles, it enters the tissues via the smallest subdivision of these vessels, known as **capillaries** (Fig. 24-3).

Veins: The deoxygenated blood returns to the heart through the venous system. The venous system extends from venous capillaries to venules to veins, increasing in size as it nears the heart.

PULMONARY CIRCULATION

The blood vessel circuit (veins, venules, capillaries, arterioles and arteries), which supplies blood to the lungs and back, composes the **pulmonary circulation** component of the cardiovascular system.

As previously noted, arteries generally carry oxygenated blood away from the heart to the capillaries. The exception to this are the **pulmonary arteries,** which carry the **deoxygenated blood** to the lungs that has been returned to the heart through the venous system.

The superior and inferior vena cava empty the returning deoxygenated blood into the **right atrium** of the heart.

The heart pumps this deoxygenated blood from the **right ventricle** through the pulmonary arteries to the lungs where oxygen and carbon dioxide are exchanged through the small air sacs or alveoli of the lungs. The **oxygenated blood** then returns through the **pulmonary veins** to the **left atrium** of the heart (Fig. 24-4).

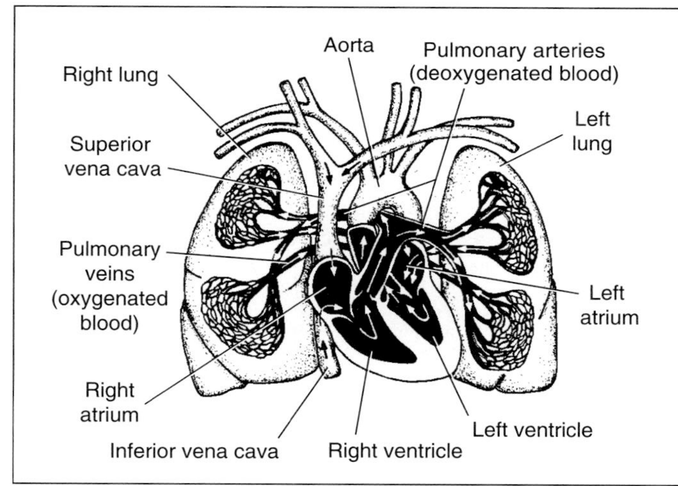

Fig. 24-4. Pulmonary circulation.

GENERAL SYSTEMIC CIRCULATION

Heart

The heart is a muscular organ that pumps blood throughout the various parts of the body. Anatomically, the heart lies within the mediastinum, or middle area of the chest, and rests on the **diaphragm** (Fig. 24-5). Cardiac tissue differs from other muscle tissues of the body in its construction and is termed myocardium. The left side of the heart is responsible for the extensive systemic circulation, thus, the left muscle wall is about three times as thick as the right side.

The heart itself is divided into four chambers. These are the **right and left atria** and the **right and left ventricles.** Each chamber functions either to receive and/or pump blood. The blood circulation is a closed system by which unoxygenated blood enters the **right atrium** from all parts of the body, is reoxygenated in the lungs and returned to the body via the **left ventricle.**

Blood returning to the heart enters the right atrium through the **superior and inferior vena cava** (Fig. 24-6). Blood in the superior vena cava originates from the head, chest, and upper extremities. The inferior vena cava serves to deliver blood into the right atrium from the abdomen and lower limbs.

From the **right atrium,** blood is pumped through the tricuspid valve to the **right ventricle**. The right ventricle contracts, moving the blood through the **pulmonary (pulmonary semilunar) valve** to the **pulmonary arteries** and on to the lungs. While in the lungs, the blood is oxygenated and then returned to the left atrium of the heart via the **pulmonary veins.** As the left atrium contracts, blood is transported through the **mitral (bicuspid) valve** to the left ventricle.

When the left ventricle contracts, the oxygenated blood exits the chamber via the **aortic (aortic semilunar) valve,** flows through the aorta and is delivered to the various body tissues by the remaining arterial vessels.

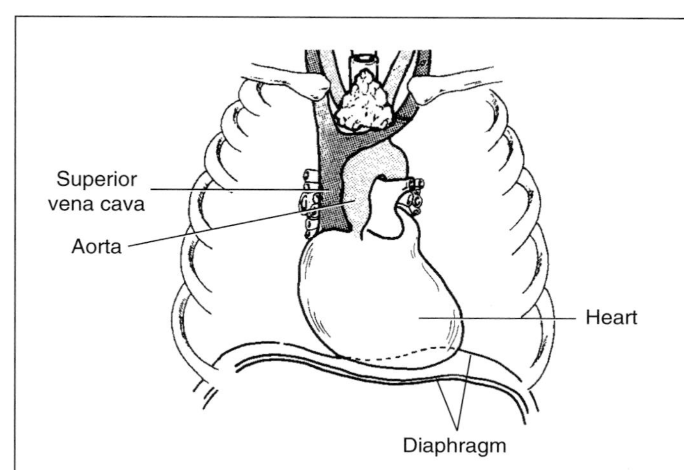

Fig. 24-5. Heart and mediastinal structures.

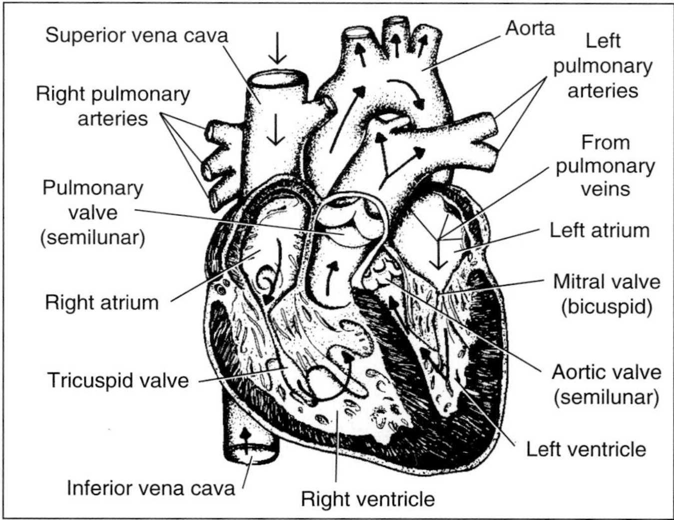

Fig. 24-6. Cross-section of heart.

Coronary Arteries

The coronary arteries are the vessels that deliver blood to the heart muscle. There are **two coronary arteries, the right and left.** Both coronary arteries originate from the **aortic bulb.** The right coronary artery arises from the right (anterior) sinuses of the aortic bulb, while the left coronary artery originates from the left (posterior) aortic bulb sinus. The right coronary artery supplies much of the **right atrium** and the **right ventricle** of the heart.

The left coronary artery supplies blood to both ventricles and the left atrium of the heart. There are many interconnections or anastomoses between the left and right coronary arteries. Blood returns to the right atrium of the heart via the coronary veins.

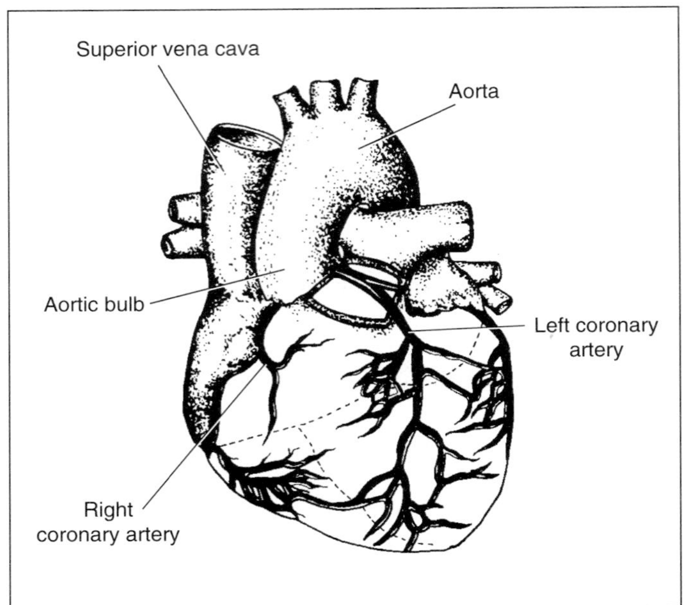

Fig. 24-7. Arteries of the heart (anterior view).

Coronary Veins

The coronary sinus system returns blood to the right atrium for recirculation. The **coronary sinus** is a large vein on the posterior side of the heart between the atria and ventricles. The coronary sinus vein has three major branches: **the great, middle and small cardiac veins.** The great cardiac vein receives blood from both ventricles and the left atrium. The middle cardiac vein drains blood from the right ventricle, right atrium and part of the left ventricle. The small cardiac vein returns blood from the right ventricle. The coronary sinus drains most of the blood from the heart. Some small veins drain directly into both atria.

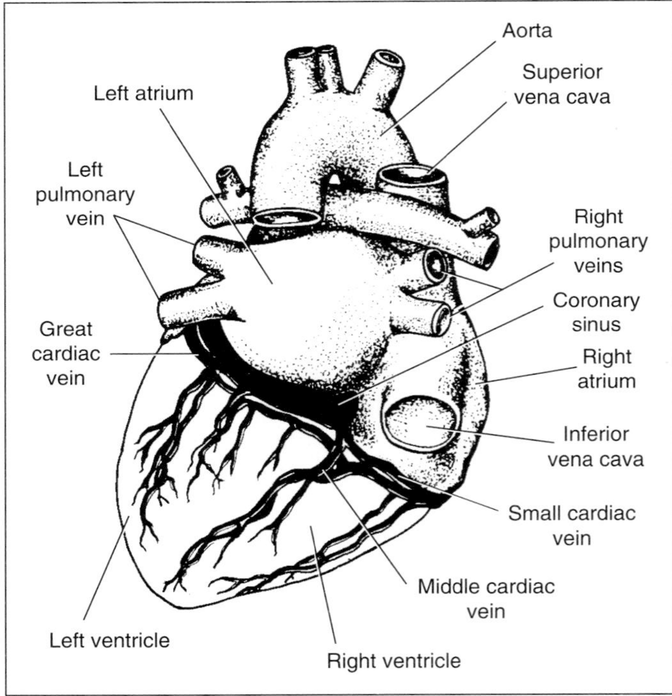

Fig. 24-8. Veins of the heart (posterior view).

CEREBRAL ARTERIES

Blood Supply to the Brain

The brain is supplied with blood by major arteries of the systemic circulation. The four major arteries supplying the brain are (Fig. 24-9):

1. **Right common carotid artery**
2. **Left common carotid artery**
3. **Right vertebral artery**
4. **Left vertebral artery**

Major branches of the two common carotids supply the anterior circulation of the brain, while the two vertebrals supply the posterior circulation. Radiographic examination of the neck vessels and entire brain circulation is referred to as a "four-vessel angiogram" since these four vessels are collectively and selectively injected with contrast medium. Another common series is the "three-vessel angiogram" in which the two carotids and only one vertebral artery are studied.

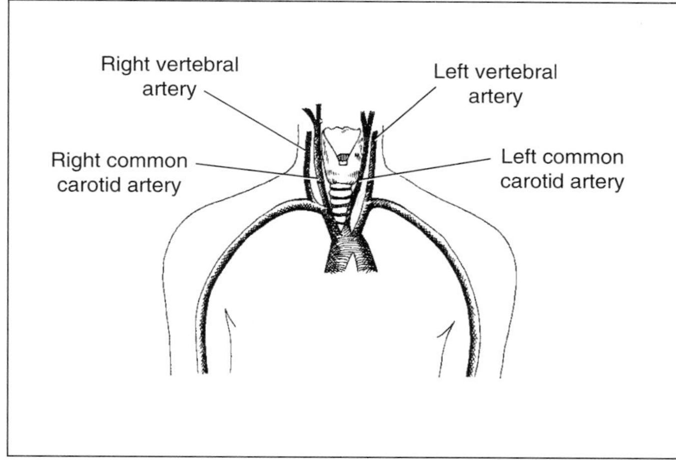

Fig. 24-9. Blood supply to brain.

Branches of the Aortic Arch

The aorta is the major artery leaving the left ventricle of the heart. There are three major branches arising from the **arch** of the **aorta**. These are (Fig. 24-10):

1. **Brachiocephalic artery**
2. **Left common carotid artery**
3. **Left subclavian artery**

The brachiocephalic trunk is a short vessel that bifurcates into the **right common carotid artery** and the **right subclavian artery**. This bifurcation occurs directly posterior to the right sternoclavicular joint. The right and left vertebral arteries are branches of the subclavian arteries on each side. Since the left common carotid artery rises directly from the arch of the aorta, it is slightly longer than the right common carotid artery.

In the cervical region, the two common carotids resemble one another. Each common carotid artery passes cephalad from its origin along either side of the trachea and larynx to the level of the upper border of the thyroid cartilage. Here, each common carotid artery divides into **external and internal carotid arteries.** The level of bifurcation of each common carotid is the level of the **fourth cervical vertebra**.

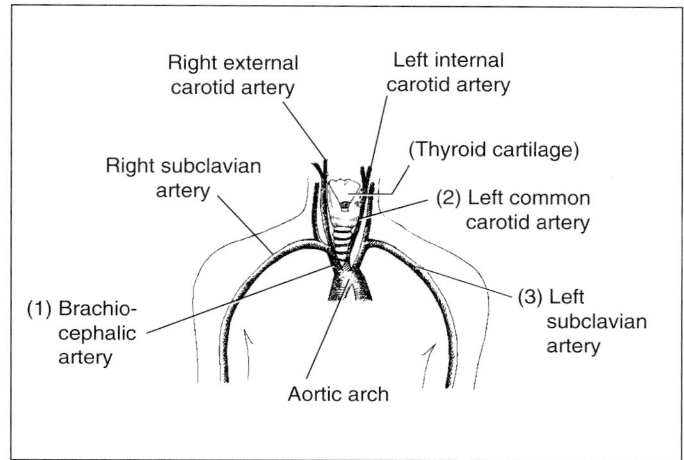

Fig. 24-10. Branches of aortic arch.

Neck and Head Arteries

The major arteries supplying the head, as seen from the right side of the neck, are shown in Fig. 24-11. The **brachiocephalic trunk artery** bifurcates into the **right common carotid artery** and the **right subclavian artery.**

The right common carotid artery ascends to the level of the fourth cervical vertebra to branch into the **external carotid artery** and the **internal carotid artery.** Each external carotid artery primarily supplies the anterior neck, the face and the greater part of the scalp and meninges (brain coverings). Each internal carotid artery supplies the cerebral hemispheres, the pituitary gland, the orbital structures, the external nose and the anterior portion of the brain.

The **right vertebral artery** arises from the right subclavian artery to pass through the transverse foramina of C6 through C1. Each vertebral artery passes posteriorly along the superior border of C1 before angling upward through the foramen magnum to enter the cranium.

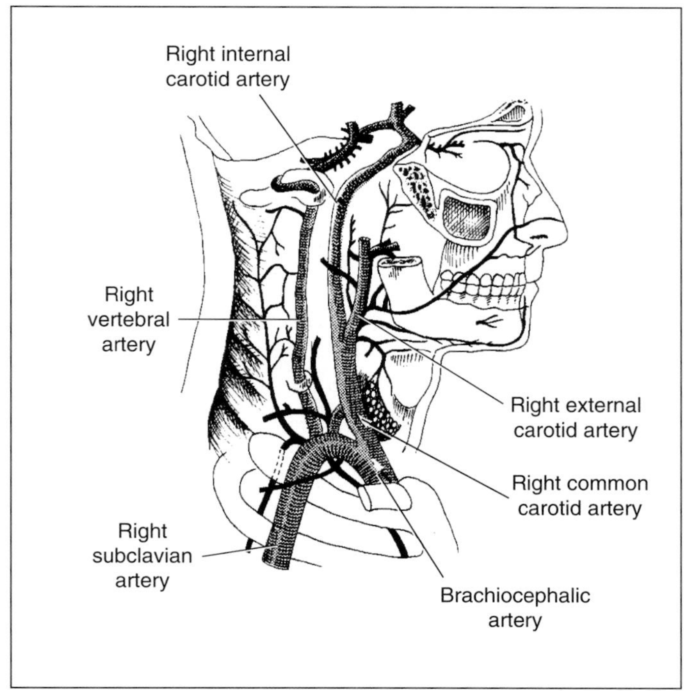

Fig. 24-11. Neck and head arteries.

External Carotid Artery Branches

The four major branches of the external carotid artery are shown in Fig. 24-12. These are:

1. **Facial artery**
2. **Maxillary artery**
3. **Superficial temporal artery**
4. **Occipital artery**

The most important branch of the maxillary artery is **the middle meningeal artery**, which has an **anterior and a posterior branch.** This middle meningeal artery enters the cranial cavity and produces a groove along the inner table of the cranium. Trauma to the squamous portion of the temporal bone, sufficient to fracture the bone, may lead to a laceration of the middle meningeal artery and a subsequent epidural hemorrhage.

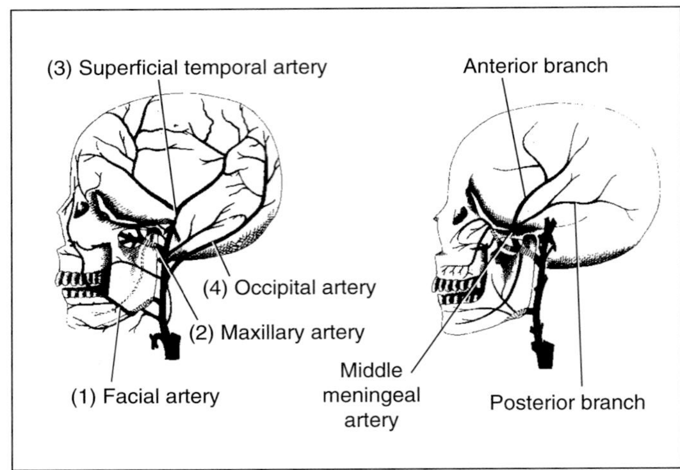

Fig. 24-12. External carotid artery branches.

Internal Carotid Artery

Each internal carotid artery ascends to enter the carotid canal in the petrous portion of the temporal bone. Within the petrous pyramid the artery curves forward and medially. Before supplying the cerebral hemispheres, each internal carotid artery passes through a collection of venous channels around the sella turcica. Each internal carotid artery passes through the dura mater, medial to each anterior clinoid process, to bifurcate into the cerebral branches.

The S-shaped portion of each internal carotid artery is termed the **carotid siphon** and is studied carefully by the radiologist (Fig. 24-13).

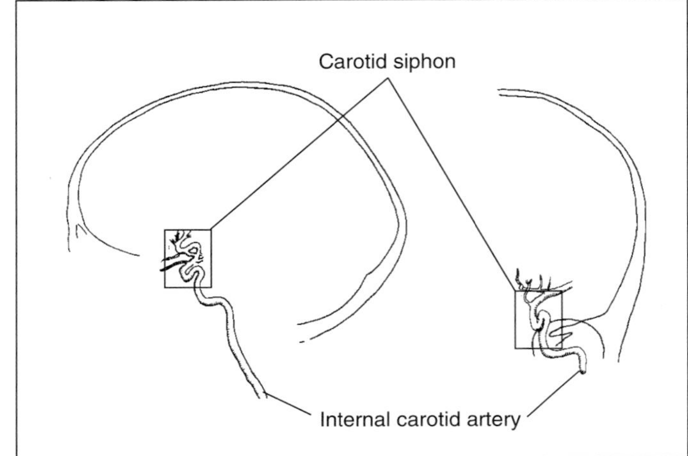

Fig. 24-13. Internal carotid artery.

Anterior Cerebral Artery

The two end branches of each **internal carotid artery** are the **anterior cerebral** and the **middle cerebral arteries.** Each anterior cerebral artery and its branches supply much of the forebrain near the midline. The anterior cerebral arteries curve around the corpus callosum, giving off several branches to the mid portions of the cerebral hemisphere (Fig. 24-14). Each anterior cerebral artery connects to the opposite one, as well as to the posterior brain circulation.

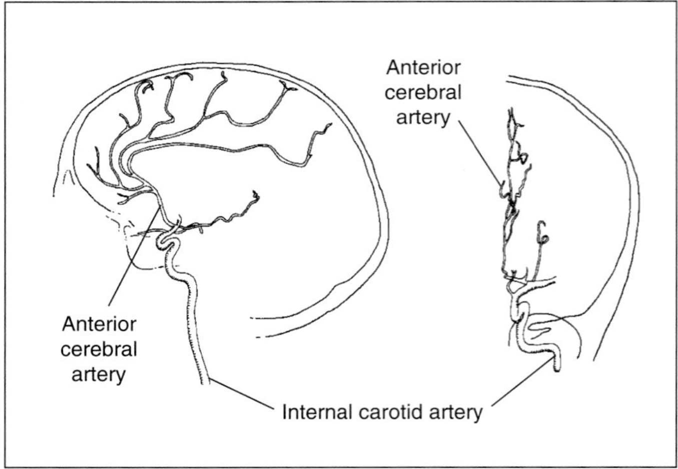

Fig. 24-14. Anterior cerebral artery.

Middle Cerebral Artery

The middle cerebral artery is the largest branch of each internal carotid artery. This artery supplies the **lateral aspects of the anterior cerebral circulation**. As the middle cerebral artery courses toward the periphery of the brain, branches extend upward along the lateral portion of the **insula or central lobe** of the brain. These small branches supply brain tissue deep within the brain (Fig. 24-15).

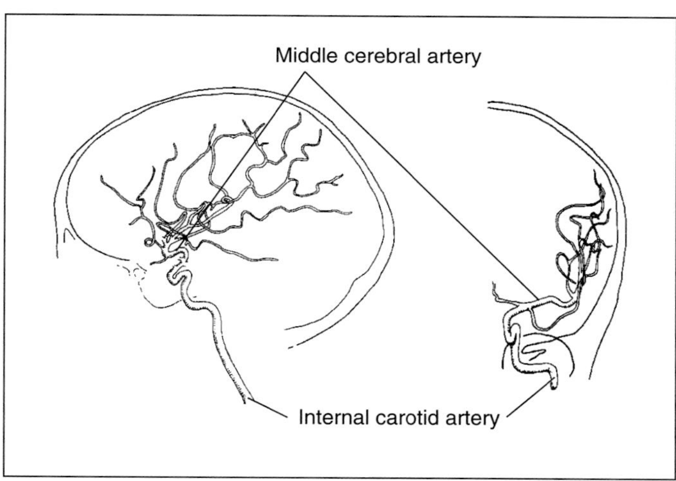

Fig. 24-15. Middle cerebral artery.

Internal Carotid Arteriogram

When one internal carotid artery is injected with contrast medium, both the anterior cerebral artery and the middle cerebral artery fill. The arterial phase of a cerebral carotid angiogram is similar to the drawings in Fig. 24-16.

In the frontal view or anteroposterior projection, there is little superimposition of the two vessels since the anterior cerebral courses toward the midline and the middle cerebral extends laterally.

In the lateral position there obviously is some superimposition. Note that the **internal carotid artery supplies primarily the anterior portion of the brain**.

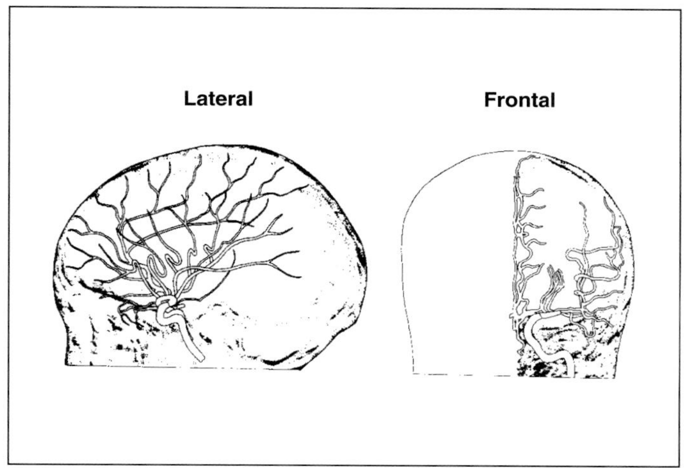

Fig. 24-16. Internal carotid arteriogram.

Vertebrobasilar Arteries

The two **vertebral arteries** enter the cranium through the foramen magnum and unite to form the single **basilar artery.** The vertebral arteries and basilar artery and their branches form the vertebrobasilar system. By omitting much of the occipital bone in Fig. 24-17, these arteries are shown along the base of the skull. Several arteries arise from each vertebral artery prior to their point of convergence to form the basilar artery. These branches supply the **spinal cord and the hindbrain**. The basilar artery rests upon the **clivus,** the portion of the occipital and sphenoid bones anterior to the foramen magnum and posterior to the dorsum sella.

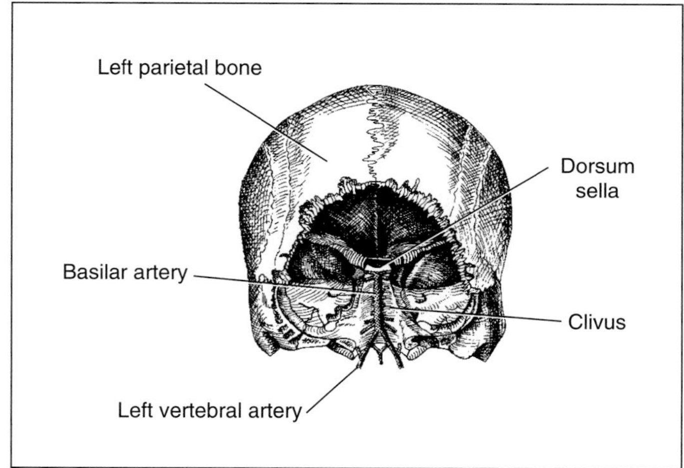

Fig. 24-17. Vertebrobasilar arteries.

Circle of Willis

The blood to the brain is supplied by the internal carotid and vertebral arteries. The posterior brain circulation communicates with the anterior circulation along the base of the brain in the arterial circle, or **circle of Willis** (as shown in Fig. 24-18). The five arteries or branches which make up the circle of Willis are (1) the **anterior communicating artery**, (2) the **anterior cerebral arteries**, (3) branches of the **internal carotid arteries**, (4) the **posterior communicating artery**, and (5) the **posterior cerebral arteries**.

Not only are the anterior and posterior circulations connected, but also both sides connect across the midline. Therefore, an elaborate anastomosis interconnects the entire arterial supply to the brain. As the basilar artery courses forward toward the circle of Willis, it gives off several branches to the hindbrain and posterior cerebrum. The posterior cerebral arteries are two of the larger branches.

Certain aneurysms may occur in these vessels making up the circle of Willis and they need to be well demonstrated on cerebral angiographic studies.

It should also be noted that the important "master" gland, the hypophysis (pituitary gland) and its surrounding bony structure, the sella turcica, are located within the circle of Willis. (See Fig. 24-17 on the preceding page for the location of the basilar artery resting on the clivus and the relationship of these structures to the dorsum sella, and also to the circle of Willis as shown in Fig. 24-18 of this page.)

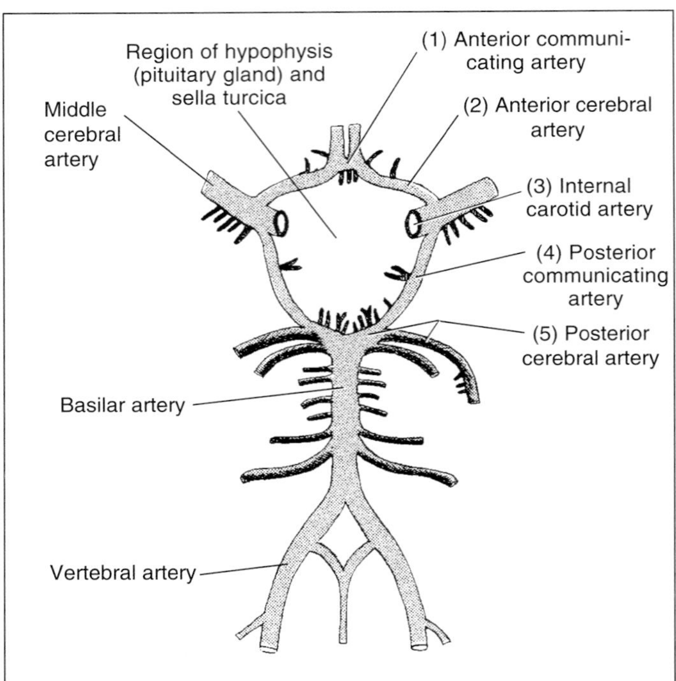

Fig. 24-18. Circle of Willis.

Vertebrobasilar Arteriogram

A standard vertebrobasilar arteriogram appears similar to the simplified drawing in Fig. 24-19. The vertebral arteries, basilar artery and posterior cerebral arteries can be seen. The several branches to the cerebellum have not been labeled on this drawing.

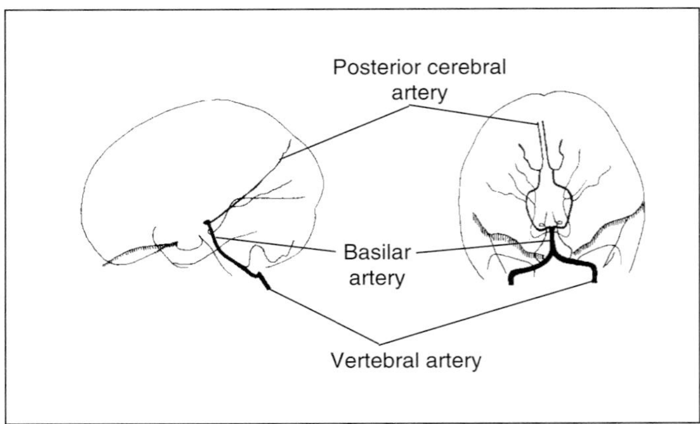

Fig. 24-19. Vertebrobasilar arteriogram.

CEREBRAL VEINS

Great Veins of the Neck

The **three pair** of major veins of the neck draining the head, face and neck region shown in Fig. 24-20 are:

1. Right and left **internal jugular veins**.
2. Right and left **external jugular veins**.
3. Right and left **vertebral veins**.

Each **internal jugular vein** drains the cranial and orbital cavities. In addition, many smaller veins join each internal jugular vein as it passes caudad to connect to the **brachiocephalic vein** on each side. The right and left brachiocephalic veins join to form the superior vena cava, which returns blood to the right atrium of the heart.

The pair of **external jugular veins** are more superficial trunks that drain the scalp and much of the face and neck. Each external jugular vein joins the respective **subclavian vein**.

The right and left **vertebral veins** form outside the cranium and drain the upper neck and occipital region. Each vertebral vein enters the transverse foramen of Cl, descends to C6 and then enters the subclavian vein.

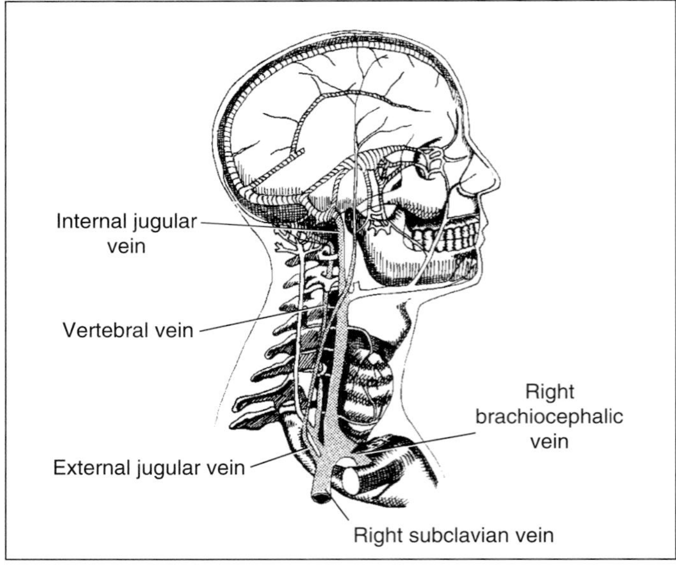

Fig. 24-20. Great veins of neck.

Dura Mater Sinuses

The sinuses of the dura mater are venous channels that drain blood from the brain (Fig. 24-21). The sinuses are situated between the two layers of the dura mater.

The **falx cerebri** is a strong membranous portion of the dura mater extending down into the longitudinal fissure between the two cerebral hemispheres. A space between the two layers of the dura, along the superior portion of the longitudinal fissure, contains the **superior sagittal sinus.** The **inferior sagittal sinus** flows posteriorly to drain into the **straight sinus.** The straight sinus and the superior sagittal sinus empty into opposite transverse sinuses.

Each **transverse sinus** curves medially to occupy a groove along the mastoid portion of the temporal bone. The sinus in this region is termed the **sigmoid sinus.** Each sigmoid sinus then curves caudad to continue as the **internal jugular vein** at the jugular foramen.

The **occipital sinus** courses posteriorly from the foramen magnum to join the superior sagittal sinus, straight sinus and transverse sinuses at their confluence.

The **confluence of sinuses** is located near the internal occipital protuberance. Other major dura mater sinuses drain the area on either side of the sphenoid bone and sella turcica.

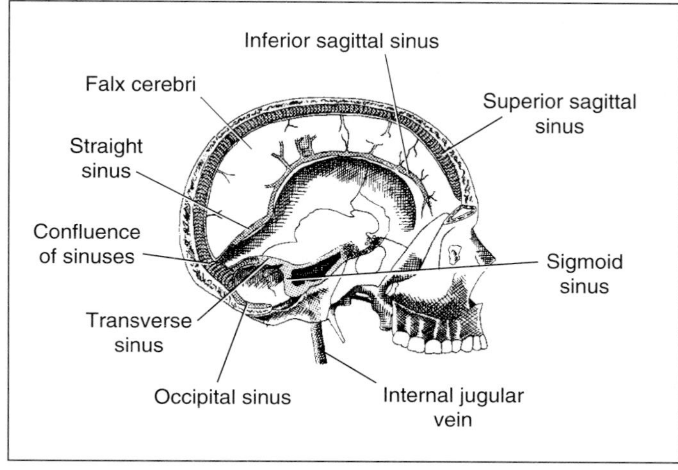

Fig. 24-21. Dura mater sinuses.

Cranial Venous System

The major veins of the entire cranial venous system are shown in Fig. 24-22. Only the most prominent veins are identified. One group not individually named is the external cerebral veins, which drain the outer surfaces of the cerebral hemispheres. Like all veins of the brain, the external cerebral veins possess no valves and are extremely thin since they have no muscle tissue.

Another important group is the deep cerebral veins that drain into the straight sinus along with the inferior sagittal sinus. These deep cerebral veins drain the area of the midbrain.

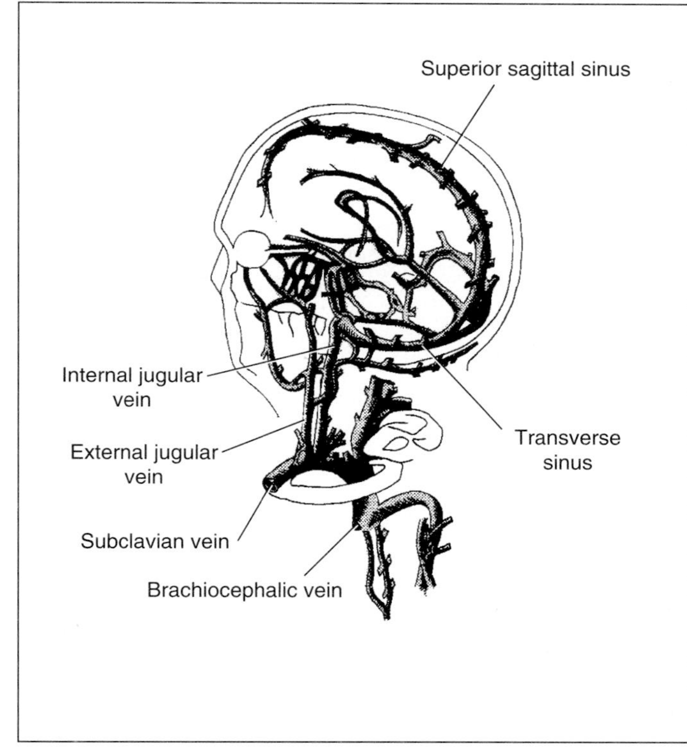

Fig. 24-22. Cranial venous system.

THORACIC CIRCULATORY SYSTEM

Thoracic Arteries

The **aorta and pulmonary arteries** are the major arteries located within the chest. The pulmonary arteries supply the lungs with blood (as shown earlier in Fig. 24-4).

The aorta extends from the heart to about the fourth lumbar vertebra and is divided into thoracic and abdominal sections. The **thoracic section** is subdivided into **four segments** (Fig. 24-23):

1. **Aortic bulb**
2. **Ascending aorta**
3. **Aortic arch**
4. **Descending aorta**

The **bulb** is at the proximal end of the aorta and is the area from which the coronary arteries originate. Extending from the bulb is the **ascending portion** of the aorta, which terminates at approximately the second sternocostal joint and becomes the **arch**. The arch is unique from the other segments of the thoracic aorta because there are three arterial branches arising from it, the brachiocephalic artery, the left common carotid, and the left subclavian artery. (This is also shown on a previous page in Fig. 24-10 under the cranial circulatory system.)

There are many variations of the aortic arch. Three more common variations sometimes seen in angiography, as shown in Fig. 24-24, are:

A. **Left circumflex aorta** (normal arch with the descending aorta downward and to the right)
B. **Inverse aorta** (arch is to the right)
C. **Pseudocoarctation** (arched descending aorta)

At its distal end, the arch becomes the **descending aorta** (Fig. 24-23). The descending aorta extends from the isthmus to the level of the twelfth dorsal vertebra. There are numerous intercostal, bronchial, esophageal, and superior phrenic arterial branches arising from the descending aorta, not shown in Fig. 24-23. These arteries transport blood to the organs for which they are named.

Thoracic Veins

The major veins within the chest are the **superior vena cava, azygos and pulmonary veins.** The superior vena cava returns the blood transported from the thorax to the right atrium. The azygos vein is the major tributary returning blood from the chest to the superior vena cava. (Fig. 24-25). The azygos vein enters the superior vena cava posteriorly. Blood from the chest enters the azygos vein from the intercostal, bronchial, esophageal, and phrenic veins.

The pulmonary veins return oxygenated blood from the lungs to the left atrium as previously shown in Figs. 24-4 and 24-6. The inferior vena cava returns blood from the abdomen and lower limbs to the right atrium as also shown in Figs. 24-4 and 24-6.

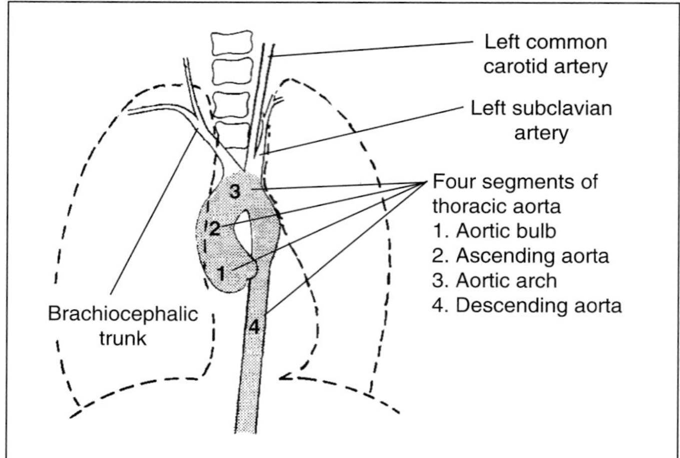

Fig. 24-23. Thoracic aorta.

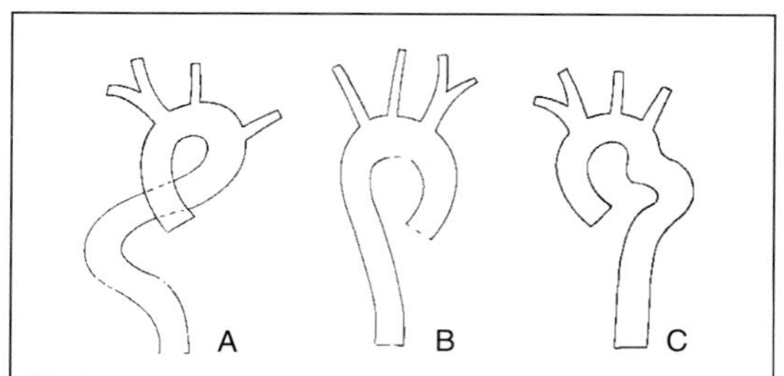

Fig. 24-24. Variations of the arch.

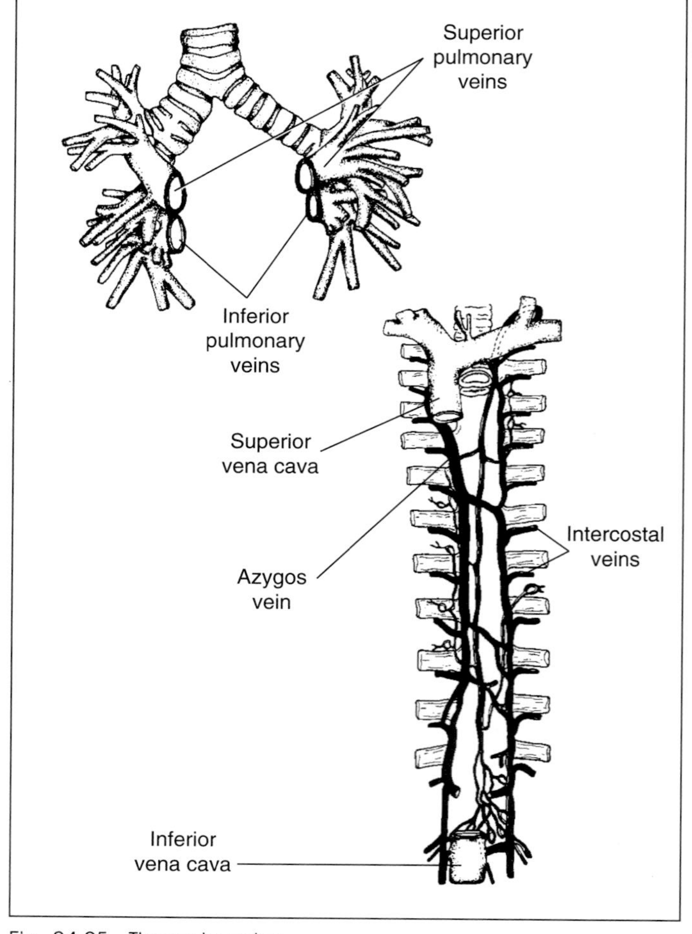

Fig. 24-25. Thoracic veins.

ABDOMINAL CIRCULATORY SYSTEM

Abdominal Arteries

The abdominal aorta is the continuation of the thoracic aorta. The abdominal aorta is anterior to the vertebrae and extends from the diaphragm to approximately L4 where it bifurcates into the right and left common iliac arteries. There are **five major branches** of the abdominal aorta that are of most interest in angiography. Any one of these branches may be selectively catheterized for study of a specific organ.
These are shown in Fig. 24-26 as follows:

1. **Celiac axis**.
2. **Superior mesenteric artery**.
3. **Left renal artery**.
4. **Right renal artery**.
5. **Inferior mesenteric artery**.

The **trunk** of the **celiac axis** arises from the aorta just below the diaphragm and about 1.5 cm above the origin of the superior mesenteric artery. Organs supplied with blood by the three large branches of the celiac trunk are the hepatic, splenic, and gastric.

The **superior mesenteric artery** supplies blood to the pancreas, most of the small intestine and portions of the large intestine, (cecum, ascending and about one-half of the transverse colon). It originates from the anterior surface of the aorta at the level of the first lumbar vertebra about 1.5 cm below the celiac artery.

The **inferior mesenteric artery** originates from the aorta at about the third lumbar vertebra (3 or 4 cm above the level of the bifurcation of the common iliac arteries). Blood is supplied to portions of the large intestine, (left half of transverse colon, descending colon, sigmoid colon and most of the rectum) by the inferior mesenteric artery.

The **right and left renal arteries** supplying blood to the kidneys originate on each side of the aorta just below the superior mesenteric artery at the level of the disk between the first and second lumbar vertebrae.

The distal portion of the abdominal aorta bifurcates at the level of the fourth lumbar vertebra into the **right and left common iliac arteries.** Each common iliac artery then divides into the **internal and external iliac arteries.** The internal iliac arteries supply the pelvic organs, (urinary bladder, rectum, reproductive organs, and pelvic muscles), with blood.

The lower limbs receive blood from the external iliac arteries. The **external iliac artery** is more significant in angiography than the internal iliac artery and is used **to study each lower limb**.

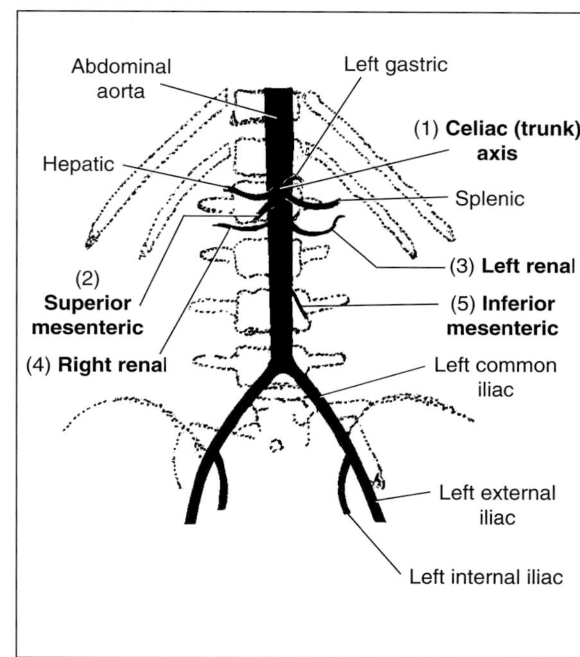

Fig. 24-26. Abdominal arteries.

Abdominal Veins

Blood is returned from structures below the diaphragm (the trunk and lower limbs) to the right atrium of the heart via the **inferior vena cava.** There are several radiographically important tributaries to the inferior vena cava. These veins include the right and left **common iliacs**, **internal iliacs**, **external iliacs**, **renal veins**, (Fig. 24-27) and the **portal system** (Fig. 24-28). The iliacs drain the pelvic area and lower limbs, while the renal veins return blood from the kidneys.

The **superior** and **inferior mesenteric veins** return blood from the small and large intestine through the **portal vein**, **hepatic vein** and into the **inferior vena cava**. This is best shown in Fig. 24-28 on the following page.

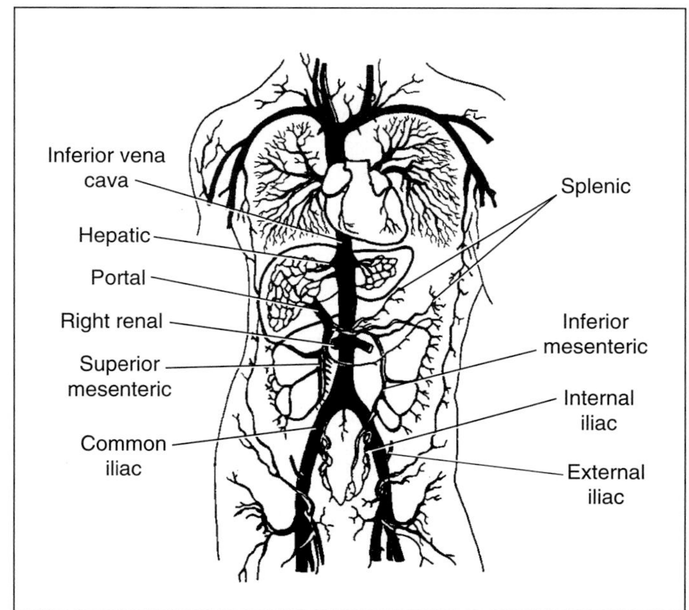

Fig. 24-27. Abdominal veins.

Portal System

The portal system includes all the veins that drain blood from the abdominal digestive track and from the spleen, pancreas and gallbladder. From these organs this blood is conveyed to the liver through the **portal vein.** While in the liver this blood is "filtered" and returned to the inferior vena cava by the hepatic veins. There are several major tributaries to the **hepatic vein** as shown in Fig. 24-28. The **splenic vein** is a large vein with its own tributaries, which return blood from the spleen.

The **inferior mesenteric vein,** which returns blood from the rectum and from parts of the large intestine, usually opens into the splenic vein but in about 10% of cases it ends at the angle of union of the splenic and superior mesenteric veins. The **superior mesenteric vein** returns blood from the small intestine and parts of the large intestine. It unites with the splenic vein to form the portal vein.

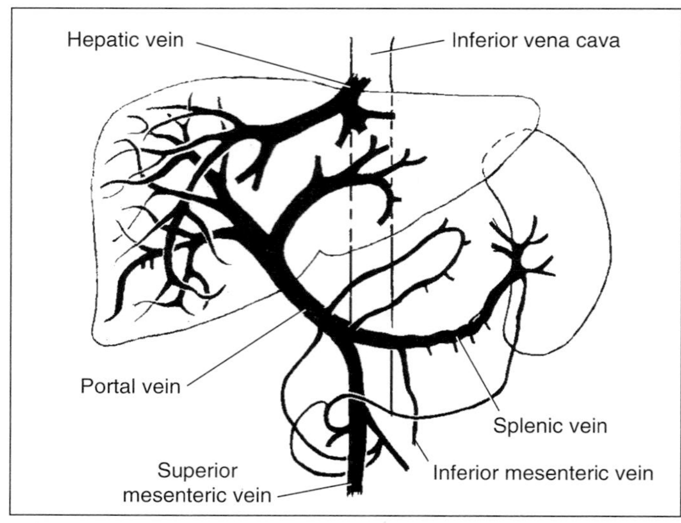

Fig. 24-28. Portal system.

PERIPHERAL CIRCULATORY SYSTEM

Upper Limb Arteries

The arterial circulation of the upper limb is generally considered to begin at the **subclavian artery**. The origin of the subclavian artery differs from the right to left side. On the right side the subclavian arises from the **brachiocephalic artery**, whereas the left subclavian originates directly from the aortic arch.

The subclavian continues to become the **axillary artery,** which gives rise to the **brachial artery**. The brachial artery bifurcates into the **ulnar** and **radial arteries** at approximately the level of the neck of the radius. The radial and ulnar arteries continue to branch until they join together to form **two palmar arches** (deep and superficial). Branches of these arches supply the hand and fingers with blood (Fig. 24-29).

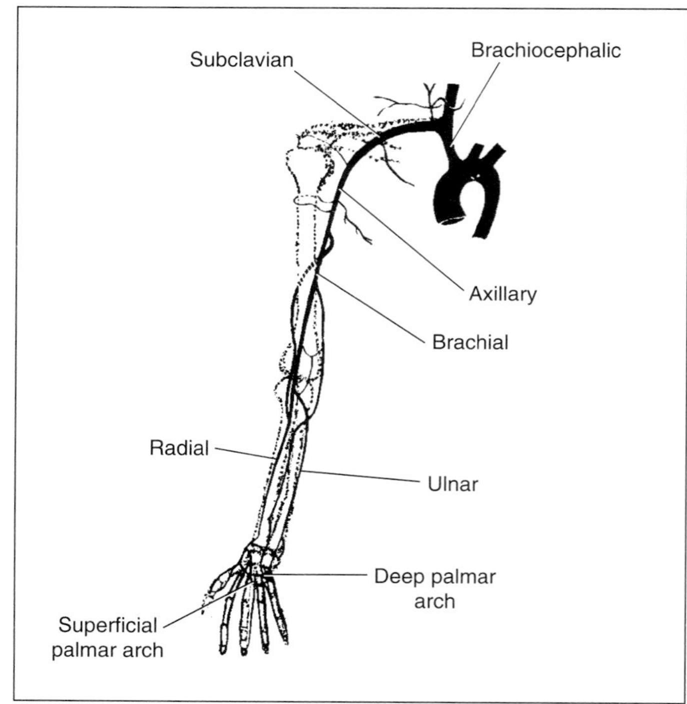

Fig. 24-29. Upper limb arteries.

Upper Limb Veins

The venous system of the upper limb may be divided into two sets, the **deep** and the **superficial veins.** They communicate with each other at frequent sites and thus form two parallel drainage channels from any single region. The **cephalic and basilic veins** are the primary tributaries of the superficial venous system. Both veins originate in the arch of the hand. Anterior to the elbow joint is the **median cubital vein** (the vein most commonly used to draw blood) , which connects the superficial drainage systems of the forearm. The upper basilic vein empties into the large **axillary vein** which then flows into the **subclavian** and eventually the **superior vena cava.** The lower basilic vein joins the median cubital vein continuing to the upper basilic vein (Fig. 24-30).

The deep veins include the **two brachial veins which** drain the **radial vein, ulnar vein and the palmar arches.** The deep brachial veins join the superficial basilic to form the axillary vein, which empties into the subclavian and finally into the **superior vena cava**.

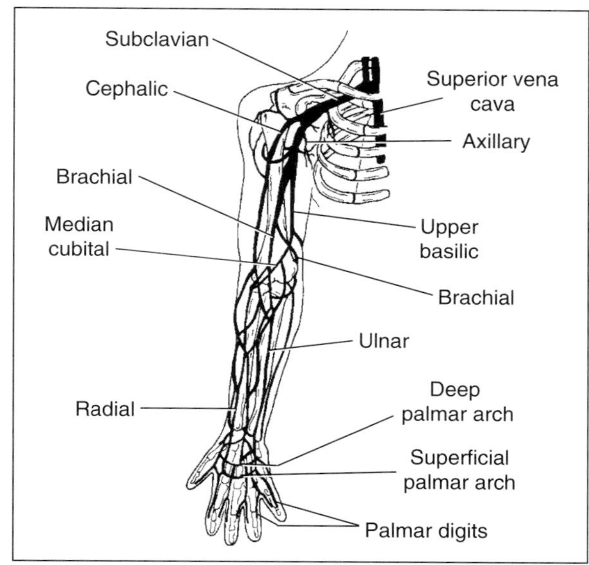

Fig. 24-30. Upper limb veins.

Lower Limb Arteries

The arterial circulation of the lower limb begins at the **external iliac artery** and ends at the veins of the foot (Fig. 24-31). The first artery to enter the lower limb is the **common femoral artery.** The common femoral artery divides into **the femoral and deep femoral arteries**. The femoral artery extends down the leg and becomes the **popliteal** artery at the level of the knee. Branches of the popliteal are the **anterior tibial, posterior tibial, and peroneal arteries**.

The **anterior tibial artery** continues as the **dorsalis pedis artery** with branches to the ankle and foot. The **peroneal artery** and the **anterior tibial artery** supply the calf and plantar surface of the foot.

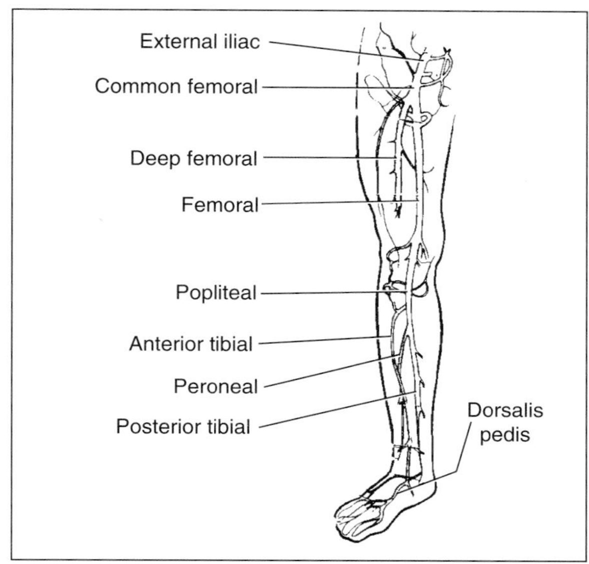

Fig. 24-31. Lower limb arteries.

Lower Limb Veins

The veins of the lower limb are similar to the upper limb in that both have a **superficial and deep venous system.** The superficial venous system contains the **great and small saphenous** veins and their tributaries and the superficial **veins of the foot.**

The **great saphenous vein** is the longest vein in the body and extends from the foot, along the medial aspect of the leg to the thigh where it opens into the **femoral vein.** The **small saphenous** originates in the foot and extends posteriorly along the leg terminating at the knee where it empties into the **popliteal vein.**

The **major deep veins** are the **posterior tibial, peroneal, anterior tibial, popliteal and femoral.** The posterior tibial vein and the peroneal vein join after draining the posterior foot and leg. The posterior tibial extends upward and unites with the **anterior tibial vein** to become the **popliteal vein** at the level of the knee. The popliteal continues upward to become the **femoral vein** before becoming the **external iliac vein** (Fig. 24-32).

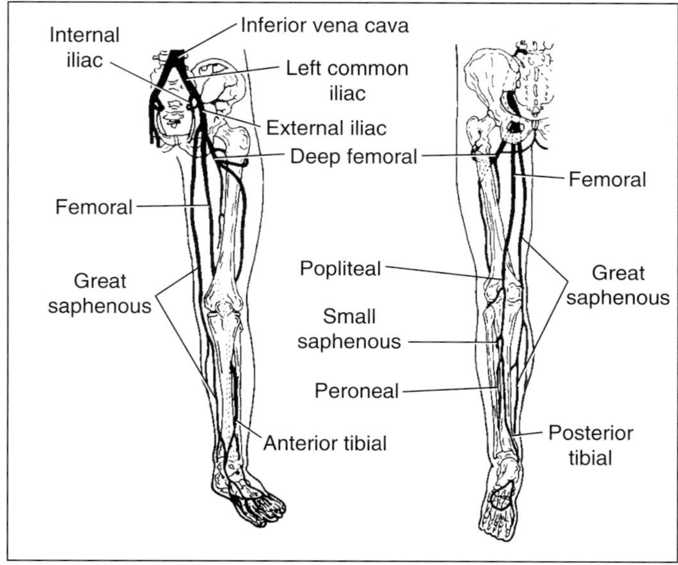

Fig. 24-32. Lower limb veins.

SUMMARY OF MAJOR ARTERIES

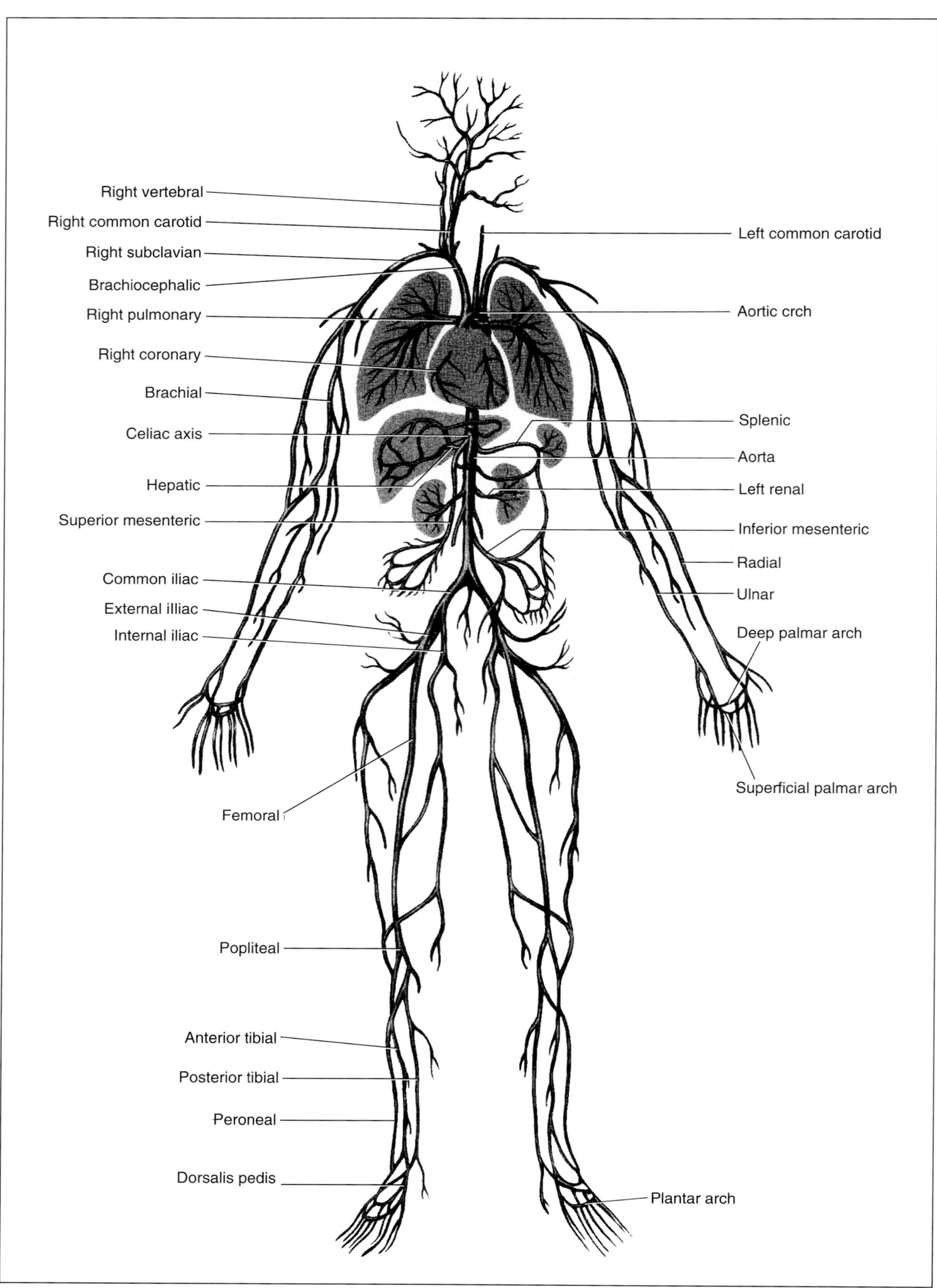

Fig. 24-33. Major arteries.

SUMMARY OF MAJOR VEINS

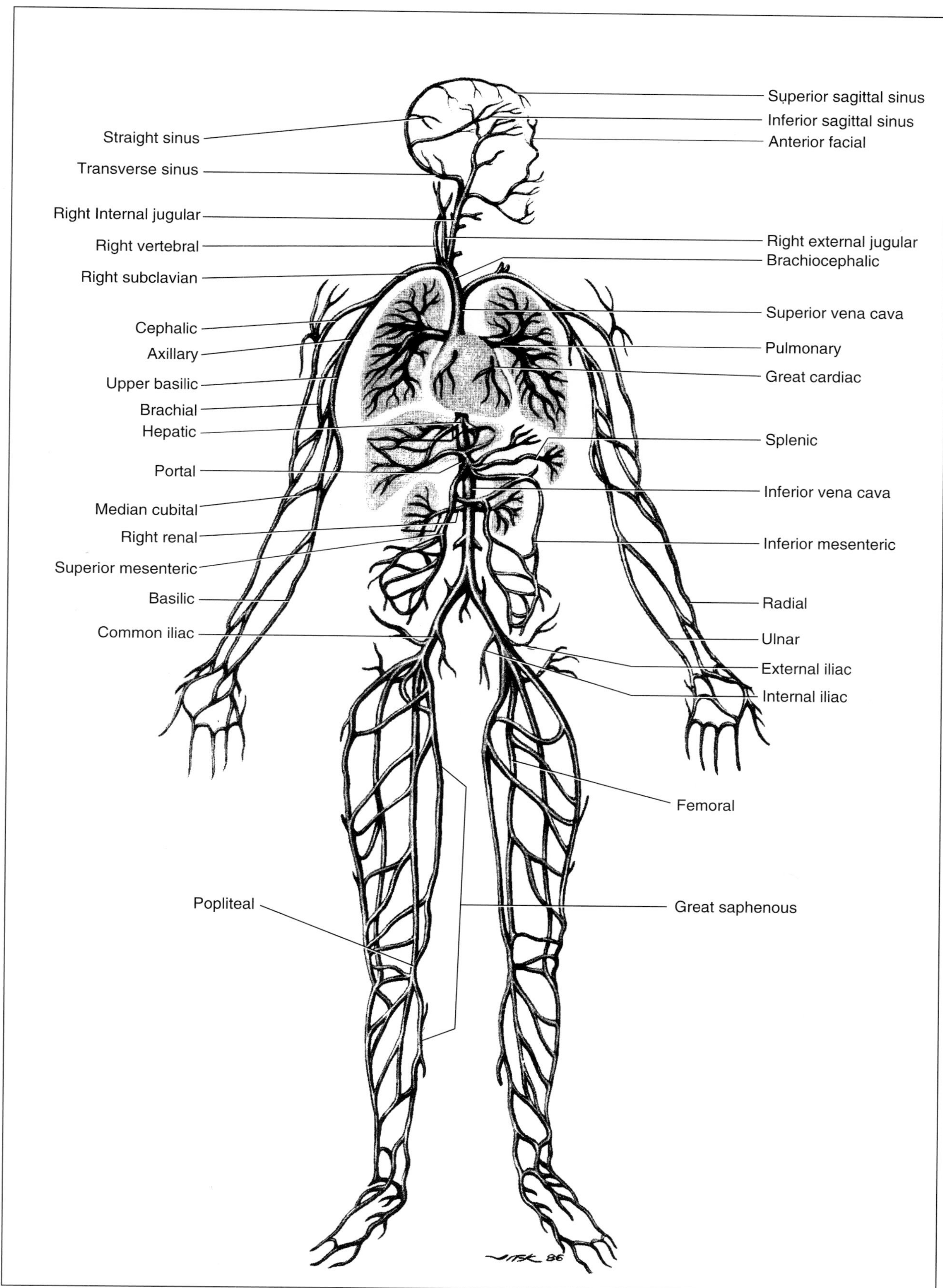

Fig. 24-34. Major veins.

LYMPHATIC SYSTEM

Lymph Drainage

The lymphatic system serves to drain interstitial fluid (fluid in the spaces between the cells) and return it to the venous system. The fluid from the **left side of the body**, **the lower limbs**, **pelvis**, and **abdomen** enters the venous system via the **thoracic duct** (largest lymph vessel in body) which drains into the **left subclavian vein** near its junction with the left jugular vein.

The upper **right side of the body**, **upper limb**, **head** and **neck region** drain lymph fluid into the venous system at the junction of the **right jugular** and **right subclavian veins** via the **right lymph duct**. (See Figs. 24-35 and 24-36.)

Functions

Functions of the lymphatic portion of the circulatory system are:

1. Fight disease by producing lymphocytes and microphages.
2. Return proteins and other substances to the blood.
3. Filter the lymph in the lymph nodes.
4. Transfer fats from the intestine to the thoracic duct and hence to the blood.

The lymphatic system has no heart to pump lymph fluid to its destination. Fluid is transported by diffusion, peristalsis, respiratory movements, cardiac activities, massage and muscular activity. The transportation of lymphatic fluid is in one direction only; away from the tissues. The sequence of fluid movement is from lymphatic capillaries to the various lymph vessels where the fluid enters the lymph nodes and is returned to the venous system by efferent lymphatic vessels.

Lymph nodes tend to form in clusters, although they may appear singularly. There are thousands of nodes throughout the body, some of which are identified in Fig. 24-36. The major collections of nodes that are seen radiographically are those in the thoracic, abdominal, pelvic and inguinal regions.

Lymphography

Lymphography *(lim-fog′ rah-fe)* is the general term describing radiographic examination of the lymphatic vessels and nodes after injection of a contrast medium. The term **lymphangiography** is often used for a radiographic study of the **lymph vessels** following injection of contrast medium. This is done by injecting an oil-based contrast medium into a lymph vessel (usually in the feet or hands) and tracking its path by taking radiographs at timed intervals.

Since the rate of circulation of the lymphatic system is very slow, the required timed film sequences are also very slow. The lymph vessels are usually visualized within the first hour after injection and the lymph nodes 24 hours later.

With the advent of computed tomography and other newer imaging modalities that can readily visualize enlarged lymph nodes, fewer lymphography examinations utilizing contrast medium as described above are being performed.

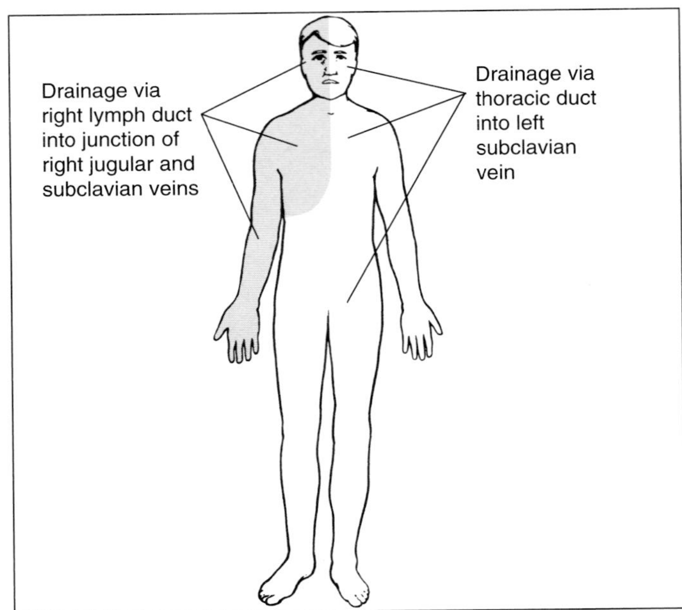

Fig. 24-35. Right and left lymph drainage.

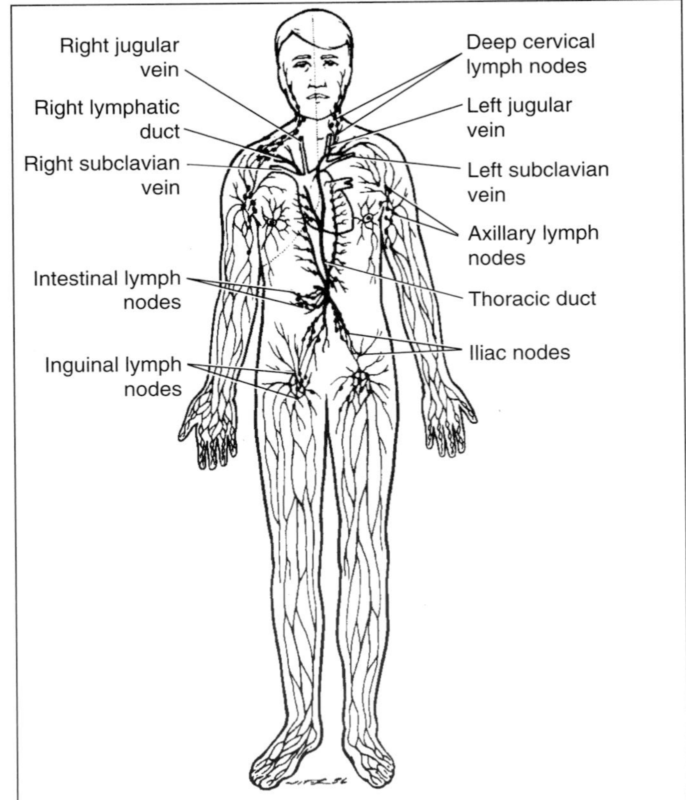

Fig. 24-36. Lymph drainage.

Radiographic Procedures & Positioning

The first part of this chapter covered the anatomy of the circulatory system which may be visualized radiographically with angiography following the injection of a positive contrast medium.

The second part of this chapter now covers the general procedure and the specific positioning required for angiography of the four anatomical regions, **cerebral**, **thoracic**, **abdominal** and **peripheral** (upper and /or lower limbs). Since angiographic procedures in each of these four body regions require the injection of contrast medium, the introduction of a needle and/or catheter into the associated blood vessel is required. A common method for this is called the **Seldinger technique**.

Seldinger Technique

The introduction of a catheter into a vessel requires puncturing through the skin, muscle, and tissue until the vessel of interest is reached. There are several methods that may be used to accomplish vessel puncture but the safest and most common method is the Seldinger technique. This technique was developed by Sven Seldinger in the 1950s and involves the use of specific catheters and guide wires. The catheters have different shapes at the distal end to permit easier access to the various vessels (Fig. 24-37). The radiographer must be familiar with the various dimensions, types, construction, tip design and radiopacity of the catheters and guide wires in use in the radiology department.

Following is a step by step description of the Seldinger technique (as shown in Fig. 24-38):

Step 1–Insertion of Needle: The needle is placed in a small incision and advanced so that it punctures both walls of the vessel.

Step 2–Placement of Needle in Lumen of Vessel: Placement of the needle in the lumen of the vessel is achieved by slowly withdrawing the needle until a steady blood flow returns through the needle.

Step 3–Insertion of Guide Wire: When the desired blood flow is returned through the needle, the flexible end of a guide wire is inserted through the needle and advanced about 10 centimeters into the vessel.

Step 4–Removal of Needle: After the guide wire is in position, the needle is removed by withdrawing it over that portion of the guide wire remaining outside the patient.

Step 5–Threading of Catheter to Area of Interest: The catheter is then threaded over the guide wire and advanced to the area of interest under fluoroscopic control.

Step 6–Removal of Guide Wire: When the catheter is located in the desired area, the guide wire is removed from inside the catheter. The catheter then remains in place as a connection between the exterior of the body and the area of interest.

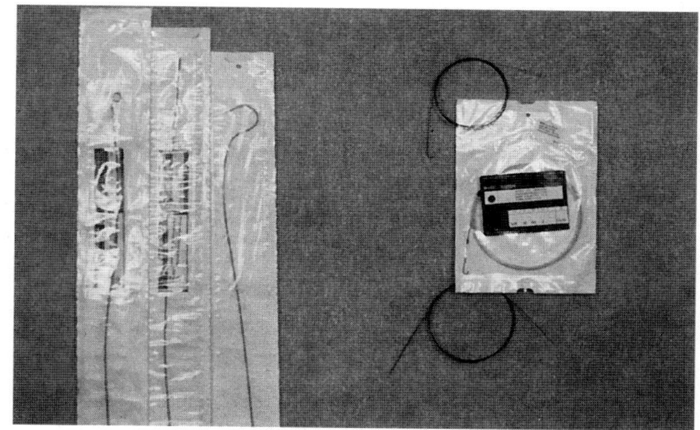

Fig. 24-37. Seldinger technique-Catheters and guide wires.

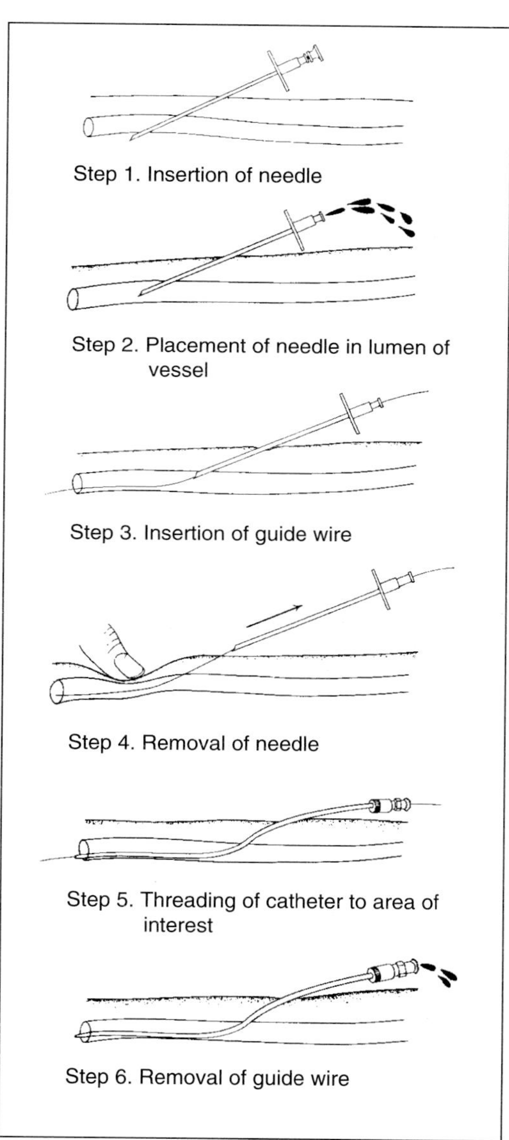

Fig. 24-38. Seldinger technique.

Special Procedure Room

The special procedure room, shown in Fig. 23-39, is equipped for all types of angiographic procedures. The angiographic room is usually considerably larger than a conventional radiographic room. An adjoining room or adjacent alcove houses the control panels, generators and computer accessory equipment. A scrub area, film processor, radiograph viewing area and adequate storage facilities should be readily accessible to the procedure room. The special procedure room should be close to, but somewhat isolated from, the general radiography department. The room location should be easily accessible to the emergency department, ambulance entrance, surgery and recovery rooms.

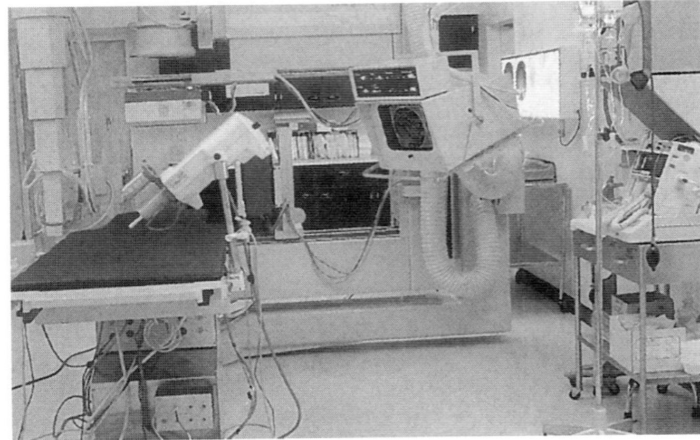

Fig. 24-39. General angiographic room.

Equipment

A modern angiography/interventional suite generally includes the following:

1. Biplane film changers capable of rapid simultaneous or alternating exposures (Fig. 24-40).
2. Changers capable of serial uniplane filming and magnification techniques.
3. Programmable automatic, electromechanical contrast media injectors.
4. Image-amplified television fluoroscopy that can rotate 180°.
5. Appropriate generators, controls and x-ray tubes.
6. Island type table with floating top.
7. Physiologic monitoring equipment.

Additional equipment may include:
1. 70 or 90 mm cine camera
2. Video tape or disk recorder

The floor should be made free of any cables or wires by utilizing subfloor conduits for necessary circuitry. The x-ray tubes and image intensifier can be a "C" or "U" arm type to further clear the working area. Outlets for oxygen and suction should be located in the room walls. The room should also have ample heating and air conditioning for optimum temperature control.

Biplane Film Changers

The typical cerebral angiographic procedure utilizes biplane film changers in conjunction with two radiographic tubes. Each unit should be independent of the other, and the two should be easily placed at right angles to one another. This arrangement allows exposure of a series of radiographs in both the lateral position and the AP projection to be exposed with a single injection of contrast medium. Blood flow through the brain is rapid, usually passing from carotid artery to jugular vein in less than 8 seconds. Consequently, the biplane film changers must be capable of multiple radiographs per second, each with superb radiographic detail. There are three basic types of changers available. They include: (1) the roll film changer, (2) the cassette changer, and (3) the cut film changer. While each has advantages and disadvantages, the cut film changer, as illustrated in Fig. 24-40, is widely used for angiography.

The internal mechanism of the film changer moves film rapidly from the supply compartment to the exposure area, and finally to the receiving bin. A program selector operates the film changer during single or serial exposures, regulating film rate and the duration of each phase of the series. Therefore, the program selector controls the number of films per second as well as the total length of time that exposures are to be made. The program selector is integrated so the contrast medium injector is synchronized with the imaging process.

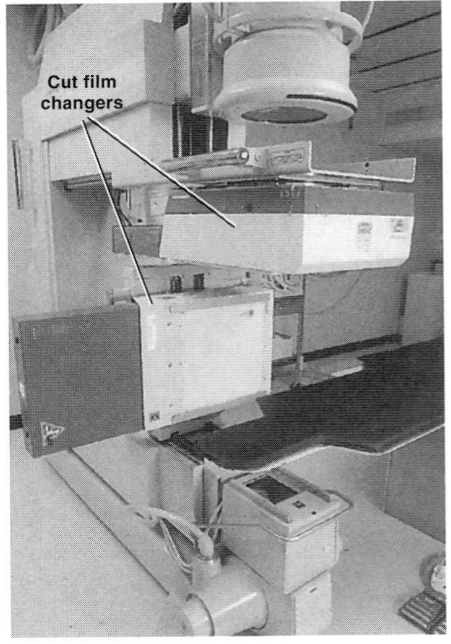

Fig. 24-40. Biplane film changers.

Automatic Electromechanical Contrast Medium Injector

As contrast medium is injected into the circulatory system, it is diluted by blood. The contrast material must be injected with sufficient pressure to overcome the patient's systemic arterial pressure and to maintain a bolus to minimize dilution with blood. To maintain the flow rates necessary for angiography, an automatic electromechanical injector is used. The flow rate is affected by many variables, such as the viscosity of contrast medium, length and diameter of the catheter, and injection pressure. Depending on these variables and the vessel to be injected, the desired flow rate can be selected prior to injection.

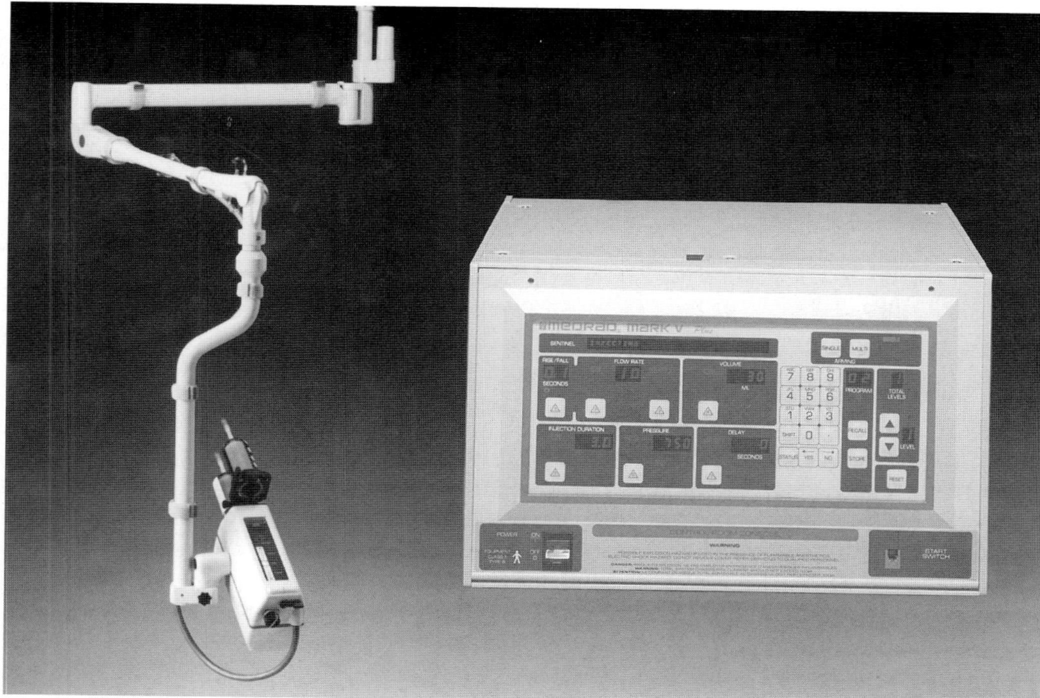

Fig. 24-41. Electromechanical contrast media injector. –Medrad Mark V Plus
(Courtesy of Medrad Inc., Indianola, PA.)

A typical automatic contrast medium injector is shown in Fig. 24-41. Every injector is equipped with syringes, a heating device, a high-pressure mechanism and a control panel. The syringes are disposable. Reusable syringes must be easily disassembled for sterilization. The heating device warms and maintains the contrast medium at body temperature, reducing the viscosity of the medium. The high-pressure mechanism is usually an electromechanical device consisting of a motor drive that moves a piston into or out of the syringe.

Additional features of an automatic mechanical injector other than safety, convenience and ease of use, and reliability of flow rate settings include: (1) ready light when armed and set for injection, (2) a slow or manual injector control to remove air bubbles from the syringe, and (3) controls to preclude inadvertent injection, or excessive pressure or volume injection.

Basic Radiographic Equipment

Island Table and Film Changers: A basic island radiographic table and two cut film changers are shown in Fig. 24-42. The island-type table is necessary for catheterization techniques and allows the radiologist to work from either side of the patient. A four-way floating top on a central pedestal permits the changers to be placed at either end of the table and still allows room for the image intensifier. The table height should be adjustable to permit magnification techniques.

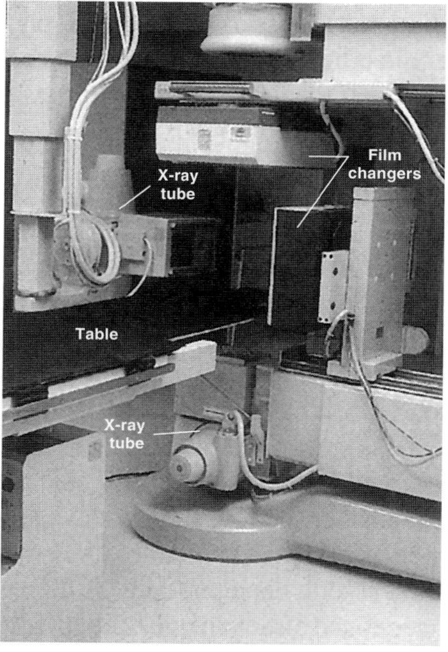

Fig. 24-42. Film changers, island table and x-ray tubes.

X-ray Tubes: The need to visualize the smaller blood vessels during angiography, and the use of magnification techniques, have resulted in specialized x-ray tubes. These x-ray tubes provide very small, effective focal spots that are the combined result of steep angle anodes and fractional focal spots.

Other modifications in the anode material and focal track, as well as high-speed anode rotation, have increased the loading capacity and the heat unit storage capabilities. The net result is an x-ray tube capable of (1) serial exposures with very high mA and short time settings and (2) superb definition production even during magnification techniques.

Collimators: Precise collimation is absolutely essential for angiography. All shutters of the collimator must be in perfect alignment to prevent degradation of the image from off-focus radiation, or unwanted secondary and scatter radiation. Aperture diaphragms may also be used to further limit the field size.

STERILE SUPPLIES

Angiographic procedures are carried out under sterile conditions. The special procedures room and equipment must be scrupulously clean. The room should be fully stocked and prepared before the patient's arrival. All radiographic and accessory equipment must be inspected and in working order. The appropriate sterile tray, catheters, guide wires and contrast medium must be assembled.

Basic Sterile Tray for Seldinger Catheterization

A sterile disposable tray, such as the one shown in Fig. 24-43, contains the basic equipment necessary for Seldinger catheterization of a femoral vessel. Basic sterile items include:

1. Hemostats.
2. Prep sponges and antiseptic solutions.
3. Scalpel blade.
4. Syringe and needle for local anesthetic.
5. Basins and medicine cup.
6. Sterile drapes/towels.
7. Bandaids.
8. Sterile image intensifier cover.

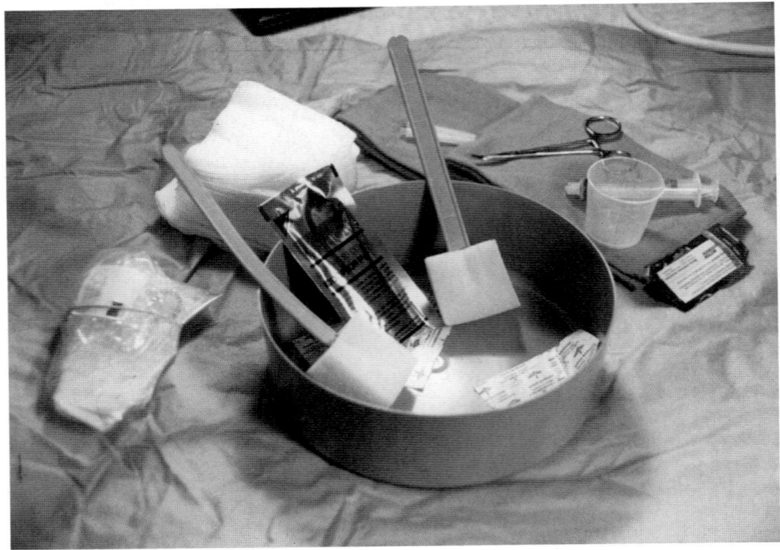

Fig. 24-43. Basic sterile tray.

Items Added to Basic Sterile Tray

Sterile items that must be supplemented to the basic tray are shown in Fig. 24-44. These include:

1. Appropriate catheters.
2. Guide wire.
3. Dilator.
4. Arterial needle.
5. Syringes.
6. Connective tubing.
7. Disposable fluids reservoir.

Additional items, not seen in Fig. 24-44, that are wrapped separate from the sterile tray are sterile gloves, gown, goggles and mask. Most catheters are supplied preformed by various companies. The guide wire is a Teflon-coated, safety wire with a J-shaped tip. The dilator shown in Fig. 24-44 is the same size as the catheter and is used to dilate the vessel to facilitate catheter introduction.

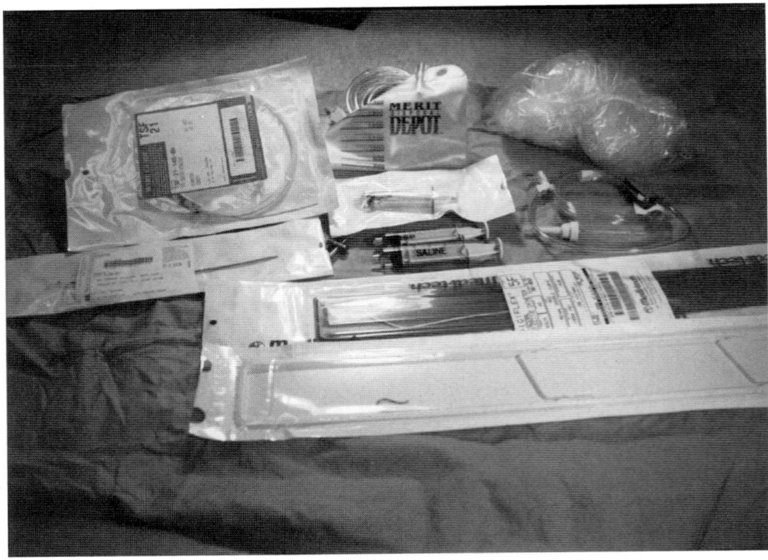

Fig. 24-44. Additional sterile supplies.

Cerebral Angiography

RADIOGRAPHIC PROCEDURE

Purpose

Cerebral angiography is the **radiographic examination of the blood vessels of the brain following injection of a positive contrast medium.** The primary purpose of cerebral angiography is to provide an exact vascular road map, enabling physicians to satisfactorily localize and diagnose certain abnormalities or pathologies.

Indications

Cerebral angiography is indicated whenever surgical or vascular interventional treatment is under strong consideration, when other imaging modalities and nonradiographic studies have not provided a precise diagnosis, or to determine the extent of vascular involvement of a positive CT or MRI examination. Cranial computed tomography or MRI is often performed prior to the angiographic study and, in many instances, provides sufficient information for diagnosis. **Vascular lesions, including arterial occlusions, aneurysms** and **arteriovenous malformations**, are best visualized by cerebral angiography.

Contraindications

There are few strict contraindications to cerebral angiography, although certain conditions make the examination more difficult for the radiologist. These conditions include the young and the aged, advanced arteriosclerosis, and especially atherosclerosis, severe hypertension and severe cardiac decompensation. A history of anaphylactoid reaction to iodinated contrast media will cause some concern, as will a strong history of thromboembolism. One absolute contraindication to use of the femoral approach is **lack of pulsation of either femoral artery**. Serious illness exists in most cases requiring cerebral angiography; therefore, the procedure is usually attempted as long as no life-threatening contraindications exist.

Contrast Media

Contrast media for cerebral angiography may be ionic or nonionic. Cerebral angiography is safest when using nonionic contrast medium. If ionic contrast medium is used, it is best to use 100 % meglumine salts at 60 % weight-to-volume concentrations. Injectable meglumine salts tend to be less toxic than the sodium salts.

Reaction to the contrast medium or the premedication is a possibility and must be kept in mind. Thus an emergency cart should be readily available.

Patient Placement

After arriving in the radiology department, the patient is placed in the supine position on a well-padded table. A pillow or sponge support placed under areas of strain, such as the small of the back and the knees, will add to patient comfort. Even though the patient is sedated, a burning sensation may be felt on injection. Head restraints may be necessary to help prevent involuntary motion during this crucial phase of the examination. The skin surface of the femoral triangle on the side to be catheterized is shaved and prepared with a germicide. Appropriate sterile drapes are then placed over the prepared area, as shown in Fig. 24-45.

Patient Preparation

Patient preparation for cerebral angiography depends on patient condition, which dictates the amount of time available before the examination. The patient may be hospitalized and, ideally, should be NPO to prevent problems associated with premature regurgitation of the stomach contents. Mild sedatives are generally prescribed so that the patient is relaxed, but able to fully cooperate.

The patient must also be psychologically prepared to undergo the examination. Ideally, the radiologist should visit the patient on the day prior to the examination to explain the procedures. This explanation must be done in language that the patient understands.

Prior to catheterization, both femoral artery pulses should be assessed and recorded. In addition, the dorsalis pedis and posterior tibial artery pulses are evaluated bilaterally and recorded before the procedure, just prior to catheter pullout and at the end of the procedure. Before, during and after the procedure, one member of the team should monitor the patient's blood pressure, pulse and level of consciousness.

Consent Form: At the time of the radiologist's visit, informed consent for the procedure is obtained from the patient or other legally authorized person. The examination is verbally described to the patient, and any complications that may occur are discussed. A printed sheet outlining relative risks and describing the procedure is presented for the patient's signature. This informed consent sheet should be placed in the patient's chart.

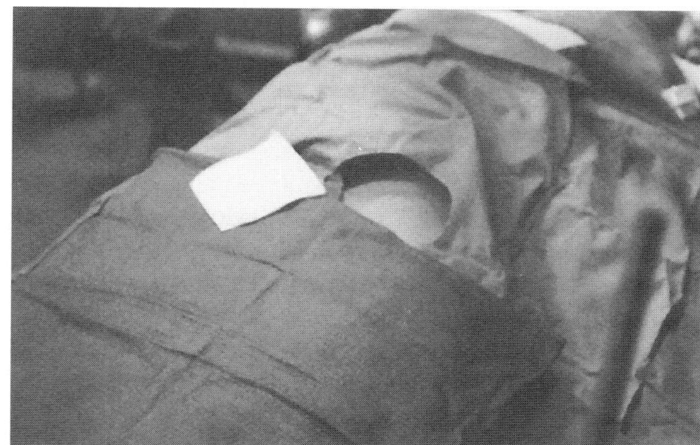

Fig. 24-45. Patient placement and preparation.

Patient with Vascular Catheter

Sterile items shown in Fig. 24-46 are prepared for the arterial puncture by the radiologist. The three-division manifold shown on the sterile sheet in this illustration is connected by lengths of tubing to (1) a transducer for vessel pressure readings, (2) a heparinized saline drip under pressure, and (3) an appropriate contrast medium. The syringe attached to the lower end of the manifold allows hand injection of medication or contrast medium, while the other end of the manifold attaches to the positioned catheter.

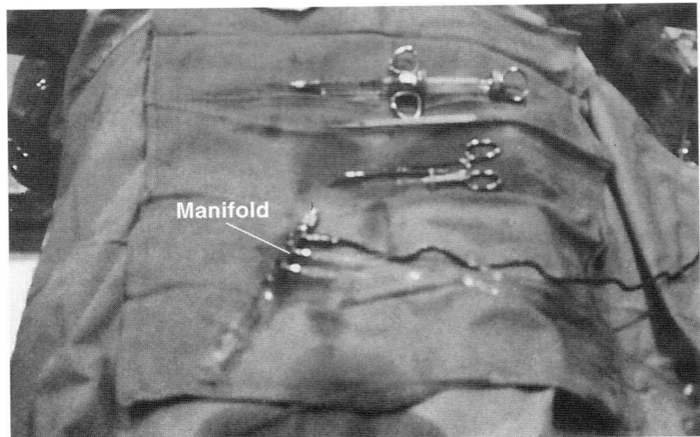

Fig. 24-46. Ready for radiologist.

Seldinger Catheterization Procedure

For cerebral angiography, the basic Seldinger technique is used to catheterize the femoral artery. The femoral approach is generally preferred and is versatile in that any of the four vessels supplying the brain, as well as the arch of the aorta or the external carotids, can be injected directly.

Arterial Puncture and Insertion of the Catheter: After localization and assessment of the femoral artery, the radiologist punctures the femoral artery with a special arterial needle. The arterial needle is placed in the femoral artery. Blood will backflow from the needle as shown in Fig. 24-47. The guide wire is immediately advanced through the needle cannula into the femoral artery. The cannula is removed and the vessel puncture site is dilated with the dilator. The dilator is removed and the catheter of choice is passed over the guide wire. Both guide wire and catheter are advanced to the desired location. Finally, the guide wire is removed and the catheter is flushed and attached to a saline drip.

The catheter is shown in place in Fig. 24-48. At this point the catheter is advanced to the ascending aortic arch and maneuvered into the vessel chosen for study. Proposed injection sites are always tested fluoroscopically following a hand injection of contrast medium. Once it is confirmed that the catheter is correctly placed, serial radiographic or DSA filming may proceed.

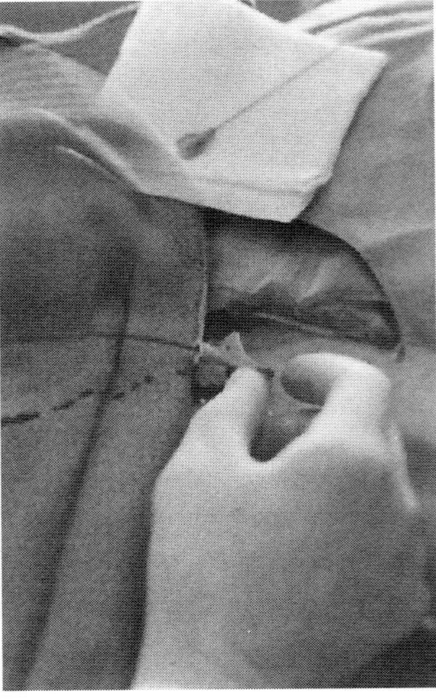

Fig. 24-47. Arterial puncture (blood backflowing from needle).

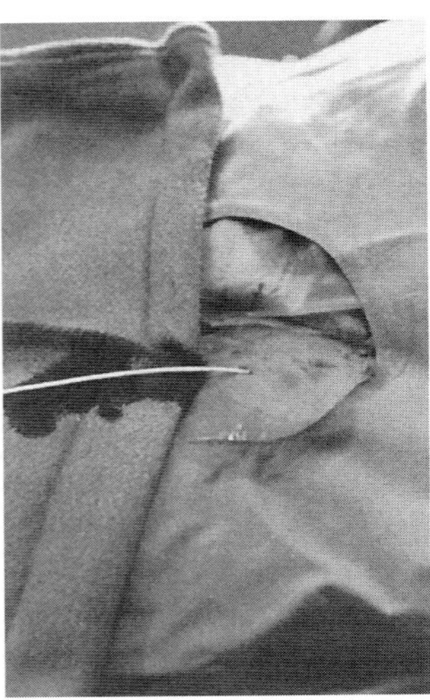

Fig. 24-48. Catheter in place.

POSITIONING ROUTINE AND EXAMINATION PROCEDURE

Positioning for Internal Carotid (Anterior Circulation) Angiography Scout

As soon as the patient is placed on the radiographic table, and prior to the catheterization process, scout radiographs are taken. Scout radiographs are necessary whenever contrast medium is injected. If the primary interest is the internal carotid artery, or anterior brain circulation, an AP axial and a lateral scout are exposed.

AP Axial Projection: Precise positioning is essential, and for the AP axial projection, the midsagittal plane is perpendicular to the frontal changer and parallel to the lateral changer. The **orbitomeatal line (OML) is positioned perpendicular to the frontal changer or image receptor**, as shown in Fig. 24-49. The primary objective for the frontal projection is to superimpose the petrous ridge and the orbital plate on each side. This positioning projects the anterior and middle cerebral arteries above the floor of the anterior fossa. The central ray is angled **10 to 15° caudad** and centered to pass through the **level of the EAM** and exit at the foramen magnum.

Lateral Position Centering: The lateral beam central ray is centered to about **1 in.** (2.5 cm) **above the EAM**. Both beams are tightly collimated.

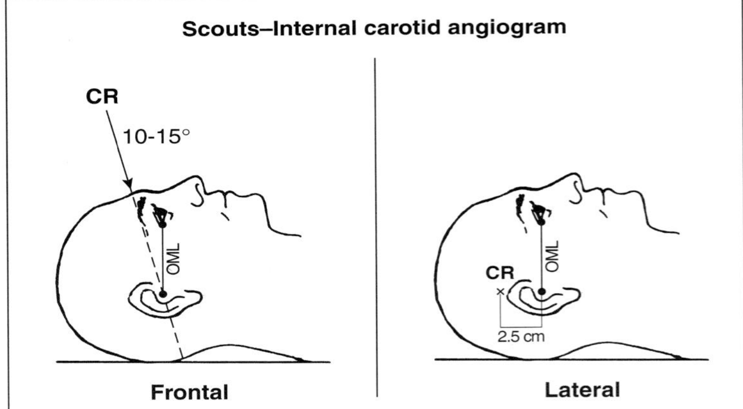

Fig. 24-49. Anterior circulation scout positioning.
–AP, CR 10-15° caudal to OML, through level of EAMs.
–Lateral, CR 1 in. (2.5 cm) above EAM.

Positioning for Vertebrobasilar (Posterior Circulation) Angiography Scout

If the primary interest is the **posterior circulation** or **vertebrobasilar system**, then slightly different positioning methods are utilized. The **midbrain** and **hindbrain** must be visualized when radiographically studying the vertebrobasilar system.

Axial AP Projection: The frontal position utilizes a caudal angle of **30 to 35° to the OML**, to pass through **at ≈1 in.** (2.5 cm) **superior to the EAM** and exit at the foramen magnum. Parallax (shape distortion) is a problem with extreme tube angles, and occasionally the neck must be hyperflexed with a sponge placed under the head with little or no tube angle (center illustration of Fig. 24-50). This modification is especially necessary for magnification techniques. The 30° angle is maintained between the central ray and the OML.

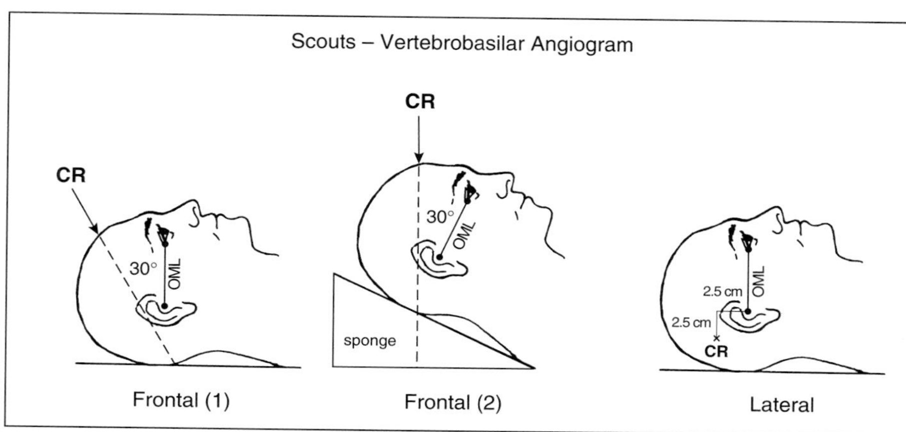

Fig. 24-50. Posterior circulation scout positioning.
-AP axial, CR 30-35° caudal to OML, through 1 in. superior to EAM.
-Lateral, CR 1 in. (2.5 cm) posterior and superior to EAM.

Lateral Position Centering: Centering for the lateral x-ray tube is to about **1 in.** (2.5 cm) **superior** and **1 in.** (2.5 cm) **posterior to the EAM**, as shown on the right in Fig. 24-50.

Position for Common Carotid Arteriography

Sometimes before a complete three- or four-vessel angiogram is done, two radiographic views of the neck to visualize each common carotid are taken. The position for a common carotid arteriogram is demonstrated in Fig. 24-51. The right common carotid artery is demonstrated in the AP projection and the lateral position to examine this artery and its bifurcation into internal and external carotid arteries. The area of bifurcation is studied carefully for occlusive disease. The left common carotid artery is studied in a similar manner during the examination.

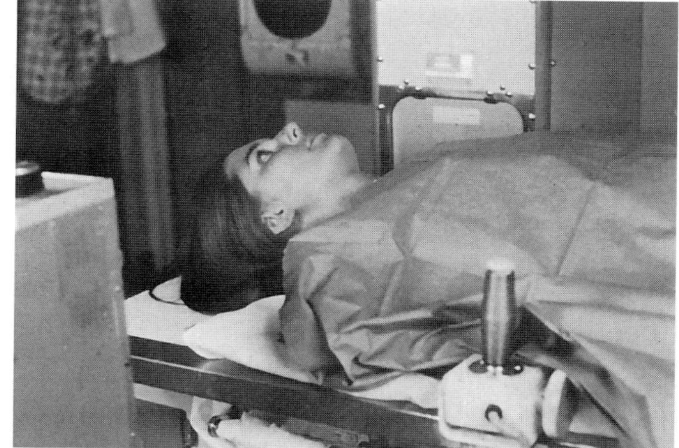

Fig. 24-51. Position for common carotid arteriography.
-AP and lateral positioning to neck region for common carotid artery.

Left Common Carotid Arteriograms

An AP and a lateral arteriogram of the left common carotid artery are shown in Figs. 24-52 and 24-53. The catheter has been placed in the most proximal portion of the common carotid artery. The area of bifurcation is of special interest to the radiologist. On the AP projection, the internal carotid artery (A) is located more laterally than the external carotid artery (B). On the lateral view to the right, the internal carotid artery courses anteriorly before ascending to the base of the brain.

Arch Aortography: In order to completely image the four major vessels leading to the brain, the radiologist may elect to do an initial arch aortogram. Arch aortography allows the radiologist to evaluate the major vessels for size, position, lumen status and anomalous origin. Arch aortography is rarely utilized during a three- or four-vessel angiogram, but is included as one of several possibilities. The arch aortogram is described later in this chapter under thoracic angiography.

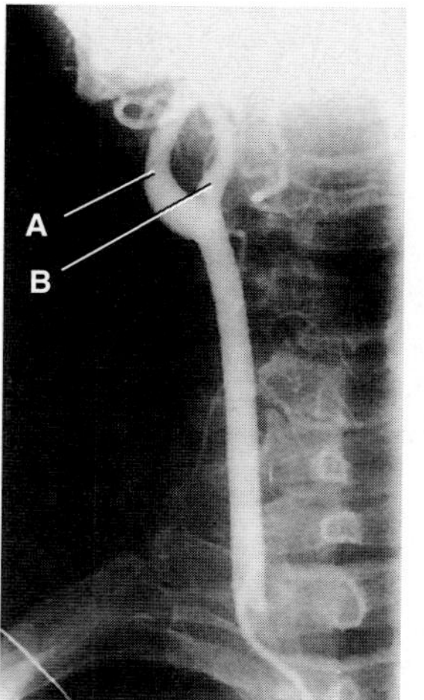

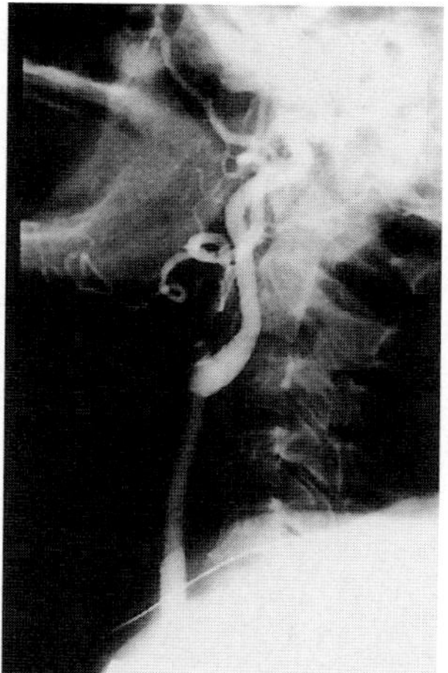

Fig. 24-52. AP. Fig. 24-53. Lateral.
Left common carotid arteriograms.

INTERNAL CAROTID ANGIOGRAPHY

Procedure and Position for Internal Carotid Angiography

If common carotid angiography is not performed, an injection of the aortic arch should occur to determine the number and type of branches off the aorta. After determining the aortic arch vessel branches, the catheter is advanced into the respective **internal carotid artery**. Hand injection of contrast medium under fluoroscopic control assures the radiologist of correct catheter placement. The anterior cerebral circulation is studied with a sufficiently long exposure run to visualize the arterial, capillary and venous phases of circulation.

Assuming a normal circulation exists, each plane is exposed at the rate of 2 exposures per second for 4 seconds followed by 1 exposure per second for 6 seconds. In biplane filming, it is best if the exposures alternate between frontal and lateral modes. Simultaneous firing of both x-ray tubes is usually not attempted as this may produce excessive cross-fogging and subsequent degradation of image quality

Positioning: Positioning for internal carotid angiography is the same as the scout imaging (Figs. 24-49 and 24-54). However, during contrast medium injection, it is very important that a strap be secured across the forehead and chin to immobilize the patient (Fig. 24-55).

For the **AP axial projection**, the frontal x-ray tube is angled **10 to 15° caudal to the OML** to pass through the **level of the EAM** and exit at the foramen magnum. **Lateral centering** is about **1 in**. (2.5 cm) **above the EAM**.

Patient Instructions: Immediately prior to injection, the radiologist must explain to the patient the necessity of holding absolutely still during the contrast medium injection even though a temporary burning sensation may be felt along the injection pathway. This warning cannot be minimized since, quite often, the burning sensation is intense and causes the patient to move.

Left Internal Carotid Arteriograms

Representative radiographs of the arterial phase of a left internal carotid angiogram are shown in these radiographs (Figs. 24-56 and 24-57). On the AP axial radiograph to the left, the floor of the anterior fossa and the petrous ridges superimpose. This allows visualization of the bifurcation of the internal carotid artery into the anterior and middle cerebral arteries.

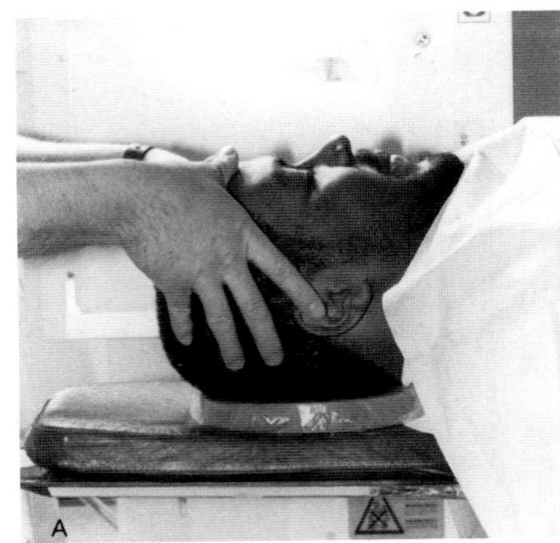

Fig. 24-54. Positioning for internal carotid angiography.

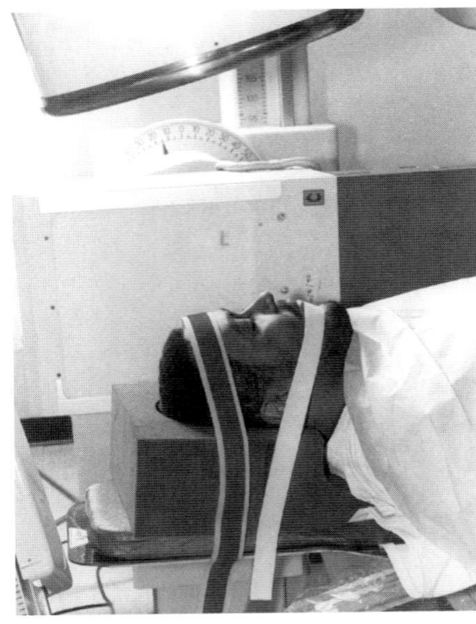

Fig. 24-55. Position for internal carotid angiography.

-AP axial, CR 10-15° caudal to OML, through level of EAM.

-Lateral, CR to 1 in. (2.5 cm) above EAM.

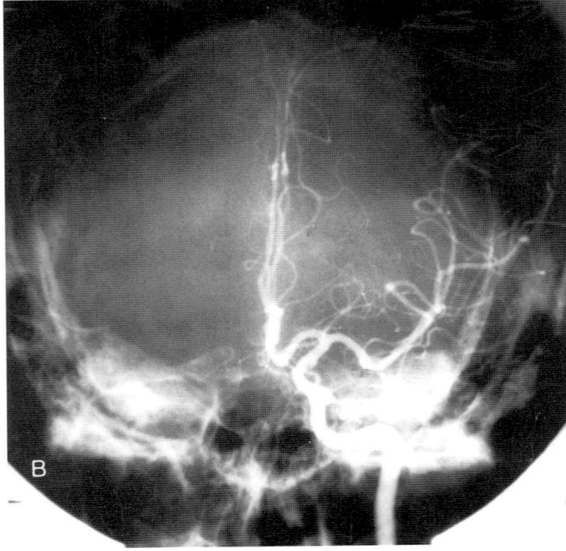

Fig. 24-56. AP axial–Left internal carotid arteriogram.

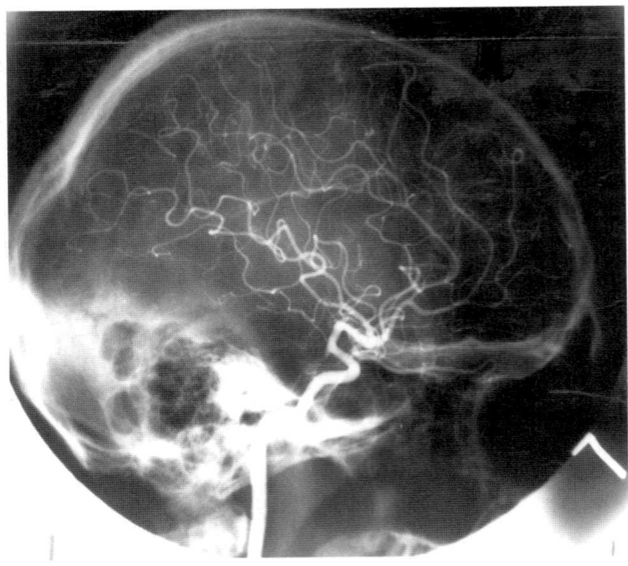

Fig. 24-57. Lateral–Left internal carotid arteriogram.

MAGNIFICATION RADIOGRAPHY

Frontal Position (2X Magnification)

Magnification filming must often be done to demonstrate small vessels. The law of image magnification states that the width of the image is to the width of the object as the distance of the image from the x-ray source is to the distance of the object from the x-ray source. In order to achieve **2X magnification** in the frontal position, the patient's head is positioned similar to the dry skull shown in Fig. 24-58. The center of the head is positioned **exactly halfway between the film and x-ray source**. (In these photos it appears the skull is closer to the tube than to the film, but remember the true x-ray source is at the target of the x-ray tube and not in the collimator.)

In 2X magnification, all anatomic structures equal to or larger than the effective focal spot size will be displayed twice their normal size on the finished radiograph.

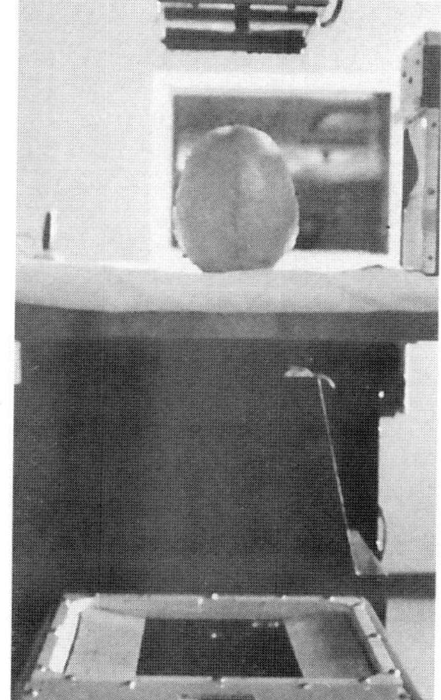

Fig. 24-58. Magnification radiography (frontal).

Lateral Position (2X Magnification)

Head placement to achieve 2X magnification in the lateral position is shown in Fig. 24-59. Again, the patient's head is exactly halfway between the film and the x-ray source. If the head were placed even closer to the x-ray tube, there would be greater magnification of the image. Rarely will magnification factors greater than 2X be attempted using a focus-film distance of 100 cm. Due to the size of the collimator, the head must be placed very close to the exit port of the collimator in order to achieve magnification factors greater than 2X.

Another limiting factor is the size of the film used in the automatic changer. The maximum field size of most larger changers is 35 cm x 35 cm. Even at 2X magnification, the entire cranium is barely demonstrated on a 35 cm x 35 cm field.

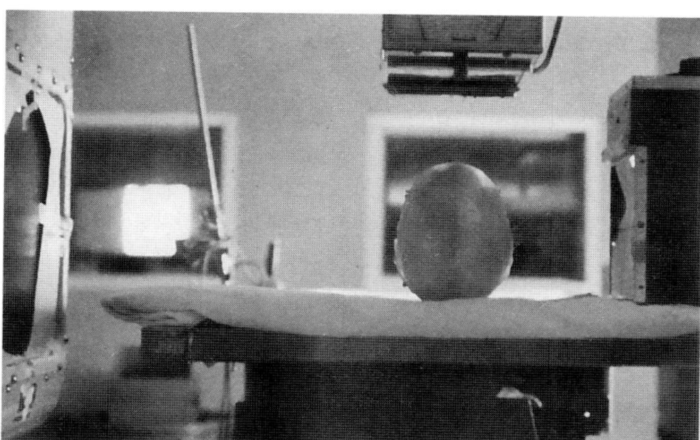

Fig. 24-59. Magnification radiography (lateral).

Position for Magnification Angiography of Internal Carotid Artery

Figure 24-60 demonstrates patient positioning for a magnified internal carotid angiogram.

Air-Gap Principle: A beneficial adjunct to magnification radiography is application of the air-gap principle. Whenever the image detection system is separated from the object by an appreciable distance, there is a remarkable decrease in the amount of secondary and scatter radiation that reaches the film surface. Much of the secondary and scatter radiation is directed away from the film. A large percentage of the weaker radiation emerging from the skull and directed toward the film is absorbed in the air and never reaches the film surface.

If two x-ray tubes are used, both beams should be closely collimated to further reduce radiation exposure to the patient. This close collimation is especially important because the short SID increases skin dosage to the radiation-sensitive areas of the head and neck.

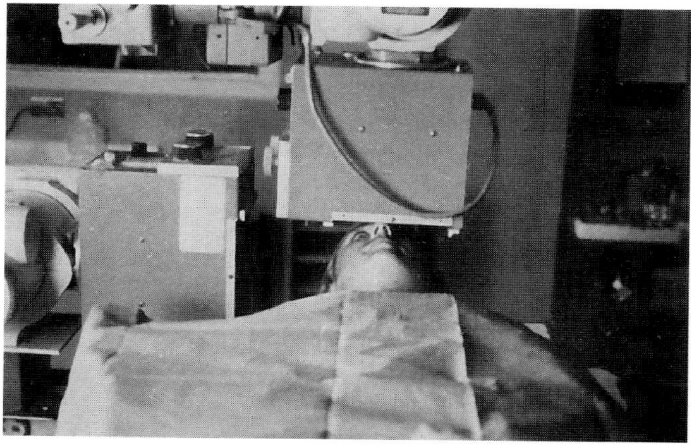

Fig. 24-60. Internal carotid magnification.

Magnified Internal Carotid Arteriograms

Magnified radiographs of an internal carotid arteriogram are shown in Figs. 24-61 and 24-62. The AP radiograph to the left and the lateral radiograph to the right visualize arteries much smaller than those seen on a nonmagnified study. Patient motion must be minimized during magnification techniques since any unsharpness due to voluntary or involuntary movement will be accentuated. Any motion unsharpness will be proportionately enlarged, depending on the magnification factor.

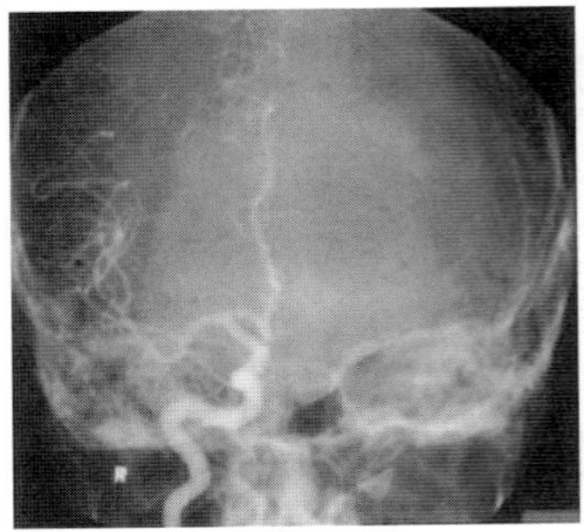

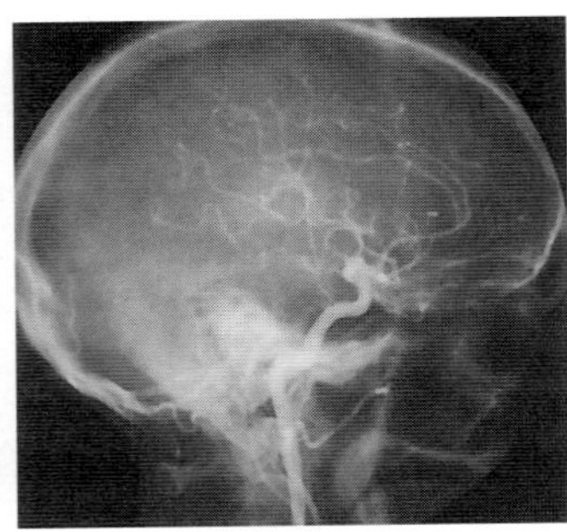

Fig. 24-61. AP. Lateral. Fig. 24-62.
Magnified internal carotid arteriograms.

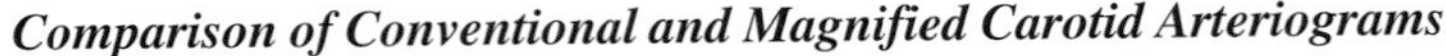

Comparison of Conventional and Magnified Carotid Arteriograms: Two lateral internal carotid arteriograms are shown for comparative purposes in Figs. 24-63 and 24-64. The routine nonmagnified study is to the left, while the 2X magnified radiograph is to the right. The phase of circulation is similar for each of these radiographs. Small arteries that cannot be delineated on the routine study are readily apparent on the magnified view.

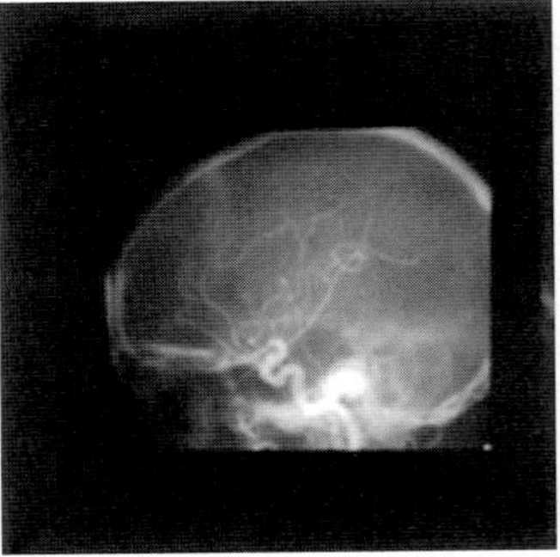

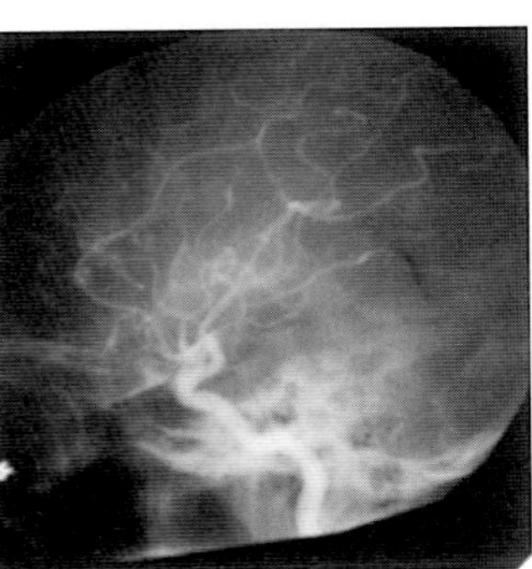

Fig. 24-63. Conventional. Magnified. Fig. 24-64.
Conventional vs. magnified carotid arteriograms.

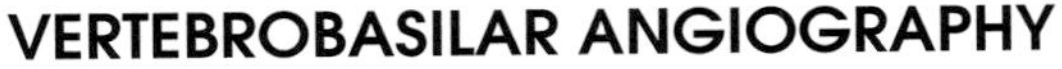

VERTEBROBASILAR ANGIOGRAPHY

Position for Vertebrobasilar Angiography

Following radiographic study of the neck and anterior circulation on both sides, the posterior circulation is studied, if it is of interest. Usually, the left vertebral artery is catheterized first. If injection volume and pressure are adequate to visualize certain branches of the opposite vertebral artery by reflux, then the right vertebral artery is usually not injected directly. Therefore, injection of both right and left internal carotid arteries and the left vertebral artery constitute the usual **three-vessel angiogram.** If both vertebral arteries are injected, the examination is termed a **four-vessel angiogram.**

Positioning for the vertebrobasilar angiogram is similar to positioning for the internal carotid angiogram (Fig. 24-65). The patient's head is immobilized, and the OML is adjusted perpendicular to the frontal changer. Frontal centering for the vertebrobasilar angiogram must include the area surrounding the fourth ventricle.

Frontal positioning involves a modified AP axial projection, maintaining a **30° caudal angl**e between the central ray and the OML. The central ray passes through the **level of the EAM**.

Lateral centering is to **about 1 in**. (2.5 cm) **superior** and **1 in**. (2.5 cm) **posterior** to the EAM.

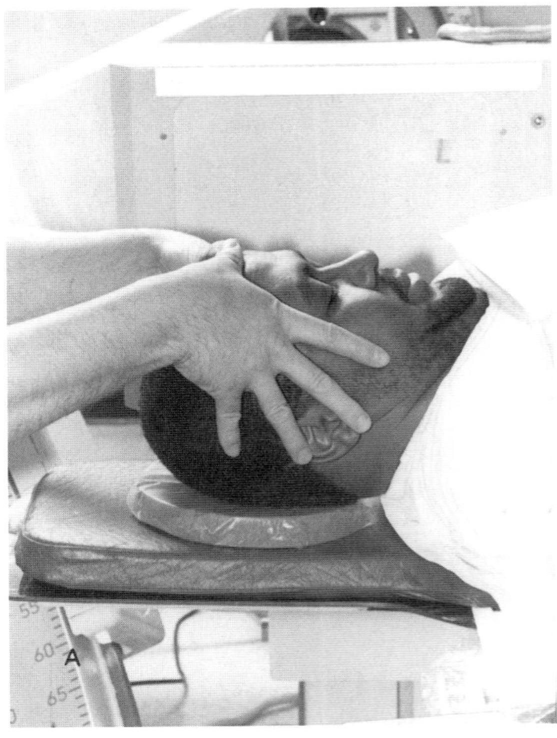

Fig. 24.65. Positioning for vertebrobasilar angiography.
-AP axial, CR 30° caudal to OML through level of EAM.
-Lateral, CR 1 in. (2.5 cm) superior and posterior to EAM.

Left Vertebrobasilar Arteriogram

Representative vertebrobasilar arteriograms are shown in Figs. 24-66 and 24-67. The AP radiograph demonstrates a left-sided injection with adequate filling of the necessary branches of the right vertebral artery.

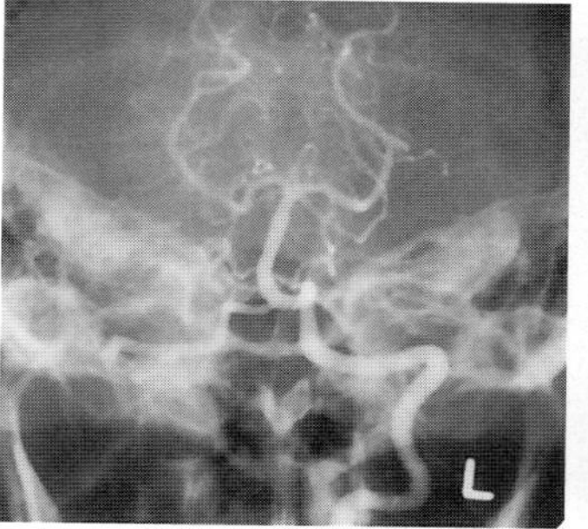

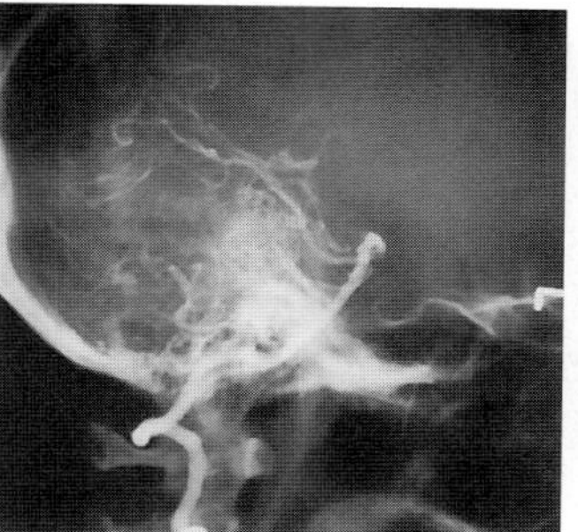

Fig. 24-66. AP. Lateral. Fig. 24-67.
Left vertebrobasilar arteriograms.

Position for Magnification Angiography of the Vertebrobasilar System

Patient position for magnification studies of the vertebrobasilar system is demonstrated in Fig. 24-68. The head is placed halfway between the focal spot and the film to achieve a 2X magnification. An angle of 30 to 35° is maintained between the OML and the central ray for the AP axial projection.

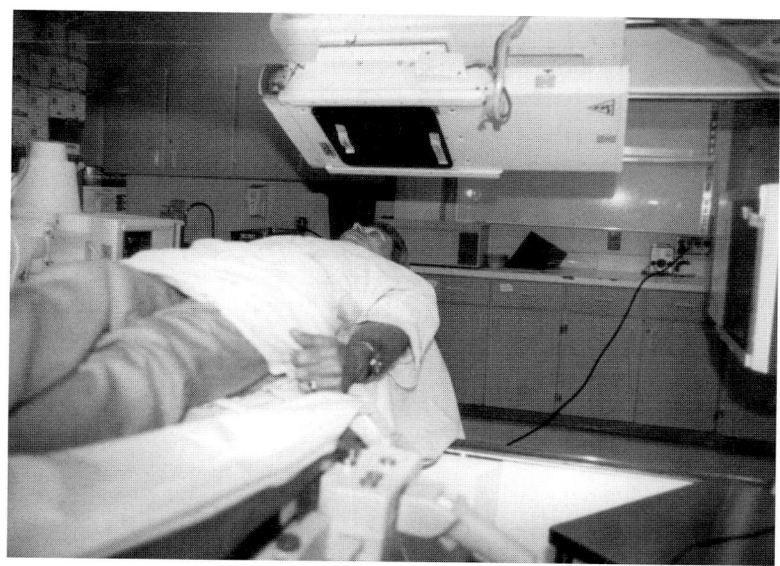

Fig. 24-68. Vertebrobasilar magnification.

Magnified Vertebrobasilar Arteriogram

Magnified vertebrobasilar arteriograms are shown in Figs. 24-69 and 24-70. The axial AP projection to the left and the lateral radiograph to the right visualize large and small arteries. Patient instructions, immobilization, close collimation and elimination of tube angulation all contribute to reduced unsharpness and, consequently result in superior quality radiographs.

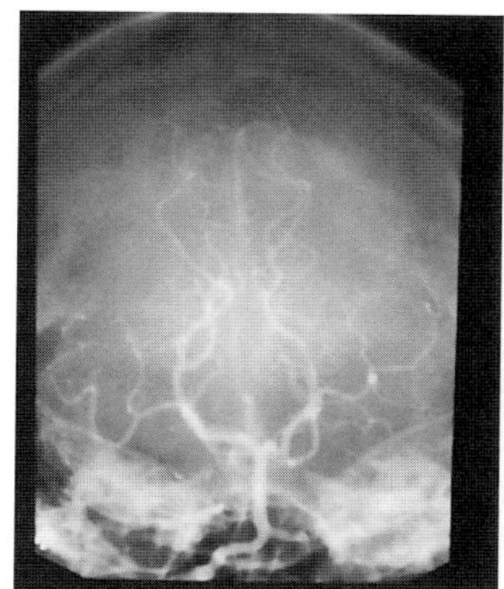

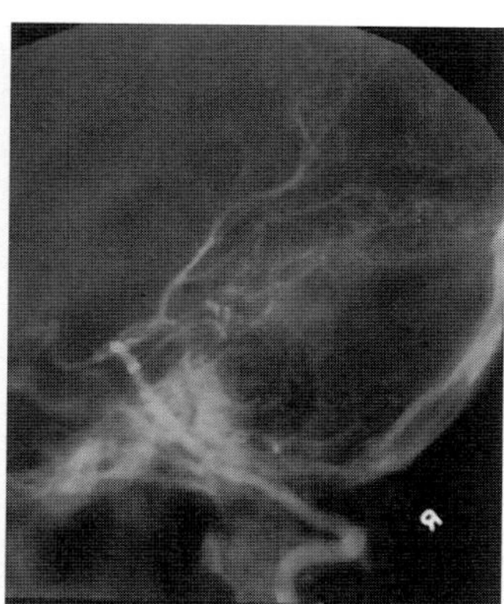

Fig. 24-69. AP. Lateral. Fig. 24-70.
Magnified vertebrobasilar arteriograms.

ANEURYSM ARTERIOGRAPHY

Special Oblique Positions

Occasionally, special oblique positions are necessary to fully evaluate aneurysms. A common site for aneurysm in the anterior circulation is near the bifurcation of the internal carotid artery into the anterior and middle cerebral arteries. The **supraorbital posterior oblique position**, as shown to the upper left in Fig. 24-71, is identical to the frontal projection for the internal carotid artery, except that the head is rotated 30° from the midsagittal plane.

The **transorbital posterior oblique position** shown to the lower right in Fig. 24-71 utilizes a 20° cephalad angulation in addition to the 30° rotation of the head. In most cases the head is rotated 30° away from the side being injected.

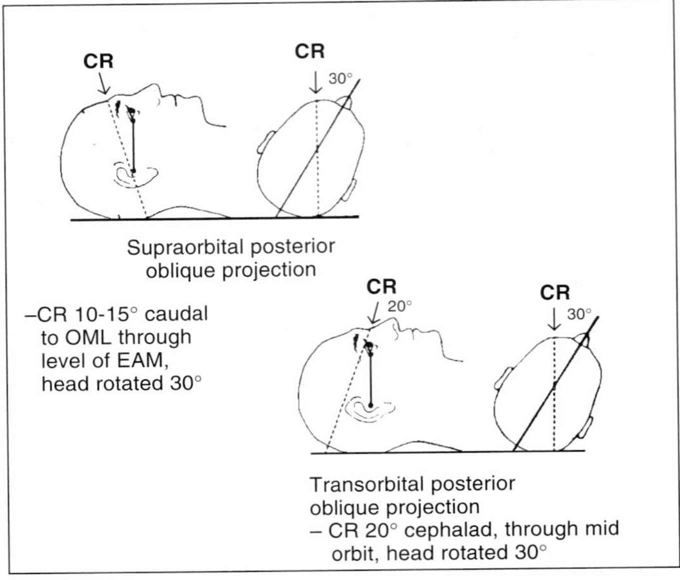

Fig. 24-71. Special oblique positions.

Oblique Position for Internal Carotid and Branches

The position for an oblique view of the left internal carotid artery and its branches is demonstrated in Fig. 24-72. This illustration could represent either a supraorbital or transorbital oblique position, depending on tube angulation. An approximate 15° caudal angulation to the feet would give the supraorbital oblique position, while a 20° cephalad angulation would produce the transorbital position. This oblique position is usually radiographed in both frontal and lateral planes. Since only the arterial phase needs to be visualized, a run of 3 to 4 seconds is usually adequate.

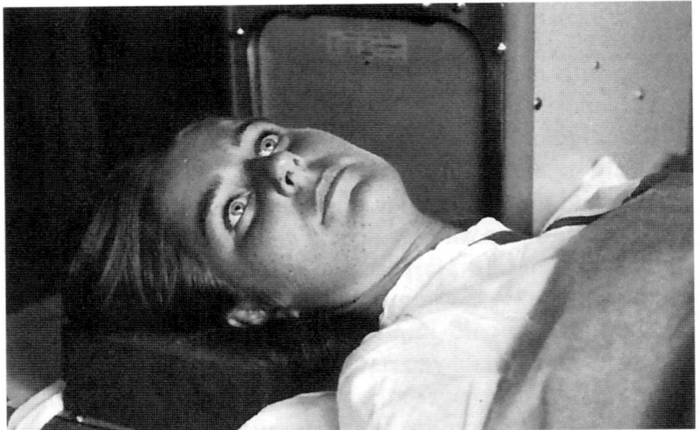

Fig. 24-72. Oblique position for aneurysm.

Transorbital Oblique Radiography

An arteriogram utilizing the transorbital oblique position is shown in Fig. 24-73. A large aneurysm is evident at the bifurcation of the anterior and middle cerebral arteries (see arrow).

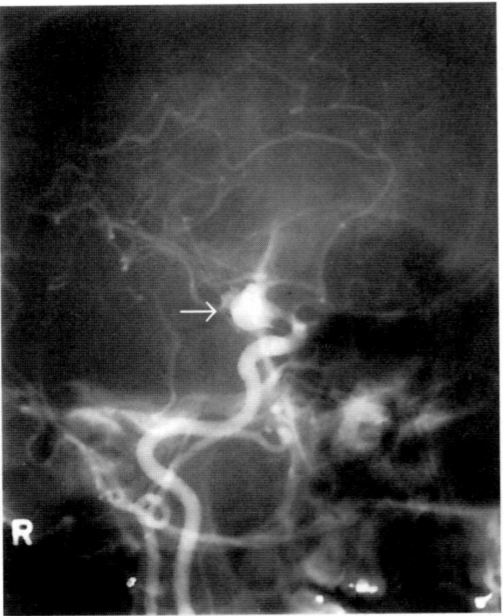

Fig. 24-73. Transorbital oblique position (aneurysm demonstrated).

PHOTOGRAPHIC SUBTRACTION

Control and Injection Radiographs

Photographic subtraction is a technique that subtracts or cancels all structures common to both a scout radiograph and an injected radiograph. In theory, this technique will produce a radiograph that shows only the opacified vessels without interference from bony structures. Both the control radiograph and the injected radiograph, as shown in Figs. 24-74 and 24-75, are obtained during the exposure series. The control radiograph is exposed immediately prior to the injection and is the first radiograph of the series. There must be no motion and no contrast medium on the control radiograph.

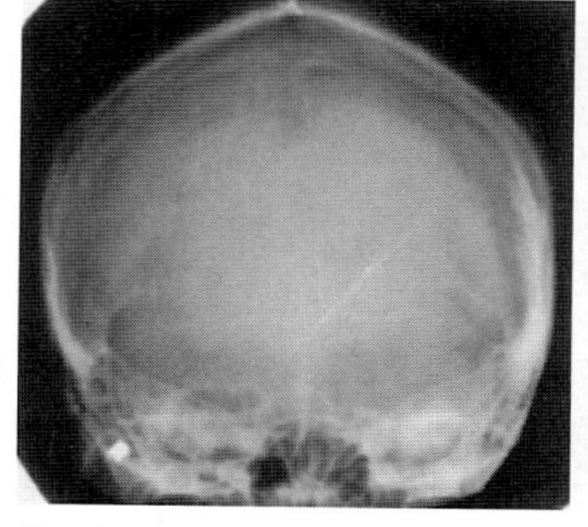
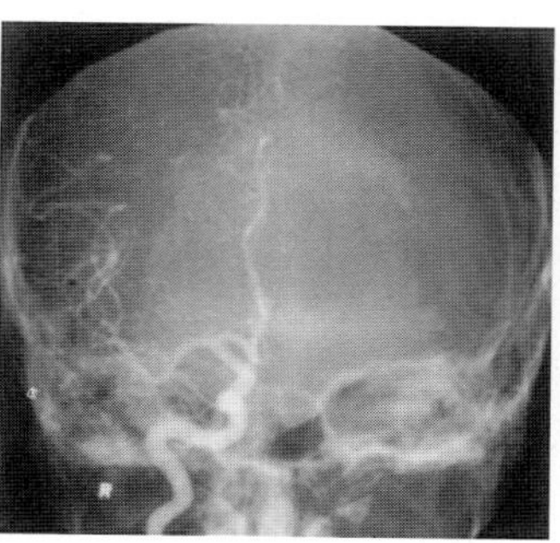

Fig. 24-74. Control and injection radiographs. Fig. 24-75.

Positive Mask and Subtraction Radiographs

A standard radiograph, one in which bone and opacified vessels appear white, is termed a negative image. The simplest method of subtraction involves first producing an exact reversal of the control radiograph. This step is accomplished in the processing room by exposing a single-emulsion film through the control radiograph. The result is a positive image, termed a positive mask or diapositive (Fig. 24-77).

A composite is then made by registration. For registration a positive mask and any radiograph in the series containing contrast medium are precisely superimposed. All bony landmarks are placed in exact register and the two radiographs are taped together. A print is made of this composite (Fig. 24-77). The positive and negative radiographs tend to cancel each other, leaving a radiograph showing only the opacified blood vessels.

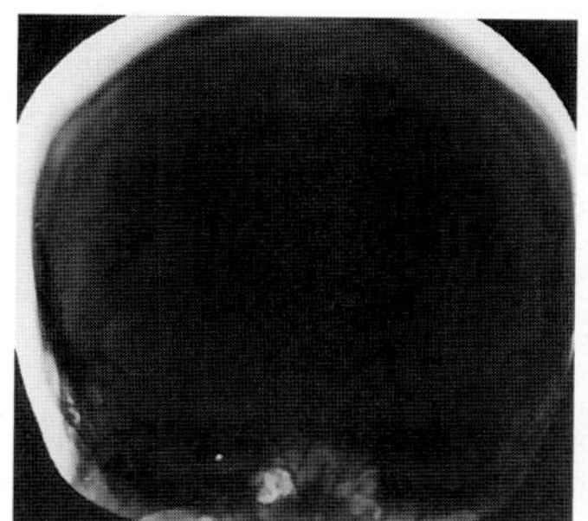
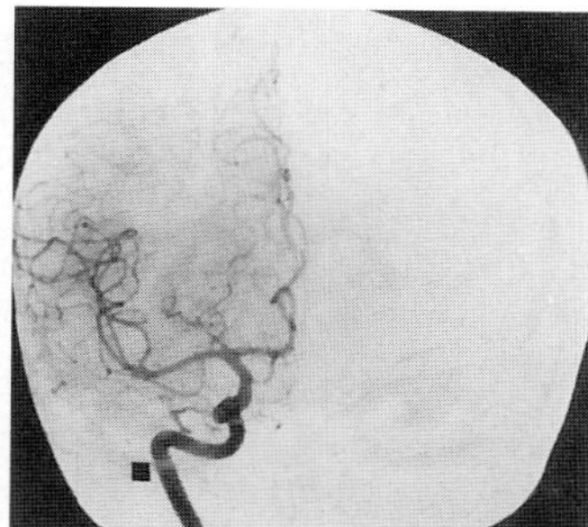

Fig. 24-76. Fig. 24-77.
Positive mask and subtraction radiographs.

Subtraction Venogram

A magnified carotid venogram and a subtraction study of the same radiograph are shown in Figs. 24-78 and 24-79. It is apparent that more diagnostic information is made available to the radiologist on the subtraction study. The two techniques of (1) direct roentgen enlargement or magnification and (2) composite mask subtraction greatly enhance the more routine methods of cerebral angiography. Techniques utilized in digital angiography allow electronic subtraction of the nonessential portion of the television image.

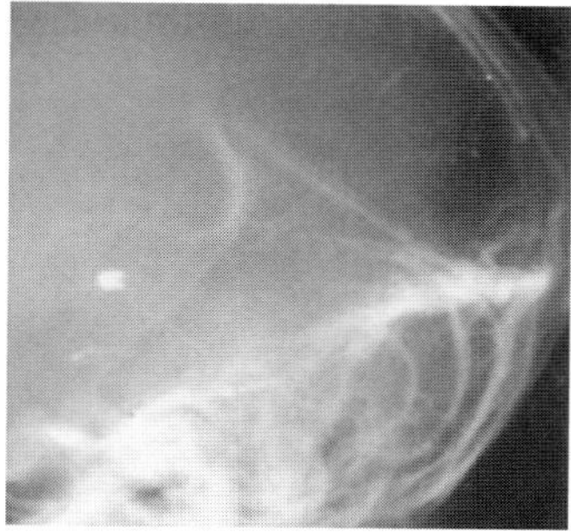
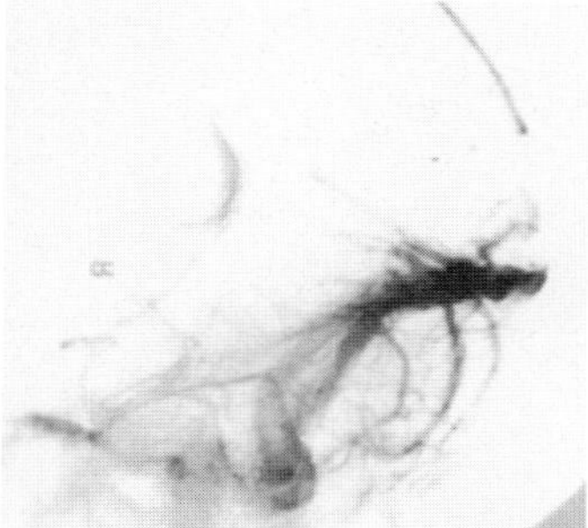

Fig. 24-78. Regular venogram vs. subtraction. Fig. 24-79.

Newer Technology - Digital Subtraction Angiography

In most modern radiology departments, the above described photographic subtraction method has been replaced (or is being replaced) with digital subtraction angiography as described on the following page.

DIGITAL SUBTRACTION ANGIOGRAPHY (DSA)

Common use of computer technology evolved during the 1970s However, it wasn't until the 1980s that this technology was applied to angiographic procedures. The most common application of computers in angiography is that of **digital subtraction angiography (DSA)**. This technology is designed to improve upon conventional photographic subtraction through use of a computer.

The type of equipment needed for DSA is very similar to conventional angiographic equipment. The basic apparatus for DSA includes, but is not limited to, image processor, generator, image intensifier, x-ray tube, television and camera, and analog to digital converter.

The image processor is equivalent to the central processing unit (CPU) of a personal computer. It controls and integrates the various processes needed to produce a DSA image. The image processor sends signals to the generator, which activates and deactivates the x-ray tube on command. The process of DSA begins when the image processor signals the generator to initiate the exposure. The radiation passes through the patient and is detected by the image intensifier. The image intensifier converts the x-ray energy to light and transmits it to the television camera, which directs it through an analog to digital converter where it is digitized and returns to the DSA imager processor. The operator uses the image processor to display, manipulate or store the images.

The images are subtracted using one of several methods. The most basic method is similar to conventional photographic subtraction in which a frame without contrast medium is used with a frame with contrast medium to produce the subtracted print. Another, more complicated method has the ability to subtract images at different frame intervals, e.g., frame 1 with 3 (interval=2), frame 2 with 4 (interval=2), etc. Additionally, unlike conventional photographic subtraction, the pixels (picture elements that make up the television monitor image) can be manipulated to help compensate for patient movement, thus assisting in proper superimposition of the frames.

Examples of DSA Radiographs

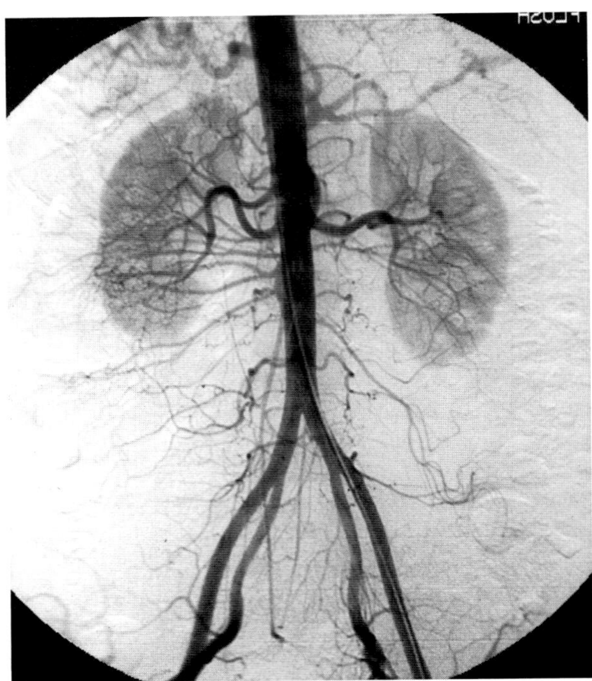

Fig. 24-80. AP spot of lower abdomen–Abdominal femoral runoff.
(Courtesy of General Electric Medical Systems, Milwaukee, WI.)

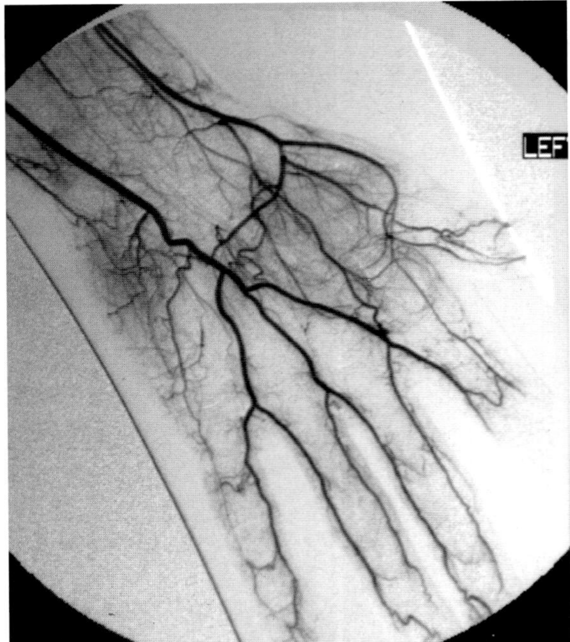

Fig. 24-81. Left hand with edge enhancement filter.
(Courtesy of General Electric Medical Systems, Milwaukee, WI.)

Thoracic Aortography

RADIOGRAPHIC PROCEDURE

Purpose

Thoracic aortography *(a″ or-tog′ rah-fe)* is a **radiographic examination of the thoracic aorta following the injection of a radiopaque contrast medium**. The contrast medium outlines the contour of the aorta and its major branches. By observing the size, shape and possible displacement of the vessels, radiologists are able to identify abnormalities. Abnormalities are frequently located in the aortic arch or its branches.

Indications

Thoracic aortography is indicated when patient symptoms suggest possible pathology of the aorta or its branches. This is especially true for patients with inconclusive pre-examinations and persistent symptoms suggesting aortic pathology. Some specific pathologies that would indicate thoracic aortography are **patent ductus arteriosus**, **aortic aneurysm**, **coarctation**, **aortic arch anomalies** or **aortic stenosis**.

Contraindications

The primary contraindication to thoracic aortography is **adverse reaction to the contrast medium**. Most patients having thoracic aortography are severely ill or have inconclusive previous test results. Thoracic aortography may be the only remaining test available to obtain conclusive evidence for proper diagnosis. This may necessitate thoracic aortography being performed under less than ideal situations, i.e., poor patient condition or possible reaction to contrast medium.

Patient Preparation

Patients having thoracic aortography are generally anxious and apprehensive about the procedure, thus a mild sedative is recommended. The type and amount of medication given the patient is the decision of the attending physician. Atropine may be administered to lessen bradycardia.

Prior to the examination the radiologist should visit the patient to explain the procedure and the risks involved. When the patient understands the procedure and potential complications, an informed consent form is signed by the patient, which outlines the procedure and explains the risks of the procedure.

To assist in the diagnosis, pre-examination tests should be performed. These would include an overpenetrated chest radiograph and the blood pressure differences between the right and left arms. The results of the tests are helpful in determining if there is any aortic pathology. If the patient has previous chest radiographs, the former radiographic diagnosis should be compared with the current diagnosis in order to determine possible changes.

Major Equipment

The major equipment needed for thoracic aortography includes:

1. Electromechanical injector.
2. Single rapid serial film changer.
3. Image intensifier with television monitor.
4. Floating table top.
5. Cineradiographic camera.

The electromechanical injector is used to deliver the contrast medium to the area of interest. Placement of the catheter in the involved area is performed under fluoroscopy. The area of interest indicates the type of recording device to be used, i.e., a rapid serial film changer or cine camera. Cineradiography is utilized if the pathology is located in the aortic valve or left ventricle. To record the aortic arch and its branches, a rapid serial film changer is used. This type of filming is achieved by moving the floating table top over the serial film changer.

Accessory Equipment

Additional equipment for thoracic aortography includes:

1. Sterile angiographic tray.
2. Vascular catheters.
3. Electrocardiograph recorder.
4. Emergency cardiopulmonary equipment (crash cart).

The sterile tray is used during insertion of the catheter in the vessel. The heart is monitored by attaching electrocardiographic leads to the patient's body. It is advisable to have an emergency cardiac cart should cardiopulmonary resuscitation become necessary.

Catheterization Method

The safest and most common method of catheterization of the aorta is through a puncture of the femoral artery using the Seldinger technique. After successful puncture of the femoral artery, a pigtail catheter or a closed-end catheter is inserted into the artery and positioned at the desired aortic location for contrast medium injection.

Contrast Medium

The amount of high-concentration contrast medium used for thoracic aortography depends on the suggested pathology. Quantities ranging from 40 cc to 80 cc may be required. The larger dose would be injected when the aorta is dilated or when visibility of the entire arch is desirable. The smaller dose is advantageous in the case of a constricted aorta or when only a section of the aorta is to be visualized.

Reaction to the contrast medium or to the premedication is always a possibility, as with any procedure using contrast medium and should be planned for in case it does occur.

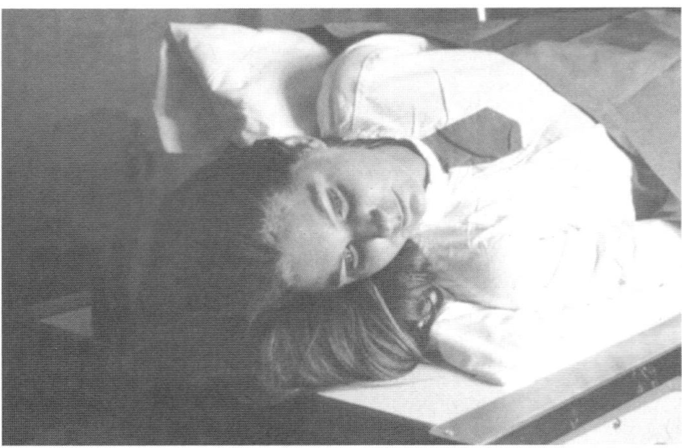

Fig. 24-82a. Position for arch aortography. (Patient obliqued over serial film changer.)

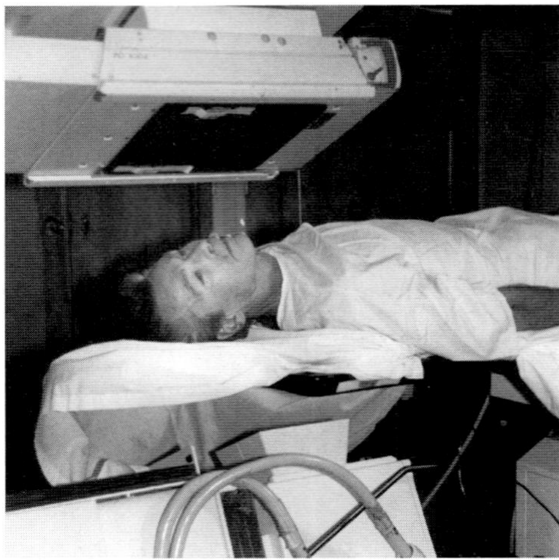

Fig. 24-82b. Position for arch aortography. (X-ray tube and image receptor angled.)

POSITIONING ROUTINE

The patient position for thoracic aortography depends on the pathology in question. Since the aorta courses posteriorly and to the left as it leaves the left ventricle of the heart, it is necessary to oblique, or angle, the imaging system or the patient to demonstrate all parts of the arch. The most commonly used patient positions are a 30-45° right or left posterior oblique (RPO or LPO). An RPO position is shown in Fig. 24-82a. With newer systems and with cineradiography or digital imaging, the entire imaging system can be angled with the patient remaining in a supine position as shown in Fig. 24-82b.

Positioning and centering for both of these imaging methods should ensure that the heart, arch and great vessels are included.

Right Posterior Oblique

The **RPO position** is most useful in visualizing **the arch** or **great vessel branch deformities,** as demontrated in Fig. 24-83.

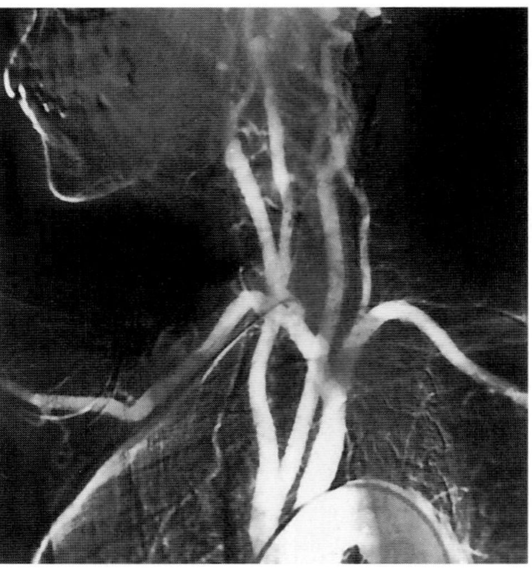

Fig. 24-83. RPO, arch aortogram.

Left Posterior Oblique

Angulation of equipment or positioning of the patient is similar to, but opposite of, the RPO position. For imaging system angulation, the angulation is to the left, with the patient's head rotated to the left. If the patient rather that the imaging system is angled, the patient is rotated into an **LPO position** with the head rotated into a left lateral position. This oblique position is used to demonstrate **ductus arteriosus** (a condition in which a vessel connects the pulmonary artery directly to the descending aorta) or **coarctation** (compressed or constricted vessels).

Filming Rate: The filming rate for the rapid film changer should be 4 films/second for the first 2 seconds, followed by 2 films/second for 3 to 5 seconds. If cineradiography is employed, the rate of filming is 30 to 60 frames/second.

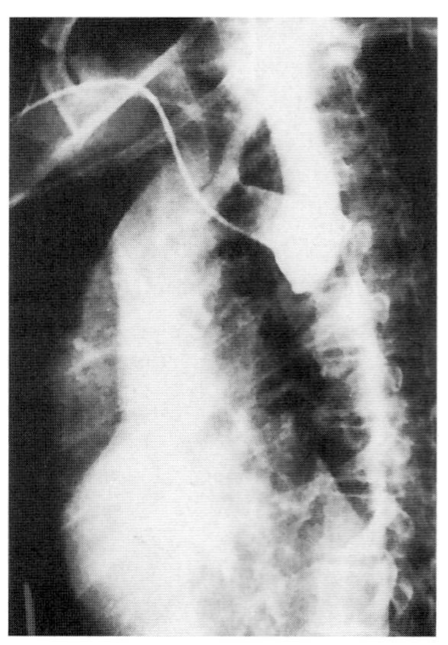

Fig. 24-84. LPO, coarctation of thoracic aorta.

Abdominal Angiography

RADIOGRAPHIC PROCEDURES

Purpose

Diagnostic abdominal angiography involves the **injection of contrast medium to demonstrate the contour, size and possible displacement of the abdominal aorta and its branches**. The shape, size and displacement of the vessels recorded on the radiographs are used by the radiologist to diagnose vascular disease.

Indications

Abdominal angiography is employed to detect **aneurysms**, **congenital anomalies**, **stenosis**, or **occlusions of the abdominal aorta**. Organs that receive blood directly from the abdominal aorta, i.e. kidneys, may be selectively catheterized to rule out any existing pathologies.

Contraindications

Abdominal angiography utilizing contrast medium should not be performed on patients having **known adverse reaction to contrast media** or allergic reactions to **iodine**. If there is an absence of a pulse in the vessel to be catheterized, a different vessel should be selected.

Patient Preparation

Patients should be premedicated prior to abdominal angiography. The type and amount of medication given the patient depends on the patient's condition. Most common prescriptions include drugs to protect against vasovagal reaction, and a mild sedative to relieve patient anxiety or stress. Anticoagulants should be withheld at least 4 hours before the procedure.

Prior to the examination, a radiologist should visit the patient to verbally explain the procedure and risks involved. When the patient understands the procedure and potential complications, an informed consent form which outlines the procedure and possible risks, is signed by the patient.

Major Equipment

The major equipment required for abdominal angiography includes:

1. Electromechanical injector.
2. Single rapid serial film changer.
3. Image intensifier with television monitor.
4. Floating table-top.

The electromechanical injector is used to deliver the contrast medium to the area of interest. Image intensification is employed during catheter positioning. Images are recorded on the single plane rapid serial film changer. The floating table-top serves to move the patient over the film for imaging.

Accessory Equipment

The accessory equipment for abdominal angiography includes:

1. Sterile angiographic tray.
2. Vascular catheters.
3. Electrocardiograph recorder.
4. Emergency cardiopulmonary equipment.

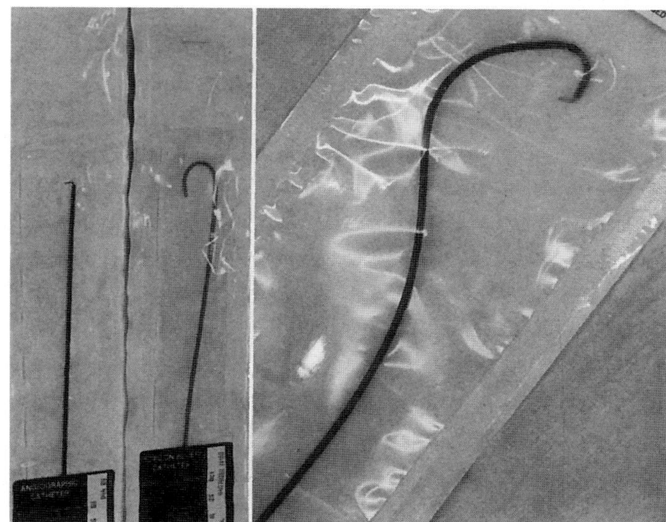

Fig. 24-85. Abdominal angiography catheters.

Catheterization of the vessel is performed using the sterile tray. The type of catheter employed for abdominal angiography depends on the area of interest. Figure 24-85 represents a variety of catheters that may be used for abdominal angiography.

The electrocardiograph recorder is used to monitor the patient's heart. Cardiopulmonary equipment should be in the room or immediately available if needed.

Catheterization Method

The most common approach to abdominal angiography is via puncture of the femoral artery using the Seldinger technique. The type and position of the catheter within the vessel depends on the area of interest.

For nonselective abdominal angiography, radiographs are taken of the abdomen. This requires the injection of a large bolus of contrast medium in a short period of time. A **straight end catheter** with side holes or a pigtail is most advantageous for delivering large quantities of contrast medium and should be used for demonstration of the abdominal aorta and its branches.

Selective abdominal angiography refers to the catheterization of one of the abdominal aortic branches. The most common branches catheterized are the renal arteries and the celiac axis. Since these vessels are small, as compared with the abdominal aorta, an end-hole-only catheter is used for injection of contrast medium.

Contrast Medium

The amount of contrast medium injected is relative to the size of the organ to be examined. For demonstration of the entire abdomen, 40 to 50 cc of a high-concentration contrast medium is delivered at a rate of 25 cc/second. Selective abdominal angiography of the celiac axis requires 35 to 45 cc of a high-concentration contrast medium injected at 8 to 12 cc/second, while selective renal angiography contrast volume range is 6 to 10 cc at a rate of 5 to 6 cc/second.

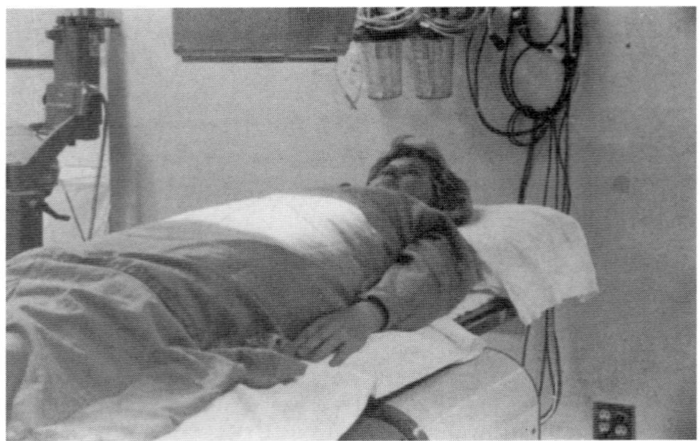

Fig. 24-86a. Position for abdominal angiogram with serial film changer, **AP projection**.

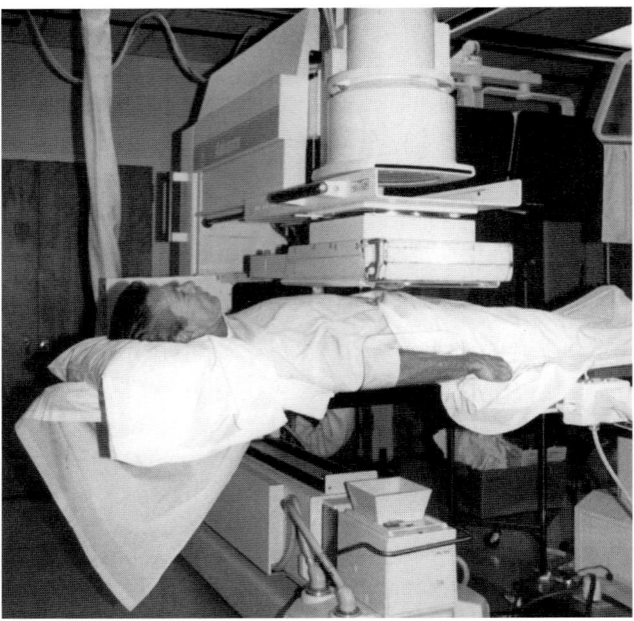

Fig. 24-86b. Position for abdominal angiogram, **PA projection**.

POSITIONING ROUTINE AND FILMING PROCEDURE

Abdominal Angiography

Filming for abdominal angiography is performed with the patient supine. The area of interest governs the size of the field to be irradiated.

To demonstrate the abdominal aorta, the patient is positioned supine for an AP projection over the serial film changer (Fig. 24-86a). Newer equipment which can also utilize digital imaging is shown in Fig. 24-86b with the patient supine but with a **PA projection** since the x-ray tube is below the patient.

The midsagittal plane is perpendicular to the film. Care should be taken with centering to ensure that both the proximal and distal ends of the pathology are recorded on the radiographs (Fig. 24-87).

Film Rate and Sequence with Serial Film Changer: A common filming sequence involves 14 radiographs. The rate used is 2 films/second for 4 seconds, followed by 1 film/second for 2 seconds; and finally 1 film every other second for 8 seconds.

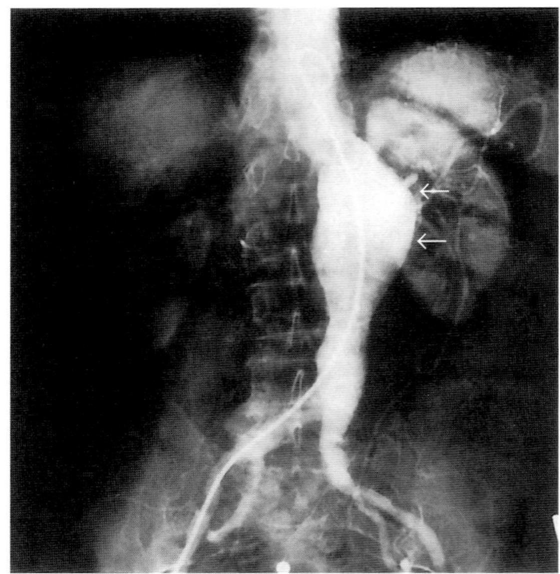

Fig. 24-87. Abdominal angiogram demonstrates an abdominal aneurysm (arrows).

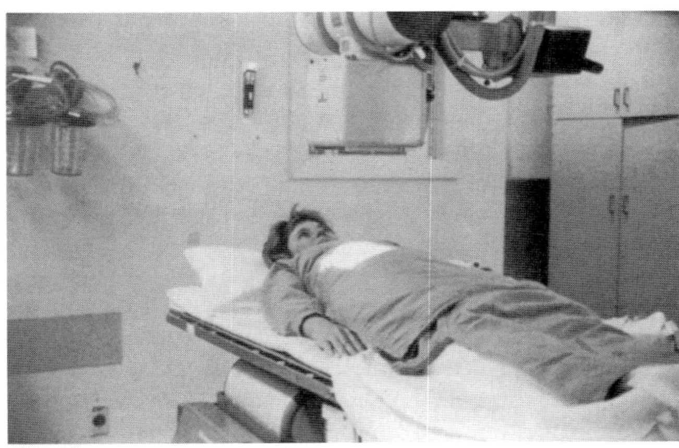

Fig. 24-88a. AP projection for renal angiogram with serial film changer.

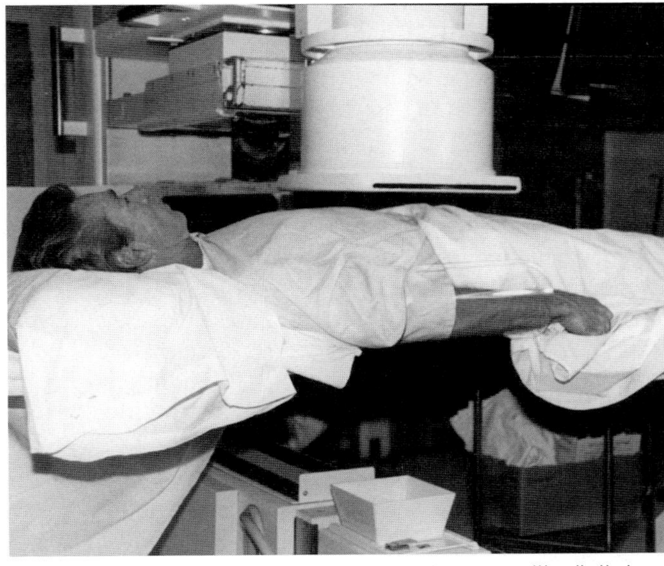

Fig. 24-88b. PA projection for renal angiogram with digital imaging.

Renal Angiography

Renal angiography uses the supine position (AP or PA projection), which demonstrates the kidney in an oblique position (Fig. 24-88a and 24-88b). Fig. 24-88b demonstrates a PA projection with positioning for digital imaging, which eliminates the need for a film changer.

In this supine position the kidneys are rotated about 30° posteriorly to the midcoronal plane. The irradiated field in renal angiography differs from abdominal angiography in that the field is limited to the upper right or left quadrant of the abdomen containing the kidney of interest (Fig. 24-89).

Filming Rate: The filming rate is 2 to 3 films/second during injection, followed by 1 film/second for 2 seconds, and 1 film every other second for 6 seconds.

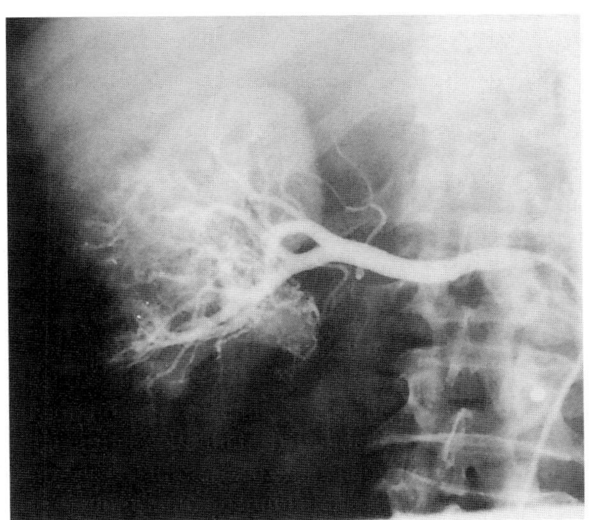

Fig. 24-89. Renal arteriogram.

Splenaportography

The AP or PA projection also best demonstrates the liver and spleen. This projection should include the lower thoracic and upper abdominal regions during mid-inspiration. (Fig. 24-90).

Filming Rate: The filming rate is 2 films/second for 4 seconds and 1 film/second for 16 to 20 seconds.

A post-injection radiograph is taken to determine if there are any extrasplenic contrast medium deposits.

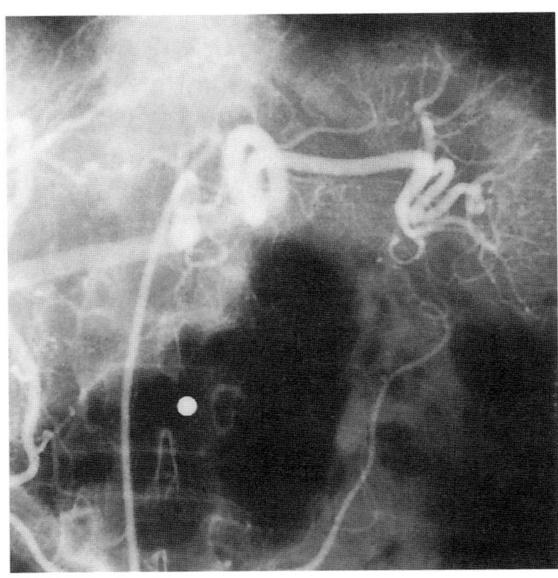

Fig. 24-90. Splenaportogram.

Peripheral Angiography

RADIOGRAPHIC PROCEDURE

Purpose

Peripheral **angiography** is a radiographic examination of the vessels of the **upper or lower limbs following the injection of contrast medium**. Upper limb angiography includes arterial examination of the shoulder, upper arm, elbow, forearm, wrist, and hand areas. Lower limb angiography includes procedures to examine the arteries called **arteriography**. *(ar″ te-re-og′ rah-fe)*; or procedures for the **veins** of the lower limb, called **venography** *(ve-nog′ rah-fe)*. Lower limb procedures involve x-rays of the abdomen, thigh, knee and leg areas.

During peripheral angiography, contrast medium flows through the vessels of interest outlining their shape and location. By observing the degree of vessel opacity and flow of the contrast medium within the system, physicians are able to identify abnormalities.

Indications

Peripheral angiography is indicated in cases of **tumors**, **emboli**, **thrombus**, **arteriovenous malformations** and **occlusions**. The majority of peripheral angiograms are performed to investigate diseases having pathological origin. However, a large percent of arteriovenous malformations result from trauma.

Contraindications

The most common contraindication to peripheral angiography is **adverse reaction to contrast medium**. For lower limb arteriography, an examination should be done to assess the presence of bruits (abnormal pulsation), scar tissue, or the absence of a femoral or iliac pulse at the puncture site. If any of these symptoms are present, then a puncture in that area should be avoided.

Caution is advised when performing lower limb venography on patients suspected of thrombosis, phlebitis, severe ischemic disease, local infection or a totally obstructed venous system as contrast medium extravasation can create complications.

Patient Preparation

Patients having peripheral angiography should be premedicated to reduce anxiety and stress. Anxiety can be alleviated by having a radiologist explain the procedure and risks involved to the patient. When the patient understands the procedure and potential risks, an informed consent form is signed by the patient.

Prior to the examination, the pulses should be assessed to determine their strength and if bruits are present. Weak pulses or the presence of bruits require that an alternate vessel be catheterized. A mixture of 2% lidocaine with the contrast medium may be given to alleviate pain during the injection.

Major Equipment

The major equipment used for arteriography includes:

1. Rapid serial film changer
2. Image intensifier with television monitor device
3. Electromechanical injector

Placement of the catheter is accomplished by viewing the catheter with the image intensifier. The rapid film changer is used to record the image. Injection of the contrast medium is the function of the electromechanical injector.

Lower extremity arteriography also requires a stepping table. This table automatically moves a predetermined distance at varying intervals so that a different part of the patient is over the film changer for each table movement (Fig. 24-91).

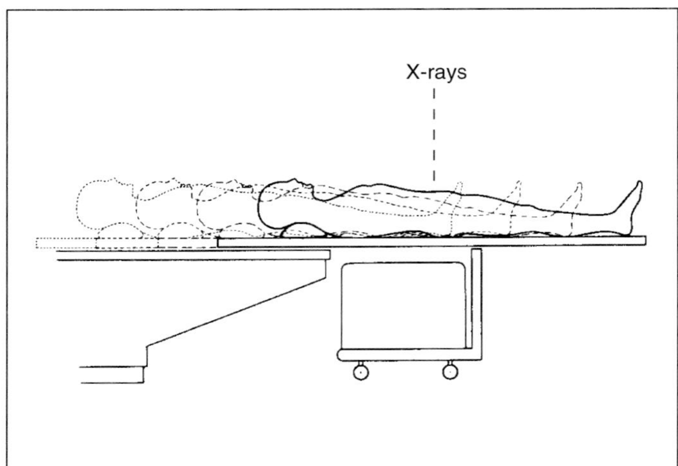

Fig. 24-91. Stepping table.

Accessory Equipment

Additional equipment needed for peripheral (upper and lower limb) angiography includes:

1. Sterile angiographic tray
2. Vascular catheters
3. Emergency cardiopulmonary equipment

The sterile tray is used during insertion of the catheter. It is recommended that an emergency cardiac cart be immediately available should cardiopulmonary resuscitation be required.

When performing lower limb arteriography both lower extremities may be examined simultaneously. Concurrent injection of the iliacs requires the use of a Y Luer Lok.

Catheterization Method

Lower limb arteriography may include the abdomen and lower limbs or involve selective catheterization of the lower limbs. If abdominal angiography is to be performed, the catheter is placed at the level of the twelfth thoracic vertebra via a femoral artery. The type of catheter employed is a pigtail, ring or straight tip catheter having multiple side holes with the end hole occluded. These catheters allow for the delivery of a large bolus of contrast medium over a short period of time.

When visualization of the iliac and lower limbs arteries is performed, an end-hold, multiple side-hole catheter is placed at the level of the fourth lumbar vertebra following femoral artery puncture. Sometimes pathology is such that the contralateral side is catheterized in place of the involved side. In these cases a selective sharp, curved catheter is used to catheterize the vessel of interest (Fig. 24-92).

Catheterization of the upper limb may be performed via the axillary, brachial or femoral arteries. The femoral approach is the safest and most common. The most common catheter used for upper limb angiography is a brachiocephalic end hole type.

Contrast Medium

The amount of contrast medium for lower limb arteriography varies with the type of filming required. When abdominal radiographs are required, 40 to 60 cc of high-concentration contrast medium is used at a rate of 10 to 15 cc/second. Selective lower limb arteriography employs a dose of 20 to 30 cc injected at a rate of 8 to 10 cc/second.

Often, patients having lower limb arteriography have poor circulation. To increase the rate of blood flow, certain drugs, i.e., tolazoline, may be administered prior to the injection of the contrast medium to dilate the vessels thereby increasing the blood flow rate. Other methods used to increase blood flow are blood pressure cuffs and exercise. Exercise decreases aortic pressure and facilitates the flow of blood to the distal parts of the body. A blood pressure cuff is used to increase blood flow by inflating it at a level above the knee for 3 minutes then deflating it, which creates a rapid flow of blood toward the feet.

Upper limb arteriography requires 15 cc of a 45 to 60 % concentration of contrast medium. The contrast medium is injected at a rate of 7 to 8 cc/second.

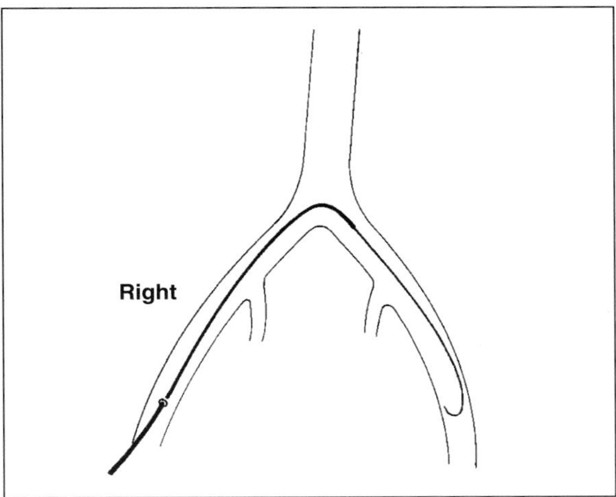

Fig. 24-92. Selective contralateral catheterization of common iliac artery.

LOWER LIMB ARTERIOGRAPHY

After catheterization and placement of the catheter in the appropriate vessel for arteriography, anterior-posterior projection radiographs are taken. The filming rate and centering for lower limb arteriography involving the abdominal aorta are the same as abdominal angiography. When radiographing the lower limbs, to ensure a true anterior-posterior projection, the patient's feet are internally rotated 15-20 degrees. The feet may be taped together or otherwise supported to prevent movement during filming.

Filming Sequence

The actual filming of arteries of the lower limbs involves the sequencing of table top movement, radiographic technique changes, and proper exposure synchronization. The great variance in the thickness of the leg requires the correct use of the anode heel effect. Thus, the cathode end of the x-ray tube should be placed toward the thickest part, the thigh.

Stepping Table

Exposures are made of the thighs, knees and lower legs (Fig. 24-93). This is achieved by activation of the stepping table top, which moves the individual parts of the patient over the rapid serial film changer automatically.

Other methods that may be used to maintain the same density through the lower limb are wedge filters, special cones, or special cassettes with varying speed intensifying screens.

UPPER LIMB ARTERIOGRAPHY

Upper limb arteriography is also performed with anteroposterior projections. The patient's arm is placed diagonally on the rapid serial film changer (Fig. 24-94).

Filming Rate: Filming Rate depends upon the area of interest. The rate for the proximal portion is 1 film/second for 20 seconds.

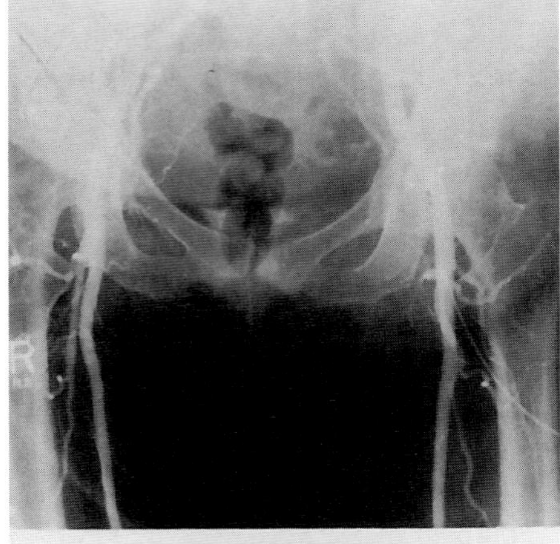

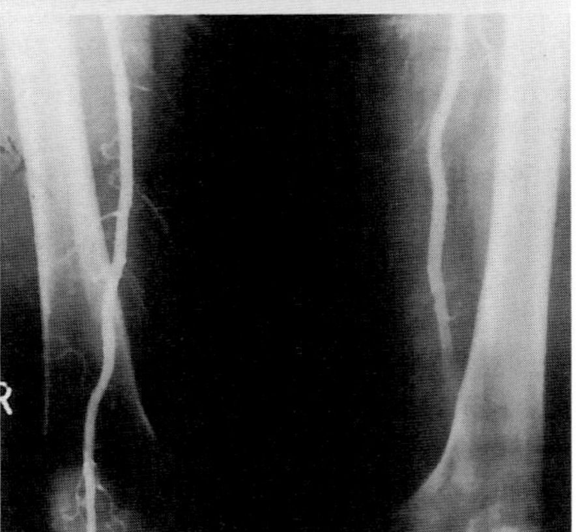

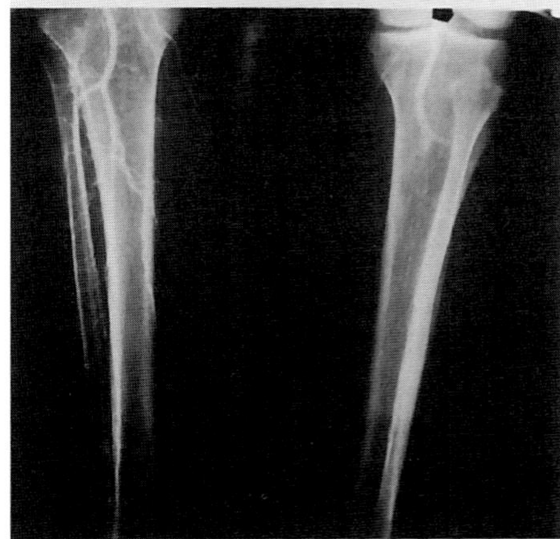

Fig. 24-93. Lower limb arteriogram.

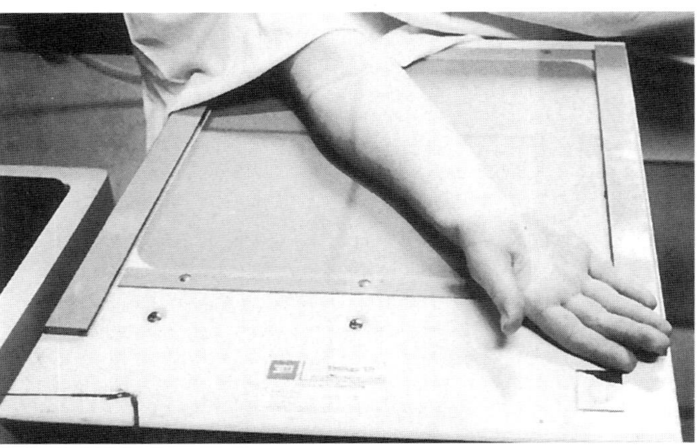

Fig. 24-94. AP projection for upper limb arteriogram.

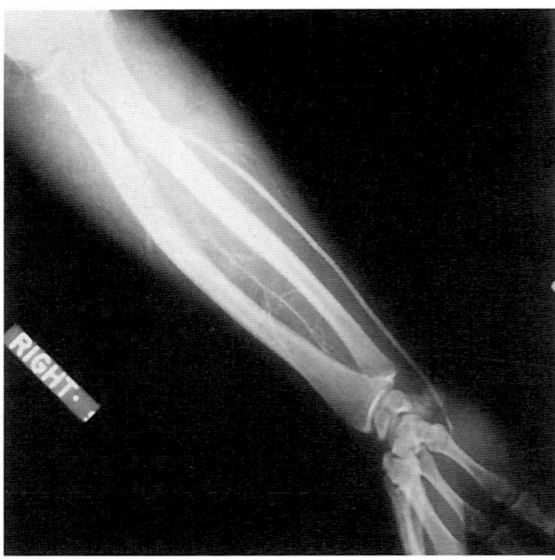

Fig. 24-95. Upper limb arteriogram.

LOWER LIMB VENOGRAPHY

Lower limb venography is a contrast medium study of the deep veins from the ankle to pelvic area. As contrast media is injected, AP and lateral radiographs of the limb are taken. Filming is accomplished by utilizing fluoroscopic spot filming on 14 in. x 14 in. (35 x 35 cm) cassette or by high speed cameras employing a 105 mm roll or 100 mm precut film.

Filming Sequence: A typical filming procedure would include:

- –AP and lateral of calf to include knee
- –AP and lateral centered at knee
- –AP and lateral of thigh
- –AP of hip to include iliac crest

Fluoroscopic control ensures that all levels of the venous circulation are visualized with contrast present.

Equipment and Procedure

In addition to a fluoroscopic unit with filming capabilities, a 90° tilting table with a foot board and a small block is needed. The contrast medium is introduced through a superficial vein on the dorsum or anterior surface of the foot. The injection begins with the table and patient semi-erect (approximately 60°). The patient stands on the block (resting on the footboard) with the unaffected leg. (See arrows, Fig. 24-96.) The affected leg is allowed to dangle (away from the block) so that it bears no weight.

As the contrast is injected, the distal aspect of the extremity is filmed. The table is slowly lowered in stages (to decrease the effect of gravity and allow flow of the contrast upward) and the mid and proximal portions of the extremity are filmed.

Filming of the hip area is performed with the table horizontal (Fig. 24-97). When the exam is completed, a flushing solution (e.g., saline or 5% dextrose in water) is used to force contrast from the lower extremity. This aids in preventing a possible phlebitis, which may be caused by the irritating effect of the contrast on the lining of the veins.

Contrast Medium

Approximately 50 to 100 cc of a water-soluble, iodine-based contrast medium of relatively low density is used for venography. Since injection is into a distal superficial vein, one or two tourniquets are applied just above the ankle to compress the superficial system and direct the contrast medium into the deep system through interconnecting veins (Fig. 24-100).

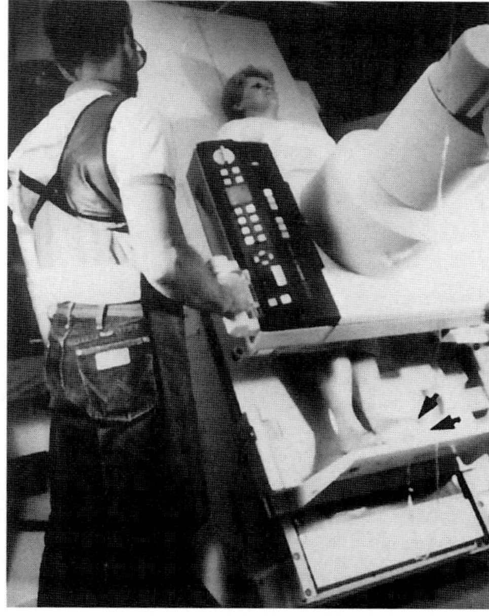

Fig. 24-96. AP knee and thigh area filming.

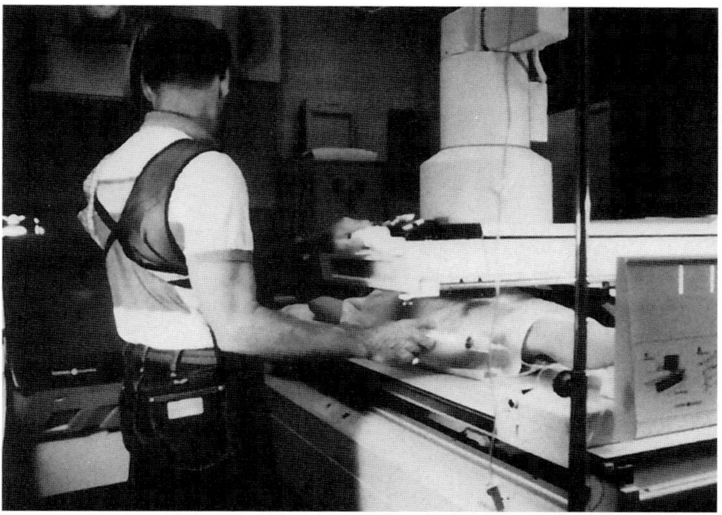

Fig. 24-97. AP hip area filming.

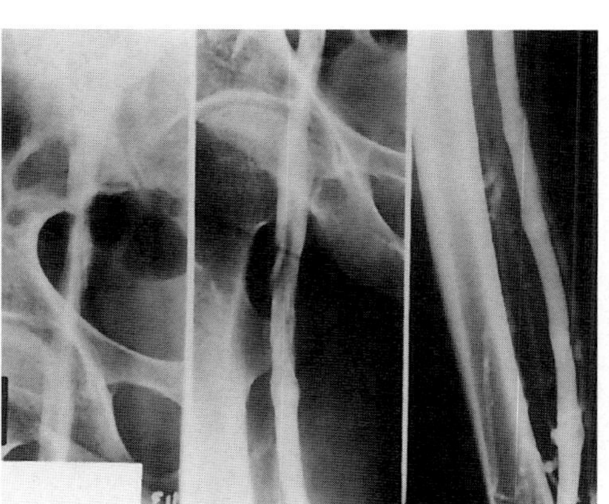

Fig. 24-98. AP lower limb venogram.

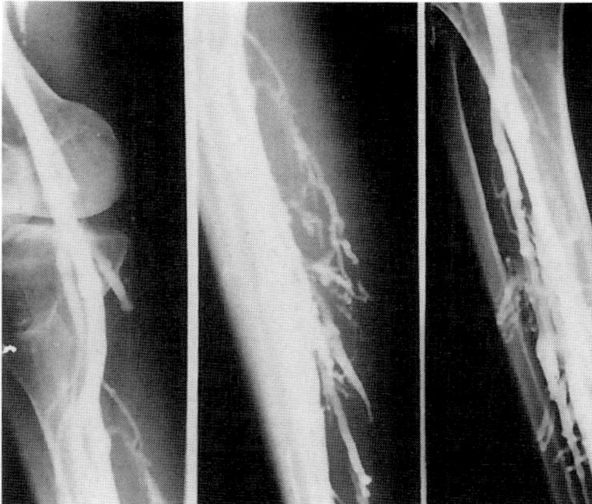

Fig. 24-99. Lateral lower limb venogram.

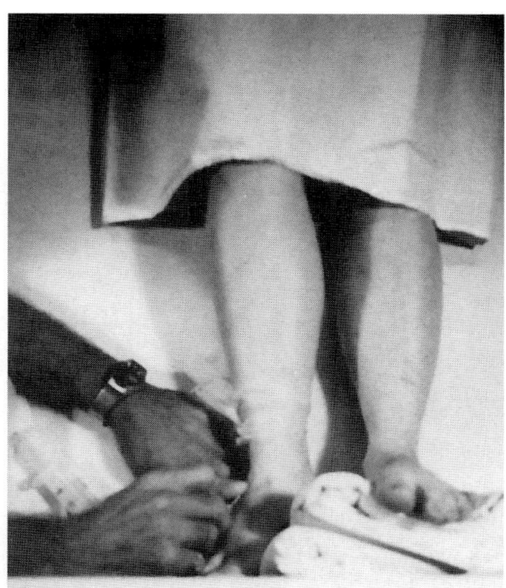

Fig. 24-100. Injection of contrast medium (2 tourniquets applied).

Interventional Angiography

Introduction

Interventional angiography employs angiographic methods primarily for the **treatment of disease** and sometimes for **diagnosis.** These procedures may use a vascular or nonvascular approach. Examples of common **vascular** procedures include infusion of chemotherapeutic agents or radioactive materials, extraction of vascular foreign bodies, transluminal angioplasty, stent, and temporary or permanent embolization of vessels.

Common **nonvascular** procedures include nephrostomy, percutaneous biliary drainage, abdominal percutaneous drainage, gastrostomy, and biopsy.

Most interventional procedures are indicated in cases for which surgery is contraindicated or hazardous, and as a preoperative tool, e.g. patients with vascular bleeding. The application of these techniques to various organs or disease processes is almost unlimited and it is nearly impossible to list all the areas in which interventional procedures can be employed. The more common vascular and nonvascular interventional procedures are described below.

VASCULAR INTERVENTIONAL ANGIOGRAPHY

Infusion Therapy

The infusion of therapeutic drugs may be via a systemic or a superselective approach. Treatment duration ranges from a few days to several weeks. The type of approach and the duration of infusion therapy is determined by the pathology present, the area to be treated, the patient's condition and the results of previous therapeutic methods. Vasoconstrictors, vasodilators, chemotherapeutic drugs and radioactive materials are employed for infusion therapy.

Vasoconstrictors are used to help control bleeding. A common vasoconstricting drug currently employed is vasopressin (Pitressin). It may be administered intravenously or intraarterially. Vasodilators are useful in the treatment of vascular spasms or constriction. Currently, sodium nitroprusside is employed for vascular spasms and papaverine relieves nonocclusive mesenteric vascular ischemia.

Infusion of drugs for chemotherapeutic reasons is employed in patients with advanced nonresectable malignancies. The percentage of patients responding to chemotherapy varies greatly.

Extraction of Vascular Foreign Bodies

Most foreign bodies found in the vascular system are limited to calculi, fragments of vascular catheters or guide wires, pacemaker electrodes and shunts. Some common instruments used to retrieve the foreign bodies include loop snares, ureteral stone basket catheters and endoscopic grasping forceps. To remove foreign bodies with a loop snare or a basket catheter, the catheter is inserted beyond the foreign body and then withdrawn to catch the foreign body. Care should be taken to avoid tearing the vascular intima lining when removing foreign bodies that are adhered to the vessel; these must be removed surgically.

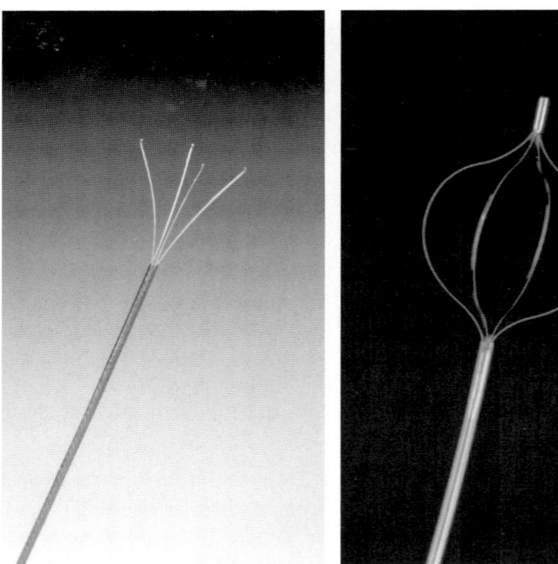

Fig. 24-101. Retrieval instruments.
-Grasping forceps. -Retrieval basket.
(Courtesy of Medi-tech/Boston Scientific Corporation)

Transluminal Angioplasty

Transluminal angioplasty is a method of vascular catheterization designed for the purpose of **dilating a stenosed vessel**, or to **cannulize (create an opening) short arterial occlusions**. This is accomplished by compressing the atheromatous material against the vessel wall.

The balloon catheter is used in conjunction with a pressure gauge. The deflated balloon is inserted into the involved vessel and positioned at the vessel stenosis or occlusion. Arterial pressures are recorded. The balloon is then filled (inflated) with contrast medium which compresses the plaque into the vessel wall dilating the lumen. After vessel dilation and withdrawal of balloon, arterial pressures are again recorded. A comparison of the pre-therapeutic and post-therapeutic pressures indicate whether the procedure was successful. Another method of verifying success is to compare the pre-dilation and post-dilation vessel angiograms.

Balloon catheter vessel dilation has been reported to be effective in maintaining vessel patency for as long as 3 to 5 years, after which another balloon dilation may be required.

Stent

A stent is **a cage-like metal device placed in a vessel to enlarge the lumen**. The stent remains in the vessel and acts as a support for the vessel wall. Stents are indicated when balloon angioplasty is unsuccessful.

Stents are constructed in one of two ways; self-expanding or balloon expandable. The type of design indicates the method used to position the stent in the vessel. As the name indicates, self expanding stents automatically expand when the cover used to compress the stent is removed. The balloon expandable stent (Fig. 24-103) requires an angioplasty type balloon to implant the stent in the vessel. To implant the stent, the compressed stent is located over the balloon and both are positioned in the area of interest. Once positioned, the balloon is inflated, expanding and implanting the stent in the vessel wall. After the stent is positioned correctly, the balloon is deflated and removed.

Thrombolysis*

If diagnostic angiographic studies demonstrate that a vessel is blocked by a thrombus (clot), a **thrombolysis procedure** may be indicated. If blood-clotting coagulation laboratory studies support this procedure, a thrombolysis may be performed wherein the clot or thrombus is lysed (disintegrated) by passing a guide wire and catheter through the clot, or as far into the clot as possible.

A **dissolving agent is then injected through the catheter** into the region of the thrombus. Various types of catheters may be used for this such as a pulse spray type (Fig. 24-104), or an infusion type (Fig 24-105). The pulse spray method involves hand injection with a syringe, whereas the infusion method generally involves a slow injection process using a pump to slowly infuse the dissolving agent over a period of hours or even several days. The catheter may be advanced during this time as the thrombus is being dissolved.

Possible complications with this procedure may be bleeding or the possibility of partially dissolved clots moving on to block other smaller vessels.

Embolization

Transcatheter embolization of vessels is employed to produce a restricted blood flow in patients with **uncontrolled hemorrhage** or highly vascular neoplasms. Special catheters are used through which embolic agents are injected into the hemorrhaging vessel. Because of the potential dangers associated with vessel occlusion, embolization should only be performed by experienced and skilled angiographers.

There are a variety of embolic agents that can be used. In general, embolic material may be classified as either temporary or permanent occlusive agents.

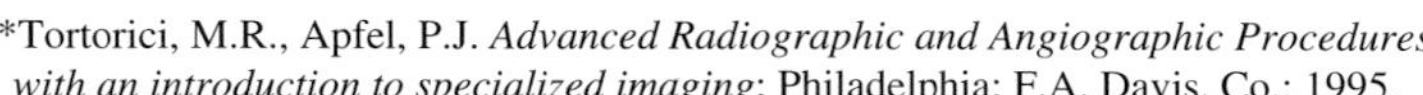

*Tortorici, M.R., Apfel, P.J. *Advanced Radiographic and Angiographic Procedures with an introduction to specialized imaging*; Philadelphia; F.A. Davis, Co.; 1995.

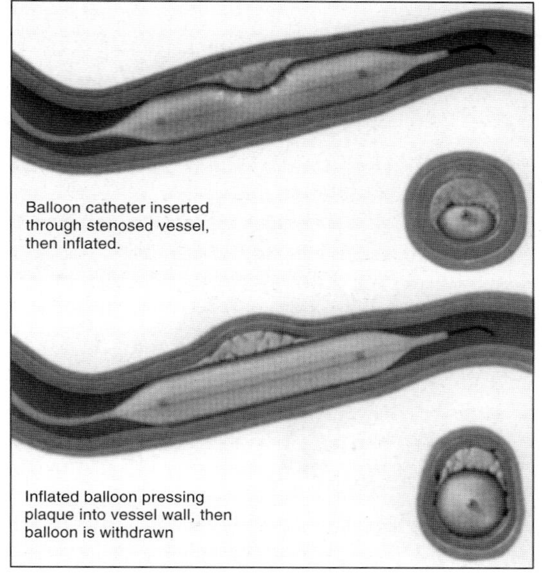

Fig. 24-102. Transluminal angioplasty–Balloon catheter.
(Courtesy of Medi-tech/Boston Scientific Corporation)

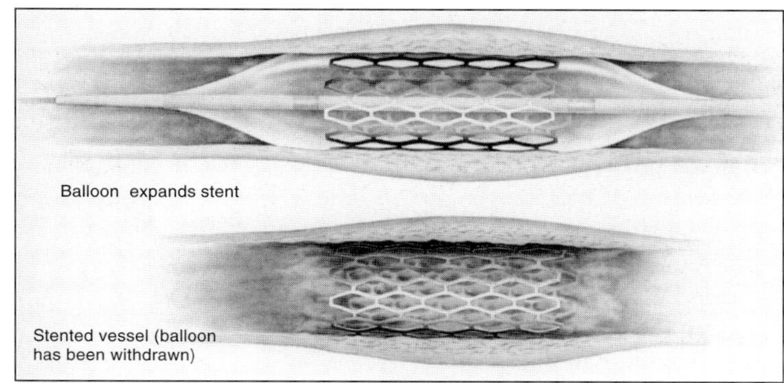

Fig. 24-103. Balloon expanding stent.
(Courtesy of Cordis Corporation, a Johnson & Johnson Company)

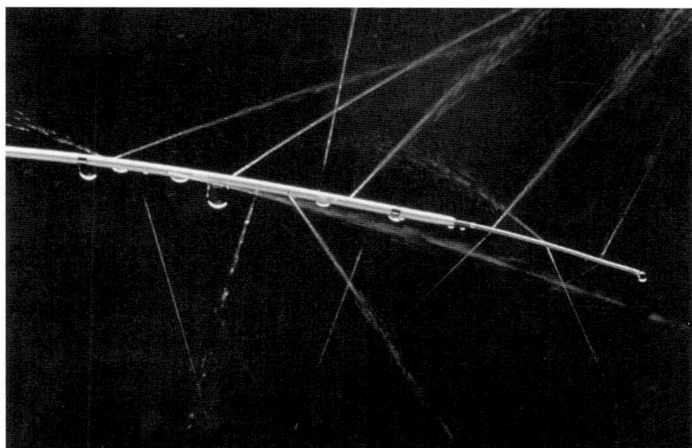

Fig. 24-104. Thrombolysis pulse spray catheter.
(Courtesy of Medi-tech/Boston Scientific Corporation)

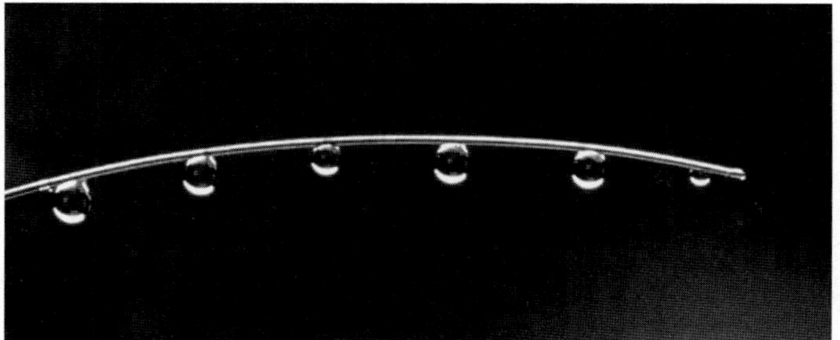

Fig. 24-105. Thrombolysis infusion catheter.
(Courtesy of Medi-tech/Boston Scientific Corporation)

NONVASCULAR INTERVENTIONAL PROCEDURES

Nephrostomy

Nephrostomy may be performed for diagnostic or therapeutic reasons. It is useful in treating several types of kidney pathologies or disorders. Nephrostomy is useful as a diagnostic procedure for renal function assessment; a urine culture; Brush biopsy; Whitaker test (determine cause of urinary tract dilation); nephroscopy; and failed retrograde pyelography. Therapeutic reasons for performing nephrostomy include stone diversion, chemolysis, and abscess drainage.

In this procedure, a catheter (Fig. 24-106) is introduced through the skin and kidney parenchyma to the renal pelvis or other target area. After proper catheter placement, the specific intervention (e.g. drainage, stone removal) occurs.

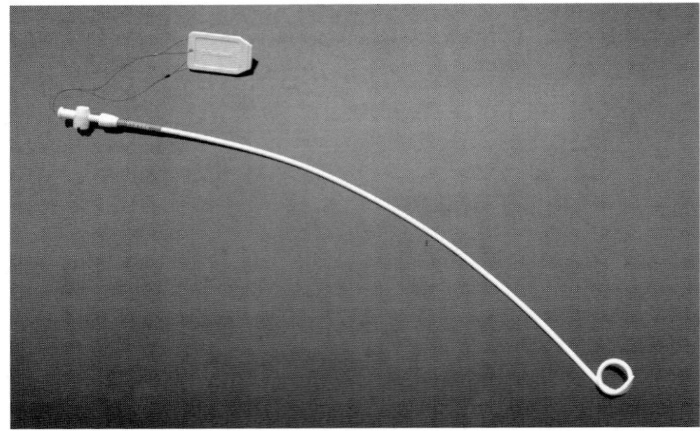

Fig. 24-106. Nephrostomy drainage catheter.
(Courtesy of Medi-tech/Boston Scientific Corporation)

Percutaneous Biliary Drainage (PBD)

Percutaneous biliary puncture (PBD) can be used for many reasons which include internal or external drainage, stone removal, dilation of obstructed bile duct, and biopsy. The most common use of PBD is as a palliative procedure for unresectable malignant disease. Less popular uses include the treatment of biliary obstruction, suppurative cholangitis, post-operative or post-traumatic biliary leakage and stone removal.

Patients undergoing PBD tend to have infected bile. To avoid the spread of infection, antibiotics should be administered at least 1 hour before the procedure.

A common treatment of PBD is internal or external drainage. External treatment usually involves placement of the catheter in the duodenum. Internal drainages use a stent or catheter. Often an external drain is in place for a couple of days and then the catheter is capped resulting in internal drainage.

Percutaneous Abdominal Abscess Drainage (PAD)

Percutaneous abdominal drainage has a 70 to 80% success rate. It is indicated when abdominal or pelvic abscess cannot be readily treated by simple incision, and if the location of the abscess is in a safe place for needle entry. If present, foreign bodies should be removed as they serve as foci of infection. If no improvement is seen in 24 to 48 hours another treatment method may be considered.

Needle Aspiration: Needle placement is performed under CT or sonography. Sonography is better for superficial abscess, abscess in solid material, and when the abscess is not surrounded by bowel. The advantage of sonography is that it allows for continuous monitoring. The procedure requires a 20 or 22g needle be positioned in the abscess and fluid withdrawn for immediate Gram's stain and other tests. If the fluid is purulent, the drainage procedure continues. If the material is sterile, the fluid is withdrawn and the needle is removed. The fluid is removed using gravity or a special suction pump. The gravity method is preferred as suction may erode the abscess wall or cause the wall to adhere to the catheter.

Catheter Drainage: Catheter drainage using the Seldinger over-the-wire technique may be used for inserting the catheter. An example of this is the Van Sonnenberg sump drain type catheter illustrated in Fig. 24-107. If a sump pump type arrangement is used, a double-lumen type catheter is required in which room air can flow into the abscess region while the suction is being applied. This simultaneous drainage and venting prevents suction, which will cause the abscess material to cling to the walls of the catheter blocking the drainage holes. The "pig tail" type design at the end of the catheter shown in Fig. 24-107 aids in retention or accidental withdrawal.

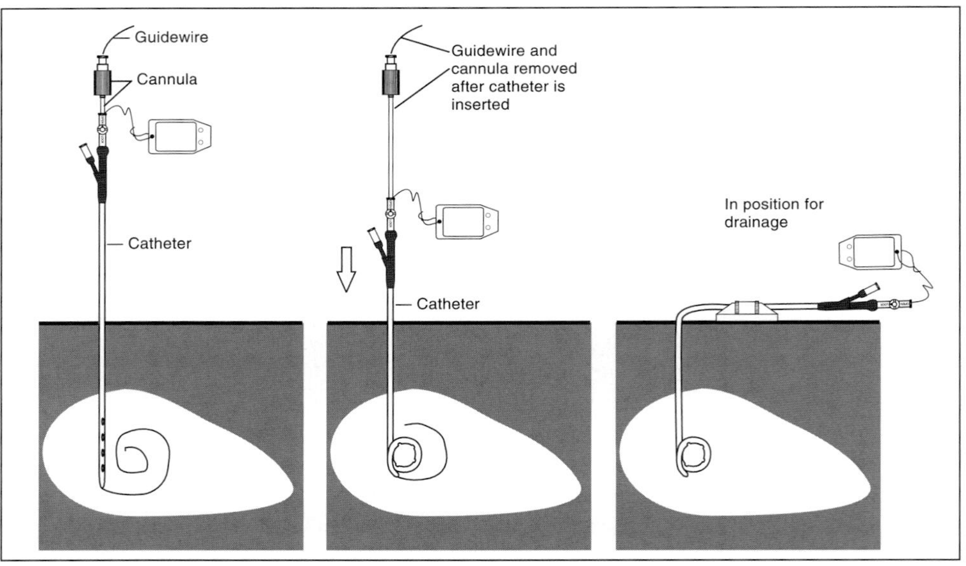

Fig. 24-107. Over-the-wire (Seldinger) technique with VanSonnenberg Sump™ drain catheter.
(Courtesy of Medi-tech/Boston Scientific Corporation)

The catheter is removed when there are no more symptoms or the signs of infection disappear (normal WBC); there is no more drainage; or a post procedural CT, or sonogram is normal.

Percutaneous Needle Biopsy

Percutaneous needle biopsy is performed when there is a suspicion of primary or metastatic malignancy. A biopsy is useful in providing information about the stage and extent of the disease, confirming if there is a tumor recurrence, and in the diagnosis of infection.

To perform a biopsy, a site and depth of the pathology is determined. Correct positioning of the needle may be achieved by monitoring needle introduction with sonography, computed tomography, or fluoroscopy. Sonography is the modality of choice for lesions in organs that differ significantly in echogenicity from adjacent structures as long as the lesion is not surrounded by gas, fat or calcified structures, e.g. liver, kidney and pelvic organs. CT is good for small, deep lesions, especially those surrounded by large vessels or bowel. The disadvantage of CT is the time needed for placement of the needle, scanning and repositioning. Fluoroscopy is best for lesions that differ significantly in radiopacity from surrounding tissue, e.g. pulmonary pleura, osseous lesions, and lymph nodes filled with contrast medium.

A tissue sample is obtained by advancing the needle to the target and alternately moving it vertically 1 to 2 cm and rotating it. The needle is then removed and the sample prepared for immediate examination. It is recommended that at least 4 samples be taken to include the center and peripheral areas.

Research indicates the following accuracy rates for biopsy–Lung: 85 to 90%; liver, kidney and pancreas: 70 to 90%; and lymph node: 50 to 75%.

Percutaneous Gastrostomy

Percutaneous gastrostomy is performed for extended feeding (greater than 4 weeks) of patients unable to eat, gastric decompression, or dilation of upper GI tract when the oral approach fails. Individuals who may be candidates for gastrostomy include those with impaired swallowing due to neurologic disease or obstructing oropharyngeal/ esophageal tumors; burn patients; trauma patients; cancer patients suffering from anorexia; or patients with pharyngeal or esophageal fistulae.

In this procedure, pre-examinations are performed to ensure no organ is located over the puncture site to avoid puncturing these organs. A nasogastric tube is placed in the stomach to inflate the stomach with 500 to 1,000 cc of air. The puncture site is at the upper or middle area of the stomach. A tube is placed and secured in the stomach. Once the tube is positioned, the patient is suctioned for 24 hours, after which feeding begins.

CHAPTER 25

Magnetic Resonance Imaging

CONTRIBUTIONS BY:
Joan Radke, BS, RT (R)
Russell Ritenour, Ph.D.

CONTENTS

Physical Principles

Definition and comparison with radiography **724**

Interaction of nuclei with magnetic fields **725**

Precession **725**

Sending radio signal to precessing nuclei **725**

Resonance **726**

Receiving signal from body tissues **726**

T1 and T2 relaxation **727**

Spin density **727**

Gradient magnetic fields **728**

Multislice imaging **728**

Pulse sequences:
- Spin-echo pulse sequence **729**
- Pulse sequence timing factors **730**

Equipment Components

Magnets:
- Resistive magnets **731**
- Permanent magnets **732**
- Superconducting magnets **732**

Gradient coils **732**

Radio frequency (RF) coils **733**

Electronic support system **733**

Computer and display **734**

Summary of MRI process and system components used **734**

Clinical Applications

Comparison with CT **735**

Basic safety considerations:
- Potential hazard of projectiles **736**
- Additional safety considerations **737**

Occupational hazards **738**

Patient history **738**

Patient preparation:
- Relieving patient anxiety **739**
- Patient monitoring **740**
- Contrast agents **740**

Positioning considerations and coil selection **741**

Imaging parameters:
- Subject contrast **742**
- Proton density image **742**
- T1-weighted images **742**
- T2-weighted images **742**
- Motion reduction techniques **743**
- Rapid imaging techniques **743**

MRI Examinations

Routine procedures **744**

Brain imaging **745**

Spine imaging **746**

Joint and limb imaging **747**

Cardiovascular system imaging **748**

Abdomen and pelvis imaging **749**

Angiography **750**

Definition of terms **751**

References **753**

Physical Principals

Definition

Magnetic resonance imaging (MRI) refers to **the use of magnetic fields and radio waves to obtain a mathematically reconstructed image.** This image represents differences among various tissues of the patient in the **number of nuclei,** and in the **rate at which these nuclei recover** from stimulation by radio waves in the presence of a magnetic field.

Comparison with Radiography

X-rays are electromagnetic waves and as such can be described in terms of their wavelength, frequency, and the amount of energy that each "wave packet" or photon carries. A typical x-ray photon used in medical imaging may have a wavelength of 10^{-9} centimeters, a frequency of 10^{19} hertz (cycles/sec) and an energy of 60,000 electron volts (Fig. 25-1).

Imaging with x-rays is possible because the photon has enough energy to ionize atoms. Thus, some photons are removed from the total number sent into the patient. The pattern of photons transmitted through the patient constitutes a radiographic image that may then be captured by an image receptor such as film. The fact that x-ray photons have enough energy to ionize atoms implies that some small biological hazard is associated with a radiographic examination.

It is possible to obtain an image of the body through the use of electromagnetic waves having energies far below that required to ionize atoms thereby reducing if not eliminating the threat of biological harm to the patient. The technique of magnetic resonance imaging (MRI) makes use of the **radio** portion of the electromagnetic spectrum in which photons have relatively long wavelengths of 10^3 to 10^{-2} meters with frequencies of only 10^5 to 10^{10} hertz. A typical photon used in MRI has an energy of only 10^{-7} electron volts (a tenth of a millionth of an electron volt). See Fig. 25-2.

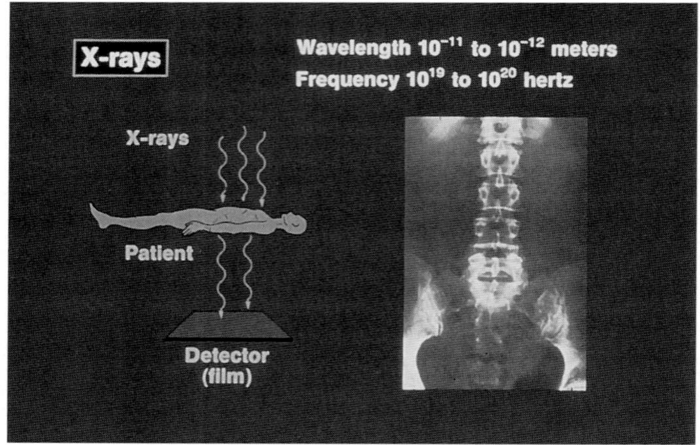

Fig. 25-1. Typical X-ray–60,000 eV energy (implies some biological hazard).

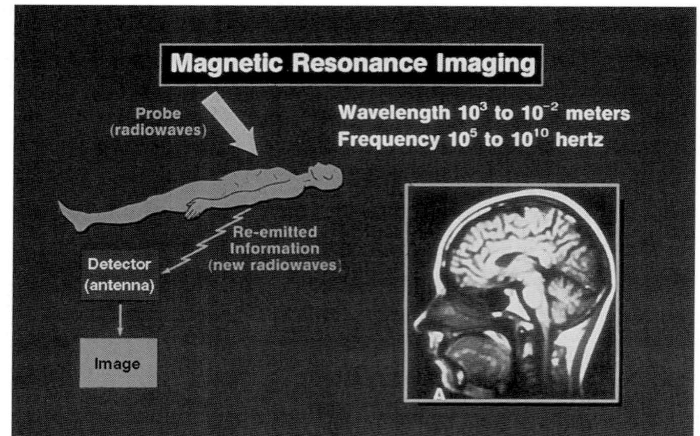

Fig. 25-2. MRI–0.0000001 eV energy.

General Principles of MRI

Certain **nuclei** in the body will receive and re-emit radio waves of specific frequencies when those nuclei are under the influence of a magnetic field. These re-emitted radio signals contain information about the patient that is captured by a **receiver** or **antenna.** The electrical signal from the antenna is transmitted through an "analog-to-digital" (A to D) converter and then to a computer, where an image of the patient is reconstructed mathematically.

The main components of the MRI system are shown in Fig. 25-3 and are discussed in more detail later in this chapter. However, before beginning a study of the components or the equipment of an MRI system, the physical principles of MR imaging will be discussed.

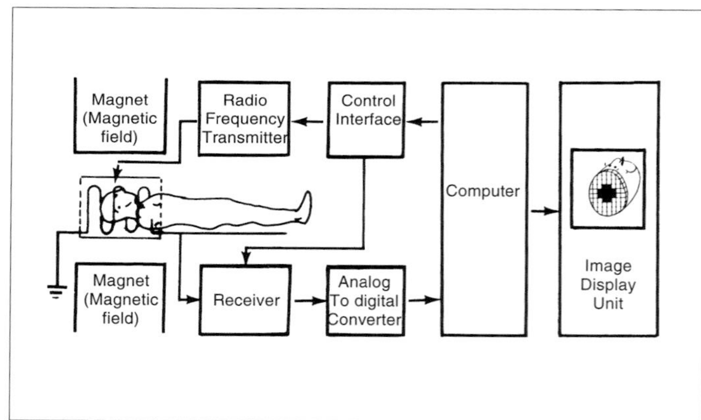

Fig. 25-3. MRI schematic.

The Interaction of Nuclei With Magnetic Fields (The Basis of MR Imaging)

Radiographic imaging involves the interaction of x-rays with the electrons surrounding the nuclei of atoms whereas, magnetic resonance imaging involves the interaction of radio waves (and static magnetic fields) with the nuclei alone. Not all nuclei respond to magnetic fields. A list of the nuclei found in the body that are magnetic themselves (those having odd numbers of protons or neutrons) and thus suitable for magnetic resonance studies is shown in Fig. 25-4. Although there are in theory a number of such suitable nuclei, at present most imaging is performed with **hydrogen nuclei (single protons).**

One reason for this preference is that there is a great deal of hydrogen present in any organism. To convince ourselves of this fact we need only recall that there are two hydrogen atoms in each water molecule and that the body is roughly 85% water. Hydrogen is also contained within many other molecules. Thus, a typical cubic centimeter of the body may contain approximately 1,022 hydrogen atoms, each of which is capable of sending and receiving radio signals. Other nuclei do not exist in such abundance and therefore will not provide such a strong signal.

Nuclei Suitable for MR	
$^{1}_{1}$H	**–Hydrogen**
$^{13}_{6}$C	–Carbon
$^{14}_{7}$N	–Nitrogen
$^{17}_{8}$O	–Oxygen
$^{39}_{19}$K	–Potassium
$^{19}_{9}$F	–Fluorine
$^{23}_{11}$Na	–Sodium
$^{31}_{15}$P	–Phosphorus

Fig. 25-4. Nuclei potentially suitable for MRI.

Precession

Magnetic resonance imaging is possible because a magnetic nucleus will **precess** about a strong **static (unchanging) magnetic field.** The phenomenon of precession **occurs whenever a spinning object is acted upon by an outside force.** Three examples of precession are shown in Fig. 25-5. A spinning top, when acted upon by the force of gravity, precesses or wobbles about the line defined by the direction of gravitational force. In MRI application, a spinning proton (hydrogen nucleus) precesses when placed in a strong magnetic field. A third example is the earth itself, which precesses because of the interplay between the forces of the sun and the planets.

The **rate of precession** of a proton in a magnetic field **increases as the strength of magnetic field increases.** The rate of precession of protons in an MRI system is difficult to imagine. Protons in a low field system may precess at 5,000,000 cycles per second. (See Fig. 25-5.)

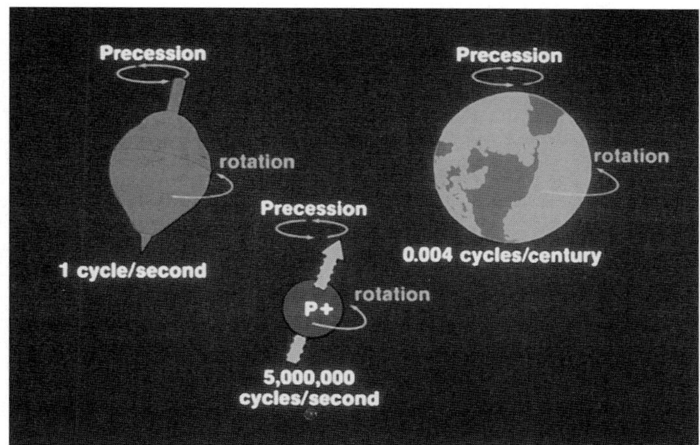

Fig. 25-5. Examples of precession.

Sending a Radio Signal to Precessing Nuclei

After the static magnetic field has been applied, the precession of nuclei in the patient can be further influenced by radio waves since a radio wave contains a time varying magnetic field. One effect of the radio wave is to cause the nucleus to precess at a greater angle. **The longer the radio wave is applied to the patient the greater the angle of precession.** In the example shown in Fig. 25-6, the radio wave has been applied long enough to cause the nucleus to change from near vertical (parallel to the static magnetic field) to horizontal (at right angles to the static magnetic field). However, even this duration of the radio waves sufficient to change the precession of the nuclei to a near horizontal position seems short in relation to events in everyday life. We say that the radio wave is applied to the patient in a "pulse" that may last for a fraction of a second during the "send" phase of the MRI process. Pulse sequences are described in more detail later in this chapter.

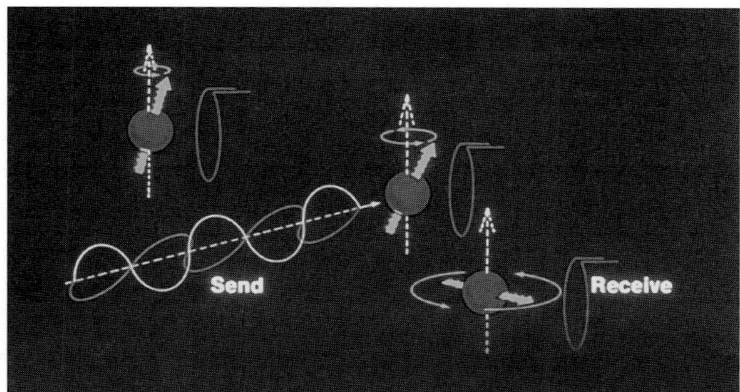

Fig. 25-6. Radio waves increase angle of precession.

Resonance

Radio waves affect the precessing nuclei because the **time varying magnetic field** of the radio wave (i.e., the radio frequency part of the electromagnetic spectrum) changes at the same rate as the nuclei precess. This means that as the nucleus rotates, the magnetic field appears at just the proper time to have maximum effect in "pushing" the nucleus away from the static magnetic field. This timing of a force and a periodically changing system is an example of the concept of **"resonance."**

Another common example of resonance is the pushing of a child on a swing. When we push a child on a swing, we naturally push the child in "resonance." That is, we apply force to the swing at a frequency that matches the frequency with which the swing returns to us. We know that if we apply our energy at any other frequency there will be no useful effect. Thus, the principle of resonance explains why we use radio frequency waves applied in pulses for MR imaging. **Radio waves** (because of their specific wavelength) **are in resonance with the precessing nuclei.** (This explains the use of radio waves in MRI rather than other electromagnetic waves such as microwaves or visible light which, because of their wavelength, would not be in resonance with the precessing nuclei.)

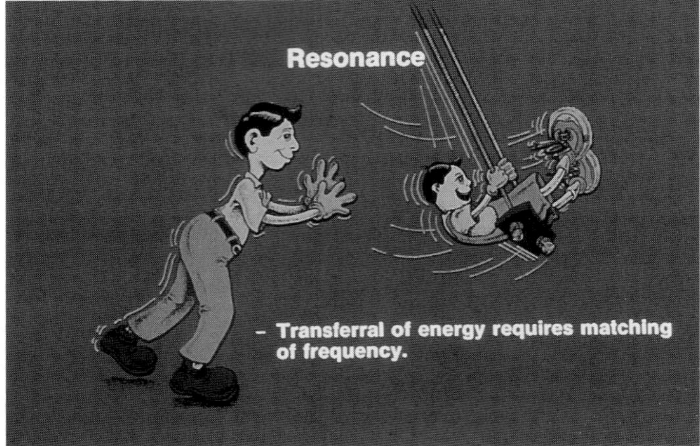

Fig. 25-7. Example of resonance.

Receiving the MRI Signal From Body Tissues

Because the nucleus is itself a tiny magnet, as it rotates it emits electromagnetic waves. These emitted waves from nuclei within body tissue are picked up by an antenna or **receiver coil during** the "receive" phase of the MRI process (Fig. 25-8). This electrical signal obtained from the receiver coil is sent to a computer. The image of the patient is then reconstructed by the computer. Various mathematical techniques may be used to build up an image from the received radio waves. Some techniques are similar to those used in computed tomography.

The received signal is described relative to random superimposed signals or noise that is also picked up by the antenna. **The signal to noise ratio** (SNR or S/N) **is used to describe the relative contribution of the true signal from the tissue and random noise**.

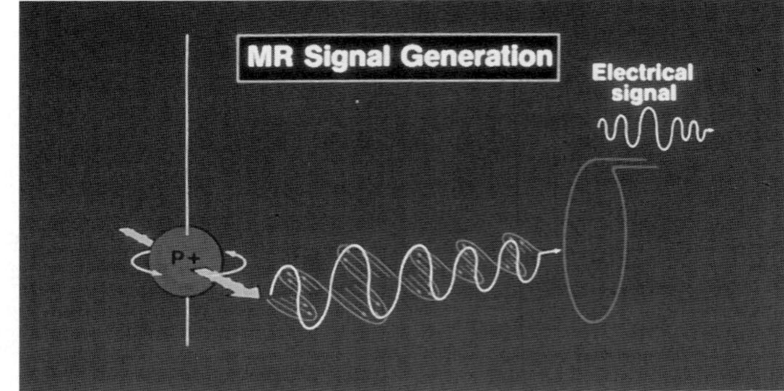

Fig. 25-8. MRI signal generation.

Relaxation

When the radio frequency pulse that was sent to the nuclei is over, the nuclei are precessing together in phase. As soon as the radio frequency pulse is turned off, the nuclei begin to return to a more random configuration in a process called **relaxation**. As the nuclei relax, the MRI signal received from the precessing nuclei diminishes. The **rate of relaxation** gives us information about normal tissue and pathologic process in the tissues. Thus, relaxation influences the appearance of the MR image. Relaxation may be divided into two categories as shown in Fig. 25-9. These are commonly referred to as **T1** and **T2 relaxation**.

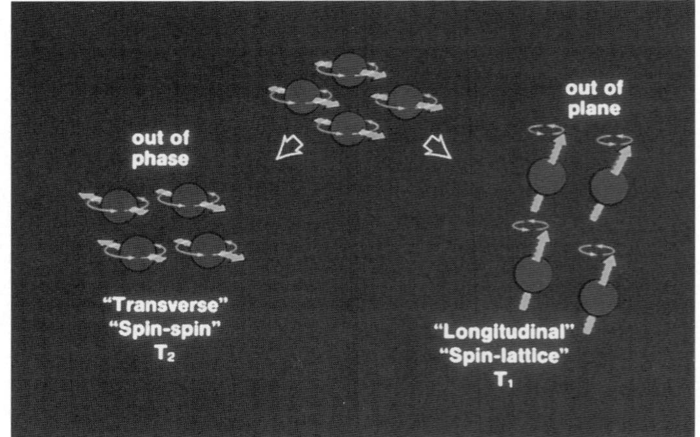

Fig. 25-9. Two categories of relaxation.

T1 Relaxation: This relaxation category occurs when the spins begin to precess at **smaller and smaller angles,** that is from a near horizontal or transverse precession to a more vertical (see Fig. 25-10). This process, referred to as **longitudinal or spin lattice** type relaxation (T1) causes the **MRI signal to decrease in strength.** We define the time required for this signal to decrease to 37% of its maximum value as T1 (See Fig. 25-10.)

T2 Relaxation: When spins begin to precess **out of phase** with each other, the result is referred to as **transverse or spin-spin type** relaxation. This is called T2 relaxation. Note in Fig. 25-11 that the nuclei along the top of the graph are shown to be "in phase" at the beginning but that they go out of phase as indicated by the direction of the arrows. As this T2 relaxation occurs, the **MRI signal will decrease in strength.** The time required for the MRI signal to decrease to 37% of its maximum value is defined as T2 (See Fig. 25-11.)

The rate of these two types of relaxation changes, T1 and T2, following exposure to the radio frequency (applied in resonance) constitutes the primary basis from which the MR image is reconstructed. However, a third factor, spin density, also plays a minor role in determining the appearance of the MR image.

Spin Density: A stronger signal will be received if the **quantity** of hydrogen nuclei that are present in a given volume of tissue **is increased.** However, this quantity, called the "proton density" or **"spin density"** is a minor contributor to the appearance of an MR image because the tissues imaged by proton (hydrogen nucleus) do not differ markedly in spin density. A more important consideration as discussed above, is that the nuclei that compose **different tissues** within the body, **respond at different relaxation rates,** T1 and T2.

Summary: The **MRI signal strength,** as received by an antenna or receiver coil, is used to define the **brightness of each point of the image of the patient.** Thus, the differences among T1, T2 and spin density of tissues produce differences in relative brightness of points in the image. The **three primary factors** that determine the signal strength and therefore the brightness of each part of the image or the image contrast are **spin density** and **T1 and T2** relaxation rates. Other factors such as flowing blood or the presence of contrast material also play a role, but are beyond the scope of this introductory discussion.

Magnetic resonance imaging is a fundamentally different way of looking at the body compared with other imaging modalities. For example, in radiography, the physical density (grams per cc) and atomic number of tissues determine the appearance of the image. The rate of recovery of atoms from their interactions with x-rays is not important in radiography. In MRI, however, the rate of recovery of nuclei following the application of radio waves (relaxation rate) is the most important factor in determining the MR image. This provides the basis for the MR image as seen in Fig. 25-12. High tissue density such as in dense bone structure does **not** result in image contrast in **MR** imaging. Soft tissues such as gray and white matter of the brain, the brain stem and the corpus callosum however, are clearly visualized because of the response of nuclei in these tissues as described above.

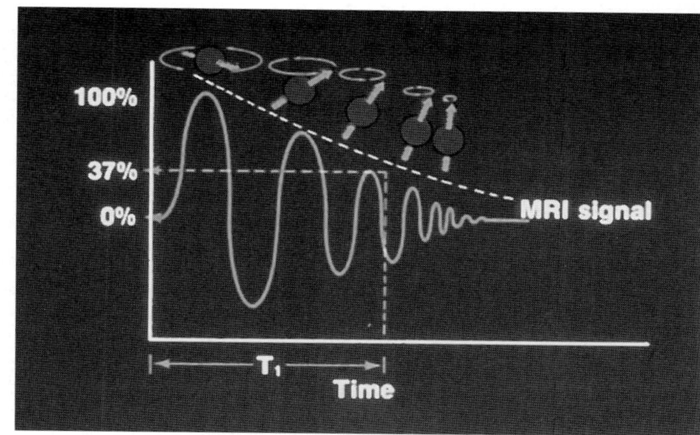

Fig. 25-10. T1 relaxation (longitudinal or spin lattice).

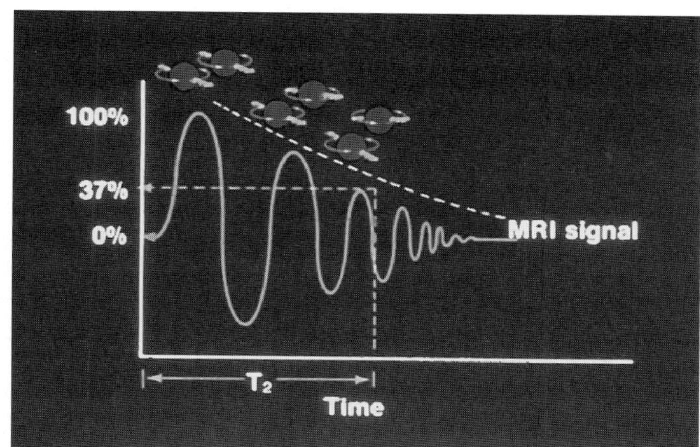

Fig. 25-11. T2 relaxation (transverse or spin-spin).

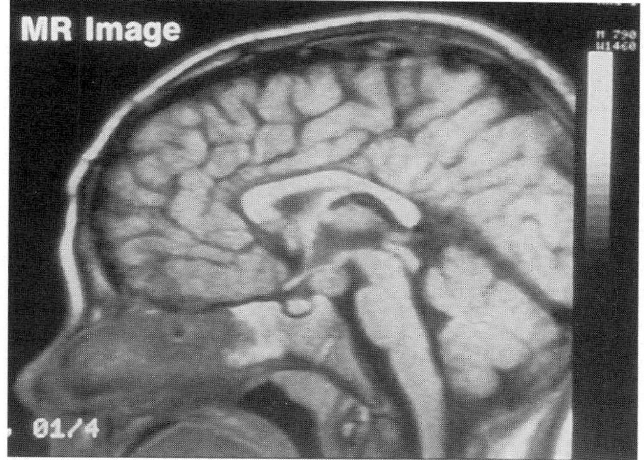

Fig. 25-12. MR image.

Gradient Magnetic Fields

To further understand the method of image reconstruction used in MRI, it is necessary to understand the concept of a **gradient, or a change of magnetic field strength through a certain region or "slice" of body tissue.** The gradient magnetic field is used to obtain information from specific regions or slices of body tissue. Knowledge of the exact location of origin of received MRI signals from within the patient allows the computer to reconstruct the MR image.

Earlier in this chapter it was shown that the strength of the magnetic field determines the **precession rate** of the nuclei. The precession rate determines the exact value of radio wave frequency that will be in resonance with the nuclei. The MRI system sends and receives radio waves from nuclei only when those nuclei are processing at the same frequency as the frequency of the radio wave, i.e., at resonance frequency. Thus an MRI system **changes the gradient** or **magnetic field strength through a certain region or slice of body tissue so that the system will only receive the MR signal from nuclei that precess within that region or slice.** The computer can decode this as well as other information such as spin density and T1 and T2 relaxation and can thereby, reconstruct the MRI image.

The use of gradient magnetic fields in MRI is similar in many ways to the use of x-ray collimators in CT (Computed Tomography) where information from specific slices of irradiated tissue is used to reconstruct the CT image. Gradient magnetic fields are produced by "gradient coils" located within the bore of the main system magnet.

The gradient magnetic fields are much weaker than the static magnetic field produced by the main MRI system magnet. The gradient field adds to or increases the strength of the static magnetic field over some regions of the patient and decreases the strength of the static field over other regions of the patient. Since the strength of the magnetic field determines the frequency of precession of nuclei, this in turn determines the frequency of the MRI signal produced from that region. Thus, gradient fields cause different regions of the patient to produce MRI signals at slightly different frequencies. (See Fig. 25-13.)

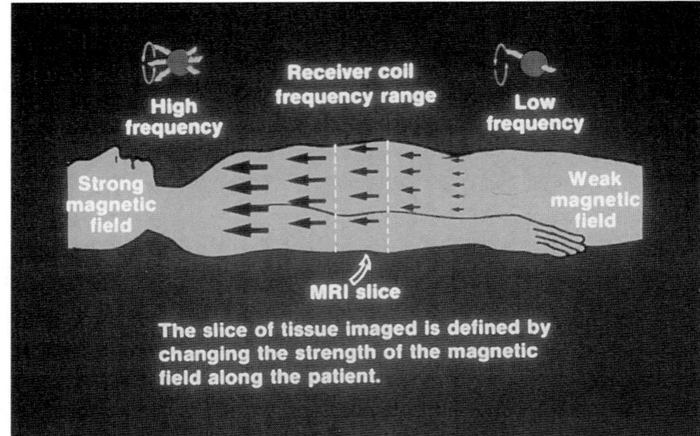

Fig. 25-13. Gradient magnetic fields (basis of MRI "slice").

Summary: The strength of the MRI signal is determined by the number of nuclei per unit volume (spin density) and the orientation of the nuclei with respect to the static magnetic field (T1 relaxation) and with respect to each other (T2 relaxation). The **location of origin** within the patient of the MRI signal may be determined by the **frequency** of the MRI signal. The application of gradient magnetic fields assures us that the frequency of the MRI signal will vary from one location to another within the patient and that the computer may therefore, produce a unique image of the patient.

The frequency of the signal is a measure of how often it varies in strength. Other techniques are used to alter the "phase" of the MR signal, whether it is large or small at a specific time. By varying the frequency in one direction, and the phase in another direction, the location of origin of MR signal may be found for each point within a slice.

Multislice Imaging

Fig. 25-14 demonstrates multislice MR imaging of the cranium. Note by the anatomical structures visualized on these various images that each image represents a reconstruction of data received by the computer through the receiving coils as the magnetic field strength was varied or changed through specific regions or slices of the body tissues.

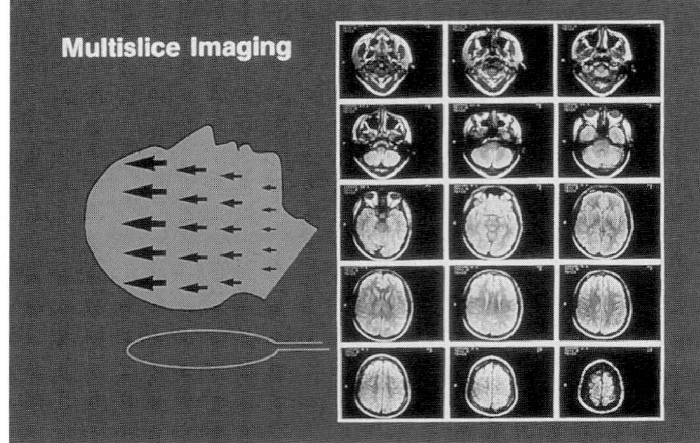

Fig. 25-14. Multislice images.

Pulse Sequences

The image produced by an MRI system is critically influenced by the exact sequence of radio wave pulses used as well as the moment at which the signal emitted by the nuclei is sampled or received. Since the duration of the radio wave pulse that is sent into the patient determines the angle at which the nucleus processes, **the length of the pulse is often specified in terms of the angle it will produce.** Fig. 25-15 illustrates 90°, 45° and 180° pulses.

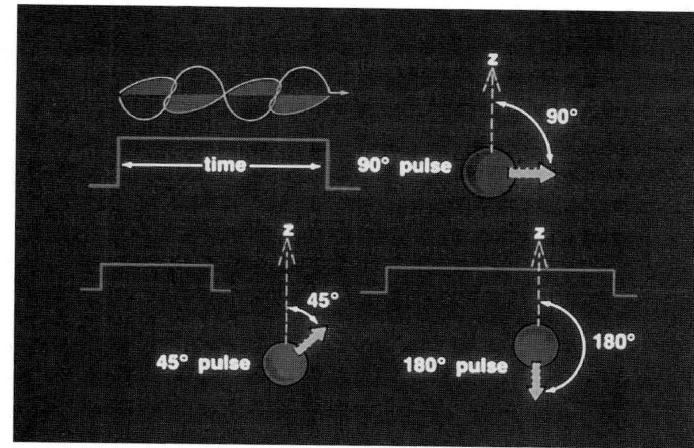

Fig. 25-15. Pulse sequences.

Spin-Echo Pulse Sequence: A typical pulse sequence is diagrammed in Fig. 25-16. The sequence contains two pulses, a 90° pulse and a 180° pulse. Radio frequency waves are sent into the patient during each pulse. The sequence is repeated again after a time, TR (repetition time), has elapsed. Typical TR values used in imaging may vary from 200 to 2000 millisec (0.2 to 2 sec). The pulse sequence changes the angle of precession of the nuclei and causes a radio frequency wave called an "echo" to be emitted from the patient.

In MRI techniques, the receiver coil listens to an echo of the signal, rather than the initial signal, which is called the FID or free induction decay. The echo is intercepted by the receiver coils of the MR system and is used to construct an image of the patient. The echo occurs at a time TE (time-to-echo) after the initial pulse of the sequence. Typical TE values used in imaging vary from 10 to 100 milliseconds. Both TR and TE are technique variables that are selected by the operator of the MR system to optimize the appearance of an image and to allow acquisition of information weighted toward T1 or T2 relaxation rates.

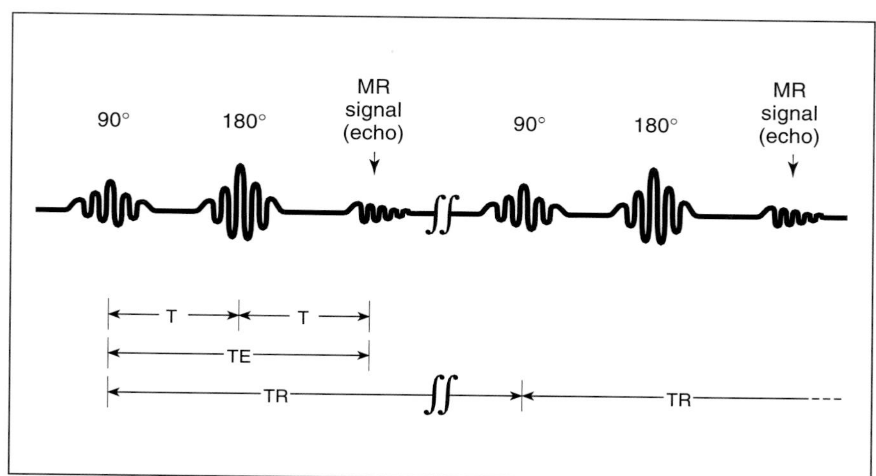

Fig. 25-16. Spin-echo pulse sequence.*

Acquisition of an image requires that gradient magnetic fields be turned on and off at appropriate times during a pulse sequence. Gradients are used to vary the phase and frequency of precession of protons throughout the patient so that the origin of the MR signal (echo) may be assigned to the appropriate locations within the image. The complete pulse sequence timing diagram for a spin-echo pulse sequence is shown in Fig. 25-17. A spin-echo pulse sequence is a commonly used pulse sequence in clinical situations and is just one of the techniques available for imaging. Gradient-echo and inversion recovery are two other types of pulse sequences. (See definitions at end of chapter.) The slice select gradient, G slice, is turned on while pulses are sent into the patient. The frequency encoding gradient, G frequency, is turned on only while the echo signal is received. The phase encoding gradient, G phase, is turned on between pulses. The entire process is repeated with different values of the phase encoding gradient (indicated by the dotted lines for G phase in Fig. 25-17).

The three gradient directions (slice, phase and frequency) correspond to the three axes of the patient, x, y and z which may be identified with slice (plane) selection. The x, y and z gradients are explained in more detail later in this chapter.

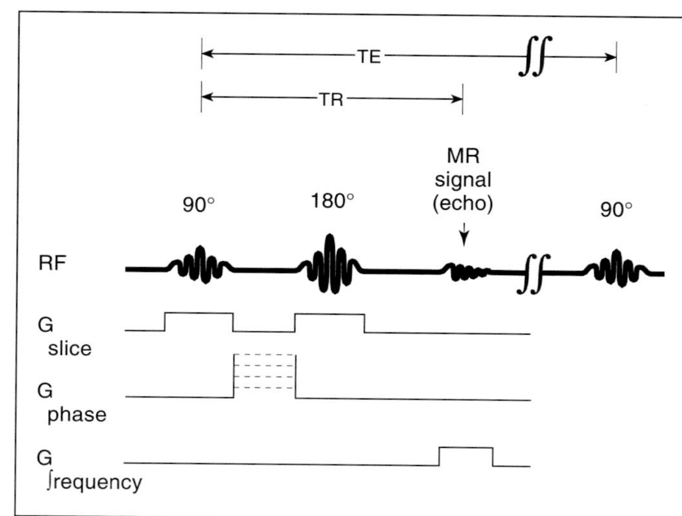

Fig. 25-17. A magnetic resonance image acquisition diagram showing a spin-echo pulse sequence along with gradient magnetic fields.*

*Hendee WR; Ritenour , ER; *Medical Imaging Physics*, 3rd ed. Mosby-Year Book, Chicago, 1992.

Pulse Sequence Timing Factors: At the present, several types of pulse sequences are used to accentuate one or more of the parameters that influence MR images. Fig. 25-18 demonstrates the differences in the appearance of the image created by changing certain pulse sequence timing factors. Notice that some areas of the image change almost completely from white to black because of the change in pulse repetition time (TR), or the time between pulse sequences. The time between the initial pulse that is sent into the patient and the time that the MR signal is sampled from the patient, the time-to-echo (TE), also influence the image. Both the TR and TE are selected by the operator and have a profound influence upon contrast in the image.

Number of Signal Averages: Another variable that is set by the operator and that influences the appearance of the image is the number of signal averages. The entire pulse sequence is repeated several times and the MR signal value is then averaged. Signal averaging reduces the effects of spurious noise but increases the time required to complete a scan.

Summary: A good understanding of the physical principles of MR imaging involving the interaction of nuclei with magnetic fields as described in this chapter provides a foundation for further study and understanding of all parameters of MRI.

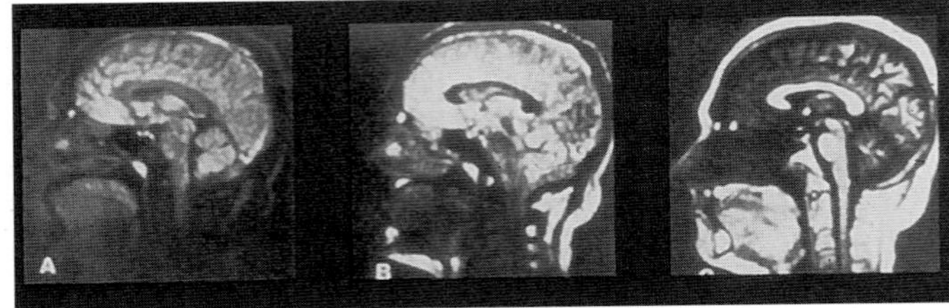

Fig. 25-18. TR (pulse sequence) variables.

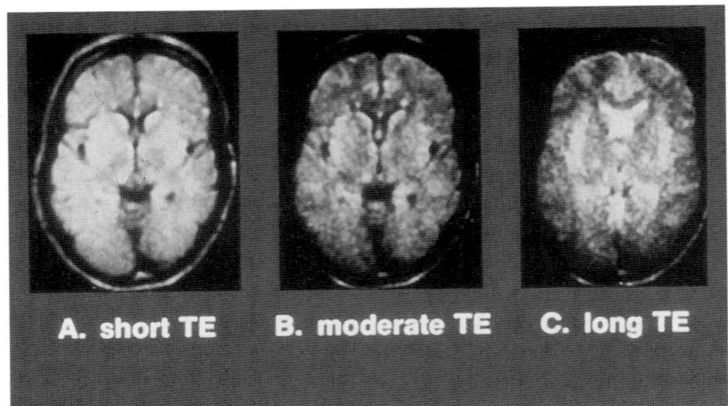

Fig. 25-19. TE (time-to-echo) variables.

Equipment Components

MRI System Components

The application of the principle of magnetic resonance in the modern hospital requires an impressive collection of "state of the art" equipment. The six main components of the MRI system are shown in Fig. 25-20 and are discussed in the following section. They are as follows:

- Magnet.
- Gradient coils.
- Radio frequency coils.
- Electronic support systems.
- Computer.
- Display.

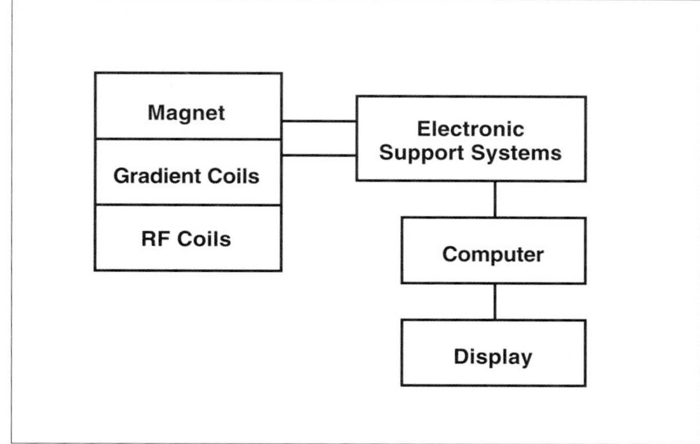

Fig. 25-20. MRI main components.

Magnets

The most visible and probably the most often discussed component of the MRI system is the magnet. The **magnet provides the powerful static** (constant strength) **magnetic field** about which the nuclei precess. At the present time there are **three** types of MRI system magnets. Not one of the three is inherently superior to the others. Each have their own unique characteristics. They share a common purpose, however, in creating a magnetic field that is measured in units of **Tesla*** *(tes′la)*. Field strengths used clinically vary from 0.1 to 2.0 Tesla. In comparison, the earth's magnetic field is approximately 0.00005 Tesla (Fig. 25-21).

Static field strengths surrounding the magnet, called fringe magnetic fields, are sometimes measured in **Gauss**† *(gous)*. One Tesla equals 10,000 Gauss.

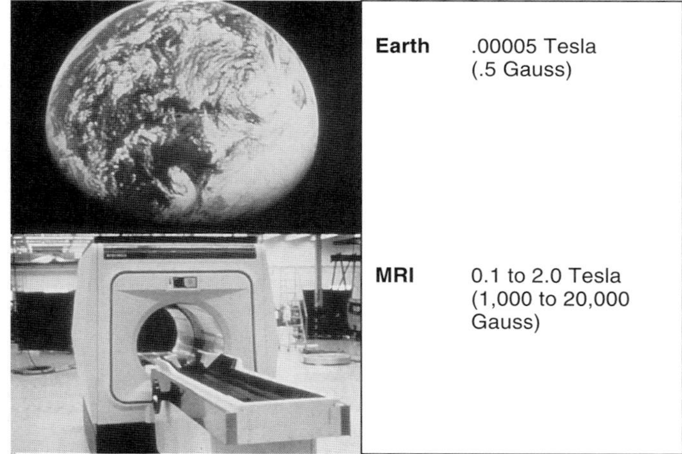

Fig. 25-21. Magnetic field strength.

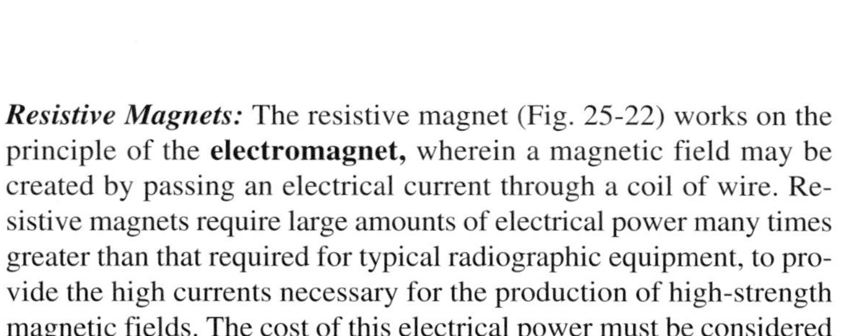

Resistive Magnets: The resistive magnet (Fig. 25-22) works on the principle of the **electromagnet,** wherein a magnetic field may be created by passing an electrical current through a coil of wire. Resistive magnets require large amounts of electrical power many times greater than that required for typical radiographic equipment, to provide the high currents necessary for the production of high-strength magnetic fields. The cost of this electrical power must be considered as part of the cost of operation of the unit.

In addition, the high electrical currents produce heat, which must be dissipated with a cooling system. The heat is produced by the resistance of the wire to the flow of electricity. This resistance acts as a type of "friction" that produces heat and ultimately limits the amount of current that can be produced. Typical resistive systems produce magnetic field strengths of up to **0.3 Tesla.**

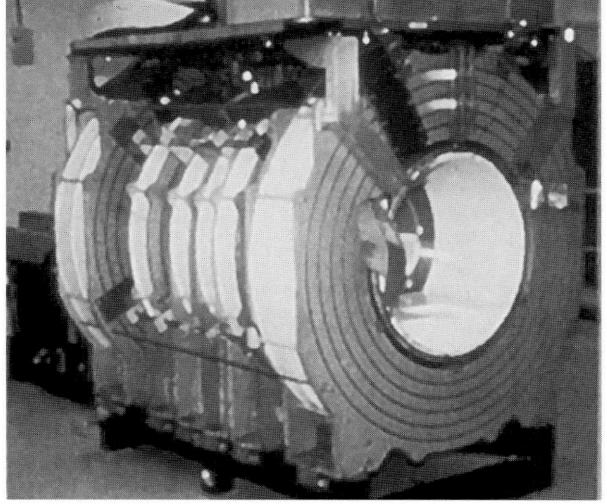

Fig. 25-22. Resistive magnet (field strength to 0.3 Tesla).

*Nikola *Tesla*, 1856-1943, U.S. (born in Croatia) researcher in electromagnetic phenomena . *Tesla* is a unit of magnetic flux density equal to one weber per square meter (SI unit of measurement).

†Carl F. *Gauss*, German physicist, 1777-1855, a measurement of magnetic flux density in lines of flux per square centimeter (GCS unit of measurement).

Permanent Magnets: The high operating costs associated with the other two types of magnets, namely the electrical power and cryogens, are avoided in the permanent magnet system (Fig. 25-23). Certain materials can be given permanent magnetic properties. An example of a very small permanent magnet of this type is the magnet used to attach notes to refrigerator doors. For MRI use, certain very large permanent magnets may be made with field strengths up to **0.3 Tesla.**

The initial cost of the permanent magnet is somewhere between the above two types. Since no electrical power is needed for this magnet, the operating cost is nearly negligible. A disadvantage, however, may be the inability to turn off the power of the magnetic field. If metal objects accidentally become lodged in the bore of the magnet, they must be removed against the full power of the magnetic field.

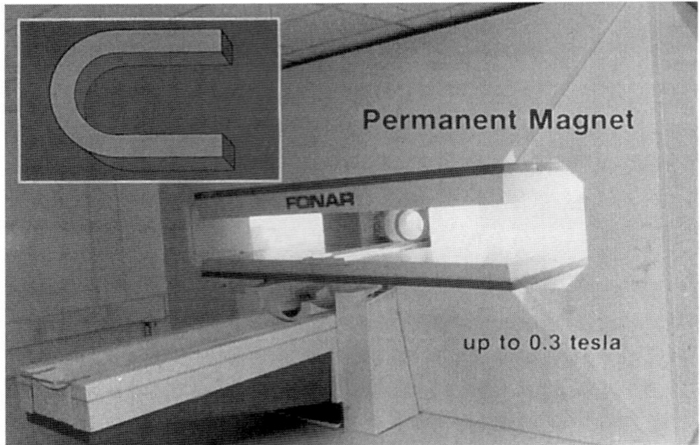

Fig. 25-23. Permanent magnet (field strength to 0.3 Tesla).

Superconducting Magnets: The superconducting magnet (Fig. 25-24) also uses the principle of the **electromagnet.** In addition, it uses a property that is demonstrated by some materials at **extremely low temperatures,** the property of **superconductivity.** A superconductive material is a material that has lost all resistance to electrical current. When this occurs, very large electrical currents may be maintained with essentially no use of electrical power. Thus, the electrical costs of running a superconducting magnet are negligible.

A significant factor, however, is the cost of providing these very low temperature cooling materials, called "cryogens" *(kri′o-jen).* The two cryogens currently employed are liquid nitrogen (-195.8° C), and liquid helium (-268.9° C). The cost of maintaining this intensive cooling system is of the same order of magnitude or even higher than the electrical costs of a resistive system. The initial cost is also the highest of the three types of magnets. Higher magnetic field strengths are possible with the superconducting magnet, with values as high as **2 Tesla** for clinical use. These are currently a common type of magnet in clinical use because of their greater magnetic field strength.

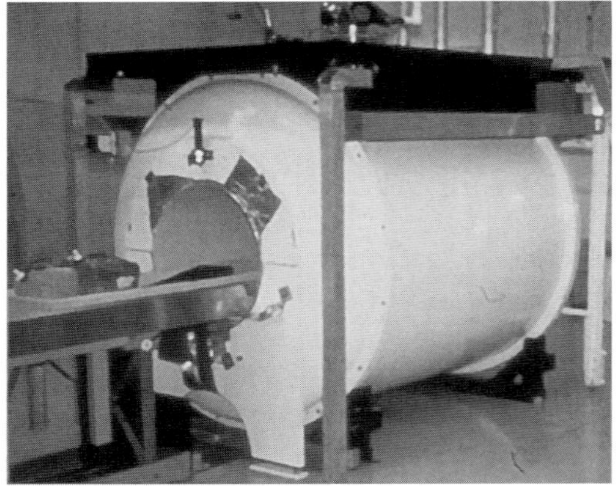

Fig. 25-24. Superconducting magnet (field strength to 2 Tesla).

Gradient Coils

In addition to the powerful magnets, a second major component of the MRI system is the gradient coil. The gradient magnetic fields **cause nuclei in different locations within the patient to precess at slightly different rates,** allowing the computer to determine the location within the patient from which the received MRI signal originated. This information is, of course, crucial to the reconstruction of an image of the patient. The **gradient fields are much weaker** than the static magnetic fields and can be produced by relatively simple coils of wire.

One typical configuration of the gradient coils is shown in Fig. 25-25. An MRI system may contain three sets of gradient coils, allowing a gradient to be applied in the three directions – x, y, and z. These coils, referred to as the x, y, and z gradient coils, are located within the bore of the main system magnet. By electronically adjusting the amount of current in these three sets of coils, it is possible to obtain a gradient in any direction. This flexibility allows a magnetic resonance imaging system to obtain images at any orientation within the patient.

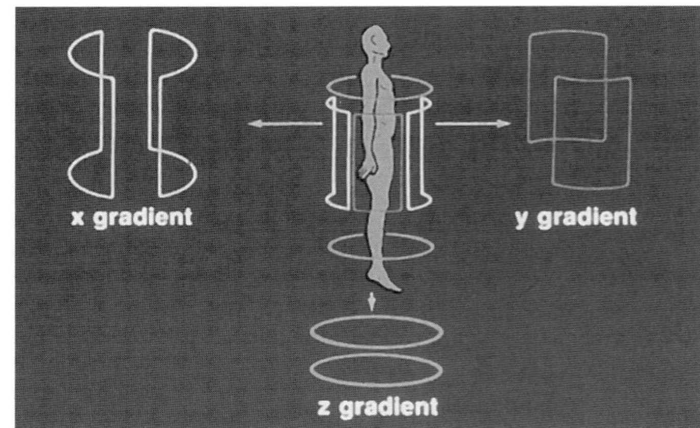

Fig. 25-25. Gradient coils.

Radio Frequency (RF) Coils

A third key component of the MRI system is the radio frequency (RF) or "send and receive" coils. These RF coils act **as antennas to produce and detect the radio waves** that are referred to as **the MRI "signal."**

A typical RF coil is encased or enclosed in the gantry of the magnet and thus is not specifically visible. These encased RF coils, sometimes referred to as body coils, **completely surround the patient** including the table on which the patient lies as indicated by the arrows in Fig. 25-26.

Designs of RF coils vary from this large, enclosed **body coil** to separate smaller **circumferential whole-volume coils**, which also encircle the part being imaged. Examples of these are the head coil and the limb (extremity) coil (Fig. 25-27).

Some **surface coils**, such as the shoulder coil, are placed on the area to be imaged. Generally, this type of surface coil is used to image more superficial structures.

These various coils will be described and demonstrated in use with specific MRI procedures later in this chapter. A display of an assortment of circumferential whole-volume and surface coils are shown in Fig. 25-27.

Another type of frequently used RF coil is the **phased array coil**. These consist of multiple coils and receivers that are grouped together. Each coil is independent of the other and has its own receiver which allows large field of view coverage for use in imaging the spine.

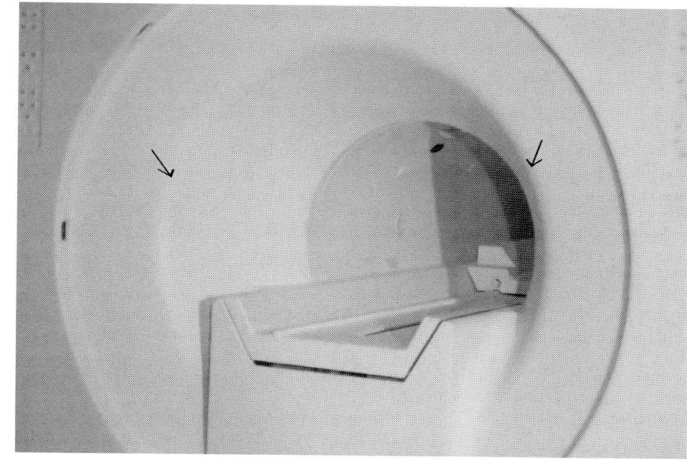

Fig. 25-26. Encased RF coils (body coils) in gantry of magnet.

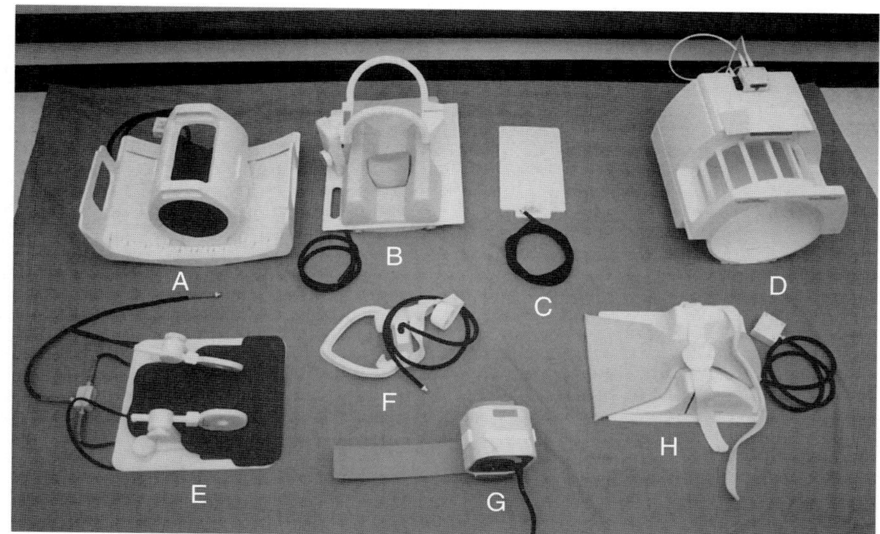

Fig. 25-27. Examples of circumferential whole-volume and surface coils
A. Limb (extremity) coil.
B. Volume neck coil.
C. Planar surface coil (license plate coil).
D. Head coil.
E. TMJ coil (bilateral).
F. Shoulder coil.
G. Wrist coil.
H. Posterior C-spine coil.

Electronic Support System

The electronic support systems, making up the fourth component of the MRI system, can be divided into two parts. The first part, the **power supply**, provides voltage and current for all parts of the MRI system that require it, such as the gradient coils, the cooling system, the magnet, and the computer. The power usage varies in different MRI systems. For example, the cooling system and magnet requirements are negligible in permanent magnet systems, but they provide the heaviest load in resistive systems. Thus, the power consumption varies from about 25 kilowatts in permanent magnet systems to over 150 kilowatts in resistive systems.

The second major part of the electronic support system is the **RF transmitter and receiver.** This part of the system performs the same functions as broadcast radio communication transmitters and receivers. It sends the radio wave pulses into the patient and receives the MRI signals from the patient. (The RF send and receive coils, as described above, are part of this system.) The RF transmitter also contains amplifiers that boost the strength of relatively weak radio signals received from deep within a patient in the bore of the magnet.

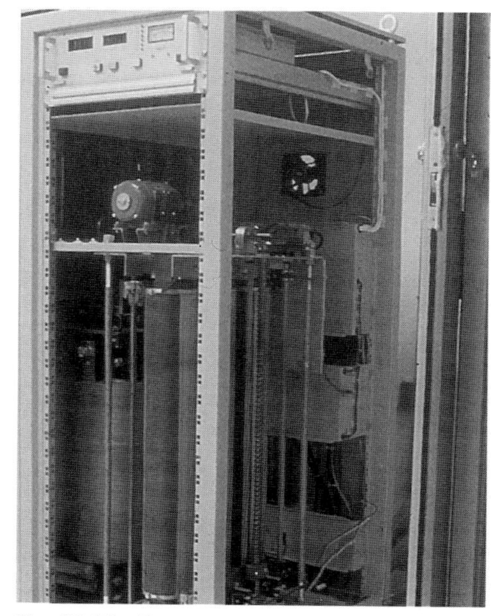

Fig. 25-28. Example of power supply (25 to 150+ kilowatts).

Computer

The fifth component of the MRI system is the computer, a key component of an MRI unit. It processes information from all parts of the MRI system. During a scan it controls the timing of pulses to coincide with changes in gradient field strengths. After a scan it reconstructs the image of the patient using techniques such as Fourier transforms that are similar to those used in computed tomography.

The computer contains both internal and external memory devices. Internal memory allows the computer to manipulate the millions of bits of information required to define an image of the patient. External memory includes the various types of magnetic storage media, such as hard disks, optical disks, and tape cartridges, that are used to store information for future use.

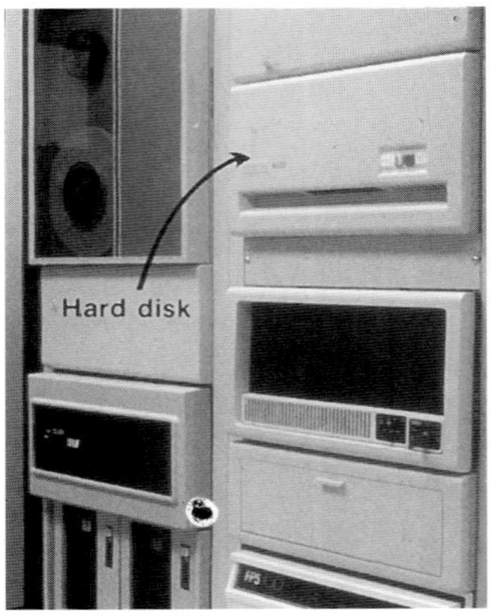

Fig. 25-29. MRI computer.

Display

The sixth and last component of the MRI system to be discussed is the display or workstation, which allows the technologist to control the operation of the system and view images as they are reconstructed. A central or system workstation, as shown in Fig. 25-30, may contain the **controls** used by the technologist to **select pulse sequences, set the various operator adjustable parameters,** such as number of signal averages and pulse repetition time (TR), and to **initiate the scan.** Controls on the display allow **brightness and contrast to be altered** to bring out significant features in the image.

Independent display stations located away from the central display station (in a separate room) are often included to allow images to be viewed while other patients are being scanned. Image processing capability is sometimes available to allow enhancement operations such as digital filtering.

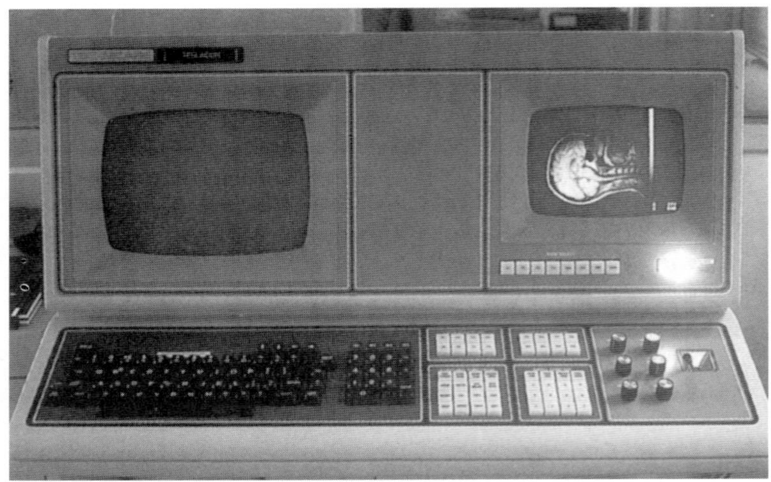

Fig. 25-30. MRI display station.

Summary of MRI Imaging Process and System Components Used

Following is a five-step summary of the entire MR imaging process identifying the component of equipment used and the results of each step:

Step	Component	Result
1. Apply static magnetic field.	Magnet	Nuclei align and precess.
2. Select slice by applying gradient magnetic field (variation of magnetic field strength over patient).	Gradient coils	Nuclei precess at a particular frequency.
3. Apply RF pulses.	RF sending coil or antenna	Nuclei in the slice area precess in phase at a greater angle.
4. Receive RF signal.	RF receiving coil or antenna	Electrical signal is received from nuclei and sent to computer.
5. Convert signal to image.	Computer	Reconstructed image is displayed.

Fig. 25-31. Summary

Clinical Applications

It has become increasingly popular to refer to radiology departments as diagnostic imaging centers. This new terminology is due in part to the increased use of magnetic resonance imaging. The need for radiographers to have a basic knowledge of MRI continues to grow as MRI continues to improve in its ability to show disease processes.

With increases in the number of MR scanners available, radiographers will continue to be called upon to assume staff positions in the MRI section of radiology. Many students of radiologic technology will have the opportunity to observe and participate in patient examinations utilizing MRI.

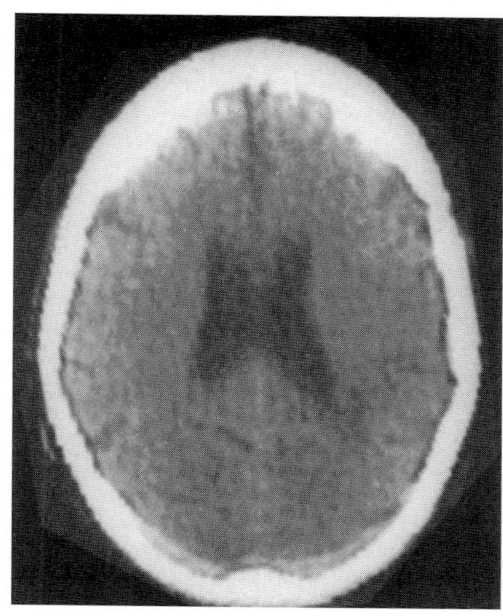

Fig. 25-32. CT axial section.

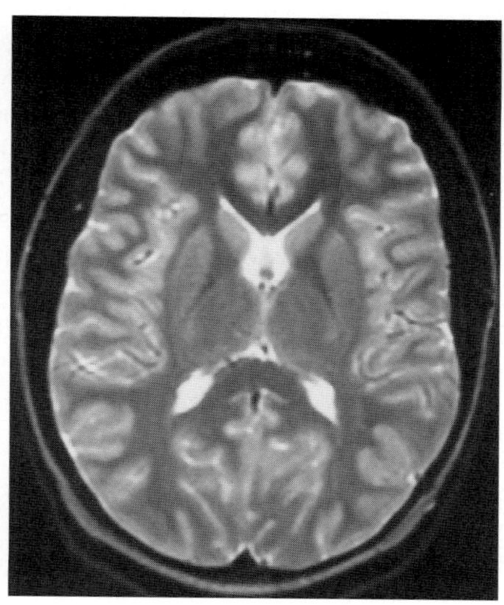

Fig. 25-33. MRI axial section.

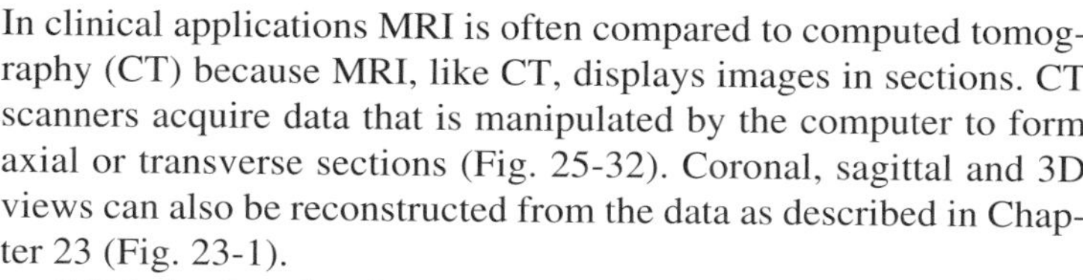

Comparison with Computed Tomography

In clinical applications MRI is often compared to computed tomography (CT) because MRI, like CT, displays images in sections. CT scanners acquire data that is manipulated by the computer to form axial or transverse sections (Fig. 25-32). Coronal, sagittal and 3D views can also be reconstructed from the data as described in Chapter 23 (Fig. 23-1).

MRI also has the diversity to image anatomy in axial or transverse, sagittal or coronal sections or planes (Figs. 25-33, 25-34, and 25-35). Oblique views of anatomical structures can also be obtained by using a combination of gradient coils.

MRI and CT technologists require an in-depth knowledge of anatomy (including sectional anatomy) for accurate viewing of images obtained from various planes or sections. A thorough knowledge of bony landmarks, organs and vessel placement will enable technologists to appropriately interpret images to determine if the scans have adequately covered the region of interest.

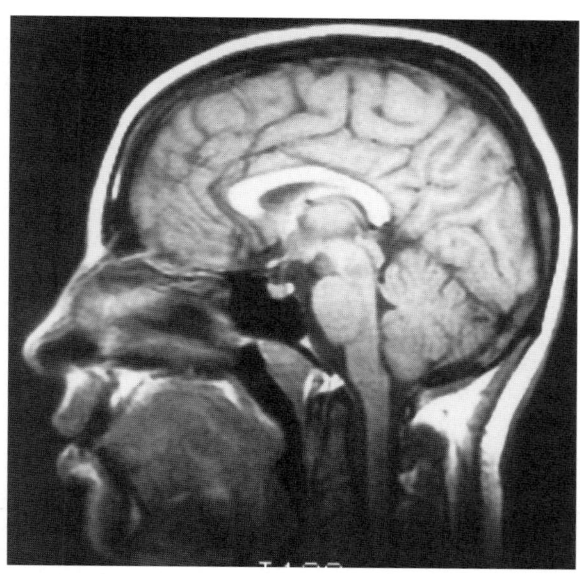

Fig. 25-34. MRI sagittal section.

CT shows an improvement in soft tissue contrast over conventional screen-film imaging. This ability to show soft tissue contrast is referred to as **contrast resolution**. The MR imaging system is more sensitive to the molecular nature of tissue and thus allows excellent contrast resolution as shown on these MRI sections. For example, MRI is sensitive to the slight difference in tissue composition of normal gray and white matter of the brain. Therefore, MRI is replacing CT as the study of choice for diseases involving the CNS, especially for examination of white matter pathology.

While CT and conventional radiography measure the attenuation of the x-ray beam, MRI uses a technique that stimulates the body to produce a radio frequency signal and uses an antenna or receiver coil to measure this signal as already discussed in Part 1 of this chapter. Technologists of MRI are required to have an understanding of how technical factors affect signal production. These technical factors impact the contrast and spatial resolution. Therefore the technologist is required to utilize these technical factors for optimum image quality.

Diagnosis of diseases such as those involving the CNS can be made with MRI by making comparisons between the signal produced in normal tissue and the signal produced in abnormal tissue.

Unlike CT, nuclear medicine and radiography, no ionizing radiation is used in MRI. Therefore MRI is deemed safer in terms of biological tissue damage. Even though the MRI scanner does not use ionizing radiation, there are safety considerations that must be identified and understood as demonstrated on the following pages.

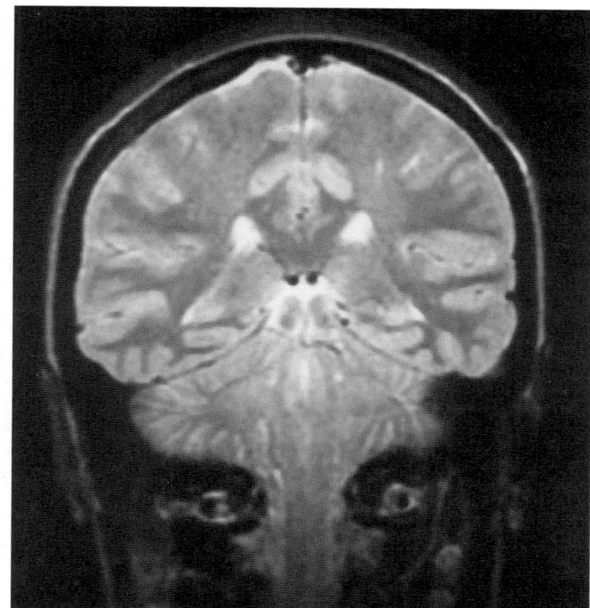

Fig. 25-35. MRI coronal section.

Basic Safety Considerations

Safety concerns for the technologist, patient and medical personnel must be recognized and are due to **the interaction of the magnetic fields with metallic objects and tissues.** During an MR scan, patients as well as other personnel in the immediate area are exposed to **static, gradient-induced** (time-varying) and **radio-frequency (RF) magnetic fields.**

Suggested maximum permissible field strengths for these fields are illustrated in Fig. 25-36. These values are to assist a hospital and review boards in assessing health consequences of operating an MR unit. It may be acceptable to operate an MR unit that exceeds these guidelines provided that the vendors of the MR equipment have shown to the satisfaction of the hospital or review board that the actual static, time varying and RF fields do not create a significant health risk.*

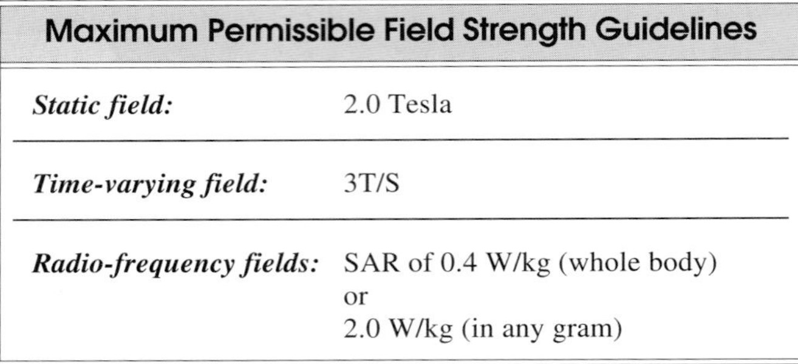

Maximum Permissible Field Strength Guidelines	
Static field:	2.0 Tesla
Time-varying field:	3T/S
Radio-frequency fields:	SAR of 0.4 W/kg (whole body) or 2.0 W/kg (in any gram)

Fig. 25-36. Guidelines by Food and Drug Administration through the publication of National Center for Devices and Radiological Health (DHHS:1982).

Safety concerns of MRI resulting from the interaction of these magnetic fields with tissues and metallic objects are as follows:

(1) Potential hazard of projectiles.
(2) Electrical interference with implants.
(3) Torquing of metallic objects.
(4) Local heating of tissues and metallic objects.
(5) Electrical interference with the normal function of nerve cells and muscle fibers.

Each of these five safety concerns will be discussed beginning with the potential hazards of projectiles.

(1) Potential Hazard of Projectiles

A static magnetic field surrounds the magnet and is referred to as the **fringe magnetic field**. Certain items are not allowed inside these fringe fields and monitoring is essential before allowing anyone to enter the magnet room. Warning posters and door security systems need to be in use to prevent unauthorized personnel from entering restricted areas within the fringe magnetic field.

The fringe magnetic fields are generally measured in Gauss (G). The fringe field strength is inversely proportional to the cube of the distance from the bore of the magnet, therefore the danger of projectiles becomes greater as one moves closer to the magnet. For example on a 1.5 Tesla imaging system, a ferromagnetic object 3 feet away will have a force 10 times that of gravity; and at 7 feet it would equal that of gravity (Fig. 25-38). If a small ferromagnetic object were released close to the magnet, it could become lethal as it attains a terminal velocity of 40 miles per hour by the time it reaches the center of the magnet.†

In the event of a code (respiratory or cardiac arrest), the patient must first be removed from the scan room and all personnel advised of the routine procedure of response to eliminate the possibility of metallic objects becoming dangerous projectiles.

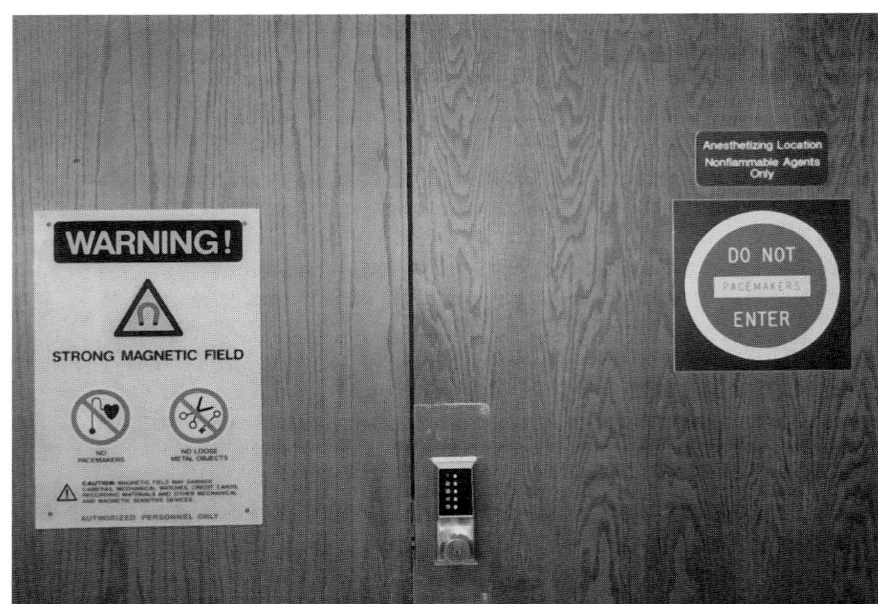
WARNING!
STRONG MAGNETIC FIELD
Anesthetizing Location
Nonflammable Agents
Only
DO NOT
PACEMAKERS
ENTER

Fig. 25-37. Warning posters and door security.
(Courtesy of University of Iowa Hospitals and Clinics)

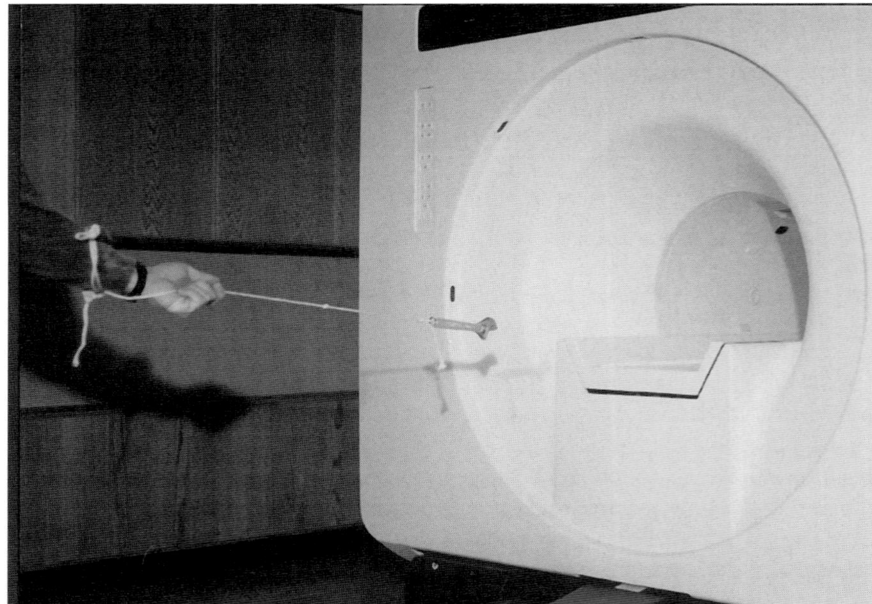

Fig. 25-38. Demonstration of potential hazard of projectiles. (A metallic object is shown in midair suspension as it is strongly attracted towards the magnet. If not securely held back by the rope, it would become a dangerous projectile. This demonstration is not recommended without adequate precautions and safety measures.)
(Courtesy of University of Iowa Hospitals and Clinics)

*Stark DD, Bradley, WG; *Magnetic Resonance Imaging*; CV Mosby; St Louis, MO: 1987
†Williams, K.D.; Drayer, B.P.; *BNI Quarterly*, Barrow Neurological Institute of St. Joseph's Hospital and Medical Center; Phoenix, AZ; 5:1 1989

As a rule, patient equipment such as 0_2 tanks, IV pumps, patient monitoring equipment, wheelchairs, and carts are **not** allowed inside the **50 Gauss line,** although some special equipment has been designed to be used specifically in MRI.

Fig. 25-39 below represents recommended minimum distances for various types of devices and/or personnel in relationship to the various Gauss line perimeters around the MRI system.

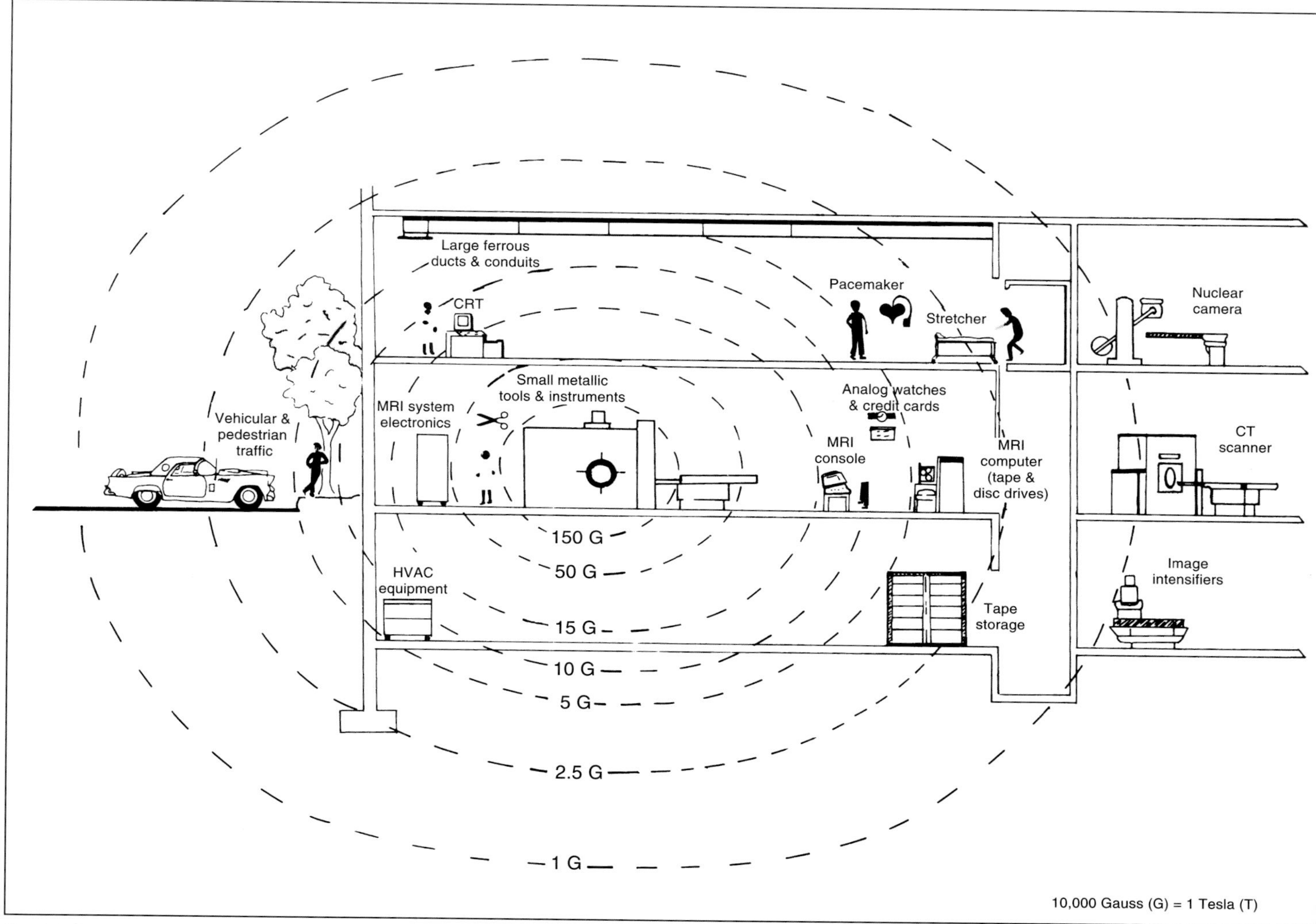

Fig. 25-39. Recommended minimum distances–Based on a non-magnetically shielded system.
(Courtesy of Picker International)

(2) Electrical Interference with Electromechanical Implants

A second major concern is possible damage to electronic components and function of cardiac pacemakers; therefore, these are not allowed within the **5 Gauss line**. Besides the static magnetic field causing possible damage to cardiac pacemakers, the RF pulses may induce voltage in the pacemaker leads.

Other devices that may be adversely affected by MRI are cochlear implants, neurostimulators, implanted drug infusion pumps and bone growth stimulators. Objects such as magnetic tapes, credit cards, and analog watches may also be affected and should therefore be kept outside the **10 Gauss line** as shown above.

(3) Torquing of Metallic Objects

The third safety concern involves metallic objects such as surgical clips located inside or on the patient's body and their interaction with the static field. The magnetic field may cause torquing or a twisting movement of the object and damage to the tissue surrounding the surgical site.

The most important contraindication in this category is for patients with intracranial aneurysm clips. Various aneurysm clips have been shown to exhibit torquing when exposed to the static magnetic field used in MRI. Aneurysm clips would be considered a contraindication unless the exact type is known and has been proven to be nonferro-magnetic.*

Caution is recommended for all patients with recent placement of surgical clips. Stapedial replacement prostheses may be considered a contraindication. Patients with metallic foreign objects such as bullets, shrapnel and especially intraocular metallic objects must be carefully screened. Conventional screening radiographs may be indicated.

(4) Local Heating of Tissues and Metallic Objects

A fourth area of concern is with local heating of tissues and large metallic objects inside the patient's body. The RF pulses that pass through the patient's body cause tissue heating. This heating is measured in W/kg (watts per kilogram) and is referred to as the **SAR** or specific absorption ratio. Technologists must be concerned with SAR limits although MR scanners may be equipped to regulate the parameters so that SAR limits are not exceeded. (See Fig. 25-36 on page 736.) Often the technologist must enter the patient's weight for this calculation to be made.

The amount of heat produced is dependent on the number of slices, the flip angle, the number of signal averages, the TR and the tissue type. The body is able to dispel the heat through the normal circulatory and evaporative processes. At the RF levels used in MR, no biologically detrimental tissue heating has been shown to occur.

This however, is one reason pregnant women are not routinely scanned. The increase in fetal temperature may be harmful. The effects of this for MRI have not been fully documented.

(5) Electrical Interference with Normal Functions of Nerve Cells and Muscle Fibers

Rapidly changing gradient-induced magnetic fields may cause electrical current in tissues. These may be great enough to interfere with the normal function of nerve cells and muscle fibers. Examples of this include sensations of flashes of light and ventricular fibrillation. The maximum gradient magnetic field change allowed in MR is at least ten times lower than the threshold value for fibrillation and has therefore not been considered a serious problem.

OCCUPATIONAL HAZARDS

To date there have been no documented long-term biological adverse effects for technologists working in the MRI department. As a precaution, some MRI centers have recommended that technologists who are pregnant remain outside the scan room when the gradients are pulsing. Radiobiologists continue to investigate the possibility and occurrence of adverse effects due to electromagnetic fields.

Summary: The primary concern is safety of the patient and medical personnel from dangers involving MRI due to interaction of the magnetic fields with tissues and metallic objects as described above. The absolute contraindications for patient scanning will be addressed in the following section.

PATIENT HISTORY

A thorough patient history must be obtained before scanning. When contrast is indicated, an allergy history must be obtained. A patient information form (Fig. 25-40) is given to the patient before the exam in preparation for the upcoming questions. The patient is questioned regarding surgical, accidental and occupational histories. If an implant is unknown, the exam may have to be delayed until an exact description can be obtained. Conventional radiographs may also need to be obtained first. Many limb prostheses are magnetic and must be removed before entering the scanning room. They may turn into projectiles. Permanent eye-liner and other types of eye makeup may contain metallic fragments and can cause discomfort.

MR Information Form

You have been referred to the Magnetic Resonance Imaging Center for an examination which your physician feels may provide useful diagnostic information about your physical condition. Magnetic resonance (MR) imaging is a technique which will provide pictures of the interior of your body. This examination consists of placing you inside a large magnet. Radio signals will be transmitted into your body. This will cause your body to emit weak radio signals which are picked up by an antenna and formed into a picture or image by a computer. The examination will take about an hour. The only discomfort will be from lying still in the confined center of the magnet for a length of time, and the examination is rather noisy.

Examining you could be hazardous if you have certain metal in your body from either surgery or an accident.

Please inform us if you have any of the following:

- *Cardiac pacemaker*
- *Electronic implant*
- *Aneurysm clip in the brain*
- *Inner ear surgery*
- *Metallic fragments*
- *Metal in and/or removed from your eye(s)*
- *Eye prostheses*
- *Pregnancy*

Nothing should enter the examination room that can be attracted to a magnet. You may or may not receive an injection of a contrast agent to improve the diagnostic capability of the examination. This agent is injected into one of your veins. Most patients experience no unusual effects from this injection.

Your radiologist will be happy to answer any specific questions you may have about the procedure, either before or at the time of the study.

At this time, please empty all of your pockets and remove your watch, earrings, necklaces, chains, and anything in your hair which contains metal. You may be asked to change into a hospital gown.

*Your name:*____________________ *Your weight:* ______

Fig. 25-40. Sample patient information form.
(Courtesy of University of Iowa Hospitals and Clinics)

*Heiken, Jay P.; Brown, Jeffery J.; *Manual of Clinical Magnetic Resonance Imaging*, 2nd ed.; Raven Press; 1991.

Contraindications

There are certain absolute contraindications to patient MR scanning, as shown in Fig. 25-41. Although not an absolute contraindication, pregnancy is also often considered a contraindication. When an MRI examination is indicated with pregnancy, an informed consent should be obtained and clinically documented.

Absolute Contraindications to MRI*
• Pacemakers
• Ferromagnetic aneurysm clips
• Metallic fragments in the eye
• Cochlear implants
• Starr-Edwards pre-6000 model prosthetic heart valve
• Internal drug infusion pumps
• Neurostimulators
• Bone-growth stimulators

Fig. 25-41. Absolute contraindications.

PATIENT PREPARATION

Each person involved in patient scheduling and preparation plays a key role in a successful MR exam. A brief form or brochure explaining the exam may be given when the appointment is scheduled (Fig. 25-42). Gaining the patient's confidence is a major concern because the more relaxed and comfortable the patient is, the more likely a successful exam. Sufficient time must be allowed to inquire about the patient's history, explain the exam in detail, remove all metal and assure that the patient is comfortable. Information to be included when preparing a patient for an MR scan may include explanations of the following:

1. A description about the MR scanner.
2. The importance of lying still.
3. The knocking sound they will hear.
4. The length of time a sequence will last.
5. The two-way communication system and the monitoring that will take place.
6. The lack of ionizing radiation.
7. The importance of removing all metal.

Certain pulse sequences generate a high-volume knocking noise that is associated with the gradient usage. The patient must be informed of this and ear protection may be required during these sequences.

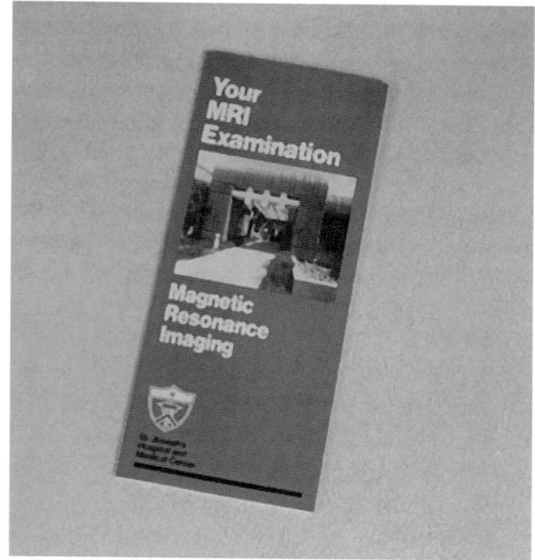

Fig. 25-42. Patient information brochure.
(Courtesy of St. Joseph's Hospital and Medical Center)

Relieving Patient Anxiety

The aperture or bore of the magnet (gantry) into which the patient is positioned on the scanning couch or table for MR imaging is shown in Fig. 25-43. This may be a rather narrow and confining space and some patients with claustrophobic tendencies may become anxious or even alarmed by this. There is some controversy over whether to tell the patient they may experience claustrophobia but in general it is considered better to not mention the potential for claustrophobia. The MR technologist, however, must be prepared if the patient mentions claustrophobia, in which case, steps can be taken to ensure the patient has as little anxiety as possible. Claustrophobia may occur quite spontaneously once the patient is in the magnet. The following options may be used to reduce anxiety and gain a successful examination:

(1) Music and relaxation techniques. Have the patient close his/her eyes and think of something pleasant.
(2) Move the patient slowly into the magnet.
(3) Allow a family member in the room during the exam. The family member can hold the patient's foot or hand reminding the patient that the scanner is open on both ends.

In some situations sedation may be required. The type of sedation and contraindications vary depending on department routines. The patient must be closely monitored if sedated and must not be allowed to travel home alone following sedation.

Summary: The major concerns in preparing a patient for an MRI examination are:

(1) Screening for contraindications.
(2) Explaining the exam, (reducing patient anxiety and fear).
(3) Removing all metal.
(4) Assuring patient comfort.

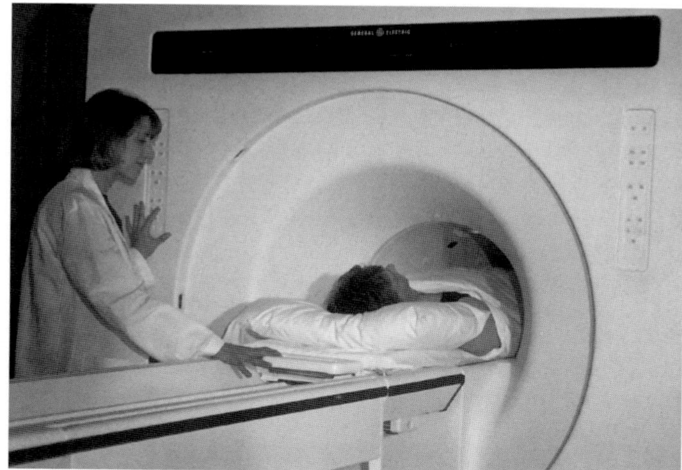

Fig. 25-43. Relieving patient anxiety (claustrophobia may occur).
(Courtesy of University of Iowa Hospitals and Clinics)

*Shellock, F.G.; Crues JV; Safety Consideration in Magnetic Resonance Imaging; *MRI Decisions*; 2:25;1988.

Patient Monitoring

Monitoring of the patient may require frequent reassurance during the scan or during the breaks between pulse sequences. If reassurance is given during the examination, the patient must be reminded to not move or talk during data acquisition.

Monitoring of the sedated patient is difficult due to the length of the bore of the magnet. The key concerns are whether the patient is breathing and whether they have enough oxygen. Observing respirations is generally sufficient to ensure breathing but a pulse oximeter may be used to ascertain whether there is adequate exchange of 0_2 and $C0_2$. Magnetic field and RF interference can cause problems in the operation of such monitoring equipment and therefore present some limitations.

Contrast Agents

Contrast agents have become increasingly popular for MR examinations. The contrast agent that is most popular is **Gadolinium-DTPA (Gd-DTPA).**[†] It is currently given in a dose of .2 ml/kg with the injection rate not to exceed 10 ml/min. The injection may be followed by a saline flush. The patient may experience a sensation at the injection site and should be observed during and after the injection for possible reaction. Gd-DTPA has lower toxicity and has fewer side effects than iodinated contrast.

After injection, a sufficient level of contrast remains in the system for approximately 60 minutes, which allows a great deal of latitude in scan time. The major route of excretion is through the kidneys, therefore renal failure would be a contraindication for its use. Pregnancy may also be a contraindication for the use of Gd-DTPA.

Gd-DTPA is considered a **paramagnetic agent** and **shortens the Tl and T2 relaxation time of water protons.** Overall Gd-DTPA quickens the rate at which water protons align with the main magnetic field. This results in greater MR signal and higher contrast, especially in areas where gadolinium crosses the blood-brain barrier (BBB). (The blood-brain barrier is the selective barrier separating the blood from the parenchyma of the central nervous system.) The contrast agent remains confined intravascularly for a period of time unless the BBB has been damaged by pathologic processes. Gd-DTPA is generally used with Tl-weighted pulse sequences.

Gd-DTPA improves visualization of small tumors and tumors of isointensity with normal brain. The most frequent use of Gd-DTPA is in evaluation of the central nervous system. Gd-DTPA is useful for evaluation of **meningionas**, **acoustic neuroma**, **Schwannomas**, **chordomas** and **pituitary tumors.** (See end of chapter for definitions.)

This contrast medium often helps identify primary disease (tumor) from secondary effects (edema). Further, it helps in the evaluation of metastasis, infection, inflammatory processes and subacute cerebral infarcts. In the spine, Gd-DTPA increases sensitivity in detecting primary and secondary tumors and can help differentiate scarring from recurrent disk disease in the postoperative spine.

Contrast use may become increasingly important in abdominal, thoracic and limb (extremity) imaging. At the present time, Gd-DTPA has been FDA approved for evaluation of the brain and CNS. It is likely that approval will also be granted for evaluation of other areas of the body besides the CNS in the future. Oral contrast agents are still under investigation but have been used with limited success in research trials.

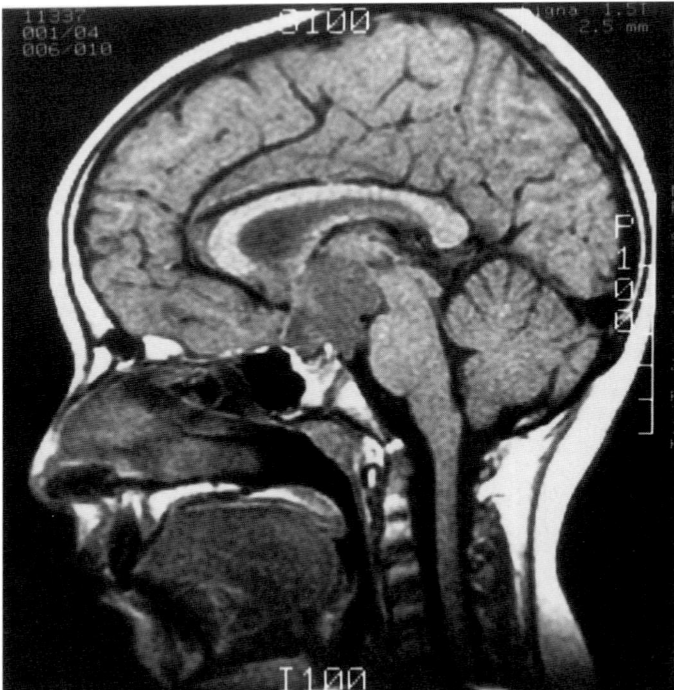

Fig. 25-44. Without contrast agent (T1-weighted image). (Pathology appears gray).

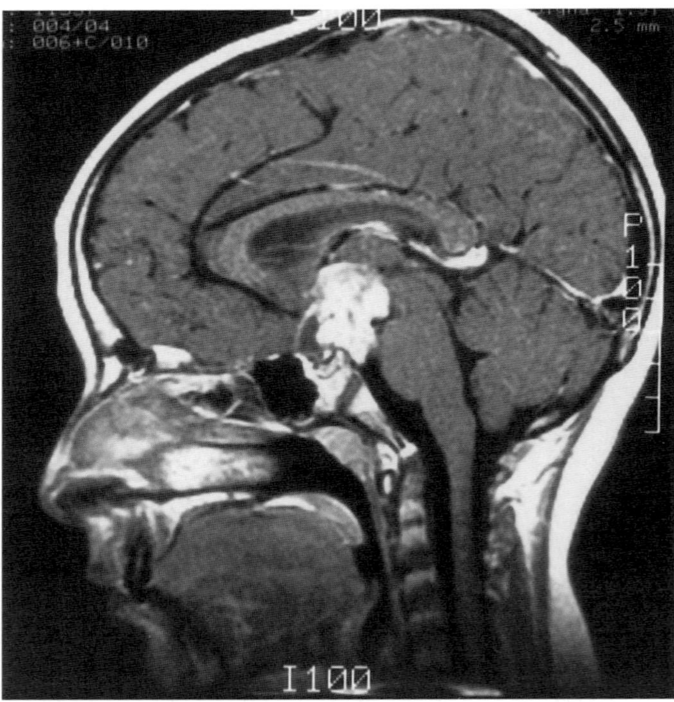

Fig. 25-45. With contrast agent, Gd-DTPA (T1-weighted image). (Pathology appears as "bright" areas in central brain.)

*Runge, Val, Clinical Magnetic Resonance Imaging; JB Lippincott Co. 1990; pp 506-507.

†Gadolinium *(gad″ o-lin′ e-um)*–A rare element which is metallic and very magnetic; symbol, Gd- DTPA (Diethylene-Triaminepentaacetic Acid).

POSITIONING CONSIDERATIONS AND COIL SELECTION

The patient lies in the bore of the magnet in the supine, prone, oblique or decubitus position. In most situations, the patient is supine with the anatomy of interest centered to the RF coil. The distinction between types of RF coils varies between manufacturers, but three of the most frequently used coil designs are the (1) **circumferential whole-body coils**, (2) **surface coils** and (3) **phased array coils**. Each of these three coil designs is described below.

Care must be taken when placing the coils. For safety reasons, the coil must be connected properly and the lines not looped as they extend from the magnet. This reduces the chance of electric "arcing" of sparks that may burn the patient.

Attention must be given to the orientation of the surface coil relative to the transmit coil. No signal will be detected unless the receiving coil **is perpendicular to the magnetic field established by the transmitter coil**. A slight tilt can result in significant loss of signal. For a superconductive system, the coil can be placed coronal or sagittal to the main magnetic field.

(1) Circumferential Whole-volume

Three of the more common circumferential whole-volume coils that surround the part being imaged are the **body coil**, the **head coil**, the **limb** (extremity or knee) **coil** and the **volume neck coil**.

The performance of an RF coil is largely determined by its filling factor, which reflects the ratio of the total coil volume to the volume of the anatomic region within the coil.

S/N ratio is enhanced by selecting a coil that most closely approximates the size of the anatomic region being studied. Therefore, smaller surface coils are sometimes chosen over the whole-volume coils for small volume imaging.*

(2) Surface Coils

Surface coils are placed directly on the body part being imaged. The greatest SNR (signal-noise-ratio) is obtained near the surface of the structure to which the coil is applied, with a fall-off in signal occurring with increasing distance from the coil.* The anatomy of interest should be centered to the middle of the coil and the coil must be kept still during data acquisition. The main advantage of surface coils is the increase in SNR. The main disadvantage is the limited field of view.

(3) Phased Array Coils

These coils consist of up to six coils and receivers which are grouped together. Each coil is independent of the other and has its own receiver and memory board. When the coils are linked together, longer areas of anatomy can be imaged without penalty of signal being received from other parts of the body. Because of this design, a large field of view coverage is possible (i.e., the entire spine) and can be obtained with the SNR comparable to that from a single coil. There is no increase in imaging time because the signal output from each coil is acquired separately within one sequence, not multiple sequences. The information is processed to form an image that represents one single larger field of view.

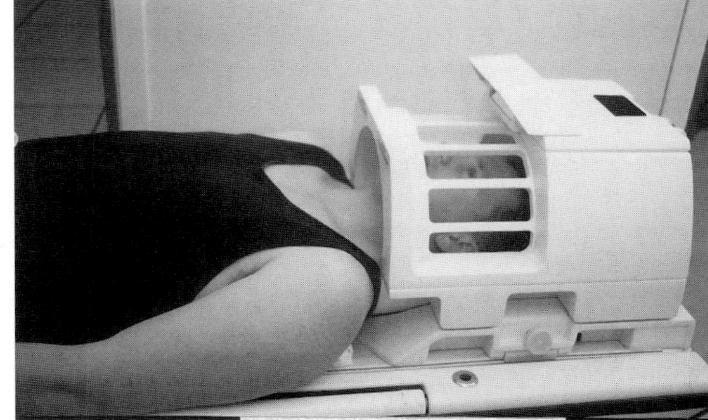

Fig. 25-46. Head coil in place.

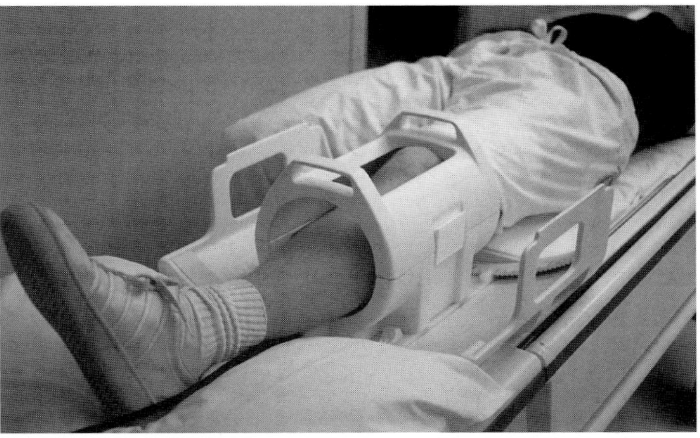

Fig. 25-47. Knee coil in place.

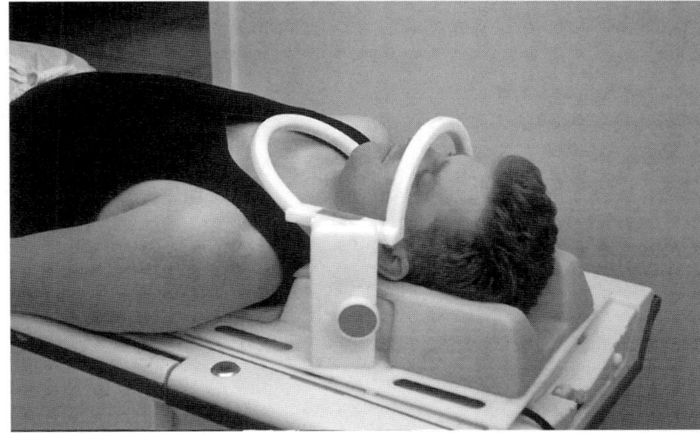

Fig. 25-48. Volume neck coil in place.

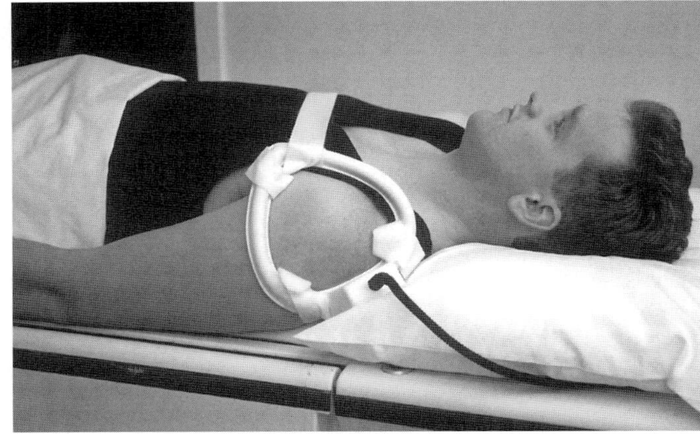

Fig. 25-49. Shoulder coil in place (surface coil).

*Heiken, Jay P.; Brown, Jeffery J.; *Manual of Clinical Magnetic Resonance Imaging*, 2nd Ed.; Raven Press; 1991.

IMAGING PARAMETERS

The MR imaging system employs many technical factors that must be considered, understood and sometimes modified at the control panel during the course of the examination. Many scanners allow these factors to be programmed into a protocol similar to CT protocol's programming. Pulse sequence parameters are designed to suppress artifacts and optimize the diagnostic quality of the specific anatomy and pathology.

The process of choosing parameters involves considerably more than selection of TR and TE. The initial decision also involves the **type of pulse sequence** to be used such as spin-echo, gradient echo or inversion recovery. Besides the type of pulse sequence, the other operator-dependent choices include **matrix size, slice thickness, interslice gap, field of view, number of data acquisitions, RF flip angle, coil selection, single or multiple slice acquisition, multislice position** and **multislice excitation order**. These factors allow the examination to be tailored for a particular area of interest and abnormality. Many of these factors are interrelated individually as well as collectively. These relationships have an impact on the S/N ratio, contrast, spatial resolution and artifact production. These factors affect imaging time, which in turn affects patient cooperation and management of scheduling.*

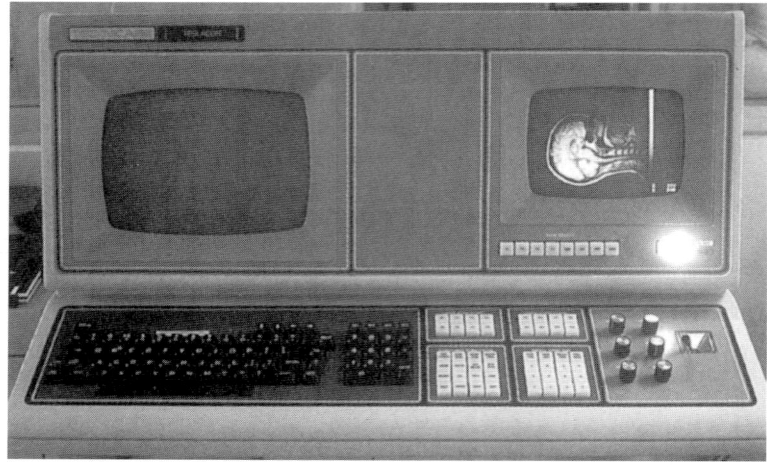

Fig. 25-50. Control panel and display station.

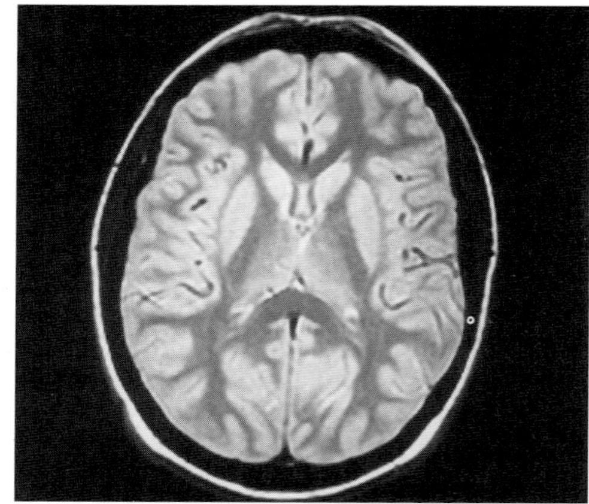

Fig. 25-51. Proton density image.

Subject Contrast

The contrast in MR arises from the relationship of operator-dependent options previously discussed and tissue factors including proton density, Tl and T2 relaxation times and tissue motion such as flow of CSF and blood. These tissue factors depend on the biochemistry of the tissue. By choosing certain pulse sequences, images can be produced that emphasize these tissue factors and allow visualization of the contrast seen in MR images.

Proton Density (Spin-Density) Images

A pulse sequence using a combination of long TR and short TE (TR 2000 ms and TE 20-30 ms) produces images with contrast resulting from the **proton density** (sometimes referred to as spin density), with the contrast effects due to Tl and T2 relaxation having been decreased. Since Tl and T2 have been suppressed, pathology that can be demonstrated by the change in Tl and T2 relaxation times may be invisible on an image produced in this manner. The use of pulse sequences with varying amounts of Tl and T2 weighting help to identify anatomy and pathology.

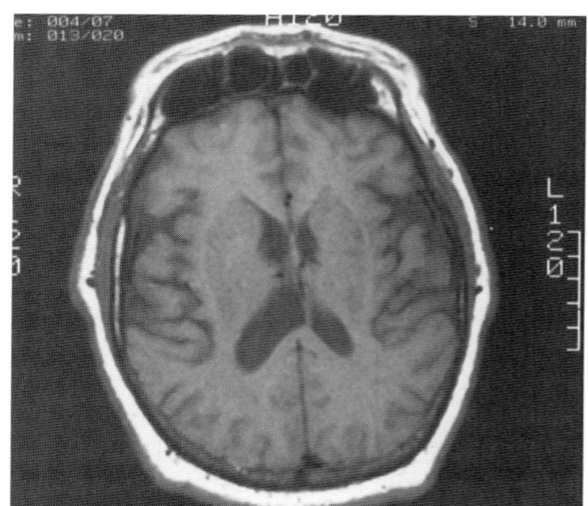

Fig. 25-52. T1-weighted image.

T1-Weighted Images

In order to maximize the difference in signal intensity based on Tl relaxation times, the TR in the pulse sequence is shortened. **A short TR, short TE sequence produces a Tl-weighted image** (TR 350-800 ms and TE of 30 ms or less). This allows structures with short T1 relaxation times to be bright (fat, proteinogenous fluids, subacute blood) and structures with long Tl to be dark (neoplasm, edema, inflammation, pure fluid, CSF). One aspect to remember with Tl-weighted imaging is that as the TR is shortened, the overall signal to noise decreases.

T2-Weighted Images

T2-weighted imaging employs a long TR and long TE pulse sequence (TR 2000 ms and TE 60-80 ms). As the TE is lengthened the T2 contrast increases; however, the overall signal to noise decreases. The structures on a T2-weighted image will show contrast reversal from the structures on the Tl-weighted image.

Structures with long T2 appear bright (neoplasm, edema, inflammation, pure fluid, CSF). Structures with short T2 appear dark (structures with iron such as blood breakdown products).

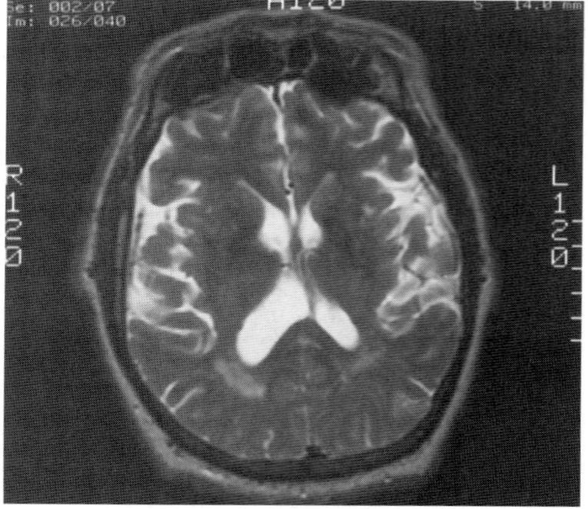

Fig. 25-53. T2-weighted image.

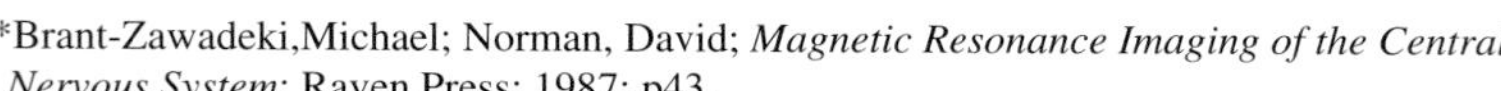

*Brant-Zawadeki,Michael; Norman, David; *Magnetic Resonance Imaging of the Central Nervous System*; Raven Press; 1987; p43.

Summary of T1 and T 2-Weighted Images

Although T1 and T2 relaxation occur simultaneously, they are independent of each other. The T1 of most biological tissue is in the range of 200 to 2000 msec. The T2 relaxation in most tissues fall in the 20 to 300 msec range, although water has a T2 in the range of 2000 msec. (See Fig. 25-54.)

Notice that the T1 is greater than or equal to the T2 relaxation times for any given tissue. The pulse sequences are generally chosen to accentuate the difference between the relaxation times of different tissues. Contrast between tissues is achieved in the final MR image by accentuating these differences. However, regardless of how the pulse sequence is changed, if there are few mobile hydrogen protons (as is the case for cortical bone and air), the image will be black.

Motion Reduction Techniques

MRI software techniques can reduce or eliminate problems related to involuntary motion and flow, or in some cases like MR angiography, enhance anatomy where flow is present. When motion causes problems that result in signal alterations, these signal alterations are referred to as **motion artifacts**.

Software methods that compensate for artifacts related to motion and flow are available, however, they usually require a trade-off of longer imaging times. These techniques include **signal averaging**, **reordered phase encoding**, **gradient moment nulling** and **presaturation**. (See definition of terms at end of chapter.) These techniques may be used individually or in combination.

The other technique used to reduce problems related to motion is **physiologic gating.** One type, **respiratory gating,** employs bellows placed around the patient's chest. These are used either to trigger data acquisition by the patient's respirations or only to accept data acquired during a certain phase of the respiratory cycle. Pulsatile arterial flow (motion related to cardiac movement) and CSF pulsations can be reduced by synchronizing the MR sequence with the cardiac cycle. This is called **cardiac gating**.

Rapid Imaging Techniques

Rapid imaging techniques continue to develop. The most widely used rapid imaging techniques are **gradient echo imaging** and **fast spin echo**.

The **gradient echo technique** uses a single RF excitation pulse (10° to 90°) and the echo is produced by reversal of the magnetic field gradient rather than a 180° RF pulse used in conventional spin echo imaging. This technique allows variations in the pulse sequence and can be manipulated to achieve T1, T2, and proton density weighting.

The **spin echo technique** has continued to develop and continues to gain in popularity. It is similar to the spin echo pulse sequence but has considerably shorter scan times. In fast spin echo, the scan time is reduced by performing more than one phase encoding step per TR and thus the data is acquired in less time. The scan time reduction is proportional to the number of phase encoding steps performed during the TR. The contrast is similar to conventional spin echo acquisitions, however fat remains bright on T2 weighted images. This is often compensated for by adding fat suppression techniques

Echo planar imaging is currently being introduced as a new method for extremely fast MR imaging.

The major advantages of rapid imaging techniques are rapid acquisition time, reduced SAR, and motion artifact. These sequences allow acquisition of data during breathholding. The use of rapid imaging techniques is likely to continue to increase as techniques are further developed. The main disadvantages are low S/N ratio and an increase in other types of artifacts (besides motion artifact).

Comparison of Representative Proton Density

Tissue	*Proton density*	*T1 (msec)*	*T2 (msec)*
CSF	10.8	2000	250
Gray matter	10.5	475	118
White matter	11.0	300	133
Fat	10.9	150	150
Muscle	11.0	450	64
Liver	10.0	250	44

Fig. 25-54. Comparison of representative proton density, T1 and T2 values for various tissue types at midfield strength.*

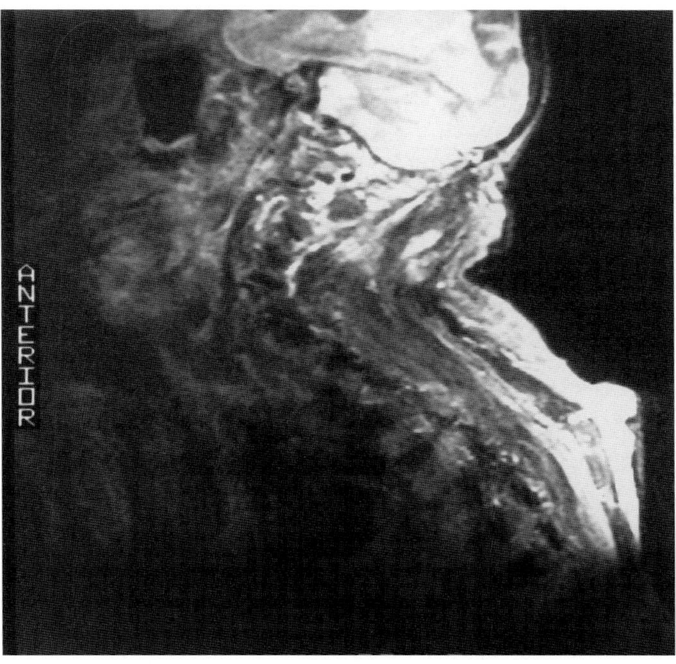

Fig. 25-55. MRI image with motion artifacts (sagittal C-spine, image quality severely degraded due to patient movement during data acquisition).

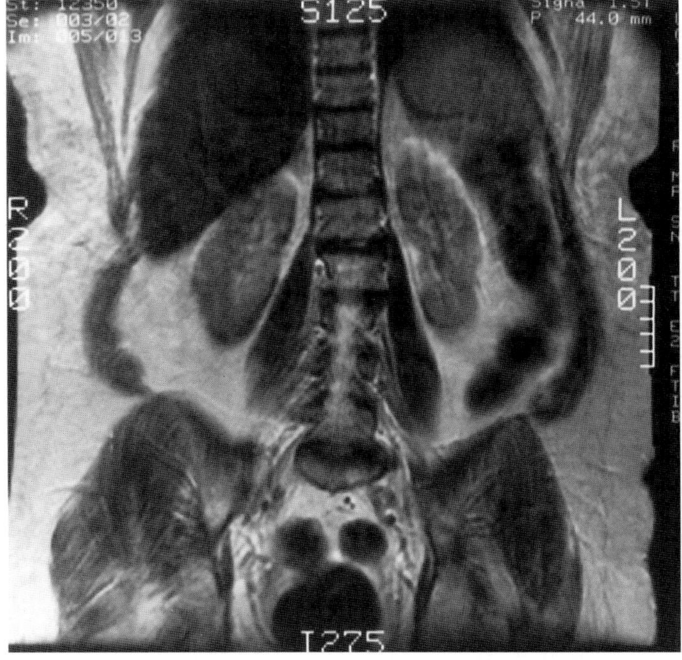

Fig. 25-56. Rapid imaging techniques (coronal section of abdomen using rapid data acquisition technique).

*Lufkin, Robert B.; *The MRI Manual*; Mosby Year Book; 1990; p 24.

MRI Examinations

The more common MRI examinations and guidelines for imaging will be described and discussed. There is an increasing number of software choices that are selected depending upon the patient and pathologic considerations. Both T1 and T2-weighted images are acquired, allowing for a complete examination and diagnosis. The main goal is **good quality images in an acceptable time limit**. When choosing software options, attention is given so that the scan time, resolution, S/N, and number of slices are within acceptable limits.

In all examinations, careful attention to patient comfort and to the positioning of the part with the magnet is of utmost importance.

The high cost of MR equipment requires that constant attention is given to efficient scheduling of patient exams. By choosing parameters carefully, positioning the patient accurately and maintaining patient comfort, the goal of good quality images within the scheduled time limit, usually 1 hour or less, can be achieved.

Brain imaging
Routine sections
- Sagittal
- Coronal
- Axial

Spine imaging
Routine sections
- Sagittal
- Axial

Limb and joint imaging
Routine sections
- Sagittal
- Coronal
- Axial

Cardiovascular system imaging
Routine sections
- Sagittal
- Coronal
- Axial
- Obliques

Abdomen and pelvis imaging
Routine sections
- Sagittal
- Coronal
- Axial

Angiography
- Time of flight method
- Phase contrast method
  –2D images
  –3D images

Brain Imaging

Brain imaging
Routine sections
• **Sagittal**
• **Coronal**
• **Axial**

Structures Best Shown

Gray matter, white matter, nerve tissue, basal ganglia, ventricles, brain stem.

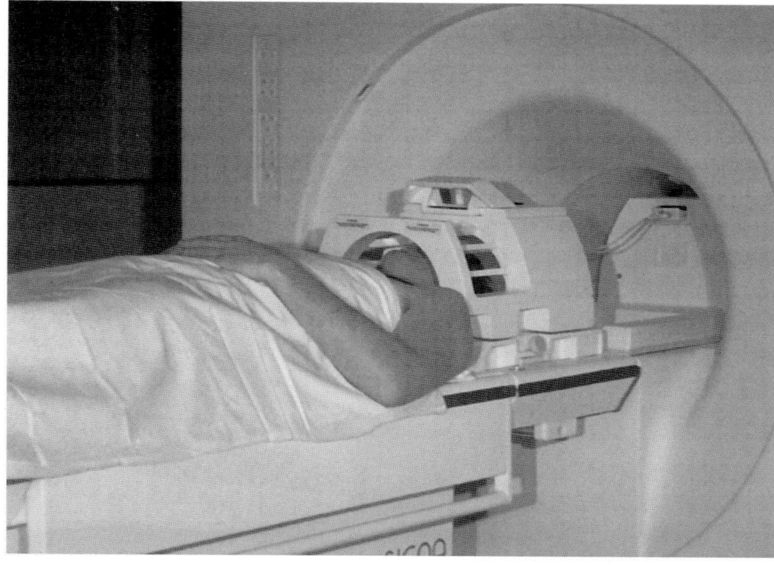

Fig. 25-57. Patient positioned in head coil (patient and coil will be moved into magnet center).

Pathology Demonstrated

White matter disease, especially multiple sclerosis and other demyelinating disorders, neoplasm, infectious diseases including those associated with AIDS and herpes, hemorrhagic disorders, CVA and ischemic disorders

Contrast Agent

- Gd-DTPA with T1-weighted images. Gd-DTPA has been proven to aid in the diagnosis for a large number of different brain abnormalities.

Technical Factors

- Standard head coil
- Surface coils are used for smaller anatomical regions such as for an orbit or TMJ study.
- T 1-weighted sequence
- T 2-weighted sequence

Part Position

- Patient supine, head first.
- Head rests comfortably in head coil.
- Head and coil centered to the main magnet.

T1-Weighted Images: T1-weighted images are used to demonstrate anatomic structure. Gd-DTPA T1-weighted studies are best utilized to improve detection and to characterize lesions identified on T1 and T2-weighted images.

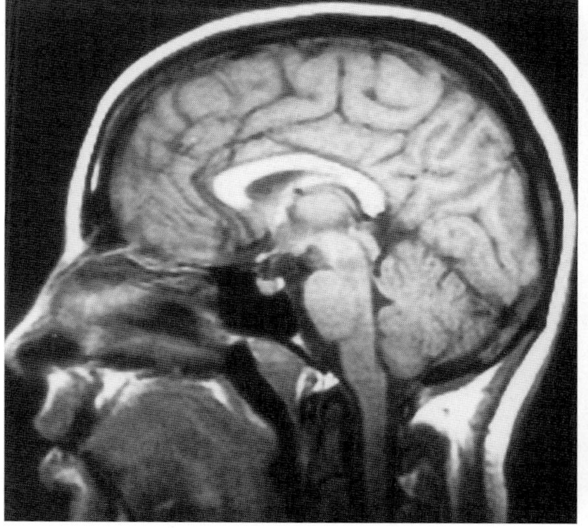

Fig. 25-58. Sagittal section (T1).

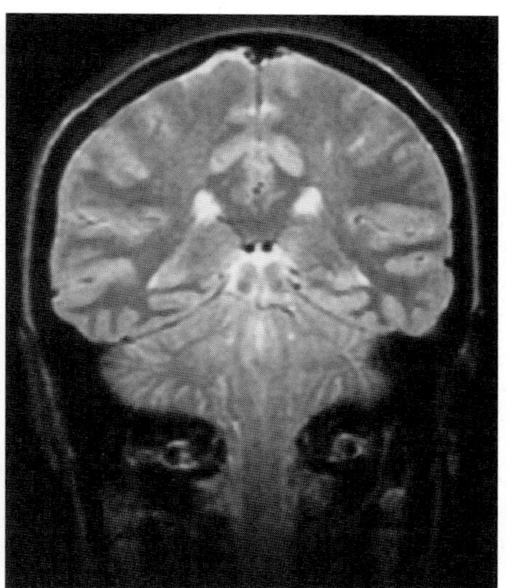

Fig. 25-59. Coronal section (T2).

T2-Weighted Images: T2-weighted images are effective in demonstrating pathology and the edema that is associated with the abnormality. Conditions demonstrated on T2-weighted image include infarction, trauma, inflammation, degeneration, neoplasm and bleeding.

Comparisons with CT: MRI has proven to have superior soft tissue contrast resolution, multi-planar imaging capabilities and no ionizing radiation as compared to CT. MRI is superior to CT in imaging of the posterior fossa and brain stem due to the lack of bone artifact, and in detecting small changes in tissue water content.

In cases where small calcifications are important to identify, CT is chosen over MRI because MRI is generally insensitive to small calcification. CT and conventional radiographs have remained the study of choice for brain imaging to diagnose fractures of the calvarium. The very ill patient with monitoring and life support equipment is often imaged in CT as is the trauma patient. This is due to the faster exam time, tolerance to patient motion, ability to monitor the patient adequately, the ability to show acute blood and fractures and the physical components of life support equipment.

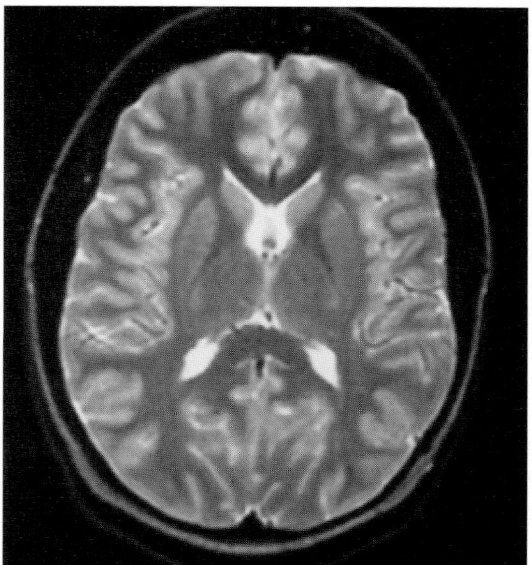

Fig. 25-60. Axial section (T2).

Spine Imaging

Spine imaging
Routine sections
- Sagittal
- Axial

Structures Best Shown

Spinal cord, nerve tissue, intervertebral disks, marrow, facet joint spaces, basivertebral vein, ligamentus flavum.

Pathology Demonstrated

Disk herniation and degeneration, bone and bone marrow changes, neoplasm, inflammatory and demyelinating disease, and congenital and developmental abnormalities.

Contrast Agent

- Gd-DTPA with T1-weighted.
- These images are acquired through the abnormal area. Gd-DTPA enhances tumors and is useful post-operatively to help differentiate scarring from recurrent disk disease.

Technical Factors

- ***C Spine:*** Planar, contour or quadrature surface coil
- ***T/L Spine:*** Planar surface coil (see arrows).
- T1-weighted sequence
- T2-weighted sequence
- Cardiac gating (when myelopathy is suspected)

Part Position

- Patient supine, head first for C spine, head or feet first for T spine and feet first for L spine.
- Anatomy of interest centered to the surface coil.
- Surface coil and patient centered to the main magnet.

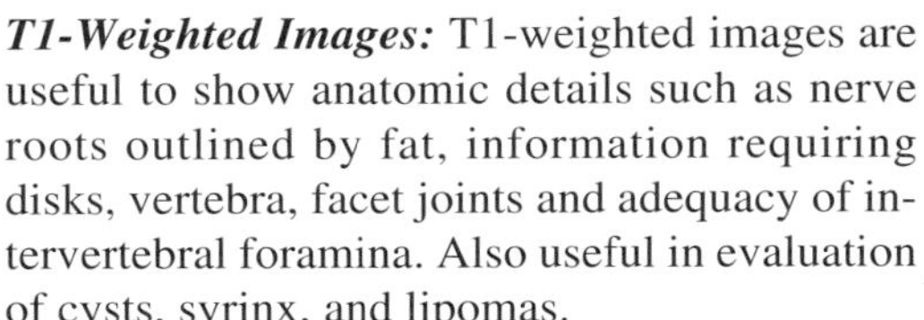

T1-Weighted Images: T1-weighted images are useful to show anatomic details such as nerve roots outlined by fat, information requiring disks, vertebra, facet joints and adequacy of intervertebral foramina. Also useful in evaluation of cysts, syrinx, and lipomas.

T2-Weighted Images: T2-weighted images are required in the evaluation of disk disease, cord abnormalities, tumor, and inflammatory changes. Gradient Echo (GE) or spin-echo images utilizing T2-weighting produce a myelographic effect showing sharp contrast between cord and CSF.

Comparison with CT: The major advantages of MR over CT are that it does not require the use of intrathecal (within a sheath) contrast material to evaluate the spinal cord and subarachnoid space, and it covers large areas of the spine in a single sagittal view. CT remains essential for evaluation of significant spinal trauma.

Even though the need for myelography has decreased, it is still useful in selected cases. Myelography combined with CT is useful when patient motion or severe scoliosis renders MR suboptimal.

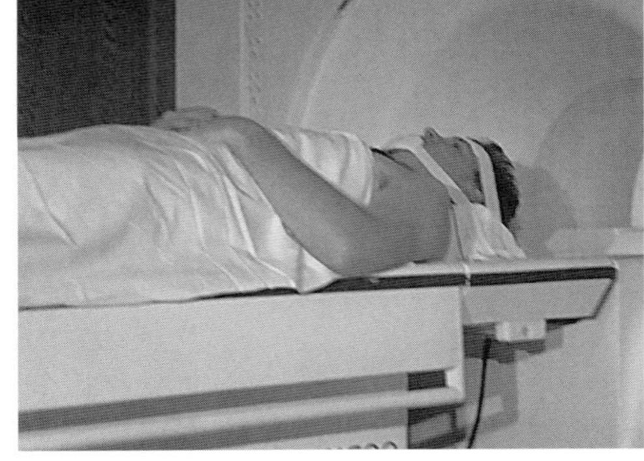

Fig. 25-61. Cervical spine (posterior C spine coil in place, will be moved to magnet center).

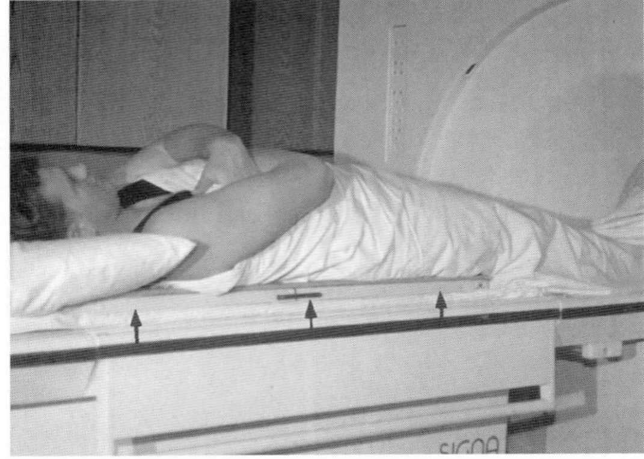

Fig. 25-62. Lumbar spine (planar surface coil under patient, will be moved to magnet center).

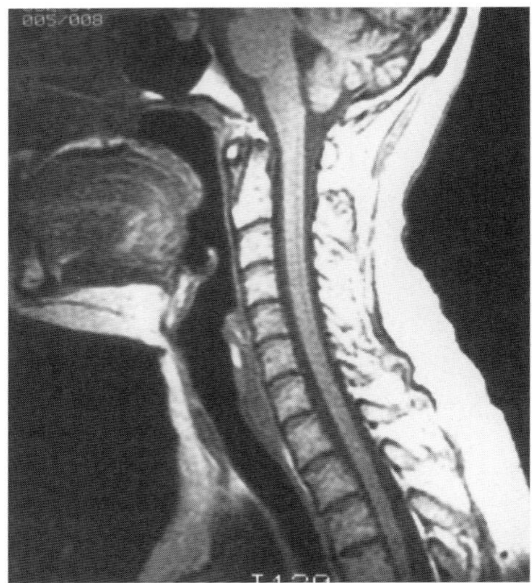

Fig. 25-63. C spine–Sagittal section (T1).

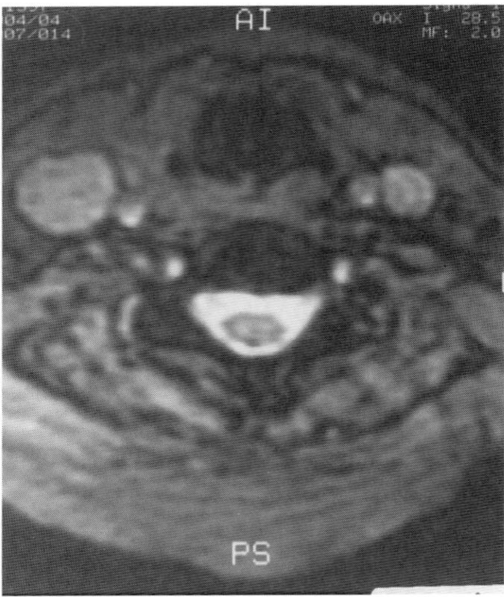

Fig. 25-64. C spine–Axial section (T1).

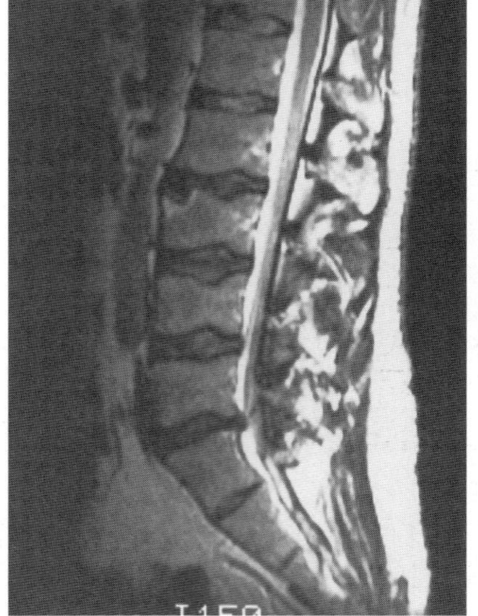

Fig. 25-65. L spine–Sagittal section (T2).

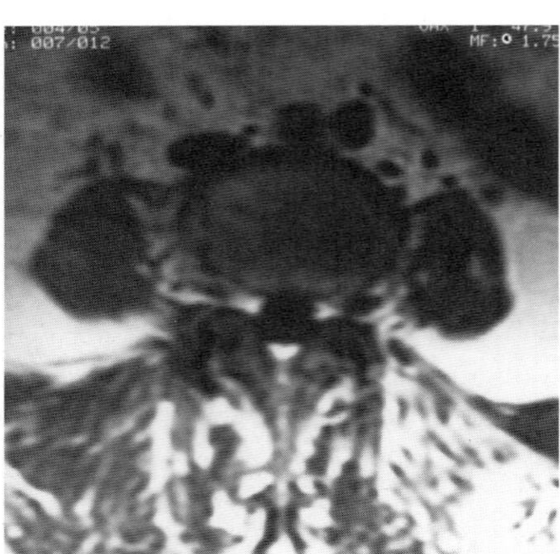

Fig. 25-66. L spine–Axial section (T1).

Joint or Limb Imaging

Limb and joint imaging
Routine sections
- Sagittal
- Coronal
- Axial

Structures Best Shown

Fat, muscles, ligaments, tendons, nerves, blood vessels, marrow.

Pathology Demonstrated

Bone marrow disorders, soft tissue tumors, osteonecrosis, ligament and tendon tears.

Technical Factors

- Limb (extremity) surface coils
- T1-weighted sequence
- T2-weighted sequence
- If the region of interest is fairly deep, then a coil that surrounds the object is chosen. If the structure is superficial, then a coil that lies on top of the anatomy is chosen.

Part Position

- Head or feet first. (Figs. 25-67 and 25-68).
- Supine or prone as most comfortable.
- Anatomy of interest centered to the coil.
- Coil centered to main magnet.

T1-Weighted Images: T1-weighted images are useful for showing anatomic detail and for evaluating articular cartilage, ligaments and tendons. T1-weighted images are also useful in depicting osteonecrosis.

T2-Weighted Images: T2-weighted images are useful to show tumors, inflammatory changes and the edema surrounding ligament and tendon tears. T2- weighted images are also useful for bone marrow disorders, bony tumors and to show the extent of lesions in muscles.

Note: MR is an increasingly effective imaging method for the musculoskeletal system. MRI is a primary method of evaluating internal derangements of the knee, meniscal abnormalities in the TMJ, avascular necrosis, soft tissue masses and bone marrow abnormalities.* Evaluation of shoulder disorders with MRI has proved useful.

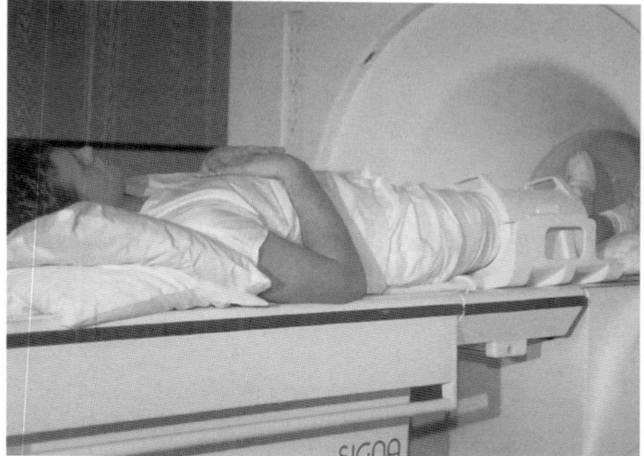
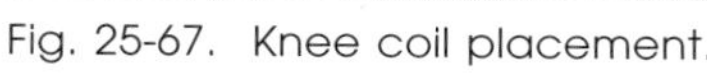

Fig. 25-67. Knee coil placement.

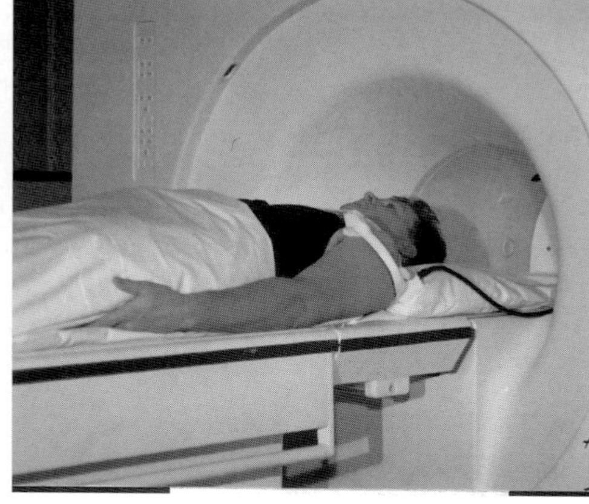

Fig. 25-68. Shoulder coil placement.
(Patient with coil in place will be moved to magnet center)

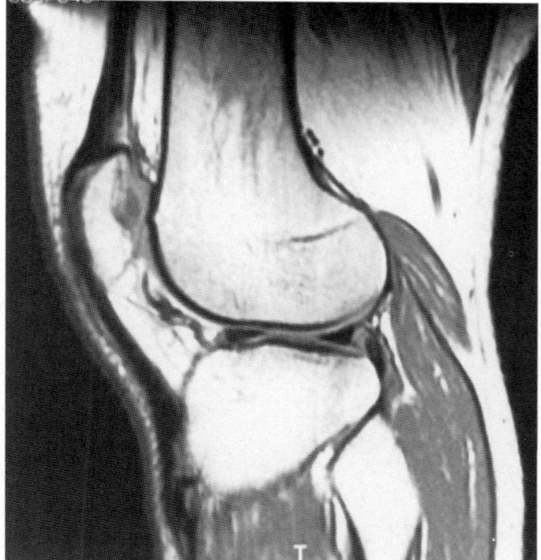

Fig. 25-69. Knee–Sagittal section (proton density).

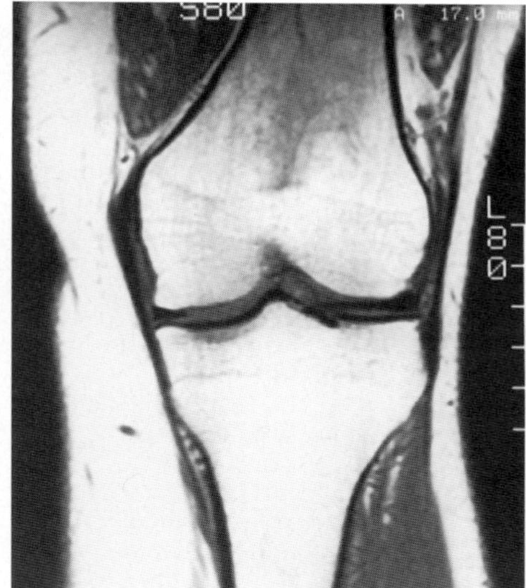

Fig. 25-70. Knee–Coronal section (T1).

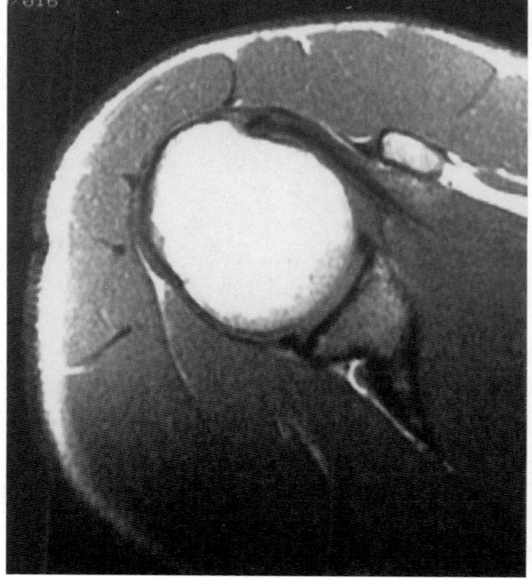

Fig. 25-71. Transaxial shoulder (T1).

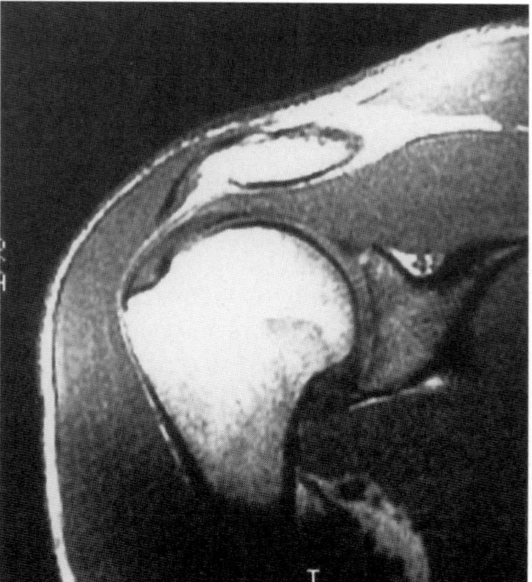

Fig. 25-72. Coronal shoulder (T1).

*Runge, Val M.; *Clinical Magnetic Resonance Imaging*; J.B.Lippincott Co.; 1990; p 403.

Cardiovascular System Imaging

Cardiovascular system imaging
Routine sections
• Sagittal
• Coronal
• Axial
• Obliques

Structures Best Shown

Great vessels, fat, myocardium, skeletal muscles, static and moving blood, valves, pericardium, coronary arteries.

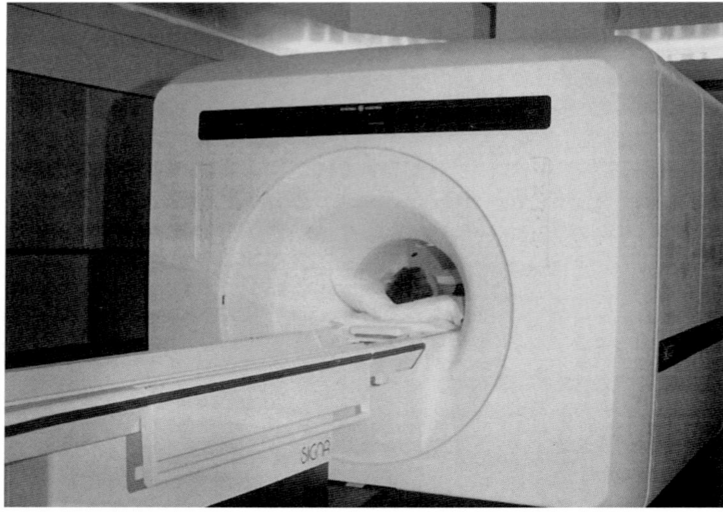

Fig. 25-73. Patient positioned for cardiovascular MRI.

PATHOLOGY DEMONSTRATED

Congenital heart disorders, graft patency, cardiac tumors, thrombi, pericardial masses, evaluation of aortic dissection and aneurysm.

Technical Factors

- Body coil
- T1-weighted sequence
- T2-weighted sequence (as needed)
- Cine (as needed)
- Gating (respiratory and cardiac)

Part Position

- Supine (or prone) feet first.
- Nipple level at magnet center.

T1-Weighted Images: T1-weighted images are useful for showing anatomic detail of the heart, great vessels and pericardium. Patent coronary artery bypass grafts, and thrombus are demonstrated with T1-weighted images.

T2-Weighted Images: T2-weighted images are useful for detection of infarction, thrombus and pericardial effusions.

Cine: Cine images allow evaluation of muscle thinning, previous infarction, wall motion and valve abnormalities. Volume measurements can be taken.

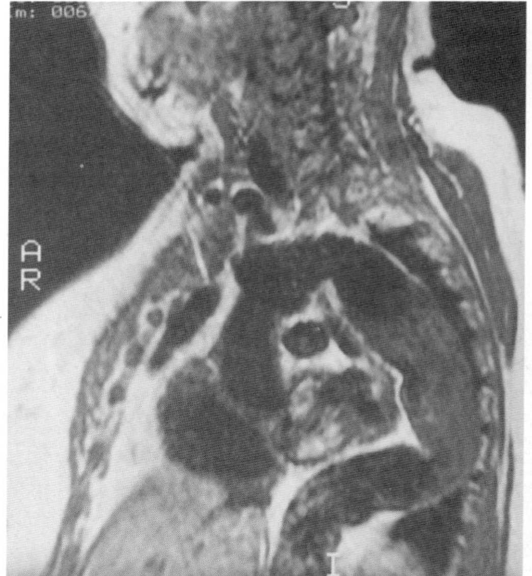

Fig. 25-74. Sagittal section (T1) (demonstrates an aortic aneurysm).

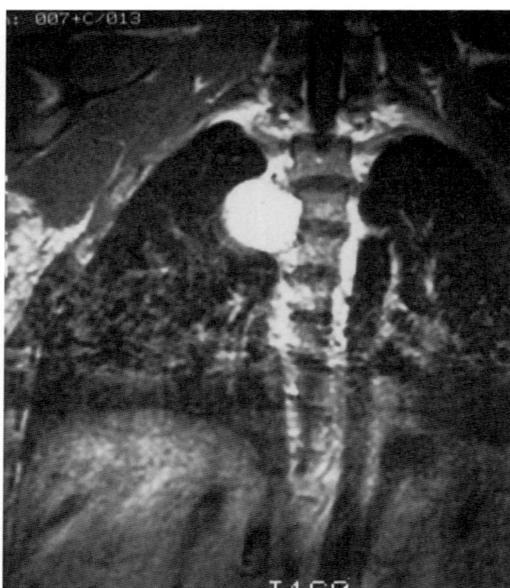
Fig. 25-75. Coronal section (T1 with GD) (aorta shown posterior to heart, paraspinal mass demonstrated).

Gating: The most widely used gating mechanism is the electrocardiogram. The heart's electrical activity bears a constant relationship to its mechanical activity. The R wave is often used to synchronize the MR sequence with the cardiac cycle. The recording of ECG is difficult due to the static and changing magnetic fields. The electrodes are placed to maximize the amplitude of the R wave. Special electrodes containing non-ferrous metals are used.

Note: MRI is unlikely to replace echocardiography but can provide a 3D view of tumors and masses, especially as to the extent of growth. MRI used as an adjunct to CT, has proven helpful in assessing mediastinal pathology and in the evaluation of aortic dissection and aneurysm. Radiographs of the thorax will continue to be used as a first tool of assessment.

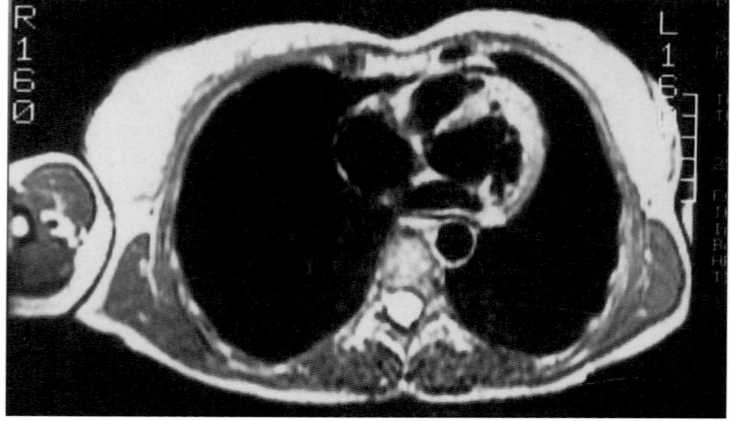

Fig. 25-76. Axial section (T2).

Note: The above sections (Figs. 25-74 to 25-76) are not on the same patient.

Abdomen and Pelvis Imaging

Abdomen and pelvis imaging
Routine sections
- Sagittal
- Coronal
- Axial

Structures Best Shown

Liver, pancreas, spleen, adrenals, gallbladder, kidney, vessels, reproductive organs.

Pathology Demonstrated

Tumor size and staging of tumors especially pediatric tumors such as neuroblastoma, and Wilm's tumor. Retroperitoneal structures and hemangioma of the liver are well demonstrated by MRI.

Pre-Exam Prep

Patients may be asked to fast or only consume clear liquids 4 hours prior to scanning. Glucagon is often administered to reduce peristalsis of the bowel.

Technical Factors

- Body coil.
- T1-weighted sequence.
- T2-weighted sequence.
- Respiratory gating.
- Breathholding in upper abdomen.
- Generally a standard body coil is utilized however, surface coils may be used for superficial structures. A transrectal coil may be used to image the prostate and reproductive organs.

Part Position

- Supine, feet first for abdomen and pelvis.
- Area of interest centered to main magnet.

T1-Weighted Images: T1-weighted images are useful for demonstrating anatomic detail. T1-weighted images also help identify tumors containing fat and hemorrhage.

T2-Weighted Images: T2-weighted images are useful to demonstrate changes in water content in the tissue associated with tumors and other abnormalities.

Notes: MRI evaluation of the abdomen has been limited due to artifacts caused by respiratory, cardiac and peristaltic motion. Lack of an acceptable oral contrast material remains a limitation in abdominal MRI. CT is still the primary method for evaluation of the liver due to motion artifacts. Sonography and CT will likely remain the imaging modality for renal cysts. MRI has proved useful in the evaluation of renal transplants.

Pelvic anatomy is well demonstrated by MRI. Ultrasound remains the screening tool for uterine, ovarian and scrotal abnormalities.

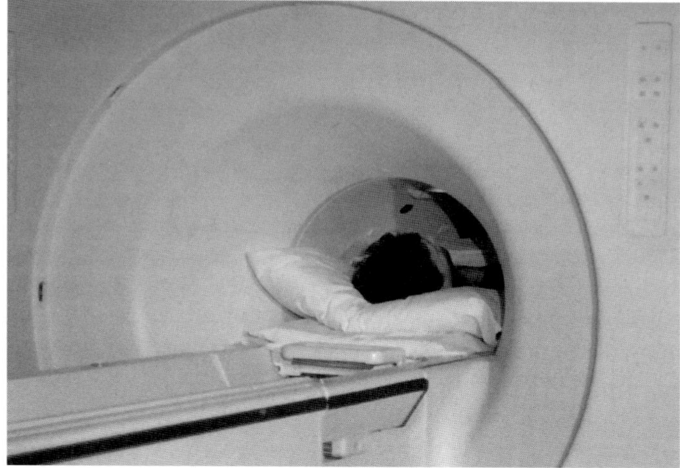

Fig. 25-77. Patient positioned for abdominal MRI.

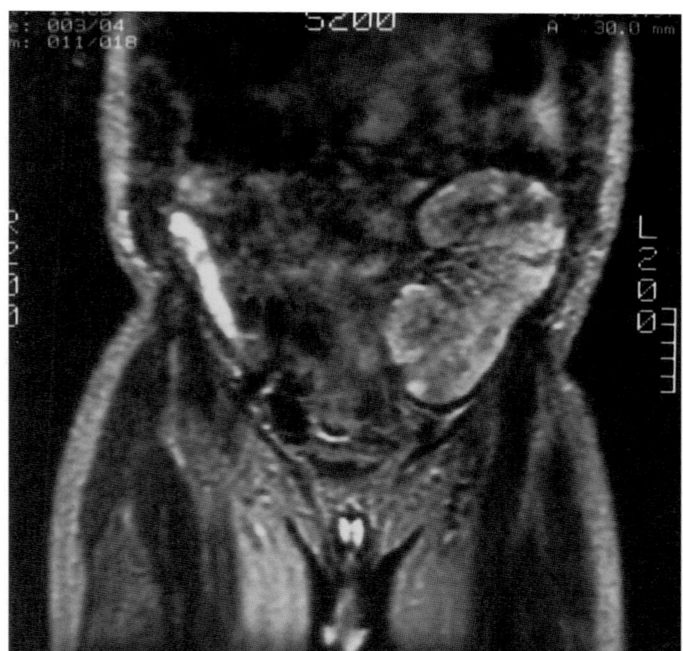

Fig. 25-78. Coronal section (T2).
(Post kidney transplant on left)

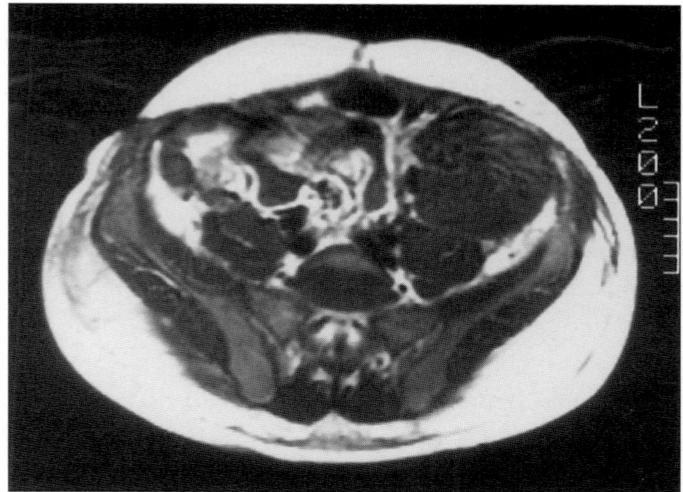

Fig. 25-79. Axial section (T1).
(Transplanted kidney on left)

Angiography

Angiography
- Time of flight method
- Phase contrast method
  - –2D images
  - –3D images

Pathology Demonstrated

Aneurysm, AVM, stenotic disease, and graft patency detection.

Angiography

MR angiography is an imaging method that exploits the physical properties of blood to generate contrast and thus allows visualization of blood vessels. These physical properties include **blood velocity**, **pulsation of blood**, **turbulent flow** or **lack of turbulent flow** and **relaxation times**. The operator-dependent choices are complex and require an understanding of hemodynamics and software options that are supplied by the manufacturer.

In general, the imaging strategies can be broken down into two fundamental approaches. They are **Time-of-Flight** (TOF) and **Phase Contrast** angiography. Further, the information can be obtained as a series of 2D images or as a 3D data set.

Time-of-Flight (TOF)

TOF angiography generally relies on the inflow of fully magnetized blood into the imaging plane. This process is described as **flow-related enhancement**. Blood that flows into the slice will not have experienced RF pulses and will therefore, appear brighter than stationary tissue. This allows themoving and stationary spins to be distinguished and thus create MR angiograms.*

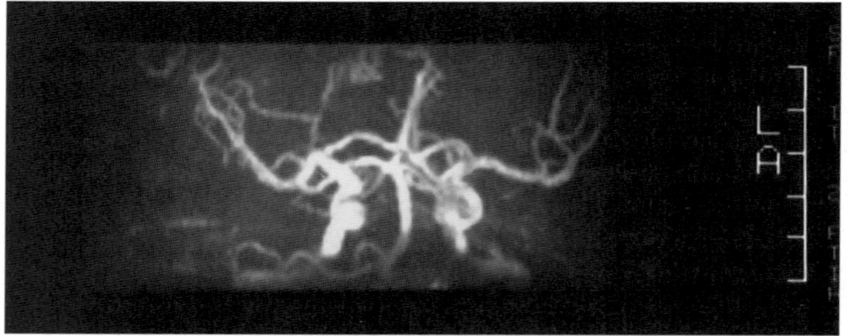

Fig. 25-80. 3D time of flight.

Phase Contrast

The phase contrast technique utilizes alterations in spin phase for image contrast. This imaging technique relies on velocity-induced phase shifts to distinguish flowing blood from stationary tissues. Two or more acquisitions with opposite polarity of the bipolar flow-encoding gradients are subtracted to produce an image of the vessels.*

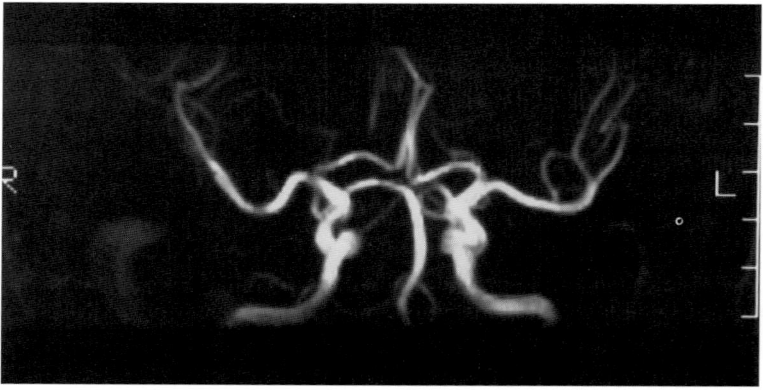

Fig. 25-81. 3D phase contrast.

2D Images

In general the 2D acquisition method will be used to image medium to slow flow areas and straight vessels. Specific applications include carotid arteries, basilar and vertebral arteries, and limbs.

3D Images

3D acquisition methods may best be used where flow is faster, especially through tortuous vessels. Both methods allow the images to be obtained in a sequential fashion, and post processing allows the images to be viewed from a variety of angles. This allows vessels to rotate around an axis and can then be viewed with reduced overlap.

Note: MR angiography is likely to become a common procedure in the screening and imaging of a known lesion. The biggest drawbacks include motion artifact and the turbulent flow, which may give a false impression of a defect. Improvements in imaging techniques, however, will continue to reduce these drawbacks.

*GE Medical Systems, Signal Applications Guide: *Vascular Magnetic Resonance Imaging*, Vol.3, pp 46,48, Aug.1990

Definition of Terms

PATHOLOGICAL TERMS

(Dorland's Illustrated Medical Dictionary, 27th ed)

Acoustic Neuroma *(nu-ro′mah):* A tumor growing from nerve cells and nerve fibers involving the sense of hearing.

Chordoma *(kor-do′mah):* A malignant tumor arising from the embryonic remains of the notochord (the rod-shaped body defining the primary axis of the embryonic body).

Meningioma *(me-nin-je-o′mah):* A hard, slow-growing vascular tumor occurring primarily along the meningeal vessels and superior longitudinal sinus invading the dura and skull causing erosion and thinning of the skull.

Osteonecrosis *(os″te-o-ne-kro′sis):* A death or necrosis of bone.

Pituitary Tumors: Tumors involving the pituitary gland.

Schwannoma *(shwon-no′mah):* A new growth of the white substance of Schwann (nerve sheath).

TERMS RELATED TO MRI

Artifacts: False features of an image caused by patient instability or equipment deficiencies.[1]

Averaging (signal averaging)*:* A SNR-enhancing technique in which the same MR signal is repeatedly acquired two or more times and then combined and averaged.[2]

Bipolar Flow-Encoding Gradients: Gradients whose polarity is inverted in order to encode velocities as changes of phase–a technique used in phase contrast angiography.[2]

Cine: In magnetic resonance imaging, acquisition of multiple images at different times in a cycle, e.g. the cardiac cycle and subsequent sequential display of the images in a manner that simulates motion.[2]

Coil: Single or multiple loops of wire designed either to produce a magnetic field from current flowing through the wire or to detect a changing magnetic field by voltage induced in the wire.[1]

Contrast Resolution: Ability of an imaging process to distinguish adjacent soft tissues from one another. This is the principal advantage of MRI.[1]

Cryogen: Atmospheric gases such as nitrogen and helium that have been cooled sufficiently to condense into a liquid.[1]

Field of View (FOV): The area (usually expressed in cm) of the anatomy being imaged; a function of acquisition matrix times pixel size.[2]

Filling Factor: Measure of the geometric relationship of the RF coil and the body. It affects the efficiency of irradiating the body and detecting MRI signals, thereby affecting the signal-to-noise ratio. Achieving a high filling factor requires fitting the coil closely to the body.[1]

Flip Angle: Amount of rotation of the net magnetization vector produced by an RF pulse, with respect to the direction of the static magnetic field B_0.[1]

Flow-Related Enhancement: A process by which the signal intensity of moving tissues, such as blood, can be increased compared with the signal of stationary tissue. Occurs when unsaturated, fully magnetized spins replace saturated spins between RF pulses.[2]

Fourier Transform (FT): Mathematical procedure to separate the frequency components of a signal from its amplitudes as a function of time. The Fourier transform is used to generate the spectrum from the FID and is essential to most imaging techniques.[1]

FOV: See field of view.

Free Induction Decay (FID): If transverse magnetization (Mxy) of the spins is produced, a transient NMR signal will result that will decay with a characteristic time constant T2. This decaying signal is the FID.[1]

Fringe Field: Stray magnetic field that exists outside the imager.[1]

Gating: An MR technique, used to minimize motion artifacts, in which conventional electrocardiography or photopulse sensing is used to trigger the acquisition of image data. It times data acquisition to physiological motion.[2]

Gauss (G): Unit of magnetic flux density in the older CGS system. The currently preferred (SI) unit is the Tesla (T) (lT = 10,000 G).[1]

Gradient Coils: Current-carrying coils designed to produce a desired gradient magnetic field. Proper design of the size and configuration of the coils is necessary to produce a controlled and uniform gradient.[1]

Gradient-Induced Magnetic Field: A magnetic field that changes in strength in a given direction. These fields are necessary to select a region for imaging (slice selection) and for encoding the location of the MR signal.

Gradient Moment Nulling: Application of gradients to correct phase errors caused by velocity, acceleration or other motion. First-order gradient nulling is the same as flow compensation.[2]

Gradient Pulse: Briefly applied gradient magnetic field.[1]

Inversion Recovery (IR): RF pulse sequence for MRI wherein the net magnetization is inverted and returns to equilibrium with the emission of an NMR signal.[1]

Magnetic Field Gradient: Device for varying the strength of the static magnetic field at different spatial locations. This is used for slice selection and determining the spatial locations of the protons being imaged. Also used for velocity encoding, flow comp, and in place of RF pulses during gradient echo acquisitions to rephase spins. Commonly measured in Gauss per centimeter.[2]

Terms Related to MRI continued

Partial Saturation (PS): Excitation technique applying repeated 90° RF pulses at times on the order of or shorter than Tl. Although partial saturation is also commonly referred to as saturation recovery, the latter term should properly be reserved for the particular case of partial saturation when the 90° RF pulses are far enough apart in time that the return of nuclear spins to equilibrium is complete.[1]

Phase Contrast (PC) Angiography: A 2D or 3D imaging technique that relies on velocity-induced phase shifts to distinguish flowing blood from stationary tissues. Two or more acquisitions with opposite polarity of the bipolar flow-encoding gradients are subtracted to produce an image of the vasculature.[2]

Phase Encoding: The act of localizing an MR signal by applying a gradient to alter the phase of spins before signal readout. In reordered PE, the sequence if localizing the signal is altered.[2]

Pixel: Acronym for a picture element; the smallest discrete part of a digital image display.[1]

Precession: Comparatively slow gyration of the axis of a spinning body so as to trace out a cone, caused by the application of a torque tending to change the direction of the rotation axis.[1]

Presaturation: See saturation.[2]

Proton Density: See spin density.[1]

Pulse Sequences: Set of RF or gradient magnetic field pulses and time spacings between these pulses.[1]

Radio Frequency (RF): Electromagnetic radiation just lower in energy than infrared. The RF used in MRl is commonly in the 10- to 100-MHz range.[1]

Radiofrequency (RF) Pulse: A burst of RF energy which, if it is at the correct Larmor frequency, will rotate the macroscopic magnetization vector by a specific angle, dependent on the pulse's amplitude and duration.[2]

Receiver Coil: Coil of the RF receiver; detects the NMR signal.[1]

Relaxation Time: After excitation, the nuclear spins will tend to return to their equilibrium position, in accordance with these time constants.[1]

Rephasing Gradient: Gradient magnetic field applied briefly after a selective excitation pulse, in the opposite direction to the gradient used for the selective excitation. The result of the gradient reversal is a rephasing of the spins, forming a spin echo.[1]

RF Coil: Used for transmitting RF pulses and or receiving NMR signals.[1]

RF Magnetic Fields: Electromagnetic radiation just lower in energy than infrared. RF magnetic fields are applied during pulse sequences.

Saturation: Repeated application of radiofrequency pulses in a time that is short compared with the T1 of the tissue, producing incomplete realignment of the net magnetization with the static magnetic field.[2]

Saturation Recovery (SR): Particular type of partial saturation pulse sequence in which the preceding pulses leave the spins in a state of saturation so that recovery to equilibrium is complete by the time of the next pulse.[1]

Signal Averaging: Method of improving SNR by averaging several FIDs or spin echoes.[1]

Signal-to-noise Ratio (SNR or S/N): Used to describe the relative contributions to a detected signal of the true signal and random superimposed signals or noise. The SNR can be improved by averaging several NMR signals, by sampling larger volumes, or by increasing the strength of the B_o magnetic field.[1]

Spin Density (SD): Density of resonating nuclear spins in a given region; one of the principal determinants of the strength of the NMR signal from that region.[1]

Spin Echo: Reappearance of an NMR signal after the FID has disappeared. The result of the effective reversal of the dephasing of the nuclear spins.[1]

Spin Echo Imaging: Any one of many MRI techniques in which the spin echo NMR signal rather than the FID is used.[1]

Static Magnetic Fields: The regions surrounding a magnet. A magnetic field produces a magnetizing force on a body within it.

Tl: Spin lattice or longitudinal relaxation time; the characteristic time constant for spins to tend to align themselves with the external magnetic field.[1]

T2: Spin-spin or transverse relaxation time; the characteristic time constant for loss of phase coherence among spins oriented at an angle to the main magnetic field owing to interactions between the spins. T2 never exceeds T1.[1]

TE Echo Time: Time between middle of 90° RF pulse and middle of spin echo.

Tesla (T): Preferred (SI) unit of magnetic flux density or magnetic field intensity. One Tesla is equal to 10,000 Gauss, the older (CSG) unit. One Tesla also equals one Newton/amp-m.[1]

Time-of-Flight (TOF) Angiography: 2D or 3D imaging technique that relies primarily on flow-related enhancement to distinguish moving from stationary spins in creating MR angiograms. Blood that has flowed into the slice will not have experienced RF pulses and will therefore appear brighter than stationary tissue.[2]

Time-varying Magnetic Field: (See gradient-induced magnetic field.)

Torque: Force that causes or tends to cause a body to rotate. It is a vector quantity given by the product of the force and the position vector where the force is applied.[1]

TR: Repetition time. The time between successive excitations of a slice—i.e., the time from the beginning of one pulse sequence to the beginning of the next. In conventional imaging, it is a fixed value equal to a user selected value. In cardiac-gated studies, however, it can vary from beat to beat depending on the patient's heart rate.[2]

Turbulence: In a flowing fluid, velocity components that fluctuate randomly, causing spin dephasing and signal loss.[2]

Two-dimensional Fourier Transform Imaging (2DFT): Form of sequential plane imaging using Fourier transform imaging.[1]

Voxel: Volume element; the element of three-dimensional space corresponding to a pixel for a given slice thickness.[1]

[1] Bushong, Stewart C.; **Magnetic Resonance Imaging Physical and Biological Principles**; 2nd ed; Mosby-Year Book; 1995.
[2] Signa Applications Guide; **Vascular Magnetic Resonance Imaging**; Vol 3; GE Medical Systems; Cat. # E8804DB; 1990.

References

BOOKS

Berquist, Ehman, Richardson; **Magnetic Resonance of the Musculoskeletal System**; Raven Press; 1987.

Brant-Zawadski, Michael; Norman, David; **Magnetic Resonance Imaging of the CNS**; Raven Press; 1987.

Bushong, Stewart C.; **Magnetic Resonance Imaging Physical and Biological Principles**; Mosby-Year Book; 1995.

Heiken, Jay P.; Brown, Jeffrey J.; **Manual of Clinical Magnetic Resonance Imaging**, 2nd Ed.; Raven Press; 1991.

Kaiser, Ramos; **MRI of the Spine: A Guide to Clinical Applications**; Theime Medical Publishers, Inc.; 1990.

Lufkin, Robert B.; **The MRI Manual;** Year Book Medical Publishers, Inc.; 1990.

Maravilla, Cohen; **MRI, Atlas of the Spine**; Raven Press; 1991.

Partain, et al; **Magnetic Resonance Imaging Volume 1 Clinical Principles**, 2nd ed.; W.B. Saunders; 1988.

Runge, Val M.; **Clinical Magnetic Resonance Imaging**; J.B. Lippincott Company;1990.

Stark DD, Bradley WG (Eds); **Magnetic Resonance Imaging**; C.V. Mosby; St. Louis, MO; 1987.

PERIODICALS

BNI Quarterly; Barrow Neurological Institute of St. Joseph's Hospital and Medical Center; Phoenix, AZ; Vol. 5:1; Winter; 1989

Brant-Zawadski, M.D., Michael; **MR Imaging of the Brain**; Radiology; Jan 1988; Vol 166; Number 1.

G.E. Medical Systems; **Signa Applications Guide, Vascular Magnetic Resonance Imaging**; Vol. 3 ; Cat. # E8804DB; 1990.

Marqulis, Higgins, Kaufman, Crooks; **Clinical Magnetic Resonance Imaging**; Radiology Research and Education Foundation; San Francisco; 1983.

Shellock, F.G.; Crues, J.V.; **Safety Considerations in Magnetic Resonance Imaging**; MRI Decisions,2:25, 1988.

Shellock, Frank; Emanual, M.D.; **Policies, Guidelines, and Recommendations for MR Imaging Safety and Patient Management**; SMRI Report Journal of Magnetic Resonance Imaging; Vol 1; Number 1; Jan/Feb 1991.

Shellock, Frank; **MR Imaging of Metallic Implants and Materials: A Compilation of the Literature**; AJR; Oct. 1985.

Underwood, Richard,; Firmin, David; **Magnetic Resonance of the Cardiovascular System**; Blackwell Scientific Publications; London; 1991.

BIBLIOGRAPHY

Ballinger, Phillip W. *Merrill's Atlas of Radiographic Positions and Radiologic Procedures*, ed. 8, vol. 1, 2, & 3. St. Louis: C. V. Mosby Co., 1995.

Becker, R.; Wilson, J.; Gehweiler, J. *The Anatomical Basis of Medical Practice*, ed. 1, Baltimore: The Williams & Wilkins Co., 1971.

Bushong, Stewart C. *Radiologic Science for Technologists*, ed. 5. St. Louis: C. V. Mosby Co., 1994.

Cahill, D.R; Orland, M.J. *Atlas of Human Cross-Sectional Anatomy*, Philadelphia: Lea & Febiger, 1984.

Carlton, R.R., Adler, A.M. *Principals of Radiographic Imaging;* Albany, NY: Delmar Publishing, Inc., 1992.

Carroll, Q.B. *Fuchs's Principles of Radiographic Exposure, Processing and Quality Control* ; ed. 4. Springfield, Illinois: Charles C. Thomas; 1990.

Christensen, E.; Curry, T.; Dowdey, J. *An Introduction to the Physics of Diagnostic Radiology*, ed. 2. Philadelphia: Lea & Febiger, 1978.

Clark, K. C. *Positioning in Radiography*, ed. 11. London: Ilford Ltd., William Heinemann Medical Books, Ltd., 1986.

Compere, W. *Radiographic Atlas of the Temporal Bone*, Book 1, ed. 1. St. Paul, Minnesota: H.M. Smyth Co., Inc., 1964.

Cullinan, Angeline M. *Optimizing Radiographic Positioning*, Philadelphia: J. B. Lippincott Co., 1992.

Egan, R. *Technologist Guide to Mammography*, ed. 1, Baltimore: The Williams & Wilkins Co., 1968.

Eisenberg, R.L.; Dennis, C.A.; May, C.R. *Radiographic Positioning*, Boston: Little, Brown and Co., 1989.

Etter, L. *Roentgenography and Roentgenology of the Middle Ear and Mastoid Process*, ed. 1. Springfield, Illinois: Charles C. Thomas, Publisher, 1965.

Gerhart, P.; Van Kaich, G. *Total Body Computed Tomography*, ed.2. Stuttgart: Georg Thieme Publishers, 1979.

Godderidge, C. *Pediatric Imaging,* Philadelphia: W.B. Saunders Co., 1995.

Gray, H. *Anatomy of the Human Body*, ed. 30. Philadelphia: Lea & Febiger, 1985.

Hendee, W.R.; Ritenour, E.R. *Medical Imaging Physics*, ed. 3; Chicago: Mosby - Year Book Inc., 1992.

Jacobi, C.; Paris, D. *Textbook of Radiologic Technology*, ed. 5. St. Louis: C. V. Mosby Co., 1972.

Kreel, L.; Steiner, R. *Medical Imaging*, ed. 1. Exeter, Great Britain: A. Wheaton & Co. Ltd., 1979.

Long, B.W., Rafert, J.A. *Orthopaedic Radiography*, Philadephia: W.B. Saunders Co., 1995

McQuillen-Martensen, K. *Radiographic Critique,* Philadelphia: W.B. Saunders Co., 1996.

Meschan, I. *An Atlas of Anatomy Basic to Radiology*, ed. 1. Philadelphia: Lea & Febiger, 1975.

Meschan, I. *Radiographic Positioning and Related Anatomy*, ed. 2 Philadelphia: W. B. Saunders Co., 1978.

New, P.; Scott, W. *Computed Tomography of the Brain and Orbit*, ed. 1. Baltimore: The Williams & Wilkins Co., 1975.

Norman, D.; Korobkin, M.; Newton, T., eds. *Computed Tomography*, ed. 1. St. Louis: C. V. Mosby Co., 1977.

Ramsey, R. *Advanced Exercises in Diagnostic Radiology, Computed Tomography of the Brain*, ed. 1. Philadelphia: W. B. Saunders Co., 1977.

Statkiewicz, M.A.; Ritenour, E.R. *Radiation Protection for Student Radiographers;* ed. 2. St. Louis: Mosby Year Book; 1993.

Taveras, J.; Wood, E. *Diagnostic Neuroradiology*, ed. 2, vol. 1, Baltimore: The Williams & Wilkins Co., 1976.

Tortora, G. R., Anagnostakos, N.P. *Principles of Anatomy and Physiology*. ed 4. New York: Harper & Row Publishers, 1984.

Tortorici, M. *Medical Imaging,* Philadelphia: W.B. Saunders Co., 1996.

Tortorici, M.R., Apfel, P.J. *Advanced Radiographic and Angiographic Procedures With an Introduction to Specialized Imaging,* Philadelphia: F.A. Davis Co., 1995.

Watkins, G.L., Moore, T.F. *Atypical Orthopaedic Radiographic Procedures;* St. Louis: Mosby Year Book, 1993

Woodburne, R.T., Burkel, W.E. *Essentials of Human Anatomy*, ed. 8 New York: Oxford University Press, 1988.

APPENDIX A – NATIONAL SURVEY RESULTS

Regional Differences

Following is a list of projections and the percent of responses for those projections for which there was a 10% or more regional difference. These were responses by clinical affiliates of accredited radiologic technology programs in the United States indicating them as either basic or special projections in their institutions, and which in their opinion were minimum essential projections for which all students should demonstrate competency prior to graduation.

The exams and/or projections not listed below, but included in this text, indicate strong agreement (less than 10% difference) among all regions within the United States. (See front pages (ix and x) of this text for more information on this survey.)

		Regions of U.S.					
		West		Mid		East	
Exam	Projection	Basic	Special	Basic	Special	Basic	Special
Chest	AP lordotic		60%		75%		72%
Acute abdomen series	PA chest (as part of series)	82%		70%		60%	
Hand	Fan lateral (vs. lat. in flex. or ext.)	96%		85%		77%	
Wrist	Scaphoid (ulnar flexion)		37%		58%		51%
	Carpal canal (Gaynor-Hart)		44%		49%		58%
Elbow	Internal oblique and/or	47%		45%		62%	
	External oblique	73%		68%		73%	
Shoulder	Posterior oblique (Grashey)	28%		27%		19%	
	Bicipital groove (tangential)		51%		45%		41%
	Apical oblique		20%		19%		10%
Ribs	PA chest	69%		56%		59%	
Foot	Lateromedial	40%		18%		19%	
Ankle	AP mortise	56%		36%		39%	
Knee-patella	Merchant method	49%		29%		18%	
Cervical spine	Swimmers (Twining)	58%		54%		44%	
Skull	PA 15° caudad (Caldwell)	75%		57%		65%	
	or PA 0°	45%		60%		44%	
Facial bones	PA modified Waters (55° to OML)	36%		25%		23%	
Optic foramina	Parieto-orbital (Rhese)	70%		79%		80%	
Zygomatic arch	Tangential (axial oblique)	72%		68%		62%	
Mandible	AP axial (Towne)	86%		79%		61%	
	Submentovertex (SMV)		24%		11%		13%
	Trauma horizontal beam axiolateral obliques		39%		31%		24%
TMJs	Tomogram laterals		47%		44%		26%
Mammogram	Laterally exaggerated craniocaudal (XCCL)		24%		17%		11%
	Ecklund technique CC and MLO implants		36%		25%		17%
	Axillary tail view (Cleopatra view)		16%		11%		9%
Gallbladder	RAO	36%		26%		17%	
	R lateral decubitus	47%		34%		29%	
	PA erect	38%		29%		28%	
	Sonography in combination with radiographs		28%		36%		26%
Intravenous urogram	AP erect post-void	75%		45%		43%	
	AP ureteric compression		47%		28%		28%
	Tomograms	90%		74%		76%	
Cystogram	AP, 10-15° caudad	86%		63%		57%	
	RPO and LPO	85%		72%		61%	
	Lateral	67%		54%		29%	
Voiding cystourethrogram	Male–RPO 30°	90%		76%		69%	
	Female–AP	91%		78%		75%	
Small bowel series	PA scout	78%		73%		68%	
	Enteroclysis		21%		11%		12%

Survey Respondents by Regions of U.S.

Region of U.S.	States	College Affiliates: More than 300 beds	College Affiliates: Less than 300 beds	Hospital Based	Total Respondents*
West	13 states	66	24	11	101
Mid	19 states	49	137	81	267
East	18 states	64	106	99	269
Totals		**179**	**267**	**191**	**637**

*Note: An additional 61 responses were received from program directors of college based programs which were not included in these totals. The reason for this was an attempt in this survey to determine what the clinical facilities themselves considered basic (routine) or special (optional) in their departments, thus indicating what students should be able to perform upon graduation to function in their departments.

Map of Three Regions

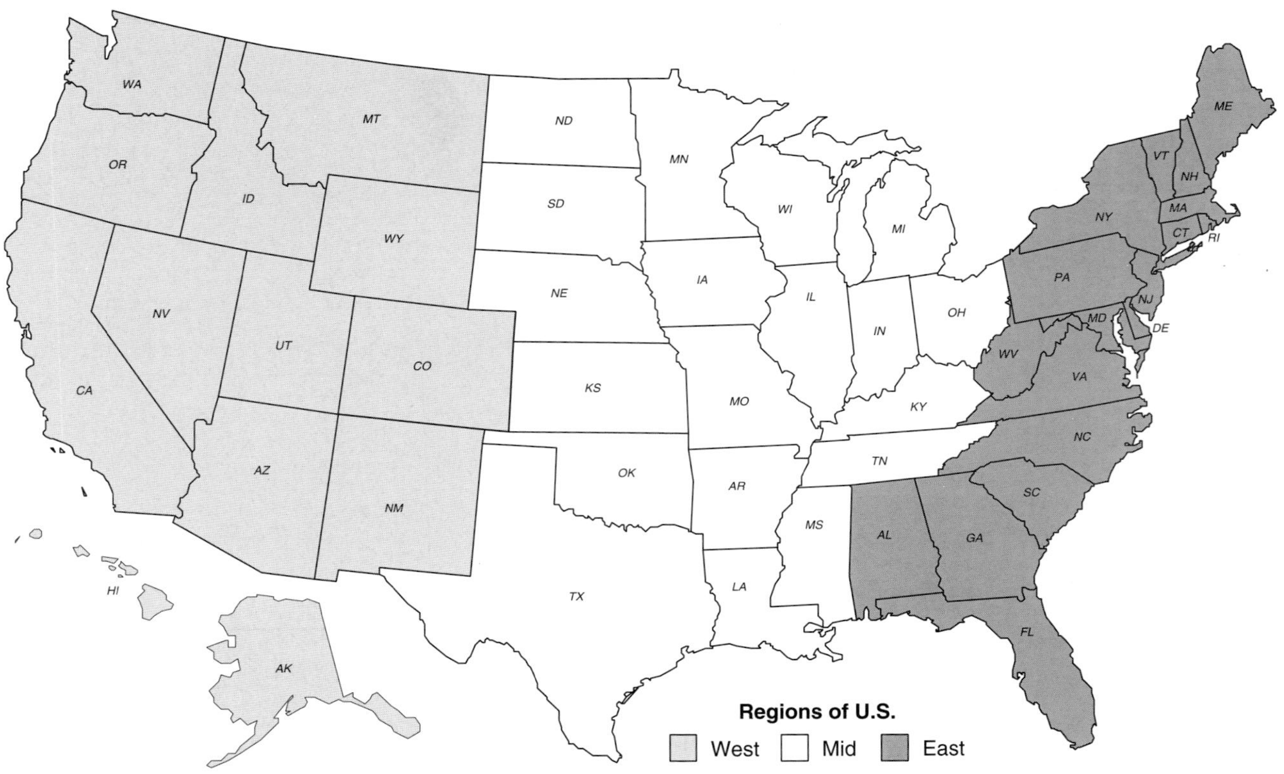

INDEX

A

Abdomen, 85-100
 anatomy of, 86-91, 667-670
 angiography of, 711-713
 anteroposterior projection of
  in erect position, 97, 99
  in supine position, 94, 99
 basic and special projections of, 93
 of child, radiography of, 600
  anteroposterior erect projection for, 602
  anteroposterior projection for, 601
  dorsal decubitus-lateral position for, 603
  KUB projection for, 601
 circulatory system of, 689-690
 computed tomography of, 659-677
  contraindications to, 674
  contrast media for, 675-676
  indications for, 673
  positioning and procedures for, 673-677
  preparation for, 674, 676
  procedure for, 677
 dorsal decubitus position for, 98
 fluoroscopic procedures of,
  pregnancy and, 44
 landmarks of, 91
 lateral decubitus position for, 98
 magnetic resonance imaging of, 749
 posteroanterior projection of,
  in prone position, 95
 positioning of, 92-99
 pseudotumors of, 674
 quadrants and regions of, 90
 radiographs of, 93, 422
 surgery of, recent, as contraindication to ureteric compression, 516
 topographic landmarks of, 91
 trauma to, as contraindication to ureteric compression, 516
 trauma and mobile radiography of, 552
  anteroposterior supine and decubitus projections for, 561
Abdomen and chest projections, decubitus, viewing radiographs of, 54
Abdominal abscess drainage, percutaneous, 720
Abdominal aorta, 63, 452, 506
Abdominal aortic aneurysm as contraindication to ureteric compression, 516
Abdominal arteries, 689
Abdominal cavity, 89
 anatomy of, 89, 451-452
 digestive organs in, 86
Abdominal mass
 as contraindication to ureteric compression, 516
 excretory urography to diagnose, 514
Abdominal muscles, 86
Abdominal organs, 86-88
 anatomical relationships of, 89
 infraperitoneal, 89
 retroperitoneal, 89
Abdominal pain as contraindication to ureteric compression, 516
Abdominal veins, 689
Abdominopelvic cavity, 453
Abducens nerve, 641
Abduction, 26
Abscess
 abdominal
  abdominal computed tomography to diagnose, 673
  percutaneous drainage of, 720
 brain, cranial computed tomography to diagnose, 655
 chest, thoracic computed tomography to diagnose, 664
 pelvic, pelvic computed tomography to diagnose, 673
Absorbed dose, radiation, 38
Absorption in intestines, 454
Abuse, child, reporting, 582
Acanthiomeatal line, 345
Acanthion, 333, 344
Acanthioparietal projection, 28
Accessory digestive organs, 88
Accessory ligaments of synovial joints, 11
Accessory organs of digestion, 3, 412
Accuracy, positioning, 29
Ace bandage for immobilization during pediatric radiography, 584
Acetabular fracture, 673
Acetabulum, 11, 223
 anterior oblique position of, 237
 union of, 228
Acoustic meatus
 external, 260, 261, 327, 345, 390, 391, 392
 internal, 327, 391
Acoustic nerve, 641
Acoustic neuroma, MRI to diagnose, 740
Acromioclavicular joint, 149
 anteroposterior projection of, 166-167
  in supine position, 167
 basic and special projections in, 155
 bilateral radiograph of, with and without weights, 166
 routine for, 154
 stress view of, with weights, 166
Acromion, 150
Acromion process, 150
Acute abdominal series, 86, 99
 basic and special projections in, 93
Adam's apple; *see* Thyroid cartilage
Adaptation, trauma, 551
Added filtration, 41
Adduction, 26
Adductor tubercle, 179
Adipose capsule, 505
Adipose tissue of breast, 531, 532
Aditus, 391
Adjustable collimator, 42
 illuminated, to restrict x-ray beam, 48
Adrenal glands, 88, 89, 452, 453
 pathology of, abdominal computed tomography to diagnose, 673
Adult
 appendicular skeleton of, bones of, 7
 axial skeleton of, bones of, 6
Adynamic ileus, small bowel series to diagnose, 455
Afferent arterioles of kidney, 507
Air
 and barium in large intestine, relative locations of, 453
 pathway for, 57
Air cells, mastoid, 391
Air enema for child, 606-607
Air-barium distribution in stomach, 417
Airway, upper, 57
 anteroposterior projection of, 82
 basic projections of, 71
 lateral position of, 81
 radiographs of, 59
  national survey norms for, 70
Ala
 of ilium, 223
 of sacrum, 281
 of scapula, 150
ALARA principles, 38
Alignment
 central ray, distortion and, 36
 of fractures, two projections to determine, 50
 object, distortion and, 35
Alimentary canal, 3, 412, 446
Aluminum for filters, 41
Alveolar process
 of mandible, 336
 of maxilla, 333
Alveoli
 of breast, 532
 of lungs, 60
Amino acids, digestion and, 419
Amphiarthrodial joints, summary of, 13
Amphiarthrosis, 10
Amplitude in tomography, 626
Ampulla
 breast, 532
 hepatopancreatic, 485
 rectal, 449
Amygdaloid nucleus, 641
Anal canal, 448, 449
Anatomic apposition of fracture, 547
Anatomical neck, of humerus, 148
Anatomical position, 14
Anatomical side marker, 30
Anatomical structures, superimposition of, two projections needed because of, 50
Anatomy
 arthrology and, 1-13
 definition of, 2
 general, 2
  principles of, 2-6
 skeletal, 6-9
 systemic, 3-6
Anatrast for defecography, 466
Anemia, sickle cell, 514
Aneurysm
 aortic, abdominal, 516
 arteriography of, 706
 cranial computed tomography to diagnose, 655
 thoracic, thoracic computed tomography to diagnose, 664
Angiography, 679-721
 abdominal, 711-713
  positioning for, 712
 cerebral, 699-708
 definition of, 680
 equipment for, 696, 697
 internal carotid, 702
 interventional, 718-721
  vascular, 718-719
 magnetic resonance, of cardiovascular system, 750
 magnification, of vertebrobasilar system, 705
 peripheral, 714-717
 procedures and positioning for, 695-717
 renal, 713
 sterile supplies for, 698
 subtraction, digital, 708
 vertebrobasilar, 704-705
Angioplasty, transluminal, 719
Angle blocks, weighted, as head clamps for immobilization during pediatric radiography, 584
"Angle finder" as positioning aid in skull radiography, 345
Angle
 costophrenic, 62
 exposure, in tomography, 626
 jaw, 260, 261
 mandibular, 336, 344
 of proximal femur, 222
 of pubic arch, 226
 of rib, 307
  inferior, 306
 of scapula, 150
 sternal, 260, 261, 306
 of Treitz, 418
Angular notch, 416
Angulation of fracture, 547
Anion, 511
Ankle, 12, 176
 anteroposterior and lateral projection for, 568
 anteroposterior mortise and lateral projection for, 568
 anteroposterior oblique mortise projection of, with 15 to 20° medial rotation, 200
 anteroposterior oblique projection of, with 45° medial rotation, 201
 anteroposterior projection of, 199
 anteroposterior stress projections of, 203
 basic and special projections for, 188
 dorsiflexion of, 25
 eversion stress of, 25
 inversion and eversion positions of, 203
 inversion stress at, 25
 lateral-mediolateral (lateromedial) projection of, 202
 mediolateral projection of, 20
 motions of, 184
 plantar flexion of, 25
 radiograph of, 177
 routine for, 187
 stress movements of, 25
Ankle, cont'd
 summary of, 183
 three projections required for, 51
 trauma and mobile radiography of, 568
Annual effective dose, 37
Annual effective dose limit, 37
Annulus fibrosus, 251
Anode heel effect, 36
Anterior arch of atlas, 253
Anterior crest of tibia, 178
Anterior cruciate ligament, 180, 181
Anterior fat pad of elbow joint, 111
Anterior horn of lateral ventricles, 637, 638
Anterior nasal spine, 333
Anterior oblique position, left and right, 18
Anterior position, erect, 20
Anterior superior iliac spine, 223, 224, 286
 as topographic landmark of abdomen, 52, 91
Anterior surface, 16
 of foot, 184
Anterior tubercle, ankle and, 176
Anteroposterior cervical spine, radiographs of, 256
Anteroposterior diameter of thoracic cavity, 64
Anteroposterior projection, 18, 19, 20
 axial (semi-axial), 21
 correct use of term, 28
 for joint, 51
 lordotic, 21
 oblique, 18, 20
 viewing radiographs of, 54
Anteroposterior thoracic spine, radiographs of, 256
Anthropological base line, 16, 345
Anthropological plane, 16
Antrum, 391
 cardiac, 415, 416
 of Highmore, 386
Anuria, 514
Anus, 86, 412, 446, 448
Aorta, 63, 89, 415, 688, 692
 abdominal, 452, 506
 on CT cross sectional image at level of T9, 61
 thoracic, 414
Aortic aneurysm, abdominal, as contraindication to ureteric compression, 516
Aortic arch, 63, 414, 688, 692
 branches of, 683
Aortic bulb, 682, 688
Aortic valve, 681
Aortography
 arch, 701
 thoracic, 709-710
Apex
 of coccyx, 282
 of fibula, 178
 of sacrum, 281
Apex angulation of fracture, 547
Apical anteroposterior projection, lordotic position, 21
Apophyseal joints, 251, 252, 255, 280, 284, 285
Appendicitis, 448
 barium enema to diagnose, 459
Appendicular skeleton, 6, 7
Appendix, 86, 448, 453
Appendolith, 459
Apposition of fracture, 547
Aprons, lead, for worker protection, 40
Aqueduct
 cerebral, 637
 of Sylvius, 637
Arachnoid, 635
Arcelin method for mastoid radiographs, 406
Arch(es)
 of aorta, 63
 of foot, 175
 palmar, 690, 691, 692
 pubic, 226
 superciliary, 325
 vertebral, 250
 zygomatic; *see* Zygomatic arch
Areola, 530, 532

INDEX

Arm(s), 22; *see also* Upper limb
bones of, 7
cross section of, 23
raised for lateral chest radiographs, 68
Artery(ies), 680, 689-692; *see also* specific artery
abdominal, 689
basilar, 684, 686
brachiocephalic, 683, 690, 692
carotid, 683, 686, 692
branches of, 684
magnification radiography of, 703
cerebral, 683-686
coronary, 682
facial, 684
inside rib, 307
lower limb, 691
major, summary of, 692
maxillary, 684
neck and head, 683
nutrient, of long bone, 8
occipital, 684
pulmonary, 63, 681, 688
renal, 506, 689, 692
subclavian, 683, 690, 692
temporal, 684
thoracic, 688
upper limb, 690
vertebral, 683
vertebrobasilar, 684
Arteriogram
internal carotid, 685
vertebrobasilar, 686
Arteriography
aneurysm, 706
common carotid, 701
lower limb, 716
upper limb, 716
Arterioles, 680
of kidney, afferent and efferent, 507
Arthrography
knee, 615-618
shoulder, 619
temporomandibular joint, 615
Arthrology, 3, 6, 10-13
anatomy and, 1-13
Articular bursa, 181
Articular capsule of knee, 181
Articular cartilage, 7
hyaline, of synovial joints, 11
Articular disk, 109, 181
Articular facets, 174, 178
Articular pillar, 252, 253
Articular process
of lumbar vertebrae, 280, 284
of sacrum, 281
of thoracic vertebrae, 255
of vertebrae, 250, 251
Articulated thorax, 308
Articulation(s)
atlanto-occipital, 253
rib, 254, 307
sternal clavicle, 306
of thorax, anatomy of, 308
Ascending aorta, 63
Ascending colon, 86, 448, 449, 452, 453
ASIS; *see* Anterior superior iliac spine
Asterions, 330
Asthenic body habitus, 53
chest radiography and, 64
gastrointestinal organs and, 420, 421
Astragalus bone; *see* Talus bone
Atelectasis, chest radiography for, 66
Atlantal ligament, transverse, 253
Atlanto-occipital articulations, 253
Atlas, 252, 253
and axis, joint between, 12
Atoms, 2
Atria of heart, 681, 682
Atrophy, brain, cranial computed tomography to diagnose, 655
Attenuation in cranial computed tomography, 652
Attic, 390, 391
Auditory meatus; *see* Acoustic meatus
Auditory ossicles, 6, 390, 392
Auditory tube, 390, 391, 414
Auricle, 390
of ear, 344
Auricular point, 16, 345
Auricular surface of sacrum, 281
Automatic electromechanical contrast medium injector, 697
Automatic positive beam limitation, 42
Autotomography, 631
Avascular necrosis, fractures and, 231
Avulsion fracture, 550
Axial image, 15
viewing, 54
Axial plane, 15
Axial projection, 21, 28
Axial sections, 15
Axial skeleton, 6
Axillary artery, 690
Axillary prolongation of breast, 530
Axillary tail, 530
Axillary vein, 691, 693
Axis, 252, 253
and atlas, joint between, 12
Axon, 634
myelinated, 640
Azygos veins, 688

B

Back of body, terms for, 16
Back scatter protection, during chest radiography, 65
Badges, film, for personnel monitoring, 38
Ball and socket joint, 13
Barium in stomach, 422
Barium enema, 446, 450, 459-463
anteroposterior axial or anteroposterior axial oblique projections for, 480
basic and special projections for, 469
"butterfly" positions for, 480, 481
for child, 606-607
clinical indications for, 459
contraindications to, 459
definition of, 459
double-contrast, 459
left lateral decubitus position (AP) for, 478
patient exposures during, 39
procedure for, 464-465
right lateral decubitus position (AP) for, 477
enema tips for, 461
insertion of, 462
equipment and supplies for, 460
lateral rectum position, lateral or ventral decub, 476
left anterior oblique position for, 474
left posterior oblique position for, 475
posteroanterior and/or anteroposterior projection for, 472
oblique, 481
post-evacuation, 479
preparation for, 460, 461
procedure for, 460-463
right anterior oblique position for, 473
right posterior oblique position for, 475
routine for, 468
safety considerations for, 467
Sims position for, 461
single-contrast, 459
procedure for, 464
types of, 459
Barium enema containers, 461
Barium sulfate, 423
air and, in large intestine, relative locations of, 453
contraindications to, 424
defecation after exam with, 424
double contrast procedures using, 424
for abdominal and pelvic computed tomography, 675, 676
thick, 423
thin, 423
Barium swallow, 412
for children, 604-605
Barton's fracture, 549
Basal ganglia, 640, 641
Base
of metatarsals, 172
of phalanx, 102
Base line, 16
Base plane of skull, 16
Baseball fracture, 549
Basilar artery, 684, 686
Basilar position and Towne method for petrous pyramid radiographs, 408
Basilic vein, 691, 693
Battery driven, battery operated mobile x-ray units, 554
Bayonet apposition of fracture, 547
Beam, x-ray, divergence of, 34
Beam limitation, positive, automatic, 42
Beam-restricting devices, 48
Bennett fracture, 549
Bezoar, upper GI series to diagnose, 431
Bicipital groove, 148
tangential projection of, 160
Bicuspid valve, 681
Bifid tip of spinous process of cervical vertebra, 252
Bile, 419
gallbladder and, 485
Bile duct, common, 485
Biliary calculi, oral cholecystogram to diagnose, 487
Biliary drainage
percutaneous, 720
stone extraction and, percutaneous transhepatic cholangiography for, 492
Biliary duct(s)
anatomy of, 485-486
basic and special projections for, 496
and gallbladder, 483-501
positioning of, 495-496
radiographs of, 486, 487
national survey norms for, 495
special procedures for, 496
Biliary stenosis, oral cholecystogram to diagnose, 487
Biliary system, radiographs of, 494
Biopsy, needle, percutaneous, 721
Biplane film changers, 696
Birth canal, 225
Bladder, urinary, 88, 89, 452, 504, 508-509
carcinoma of, pelvic computed tomography to diagnose, 673
functions of, 509
size and position of, 509
term pregnancy relationship to, 509
Blood in urine, 514
Blood cells, 680
production of, 8
Blood pressure, very low, from urologic contrast media, 513
Blood vessels
great, axial (cross-section) image of, 60
renal, 506
Blowout fracture, 339, 550
Blur, 33
in tomography, 626, 629-630
Blur margin in tomography, 626
Blurring patterns in conventional tomography, 626
Blurring principle in conventional tomography, 628
Body
of axis, 253
of cervical vertebra, 252
of clavicle, 149
of compact bone, 8
of femur, 179, 222
of fibula, 178
of gallbladder, 485
of humerus, 107, 148
of ilium, 223
of ischium, 224
of lateral ventricles, 637, 638
lines of, 16
long bones, 7
of lumbar vertebra, 280
of mandible, 336
of maxilla, 333
of metatarsals, 172
of phalanx, 102
planes of, 15
of pubis, 224
of radius, 106
of rib, 307
of scapula, 150
sections of, 15
of sternum, 56, 260, 306
of stomach, 416, 417
structural organization of, 2
surfaces and parts of, 16
of tibia, 178
of vertebra, 250
Body habitus, 53
chest radiography and, 64
gastrointestinal organs and, 420, 421
Body part
placement of, on film holder, 29
positioning of, 49
thickness of, measuring, 49
Body planes, cranial topography and, 344
Body positions, 17-19
Body section radiography, 626
Body systems, 3-6
Bone marrow, 8
Bones, 3, 6, 7-8; *see also* specific bone
classification of, 7-8
cranial
anatomy of, 324-329
radiographs of, 331
skull and, 323-358
positioning of, 343-357
development of, 9
pediatric radiography and, 586
facial; *see* Facial bones
formation of, kinds of, 9
frontal, coronal section through, 643
growth of, radiograph demonstrating, 9
hand and wrist, 102
hip, 223
hyoid, 57, 58
metatarsal, 172
joints of, 173
nasal, radiographs of
basic and special projections for, 362
routine for, 361
of vertebral column, 248
palatine, 333
pelvic, 8
anterior, anteroposterior axial projection of, 236
sesamoid, of feet, 173
study of; *see* Arthrology
sutural (Wormian), 330
temporal; *see* Temporal bones
wrist, 104
Bony labyrinth, 392-393
Bony landmarks, positioning, 52
Bony nasal septum, 332, 335
Bony thorax, 23
anatomy of, 56, 306
anteroposterior oblique and lateral sternum projection for, 559
anteroposterior and oblique ribs projection for, 560
sternum and ribs, 305-322
trauma and mobile radiography of, 552, 559, 560
Bowel, small, 89; *see also* Intestine
Bowman's capsule, 507
Boxer's fracture, 549
Brachial artery, 690, 692
Brachial vein, 691, 693
Brachiocephalic artery, 683, 690, 692
Brachiocephalic trunk artery, 683
Brachiocephalic vein, 686, 693
Brachycephalic skull, 343
Brain, 634
blood supply to, 683
coverings of, 635
disorders of, cranial computed tomography to diagnose, 655
divisions of, 635
inferior surface of, 641
magnetic resonance imaging of, 745
sectional anatomy of, 643-648
Brain stem, 635, 639, 641
Breast
anatomy of, 530-532
classifications of, 533
front view of, 532
imaging modalities for, 535
new, 536-537
localization on, 531
mammography of, positioning for, 534-535
sagittal sections of, 531
shielding, 43
with cranial radiography, 346
for humerus and shoulder girdle radiographs, 154
sonography of, 535
tissue of, types of, 532
Breast dose, calculation of, 45
Breast implants, MRI to diagnose problems related to, 536

Breast shadows on posteroanterior chest radiographs, 67
Breastbone, 56
Breathing, difficulty in, from urologic contrast media, 513
Breathing exercises to prevent esophageal reflux, 429
Breathing instructions for patients, 41
for abdominal radiographs, 92
for chest radiography, 66
for sternal radiographs, 310
Breathing mechanism, 61
Breathing movements, chest radiography and, 64
Bregma, 330
Brim, pelvic, 225, 508
Bronchioles, 60
Bronchus (bronchi), 57, 60, 63
axial (cross-section) CT image of, 60
main stem, axial (cross-section) image of, 60
primary, 414
Bruise, 547
Buccal cavity, anatomy of, 413
Bucky grid in x-ray table, 48
Bucky slot shield for worker protection, 40
Bulb of eye, 642
Bursa (bursae), 181
omentum, 451
Burst fracture, 550
Butterfly fracture, 548

C

C1 and C2, relationship of, 253
C1-2 joint, 12
anteroposterior or posteroanterior projection for, 273
C4-T3 region, radiography of, Twining method for, 270
C7-T1, radiography of, alternate methods of visualizing, 271
C-arm digital fluoroscopy systems, mobile, 555-556
ALARA principles and, 38
radiation protection with, 557
Calcaneal sulcus, 174
Calcaneus bone, 174
basic and special projections for, 188
lateral-mediolateral projection of, 198
plantodorsal (axial) projection of, 197
routine for, 187
Calcium citrate to produce carbon dioxide gas, 424
Calculations, dose, for patient protection, 45
Calculi
biliary, oral cholecystogram to diagnose, 487
renal or ureteral, excretory urography to diagnose, 514
small, ultrasound to detect, 489
ureteral, as contraindication to ureteric compression, 516
Caldwell method
for cranial radiography, 350
for facial bone radiographs, 365
for paranasal sinus radiographs, 398
Caldwell projection
anteroposterior reverse, for pediatric radiography of skull, 598
of cranial bones, 331
modified
for internal acoustic meatus radiographs, 391
for paranasal sinus radiographs, 394
reverse, for trauma and mobile radiography of skull, 576-577
Calvarium, 8, 324
Calyces, kidney, 507
Camp Coventry method for knee, 210
Cancellous bone, 8
Canthi, 344
Cap
duodenal, 86
knee; *see* Patella
Capacitor-discharge mobile radiographic x-ray units, 554
Capillaries, 680
Capitate bone of wrist, 103, 104
Capitellum; *see* Capitulum
Capitulum, 107
Capsule
articular, of knee, 181
Capsule, cont'd
fibrous, 11
glomerular (Bowman's), 507
Carbohydrates, chemical digestion of, 419
Carbon dioxide gas as contrast medium, 424
Cardiac antrum, 415, 416
Cardiac arrest from urologic contrast media, 513
Cardiac gating in MRI, 743
Cardiac muscle, 5
Cardiac notch, 416
Cardiac orifice, 415, 416
Cardiac series, 430
Cardiac veins, 682, 693
Cardiovascular organs, 3
Cardiovascular system, 680
computed tomography of, 650
functions of, 680
magnetic resonance angiography of, 750
magnetic resonance imaging of, 748, 750
Care, patient, professional ethics and, 46
Carina, 60, 62
Carotid artery, 683, 684, 686, 692
angiography of, 702
magnification radiography of, 703
Carotid siphon, 684
Carpal bones, 8, 102, 104
Carpal canal, radiograph of, 105
Carpal sulcus, 104
Carpometacarpal joints, 11, 12, 103
Cartilage, 6
articular, 7, 11
cricoid, 58, 414
hyaline, 7, 11
rib, 307
septal, 335
thyroid, of larynx, 57, 58, 260, 261
Cartilaginous joints, 10, 11
summary of, 13
Cassette tray in x-ray table, 48
Cast
lower limb, conversion chart for radiographs with, 186
on upper limb, conversion chart for radiographs with, 112
Central ray icon, 49
Cathartics, 460
Cation, 511
Caudad, 22
Caudad central ray angle, 22
Caudate lobe of liver, 484
Caudate nucleus, 641
Cavity (cavities)
abdominal, 89
digestive organs in, 86
abdominopelvic, 453
buccal, anatomy of, 413
of cerebral ventricles, 636
communicating with pharynx, 414
facial, 338
glenoid, 150
Grashey method for, 159
joint, 11
medullary, 8
nasal, 57, 386, 414
oral, 57, 412, 413
orbital, 642
peritoneal, 89, 451
pleural, 61
synovial, of knee, 181
thoracic, breathing movements and, 64
tympanic, 390, 391, 414
Cecum, 86, 448, 453
Celiac axis, 689, 692
Cell body, 634, 640
Cells, 2
air, mastoid, 391
blood, 680
production of, 8
Centering, film, 49
Centers of endochondral ossification, 9
Centi-, 37
Central gyri, 636
Central lobe of cerebral hemisphere, 636
Central nervous system, anatomy of, 634-635
Central ray, 20
alignment of, distortion and, 36
angling of, in trauma radiography, 551, 553
caudad angle of, 22
centering of, in trauma radiography, 551, 553
cephalad angle of, 22
and chest and lung measurement study, 84
Central ray, cont'd
chest positioning method for, 69-70, 84
positioning and, 49
Central sulcus, 636
Centrum semiovale, 640
Cephalad, 22
Cephalad central ray angle, 22
Cephalic vein, 691, 693
Cephalocaudad projection, axial, 21
Cephalopelvimetry, 225
Cerebellar notch, 640
Cerebellum, 635, 639, 640, 641
coronal section through, 645
Cerebral angiography, 699-708
positioning for, 700-701
procedure for, 699-700
Cerebral aqueduct, 637
Cerebral arteries, 683-686
Cerebral cortex, 636, 640
Cerebral hemispheres, 636, 640
axial section through, 645, 646
Cerebral nuclei, 640, 641
Cerebral peduncle, 641
Cerebral veins, 686-687
Cerebral ventricles, 636
axial section through, 646, 647
Cerebrospinal fluid, 635
Cerebrum, 635, 636
Cervical curve, 249
Cervical region, myelography of, 623
Cervical spine
anatomy of, 248-259
anteroposterior axial projection of, 266
anteroposterior "chewing" or "wagging jaw" projection of, 274
anteroposterior and lateral projection for, 572
anteroposterior "open mouth" projection of, C1 and C2, 265
anteroposterior or posteroanterior projection for C1-2 of, 273
basic and special projections of, 264
biplanar angulation method for, 573
cervicothoracic (swimmer's) lateral position for, 270
discogram of, 625
lateral horizontal beam position for, 269
lateral position for, 268, 572
in hyperflexion and hyperextension, 272
Ottonello method for, 274
overhead oblique projection for, 573
positioning of, 260-277
posteroanterior or anteroposterior oblique projections of, 267
radiographs of, 256, 257, 258
national survey norms for, 263
routine for, 263
topographical landmarks of, 260, 261
trauma and mobile radiography of, 572, 573
Cervical spine skeleton, 258
Cervical vertebra, 248
axial CT image of, 58
characteristics of, 252-253
joint between, 12
7th; *see* Vertebra prominens
subluxation of, 546
Cervicothoracic vertebrae, radiography of alternate methods for, 271
swimmer's lateral position for, 270
Cervix, carcinoma of, pelvic computed tomography to diagnose, 673
Chassard-Lapine axial projection, 468
Chauffeur's fracture, 549
Chemical digestion, 419
Chemical level of organization, 2
Chemotoxic theory, 511
Chest, 55-84; *see also* Thorax
anatomy of, 56-63
anterior oblique positions of, 79
anteroposterior projection of, 20, 558
lateral decubitus position for, 77
lordotic, 21, 78
supine or semierect, 76
topographical landmarks for, 70
axial sections of, 661-663
basic and special projections of, 71
central ray location positioning method for, 69-70, 84
central ray and lung measurement study and, 84
of child, radiography of anteroposterior/posteroanterior projection for, 588-589
Chest, cont'd
lateral position for, 590-591
decubitus position for, 312
viewing radiographs of, 54
during inspiration and expiration, 66
lateral position of, 62, 68, 81
for ambulatory patient, 74
for nonambulatory patient, 75
positioning of, 64-70
posterior oblique positions of, 80
posteroanterior projection of, 20, 62, 65, 67
of ambulatory patient, 72
in erect position, 99
in lateral position, 62
of nonambulatory patient, 73
ribs visible on, 64
topographical landmarks for, 69
radiographs of, 312
breathing instructions for, 66
evaluation criteria for, 67-68
national norms for, 70
viewing, 54
routine for, 70
semi-axial anteroposterior lordotic projection of, 78
semierect anteroposterior projection of, 76
supine anteroposterior projection of, 76
trauma and mobile radiography of, 552, 558
two projections required for, 51
Chiasma, optic, 639, 641, 642
Chiasmatic cistern, 638
Chiasmatic groove, 328
Child (children)
abuse of, reporting, 582
age of understanding and cooperation from, 582
radiography for, 581-610; *see also* Pediatric radiography
Chin, extending, on posteroanterior chest radiographs, 67
Chip fracture, 550
Cholangiogram (cholangiography), 487
laparoscopic, 491
laparoscopic surgery with, 491
operative, 490
anteroposterior and/or right posterior oblique projection for, 501
operative, routine, 495
summary of, 494
T-tube (postoperative or delayed), 491
basic and special projections for, 496
national survey norms for, 495
transhepatic, percutaneous, 492
basic and special projections for, 496
national survey norms for, 495
Cholangiopancreatography, retrograde, endoscopic, 493
basic and special projections for, 496
national survey norms for, 495
Cholecystectomy, laparoscopic surgery with, 491
Cholecystitis, oral cholecystogram to diagnose, 487
Cholecystogram (cholecystography), 487
oral; *see* Oral cholecystogram
summary of, 494
Cholecystokinin, 485
Cholecystopaques, 487
Cholelithiasis, oral cholecystogram to diagnose, 487
Chordomas, MRI to diagnose, 740
Chronic gastritis, upper GI series to diagnose, 431
Chyme, 419
Cinefluorography, 425
Circle of Willis, 686
Circulation
pulmonary, 681
systemic, 680
Circulatory system, 3, 680
abdominal, 689-690
peripheral, 690-691
thoracic, 688
Circumduction, 27
Circumferential whole-volume coils for MRI, 741
Circumflex aorta, 688
Cistern(s)
chiasmatic, 638
subarachnoid, 638
Cisterna magna, 637, 638

Cisterna pontis, 638
Clamps, head, for immobilization during pediatric radiography, 584
Claustrum, 641
Clavicle, 56, 148, 149, 307
  anteroposterior and anteroposterior axial projections of, 165
  anteroposterior and lateral projections for, 566
  anteroposterior radiograph of, 149
  basic and special projections in, 155
  radiograph of, 149
  routine for, 154
  trauma and mobile radiography of, 566
Clavicle sternum articulation, 306
Clavicular notch, 307
Cleaves method, modified, for pelvis, 235
Clements-Nakayama method for hip and proximal femur, 241
Clinoid processes, 328, 329, 684
Clivus, 328, 684
Closed fracture, 548
"Closed" joint spaces, 35
Closed mouth position, 337
Closed reduction of fracture, radiographs following, 551
Clubfoot, congenital, Kite method for, 595
Coccygeal segments, 248
Coccyx, 223, 248, 286
  anatomy of, 282
  anteroposterior axial projection for, 300
  basic and special projections in, 288
  lateral position for, 302
  sacrum and lumbar spine, 279-303
    positioning of, 286-302
Coccyx and sacrum exam, pregnancy and, 44
Cochlea, 392, 393
Cochlear window, 392, 393
Code of ethics, 46
Colcher-Sussman ruler, 225
Colic flexure, 86, 448
Colitis, barium enema to diagnose, 459
Collar bone; *see* Clavicle
Collar extensions, raised, for lead apron, 40
Collateral ligaments
  of knee, 180-181
  of wrist, 109
Collecting tubule, 507
Colles fracture, 549
  reverse, 549
Collimation, 42
Collimator, adjustable, 42
  illuminated, to restrict x-ray beam, 48
  x-ray beam divergence controlled by, 34
Colon, 86, 89, 448, 449, 452, 453
  large intestine vs., 448
Comminuted fracture, 548
Common bile duct, 485
Common carotid artery, 683, 692
  arteriography of, 701
Compact bone, 8
Comparison chest radiographs, 66
Compensatory curve, 249
Complete fracture, 548
Compound fracture, 548
Compression
  of breast for mammography, 534
  ureteric, 515-516, 525
    intravenous urogram with, 517
Compression bands for immobilization during pediatric radiography, 584
Compression fracture, 550
Compression technique to prevent esophageal reflux, 429
Computed gray scale in cranial computed tomography, 653
Computed myelography, 625
Computed tomography
  abdominal, 659-677; *see also* Abdomen, computed tomography of
  cardiovascular, 650
  changes and advances in, 649
  comparison of magnetic resonance imaging with, 735
  cranial, 633-658; *see also* Cranial computed tomography
  definition of, 660
  helical scanners for, 650
  kidney cross-section with, 505
  of neck through larynx, axial (cross) section at level of C5, 58
Computed tomography, cont'd
  of pelvis; *see* Pelvis, computed tomography of
  pregnancy and, 44
  thoracic; *see* Thorax, computed tomography of
  viewing images of, 54
Computed tomography scanograms for long bone measurement, 612
Computer for MRI, 734
Concave, 249
Conchae, nasal, 329, 332, 335
Condylar portion of occipital bone, 326
Condyles
  of condyloid process, 336, 337
  of femur, 179, 180
  humeral, 107
  occipital, 326
  of tibia, 178
Condyloid joints, 12, 13
  of hand and wrist, 108
Condyloid process, 336
Cones, metal, to restrict x-ray beam, 48
Congenital anomalies of gallbladder, oral cholecystogram to diagnose, 487
Congenital clubfoot, Kite method for, 595
Congenital hip dislocation, radiography of, 231
Congestive heart failure as contraindication to excretory urography, 514
Connective tissue, 2
  of breast, 532
Consciousness, loss of, from urologic contrast media, 513
Contact shields, gonadal, 43
Contralateral, 23
Contrast, 32
  in chest radiography, 65
Contrast media
  for abdominal angiography, 711
  for barium enema, preparation of, 461
  for cerebral angiography, 699
  for cranial computed tomography, 655
  for defecography, 466
  iodinated, water-soluble, 424
  for knee arthrography, 616
  for magnetic resonance imaging, 740
  for myelography, 622
  in pediatric radiography, patient preparation for, 600
  for shoulder arthrography, 619
  for thoracic aortography, 709
  for thoracic computed tomography, 665
  for upper gastrointestinal system, 423-424
  urologic, 511-513
Contrast medium injector, automatic electromechanical, 697
Contrast scales in thoracic computed tomography, 666
Contusion, 547
Conus medullaris, 248, 634
Conventional tomography, 626-631
  blurring principle in, 628
  variable vs. fixed fulcrum in, 628
  variations of, 631
Conversion table, traditional to SI units, 37
Conversions, SI, 37
Convex, 249
Convoluted capsule, proximal and distal, 507
Convulsions from urologic contrast media, 513
Cooper's ligaments, 532
Coracoid process, 150
Cord(s)
  spinal; *see* Spinal cord
  vocal, 58
    during swallowing, 414
Cornua, sacral, 281
Coronal image, 15
  viewing, 54
Coronal plane, 15
Coronal suture, 330
Coronary arteries, 682, 692
Coronary sinus, 682
Coronary veins, 682
Coronoid fossa, 107
Coronoid process
  of forearm, 106
  of mandible, 336
Coronoid tubercle, 106
Corpus
  of sternum, 306
  of stomach, 416, 417
Corpus callosum, 636, 640, 641
Cortex
  cerebral, 636, 640
  kidney, 507
  of long bones, 8
Costal margin of rib, 286, 306
  as topographic landmark of abdomen, 52, 91
Costocartilage, 307
Costochondral union (junction), 308
Costophrenic angle, 62
Costotransverse joints, 254, 308
Costovertebral joints, 254, 308
Coulombs, 37
Coyle method for elbow, 140
CR; *see* Central ray
Cranial bones
  anatomy of, 324-329
  radiographs of, 331
  and skull, 323-358
    positioning of, 343-357
Cranial computed tomography, 633-658
  advantages of, over conventional radiography, 649
  attenuation in, 652
  basic principles and procedures for, 649-658
  computed gray scale in, 653
  contraindications to, 655
  contrast media for, 655
  CT scanning unit for, 654
  degree of attenuation of voxel in, 653
  differential absorption in, 653
  exposure factors in, 652
  image manipulation in, 653
  image reconstruction in, principles of, 651-653
  indications for, 655
  picture reconstruction in, 652
  positioning for, 656-658
  preparation for, 655, 656
  procedure for, 655-656
  source and detector collimation in, 651
  summation in, 652
  viewing images in, 54
  x-ray transmission and collection of data in, 651
Cranial nerves, 641
Cranial venous system, 687
Cranium, 324, 635
  adult, 330
  anteroposterior axial projection for, 356
  base of, bones of, 8
  basic and special projections for, 348
  basilar position for, 354
  Caldwell method for, 352
  computed tomography of; *see* Cranial computed tomography
  exposure factors for, 346
  Haas method for, 350, 357
  infant, 330
  joints of, 330
  lateral position for, 351, 355
  medial sectional view of, 329
  positioning considerations for, 346
  positioning errors for, 346
  posteroanterior axial projection for, 350, 352, 357
  posteroanterior projection for, 353
  projections required for, 51
  radiographs of, national survey norms for, 347
  submentovertex projection for, 354
  surface landmarks of, 344-345
  Towne method for, 349, 356
Crest
  anterior, of tibia, 178
  iliac, 223, 224
  intertrochanteric, 222
Cribriform plate, 329, 335
Cricoid cartilage, 58, 414
Crista galli, 329, 335
Crohn's disease, enteroclysis to diagnose, 457
Cross-sectional image, 15
  viewing, 54
Cross-sectional sections, 15
Cruciate ligaments, 180, 181
Cubital vein, 693
Cuboid bone, 175
Cuneiform bone, 175; *see also* Triquetrum bone of wrist
Curvatures
  of stomach, 416
  vertebral (spinal), 249
Cyanosis from urologic contrast media, 513
Cystic duct, 485
Cystogram (cystography), 518
  anteroposterior projection for, in LPO and RPO position, 527
  basic and special projections in, 520
  retrograde, 518
  routine, 520
Cystourethrogram (cystourethrography), voiding, 510, 519
  anteroposterior projection for (female), 528
  basic and special projections in, 520
  for child, 608-609
  right posterior oblique position for (male), 528
  routine, 520

D

Danelius-Miller method
  for hip and proximal femur, 239
  for trauma and mobile radiography of pelvis, 571
Deca-, 37
Deci-, 37
Decub. position, 19
Decubitus chest and abdomen projections, viewing radiographs of, 54
Decubitus position, 19
  markers for, 30
Decubitus projections, 19
Deep, 23
Defecation, 454
  post-exam, 424
Defecogram (defocography), 459; *see also* Barium enema
  procedure for, 466-467
Deglutition, 413, 414, 419
Delayed cholangiography, 491
Demifacets of thoracic vertebrae, 254
Dendrites, 634, 640
Dens
  of atlas, 253
  of axis, 253
  radiography of, anteroposterior or posteroanterior projection for, 273
Density, 31
  proton, 727
  spin, 727
Density change rule, 31
Depressed fracture, 550
Depression, 27
  of distal humerus, 107
Descending aorta, 63
Descending colon, 86, 448, 449, 452, 453
Detail, 33
Development of bones, 9
Deviation, ulnar and radial, 24, 110
Diabetes mellitus as contraindication to excretory urography, 514
Diagnostic gastrointestinal intubation, 457
Diagnostic procedures, general, protocol and order for, 47
Diaphragm, 57, 62, 63, 86, 681
  esophagus passing through, 415
  fixation or lack of movement of, chest radiography for, 66
  on lateral chest radiograph, 62
  openings in, 415
Diaphysis
  bone development and, 586
  of compact bone, 8
  of long bones, 7
Diarthrodial joints, summary of, 13
Diarthrosis, 10
Digested substances, 419
Digestion, 419-420
  accessory organs of, 3, 412
  chemical, 419
  in intestines, 454
  mechanical, 419
Digestive functions, 454
Digestive organs
  in abdominal cavity, 86
  accessory, 88
Digestive system, 3, 86
  anatomy of, 412, 446
  movements of, 454
Digital fluoroscopy systems, C-arm, mobile, 555-556
  ALARA principles and, 38
  radiation protection with, 557

Digital fluoroscopy, 426
Digital mammography, 536
Digital subtraction angiography, 708
Digits
  of foot, 172
  of hand, 102
Diploe, 8
Discography, 625
Disk(s)
  articular, 109, 181
  intervertebral, 11, 248, 251
  slipped, 251
Dislocation, 546
  hip, congenital, radiography of, 231
Display for MRI, 734
Distal, 22
Distal convoluted tubule, 507
Distal interphalangeal joints
  of fingers, 103
  of toes, 173
Distal phalanges, 102
Distal radioulnar joint, 105, 109
Distal tibiofibular joint, 183
Distance, source image receptor, density and, 31
Distortion, image quality and, 34-36
Distraction, fracture, 547
Divergence, x-ray beam, 34
Diverticulae, upper GI series to diagnose, 431
Diverticulitis, barium enema to diagnose, 459
Diverticulosis, barium enema to diagnose, 459
Diverticulum, 459
Dolichocephalic skull, 343
Dorsal decubitus left lateral position, 19
Dorsal decubitus position, 19
Dorsal radiocarpal ligament of wrist, 109
Dorsal recumbent position, 17
Dorsal surface, 16
Dorsalis pedis artery, 691, 692
Dorsiflexion, 184
  ankle, 25
  wrist, 24
Dorsoplantar projection, 184, 193
  of foot, 28
Dorsum, 16
  of foot, 184
Dorsum pedis, 184
Dorsum sellae, 328, 329
Dose
  absorbed, radiation, 38
  annual effective, 37
  breast, calculation of, 45
  calculations of, for patient protection, 45
  effective, 38
  gonadal, calculation of, 45
  lifetime effective, 37
  limit on, annual effective, 37
  midline, calculation of, 45
  patient
    chart of, 39
    per exam, patient protection and, 45
    of radiation, 38-39
  radiation, units of, 37
  skin, calculation of, 45
  thyroid, calculation of, 45
  tissue, collimation and, 42
  whole body effective, 37
Dose limit, annual effective, 37
Dose-limiting recommendations for radiographers, 37
Double-contrast barium enema, 459; *see also* Barium enema
  for child, 606-607
  left lateral decubitus position (AP) for, 478
  patient exposures during, 39
  procedure for, 464-465
  right lateral decubitus position (AP) for, 477
Double contrast procedures, 424
Drainage
  abdominal abscess, percutaneous, 720
  biliary
    percutaneous, 720
    stone extraction and, percutaneous transhepatic cholangiography for, 492
Drape shields, tower, for worker protection, 40
Drum crest, 390
Drum spur, 390
Duct(s)
  bile, common, 485
  biliary; *see* Biliary ducts
  of breast, 532

Duct(s), cont'd
  cystic, 485
  endolymphatic, 392
  hepatic, 485
  lymphatic, 694
  pancreatic, 485
  thoracic, 694
  of Wirsung, 485
Ductless glands, 5
Duodenal bulb (cap), 86, 418
Duodenal papilla, 485
Duodenal ulcer, 422
Duodenojejunal flexure, 418
Duodenojejunal junction, 447
Duodenoscope, 493
Duodenum, 86, 447, 452, 453
  anatomy of, 418
  parts of, 418
  polyp in, upper GI series to diagnose, 431
  posteroanterior projection of, 418
  radiographs of, 418
  tumors in, upper GI series to diagnose, 431
Dura mater, 635
  sinuses of, 687

E

E; *see* Effective dose
EAM; *see* External acoustic meatus
Ear, 390-393
  external, 390
  internal, 392-393
  middle, 390-392
  positioning landmarks of, 344
  structures of, tomography of, 395
Echo planar imaging in MRI, 743
Ecklund technique for implant mammography, 542
ED; *see* Effective dose
Edema, laryngeal, from urologic contrast media, 513
Effective dose, 37, 38
Effective dose limit, annual, 37
Efferent arterioles of kidney, 507
Effusion, sphenoid, 387
Elbow, 12, 109
  acute flexion projections of, 140
  anteroposterior oblique projection of
    with lateral (external) rotation, 137
    with medial (internal) rotation, 138
  anteroposterior projection of, 108, 136
  basic and special projections of, 114
  Coyle method for, 140
  fat stripes of, 111
  flexion and extension of, 24
  "jerked," 549
  Jones method for, 140
  lateral radiograph of, 108
  lateral-lateromedial projection of, 139
  radial head lateral-lateromedial projections of, 142
  rotational movements of, 110
  routine for, 113
  summary of, 109
  three projections required for, 51
  trauma axial lateral-axial lateromedial projections of, 141
  trauma and mobile radiography of, 564
  true lateral, 107
Electrical interference of MRI with electromechanical implants, 737
Electromechanical implants, electrical interference of MRI with, 737
Electron beam tomography, 650
Electronic support system for MRI, 733
Elevation, 27
Elimination, 454
  post-exam, 424
Ellipsoidal joints, 12, 13
  of hand and wrist, 108
Embolization, 719
Emphysema, pulmonary, 61
Encephalitis, 391
Encephalon; *see* Brain
Endochondral ossification, 9
Endocrine system, 5, 88
Endolymphatic duct, 392
Endoscopes, video, 493
Endoscopic retrograde cholangiopancreatography, 493

Endoscopic retrograde, cont'd
  basic and special projections for, 496
  national survey norms for, 495
Endoscopy, 493
Ends of long bones, 7
Enema, barium; *see* Barium enema
Enema tips, 461
  insertion of, 462
Engorgement of pulmonary vessels, 66
Enteritis, small bowel series to diagnose, 455
Enteroclysis, 457, 468
Entrance skin exposure, 38
Enzymes, chemical digestion and, 419
Epicondyles, 107, 179, 180
Epidural hematoma, cranial computed tomography to diagnose, 655
Epidural space, 635
Epidural venography, 625
Epigastric region of abdomen, 90
Epiglottis, 57, 58, 413
  during swallowing, 414
Epiphyseal fracture, 550
Epiphyseal fusion of long bones, 9
Epiphyseal plates, 9, 11
  bone development and, 586
Epiphysis
  bone development and, 586
  endochondral ossification and, 9
Epithelial tissue, 2
Epitympanic recess, 390, 391
Equalization filter in digital fluoroscopy, 426
Equilibrium, organs of, anatomy of, 390-393
Equipment
  fluorography, 425-426
  magnetic resonance imaging, 731-734
ERCP; *see* Endoscopic retrograde cholangiopancreatography
Erect anterior position, 20
Erect chest radiographs, 66
Erect left posterior oblique position, 18
Erect marker, 30
Erect position, 17
Erect posterior position, 20
Erect right lateral position, 18
Erect right posterior oblique position, 18
Erythrocytes, 680
Escherichia coli causing urinary tract infections, 514
ESE; *see* Entrance skin exposure
Esophageal reflux
  esophagram to diagnose, 427
  during fluoroscopy, 429
Esophageal varices, esophagram to diagnose, 427
Esophagogastric junction, 415, 416
Esophagram, 412, 415, 427-430
  anteroposterior (posteroanterior) projection for, 437
  contraindications to, 427
  definition of, 427
  lateral position for, 436
  left anterior oblique position for, 438
  preparation for, 427-428
  procedure for, 428
  purpose of, 427
  right anterior oblique position for, 435
  routine views in, 434
  soft tissue lateral position for, 439
Esophagus, 57, 63, 86, 412, 413, 414
  anatomical anomalies of, esophagram for, 427
  anatomy of, 414-415
  axial (cross-section) image of, 60
  on CT cross sectional image at level of T9, 61
  through diaphragm, 415
  foreign bodies in, esophagram to diagnose, 427
  indentations in, 414
  in mediastinum, 414
  swallowing and peristalsis and, 415
Ethics
  code of, 46
  professional, and patient care, 46
Ethmoid bone, 324, 329, 335
  orbits and, 338
Ethmoid sinuses, 387
Ethmoidal notch, 325
Eustachian tube, 390, 414
Evacuative proctography; *see* Defecography
Evaluation criteria for radiograph, 29

Eversion, 25
  of ankle, 25
  of foot, 184
Eversion stress of ankle, 25
Examination, radiographic, 14
Excretory urogram (urography), 89, 510, 514-515; *see also* Intravenous urography
  basic and special projections in, 520
  contraindications to, 514
  indications for, 514
  pregnancy precautions with, 515
  preparation for, 515
Exercises, breathing, to prevent esophageal reflux, 429
Exocrine system, 88
Expiration
  full, chest radiograph during, 66
  thoracic cavity during, 64
Expiration marker, 30
Exposure
  entrance skin, 38
  fluoroscopy, patterns of, tower drape shields and, 40
  patient, during fluoroscopic procedures, 39
  radiation
    patient, minimizing, 45
    units of, 37
  sample, explanations of, 45
  skin entrance, 38
Exposure angle in tomography, 626
Exposure factors, 31
  optimum, for patient protection, 44
Exposure patterns, worker protection and, 40
Exposure rates, fluoroscopy, limits for, 41
Exposure time
  for chest radiography, 65
  control of, 31
Exposure variables, 31
Extension, 24
  excessive, in cranial radiography, 346
Exterior, 23
External, 23
External acoustic meatus, 16, 260, 261, 327, 345, 390, 391, 392
External ear, 390
External marker, 30
External occipital protuberance, 326
External rotation, 25
  of hip, 228
  of humerus, 153
Extraction of vascular foreign bodies, 718
Extravasation from urologic contrast media, 513
Extremity, upper; *see* Upper limb
Eyes
  coronal section through, 643
  positioning landmarks of, 344

F

Facet(s)
  articular, 174, 251
    of tibia, 178
  superior, of atlas, 253
  of thoracic vertebrae, 254
Facial artery, 684
Facial bones, 8, 359-384
  anatomy of, 332-336
  basic and special projections for, 362
  Caldwell method for, 365
  lateral and anteroposterior acanthioparietal projection for, 578
  lateral position for, 363
  parietoacanthial (Waters) projection for, 360, 364
    modified, 366
  positioning considerations for, 360
  posteroanterior axial projection for, 365
  posteroanterior skull projection for, 360
  projections required for, 51
  radiographs of, national survey norms for, 361
  review of, 340-342
  routine for, 361
  trauma and mobile radiography of, 578
  Waters method for, 360, 364
    lateral reverse, 578
    modified, 366
    modified reverse, 578
Facial cavities, 338

Facial nerve, 641
Facial vein, 693
Falciform ligament, 484
False pelvis, 225
False ribs, 307
Falx cerebelli, 640
Falx cerebri, 636, 687
Fast spin echo in MRI, 743
Fat(s)
breast, 532
chemical digestion of, 419
orbital, 642
perirenal, 505
Fat bands of wrist joint, 109
importance of visualizing, 111
Fat pads
infrapatellar, 181
of wrist joint, 109
importance of visualizing, 111
Fat stripes of wrist joint, 109
importance of visualizing, 111
Fatigue fracture, 550
Fatty acids, digestion and, 419
Fatty breast, 533
Feces, elimination of, 454
Female
breasts of, shielding, for humerus and shoulder girdle radiographs, 154
gonadal dose for, 45
gonadal shields for, 43
pelvic organs of, 509
pelvis of, 226
anatomy of, 672
reproductive organs of, 4
voiding cystourethrogram in, 519
Femoral artery, 691, 692
Femoral vein, 691, 693
Femorotibial joint, 183
Femur, 179-180, 222-223
basic and special projections for, 188
correct central ray for, 36
development of, 586
mid and distal
anteroposterior projection of, 217
lateral-mediolateral and lateromedial projections, 218, 219
patella and, 180
and pelvic girdle, 221-245
anatomy of, 222-228
basic and special projections for, 233
positioning of, 229-244
radiographs of, national survey norms for, 232
proximal, 227
in anatomical position, 228
angles of, 222
and hip; *see* Hip and proximal femur
spiral fracture of, 548
trauma and mobile radiography of, 570, 571
two projections required for, 51
Ferguson method, AP, for scoliosis series, 296
Fibro-fatty breast, 533
Fibro-glandular breast, 533
Fibrous breast tissue, 532
Fibrous capsule, 11
of kidney, 507
Fibrous joints, 10
summary of, 13
Fibula, 178, 180
ankle and, 176
anteroposterior and lateral projection for, 568
anteroposterior mortise and lateral projection for, 568
compound fracture of, 548
Pott's fracture of, 549
trauma and mobile radiography of, 568
two projections required for, 51
Fibular collateral ligament, 180, 181
Fibular notch, 178
Film
centering, 49
x-ray, 14
Film badges for personnel monitoring, 38
Film holders
for lower limb radiographs, 186
part placement on, 29
placement of, for chest radiography, 70
Film markers, 30
for abdominal radiographs, 92
for chest radiography, 65
Film markers, cont'd
for lower limb radiographs, 186
for upper limb radiographs, 112
Film object alignment, distortion and, 35
Film positioning, 49
Filming, spot, patient exposures during, 39
Film-screen combinations, optimum speed, for patient protection, 44
Film-screen mammography, 532, 535
Filtration, 41
Fingers, 102
abduction and adduction of, 26
anteroposterior (PA) oblique and lateral projection for, 562
interphalangeal joints of, 12
joints of, 103
lateral lateromedial or mediolateral projections of, 117
metacarpophalangeal joints of, 12
posteroanterior oblique projection of, medial or lateral rotation, 116
posteroanterior projection of, 115
three projections required for, 51
and thumb, routine for, 113, 114
trauma and mobile radiography of, 562
Fisk method for shoulder, 160
Fissures
of cerebral hemispheres, 636
of lungs, 61
orbital, 328, 339
Fixed table-top x-ray table, 48
Fixed vs. variable fulcrum in conventional tomography, 628
Flank pain, excretory urography to diagnose cause of, 514
Flat bones, 8
Flexion, 24
excessive, in cranial radiography, 346
plantar, 25, 184
radial, 24, 110, 130
radiograph of, 105
ulnar, 24, 110
radiograph of, 105
Flexure
colic (hepatic), 86, 448
splenic, 86
Floating ribs, 307
Floating table-top x-ray table, 48
Fluorography equipment, 425-426
Fluoroscopic procedures
patient exposure during, 39
pregnancy and, 44
Fluoroscopy exposure patterns, tower drape shields and, 40
Fluoroscopy exposure rates limits, 41
Fluoroscopy room, 422, 425
Fluoroscopy unit(s)
general, 425
mobile C-arm digital; *see* Mobile C-arm digital fluoroscopy systems
Fluoroscopy
with barium enema, 463
digital, 426
mobile C-arm systems for; *see* Mobile C-arm digital fluoroscopy systems
esophageal reflux during, 429
film badges and, 38
gastrointestinal, 422
on child, 604-607
routine projections for, 430
oral cholecystogram with, 489
patient exposures during, 39
procedure after, 430
pulsed, 39
scatter radiation from, 40
and spot filming
in knee arthrography, 616, 617
in myelography, 622
television, 425
upper GI, positioning for, 433
worker protection during, 40-41, 425
Focal plane in tomography, 626
Focal spot size, 33, 35
Fontanels, 330
Foot, 172-173
anteroposterior and lateral projections for, 567, 595
weight-bearing, 196
anteroposterior oblique projection of, 20
with medial (lateral) rotation, 194
anteroposterior projection of, 193
Foot, cont'd
arches of, 175
basic and special projections for, 188
bones of, 172
of child, 595
dorsoplantar projection, 28, 193
inward stress movement of, 25
joints of, summary of, 183
Kite method for, 595
lateral-mediolateral (lateromedial) projections of, 195
motions of, 184
outward stress movement of, 25
plantodorsal projections of, 28
radiograph of, 177
routine for, 186
surfaces of
and projections of, 184
terms for, 16
three projections required for, 51
trauma and mobile radiography of, 551, 567
Foramen (foramina)
interventricular, 637, 638
intervertebral, 250, 251, 252, 255, 280
vs. zygapophyseal joints, 258-259, 285
jugular, 327
of Luschka, 637
mental, 336
of Monro, 637
nutrient, of long bone, 8
obturator, 224
optic; *see* Optic foramen
sacral, posterior 281
transverse, 252, 253
vertebral, 250
Foramen magnum, 326
coronal section through, 644
Foramen ovale, 328
Foramen rotundum, 328
Foramen spinosum, 328
Forearm, 102, 106-107
anteroposterior projection of, 110, 134
joints of, summary of, 109
lateral
correct positioning of, 29
evaluation criteria for, 29
lateral and medial rotation of, 25
lateral-lateromedial projection of, 135
rotational movements of, 110
routine for, 113, 114
trauma and mobile radiography of, post reduction, 563
two projections required for, 51
Forebrain, 635, 636-639
Foreign bodies
in esophagus, esophagram to diagnose, 427
localization of, two projections for, 50
in thorax, chest radiography for, 66
vascular, extraction of, 718
Fossa
coronoid, 107
glenoid, 150
infraspinous, 150
intercondylar, 179, 180
intercondyloid
anteroposterior axial projection of, 211
basic and special projections for, 188
posteroanterior axial projection of, tunnel view, 210
nasal, 386
olecranon, 107
radial, 107
subscapular, 150
supraspinous, 150
temporomandibular, 327, 337
Four-sided collimation, 42
Fourth ventricle of cerebrum, 636, 637-638
Fovea capitis, 222
Fowler's position, 17
Fracture(s)
acetabular, 673
alignment of
terminology related to, 547
two projections to determine, 50
definition of, 547
hip
clinical indicators for radiography of, 231
evidence of, 228
typical rotation with, 230
orbital, 339
Fractures, cont'd
pelvic ring, radiography of, 231
reduction of, radiographs following, 551
terminology related to, 112, 546-550
types of, 548-549
Frankfort horizontal plane, 16
Fringe magnetic field, 736
Front of body, terms for, 16
Frontal bone(s), 324, 325, 329
coronal section through, 643
orbits and, 338
Frontal horn of lateral ventricles, 637
Frontal lobe of cerebral hemisphere, 636
Frontal plane, 15
Frontal process of maxilla, 333
Frontal sinus, 329, 387
Frontal tuberosity, 325
Fuch method for cervical spine radiography, 273
Fulcrum in tomography, 626, 628
Fulcrum level in tomography, 626
Functional classification of joints, 10
Fundus
of gallbladder, 485
of stomach, 416, 417
Fusion, epiphyseal, of long bones, 9

G

Gallbladder, 88, 412, 453
anatomy of, 484, 485-486
basic and special projections for, 496
and biliary ducts, 483-501
positioning of, 495-496
body habitus and position of, 420, 421
congenital anomalies of, oral cholecystogram to diagnose, 487
exam of, pregnancy and, 44
functions of, 485
left anterior oblique position for, 498
location of, variation in, 486
neoplasms of, oral cholecystogram to diagnose, 487
posteroanterior projection for, 497
in erect position, 500
in right lateral decubitus position, 499
radiographs of, 486, 487, 494
national survey norms for, 495
scout, 497
right lateral decubitus position for (posteroanterior projection), 499
ultrasound (sonography) of, 489
Gallstones, oral cholecystogram to diagnose, 487
Ganglia, basal, 640, 641
Garth method for shoulder, 164
Gadolinium-DTPA, 740
Gastric canal, 417
Gastric folds, 417
Gastritis, upper GI series to diagnose, 431
Gastrografin, 424
Gastrointestinal fluoroscopy, on child, 604-607
Gastrointestinal intubation, diagnostic, 457
Gastrointestinal system, 86
upper, 411-444
Gastrointestinal tract, 86
Gastrostomy, percutaneous, 721
Gating in MRI, 743
Gauss, 731
Gaynor-Hart method for wrist, 131
General anatomy, 2
principles of, 2-6
General diagnostic procedures, protocol and order for, 47
General fluoroscopy unit, 425
General patient positioning, 49
Genital system, 4
Genitourinary system, pediatric radiography of, 608-609
GI series; *see* Lower GI series; Upper GI series
Giga-, 37
Ginglymus joints, 12, 13
of hand and wrist, 108, 109
Girdle, shoulder; *see* Shoulder girdle
Glabella, 325, 344
Glabelloalveolar line, 345
Glabellomeatal line, 345
Gladiolus of sternum, 306
Gland(s)
ductless, 5

Gland(s), cont'd
lacrimal, 642
parathyroid, 59
parotid, 413
pineal, 637, 639
pituitary, 328, 639, 641
coronal section through, 644
prostate, 508, 509
salivary, 412, 413
sublingual, 413
submandibular, 413
suprarenal (adrenal), 88, 89, 452, 453, 504
pathology of, abdominal computed tomography to diagnose, 673
thymus, 59, 63
thyroid, 57, 59
Glandular breast tissue, 531, 532
Glenohumeral joint, 150, 152
Glenoid cavity, 150
Grashey method for, 159
posterior oblique radiograph of, 159
Gliding joints, 11, 13
of hand and wrist, 108
Glioma, cranial computed tomography of, 658
Glomerular capsule, 507
Glomeruli, 507
Glossopharyngeal nerve, 641
Glycerol, digestion and, 419
Gomphosis, 10
Gonadal dose, calculation of, 45
Gonadal shielding, 43-44
for abdominal radiographs, 92
for cervical and thoracic spine radiographs, 262
for chest radiography, 65
or cranial radiography, 346
for humerus and shoulder girdle radiographs, 154
for lower limb radiographs, 185, 231
for lumbar spine, sacrum and coccyx radiographs, 287
for pediatric radiography, 587
for upper limb radiographs, 112
Gonion, 260, 261, 336, 344
Gradient coils for MRI, 732
Gradient echo imaging, 743
Gradient echo technique in MRI, 743
Gradient magnetic fields, 728
Gradient moment nulling in MRI, 743
Grashey method for glenoid cavity, 159
Gray, 37
conversion of rad to, 37
Gray matter, 640, 641
Gray scale, computed, in cranial computed tomography, 653
Great blood vessels, axial (cross-section) image of, 60
Great veins of neck, 686
Great vessels, 63
Greater curvature of stomach, 416
Greater multangular bone; *see* Trapezium bone of wrist
Greater omentum, 452
Greater pelvis, 225
Greater sac, 451
Greater sciatic notch, 224
Greater trochanter of femur, 222, 224, 286
as topographic landmark of abdomen, 52, 91
Greater tubercle, 148
Greater wings of sphenoid bone, 328
Greenstick fracture, 548
Grids in trauma radiography, 553
Groove
bicipital, 148
chiasmatic (optic), 328
intertubercular (bicipital), 148
tangential projection of, 160
supraorbital, 325, 344
trochlear, 107, 179
Growth, bone, radiograph demonstrating, 9
Gullet; *see* Esophagus
Gyrus, 636

H

Haas method
for cranial radiography, 350, 357
for sella turcica radiographs, 356
Habitus, body; *see* Body habitus
Hamate bone of wrist, 103, 104
Hamulus(i)
of hamate bone, 104
pterygoid, 328, 329, 333
Hand(s)
anteroposterior (posteroanterior) oblique and lateral projection for, 562
"fan" lateral-lateromedial projection of, 123
joints of, 103
summary of, 109
lateral, 22
in extension and flexion-lateromedial projections of, 124
lateromedial projection of, 20
movements of, 26
posteroanterior oblique projection of, 20
with lateral rotation, 122
posteroanterior projection of, 103, 121
positioning of, with joints open, 35
routine for, 113, 114
surfaces of, terms for, 16
three projections required for, 51
trauma and mobile radiography of, 562
and wrist, 102-104
joints of, 108-109
Hand spread method for locating CR on posteroanterior chest radiograph, 69
Hangman's fracture, 549
Hard palate, 57, 333, 413
Haustrum, 449
Head
arteries of, 683
of condyloid process, 336
of femur, 222
of fibula, 178
of humerus, 148
of metatarsals, 172
of pancreas, 418
of phalanx, 102
of radius, 106, 107
of rib, 307
of scapula, 150
trauma radiography of, 552
of ulna, 106
Head clamps for immobilization during pediatric radiography, 584
Hearing, organs of, anatomy of, 390-393
Heart, 63, 414, 681
anatomy of, 63
axial (cross-section) image of, 60
chambers of, axial (cross-section) image of, 60
on computed tomography cross sectional image at level of T9, 61
cross section of, 61
disease of, thoracic computed tomography to diagnose, 664
on posteroanterior chest radiograph, 62
valves of, 681
Heart failure, congestive, as contraindication to excretory urography, 514
Heating of tissues and metallic objects during MRI, 738
Hecto-, 37
Heel effect, anode, 36
Helical CT scanners, 650
Hematoma(s)
epidural and subdural, cranial computed tomography to diagnose, 655
hepatic or splenic, abdominal computed tomography to diagnose, 673
subdural, cranial computed tomography of, 658
Hematuria, excretory urography to diagnose, 514
Hemidiaphragm, 57
on lateral chest radiograph, 62
Hemispheres, cerebral, 636, 640
axial section through, 645, 646
Hemorrhage, intracranial, cranial computed tomography to diagnose, 655
Hemothorax, 61
Henle, loop of, 507
Hepatic artery, 692
Hepatic ducts, 485
Hepatic flexure, 86, 448
Hepatic vein, 689, 690, 693
Hepatopancreatic ampulla, 485
Hepatopancreatic sphincter, 485
Hernia, hiatal, upper GI series to diagnose, 431
Herniated nucleus pulposus, 251
Hiatal hernia, upper GI series to diagnose, 431
Hickory stick fracture, 548
Highmore, antrum of, 386
Hilar lesions, thoracic computed tomography to diagnose, 664
Hilum
of kidney, 506
of lungs, 62
Hindbrain, 635, 639-640
Hinge joints, 12, 13
of hand and wrist, 108, 109
Hip, 13, 228
congenital dislocation of, radiography of, 231
Danelius-Miller method for trauma and mobile radiography of, 571
evaluation of, pelvic computed tomography for, 673
external rotation of, 228
female, flat contact shield for radiograph of, 43
fracture of
clinical indicators for radiography of, 231
evidence of, 228
typical rotation with, 230
lateral, 227
proximal, fractures of, radiography of, 231
and proximal femur
anteroposterior unilateral projection of, 238
axiolateral (inferosuperior) projection of, 239
modified, for possible trauma, 241
basic and special projections for, 233
Clements-Nakayama method for, 241
Danelius-Miller method for, 239
exam of, pregnancy and, 44
modified Lauenstein and Hickey method for, 240
routine for, 232
unilateral "frog-leg" projection of, mediolateral, 240
Sanderson method for trauma and mobile radiography of, 571
trauma and mobile radiography of, 571
two projections required for, 51
pediatric radiography of, anteroposterior and lateral projections for, 596-597
Hip bone, 223-224
Hip pointer, 547
Hives from urologic contrast media, 513
Holmblad method for knee, 210
Homeostasis, disruption of, with urologic contrast media, 511
Horizontal plane, 15
Frankfort, 16
Hormones, 5
Horns, sacral, 281
Humeral condyle, 107
Humerus, 7, 23, 102
anatomy of, 148
anteroposterior projection of, 143
with external rotation, 153
distal, 107
lateral projection of, with internal rotation, 153, 157
oblique projection of, with neutral rotation, 153
proximal, 148-152
anteroposterior projection of, with external rotation, 156
frontal view of, 148
inferosuperior (axiolateral) projection of, 151
positioning of, 153-169
radiographs of, 153
rotation of, 153-154
and shoulder girdle, 147-170
rotational lateral-lateromedial or mediolateral projections of, 144
routine for, 114
and shoulder girdle, radiographs of, 154-155
trauma cross table lateral-lateromedial projection of, 145
trauma and mobile radiography of, 565
two projections required for, 51
Hutchinson's fracture, 549
Hyaline articular cartilage of synovial joints, 11
Hyaline cartilage, 7
of synchondroses, 11
Hydrocephalus, 638
cranial computed tomography of, 658
Hyoid bone, 6, 57, 58
Hyperemia of pulmonary vessels, 66
Hyperextension, 24
Hypersthenic body habitus, 53
chest radiography and, 64
gastrointestinal organs and, 420, 421
Hypertension, excretory urography to diagnose, 514
Hypertensive intravenous urogram, 517
Hypochondriac region of abdomen, 90
Hypogastric region of abdomen, 90
Hypoglossal nerve, 641
Hypopharynx, 413
Hypophysis, 328, 639
Hyposthenic body habitus, 53
chest radiography and, 64
gastrointestinal organs and, 420, 421
Hypothalamus, 635, 639

I

Identification, patient, and date, 30
Ileocecal valve, 86, 448
spot film of, 450
Ileum, 86, 447
terminal, 448
Ileus, small bowel series to diagnose, 455
Iliac arteries, 689, 691, 692
Iliac crest, 223, 224, 286
as topographic landmark of abdomen, 52, 91
Iliac regions of abdomen, 90
Iliac spines, 223, 224
anterior superior, 286
as topographic landmark of abdomen, 52, 91
Iliac veins, 689, 693
Ilium, 223
Illuminated adjustable collimator to restrict x-ray beam, 48
Image intensification in fluoroscopy, 425
Image manipulation in Cranial computed tomography, 653
Image quality, technique and, 31-37
Image reconstruction, principles of, in cranial computed tomography, 651-653
Image unsharpness, focal spot size and, 35
Images
computed tomography, viewing, 54
magnetic resonance imaging, viewing, 54
sagittal, coronal and axial, 15
Imaging
basic principles of, 29-36
magnetic resonance; *see* Magnetic resonance imaging
multislice, in MRI, 728
Immobilization for pediatric radiography, 583-586
Impacted fracture, 549
Implants
breast, MRI to diagnose problems related to, 536
electromechanical, electrical interference of MRI with, 737
Incisura angularis, 416
Incisura cardiaca, 416
Incomplete fracture, 548
Incontinence, 509
Incus, 392
Infections, urinary tract, excretory urography to diagnose, 514
Inferior, 22
Inferior angle of scapula, 150
Inferior articular process, 251, 252, 253, 255
Inferior costal margin as topographic landmark of abdomen, 52, 91
Inferior horn of lateral ventricles, 637, 638
Inferior nasal conchae, 335
Inferior orbital fissure, 339
Inferior ramus of pubis, 224
Inferior vena cava, 63
Inferior vertebral notch, 250
Inferosuperior axial projection, 28
Inframammary crease, 530, 531
Infraorbital margin, 344
Infraorbitomeatal line, 16, 345
Infrapatellar bursa, 181
Infrapatellar fat pad, 181
Infraperitoneal abdominal organs, 89

Infraperitoneal organs, 452
Infraspinatus fossa; *see* Infraspinous fossa
Infraspinous fossa, 150
Infundibulum, 639, 641
Infusion therapy, 718
Inguinal region of abdomen, 90
Inherent (built-in) filtration, 41
Inion, 326, 345
Inlet, pelvic, 225, 226, 281
Inner canthus, 344
Innominate bones, 223
Inside, 23
InSight wafer grid, 553
Inspiration
  full, chest radiograph during, 66
  degree of, for chest radiography, 64
  thoracic cavity during, 64
Inspiration marker, 30
Instructions, patient, to avoid repeat radiographs, 41
Insula, 636
Integumentary system, 6
Intensifier tower, worker protection and, 40
Intercarpal joint, 11
Interchondral joint, 308
Intercondylar fossa, 179, 180
Intercondylar notch, 180
Intercondylar sulcus, 179
Intercondyloid eminence, 178
Intercondyloid fossa
  anteroposterior axial projection of, 211
  basic and special projections for, 188
  posteroanterior axial projection of, tunnel view, 210
Intercondyloid tubercles, 178
Interior, 23
Intermetacarpal joint, 11
Internal, 23
Internal acoustic meatus, 327, 391
  anterior oblique projection for, 391
  modified posteroanterior (Caldwell) projection for, 391
Internal carotid angiography, 702
Internal carotid artery, 684; *see also* Carotid artery
  arteriogram of, 685
Internal ear, 392-393
Internal marker, 30
Internal rotation, 25
  of humerus, 153
  of leg, positioning and, 228
Internal secretion system, 88
Interorbital line, 344
Interphalangeal joints, 12, 103, 108, 173, 183
  open, positioning for, 35
Interpupillary line, 344
Intertarsal joints, 183
Intertrochanteric crest, 222
Intertubercular (bicipital) groove, 148
  tangential projection of, 160
Interventional angiography, 718-721
  vascular, 718-719
Interventricular foramen, 637, 638
Intervertebral disks, 11, 248, 251
Intervertebral foramina, 250, 251, 252, 255, 280
  vs. zygapophyseal joints, 258-259, 285
Intervertebral joint(s), 11
  of lumbar vertebrae, sacrum and coccyx, 284
Intervertebral spaces, 257
Intestine; *see also* Bowel
  large; *see* Large intestine
  neoplasms of, small bowel series to diagnose, 455
  small; *see* Small intestine
Intracartilaginous ossification, 9
Intracranial hemorrhage, cranial computed tomography to diagnose, 655
Intramembranous ossification, 9
Intravenous pyelogram; *see* Excretory urogram
Intravenous urogram, 89, 514-515, 516-517
  anteroposterior projection for (scout and series), 521
    post-void, 524
    for ureteric compression, 525
  basic and special projections in, 520
  on children, 600, 609-610
  hypertensive, 517
  nephrotomogram (tomogram) and nephrogram in, 522
Intravenous urogram, cont'd
  right posterior oblique and left posterior oblique positions for, 523
  routine, 520
Intubation, gastrointestinal, diagnostic, 457
Intussusception, barium enema to diagnose, 459
Inverse aorta, 688
Inversion, 25
  of ankle, 25
  of foot, 184
Inversion stress at ankle, 25
Involuntary motion, control of, 33
Involuntary muscle, 5
Involution, breast, 533
Inward stress movement of foot, 25
Iodides, organic, for urology, 511
Iodinated contrast media, water-soluble, 424
IOML; *see* Infraorbitomeatal line
Ionic organic iodides for urology, 511
Ipsilateral, 23
Irregular bones, 8
Ischial tuberosity, 224
  as topographic landmark of abdomen, 52, 91
Ischium, 223, 224
Itching from urologic contrast media, 513
IVP; *see* Excretory urogram
IVU; *see* Intravenous urogram

J

Jaundice, obstructive, percutaneous transhepatic cholangiography to diagnose, 492
Jaw
  angle of, 260, 261
  protraction and retraction of, 26
Jejunum, 86, 418, 447
"Jerked elbow," 549
Joint(s); *see also* specific joint
  acromioclavicular; *see* Acromioclavicular joints
  amphiarthrodial, summary of, 13
  ankle; *see* Ankle
  C1-2, 12
  carpometacarpal, of thumb, 11, 12, 103
  cartilaginous, 10, 11
    summary of, 13
  classification of, 10-13, 108-109
  costotransverse, 254, 308
  costovertebral, 254, 308
  cranial, 330
  diarthrodial, summary of, 13
  elbow; *see* Elbow
  ellipsoidal (condyloid), 12, 13
  femorotibial, 183
  fibrous, 10
    summary of, 13
  ginglymus (hinge), 12, 13
  glenohumeral, 150, 152
  hand and wrist, 103, 108-109
  hip; *see* Hip
  intercarpal, 11
  interchondral, 308
  intermetacarpal, 11
  interphalangeal; *see* Interphalangeal joint(s)
  intertarsal, 183
  intervertebral, 11
    of lumbar vertebrae, sacrum and coccyx, 284
  knee; *see* Knee
  lower limb, classification of, 183, 228
  of lumbar spine, sacrum and coccyx, classification of, 284
  magnetic resonance imaging of, 747
  metacarpophalangeal, 12, 103, 108
  of metatarsals, 173
  metatarsophalangeal, 12, 173, 183
  occipito-atlantal, 326
  patellofemoral; *see* Patellofemoral joints
  plane (gliding), 11, 13
  radiocarpal, 109
  radioulnar, 12, 105, 109
  sacroiliac; *see* Sacroiliac joints
  scapulohumeral, 150, 152
  sellar (saddle), 12, 13
  shoulder; *see* Shoulder
  of shoulder girdle, 152
  of skull and mandible, classification of, 337
  spheroid (ball and socket), 13
Joints, cont'd
  sternoclavicular; *see* Sternoclavicular joints
  sternocostal, 308
  study of; *see* Osteology
  subtalar, 174
  synarthrodial, summary of, 13
  synovial, 10, 11-13
  talocalcaneal, 174
  tarsometatarsal, 173, 183
  temporomandibular; *see* Temporomandibular joints
  three projection minimum for, 51
  tibiofibular, 10, 180, 183
  of toes, 173
  trauma radiography of, 552
  trochoid (pivot), 12, 13
  wrist, 12
  zygapophyseal (apophyseal), 251, 252, 255, 280, 284, 285
    intervertebral foramina vs., 258-259, 285
Joint cavity, 11
Joint spaces, open and closed, 35
Jones method for elbow, 140
Judd method for cervical spine radiography, 273
Jugular foramen, 327
Jugular notch, 149, 260, 261, 306
  for central ray positioning on chest radiograph, 70
  as positioning landmark, 52, 56
Jugular vein, 686, 687, 693, 694

K

Kidney, 88, 89, 452, 453, 504, 505-507
  angiography of, 713
  blood vessels of, 506
  cross-sectional view of, 505
  disease of, 514
  lesions of, abdominal computed tomography to diagnose, 673
  location of, 506
  macroscopic structure of, 507
  microscopic structure of, 507
  movement of, 506
  orientation of, 505
  trauma to, excretory urography to diagnose, 514
Kidney failure, excretory urography to diagnose, 514
Kidney stones, excretory urography to diagnose, 514
Kidney, ureter and bladder (KUB) radiograph, 86, 511
  anteroposterior projection, supine position, 94
  basic and special projections in, 93
  national norms for, 93
Kilo-, 37
Kilovoltage
  for chest radiography, 65
  contrast and, 32
  control of, 31
Kite method for pediatric radiography of foot, 595
Knee, 12, 180-181
  anteroposterior, correct central ray for, 36
  anteroposterior axial projection of, 211
  anteroposterior oblique projection of, with medial (lateral) rotation, 207
  anteroposterior (posteroanterior) weight-bearing bilateral projection of, 209
  anteroposterior projection of, 206
  arthrography of, 181, 615-618
    anteroposterior projection for, 615, 617
    horizontal beam projections for, 618
    lateral projection for, 615, 617
    positioning for, 617-618
  basic and special projections for, 188
  Camp Coventry method for, 210
  of child, 9
  flexion and extension of, 24
  Holmblad method for, 210
  lateral-mediolateral projection of, 208
  ligaments of, 180
  mediolateral projection of, 28
  posteroanterior axial projection of, tunnel view, 210
  radiographs of, 182
  routine for, 187
  summary of, 183
  three projections required for, 51
Knee, cont'd
  trauma to, 181
  trauma and mobile radiography of, 569
Knee cap, 179, 180
Kuchendorf method for patella, 216
Kyphosis, 249

L

Labyrinths of ethmoid bone, 329
Lacrimal bones, 332, 334
  orbits and, 338
Lacrimal gland, 642
Lambda, 330
Lambdoidal suture, 330
Lamina of vertebrae, 250, 255, 280
LAO; *see* Left anterior oblique position
Laparoscopic cholangiography, 491
Large intestine, 86, 87, 412, 446
  air and barium in, relative locations of, 453
  anatomy of, 448-449
  barium enema of, 446
  body habitus and position of, 420, 421
  characteristics of, 449
  colon vs., 448
  digestive functions in, 454
  digestive movements in, 454
  neoplasms in, barium enema to diagnose, 459
  polyps in, barium enema to diagnose, 459
Laryngeal edema from urologic contrast media, 513
Laryngeal prominence, 58
Laryngopharynx, 57, 413, 414
Larynx, 57, 58, 414
  axial (cross-section) image of, 58
  axial CT image of, 58
  opening of, CT image of, 58
  on posteroanterior chest radiograph, 62
  thyroid cartilage of, 57, 58
Lateral, 22
Lateral abdomen, 22
Lateral angle of scapula, 150
Lateral arm, 22
Lateral border of scapula, 150
Lateral cervical spine, radiographs of, 257
Lateral chest positioning, 68
Lateral condyles
  of femur, 179, 180
  of tibia, 178
Lateral elbow, true, 107
Lateral epicondyles, 107, 179, 180
Lateral forearm
  correct positioning of, 29
  evaluation criteria for, 29
Lateral hand, 22
Lateral hip, 227
Lateral intercondyloid tubercle, 178
Lateral malleolus, 176, 178
Lateral mass of cervical vertebra, 252, 253
Lateral menisci, 181
Lateral planes to divide abdomen into regions, 90
Lateral positions, 18, 19
Lateral process of calcaneus, 174
Lateral projection, 20
  for joint, 51
  viewing radiographs of, 54
Lateral recess of fourth ventricle, 637
Lateral recumbent position, 17
Lateral region of abdomen, 90
Lateral rotation, 25
Lateral sinuses, radiographs of, 388
Lateral thoracic spine, radiographs of, 256
Lateral ventricles of cerebrum, 636, 637
Lateromedial projection, 20, 28
Lauenstein and Hickey method, modified, for hip and proximal femur, 240
Law method, modified
  for mastoid and petrous pyramid radiographs, 389
  for mastoid radiographs, 389, 393, 394, 402
  for temporomandibular joint radiography, 380
Lawrence method for shoulder, 158, 163
Lead aprons for worker protection, 40
Left anterior oblique position, 18
Left colic flexure, 86
Left hypochondriac region of abdomen, 90
Left iliac region of abdomen, 90
Left inguinal region of abdomen, 90
Left lateral chest positioning, 68
Left lateral decubitus position, 19

Left lateral plane to divide abdomen into regions, 90
Left lateral position, 19, 28
Left lateral region of abdomen, 90
Left lower quadrant of abdomen, 90
Left lumbar region of abdomen, 90
Left marker, 30
Left posterior oblique position, 18, 28
Left primary bronchus, 60
Left upper quadrant of abdomen, 90
Leg, 178
  anteroposterior and lateral projection for, 568, 595
  anteroposterior mortise and lateral projection for, 568
  anteroposterior projection of, 204
  basic and special projections for, 188
  bones of, 7
  of child, 595
  discrepancies in length of, orthoroentgenography for, 612, 613
  internal rotation of, positioning and, 228
  joints of, summary of, 183
  lateral-mediolateral projection of, 205
  lower, radiographs of, routine, 187
  radiographs of, 182
  trauma and mobile radiography of, 568
  trauma radiography of, 552
  two projections required for, 51
Lentiform nucleus, 641
Lesions, localization of, two projections for, 50
Lesser curvature of stomach, 416
Lesser multangular bone; *see* Trapezoid bone of wrist
Lesser omentum, 452
Lesser pelvis, 225
Lesser sac, 451
Lesser sciatic notch, 224
Lesser trochanter, 222
Lesser tubercle, 148
Lesser wings of sphenoid bone, 328
Leukocytes, 680
Lifetime effective dose, 37
Ligament
  accessory, of synovial joints, 11
  atlantal, transverse, 253
  Cooper's, 532
  falciform, 484
  knee, 180-181
  patellar, 181
  radiocarpal, of wrist, 109
  sutural, 10
  of Treitz, 418, 447
Limb
  lower; *see* Lower limb
  magnetic resonance imaging of, 747
  upper; *see* Upper limb
Line
  acanthiomeatal, 345
  anthropological base, 345
  body, 16
  glabellomeatal, 345
  infraorbitomeatal, 345
  interpupillary (interorbital), 344
  mentomeatal, 345
  orbitomeatal, 345
  positioning, skull, 345
  Reid's base, 345
Lipids, chemical digestion of, 419
Lips-meatal line, 345
Lithotomy position, 17
Liver, 87, 88, 89, 412, 453
  anatomy of, 484
  disease of, 514
  function of, 484
  lesions of, abdominal computed tomography to diagnose, 673
  lobes of, 484
  metastasis to, 673
Lobes
  of breast, 532
  of cerebral hemispheres, 636
  of liver, 484
  of lungs, 60, 61, 63
    axial (cross-section) image of, 60
    on lateral chest radiograph, 62
Lobules of breast, 532
Local heating of tissues and metallic objects during MRI, 738
Localization of lesions or foreign bodies, two projections for, 50
Long bones, 7-8
  composition of, 8
  epiphyseal fusion of, 9
  of lower limbs, measurement of, 613
  measurement of, 612
  of upper limbs, measurement of, 614
Long scale contrast, 32
Longitudinal arch of foot, 175
Longitudinal fissure of cerebral hemispheres, 636
Longitudinal relaxation, 727
Longitudinal sections, 15
Loop of Henle, 507
Lordosis, 249
Lordotic position, apical anteroposterior projection, 21
Lower gastrointestinal examinations, types of, 464-467
Lower gastrointestinal series, 446
  on children, 600
Lower gastrointestinal system, 445-481
  radiographs of, 455
    national survey norms for, 468-469
  study of, for child, 606-607
Lower limb(s), 171-220
  anatomy of, 172-184
  anteroposterior and lateral projections for, 594, 595
    for ankle and leg, 568
    for femur, 570
    for knee, 569
    of toes and foot, 567
  anteroposterior mortise and lateral projection for, for ankle and leg, 568
  anteroposterior pelvis and proximal femora projection for, 570
  arteries of, 691
  arteriography of, 716
  basic and special projections for, 188
  bones of, 7
  of child, 595
  discrepancies in length of, orthoroentgenography for, 612, 613
  joints of, classification of, 183, 228
  positioning of, 185-219
  radiographs of, national survey norms for, 186-187
  rotation of, effect of, on radiographs, 230
  trauma and mobile radiography of, 552, 567-570
  veins of, 691
  venography of, 717
  viewing radiographs of, 54
Lower quadrants of abdomen, 90
LPO; *see* Left posterior oblique position
Lumbar curvature, 249
Lumbar region of abdomen, 90
  myelography of, 624
Lumbar spine
  anatomy of, 280
  anteroposterior axial L5-S1 projection for, 293
  anteroposterior and horizontal beam lateral projection for, 574
  anteroposterior or posteroanterior projection for, 287, 289
  basic and special projections in, 288
  exam of, pregnancy and, 44
  lateral L5-S1 position for, 292
  lateral position for, 291
  oblique position for, 290
  sacrum and coccyx, 279-303
    basic and special projections for, 288
    positioning of, 286-302
    radiographs of, national survey norms for, 288
  summary of joints of, 285
  trauma and mobile radiography of, 574
Lumbar vertebrae, 248
  anatomy of, 280
  oblique, radiograph of, 284
  radiographs of, 283, 284
Lumbosacral spine
  radiographs of, 284
  routine for, 288
Lunate bone of wrist, 104
Lung contrast scale, 666
Lungs, 57, 63
  alveoli of, 60
  anatomy of, 61-62
  apex of, 62
Lungs, cont'd
  average measurements of, 84
  axial (cross-section) CT image of, 60
  base of, 62
  chest central ray and, measurement study of, 84
  on computed tomography cross sectional image at level of T9, 61
  cross section of, 61
  dimensions of, 70
  fissures of, 61
  foreign body in, chest radiography for, 66
  hilum of, 62
  on lateral chest radiograph, 62
  left, medial, 62
  lobes of, 60, 61, 63
    axial (cross-section) image of, 60
    on lateral chest radiograph, 62
  lower mediastinum and, cross section of, 61
  parts of, 62
  on posteroanterior chest radiograph, 62
  right and left, 61
  root region of, 62
  shielding of, for humerus and shoulder girdle radiographs, 154
Luschka, foramen of, 637
Luxation, 546
Lymph drainage, 694
Lymph nodes, 694
Lymphatic ducts, 694
Lymphatic system, 3, 88, 680, 694
Lymphography, 694

M

Magnesium citrate to produce carbon dioxide gas, 424
Magnetic field, fringe, 736
Magnetic resonance angiography of cardiovascular system, 750
Magnetic resonance imaging, 723-752
  of abdomen, 749
  basic safety considerations with, 736-738
  basis of, 725
  of brain, 745
  of breast, 536
  of cardiovascular system, 748, 750
  of cervical spine, 257
  clinical applications for, 735-743
  comparison of
    with computed tomography, 735
    with radiography, 724
  contraindications to, 739
  contrast agents for, 740
  equipment for, 731-734
  examinations in, 744-750
  general principles of, 724
  imaging parameters for, 742-743
  information form for, 738
  of joints, 747
  of limbs, 747
  occupational hazards of, 738
  patient history before, 738
  patient monitoring during, 740
  of pelvis, 749
  physical principles of, 724-730
  positioning guidelines and coil selection for, 741
  precession in, 725
  preparation for, 739-740
  of spine, 746
  terminology related to, 751-752
  viewing, 54
Magnets for MRI, 731
Magnification, 34
Magnification angiography of vertebrobasilar system, 705
Magnification radiography of internal carotid artery, 703
Main stem bronchi, 60
  axial (cross-section) image of, 60
Major calyx, 507
Malabsorption syndrome
  enteroclysis to diagnose, 457
  small bowel series to diagnose, 455
Malar bone, 334
Male
  gonadal dose for, 45
  gonadal shields for, 43
  pelvic organs of, 509
  pelvis of, 226
Male, cont'd
    anatomy of, 670-671
  reproductive organs of, 4
  retrograde urethrogram in, 519
Malleolus, 176, 178
Mallet fracture, 549
Malleus, 392
Mammography, 529-543
  ACR terminology for, 537
  basic and special projections for, 537
  craniocaudal (CC) projection for, 538
  digital, 536
  film-screen, 532, 535
  implant procedure with Ecklund technique, 542
  laterally exaggerated craniocaudal projection for, 540
  mediolateral lateral (ML)-true lateral projection for, 541
  mediolateral oblique (MLO) projection for, 539
  superomedial-inferolateral oblique projection for, 539
Mammography Quality Standards Act, 530
Mandible, 332, 336
  angle of, 336, 344
  anteroposterior axial, anteroposterior and axiolateral oblique projections for, 579
  axiolateral projection for, 373
  basic and special projections for, 362
  basilar position for, 376
  joints of, classification of, 337
  panorex of, 377-378
  posteroanterior axial projection for, 374, 375
  posteroanterior projection for, 374
  routine for, 361
  submentovertex (SMV) projection for, 336, 376
  Towne method for, 375
  trauma and mobile radiography of, 579
Mandibular notch, 336
Manual collimation, 42
Manubrial notch; *see* Jugular notch
Manubrium, 56, 260, 306
"March" fracture, 550
Markers, film, 30
  positioning and, 49
Marrow, bone, 8
Mastication, 413, 419
Mastoid air cells, 391
Mastoid fontanels, 330
Mastoid portion of temporal bones, 327, 389
Mastoid process, 327
Mastoid tip, 260, 261, 327, 390
Mastoids, 391
Mastoids
  anteroposterior axial oblique projection for, 407
  anteroposterior axial projection for, 389, 404
  Arcelin method for, 406
  axiolateral 15° oblique, 389
  axiolateral oblique projection for, 394, 402
    anterior profile projection for, 406
    posterior profile position for, 403
  axiolateral projection for, 393, 405
  basic and routine projections for, 396
  Mayer method and Owen modification for, 407
  modified Law method for, 389, 393, 402
  posterior profile projection for, 393
  radiographs of, 389
    national survey norms for, 396
    positioning for, 394
  routine for, 396
  Schuller method for, 405
  Stenvers method for, 393, 403
    reverse, 406
  temporal bone, and paranasal sinuses, 385-409
  Towne method for, 389, 404
Maturity, full, 9
Maxilla(e), 332-333
  orbits and, 338
Maxillary artery, 684
Maxillary bones, 332-333
Maxillary processes, 333
Maxillary sinus, 333, 386

Mayer method and Owen modification for mastoid radiographs, 407
MD-Gastroview, 424
Measurement study, chest CR and lung, 84
Mechanical digestion, 419
Mechanical ileus, small bowel series to diagnose, 455
Medial, 22
Medial arm, 22
Medial border of scapula, 150
Medial condyles
  of femur, 179, 180
  of tibia, 178
Medial epicondyle, 107, 179, 180
Medial intercondyloid tubercle, 178
Medial malleolus, 176, 178
Medial menisci, 181
Medial plane, 22
Medial process of calcaneus, 174
Medial rotation, 25
Median cubital vein, 691
Median plane, 15, 344
Mediastinal contrast scale, 666
Mediastinum, 63
  anatomy of, 63
  esophagus in, 414
  lesions of, thoracic computed tomography to diagnose, 664
  lower, and lungs, cross section of, 61
Mediolateral ankle projection, 20
Mediolateral projection, 20, 28
Medulla
  brain, 635
  of hindbrain, 639
  kidney, 507
Medulla oblongata, 248, 635
Medulla spinalis, 634
Medullary cavity, 8
Mega-, 37
Membrane
  synovial, of knee, 181
  tympanic, 390
Membranous labyrinth, 392
Meningeal spaces, 635
Meninges, brain, 635
Meningiomas, MRI to diagnose, 740
Menisci, 181
Mental foramina, 336
Mental point, 336, 344
Mental protuberance, 336
Mentomeatal line, 345
Mentum, 336
Mesenteric arteries, 689, 692
Mesenteric veins, 689, 690, 693
Mesentery, 89, 451
Mesial, 22
Mesocephalic skull, 343
Mesocolon, transverse, 451, 452
Metacarpals, 102
Metacarpophalangeal joints, 12, 103, 108
Metal cones to restrict x-ray beam, 48
Metallic objects
  local heating of, during MRI, 738
  torquing of, during MRI, 738
Metastases, brain, cranial computed tomography to diagnose, 655
Metatarsal bones, 172
  joints of, 173
Metatarsophalangeal joints, 12, 173, 183
Micro-, 37
Micturition, 509
Mid thorax, locating, 56
Midbrain, 635, 639-640, 641
Midcoronal plane, 15
Middle ear, 390-392
Middle phalanges, 102
Midlateral orbital margin, 344
Midline dose, calculation of, 45
Midsagittal plane, 15, 344
  to divide abdomen into quadrants, 90
Mild reaction to urologic contrast media, 512, 513
Milli-, 37
Milliamperage, 31
Millisievert, conversion of rem to, 37
Minerals, chemical digestion of, 419
Minimum repeat radiographs for patient protection, 41
Minimum total filtration, 41
Minor calyx, 507
Minors, radiation protection for, 38; *see also* Child
Mitral valve, 681
Mobile C-arm digital fluoroscopy systems, 555-556
  ALARA principles and, 38
  maintaining sterile fields in, 556
  radiation protection with, 557
Mobile radiography, trauma radiography and, 545-579; *see also* Trauma and mobile radiography
Mobile x-ray equipment, 554-557
Moderate reaction to urologic contrast media, 513
Molecules, 2
Molybdenum for filters, 41
Monitoring, personnel, 38
Monro, foramen of, 637
Monteggia's fracture, 549
Mortise for ankle, 176
Mortise position, 176
Motion
  image detail and, 33
  involuntary, control of, 33
  voluntary, control of, 33
Motion artifacts in MRI, 743
Motoneuron, multipolar, 634
Mouth, 86, 412
  accessory organs in, 413
  anatomy of, 413
  mechanical digestion in, 419
Movement
  breathing, chest radiography and, 64
  elbow rotational, 110
  forearm rotational, 110
  hand, 26
  inward stress, of foot, 25
  outward stress, of foot, 25
  rotational, 25
  shoulder, 27
  terminology related to, 24-27
  wrist joint, terminology for, 110
Movement types of synovial joints, 11-13
Mueller maneuver to prevent esophageal reflux, 429
Multangular bones; *see* Trapezium bone of wrist; Trapezoid bone of wrist
Multiple myeloma, 514
Multipolar motoneuron, 634
Multislice imaging in MRI, 728
"Mummifying" for immobilization during pediatric radiography, 585
Mumps, 413
Muscle, 5; *see also* specific muscle; specific muscle type
  abdominal, 86
  ocular, 642
  pectoralis major, 531
  psoas major, 505
Muscular system, 5
Muscular tissue, 2
Myelinated axons, 640
Myelography, 620-625
  computed, 625
  contraindications for, 620
  contrast media for, 622
  equipment for, 621
  fluoroscopy and spot filming in, 622
  indications for, 620
  needle placement and injection process for, 621
  positioning routines for, 622-624
  preparation for, 620
Myeloma, multiple, 514

N

Nano-, 37
Nasal bones, 332, 334
  basic and special projections for, 362
  lateral position for, 367
  routine for, 361
  superoinferior tangential (axial) projection for, 368
Nasal cavity, 57, 386, 414
Nasal conchae, 329, 332, 335
Nasal fossae, 386
Nasal septum, bony, 332, 335
Nasal spine, 325, 333
Nasal turbinates, 329, 335
Nasion, 334, 344
Nasopharynx, 57, 413, 414
Nausea and vomiting from urologic contrast media, 513
Navicular bone, 175
Neck
  arteries of, 683
  of condyloid process, 336
  of femur, 222
  of fibula, 178
  of gallbladder, 485
  great veins of, 686
  of humerus, 148
  of radius, 106, 107
  of rib, 307
  of scapula, 150
Necrosis, avascular, fractures and, 231
Needle biopsy, percutaneous, 721
Neer method for shoulder, 162
Neoplasms
  brain, cranial computed tomography to diagnose, 655
  gallbladder, oral cholecystogram to diagnose, 487
  intestinal, small bowel series to diagnose, 455
  in large intestine, barium enema to diagnose, 459
Nephrogram, 517, 522
Nephron, 507
Nephroptosis, 506
Nephrostomy, 720
Nephrotomogram, 517, 522
Nerve(s)
  inside rib, 307
  ocular, 642
  optic, 641
Nervous system, 5
  central, anatomy of, 634-635
Nervous tissue, 2
Neurohypophysis, 639
Neuroma, acoustic, MRI to diagnose, 740
Neurons, 634
Neutral rotation of humerus, 153
Nipple, 530, 531, 532
Nonaccidental trauma, reporting, 582
Nonionic organic iodides for urology, 511
Nonlinear wafer type portable grid for trauma radiography, 553
Nonvascular interventional procedures, 720-721
Notch
  angular, 416
  cardiac, 416
  cerebellar, 640
  clavicular, 307
  ethmoidal, 325
  fibular, 178
  intercondylar, 180
  jugular, 260, 261, 306
  mandibular, 336
  manubrial, 306
  scapular, 150
  sciatic, 224
  supraorbital, 325
  suprasternal, 306
  trochlear (semilunar), 107
  vertebral, 250
Nucleus
  amygdaloid, 641
  caudate, 641
  cerebral, 640, 641
  lentiform, 641
Nucleus pulposus, 251
Nursemaid's fracture, 549
Nutrient artery of long bone, 8
Nutrient foramen of long bone, 8

O

Object film alignment, distortion and, 35
Object image receptor distance
  detail and, 33
  distortion and, 35
Objective plane in tomography, 626
Oblique cervical spine, radiographs of, 257
Oblique fracture, 548
Oblique planes, 15
Oblique position, 18
Oblique projection
  correct use of term, 28
  for joint, 51
  anteroposterior and PA, 18, 20
Oblique sections, 15
Obstructive jaundice, percutaneous transhepatic cholangiography to diagnose, 492
Obturator foramen, 224
Occipital artery, 684
Occipital bone, 324, 326, 329
Occipital condyles, 326
Occipital horn of lateral ventricles, 637
Occipital lobe of cerebral hemisphere, 636
Occipital protuberance, external, 326
Occipital sinus, 687
Occipito-atlantal joint, 326
OCG; *see* Oral cholecystogram
Ocular muscles, 642
Ocular nerves, 642
Ocular orbits, axial section through, 648
Oculomotor nerve, 641
Oddi, sphincter of, 485
Odontoid process, 253
OEC mini 6600 digital mobile C-arm system, 555
OEC 9600 C-arm system, 556
OID; *see* Object image receptor distance
Olecranon fossa, 107
Olecranon process, 106
Olfactory nerve, 641
Omentum, 89, 452
Omentum bursa, 451
Open fracture, 548
"Open" joint spaces, 35
Open mouth position, 337
Open mouth radiograph, 253
Open reduction of fracture, radiographs following, 551
Operative cholangiogram, 490
  anteroposterior and/or RPO projection for, 501
  routine for, 495
Optic canal, 328
Optic chiasma, 639, 641, 642
Optic foramen (foramina), 328, 338, 339
  basic and special projections for, 362
  parieto-orbital projection for, 27, 372
  Rhese method for, 372
  routine for, 361
Optic groove, 328
Optic nerve, 641
Optic radiations, 640, 642
Optic tracts, 641, 642
Oral cavity, 57, 412
  accessory organs in, 413
  anatomy of, 413
Oral cholecystogram, 487-489
  contraindications to, 487
  fluoroscopy with, 489
  indications for, 487
  left anterior oblique position for, 498
  posteroanterior projection for, 497
    in erect position, 500
    in right lateral decubitus position, 499
  procedure for, 488-489
  purpose of, 487
  right lateral decubitus position for, 489, 499
  routine for, 495
  scout, 497
Oral Hypaque, 424
Orbital cavity, 642
Orbital fat, 642
Orbital fissure, 328, 339
Orbital margins, 344
Orbital plate, 325, 338
Orbital portion of frontal bone, 325
Orbital scanning, positioning for, 657
Orbitomeatal line, 345
Orbitoparietal projection, 28
Orbits, 338-339
  basic and special projections for, 362
  bones of, 340
  bony composition of, 338
  fractures of, 339
  ocular, axial section through, 648
  openings of, 340
  parieto-orbital projection of, 340
  posterior, openings in, 339
Organic iodides for urology, 511
Organism, 2
Organization of body, structural, 2
Organs, 2
  abdominal, 86-88
    anatomical relationships of, 89

Organs, cont'd
  cardiovascular, 3
  of digestion
    in abdominal cavity, 86
    accessory, 3, 88, 412
  of hearing and equilibrium, anatomy of, 390-393
  in oral cavity, accessory, 413
  pelvic
    female, 509, 452
    male, 452, 509
    retroperitoneal and infraperitoneal, 452
  reproductive, 4, 452
Orifice
  cardiac, 416
  pyloric, 416
Oropharynx, 57, 413
Orthoroentgenography, 612-614
  on lower limb, 613
  on upper limb, 614
Os calcis; *see* Calcaneus bone
Os magnum; *see* Capitate bone of wrist
Osmolality, increase in, with urologic contrast media, 511
Ossa coxae, 223
Osseous labyrinth, 392-393
Ossicles, auditory, 6, 390, 392
Ossification, 9
  endochondral, 9
  intracartilaginous, 9
  intramembranous, 9
  pediatric radiography and, 586
Osteology, 3, 6-7
Osteoporosis, fractures and, 231
Ottonello method for radiography of cervical spine, 274
Outer, 23
Outer canthus, 344
Outlet of true pelvis, 225
Outward stress movement of foot, 25
Oval window, 392
Ovary, 509
  carcinoma of, pelvic computed tomography to diagnose, 673
Owen modification of Mayer method for mastoid radiographs, 407

P

Pain
  abdominal, 516
  flank, excretory urography to diagnose cause of, 514
Palate
  hard, 57, 333, 413
  soft, 57, 413
    during swallowing, 414
Palatine bones, 332, 333, 335
  orbits and, 338
Palatine process of maxilla, 333
Palatine uvula, 413
Palm of hand, 102
Palmar arches, 690, 691, 692
Palmar radiocarpal ligament of wrist, 109
Palmar surface, 16
Palpation to locate positioning landmarks, 52, 91
Pancreas, 86, 88, 412, 418, 452, 453
  ducts of, 485
  lesions of, abdominal computed tomography to diagnose, 673
Pancreatic duct, 485
Pancreatitis, abdominal computed tomography to diagnose, 673
Panoramic tomography of mandible, 377-378
Panorex radiography of mandible, 377-378
Panorex unit, 631
Pantomography, 631
Papilla
  duodenal, 485
  renal, 507
Paralytic ileus, small bowel series to diagnose, 455
Paranasal sinuses
  anatomy of, 386-387
  basic and routine projections for, 396
  basilar position for, 388, 400
  Caldwell method for, 398
  lateral position for, 397
  mastoids and temporal bone, 385-409
  open-mouth Waters method for, 388, 401
Paranasal sinuses, cont'd
  parietoacanthial projection for, 399
  posteroanterior (Caldwell) projection for, 388, 398
    modified, 394
  posteroanterior axial transoral projection for, 388, 401
  radiographs of, 388
    national survey norms for, 396
    positioning for, 394-395
  routine for, 396
  submentovertex projection for, 388, 400
  Waters method for, 399
Parathyroid glands, 59
Parenchyma
  lung, 61
  renal, 507
Parent, role of, in child's radiography, 582
Parietal bones, 324, 326, 329
Parietal lobe of cerebral hemisphere, 636
Parietal peritoneum, 89, 451
Parietal pleura, 61
Parietal tubercles, 326
Parietoacanthial projection, 28
Parieto-orbital projection, 28
  for optic foramen, 27
  of orbits, 340
Parotid glands, 413
Pars interarticularis, 280, 284
Pars petrosa, 327, 389
Part placement on film holder, 29
Partial fracture, 548
Patella, 179, 180
  axial oblique view of, 216
  basic and special projections for, 188
  femur and, 180
  Kuchendorf method for, 216
  Hughston method for, 215
  lateral-mediolateral projection of, 213
  Merchant bilateral method for, 214, 215
  posteroanterior oblique projections of, with internal and external rotation, 216
  posteroanterior projection of, 212
  routine for, 187
  Settegast method for, 215
  stellate fracture of, 550
  tangential (axial or sunrise/skyline) projections of, 21, 214, 215
Patellar ligament, 181
Patellofemoral joint, 180, 183
  basic and special projections in, 188
  Merchant bilateral method for, 214, 215
  tangential (axial or sunrise/skyline) projections of, 182, 214, 215
Pathologic fracture, 550
Patient
  care of, professional ethics and, 46
  dose chart for, 39
  dose icon boxes for, sample, 45
  exposure of, to radiation
    during fluoroscopic procedures, 39
    during fluoroscopy and spot filming, 39
    minimizing, 45
  general positioning for, 49
  identification of, 30
  instructions to, to avoid repeat radiographs, 41
  preparation of
    for abdominal radiograph, 92
    for chest radiography, 65
  protection of, 41-45
    from radiation during chest radiography, 65
Patient radiation doses, 38-39
Patient doses per exam, patient protection and, 45
PBL; *see* Positive beam limitation
Pectoralis major muscle, 531
Pediatric radiography, 581-610
  of abdomen
    anteroposterior erect position for, 602
    anteroposterior projection for, 601
    dorsal decubitus projection for, in lateral position, 603
    KUB, 601
    preparation for, 600
  age of child and, 582
  bone development and, 586
  of chest
    anteroposterior/posteroanterior projection for, 588-589
    lateral position for, 590-591
Pediatric radiography, cont'd
  contrast media in, patient preparation for, 600
  gastrointestinal fluoroscopy in, 604-607
  of genitourinary system, 608-610
  gonadal shielding during, 587
  immobilization for, 583-586
  intravenous urogram in, 600
  on lower gastrointestinal tract, 600
  of lower limbs
    anteroposterior and lateral projections for, 594, 595
    Kite method for, 595
  parent protection during, 587
  of pelvis and hips, anteroposterior and lateral projections for, 596-597
  pre-exam introduction and child/parent evaluation in, 582
  preparation for, 587
  radiation protection during, 587
  of skull
    anteroposterior, anteroposterior reverse Caldwell and anteroposterior Towne projections for, 598
    lateral position for, 599
  on upper gastrointestinal tract, 600
  of upper limbs, anteroposterior and lateral projections for, 592-593
Pedicles of vertebrae, 250, 252, 255, 284
Peduncle, cerebral, 641
Pelvic bones, anterior, anteroposterior axial projection of, 236
Pelvic brim, 508
Pelvic curve, 249
Pelvic girdle, 223
  bones of, 7
  proximal femur and, 221-245
    anatomy of, 222-228
    positioning of, 229-244
Pelvic inlet, 281
Pelvic mass, excretory urography to diagnose, 514
Pelvic organs
  female, 452, 509
  male, 452, 509
  retroperitoneal and infraperitoneal, 452
Pelvic ring fractures, radiography of, 231
Pelvis, 223, 227
  anterior oblique position of, 237
  anteroposterior axial projection of, 236
  anteroposterior bilateral "frog-leg" projection of, 235
  anteroposterior and lateral projections for, 596-597
  anteroposterior projection of, 234
  basic and special projections for, 233
  bones of, 8
  of child, 596-597
  computed tomography of, 659-677
    contraindications to, 674
    contrast media for, 675-676
    indications for, 673
    positioning and procedures for, 673-677
    preparation for, 674, 676
    procedure for, 677
  Danelius-Miller method for trauma and mobile radiography of, 571
  development of, 586
  exam of, pregnancy and, 44
  female, 672
  greater or lesser, 225
  lateral projection for, for proximal femur and hip, 571
  lead shields in place over, 43
  magnetic resonance imaging of, 749
  male, 670-671
    vs. female, 226
    flat contact shield for radiograph of, 43
  modified Cleaves method for, 235
  radiographs of, decision guide for, 233
  renal, 507
  routine for, 232
  Sanderson method for trauma and mobile radiography of, 571
  Taylor method for, 236
  Teufel method for, 237
  trauma and mobile radiography of, 570, 571
  true and false, 225
Peptic ulcers, upper GI series to diagnose, 431
Percutaneous abdominal abscess drainage, 720
Percutaneous biliary drainage, 720
Percutaneous gastrostomy, 721
Percutaneous needle biopsy, 721
Percutaneous transhepatic cholangiogram (cholangiography), 492
  basic and special projections for, 496
  national survey norms for, 495
Pericardial disease, thoracic computed tomography to diagnose, 664
Pericardial sac, 61, 63
Periosteum, 8
Peripheral angiography, 714-717
Peripheral circulatory system, 690-691
Perirenal fat, 505
Peristalsis, 415, 419
  esophagus and, 415
Peristaltic activity, 419
Peritoneal cavity, 89, 451
Peritoneum, 89, 451
Peritonitis, 448
Permanent magnets for MRI, 732
Peroneal artery, 691, 692
Peroneal trochlea, 174
Peroneal vein, 691
Perpendicular plate of ethmoid bone, 329
Personnel monitoring, 38
Petromastoid portion of temporal bones, 327
Petrous portion of temporal bones, 327, 389
Petrous pyramid, 327, 389
  anteroposterior axial projection and submentovertex projection for, 408
  basic and routine projections for, 396
  radiographs of, 389
  routine for, 396
  Towne method and basilar position for, 408
Petrous ridges, 327, 389
Phalanx (phalanges)
  of foot, 172
  of hand, 102
  tuft fracture of, 550
Pharynx, 57, 86, 412, 413
  anatomy of, 413-414
  cavity communicating with, 414
Phase encoding, reordered, in MRI, 743
Phased array coil for MRI, 733, 741
Pheochromocytoma as contraindication to excretory urography, 514
Phillips BV29 C-arm digital fluoroscopy system, 555
Photographic subtraction, 707
Photospot images, 425
Physiologic gating in MRI, 743
Physiology, definition of, 2
Pia mater, 635
Picker Explorer II mobile x-ray system, 554
Picture reconstruction in cranial computed tomography, 652
Pigg-O-Stat, 583
  erect lateral chest radiograph with, 591
  erect posteroanterior chest radiograph with, 589
Pineal gland, 637, 639
Ping-pong fracture, 550
Pinna, 344, 390
Pisiform bone of wrist, 104
Pituitary gland, 328, 639, 641
  coronal section through, 644
  tumors of, MRI to diagnose, 740
Pivot joints, 12, 13
  of wrist, 108
Pixels, two-dimensional, converting three-dimensional voxels to, 653
Plain films of abdomen, 86, 511
Plane
  anthropological, 16
  base, of skull, 16
  body, 15
    cranial topography and, 344
  horizontal, Frankfort, 16
  medial, 22
Plane joints, 11, 13
  of hand and wrist, 108
Plantar arch, 692
Plantar flexion, 25, 184
Plantar surface, 16
  of foot, 184
Plantodorsal projection, 28, 184
Plasma, 680
Plastic fracture, 548
Platelets, 680

Pleura, 61
Pleural cavity, 61
Pleural sac, 61
Pleurisy, 61
Plexiglass hold-down paddle for pediatric radiography, 583
Pneumothorax, 61
  chest radiography for, 66
Polibar Plus for defecography, 466
Polyps
  large intestine, barium enema to diagnose, 459
  in stomach or duodenum, upper GI series to diagnose, 431
Pons, 635, 638, 639, 641
Popliteal artery, 691, 692
Popliteal region, 180
Popliteal vein, 691, 693
Portable grid, nonlinear wafer type, for trauma radiography, 553
Portal system, 689, 690
Portal vein, 689, 690, 693
Position(s); *see also* specific body part
  anatomical, 14
  body, 17-19
  correct use of term, 28
  mortise, 176
Positioning, 17-19
  of abdomen, 92-99
  accuracy in, 29
  anode heel effect and, 36
  to avoid repeat radiographs, 41
  bony landmarks for, 52
  chest, 64-84
    lateral, 68
    posteroanterior, 67
  errors in, with cranial radiography, 346
  for facial bone radiography, 360
  film, 49
  methods and steps for, 48-49
  patient, general, 49
  principles for, 46-54
  routines for, principles for determining, 50-51
  sequence and routine for, 49
  for sternal radiographs, 310
  topographic landmarks for, 52
  of upper limb, 112-145
Positioning lines, skull, 345
Positive beam limitation, automatic, 42
Posterior arch of atlas, 253
Posterior cruciate ligament, 180, 181
Posterior fat pad of elbow joint, 111
Posterior horn of lateral ventricles, 637
Posterior malleolus, 176
Posterior oblique position, left and right, 18
Posterior position, erect, 20
Posterior sacral foramina, 281
Posterior superior iliac spine, 223
Posterior surface, 16
Posterior tubercle of atlas, 253
Posteroanterior chest positioning, 67
posteroanterior oblique projections, 18, 20
Posteroanterior projection, 18, 19, 20
  correct use of term, 28
  for joint, 51
  viewing radiographs of, 54
Posteroanterior Waters skull projection, special, 28
Postoperative cholangiogram (cholangiography), 491
  T-tube
    basic and special projections for, 496
    national survey norms for, 495
Post-traumatic abnormalities of brain, cranial computed tomography to diagnose, 655
Pott's fracture, 549
Precession, 725
Prefixes, SI, 37
Pregnancy
  excretory urography during, precautions with, 515
  protection for, 44
  small bowel series and, 458
  term, relationship to bladder of, 509
  upper GI series and, 432
Pregnant radiographers, 38
Presaturation in MRI, 743
Primary bronchus (bronchi), 60, 414
Primary center of endochondral ossification, 9
Primary curves, 249
Principles
  ALARA, 38
  arthrology, 10-13
  basic imaging, 29-36
  general anatomy, 2-6
  positioning, 46-54
  skeletal anatomy, 6-9
Process
  alveolar, of mandible, 336
  articular
    of sacrum, 281
    of vertebrae, 250, 251, 255, 280, 284
  of calcaneus, 174
  clinoid, 328, 329
  condyloid, 336
  coronoid
    of forearm, 106
    of mandible, 336
  mastoid, 327
  maxillary, 333
  odontoid, 253
  olecranon, 106
  pterygoid, 328, 329
  spinous; *see* Spinous process
  styloid, 106, 178, 327, 390
  transverse; *see* Transverse process
  vermiform, 448
  xiphoid, 260, 306
  zygomatic, 327
Proctography, evacuative; *see* Defecography
Professional ethics and patient care, 46
Projectiles in MRI, potential hazard of, 736-737
Projections, 18, 20-21, 28
  anteroposterior (AP), 18, 19, 20
    viewing radiographs of, 54
  basic, of chest, 71
  correct use of term, 28
  decubitus, 19
  decubitus chest and abdomen, viewing radiographs of, 54
  definition of, 20
  dorsoplantar, 184, 193
  essential, positioning and, 50
  joint, 51
  lateral, viewing radiographs of, 54
  minimum of three, for joints, 51
  minimum of two, studies requiring, 50
  oblique, anteroposterior and PA, 18
  parieto-orbital, for optic foramen, 27
  plantodorsal, 184
  posteroanterior (PA), 18, 19, 20
    viewing radiographs of, 54
  special positioning uses of term, 28
  special use, 21
  tangential, for zygomatic arch, 27
Promontory, sacral, 281
Pronation, 26
Pronator fat stripe, 111
Prone position, 17
Prostate gland, 508, 509
  carcinoma of, pelvic computed tomography to diagnose, 673
Protection
  patient, 41-45
  for pregnancies, 44
  radiation, 37-45
    for minors, 38
    principles and terminology and, 1-54
  worker
    exposure patterns and, 40
    during fluoroscopy, 40-41
    practices of, 40-41
Proteins, chemical digestion of, 419
Protocol for general diagnostic procedures, 47
Proton density, 727
Proton density images, 742
Protraction, 26
Protuberance
  mental, 336
  occipital, external, 326
Proximal, 22
Proximal convoluted tubule, 507
Proximal femur, 227
  in anatomical position, 228
  angles of, 222
  hip and; *see* Hip and proximal femur
  and pelvic girdle, 221-245
Proximal hip, fractures of, radiography of, 231
Proximal humerus; *see* Humerus, proximal
Proximal interphalangeal joint, 103, 173
Proximal phalanges, 102
Proximal radioulnar joint, 105
Proximal tibiofibular joint, 180, 181
Pseudocoarctation, 688
Pseudotumors of abdomen, 674
Psoas major muscles, 86, 505
PTC; *see* Percutaneous transhepatic cholangiography
Pterions, 330
Pterygoid hamuli, 328, 329, 333
Pterygoid process, 328, 329
Pubic arch, angle of, 226
Pubic bone, 224
Pubic region of abdomen, 90
Pubis, 223, 224
Pulmonary arteries, 63, 681, 688, 692
Pulmonary circulation, 681
Pulmonary emphysema, 61
Pulmonary pleura, 61
Pulmonary valve, 681
Pulmonary veins, 63, 681, 688, 693
Pulmonary vessels, engorgement or hyperemia of, 66
Pulse repetition time, 730
Pulse sequence timing factors, 730
Pulse sequences in MRI, 729
Pulsed fluoroscopy, 39
Pyelogram
  anteroposterior projection for, 526
  intravenous; *see* Excretory urogram; Intravenous pyelogram
  retrograde, 510
Pyelonephritis, 514
Pyloric canal, 416
Pyloric orifice, 416
Pyloric portion of stomach, 416, 417

Q

Quadrants, abdominal, 90
Quadrate lobe of liver, 484
Quality, image, technique and, 31-37

R

R; *see* Roentgen
Rad, 37, 38
  conversion of, to gray, 37
Radial artery, 690, 692
Radial collateral ligament of wrist, 109
Radial deviation, 24, 110
Radial flexion, 24, 110, 130
  radiograph of, 105
Radial fossa, 107
Radial notch, 106
Radial tuberosity, 106, 107
Radial vein, 691, 693
Radiation absorbed dose, 38
Radiation
  doses of
    patient, 38-39
      per exam, patient protection and, 45
    units of, 37
  exposure to, units of, 37
  patient exposure to, minimizing, 45
  protection from, 37-45
    during chest radiography, 65
    with cranial radiography, 346
    with mobile C-arm digital fluoroscopy systems, 555-556
    for abdominal radiographs, 92
    for minors, 38
    principles and terminology and, 1-54
  optic, 640, 642
  scatter
    fluoroscopy and, 40
    minimizing effect of, for cervical and thoracic spine radiographs, 262
    worker protection and, 40
  units of, 37
Radio frequency coils for MRI, 733
Radiocarpal joint, 109
Radiocarpal ligaments of wrist, 109
Radiograph (radiography), 14
  body section, 626
  bone growth demonstrated on, 9
  comparison of magnetic resonance imaging with, 724
  evaluation criteria for, 29
  repeat, minimum, for patient protection, 41
  underexposure of, 31
  viewing, 14, 28, 54
Radiographer(s)
  code of ethics for, 46
  initials of, as markers, 30
  pregnant, 38
  protection of, 37-38
Radiographic examination, 14
Radiographic procedures, diagnostic, general, protocol and order for, 47
Radiographic technique and image quality, 31-37
Radiologic technologist, code of ethics for, 46
Radioulnar joints, 12, 105, 109
Radius, 105
  Colles fracture of, 549
  distal humerus and, 107
  impacted fracture of, 549
Raised collar extensions for lead apron, 40
Ramus
  of ischium, 224
  mandibular, 336
  of pubis, 224
RAO; *see* Right anterior oblique position
Rapid imaging techniques in MRI, 743
Reabsorption in intestines, 454
Recess, epitympanic, 390
Reclining position, 17
Recorded detail, 33
Rectal ampulla, 449
Rectum, 86, 89, 448, 449, 452, 509
Recumbent left posterior oblique position, 18
Recumbent position, 17
Recumbent right anterior oblique position, 18
Recumbent right lateral position, 18
Red blood cells, 680
  production of, 8
Red bone marrow, 8
Reduction of fracture, radiographs following, 551
Reflux, esophageal
  esophagram to diagnose, 427
  during fluoroscopy, 429
Region(s)
  abdominal, 90
  popliteal, 180
Reid's base line, 16, 345
Relationship terms, 22-23
Relaxation in MRI, 726
Rem, 37
  conversion of
    to millisievert, 37
    to Sievert, 37
Renal angiography, 713
Renal artery, 506, 689, 693
Renal calculi, excretory urography to diagnose, 514
Renal columns, 507
Renal cortex, 507
Renal failure, excretory urography to diagnose, 514
Renal hypertension, excretory urography to diagnose, 514
Renal medulla, 507
Renal papilla, 507
Renal parenchyma, 507
Renal pelvis, 507
Renal pyramids, 507
Renal sinus, 507
Renal veins, 506, 689, 693
Reordered phase encoding in MRI, 743
Reproductive organs, 452
Reproductive system, 4
Resistive magnets for MRI, 731
Resonance in MRI, 726
Respiratory arrest from urologic contrast media, 513
Respiratory gating in MRI, 743
Respiratory system, 4
  anatomy of, 57-62
  parts of, 58-61
Retention, urinary, 509
Retention catheters for barium enema, 461
Retraction, 26
Retrograde cholangiopancreatography, endoscopic, 493
  basic and special projections for, 496
  national survey norms for, 495
Retrograde cystography, 518
Retrograde pyelogram, 510
Retrograde urethrography, 519

Retrograde urogram (urography), 518
  anteroposterior projection for, 526
  basic and special projections in, 520
  routine, 520
  scout, anteroposterior projection for, 526
Retromammary space, 531
Retroperitoneal organs, 89, 452
Reverse Colles' fracture, 549
Reverse Waters skull projection, 28
Rhese method, 28
  for optic foramina radiographs, 372
Rhese oblique projection, 28
Rhythmic segmentation, 419
Rib angle, inferior, 306
Rib cage, 308
Rib margin as topographic landmark of abdomen, 52, 91
Ribs, 8, 56, 306, 307
  anatomy of, 307
  angle of, 307
  anterior, radiographs of, posteroanterior projection for, 319
  articulations of, 254, 307
  axillary, radiographs of, posterior or anterior oblique positions for, 320-321
  basic and special projections in, 313
  cartilages of, 307
  in chest radiograph, 64
  exterior and interior surfaces of, 23
  injuries to, 307
  photograph of, 309
  positioning considerations for, 311-312
  posterior, radiographs of, anteroposterior projection for, 318
  routine for, 313
  and sternum
    and bony thorax, 305-322
    radiographs of
      basic and special projections for, 313
      national survey norms for, 313
  trauma and mobile radiography of, 560
  tubercles of, 307
  typical, 307
  visible on posteroanterior chest radiograph, 64
Right angle radiograph, 612; *see also* Orthoroentgenography
Right anterior oblique position, 18
Right colic flexure, 86
Right hypochondriac region of abdomen, 90
Right iliac region of abdomen, 90
Right inguinal region of abdomen, 90
Right lateral decubitus position, 19
Right lateral plane to divide abdomen into regions, 90
Right lateral position, 19
Right lateral region of abdomen, 90
Right lateral shoulder position, 21
Right lower quadrant of abdomen, 90
Right lumbar region of abdomen, 90
Right marker, 30
Right posterior oblique position, 18
Right primary bronchus, 60
Right upper quadrant of abdomen, 90
Ring, Schatzke's, 418
Roentgen, 37
Room air as contrast medium, 424
Rotation, 27
  in cranial radiography, 346
  external, of hip, 228
  internal, of leg, positioning and, 228
  lateral (external), 25
  on lateral chest radiographs, 68
  of lower limb, effect of, on radiographs, 230
  medial (internal), 25
  positioning accuracy and, 29
  on posteroanterior chest radiographs, 67
  proximal humerus, 153-154
  37°, from PA, 27
Rotational movements, 25
  elbow, 110
  forearm, 110
Round window, 392, 393
RPO; *see* Right posterior oblique position
Rugae of stomach, 417

S

Sacral canal, 281
Sacral crest, 281
Sacral curve, 249
Sacral foramina, posterior, 281
Sacral horns, 281
Sacral promontory, 281
Sacral segments, 248
Sacroiliac joints, 11, 281, 228
  anterior oblique positions of, 244
  anteroposterior axial projection of, 242
  basic and special projections for, 233
  posterior oblique positions of, 243
  routine for, 232
Sacrum, 223, 248, 449
  anatomy of, 281
  anteroposterior axial projection for, 299
  basic and special projections in, 288
  and coccyx
    exam of, pregnancy and, 44
    and lumbar spine and, 279-303
      positioning of, 286-302
    routine for, 288
  lateral position for, 301
Saddle joint, 12, 13
  of hand and wrist, 108
Sagittal image, 15
  viewing, 54
Sagittal plane, 15
Sagittal sinus, 687, 693
Sagittal suture, 330
Saliva, 413
Salivary glands, 412, 413
Sandbags for pediatric radiography, 584
Sanderson method for trauma and mobile radiography of pelvis, 571
Saphenous vein, 691, 693
Scale contrast, 32
Scanning, orbital, positioning for, 657
Scanograms, computed tomography, for long bone measurement, 612
Scaphoid bone
  of foot, 175
  of wrist, 104
Scaphoid fat stripe, 111
Scapula, 8, 56, 148, 149, 150-151
  anteroposterior projection of, 151, 168, 566
  basic and special projections in, 155
  inferosuperior (axiolateral) projection of, 151
  lateral projection of, 151, 566
    in RAO or LAO body position, 169
  routine for, 154
  trauma and mobile radiography of, 566
Scapular notch, 150
Scapulohumeral joint, 150, 152
Scatter radiation
  fluoroscopy and, 40
  minimizing effect of, for cervical and thoracic spine radiographs, 262
  worker protection and, 40
Schatzke's ring, 418
Schuller method
  for mastoid radiographs, 405
  for temporomandibular joint radiography, 381
Schwannomas, MRI to diagnose, 740
Sciatic notch, 224
Scoliosis, 249
  radiograph for, shielding for, 43
Scoliosis series, 294-297
  anteroposterior Ferguson method for, 296
  anteroposterior (posteroanterior) projection for, with right and left bending, 297
  basic and special projections in, 288
  erect lateral position in, 295
  posteroanterior (anteroposterior) projection in, 294
"Scotty dog" on oblique lumbar vertebra radiograph, 284
Scout radiograph for oral cholecystogram, 488
Screen-film combinations, optimum speed, for patient protection, 44
Screen-film rule, 44
Secondary bronchi, 60
Secondary center of endochondral ossification, 9
Sectional thickness in tomography, 626
Sections, body, 15
SEE; *see* Skin entrance exposure
Segmental fracture, 548
Segmentation, rhythmic, 419
Seldinger technique for vessel puncture, 695
Sella turcica, 328, 329, 639
Sella turcica, cont'd
  anteroposterior axial projection for, 356
  axial section through, 648
  basic and special projections in, 348
  Haas method for, 357
  lateral position for, 355
  posteroanterior axial projection for, 357
  routine for, 347
  Towne method for, 356
Sellar joint, 12, 13
  of hand and wrist, 108
Semi-axial projection, 28
  anteroposterior axial, 21
Semicircular canals, 392, 393
Semilunar bone; *see* Lunate bone of wrist
Semilunar notch, 106, 107
Semilunar valves, 681
Septal cartilage, 335
Septum, nasal, bony, 332, 335
Sesamoid bones, of feet, 173
  tangential projection of, 192
Severe reaction to urologic contrast media, 513
Shadow shields, gonadal, 43
Shaft; *see* Body
Sheets, wrapping child with, for immobilization during pediatric radiography, 585
Shield (shielding)
  Bucky slot, for worker protection, 40
  for cervical and thoracic spine radiographs, 262
  contact, gonadal, 43
  gonadal; *see* Gonadal shielding
  for lower limb radiographs, 231
  with mobile C-arm digital fluoroscopy systems, 555-556
  shadow, gonadal, 43
  specific area, for patient protection, 43-44
  thyroid, for worker protection, 40
  tower drape, for worker protection, 40
Shock, profound, from urologic contrast media, 513
Short bones, 8
Short scale contrast, 32
Shoulder blade; *see* Scapula
Shoulder girdle, 102, 148-152
  anteroposterior and lateral projections for, 566
  anteroposterior radiograph of, external rotation, 148
  bones of, 7
  and humerus, radiographs of, 154-155
  joints of, 152
  positioning of, 153-169
  proximal humerus and, 147-170
  trauma and mobile radiography of, 566
Shoulder, 13, 150, 152
  anteroposterior apical oblique axial projection of, in RPO or LPO position, 164
  anteroposterior oblique projection of, in LPO or RPO position, 159
  anteroposterior projection of
    with external rotation, 156
    with internal rotation, 157
    and lateral projection, 566
    with neutral rotation, 161
  arthrography of, 619
  basic and special projections in, 155
  dislocation of, 546
  elevation and depression movements of, 27
  Fisk method for, 160
  Garth method for, 164
  inferosuperior axiolateral projection of, 158
  Lawrence method for, 158, 163
  Neer method for, 162
  non-trauma routine for, 156-160
  right lateral position of, 21
  routine for, 154
  scapular Y lateral-posteroanterior oblique projection (RAO or LAO) of, 162
  supraspinatus outlet tangential projection of, 162
  tangential projection of, 160
  transthoracic lateral projection of, in right or left lateral position, 163
  trauma and mobile radiography of, 566
  trauma routine for, 161-164
Shoulders-forward method for cervicothoracic vertebrae radiography, 271
SI; *see* System Internationale
Sickle cell anemia as contraindication to excretory urography, 514
SID; *see* Source image receptor distance
Side marker, anatomical, 30
Siemens Mobilett Plus, 554
Sievert, 37
  conversion of rem to, 37
Sigmoid colon, 86, 448, 449, 453
Sigmoid sinus, 687
Signal averaging in MRI, 743
Simple fracture, 548
Simple sugars, digestion and, 419
Sims position for barium enema, 461
Single-contrast barium enema, 459; *see also* Barium enema
  for child, 606-607
  procedure for, 464
Sinus(es)
  coronary, 682
  dura mater, 687
  ethmoid, 387
  frontal, 329, 387
  lateral, radiographs of, 388
  maxillary, 333, 386
  occipital, 687
  paranasal; *see* Paranasal sinuses
  renal, 507
  sagittal, 687, 693
  sigmoid, 687
  sphenoid, 329, 387
  straight, 687, 693
  transverse, 687, 693
  venous, 635
Sinus tarsi, 174
Skeletal anatomy, 6-9
Skeletal muscle, 5
Skeletal system, 3
Skeleton
  appendicular, 6, 7
  axial, 6
  cervical spine, 258
  thoracic spine, 259
Skin, 6, 23
Skin dose, calculation of, 45
Skin entrance exposure, 38
Skin exposure, entrance, 38
Skull, 386-389, 635
  anatomy of, 324
  anteroposterior projection for, 576-577
    anteroposterior reverse Caldwell and anteroposterior Towne projections for, 598
  base plane of, 16
  bones of, 6
  brachycephalic, 343
  of child, 598, 599
  classification of, by shape and size, 343
  and cranial bones, 323-358
    positioning of, 343-357
  dolichocephalic, 343
  joints of, classification of, 337
  lateral and horizontal beam projection for, 575
  lateral position for, 599
  mesocephalic, 343
  morphology of, 343
  positioning aids for, 345
  positioning considerations for, 343, 346
  positioning lines for, 345
  posteroanterior projection for, 360
  projections required for, 51
  radiographs of, 343-348
  reverse Caldwell projection for, 576-577
  suture of, 10
  tangential projection of, 21
  Towne projection for, 576-577
  trauma and mobile radiography of, 575-577
  trauma radiography of, 552
  Waters and reverse Waters projections of, 28
Skull series
  anteroposterior axial projection in, 349
  basic and special projections in, 348
  basilar position for, 354
  Caldwell method for, 352
  Haas method for, 350
  lateral position for, 351
  posteroanterior axial projection for, 350, 352
  posteroanterior projection for, 353
  routine for, 347
  submentovertex projection for, 354
  Towne method for, 349
Slipped disk, 251
Small bowel, 89

Small bowel series, 446, 455
basic and special projections for, 469
imaging for, 458
posteroanterior projection for, 470-471
pregnancy precautions for, 458
preparation for, 458
procedures for, 456-458
routine for, 468
upper gastrointestinal system combined with, 456
for child, 604-605
Small intestine, 86, 87, 412, 446
anatomy of, 447
digestive functions in, 454
digestive movements in, 454
obstruction of, enteroclysis to diagnose, 457
radiograph of, 86, 450; *see also* Small bowel series
sectional differences in, 447
Smith's fracture, 549
Smooth muscle, 5
Sneezing from urologic contrast media, 513
SOD; *see* Source object distance
Soft palate, 57, 413
during swallowing, 414
Sonography
breast, 535
gallbladder, 489
Source image receptor distance
density and, 31
detail and, 33
distortion and, 34
minimum 40 inch, 34
Source object distance, minimum, 34
Space
epidural, 635
intervertebral, 257
meningeal, 635
retromammary, 531
subarachnoid, 635
subdural 635
Special (alternate) projections, 50
Special use projection terms, 21
Specific area shielding for patient protection, 43-44
Sphenoid bone, 324, 328-329
orbits and, 338
Sphenoid effusion, 387
Sphenoid fontanels, 330
Sphenoid sinus, 329, 387
Sphenoid strut, 339
Spheroid joint, 13
Sphincter
hepatopancreatic, 485
of Oddi, 485
Spin density, 727
Spin-density images, 742
Spin echo technique in MRI, 743
Spin-echo pulse sequences in MRI, 729
Spin lattice relaxation, 727
Spin-spin relaxation, 727
Spina bifida, 280
Spinal accessory nerve, 641
Spinal canal, 248, 251
Spinal cord, 248, 251, 634, 635
axial (cross-section) image of, 60
axial CT image of, 58
Spinal curvatures, 249
Spinal fusion series, 297-298
anteroposterior (posteroanterior) projection for, with right and left bending, 297
basic and special projections in, 288
lateral positions for, in hyperextension and hyperflexion, 298
Spine
cervical; *see* Cervical spine
flexion, extension and hyperextension of, 24
iliac, 223, 224
anterior superior, 286
as topographic landmark of abdomen, 52, 91
lumbar; *see* Lumbar spine
lumbosacral, radiographs of, 284
magnetic resonance imaging of, 746
nasal, 325, 333
of scapula, 150
scoliosis of, radiograph for, shielding for, 43
thoracic; *see* Thoracic spine
tibial, 178
trauma radiography of, 551, 552
Spinous process, 250
of axis, 253
of cervical vertebra, 252
of lumbar vertebrae, 280
of thoracic vertebrae, 255
Spiral fracture, 548
Spiral valve, 485
Spleen, 86, 88, 453
lesions of, abdominal computed tomography to diagnose, 673
Splenaportography, 713
Splenic artery, 692
Splenic flexure, 86
Splenic vein, 693
Splintered fracture, 548
Spondylolisthesis, 280
Spongy bone, 8
Spot, focal; *see* Focal spot
Spot filming, patient exposures during, 39
Sprain, 547
Squamosal suture, 330
Squamous portion
of frontal bone, 325
of occipital bone, 326
of temporal bones, 327, 329, 389
Stapes, 392
Stellate fracture, 550
Stenosis, biliary, oral cholecystogram to diagnose, 487
Stents, balloon expanding, 719
Stenvers method for mastoid radiographs, 393, 403
reverse, 406
Stenvers projection for internal acoustic meatus radiographs, 391
Sterile fields, maintaining, in Mobile C-arm digital fluoroscopy systems, 556
Sternal angle, 260, 261, 306
as bony positioning landmark, 52
Sternal clavicle articulation, 306
Sternal rib articulations, 307
Sternoclavicular joint, 149, 152, 306, 307, 308
anterior oblique positions for, 317
basic and special projections in, 313
posteroanterior projection of, 316
routine for, 313
Sternocostal joint, 308
Sternum, 8, 56
anatomy of, 306
basic and special projections in, 313
lateral position for, 315
positioning considerations for, 310
radiographs of, 309
and ribs
basic and special projections for, 313
and bony thorax, 305-322
radiographs of, national survey norms for, 313
right anterior oblique position for, 314
routine for, 313
topographical landmarks of, 260, 261
trauma and mobile radiography of, 559
Sthenic body habitus, 53
chest radiography and, 64
gastrointestinal organs and, 420, 421
Stockinette for immobilization during pediatric radiography, 584
Stomach, 86, 87, 89, 412, 453
air-barium distribution in, 417
anatomy of, 416-417
barium in, 422
body habitus and position of, 420, 421
coronal section of, 417
curvatures of, 416
empty, orientation of, 417
emptying of, 419
folds within, 417
mechanical digestion in, 419
openings and curvatures of, 416
peristalsis in, 419
polyp in, upper GI series to diagnose, 431
position of, 417
posteroanterior projection of, 418
radiograph of, 86, 418, 422
subdivisions of, 416
tumors in, upper GI series to diagnose, 431
Stones
extraction and biliary drainage for, percutaneous transhepatic cholangiography for, 492
ureteric, 516
Straight radiograph, 612; *see also* Orthoroentgenography
Straight sinus, 687, 693
Straightedge as positioning aid in skull radiography, 345
Stress
eversion, of ankle, 25
inversion, at ankle, 25
valgus, 25
varus, 25
Stress fracture, 550
Stress movement of foot, 25
Striated muscle, 5
Structural classification of joints, 10-13
Structural organization of body, 2
Styloid process, 106, 178, 327, 390
Subarachnoid cisterns, 638
Subarachnoid space, 635
Subclavian artery, 683, 690, 692
Subclavian vein, 686, 687, 693, 694
Subdural hematoma, cranial computed tomography to diagnose, 655, 658
Subdural space, 635
Sublingual glands, 413
Subluxation, 546
Submandibular glands, 413
Submentovertex (SMV) projection, 28
of mandible, 336
Subscapular fossa, 150
Subtalar joint, 174
Subtraction, photographic, 707
Subtraction angiography, digital, 708
Subtraction venogram, 707
Sugars, simple, digestion and, 419
Sulcus, 179
calcaneal, 174
carpal, 104
central, 636
intercondylar, 179
trochlear, 107
Summation in cranial computed tomography, 652
Superciliary ridge, 325, 344
Superconducting magnets for MRI, 732
Superficial, 23
Superimposition of anatomical structures, two projections needed because of, 50
Superior, 22
Superior angle of scapula, 150
Superior articular process, 251, 252, 253, 255
Superior border of scapula, 150
Superior facet of atlas, 253
Superior orbital fissures, 328, 339
Superior ramus of pubis, 224
Superior vertebral notch, 250
Superoinferior axial projection, 21, 28
Supination, 26
Supinator fat stripe of elbow joint, 111
Supine position, 17
Support devices to control unsharpness, 33
Supraorbital groove, 325, 344
Supraorbital margin, 325, 344
Supraorbital notch, 325
Suprapatellar bursa, 181
Suprarenal glands, 88, 89, 504
Supraspinatus fossa; *see* Supraspinous fossa
Supraspinous fossa, 150
Suprasternal notch; *see* Jugular notch
Surface coils for MRI, 741
Surfaces, body, 16
Surgical neck of humerus, 148
Suspensory ligaments of breast, 532
Sustentaculum tali, 174
Sutural bones, 330
Sutural ligament, 10
Sutures, 10
cranial, 330
cross-sectional view of, 10
Swallow, barium, 412
Swallowing, 413, 414
esophagus and, 415
impaired, esophagram to diagnose, 427
Swimmer's lateral position
for cervicothoracic vertebrae radiography, 270
horizontal beam, for myelography, 623, 624
Swimmer's method, modified, for cervicothoracic vertebrae radiography, 271
Sylvius, aqueduct of, 637
Symphyses, 11
Symphysis menti, 336
Symphysis pubis, 11, 224, 286, 504, 509
joints of, 228
as topographic landmark of abdomen, 52, 91
Synarthrodial joints, summary of, 13
Synarthrosis, 10
Synchondroses, 11
Syndesmoses, 10
Synovial cavity of knee, 181
Synovial fluid, 11
Synovial joints, 10, 11-13
Synovial membrane of knee, 181
System, 2
body, 3-6
cardiovascular
magnetic resonance angiography of, 750
magnetic resonance imaging of, 748, 750
circulatory, 3
digestive, 3, 86
endocrine, 5, 88
exocrine, 88
gastrointestinal, 86
genital, 4
integumentary, 6
lymphatic, 3, 88, 694
muscular, 5
nervous, 5
reproductive, 4
respiratory, 4
skeletal, 3
urinary, 4, 88-89
System Internationale prefixes and conversions, 37
System Internationale units, 37
Systemic anatomy, 3-6
Systemic circulation, 680
general, 681-682

T

T1 relaxation, 726, 727
T1-weighted images, 742, 743
T2 relaxation, 726, 727
T2-weighted images, 742, 743
T5 to T8, 254
T10 to L2, 254
T-tube cholangiography, 491
basic and special projections for, 496
postoperative, national survey norms for, 495
Tachycardia from urologic contrast media, 513
Taeniae coli, 449
Tail of breast, 530
Tailbone; *see* Coccyx
Talocalcaneal joint, 174
Talus bone, 174
ankle and, 176
Tangential projection, 21, 28
for zygomatic arch, 27
Tape for immobilization during pediatric radiography, 584
Tarsal sinus, 174
Tarsals, 8, 174-175
Tarsometatarsal joints, 173, 183
Tax-em Board, 583
Taylor method for pelvis, 236
Technologist, radiologic, code of ethics for, 46
Teeth, 413
Tegmen tympani, 391
Television fluoroscopy, 425
Temporal artery, 684
Temporal bones, 324, 327, 329
anatomy of, 389-392
mastoids, and paranasal sinuses, 385-409
paranasal sinuses and, 386
positioning for, 394
radiographs of, national survey norms for, 396
tomography of, 395
Temporal horn of lateral ventricles, 637
Temporal lobe of cerebral hemisphere, 636
Temporomandibular fossa, 327, 337
Temporomandibular joint(s), 327, 336, 337
anteroposterior axial projection of, 379
arthrography of, 615
axiolateral oblique projection of, 380
axiolateral projection for, 381
basic and special projections for, 362
modified Law method for, 380
modified Towne method for, 379
motion of, 337
routine for, 361
Schuller method for, 381
tomography of, 382-383

"Ten-day rule" for protection of
pregnancies, 44
Term pregnancy, relationship to bladder of, 509
Terminal bronchioles, 60
Terminal ileum, 448
Terminology, 14-28
fracture alignment, 547
magnetic resonance imaging, 751-752
movement, 24-27
pathological, 751
projection, special use, 21
relationship, 22-23
trauma and fracture, 546-550
wrist joint movement, 110
Tesla, 731
Test, water, to prevent esophageal reflux, 429
Teufel method for pelvis, 237
Thalamus, 635, 639, 641
coronal section through, 644
Therapeutic intubation, 457
Therapy, infusion, 718
Thermoluminescent dosimetry badges for
personnel monitoring, 38
Thick barium, 423
Thigh bone; *see* Femur
Thin barium, 423
Third ventricle of cerebrum, 636, 637, 638
Thoracic aorta, 414
Thoracic aortography, 709-710
Thoracic arteries, 688
Thoracic cavity, breathing movements and, 64
Thoracic curve, 249
Thoracic duct, 694
Thoracic region, myelography of, 623-624
Thoracic spine, 247-278
anatomy of, 248-259
anteroposterior and horizontal beam
lateral projection for, 574
anteroposterior projection of, 275
basic and special projections of, 264
computed tomography of, 659-677
lateral position for, 276
oblique position for, 277
positioning of, 260-277
radiographs of, 256, 259
routine for, 263
topographical landmarks of, 260, 261
trauma and mobile radiography of, 574
Thoracic spine skeleton, 259
Thoracic veins, 688
Thoracic vertebra(e), 56, 306
axial (cross-section) image of, 60
characteristics of, 254-255
9th or 10th, 56
typical, 255
Thorax; *see also* Chest
anatomy of, 661-663
articulated, 308
articulations of, anatomy of, 308
bones of, 6
bony
anatomy of, 56, 306
anteroposterior oblique and lateral
sternum projection for, 559
anteroposterior and oblique ribs
projection for, 560
exterior and interior of, 23
sternum and ribs, 305-322
trauma and mobile radiography of, 559, 560
trauma radiography of, 552
circulatory system of, 688
computed tomography of, 664-665
axial image of, viewing, 54
positioning and procedures for, 664-666
lower
computed tomography cross sectional
image of, 61
computed tomography image of, 61
mid, locating, 56
on posteroanterior chest radiograph, 62
viscera in, 56
Three-way abdominal series, 86, 99
Thrombolysis, 719
Thumb, 102
anteroposterior (PA) oblique and lateral
projection for, 562
anteroposterior projection of, 118
carpometacarpal joint of, 12
dislocation of, 546
and finger, routine for, 113, 114
joints of, 103
Thumb, cont'd
lateral position for, 120
posteroanterior oblique projection of,
with medial rotation, 119
trauma and mobile radiography of, 562
Thymus gland, 59
anatomy of, 63
Thyroid cartilage of larynx, 57, 58, 260, 261
Thyroid dose, calculation, 45
Thyroid gland, 57, 59
Thyroid shielding
with cranial radiography, 346
for humerus and shoulder girdle
radiographs, 154
for worker protection, 40
Tibia, 178, 180
ankle and, 176
anteroposterior and lateral projection for, 568
anteroposterior mortise and lateral
projection for, 568
comminuted fracture of, 548
compound fracture of, 548
Pott's fracture of, 549
trauma and mobile radiography of, 568
two projections required for, 51
Tibial artery, 691, 692
Tibial collateral ligament, 180, 181
Tibial plateau, 178
Tibial spine, 178
Tibial tuberosity, 178
Tibial vein, 691
Tibiofibular joint, 180
distal, 10, 183
Tilt, 27
in cranial radiography, 346
15°, 27
on lateral chest radiographs, 68
Time, exposure, control of, 31
Time indicators on radiograph, 30
Time-to-echo variables, 730
Tissue(s), 2
adipose, of breast, 531
glandular, of breast, 531
joint classification based on, 10
local heating of, during MRI, 738
Tissue dose, collimation and, 42
TLD badges for personnel monitoring, 38
Toe-touch maneuver to prevent esophageal
reflux, 429
Toes, 172
abduction and adduction of, 26
anteroposterior and lateral projection for, 567
anteroposterior oblique projection of,
with medial or lateral rotation, 190
anteroposterior projection of, 189
basic and special projections for, 188
interphalangeal joints of, 12
joints of, 173
lateral-mediolateral or lateromedial
projections of, 191
metatarsophalangeal joints of, 12
routine for, 186
tangential projection of, 192
three projections required for, 51
trauma and mobile radiography of, 567
Tomogram (tomography), 522, 626
computed; *see* Computed tomography
conventional, 626-631; *see also*
Conventional tomography
tube trajectories in, 626, 627
electron beam, 650
panoramic, of mandible, 377-378
for sternal radiographs, 310
of temporal bone, 395
temporomandibular joint, 382-383
Tongue, 413
during swallowing, 414
Top of ear attachment, 327, 344, 391
Topographic positioning landmarks, 52
Torquing of metallic objects during MRI,
738
Torus fracture, 548
Towels, wrapping child with, for
immobilization during pediatric
radiography, 585
Tower, intensifier, worker protection and, 40
Tower drape shields for worker protection, 40
Towne method
and basilar position for petrous pyramid
radiographs, 408
of cranial radiography, 349, 356
Towne method, cont'd
for mandible radiographs, 375
for mastoid and petrous pyramid
radiographs, 389
for mastoid radiographs, 404
modified
for temporomandibular joint
radiography, 379
for zygomatic arch radiographs, 371
for sella turcica radiographs, 356
Towne projection
anteroposterior, pediatric radiography of
skull, 598
for trauma and mobile radiography of
skull, 576-577
Trabeculae of breast, 532
Trachea, 57, 58, 59, 413
anatomy of, 63
axial (cross-section) computed
tomography image of, 59
axial (cross-section) image of, 59
on posteroanterior chest radiograph, 62
radiographs of, 59
Traditional radiation units, 37
Tragus of ear, 344
Transhepatic cholangiography, percutane-
ous, 492
basic and special projections for, 496
national survey norms for, 495
Transluminal angioplasty, 719
Transorbital oblique radiography, 706
Transpyloric plane to divide abdomen into
regions, 90
Transthoracic projection, 21, 28
Transtubercular plane to divide abdomen
into regions, 90
Transverse arch of foot, 175
Transverse atlantal ligament, 253
Transverse colon, 86, 89, 448, 449, 453
Transverse diameter of thoracic cavity, 64
Transverse foramen, 252, 253
Transverse fracture, 548
Transverse images, viewing, 54
Transverse mesocolon, 451, 452
Transverse plane, 15
Transverse process, 250
of cervical vertebrae, 252
of coccyx, 282
of lumbar vertebrae, 280, 284
of thoracic vertebrae, 255
Transverse sections, 15
Transverse sinus, 687, 693
Trapezium bone of wrist, 103, 104
Trapezoid bone of wrist, 103, 104
Trauma
abdominal, as contraindication to ureteric
compression, 516
adaptation for, 551
knee, 181
nonaccidental, reporting, 582
terminology related to, 546-550
Trauma and mobile radiography, 545-579
of abdomen, 561
of bony thorax, 559-560
of cervical spine, 572-573
of chest, 558
of facial bones, 578
of lower limb, 567-570
of mandible, 579
of pelvis, 571
positioning in, 558-579
positioning principles for, 551-553
of shoulder girdle, 566
of skull, 575-577
of thoracic and lumbar spine, 574
two projections for, 551
of upper limb, 562-565
use of grids in, 553
x-ray equipment for, 554-557
Treitz
angle of, 418
ligament of, 418, 447
Trendelenburg position, 17
for intravenous urogram, 516
Triangular bone; *see* Triquetrum bone of
wrist
Tricuspid valve, 681
Trigeminal nerve, 641
Trigone, 508
Trimalleolar fracture, 550
Tripod fracture, 550
of orbit, 339
Triquetrum bone of wrist, 104
Trochanter(s)
greater, 222, 224, 286
as topographic landmark of abdomen,
52, 91
lesser, 222
Trochlea, 107, 179
peroneal, 174
Trochlear nerve, 641
Trochlear notch of ulna, 106, 107
Trochlear process of calcaneus, 174
Trochlear sulcus (groove), 107, 179
Trochoid joints, 12, 13
Trochoidal joints of wrist, 108
True anteroposterior projection, 20
True lateral elbow, 107
True posteroanterior projection, 20
True pelvis, 225
True ribs, 307
True vocal cords, 58
Tube, eustachian or auditory, 390, 391, 414
Tube movement in tomography, 626
Tube shift in tomography, 626
Tube trajectories in conventional
tomography, 626, 627, 630
Tubercle
adductor, 179
anterior, ankle and, 176
coronoid, 106
greater, 148
intercondyloid, 178
lesser, 148
parietal, 326
posterior, of atlas, 253
rib, 307
Tuberosity
of calcaneus, 174
of fifth metatarsal, 172
frontal, 325
ischial, 224
as topographic landmark of abdomen,
52, 91
radial, 106, 107
tibial, 178
Tubule
collecting, 507
convoluted, proximal and distal, 507
Tuft fracture, 550
Tumors
pituitary, MRI to diagnose, 740
in stomach or duodenum, upper GI series
to diagnose, 431
Turbinates, nasal, 329, 335
Twining method for radiography of C4-T3
region, 270
Two-way abdomen series, 86, 99
Tympanic cavity, 390, 391, 414
Tympanic membrane, 390

U

UGI; *see* Upper gastrointestinal series
Ulcer(s)
duodenal, 422
peptic, upper GI series to diagnose, 431
Ulcerative colitis, barium enema to
diagnose, 459
Ulna, 105
distal humerus and, 107
greenstick fracture of, 548
Monteggia's fracture of, 549
trochlear notch of, 107
Ulnar artery, 690, 692
Ulnar collateral ligament of wrist, 109
Ulnar deviation, 24, 110
Ulnar flexion, 24, 110
radiograph of, 105
Ulnar notch, 106
Ulnar vein, 691, 693
Ultrafast CT, 650
Ultrasound; see sonography
of birth canal, 225
gallbladder, 489
Umbilical region of abdomen, 90
Unciform bone; *see* Hamate bone of wrist
Underexposure of radiograph, 31
Units
of radiation, 37
of radiation dose, 37
of radiation exposure, 37

Unsharpness, 33
focal spot size and, 35
Upper airway, 57
anteroposterior projection of, 82
basic projections of, 71
lateral position of, 81
radiographs of, 59
national norms for, 70
routine for, 70
Upper digestive tract, 86
Upper gastrointestinal series, 412, 431-433
anteroposterior projection for, 444
basic and special projections for, 434
on children, 600
double-contrast radiographs of, 424
left posterior oblique position for, 443
patient exposures during, 39
positioning for, 434
posteroanterior projection for, 441
procedure for, 433
radiographs in, national survey norms for, 434
right anterior oblique position for, 440
right lateral position for, 442
routine for, 434
Upper gastrointestinal system, 411-444
contrast media for, 423-424
fluoroscopy of, 422
radiographs of, similarities in, 422
small bowel study combined with, 456
for child, 604-605
Upper gastrointestinal system study for children, 604-605
Upper GI; *see* Upper gastrointestinal series
Upper limb, 101-146
anatomy of, 102-111, 148-152
anteroposterior and lateral projections for, 592-593
forearm, 563
humerus, 565
anteroposterior (posteroanterior) oblique and lateral projections for, 562
arteries of, 690
arteriography of, 716
bones of, 7
of child, 592-593
discrepancies in length of, orthoroentgenography for, 614
positioning of, 112-145
post reduction of forearm and wrist, 563
posteroanterior and lateral elbow projection for, 564
radiographs of
cast conversion chart for, 112
national survey norms for, 113
trauma and mobile radiography of, 552, 562-565
veins of, 691
viewing radiographs of, 54
Upper quadrants of abdomen, 90
Upright marker, 30
Ureterogram, anteroposterior projection for, 526
Ureteropelvic junction, 508
Ureterovesical junction, 508
Ureters, 88, 89, 452, 504, 508
calculi in, 516
excretory urography to diagnose, 514
compression of, 515-516, 525
intravenous urogram with, 517
size of and points of constriction of, 508
Urethra, 88, 504, 508
female, 509
male, 509
Urethrography, retrograde, 519
Urinary bladder, 88, 89, 452, 504, 508-509
carcinoma of, pelvic computed tomography to diagnose, 673
functions of, 509
size and position of, 509
term pregnancy relationship to, 509
Urinary system, 4, 88-89, 503-528
anatomy of, 504-509
basic and special projections in, 520
functions of, 506
national survey norms for, 520
radiographic procedures for, 511-519
Urinary tract infections, excretory urography to diagnose, 514
Urination, 509
Urine
blood in, excretory urography to diagnose cause of, 514
production of, 506
Urogram (urography), 511
excretory, 89, 510, 514-515
basic and special projections in, 520
intravenous; *see* Intravenous urography
retrograde; *see* Retrograde urography
Urology, contrast media for, 511-513
Urticaria from urologic contrast media, 513
Uterus, 89, 509
Uvula, 57, 413

V

Vagina, 509
Vagus nerve, 641
Valgus, 25
Valgus deformity, 547
Valgus stress, 25
Valsalva's maneuver to prevent esophageal reflux, 429
Valve(s)
heart, 681
ileocecal, 86, 448
spot film of, 450
spiral, 485
Variable vs. fixed fulcrum in conventional tomography, 628
Variables, exposure, 31
Varices, esophageal, esophagram to diagnose, 427
Varus, 25
Varus deformity, 547
Varus stress, 25
Vascular foreign bodies, extraction of, 718
Vascular interventional angiography, 718-719
Vasovagal response from urologic contrast media, 513
Veins, 680, 686, 689, 691, 693
azygos, 688
cardiac, 682, 693
cerebral, 686-687
coronary, 682
hepatic, 689, 690, 693
inside rib, 307
jugular, 686, 687, 693, 694
major, summary of, 693
mesenteric, 689, 690, 693
portal, 689, 690, 693
pulmonary, 63, 681, 688, 693
renal, 506, 689, 693
subclavian, 686, 687, 693, 694
thoracic, 688
Vena cava, 63, 415, 452, 484, 506, 681, 688, 689, 691, 693
Venogram (venography)
epidural, 625
lower limb, 717
subtraction, 707
Venous sinuses, 635
Ventral decubitus position, 19
Ventral recumbent position, 17
Ventral surface, 16
Ventricles
cerebral, 636
axial section through, 646, 647
of heart, 681, 682
Vermiform process, 448
Vermis, 640
Vertebra(e), 8, 248
cervical; *see* Cervical vertebra(e)
7th; *see* Vertebra prominens
cervicothoracic
radiography of, alternate methods for, 271
swimmer's lateral position for, 270
compression fracture of, 550
lumbar; *see* Lumbar vertebra(e)
thoracic; *see* Thoracic vertebra(e)
typical anatomy of, 250-251
Vertebra prominens, 252, 260, 261
for central ray positioning on chest radiograph, 69
collimation guidelines and, 70
as positioning landmark, 52, 56
Vertebral arch, 250
Vertebral artery, 683, 692
Vertebral body, 11
Vertebral canal, 250
Vertebral column, 248
bones of, 6
divisions of, 248
Vertebral curvatures, 249
Vertebral foramen, 250
Vertebral notch, 250
Vertebral veins, 686, 693
Vertebrobasilar angiography, 704-705
Vertebrobasilar arteries, 684
Vertebrobasilar arteriogram, 686
Vertebrobasilar system, magnification angiography of, 705
Vertical diameter of thoracic cavity, 64
Vertical plane, 15
Verticosubmental projection, 28
Vessels
great, 63
pulmonary, engorgement or hyperemia of, 66
Vestibule, 392
Video endoscopes, 493
View, correct use of term, 28
Viewing radiographs, 54
Viscera, thoracic, 56
Visceral muscle, 5
Visceral peritoneum, 89, 451
Visceral pleura, 61
Visual centers, 642
Visual pathway, 642
Vitamins, chemical digestion of, 419
Vocal cords, 58
during swallowing, 414
true, 58
Voice box; *see* Larynx
Voiding cystourethrogram (cystourethrography), 510, 519
anteroposterior projection for (female), 528
basic and special projections in, 520
for child, 608-609
right posterior oblique position for (male), 528
routine, 520
Voiding, 509
Volar surface, 16
Volume element, 651
Voluntary motion, control of, 33
Voluntary muscle, 5
Volvulus, barium enema to diagnose, 459
Vomer, 335
Vomiting from urologic contrast media, 513
Voxel, 651
degree of attenuation of, in cranial computed tomography, 653
three-dimensional, converting, to two-dimensional pixels, 653

W

Wafer grid for trauma radiography, 553
Water, chemical digestion of, 419
Water test to prevent esophageal reflux, 429
Water-soluble iodinated contrast media, 424
Waters method
for facial bone radiograph, 364
lateral reverse, for trauma and mobile radiography of facial bones, 578
modified, for facial bone radiographs, 366
modified reverse, for trauma and mobile radiography of facial bones, 578
open-mouth, for paranasal sinus radiographs, 388, 401
for paranasal sinus radiographs, 399
Waters skull projection
reverse, 28
special PA, 28
Weighted angle blocks as head clamps for immobilization during pediatric radiography, 584
White blood cells, 680
White matter, 640
Whole body effective dose, 37
Whole body scanner, 660
Willis, circle of, 686
Willow stick fracture, 548
Windpipe; *see* Trachea
Wing(s)
of ilium, 223
of sacrum, 281
of scapula, 150
of sphenoid bone, 328
Wirsung, duct of, 485
Worker protection
exposure patterns and, 40
during fluoroscopy, 40-41
Worker protection practices, 40-41
Wormian bones, 330
Wrapping child with sheets or towels for immobilization during pediatric radiography, 585
Wrist, 12
anteroposterior (posteroanterior) oblique and lateral projection for, 562
anteroposterior projection of, 125
basic and special projections in, 114
bones of, 104
carpal bridge-tangential projection of, 133
carpal canal of
alternate superoinferior projection of, 132
tangential inferosuperior projection of, 131
dorsiflexion of, 24
fat stripes of, 111
Gaynor-Hart method for, 131
and hand
anatomy of, 102-104
joints of, 108-109
lateral radiograph of, 105, 111
lateral-lateromedial projection of, 127
movements of, 24
terminology for, 110
oblique radiograph of, 111
post reduction, 563
posteroanterior and oblique projection of, 111
with lateral rotation, 126
posteroanterior projection of, 105, 111, 125
with radial flexion, 130
posteroanterior scaphoid projection of
with central ray angle and ulnar flexion, 128
with hand elevated and ulnar flexion, 129
routine for, 113
summary of, 109
tangential superoinferior projection of, 132
three projections required for, 51
trauma and mobile radiography of, 562, 563

X

X-ray beam divergence, 34
X-ray beam restricting devices, 48
X-ray film, 14
X-ray systems, mobile, types of, 554-556
X-ray table
cassette tray and Bucky grid in, 48
fixed vs. floating, 48
Xiphoid process, 56, 260, 306
as topographic landmark of abdomen, 52, 91
Xiphoid tip, 56, 260, 261, 286, 306

Y

Yellow bone marrow, 8

Z

Zygapophyseal joints, 251, 252, 255, 280, 284, 285
vs. intervertebral foramina, 258-259, 285
Zygoma, 332, 334
Zygomatic arch, 327, 334
anteroposterior axial projection of, 371
basic and special projections for, 362
basilar position for, 369
modified Towne method for, 371
oblique inferosuperior (tangential) projection for, 370
routine for, 361
submentovertex (SMV) projection for, 369
tangential projection of, 21
Zygomatic bone, 334
orbits and, 338
Zygomatic process, 327, 333
Zygomatic prominence, 334